principles of
ANESTHESIOLOGY
general and
regional anesthesia

VINCENT J. COLLINS, M.D.

Professor Emeritus of Anesthesiology
Northwestern University School of Medicine
Chicago, IL

Professor Emeritus of Anesthesiology
University of Illinois College of Medicine
and University Hospital
Chicago, IL

principles of ANESTHESIOLOGY

general and regional anesthesia

THIRD EDITION

Volume 1

1993

LEA & FEBIGER
Philadelphia

Lea & Febiger
200 Chester Field Parkway
Box 3024
Malvern, Pennsylvania 19355-9725
U.S.A.
(215)251-2230

Executive Editor: Carroll C. Cann
Project Editor: Dorothy A. DiRienzi
Production Manager: Michael DeNardo

First edition 1966
  Reprinted 1970, 1972
Second edition 1975
  Reprinted 1978, 1979, 1980
Third Edition 1993

Library of Congress Cataloging-in-Publication Data

Collins, Vincent J. (Vincent Joseph), 1914-
    Principles of anesthesiology : general and regional anesthesia /
  Vincent J. Collins.—3rd ed.
      p.   cm.
    Includes bibliographical references and index.
    ISBN 0-8121-1322-5
    1. Anesthesiology. 2. Anesthesia.   I. Title.
    [DNLM: 1. Anesthesia.   WO 200 C713pe]
  RD81.C65 1991
  617.9'6—dc20
  DNLM/DLC   91-7038
  for Library of Congress   CIP

Reprints of chapters may be purchased from Lea & Febiger in quantities of 100 or more.
Contact Sally Grande in the Sales Department.

Copyright © 1993 by Lea & Febiger. Copyright under the International Copyright Union. All Rights Reserved. This book is protected by copyright. *No part of it may be reproduced in any manner or by any means without written permission from the publisher.*

PRINTED IN THE UNITED STATES OF AMERICA

Print number: 5 4 3 2 1

This work is dedicated to my wise and patient wife, Florence, and to my loving and understanding children, Katherine, Patricia, Michael, Gregory, Peter, Delia, Mary-Claire, and Vincent Jr.

PREFACE

I have largely pursued, with some modifications, the concept of a single volume with single authorship, as originally intended. First, it has been necessary to produce initially two separate volumes entitled (I) *Principles of Anesthesiology: General Anesthesia* and (II) *Principles of Anesthesiology: Regional Anesthesia*. A third volume, entitled *Principles of Anesthesiology: The Physiologic and Pharmacologic Basis of Anesthesia*, is forthcoming.

The explosion in knowledge and the refinements in techniques that have occurred in the last 15 years have made it difficult to select the most important and basic information of lasting value. Accommodation of the sheer volume of new and valuable information has made division of the book necessary.

In addition, I have made some modifications by choosing clinicians of a similar philosophy to aid in the preparation of certain chapters. Thus, John Thomas Martin has revised my original chapters on Physiology of Posture, Positioning of Patients, and Complications of Position. Likewise, Theodore Smith of Loyola University has been enormously helpful in our revision of the chapter on Equipment. Jerry Calkins and Gerald Maccioli have been co-contributors to the chapter on Monitoring. For Spinal-Subarachnoid and Epidural Opiates, a former resident and now a leader in the field of spinal opioids—namely Florella Magora—has contributed a superbly informative chapter. Lastly, Beverly Phillips has added a succinct and practical chapter on Anesthesia for Ambulatory Surgery.

With the exception of these contributors, the remainder of the 63 chapters are of my doing and I take responsibility for the contents and the selection of the material. I have approached the task by asking myself as a practicing and "teaching" anesthesiologist, the following questions. What new ideas and techniques are important and will be likely to find a permanent place in practice? What would I acquire and add to my knowledge? Will this add to the safe, humane care of patients? After 48 years of clinical experience and teaching, which ideas and techniques should be added to my practice? The answers to such questions have been my quest.

Vincent J. Collins
Chicago, Illinois

ACKNOWLEDGMENTS

My gratitude is extended particularly to Dr. Alon Winnie for encouraging and enabling me to devote 3 years, almost exclusively, to literature review and library research in the selection of new material for this third edition. Special mention is made to Dr. Zairo Vieira of Rio de Janeiro, Brazil, formerly an associate at Cook County Hospital and recently my close associate at the University of Illinois Hospital and College of Medicine. He has greatly contributed to my efforts in dealing with advances in endotracheal anesthesia.

Special thanks are due to Mary Gorney for much secretarial help and library assistance. To Melissa Goldin, my secretary from 1989 to 1991, goes a meritorious award for adjusting to my composing techniques. Above all, her talents at preparing references were outstanding, as was her patience.

The personnel of Ruttle, Shaw and Wetherill of Fort Washington, Pennsylvania, particularly Peg Markow, are commended for their editorial reviews of chapters, and the personnel of Lea & Febiger, especially Carroll Cann, are to be commended for the remarkable transformation of my efforts into the printed book.

VJC

CONTRIBUTORS

MARK V. BOSWELL, Ph.D., M.D.
Assistant Professor
Case Western Reserve University and University Hospitals
Cleveland, Ohio

JERRY M. CALKINS, Ph.D., M.D.
Chairman, Department of Anesthesiology
Lovelace Medical Center
Albuquerque, New Mexico

ADEL A. EL-ETR, M.D.
Professor of Anesthesiology
University of Miami School of Medicine
Miami, Florida

STUART R. HAMEROFF, M.D.
Associate Professor
Department of Anesthesiology
University of Arizona College of Medicine
Tucson, Arizona

MICHAEL F. JAMES, M.D.
Staff Anesthesiologist
Department of Anaesthetics
Hillbrow Hospital
Johannesburg, South Africa

BRUCE KLEINMAN, M.D.
Attending Anesthesiologist
Illinois Masonic Medical Center
Chicago, Illinois
Clinical Professor of Anesthesiology
University of Illinois College of Medicine
Chicago, Illinois

FLORELLA MAGORA, M.D.
Professor of Anesthesiology
Department of Anesthesiology
Director, Pain Clinic
Hadassah Medical Organization
Kiryat Hadassah
Jerusalem, Israel

GERALD A. MACCIOLI, M.D.
Staff Anesthesiologist and Staff Intensivist
Raleigh Community Hospital and Rex Hospital
Raleigh, North Carolina

JOHN T. MARTIN, M.D.
Professor (Emeritus)
Department of Anesthesiology
Medical College of Ohio
Toledo, Ohio

RICHARD McCAMMON, M.D.
Associate Professor
Department of Anesthesiology
University of Indiana Medical Center
Indianapolis, Indiana

JONATHAN MOSS, M.D., Ph.D.
Professor and Vice Chairman for Research
Department of Anesthesia and Critical Care
University of Chicago, Pritzker School of Medicine
Chicago, Illinois

BRIAN OLSHANSKY, M.D.
Assistant Professor of Cardiology
Division of Cardiology
Department of Medicine
Loyola University Medical Center
Maywood, Illinois

TADIKONDA L.K. RAO, M.D.
Professor and Chairman
Department of Anesthesiology
Loyola University of Chicago
Maywood, Illinois

MICHAEL F. ROIZEN, M.D.
Professor and Chairman
Department of Anesthesiology
University of Chicago
Division of the Biological Sciences
Pritzker School of Medicine
Chicago, Illinois

MOHAMED RAMEZ SALEM, M.D.
Professor and Chairman
Department of Anesthesiology
Illinois Masonic Medical Center
Chicago, Illinois

THEODORE C. SMITH, M.D.
Professor of Anesthesiology
Department of Anesthesia
Loyola University of Chicago
Maywood, Illinois

ZAIRO E.G. VIEIRA, M.D., FFARCS
Professor of Anesthesiology
University of Brasilia
Brasilia, Brazil
Visiting Professor of Anesthesiology
University of Illinois College of Medicine at Chicago
Chicago, Illinois

CONTENTS

section I
GENERAL ANESTHESIA

Volume 1

1. THE HISTORY OF ANESTHESIOLOGY — 3
2. RECORDS, MORTALITY, OPERATIVE RISK, AND MEDICOLEGAL CONSIDERATIONS — 29
3. MONITORING THE ANESTHETIZED PATIENT — 67
4. FUNDAMENTAL PHYSICS — 100
5. ANESTHESIA MACHINES AND COMPONENTS — 118
6. THE PHYSIOLOGY OF PATIENT POSTURE — 163
7. TECHNICAL ASPECTS OF PATIENT POSITIONING — 174
8. COMPLICATIONS OF PATIENT POSITIONING — 192
9. PREANESTHETIC EVALUATION AND PREPARATION — 207
10. DRUG INTERACTIONS — 253
11. PRINCIPLES OF PREANESTHETIC MEDICATION — 284
12. GENERAL ANESTHESIA—FUNDAMENTAL CONSIDERATIONS — 314
13. GENERAL ANESTHESIA—CLINICAL SIGNS — 360

#	Chapter	Page
14.	GENERAL ANESTHESIA—SPECIAL CONSIDERATIONS	375
15.	INHALATION ANESTHESIA—BREATHING SYSTEM	387
16.	INHALATION ANESTHESIA—PROCEDURAL CONSIDERATIONS	423
17.	CLIMATE, ALTITUDE, AND ANESTHESIA	444
18.	CARBON DIOXIDE ABSORPTION TECHNIQUE	452
19.	ENDOTRACHEAL ANESTHESIA: I. BASIC CONSIDERATIONS	460
20.	ENDOTRACHEAL ANESTHESIA: II. TECHNICAL CONSIDERATIONS	518
21.	ENDOTRACHEAL ANESTHESIA: III. COMPLICATIONS	565
22.	ENDOBRONCHIAL TECHNIQUE	597
23.	CONTROL OF BREATHING BY ARTIFICIAL METHODS	618
24.	BARBITURATE INTRAVENOUS ANESTHETIC AGENTS: THIOPENTAL	653
25.	INTRAVENOUS ANESTHESIA: THIOPENTAL SUBSTITUTES	689
26.	INTRAVENOUS ANESTHESIA: NARCOTIC AND NEUROLEPTIC–NARCOTIC AGENTS	701
27.	INTRAVENOUS ANESTHESIA: NONBARBITURATES—NON-NARCOTICS	734
28.	INTRAVASCULAR LOCAL ANESTHETICS AND REGIONAL BLOCK	787

Volume 2

#	Chapter	Page
29.	RELAXANTS—FUNDAMENTAL CONSIDERATIONS	809
30.	RELAXANTS—CLINICAL CONSIDERATIONS	847
31.	RELAXANTS—PHARMACOLOGY AND USE	938
32.	REVERSAL OF RELAXATION; ANTAGONISTS TO RELAXANT DRUGS	1023
33.	CONTROLLED HYPOTENSION	1056
34.	DELIBERATE, CONTROLLED TOTAL-BODY HYPOTHERMIA AND HYPERTHERMIA	1096
35.	REGIONAL HYPOTHERMIA (REFRIGERATION ANESTHESIA)	1116
36.	ELECTROANESTHESIA	1119
37.	HYPNOSIS	1125
38.	HYPERBARIC OXYGENATION	1134
39.	HAZARDS IN ANESTHESIA PRACTICE	1149
40.	AUTONOMIC REFLEXES DURING ANESTHESIA AND SURGERY	1179

section II
REGIONAL ANESTHESIA

#	Chapter	Page
41.	PRINCIPLES GOVERNING REGIONAL ANESTHESIA	1199
42.	LOCAL ANESTHETICS	1232
43.	POTENTIATION OF ACTION	1282
44.	TOXICOLOGIC BASIS FOR LOCAL ANESTHETIC REACTIONS	1291
45.	REACTIONS TO LOCAL ANESTHETICS	1302
46.	MECHANISMS OF PAIN AND CONTROL	1317
47.	BLOCK OF CRANIAL NERVES	1350
48.	BLOCKS OF CERVICAL SPINAL NERVES	1363
49.	BLOCKS OF NERVES OF THE UPPER EXTREMITIES	1385
50.	BLOCKS OF NERVES OF LOWER EXTREMITIES	1395
51.	BLOCKS OF THE TRUNK, ABDOMEN, AND PERINEUM	1413
52.	PARAVERTEBRAL BLOCKS	1429

53.	TESTS OF SYMPATHETIC FUNCTION	1438
54.	SPINAL ANESTHESIA—PRINCIPLES	1445
55.	SPINAL ANALGESIA—PHYSIOLOGIC EFFECTS	1498
56.	SPINAL ANESTHESIA TECHNIQUE	1521
57.	COMPLICATIONS DURING SPINAL ANESTHESIA	1540
58.	POSTOPERATIVE COMPLICATIONS PECULIAR TO SPINAL ANESTHESIA	1555
59.	EPIDURAL ANESTHESIA	1571
60.	CAUDAL ANALGESIA	1611
61.	SUBARACHNOID AND EPIDURAL OPIOID ANALGESIA	1622
62.	ACUPUNCTURE	1634
63.	ANESTHESIA FOR AMBULATORY SURGERY	1641

section I

GENERAL ANESTHESIA

In man's struggle to survive, perhaps his greatest and indeed his constant battle is against physical pain. The story is a dramatic one, and the present state of achievement in the control of pain is a culmination of many disheartening experiments and isolated triumphs. Men have made this story. To understand pain control and anesthesia, we are obligated, therefore, to report the contributions of men, and we will follow the history of anesthesia in terms of many men of vision and of courage.[1-4]

Prior to 1842, an operative procedure was a struggle for the surgeon and an ordeal for the patient. The most important attribute of the surgeon was not his skill but his speed. Numerous agents had been used with the purpose of relieving pain, but all were attended with minimal success.

ANESTHESIA IN ANTIQUITY

At the beginning of historic time man is found seeking means to dull the morbid and even lethal edge of pain. In the dark ages, memorable battles against pain were fought without much success. The first attempts at deadening human pain began with the use of the poppy, mandrake root, henbane, and alcohol.[5] A sponge impregnated with a preparation of opium, henbane, and mandrake was known as the "soporific sponge" and employed by Hippocrates and Galen. It was used to produce inhalant anesthesia. When actually tested it was found not to "even make a guinea pig nod." One can well imagine the witchcraft and quackery associated with the preparation of "soothing brews," most of which had little scientific value.

We know that the Greeks used infusions of herbs and various drugs to induce sleep as recounted in Homer's Odyssey. One can speculate on the ingredients of such infusions. Perhaps the lotus, which hypnotized with lethean forgetfulness the navigators of Odysseus, was part of the potion. The lotus referred to was probably the fruit of the African jujube or the nettletree of southern Europe.

THE POPPY. The occasion when the poppy was first employed as a means to alleviate pain is lost in the

THE HISTORY OF ANESTHESIOLOGY

mists of time. The people of Asia were certainly among the first to use concoctions to relieve pain, and opium constituted the basic ingredient. In addition, "hashish" was used for centuries by oriental peoples to produce euphoria, forgetfulness, and inebriation.

TEARS OF POPPY. The sap exuding from scratches on the unripe seed pod was actually opium. It was known to many as an effective drug. Dioscorides, Galen, Paré, Celsus, and others mentioned opium and recognized narcotic action. Celsus was especially interested in providing sleep. Among his several formulas for anesthesia is the following pill containing poppy:

> Those pills which alleviate pain by causing sleep are called anodynes in Greek. It is bad practice to employ them except in cases of urgent necessity, for they were compounded of powerful drugs and are bad for the stomach. However, one may be used, which contains a denarius (about 3i) each of tears of poppy and galbanum, and two denarii each of myrrh, castoreum, and pepper. It is enough to swallow a piece of the size of a bean.

HENBANE (HYOSCYAMUS). In the fifth century before Christ, the physicians of Cos and Cretona used many and varied medicinal substances, and actually had a pharmacologic classification of drugs, according to their effects. One group, the refrigerants, was considered to be soporific or narcotic. They were named *frigidi*, *frigidiori*, and *frigidissimi*, according to their intensity. (It was considered that relief of pain or suffering was the result of "cooling.") Henbane was called herba frigidissima—it was quite effective; wild lettuce was only slightly effective.

The seeds of henbane were used to eliminate pain. Dioscorides knew its actions and its poisonous effect. It was used to catch mice, to catch birds, and to produce sleep. Celsus, the surgeon, used a concoction to relieve toothache and to provide a sleepy, forgetful patient for his surgery. Generally, in most potions, henbane was combined with opium, and Celsus had several formulas containing both.

MANDRAKE (MANDRAGORA OFFICINARUM). The third most popular drug of antiquity was Mandrake root. The mandrake, or mandragora, sometimes called the "May apple," has been sought after for thousands of years for its magical and medical properties. The mandrake root was said to grow in the shape of human beings and to "bleed" when cut or broken. When pulled from the ground it would emit a scream, which was immediately fatal to those who heard it. It was thus common to employ a half-starved dog to do the actual pulling from the ground. The rind of the root was preferred for its potency and was recognized as an anesthetic, an aphrodisiac, and a soporific. As a poultice, it was used to "draw phlegm or black bile" from any site where it was applied. The Persians named the plant *merdomgia* (man-like plant) or *segken* (dog dug). The Greeks, likewise, named the plant *kynospastos* (dog dragged).

The mandrake was especially favored by the Romans as a surgical anesthetic and was mentioned by Pliny in his works.

Dioscorides wrote of mandrake

> It is an herb whose rind mixed with wine, is given to drink, to those whose cure must be surgical, so that they will fall asleep and feel no pain.

At the famed University of Bologna, the Dominican friar Theodoric of Lucca (1205–1298) was known for his surgery and his admonitions. In surgery, he advocated the use of sponges drenched with a narcotic or mandragora that were applied to the patient's nose; cutting was not to begin until the patient was asleep.

Priority in the usage of the word *anesthesia* in its modern connotation belongs to Dioscorides. In describing the effects of mandragora he used the word exactly as one would today.[5,6]

ALCOHOL. For centuries alcoholic preparations were employed prior to operations and to the reduction of dislocations and fractures. Wine was a favorite. Only when it was given in large quantities was there material relief of pain. In the eighteenth and nineteenth centuries it was rather popular. Usually, the patient drank quantities of the beverage until a stuporous state was reached, whereupon the surgeon proceeded. Dr. Philip Syng Physick of Philadelphia (1768–1837) recommended the use of intoxicating amounts of alcoholic preparations for the purpose of relaxing muscles before manipulating fractures.

STRANGE METHODS OF ANESTHESIA. One strange method of pain relief for surgery was that of strangulation, used by the Assyrians for circumcision of their children. The asphyxia and attendant unconsciousness obviously relieved the pain of the moment and allowed the surgeon to proceed with his operation. Anesthesia by strangulation to the point of unconsciousness was practiced in Italy as late as the seventeenth century. Another method was that of cerebral concussion, achieved by placing a wooden bowl over the head of the patient and striking it until the patient became unconscious. The directions were simple: Strike the bowl with sufficient strength to crack an almond but leave the skull intact.

Some diminished pain by application of intense cold or compression of the nerve roots. Such methods were used by the Romans, apparently learned from the Assyrian monks. Revived in 1700 by Moore, it was used in Italy by Ruggieri.

PRECURSORS

In the latter part of the eighteenth century, study on the chemistry of gases fired the work of many men. In 1750 J. Black studied carbon dioxide, which he called "fixed air." Cavendish identified hydrogen in 1776 and described it as "inflammable air." In this period Lavoisier discovered both nitrogen and oxygen. Rutherford called nitrogen "phlogisticated air." In 1774 Joseph Priestley prepared oxygen, which he called "dephlogisticated air," and in 1776 he discovered nitrous oxide. In these findings lay some hope for man in his struggle to alleviate pain. To explore the possibilities other men with imagination were needed, and they soon appeared.

A FOUNDER: SIR THOMAS BEDDOES (1760–1808). Beddoes began the study of the action of gases on man in Bristol, England. In collaboration with James Watt he published a work entitled Considerations on the Medicinal Use and Production of Factitious Airs. He founded the famous Pneumatic Institute in Clifton. In the annex to the laboratory sick people were treated with various gases. Oxygen was especially popular, but the expectations were too great and the venture fell into disrepute. Beddoes published a case report of deep sleep produced by ether.

DISCOVERY: HUMPHREY DAVY. In 1799 this young man was placed in charge of Beddoes' laboratory and instructed to do research on the actions of carbon dioxide and nitrous oxide. Both animals and men were used for these experiments.

He wrote a book on his work and had it published under the title of *Researches, Chemical and Philosophical—Chiefly Concerning Nitrous Oxide and Respiration*. In it he described methods of obtaining the gas and the effects of the gas on human beings. The subjects included Davy himself and many of his distinguished visitors. The central effects were readily appreciated, especially the pleasant inebriation and the associated relief of pain. Because of the exhilarating property of nitrous oxide he called the substance "laughing gas." Recognizing the practical possibilities of his discoveries, and he wrote

> As nitrous oxide ... appears capable of destroying physical pain, it may probably be used to advantage during surgical operations in which no great effusion of blood takes place.

This statement went unheeded.

OBSCURITY: HENRY HILL HICKMAN. A young English doctor from Ludlow was driven by the terrors of the operating room to seek a remedy for pain. Hickman pursued further the researches of Davy and in 1824 successfully anesthetized animals placed under bell jars with a mixture of nitrous oxide and oxygen. The animals remained unconscious long enough to have amputations performed, and most important, they recovered. These results were published in a book on suspended animation.

Hickman was opposed in his desire to try the gases on human beings. In 1828 he demonstrated his experiments before the French Academy. Only Baron Larrey recognized the possibilities and offered himself as a subject, but even his enthusiasm was dampened by the general skepticism. Hickman was soon discouraged and returned to England to die within a few months.

MICHAEL FARADAY. In 1818, Faraday wrote about the stupefying effects of ether. He noted that when the vapor of ether was mixed with air it produced effects similar to those of nitrous oxide. Physicians, especially in America, were familiar with these effects in producing inebriation and sleep.

Although the drug was considered dangerous in medical practice, it was considered safe enough to be used by medical students at their parties. These ether frolics were called "jags" and were attended by many, including Crawford Long.

MESMERISM. The use of hypnotism is a strange chapter in the story of anesthesia. Operations were performed painlessly during mesmeric trances—and are being performed today. In 1779, Friedrich A. Mesmer of Vienna startled the world by publishing his "pretensions concerning animal magnetism" and by demonstrating his capacity to bring certain subjects under hypnotic influence. It appears that the first surgical procedure under mesmerism was performed by J. Cloquet, a French surgeon, in 1829. In England, mesmerism as a medical tool was introduced and popularized by John Elliotson, a physiologist. At his demonstrations many famous men were observers, including Charles Dickens and Thomas Moore. He used the technique to manage epilepsy and other medical problems as well as to provide pain relief. Elliotson gave lectures on the subject at University College Hospital. His advocacy between 1830 and 1840 aroused strong resentment among his rivals.

In the meantime, James Esdaile (from Perth, England), in charge of the Native Hospital in Hooghly, India, read of Elliotson's activities and was inspired to try mesmerism on a surgical case. The results encouraged him to try the technique on others, and he reported 73 operations in 1846 done under hypnosis.

But a new star was in ascendance. Opposition to mesmerism on philosophical grounds was one thing, but competition with a more effective method was another. Mesmerism failed because it was less efficient than ether and chloroform. An advocate of mesmerism commented that "the more tangible agents, ether and its fellows, possess one advantage, namely, that of superior certainty." Furthermore, the process was time-consuming and not suited to surgery. In another hundred years, however, its proper niche in the field of anesthesia would be found (See Chapter 37, Hypnosis).

THE DISCOVERY OF ANESTHESIA AND THE ETHER CONTROVERSY

The introduction of surgical anesthesia is an American contribution and has been called America's greatest contribution to medicine. The significance of this discovery is of such a nature, however, that it might be called one of the greatest contributions to mankind. At the semicentennial anniversary of the discovery of ether as an anesthetic, Weir Mitchell, a poet-physician, wrote

> Whatever triumphs still shall hold the mind,
> Whatever gift shall yet enrich mankind,
> Ah! here no hour shall strike through all the years,
> No hour as sweet, as when hope, doubt, and fears,
> 'Mid deepening stillness, watched one eager brain,
> With Godlike will, decree the Death of pain.

Events in the period between 1842 and 1846 were the culmination of a long series of experiments and frustrations, of researches and discoveries.[3] About discoveries in every sphere one always asks two questions: How long must the world wait to be convinced? What event triggers the universal acceptance of an idea? Three men lay claim to be called inventors of surgical anesthesia, but only one got full credit, and all, in their attempts to gain contemporary recognition, ended in some tragedy or met a violent fate, and their characters were tarnished.[8]

THE DENTIST—HORACE WELLS. In Hartford, Connecticut, Horace Wells, a dentist, attended a sideshow in which Colton, a chemist, demonstrated the exhilarating effects of nitrous oxide. A subject accidentally injured his shins, but he did not cry out or recall having any pain. Wells was so impressed by the insensibility produced by the gas that he decided to use it in dental extractions. On December 10, 1844, another dentist, Dr. Riggs, painlessly extracted a tooth from Wells, who was under the influence of nitrous oxide.

Wells continued to use the agent in his practice and become well known for his painless dentistry. Eventually he was invited to demonstrate his work before a group of colleagues at Massachusetts General Hospital in Boston for a major surgical operation. The demonstration was a failure. Ridicule followed, and nitrous oxide fell into disrepute. Wells became deranged and an ether addict. He committed suicide in a New York City prison cell by cutting his cubital vein while his arm was in a hot water bath. An ironic touch to the suicide act was the simultaneous inhalation of the vapor of ether. Perhaps to relieve the pain of the incision?

FIRST USE—LONG. In his youth, Crawford W. Long first witnessed the effects of ether at "jags" in Philadelphia. He came to appreciate the possibilities of ether in surgery. In January 1842 he administered the vapors of ether to James Venable in Jefferson, Georgia. The method was successful, and he removed a large tumor from Venable's neck. Thereafter he often used the method for minor surgery. Long's use of ether threw the neighborhood of Jefferson into excitement, and the population threatened to lynch him. He, therefore abandoned operations under ether and moved his office to Athens, Georgia. He never became acutely involved in the vexatious disputes about priority and was the only character in the controversy to escape real tragedy. Furthermore, his work received little recognition until publicized by Marion Sims. Long has been honored by a statue in the Statuary Hall in Washington, D.C. The inscription written by men of strong belief reads, "Discoverer of the use of sulphuric ether as an anesthetic in surgery on March 30th, 1842, at Jefferson, Jackson County, Georgia."

A curious sequel to Long's first use of ether occurred in Texas. Dr. George Pascal related that "a practicing physician in San Antonio by name, George Venable, recently removed a tumor from the arm of a Mrs. Long who was under ether anesthesia." Both were descendants of the original parties to the use of ether, but the roles were reversed in this later episode.

FIRST DEMONSTRATION—MORTON. Born in Charleston, Massachusetts, William T.G. Morton had the consuming ambition to be a physician. His father could not afford the schooling, so William entered dentistry. He began his practice in Farmington, Connecticut, and while there became acquainted with Wells. The two aspired to open an office in Boston, but Wells was discouraged and only Morton persisted. He established a good practice, but he was inwardly driven to seek a means for alleviating the pain of dental operations, and he decided to undertake medical studies at Harvard.

Meanwhile, he consulted with Professor Charles T. Jackson and learned that sulfuric ether had some effect in producing unconsciousness. Morton then experimented on his dog, on fish, on himself and his friends, and finally extracted a tooth painlessly under ether.

As a second-year medical student he secured permission from John Collins Warren, professor of surgery at Harvard, to make a public trial of ether for a major operation. The demonstration was set for October 16, 1846. It was the turning point in the history of anesthesia.

The event was brief but dramatic and world-shaking. Morton was late because he was developing an inhaler (Fig. 1–2), but he finally arrived in the amphitheater of Massachusetts General Hospital, now the ether dome, and proceeded to anesthetize Gilbert Abbott. When the patient was unconscious Morton said to Dr. Warren, "Sir, your patient is ready." The operation proceeded quietly; there was no struggle or screaming. At the conclusion of the operation, Warren turned to the audience and said, "Gentlemen, this is no humbug." Henry J. Bigelow, an eminent surgeon, declared, "I have seen something today which will go around the world." In fact, Bigelow's father helped to promote worldwide knowledge of the event, for in a letter to Dr. Bott of London the following month he inspired English surgeons to try ether anesthesia. The earliest printed reference of the first demonstration appeared in the Boston Daily Journal on October 17. A paper by Bigelow dated November 18, 1846 was the original medical announcement.

These and other papers and communications establish Morton as discoverer of surgical anesthesia. Following Morton's demonstration of the effectiveness and comparative harmlessness of ether anesthesia, the practice was generally accepted. Prior to this, "the profession had never dared to use ether in this way,"[8] but Morton's youthful recklessness and disregard for the status quo convinced the world, and the idea became sustained practice.

Morton went through many trials and hardships thereafter. He was maligned by the public. He was ridiculed one day and honored the next. He was on the verge of wealth, but really poverty-stricken. He was the subject of a Congressional inquiry and even denoted as the "Benefactor of Mankind." President Pierce was about to settle the controversy when he wavered on a technicality. Only in two circumstances did Morton appear content and happy—one was as a farmer on his place in Needham, Massachusetts; the other as a physician administering anesthesia to soldiers of the Union Army.

Dr. Oliver Wendell Holmes, in a letter to Morton, said, "I think this state should be called anesthesia. This signifies insensibility, more particularly to objects of touch." Holmes did not coin the word—it had already been used by Greek philosophers and had appeared in Bailey's English Dictionary in 1721.[9]

After the Civil War, Morton returned to Massachusetts. But one day he received a copy of an article written by Jackson in a monthly magazine. It was full of hatred and claimed that Morton had nothing to do with the discovery of ether. Morton was enraged and suffered a mild stroke, but he recovered sufficiently to go to New York City to refute the article. Summer had come to the city, and on July 15 it was a furnace, especially the Riverside Hotel, where Morton was staying. So he drove through Central Park in the evening to steady his nerves.

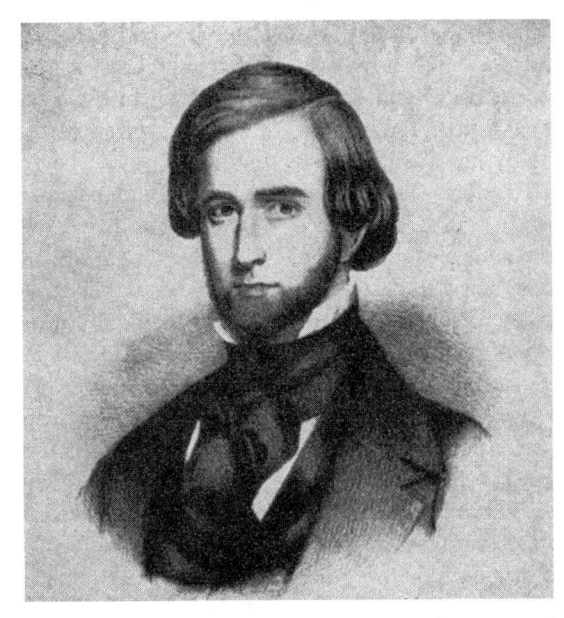

FIG. 1–1. William T.G. Morton. From Fulton, J.F.: *An Annotated Catalogue of Books and Pamphlets Bearing on Early History of Surgical Anesthesia.* New York, Henry Schuman, 1946.

Part way through he grew giddy and weak. Then, just before the carriage reached the park gates he reined up the horses, jumped to the ground, and soon fell unconscious in his wife's arms beneath a tree. He was taken to St. Luke's Hospital and there died of his apoplexy. Peace had come at last. Though rejected in 1868, his place in history is secure forever.

In all this controversy, only the reflection of later generations can distinguish values. The point of history is not who was first but rather who helped to integrate an idea into acceptable medical practice.

THE OTHERS. Crawford W. Long served as a physician with the Confederate forces. After Appomattox he was a ruined man, ever plagued by "ifs" and disappointment. One evening he went to deliver a farmer's wife, and while inducing ether anesthesia he fell across the patient's bed—dead.

Consuming jealousy and hate ended Jackson's career. After Morton's death, he continued his efforts to discredit him, but death has a way of immortalizing men. It was impossible to answer every reference to Morton. Bitterness was drowned in whiskey. One afternoon he wandered to the Mount Auburn Cemetery and caught sight of the monument erected by the citizens of Boston to Morton. On reading the inscription he became enraged and thenceforth was a frenzied maniac. He was committed to a lunatic asylum and died there in 1880.

The inscription read by Jackson on Morton's memorial is simple and true.

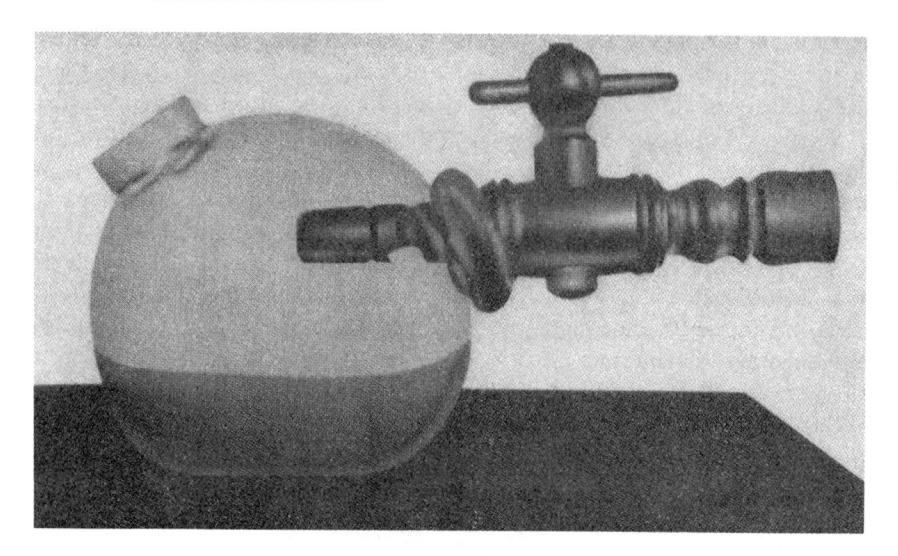

FIG. 1–2. The original Morton inhaler, with which operations were performed at Massachusetts General Hospital. From Fülöp-Miller, R.: *Triumph Over Pain.* New York, Bobbs-Merrill, 1938.

Inventor and revealer of anesthetic inhalation
By whom pain in surgery was averted and annulled;
Before whom in all time, surgery was agony
Since whom Science has control of Pain.

EARLY MILITARY USE OF ANESTHESIA

Perhaps the urgency of surgery of wounded men during wartime maneuvers gave great impetus to the use of the new pain-relieving technique of ether inhalation. It certainly was quickly appreciated by the men and widely used by the medical personnel.

The first use of anesthesia in military surgery occurred under the direction of Dr. Edward H. Barton during the Mexican-American War of 1846–1848, as the occupation army of the United States crossed the Rio Grande (Bravo), captured Monterrey, and proceeded to Vera Cruz. Ether was provided to the army in spring of 1847, and in late March the first administration of anesthesia during an armed conflict was to a teamster at Vera Cruz, Mexico.[10]

Subsequently anesthesia was administered to wounded soldiers in other armed conflicts. Chloroform was the agent used in the Crimean war (1848) and the German-Danish conflict (1848).[11]

EARLY DEVELOPMENT OF ANESTHESIA: 1846 TO 1920

The period from 1846 until the end of World War I can be considered one of early development and sporadic discovery.[4] During this time, several men stand out prominently along with their discoveries.

JOHN SNOW OF LONDON (1813–1857). The first qualified physician to devote his full time to anesthesia was John Snow.[12,13]

After his education he became interested in gases, and in 1841 he developed an early "pulmotor" for asphyxiated infants. When news arrived from America in late 1846 that surgery could be performed without pain by having the patient inhale the vapors of ether, he decided to enter the clinical practice of anesthesia and to investigate the method. He overcame the initial distrust held by many surgeons by developing an inhaler assembly that made ether administration efficient. This device was described to the medical profession at the Westminster Medical Society in 1847.

Besides being a practicing anesthetist, Snow was an investigator and teacher. He was endowed with intellectual curiosity and sought to understand the process of anesthesia. He appreciated the need for measuring the amount of agent administered, the significance of oxygen lack, and the problem of carbon dioxide. For the guidance of clinicians he divided the progress of anesthesia into five stages, now well known as the clinical signs of anesthesia. All this material and various researches were gathered together into a monograph in 1847 entitled On the Inhalation of the Vapour of Ether.[14] It is a classic in medicine and anesthesia.

Fame came to Snow in 1853 when he successfully administered chloroform to Her Majesty Queen Victoria at the birth of Prince Leopold. The event is memorialized in the phrase "anesthesie à la reine." Actually, obstetric inhalation analgesia, as the phrase could be defined, was first employed in 1847 by N.C. Keep, first dean of Harvard Dental School.[15]

Cholera hit London severely in 1854. Snow turned his attention to the epidemic and demonstrated that this dreaded disease was transmitted by water. Recognition of this aspect of the disease resulted in the institution of water purification by boiling; thus was this epidemic overcome and subsequent epidemics limited.

A second book was written by Snow: On Chloroform and Other Anesthetics.[16] It was really completed by his good friend Benjamin Richardson. This treatise is a textbook of anesthesia of the time. Included are chapters on methods, pharmacology, clinical applications, medical uses, and complications. A collection of fatal cases is included, and "cardiac arrest" is discussed for the first time.

Indeed, John Snow was not only the first anesthesiologist, he was a medical giant of the times. He has bequeathed a great legacy to anesthesiologists.

USE OF ANESTHESIA IN OBSTETRICS. In Edinburgh, James Y. Simpson held the chair of obstetrics from 1842 to 1864, and his ability as a teacher attracted students from every country. On learning of the Morton demonstration, he quickly introduced the use of ether anesthesia in obstetrics for the relief of pain of childbirth. There was immediate opposition from the clergy and the public. But Simpson was not concerned; he was merely dissatisfied with the side effects of ether and sought other drugs to accomplish the task. Waldie, a Liverpool chemist, suggested chloroform, which had been synthesized by Sam Guthrie of Brimfield, Massachusetts, in 1831 (also by Soubierain, a French chemist, at the same time). A French physiologist, Flourens, had described the properties of chloroform, and these so impressed Simpson that he investigated the effects on himself and other chemists. It not only produced anesthesia but was pleasant. In a short time he published a report of results of 50 surgical operations under chloroform. From that time on the surgical world centered its attention on ether and chloroform.

Chloroform also proved to be the agent Simpson wanted for his obstetric practice, and he proceeded to use the drug extensively and to extol the value of painless childbirth. Opposition grew to this heresy and to Simpson's "satanic activities." But conviction held the day. Simpson quoted from the Bible in noting for the moralists that God Himself introduced the practice of anesthesia to relieve pain when he induced a profound sleep in Adam for removal of a rib from which He created Eve. When Queen Victoria accepted chloroform for the delivery of Leopold, the opposition was broken. Thenceforth, women throughout the world unhesitatingly accepted the anesthesia.

Classic Aphorisms. In London, when chloroform was being used the dictum was "watch the pulse." In Edinburgh, James Syme, a leading surgeon of the day, coined an aphorism about ether, to wit, "attend to the respiration, never mind the pulse."

REVIVAL OF NITROUS OXIDE. In 1863, Colton, an itinerant chemist, arrived in New Haven, Connecticut, to demonstrate the effects of laughing gas. He be-

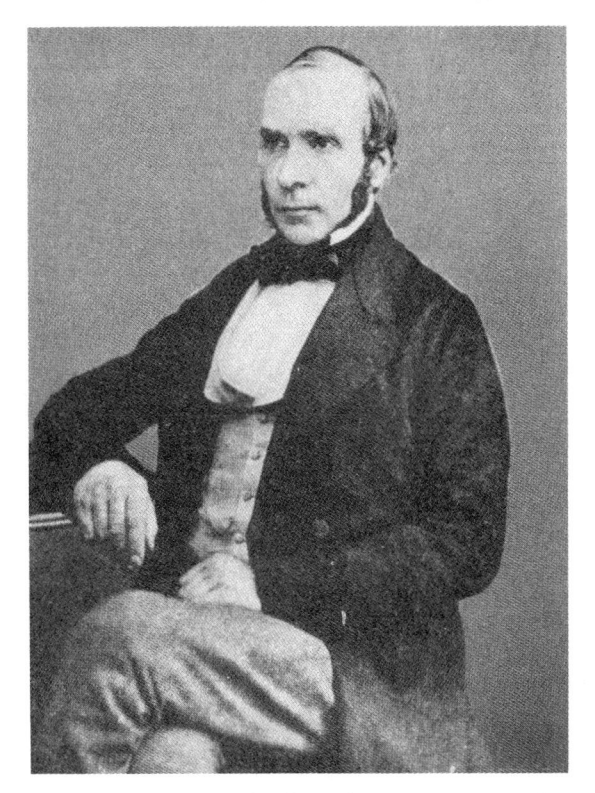

FIG. 1–3. John Snow, the first physician to specialize in anesthesia.

lieved that the gas could be put to good use, but he confined his presentations to pleasure-seeking audiences. A dentist, J.H. Smith, was stirred by the story of Wells that Colton always related, and he reinvestigated the gas. He found it effective and in the magic numbers lay success: after 20,000 painless dental extractions the use of nitrous oxide in dentistry spread throughout the United States and the gas was on the verge of being used in surgery.

To enable one to administer nitrous oxide continuously, a Chicago surgeon, Edmund W. Andrews, in 1868 introduced the use of oxygen with nitrous oxide to make a 10% mixture and demonstrated its reliability and safety.[17] He also adequately described the proper technique of administration, which he called "interval narcosis," or the prolonged administration of laughing gas. Asphyxia was no longer feared. Soon the method was preferred in America because nitrous oxide–oxygen appeared to be less toxic than ether or chloroform and was more pleasant for patients, who recovered promptly from its effects.

The method of delivery of nitrous oxide–oxygen was directly to the respiratory system. It was a high-flow and high-pressure technique. Subsequently, as a means of providing a reservoir and point of delivery of gases to the respiratory system, Joseph Clover introduced a semi-elastic bag, which was the forerunner of rubber rebreathing bags.

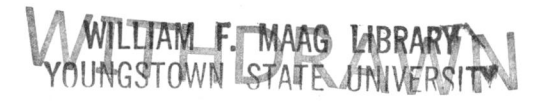

PAUL BERT AND NARCOSIS (1887). The state of anesthesia naturally attracted the curiosity of physiologists. Paul Bert, a pupil of Claude Bernard, contributed much to the physiology of narcosis. He showed that the depth of anesthesia was related to the content of nitrous oxide in the alveolar space; an increased concentration provided deeper anesthesia and even muscular relaxation. Unaware of Andrews' work, Bert also found that nitrous oxide could not be administered in pure form without asphyxia and found that oxygen was necessary. Being an experimentalist of the Bernard school, Bert naturally carried out his investigations first in the laboratory; after sufficient successes with animals, he finally recommended nitrous oxide–oxygen for human patients.

Bert carried out other researches on gases. Carbonic acid gas occupied his attention in 1874. While studying its toxic action, he noted its anesthetic action and showed experimentally that in concentrations of 40% and 60% it produced narcosis. However, he cautioned that application in dogs was one thing, but to use the gas on humans was not authorized. In 1878 he demonstrated that mountain sickness was caused by a decrease in the partial pressure of oxygen, and he described much of what is known today about disturbed physiology at high altitudes. In addition, he described the symptoms of oxygen toxicity and demonstrated that breathing oxygen in high concentrations could produce toxic effects.

LOCAL ANESTHESIA AND HALSTED. In 1836, La Fargue of France devised a needle trocar for depositing morphine in paste form. Up to this time, drugs were administered by rubbing them into a previously made skin incision.

In 1844, F. Rynd of Ireland invented a hollow metal needle that he used for hypodermic medication. In 1851, Charles Gabriel Pravaz, a Frenchman, invented the hypodermic syringe, the tool destined to fill an essential role in regional anesthesia. Alexander Wood improved the syringe in 1854.

In 1884, Carl Koller of Bohemia instilled a few drops of cocaine solution into the eyes of some patients and found complete anesthesia of the cornea and conjunctiva. He published the first description of the physiologic action of cocaine, and besides using this drug as a surface anesthetic in his ophthalmologic practice, he lectured extensively on the value of cocaine for local anesthesia. In 1888 Koller came to the United States and began his ophthalmologic practice in New York.

With the stage now set, William Halsted, in 1885, introduced the concept and use of nerve block and infiltration anesthesia by the injection of cocaine. Together with R.J. Hall, he used the principle of nerve blocking by intraneural injection of cocaine solutions to provide surgical anesthesia. The nerve he blocked first was the mandibular nerve.

Halsted relates these experiments in 1884 and 1885. Much of the work was done in a large tent erected near Bellevue Hospital because it was "impossible to carry out anti-septic precautions in the general amphitheater at Bellevue, where numerous anti-Lister surgeons dominated and predominated." On the basis of his experience, Halsted was able to evolve the principles of regional anesthesia. In the course of this work Halsted and his colleagues became addicted to cocaine. Only Halsted was able to overcome the habit. After 2 years he was able to regain his old energy, which carried him to commanding heights in surgery and medical education.

EPIDURAL ANESTHESIA AND LEONARD CORNING. Leonard Corning, a New York neurologist, in 1885 experimented on dogs with the idea of producing anesthesia of the spinal nerves. He injected cocaine hydrochloride solutions between the spinous processes of the inferior dorsal vertebrae. From a description of his results and the manner of onset of anesthesia, there is little doubt that epidural anesthesia was produced. He later repeated the procedure on a man suffering from a spinal pain syndrome and obtained anesthesia and pain relief. Details are lacking, but again epidural anesthesia was probably produced.

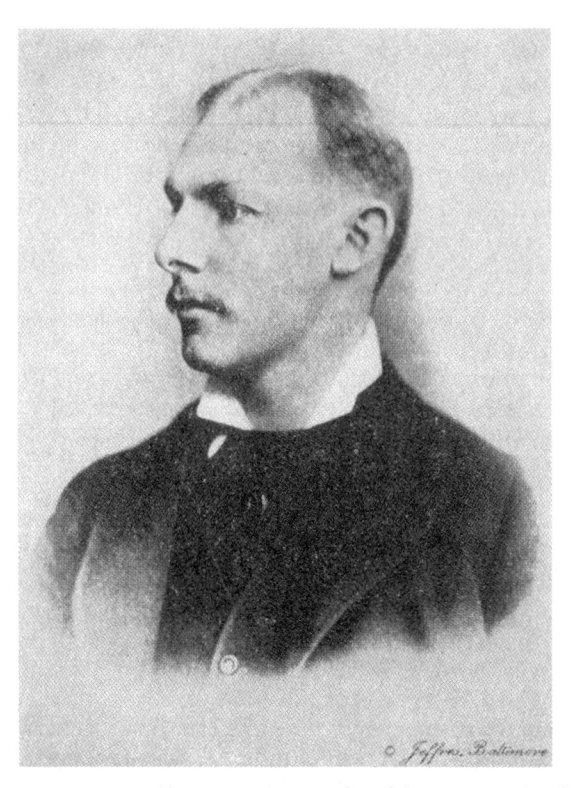

FIG. 1–4. William Stewart Halsted (1852–1922). The father of nerve blocking, Halsted established the principles of regional anesthesia.

It remained for Quincke in 1891 to demonstrate the usefulness and practicality of spinal puncture as a diagnostic procedure and to outline the proper technique of introducing a needle through the dura to obtain spinal fluid.

SPINAL ANESTHESIA AND AUGUST BIER. Using previous knowledge of anesthetic action and the technique of spinal puncture of Quincke, August Bier produced true spinal anesthesia in animals and man in 1898. To him belongs the credit of introducing spinal anesthesia and of demonstrating its merits for surgery. He not only injected his assistant, but submitted to the anesthesia himself. On August 16, 1898, he had to amputate the foot of a tuberculous patient who was a poor risk. He decided to inject 3 mL of 0.5% cocaine solution into the dural sac. Complete anesthesia of the lower limbs occurred that lasted an hour. Recovery was uneventful and thenceforth he used the technique in his surgical practice. After 6 cases he tried the anesthesia on his assistant and on himself. They were both rather sick for several days.

The subsequent story of spinal anesthesia is that of newer drugs, modifications of the basic method, popularizing its use, management of complications, and increasing the safety of the method.

CAUDAL ANALGESIA AND CATHELIN. The introduction of agents through the sacrum to each of the spinal nerves seemed a natural development from Corning's work. In 1901, M. Cathelin deliberately produced epidural anesthesia by this means.

TECHNIQUES AND APPARATUS

MONITORING BY RECORDS. Cushing and Codman introduced the use of ether charts in 1895.[18] In 1901, after his visit with Riva-Rocci in Italy, Cushing brought the pneumatic blood pressure cuff to America to be used in measuring blood pressure. This valuable observation was added to observations of the pulse and respiratory rates to complete the anesthesia record.

McKESSON'S CONTRIBUTIONS. E.I. McKesson (1881–1935) of Toledo, Ohio, further developed the use of blood pressure testing and charting during anesthesia and surgery.[19,20] His studies of blood pressure records enabled him to devise a clinical evaluation of circulation and a clinical means of making the diagnosis of shock. McKesson's rule for shock included the following criteria: pulse greater than 100, systolic pressure less than 100 mm Hg, and pulse pressure less than 20 mm Hg. Practical record-keeping was a crusade for McKesson; popularizing of routine observations in surgical anesthesia was largely due to his efforts.

In the first decade of the twentieth century, Boothby developed the first valve for anesthesia based on the valves he observed on kegs at breweries. He introduced the first apparatus for the intermittent flow of nitrous oxide and oxygen. Using this type valve, McKesson in 1910 developed the first practical intermittent-flow nitrous oxide–oxygen anesthesia machine.[21] In the same year he introduced the principle of fractional rebreathing. By this means the first part of each exhalation was saved in the breathing bag for rebreathing. An expiratory valve allowed the latter part of the exhalation to escape to the air.

HEIDBRINK AND HIS MACHINES. Jay A. Heidbrink (1875–1957) became interested in anesthesia because of personal experiences with surgery on his teeth and tonsils. He graduated from dental college at the University of Michigan and entered the private practice of dentistry in Wisconsin in 1901. His experiences with cocaine infiltration were not happy, and he soon purchased a primitive gas machine, but he was dissatisfied with the unit and proceeded to develop a better machine for the administration of nitrous oxide–oxygen.[22] When C. Teter of Cleveland introduced an effective machine in 1903, Heidbrink immediately secured one and proceeded to devise means to adjust gas mixtures. He incorporated reducing valves as part of a flowmeter arrangement. Heidbrink was a careful observer and found that in most cases the state of anesthesia developed uniformly and in about the same time. He advocated so-called "timed anesthesia." By 1913 he had remarkably improved the Teter machine and went into the manufacturing business. He had a machine shop build his first good working model—Model A—quite inexpensively. It cost 1 dollar per pound or 32 dollars. This was the first large-scale production of an inexpensive workable anesthetic machine. After 20 changes it was called the Model T. This model was used primarily for dental anesthesia, and Heidbrink trained many people in its use. In 1940 his company became part of the Ohio Chemical Company.

DENNIS E. JACKSON—THE INVENTOR. An Indiana man who became a PhD. in pharmacology and also received his M.D., Jackson maintained his first interest by becoming professor of pharmacology at Cincinnati. In 1914 he carried out his work on carbon dioxide absorption in animals and men. Much of this was related to the problems of submarine conditions existing during World War I.[23,24] In 1923 Dr. Ralph Waters was inspired by Jackson's work. He conferred with Jackson about application to surgical anesthesia and proceeded to outline the basic concepts of carbon dioxide absorption in clinical anesthesia practice. Jackson continued to do pharmacologic research on anesthetic drugs (trichloroethylene and vasopressors) and to develop gadgets for instrumentation for use in the laboratory and clinic. Many of these have complex counterparts today, such as the ballistocardiograph, which originally consisted of two pie-plates called a "vibrograph."[25]

RICHARD VON FOREGGER. In 1914 Foregger built a nitrous oxide–oxygen machine without reducing valves. This was a different approach from the Heidbrink concepts. The first Gwathmey apparatus was built without reducing valves but had control valves. Boyle modified the Foregger unit, and with a few other changes it is the standard anesthesia machine used in England.

Through the years, Foregger improved the to-and-fro system. The company was always ready to make and supply new instruments and anesthesia accessories, and the tooling skill of the company were appreciated by inventive anesthesiologists for many years. In 1928 Foregger constructed the first modern carbon dioxide absorption canister. It should be mentioned that Foregger in 1915 was not only interested in the carbon dioxide absorption problem, but was also stimulated by submarine living conditions to use sodium peroxide and water to produce oxygen. With this source of oxygen he was "buried alive" in sideshow demonstrations on Times Square in New York City.

KARL CONNELL. From the Department of Surgery at the College of Physicians and Surgeons of Columbia came a new anesthesia machine in 1913 called the "anesthesiometer" devised by Karl Connell. This apparatus could automatically measure and mix vapors and gases, and it was shown that the tension of ether vapor necessary to produce narcosis in man was about 50 mm Hg. Later Connell reported on the use of a high-resistance intercoupling for the prevention of fires and explosions due to static electricity.

THE CIRCLE SYSTEM. About 1926 Brian C. Sword investigated the possibilities of a circle filter system. Up to then, closed systems of anesthesia were essentially the to-and-fro type as devised by Jackson and Waters. For many this technique was awkward. Sword consulted with Y. Henderson of Yale and then had an apparatus based on the circle concept constructed by Foregger. About the same time Ben Morgan also devised a circle system. These were called "round trip" absorbers.

THE PHARYNGEAL AIRWAY AND HEWITT. One of the most useful anesthetic devices is the pharyngeal airway. It was introduced in 1913 by Hewitt. Modification and improvement of the airway were accomplished by many men. These include Joseph Lumbard, Karl Connell, and R. C. Coburn in the early days, and subsequently Arthur Guedel and Ralph Waters.

HISTORICAL DEVELOPMENT OF ANESTHESIA APPARATUS*

ANESTHETIC ON A CLOTH. Between 1846 and 1850 ether was administered using a folded towel and chloroform on a folded handkerchief.

ERA OF CONE INHALERS, 1850 TO 1876. The earliest cone was a pinned-up towel containing a marine sponge. Cones were then made with walls of domet (Guy's circa 1870), leather (Rendle's circa 1870) or the Hyderabad cone of 1890[1]; a cone entirely of metal (Sudek's cone circa 1900).

ERA OF "CLOSED" INHALERS, 1876 TO 1906. Chloroform was too potent an anesthetic to be given by a "closed" method, but the desire for greater anesthetic potency led to the "closed" administration of ether. The best known of such inhalers was Clover's, which (in its original form or in modifications by Hewitt, Probyn Williams, Ombredanne, and others) dominated European practice for a generation. These "closed" inhalers presented ether at its worst, with all the drawbacks of excessive concentration, salivation, mucous secretion, deficiency in oxygen supply, and excessive accumulation of carbon dioxide.[26]

ERA OF "OPEN" METHODS OF ADMINISTRATION, 1895 TO 1945. "Open" ether anesthesia was reintroduced in 1895 but did not gain general acceptance until about 1905 to 1910. The method was very satisfactory and is still in use, although it is now being challenged by the wide-bored "inhalational" vaporizers of the Oxford type. The wire-framed, gauze-covered masks of Schimmelbusch, Ballamy Gardner, and Ochsner have been used continuously. Chloroform was always given by the "open" method. The wire-framed, domet-covered masks of Esmarch and Murray are still in use. The screen mask of Yankauer was popular and is used in many third world countries.

REGRESSION TO "SEMI-OPEN" METHODS, 1905 TO 1941. Anesthetists have attempted, from time to time, to gain anesthetic potency by concentrating the vapor. To this end, a dome of more or less impervious material was erected around the "open" mask. The method is really a regression to the old "cone" inhaler and has the same faults, namely, restriction of oxygen supply and accumulation of carbon dioxide. Examples include the original semi-closed mask of Ferguson (1905), that of Coutts (circa 1930), and an appalling example used by the Italian army in Libya (1941).

"VAPOR" METHODS, 1867 TO 1941. Vapor methods, that is, the delivery to the patient of an anesthetic vapor generated in a mechanical vaporizer, began with

---

* Material in this section comes from a historical exhibition of the Australian Society of Anesthetists by Geoffrey Kaye.

Junker's chloroform inhaler (1867). The best known ether vapor apparatus was Shipway's (1915), used by the British army in the first German war. Vernon Harcourt's chloroform inhaler (1902) had the inadequate size of the valves and channels then thought appropriate. For comparison, a modification of Marrett's apparatus (1942) presents the wide-bore channels and effortless valves that are characteristic of the modern inhalational vaporizer. The most refined example of this class of apparatus is the Oxford vaporizer (1941); it is designed with wide-bore valves to replace the unduly small valves supplied commercially, which are inappropriate to an inhalational system with a vaporizer.

ENDOTRACHEAL ANESTHESIA, 1871 TO 1945. Trendelenburg's tampon canula (1871) was one of the earliest attempts at endotracheal anesthesia. Had it not been forgotten, it might have evolved into endotracheal inhalational anesthesia as understood today and as rediscovered by Magill in 1920. When the endotracheal method entered general use in 1909, however, the technique was insufflational: a small-bore catheter and a positive pressure of delivery were used. Boyle's endotracheal apparatus (1912) used the drip-feed method of generating ether vapor. His gum-elastic catheter and Jackson's laryngoscope were typical of the period.

In 1920, Magill introduced the wide-bore rubber tube, the exhalation valve, the effective pharyngeal pack, and the technique of semiclosed administration at low pressure.

GAS ANESTHESIA, 1894 TO 1945. Modern gas anesthesia began when effective control could be exercised over the percentage mixture of anesthetic gas and oxygen. Hewitt's apparatus (circa 1895) was the earliest English gas-oxygen apparatus. The apparatus most used in England to this day is Boyle's, which has been continually improved. An example of the original form (1915), used in the British army in World War I, is part of the Kaye and Wood collections. It has the pioneer Gwathmey water flowmeters and once belonged to the eminent Howard Jones of London. An Australian army gas anesthesia apparatus (1939) illustrates the development of the water flowmeter since Gwathmey's day. McKesson's "Nargraf" apparatus (1929) illustrates the intermittent flow technic with positive pressure; the Austox "D-M" Apparatus (1931) was an Australian variation using McKesson's principles. Appliances for carbon dioxide absorption anesthesia after the method of Waters (1932) are included in the equipment of the army gas apparatus, whereas the McKesson apparatus is fitted with circle absorber, an appliance first introduced by Sword (1928). The application of the Waters absorber to "controlled respiration" in thoracic surgery is illustrated by appliances in use by Orton in the thoracic surgical unit, Alfred Hospital.

MODERN ANESTHESIA: 1920 TO 1940

Great strides were made in the development of anesthesia between 1920 and 1940. This was due to the pioneering efforts of individuals. From 1940 onward, anesthesiology, becoming recognized and accepted as a scientific and medical specialty, advanced through the contributions of anesthesiologists in organized groups and in organized departments of anesthesiology.[27]

THE MODERN PIONEERS

GWATHMEY—FIRST OF THE MODERN TITANS. The influence of James T. Gwathmey on the specialty of anesthesia was extensive and profound for almost 40 years, and it has continued.[28,29] He was a respected physician, a true scientist, and an organizer. He demonstrated to the New York Academy of Medicine that oxygen increased the safety of all anesthetics without decreasing their anesthetic effect. In 1903 he introduced the technique of rectal administration of anesthesia in the form of an ether-oil mixture.[30] This method was especially applied in the relief of pain of childbirth. Improvements in anesthesia machines was his hobby, and he developed the flowmeter as a means to regulate the proportion of gases. In 1914 he published one of the first useful textbooks in anesthesia in the United States.

In the meantime he was most active in organizing anesthetists, and in 1912 he became President of the New York Society of Anesthetists, the forerunner of the American Society of Anesthesiologists. In World War I he directed his energies as Chief Anesthetist of the European Theater and succeeded in obtaining approval for gas-oxygen-ether machines as standard equipment for the American Expeditionary Force.

BUCHANAN AND THE FIRST DEPARTMENT OF ANESTHESIA. At the beginning of the twentieth century among the few devoting their entire practice to anesthesia was Thomas Drysdale Buchanan. Through his efforts a department of anesthesia was created at New York Medical College (then called New York Homeopathic Hospital) in 1904. He was appointed professor of anesthesia and later received the same title from the New York Postgraduate Medical School (1919) and in 1918 was made clinical professor of anesthesiology at College of Physicians and Surgeons of Columbia.

Buchanan indeed raised the standards of the specialty. He inaugurated regular residency training programs, worked to increase educational facilities in medical schools, and fostered the creation of certifying boards.

In 1934 he set up a model department of anesthesia at the request of the Hospital Superintendent's Association of New York.

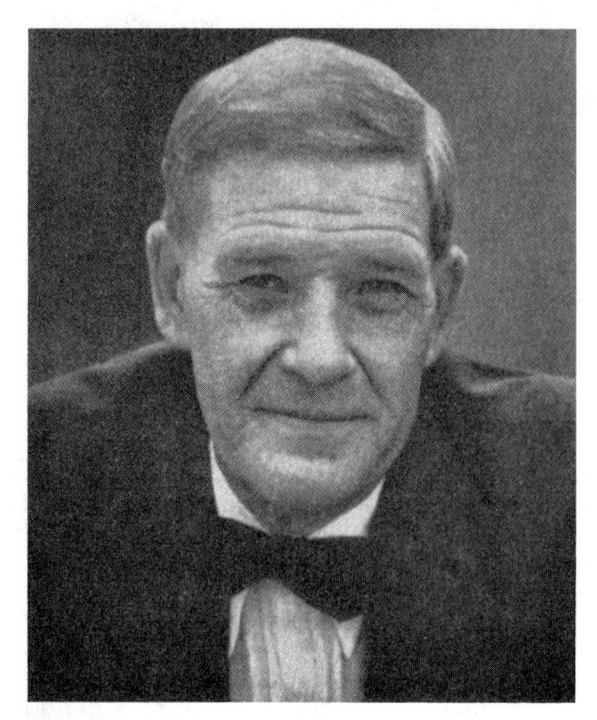

FIG. 1–5. Arthur E. Guedel.

GUEDEL AND THE SIGNS OF ANESTHESIA. Arthur E. Guedel was one of the pioneers in anesthesia and is particularly identified with the clear description of the signs of anesthesia.[30] He was an intense and impressive man who maintained a continuing interest in athletics as well as his profession. He was born in Indiana and was graduated from the Indiana University School of Medicine in 1908. His interest in anesthesia began at this time. He devised a technique of self-administration of nitrous oxide and air for obstetrics and then devoted a good deal of his time to the development of newer anesthetic agents. Throughout his practice he was interested in clinical factors. He was especially interested in the physiologic effects of disease, particularly emphysema, on the conduct of anesthesia.

As an officer in World War I, he had many responsibilities in France for anesthesia coverage; indeed he taught many the techniques of anesthesia then available. While engaged in this task he recorded and collected voluminous notes on the reactions and responses of patients to the induction and the maintenance of the anesthetic state.

In consequence of this work he elaborated on the stages of anesthesia as suggested by John Snow. Guedel's further classification and elucidation of the progressive changes in the clinical condition of a patient resulted in the now classic description of the stages and signs of anesthesia, published as a monograph entitled *Inhalation Anesthesia*.

Many honors came to Arthur Guedel. In 1941 he received the third Henry Hickman Medal from the Royal College of Medicine in London. He received the Distinguished Service Award from the American Society of Anesthesiologists in 1950. He spent the latter years of his life in California, where he died in 1956.

WATERS—THE VISIONARY. One of the grand men of anesthesiology was Ralph Waters, who was born in Bloomfield, Ohio, in 1883.[31] He completed his graduate and medical education at Western Reserve University, after which he moved westward to Sioux City, Iowa, where he was engaged for a brief time in general practice. During this time he became interested in anesthesia, and in 1916 he decided to limit his work to anesthesia.

To prepare himself for this field he studied avidly pharmacology, physiology, and pathology. In truth, Waters was a self-taught anesthesiologist using the word in its current sense. In 1927 he visited the state hospital at the University of Wisconsin, and the challenge of organizing an anesthesia department caused him to stay for over 25 years. In 1933 he was appointed professor of anesthesiology and chairman of the department. This was the first such appointment in a university, although the title Professor of Anesthesia had been conferred on Buchanan in 1919.

During the period at Wisconsin, Waters made many significant contributions to the practice of anesthesia. Perhaps the greatest was his organization of training programs. He envisioned an integrative, progressive training course, including work in the laboratory. To a large extent this was influenced by the Hopkins philosophy, then prominent, and this made the University of Wisconsin famous for its training in anesthesiology.

One of the first and continuing interests of Waters was the subject of carbon dioxide absorption and the closed system of anesthesia. In 1924 he developed the to-and-fro closed system technique practiced today. Waters then became interested in a new anesthetic agent called cyclopropane. Together with Emery Rovenstine and W.B. Neff, he was instrumental in introducing this agent as an anesthetic. The insistence on meticulous records was characteristic of Waters and his department. Their record system was standardized by a special committee of the American Society of Anesthetists in 1937. In 1940 Waters persuaded a subcommittee on anesthesia in the National Research Council to prepare a book entitled *Fundamentals of Anesthesia*. This was published under the auspices of the American Medical Association and was a bible for anesthetists during World War II. In the later years of his tenure at Wisconsin, Waters reinvestigated the use of chloroform. Together with Orth and others he published a book in 1951 negating the established opinion expressed in 1914 that "chloroform anesthesia was too dangerous to use."

Many honors came to Waters during his career. He was president of the American Society of Anesthesiologists and was the first chairman of the section on anesthesiology of the AMA in 1941. In 1944 he received the Hickman medal of the Royal Society of Medicine in England, and in 1947 he was honored by King Gustaf of Sweden.

WESLEY BOURNE—THE CLASSICIST. An affable physician, Wesley Bourne rose to world prominence in anesthesia through his leadership in the field in Canada.[32] He was born in the Barbados in 1886 and received his education at McGill, where he was graduated with the degree of medicine in 1911. He was ever afterwards identified with the McGill Faculty of Medicine. Though desirous of being a surgeon, he began his career in anesthesia within a year after graduation when asked to try his hand at "dropping ether."

Bourne always believed that adequate time should be spent in the pharmacology laboratory exploring the effects of anesthetic agents. He maintained a close association with pharmacology throughout his career. In 1921 he was lecturer in pharmacology at McGill. In 1946 a department of anesthesia was established at McGill and Bourne became a full professor. He was president of the International Anesthesia Research Society in 1925 and again in 1940. In 1942 he was elected president of the American Society of Anesthesiologists and has been the only man outside of the United States so honored. In 1935 he received the Hickman medal of the Royal Society of Medicine.

Bourne was eminent in all fields related to the medical practice of anesthesia. He was a capable clinical practitioner; he was devoted to laboratory research; and his teaching was always sparked by wit and classic quotations. His contributions to organization were many. He was a writer in the classic manner, and his works are always delightful. *Mysterious Waters to Guard* is a collection of essays on anesthesia that are full of wisdom. As a professor emeritus, Wesley Bourne was a youthful-minded person with a spry physical manner and was regarded with affection by all his colleagues. He died in 1965.

MAGILL OF WIMPOLE STREET. Besides the Barretts, Wimpole Street stands out in the field of medicine and in anesthesia particularly, for the family Ivan Magill.[33] For many years he was a prominent figure in Westminster Hospital of London, and the profundity of his contributions to safe anesthesia and the emphasis on the provision of adequate airways are immortalized in the lives that have been saved. He developed the wide-bore endotracheal tube, which enabled anesthetists to provide safe anesthesia for surgery of the head, neck, and thorax.

An Irishman, he was born in County Antrim on July 23, 1888. He received his education at the University of Belfast. In England, he succeeded in having anesthesia accepted as a specialty, and he struggled to establish the Diploma in Anesthetics. He served in both world wars and in the second conflict was advisor to the Minister of Health. During the London blitz he narrowly escaped death when his apartment on Wimpole Street was destroyed while he was dining out.

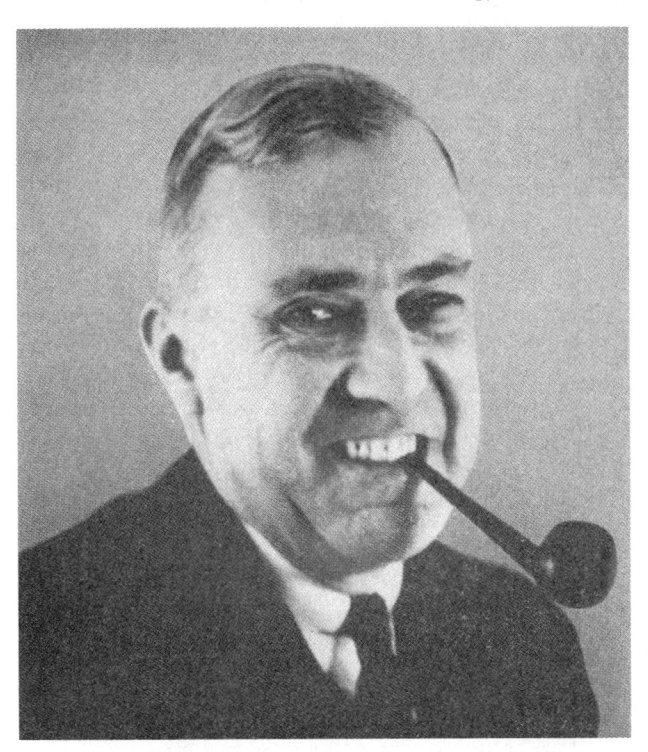

FIG. 1–6. Ralph M. Waters.

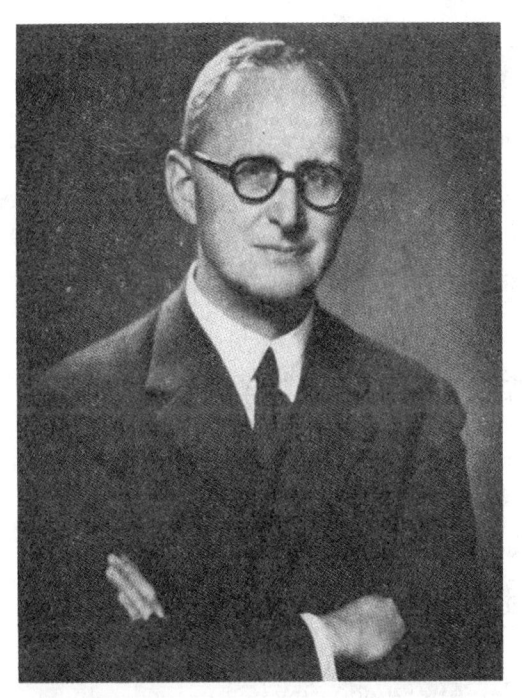

FIG. 1–7. I.W. Magill.

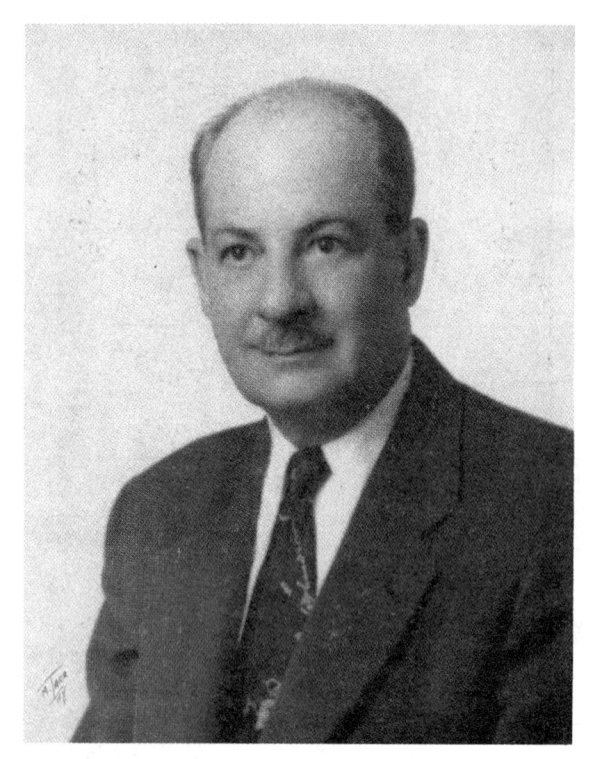

FIG. 1–8. Emery Andrew Rovenstine (1895–1960), the physician who applied regional anesthesia to the therapy of pain and who popularized nerve blocking.

Many honors came to Magill. In 1938 he received the Hickman medal for his contributions to anesthesia. Having served the Royal Family for many years he was invested in 1946 with the title Commander of the Royal Victorian Order.

ROVENSTINE OF BELLEVUE. Versatility, dedication to teaching, the investigative approach, and the conviction that anesthesiology is a dignified branch of the practice of medicine are phrases to be associated with Rovenstine.[34]

Emery A. Rovenstine (Rovey to his close associates) was born in Atwood, Indiana. He was a versatile athlete in high school and a typical mid-western farmboy. His introduction to anesthesia occurred early. While playing school basketball he ran into the referee, Dr. Arthur E. Guedel, and was properly reprimanded. After graduating from highschool he taught in a one-room grammar school.

In World War I he served as a sergeant and as a second lieutenant. His assignment, dispatch-riding to the front, enabled him to view the lethal effects of wound shock, and this aroused his interest in medicine. After another stint as a highschool teacher of mathematics and chemistry in Michigan, he decided to enter medicine and matriculated at the University of Indiana Medical School, where he took all available courses in anesthesia under Arthur Guedel. After graduating he interned at Indianapolis and pursued a general practice for more than a year, when he decided to learn all about anesthesia. This meant taking a special course with McKesson of Toledo. About this time, Guedel, recognizing the young man's worth, arranged for an appointment with Ralph Waters, one of the great anesthetists of the time and of this century. The Waters approach was in the tradition of the Hopkins system. Rovenstine actually became the first physician to serve a full apprenticeship in a residency program. He stayed with Waters for 5 years as instructor and as assistant; 1 full year was in the laboratory.

Other medical schools decided to adopt the Wisconsin plan. In 1935 New York University asked Waters to suggest someone, and Rovenstine was proposed. It was a fortuitous combination. The New York University Hospital was Bellevue, and the opportunities for medical training were unparalleled.

From 1935 to 1960 the influence of Rovenstine and of Bellevue was far-reaching and deep. The teaching philosophy of graded responsibility with minimal supervision was expounded, and the idea that men must participate in laboratory experience and in clincial research was fostered. The medical approach rather than the technical approach to the practice of anesthesia was developed. The consequence has been the development of outstanding men in anesthesia in its blossoming years. Some 34 students became heads of medical school departments of anesthesiology.

In addition, Bellevue became known as the cyclopropane school—nowhere was its everyday clinical use better taught. A nerve block clinic, the first of its kind, was organized, and this was fitting because Halsted introduced the concept of nerve blocking in surgery at Bellevue and Labat perfected many of the techniques at Bellevue—and now Rovenstine applied the knowledge for the relief of pain problems of mankind.

In 1938 Rovenstine was among the seven founders of the American Board of Anesthesiology. In 1940 he was president of the Board. In 1943 and 1944 he was president of the American Society of Anesthetists.

In 1937 he was invited by Sir Robert MacIntosh to help organize the new department of anesthetics at Oxford. This was made possible through Jack Morris, later Lord Nuffield, who established five chairs at Oxford, one in anesthesia. The department was set up in the Radcliffe Infirmary and was patterned after the Bellevue department, incorporating many of the ideals Rovenstine envisioned but had not achieved in his own. Oxford's anesthesia department is the paragon of departments in England.

In World War II, Rovenstine conducted almost singlehandedly one of the most effective and brilliant courses in practical anesthesia for physicians in the military service. Many of these men became heads of departments in general hospitals.

Honors were many. In 1960 Rovenstine was awarded the New York University Presidential Citation at the alumni meeting, which also saw honors bestowed on the developer of the attenuated polio vaccine, Dr. Sabin, and on Severo Ochoa, who received the Nobel Prize in 1959 for work on cell mechanisms and nucleic acids.

In 1957, he was given the Distinguished Service Award of the American Society of Anesthesiologists, Inc. Since 1935, meetings on clinical anesthesia have been conducted on Monday nights at Bellevue. This is the longest known formal case discussion conference in anesthesia. It was most popular and was attended by over 50 people, including the residents, anesthetists from the city, and many visitors from around the world. Perhaps this is the greatest tribute to any man and his concept.

In 1946 and 1947 Rovenstine served as one of the seven physicians on the Unitarian mission to Czechoslovakia to bring that country up to date medically. His teaching was such a brilliant success that he received the Order of the White Lion, the highest honor the Czechoslovak government bestows on foreigners. He retired in 1960 and died the same year.

LUNDY OF MAYO CLINIC. An amiable modern leader in the specialty of anesthesia, John Lundy was always known as the man who was willing to do hard jobs.[35] Born in North Dakota in 1894, he received his medical degree from Rush Medical College in 1920. After graduation he moved to Seattle, where in 1921 he specialized in anesthesia. Interest in anesthesia was growing through the country, and as ever the Mayo Clinic was in the forefront of institutions to recognize the budding specialty. In 1924 Lundy was invited to run the department of anesthesia, and he stayed until 1952.

Lundy was a prolific writer. He published a book on clinical anesthesia and established a digest entitled Anesthesia Abstracts. In the field of clinical anesthesia, he introduced the practice of the intravenous pentothal technique on June 18, 1934. In 1935 he developed a forerunner of the modern blood bank. In 1942 the first postanesthesia recovery unit was established.

His contributions to teaching have been far-reaching. He trained many men at the Mayo Clinic in the fellowship program. During World War II he trained over 250 physicians to supply the military with proper anesthesia personnel.

His contributions as a leader have been many. He was one of the founders and president of the American Board of Anesthesiology; he was president of the American Society of Anesthesiologists and helped to establish the Section on Anesthesia of the American Medical Association. In this organization he became known as the perennial secretary. Finally in 1955 he became the chairman of the section. The American Society of Anesthesiologists conferred on him the Distinguished Service Award in 1948.

Besides his contributions directly to anesthesia,

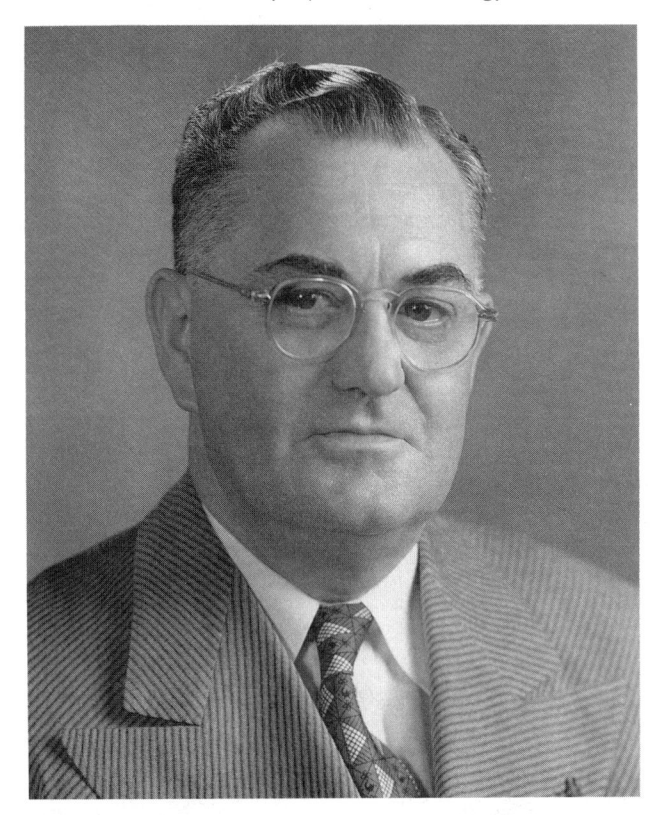

FIG. 1–9. John Lundy.

Lundy was instrumental in establishing, in 1956, the Anesthesia Memorial Foundation. This is a revolving loan fund for young men, and the indirect influence that this is having and will have cannot be estimated. Lundy died in 1973.

GRIFFITHS AND THE WORLD FEDERATION. Harold R. Griffiths, who was born in Montreal in 1894, profoundly affected the specialty of anesthesia.[36] He was the son of a physician and received medical degrees from the University of Ontario and Hahnemann Medical College in Philadelphia. He served as surgeon in World War I and as consultant in anesthesia in the Royal Canadian Air Force in World War II.

Griffiths was known as an outstanding clinical anesthetist. He wrote many papers on the practice of anesthesia, but his outstanding contribution in the scientific field was pioneering work on the clinical use of curare. Equally important was his extensive work on the clinical application of cyclopropane. In 1946 Griffiths became lecturer in anesthesia at McGill University Faculty of Medicine, and in 1950, with the retirement of Wesley Bourne, he became head of the department.

Many honors came to Harold Griffiths. He was president of the Canadian Anesthetists Society as well as president of the International Anesthesia Research Society. For some time he was chairman

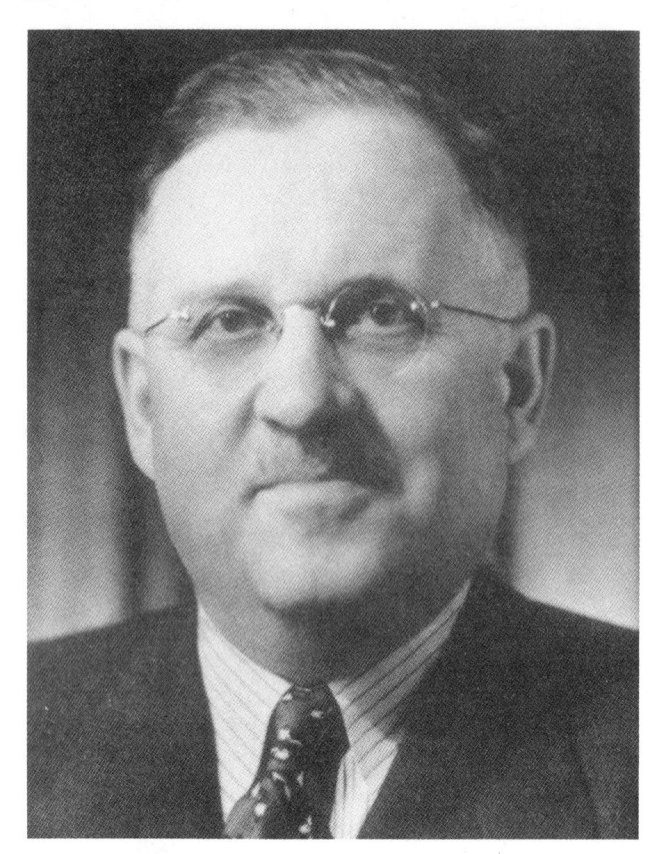

FIG. 1–10. Harold R. Griffiths.

of the committee on anesthesia of the Royal College of Physicians and Surgeons in Canada. In 1956 he received the Hickman medal for outstanding contributions to his specialty.

Throughout his career Griffiths preached the art of anesthesia and emphasized that anesthesiologists are physicians first. This consuming philosophy led to a dedication of purpose to spread the practice of anesthesia throughout the world. To this end he helped to establish the World Federation of Societies of Anesthesiologists and planned the first World Congress in The Netherlands in 1955. He served as first president of the World Federation, and in 1960, when the American Society of Anesthesiologists became one of the federated members, his full dream for anesthesia was realized.

BOOKS

The first comprehensive books on anesthesia were published during and following World War I. In 1914 Gwathmey published the first edition of his book *Anesthesia*; in 1916 Flagg published *The Art of Anesthesia*, in 1920 Arthur E. Guedel published *Signs of Anesthesia*, and in 1922 Gaston Labat published his classical treatise *Regional Anesthesia*. Later, in 1937, Guedel published a more extensive book entitled *Inhalation Anesthesia*; in 1938 Henry K. Beecher published his *Physiology of Anesthesia*; in 1941 Adriani's *Pharmacology of Anesthetic Drugs* was available; and in 1942 Lundy's *Clinical Anesthesia* was published. Many others also have been published, but those mentioned can rightfully be called classics.

Several journals influenced the development of anesthesia. Among these journals were The British Journal of Anesthesia (1923), Current Researches in Anesthesia and Analgesia (1923), Narkose und Anesthesia in Germany (1928), Bulletin of National Association of Nurse-Anesthetists, (1933, now the Journal of the American Association of Nurse Anesthetists), Anesthetic et Analgesia in France (1935), Anesthesia Abstract (1937), and finally Anesthesiology (1940).

NEW AGENTS AND TECHNIQUES

Ethylene was introduced in 1923 by Luckhardt.[37] Cyclopropane was introduced experimentally in 1929 and used clinically for the first time in 1933.[38] Its development and use were due to the group of Wisconsin anesthetists under Ralph M. Waters, W.B. Neff, and E.A. Rovenstine.[39] Vinethene was introduced in 1930 by Leake.[40] Pontocaine was introduced in 1930. In 1934 Lundy introduced the use of sodium pentothal for intravenous anesthesia.[41]

In 1920 I.W. Magill of England developed endotracheal anesthesia.[42] About the same time Labat brought regional anesthesia to the point of an exact science. In 1923 Ralph M. Waters perfected a closed system of anesthesia and developed the use of soda lime for carbon dioxide absorption.[43] Richard Von Foregger constructed an apparatus for the administration of numerous anesthetic agents.

In 1926 rectal anesthesia was given a great impetus by the introduction of tribromoethanol (Avertin) in Germany.[44] Finally in 1934 intravenous anesthesia reached a high degree of technical perfection through the efforts of John S. Lundy at Mayo Clinic.

ORGANIZATIONS

As the development of anesthesia progressed, the need for men to meet, to communicate, and to grow was pressing. The time was ripe to get together and to organize an anesthesia society.[45] The London Society of Anesthetists was founded in 1893. In the United States, two men stand out in their attempts to organize anesthesia. One was successful.

THE ASA. In 1905 the first anesthesia society in the United States was organized in Brooklyn and called the Long Island Society of Anesthetists. The object of the new society was "to promote the art and science of anesthetics." The annual fee was $1.00 for any regularly qualified physician whose interest centered in anesthesia. In 1911 this group combined with men from Manhattan, and the New York Society of Anesthetists was formed. At their organizing meeting in the old New York Academy of Medicine, Yandell Henderson spoke on the relation of the physiologic chemist to the anesthetist. Later in the same evening the celebrated Verworn spoke on "narcosis."

In 1932 the society was presented with the central seal designed by Paul M. Wood, (Fig. 1–9).

The significance of this seal is as follows: "The ship represents the patient sailing the troubled sea of unconsciousness with clouds of doubt and waves of terror. The ship is guided by the skillful pilot (the anesthetist) with constant and eternal (stars) vigilance (the motto) by his dependable (lighthouse) knowledge of the art of sleep (moon) to a safe (shield) and happy outcome of his voyage into the realms of the unknown."

By 1935 this organization became national in scope with the energetic Paul Wood as secretary; the title was changed in 1936 to the American Society of Anesthetists and the society was incorporated in the state of New York.[37]

In 1944 Paul Wood proposed that the name be changed to the American Society of Anesthesiologists, Inc.[46] Wood disclaimed coining the word "anesthesiology" and stated that it had been used long before he entered medical school. Lexicographers defined the term as the "study and practice of the art and science of anesthesia in all its forms and all that pertains thereto (i.e., gas therapy, resuscitation)." Wood made public in 1945 a letter received from Dr. M.J. Siefert that read as follows: "In 1902 while teaching at the University of Illinois, I coined the word *anesthesiology* and defined it as follows: The Science that treats of the means and methods of producing various degrees of insensibility to pain with or without hypnosis. An *anesthetist* is a technician and an *anesthesiologist* is the scientific authority on anesthesia and anesthetics. I cannot understand why you do not term yourself the American Society of Anesthesiologists." On April 12, 1945, the certificate of change of name was received.

FRANK MCMECHAN AND THE CONGRESSES. The American Association of Anesthetists was formed by James Gwathmey and Frank McMechan in 1919. McMechan was a zealot for anesthesia.[47] Though an arthritic cripple most of his adult life, he profoundly influenced thoughts from his wheelchair. He organized several regional societies such as the Associated Anesthetists of the United States and Canada in 1926. In 1919 he founded with McKesson the National Anesthesia Research Society to include manufacturers of drugs and apparatus and other laymen interested in anesthesia. By 1922 the International Research Society was formed by Dr. McMechan and its first "congress" held the same year.

In 1923 the American Society of Regional Anesthetists was formed. It was founded to honor Gaston Labat, who resisted efforts to have the society named after him. Only four of the members were anesthetists; the majority were neurosurgeons. Labat crusaded for anesthesia to be recognized as a medical discipline and outlined the responsibilities of the anesthetist that would justify a physician entering the field.

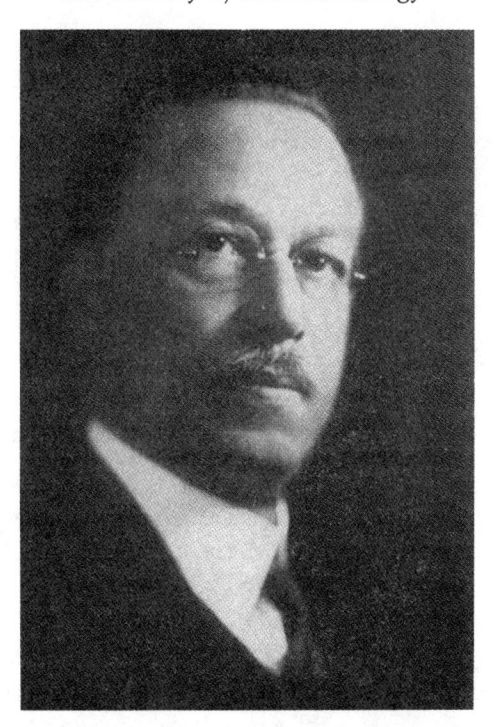

FIG. 1–11. Gaston Labat (1877–1934), the developer of techniques in regional anesthesia.

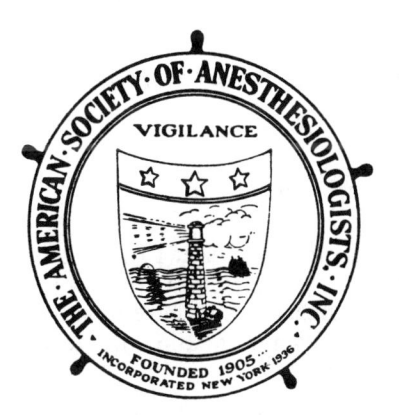

FIG. 1–12. Seal of the American Society of Anesthesiologists, designed by Paul M. Wood.

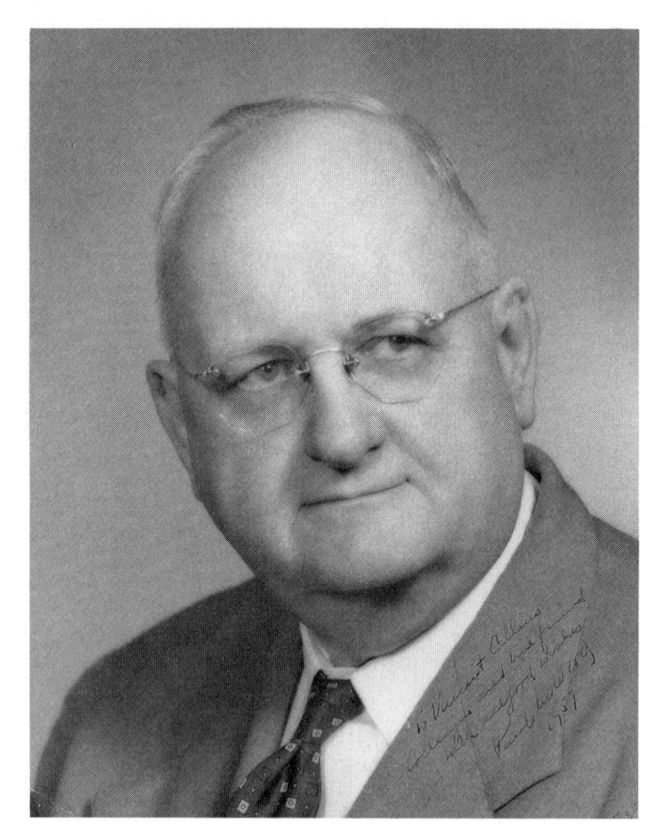

FIG. 1–13. Paul M. Wood.

ANESTHESIA—A SPECIALTY

With the introduction of so many agents and so many techniques for the alleviation of pain and with the recognition that good anesthesia could be performed only with a thorough knowledge of physiology and pharmacology, it became readily apparent that anesthesia was a specialty in medicine. As a result, numerous hospitals, especially those associated with medical schools and universities, began the organization of departments of anesthesiology. In 1937 the American Board of Anesthesiology was formed, and in the same year anesthesiology was recognized as a specialty by the American Medical Association. The first section meeting under the American Medical Association was held in Chicago in 1941.

MILITARY ASPECTS

From 1846 until World War I there is little of note. During the Civil War, sporadic surgical cases received ether anesthesia at base hospitals. Instances of ether anesthesia were likewise recorded for the Spanish war in 1899.

With the advent of World War I, a great impetus was given to anesthesia and to the subject of transfusions. During this war, open drop inhalation and local anesthesia were used quite extensively. There was some spinal anesthesia, and later in the war a closed system of inhalation anesthesia was introduced.

During this period, methods were introduced for the preservation of whole blood and for direct and indirect transfusion. World War I stimulated many studies on the use of blood substitutes in shock, such as gum acacia in saline, and on the mechanisms of shock.

The military, influenced by outstanding civilian pioneers, was quick to recognize the importance of anesthesia, and in 1939 the Surgeon General's office recognized anesthesiology as a medical specialty and proceeded to organize a section of anesthesia.[48] Eventually, it planned to have anesthesiologists with officer status in all the larger medical installations. Much of the work on organization was due to the efforts of Ralph M. Tovell. The various echelons of medical service as organized by the Army were investigated and analyzed with the purpose of providing the appropriate anesthetic agents and techniques for each individual unit.[49,50]

About the same time that Army anesthesia was being organized in its broad aspect, the first organized course in anesthesia in the history of the Army was developed at Tilton General Hospital, in July 1941, through the efforts of Major Stevens J. Martin.[51] One year later a school of anesthesia was officially authorized by the War Department, as were several schools of anesthesia in various civilian hospitals throughout the country, among these being the School of Anesthesia at Bellevue Hospital, New York, and the School of Anesthesia at Mayo Clinic under John S. Lundy.

ANESTHESIA IN ITS MATURING YEARS

It is now well recognized that anesthesiology is first of all a medical discipline.[52] It has long been recognized by major medical associations as a practice of medicine.[53-55] The traditional activity of an anesthetist was the routine administration of an anesthetic. Today, however the scope of the anesthesiologist's activities is significantly broader. He is now concerned with all the medical problems to which the human being is heir, as they might be encountered in the operating room and during anesthesia.[56] Accordingly, the anesthesiologist should have five attributes:

1. He must be a fairly good diagnostician, familiar with the prevention and treatment of common medical conditions.
2. He must have surgical awareness. He should be cognizant of most common surgical procedures

so that he can anticipate the steps demanded of the surgeon.
3. He must be a good pharmacologist, familiar not only with analgesic and anesthetic drugs, but also with the resources used by the general practitioner of medicine, who is faced with many emergency situations.
4. He must be a good physiologist. To this end, he must be particularly familiar with respiratory mechanisms, respiratory gas exchange, cardiovascular hemodynamics, and renal and hepatic functions.
5. Finally, he must be a good technician.

Outside the operating room, the endeavors and responsibilities of the anesthesiologist have extended into three areas of medical care. These include diagnostic and therapeutic nerve blocking; the management of fluid therapy, including blood bank supervision and the management of transfusion problems; and the supervision of inhalation therapy and resuscitation. In all these activities one recognizes the application of the team concept in medical management. It is obvious that the practice of medicine is more and more a cooperative endeavor, and this is truly apparent in the practice of anesthesiology.

The anesthesiologist is a consultant. He is particularly a consultant to the surgeon in respect to problems of pharmacology and physiology. He is, in fact, the medical internist in the operating room. As the internist in the operating room, he advises the surgeon concerning physiologic dysfunction, pharmacologic aspects, and the treatment of medical complications that arise in the patient during the course of anesthesia and surgery. His sphere of activity is thus clearly defined. It is to care for the physiologic functions of the patient, thereby permitting the surgeon to devote and concentrate his entire attention and skill to the correction of anatomic abnormalities. Thus the surgeon's skills are directed more toward anatomy, whereas the anesthesiologist's skills are directed more toward physiology.

RECOGNITION

Anesthesiology as a medical discipline was rapidly recognized in the United States.[57] In general, its development was analogous to the development of the medical discipline of obstetrics. Obstetrics had progressed from a fertile field for midwives in the year 1920 to an exact science with untold advantages for women by about 1950. Whereas, prior to 1920, some 75% of the deliveries in the United States were furnished by other than physicians, in the year 1950, the reverse was true.

In 1935 the American Society of Anesthesiologists was formed with 300 members. In 1940 the American Medical Association endorsed the formation of a Section of Anesthesiology. By 1950 or 15 years after the formal organization in the United States of a Society of Anesthesiology, there were 4000 members. Thus, in 15 years, there was a 15-fold increase in the number of specialists engaged in the practice of anesthesia.[58] Today, in 1990 there are over 26,000 anesthesiologists.

THE DEPARTMENT OF ANESTHESIOLOGY

The well organized and coordinated department of anesthesiology can and should supply assistance and consultation to all the other medical services in a hospital.[56]

Besides the inherent responsibilities in the operating room, the scope of activity of the anesthesiologist includes a group of ancillary services in which his knowledge and capabilities can be put to use for the benefit of the patient. Such services include

1. Alleviation of various pain states and establishment of nerve block clinics.
2. Management and supervision of inhalation therapy including all the aspects of oxygen and helium applications and the techniques of aerosol administration.
3. Resuscitation, including resuscitation of the newborn; management of drug poisoning cases, such as barbiturate and morphine intoxication; and team management of chronic respiratory diseases.[59,60]
4. Supervision and responsibility of intravenous fluid therapy, especially during surgical procedures; and in some institutions, the supervision and running of a blood bank.

TRAINING IN ANESTHESIOLOGY

The best clinical anesthesiologists are those who have trained in the school of purism. By this is meant that the trainee has learned various anesthetic techniques and the use of various agents by observing the use of each one alone and by practicing the use of each one separately and unadulterated by a host of other anesthetics or adjuncts. Probably, anesthesiologists can progress best by learning simple sequences of agents and techniques. For example, experience can be acquired first in open-drop ether-oxygen anesthesia and in simple gas-oxygen semiclosed system anesthesia. This can be followed by gas oxygen-ether technique by closed system and then techniques of pentothal-oxygen administration. The basic experience would be completed by a variety of simple regional anesthetic procedures including epidural and spinal methods.

Subsequently, a combination of agents can be used

when proper indications are presented. Thus, in the course of a cyclopropane and oxygen anesthesia it might be wise and proper to administer a relaxant. If the trainee begins by being exposed to the combination or balanced type of anesthetics, however, he never quite comes to know the reactions of a patient to any specific agent, but is always faced with a confusion of pharmacologic stress. Once having mastered the use and learned the pharmacology by observation of the available agents, he can then complicate his anesthetic situation.

Most residents who enter the field of anesthesia seem to progress through three distinct phases.[61] First, he is the novice. He enters this specialty and is quickly presented with an overwhelming need for knowledge of anesthesiology and physiology and pharmacology as well as a multiplicity of technical procedures. If his preceptor is a mature and able individual, some order can be quickly derived.

Soon the budding anesthesiologist learns to handle a few anesthetic methods acceptably, and with a little further knowledge he enters the second phase, which is designated as the stage of unfounded confidence. This phrase was borrowed from Dr. Artusio at New York Hospital. At this stage, the man having mastered several simple techniques and a smattering of knowledge regarding agents, he blithely goes on his way producing anesthesia that is relatively acceptable. Sometimes this phase lasts for many years and some anesthesiologists actually never achieve the final goal that really labels him as an expert.

Often, however, some complication or mishap occurs that disturbs our young man considerably. A patient's life might actually be lost. If our man is conscientious, a period of remorse and introspection will ensue, and the stage of unfounded confidence will be climaxed by a period of uncertainty. If, at this time, there is again a mature and wise counselor, the young man can be assured and can thereby become, as a result of his experience, a more competent and moral physician. When this occurs the third stage is achieved, which is the phase of calm assurance. The man can now be called an expert.

In many training programs new residents observe for a period of 2 full weeks. Nothing is performed. Few technical responsibilities are given to the man. At the end of this period the simple and pure techniques are begun, and with the presentation of basic knowledge a firm foundation is gradually developed. It is undesirable to plunge young physicians into significant anesthesia responsibilities early in their period of exposure.

Men entering the field of anesthesiology should be encouraged to broaden their interests and their knowledge of problems in general medicine, particularly those in the field of cardiology and respiratory diseases. They should be thoroughly trained in the theoretic and practical aspects of fluid and electrolyte balance. New developments in basic physiology must ever be an integral part of the education syllabus.

PROFILES OF ANESTHESIOLOGISTS IN THE MATURING YEARS: 1950 TO 1980

HENRY K. BEECHER—EDUCATOR, RESEARCHER, AND ETHICIAN. To many anesthesiologists, Massachusetts General Hospital and Harvard Medical School meant Henry K. Beecher.[62] After his early education in Kansas and receipt of a B.A. and an M.A. he went to Harvard University School of Medicine, from which he graduated with the M.D. degree in 1932. During a 2-year surgical house officer appointment, he was persuaded to engage in research by Churchill and then began a 2-year program under August Krogh in Copenhagen studying the capillary circulation and absorption of insulin.[63] On returning to Boston in 1936, Beecher was appointed anesthetist-in-chief at Massachusetts General Hospital. His fellowship and research led to the publication of a textbook, The Physiology of Anesthesia,[64] and he was appointed as the Henry Isaiah Dorr Professor of Research in Anesthesia.

With the entrance of the United States into World War II, Beecher joined the Army and was appointed by Churchill to the position of Consultant in Resuscitation and Anesthesia for the Mediterranean theatre.[65,66]

The contributions of Beecher to the rapidly growing science of anesthesiology, as well as its practice both before the war and after, are evident in the publications of his wide-ranging interests in medicine and research. At the same time, he designed an outstanding residency program and trained over 350 anesthesiologists, many of whom became professors and eminent anesthesiologists.

The Physiology of Anesthesia (1938)[64] dealt with the fundamental aspects of anesthesia; Beecher was concerned with the effects of anesthetics, not techniques.

Beecher wrote Resuscitation and Anesthesia in the Wounded (1946)[67] as a result of his experience in World War II.

An important aspect of his war experience was to identify the dangers of morphine in wounded subjects. This led to many studies of the precise pharmacology of morphine, as well as concepts of pain.[68,69]

Together with D.P. Todd, Beecher wrote A Study of the Deaths Associated with Anesthesia (1954)[70] which dealt with methods of statistical evaluation.

In Experimentation in Man,[71] Beecher presented some of the earliest methods allowing objective measurements of subjective responses. The double-blind technique provided a scientific basis for evaluation of the subject's human responses of the drugs.[72,73] This replaced the crude "clinical impression" concept.

Research and the Individual: Human Studies (1970)[74] entered into the field of moral and ethical problems related to medical care. Programs were presented and analyzed with regard to the protection of the rights of patients and of research volunteers.

A base for this book appeared in the New England Journal of Medicine in 1966, entitled Ethics and Clinical Research.[75] This is a classic report and is must reading for clinical investigators.

Criteria for Definition of Death: Irreversible Coma was produced by a committee set up by the Harvard Medical School with Beecher as chairman. It established medical guidelines for determination of brain death as a form of death, in addition to the traditional absence of respiration and heartbeat. The flat electroencephalogram and the absence of neurological responses were essential criteria.

Henry Beecher was an active member in many anesthesia organizations as well as allied medical societies, and he was *continued* as a consultant in anesthesia and research to all branches of the armed services. He was president of the Association of University Anesthetists.

Among the honors he received are the following: Ralph M. Waters Award, Distinguished Service Award of the American Society of Anesthesiologists, Chevalier of the French Legion of Honor, and Knight of the Royal Order of Dannenborg of Denmark.

On retirement in 1969 Beecher spent his time in the Gountway Library in Boston and pursued his hobby of cultivating prize camellias at home until his death in 1976.

VIRGINIA APGAR—PIONEER OBSTETRIC ANESTHESIOLOGIST AND NEONATOLOGIST. Early in her life, Virginia Apgar became interested in science due to her father's experiments in electricity and his work in astronomy. By the time she graduated from highschool she had decided to become a physician—a fortuitous decision for all of medicine. She attended Mt. Holyoke College, where she was an outstanding student, both academically and in many extracurricular activities. After her graduation in 1929 she maintained a close association with Mt. Holyoke as an alumna, and eventually her papers, letters, and personal diary became part of the College Library Archives. With graduation, she matriculated at the College of Physicians and Surgeons of Columbia University, was elected a member of the AOA, and received her M.D. degree in 1933.

Apgar's postgraduate education started with a surgical internship at Columbia-Presbyterian Hospital, and although she performed brilliantly, she was persuaded to enter the field of anesthesia by Alan Whipple, the chairman of the department of surgery. After completing her internship she continued at Columbia-Presbyterian, working with the head nurse anesthetist, Anne Penland.[76]

Meanwhile she sought information about training programs in anesthesia from Frank McMechan (Secretary of Associated Anesthetists of the U.S. and Canada) and received a list of 13, of which fewer than 6 were of any quality or breadth.[77] At the beginning of 1937 she visited Ralph Waters and the Department of Anesthesia at Madison, Wisconsin—the preeminent training program at the time—and stayed for 6 months. She then returned to New York City to Bellevue Hospital and continued her training with Emery Rovenstine, who had recently completed the program at Madison, and an appointment as Dr. Waters' Associate. Rovenstine had gone to Bellevue to establish a residency in anesthesia based on Waters' concepts.

In 1938, with completion of her formal training in anesthesia, Apgar returned to Columbia University and was appointed Director of the Division of Anesthesia and Attending Anesthetist at Columbia-Presbyterian Medical Center. It is difficult to imagine the overwhelming obstacles to be surmounted by anyone attempting to establish the specialty of anesthesiology in a hospital or medical school at this time, with the additional obstacle of the attitude of men physicians toward the few women in medicine.

But Apgar's diligence, enthusiasm, skill, and knowledge prevailed. She was an outstanding teacher, with an overwhelming ambition to impart every speck of knowledge about the specialty to any

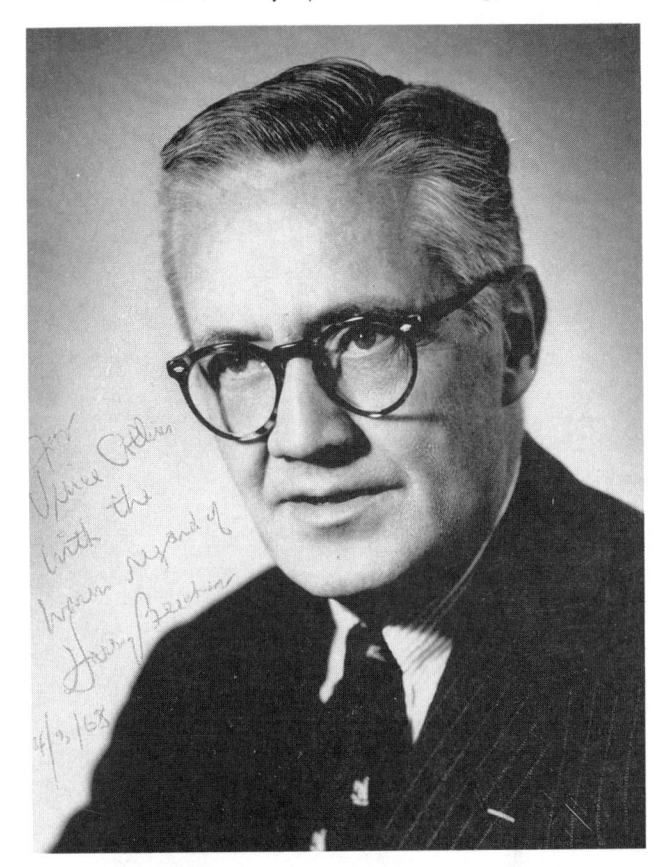

FIG. 1–14. Henry K. Beecher.

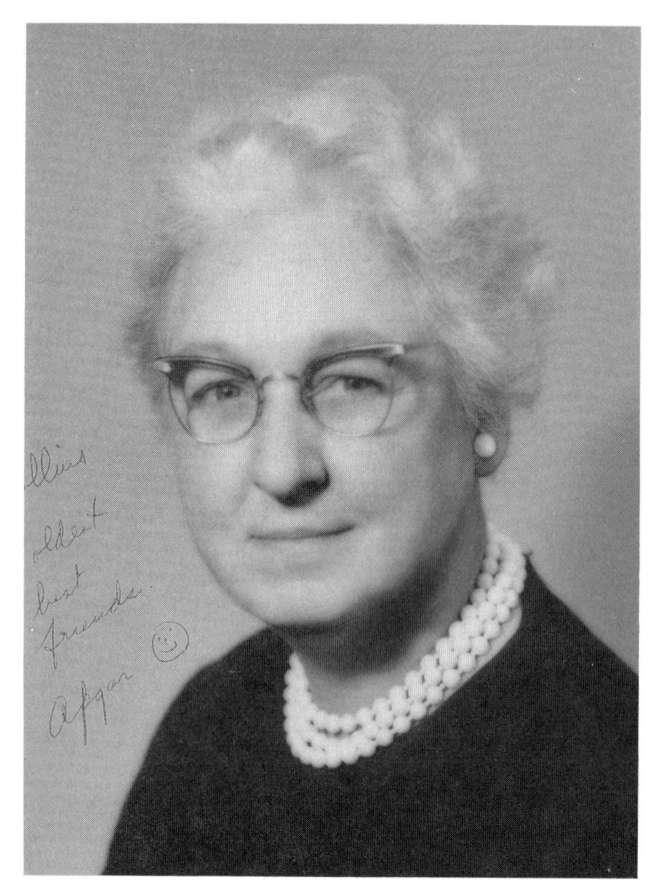

FIG. 1–15. Virginia Apgar.

student. She was a role model and convinced many new and older physicians to enter the young specialty.

In 1949, after World War II, anesthesiology was emerging as a vigorous specialty, with young men returning to civilian practice and not to be denied. It is to Apgar's credit and foresight that she desired to have more fundamental research and fuller input into the medical school and hospital administrative structure. To this end, Dr. E.M. Papper was appointed as chairman of the Department of Anesthesiology, and both he and Apgar were appointed full professors of anesthesiology—she being the first full professor of anesthesiology at Columbia University.

Obstetric Anesthesia. With Papper assuming the responsibilities of administration, Apgar was free to pursue her ambition to improve the anesthetic care of women in labor, and she pioneered the development of the subspecialty of obstetric anesthesiology.[78,79] Her work in this field credits her to the title of Mother of Obstetric Anesthesiology.

The Apgar Score for the Newborn. Until 1949 no evaluation of the newborn had been standardized. The idea of a score came to Apgar when a medical student wondered how the condition of a newborn could be assessed. Apgar responded, "That's easy! You do it this way," whereupon she wrote down on a piece of paper the five points that became the Apgar Score. It was quickly applied and was found to be simple, practical, and reliable as an index. It was first published in 1953 and again in JAMA in 1958.[78,80]

As a method of evaluation at 1 minute and at 5 minutes, it has become the base to correlate the effects of labor, delivery, drugs, and anesthetics on the physiologic condition of the baby. It was found to serve as a guide for instituting appropriate resuscitation measures and to correct abnormal conditions such as hypoxia and birth trauma. It is also a predictor of neonatal survival and neurologic development.[81]

Two research associates of Apgar, namely Duncan Holaday and Stanley James, introduced new technology for the monitoring of the newborn and enable physician to accurately correlate clinical states with biochemical conditions. Indeed, these studies formed the basis of a new subspecialty to be named Neonatology, mothered by Virginia Apgar.

New Horizons. To further her knowledge of the impact of birth events on outcome, Apgar went to Johns Hopkins University and obtained a master's degree in public health. Because of her research on factors producing birth defects and congenital abnormalities, she was appointed to the research staff of the National Foundation (March of Dimes) and headed the Division of Congenital Malformations.[82] In 1967 she became vice-president and director of basic research of the Foundation. About this time (1965) she was appointed professor of pediatrics (teratology), the first appointment covering birth defects as a subspecialty.

Societies and Honors. Apgar's innumerable honors included the ASA (American Society of Anesthesiology) Distinguished Service Award (1961); she was awarded an honorary Doctor of Science degree by Mt. Holyoke College in 1965; memberships in societies other than those in anesthesia and medicine included the AAAS, the American Society of Human Genetics, the Teratology Society, the American Public Health Association; she held fellowships in the New York Academy of Medicine, the New York Academy of Science, the American College of Obstetrics and Gynecology, and the Harvey Society.

But Apgar's life was not all medicine and science. She was an accomplished musician and played the cello in the Teaneck Symphony Orchestra. Her hobby was making stringed instruments; this work was recognized by outstanding musicians, and she was elected a member of the exclusive Catgut Acoustical Society.[76,83]

Apgar co-authored a book entitled *Is My Baby All Right?*[84] with Joan Beck, and it became a bestseller for pregnant women during the 1970s.

Virginia Apgar contributed much. She will be

missed by many, and she was an inspiration to all whom she touched.

JOHN ADRIANI—EDUCATOR, AUTHOR, AND POLITICIAN. The phrase "Connecticut Yankee in the South" well describes John Adriani. He was born in Bridgeport, Connecticut, where he had his elementary education. Medicine was in his blood, and he pursued courses in premed, as well as his medical education, at Columbia University. Subsequently he served his residency in anesthesiology under E.A. Rovenstine at Bellevue Hospital.[84,85]

In 1939, the New Charity Hospital, under the influence of Dr. C.B. Odom (who was in charge of surgical affairs and who developed the Odom technique for epidural anesthesia), decided that physician anesthesia was necessary. John Adriani was appointed to the position in March 1941 after brief negotiations and no interview.[86,87]

Adriani was an involved member of the American Society of Anesthesiology. He was a "politician" in this regard, but he was also a worker and held many positions. He actively participated in the American Medical Association. He was the chairman of the Advisory Committee on Anesthetics for the revision of the U.S. Pharmacopeia XVIII.

Also expert in clinical pharmacology, Adriani was an advocate of generic terminology and prescription writing. His esteem and knowledge in this regard placed him on the American Medical Association Council on Drugs, where he served as chairman. In such efforts he was a professional protagonist for the consumer as well as for lower prices of drugs.[84]

His interest in pharmacology led him into many governmental and specialty organizations requiring in-depth knowledge of drugs. He was nominated for the position of Director of the Bureau of Medicine in the United States Food and Drug Administration in 1969, but political pressure from the pharmaceutical industry resulted in the withdrawal of his appointment.[87]

In organizing his department of anesthesia from a nonexisting-to-chaotic service to an outstanding clinical service that was well equipped with machines and instruments, he followed and enhanced the dictums of Rovenstine. These were: anesthesiology as a medical specialty to be engaged in *only* by trained personnel, training programs to emphasize basic physiology and pharmacology and a residency for young physicians. His first three residents were female graduates of Louisiana State University. As a result of this residency program, the South particularly and many other areas of the country were supplied with outstanding anesthesiologists.

To implement his educational program, Adriani authored many books, which became major sources of anesthesia information throughout the United States and even abroad. Outstanding among these texts was The Pharmacology of Anesthetic Drugs (1942), which was a concise, tabular type of presentation and a classic source for educators and residents alike from 1942 to 1955. Also outstanding was the Chemistry of Anesthesia (1946), which was followed by a more comprehensive book entitled The Physics and Chemistry of Anesthesia. Techniques and Procedures was also a major reference source. All these books were published by Charles C Thomas of Springfield, Illinois—an author-publisher marriage of renown.

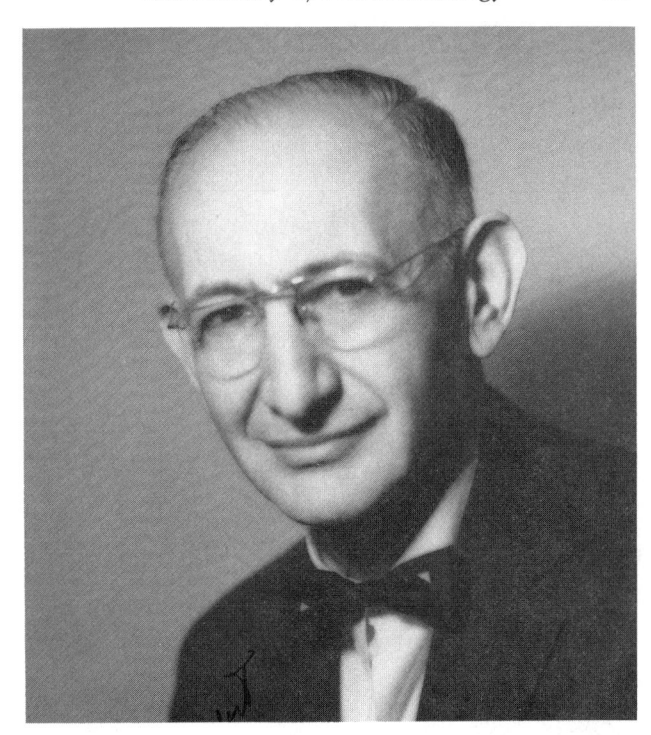

FIG. 1–16. John Adriani.

Disqualified for military service by a heart murmur, Adriani conducted a training program for all medical students and for assigned medical officers. He was appointed to professorships at both Louisiana State University and Tulane and quickly became involved in the administration of the hospital. Later in his career he became the associate director of Charity Hospital in New Orleans.

Many awards came to John Adriani including the ASA Distinguished Service award and the Ralph Waters award. All knew him as a gifted, incisive teacher and lecturer, but he was also recognized for being direct, for his critical witticisms, and for his bow tie.

ROBERT D. DRIPPS. In 1939, Dr. Dripps—with a widening interest in physiology and pharmacology due to Julius Comroe and Carl Schmidt—was persuaded by Dr. H.K. Beecher of Harvard to enter the specialty of anesthesiology. Dr. Dripps sought his training under Dr. R.M. Waters at the University of Wisconsin and, after 9 months, returned to the University of Pennsylvania in 1941. He spent his time working both in the area of laboratory research and in clinical anesthesia. From a small beginning of four nurse

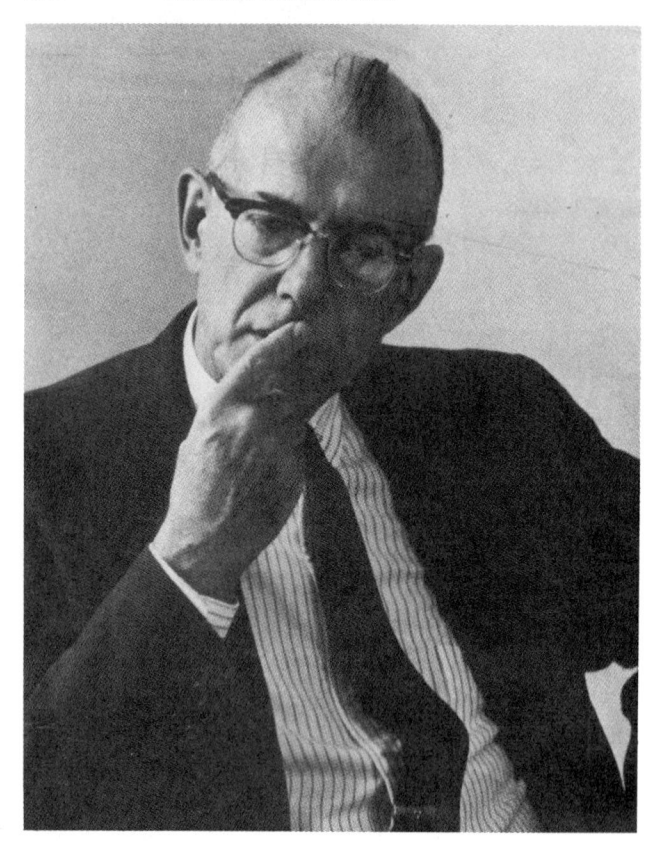

FIG. 1–17. Robert D. Dripps

anesthetists and Dr. Margery Van N. Deming, the first resident, prior to World War II to a suddenly expanded postwar staff of physicians, some with previous training and combined war anesthesia experience, a department developed that was based on the triad of education as expounded by Dr. Waters: basic science education, laboratory research, and clinical care of patients. These principles were avidly pursued. Among the veterans with war experience who began more formal training in anesthesiology was James Eckenhoff, who started with pharmacology.

Dr. Dripps was imbued with the philosophy that anesthesia is a medical specialty and that physicians in anesthesiology should act as physicians and not technicians. Dripps felt that they should act in the Waters and Rovenstine model and that they should consult with other physicians not only during surgery but also during the preoperative and postoperative periods. By 1950, the Department was flooded with many talented applicants from good medical schools in the United States and in Europe; by this time, Dripps also required that all junior medical students spend a week's rotation in the anesthesiology service. Elective courses also became available for fourth year students, interns, and residents.

With a competent and dedicated staff of teachers and clinicians, Dr. Dripps became active in broad organizational, educational, and research programs. This was exemplified by many appointments: membership in and chairmanship of the National Research Council (Subcommittee on Anesthesiology); as an active member of the American Board of Anesthesiologists in the 1950s and early 1960s and as president of the Board for a year. He served as Chairman of the World Health Organizations Scientific Group on the Evaluation of Drugs. Dr. Dripps was also an organizing member of the Association of University Anesthetists.

Among his many honors, Dr. Dripps was granted the Distinguished Service Award of the American Society of Anesthesiologists, a fellowship in the Royal College of Surgeons in England and of Ireland, and election to membership in the American College of Surgeons and in the elite Halsted Society. His recognition as an outstanding physician resulted in the endowment of the Robert Dunning Dripps Chair in Anesthesia at the University of Pennsylvania. As a teacher and researcher, he was meticulous in seeing that the papers published by the department members were short, concise, and oriented to the basic sciences. This description fits one of the first and most popular books, entitled *Introduction to Anesthesia*, for medical students and residents, and a reference for senior faculty as well.

In 1970, Dr. Dripps was invited by Julius Comroe to work on a project at the Cardiovascular Research Institute at the University of California in San Francisco to document how the results of research impacted on medicine. A book entitled *Retrospectroscope: Insights into Medical Discovery* (Comroe, J.H.; Menlo Park, California, VonGehr Press, 1977) resulted from this work. In 1972, Dripps returned to Philadelphia a "refreshed" man.

How would one summarize Robert Dripps' contribution to anesthesia? He was an excellent physician and a competent scientist: clear-thinking and intuitive in planning for the future. He was a visionary, a teacher of great merit, and a challenging, superb lecturer. Dr. Dripps was also a fine administrator and a respected leader who developed a generation of leaders to follow. Julius Comroe, a great scientist and teacher in his own right, considered Dr. Dripps' great professional achievement to be "his role in developing anesthesia as a scientific academic discipline."

REFERENCES

1. Fulop-Miller, R.: Triumph Over Pain. Hamish, London, 1938.
2. Keys, T.E.: The History of Surgical Anesthesia. New York, Schuman's, 1945.
3. Journal of the History of Medicine: Anesthesia Centennial Number, New York, Henry Schuman, October, 1946.
4. Keys, T.E.: The Development of Anesthesia. Anesthesiology, 3:11, 282, 560, 1942.
5. Mitchell, S.W.: The birth and death of pain; a poem read October 16, 1896 at the commeration of the fiftieth anni-

versary of the first public demonstration of surgical anesthesia. New York, Vreeland Advertising Press 1896.
6. Horine, E.F.: Episodes in the History of Anesthesia. J. Hist. Med., 1:521, 1946.
7. Rosen, G.: Mesmerism and Surgery. J. Hist. Med., 1:527, 1946.
8. Fulton, J.F., Stanton M.E.: The Centennial of Surgical Anesthesia. An annotated catalogue (Yale Library). New York, Henry Schuman Pub., 1946.
9. Miller, A.H.: The Origin of the Word "Anesthesia." Boston Med. Surg., 197:1218, 1927.
10. Aldrete, J.A., Marron, G.M., and Wright, J.: The first administration of anesthesia in military surgery: On occasion of the Mexican-American War. Anesthesiology, 61:585, 1984.
11. Secher, O.: Introduction of chloroform into Denmark. Acta Chir. Scand. (Suppl.), 433:42, 1973.
12. Waters, R.M.: John Snow, First Anesthetist. Bios, 7:25, 1936.
13. Keys, T.E.: John Snow, M.D., Anesthetist. J. Hist. Med., 1:551, 1946.
14. Snow, J.: On the Inhalation of Vapour of Ether. London, John Churchill, 1847.
15. Thomas, H.: Anesthesie à la Reine. Am. J. Obstet. Gyn., 40:340, 1940.
16. Snow, J.: On Chloroform and Other Anesthetics, Edited by B.W. Richardson. London, 1858.
17. Andrews, E.: The Oxygen Mixture: A New Anesthetic Combination. Chicago Med. Exam., 9:656, 1868.
18. Fulton, J.F.: The Biography of Harvey Cushing. Springfield, IL, Charles C Thomas, 1946.
19. McCarthy, K.C., Editor: Some Papers on Nitrous Oxide-Oxygen Anesthesia by E. I. McKesson. Priv. Printing, 1953.
20. McKesson, E.I.: Blood Pressure in General Anesthesia. Am. J. Surg. Anesth. (Suppl.):30, 2, 1916.
21. McKesson, E.I.: Nitrous oxide–oxygen anesthesia with a description of the new apparatus. Surg. Gynec. Obstet., 13:456, 1911.
22. A.S.A. Newsletter, 18:1, 1954.
23. Jackson, D.E.: Anesthesia equipment from 1914 to 1954 and experiments leading to its development. Anesthesiology, 16:953, 1955.
24. Jackson, D.E.: A new method for the production of general analgesia and anesthesia with a description of the apparatus used. J. Lab. Clin. Med., 1:1, 1915.
25. Jackson, D.E.: A special method for recording the actions of the heart: The cardiovibrograph and the vibrogram. Anesthesiology, 16:536, 1955.
26. Kaye, G.: If Embly were to return. Med. J. Aust., 18:197, 1945.
27. Betcher, A.M.: The jubilee year of organized anesthesia. Anesthesiology, 17:226, 1956.
28. Foregger, R.: Gwathmey. Anesthesiology, 5:296, 1944.
29. Gwathmey, J.T.: Oil-ether Anesthesia. Lancet, 2:1756, 1913.
30. [Editorial]: Obituary—A. E. Guedel. A.S.A. Newsletter, 20, 28, 1956.
31. [Editorial]: We salute Ralph Waters. Anes. Analg., 36:81, 1957.
32. [Editorial]: We salute Wesley Bourne. Anes. Analg., 37:23, 1958.
33. [Editorial]: We salute Ivan Magill. Anes. Analg., 37:21, 1958.
34. [Editorial]: We salute Emery A. Rovenstine. Anes. Analg., 39:24, 1960.
35. [Editorial]: We salute John Lundy. Anes. Analg., 36:79, 1957.
36. [Editorial]: We salute Harold Griffiths. Anes. Analg., 36:71, 1957.
37. Luckhardt, A.B., and Carter, J.B.: Ethylene as a gas anesthetic. JAMA, 80:1440, 1923.
38. Lucas, G.H.W., and Henderson, V.E.: New anesthetic gas: Cyclopropane. Canad. Med. Assoc. J., 21:173, 1929.
39. Stiles, J.A., et al.: Cyclopropane as an anesthetic agent. Anes. Analg., 13:56, 1934.
40. Leake, C.D., and Chen, M.Y.: Anesthetic properties of certain unsaturated ethers. Proc. Soc. Exp. Biol. Med., 28:151, 1930.
41. Lundy, J.S., and Tovell, R.M.: Annual report for 1934 of Section on Anesthesia: Including data on blood transfusions. Proc. Staff Meetings, Mayo Clin., 10:257, 1935.
42. Magill, I.W.: Development of endotracheal anesthesia. Proc. R. Soc. Med., 22:1928.
43. Waters, R.M.: Clinical scope and utility of carbon dioxide filtration in inhalation anesthesia. Anesth. Analg., 3:20, 1924.
44. Butzengeiger, O.: Klinische Erfahrungen mit Avertin (E107). Deutsche Med. Wchnschr., 53:712, 1927.
45. Waters, R.M.: Organization and anesthesiology [editorial]. Anesthesiology, 7:198, 1946.
46. Anesthesiology. American Society of Anesthesiologists, A.S.A., 1945.
47. [Editorial]. Frank McMechan, Anesth. Analg., 1954.
48. Martin, S.J.: Current considerations of the Army anesthesiologist. N. Engl. J. Med., 229:893, 1943.
49. Tovell, R.M.: Problems in training in and practice of anesthesiology in the European theater of operations. Anesthesiology, 8:62, 1947.
50. Tovell, R.M.: Problems in supply of anesthetic gases in the European theater of operations, U.S. Army. Anesthesiology, 8:303, 1947.
51. Martin, S.J.: Instruction in anesthesiology at Tilton General Hospital. Anesthesiology, 3:433, 1942.
52. Rovenstine, E.A.: Anesthesia and its maturing years. Med. Clin. North Am., 37:671, 1957.
53. Relation of physicians and hospitals. JAMA, 147:1684, 1951.
54. Report of joint committee on hospital-physician relationship of board of trustees of American Medical Association and American Hospital Association. JAMA, 152:729, 1953.
55. Report of committee on voluntary health insurance. JAMA, 154:66, 1954.
56. Collins, V.J.: Concepts in anesthesiology. JAMA, 182:105, 1962.
57. Bishop, H.F. [Editorial]: Progress and scope in anesthesiology. Westchester Med. Bull., 22:24, 1954.
58. Lorhan, P.: Booklet of Information—Published by American Society of Anesthesiologists, 1954.
59. O'Brien, W.A., et al: The anesthesiologist, the poliomyelitis team and the respirator. JAMA, 156:27, 1954.
60. Davis, H.S., and Bishop, H.F.: Airway management in patients wth poliomyelitis. JAMA, 149:1175, 1952.
61. Artusio, J.: The anesthesiologist. Bull. NY State Soc. Anes., 6:2, 1954.
62. [Editorial]: We salue Henry K. Beecher, M.D. Anesth. Analg., 38:22, 1959.
63. [Editorial]: Henry K. Beecher, M.D. N. Engl. J. Med., Sept. 23, 1976.
64. Beecher, H.K.: The Physiology of Anesthesia. New York, Oxford, 1938.
65. Beecher, H.K.: The internal state of the severely wounded man on entry to the most forward hospital. Surgery, 22:672, 1947.
66. Beecher, H.K.: Resuscitation and Anesthesia For Wounded Men. Springfield, IL, Charles C Thomas, 1949.
67. Beecher, H.K.: Resuscitation and Anesthesia in the Wounded.
68. Lasagna, L., and Beecher, H.K.: The optimal dose of morphine. JAMA, 156:230, 1954.
69. Gravenstein, J., and Beecher, H.K.: The effect of preoperative

medication with morphine on postoperative analgesia with morphine. J Pharmacol Exper Ther, *119:*506, 1954.
70. Beecher H.K., and Todd, D.P.: A Study Of the Deaths Associated with Anesthesia and Surgery Based on a Study of 599,548, Anesthesias in 10 Institutions, 1948–1952 Inclusive. Springfield, IL, Charles C Thomas, 1954.
71. Beecher, H.K.: Experimentation in Man. Springfield, IL, Charles C Thomas, 1959.
72. Beecher, H.K.: Appraisal of drugs intended to alter subjective responses. JAMA, *158:*399, 1955.
73. Beecher, H.K.: Ethics and clinical research. N. Engl. J. Med., *174:*1354, 1966.
74. Beecher, H.K.: Research and the Individual: Human Studies. Boston, Little, Brown, 1970.
75. Ethics and clinical research. N. Engl. J. Med., *274:*1354, 1966.
76. Zoffer, B. (ed.): Sphere, *32:* 1974.
77. Apgar Papers, Mount Holyoke College Library Archives: Box 1, Folders 1,3,4; Box 4, Folders 1,21; Box 5, Folders 21,23.
78. Apgar, V.: Proposal for a new method of evaluation of the newborn infant. Curr Res Anes, *32:*260, 1953.
79. Apgar, V., Holaday, D.A., and James, L.S.: Comparison of regional and general anesthesia in obstetrics. JAMA, *165:*2155, 1957.
80. Apgar, V., et al.: Evaluation of the newborn infant—second report. JAMA, *168:*1985, 1958.
81. Drage, J.S., Kennedy, C., and Schwartz, B.K.: The Apgar score as an index of neonatal mortality. Obstet. Gynecol., *24:*222, 1964.
82. National Foundation of March of Dimes. New York (July), 1959.
83. Apgar, V., and Beck, J.: Is My Baby All Right? New York, Trident Press, 1972.
84. ASA News Letter. American Society of Anesthesiology, Inc. August, 1988.
85. Bridgeport Sunday Post. May 13, 1986.
86. Collins V.J.: Personal Communication. May 27, 1968.
87. Zepernick R.G., Hyde E.G., Naraghi M.H.: John Adriani. In: Genesis of Contemporary American Anesthesiology.

"Thorough charts should always be maintained with factual documentation of all the aspects of anesthesia. An inadequate chart may be prima facie evidence or negligence or fraudulent concealment."

—J. E. CAMPBELL

ANESTHESIA RECORDS

Good records are essential to the development of any science, and this applies particularly to the discipline of anesthesia. The first step in evaluation of a situation and in the patient assessment is the recording of events. To this end the anesthesia record is an integral part of the patient's clinical hospital chart. All vital function measurements, all procedures, and all drugs should be charted in time sequence. The accuracy of clinical anesthesia diagnosis depends on the quality and sufficiency of these recorded observations.

PURPOSES OF KEEPING RECORDS

The purposes for which a record is kept during anesthesia are:

1. To facilitate the care of the patient:
   a. By insuring frequent attention to the patient's condition
   b. By providing information regarding the patient's general condition
   c. By establishing the sequence of events leading to reactions and complication
2. To provide material for teaching, for study, and for statistical information
3. To establish a medicolegal record

HISTORY OF ANESTHETIC RECORDS

The introduction of records in anesthesia is attributed to Harvey Cushing in 1895.[1] At this time he and Amory Codman were second-year medical stu-

RECORDS, MORTALITY, OPERATIVE RISK, AND MEDICOLEGAL CONSIDERATIONS

dents and were frequently delegated to administer ether at Massachusetts General Hospital. They were dissatisfied with the procedure and worked out a system of continuous recording of pulse and respiration whereby the anesthetist and surgeon could see the patient's condition.[2] These records became known as "ether charts." In 1902, after Cushing returned from Pavia, Italy, where he saw Riva-Rocci's instrument for measuring blood pressure, he developed a new chart providing space for continuous graphic recording of blood pressure as well as pulse and respiration. Thus was established the anesthetic record essentially as it is today. Cushing fully realized the value of blood pressure readings and insisted on recording of observations. He published an important paper on the subject entitled "On routine determination of arterial tension in operating room and clinic."[3] Today, apparatus and methods are available for the automatic recording of pressures and other physiological phenomena.[4]

CHARACTER OF RECORDS

One of the important functions of a good anesthetist and of a department of anesthesiology is the keeping of records.[5] These records should be *vital, available,* and *accurate*.

To be *vital* (or alive) and representative of the actual progress of a particular anesthesia and surgical operation, a record must be complete; it must be a stark observational picture of the situation; every physiologic parameter possible should be measured continuously and recorded; changes in technique, in agents, in position, or in the surgical procedure must be noted; all complications should be identified; and the final condition must be assessed.

To be *available*, a record should be kept moment to moment to serve as a possible diagnostic and prognostic element in the operative course; delays between observations and recording lead to errors. The record must be neat and legible; sloppy and illegible records are worthless medically and legally.

To be *accurate*, the data should be obtained from observation of the patient—not by guessing—and should be immediately recorded. To err is human; to guess, despicable. Above all it is easy to forget figures and statistics, so write them down immediately.

TYPES OF ANESTHESIA CHARTS

Records may be written, graphic, or carded. These are the three systems in current use. The old Army medical department record was a written one. Blood pressure figures were written down as well as the figures of the other vital signs. This is laborious and does not lend itself to good illustration or interesting analysis. Also the exact course, concentration of agent, and depth of anesthesia are difficult to include.

Most of the bad features of written records have been obviated by the graphic record[2,6–8] (Figs. 2–1; 2–2). Vital signs are noted by means of checks (for blood pressure), dots (for pulse), and circles (for respiration). Space is provided for indicating the agent in use at particular times and also for estimating the degree of depth of anesthesia. When such a completed record is observed, one has at a glance a complete picture of the physiology throughout the particular study. For the recording of positions,[9] diagrams should be used (Fig. 2–3).

PUNCH CARD SYSTEMS. For file tabulation and statistical purposes the punch card system has been used. All data are either coded or a marginal perforation is made corresponding to the information that is positive. There are three varieties of such punch card systems: the direct punch keyport card,[10] the coded keyport card,[11] and the Hollerith punch card.[5] The latter is an excellent adjunct to the graphic teaching record and supplements this form for statistical analysis.

Where codes are used, each operation technique and agent is represented by a numerical equivalent; when a particular operation is performed the number of the operation is punched on the card along with the numbers for the technique of anesthesia, complications, and all other pertinent information.

AUTOMATED RECORD-KEEPING SYSTEMS. Since 1970 the amount of information available has increased dramatically because of the increase in sophisticated monitoring systems. The current manual record can thus lack completeness, accuracy, and legibility. Events transpire so quickly, especially during induction and termination of anesthesia or when a crisis arises in the intraoperative period, that it is difficult for one person to have a complete record. Furthermore, the administration of various anesthetic drugs and supportive agents can have a transient but extremely strong stress and cardiovascular effect. In 1973 Hallen described computerized anesthesia record-keeping,[13] and in 1977 Zollinger proposed that computer-generated records were better than handmade records.[14a] In 1985 a commercial automated and computerized anesthesia record-keeping system became available[14b] and was used by Gravenstein.[15]

Advantages.[15] Transient events can be quickly recorded, there is immediate feedback with regard to a patient's response, and during crises a record becomes available and a centralized display of vital events can help the anesthesiologist to make decisions. However, there are several features in the administration of anesthesia or interventions performed by either the anesthesiologist or surgeon that require entry by the anesthesiologist. Three entry systems are available: (1) a keyboard data entry

FIG. 2–1. Anesthetic record (see Fig. 2–2 for reverse side).

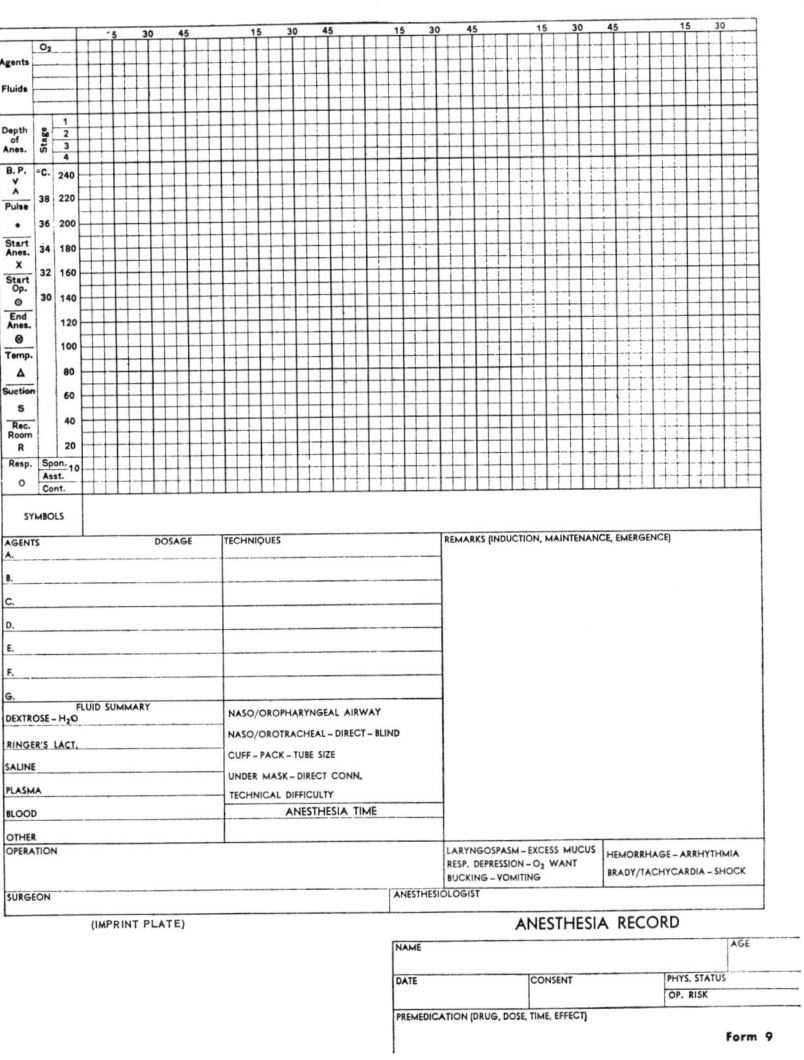

system; (2) the CRT screen, which responds to touch; and (3) the newer voice entry system.

Types. Four automated entry systems are currently available. The oldest was developed by Gravenstein and is known as the Datatrac system.[16] This system was made available in July 1985. It is an electronic clipboard designed to resemble the manual record. The system is designed automatically to gather valid data from any and all connected monitors, so that the heart rate, blood pressure, temperature, inspired oxygen, end-tidal CO_2, respiratory rate, cardiac output, and the time can be graphically printed on one part of a record, usually the left side. The timing is at each minute. On the right side of the record the anesthesiologist can make hand notations of special events.

The second automated record system is known as CARIN (Computerized Anesthesia Recording and Information Network). It became available in August 1985. This system runs on the Apple-Macintosh computer. It can interface with seven different operating room monitors and is compatible with the equipment of many manufacturers. The anesthesiologist can select a variety of drugs on a list presented on a computer screen, which can then be entered into the permanent record.

The third system is manufactured by Ohmeda. It is designed for use with the Moduless II Anesthesia System. All the monitors installed on this anesthesia machine are connected internally with the record-keeper. At the present time a total of 16 different monitors can be used with the system, and all data electronically monitored are entered into the system and into the record.

The fourth system is in the process of development. It has a touch screen for the selection of drugs and also a voice-recognition system. All electronically monitored physiologic parameters can be recorded, and in addition the anesthesiologist can talk

PRE-OPERATIVE EVALUATION

NAME OF PATIENT..........AGE..........SURGERY..........
HABITUS: Asthenic..........; Athletic..........; Pyknic..........; Height.......... Weight..........; Wt loss..........
HABITS: Tobacco.......... packs/day; Alcohol..........; Narcotics..........
ALLERGY: Asthma..........; Hayfever..........; Specific (drugs, etc.)..........
DENTITION: Edentulous..........; Deciduous teeth; Other dental problems..........
CARDIOVASCULAR: BP..........; Pulse..........; Rhythm..........
History: Pain..........; Dyspnea..........; Orthopnea..........; Edema..........; Digitalis..........
Physical: Cardiomegaly..........; Murmurs..........; Arrhythmias..........; ECG..........
RESPIRATORY: Rate..........; Character of Respirations..........
History: Cough..........; Sputum..........; Hemoptysis..........; URI..........; Fever..........; X-ray..........
Physical: A-P diameter..........; Rales..........; Cyanosis..........; Clubbing..........; Pallor..........
Bedside Tests: Breath holding..........sec; Valsalva..........; Induced cough..........
Pulmonary Function: VC..........%; TVC; ½ sec..........%; 1 sec..........%; 2 sec..........%; 3 sec..........%
MBC..........%; MEFR..........L/minute
LABORATORY DATA: Blood volume: Plasma..........; RBC Mass..........; Total..........
Hemoglobin..........gm; (..........%); Hematocrit..........%
Total protein..........; A/G ratio..........
Renal profile: BUN..........; Sp. G..........; Sugar..........; Protein..........; Acetone..........
Liver profile: Alk phos..........; Ceph..........; Thymol..........; GGT..........; BSP..........
Electrolytes: Na......: K..........; C1..........; CO_2..........;
Endocrine studies:..........
DRUG THERAPY:..........
ANESTHETIC HISTORY: Regional..........; General..........
SUMMARY OF PREOPERATIVE CONDITION:..........

PHYSICAL STATUS 1 2 3 4 5 ....E; OPERATIVE RISK..........
ANESTHETIC PRESCRIPTION: General..........; Endotracheal..........; Regional (specify)..........
1) HS sedation..........; Premedication..........; Regional (specify)..........
2) Anesthetic agents: Induction..........; Maintenance..........
3) Relaxants..........

....
Signature

INTRA-OPERATIVE COMPLICATIONS

POST-OPERATIVE COMPLICATIONS

FIG. 2–2. Anesthetic record—reverse side of Figure 2–1.

to the automated record system and state interventions that have been carried out and make comments as well; the comments then become part of the permanent record. Each anesthesiologist must program his voice into the system's voice-recognition program.

Comment.[17,18] The automated record is simply a record. The interpretation of the data in this record, both at the time and subsequently for study, still depends upon the anesthesiologist. The capacity to make differential diagnoses and to decide on a proper course of action still remains the essence of safe anesthesiology. The final record, of course, should always be edited, and any unusual events that were missed should be entered into the final record. A semiautomated record system is probably the most useful. The monitoring devices collect and record the data to assist in interventions and the decision-making process, but decisions still depend on the judgment, experience, and skill of the anesthesiologist.

NERVE BLOCK CLINIC AND RECORDS

An interesting development in anesthesia is that of the nerve block clinic.[19a] This clinic is organized not only for purposes of anesthesia but also for diagnosis and therapeutics. Cooperation among the various hospital services is a prerequisite. This is the multidisciplinary approach brought to a high level of organization and promoted by Bonica.[19b] The specialty services present pain problem patients, and the overall management is discussed by the members from all the services.

If nerve blocking is considered to be one of the technics for diagnosis or therapy, the patient is re-

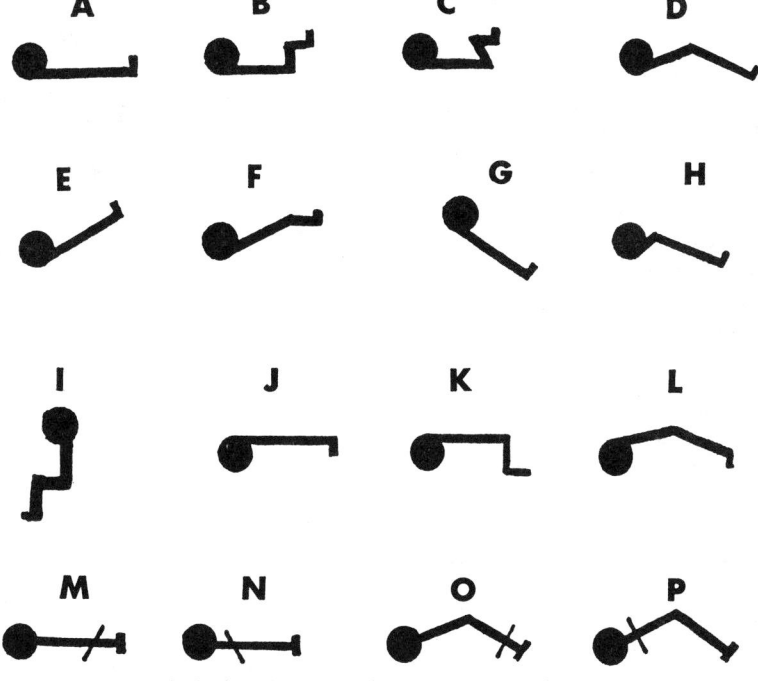

FIG. 2–3. Symbols for charting of some commonly used operative positions.

A. Supine—Reflex Abdominal
B. Supine–Lithotomy
C. Supine—Advanced Lithotomy
D. Supine—Gall Bladder Rest
E. Supine—Head Down (Scultetus)
F. Supine—Trendelenburg
G. Supine—Head Up (Fowler)
H. Supine—Thyroid
I. Sitting
J. Prone
K. Prone—Hips Flexed Jack-Knife
L. Prone—Lift Under Pelvis
M. Lateral—Straight Right (Kidney or Chest)
N. Lateral—Straight Left
O. Lateral—Flexed Right
P. Lateral—Flexed Left

ferred to the Pain Control Center Nerve Block Unit. Members of the nerve block unit are specially trained in the technical aspects of regional anesthesia by anatomical dissection, practice on cadavers, demonstrations on patients, and then performance.

The practice of "trying a block" is frowned on. Accurate diagnosis is insisted on preanesthetically, and technical proficiency is maximum when the block is performed. As a result blocks are not hit-or-miss procedures but accurate and attended with excellent results. Toward this end the function of record-keeping is emphasized. Individual case records are started as each block is performed, and index cards are filed with the information from the individual records. From these index cards a monthly report is made.

A numerical code of classification similar to that for general anesthesia is used and a record form completed. Cases are considered in four categories, within each of which the case is assigned a numerical equivalent: (1) diseases and disorders; (2) nerve block procedure; (3) indication; and (4) drugs employed.

A schematic drawing of the distribution of sensory nerves or skin dermatome should be available as well as a chart for recording skin temperatures when this is desirable.

TRANSFUSION RECORDS

Besides basic data such as name, age, blood type, compatibility, blood count, and indication for transfusion, certain additional information should be noted on a transfusion record.[20] This concerns the donor on the one hand and the recipient on the other. With respect to the donor, one should like to know how long the donor had been fasting before blood was drawn, the time of day blood was taken, the dates of previous donations, a history of allergy, a short physical examination, and finally any reaction the donor might have had while in the process of donating blood. (About 5% of new donors exhibit untoward reactions either before or while blood is being drawn.)

As regards the recipient, notes should be made of the age of the blood, time of transfusion, rate of drops, length of time required for transfusion, gauge of intravenous needle, vein used, ease of venipuncture, and, any reactions, whether immediate or delayed. If reactions do occur, laboratory data should be included, such as various urine tests for hemoglobinuria, hemoglobin in the serum, and a recheck of the serology and blood type of the patient. Finally, the type of treatment given should be included.

RESUSCITATION AND INHALATION THERAPY RECORDS

Resuscitation and inhalation therapy records should include diagnosis, indication for therapy, technique of administration of therapy, type of therapy, duration of therapy, rate of flow of gases, relief of indication, and whether the technique was suitable to the patient's comfort. Finally, the outcome should be noted.[21,22]

OPERATING ROOM DEATHS

Death can be defined as the cessation of integrated life functions.[23] Life depends on the integration of the following physiologic mechanisms: ingestion, digestion, and absorption; respiration, circulation, and coordination (nervous and endocrine systems); and metabolism, excretion, and elimination. Death occurs if any of these functions is much impaired or arrested. One can distinguish between clinical and biologic death. In clinical death essential or vital functions are arrested and the subject is without apparent life. This is at times reversible, as in acute cardiorespiratory arrest. Biologic death exists when no amount of resuscitative therapy can restore a patient to even a vegetative existence.[24]

When death is due to impairment of the first or last three of the listed life functions, a long period of symptoms usually precedes the event. Thus, chronically ill patients with prolonged intestinal obstruction and those with peritonitis might have passed the stage of reversibility and hence die as a consequence of their disease and not of anesthesia and surgery. On the other hand, disturbance of the middle three functions generally precipitates the so-called sudden deaths. These are basically concerned with deprivation of oxygen to tissues.

In the operating room morphologic causes of death are secondary. They contribute to the extent that they distort physiologic function. One must recognize that physiologic mechanisms often kill without positive findings and that, in many instances, there are no demonstrable findings at autopsy. No presumption as to the cause of death is justified without thorough postmortem studies. In addition to tissue pathology studies, considerable basic biochemical information should be obtained. The following data are desired:

1. Distribution of agents in tissues
2. Acid-base balance
3. Electrolyte studies
4. Catecholamine levels
5. Hormonal levels

CAUSES. In analyzing the cause of death, one must have two objectives in mind:

1. To list the sequence of operative events preceding death and
2. To list in the order of significance the role each pathophysiologic entity played in shortening the life of the patient

Analysis of operative mortality requires that, exclusive of intrinsic patient disease, one must identify the lethal hazards imposed on a patient. These are best considered as being *human errors* in anesthesia or in surgery. Such errors are:

1. Errors in diagnosis
2. Errors in judgment
3. Errors in technique

CLASSIFICATION.[24-26] Intraoperative deaths have multiple causes which may be separated into three categories, namely surgical factors, anesthesia factors, and patient factors (Table 2–1). One should always be alert to the occurrence of natural causes of death during surgery. These are distinct from the surgical disease. In any event, every factor must be assessed as to its contribution in shortening the life of the patient.

It is evident that in the operating room anesthesia and surgery are inseparable. Surgery is performed for two reasons: to prolong life and improve health or to save life. Anesthesia is the handmaiden of surgery and a necessary hazard. It profoundly modifies the integrative action of the nervous system, but this is usually a reversible phenomenon. By modifying nervous system response to the trauma and stress of surgery, anesthesia actually protects the organism.

A careful analysis of 645 operating room deaths by Campbell[30,31] reveals the following:

In only 5.1% was anesthetic misadventure the sole major factor

In 5.6% both anesthesia and surgery were major factors

In 25% anesthesia was a minor factor

In 65% anesthesia was an incidental concomitant of surgery, and these deaths were completely due to surgical misadventure

In some instances either anesthesia or surgery is the *major* contributing element responsible for the fatal result. In many instances both anesthesia and surgical factors share major roles in causing the patient's death. Thus a more complete breakdown in classification of deaths is necessary:

1. Anesthesia sole factor
2. Surgery sole factor
3. Anesthesia major factor—surgery minor factor
4. Anesthesia minor factor—surgery major factor
5. Patient's disease major factor
6. Indeterminate

DEATHS ASSOCIATED WITH ANESTHETIC MANAGEMENT.[27-29] The continual broadening of surgical horizons demands the highest skill from the anesthesiologist with minimal physiologic trespass in order to ensure patient survival. Deaths related to anesthesia should be recognized and identified. It is not sufficient to use anesthesia as a catchall for surgical deaths. Certain positive features define an anesthetic hazard and indicate that it is lethal in the given circumstances. As with other categories these are often human errors in diagnosis, judgment, and technique.

Among the events where it is reasonably certain that death is caused by the anesthetic management are the following:

1. Death during induction
2. Explosion
3. Pulmonary aspiration
4. Failure to secure airway
5. Hypoxia
6. Overdose of agent
7. Technical mismanagement
8. Maladministration of fluids (an embolism)

It is paramount to recognize that agents *per se* are rarely at fault. It is the administration, the choice, or the dose that plays the lethal role.[27,28,29]

EQUIPMENT FAILURE. Equipment failure is a rare cause of death during anesthesia.[29] In a review of 236 deaths possibly related to errors in anesthetic management, only four instances could be considered related to equipment failure. In two of these instances the cause could have been recognized in sufficient time to prevent either a cardiac arrest, permanent damage, or death. Even in the instances in which hospital construction of a piping system was at fault with a transfer of oxygen to a nitrous oxide outlet and vice versa, the hazard could have been identified by early clinical diagnosis and appropriate steps taken to eliminate it. Back-up cylinder oxygen could have been used, or even an air mask resuscitation technique.

The incidence of equipment failure without death varies between 3% and 5%.

DEATHS ASSOCIATED WITH SURGICAL FACTORS.[30-32] The determinants of an operating room death are limitless and entwined with local conditions. One need merely consider the type of patient submitted to surgery in some institutions, the venturesome-

TABLE 2–1. CLASSIFICATION OF OPERATING ROOM DEATHS

I. Anesthetic deaths: those associated with anesthetic management and anesthetic agents
  1. Overdose of anesthetic agents
  2. Deaths during induction
  3. Massive vomiting and aspiration
  4. Errors in technical management
II. Surgical deaths—stress imposed by surgery
  1. Sudden overwhelming hemorrhage
  2. Continuous prolonged bleeding
  3. Wear and tear of trauma—prolonged surgery
  4. Reflex stresses
III. Disease of patient: physical condition of patient
  1. Patients whose condition precludes tolerance to minimal surgical stress or minimal anesthetic stress
  2. General debility, moribund patients

ness of the surgical team, the importance of the type of surgical procedure (e.g., intrathoracic *vs.* peripheral surgery; intracranial *vs.* orthopedic), the time characteristic of surgery (e.g., the rapid, expeditious surgery taught in some clinics *vs.* the meticulous, time-consuming surgery in others) and the level of training and experience of surgeon and anesthesiologist.

Recommendations. The following principles and lessons can be derived:

1. No last resort surgery.
2. Operations of necessity should be performed only if the patient is not in extremis.
3. Surgery should be careful but expeditious, even in elective surgery in good risk patients. Mortality increases rapidly after the first 6 to 8 hours in adults. In infants and in geriatric patients mortality advances quickly after the first 4 hours of surgery.
4. The greater the operative risk the greater the need for a skillful and experienced surgical and anesthetic team. In a teaching clinic this team should perform and teach by example, not by direction from the sidelines.
5. The greater the operative risk the shorter the time the patient should be subjected to the trauma of surgery and the depression of anesthesia. The quantity of both surgery and anesthesia should be proportionally reduced.
6. Eliminate all unnecessary delays in preparing the patient for surgery. Improve the skill and the number of personnel trained in the care of unconscious patients.

DEATHS RELATED TO PATIENT DISEASE. These are related to the following circumstances:

1. Deaths related to the surgical disease
2. Deaths due to associated medical disease
3. Deaths related to unforeseeable medical events

The patient's disease can progress during anesthesia and surgery. Neither administration of anesthesia nor embarking on a surgical procedure arrests the existing diseases.

Indeed, certain surgical conditions (e.g., severe general peritonitis) are conducive to inevitable death at the present time. Further, a patient can have underlying intrinsic heart disease and suffer a coronary occlusion or progressive myocardial failure. Last, unanticipated catastrophes can occur such as pulmonary embolism or cerebral accident.

ACCIDENTAL AND INCIDENTAL CAUSES OF DEATH. The medical causes of death deserve separate attention because their importance is increasing with the frequency of medicolegal and professional criticism based on the too-ready assumption that every death under anesthesia is caused by anesthesia or the anesthetist in the absence of an obvious catastrophic event such as uncontrollable hemorrhage. Furthermore, these difficult diagnostic problems have been largely disregarded or slighted by investigators of death under anesthesia in spite of the prudence of having such findings recorded and remembered, especially by anesthesiologists. Awareness of these possibilities serves as an incentive to obtain an autopsy or, at least, a postmortem radiograph of the chest or spine, or a postmortem puncture of the subarachnoid peritoneal or thoracic cavity, as circumstances warrant and permit.

Accidental or incidental causes of death under anesthesia that have come to the attention of the Anesthesia Study Committee include the following:

1. Fracture of a cervical vertebra with compression of the spinal cord in an infant under anesthesia for repair of cleft palate. The neck was excessively hyperextended by the surgeon to have the infant's head rest in the operator's lap. The fracture was revealed by a postmortem radiograph ordered by the anesthesiologist.
2. Acute adrenal insufficiency. Abrupt respiratory and circulatory failure occurred in a middle-aged white female under an initial small dose of dilute intravenous thiopental. The intended laparotomy was never started. Autopsy showed complete replacement of both adrenal glands by metastatic carcinoma.
3. Acute hypertensive crisis and pulmonary edema due to pheochromocytoma. Under general anesthesia the unknown "renal mass" was repeatedly palpated by several observers before operation, initiating the rapidly fatal chain of events.
4. Pulmonary embolus arising from thrombosed pelvic or femoral veins during unrelated procedures.
5. Spontaneous pneumothorax during pelvic laparotomy.
6. Massive pulmonary atelectasis during spinal anesthesia for subtotal gastrectomy.
7. Myocardial infarction during an entirely normal general anesthesia for colporrhaphy.
8. Air embolism during vaginal and cesarean deliveries.
9. Amniotic fluid embolism during delivery.
10. Fat embolism during surgical trauma to fat-containing tissues.
11. Intracranial hemorrhage during a normal anesthetic course for minor surgery.

CASE STUDY CONFERENCES.[33] The clinical anesthesia conference (CAC) offers the most instructive method for the analysis of anesthetic and operating room complications and deaths.

It was actively developed by the Anesthesia Study Committee of the New York State Society of Anesthesiologists, and their cases are published in the New York State Journal of Medicine. The conference is patterned after the clinical pathologic conference (CPC), in which case histories are presented and pertinent data noted in a challenging manner. Staff discussion ensues, diagnoses are made, and after the actual outcome is determined clinical conclusions are reached. This conference can be logically organized by the anesthesiologist and should be at any level at which an educational need will be filled.

Throughout the conference the importance of medicine in its broad aspects is applied to the patient under anesthesia. Emphasis is on the "practice of medicine" in the operating room and not on the technical features of anesthesia. Unusual mechanisms producing complications and fatalities are selected.

The special purpose of this conference group of reports is to analyze abnormal physiologic changes and signs exhibited by patients during surgery and to diagnose the medical conditions represented. Many of these are medical problems met by the internist. The anesthesiologist, in his role of internist in the operating room unit, must diagnose these same pathologic states and distinguish them from other attendant conditions related more specifically to anesthesia or surgery. For example, such problems as diabetic acidosis, insulin hypoglycemia, status asthmaticus, coronary occlusion, pulmonary edema, cardiac failure, pneumothorax, and atelectasis must be differentiated from the toxic effects of anesthetics, shock, hypoxia, and respiratory acidosis. Prompt and precise diagnosis is necessary for proper treatment. Delayed diagnosis or treatment can result in death.

The tragedy of death during anesthesia focuses attention on the second special purposes of these conferences, namely, to assess the mechanisms and causes of death during anesthesia administered by expert anesthesiologists using methods that conform to generally accepted standards. The conference therefore has two purposes:

1. To emphasize the vital importance of the clinical practice of "operating room medicine" by the anesthesiologist

2. To focus attention on the problems in anesthesiology practice that continue to contribute to death during anesthesia even in expert hands

STUDY COMMISSIONS.[33] To complement the clinical anesthesia conference it is necessary to develop study commissions for the operating room in each state. The commission should organize study committees, mainly at county levels. It should be the primary objective of this commission to secure statistics on deaths, to analyze the case reports, and to classify according to an agreed-upon system.

The organization of this commission should be as follows: It should be under the aegis of the state medical society, and in turn each functioning component (district or county medical society) should have a working committee.

These commissions should be the responsibility of all physicians, not only anesthesiologists. They should be composed of three primary specialists: the anesthesiologist, the surgeon, and the pathologist. The chairmanship should be rotated each year.

This commission should be an official committee of the medical society, and the society should enlist the support and help of the medical examiner's office as well as the local bureau of vital statistics. Copies of death certificates representing deaths occurring in hospitals consequent to some medical procedure should be sent to the commission. Those that are pertinent would be analyzed and classified.

Pertinent deaths are considered to be those occurring chiefly in the intraoperative period. This period is defined as the entire period of preparation, preanesthetic medication, anesthesia, surgery, and postanesthetic and operative recovery up to 12 hours. Other deaths may be considered that are related to operation but are delayed.[34]

NEED FOR ACCURATE RECORDS OF DEATH DURING ANESTHESIA. The infrequency of autopsies seriously limits the definitive conclusions of anesthesia study committees. This situation could be readily corrected if every death under anesthesia were subjected to postmortem examination as regularly as is the practice in deaths due to accidental or unknown causes.

DEATH CERTIFICATE DEFINITIONS. For proper completion of a death certificate, one must distinguish five features of the cause of a death (Table 2–2).[35] One first identifies the underlying or primary cause of death that initiated the sequence of events resulting in death. It is etiologically specific and is "antecedent to all other causes with respect to time and pathologic relationships." The immediate cause is that which immediately precedes death; it is the final consequence of the primary cause of death. One must then identify contributing events that intervene between the primary cause and the immediate cause. The mechanisms need to be identified and are essentially the physiologic derangements produced by the primary cause. They are not etiologically specific. Last, the manner of death should be determined, because it explains how the cause is either natural or unnatural.

ANESTHESIA PERSONNEL. Not only are the skill and training of the anesthesiologist essential in the avoidance of anesthetic deaths, but also the conscientiousness of the individual. In addition, another personal factor must be recognized, namely, *anesthetist fatigue*. It should be appreciated that physicians in active clinical practice of anesthesia are usually exposed to a daily unvarying schedule devoted in large measure to a monotonous repetition of the same technical acts in the same environment of an operating room. This frequently begins at 7:00 A.M. and continues through late afternoon. Time for breaks is limited, especially when the staff is shorthanded. It is also likely that one anesthesiologist is on call through the night, and is up part of the night, only to face another day of a regular full schedule. All these features and many more lead to operating room hypnosis.

The lack of alertness unquestionably leads to substandard anesthesia and a higher complication rate.

At least two recommendations are evident. First, a definite midday break is necessary, "just to get out

TABLE 2–2. THE FIVE FEATURES OF THE CAUSE OF DEATH

Term	Definition	Comment
Underlying cause of death (synonyms: primary, proximate)	The disease or injury that initiated the train of morbid events resulting in death, or the circumstances or violence that produced the fatal injury	In the absence of the underlying cause, the patient would be alive today
Immediate cause of death	The disease, injury, or complication that directly precedes death	The ultimate and final consequence of the underlying cause
Intervening cause(s) of death	Other conditions that contribute to death and are a result of underlying cause	The conditions are listed in physiologic sequence
Mechanism of death (synonym: mode)	A physiologic derangement or biochemical disturbance produced by a cause of death	The means by which cause exerts its effect
Manner of death	Explanation of how the cause of death arose	Natural or unnatural

From Kircher, T., and Anderson, R.E.: Cause of death: Proper completion of the death certificate. JAMA, 258:349, 1987.

of the operating rooms," and second, personnel on call the previous night should be off at least the succeeding half day.

The role of anesthetic drugs inhaled or absorbed by the anesthesiologist has not been determined.

OPERATIVE RISK

Operative risk involves many variables and some intangibles. Such variables fall into four categories: (1) those related to the patient, (2) factors related to the surgical procedure, (3) considerations of the anesthesia, and (4) operating room conditions.

PHYSICAL STATUS CLASSIFICATION. In assessment of operative risk only the patient is the *constant factor*.[36] The patient is presented to the surgical team "as is." Both surgeon and anesthesiologist minister to the patient. The patient cannot withstand a poor anesthetic or a poor operation, and only the physicians concerned provide poor surgery or administer a poor anesthetic. As a result of such considerations patients have been graded for surgical procedures into several classes of physical condition termed *physical status*. This classification (below) was prepared by Saklad[36] and was modified and adopted in 1963 by a committee[2] of the American Society of Anesthesiologists[37] and approved by the House of Delegates as a uniform system of patient classification.[38]

Class 1. A normal healthy patient.
No disease other than surgical pathology.
No systemic disturbances
Class 2. A patient with mild systemic disease.
Systemic disturbance due to (a) general disease or (b) surgical condition.
Class 3. A patient with moderate to severe systemic disease.
Systemic disturbance due to
(a) general disease or (b) surgical condition that limits activity but is not incapacitating.
Class 4. A patient with a severe systemic disease that is incapacitating and which is an imminent threat to life.
Class 5. A moribund patient not expected to survive more than 24 hours with or without operation.

Emergency: Precede the number with "E".

Note that the system adopted as the ASA Classification in 1963 uses the word *class* and the *Arabic* numbering (not Roman numerals).

A distinction is noted here between the total operative risk and physical status of the patient. Physical status refers to the medical condition of the patient (presence or absence of disease) (Table 2–3) and the overall efficiency and function of his organ systems. It is concerned with the "state" of the patient and is independent of the type of surgery. It also refers to some extent to reserve of the systems specifically to withstand stress. Optimal physical condition is observed in the athlete in the pink of condition as the result of training. Many patients can have their various physiologic mechanisms brought to a point of optimal efficiency by appropriate and interested medical therapy or conditioning. They will be more ready to survive the insults of anesthesia and surgery.

In determining physical status, one must rely on the examination and reports of the internist. The anesthesiologist should note not only diseases and disabilities, but also should learn whether the internist believes that any derangements can be corrected or whether functional preparation is optimal. If no further improvement can be reasonably expected, one should consider the patient prepared medically.

It is axiomatic that sicker patients are more likely to die. All studies indicate that patients at the extremes of age—infants under 6 months and those over 70 years—are at greater risk and have a higher mortality. Males show a higher mortality rate throughout all decades after puberty. This can be attributed to greater trauma and to a higher prevalence of cardiovascular disease.

Psychological factors also play a role. A depressed patient is a poor candidate for anesthesia and surgery (death wish), and the overanxious patient is more vulnerable to sudden death. Evaluation of the emotional state of patients has had value in identifying those likely to die following cardiac surgery.

Some important factors contributing to risk are[39]

1. Poor physical state (presence of diseases)
2. Poor physical fitness (absence of disease but no reserve)
3. Cardiac abnormalities, American Heart Association classification; ECG abnormalities, angina, congestive failure
4. Extremes of age
5. The adult male
6. Psychological depression or extreme anxiety
7. Race—nonwhites
8. Long duration of anesthesia and surgery (time factor)
9. Surgery of vital organs
10. Complex surgery
11. Emergency surgery
12. Lack of skill and infrequent performance and excessive aggressiveness

SURGICAL FACTORS IN RISK. In the estimation of operative risk the magnitude of the surgical procedure[40] (Table 2–4) and the skill of the operating surgeon must be considered.

Major surgical procedures and complex proce-

TABLE 2-3. PHYSICAL STATUS CLASSIFICATION—ASA EXAMPLES OF DISEASE STATES

Status	Disease State	Status	Disease State
ASA Class 1	Fractures (unless shock) Blood loss Emboli Systemic signs of an injury Congenital deformities (unless they cause systemic disturbance) Localized infections (unless they cause fever) Osseous deformities Uncomplicated hernias		Complicated or severe diabetes Complete intestinal obstruction that has existed long enough to cause serious physiological disturbance Pulmonary disease that has reduced vital capacity sufficiently to cause tachycardia or dyspnea Patients debilitated by prolonged illness with weakness of all or several systems
ASA Class 2	Heart disease—functional capacity I or IIa—slight limitation of activity Hypertension Psychotic patients unable to care for themselves. Mild diabetes Mild acidosis Anemia moderate Septic or acute pharyngitis Sinusitis—acute; chronic with postnasal discharge Minor or superficial infections that cause a systemic reaction Nontoxic adenoma of thyroid that causes partial respiratory obstruction Mild thyrotoxicosis Osteomyelitis (acute or chronic) Pulmonary disease with involvement of pulmonary tissue insufficient to embarrass activity and without other symptoms Chronic bronchitis Morbid obesity	ASA Class 4	Severe trauma from accident resulting in shock that may be improved by treatment Pulmonary restrictive disease Cardiac disease—functional capacity III—(Cardiac Decompensation) Advanced cardiovascular—renal or hepatic disease with markedly impaired function A combination of cardiovascular, renal, and/or hepatic disease with moderate dysfunction of each Severe trauma with irreparable damage Complete intestinal obstruction of long duration Debilitated patients
		ASA Class 5	Multiple-organ trauma Uncontrolled hemorrhage from ruptured aneurysm Coma from cerebral trauma Pulmonary embolus Last-resort surgery
ASA Class 3	Cardiac disease—functional capacity IIb—with limitations of activity Essential hypertension Combinations of heart disease and respiratory disease or others that impair normal functions severely	Emergency Operation (E)	An emergency operation is arbitrarily defined as a surgical procedure that, in the surgeon's opinion, should be performed without delay.

dures are associated with higher morbidity and mortality. This is correlated with the organ involved. Operations on the more vital organs result in a higher mortality. Operations on the brain and cardiac or pulmonary systems show a higher death rate than those on the gastrointestinal tract. An order of risk appears to be brain, heart, pulmonary, gastrointestinal tract, hepatic system, renal, genital, muscle, skeletal. Further, emergency operations result in greater mortality than elective ones.

Skill of the surgeon is a matter of consensus. It has not or cannot be quantitated. But some qualities can be recognized: applied anatomic knowledge, manual dexterity, decisiveness, and speed. Aggressiveness of the surgical team is important. In addition, overall experience and the frequency that a surgeon operates are important in establishing and maintaining skill. This may be exemplified by studies showing that the mortality for various cardiac surgical procedures is twice as high in small hospitals (where the procedure is infrequent) as in large teaching hospitals. In selected radical operations, mortality among surgeons ranges from 0.5 to 5%—a tenfold variation. Variations in skill can therefore play a prominent role in increasing or decreasing the chances of a patient's survival. These chances and the morbidity and mortality associated with particular procedures are best known to the surgeon, who must acquaint his teammate, the anesthesiologist, with the plan of surgery. Such requirements as relaxation, position, the need for respiratory control, and probable blood needs should be reviewed.

Part of the risk involves the actual operating conditions. Thus the excellence of physical facilities and equipment as well as the expertness of the nursing personnel play a part in patient safety.

There are two surgical intangibles. The first intangible is related to surgical procedures; duration

TABLE 2–4. EXTENT OF SURGICAL TRAUMA—
A Semiquantitative Framework for Grading of Stress and the Metabolic Response

Scale	Examples
1	Sprained ankle
	Operative counterpart
2	Simple procedures
	Tonsillectomy
3	Appendectomy
	Thyroidectomy
4	Hysterectomy
	Cholecystectomy
5	Common duct exploration
	Prostatectomy, GI surgery
6	Nephrectomy
	Lobectomy
7	Multiorgan surgery
8	Pulmonary surgery
9	Multiple wounds
	Compound fractures
10	Burns 25% or more

From Moore, F.D.: *Metabolic Care of the Surgical Patient.* Philadelphia, W.B. Saunders, 1959.

of this was clearly identified by Vandan.[41] Furthermore, I surmise but it is not admitted that surgical morbidity and mortality increase in a progressive manner after an initial period of about 4 hours. Patients cannot be operated on indefinitely—some cardiovascular changes, for example, are time-related. The *other* intangible is related to insight. Many surgeons fail to recognize their ineptness or indecision; they also underestimate such an important factor as blood loss. Failure to admit their deficiencies extracts its toll on patients.

ANESTHESIA FACTORS IN RISK. The anesthetic and the anesthetist enter into the determination of risk; when either is deficient the hazards are increased out of proportion to the situation. The improper choice of either the anesthetic technique or the agent enhances total risk. By relating the surgical needs to the physical state of the patient the anesthesiologist can arrive at the proper selection of an anesthetic method that is going to be safe and adequate in his hands.

Duration of anesthesia contributes to morbidity and mortality, just as duration of surgery does. More important than the continued pharmacologic stress is the factor of *fatigue*. Prolonged operations and anesthesia lead to inattention and errors. This adverse condition affects all participants.

PHYSICAL STATUS AND MORTALITY. A direct correlation of physical state with anesthesia and surgical mortality is a logical concept. As patients' physical conditions worsen, deaths related to overall surgical mortality increase, and specifically deaths related to anesthesia increase. One of the first studies correlating ASA physical status grades with mortality was that of Dripps (Table 2–5).[42]

For mortality due to anesthesia in patients with PS1 only an estimate can be made. This has been variously placed as 1 death in 25,000 to 1 death in 100,000. Though little difference can be noted in the reported figures between patients given spinal or general anesthesia, nevertheless, extrapolation from the present figures would indicate a lesser mortality for spinal anesthesia in similar surgical procedures where the choice is apparently equally good.

In patients with PS2 the mortality clearly related to spinal anesthesia is about 1 in 3500; the mortality related to general anesthesia is about 1 in 1000. When the definitely related anesthetic deaths are combined with possibly related deaths the ratios are 1 in 2,000 for spinal and 1 in 600 for general. In either case the mortality in patients given spinal anesthesia is 3 to 4 times lower than in those given general anesthesia.

Significantly greater safety is also noted for patients in PS3 given spinal anesthesia when both definite and possible anesthetic causes of death are considered. The approximate rates are 1 in 220 (spinal) and 1 in 150 (general).

Only in PS4 and 5 is there a reverse in the mortality ratios for general and spinal anesthesia. In patients so assessed, the mortality from spinal becomes greater than that for general. One might consider that strict regional anesthetic techniques and local infiltration would provide a greater margin of safety, but this is an assumption. Indeed, light inhalation anesthesia in appropriate doses with abundant oxygen and ventilation has in many clinics been associated with better surgical working conditions and lower immediate mortality than local infiltration. A working rule therefore appears to be *the sicker the patient, the greater the indication for an inhalation anesthetic.* Inhalation drugs are employed to produce general anesthesia because they are "retrievable," as opposed to regional anesthetics, which must be detoxified.

In 1973 Marx[43] confirmed the correlation of ASA grades with mortality. The contribution of emergency surgery to mortality was also identified (Fig. 2–4). In 1970 Vacanti also correlated the ASA PS grades with mortality rates for both elective and emergency operations.[44] The rates are lower than in Marx's study but somewhat higher than Dripps' (Table 2–4) due to the inclusion of emergency procedures (Table 2–6). More recent studies since 1980 establish an anesthesia mortality rate of 1 per 10,000.[44b,49a]

ROLE OF RELAXANTS. Muscle relaxants can also contribute to morbidity and mortality among patients. A direct relationship with the patient's physical status was identified, and Dripps' data appear to indicate a higher risk in general anesthesia with relaxants. That is, relaxants might be contributory in only half of the patients undergoing general anesthesia. In Beecher and Todds' study a greater role of relaxants in contributing to mortality was proposed.[45a]

The understanding of relaxant action and the advent of newer relaxants have minimized the role of these drugs in toxicity.[45b] Advances in monitoring to indicate physiologic changes, the emphasis on continuous observation in the entire perioperative period, and the use of newer modes of resuscitation and application of drug antagonists have largely eliminated many of the concerns and dangers expressed in the earlier studies of mortality. On balance, muscle relaxants as currently used provide a major advance and unquestionably improve the safety of major surgery and anesthesia.

RACE AND ANESTHETIC RISK.[46,47] It has often been stated that blacks are greater anesthetic risks than whites. The surgical and anesthetic death rate has been reported as 3 to 6 times greater than in the white population. The difference is not based on factors peculiar to blacks in contrast to whites, but to the greater frequency of certain economic, hygienic, and sociologic disadvantages. These same factors exist in whites of comparable social levels.

The determinants of anesthetic risk, drug intolerance, over-reaction to stress, and toxicity in blacks are the same as in whites and are modified by the same factors. These include psychological background, presence of cardiovascular disease, pulmonary reserve, and nutritional states. In general, one must recognize the existence of special hazards in a higher proportion of minorities or the disadvantaged.

Patients of minority status tend to exhibit many reactions of insecurity. Fear dominates the picture, and appearance of agreeableness often masks an inner distrust. A psychic shock reaction can often be noted.

It has been pointed out that peculiarities of mesodermal structures explain many reactions to disease. (Blacks exhibit a relative immunity to ectodermal and nervous system involvement.) Thus, blacks are more likely to be vasomotor hyperreactors and have an increased peripheral resistance. Hypertension is more frequent and more fulminating. Myocardial and endocardial disease is more prevalent in blacks, whereas coronary artery disease, especially angina, is infrequent or rare.

Quantitative differences in the blood pressure reactions to a standard vasomotor stimulus are evident in blacks. There is an excessive autonomic response; the hypertension is labile. Stabilizing pressure is quite difficult. Sudden constriction of skin veins is a common phenomenon.

Because of their nutritional status, blacks are more likely to exhibit hypoproteinemia, liver damage, and anemia. Plasma volume is diminished. Vitamin deficiency affects carbohydrate metabolism; the endocrine responses to stress and prothrombin formation are decreased. Hemoglobinopathies are prevalent. Sickle cell disorders (Hb·S-A) occur in about 8% of the Afro-American population. The prevalence of sickle cell anemia (Hb·S-S) is 1 in 625.

Malnutrition and lowered protein levels increase the sensitivity to morphine, barbiturates, and other drugs. Smaller amounts than usual produce the desired effects. One exception has been noted namely that blacks are less susceptible than whites to the central effects of atropine.

Biochemical differences of a quantitative nature have been shown to exist. For example, the mean 24-hour urinary 17-keto-hydroxysteroid excretion in blacks is about one-half that of Europeans of the same status. This suggests a relative adrenal cortical hormone deficiency. It is not necessarily environmental, because it is similar in blacks in London

TABLE 2–5. MORTALITY RELATED TO PHYSICAL STATUS

Physical Status Grade	Spinal Anesthesia Frequency	General Anesthesia and Relaxants Frequency
DEFINITELY RELATED TO ANESTHESIA		
1	1:100,000*	1:25,000*
2	1:3,500	1:1,000
3	1:400	1:350
4	1:35	1:46
5	1:16	1:24
POSSIBLY RELATED TO ANESTHESIA		
1	0:10,164	0:6,028
2	1:2,260	1:600
3	1:228	1:150
4	1:19	1:23
5	1:16	1:10

*Estimated
From Dripps R.D., Lamont, A., and Eckenhoff, J.E.: The role of anesthesia in surgical mortality. JAMA, *178*:263, 1961.

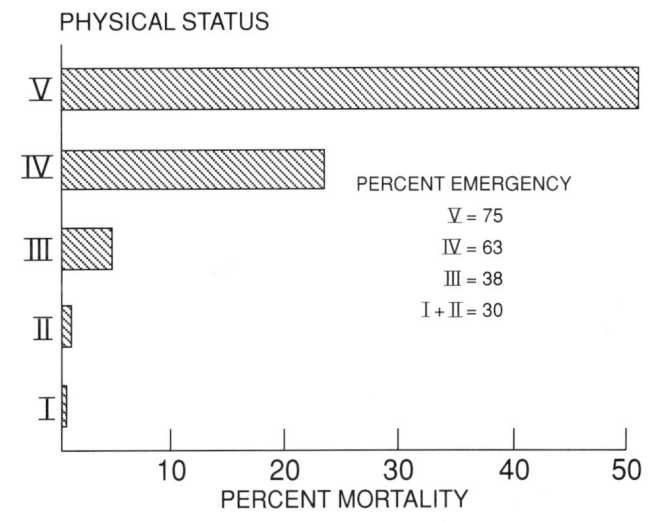

FIG. 2–4. The death rate increases with increasing physical status class for elective operations, and the percentage of deaths in emergency operations increases in a similar manner. (Marx[43]).

TABLE 2–6. PERIOPERATIVE MORTALITY RATES FOR EACH ASA PHYSICAL STATUS GRADE INCLUDES BOTH EMERGENCY AND ELECTIVE SURGERY

ASA Physical Status Grade	Anesthetic Procedures	Deaths	Mortality Rate/1000
1	50,703	43	0.8
2	12,601	34	2.7
3	3,626	66	18.2
4	850	57	77.6
5	606	266	93.8
Total	68,386		3.9

From Vacanti, C.J., Van Houten, R.J., and Hill, R.C.: A statistical analysis of the relationship of physical status to postoperative mortality in 68,386 cases. Anesth. Analg., *49*:564, 1970.

and in Nigeria. There is a poorer response to stress. The response to stress is a predominant epinephrine release. Blood glucose changes are usually excessive. The blood sugar rises 70% in response to the anesthetic stress of nitrous oxide, oxygen, and meperidine, whereas the rise is only 10% in whites.

Any patient, regardless of race, who exhibits any of the aforementioned biochemical abnormalities is expected to have a decreased tolerance to anesthetic drugs, a diminished reaction to stress, and an unstable cardiovascular system. Such a patient is a poorer risk.

MORBIDITY AND MORTALITY

The physical status (PS) classification of patients developed by Saklad in 1941 and updated by the American Society of Anesthesiologists in 1963 has been found to be a simple and easily applied system relating to perioperative morbidity and mortality. It has served as a common language worldwide for the assessment of both surgical and anesthetic outcome. Despite minor drawbacks, this grading has proven to be a powerful, practical, and dependable predictor of perioperative and postoperative complications and mortality. It is a reliable predictor of outcome for both the surgical and anesthetic factors.[44,48–50] A direct correlation of ASA PS grades with morbidity and mortality rates due to both anesthesia and surgery has been documented by these reports.

In studies of patients with cardiac disease, Goldman[51] has developed a more precise index of risk and cardiac mortality. He has correlated this index with the ASA PS grading (vide infra) and has pointed out that the ASA grading is probably the best predictor of noncardiac deaths and a fair predictor of cardiac deaths. The cardiac risk index is a more accurate predictor of outcome in patients with known cardiac or ischemic heart disease.[52]

MORBIDITY (COMPLICATIONS)

A *major complication* is defined as any misadventure, mishap, or accident that is life-threatening or produces severe sequelae.[49] Not all complications are followed by death or coma. Major complications collectively form the basis for morbidity and mortality rates and for the assessment of risk.

Anesthesia morbidity includes any problem occurring in the perioperative period. The rate of all perioperative complications increases with ASA physical status classification. The rate of complications due to anesthetics, partially or alone, and considered separately, also increases with the higher physical status grades (Fig. 2–5).[50]

The outcome of complications should be assessed 24 hours after operation as (1) death within 24 hours; (2) persistent coma at the 24th hour; or (3) survival. Overall morbidity and mortality rates have been estimated in the first 24 hours.[50,53] The frequency of all complications partially or totally related to anesthesia is 1 in about 750 operations. Many of these are self-limited and minor or are easily corrected.

Death during anesthesia or within 24 hours attributed totally to anesthesia occurs once in about every 13,000 operations. Coma (usually fatal) and death within 24 hours directly and totally attributed to anesthesia occurs once in every 8000 to 10,000 operations (Table 2–7).[50] The crude overall mortality rate is approximately 1 per 1000 operations.

THE CRITICAL INCIDENT FACTOR.[54] A study of errors in anesthesia practice reveals that certain events are critical in the process of developing complications leading to morbidity and mortality. The authors define a critical incident as "an occurrence due to human error or equipment failure that could have led without discovery and timely correction, or did so lead, to an undesirable outcome, i.e., morbidity or mortality."[54] Included in undesirable outcomes

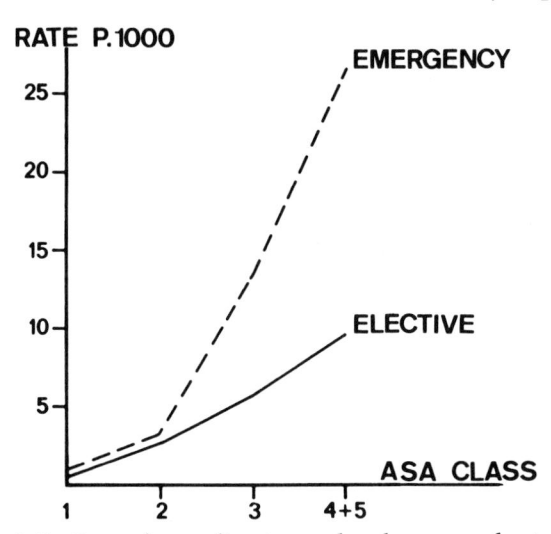

FIG. 2-5. Rate of complications related to anaesthesia according to physical status for elective and emergency procedures occurring in the first 24 hours. From Tiret, L., et al. Complications Associated With Anaesthesia. Can. Anaesth. Soc. J., 33:3, 336-44, 1986. With permission.

are increased length of stay in the recovery room or lengthened hospital stay.

The most common incidents are listed in order of decreasing frequency in Table 2-8.

CAUSES OF INCIDENTS. Human error (see Table 2-9) appears to be at fault in about 80% of the critical incidents; only 20% are caused by actual equipment failure.[55-57]

A prospective survey of mishaps during anesthesia confirms the estimate that human error accounts for 80% of the incidents.[57] In this study, mishaps were frequently due to failure to perform a normal check of machine and equipment, lack of familiarity with equipment, and lack of experience with the anesthetic technique. On the basis of this information, an anesthesia equipment checklist was introduced into anesthetic management. Use of the checklist decreased the number of incidents by half, although human error still accounted for 80% of the mishaps and about 10% were due to equipment failure. Critical incidents were summarized into three categories: transmission of anesthetic gases and vapors, drug administration, and miscellaneous (Table 2-10). Errors in transmission of anesthetic gases were the most common causes, and errors in drug administration were the second most common group of causes. Of those causes related to transmission of anesthetic gases, disconnections, leaks, and problems with ventilator and tracheal tubes were frequent.

A most common factor associated with these critical incidents is inadequate experience or skill of the anesthesiologist[58] or failure to follow standards of practice.

TABLE 2-7. FREQUENCY OF COMPLICATIONS PARTIALLY OR TOTALLY RELATED TO ANESTHESIA (NUMBER OF ANESTHETICS: 198,103)

Complication	Partially related	Totally related	Total
Death	1:3810	1:13207	1:1957
Death and coma	1:3415	1:7924	1:2387
All complications	1:1887	1:1215	1:739

From Tiret, L., et al.: Complications associated with anesthesia—a prospective survey in France. Can. Anaesth. Soc. J., 33:336, 1986.

TABLE 2-8. THE MOST COMMON CRITICAL INCIDENTS

Breathing circuit disconnection
Syringe swap
Gas flow control technical error
Loss of gas supply
Intravenous line disconnection
Vaporizer off unintentionally
Drug ampule swap
Drug and inhalation agent overdose
Breathing circuit leak
Unintentional extubation
Misplaced tracheal tube
Breathing circuit misconnection
Inadequate fluid replacement
Premature extubation
Ventilator malfunction
Misuse of blood pressure monitor
Breathing-circuit control technical error
Wrong choice of airway management technique
Laryngoscope malfunction
Wrong intravenous line used
Hypoventilation
Wrong choice of drug

From Cooper, J.B., Newbower, R.S., and Kitz, R.J.: An analysis of major errors and equipment failure in anesthesia management: Considerations for prevention and detection. Anesthesiology, 60:34, 1984.

TABLE 2-9. HUMAN FACTORS ASSOCIATED WITH MISHAPS

	A	B
Failure to perform a normal check	24	9
Lack of experience or familiarity with equipment	19	7
Inattention or carelessness	19	6
Distraction	12	5
Haste	10	7
Lack of experience with technique	5	3
Difficult or demanding case	3	5
Emergency case	3	3
Fatigue	3	1
Poor labeling of drugs	3	0
Miscellaneous—e.g., lengthy procedure, boredom, poor communication	8	6

A, inexperienced residents in training. B, experienced anesthesiologists. From Kumar, V., et al.[57]

44 General Anesthesia

TABLE 2–10. MISHAPS DURING ANESTHESIA

Category	Type of Incident	Details of Incident	A	B
Transmission of anesthetic gases and vapors	Vaporizer problems	Cooper kettle control error	9	1
		Forgot to turn on vaporizer	2	1
		Fresh gas flow not connected to vaporizer	2	
		Inaccurate calibrations	2	
		Selector valve problems	2	2
		Vaporizer left on accidentally		1
	Disconnections	Common gas outlet	3	1
		Humidifier	3	
		Fresh gas supply to Bain system	1	
		Pipe gas supply	1	
		Tracheal tube and breathing system		1
	Inadvertent gas flow changes	66% O_2, 33% N_2O	2	
		Accidentally switched off N_2O	1	
		100% N_2O for preoxygenation	1	
	Malfunctioning evacuation	Disconnection at vacuum source	4	1
		Reservoir bag missing		1
	Leaks	Soda lime canister	2	1
		Ventilator bellows	2	
		Humidifier		1
		Broken pressure gauge		1
	Ventilator problems	Pediatric bellows for adult case	1	
		Malfunctioning ventilator	1	3
	Problem with ventilation	Trying to ventilate manually with switch on machine mode	2	1
	Tracheal tube problems	Right main stem intubation	3	
		Obstruction	2	
		Accidental extubation	2	1
		Cuff failure	2	
		Difficult intubation—mediastinal emphysema	1	
Drug administration	Syringe swap	Wrong drug given	15	5
		Intravenous infusion swap	1	
	Relative overdosage	Prolonged neuromuscular blockade	4	1

TIMING OF INCIDENTS. Most critical incidents occur during maintenance of anesthesia.[54] It has been estimated that 60% of the complications occur at this time and that 40% occur postanesthetically (Fig. 2–6).[50] Lack of skill probably accounts for the incidents occurring during induction and emergence.

MORTALITY RATE

The overall mortality rate from anesthesia in the United States and in western nations is about 1 death per 10,000 anesthetics (Table 2–11).[49] This is the risk of death due to anesthesia for a patient in ASA physical status grades 1 and 2 undergoing elective surgery.

SEVEN-DAY PERIOPERATIVE MORTALITY.[59] Four factor groups have been assessed for elective surgery to ascertain which variables are predictive of 7-day operative mortality. Variables in these groups found by Cohen as clearly predictive of mortality include

1. Patient factors
   a. Increasing surgical/anesthesia mortality with increasing age after 30 years[43] and advanced age (over 80 years)[59]
   b. Mortality rates are twice as high for males

TABLE 2–10. MISHAPS DURING ANESTHESIA (continued)

Category	Type of Incident	Details of Incident	A	B
Miscellaneous	Other	CNS side effect following axillary block	2	
		Postoperative respiratory depression		1
		1:20,000 adrenaline		1
		Overdose of aminocaproic acid		1
		Ephedrine for normal blood pressure		1
		Hypotension following vancomycin		1
		Vomiting/aspiration on induction	3	1
		Intravenous disconnection	2	2
		Significant hypotension after induction	2	
		Epidural catheter without holes	1	
		Subcutaneous lignocaine via epidural catheter	1	
		Patient awakened during surgery	1	
		Exhaustion of soda lime	1	
		Tooth damage	1	2
		Laryngoscope failure	1	
		Intraoperative myocardial infarction		1
		Death 6 hours after surgery		1
		Significant leak around tracheal tube resulting in ventricular tachycardia		1
		Oxygen sensor failure		1
		Humidifier too hot		1
		Blood warmer malfunction		1
		High spinal		2
		Intravascular placement of epidural catheter		1
		Epidural catheter in subarachnoid space		1
	Total number of incidents		86	43

From Kumar, V., et al.: Forum: An analysis of critical incidents in a teaching department for quality assurance. A survey of mishaps during anaesthesia. A, inexperienced and B, anesthetist with more than 2–3 years' experience. Anaesthesia, 43:879, 1988.

    c. Physical status classification proved to be the powerful predictor of postoperative mortality; rates are low for healthy patients but increase dramatically with higher PS grades
2. Surgical complexity
    a. Intermediate surgery and emergency surgery
    b. Monitored anesthesia care or standby requests had the highest rate of mortality (200 per 10,000 patients in Cohen's study)
3. Anesthesia factors
    a. Experienced anesthesiologists (over 8 years) had lower mortality rates than those with less experience (< 600 procedures for 8 years)
    b. Narcotic anesthetic techniques and administration of multiple drugs were associated with higher mortality rates
4. Intraoperative complications
    a. Anesthetic
    b. Surgical

Anesthesia factors are less important than patient or surgical risk factors.

CORRELATION BETWEEN ASA GRADE AND MORTALITY.[59]
The experience in a single large teaching hospital provides a prototype of audit of morbidity and mortality. Medical records departments should provide the basic information. This can be coded according

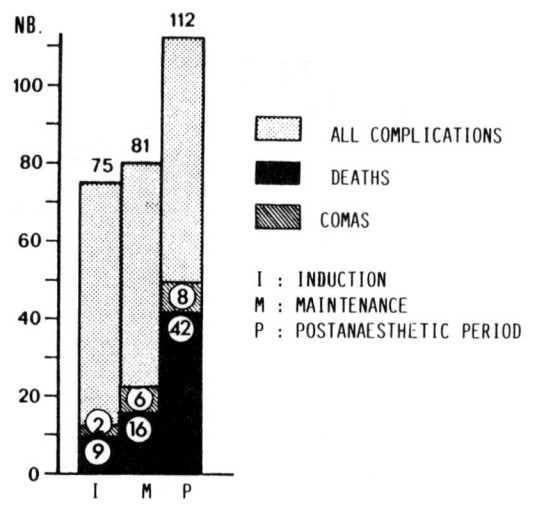

FIG. 2–6. Time of occurrence of complications. From Tiret, L., et al. Can. Anaesth. Soc. J., 33:338, 1986. With permission.

to patient condition and to surgical and anesthetic detail. One mortality audit of combined emergency (20%) and elective (80%) surgery showed 2.4 operative deaths per 1000 in the first 24 hours and 4.3 deaths per 1000 in the 7-day period after anesthesia for a 7-day rate of 6.8 deaths per 1000. The ASA PS grade system provided the single most valuable predictor of outcome. No patients in ASA grade 1 died; at the higher grades, mortality per 1000 patients progressed from 2.5 ASA (grade 2) to 7.3 (grade 3), 56 (grade 4), and 287 (grade 5) (Table 2–11).[60]

A similar audit by Cohen of the experience at the University of Manitoba demonstrates the high predictability of complication and outcome as related to the ASA grading of patients. The higher ASA scores show a dramatically increased mortality rate (Table 2–12).[59]

A COMPOSITE PREDICTION OF OUTCOME. From the recent comprehensive reports on morbidity and mortality of Cohen[59] and Tiret[50] and from analysis of specific contributing factors (vide infra), a prediction of outcome from the administration of anesthesia can be made from five preoperative factors:

1. Age of patient
2. ASA physical status grade
3. Complexity of the surgery
4. Nature of the Surgery (elective or emergency)
5. American Heart Association's functional classification and the Cardiac Index

Supplementing these primary factors is a knowledge of the specific factors below. Finally, there is the subtle factor of clinical intuition, which takes into consideration experience and the nuances of anesthesia and surgical skills, usually unspoken.[53]

FACTORS AFFECTING MORBIDITY AND MORTALITY

Age

Morbidity and mortality are significantly greater at the extremes of age, as is seen in many studies. In Tiret's audit, the following rates for complications were determined: in infants a rate of 3/1000 was reported; in ages 1 to 15 a rate of 0.5/1000; and in ages 15 to 45 a rate of 0.6/1000.[61] Thereafter, from 45 to 75, a steady significant rise in rate occurred, from 1/1000 to over 5 per 1000 (Table 2–13).[50] Similar increases in mortality rates in older patients have been reported from the Mayo Clinic. In the

TABLE 2–11. STUDIES OF ANESTHETIC MORTALITY IN HOSPITALS

Year	Author(s)	Procedures	Anesthetic Deaths	Anesthetic Deaths/ 10,000
1954	Beecher and Todd (Boston)	599,584	224	3.7
1956	Hingson et al. (Cleveland)	136,043	23	1.7
1963	Clifton and Hotten (Sydney)	205,640	34	1.6
1970	Vacanti et al. (US Navy)	68,388	27	4.00
1973	Marx, Matteo, and Orkin (NY)	34,145	7	1.1
1975	Bodlander (Australia)	211,130	15	0.7
1978	Harrison (Goote-Schuur)	240,483	53	2.2
1980	Hori-Viander (Finland)	339,000	18	0.6
1980	Turnbull (British Columbia)	195,000	20	1.1
1982	Lunn and Mushin (UK)	1,147,362	115	1.0
1985	Keenan and Boyan (US)	163,240	14	0.9
1986	Tiret et al. (France)	198,100	67	0.8
1987	Derrington and Smith review	2,500,000	250	1.0

Data from Derrington, M.C., and Smith, G.: A review of studies of anaesthetic risk, morbidity and mortality. Brit. J. Anaesth., 59:815, 1987; Tiret, L., et al.: Complications associated with anaesthesia—a prospective survey in France. Can. Anaesth. Soc. J., 33:336, 1986; and original reports.

sixth decade, crude mortality was about 7/1000; in the seventh decade, 10/1000; in the eighth decade, 13/1000;[59] and at 80 years or beyond, over 22/1000.

COMPLICATIONS OF ANESTHESIA IN INFANTS AND CHILDREN.[61] A prospective survey of over 40,000 anesthetics administered to patients younger than 15 years revealed a rate of major complications of 0.71/1000. The risk of complications was found to be higher in infants (4.3 per 1000) than in children aged 2 to 15 years (0.5 per 1000). The rate of complications showed a strong correlation with the ASA physical status classifications. As the ASA class progressed from PS I to PS IV–V, the rate per 1000 complications increased from 0.4/1000 to over 16/1000[61] (Table 2–14). These results further emphasize the value of the ASA PS system as a predictor of complication and risk. Additional features of morbid events included the following:

1. Accidents to infants occurred mainly during maintenance of anesthesia and were largely those of respiratory failure.
2. In children, misadventures were equally divided between cardiocirculatory failure and respiratory failure. The time of occurrence was more frequently observed during induction and in the recovery period.
3. The rate of complications increased in proportion to the number of coexisting diseases.
4. Other factors contributing to increased morbidity included emergency procedures, duration of fasting less than 8 hours, and history of previous anesthetics.

Nearly all studies indicate that morbidity rates are higher at the extremes of age. One study, however, showed a greater risk of postoperative complications in older children submitted to certain operative procedures than in infants.[62] ENT procedures including complicated orotracheal procedures such as tonsillectomy, tracheostomy, and bronchoscopy were associated with the highest complication rate (about 20%). A second procedure associated with a high complication rate (14%) was the placement of a permanent indwelling central venous catheter. Complicated ear operations had a complication rate of 12%. Thus the type of surgical procedure must be considered in estimating morbidity risk along with ASA classification. Further, a standard of vigilance must be applied in the postanesthetic period similar to that in the operating room.

MORBIDITY AND MORTALITY IN THE GERIATRIC PATIENT. At present a geriatric patient is considerd to be one 75 years of age or chronologically older. Physiologic and general fitness factors modify this arbitrary age.[63]

Physiologic changes of significance with respect to general physical fitness occur during the aging process, and some are listed as follows:

1. Cardiac output decreases[64]
2. Hepatic (portal) and renal blood flow decrease,[64] with
    a. Reduced hepatic enzyme activity
    b. Reduced glomerular filtration and tubular secretion

TABLE 2–12. MORTALITY (Crude) PER 1000 OPERATIONS WITHIN 7 DAYS OF OPERATION RELATED TO ASA PHYSICAL STATUS GRADE

ASA GRADE		COHEN et al.* (Manitoba)	BRADLEY et al.† (Australia)
I	1.	0.8/1000	0
II	2.	2/1000	2.5/1000
III	3	11/1000	7/1000
IV	4	76/1000	56/1000
V, E	5E	335/1000	287/1000

Data from Cohen, M.M., et al.: Does anesthesia contribute to operative mortality? JAMA, 260:2859, 1988.
Bradley, J.P., et al.: Mortality audit in a large teaching hospital. Anaesth. Intens. Care, 16:94, 1988.
* Audit of 100,000 anesthetics.
† Audit of 12,000 anesthetics.

TABLE 2–13. RELATIVE RISK* OF COMPLICATIONS ACCORDING TO DIFFERENT RISK FACTORS

Risk Factor	Rate of Complications (per 1000)	Relative Risk	Significance
ASA physical status class			
I	0.5	1.0	p < 0.001
II	2.9	5.8	
III	7.2	14.4	
IV, V	18.7	37.4	
Emergency			
No	1.1	1.0	p < 0.001
Yes	2.9	2.6	
Age (years)			
<1	3.5	8.7	p < 0.001
1–14	0.4	1.0	
15–44	0.6	1.5	
45–54	1.3	3.2	
55–64	1.9	4.7	
65–74	3.2	8.0	
>75	5.2	13.0	
Duration of procedure (hours)			
<½	0.4	1.0	p < 0.001
½–1	0.9	2.3	
1–2	2.0	5.0	
2–4	3.4	8.5	
4–6	5.2	13.0	
6–8	8.0	20.0	

* Relative risk = ratio between the rates of complications observed in one class of risk and the class of lowest risk of the same factor. RR = 1 in the class of lowest risk.
From Tiret, L., et al.: Complications associated with anesthesia—a prospective survey in France. Can. Anaesth. Soc. J., 33:336, 1986.

TABLE 2-14. INCIDENCE OF ANESTHETIC COMPLICATIONS (NUMBER AND RATE PER 1000) ACCORDING TO RISK FACTORS (INFANTS AND CHILDREN GROUPED TOGETHER)

Risk Factor	No. Anesthetics	Major Complications No.	Rate	P
ASA class				
I	36,903	14	0.4	
II	1,461	5	3.4	0.001*
III	518	6	11.6	
IV + V	122	2	16.4	
Number of co-existing diseases				
0	36,544	18	0.5	
1	3,064	4	1.3	
2	490	2	4.1	0.001†
≥ 3	142	3	21.1	
Previous anesthetic				
No	27,517	14	0.5	0.05
Yes	11,343	13	1.1	
Duration of preoperative fasting (h)				
< 8	5,189	8	1.5	0.05
≥ 8	34,067	19	0.6	
Emergency				
No	33,391	18	0.5	0.05
Yes	5,918	9	1.5	

From Tiret, L., et al., Complications related to anaesthesia in infants and children. Brit. J. Anaesth., 61:263, 1988.
* Group ASA I vs. groups ASA II, III, IV, and V.
† Groups with 0 or 1 coexisting disease vs. groups with 2 or 3 coexisting diseases.

3. Cerebral, coronary, and skeletal muscle blood vessels receive a greater percent of the cardiac output, and blood flow increases[65]
4. Total body weight decreases, with a relative increase in adipose tissue
5. In females, lean body mass decreases about 5 kg by 65 years of life; in males, a decrease of about 12 kg is usual by 65 years[66]

As a consequence of the aging process, the crude morbidity and mortality rates are higher than in the age groups under 50 years; crude mortality rates tend to rise after 50 years.[67] In Cohen's Mayo Clinic report, the age groups over 60 years were found to have a significant increased operative risk. Thus, the odds of dying within 7 days of surgery in two age groups is reported as follows:

For those 60 to 79 years of age compared with those under 60 years of age, the relative odds are 2.3:1; that is, the chance of dying is twice as great

For those 80 years plus of age compared with those under 60 years of age, the relative odds are 3.2:1; the chance of dying is three times as great

MORBIDITY AND MORTALITY AT ADVANCED AGE (OVER 90 YEARS) (TABLE 2-15).[68] The surgical population in patients over 90 years of age has increased nearly five-fold since 1975. Serious morbidity within 48 hours after surgery has been reported to be 9.4% and mortality 1.6%. Perioperative morbidity and both short- and long-term mortality were found to be highly associated with the ASA physical status classification of the patient. The PS grading system proves to be reliable for predicting outcome. Factors found to increase the risk of a poor outcome include male sex and perioperative renal, liver, and CNS impairment, which are included in the ASA classification. Surgery of the mouth, nose, and pharynx represented a significant increased risk factor.

Sex

Beecher was the first to indicate that males present a greater anesthetic risk than females,[45] and this finding was corroborated by Pederson.[69] It appears from Cohen's studies that the mortality for males is about twice that of females.[59] Reasons for this difference relate to the greater number of minor gynecologic procedures in females as compared with the greater number of urologic procedures at an older age for males and the presence of more severe heart and lung disease in males.[42]

Duration of Procedure

The risk of complications and of mortality increases with the duration of surgery and anesthesia (Fig. 2-7).[48,50] The morbidity rate is low for short operations. For those lasting up to 1 hour one major complication can be expected per 1000 procedures. Procedures lasting for 3 hours or more have a perioperative pulmonary complication rate twice that for shorter operations.[42] Complication rates approximately double for each 2-hour interval exposure to operation,[50] and in patients in ASA physical status grades III to V, the use of spinal anesthesia or pure opioid techniques places a further risk of complications.[48]

Overall hospital mortality rates for surgery and anesthesia have also been analyzed with respect to duration of the surgery. For operations

less than 2 hours in duration the mortality rate was reported as 1.6%, for those lasting 2 to 6 hours the rate was about 7%, and for those lasting 6 to 10 hours the rate was about 15%.

Cardiovascular and pulmonary difficulties were primarily responsible for these mortality rates. In this analysis of operative mortality and in others the anesthesia factors were found to be of lesser importance.[59]

It is evident that the duration of an operation is largely related to the complexity of the surgery, but inexperienced surgeons and anesthesiologists also contribute to longer duration of procedures and to poor outcome.

Complexity of Surgery

A relationship between complexity as a factor separate from duration has been established for mortality. Minor surgical procedures are associated with a crude mortality rate of about 30/10,000; mortality is doubled for those of intermediate complexity, with a mortality rate of 87/10,000. Major surgery is accompanied by a mortality rate of over 300/10,000. Procedures with the highest operative mortality were in the intracranial and intrathoracic cavities and in major vascular surgery.[50,59]

Associated Diseases

Complication rates increase with the number of coexisting diseases. The rates are high when three or more diseases coexist.[50]

Emergency Operations

Patients undergoing emergency anesthesia and surgery have a threefold greater risk of major anesthetic complications compared with the risks in elective surgery (Fig. 2–4).[50]

The higher frequency of critical incidents and morbid events increases the overall odds of dying. In the Mayo Clinic study the odds of dying within 7 days of emergency surgery were assessed at 4.4 times those of elective surgery. The crude mortality rate for patients in ASA physical status grades and undergoing emergency procedures was found to be about 350 per 10,000 procedures within 7 days of operation versus an overall 7-day mortality rate of only 35 per 10,000 elective procedures[59] or a tenfold greater mortality for emergency operations.

Similar overall rates were found by Bradley.[60] In his audit, overall operative mortality was determined at 30 deaths per 1000 emergency procedures, in contrast to 3 deaths per 1000 elective procedures due to both surgical and anesthesia factors.

In Vacanti's study in 1970 of ASA grade 5 patients (emergencies) a mortality rate of 940 per 10,000 procedures was reported, compared with a mortality rate of approximately 40/10,000 elective procedures in patients of grades 1 to 3.[44]

From these studies it is evident that the factor of emergency anesthesia and surgery imposes a significantly greater risk of death than do elective procedures.

It is estimated that mortality due indirectly or directly to anesthesia alone is about one-tenth the crude mortality rate for anesthesia and surgery combined.

TABLE 2–15. SERIOUS MORBIDITY AND MORTALITY WITHIN 48 HOURS OF SURGERY IN PERSONS 90 YEARS OF AGE AND OLDER (1975–1985)
Correlated with ASA Physical Status Grade: 795 Patients Undergoing 1063 Operations at Mayo Clinic

ASA Physical Status Class	No. Patients	Morbidity (%)	Mortality (%)
2	158	3.2	1.3
3	494	8.5	0.8
4	137	18.3	2.2
5	6	50.0	66.7

Data from Hosking, M.P., et al.: Outcomes of surgery in patients 90 years of age and older. JAMA, 261:1909, 1989.

Natural Death Factor

An obligatory death rate is recognized. In a given year 20 to 25 million persons have an operation in the U.S. (1980), spending a total of 80 to 100 million man days in the hospital. Some of these patients die as a normal course of life. A significant percentage of persons die of myocardial infarction in the first 24 hours who have no symptoms of coronary artery disease.[43] It is estimated that over 350,000 Americans in good health die annually of the sudden death syndrome, defined as unexpected or unexplained natural death within 1 hour after collapse. Some of these deaths occur in the perioperative period.[58]

Traumas

To define the risk for trauma patients, several scores have been proposed. These include the Glasgow Coma Scale and the Trauma Score, which are physiologic scores and have limited applicability. The Injury Severity Score, an anatomic severity score, has been identified as being useful in retrospective evaluation; too often the extent of injury is not evident until surgery has begun. Koch has applied the ASA physical classification system and has demonstrated its practicality and reliability in predicting risk and outcome in blunt-trauma patients treated as

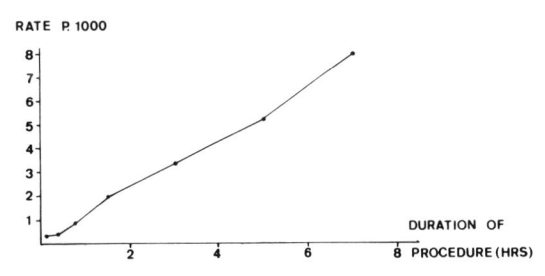

FIG. 2–7. Rate of complications related to anaesthesia according to the duration of procedure. From Tiret, L. Desmonts, J.M., Hatton, F., et al. Complications associated with anaesthesia—a prospective survey in France. Can. Anaesth. Soc. J., 33:336–44, 1986. With permission.

General Anesthesia

TABLE 2–16. PATIENTS OUTCOME AND ASA CLASS
for Emergency Operations in Patients following Blunt Trauma

Class	Percent of Total	Outcome Survivors (% of Class)	Deaths (% of Class)
1E	0		
2E	15	97	3
3E	40	94	6
4E	33	90	10
5E	12	8	92

From Koch, J.P.: ASA Status: Predictor of outcome in blunt trauma surgery. Presentation at ASA Annual Convention, Atlanta, 1987.

emergencies (Table 2–16).[70] In a study of such patients the predictive accuracy was 93%.

The ASA physical status classification correlates not only with the severity of injury score but is also more predictive of risk and outcome. Hence it is an uncomplicated and practical score system.

Emergency procedures were associated with a greatly increased risk of complication and a high risk of mortality for emergency operations in patients following blunt trauma.

Ambulatory Anesthetic Morbidity and Mortality

In the ambulatory surgical center setting, minor procedures are performed on healthy patients. It is expected that the frequency of anesthetic deaths would be low and in a large series collected by the Ambulatory Surgical Association, the frequency was recorded as 2.7 per million procedures (0.027/10,000).[71] This is one-fortieth that for inhospital patients. For office or clinic dental procedures, the anesthetic mortality is the same.[72] An even lower mortality for outpatient dental procedures has been reported since 1980 (Table 2–17).[73,74] This is significantly lower than the average current inhospital mortality rate reported since 1980 of about 1 death in 10,000 anesthetics.[75]

In a study of over 9500 adult patients undergoing ambulatory surgery, 100—or about 1% of the patients—were admitted to hospital (PS I and II).[76] The common reasons for admission were found to be pain, excessive bleeding, and intractable vomiting. Factors independently associated with the likelihood of admission were

General anesthesia (odds ratio 5.2)
Postoperative emesis (odds ratio 3.0)
Lower abdominal and urologic surgery (odds ratio 2.9)
Time in operating room greater than 1 hour (odds ratio 2.7)
Age (average 37 years) (odds ratio 2.6)

Aspiration

Inhalation of gastric contents during anesthesia poses a high risk of morbidity and mortality. Mendelson described the syndrome consequent to the aspiration of stomach contents during obstetric anesthesia in 1946.[77] Since then, the clinical course and pathophysiology have been studied in depth.[78,79] Aspiration has also been found to occur frequently in nonobstetric situations, as in adults with intestinal obstruction, in anesthesia for pediatric patients,[80] and in the elderly.

The occurrence of regurgitation and aspiration is clearly a major problem in administration of any anesthetic, not just in the obstetric setting. It is one of the major causes of morbidity and mortality in clinical anesthesia.[81–83] The frequency of aspiration during all types of anesthesia has been recorded by Olsson as about 5 per 10,000 procedures of 1/2000 anesthetics.[84] Development of aspiration pneumonitis as confirmed by radiographs is about half the frequency of aspiration, or 1 in 4500 anesthetics. Perioperative mortality due to aspiration is estimated at less than 10% of all anesthetic/surgical deaths.[85] Frequency of deaths due to aspiration during nonobstetric anesthesia is 2/100,000 anesthetics.

The important factors, increasing the risk of aspiration and indicators of this complication, are emergency operations (44%) and upper abdominal surgery (16%). In conditions of delayed gastric emptying there is a 60% chance of aspiration.[84] Delayed gastric emptying occurs in patients with a history of peptic ulcers, gastritis, pregnancy, obesity, pain or unusual stress, and elevated intracranial pressure.[84] Administration of narcotics slows emptying. Difficulties in airway management are associated with an increased risk of regurgitation and aspiration.[86,87] Pediatric patients are more vulnerable to aspiration than any other age group.[80] Infants and children under 10 years of age are especially at risk.[88]

The maternal mortality rate is reported at 3.3 per 10,000 births, and anesthesia accounts for about 10% of these deaths.[85] About half of the obstetric anesthesia deaths are due to aspiration pneumonia. The mortality rate for aspiration pneumonia (Table

TABLE 2–17. STUDIES OF AMBULATORY ANESTHETIC MORTALITY

Year	Author(s)	Anesthetics	Deaths	Deaths/10,000
1974	Driscoll[72]	2,445,570	7	0.029
1980	Lyttle, and Yoon[73]	2,580,000	3	0.012
1982	Bruns[71]	369,528	1	0.027
1984	Green and Taylor[74]	598,000	1	0.016

From Keenan, R.L.: Anesthesia disasters: Incidences, causes and preventability. Semin. Anesthesia, 5:175 1986.

TABLE 2–18. ASPIRATION DEATH IN ALL TYPES OF ANESTHESIA AND SURGERY

Author(s)	Material	Cases	Deaths	Deaths per 100,000 Anesthetics
Greene (1959)[85A]	Anesthesia (all kinds) in Connecticut	120,935	3	2.5
Harrison (1978)[85B]	Anesthesia (all kinds) in S. Africa	240,483	2	0.8
Hovi-Viander (1980)[85C]	Anesthesia (all kinds) in Finland	338,934	5	1.5
Olsson (1986)[85]	Anesthesia (all kinds) in Stockholm	185,358	4	2.2

From Olsson, G.L., Hallen, B., and Hambraeus-Jonzon, K.: Aspiration during anesthesia: A computer-aided study of 185,358 anesthetics. Acta Anaesthesiol. Scand., 30:84, 1986.

2–19) in the obstetric patient is thus less than 1/100,000 anesthetics.

Smoking

A smoking history has a profound adverse effect on morbidity and mortality related to surgery and anesthesia. It is associated with significant respiratory and cardiovascular complications. These are defined as problems requiring more definitive postoperative therapy than usually given.[89] Included are

Purulent sputum
Temperature greater than 38.3°C
Retention of secretions requiring inhalation therapy and/or chest physical therapy (not a routine)
Bronchospasm requiring bronchodilators
Paroxysmal coughing
Pleural effusions or pneumothoraces requiring chest drainage
Segmental pulmonary collapse

In a retrospective analysis of patients undergoing CAB (coronary artery by-pass) surgery who continued to smoke to the time of surgery (10 cigarettes per day or more) or who abstained from smoking for less than 8 weeks prior to surgery, the pulmonary complications rate was 39% for smokers and 11% for nonsmokers.[89] Those who abstained from smoking for more than 2 months prior to surgery had a postoperative pulmonary complication rate of about 15%—less than half the rate of those who continued to smoke and close to the rate for nonsmokers.

The reduction appears to be related to improved ciliary function[90] and small-airway conductance[91] and decreased sputum production.[92] In a prospective Mayo Clinic analysis the postoperative pulmonary complication rate for current smokers was about 33%, whereas for smokers abstaining briefly for periods less than 8 weeks the rate was greater (about 58%) or almost doubled. That smoking continued during the 8 weeks prior to surgery was verified by the presence of cotinine (the breakdown product of nicotine) at levels greater than 0.5 μg/mL. In contrast, for those abstaining for more than 8 weeks the rate was about 12%, a dramatic reduction and a percentage comparable with that of those who had never smoked.

Significant predictors for development of postoperative pulmonary complications by univariate analysis were few smoke-free days prior to surgery, low forced expiratory volumn at 1.0 second FEV_1, and low forced expiratory volumn in the mid-thoracic volume range. FEV at 25 to 75%. Other predictors included high number of "pack years," high peak expiratory flow, prolonged surgery, the use of enflurane, and a high postoperative hemoglobin level reflecting dehydration. Severe dyspnea and elevated left ventricular end-diastolic pressure and low left ventricular ejection fraction were also relative predictors.[93]

Mode of Anesthesia

Monitoring is an essential standard of anesthesia practice and is usually standardized during general anesthesia. It appears that when regional anesthesia is selected, however, the level of monitoring is sometimes minimized. This practice is a factor in morbidity and mortality and is unacceptable. All appropriate modalities of monitoring must be used during regional anesthesia.[94]

Similarly, during "monitored anesthesia care" (M-A-C), some standard monitoring modalities are often omitted. Unfortunately, this type of anesthesia care is requested for seriously ill patients for short

TABLE 2–19. ASPIRATION DEATH IN OBSTETRIC ANESTHESIA

Author(s)	Material	Cases	Deaths	Deaths per 100,000 Anesthetics
Crawford (1970)[88a]	Obstetric anesthesia	2,630,150	18	0.7
Hunter et al. (1983)[88b,c]	Obstetric anesthesia	1,500,000	11	0.7

From Olsson, G.L., Hallen, B., and Hambraeus-Jonzon, K.: Aspiration during anesthesia: A computer-aided study of 185,358 anesthetics. Acta Anaesthesiol. Scand., 30:84, 1986.

or minor surgical procedures on the mistaken assumption that a local anesthetic is the least risky. The lack of vigilance is also a contributing element. In the Mayo Clinic study of operative mortality, the use of M-A-C was found to be associated with one of the higher mortality rates—over 200 deaths per 10,000 procedures.[59]

Anesthetist Fatigue

TEST OF ALERTNESS. In the practice of anesthesia, it is necessary to maintain a state of vigilance for long periods of time. Cooper investigated "near misses" during anesthesia and suggests that tiredness and relaxed vigilance are contributory to morbidity and mortality.[95] In another study anesthesiologists were tested for psychomotor functions during the evening and night while on call.[96] Critical flicker fusion frequency (CFFF) and choice reaction time (CRT) were used as sensitive tests for level of arousal and psychomotor performance (level of sensori-motor coordination), respectively. The endpoint of CFFF is set at the time that the flicker becomes a continuous light. A decrease in flicker fusion frequency demonstrated an impairment of alertness by 11:00 P.M. (2300 h), which continued at this level through the night. On the other hand, the performance of most anesthesiologists was not significantly impaired, indicating that many could work even though suffering from fatigue, but at a decreased level of alertness. Experience and habit might well provide an explanation for continued performance in the face of decreased alertness.

In comparison, the benzodiazepines and single doses of meperidine greatly decrease alertness (CFFF) in patients and volunteers, as do injections of lidocaine for anesthesia.[97]

FATIGUE IN ANESTHESIA PRACTICE. Fatigue of anesthesiologists has been identified in the past, and I have stated in this text that it affects performance. Attention to monitoring vital signs suffers, and errors in judgment and decision-making occur. The seriousness of this aspect of practice in leading to mishaps has been clearly supported in many recent studies. The stress of anesthesia practice and the impact of the fatigue factor on performance have been reviewed by Parker,[98] who cites the following findings:

- Fatigue is related to work load, duration of work, and sleep loss. Decreased efficiency and quality of performance and increased incidence of errors have been documented when preceded by a 24-hour work period.[99]
- When duration of work exceeds 18 hours and is preceded by sleep deficit, the quality of performance deteriorates and errors increase.[100]
- A significant deterioration of reasoning occurs with sleep loss greater than 8 hours.[101]
- Fatigue and sleep loss result in deterioration, (measured by sensory-perception and sensori-motor tests) of the following specific performance characteristics:[102]
  a. Ability to collect and process information and the use of short-term memory to use the information (e.g., monitoring data)
  b. Cognitive function and interpretation of data are affected and decision making or judgment is faulty.
- Stimulus deprivation has been associated with increased stress and reduced attention. Failure to have break periods or dependable relief and the windowless environment of the entire surgical theater contribute to boredom and loss of alertness.
- Recovery from sleep loss is incomplete until a worker has two normal sleep periods. It requires this time to return to a fairly normal diurnal sleep–work cycle after loss of more than 8 hours of regular sleep.[100]
- The impact of fatigue and lack of vigilance on safety has been documented by Cooper.[101] Dangerous incidents are fairly common but are usually detected and corrected by the vigilance of an alert anesthesiologist. Forty percent are technical errors, 30% are errors in judgment, and 20% are errors in monitoring and vigilance.
- There is evidence that fatigue and sleep loss are deleterious to the function of a physician. "Deviation from a standard of 8 hours of work—even for physicians—followed by the 16 hours of rest and recovery (or some variation of these two norms) results in disruption of human efficiency and reliability in task performance.[103]

CONCLUSIONS. Fatigue seriously and adversely affects (1) the ability to perform tasks requiring problem-solving; and (2) vigilance—the ability to detect changes in normal physiology or detect abnormal events.[98]

RECOMMENDATIONS. These recommendations are quoted from Parker[98] and should be considered standard.

1. Effectiveness and safe performance are highest under moderate work loads.
2. Any anesthesiologist working with a procedure lasting for more than 3 hours should be relieved for short periods every 2 to 3 hours.
3. No anesthesiologist should regularly work more than a 16-hour work day without a full 12-hour recovery period.
4. No anesthesiologist should be on call for more than 24 hours without a full 24-hour recovery period.
5. Anesthesiologists in small or solo practices must learn to say no to unreasonable work load demands. They must resist pressures that are

stressful and affect their own and their patients' well-being.

6. State departments of health should promulgate regulations to ensure that interns and residents are supervised contemporaneously and in person by attending physicians.[104]
7. State departments of health should promulgate regulations to limit consecutive working hours for interns and junior residents in teaching hospitals.[114]
8. The work of anesthesiologists is as taxing and as important as that of airline pilots or truck drivers.[105] Since work hours are strictly regulated for pilots and for truck drivers (California), standards of work time and shift work should be established. (These should become part of the standards of the Joint Commission on Accreditation of Healthcare Organizations.—V.J.C.)

The "Relief" Anesthetist[106]

Substitution of a primary anesthetist by a relief anesthetist is a common procedure and represents a special problem. The practice assumes that the relief anesthetist is as competent as the first and that information about the patient's medical condition and intraoperative events will be transferred adequately to the substitute. Both of these assumptions are flawed, as observed in large institutional schedules. It is also presumed that a short break will increase the alertness, mental acuity, and vigilance of the initially responsible anesthetist. No experimental proof supports this concept.

Task studies in industrial engineering do reveal, however, that performance decreases with time, much of the decrease occurring in the first 10 minutes. Significantly, large decreases are not usually seen until after 24 hours.[107] A Navy study found that 15-minute breaks every 2 hours resulted in better performance. One can extrapolate from these studies that vigilance and performance would be increased with relief every 2 hours and that, as recommended by industrial psychologists, the maximum duration of work without a break or relief be 4 hours.[108] Of course the individual anesthetist must seek relief when he realizes he is fatigued. A report by Cooper is a realistic review of the factors relating to the value of breaks or relief.[109] If a relief anesthetist is to take over, then an exchange protocol should be followed as recommended by Cooper.

Cardiac Arrest Due to Anesthesia[110]

In a study of cardiac arrest due to anesthesia it was estimated that the frequency is about 1.7 per 10,000 anesthetics. The death rate was determined to be 1 in approximately 10,000 anesthetics. Analysis of the deaths revealed that the pediatric age group had a threefold higher risk than adults in developing cardiac arrest and that the risk for emergency patients was six times that for elective surgical patients.

Failure to provide adequate ventilation was the apparent cause in more than half of the anesthetic cardiac arrests due to hypoxemia.[110–112] In one-third of the patients studied, the occurrence of cardiac arrest was attributed to absolute overdose of an inhalation agent.[110] Hemodynamic instability in very ill patients was associated with cardiac arrest in 22% of the patients studied. Aspiration was a low risk factor for cardiac arrest. In brief, specific errors in anesthesia management on the part of anesthesia personnel could be identified in 75% of the cardiac arrests and deaths.

As a warning sign, progressive bradycardia preceding cardiac arrest was observed in all cases except one.

Children have a higher incidence of cardiac arrest, as shown by Salem, with a reported rate of 2.8/10,000.[113]

CARDIAC ARREST IN SPINAL ANESTHESIA. In a study of major anesthetic mishaps gathered from a review of malpractice claims, Caplan and associates identified two clinical management patterns contributing to cardiac arrest.[114] The analysis was carried out in the context of quality of care and the concept of a *sentinel event*. Such an event is defined as an unusual or unexpected outcome that should not occur under the prevailing conditions of care wherein some warning signal was overlooked.[115]

The quality of care in all instances was the overall adequacy of basic anesthetic care, both for conduct of anesthesia and the pursuit of current cardiopulmonary resuscitation guidelines. The type I pattern of occurrence was

1. Healthy patient (PSI and II)
2. Spinal anesthesia
3. Sedation sufficient to produce a sleeplike state without spontaneous verbalization
4. Unappreciated respiratory insufficiency, usually with detectable cyanosis (with or without supplemental oxygen inhalation)

The type II pattern was

1. Healthy patient
2. High spinal anesthesia
3. Failure to appreciate the interaction between high spinal anesthesia sympathetic blockade and the mechanism of cardiopulmonary resuscitation

In the first pattern, the sedation produced *subtle* respiratory changes, and presumably hypoxemia, and contributed to the cardiac arrests. The respiratory insufficiency was clinically not recognized. Major hypoxemia can occur with $Sa_{O_2} < 85\%$ without obvious changes in respiration or cyanosis.[116] With regard to spinal anesthesia, it has been reported that the administration of fentanyl to patients with high spinal and sympathetic blockade can account for sudden serious bradycardia and cardiac arrest.[117] Droperidol, a neuroleptic with alpha-adrenergic blocking action, has been reported to produce severe hypotension and cardiac arrest during spinal anesthesia.[118] In these instances, peripheral sympathetic blockade is combined with central blockade or adrenergic blockade although droperidol does not affect CO_2 response curves and appears to increase sensitivity of the hypoxic ventilatory response; when sleep is produced, respiration is depressed.[119]

RECOMMENDATIONS. Three specific recommendations for management of spinal anesthesia have emerged:[114]

1. A pulse oximeter should be used whenever sedative agents (including narcotics and neuroleptics) are administered or ability to communicate with the patient is impaired.
2. When bradycardia suddenly occurs, conventional doses of both atropine and ephedrine should be immediately administered intravenously; if not effective within 1 to 2 minutes, the administration of epinephrine should be considered.[120,121]
3. When cardiac arrest is recognized, a full resuscitation dose of *epinephrine* should be given.[114,122]

COMMENT. Keats[122] has pointed out several misconceptions: 1. too often anesthesiologists, in the presence of cardiocirculatory collapse, consider volume to be actually deficient when in fact the circulatory bed is too large for the volume.

2. Failure to differentiate between vasoconstriction of the extremities and that of the viscera and holding to the concept that high systemic vascular resistance from any cause is undesirable. Hypotension in some circumstances can occur with a high calculated vascular resistance, and administration of epinephrine could be the right choice.

3. Institution of cardiopulmonary resuscitation (CPR) within 3 minutes of circulatory failure should ensure sufficient brain blood flow. But Keats states that under many circumstances CPR does not produce adequate brain flow. CPR requires adequate volume and adequate cardiac filling—epinephrine can improve venous return and promote cardiac filling. This applies to such conditions as massive blood loss, anaphylaxis, air embolism, and massive vasodilatation due to combined sympathetic adrenergic block and the hypoxia–hypercarbia of respiratory insufficiency.

4. One must appreciate that in high spinal block there is decreased proprioceptive input to the respiratory center, and if wakefulness is simultaneously diminished by sedation there is relatively little drive to the respiratory centers. The gradually ensuing respiratory insufficiency produces hypoxemia and hypercarbia.

Narcotics (morphine sulfate, fentanyl, etc.), together with sleep doses of thiopental or diazepam, decrease exaggerated responsiveness to CO_2. Similarly, sleep doses of thiopental markedly diminish the respiratory response to hypoxia. Patients who fall asleep when receiving narcotics have a doubling of their respiratory depression over those remaining awake.[123]

EFFECT OF BENZODIAZEPINES ON SLEEP RESPIRATORY PATTERNS.[124] It has been observed that small intravenous doses of diazepam (0.15 mg/kg) or midazolam (0.05 µg/kg) administered slowly and in the absence of prior opioids cause healthy subjects to fall asleep. Apnea lasting 15 to 30 seconds also occurred in these subjects, and the breathing pattern was altered. After midazolam, a decrease of 15 to 19% in V_T occurred; after diazepam, V_T decreased 23 to 27%. Accompanying this change was a significant increase in arterial P_{CO_2}. Changes in respiratory rate were not pronounced. One concludes that small doses of these benzodiazepine tranquilizers must be used cautiously and the patient observed for several hours. The sleep produced is obviously not that of normal sleep and is associated with respiratory depression, which can be dangerous.[124]

PSYCHOGENIC CARDIAC ARREST. It is evident from the reports on unexpected cardiac arrest in spinal anesthesia that an imbalance in the two components of the autonomic nervous system, the sympathetic and parasympathetic, is fundamental.[125] With spinal or epidural anesthesia, there is extensive sympathetic block with a dominance of parasympathetic tone. Any further increase in parasympathetic tone is likely to produce excessive vagal activity. Factors other than drugs can also increase parasympathetic activity. A resting high vagal activity in those in top physical condition, such as athletes, is usually termed "vagotonia," and it is estimated that 7% of the population have an intrinsic resting bradycardia and often varying degrees of atrioventricular block.[126,127]

Psychological stress can produce either a sympathetic or parasympathetic response. If the stress is imposed in a passive-coping stiuation in which a patient cannot respond by either fight or flight, he will probably give up, and this response enhances vagal tone.[125] Fredrichs[128] has reported the effect on an athlete of being informed during surgery under epidural that he would have to discontinue all athletic activity. This prognosis obviously disheartened the patient, who lost consciousness. A Holter monitor revealed that the patient had a resting heart rate of 35 bpm and episodes of bradycardia below 35 bpm. In this instance the discussion of a poor prognosis with the patient in the presence of extensive sympathetic blockade was the etiologic precipitant.

Beecher[129] has noted that there are some preoperative warnings of potential operating room deaths, noteworthy being the attitude of the patient, a flat affect, and statements about dying. Weisman has reviewed the factors on *predilection to death*,[130] and premonitions of death have been recorded.[131,132] These reports emphasize that death from psychic causes can occur.[132,133]

One is reminded of the Freudian death wish,[134] exemplified in mutilated military personnel in World Wars I and II. These patients had little hope of living any semblance of a normal life and often expressed the wish to die before surgery or during surgery under regional anesthesia. Emphasis has been placed on conditions fostering depression or hopelessness, and inappropriately timed discussion should be avoided.[135] As Frankl has said, "Those who know how close the connection is between the state of mind of a man—and his courage and hope, or lack of them—and the state of immunity of his body will understand that the sudden loss of hope and courage can have a deadly effect."[136]

PREVENTABILITY

Three anesthesia study commissions have approached the problem of operating room deaths.[137–139] In the analysis of cases, cause of death was identified followed by an assessment of whether the cause was preventable or not preventable or unknown. The three commissions estimated that 50% of deaths are preventable. Hamilton claimed that more than 50% of anesthesia related deaths are probably preventable.[140] As information accumulates and reveals undisclosed entities to explain mechanisms of death, a greater percentage will indeed be recognized as preventable.

There has been some difference of opinion with regard to adverse reactions. Keats has stated that only 10% of anesthesia deaths related to drug reaction are preventable.[141] However, this involves a matter of judgment in the choice of agents and avoidance of those drugs likely to precipitate an adverse reaction when clinical clues of susceptibility are evident. Briefly, judgment as a factor based on applied pharmacologic knowledge would avoid many of the reactions, especially anaphylaxis and overdoses, the two most common forms of anesthetic drug complications. Hence the view of Hamilton is probably correct.

One of the pressing problems in anesthesia practice is "the diversion from the mainstream of effort in the care of patients resulting when expensive ritual and reliance on gadgetry are allowed to substitute for direct attention to the patient."[142]

The screen of the ECG monitor is the wrong place to look for trouble. The chief threats to anesthetized patients are (1) overdosage of drugs; (2) hypovolemia; and (3) inadequate management of airway.

PRACTICE STANDARDS

To avoid mishaps and prevent disasters, *the anesthesiologist must be vigilant* in the care of his patient.[143] He must follow the Guidelines for Patient Care in Anesthesiology as promulgated by the American Society of Anesthesiology[144] and the Standards for Anesthesia Care of the Joint Commission on Accreditation of Healthcare Organizations.[145] The care rendered must be documented (Table 2–20).

Many of the mishaps and mortality can be traced to basic failures

1. To assess the physical status of the patient and determine pathophysiologic conditions preoperatively
2. To obtain consultation
3. To follow a machine and equipment checkout
4. To follow recommended dose schedules
5. To apply minimal monitoring standards in all patients and advanced invasive monitoring for high-risk patients[146]

OPERATIVE RISK FOR CARDIAC COMPLICATIONS

CARDIAC RISK INDEX[51]

To estimate the risk of cardiac complications developing during anesthesia and noncardiac surgery more precisely than the ASA physical status grad-

TABLE 2–20. RECOMMENDED DOCUMENTATION OF ANESTHESIA CARE
(Approved by House of Delegates on October 12, 1988)

I. Preanesthesia evaluation
  A. Patient interview to review:
    1. Medical history
    2. Anesthesia history
    3. Medication history
  B. Appropriate physical examination
  C. Review of objective diagnostic data (e.g., laboratory, ECG, radiographs)
  D. Assignment of ASA physical status
  E. Formulation and discussion of an anesthesia plan with the patient and/or responsible adult
II. Perianesthesia (time-based record of events)
  A. Immediate review prior to initiation of anesthetic procedures:
    1. Patient re-evaluation
    2. Check of equipment, drugs, and gas supply
  B. Monitoring of the patient (e.g., recording of vital signs)
  C. Amounts of all drugs and agents used and times given
  D. The type and amounts of all intravenous fluids used, including blood and blood products, and times given
  E. The technique(s) used
  F. Unusual events during the anesthesia period
  G. The status of the patient at the conclusion of anesthesia
III. Postanesthesia
  A. Patient evaluation on admission and discharge from the post-anesthesia care unit
  B. A time-based record of vital signs and level of consciousness
  C. All drugs administered and their dosages
  D. Type and amounts of intravenous fluids administered, including blood and blood products
  E. Any unusual events including postanesthesia or postprocedural complications
  F. Postanesthesia visits

ing, Goldman and colleagues studied multiple preoperative factors. By discriminant analysis, nine variables were found to have significant independent correlation with life-threatening and fatal cardiac complications. A functional coefficient was assigned to each variable, and a point value for each was established.[52]

The discriminant-function coefficient and the point value for each factor are shown in Table 2–21. From these factor point values, the Cardiac Risk Index can be computed. Depending on the total score, patients can be separated into four categories of risk (Table 2–22). The two highest risk factors predictive of life-threatening complications were the presence of a third heart sound (S_3) or jugular vein distension (11 points) and a myocardial infarction in the previous 6 months (10 points). The second factor is related to abnormal electrocardiographic findings of (1) atrial rhythms other than sinus or premature atrial contractions on a recent ECG or (2) more than 5 premature ventricular contractions per minute at any one time (7 points).

Other important factors found to independently predict greater risk of cardiac complications included emergency operations (4 points), type of operation (thoracic, intraperitoneal, and vascular) (3 points), and general status ill health evidenced by biochemical abnormalities and/or signs of liver disease or a bedridden state due to noncardiac causes (3 points).

CORRELATION WITH ASA GRADE. ASA physical status grades have a strong univariate correlation with cardiac complications and risk of adverse outcome. The Cardiac Risk Index score provides analysis of factors predicting cardiac outcome. In general, the four ASA grades correspond to the four Cardiac Risk Index categories. Most current reviews reveal that the ASA classification predicts overall complications of anesthesia and surgery, including cardiac complications.[49–51,59,60] For patients with known cardiac disease, the Goldman Risk Index should also be used to more accurately determine cardiac risk.

PREDICTIVE VALUE OF CARDIAC RISK INDEX. In one study the Cardiac Risk Index correctly predicted cardiac complications of a life-threatening or fatal type in 81% of patients.[51]

The Cardiac Risk Index has been found valid for assessing risk of cardiac complications and predicting outcome using data from a period of 10 years.[147]

RISK IN CARDIAC PATIENTS FOR NONCARDIAC SURGERY. Several modifications of the Cardiac Risk Index have been proposed, such as that of Detsky.[148] This proposal has been equally valuable for estimating cardiac risk. Goldman[149] has taken the actual unpublished raw data provided by Detsky[148] and has incorporated these numbers into the original multifactorial index classes.[51] Also, Goldman

TABLE 2–21. COMPUTATION OF THE CARDIAC RISK INDEX

Criteria*	Multivariate Discriminant-Function Coefficient	"Points"
1. History		
a. Age > 70 yr	0.191	5
b. MI in previous 6 mo	0.384	10
2. Physical examination:		
a. S_3 gallop or jugular vein distension	0.451	11
b. Important VAS	0.119	3
3. Electrocardiogram		
a. Rhythm other than sinus or premature atrial contractions on last preoperative ECG	0.283	7
b. > 5 premature ventricular contractions/min documented at any time before operation	0.278	7
4. General status	0.132	3
P_{O_2} < 60 or P_{CO_2} > 50 mm Hg, K < 3.0 or HCO_3 < 20 mEq/L, BUN > 50 or Cr > 3.0 mg/dl, abnormal SGOT, signs of chronic liver disease or patient bed ridden from noncardiac causes		
5. Operation		
a. Intraperitoneal, intrathoracic, or aortic operation	0.123	3
b. Emergency operation	0.167	4
Total possible points		53

* MI denotes myocardial infarction, JVD jugular-vein distention, VAS valvular aortic stenosis, PACs premature atrial contractions, ECG electrocardiogram, PVCs premature ventricular contractions, P_{O_2} partial pressure of oxygen, P_{CO_2} partial pressure of carbon dioxide, K potassium, HCO_3 bicarbonate, BUN blood urea nitrogen, Cr creatinine, and SGOT serum glutamic oxalacetic transaminase.

From Goldman, L., et al.: Multifactorial index of cardiac risk in non-cardiac surgical procedures. New Engl. J. Med. 297:845, 1977.

TABLE 2–22. CARDIAC RISK INDEX

Class	Point Total	No Or Only Minor Complication (N = 943)	Life-Threatening Complication* (N = 39)	Cardiac Deaths (N = 19)
I (N = 537)	0–5	532 (99)†	4 (0.7)†	1 (0.2)†
II (N = 316)	6–12	295 (93)	16 (5)	5 (2)
III (N = 130)	13–25	112 (86)	15 (11)	3 (2)
IV (N = 18)	> 26	4 (22)	4 (22)	10 (56)

* Documented intraoperative or postoperative myocardial infarction, pulmonary edema, or ventricular tachycardia without progression to cardiac death.
† Figures in parentheses denote %.
From Goldman, L., et al.: Multifactorial index of cardiac risk in non-cardiac surgical procedures. New Engl. J. Med., 297:845, 1977.

has pooled the data of Zeldin[150] and of Jeffrey[151] to construct a composite risk index (Table 2–23); this index is not significantly different from the original Cardiac Risk Index.[51,149]

This composite risk index also divides patients into four cardiac classes, and then predicts approximate risk of major cardiac complications for noncardiac. For example, in unselected consecutive patients who have major noncardiac surgery, those risks as predicted by the pooled data are 1.6% in class I patients, 5% in class II, 16% in class III and 5.6% in class IV.

It is concluded that the original Cardiac Risk Index "has been evaluated more widely and appears able to provide prognostic stratification in a wide variety of settings" in noncardiac surgery.[147]

Type of anesthesia (spinal versus general) has not been shown to affect outcome. The peak for perioperative myocardial infarction occurs on the third postoperative day. Continuous ECG monitoring and frequent creatine phosphokinase sampling might detect earlier non-Q-wave MIs. At least 50% of postoperative MIs are painless.

PREDICTING CARDIAC COMPLICATIONS IN THE ELDERLY

Cardiac complications represent major causes of perioperative morbidity and mortality, especially in the elderly patient undergoing abdominal and noncardiac thoracic surgery. To identify patients at high risk, Gerson and associates compared rest and exercise radionuclide venticulography.[152] In an analysis of a group of patients, the only independent predictor of perioperative cardiac complications or death was the exercise-testing procedure. They noted that a larger study might identify other specific predictors of perioperative cardiac morbidity and mortality. The test had a significant sensitivity of about 80%, and it was specific for outcome in 53% of the patients studied.

PERIOPERATIVE MYOCARDIAL INFARCTION

The risk of developing a myocardial infarction during the perioperative period has been recognized since about 1930.[153,154] One of the first studies on the frequency in patients without a history of prior infarction or of coronary artery disease showed an infarction rate of 0.12%.[155] This rate was further confirmed by Driscoll in 1961.[156] Subsequent studies reported varying low rates from 0.12 to 0.66%.[157–159] From these reports Haagensen and Steen calculated a composite rate of about 0.25% or a risk of about one myocardial infarction per 4000 to 5000 operations (Table 2–24).[161] Mortality rates varied from 27 to 70% in these reports.[157,158,160,162]

TABLE 2–23. MAJOR COMPLICATION RATES IN FOUR STUDIES THAT HAVE ANALYZED THE MULTIFACTORIAL CARDIAC RISK INDEX. COMPLICATIONS INCLUDE DOCUMENTED MYOCARDIAL INFARCTION, CARDIOGENIC PULMONARY EDEMA, VENTRICULAR TACHYCARDIA, OR CARDIAC DEATH

Type of patient	Goldman et al.[51] Unselected noncardiac surgery > 40 yr	Zeldin[150] Unselected noncardiac surgery > 40 yr	Detsky et al.[148] Preoperative medical consultations	Jeffrey et al.[151] Abdominal aortic aneurysm surgery	Pooled	Pooled Likelihood Ratio†
Overall complication rate	58/1001 (6%)	35/1140 (3%)	27/268 (10%)	11/99 (11%)	131/2508 (5.2%)	
Complication rate by class						
Class I (0–5 points)	5/537 (1%)	4/590 (1%)	8/134 (6%)	4/56 (7%)	21/1317 (1.6%)	0.29
Class II (6–12 points)	21/316 (7%)	13/453 (3%)	6/85 (7%)	4/35 (11%)	44/889 (5%)	0.94
Class III (13–25 points)	18/130 (14%)	11/74 (15%)	9/45 (20%)	3/8 (38%)	41/257 (16%)	3.4
Class IV (≥ 26 points)	14/18 (78%)	7/23 (30%)	4/4 (100%)	0	25/45 (56%)	22.7

From Goldman, L.: Assessment of the patient with known or suspected ischemic heart disease for non-cardiac surgery. Br. J. Anaesth., 61:38, 1988.
* Actual unpublished numbers provided by Dr. Detsky.
† Sensitivity ÷ (1 − specificity).

TABLE 2-24. PERI/POSTOPERATIVE MYOCARDIAL INFARCTIONS IN PATIENTS WITHOUT PREVIOUS INFARCTIONS

Author(s)	Year(s)	Patients	Operations	PMI (%)	Mortality (%)
1954 Etsten[155]	1946–1952	All > 40 yr	8,200	0.12	28
1964 Topkins and Artusio[157]	1959–1963	M > 50 yr	12,054	0.65	27
1972 Tarhan et al.[158]	1967–1968	All > 30 yr	32,455	0.13	69
1981 von Knorring[160]	1975–1977	?	12,497	0.20	36
1983 Schoeppel et al.[159]	1980	All > 40 yr	928	0.40	

From Haagensen, R., and Steen, P.A.: Perioperative myocardial infarction. Brit. J. Anaesth., 61:24, 1988.

SILENT INFARCTION. A large number of infarcts in patients without a history of heart disease or an abnormal electrocardiogram are silent. The percentage has varied from 20%[158] to over 60%.[156,163] Clinical evidence of a developing myocardial infarction is usually cardiovascular collapse, hypotension, or arrhythmia. About 25% are discovered during anesthesia and the rest in the postoperative period with a peak incidence on the third postoperative day.[158,164]

PERIOPERATIVE MORTALITY IN PATIENTS WITH CORONARY DISEASE

In patients with known coronary artery disease, the *overall* perioperative (surgical/anesthesia) mortality from all causes is about 3% compared to less than 2% in the absence of cardiac disease and with a normal electrocardiogram. About half of these deaths in the patients with coronary artery disease who are anesthetized die primarily from cardiac causes (1.28%). The mortality in patients with an abnormal electrocardiogram and unknown coronary artery disease is significantly greater (3.6%). Abnormal nonspecific electrocardiograms should not be ignored.

In patients with known coronary disease, 38% have ST-segment depression;[164] of patients with arteriosclerosis, about 23% have fresh ischemic changes;[156] and of patients with disease of three coronary arteries, 20% have intraoperative myocardial infarction.[165]

Factors that increase the frequency of ischemia are abdominal surgery, duration of 3 hours or more, and hypotensive episodes.[166]

PERIOPERATIVE REINFARCTION

Patients with a history of previous infarction have a great risk of reinfarction and death. The overall rate for reinfarction in these patients from early studies varies from 3.2%[159] to over 7.5%[161,164] (Table 2–25). The overall expected reinfarction rate is about 4.5 to 6.5%, and the overall mortality after reinfarction is about 70%.[157,158,167] The rate of reinfarction (and death) varies with the interval from the first infarction to the time of surgery. From Tarhan's report, a composite table of morbidity and mortality has been constructed (Table 2–26). If anesthesia and surgery are performed in the first 6 weeks, they are associated with a reinfarction rate of 100% and a mortality rate of about the same. In operations performed after 3 months up to 6 months, the reinfarction morbidity drops dramatically to 16% with a 40% mortality. After 6 months, the rate of reinfarction stabilizes at 6.0% but mortality remains high above 30% (20%). If no reinfarction occurs, mortality is about 1%.[163]

Characteristics of Reinfarction Mortality

Most deaths (80%) from perioperative reinfarction occur within 48 hours. There is a positive correlation with the duration of surgery with a higher frequency, a doubling, of reinfarction after 3 hours. A positive correlation is also noted with the site of surgery: reinfarction and mortality associated with intrabdominal intrathoracic surgery are three times greater than in extracavitary procedures. The frequency of reinfarction also doubles in hypertensive patients.[163]

Risk Factors for Reinfarction

In the study by Rao et al.[164] on the management of patients for noncardiac surgery, several major factors were found to have a critical influence on reinfarction and mortality (Table 2–27). The study contrasted the following:

- Routine versus extensive preoperative preparation and stabilization of the patient:
    Patients with a history of congestive heart failure, angina, or hypertension had a higher reinfarction rate than those without these specific medical problems. But the patients with these problems, when vigorously managed peri-operatively, had a lower incidence of reinfarction.
- Routine perioperative management versus aggressive hemodynamic invasive monitoring:
    The latter approach sharply reduced the reinfarction rate.
- Vasopressor drugs versus vasodilator drugs:
    Vasopressor drug therapy was sharply curtailed. Hemodynamic variables were monitored extensively and in the situation of hypotension with left ventricular failure, inotropic and vasodila-

TABLE 2–25. PERI/POSTOPERATIVE MYOCARDIAL INFARCTIONS IN PATIENTS WITH PREVIOUS INFARCTIONS.

Authors	Years	Operations	PMI (%)	Mortality (%)	Type of Study
1964 Topkins and Artusio[157]	1959–1963	658	6.5	70	Prospective
1972 Tarhan et al.[158]	1967–1968	422	6.6	54	Retrospective
1978 Steen, Tinker, and Tarhan[163]	1974–1975	587	6.1	69	Retrospective
1981 von Knorring[160]	1975–1977	157	15.9	28	Prospective
1983 Schoeppel et al.*[159]	1980	63	3.2	50	Prospective
1983 Rao, Jacobs, and El-Etr[164]	1973–1976	364	7.7	54	Retrospective
	1977–1982	733	1.9	36	Prospective

* 27% of these patients had previously undergone CABG. None of these suffered PMI. If these are excluded, the reinfarction rate was 4.3%.

From Haagensen, R., and Steen, P.A.: Perioperative myocardial infarction. Brit. J. Anaesth., 61:24, 1988.

tor agents were administered instead of vasopressor drugs.
- Narcotic anesthetic techniques versus inhalation agents:
    The use of volatile anesthetics (halothane or enflurane) as primary anesthetics was associated with a significantly lower occurrence of reinfarctions.
- Routine postanesthetic monitoring versus extended intensive monitoring for 3 to 4 days:
    Extended monitoring and intensive care decreased the reinfarction rate to 1.4%, in contrast to a rate of 3.8% without extended monitoring.[164]

Interval From Previous Infarction—Effect on Mortality

Previous studies have determined that the rate of myocardial reinfarction in the perioperative period decreased progressively as the interval from the first infarction lengthened. This principle was established by the early reports[158,162] and an overall reinfarction rate of 7% has been approximated (see Table 2–25).

A high reinfarction rate of 37% was reported for operations performed within 3 months of the initial myocardial infarction; after 4 to 6 months, anesthesia and surgery were accompanied by a lower reinfarction rate of 16%. After 6 months, the reinfarction rate plateaued at about 6%.

Consequent to publication of the findings of Rao and associates, guidelines for the management of anesthesia were established (Table 2–28). A marked overall reduction in reinfarction from 5.8%[150,163] to 1.9% followed the implementation of these guidelines, especially in the application of aggressive and invasion monitoring and the use of newer inotropic drugs.

The Rao protocol significantly reduced the rate of reinfarction at each interval from the initial MI (Table 2–29). For the time interval up to 3 months from the first infarction to the time of anesthesia and surgery, the reinfarction rate was reduced to 5.8% (from 37%). But a mortality of 66% was reported mostly in the first 6 weeks. Thereafter mortality from reinfarction was significantly lower than in all earlier studies.

SOME CONTRIBUTING FACTORS TO REINFARCTION CONFIRMED

AGE EFFECT. A significant difference was found in morbidity and mortality between patients older than 65 years and those younger. In routine management the reinfarction rate was about three times greater in the older patients (11.3% versus 3.6%). In the modified but aggressive management protocol, reinfarction was significantly less in both age groups; the rate was even less in patients over 65 than in the younger group: 1.6% versus 2.5%.

DURATION OF SURGERY. When intrathoracic or upper abdominal surgery lasted more than 4 hours, a higher frequency of reinfarction occurred.[163] With the aggressive monitoring and management protocol changes, however, duration of surgery did not affect the incidence of reinfarction.

INTRAOPERATIVE MEDICAL PROBLEM. Persistent intraoperative hypotension was associated with an incidence of reinfarction between 24% and 75% (even a decrease of only 30%). Hypertension and tachycardia also greatly increased the risk of reinfarction.[162] Rapid and early treatment is apparently nec-

TABLE 2–26. EFFECT OF TIME INTERVAL AFTER INFARCTION ON REINFARCTION AND MORTALITY
(Patients over 30 years of age Submitted to Anesthesia and Surgery)

Interval from Previous MI	Reinfarction (%)	Mortality (%)
0–6 wk	100	100
6 wk–3 mo	37 (27)	60
3 mo–6 mo	16 (11)	40
6 mo–12 mo	6.5	20

Data from Tarhan, S., et al.: Myocardial infarction after general anesthesia. JAMA, 220:1451, 1972.

TABLE 2–27. RISK FACTORS FOR REINFARCTION FOLLOWING ANESTHESIA FOR NONCARDIAC SURGERY

MI-associated congestive failure
Medical problems: Jugular venous pulse
   Angina
   JVP
   Wedge pressure high
Type of surgery:
   Intrathoracic
   Upper abdominal
Routine vs. aggressive invasive monitoring
Intraoperative hemodynamic abnormalities:
   Hypotension
   Hypertension
   Tachycardia
Time interval after a first infarction to operation:
   0–3 months, 36% vs. 5.7%
   4–6 months, 26% vs. 2.3%
Postoperative monitoring duration
Possible anesthetic relation: higher with narcotic technique
Use of vasopressors vs. inotropic plus dilators
Emergency operations

From Rao, T.L.K., Jacobs, K.H., and El-Etr, A.A.: Reinfarction following anesthesia in patients with myocardial infarction. Anesthesiology, 59:499, 1983.

essary, and these hemodynamic abnormalities should not be allowed to continue for 10 minutes or more.

EMERGENCY SURGERY. This was associated with a higher incidence (16%) of reinfarction in patients in the routinely managed group, but in the aggressively managed group, the incidence was only 3%.[164]

INFARCTION AFTER BYPASS SURGERY

Several independent predictors associated with bypass cardiac surgery have been identified:[161]

1. Unstable angina did not appear to increase the incidence of postoperative myocardial infarction (PMI) compared with stable angina in some studies,[168] but was associated with a significant higher incidence in others[169,170]
2. Patients with severe pathology of the coronary vasculature and decreased ventricular performance have a higher risk of developing PMI[171,172]

TABLE 2–28. GUIDELINES FOR ANESTHESIA AND SURGERY IN PATIENTS WITH HISTORY OF MYOCARDIAL INFARCTION

Preoperative optimization of physiologic status
Use of vasoactive drugs intraoperatively—vasodilators
Aggressive invasive monitoring for 3–4 days
Immediate treatment of abnormalities
Avoidance of stress
Stress-free anesthesia
Narcotic technique 6% vs. inhalation 1.5%

From Rao, T.L.K., Jacobs, K.H., and El-Etr, A.A.: Myocardial infarction following anesthesia in patients with myocardial infarction. Anesthesiology, 59:499, 1983.

3. The intraoperative technique of cold potassium cardioplegia for myocardial preservation during aortic cross-clamping appears to provide a measure of protection against PMI[173]
4. The PMI rate increases with the duration of cardiopulmonary bypass.[172] An arrest time of more than 40 minutes increases the incidence of MI[174]
5. The quality of distal anastomosis has been an independent predictor of PMI.[174]

SUMMARY OF ANESTHESIA CARE OF MI PATIENTS

Several important conclusions have been reached with regard to patients with known or suspected ischemic heart disease[161,164] or with a previous infarction:

1. If a patient who has suffered a myocardial infarction needs an elective surgical procedure, the procedure should be delayed until the patient's cardiac risk has returned to the lowest possible level, which is considered to entail a full 6 months after the infarction[48,163]
2. If an emergency operation is indicated, there should be intensive monitoring beginning in the perioperative period and continuing through the fourth postoperative day. The rate of reinfarction within 3 months of a preoperative infarction is about 6%[164,166]; within 3 months, reinfarction is reduced to about 2%[164]
3. Anti-anginal medications, especially beta-blockers, are safely continued up to the time of operation
4. Intraoperative administration of calcium channel blockers (nifedipine) and nitroglycerin may be administered to manage ischemia[161]

TABLE 2-29. INCIDENCE OF REINFARCTION AND MORTALITY IN RELATION TO INTERVAL FROM PREVIOUS INFARCTION

Interval between Infarction and Anesthesia (months)	Number of Postanesthetic Reinfarctions (%)		Reinfarction Mortality (%)	
	Group 1	Group 2	Group 1	Group 2
0–3	4 (36)	3 (5.8)*	75	66
4–6	8 (26)	2 (2.3)	60	—
7–12	6 (5)	1 (1)	—	—
13–24	6 (5)	4 (1.56)	—	—
25	4 (5)	4 (1.7)	—	—
Total	28 (7.7)	14 (1.9)†	57	36

Incidence of postanesthetic reinfarctions compared with group 1: *$P < 0.05$; †$P < 0.005$.
From Rao, T.L.K. Jacobs, K.H., and El-Etr, A.A.: Reinfarction following anesthesia in patients with myocardial infarction. Anesthesiology, 59:499, 1983.

5. Most postoperative MIs occur within 6 days and actually peak in incidence at the 3rd day. Non-Q-wave infarctions may occur earlier. It is estimated that 50% or more of postoperative infarctions are painless and often present with unexpected alteration of vital signs[161]
6. Inhalation agents appear to have a better safety record than narcotic techniques.[164]

MEDICOLEGAL ASPECTS

DEFINITION OF MALPRACTICE (BLACK'S LAW DICTIONARY)[175]

Failure of one rendering professional services to exercise that degree of skill and learning commonly applied under all the circumstances in the community by the average prudent reputable member of the profession with the result of injury, loss or damage to the recipient of those services or to those entitled to rely upon them.

Like other physicians, anesthesiologists are responsible for their acts.[176] They are also accountable as physicians for making the decision as to *what* and *how* they prescribe and administer.

The anesthesiologist is in the eyes of the law an independent contractor. His judgment and actions will be on trial in the event of an anesthetic mishap—not the surgeon's. This is in contrast to the nurse anesthetist who has been considered the agent of the physician or surgeon.[177]

DUTIES OF A PHYSICIAN. Dornette has stated that a physician has five duties in the performance of his work.[178] These have been listed as follows:

1. Care—he must provide medical care conforming to accepted medical practices and bring to the task a reasonable degree of competence
2. Confidentiality—this is demanded by the patient–physician relationship and ethics
3. Consent—he must provide full and appropriate disclosure. The greater the risk and the uniqueness of a procedure, the greater the duty to inform.[179] One must provide that information one would expect for one's own family. Consent may be
   a. implied
   b. expressed, either verbally or in writing
   c. constructive—this is a creation of the law: a person, and especially a physician, has a duty to save life or limb and prevent pain. This is also represented as the Good Samaritan statute
4. Consultation—for specialized problems, i.e., sophisticated medical diseases
5. Continuing care—this must be provided, especially as regards the emergence and postoperative care.

All these duties must be completed in accordance with good medical practice, usually referred to as Standards of Care.

In general, the law has held that a physician must (1) perform his work in accordance with accepted medical practices and standards current in the community; (2) bring to the task a reasonable degree of skill and knowledge; and (3) exercise reasonable care.

When any of these principles are abrogated then negligence may exist. The anesthetist is liable if he fails to take those steps to satisfy himself that all is correct and those steps which a careful and prudent anesthetist would ordinarily take.[180]

BREACH OF DUTY. Generally, if an injury occurs, four elements must be present for a malpractice suit to ensue:[178,180]

1. Duty of physician with respect to standards of care must be present.
2. A breach of duty must be established. The "res ipsa loquitur" doctrine is not applied simply because some harm has occurred (requires expert testimony).
3. Causation, which means the harm or injury must be related to the breach of duty (requires expert testimony).
4. The extent of damages must be assessed (a judicial concept).

CONCLUSION. A negligent action may exist when a breach of duty is manifest. Because of such breach of duty in providing care, a harm must ensue; the nature of the harm must be assessed; the proximate causation must be recognized and, lastly, the extent of the damage estimated.

In cases where death or injury results from the injection of the wrong drug or of an actual overdose of one, it is difficult to establish a good defense. However, if the claim is based on hypersensitivity the doctor is liable only if he knew or ought reasonably to have known of the patient's undue sensitivity.

Another important court decision arose in connection with loss of teeth during administration of anesthesia.[181] Malpractice was claimed and the doctine of "res ipsa loquitur" applied. However, the court ruled that there was no evidence of negligence and stated:

"A physician is not required to exercise the highest degree of skill and care possible but only that degree ordinarily employed by members in good standing in the same community."[182]

Litigation can be avoided by anesthesiologists pursuing the following policies in addition to performing careful accepted anesthesia:

1. See the patient preoperatively and postoperatively. Evaluate the patient's condition, help manage or prevent postoperative complications.
2. Once the immediate anesthetic recovery is over, the anesthesiologist must keep posted on any complications by continued followup.
3. When consultants are brought into the situation, have them emphasize that many conditions do not mean negligence, *i.e.*, neurologists and laryngologists.

REFERENCES

1. Fulton, J.F.: *Harvey Cushing, A Biography*. Springfield, IL, Charles C Thomas, 1946.
2. Beecher, H.K.: The First Anesthesia Records. Surg. Gynec. Obst., 71:689, 1940.
3. Cushing, H.: On routine determinations of arterial tension in operating room and clinic. Boston Med. Surg. J., 148:250, 1903.
4. Slocum, H.C.: An apparatus for the automatic recording of diastolic and systolic blood pressure in clinical practice. Anesthesiology, 3:141, 1942.
4a. Blitt, C.D.: Monitoring in anesthesia and critical care medicine. New York: Churchill Livingstone, 1985.
4b. Newbower J.S., Ream, R.S., et al.: Essential non-invasive monitoring. New York: Grune & Stratton, 1980.
5. Committee on Clinical Anesthesia Study, American Society of Anesthesiology. A comprehensive simple anesthesia record. Anesthesiology, 21:557, 1960.
5a. Committee on Clinical Anesthesiology Study, American Society of Anesthesiologists, Inc. A comprehensive simple anesthesia record. Anesthesiology 21:557, 1960.
6. Saklad M.: Criteria in choice of anesthesia. Anesthesiology, 2:172, 1941.
7a. Seckzer, P.H.: Anesthesia documentation and evaluation. Quart Rev. Bull. 7:28, 1981.
7b. Apple, H.P., et al.: Design and evaluation of a semiautomatic anesthesia record system. Med. Instrum. 16:69, 1982.
8. Saunders, P.: An analysis of inhalation anesthesia by graphic means. Anesthesiology, 5:274, 1944.
9a. Miller, A.H.: Surgical posture: With symbols for its record on the anesthetist's chart. Anesthesiology, 1:241, 1940.
9b. AMA Fundamentals of Anesthesia, 3rd ed. W.B. Saunders Co., Philadelphia, 1954.
10. Conroy W.A., Cassels, W.H., and Stodsky, B.: Tabulation of anesthetic data. Anesthesiology, 9:121, 1948.
11. Pender, J.W.: A combined anesthesia record and statistical card. Anesthesiology, 7:606, 1946.
12. Committee on Clinical Records, American Society of Anesthesiology. News Letter Aug. and Sept. 1949.
13. Hallen, B.: Computerized anaesthetic record-keeping. Acta Anaesthesiol. Scand. (Supp.), 52:1, 1973.
14. Zollinger, R.M., Kreul, J.F., and Schneider, A.J.L.: Man-made versus computer generated anaesthesia records. J. Surg. Res., 22:419, 1977.
15. Gravenstein, J.S.: The automated anesthesia record. Int. J. Clin. Monit. Comput., 3:131, 1986.
16. Paulus, E.A., et al.: A semiautomated anesthesia record keeper: A clinical evaluation. J. Clin. Monit., 1:286, 1985.
17. Gravenstein, J.S., and Paulus, D.A.: A semi-automatic anesthesia record. Int. J. Clin. Monit. Comput., 2:251, 1986.
18. Roessler, P., Brenton, M.W., and Lambert, T.F.: Problems with automating anesthetic records. Anaesth. Intens. Care, 14:443, 1986.
19a. Rovenstine, E.A., and Hershey, S.G.: Therapeutic and diagnostic nerve blocking: A plan for organization. Anesthesiology, 5:574, 1944.
19b. Bonica, J.: The Management of Pain. Philadelphia, Lea & Febiger, 1990.
20. Soutter, L.: Procedures of the blood bank at the Massachusetts General Hospital. New Engl. J. Med., 230:157, 1944.
20a. Borucki, D.T., ed.: Blood Component Therapy. A Physician's Handbook. Washington, D.C., American Association of Blood Banks, 1981.
20b. Snyder, E.L., Kennedy, M.S.: Blood Transfusion Therapy: A Physician's Handbook. Arlington, Va.: American Association of Blood Banks.
21. Martin, S.J., and Makel, H.P.: Organization of a section of resuscitation and oxygen therapy. Army Med. Bull., 61:124, 1942.
22a. Saklad, M., Gillespie, N., and Rovenstine, E.A.: Inhalation therapy: Method for collecting and analysis of statistics. Anesthesiology, 5:359, 1944.
22b. Burton, G.G., Hodgkin, J.E.: Respiratory Care, 2nd ed. Philadelphia, J.B. Lippincott, 1984.
22c. Dripps, R.D., Eckenhoff, J.A., Vandam, L.: Inhalation therapy and pulmonary physiotherapy. In Introduction to Anesthesia, 3rd ed., pp. 469–476. Philadelphia, W.B. Saunders, 1980.
23a. Collins, V.J.: Fatalities in anesthesia and surgery: Fundamental considerations. JAMA, 172:549, 1960.
23b. Angrist, A.: Certified cause of death. Analysis and recommendations. JAMA, 166:2148, 1958.
24. Hingson, R.A., Holden, W.D., and Barnes, A.C.: Mechanisms involved in anesthetic deaths: Survey of operating room and obstetric delivery room related mortality in university hospitals of Cleveland. New York J. Med., 56:230, 1956.
25. Collins, V.J.: Operating Room Mortality, Proceedings, House of Delegates, New York Medical Society. New York J. Med., 58:55, 1958.

26. Resolution 28: Operating Room Mortality, Proceedings, House of Delegates, 107th Annual Session, American Medical Association, San Francisco, June 23–27, 1958, p. 48.
27. Beecher, H.K., and Todd, D.P.: A study of the deaths associated with anesthesia and surgery based on a study of 599,548 anesthesias in 10 institutions 1948–52. Ann. Surg., 140:2, 1954.
28a. Waters, R.M., and Gillespie, N.A.: Deaths in operating room. Anesthesiology, 5:113, 1948.
28b. Bishop, H.T.: Operating room deaths. Anesthesiology, 7:651, 1946.
29a. Cooper, J.B., Newbower, R.S., Kitz, R.J.: An analysis of major errors and equipment failures in anesthesia management: Considerations for prevention and detection. Anesthesiology, 60:34, 1984.
29b. Craig J., Wilson, M.E.: A survey of anaesthetic misadventures. Anaesthesia, 36:933, 1981.
30. Campbell, J.E.: Deaths associated with anesthesia. J. Forensic Sci., 5:501, 1960.
31. Campbell, J.E., Weiss, W.A., and Rieders, F.: Evaluation of deaths associated with anesthesia. Anes. Analg., 40:54, 1961.
32. Weiss, W.A.: Symposium: Deaths due to anesthesia. J. Forensic Sci., 5:523, 1960.
33a. Ruth H.S.: Anesthesia Study Commissions. JAMA 127:514, 1945.
33b. Clinical Anesthesia Conference: Series of Conferences on Medical Emergencies in Operating Room Including Causes of Death During Anesthesia. Prepared by Anesthesia Study Committee of New York State Society of Anesthesiologists, B.A. Greene (Chairman), V.J. Collins (Secretary), N.Y. State J. Med. 56:Jan. 1–June 15, 1956; M.H. Harmel, Chairman, N.Y. State J. Med. 56:July 1–Dec., 1958.
33c. Mark, L.C. (Ed.): Clinical Anesthesia Conferences. Boston, Little, Brown and Co., 1967.
34. Edwards, G., et al.: Deaths associated with anesthesia: Report on 1,000 cases. Anesthesia, 11:194, 1956.
35. Kircher, T., and Anderson, R.E.: Cause of death: Proper completion of the death certificate. JAMA, 258:349, 1987.
36. Saklad, M.: Grading for patients for surgical procedures. Anesthesiology, 2:201, 1941.
37. Committee on Records, American Society for Anesthesiology. Newsletter, 27:4, 1963.
38. Committee on Records, American Society for Anesthesiology: New classification of physical status. Anesthesiology, 24:111, 1963.
39. Goldstein, A., and Keats, A.S.: The risk of anesthesia. Anesthesiology, 33:310, 1970.
40. Moore, F.D.: Metabolic Care of the Surgical Patient. Philadelphia, W.B. Saunders, 1959.
41. Vandam, L.D.: The unfavorable effects of prolonged anesthesia. Can. Anaesth. Soc. J., 12:107, 1965.
42. Dripps, R.D., Lamont, A., and Eckenhoff, J.E.: The role of anesthesia in surgical mortality. JAMA, 178:261, 1961.
43. Marx, G.F., Matteo, C.V., and Orkin, L.R.: Computer analysis of post anesthetic deaths. Anesthesiology, 39:54, 1973.
44a. Vacanti, C.J., Van Houten, R.J., and Hill, R.C.: A statistical analysis of the relationship of physical status to postoperative mortality in 68,386 cases. Anesth. Analg., 49:564, 1970.
44b. Davies, J.M., Stranin, L.: Anesthesia in 1984: How safe is it? Can. Med. Assoc. J., 131:437, 1984.
45a. Beecher, H.K., and Todd, D.P.: A study of the deaths associated with anesthesia and surgery based on a study of 599,548 anesthesias in ten institutions 1948–1952, inclusive. Ann. Surg., 140:2, 1954.
45b. Bevan, D. R., Bevan, J.C., Donati, F.: Muscle Relaxants in Clinical Anesthesia. Chicago, Year Book Medical Publishers, Inc., 1988.
46. Hingson, R.A.: Comparative negro and white mortality during anesthesia, obstetrics and surgery. Nat. Med. Assoc., 49:203, 1957.
47. Poe, M.F.: The negro as an anesthetic risk. Anesthesiology, 14:84, 1953.
48. Cohen, M.M., et al.: A survey of 112,000 anaesthetics at one teaching hospital. Can. Anaesth. Soc. J., 33:22, 1986.
49a. Derrington, M.C., and Smith, G.: A review of studies of anaesthetic risk, morbidity and mortality. Brit. J. Anaesth., 59:815, 1987.
49b. Hingson, R.A., Holden, W.D., and Barnes, A.C.: Mechanisms involved in anesthetic deaths: A survey of operating room and obstetric delivery room related mortality in the University Hospitals of Cleveland, 1945–1955. N.Y. State J. Med., 56:230, 1956.
49c. Clifton, B.S., and Hotten, W.J.T.: Deaths associated with anaesthesia. Brit. J. Anaesth., 35:250, 1963.
49d. Bodlander, F.M.S.: Deaths associated with anaesthesia. Brit. J. Anaesth., 47:36, 1975.
49e. Hovi-Viander, M.: Death associated with anaesthesia in Finland. Brit. J. Anaesth., 52:483, 1980.
49f. Turnbull, K.W., Fancourt-Smith, P.F., and Banting, G.C.: Deaths within 48 hours of anaesthesia at the Vancouver General Hospital. Can. Anaesth. Soc. J., 27:159, 1980.
49g. Lunn, J.N., and Mushin, W.W.: Mortality associated with anaesthesia. Anaesthesia, 37:856, 1982.
49h. Keenan, R.L., and Boyan, C.P.: Cardiac arrest due to anesthesia: A study of incidence and causes. JAMA, 253:2373, 1985.
50. Tiret, L., et al.: Complications associated with anaesthesia—a prospective survey in France. Can. Anaesth. Soc. J., 33:336, 1986.
51. Goldman, L., et al.: Multifactorial index of cardiac risk in non-cardiac surgical procedures. New Engl. J. Med., 297:845, 1977.
52. Goldman, L., et al.: Cardiac risk factors and complications in non-cardiac surgery. Medicine (Baltimore), 47:357, 1978.
53. Urzua, J., et al.: Preoperative estimation of risk in cardiac surgery. Anesth. Analg., 60:625, 1981.
54. Cooper, J.B., Newbower, R.S., and Kitz, R.J.: An analysis of major errors and equipment failure in anesthesia management: Considerations for prevention and detection. Anesthesiology, 60:34, 1984.
55. Cooper, J.B., et al.: Preventable anesthesia mishaps: A study of human factors. Anesthesiology, 49:399, 1978.
56. Craig, J., and Wilson, M.E.: A survey of anaesthetic misadventures. Anaesthesia, 36:933, 1981.
57. Kumar, V., et al.: Forum: An analysis of critical incidents in a teaching department for quality assurance. A survey of mishaps during anaesthesia. Anaesthesia, 43:879, 1988.
58. Goldman, H.S.: Anesthetic mistakes, mishaps, and misadventures. Curr. Rev. Clin. Anesth., 8:115, 1988.
59. Cohen, M.M., Duncan, P.G., and Tate, R.B.: Does anesthesia contribute to operative mortality? JAMA, 260:2859, 1988.
60. Bradley, J.P., et al.: Mortality audit in a large teaching hospital. Anaesth. Intens. Care, 16:94, 1988.
61. Tiret, L., et al.: Complications related to anaesthesia in infants and children. Brit. J. Anaesth., 61:263, 1988.
62. Bell, C.: Anesthesia complications in children related to surgical procedures. Yale–New Haven Hospital Communication, 1988.
63. Farrow, S.C., et al.: Epidemiology in anaesthesia. II. Factors affecting mortality in the hospitals. Brit. J. Anaesth., 54:811, 1982.

64. Leithe, M.E., et al.: The effect of age on central and regional hemodynamics. Gerontology, 30:240, 1984.
65. Bender, A.D.: The effect of increasing age on the distribution of peripheral blood flow in man. J. Am. Geriatr. Soc., 13:192, 1965.
66. Ouslander, J.G.: Drug therapy in the elderly. Ann. Intern. Med., 95:711, 1981.
67. Farrow, S.C., et al.: Epidemiology in anesthesia: A method for predicting hospital mortality. Eur. J. Anaesth., 1:77, 1984.
68. Hosking, M.P., et al.: Outcomes of surgery in patients 90 years of age and older. JAMA, 261:1909, 1989.
69. Pederson, T., et al.: Risk factors, complications and outcome in anaesthesia: A pilot study. Eur. J. Anaesth., 3:225, 1986.
70. Koch, J.P.: ASA Status: Predictor of outcome in blunt trauma surgery. Presentation at ASA Annual Convention, Atlanta, 1987.
71. Bruns, K.: Postoperative care and review of complications. Int. Anesthesiol. Clin., 20:27, 1982.
72. Driscoll, E.J.: American Society of Oral Surgeons: Anesthesia morbidity and mortality survey. J. Oral Surg., 32:733, 1974.
73. Lyttle, J.J., and Yoon, C.: Anesthesia morbidity and mortality survey: Southern California Society of Oral and Maxillofacial Surgeons. J. Oral. Surg., 38:814, 1980.
74. Green, R.A., and Taylor, T.H.: An analysis of anesthesia medical liability claims in the United Kingdom 1977–1982. Int. Anesthesiol. Clin., 22:73, 1984.
75. Keenan, R.L.: Anesthesia disasters: Incidences, causes and preventability. Semin. Anesthesia, 5:175, 1986.
76. Gold, B., et al.: Unanticipated admission to the hospital following ambulatory surgery. JAMA, 262:3008, 1989.
77. Mendelson, C.L.: The aspiration of stomach contents into the lungs during obstetric anesthesia. Am. J. Obstet. Gynecol., 52:191, 1946.
78. Wynne, J.W., and Modell, J.H.: Respiratory aspiration of stomach contents. Ann. Int. Med., 87:466, 1977.
79. Modell, J.H.: Aspiration pneumonitis. In Refresher Course in Anesthesiology, Vol. 10. American Society of Anesthesiologists, 1982.
80. Salem, M.R., Wong, A.Y., and Collins, V.J.: The pediatric patient with a full stomach. Anesthesiology, 39:435, 1973.
81. Cotton, B.R., and Smith, G.: The lower esophageal sphincter and anaesthesia. Brit. J. Anaesth., 58:37, 1974.
82. Smith, G., Dalling, R., and Williams, T.I.R.: Gastroesophageal pressure gradient changes produced by induction of anaesthesia and suxamethonium. Brit. J. Anaesth., 50:11, 1978.
83. Edwards, G., et al.: Deaths associated with anaesthesia: Report of 1,000 cases. Anaesthesia, 11:194, 1956.
84. Olsson, G.L., Hallen, B., and Hambraeus-Jonzon, K.: Aspiration during anaesthesia: A computer-aided study of 185,358 anaesthetics. Acta Anaesth. Scand., 30:84, 1986.
85. Roberts, R.B., and Shirley, M.A.: Reducing the risk of acid aspiration during cesarean section. Anesth. Analg., 53:859, 1974.
85a. Greene, N.M., et al.: Survey of deaths: Associated with anesthesia in Connecticut. Connecticut Med. J., 23:512, 1959.
85b. Harrison, G.G.: Death attributable to anaesthesia. Brit. J. Anaesth., 50:1041,1046, 1978.
85c. Hovi-Viander, M.: Death associated with anaesthesia in Finland. Brit. J. Anaesth., 52:483, 1980.
86. Culver, G.A., Makel, H.P., and Beecher, H.K.: Frequency of aspiration of gastric contents by the lungs during anesthesia and surgery. Ann. Surg., 133:289, 1951.
87. Berson, W., and Adriani, J.: Silent regurgitation and aspiration during anesthesia. Anesthesiology, 15:644, 1954.
88. Cote, C.J., et al.: Assessment of risk factors related to the acid aspiration syndrome in pediatric patients—gastric pH and residual volume. Anesthesiology, 56:70, 1982.
88a. Crawford, J.S.: The anaesthetist's contribution to maternal mortality. Brit. J. Anaesth., 42:70, 1970.
88b. Hunter, A.R., and Moir, D.D.: Editorial: Confidential enquiry into maternal deaths. Brit. J. Anaesth., 55:367, 1983.
88c. Lunn, J.N., Hunter, A.R., and Scott, D.B.: Anaesthesia-related surgical mortality. Anaesthesia, 38:1090, 1983.
89. Warner, M.A., Divertie, M.B., and Tinker, J.H.: Preoperative cessation of smoking and pulmonary complications in coronary artery bypass patients. Anesthesiology, 60:380, 1984.
90. Camner, P., and Philipson, K.: Some studies of tracheobronchial clearance in man. Chest, 63:235, 1973.
91. Buist, A.S., et al.: The effect of smoking cessation and modification on lung function. Am. Rev. Respir. Dis., 114:115, 1976.
92. Mitchell, C., Garrahy, P., and Peake, P.: Postoperative respiratory morbidity: Identification and risk factors. Aust. N.Z. J. Surg., 52:203, 1982.
93. Bode, F.R., et al.: Reversibility of pulmonary function abnormalities in smokers. Am. J. Med., 59:43, 1975.
94. Civetta, J.M.: Perioperative effects of anesthesia. Personal communication, 1985.
95. Cooper, J.B., et al.: Preventable anesthesia mishaps: A study of human factors. Anesthesiology, 49:399, 1978.
96. Narang, V., and Laycock, J.R.D.: Psychomotor testing of on-call anaesthetists. Anaesthesia, 41:868, 1986.
97. Korttila, K., and Linnoila, M.: Psychomotor skills related to driving after intramuscular administration of diazepam and meperidine. Anesthesiology, 42:685, 1975.
98. Parker, J.B.R.: The effects of fatigue on physician performance—an underestimated cause of physician impairment and increased patient risk. Can. J. Anaesth., 34:489, 1987.
99. Goldman, L.I., McDonough, M.T., and Rosemond, G.P.: Stresses affecting surgical performance and learning. J. Surg. Res., 12:83, 1972.
100. Williams, H.L., Lubin, A., and Goodnow, J.J.: Impaired performance with acute sleep loss. Psychol. Monogr., 73:1, 1959.
101. Poulton, E.C.: Arousing environmental stresses can improve performance, whatever people say. Aviat. Space Environ. Med., 47:1193, 1976.
102. Cooper, J.B., Newbower, R.S., and Kitz, R.J.: An analysis of major errors and equipment failures in anesthesia management: Considerations for prevention and detection. Anesthesiology, 60:34, 1984.
103. Naitoh, P., and Townsend, R.E.: The role of sleep deprivation research in human factors. Hum. Factors, 12:575, 1970.
104. Lees, D.E.: N.Y. would limit work hours, mandate patient monitoring. Anesthesia Patient Safety Foundation Newsletter, 2:22, 1987.
105. Frumin, M.J.: Fatigue dangers provoke questions (Letter). APSF Newsletter, June 1987.
106. Cooper, J.B., et al.: Critical incidents associated with intraoperative exchanges of anesthesia personnel. Anesthesiology, 56:456, 1982.
107. Morgan, B.B., Brown, B.R., and Alluisi, E.A.: Effects on sustained performance of 48 hours of sleep loss. Hum. Factors, 16:406, 1974.
108. Grether, C.B.: Engineering psychology. In The Human Side of Accident Prevention. Edited by B.L. Margolis and W.H. Kroes. Springfield, IL, Charles C Thomas, 1975.

109. Cooper, J.B.: Do short breaks increase or decrease anesthetic risk? J. Clin. Anesth., *1*:228, 1989.
110. Keenan, R.L., and Boyan, C.P.: Cardiac arrest due to anesthesia. JAMA, *253*:2373, 1985.
111. Davies, J.M., and Strunin, L.: Anesthesia in 1984: How safe is it? Can. Med. Assoc. J., *131*:437, 1984.
112. Utting, J.R., Gray, T.C., and Shelley, F.C.: Human misadventure in anaesthesia. Can. Anaesth. Soc. J., *26*:472, 1979.
113. Salem, R., et al.: Cardiac arrest related to anesthesia: Contributing factors in infants and children. JAMA, *233*:238, 1975.
114. Caplan, R.A., et al.: Unexpected cardiac arrest during spinal anesthesia: A closed claims analysis of predisposing factors. Anesthesiology, *68*:5, 1988.
115. Rutstein, D.D., et al.: Measuring the quality of medical care: A clinical method. New Engl. J. Med., *294*:582, 1976.
116. Cote, C.J., et al.: A single-blind study of pulse oximetry in children. Anesthesiology, in press.
117. Hilgenberg, J.C., and Johantgen, W.C.: Bradycardia after intravenous fentanyl during subarachnoid anesthesia (Letter). Anesth. Analg., *59*:162, 1980.
118. Fortuna, A.: Droperidol and spinal anesthesia (Letter). Anesth. Analg., *63*:782, 1984.
119. Ward, D.S.: Stimulation of hypoxic ventilatory drive by droperidol. Anesth. Analg., *63*:106, 1984.
120. Pearson, J.W., and Redding, J.S.: Influence of peripheral vascular tone on cardiac resuscitation. Anesth. Analg., *44*:746, 1965.
121. Brown, C.G., et al.: Comparative effect of graded doses of epinephrine on regional brain blood flow during CPR in a swine model. Ann. Emerg. Med., *15*:1138, 1986.
122. Keats, A.S.: Anesthesia mortality—a new mechanism. Anesthesiology, *68*:2, 1988.
123. Forrest, W.H. Jr., and Bellville, J.W.: The effect of sleep plus morphine on the respiratory response to carbon dioxide. Anesthesiology, *25*:137, 1964.
124. Berggren, L., et al.: Changes in respiratory pattern after repeated doses of diazepam and midazolam in healthy subjects. Acta Anaesth. Scand., *31*:667, 1987.
125. Obrist, P.A., et al.: The relationship among heart rate, carotid dP/dt and blood pressure in humans as a function of the type of stress. Psychophysiology, *15*:102, 1978.
126. Graboys, T.B.: Stress and the aching heart. New Engl. J. Med., *311*:594, 1984.
127. Zeppilli, P., et al.: Wenckebach second-degree AV block in top-ranking athletes: An old problem. Am. Heart J., *100*:281, 1980.
128. Fredrichs, R.L., Campbell, J., and Bassell, G.M.: Psychogenic cardiac arrest during extensive sympathetic blockade. Anesthesiology, *68*:943, 1988.
129. Beecher, H.K.: Some preoperative warnings of potential operating room death. New Engl. J. Med., *255*:1075, 1956.
130. Weisman, A.D., and Hackett, T.P.: Predilection to death. Psychosomatic Med., *23*:3, 1961.
131. Hardison, J.E.: Premonitions. JAMA, *251*:1423, 1984.
132. Von Lerchenthal, E.: Death from psychic causes. Bull. Menninger Clin., *12*:31, 1948.
133. Walters, M.: Psychic death: Report of a possible case. Arch. Neurol. Psychiatry *52*:84, 1944.
134. Freud, S.: Thoughts for the times on war and death. Collected Papers, Vol. 4. London, Hogarth Press, p. 288, 1948.
135. Ruberman, W., et al.: Psychosocial influences on mortality after myocardial infarction. New Engl. J. Med., *311*:552, 1984.
136. Frankl, V.E.: Man's Search for Meaning. New York, Washington Square Press, 1963.
137. Vandam, L.D.: Cardiac arrest: Signal of anesthetic mishap. JAMA, *253*:2415, 1985.
138. Keenan, R.L., and Boyan, C.P.: Cardiac arrest due to anesthesia: A study of incidence and causes. JAMA, *253*:2373, 1985.
139. Nagel, E.L., Editorial Board: Death during general anesthesia. J. Health Care Technol. Anesth. *1*:155, 1985.
140. Hamilton, W.K.: Unexpected deaths during anesthesia: Wherein lies the cause? Anesthesiology, *50*:381, 1979.
141. Keats, A.S.: What do we know about anesthetic mortality? Anesthesiology, *50*:387, 1979.
142. Bruner, J.M.R.: Biomedical Safety and Standards: Special Supplement No. 2. Brea, CA, Quest Publishing Company, 1984.
143. Goldman, H.S.: Anesthetic mistakes, mishaps, and misadventures. Curr. Rev. Clin. Anesth., *8*:115, 1988.
144. Standards of Anesthesia Practice. American Society of Anesthesiologists. Directory of Members, 54th Edition. Park Ridge, Illinois, 1989.
145. Joint Commission on Accreditation of Healthcare Organizations: Manual Standards for Anesthesia Service. Chicago, 1988.
146. Orkin, F.K.: Practice standards: The midas touch or the emperor's new clothes? Anesthesiology, *70*:567, 1989.
147. Goldman, L.: Multifactorial index of cardiac risk in noncardiac surgery—a 10 year status report. J. Cardiothoracic Anesth., *1*:237, 1987.
148. Detsky, A.S., et al.: Predicting cardiac complications in patients undergoing non-cardiac surgery. J. Gen. Intern. Med., *1*:211, 1986.
149. Goldman, L.: Assessment of the patient with known or suspected ischemic heart disease for non-cardiac surgery. Brit. J. Anaesth., *61*:38, 1988.
150. Zeldin, R.A.: Assessing cardiac risk in patients who undergo noncardiac surgical procedures. Can. J. Surg., *27*:402, 1984.
151. Jeffrey, C.C., et al.: A prospective evaluation of cardiac risk index. Anesthesiology, *58*:462, 1983.
152. Gerson, M.C., et al.: Cardiac prognosis in noncardiac geriatric surgery. Ann. Intern. Med., *103*:832, 1985.
153. Butler, S., Feeney, N., and Levine, S.A.: Patient with heart disease as surgical risk. JAMA, *95*:84, 1930.
154. Randall, O.S., and Orr, T.G.: Post-operative occlusion. Ann. Surg., *92*:1014, 1930.
155. Etsten, B.E., et al.: Appraisal of the coronary patient as an operative risk. N.Y. State J. Med., p. 2065 (July 15), 1954.
156. Driscoll, A.C., et al.: Clinically unrecognized myocardial infarction following surgery. New Engl. J. Med., *264*:633, 1961.
157. Topkins, M.J., and Artusio, J.F.: Myocardial infarction and surgery, a five-year study. Anesth. Analg., *43*:716, 1964.
158. Tarhan, S., et al.: Myocardial infarction after general anesthesia. JAMA, *220*:1451, 1972.
159. Schoeppel, S.J., et al.: Effects of myocardial infarction on perioperative cardiac complications. Anesth. Analg., *62*:493, 1983.
160. von Knorring, J.: Postoperative myocardial infarction: A prospective study in a risk group of surgical patients. Surgery, *90*:55, 1981.
161. Haagensen, R., and Steen, P.A.: Perioperative myocardial infarction. Brit. J. Anaesth., *61*:24, 1988.
162. Eerola, M., et al.: Risk factors in surgical patients with verified preoperative myocardial infarction. Acta Anaesth. Scand., *24*:219, 1980.
163. Steen, P.A., Tinker, J.H., and Tarhan, S.: Myocardial reinfarction after anesthesia and surgery. JAMA, *239*:2566, 1978.

164. Rao, T.L.K., Jacobs, K.H., and El-Etr, A.A.: Reinfarction following anesthesia in patients with myocardial infarction. Anesthesiology, 59:499, 1983.
165. Mahar, L.J., et al.: Perioperative myocardial infarction in patients with coronary artery disease with and without aorta–coronary artery bypass grafts. J. Thorac. Cardiovasc. Surg., 76:533, 1978.
166. Kaplan, J., and King, S.B.: The precordial electrocardiographic lead in patients who have coronary artery disease. Anesthesiology, 45:570, 1976.
167. Arkins, R., Smessaert, A.A., and Hicks, R.G.: Mortality and morbidity in surgical patients with coronary artery disease. JAMA, 190:485, 1964.
168. Blackburn, H., et al.: The Exercise Electrocardiogram. Edited by M. Karlomen. Springfield, IL, Charles C Thomas, 1966.
169. Gersh, B.J., et al.: Coronary arteriography and coronary artery bypass surgery: Morbidity and mortality in patients aged 65 years or older. Circulation, 67:483, 1983.
170. Fennell, W.H., et al.: Detection, prediction and significance of perioperative myocardial infarction following aorta-coronary bypass. J. Thorac. Cardiovasc. Surg., 78:244, 1979.
171. Baur, H.R., et al.: Predictors of perioperative myocardial infarction in coronary artery operation. Ann. Thorac. Surg., 31:36, 1980.
172. Guiteras Val, P.G., et al.: Diagnostic criteria and prognosis of perioperative myocardial infarction following coronary bypass. J. Thorac. Cardiovasc. Surg., 86:878, 1983.
173. Kirklin, J.W., Conti, V.R., and Blackstone, E.H.: Prevention of myocardial damage during cardiac operations. New Engl. J. Med., 301:135, 1979.
174. Slogoff, S., and Keats, A.S.: Does perioperative myocardial ischemia lead to postoperative myocardial infarction? Anesthesiology, 62:107, 1985.
175. Black's Law Dictionary. 5th Edition, 1979.
176. Wasmuth, C.E.: Anesthesia and the Law. American Lecture Series. Springfield, IL, Charles C Thomas, 1961.
177. Hawkins, W.C.: Medico-legal hazards of anesthesia. JAMA, 165:746, 1957.
178. Dornette, W. (Ed.): Legal Aspects of Anesthesia. Philadelphia, F.A. Davis, 1972.
179. Peters, J.D., et al.: Anesthesiology and the Law. Health American Press, 1983.
180. Gild, W.M.: Medical malpractice. Progr. Anesthesiol., 11:1, 1987.
181. Medico-Legal Abstracts: Loss of teeth during tonsillectomy. JAMA, 158:777, 1955.
182. Mackauf, S.H.: (Abstr.), ASA Newsletter, 48(12)8, 1984.

"In somno securitas" and "Vigilance." These phrases are the mottos of the Association of Anaesthetists of Great Britain and Ireland and the American Society of Anesthesiologists, respectively. Each word or phrase reminds us of the necessity of constant care; together they represent the method—vigilant attention—and the goal—a safe anesthetic. Hence, these are the essence of monitoring. It is indisputable that improved patient safety has come largely from advances in monitoring technology.

"It is incident upon physicians,
I am afraid, beyond all other men,
to mistake subsequence for consequence."—Samuel Johnson

Anesthesiologists, perhaps among all physicians, must differentiate between subsequence and consequence. This confusion exists because the anesthetized condition is unique; it is monitored externally, rarely recalled, and still not completely understood. During the last half-century, awareness of anesthetic morbidity and mortality has moved to the forefront. The "eternal triangle" as depicted in Figure 3–1 represents the interactive triad of a dynamic system that forms the basis for our concern with monitoring.[1]

In concert, this dynamic system ebbs and flows. Despite any change, the anesthesiologist functions as the decision maker who remains at the top of the triangle, always evaluating, adjusting, and reacting to the situation.

Catastrophe occurs with failure of either the equipment, the anesthesiologist, the patient, or the respective interactions. In a mishap that is caused by the delivery of anesthesia in which the performance of the equipment or the anesthesiologist fails, the patient is the victim; but how and when does this occur? More importantly, can mishap related to anesthesia delivery be avoided?

To answer these questions, the ergonomics of the practice of anesthesia delivery must be reviewed. More specifically, the common denominator(s) in catastrophes related to anesthesia must be elucidated and corrected. This background forms the paradigm for the development of a monitoring philos-

3

Gerald A. Maccioli
Jerry M. Calkins
Vincent J. Collins

MONITORING THE ANESTHETIZED PATIENT

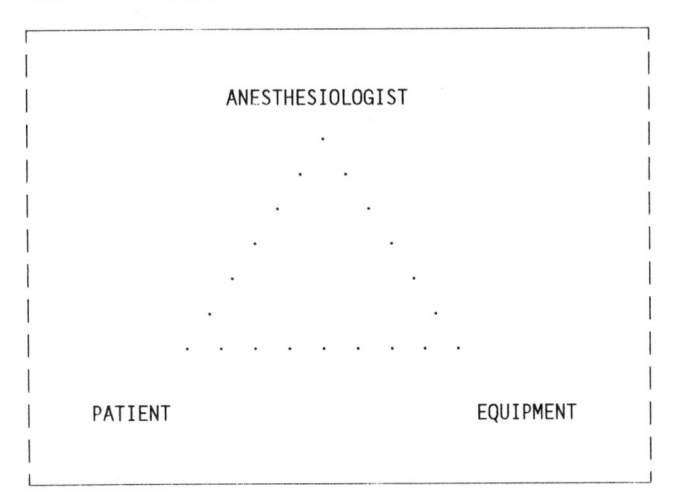

FIG. 3–1. The eternal triangle. From Calkins, J.M.: Why new delivery system? *In* FADS: The Future of Anesthetic Delivery Systems. Contemporary Anesthesia Practice, vol. 8. Edited by B.R. Brown. Philadelphia, F.A. Davis, 1984.

ophy, i.e., the why, when, where, and pitfalls of monitoring.

Duri et al. studied the interaction between the anesthesiologist and equipment for anesthesia delivery.[2] A notable finding was approximately 50% of the time, the anesthesiologist is in a mode requiring significant mental activity where gross physical activity is not required. This study of anesthesia ergonomics revealed that the anesthesiologist's time is equally divided between activities related to the patient and equipment. Unfortunately the Duri study did not define the percentage of "equipment-activities" time devoted to direct patient monitoring versus monitoring the equipment. Most ergonomic studies focus on the anatomy of catastrophes related to anesthesia rather than general mental or physical workloads. Let us evaluate the anesthesia-related catastrophe in light of Duri's time framework.

Before such an evaluation can be made, the definition of anesthesia-related catastrophe must be established. Cooper et al. used a "critical incident" method for defining anesthesia-related misadventures.[3] A "critical incident" in brief was defined as "a human error or equipment failure that could have led (if not discovered or corrected in time) or did lead to an undesirable outcome, ranging from increased length of hospital [or recovery room/ICU] stay to death."

Using a format of voluntary reporting, supplemented by interview follow-up, Cooper and his colleagues attributed approximately 70% of critical accidents to human error. Further analysis classified human error as inappropriate drug administration (24%); improper use of the anesthesia machine (22%); and airway management errors (16%). Errors in judgment occur during both patient care and equipment use. From this analysis, it was estimated that approximately 50% of anesthesia-related mortality is preventable. These findings are consistent with other studies in which human error was a factor in 87% of 80 deaths,[4] 65% of 52 deaths,[5] and 83% of 589 deaths.[6]

These data can be re-examined from the case-time perspective of the anesthesiologist during the intraoperative anesthesia procedure, i.e., induction, maintenance, and emergence. During induction and emergence, airway maintenance, which requires significant physical activity but minimal concomitant mental activity, is of primary concern. Intuitively the data suggest that if contemporaneous nonessential tasks were delayed to another time, or essential tasks delegated to others, the percentage of preventable critical incidents related to airway management would be reduced or eliminated. Similarly, the maintenance period requires significant mental activity with minimal physical activity, principally drug administration and machine utilization. Techniques decreasing the mental workload such as improved syringe labeling and equipment education might reduce or possibly eliminate these errors.

The total avoidance of anesthesia-related mishap is possibly an unobtainable goal as the delivery of anesthesia is conducted today. Intuitively improved monitoring, however, a more appropriate distribution of anesthesia-related tasks, and continuing education with critical self-analysis will help accomplish this goal of reduced risk.

The word monitor comes from the Latin "monere," meaning to warn. Functionally, monitoring anesthesia delivery can be classified into two major categories.[7] The first category consists of those devices and techniques that assess the function and performance of the anesthetic delivery system (e.g., the machine, breathing circuit, or ventilator). The second category is patient monitoring. Regardless of which major monitoring category is being considered, monitoring anesthesia delivery can provide information on three planes: vigilant, physiology, and anesthetic depth. The focus of vigilant monitoring is to avoid catastrophe. Physiologic monitoring assesses the effects of surgery and anesthetic techniques on the homeostatic mechanisms of an organ system. The assessment of cumulative agent effects is the goal of depth monitoring.

This chapter focuses on patient monitoring, which consists primarily of physiologic monitoring with the implications of vigilant monitoring. For example, an end-tidal CO_2 measurement value can be related to the physiologic status of the respiratory system. This same value for respiratory CO_2 can be used with vigilance for accessing airway integrity against interruptions, i.e., disconnections, esophageal intubations, and so forth. For the purposes of this chapter the discussion is limited to the cardiovascular, respiratory, central nervous, and genitourinary systems.

PRINCIPLES OF MONITORING PHILOSOPHY

As summarized by Hope and Morrison, monitoring is a process composed of five basic components: signal generation, data acquisition, data transmission, data processing, and data display.[8] Anesthesia monitoring includes the additional components of data analysis and clinical decision making. Regrettably, this chapter cannot address itself to equipment operation; however, it is imperative that each practitioner familiarize himself with the limitations of each device employed. Remember, while the patient serves as the source of all signal generation, the physician alone determines which signals are received and analyzed.

In each preoperative evaluation, the anesthesiologist's knowledge formulates a three-tiered plan. The preoperative plan includes further work-up necessary prior to anesthesia, premedication, or other adjunct therapies. The intraoperative plan includes two components. The anesthetic management plan and the anesthetic monitoring strategy. Furthermore, the monitoring decision must include monitors for the **vigilant, physiology,** and **depth** planes. The aforementioned studies stressed the necessity of thoughtful and careful selection of monitors appropriate to each plane for every anesthetic. Finally, a postoperative plan made in conjunction with surgical colleagues is designed.

Many preoperative anesthetic notes contain the phrase "routine" monitoring. What constitutes "routine" monitoring? In a practice environment where new technology provides more and more options and malpractice judgments continue to escalate, the phrase "routine" has little meaning. In reality there is no such thing as "minor" general anesthesia. In late 1986, Eichhorn and his Harvard colleagues published a landmark article, "Standards for Patient Monitoring during Anesthesia at Harvard Medical School."[9] The article represents a milestone not for its content (see below) but rather its premise: the first published standards of anesthesia monitoring practice in the English-speaking world. Their standards include monitoring for

- Blood pressure and continuous circulation
- Heart rate
- Electrocardiogram
- Ventilation, continuous and disconnection
- Oxygen analysis
- Temperature

In addition, on October 21, 1986, the American Society of Anesthesiologists House of Delegates approved "Standards for Basic Intra-Operative Monitoring."[10] These recommendations included the continuous presence of qualified anesthesia personnel and monitoring for

- Oxygenation
- Ventilation
- Circulation
- Temperature

While these efforts are applauded, and we realize the protean tasks accomplished, we must view these monitoring strategies as at times inadequate. Certain monitors can be categorized as vigilant or physiologic based on the interpretation of the variable. The following is a comprehensive collection of the necessary standards for patients undergoing general anesthesia.

Vigilant monitors
  Stethoscope (precordial or esophageal)
  Oxyhemoglobin saturation (pulse oximetry)
  Anesthetic and respiratory gas concentrations
  The anesthesiologists senses as monitors
Physiologic monitors
  Arterial blood pressure
  Temperature
  Neuromuscular blockade (if relaxants used)
  Electrocardiography
  Respirometry and airway/circuit pressures
Depth monitors
  No one monitor of "depth" is available at present; however, several are under clinical trial (see below). Currently clinical signs are used to access depth.

Monitoring the anesthetized patient demonstrates three crucial caveats: (1) monitoring technology is in a constant state of change; (2) no monitor can replace the well-informed, vigilant anesthesiologist; and (3) monitoring involves a multivariable situation.

The remainder of this chapter is devoted to physiologic monitoring using an organ-system approach. Anesthetic depth and neuromuscular blockade monitoring are addressed in other chapters.

MONITORING THE CARDIOVASCULAR SYSTEM

The cardiovascular system represents a significant organ system to the anesthesiologist because of (1) the increased frequency of cardiovascular disease; (2) the importance of continuous perfusion of the brain; and (3) the frequent depression of cardiovascular function during surgery and anesthesia. Over the past three decades, atherosclerotic coronary vascular disease (ASCVD) has become the primary cause of death in western societies. This epidemiologic fact, coupled with therapeutic advances that have led to an aging patient population, have made monitoring for cardiac ischemia and dysfunction a priority. Continuous perfusion of the brain and the remainder of the viscera is necessary for functional human survival. While acute, transient interruptions are tolerated, it is generally agreed the absence of perfusion for more than 4 minutes leads to ischemic central nervous system damage. Anesthesiologists frequently depress cardiovascular function with inhalational anesthetic agents and selected techniques; therefore, assessment of these effects (i.e., physiologic monitoring) is essential. Electrical and mechanical monitoring of cardiac activity makes this assessment possible.

MONITORING ELECTRICAL CARDIAC ACTIVITY

The electrocardiogram (ECG) is a necessary monitor of electrical cardiac activity for all anesthetized patients. The purpose of ECG monitoring is the detection of cardiac dysrhythmias and ischemia. This is easily accomplished with the standard three-limb lead configuration using Einthoven's triangle. Improved monitoring for ischemia can be obtained with application of precordial lateral leads.

In 1960, Cannard et al. used lead II to demonstrate the efficacy of the ECG in dysrhythmia diagnosis.[11] At present, limb lead II, as seen in Figure 3–2, continues to be the most popular configuration for intraoperative monitoring. Lead II derives its primary value from well-defined P waves facilitating rhythm diagnosis. This assumes further impact when one considers 60% or more of anesthetized patients experience cardiac dysrhythmias.[12] The vast majority of these disturbances, however, do not require therapy.

Regrettably, while lead II handily meets the necessity for rhythm disturbance detection, it is less sensitive as a monitor of ischemic events. Leads I and III have poorly defined P-wave morphology, making dysrhythmia diagnosis difficult. The precordial V leads, in particular lead V_5, are most suitable for monitoring coronary insufficiency.[13] If the anesthesiologist accomplishes the two primary monitoring goals, dysrhythmia detection and ischemia detection, it appears two different lead systems are necessary.

Usually, ECG systems consist of three, four, or five electrodes. The following configurations can be used intraoperatively:

1. Lead II, as previously stated, is the primary system used intraoperatively. It offers excellent P-wave morphology for rhythm detection but poor QRS and ST definition. In healthy patients without ASCVD, it is a sufficient system.
2. V_1 uses four limb electrodes and a fifth electrode at the fourth intercostal space at the sternal junction. With this configuration, little diagnostic information is gained over lead II.
3. V_5 uses four limb electrodes and a fifth electrode at the anterior axillary line in the fifth intercostal space. Its primary disadvantage is the use of five electrodes.
4. MCL_1 (modified chest lead I) is a simple variation of V_1 with the negative electrode located at the left clavicle. It is useful for both dysrhythmia and ischemia detection.[14] Its central disadvantage is the necessity of five electrodes.
5. Esophageal electrocardiac lead systems have been shown to be 100% accurate in dysrhythmia diagnosis.[15] A limited value in ischemia detection and concern about potential thermal patient injury have minimized the popularity of this system.
6. Endotracheal electrocardiography has been shown suitable for dysrhythmia detection.[16] The usefulness of this configuration for ischemia detection is unknown.
7. CB_5 is a relatively new lead configuration described by Bazaral and Norfleet that permits both rhythm observation and ischemia monitoring.[17] A standard three-electrode system is designed as

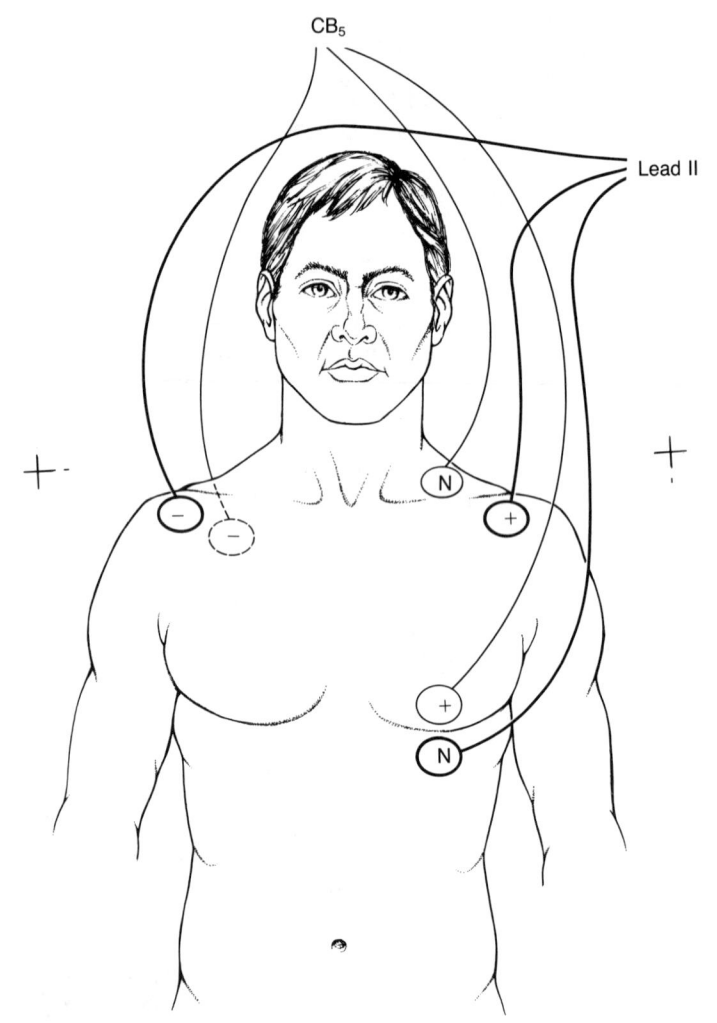

FIG. 3–2. Comparison of lead II (*thick lines*) and CB_5 (*thin lines*). One configuration is easily transformed to the other with simple electrode rearrangement. Note— the negative electrode in CB_5 is over the right scapula.

follows: a negative electrode to the right scapula, a positive electrode to the fifth intercostal space at the anterior axillary line, and the reference electrode in any convenient location. After comparing the CB$_5$ configuration with the V$_5$ configuration in patients undergoing coronary artery bypass grafting with the chest closed, ventricular deflections were 20% larger in CB$_5$ and had a correlation of r = 0.95 to 0.98. Also, the mean P-wave voltage was 90% greater in CB$_5$. Similar findings were made with the chest open.

Given these comparative findings, the CB$_5$ configuration, as seen in Figure 3–2 potentially offers the best combination of rhythm and ischemia monitoring and requires only three electrodes.

MONITORING MECHANICAL CARDIAC ACTIVITY

Arterial Blood Pressure

Mechanical cardiac activity can be assessed by arterial blood pressure observations. The frequency with which such observations should be made may be debated, but when indirect measuring techniques are used under ordinary circumstances about every 4 to 5 minutes seems appropriate.

Arterial blood pressure remains central to patient monitoring for several reasons: (1) each patient has a baseline value, thus serving as their own control; (2) measurements are readily reproduced; and (3) it represents the potential perfusion of the body. It should be understood that pressure does not imply flow in all circumstances.

Arterial blood pressure can be monitored either noninvasively (indirectly) or invasively (directly).

ORIGINS OF BLOOD PRESSURE MEASUREMENT. Historically the adoption of arterial blood pressure measurement has developed slowly and many great people have contributed to its present practice.[18,19]

During the early seventeenth century William Harvey described the essentials of human circulation.[21] Over a century later Hales in 1733 attempted direct measurement of the blood pressure.[21]

Hérrison in 1834 was the first to attempt indirect arterial pressure measurement, and he developed the first instrument known as a sphygmomanometer.[22] He observed the oscillations of a mercury column produced by pressure changes in the radial artery. Vierordt devised a similar instrument in 1855 which used a cumbersome system of balanced weights applied to the radial artery until the pulse was obliterated to palpation.[23]

The first practical system of measuring blood pressure indirectly was that of von Basch in 1880 who became known as the father of clinical sphygmometry. His instrument was used in the clinics to measure blood pressure.[24]

In 1896 a significant advance was made with the introduction of a new technique by Riva-Rocci of Italy using an armlet to occlude the arterial pressure.[25,26] The device consisted of an inflatable cuff attached to a mercury manometer and to an inflating bulb. Systolic pressure was measured at the time the pulse disappeared to palpation as the armlet was inflated. The observation of blood pressure during surgery at Pavian and other Italian hospitals by this means became rather routine. This was the first clinically useful instrument for measuring blood pressure, and the apparatus is basically the same as used today.

Meanwhile in 1894 Codman, while a medical student and assigned to provide anesthesia at the Massachusetts General Hospital, began to make individual charts of patients during anesthesia and surgery.[27] Harvey Cushing was also convinced of the importance of keeping individual records to aid in the technical administration of anesthesia as a means of foretelling critical events.[28] As medical students both men continuously recorded their observations and stressed the importance of pulse, respiration and temperature, which they recorded.[27] These charts represented the origin of the anesthesia record.* After graduation from Harvard, Cushing when to Johns Hopkins Hospital and served under William Halsted, one of the great surgeons and teachers of the time. While on a trip to Italy in 1901, Cushing learned of the work of Riva-Rocci. On his return to Hopkins, Cushing introduced Riva-Rocci's new device and brought it to the attention of G.W. Crile of Cleveland.[29] Blood pressure measurement by this indirect method and the recording of observations were popularized by these men and became routine not only in surgery but in general medical practice as well.[29,30]

Cushing now devised a new anesthesia chart that included blood pressure determinations as well as pulse and respiration recordings. This chart formed the basis for all subsequent monitoring in the operating room.[28,31] It is ironical that the Medical staff at Harvard and Massachusetts General Hospital appointed a committee to study this new technique and concluded that continual monitoring of blood pressure was not necessary since the "skilled finger" was considered more valuable than an instrument.[28,31]

In 1905, the Russian N. Korotkoff used the cuff technique for measuring blood pressure and described the nature of sounds heard over the artery at a point distal to the compression cuff using a stethoscope. This quickly became the method for observing the systolic and diastolic blood pressure, and the auscultatory indirect method is the most widely used technique today.[32,33]

---

*Beecher retrieved some early anesthesia charts from the archives of Massachusetts General Hospital: one dated November 30, 1884, is ascribed to Codman; the second, dated April 2, 1885, was signed by Cushing.

SOUNDS OF KOROTKOFF.[32,33] The sounds of Korotkoff are produced by changes in the rate of blood flow through partially constricted tubes. The sounds have four audible phases, starting with a period of silence when the blood flow through the artery is completely arrested by the compression of the manometer cuff and ending with silence represented as phase 5 as described by the American Heart Association (Fig. 3–3).[34–36]

Phase 1 As the pressure in the cuff is released just enough to permit a jet of blood to enter the constricted point, a sharp, light tap or thud sound is detected. Such taps or thuds in the normal person are heard over a range of 10 mm Hg. Initially the sounds are faint but as the pressure in the cuff is further lowered intense clear tapping sounds are generated in the blood vessel below the partially occluded point; these sounds result from the opening and closing of the blood vessels with each cardiac contraction; the walls may touch during the low pressure phase.

Phase 2 The second sound of Korotkoff is denoted by the appearance of soft but rather inconstant murmurs. The range over which these murmurs are heard is approximately 10 mm Hg.

Phase 3 When the murmuring sounds become loud, long, crisp, and clear, phase 3 is entered, and such sounds will be heard over a range of 15 to 20 mm Hg.

Phase 4 This phase begins when the crisp, clear sounds become quite muffled and dull and can be heard over a range of less than 10 mm Hg.

Phase 5 At point 5 there is no audible sound, referred to as the period of silence. In the United Kingdom the period of silence is taken as the diastolic pressure.

Interpretation. The first sound to appear on deflation is taken as the index of systolic pressure when the tapping is clear and most intense. However, the second phase may be more properly called the systolic pressure because it is at this point that blood actually travels completely under the cuff.

The fourth or final sound, just at the time before the disappearance of all audible sound, is taken as the index of the diastolic pressure in the United States. This final sound represents the most consistently reproducible and identifiable value among multiple observers.

Occasionally, instead of the first sound being followed by a murmur, there may be no sound until the third phase or the beginning of the diastolic level is reached. This is called the auscultatory gap and is sometimes misleading.[37]

INDIRECT MEASUREMENT OF BLOOD PRESSURE. Noninvasive measurement can be conducted mechanically or electromechanically.[19,38] These techniques are easily accomplished manually or automatically with today's technology. The common noninvasive techniques include the auscultatory, oscillometric, and palpatory methods of observation. Photoplethysmography is a recent sophisticated technique relying on oscillometric changes in pressure in a finger cuff.[38,39]

Auscultatory Method. This noninvasive method of arterial pressure monitoring is most common. The principle of auscultation involves use of external pressure by an inflatable cuff about the arm to interrupt the pulsatile flow of arterial blood. After complete interruption of flow, the occluding pressure is gradually released, resulting in turbulent flow that in turn produces noise. Auscultation requires detection of Korotkoff's sounds and the technique is properly referred to as the Riva-Rocci method (see above). The key to accurate measurement is adequate hearing acuity and matching the appropriate cuff width size to the circumference of the patient's arm. If the cuff width is too narrow,

Pressure	Sounds of Korotkoff
mm Hg	Silence
120	Point 1
115	Phase 1 — Little taps or thuds
110	Range 10 mm Hg — Point 2
105	Phase 2 — Soft murmurs, inconstant
100	Range 5–10 mm Hg — Point 3
95	Loud clear sounds
90	Phase 3 — Range 15–20 mm Hg
85	Point 4 — Dull and muffled
	Phase 4 — Range 5–10 mm Hg
80	Point 5 — Silence

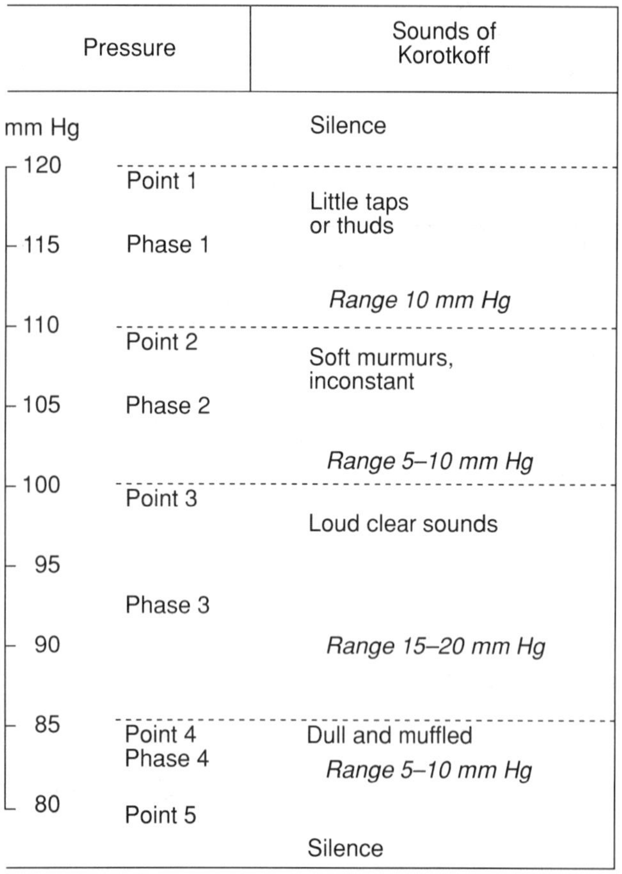

FIG. 3–3. Sounds of Korotkoff. Four sound phases are identified as one progresses from a completely constricted blood flow to a moment of unrestricted blood flow. Beyond these two end points there is silence.

measurements will be artificially high; if too wide, the readings will be falsely low. Just as important is proper application of the cuff: a loose fit leads to artificially high readings. The diaphragm of the stethoscope should be placed directly over the arterial listening site (Fig. 3–4).

After the selection and application of the proper cuff, the cuff bladder is distended to 20 mm Hg above the palpated systolic pressure. Auscultation should now reveal silence. The cuff is then decompressed at 2 to 4 mm Hg · sec^{-1} while Korotkoff sounds are auscultated.

1. On appearance of the first clear, distinct (tapping) sound the pressure in the manometer is read and recorded. This correlates with the systolic pressure.
2. On continued deflation of the cuff, sounds of phases 2 and 3 are heard. When the long, loud sounds of phase 3 become muffled and dull phase 4 has been reached and careful observation of the manometer is necessary to detect the pressure when the last sound is heard. This pressure correlates best with the diastolic pressure.
3. The silent period that follows is associated with lower pressures that are not truly representative of the diastolic pressure. There is greater observer variability in identifying the absence of sound.

Automated auscultatory measurements can be made with devices employing the Doppler principle or piezoelectric microphones. Doppler-based equipment detects arterial blood flow using an ultrasound beam, while "microphone" devices measure and convert the subaudible frequencies of arterial wall motion into audible signals.

Oscillometric Method.[40] This method of arterial blood pressure measurement involves determination of the amplitude of pulsations in the blood pressure cuff that are transmitted to a detecting device. Basically, a standard cuff is applied to the arm and connected to an oscillometer. The simplest oscillometer is an aneroid manometer, but a mercury manometer may be used. When the cuff is rapidly inflated to a pressure 20 mm Hg above the systolic pressure, the radial pulse is obliterated and only small oscillations are appreciated. The cuff is then deflated slowly; the release valve of the sphygmomanometer is opened slightly to cause a pressure drop of 2 to 3 mm Hg · sec^{-1}. The indicator needle of the aneroid manometer will pause periodically as it descends the scale of a falling cuff pressure. Such pauses are synchronous with the heart beat. The oscillations increase in amplitude with decreasing cuff pressure. This is evident by the flickering of the aneroid needle. Finally as the cuff is deflated and there is little or no pressure in the cuff, the needle movements disappear. The systolic pressure observed by this means is usually the highest of the recordings obtained by indirect methods.

A mercury manometer may be used as a detecting device. After the cuff has been inflated to obliterate the pulse, careful observation at eye level of the meniscus top of the convex mercury column is started as the cuff is deflated. The point at which the first pulsations are observed is noted. The systolic pressure is recorded at the point where the oscillations show their greatest excursion.

The obtaining of the systolic, mean, and diastolic pressure is not clearly defined from the pattern of the oscillation (Fig. 3–5). It is generally agreed, however, that the mean arterial pressure (MAP) is the lowest pressure in the cuff that will produce maximal oscillations.[41] The systolic pressure is the highest cuff pressure at which a large increase in the amplitude of oscillations first occurs,[42] while the

FIG. 3–4. Demonstration of the auscultatory method of arterial pressure monitoring. From Shepard, J.T., and Vanhoutte, P.M.: The Human Cardiovascular System. New York: Raven Press, 1979.

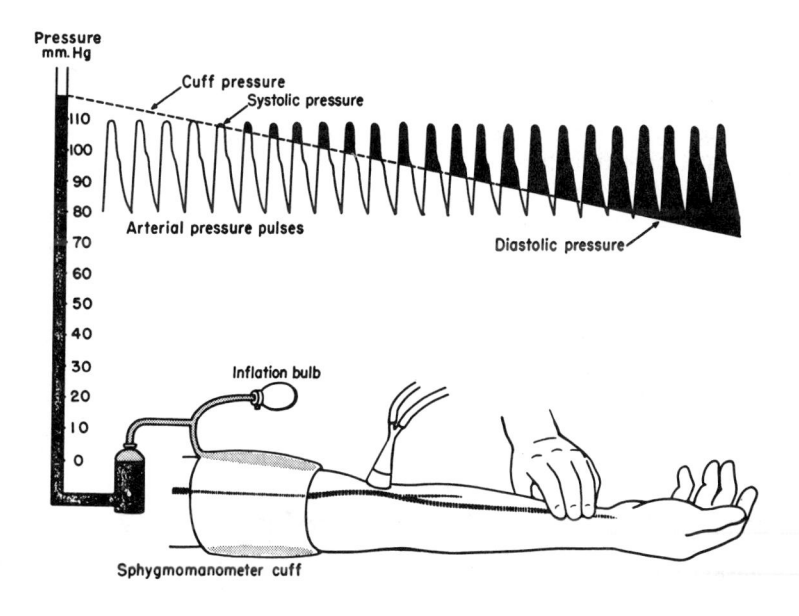

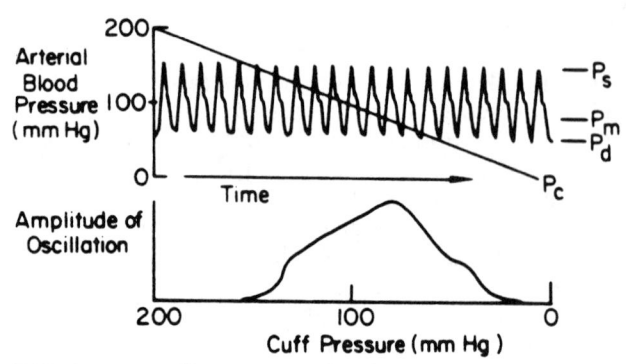

FIG. 3–5. Oscillometry amplitude during the arterial waveform. From Miller, R.: Anesthesia.

diastolic pressure is the lowest cuff pressure before the oscillations disappear.[43]

Automated Oscillometers Automated oscillometers of the Dinamap type contain two pressure indicators: one measures the main arterial blood pressure; the second quantifies the accompanying pulsation amplitude. The cuff is inflated to a standard level so the MAP and accompanying pulsation amplitude can be determined. A microprocessor continually adjusts the cuff pressure until the lowest pressure accompanying the maximal oscillation is found. This value is taken as the mean arterial blood pressure. An algorithm then estimates the systolic and diastolic pressures based on the rate of change of the measured oscillations. Some techniques utilize algorithms to cross-correlate between calculated and acoustically measured systolic and diastolic values. While the systolic and mean pressures determined by oscillometry correlate well with invasively measured values, the diastolic values tend to be markedly higher.[40] These discrepancies may relate to noninvasive measurements being flow dependent while invasive measurements are pressure dependent.

Today manual oscillometric devices are rarely used in the United States; however, the use of automated oscillometers has become widespread. The advantages of these devices include an adjustable measurement interval, freedom for the busy anesthesiologist, and the display of systolic, diastolic, and mean arterial blood pressure along with heart rate.

Palpatory Method. Palpation of the pulse is the simplest method of blood flow detection and for observation of blood pressure. Obliteration of arterial pulsation by means of an inflated arm cuff connected to an manometer is carried out and the point at which a peripheral arterial pulse is first detected by palpation of the radial artery as the cuff is deflated represents the systolic pressure level. The technique involves the application of a standard blood pressure cuff, which is inflated to 20 mm Hg above the point of disappearance of a palpated pulse. The cuff is then deflated 2 to 4 mm Hg · sec^{-1}. The point of return of a pulse observed either by palpation or by Doppler ultrasound is taken as the systolic pressure. This method is only accurate for systolic values.[43]

Photoplethysmography. This is a recently introduced technique of noninvasive blood pressure measurement. In principle the blood volume of the digits varies with systole and diastole. In photoplethysmography, also known as the Peñaz method, a small blood pressure cuff is placed around a finger. The cuff is inflated and deflated in conjunction with systole and diastole so that the transarterial pressure is zero. In this manner, the operator is provided with a continuous arterial blood pressure waveform, from which mean, systolic, and diastolic pressures are determined. In an early study comparing Peñaz monitoring to direct artery pressures, the correlation was r = 0.96.[44] Further investigation is necessary to determine the accuracy of this device in hypotensive, hypothermic, or vasoconstrictive states, and any potential injuries that may result from the use of this technique.

Comment. As stated earlier, it is essential to monitor arterial blood pressure. Any of these noninvasive methods can be used when invasive monitoring is not indicated. Complacency must not supervene in this situation—an inadequately deflated cuff leads to venous engorgement and possible intravenous infiltration or thrombosis; neurologic injury can also occur with automated devices.[45]

Standards For Sphygmomanometry

In order to reproduce reliable and accurate readings of blood pressure by the commonly used auscultatory method the American Heart Association has prepared certain recommendations.[35,36,46]

1. *The apparatus* should consist of a mercury manometer with a compression bag approximately 20% wider than the diameter of the arm (one third the circumference). Thus, the width of the arm cuff employed varies with the age and physical build of the patient.

   Standard bladder sizes and lengths are

	Width (cm)	Length (cm)
Obese adult arm	18–20	30–35
Adult's thigh	18.0	35.0
Adult's arm	12.5	35.0
Child (aged 4–10)	9.5	23.0
Child (aged 1–4)	6.0	15.0
Infant (1 year)	4.0	12.0
Newborn (<1 month)	2.5	5.0

   The bag itself should at least *half*-encircle the arm and should be over the artery. It should be covered by a cuff of inextensible material of such

a nature that an even pressure is exerted throughout the bag width on inflation.
2. *The patient* should be comfortable and relaxed; clothing should not constrict the arm.
3. *The stethoscope* should be applied over the previously prepared brachial artery. Generally, this is over the antecubital space but in the operating room should be the medial side of the upper arm. Properly, the stethoscope should not be in contact with the manometer cuff. However, for security reasons in anesthesia practice the stethoscope is placed under the mid-point of the cuff. Hence, the values are usually higher in the operating room by 1 to 2 mm Hg over those obtained in standard medical practice.
4. *Cuff inflation* should be rapid until the pulse is obliterated and no sounds are audible. Then the pressure should be allowed to fall at the following rate: namely, 2 to 3 mm Hg per heart beat or approximately 2 mm Hg $\cdot$ sec^{-1}. The systolic pressure is recorded at the time that the first clear thumping sound appears. In the event that the systolic pressure determined by the palpatory method is at a higher level than the auscultatory reading, the palpatory value should be considered to be the more accurate systolic level.
5. The *diastolic pressure* is recorded at the time that the sounds are dull and muffled, i.e., phase 4 of Korotkoff and not the period of silence.
6. *Repeat determinations* should be made only after the cuff has been completely deflated. One must avoid congestion of the arm as accuracy is decreased by venous stagnation.

Comparison of Indirect Methods.[47] Indirect methods of determining blood pressure measure lateral pressure on vessel walls, while direct methods measure the onward thrust of a fluid column against the diaphragm of the recording device. In general, the indirect readings are lower than the direct measurements. The deficit of indirect readings tends to become greater than the direct measurement as the patient's blood pressure rises.[48]

Indirect methods compared with direct arterial pressure readings are obviously less accurate and are subject to greater variability. Generally, the oscillometric method when carefully performed can be considered as the most accurate method but clinically it is time consuming and not practical.

The auscultatory method shows varying degrees of differences from direct values. Generally, the systolic pressure is an average of 3 to 4 mm Hg lower and the diastolic pressure 3 to 4 mm higher than the actual or direct value. The palpatory method is the least accurate because of several wide variables, many of which are subjective.

Clinical Limitation The indirect measuring systems presented perform with simplicity, reliability, and safety on healthy subjects. However, in shock, hypothermia, deliberated hypotension, and space monitoring they are difficult and inaccurate. Since sounds and pulse appearance are dependent on opening and closing of blood vessels and on blood flow, they are attenuated or fail to appear in presence of altered blood volume, cardiac action, or vessel integrity.

SPHYGMOMANOMETRY IN ANESTHESIA[42,46,49]

Selection of Arm. That arm which will be disturbed the least during surgery should be selected. It should be protected from pressure or manipulation by other personnel. It should neither be compressed by positioning nor should it be dependent. In the lateral position, the upper arm should be used, but it should not be elevated above chest level or else the diastolic readings will be low.

Application of Stethoscope. In general medical practice the stethoscope is placed in the antecubital fossa and free of the inflatable cuff. This is unsatisfactory in anesthesia and should be avoided, especially since flexing the arm is likely to cause displacement. Two positions are recommended (Fig. 3–6):

1. Over the brachial artery just above the bend in the elbow
2. Over the brachial artery on the medial side of the arm

In each case, the stethoscope diaphragm is secured to the arm by fastening the holding-strap *snugly*, not tightly (Fig. 3–7). The use of adhesive straps, the tying of the holding straps, and tight fastening are condemned for obvious reasons. It is especially important that venous congestion be avoided since diastolic readings will be high and inaccurate (20 mm Hg or more). Occasionally, venous stasis may result in high systolic readings.

Application of Cuff. The cuff should be applied so that the rubber inflatable bag is over the artery. Thus, it should be chiefly over the inner aspect of the arm. The lower part of the cuff should just cover the diaphragm of the stethoscope when the latter is placed in the first position. When the stethoscope is on the medial side of the mid-arm, the cuff will be applied so that the stethoscope is under the mid-point. This position provides maximum security with accurate readings. The cuff should also be placed so that the tubings lead to the anesthetist's position.

The cuff should be wound around the arm in such a manner that the upper edge of the inflatable bag is just covered by the first turn of the cloth cuff and the lower edge of rubber bag just covered by the second turn. This will prevent bulging and displacement. These windings should be firm but not tight enough to cause obstruction to venous flow. They

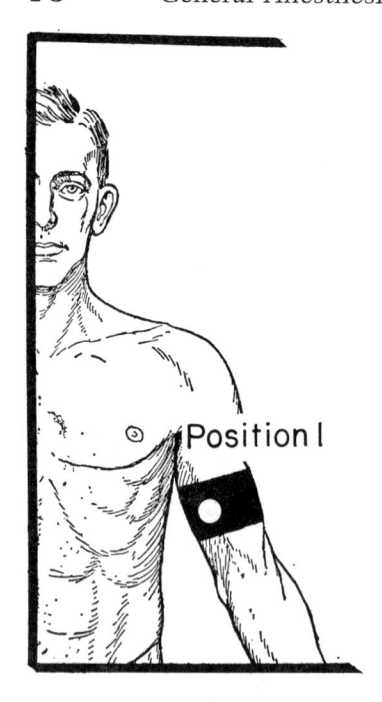

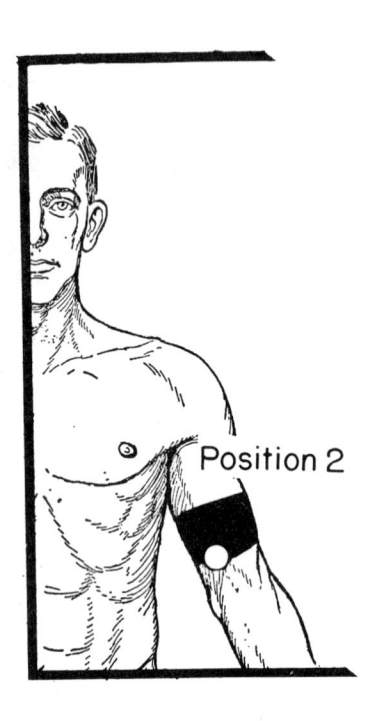

FIG. 3–6. Positions for placement of stethoscope, as commonly employed in anesthesia practice. Position 1 has been found the most favorable. From Collins, V.J., and Magora, F.: Sphygmomanometry: The indirect measurement of blood pressure. Anesth. Analg., *42*:443, 1963.

should also be smooth so that on inflation of the bag an even pressure is exerted throughout.

Inflation and Deflation of the Cuff. The cuff should be inflated rapidly to a level about 20 mm Hg above the anticipated systolic pressure or above the palpated systolic pressure. Pressure should be reduced about $2-4$ mm Hg $\cdot$ sec^{-1} while auscultating over the arterial site.

Observations. These should be made initially by both ascultation and palpation. The palpatory method gives about 4 to 6 mm Hg lower readings. The auscultatory readings are made according to the sounds of Korotkoff. The systolic pressure is read at the time when the first clear thumping sound is heard. The diastolic pressure is read when the clear-cut sounds suddenly change and become muffled, not at the moment of silence.

Pitfalls. [37] The commonest source of inaccurate readings is the size of the blood pressure cuff in relation to the size of the arm. If the width of the cuff is smaller than the recommended guides, the systolic pressure readings will be inordinately high. Thus, if a standard adult cuff of 12 to 13 cm is used in obese patients high readings will be obtained, and the same cuff in children will give quite low values. It is a general principle that there is a loss of pressure across compressible substances that results in high pressure. Thus the type of tissue is an important factor. Muscular arms of large circumference may not give false readings, but arms enlarged by fatty tissue as in the obese will be most inaccurate.[51] Generally, arms larger than 30 cm in circumference should be assessed carefully and values scrutinized.

If the cuff cannot encircle half the arm or the arm is flabby, it is recommended that pressure be observed in the lower arm.

Effect of Arm Size. The error incurred by measuring the blood pressure in large arms with a standard 13 cm cuff was demonstrated by Ragan and Bordley.[37] An arm circumference of 25 to 35 cm is considered in the normal adult range; when greater than 38 cm, inaccuracies are frequent. As the arm circumference is increased the systolic pressure increase is directly proportional (Fig. 3–8).[51]

Errors in Anesthesia Practice. Among the errors to be noted are:

1. Improper size of cuff (see above).
2. A second common error in anesthesia practice occurs when the cuff is deflated too fast. Readings will be grossly inaccurate. If the pulse pressure is small no sounds will be heard and an erroneous diagnosis of shock or cardiac arrest may be entertained. Some large vessel such as the carotid in the neck should be palpated or the surgeon requested to palpate a branch of the aorta, if he is in one of the major body cavities, to ascertain if pulses are present.
3. Leaving a cuff inflated for any length of time results in venous stasis and the diastolic pressure will be observed at levels higher than the actual value.
4. Selection of arm and position of arm. That arm which will be disturbed the least should be used. Surgeons leaning on arm will distort readings. A dependent or compressed arm causes compression of artery and the auscultatory

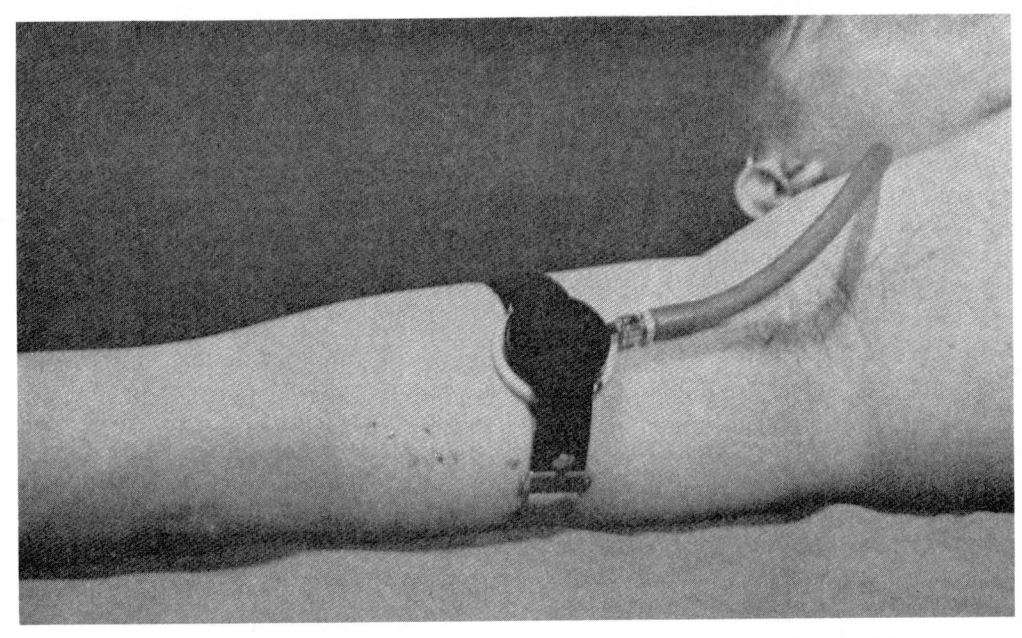

FIG. 3–7. Proper method of application of stethoscope. Tape is wrapped smoothly, and simple hook-on assembly is used. From Collins, V.J., and Magora, F.: Sphygmomanometry: The indirect measurement of blood pressure. Anesth. Analg., *42:*443, 1963.

sounds will be indistinct or inaudible. In addition, venous stasis occurs. Thus, in the lateral positions especially, the under-arm should not be used for blood pressure readings. If this is absolutely necessary—a firm but soft sheet roll should be placed under the chest just below the axilla. Occasionally, when a stethoscope is placed on the left arm with patient in lateral position, the heart sounds may be transmitted.

5. Premature ventricular beats introduce some inaccuracy. Those beats which occur after a compensatory pause are usually at a higher pressure and should be ignored.
6. Respiratory effects on blood pressure should be appreciated. A phasic variation is to be observed. During spontaneous inspiration the systemic systolic pressure is slightly elevated; during expiration the systemic systolic pressure tends to be slightly decreased.
7. Faulty apparatus. Zero levels should be checked. Aneroid barometers are easily damaged. The air vents of a mercury column tube should be free of dust or obstruction. Tubing and connections should be tight.
8. Insecure application of stethoscope or of inflatable cuff will cause slipping and elevated or variable readings.
9. Improper winding of cuff will allow bulging and displacement. This is avoided by covering edges.
10. Placement of inflatable cuff. This should be on the side of the compressible artery.

Comments on the Stethoscope. [52,53] The stethoscope has changed little since 1819, when René Laënnec "rolled a quire of paper into a kind of cylinder and applied it to my ear" to observe the heart sounds of an obese patient. Flexible tubes were used to replace the cyclinder and thence connection made directly to the ears. Thus, developed the stethoscope. The usual tubing has $\frac{3}{16}$ inch lumen. Rapaport and Sprague have found that on physical grounds and proper controlled clinical application, this is too large for heart sounds and too·small for chest sounds. They measured the sound pressures at various frequencies in the traditional stethoscope and found that for the range between 20 to 115 cycles the $\frac{3}{16}$ inch tubing is too large. This is the pitch at which the three heart sounds and the mitral murmurs occur. Even for 250 to 750 cycles where medium and high pitch murmurs occur narrow tubing is better.

On the other hand, the high-pitched rales and most pathologic breath sounds are best transmitted by larger bore tubing, *i.e.,* 0.25 inch. The lower pitched normal breath sounds are adequately transmitted by smaller tubing.

Moreover, excessively long tubes introduce energy losses in sound. For each added inch in length there is a proportionate reduction in the sound transmitted.

Precordial Stethoscope Monitoring. A precordial stethoscope with a molded earpiece enables one to continuously monitor the quality of the heart sounds and heart rhythm; it is also a means to observe respiration. The use of a precordial stethoscope during surgery must be credited to Harvey Cushing (1909),[50] who employed this technique to monitor patients during neurosurgical procedures.

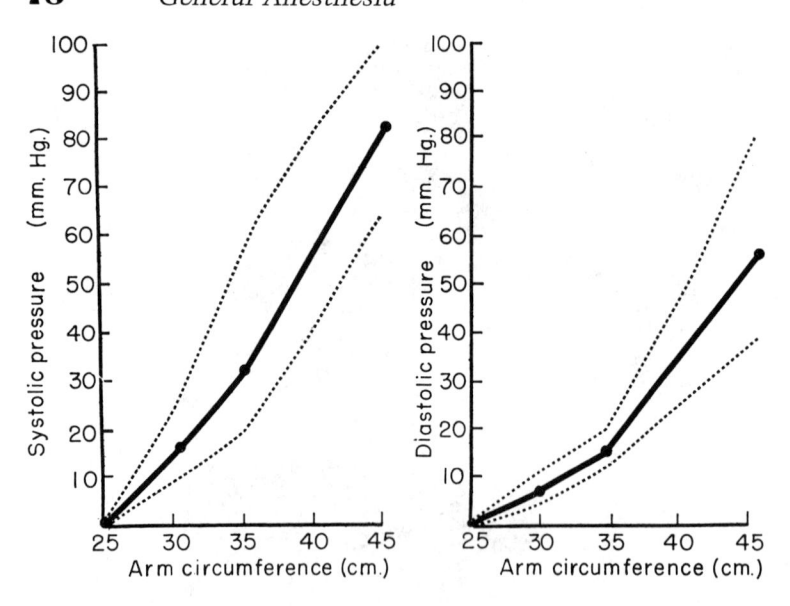

FIG. 3–8. Effect of increased arm circumference on blood pressure. The zero point represents the normal pressure and normal girth. The abscissa represents increases in cm in arm circumference over normal. Errors in systolic pressure caused by wrapping the arm with compressible cotton are illustrated in left graph and diastolic errors in right graph. From Collins, V.J., and Magora, F.: Sphygmomanometry: The indirect measurement of blood pressure. Anesth. Analg., *42*:443, 1963. Data from Trout et al.: Measurement of blood pressure in obese persons. JAMA, *162*:170, 1956.

Direct Arterial Monitoring[53]

Invasive or direct monitoring of arterial blood pressure is a technique commonly used by modern anesthesiologists.[53] The method utilizes an indwelling arterial catheter with appropriate electromechanical transducers and electronic signal processing. Because this technique involves violation of body integrity, one should be able to justify its use over noninvasive methods. In fact, it would be prudent to elaborate the rationale on the preoperative consultation sheet. Like many other areas in medical practice, selecting one technique over another means taking various factors into account. Table 3–1 lists the indications for arterial cannulation.

Invasive monitoring of arterial blood pressure also allows ready access for blood analysis in addition to beat-to-beat pressure measurement. A discerning clinician can gather other data from visual analysis of the arterial waveform (Table 3–2).

INSTRUMENTS AND EQUIPMENT. Most techniques of invasive monitoring require a transducer, fluid-mechanical coupler, and a signal processing unit. A thorough knowledge of function and calibration of these systems is essential to sound clinical practice. It is important to emphasize a few simple caveats with regard to arterial blood pressure. In general, the more distal the point of measurement, the more narrow the waveform. At the radial artery, the systolic pressure will be greater than the central aortic pressure in proportion to their distance apart. Despite this, the mean arterial blood pressure (MAP) will remain constant. Thus, after placement of an arterial cannula, a comparison cuff pressure may vary by 20 mm Hg. Brunner et al.[47] found the correlation of direct measurements to Riva-Rocci measurements to be r = 0.68 systolic and r = 0.60 diastolic.[47] Remember, flow and pressure are different entities. Because they do not measure the same physical phenomena, the results may not correlate. A second point involves extension tubing. In general, the greater the length of tubing the greater the augmentation of the pressure reading.[47]

SELECTION OF ARTERY AND ALLEN TEST. When planning to use direct arterial blood pressure monitoring, the nondominant hand is preferred as the site. On the preoperative anesthesic consultation, one should make a habit of documenting the Allen's test result.[54] Many have described the interpretation of Allen's test; however, Bedford's technique appears to be the most appropriate.[55] It is effective to have the patient make a fist, then occlude the radial and ulnar arteries with index fingers. At this point, release the ulnar artery and watch the hand. Full color should return in 5 seconds. If not, another site should be selected. Despite evidence of adequate collateral circulation, radial artery cannulation has been associated with distal vascular ischemia.

CHOICE OF CATHETER. The choice of catheter is also significant. Catheter consistency is rapidly becoming a moot point as virtually all catheters are now made of tissue-compatible materials. Catheter size, however, is within the clinician's prerogative and has important consequences. It appears the smaller the catheter relative to the artery, the lower the incidence of vessel thrombosis.[55] Duration of placement also correlates directly with subsequent thrombosis; however, this is rarely a preoperative issue. The 20-gauge catheters routinely offer the best compromise between size and subsequent thrombosis.

TECHNIQUE OF ARTERY CANNULATION. For achieving invasive arterial blood pressure monitoring, Barr's description of the catheter-over-the-needle insertion technique is the most commonly used in anesthesia practice.[56] While this description refers to the radial artery, it can be used for any palpable artery. Invasive monitoring of arterial blood pressure is most commonly performed from the radial artery.

Wrist technique. The wrist technique requires that the wrist be dorsiflexed, immobilized, and aseptically cleaned prior to catheter insertion. Periarterial infiltration with local anesthetic is recommended to prevent vasospasm and provide local analgesia. The needle and catheter are introduced percutaneously either with the "through and through" or the superficial puncture method. Thus the artery is perforated, the catheter is inserted, and the needle is withdrawn. Neither differs with regard to postcannulation thrombosis.[57] In addition, a guide wire may or may not be used for ease of insertion of the catheter into the artery.

COMPLICATIONS. Other potential complications of arterial cannulation include hemorrhage, infection, nerve injury, and ischemic necrosis of the skin. Hemorrhage can occur by simple disconnection of the pressure transducing system from the cannula. The literature on infection is skewed by the studies, most of which were performed on intensive care unit (ICU) patients who had indwelling monitors for several days. One study of ICU patients found no infection after 1 day's duration. Current practice is to place iodophor ointment on all intravascular cannulation sites.[59] Stopcocks however, represent the main system route of bacterial access and should be used sparingly.[60] Be aware that the cutdown approach to radial artery cannulation has been associated with a 30% incidence of infection.[61a]

Median nerve injury following radial artery cannulation has been reported.[61b] This injury may result from prolonged hyperextension of the wrist. A good practice may be to return the wrist to a more neutral position after cannulation has been established. Finally, the most common complication associated with radial artery cannulation is ischemic necrosis of the skin. This usually happens immediately superficial to the cannula with frequency of 0.5 to 3%.[62] The resulting lesion heals by itself, usually over many weeks.

The most prudent course of action to follow when using direct measurement of arterial blood pressure involves sound indication, good technique, use of the smallest acceptable catheter, minimal duration, and constant, vigilant sterile precautions.

Venous Pressure Monitoring

Central venous pressure (CVP) is the blood pressure measured at the junction of the right atrium and the vena cavae. From a utilitarian point of view, the terms central venous pressure and right atrial pressure (RAP) are interchangeable; however, there obviously is a small pressure gradient present.

With the advent of pulmonary artery catheters, many clinicians now believe if the decision to measure central circulatory pressures is made, full pulmonary artery catheterization should be performed. This represents, however, a serious error in understanding of the value of CVP measurement.

In an individual with normal function of all cardiac chambers and valves, the CVP represents the balance between venous capacitance, intravascular volume, and cardiac function. If one considers the right side of the heart as an independent entity, the relation between CVP and cardiac output is represented by the Frank-Starling curve. Stated another way, cardiac output depends on venous return. While generally ignored, the concept of venous return (VR) represents a crucial premise of cardiac physiology.

$$VR = \frac{Pms - RAP (CVP)}{RVR}$$

Pms is the mean systemic filling pressure, i.e., the pressure at which venous return ceases. Pms is a static measurement representing the balance between blood volume and total vascular capacity. RVR is the resistance to venous return—*not* systemic vascular resistance. This represents a balance between the resistance and capacitance of the circulation.[63,64] In light of these relationships, it is intuitive that a given volume bolus will not lead to a desired change (e.g., increased cardiac or urine output) in all situations.

TABLE 3–1. INDICATIONS FOR INVASIVE ARTERIAL PRESSURE MONITORING DURING SURGERY

Operative indications
  Cardiac surgery
  Thoracic surgery (1-lung ventilation)
  Intracranial neurosurgery
  Major vascular surgery (carotid, aorta)
  Extensive surgical procedures (burns)
  Trauma surgery
  Mechanical interference with indirect measurement sites
Patient indications
  Cardiovascular disease (NYHA III or IV)
  Pulmonary disease (COPD or other V/Q mismatch)
  Insulin-dependent diabetes mellitus (major surgery)
  Uncontrolled preoperative hypertension/hypotension
  Pregnancy-induced hypertension

TABLE 3–2. DATA FROM VISUAL ANALYSIS OF THE ARTERIAL WAVEFORM

Myocardial function:
  Steeper upstroke corresponds to a stronger left ventricle
Stroke volume:
  Area under systolic ejection phase
Peripheral Vascular Resistance:
  Location of dicrotic notch; slope of downstroke

A primary goal of invasive central monitoring is assessment of left ventricular function. Patients with cardiac disease frequently confront the anesthesiologist, and a decision whether to employ CVP or pulmonary artery monitoring must be made. While many variables influence the decision, the study of Mangano is worth noting for its value as a guide.[65] The study involved the relationship between CVP and pulmonary artery occlusion pressure (PAOP) in patients undergoing myocardial revascularization. Mangano found CVP and PAOP had a correlation of r = 0.89 in patients with an ejection fraction (EF) greater than 50% and no ventricular dyssynergy. In patients with an EF less than 40% or ventricular dyssynergy the correlation between CVP and PAOP was r = 0.24. To summarize, with good left ventricular function (e.g., EF > 50% and no wall motion abnormalities) the PAOP was of no greater value than the CVP. For patients with poor ventricular function, (e.g., EF < 40% *or* wall motion abnormalities) adequate assessment of cardiac filling required a pulmonary artery catheter.

The CVP tracing, containing a, c, v, x and y waves, reveals information about cardiac function as illustrated in Figure 3–9. The increase in RA pressure during atrial contraction is represented by the a wave. The c wave is caused by elevation of the tricuspid valve during early systole. The x descent corresponds to systolic ejection of ventricular blood. The v wave is the intraatrial increase in pressure secondary to continued venous return against a closed tricuspid valve. The fall in atrial pressure following blood flow from the atrium to the ventricle is shown by the y descent. Changes in waveform morphology can be analyzed and the pathologic condition evaluated.

Numerous indications for CVP line placement exist. Table 3–3 list the commonly accepted indications pertinent to anesthesia.

The basilic, external jugular, internal jugular, subclavian, and femoral veins may be used for CVP monitoring. Our discussion will be limited to the basilic, external jugular, and internal jugular techniques, as these are selected most frequently by anesthesiologists.

The basilic vein offers the greatest safety with regard to complications. This vein principally has a 2 to 10% rate of thrombophlebitis, coupled with the least successful rate of placement, 60 to 75%.[66-69] Prepared kits, including an introduction catheter over the needle and CVP line, are available from many manufacturers. The introducer may be placed in either the basilic vein proper or in the median cubital vein. Potential difficulties from catheter passage result from venous valves. A gentle external message coupled with a low-volume fluid infusion will usually overcome this problem. This location is relatively unsuitable for placement of pulmonary artery catheters.

The external jugular vein is easily visualized in most patients because it crosses obliquely over the sternocleidomastoid muscle. Because of its superficial location, complications with this approach are minimal. Success rates in the literature vary from a low of 50% to a high of 95%.[70,71] The success rate directly correlates with utilization of a J-wire to facilitate reduction of external jugular–subclavian vein valve junction obstruction.

For insertion, the patient is placed in Trendelenberg position with the head turned contralateral to the site of cannulation. Digital pressure at the vein–clavicle junction facilitates distension. An 18- or 20-gauge catheter over the needle is utilized for venipuncture. Upon location, the needle is withdrawn, the J-wire is inserted, and, following successful passage, the CVP catheter is threaded into place. This is referenced as the Blitt technique.[72]* This site is also suitable for pulmonary artery catheterization; however, difficulty will be encountered where the external jugular vein meets the subclavian vein.

The internal jugular vein probably represents the most common site for central venous catheteriza-

---

* For a complete description of techniques, the reader is referred to "Catheterization Techniques for Invasive Cardiovascular Monitoring" by C.D. Blitt.[73]

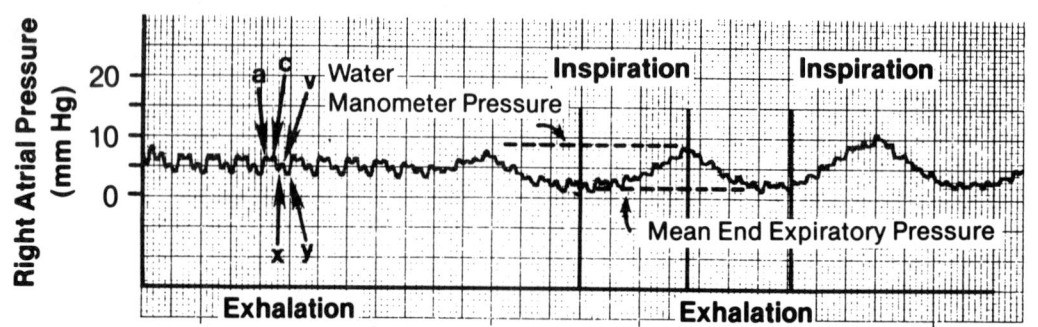

FIG. 3–9. Typical CVP wave tracing. See text for details. From Charles W. Otto: Central Venous Pressure Monitoring. p. 175 *In* Blitts, C.D.: Monitoring in Anesthesia and Critical Care Medicine. 2nd ed. New York, Churchill Livingstone, 1990.

tion by the anesthesiologist. The combination of a success rate between 90 and 98% and minimal complications have no doubt fostered this popularity.[70] While a variety of unusual complications have been infrequently reported, the most frequent complication is carotid artery puncture occuring with approximately 2% of cannulations with minimal sequelae.[71]

As with external jugular vein cannulation, the patient is placed in the Trendelenberg position, head contralateral to the site of insertion. The path of the internal jugular vein is easily imagined by drawing a straight line from the mastoid process to the medial side of the clavicular head of the sternocleidomastoid muscle. Any point along this line can be used for puncture; however, the apex of the muscular triangle represents an easily denoted point and does not necessitate muscle puncture. A 22-gauge "seeker" needle is utilized with insertion 45° to the skin, aiming at the ipsilateral hip. Following location, an 18-gauge catheter over the needle is inserted along the same path. Again, following location, the needle is removed, with the catheter in place. Next, a flexible J wire is inserted, and the catheter is withdrawn. A No. 11 scalpel blade is used to widen the puncture site. Finally, the CVP catheter itself is passed and secured into place. This site also represents a convenient location for later flotation of the pulmonary artery catheter.

Pulmonary Artery Pressure

The pulmonary artery catheter represents one of the most important developments in the history of monitoring. As recently as 1970, routine clinical measurement of intracardiac pressures, cardiac output, and gradient determinations represented significant tasks. Today, however, hemodynamic monitoring is a routine bedside procedure in the intensive care unit and the operating room. Anesthesiologists adopted pulmonary artery monitoring and their adaptation of it is supported by its co-developer, Swan, who stated, "Hemodynamic monitoring has found its greatest application in the operating room."[74]

A variety of modified pulmonary artery catheters exists. Each of these catheters is 7.5 French (French units indicate outside diameter; 1 French unit = 0.33 mm), 110 cm in length, with 10 cm band markings. Additional specifications depend on the individual manufacturer.

Indications for operative utilization are in a state of evolution but a study by Rao et al. merits individual commentary.[75] By using pulmonary artery catheterization to access myocardial function, these investigators demonstrated a reduction in perioperative reinfarction from 36 to 5.8% when surgery occurred within 3 months of previous infarction. Clearly, individuals within 3 months of myocardial infarction benefit from operative pulmonary artery catheterization, but when else is this monitor in-

TABLE 3–3. INDICATIONS FOR UTILIZATION OF CENTRAL VENOUS PRESSURE MONITORING

Operations necessitating major fluid and blood shifts
Operations with potential for air embolism
Autologous transfusion procedure
Trauma patients
Insertion of pulmonary artery catheter
Pregnancy-induced hypertension (mild)

dicated? Table 3–4 lists suggested indications; however, individual anesthesiologists will vary these criteria.

Insertion of the catheter begins with central venous catheterization from a variety of sites. When one evaluates the physical relationship of the anesthesiologist to the patient and anatomic considerations, the right internal jugular vein is the most logical insertion point. The pulmonary artery catheter introducer is placed in the right internal jugular vein as described in the section on CVP monitoring. Having reached this point, the pulmonary artery catheter can be "floated" into position. This catheter has an inflatable balloon attached around the tip and is inserted with the balloon deflated until the right atrial wave pattern is seen in Figure 3–10.

At this point, the balloon is inflated and the catheter is advanced through the right atrium, tricuspid valve, right ventricle, pulmonic valve, and into the pulmonary artery to the wedge position. The wedge position is confirmed by (1) characteristic waveform; (2) PAOP less than PAP; and (3) the ability to withdraw arterialized blood. After wedge positioning, deflate the balloon and verify a PA tracing, as seen in Figure 3–11.

Next, reinflate the balloon and confirm a wedge tracing. If any doubt exists, deflate the balloon and withdraw the catheter. Once the catheter is safely positioned, secure its location. Table 3–5 gives approximations of chamber distances for other loca-

TABLE 3–4. INDICATIONS FOR UTILIZATION OF PULMONARY ARTERY PRESSURE MONITORING

Noncardiac surgery
  Cardiac disease (NYHA III or IV)
  Pulmonary disease (impaired oxygenation)
  Circulatory instability, including:
    Sepsis
    Hemorrhage
    Trauma
    Need for inotropic, or mechanical support
  Pulmonary hypertension
  IHSS
  Pregnancy-induced hypertension (severe)
Cardiac surgery
  Coronary artery bypass graft, specifically if:
    LV dysfunction: EF < 0.4, PAOP > 18 mm Hg
    Recent (< 6 mo) myocardial infarction
  Mitral or aortic valve replacement

Abbreviations: LV = left ventricular; EF = ejection fraction; PAOP = pulmonary artery occlusion pressure.

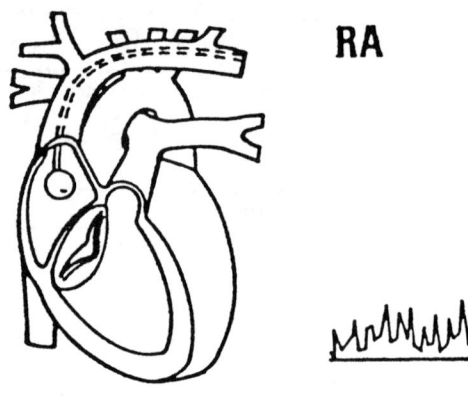

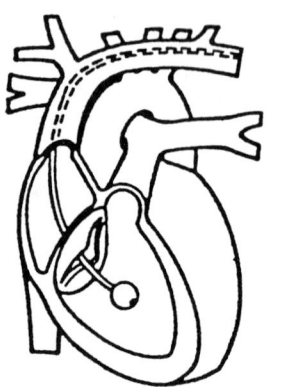

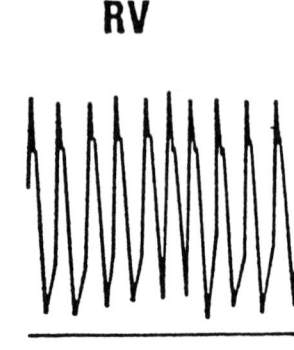

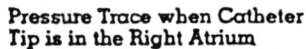

FIG. 3–10. Typical tracings with regard to catheter location during flotation. See text for details. From "Understanding hemodynamics measurements made with the Swan-Ganz catheter." American Edwards Laboratories, 1981.

tions that may prove necessary for introduction. If the catheter has not passed into the pulmonary artery within 15 cm from the right ventricle, consideration should be given to withdrawing and reinserting, because the catheter may be coiling in the ventricle.

Information derived from the pulmonary artery catheter can be divided into two categories: directly measured data (Table 3–6) and derived (calculated) data (Table 3–7). Normal ranges and formulas are also included in these tables.

It cannot be emphasized enough that an incomplete understanding of the physiologic principles involved in data interpretation constitutes one of the most significant deficiencies of PA catheter utilization. The pulmonary artery catheter allows estimation of left-sided vascular pressures from catheterization of the right side of the heart. At end diastole, the aortic and pulmonary valves are closed and the mitral valve is open. Thus, in the absence of valvular pathology, a common fluid chamber is created from the pulmonary artery to the aortic valve, as illustrated in Figure 3–12. At equilibration, during end ventricular diastole, the pressure relationships are PAEDP ≈ PVP ≈ LAP ≈ LVEDP and PAEDP ≈ PAOP ≈ PVP ≈ LAP ≈ LVEDP. Several pathologic conditions can lead to a discrepancy between PAEDP and PAOP. Nadeau and Noble have recently reviewed misinterpretation of PA catheter data; from their presentation, the pitfalls can be easily categorized, as in Table 3–8.[76]

Abbreviations:

PAEDP—Pulmonary artery end-diastolic pressure
PAP—Pulmonary artery pressure

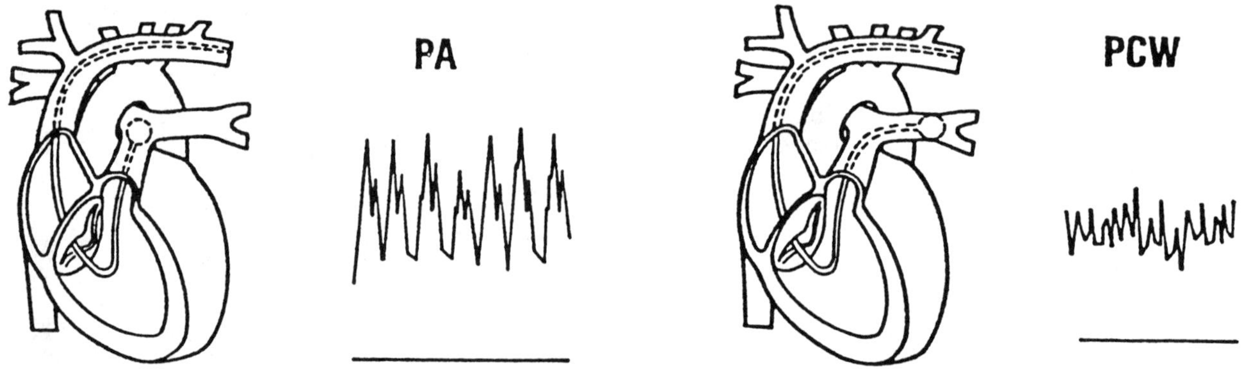

FIG. 3–11. Typical tracings with regard to catheter location during placement. See text for details. From "Understanding hemodynamic measurements made with the Swan-Ganz catheter." American Edwards Laboratories, 1981.

TABLE 3–5. APPROXIMATE DISTANCE (cm) OF CHAMBER LOCATION FROM VARIOUS INSERTION SITES

Insertion Site	Chamber Location		
	RA	RV	PA
IJV, right	20	30	45
IJV, left	25	35	50
ACV, right	50	65	80
ACV, left	55	70	85
FV	40	50	65
SC	10	25	40

Abbreviations: RA = right atrium; RV = right ventricle; PA = pulmonary artery; IJV = internal jugular vein; FV = femoral vein; SC = subclavian vein.

PVP—Pulmonary venous pressure
LAP—Left atrial pressure
LVP—Left ventricular pressure
LVEDP—Left ventricular end-diastolic pressure
PAOP = PCWP—Pulmonary artery occlusion pressure or pulmonary capillary wedge pressure

If one thinks of Figure 3–12 as a conduit, this schema merely represents malfunction of either orifices or channels of flow. One should pay particular attention to the measurement period with regard to the respiratory cycle. Anesthesia machines use intermittent positive pressure ventilators, which can change functional lung zone 3 to zone 2 or 1 during inspiration; therefore, all measurements should be made at end-expiration. The same relationships are true for spontaneous ventilation. Synchronization of measurement to the same point in the ventilatory cycle significantly improves reproducibility.[77] Positive-end expiratory pressure (PEEP) may also affect measured values, and recently Guyton and colleagues have proposed a correction formula.[78] Guyton et al. determined the change in intrapericardial pressure (in mm Hg) may be estimated by multiplying the change in PEEP (in cm H_2O) by 0.4 and subtracting the obtained value from the monitored PAOP to determine the actual change. For example, if 10 cm H_2O PEEP is added to a patient's ventilator circuit, enough fluid should be infused to maintain the PAOP at the pre-PEEP value (example, 10 mm Hg) plus 4 (i.e., 10 × 0.4) or 14 mm Hg. The primary effect of PEEP is to shift the intraventricular septum into the left ventricle, thus decreasing stroke volume. Decreased venous return is a secondary effect. Generally, up to 10 cm H_2O PEEP is tolerated with minimal hemodynamic changes.[79]

The interpretation of pulmonary artery catheter data is based on the values of the CVP, PAOP, and CO. For example, low cardiac output can be related to right ventricular or left ventricular failure. In either case the CO is low; however, in right ventricular failure, the CVP is elevated while the PAOP is normal or low. With left ventricular failure, the PAOP is high and the CVP is normal to elevated. Essentially, one evaluates not only each ventricle independently, but also their relationship to each other and the cardiac contractility. By approaching data analysis in this fashion, the anesthesiologist will develop a consistent and practical methodology.

Complications related to PA catheterizations can be grouped into four categories: (1) venous cannulation; (2) catheter flotation; (3) postcatheter insertion; and (4) value misinterpretation. Complications associated with venous cannulation are described elsewhere.

The most frequent complication occurring during catheter flotation is dysrhythmias. In their original series, Swan et al. reported a 13% incidence of premature ventricular beats.[80] Various studies have reported a frequency range of 12 to 48%. In one series, 5% of patients developed a new, sustained right bundle branch block (RBBB).[81] Therefore, in patients with a pre-existing left bundle branch block, a PA catheter with pacing capabilities should be consid-

TABLE 3–6. DIRECT PARAMETERS VIA PULMONARY ARTERY CATHETER

Variable	Abbreviation	Pressure (Mean)	mm Hg Range
Central venous pressure	CVP	5	1–10
Right ventricle			
Systolic	RVs	24	15–28
Diastolic-end	RVEDP	4	0–8
Pulmonary artery			
Systolic	PAsP	24	15–28
Diastolic	PAdP	10	5–16
Mean	PAP	16	10–22
Occlusion/wedge	PAOP or PCWP	9	6–15
Cardiac output (L/min)	CO	—	4–8
Mixed venous oxygen saturation (%)	Sv_{O_2}	75	72–77
Core temperature (° C)	T	37	—

TABLE 3-7. DERIVED PARAMETERS VIA PULMONARY ARTERY CATHETER

Variable	Formula	Units	Range Value
Cardiac index	$\dfrac{CO}{BSA}$	L/min/m²	≥ 2.2
Stroke volume	$\dfrac{CO}{hr} \times 1000$	ml/beat	60–90
Stroke index	$\dfrac{SV}{BSA}$	ml/beat/m²	40–60
Left ventricular stroke work index	$\dfrac{1.36(MAP - PAP)}{100} \times SI$	gm·m/m²	45–60
Right ventricular stroke work index	$\dfrac{1.36(PAOP - CVP)}{100} \times SI$	gm·m/m²	5–10
Total peripheral resistance	$\dfrac{MAP - CVP}{CO} \times 80$	dynes·s·cm⁻⁵	900–1500
Pulmonary vascular resistance	$\dfrac{PAP - PAOP}{CO} \times 80$	dynes·s·cm⁻⁵	50–150

BSA = body surface area; CO = cardiac output; SV = stroke volume; MAP = mean arterial pressure; PAP = pulmonary artery pressure; SI = stroke index; PAOP = pulmonary artery occlusion pressure; CVP = central venous pressure.

ered. The other major problem during flotation is intracardiac knotting of the catheter. It is hypothesized that most knots occur with coiling in the right atrium or right ventricle. Occasionally, operative removal is necessary.

Complications during postcatheter insertion have been reported 19 different times as of this writing. Unquestionably, the most catastrophic event that can occur is rupture of the pulmonary artery. Quickly one realizes the ensuing result. The principal risk factor for this complication is preexisting pulmonary artery hypertension.[82] Additional complications secondary to in-site catheters include pulmonary infarction, thrombosis, and infection.

Finally, value misinterpretation may represent the greatest danger of all. All too often attention is focused on the procedure (e.g., "floating the Swan") rather than data utilization. It is incumbent upon the anesthesiologist to be thoroughly familiar with normal cardiac physiology and the influence of vasoactive agents prior to catheter utilization. If not, catastrophe will result.

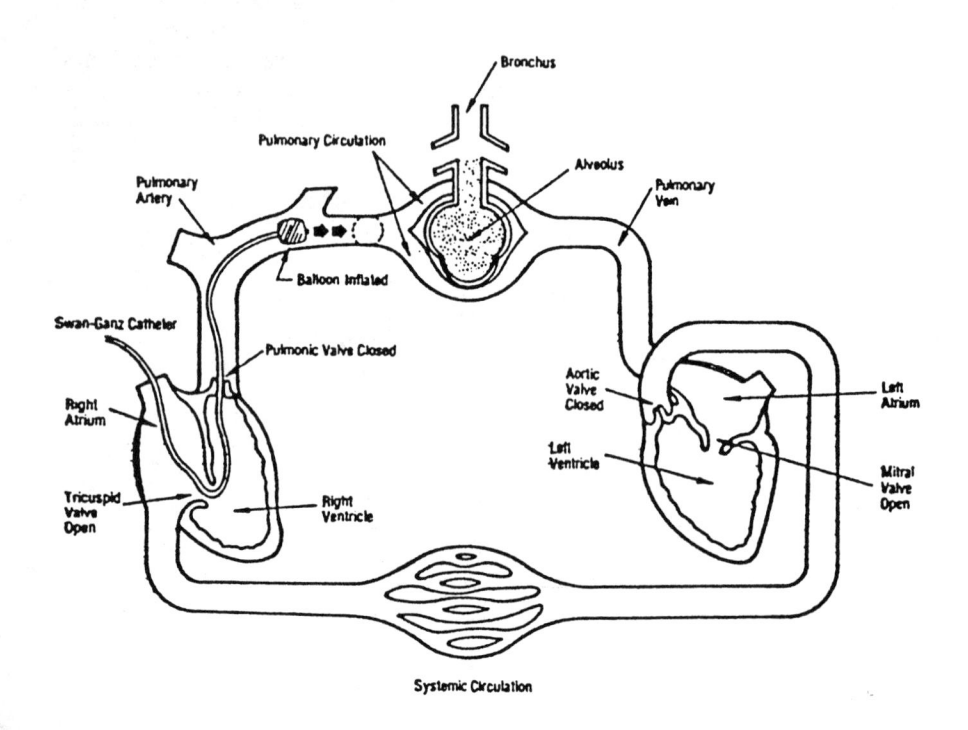

FIG. 3-12. The circulatory conduit for measurement of pulmonary artery pressures. From "Understanding hemodynamic measurements made with the Swan-Ganz catheter." American Edwards Laboratories, 1981.

Cardiac Output

As mentioned in the previous section, cardiac output (CO) is routinely measured directly via the pulmonary artery catheter. Cardiac output is defined as the volume of blood ejected by the heart per unit time. The term cardiac index (CI) is also used; CI is the CO divided by body surface area (BSA). Intraoperatively, CO and its derived hemodynamic indices are useful in selecting appropriate vasoinotropic therapy.

Many techniques, derived from the conservation of mass around the pulmonary capillary, are available to measure CO.[83] The Fick method described in 1870 is based on the principle that total uptake or release of any substance by an organ is the product of the blood flow to the organ and the arterial–venous difference of the substance. Using oxygen consumption as an example, the equation would be: O_2 consumption = CO × (arterial–venous O_2 content). Using simple algebra, the equation can be rearranged to solve for CO. In general, the Fick method is the standard by which other techniques are compared. Indicator dilution techniques involve the introduction of dye or saline at a specified proximal location in the cardiovascular system and measuring the effected change distal to the point of injection. If a dye is used, either an arterial sample is withdrawn for concentration analysis, or a densiometer employing the principles of oximetry (see below) is attached to the skin. The saline conductivity method is based on sensing the change in electrical conductivity of flowing blood. This technique is seldom used intraoperatively.

At the present time, the thermodilution method is the most common in intraoperative use and as such we shall explore it in greater detail. As stated, the thermodilution method involves the introduction of saline into the right atrium via the proximal injection port of the flow-directed thermodilution pulmonary artery (Swan-Ganz) catheter. The resultant temperatue change is measured downstream by a thermistor located near the end of the PA catheter. The change in blood temperature leads to a change in thermistor resistance, which with the volume of injectate allows computation of the CO using the equation:

$$CO = V_i (T_B - T_i) K_1 K_2 / \Delta T_B(t) \, dt$$

where: V_i = the injectate volume; T_B = the blood temperature; T_i = the injectate temperature; K_1 = a density constant for specific heat and gravity; K_2 = a computation constant for catheter dead space; and $\Delta T_B(t)dt$ = the change in blood temperature as a function of time.

Thermodilution CO has shown good correlation with the Fick method.[84] Recently, Nadeau and Noble have reviewed the limitations of CO as determined by thermodilution.[85] Technical sources of error included variation in injectate temperature, variation in injectate volume, timing and duration of injection, and electrocautery interference. Patient-related sources of error included shunts, pulmonic insufficiency, tricuspid insufficiency, and extremely low CO. Additionally, the shape of the thermodilution output curve can be utilized in the assessment of cardiac function. Any variation from the normal rapid peak followed by exponential decay may indicate unsuspected technical error (see above) or abnormal (re)circulation.

TABLE 3–8. MISINTERPRETATION OF PULMONARY ARTERY CATHETER DATA

Physiologic
  Tachycardia > 115/min
  Increased peripheral vascular resistance
  Dyskinetic left ventricle
  Hypokinetic left ventricle
  Right bundle branch block
Anatomic
  Aortic regurgitation
  Mitral stenosis
  Mitral regurgitation

The electromagnetic flow probe represents another invasive technique for determination of CO. This method incorporates blood velocity measurements with Faraday's law, so that a conductor moving through a magnetic field produces voltage proportional to its velocity. In these instances, the conductor is plasma, and the voltage produced depends on blood flow through the field. Surgeons often employ such probes after vessel reconstruction. A recent study has shown electromagnetic flow methods to have a wider range of accuracy than thermodilution catheters in a pulsatile flow simulator.[86]

Thus far, all techniques presented for the determination of CO involve the violation of body integrity, i.e., invasive monitoring. At the present time, multiple techniques are becoming available for the clinician to monitor CO noninvasively. Impedance cardiography determines CO by measuring changes in electrical conductivity due to blood flow in the chest. The technique involves two sets of electrodes located over the thorax. One pair of electrodes generates a constant current while the second measures change in impedance via voltage signals. The measured variation with electrical impedance reflects the change in thoracic blood volume during systole. In one study CO as determined by impedance cardiography had a correlation of r = 0.97 with the thermodilution method after coronary artery bypass.[87]

Doppler ultrasound techniques combine the Doppler frequency-shift effect and two-dimensional image of vessel cross-sectional area. Recalling the Doppler principle, the effect of velocity on frequency is directly proportional to the relative velocity between the observer and the observed. Stated another way, an object moving toward or away from a stationary point will reflect the signal at different frequencies. This method correlates well (r = 0.94) with thermodilution techniques; however, technical difficulties may exclude up to 15% of patients from this method.[88] Recently, a transesophageal Doppler device has been developed that may overcome the aforementioned technical difficulties.[89]

Echocardiography employs high-frequency sound waves that are transmitted and received by piezoelectric crystals. The reflected sound waves produce an electrical signal that is converted into a picture of valvular–chamber activity. In addition to providing CO data, ventricular dimensions, velocity of fiber shortening, septal wall motion, and ejection fraction can be determined. Recently, these techniques have been produced in a transesophageal system for intraoperative use.[90,91] A good correlation (r = 0.72) was found between transesophageal echocardiography (TEE) and dye dilution CO determinations. Perhaps of greater importance is the demonstration of TEE-detected segmental wall motion abnormalities. These abnormalities are more sensitive than changes in pulmonary or systemic hemodynamics and electrocardiography in the detection of new myocardial ischemia.[92,93] Additionally, TEE may be more sensitive than precordial Doppler monitoring for the detection of venous air embolism.[94]

Currently numerous CO techniques, including intravascular heating-thermistor recording, thermodilution ejection fraction, and magnetic susceptibility plethysmography, are being investigated.[83] Their clinical validity and acceptance remains to be demonstrated.

MONITORING THE RESPIRATORY SYSTEM

Respiratory monitoring has advanced far beyond the simple presence or absence of breath sounds, yet these easily detected sounds have remained in the anesthesiologist's armamentarium.

Perhaps the most spectacular change concerns anesthetic and respiratory gas monitoring. Not only has patient safety been improved, but the delivery of anesthesia has been further quantified. Any change that improves patient safety and educates the practitioner simultaneously serves us all.

THE STETHOSCOPE

The continuous introduction of new technology creates a constantly changing environment for the anesthesiologist. In spite of these advances, the stethoscope, simple and economical as it is, remains a central part of the monitoring process.

Use of a stethoscope allows the busy anesthesiologist to continually monitor cardiac and respiratory sounds and possibly to discern changes in advance of any electromechanical monitor. Depending on the patient's position, the precordial stethoscope can be placed over the anterior or posterior thorax. In fact, general anesthesia should not be induced until a precordial stethoscope is positioned.

Methodically, changing to an esophageal stethoscope after induction is recommended because the device offers better acoustics. Esophageal stethoscopes come in sizes for neonatal, pediatric, and adult patients. Complications of their use are minimal and include soft tissue hemorrhage, especially if introduced in a vigorous manner from the nasal route, and tracheal placement. Presently, esophageal stethoscopes are being evaluated as potential multichanneled probes for monitoring. Monitoring modalities from this site include electrocardiography, echocardiography, temperature, and esophageal motility.[15,90,95,96] In the next few years, a multifunctional esophageal probe may become a minimally invasive device that provides maximal information.

Blitt succinctly defined the necessity and import of stethoscope monitoring: "A failure to employ a precordial or esophageal stethoscope, except in extremely unusual circumstances, constitutes a serious breach of good medical care."[97] The newly adopted American Society of Anesthesiologists' Standards agree.

ANESTHETIC AND RESPIRATORY GAS MONITORING

Within the past few years, technologic advancements have dramatically improved the ability to monitor anesthetic and respiratory gases in the operating room. Until recently, the measurement of inspired oxygen concentration was the only readily available gas monitoring technique. Today we can measure inspired and expired concentrations of oxygen, nitrous oxide, carbon dioxide, nitrogen, and volatile agents. Anesthetic and respiratory gas monitoring are currently vigilant monitors. Possibly, the ultimate vigilant monitor as the final common pathway for the majority of anesthetic catastrophes is hypoxemia with resultant cellular hypoxia.[3] By choosing a different monitoring schema, the individual anesthesiologist can use anesthetic and respiratory gas analysis as physiologic or depth monitors. For example, a physiologic value such as oxygen consumption or a depth measure like the ventilatory response to carbon dioxide can easily be obtained.

Free-standing oxygen analyzers are generally located in the proximal inspiratory limb of the breathing circuit. Most commonly, Clark polarographic electrodes are used. The operation of this device is described in the section on oximetry. An alternative is the Pauling paramagnetic analyzer. This technique utilizes oxygen's paramagnetic property by attracting O_2 to a nonuniform magnetic field. The original device used a dumbbell with two gas spheres of nitrogen suspended by a filament. Any change in O_2 concentration leads to a deflection of the dumbbell, which is measured by the light reflected from a mirror attached to the dumbbell. A third method of O_2 analysis is the galvanic fuel cell. This unit contains a gold mesh cathode that consumes O_2 in direct proportion to the inspired O_2. Electrons are consumed in the reaction: $O_2 + 4e^- + 2H_2O \rightarrow 4OH^-$. In the lead–potassium hydroxide anode, electrons are produced in the reaction: $Pb + 2(OH)^- \rightarrow PbO + H_2O + 2e^-$. A voltmeter displays O_2 proportional to the current produced.

The availability of mass spectrometry and infrared analysis has enhanced our monitoring capability. Infrared analysis uses molecular absorption of infrared radiation to differentiate gases. Each molecular combination absorbs at characteristic wavelengths; therefore, by selecting wavelengths sensitive to the monitored gases, one obtains the desired data. In practice, infrared radiation is emitted and the desired wavelength obtained by passing the radiation through a filter. From the filter, the radiation passes through the analyzing chamber. Distal to the chamber, a semiconductor detector measures the amount of transmitted radiation at each wavelength. This information is then converted to a digital readout of gas concentrations. Please note that infrared can measure all volatile agents, nitrous oxide, and carbon dioxide. Gases with similar molecular weight, such as CO_2 and N_2O, can be differentiated by careful wavelength selection.

The magnetic sector mass spectrometer has an ionizing chamber where gas samples are bombarded by electrons passing from the cathode to the anode. Some molecules of the sample become positively charged ions removed from the chamber by accelerating and focusing plates. The stream of accelerated ions next passes through a magnetic field that leads to deflection in the ions' path. The arc of the deflection is inversely proportional to the weight of the ion, i.e., the lighter the gas, the greater the deflection. The deflected, accelerated ions proceed to strike a detector plate that uses a microprocessor to convert the number of arriving ions into gas concentrations. Variation of the focusing plate voltage allows different gases to be analyzed.

Additional techniques for the analysis of anesthetic gases include ultraviolet analyzers, gas chromatography, silicone rubber absorption, and Ramon laser scattering. Each of these methods offers useful information; however, most on-line anesthetic and respiratory gas monitoring systems currently consist of a mass spectrometer or a combined infrared, oxygen analyzer.

In addition to digital readout of anesthetic and respiratory gas concentrations, waveforms can be displayed. Perhaps the most useful of all waveforms is that of CO_2, e.g., the capnogram shown in Figure 3–13.

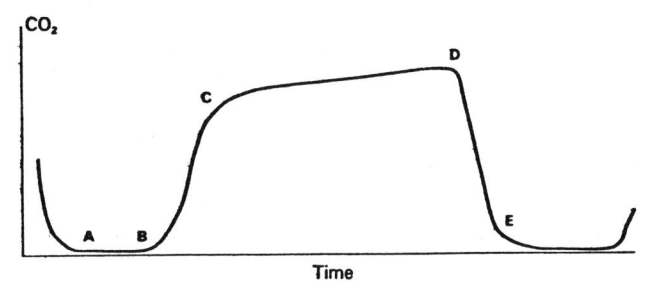

FIG. 3–13. The normal capnographic waveform. Segments are described in text. From Swedlow, D.B.: Mass spectrometers and respiratory gas monitoring. Refresher Courses in Anesthesiology, 13: 1985.

During early exhalation, the CO_2 concentration (segment A–B) is nil as tracheal (dead space) gas empties. As exhalation continues (segment B–C), increasing amounts of alveolar, CO_2-containing gas mix with dead space gas. Near end exhalation (segment C–D), an alveolar gas plateau occurs that represents nearly pure alveolar gas. Point D represents the highest concentration of alveolar CO_2. During inspiration (segment D–E) CO_2 free gas is taken in and the process begins again. The construction of such curves for inhalational agents is more complex because of ongoing agent uptake.

Additionally, the absolute value of end-tidal CO_2 (Et_{CO_2}) and the shape of the capnogram provide valuable monitoring information with regard to metabolic status (e.g., malignant hyperthermia), air embolism, neuromuscular blockade, and anesthetic mishap. For example, esophageal intubation or patient–circuit disconnect would be immediately recognized by loss of the capnogram and Et_{CO_2} value.*

CLINICAL EVALUATION OF VENTILATION AND AIRWAY PRESSURE

Respiration comprises two goals: ventilation and oxygenation. The anesthesiologist may elect to achieve these goals through a range of modalities from spontaneous to high-frequency mechanical ventilation. Regardless of the option selected clinical respiratory parameters, e.g., tidal volume, minute ventilation, and airway pressures (peak, mean, and PEEP) should be monitored.

---

*For a detailed analysis of capnographic waveform interpretation, the reader is referred to "Atlas of Capnography" by Smalhout and Kalenda.[98]

When monitoring tidal volume, one of many spirometer devices may be used (see below); however, let us first address the location of this monitor in the anesthesia circuit. Under ideal conditions, measurements would be made directly at the patient airway. For reasons related to equipment size, sterilization, logistics, and replacement after each case, this is not done routinely. Therefore, either the inspiratory or expiratory limb is used. If the flow sensor is placed in the expiratory limb, the volume measured can safely be assumed to have come from the patient's lungs.[99] With the monitor located just proximal to the CO_2 absorber, the transmission of respiratory microbes is probably minimal. If the monitor is left to the inspiratory limb, one is potentially only measuring that volume which is delivered to the circuit, *not* the volume delivered to the patient. Potential sources of error include a circuit leak distal to the sensor and volume lost secondary to circuit compliance. A standard adult circle system has a compliance of 3 to 6 ml/cm H_2O.[100] Therefore, if the flow sensor measured an **inspiratory** volume of 700 ml with a peak inspiratory pressure of 15 cm H_2O, then 45 to 90 ml of the tidal volume will be lost to the circuit due to compliance alone. Until disposable or easily reusable devices are developed for use at the patient airway, the expiratory limb flow sensor has provided a rational but incomplete compromise. Utilizing a dog model, Waterson and associates simulated 21 mechanical ventilation mishaps.[101] They demonstrated monitoring of *both* inspiratory and expiratory tidal volumes, along with airway pressures (see below), permitted more rapid identification of mishaps than did monitoring of hemodynamic variables.

Respirometers measure gas flow via a spindle connected through a geared system to turn a vane on a calibrated dial.[102,103] Pneumotachographs use a mechanical resistance placed in the circuit coupled with a pressure transducer.[104,105] The pressure difference produced is proportional to flow and is integrated to a volume measurement. Other devices employ ultrasound or heat-sensing methods. One must remember that these devices are subject to relative error and only gross values are given.

Monitoring of airway pressure is generally limited to the peak inspiratory pressure measured in cm H_2O. Anesthesia ventilators, however, also contain alarms for low pressure (e.g., circuit disconnection), high pressure (e.g., blocked endotracheal tube), continuous pressure (e.g., closed pop-off valve), and subambient pressure (e.g., interrupted fresh gas flow).[106] Rather than digress into a discussion of parenchymal versus thoracic compliance, the term compliance will be used in a generic sense. Furthermore, one must realize when compliance is viewed in this way (e.g., compliance = Δ volume/Δ pressure, the mechanical resistance of the circuit is not differentiated from patient-related factors. As a rule, the anesthesia record should document the initial peak inspiratory pressure on commencement of mechanical ventilation. One may make a mental note of the compliance. Should any change in ventilatory status occur, one may recalculate the compliance and use this information in the differential diagnosis.

LABORATORY EVALUATION OF VENTILATION (BLOOD GAS ANALYSIS)

Previously, multiple methods of ventilatory evaluation ranging from a simple stethoscope to end-tidal CO_2 via mass spectrometry have been discussed; however, arterial blood gas tension (ABG) analysis remains the gold standard.

While characterizing the ABG analysis as the gold standard, one must realize the amount of oxygen dissolved in plasma is quite small. Specifically, the Bunsen solubility coefficient for oxygen in plasma at 37° C is 0.003 ml/mm Hg.[107] The overwhelming majority of oxygen is combined with hemoglobin and O_2 saturation must be specifically measured to determine the content of whole blood oxygen. Total oxygen content (CaO_2) as measured in volume percent (vol %) uses the following equation:

$$CaO_2 = \{Hgb\ (g/dl) \times O_2\ \text{saturation}\ (\%) \times 1.34\ (ml\ O_2/dl)\} + Pa_{O_2}\ (mm\ Hg) \times .003\ (ml\ O_2/mm\ Hg)$$

Therefore, for a 25-year-old man with a hemoglobin (Hgb) of 15 g/dl, Pa_{O_2} of 95 mm Hg, and O_2 saturation of 98%;

$$CaO_2 = (15\ g/100\ ml \times 1.34 \times 0.98) + 95 \times .003 = 20\ ml/100\ (vol\ \%)$$

The correction factor of 1.34 ml O_2/g Hgb/100 ml was determined by Hufner in 1894.[108] It is important to understand the above relationship because situations may exist where Pa_{O_2} is normal but CaO_2 is not, e.g., carbon monoxide poisoning, and methemoglobinemia.

Previously, we discussed the principle of tissue oximetry under cardiovascular monitoring. While pulse oximetry is considered by many a necessary monitor, the sigmoidal shape of the oxyhemoglobin dissociation curve makes it insensitive to dramatic changes in Pa_{O_2} that can occur with anesthetic misadventure.

Arterial oxygen tension (Pa_{O_2}) is measured via a Clark polarographic electrode, as discussed in the next section, and is based on Henry's Law, i.e., the volume of a gas that dissolves in a liquid is directly proportional to the partial pressure of the gas in equilibrium with the liquid.[109]

The Severinghaus electrode is used to measure the Pa_{CO_2}.[110] Briefly, this apparatus uses a mercury-mercurous chloride pH-sensitive electrode and silver-silver chloride reference and measuring electrodes. A gas-permeable membrane separates the sample to be measured from the bicarbonate electrolyte bath containing the measuring electrode. Carbon dioxide diffuses across the membrane and hydrates in the reaction: $CO_2 + H_2O \longleftrightarrow H_2CO_3 \longleftrightarrow H^+ + HCO_3$. The resulting pH change is proportional to the Pa_{CO_2} of the sample. Lastly, ABG analysis yields a value for pH via an electrode–electrolyte bath system similar to the Severinghaus electrode.[111] While other ABG analysis techniques exist, the aforementioned methods are the most common in clinical practice.

Given the periodic battles waged in the anesthesia literature concerning whether or not to "temperature correct" ABG values, it would be remiss to not address this point. Briefly, as a general rule, Pa_{O_2} and Pa_{CO_2} decrease and pH increases with decreasing temperature. Conversely, with increasing temperature Pa_{O_2} and Pa_{CO_2} increase while pH falls.[112] As the solubilities of oxygen and carbon dioxide increase with hypothermia, the aforementioned rule appears contradictory, but other factors must be considered. Hypothermia shifts the oxyhemoglobin dissociation curve to the left and also depresses metabolic rate.[113] Thus, it is possible the effects on hemoglobin–oxygen affinity and metabolism are proportionally greater than the changes in solubility. The temperature correction of ABG values is an individual opinion left to the anesthesiologist.

OXIMETRY AND TRANSCUTANEOUS OXYGEN MONITORING

Oximetry, the measurement of hemoglobin oxygen saturation in either blood or tissue, is a principle that has recently been introduced into clinical anesthesia practice. At present, numerous corporations are marketing devices that can be used to monitor mixed venous oxygen saturation, oxyhemoglobin saturation, and transcutaneous oxygen content. The value of these new monitoring systems is still being defined, and as noted in the introduction, the oxyhemoglobin saturation (e.g., oximetry) monitor is a necessary vigilant monitor. Over the course of the 1990s, each of these systems will find some clinical usefulness, so they are worthy of noting.

With regard to mixed venous oxygen (Sv_{O_2}) and oxyhemoglobin saturation monitoring, Beer's law prevails. This law exponentially relates the concentration of a suspended solute to the intensity of light transmitted through the solution. Information can be obtained from the relative absorption of light by hemoglobin and oxyhemoglobin at different wavelengths.[114,115] Classically, this involved the use of red light (650 nm), which is principally absorbed by oxyhemoglobin, and infrared light (800 nm), which is an isobestic point, i.e., the absorption coefficient for hemoglobin and oxyhemoglobin is identical. Oxyhemoglobin saturation, however, does not utilize an isobestic wavelength. Light absorption and scattering by tissue, dark skin, and other forms of hemoglobin, make modifications with pulse oximetry necessary. Specifically, pulse oximetry functions by placing a *pulsatile* vascular bed between a two-wavelength (660 and 940 nm) source and a detector. To discriminate arterial saturation from artifact, a microprocessor program is employed. The algorithm uses the signal transmitted during diastole as its reference and measures oxyhemoglobin saturation as any deviation.[116] Arterial pulsations provide this deviation, and also allow determination of heart rate.

Mixed venous oxygen is measured in the classic sense with a third wavelength added to filter optical artifact. The wavelengths are directed on the passing red blood cells by one fiberoptic bundle. The subsequently reflected light is transmitted by an adjacent fiberoptic bundle to the photodetector. The reflected light is converted by microprocessor technology to a digital readout of Sv_{O_2} that is updated every 5 seconds.[117]

Transcutaneous oxygen tension monitoring uses a heated Clark polarographic oxygen electrode to measure oxygen that diffuses to the skin surface from dermal capillaries beneath it.[118] The electrode consists of a platinum cathode and a silver anode connected to a battery and a current meter. The electrodes are surrounded by an electrolyte bath. The presence of oxygen leads to the following reaction at the cathode: $O_2 + 2H_2O + 4e^- \rightarrow 4OH^-$. The current generated by oxygen reduction corresponds to the partial pressure of oxygen (oxygen tension) measured.

Presently Sv_{O_2} is measured via a modified pulmonary artery catheter introduced in 1982. Under normal circumstances Sv_{O_2} is approximately 75%, representing a normal 22% decline in oxygen saturation from physiologic extraction. When oxyhemoglobin is fully saturated (e.g., Sa_{O_2} = 100%), then $1 - Sv_{O_2}$ equals the oxygen extraction ratio. Sv_{O_2} represents the balance between O_2 supply and overall tissue demand. This point has led to an argument that Sv_{O_2} in a nonspecific measurement confuses rather than clears the picture.[117] Others believe this device, because of its reflection of global O_2 balance, represents the best early warning system available. Sv_{O_2} measurement is clinically useful in anesthesia practice, and this type of modified catheter is used whenever pulmonary artery catheterization is necessary.

Oxyhemoglobin saturation and transcutaneous oxygen tension (Ptc_{O_2}) monitoring are relatively unique monitoring devices in that they measure distal O_2 delivery without invasion of body integrity. The two devices are slightly different in end point measurement and each may find separate utility. Presently, they are employed in similar fashion, and the relative advantages and disadvantages are shown in Table 3–9.[119]

The potential problems of Ptc_{O_2} monitoring, i.e.,

TABLE 3–9. COMPARISON OF PULSE OXIMETRY AND TRANSCUTANEOUS OXYGEN TENSION MONITORING

Criteria	Ptc$_{O_2}$	Pulse Oximetry
Advantages	Continuous and noninvasive measure of O_2 tension	Continuous and noninvasive measure of O_2 saturation
	Provides trend of O_2	No calibration
	Detects low cardiac output	No site changes as a function of temperature or time
Disadvantages	Requires calibration	Provides no trend of Pa$_{O_2}$ until < 70 mm Hg
	Minimum 10-minute warm up	Provides no information about peripheral blood flow
	Frequent membrane changes	Empirical calibration
	Site change every 4 to 6 hours to avoid burns	

warm-up, burns, and most importantly, on-going evaluation of normal range and data interpretation with Ptc$_{O_2}$ monitors, are not apparent with pulse oximetry. In a 1986 clinical comparison, the correlation coefficient between Ptc$_{O_2}$ and Pa$_{O_2}$ varied with the patient's ASA classification. The relationship between pulse oximetry (Sa$_{O_2}$) and the laboratory-measured Sa$_{O_2}$, however, remained consistent.[120] Remember that different variables are being measured when comparing the techniques; hence, differences in the significance of variable changes and interpretations are important.

MONITORING THE CENTRAL NERVOUS SYSTEM

Postoperative neurologic complications, specifically brain damage, can be devastating for both the patient and the anesthesiologist. Regrettably, there are no reliable data on the incidence of primary neurologic problems caused by or associated with anesthesia. Estimates, however, vary between 0.5 and 40%. As might be expected, procedures involving cardiopulmonary bypass and the extracranial cerebrovascular system have the highest frequency.[121] Even more tragic are those sporadic and possibly preventable complications in previously healthy individuals undergoing elective procedures.[122] Electroencephalography is not a necessary monitor for all anesthetics, but it may offer valuable information in high-risk situations.

As presented, temperature remains the only commonly monitored CNS variable. Barring dramatic change in the delivery of anesthesia, it will always be important to the anesthesiologist.

ELECTROENCEPHALOGRAPHY

DEFINITION. Electroencephalography (EEG) refers to the study, observation, and recording of brain waves or the electrical potentials of the brain, which are a measurable expression of the electrical activity of the brain. All living tissues possess an electrical potential.[123] These potentials are measured in terms of voltage referred to a near point, as on the scalp or on the brain—this is a bipolar recording. If the reference point is a fixed point remote from the brain, a unipolar recording is obtained.

Despite the fact that electroencephalography is a noninvasive, real-time monitor of cerebral function, it has not been widely employed in the intraoperative period. Many independent forces have contributed to this trend, but none are insurmountable.

HISTORY OF EEG IN ANESTHESIA.[126–136] As noted in Table 3–10, which summarizes the significant developments in the history of the EEG in anesthesia, Adrian and Matthews were the first to study the effects of anesthesia on EEG.[125] They reported the slowing of brain waves with increasing depth of anesthesia. Other investigators studied the EEG with specific anesthetic agents.[126–128] A consistent finding in each of these studies was a marked patient-to-patient variability in the anesthetic agent concentration that correlated with an anesthetized EEG pattern. The wave changes occur in a relatively predictable manner with different activities and according to different drugs.[129,130]

MEASUREMENT SYSTEMS. Scalp electrode systems can be set up to record from several areas of the brain simultaneously. This is the method in diagnostic work. The standard electroencephalogram shows a set of 8 to 12 wave lines, each being a graph of the electric signals from one region of the head and designated as a channel.

A simplified device consisting of a single channel is used in the operating room. Investigations indicate that the variables encountered during surgery will produce characteristic changes in all parts of the cortex, although the changes will be maximal precentrally. In practice, the frontal to occipital derivation is observed. Second, the principle of frequency discrimination has been applied in order to eliminate interfering currents. A filter to remove the high-frequency artifacts and to dampen 60-cycle or background electrical interference is introduced into the circuit.

Frequency analyzers are available to permit quantitative analysis of the brain waves recorded. This device records the amount of activity at each frequency over a 10-second period. A special band amplifier is tuned to a specific frequency and the total electrical potential at this frequency is algebraically summed.

The strict interpretation of the EEG for diagnostic purposes involves quantification and pattern recognition. These areas of expertise are usually alien to the anesthesiologist.[136]

Essentially, EEG waves are the summation of electrical potentials generated by brain activity. Utilizing electrodes for data acquisition and amplifiers for transmission, the summed electrical potentials are displayed.[137] As with all monitored variables, a range of potentials exists. Scalp electrodes primarily record superficial cortical events, whereas special sites, e.g., nasopharyngeal electrodes, can generate additional information, in this case uncal and anterior hippocampal potentials.[138] A standardized placement system (International 10–20) has been developed.

SIGNIFICANCE OF EEG WAVES. Controversy exists over the ultimate significance of EEG waves and patterns. Nevertheless, an analogy has been drawn with the electrocardiogram:[139] much like the sinoatrial node in the heart, the nonspecific thalamic nuclei may act as a pacemaker for brain wave function.

CONSTRUCTION OF WAVES. The signals or waves recorded on a graph are usually analyzed according to five characteristics:

1. Frequency
2. Amplitude
3. Rhythmicity
4. Waveforms
5. Location

Frequency. This is the number of electrical pulsations that occur per unit of time, expressed as cycles per second (cps). In electroencephalographic work, the observed frequencies are of the order of ½ to 100 cps. According to the pattern of appearance of different frequencies, various rhythms can be identified. These are classified simply by Greek letter designators that represent ranges or bands of the number of oscillations.

Delta rhythm: the appearance of oscillations in the range of 4 cps or less; such slow waves of large amplitude and regular occurrence are seen during sleep.

TABLE 3–10. SIGNIFICANT DEVELOPMENTS IN HISTORY OF EEG IN ANESTHESIA[123]

1875—Richard-Caxton detected electric potentials on surface of scalps of animals.
1924—Hans Berger of Jena, father of electroencephalography, made first recording of human brain potentials. In 1929, Berger published the results of his work.[124]
1934—Adrian and Matthews published the first study of the effects of anesthesia on EEG.[125]
1936—Bergen reported the effects of *chloroform* as recorded on the electroencephalogram.
1936—Derbyshire, Rempel, Forbes and Lambert reported the effects of Avertin, pentobarbital, and diethyl ether as recorded on the electroencephalogram.
1937—Gibbs, Gibbs and Lennox described effects of diethyl ether on the brain and stated that *"a practical application of these observations might be the use of the electroencephalogram as a measure of the depth of anesthesia during surgical operations."*[126a]
1938—Beecher, McDonough, and Forbes studied the effects of hypotension and anoxia on brain waves.[127]
1940—Rubin and Freeman reported the changes in electric potentials of the brain during cyclopropane anesthesia. A tentative classification of the pattern of changes with depth of anesthesia was offered.[128]
1945—Brazier and Finesinger reported their investigations of the effects of intravenous barbiturates on the electric activity of the brain.[130b]
1949—Pender, Bickford and Faulconer reported the effects of high tensions of nitrous oxide on the human brain.[93a]
1950—Courtin, Bickford and Faulconer reported the observations on the brain waves as affected by nitrous oxide-oxygen-ether anesthesia for surgery. They presented a classification of the patterns of the brain waves according to depth of anesthesia by clinical signs.[131]
1950—Bickford reported a method of *automatic* anesthesia controlled by electroencephalography.[131]
1951—Kiersey, Bickford and Faulconer described and classified the EEG patterns for intravenous Pentothal sodium in humans.[132]
1952—Faulconer correlated EEG patterns with concentrations of ether in blood.[133]
1953—Possati, Bickford and Faulconer related changes in EEG to concentration of cyclopropane in arterial blood.[134]
1953–1955—Patrick reported the use of EEG in the diagnosis of hypercarbia in human patients.[135]

Theta rhythm: the appearance of oscillation in the range of 4 to 8 cps.
Alpha rhythm (Fig. 3–14): the appearance of oscillations in the frequency band of 8 to 12 cps; this was the first rhythm described by Berger.[124] This rate is about as fast as one can move a finger. The amplitude or size is variable but is largest at the back of the head where the optic centers are located. These waves are larger and more regular when a person has his eyes shut and is not thinking. One person in five shows no alpha rhythm, only complex irregular pulsations without fixed frequency. It is believed by some that the alpha waves represent a physiologic scanning mechanism.
Beta rhythm: the occurrence of pulsations in the frequency band of 13 to 35 cps

92 *General Anesthesia*

NORMAL ALPHA AND SLEEP RHYTHMS

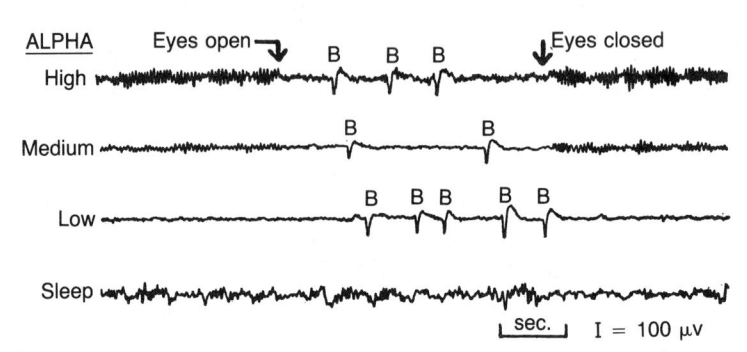

FIG. 3–14. Normal variation in amplitude of alpha rhythm as encountered in different normal persons and taken on fronto-occipital electrodes prior to anesthesia. The appearance during eye blinks is shown at B. The bottom tracing shows the recording from a normal person asleep without anesthesia: note the mixture of fast and slow waves, the pattern being different from any encountered during anesthesia, although sleep rhythms may be encountered during the recovery from anesthesia. From Faulconer, A., and Bickford, R.G.: Electroencephalography in Anesthesiology. *American Lecture Series.* Springfield, IL, Charles C Thomas, 1960.

Gamma rhythm: the occurrence of pulsations in the frequency band of 40 to 50 cps

Amplitude. This is the maximum departure of an alternating current from an average base value. It is measured as a peak to peak voltage. The amplitude of the changes in voltage seen in electroencephalograms is of the order of 10 to 100 microvolts.

Waveforms. The form of the various waves observed on a graph is simply a contour of the wave. The more commonly encountered forms are illustrated in Figure 3–15.

OBSERVATIONS DURING ANESTHESIA. Changes in the pattern of the brain waves occur during anesthesia.[123,129] A progression from the pattern seen in the waking state to that of marked depression of electrical activity seen in clinical stage IV of anesthesia can be observed (see Chapter 13).[129a,129b] The electroencephalograph obtained during this period represents a continuum of progressing cerebral depression. As the cortex is depressed by administration of increasing amounts of anesthetic or of carbon dioxide (or anoxia), characteristic EEG patterns are produced.[126b] Although each agent produces minor pattern differences, there is enough similarity in the general pattern so that a composite picture of anesthetic depth can be formed that can be correlated with clinical signs and blood levels of the anesthetic agents.[131] These patterns are relatively stereotyped but reproducible and serve to monitor the depth of anesthesia (Fig. 3–16).

CLASSIFICATION OF PATTERNS. Classification of the progressing waveforms has been accomplished by Faulconer and coworkers.[123,140] Four distinct patterns may be identified, using the conscious pattern (eyes closed; relatively fast frequency and low voltage [8–13 cps; 75 microvolts or less]) as a baseline.

Pattern 1: *Fast frequency*—Low-voltage activity seen in the waking and semiconscious state (frequency = 15 to 30 cps; voltage = 50 microvolts or less)
Pattern 2: *Rhythmic pattern*—consists of regular waves with slow frequency and high voltage (frequency = 2 to 8 cps; voltage = 150 to 300 microvolts)
Pattern 3: *Mixed pattern*—fast-frequency, low-voltage waves 10 to 20 cps; 50 to 75 microvolts are *superimposed* on high-voltage low-frequency waves (frequency = 2 to 4 cps; voltage = 100 to 200 microvolts)

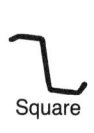

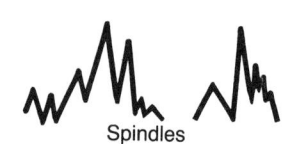

FIG. 3–15. Schematic presentation of commonly encountered waveforms.

FIG. 3–16. The *continuum* of progressing cerebral depression during anesthesia. The four patterns shown here are free-hand drawings which, in effect, compress the time element of the various stages into a form suitable for graphic presentation. (Courtesy of Verne L. Brechner and Edin Division of Epsco Inc.)

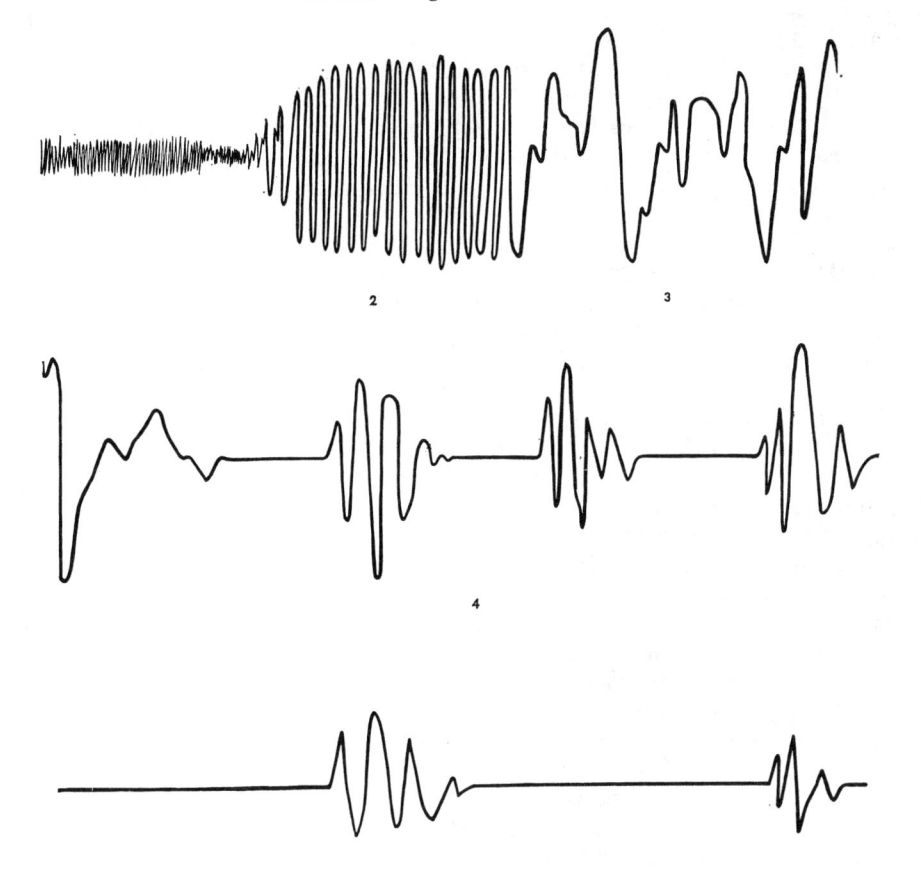

Pattern 4: *Suppression pattern*—periods of cortical inactivity separate periods of activity (so-called burst suppression). As depth of anesthesia and cortical depression continue the duration of burst suppression increases. As depression progresses the cortical activity shows decrease in voltage and frequency of waves. Four phases are recognized:
  a. Suppression less than 3 seconds' duration
  b. Suppression from 3 to 10 seconds' duration
  c. Suppression longer than 10 seconds' duration
  d. Complete cortical suppression

APPLICATIONS. The following are the clinical applications as summarized by Patrick.[135]

1. To monitor depth of anesthesia during
   a. Any anesthesia
   b. Clinical trials of new drugs
   c. Period when clinical signs of depth are not available
2. To evaluate adequacy of cerebral perfusion during
   a. Extracorporeal circulation
   b. Intracranial procedures
   c. Hypothermia
   d. Controlled hypotension
   e. Manual cardiac systole
3. To aid in diagnosis of hypercarbia
4. To aid in diagnosis of anoxia

EEG AS A MONITOR.[141] Patients with cerebral ischemia, anoxia, deep anesthesia, and sudden decrease in temperature of arterial blood display abnormal electroencephalographic patterns. Adequate cerebral perfusion results in a normal electroencephalogram.

Among the specific situations that can produce abnormal patterns, particularly suppression of electrical activity, are the following:

1. *Loss of blood*, decreased cardiac output, and hypotension—all decrease cerebral blood flow. Waves of low-frequency, high-amplitude appear.
2. *Vena caval obstruction*—causes a decreased cerebral blood flow and results in a flat EEG.
3. *Surgical manipulation*—rotation of heart causes waves of low frequency and high amplitude.
4. *Excessive anesthesia*—results in waves of low frequency, high amplitude (slow, large waves), and periods of suppression.
5. *Cerebral anoxia*—decreased oxygen saturation resulting from respiratory obstruction, decreased atmospheric oxygen, or decreased oxygen tension will diminish cerebral oxygen activity. This is especially marked when saturation of the blood reaches levels of 65% or less.

6. *Cool blood*—during open cardiac surgery blood tends to be below body temperature and hypothermia occurs. The cool blood causes alteration of cerebral electrical activity. This is pronounced when temperature of blood is 28.5° C or less. If blood is warmed to 32.5° C, no EEG changes occur.

LIMITATIONS OF STANDARD EEG MONITORING. Intraoperatively, EEG monitoring can be used for any procedure where the adequacy of cerebral perfusion is questionable, e.g., carotid endarterectomy and procedures involving cardiopulmonary bypass. Major difficulties in the intraoperative use of EEG, aside from a lack of anesthesiologist knowledge, are (1) multiple anesthetic agents; (2) changes in Pa_{CO_2} and cerebral blood flow; (3) body temperature; and (4) changes in oxygen content.

Because of space limitations, it would not be possible to review the literature with regard to the effect of a specific anesthetic agent on the EEG in this chapter. One can summarize by stating that each agent classification, and similar compounds within that same class, have profoundly different effects on the EEG. It is therefore imperative for the anesthesiologist to familiarize himself with the specific effects of the selected anesthetic regimen.

Cerebral blood flow influences EEG activity. Also, Pa_{CO_2} is routinely manipulated during anesthesia to alter the size of intracranial structures.[142,143] Finally, hypothermia, a common occurrence during anesthesia, changes the EEG.[144]

In an effort to provide meaningful patient data while minimizing the aforementioned problems, several devices using computer processing of raw EEG data have been developed. Compressed spectral array displays power versus frequency.[145] The result is a serial view of the power plotted one above the other, which is updated every 4 to 32 seconds. Another technique, cerebral function monitoring, involves a single- or dual-channel processor for recording EEG amplitude and amplitude variability. Global power and frequency are displayed in a digital fashion. While many of these devices have been introduced commercially, their value as an intraoperative monitor is still under investigation.[146]

EVOKED POTENTIALS. Depth of the general anesthetic state can also be assessed by monitoring evoked potentials. Such monitoring involves quantitation of the nervous system response to an externally administered stimulus. Three types of stimuli are usually employed during anesthesia and surgery to assess brain function: somatosensory, auditory brain stem, and visual.

Method Appropriate scalp electrodes are appropriately placed as follows: for *somatosensory* potentials (SSEP), one electrode is placed in the mid-scalp area (referred to as the midfrontal locus) over the primary sensory cortical hand area and over the fifth cervical vertebra. For *auditory* potentials, the electrodes are attached to the vertex and the mastoid and record brain stem auditory evoked potentials (BAEP); for *visual* potentials, one electrode is placed 5 cm above the inion in the midline and referred to a midfrontal locus.

For somatosensory stimulation, the median nerve is stimulated with a 100 μs constant-current pulse generator (useful in spinal cord procedures). For auditory responses, a stimulus of 10 Hz square wave click of 100 μs duration delivered at 80 dB via headphones has been used (during hypothalamic procedures). The visual stimulus is a light flash delivered by a photic stimulator at 2 Hz, repeated at least 128 times, which can be employed during posterior fossa procedures.

Evoked responses must be carefully measured. Coordination of the time of application of the stimulus to the time of the appearance of the electroencephalographic response is needed. The interval between the stimulus and response is designated as the latency period. The amplitude of the response must also be measured.

Influence of Anesthetic Agents Volatile agents all profoundly affect the cortical component of all three stimulus modalities in a graded, nonagent-specific, and reversible manner. In dosages in the clinical range, enflurane, isoflurane, and halothane all increase the latency period of the cortical component as well as markedly decrease the amplitude of the potential. There is also an increase in the latency of the early and middle brain stem component of the auditory response.

Nitrous oxide up to 50% produces graded decreases in amplitude of the visual and somatosensory evoked cortical potentials with increasing concentrations. However, there is no alteration in the latency of the auditory evoked cortical potential.[147,148] Althesin, etomidate, and fentanyl have been found to have no effect on brain stem responses.

TEMPERATURE

In today's practice of high-tech anesthesiology, it is easy to overlook the simply acquired body temperature measurement; however, one must never lose sight of this **vital sign**. Presented in its simplest schema, body temperature represents the relationship of heat production and environmental losses. Each day anesthesiologists deal with hypothermia, i.e., core temperature ≤36° C, more than any other medical specialty. Body heat is lost via either one or a combination of four mechanisms: radiation, conduction, convection, or evaporation.

Radiation, loss of heat by infrared rays, is the primary heat loss mechanism in the operating room, accounting for almost 50%.[149] Conduction heat loss occurs when heat moves from the patient to the object(s) he physically contacts. This accounts for a minimal amount of losses. Convection, i.e., heat loss to surrounding air, accounts for approximately 35% of losses.[150] Evaporation from the skin surface and the lungs accounts for the remainder of heat loss. Coupled with this normal balance, anesthesia produces a considerable shift to the loss column. Anesthesia interferes with thermal regulation via a direct inhibition of hypothalamic responses as well as peripheral vasodilation.[151,152] Therefore, if we are going to facilitate potentially dangerous loss of body heat, we must monitor the patient.

While not addressing specific anesthetic complications, our premise is that appropriate monitoring will decrease the incidence of complications. The consequences of hypothermia include decreased cardiac output, prolonged neuromuscular blockade, decreased agent metabolism, and a postoperative increase in oxygen consumpton.[153] The magnitude of the problem of postoperative hypothermia was revealed in a study by Vaughan et al.[154] They demonstrated 60% of patients admitted to the recovery unit had a core temperature of <36° C. No difference was noted between patients who had general or regional anesthesia. Finally, this study revealed that 18% of the patients were returned to the unit still hypothermic, a problem more common in patients 60 years of age or older.

Previously, many considered malignant hyperthermia the primary reason to monitor temperature intraoperatively. Recent evidence has demonstrated the first sign of impending malignant hyperthermia to be an increase in end-tidal carbon dioxide production.[155] Clearly, the well-informed anesthesiologist uses temperature monitoring to avoid hypothermia except in deliberate instances.

Once a decision has been made to monitor temperature, one must decide which of the potential sites to use. Benzinger clearly demonstrated that tympanic membrane measurements most closely reflect core temperature.[156] A concern over potential tympanic membrane damage lead Cork and associates to undertake an elaborate study of multiple sites with regard to precision and accuracy of perioperative temperature monitoring.[96] They concluded either the nasopharynx, esophagus, or bladder represents the most accurate monitoring site.

Finally, the question of liquid crystal thermography must be addressed. Generally, these devices are marketed as a tape that, when applied to the patient's forehead, changes color as temperature changes. In studies comparing this technology with tympanic membrane temperature, tape was revealed to be less sensitive with regard to absolute temperature and temperature trends.[157]

MONITORING THE GENITOURINARY SYSTEM

Compromise of the genitourinary system, i.e., acute renal failure (ARF), is a grave complication in surgical patients.[158] Oliguric or anuric ARF has a 60 to 90% mortality rate while nonoliguric ARF has a 40 to 50% mortality rate. A complication with such protean implications must be monitored, but not every anesthetized patient requires bladder catheterization. In general, any patient scheduled for intra-abdominal or intrathoracic surgery should be catheterized. Additionally, a peripheral procedure exceeding 2 hours in length, or *any* procedure necessitating blood transfusion suggests catheterization. Remember, the signs of a transfusion reaction may be masked in the anesthetized patient. A hemoglobin-tinged urine may be the anesthesiologist's first indication of a problem.

The kidneys are modulated by a variety of highly sophisticated controls including the renin-angiotensin-aldosterone system, antidiuretic hormone, ANP, and parathormone. Additionally, renal function is greatly influenced by the status of extracellular hydration.

Urine output, the principal measure of intraoperative renal function, is determined by the glomerular filtration rate (GFR) and tubular fluid reabsorption. While numerous reports of highly sensitive tests of GFR and tubular function exist, the results are not applicable to a discussion of intraoperative monitoring. Often, a specific value for intraoperative urine output is targeted. While values of less than $0.5 \text{ ml} \cdot \text{kg}^{-1} \cdot \text{hr}^{-1}$ are consistently associated with a low GFR, urine output greater than this can also be associated with a low GFR.[159] Despite these obvious shortcomings, urine output provides a gross estimate of cardiovascular function, in the absence of renal parenchymal disease, and alerts one to impending ARF.

MONITORING SYSTEMS OF THE FUTURE

New technology is continually being applied to monitoring techniques. New devices being introduced commercially include transesophageal echocardiography and digital arterial blood pressure monitors. Many other devices are undergoing clinical trials, including those that use lower esophageal contractility as a measure of anesthetic depth.[95]

With each new monitor introduced, the anesthesia workstation grows larger and more confusing. It seems as though we have become prisoners of our own advances, our workstation a maze rather than a clear path. Consequently, we are left with one more noise to seek out amid the cacaphony of alarms, and one more variable to track.

Presently, approximately 100 variables can be potentially monitored from an anesthetized patient. No anesthesiologist, no matter how competent, can accurately record, analyze, and act on so much information. During the discussion of anesthesia ergonomics in the introduction, it was noted that 22% of critical incidents relate to the misuse of equipment. It is also noted that much less than 1.0% of critical incidents is related to equipment failure.

Ideally, any new devices will provide both physical and functional integration as recently described by Waterson and Calkins.[160] Physical integration deals with the arrangement of devices in the workstation. Functional integration addresses the arrangement of device control and display. Studies of anesthesia mishaps will hopefully provide data to help the anesthesiologist prioritize the monitoring strategy in specific operative or patient-related situations.

SUMMARY

Standards for monitoring during the intraoperative period have been adopted by the American Society of Anesthesiologists, Inc. as basic procedures. They are presented as essentials for current practice in the *Directory of the American Society of Anesthesiologists*, Park Ridge, Illinois, 1991.

REFERENCES

1. Calkins, J.M.: Why new delivery systems? In FADS: The Future of Anesthetic Delivery Systems: Contemporary Anesthesia Practice, vol. 8. Edited by B.R. Brown. Philadelphia, F.A. Davis, 1984.
2. Duri, A.B., Behm, R.J., and Martin, W.E.: Predesign investigation of anesthesia operational environment. Anesthesiology 52:584, 1973.
3. Cooper, J.B., Newbower, R.S., and Kitz, R.J.: An analysis of major errors and equipment failures in anesthesia management: Considerations for prevention and detection. Anesthesiology, 60:34, 1984.
4. Boquet, G., Bushman, J.A., and Davenport, M.T.: The anesthesia machine—a study of function and design. Br. J. Anaesth. 52:61, 1980.
5. Clifton, B.S., and Hotten, W.I.T.: Deaths associated with anesthesia. Br. J. Anaesth., 35:250, 1963.
6. Edwards, G., Morton, M.J.V., and Pask, E.A.: Deaths associated with anesthesia: Report on 1,000 Cases. Anesthesiology, 11:194, 1956.
7. Calkins, J.M.: Anesthesia equipment: Help or hinderance? *In* Advances in Anesthesia, vol 2. Edited by R.K. Stoelting, P.G. Barash, and T.J. Gallagher. Chicago, Yearbook Medical Publishers, 1985.
8. Hope, C.E., and Morrison, D.L.: Understanding and selecting monitoring equipment in anaesthesia and intensive care. Can. Anaesth. Soc. J., 33:670, 1986.
9. Eichhorn, J.H., et al.: Standards for patient monitoring during anesthesia at Harvard Medical School. JAMA, 256:1017, 1986.
10a. American Society of Anesthesiologists: ASA Newsletter, 50:Dec, 1986.
10b. Vandam, L.R.: The seuses as monitors in blitt monitoring in anesthesia and critical care medicine, p5–24 New York, Churchill Livingstone, 1985.
11. Cannard, T.H., et al.: The ECG during anesthesia and surgery. Anesthesiology, 21:194, 1960.
12. Kuner, J., et al.: Cardiac arrhythmias during anesthesia. Dis. Chest, 52:580, 1967.
13. Kaplan, J.A. and King, S.B.: The pre-cordial electrocardiographic lead (V_5) in patients who have coronary-artery disease. Anesthesiology, 45:570, 1976.
14. Advanced Cardiac Life Support Text. Dallas, American Heart Association, 1983.
15. Kates, R.A., Zaidan, J.R., and Kaplan, J.A.: Esophageal lead for intraoperative electrocardiographic monitoring. Anesth. Analg., 61:781, 1982.
16. Mylrea, K.C., et al.: ECG lead with the endotracheal tube. Crit. Car. Med. 11:199, 1983.
17. Bazaral, M.G., and Norfleet, E.A.: Comparison of CB_5 and V_5 leads for intraoperative electrocardiographic monitoring. Anesth. Analg. 60:849, 1981.
18. Janeway, T.C.: Important contributions to clinical medicine during the past thirty years from the study of human blood pressure. Johns Hopkins Hosp. Bull., 26:341, 1915.
19. Master, A.M., Goldstein, I., and Walters, M.G.: New and old definition: Normal blood pressure. Bull. N.Y. Acad. Med., 27:452, 1951.
20. Harvey, W.: Origins of Blood Pressure Measurement. From Exercitatio Anatomica De Motu Cordis et Sanguinis in Animalibus, 3rd ed. English translation by Chauncey D. Leadke. Springfield, IL, Charles C Thomas. 1949.
21a. Hales, Stephen: Statistical Essays—Containing Haemastaticks. W Innys and R Manby St. Pauls London 1733. Reprint of original under auspices N.Y. Academy of Medicine, Hafner Publishing Co. New York 1964.
21b. Clark-Kennedy, A.E. (ed.): Stephen Hales: Physiologist and Botanist. Cambridge, England, Cambridge University Press, 1977.
22. Hérrison, J.: Le Sphygmonètre: Origins of blood pressure measurement. Paris, Crochard, 1834.
23. Von Vierordt, K.: Measurement of blood pressure by the sphygmograph quantitative studies of circulation, 1855. Cited in January.
24. von Basch, S.: Über die Messung des Blutdrucks am Menschen. Z. Klin. Med., 2:79, 1880.
25. Riva Rocci, S.: Un nuvo sfigmomanometro. Gaz. Med. Torino, 47: 981, 1896.
26. Riva Rocci, S.: Gaz. Med. di Torino, 1896. In Foundations of Anesthesiology. Edited by A. Faulconer and T.E. Keys. Springfield, IL, Charles C Thomas, 1965.
27. Beecher, H.K.: The first anesthesia records (Codman, Cushing). Surg. Gynecol. Obstet., 71:689, 1940.
28. Fulton, J.F.: Harvey Cushing: A biography. Springfield, IL, Charles C Thomas, 1940.
29. Crile, G.W.: Blood pressure in surgery. Philadelphia, J.B. Lippincott, 1903.
30. Cushing, H.W.: On routine determination of arterial tension in operating room and clinic. Boston Med. and Surg. J., 148:250, 1903.
31. Hirsch, N.P. and Smith, G.B.: Harvey Cushing: His contribution to anesthesia. Anesth. Analg, 65:288, 1986.

32. Korotkoff, N.S.: Izvest. imp. St. Petersburg, Voyenno-med. Acad., 1905.
33. Korotkoff, N.S.: Berichte der. St. Petersburg, diserlichen Militartzlichen Akademia, 1905.
34. American Heart Association: Standardization of blood pressure reading. Am. Heart J., *18*:95, 1939.
35. American Heart Association: Recommendations for human blood pressure determinations by sphygmomanometers. Dallas, American Heart Association, 1980.
36. American Heart Association: Recommendations for human blood pressure determination by sphygmomanometers: American Heart Association report, fifth edition. Circulation, *77*:501, 1988.
37. Ragan C., and Borderly, J.: Accuracy of clinical measurements of arterial blood pressure with note on auscultatory gap. Bull. Johns Hopkins Hosp., *69*:504, 1941.
38. Brunner, J.M.R.: Handbook of blood pressure monitoring. Littleton, MA, PSG Publishing, 1978.
39. Smith, N.T., Wesseling, K.M., and de Wit, B.: Evaluation of two prototype devices producing noninvasive, pulsative, calibrated blood pressure measurement from a finger. J. Clin. Monit., *1*:17, 1985.
40. Green, M., et al.: Comparison between oscillometric and invasive blood pressure monitoring during cardiac surgery. Int. J. Clin. Monit. Comput., *1*:21, 1984.
41. Posey, J.A., et al.: The meaning of the point of maximum oscillations in cuff pressure in the indirect measurement of blood pressure. Cardiovasc. Res. Cent. Bull., *8*:15, 1969.
42. Yelderman, M., and Ream, A.K.: Indirect measurement of mean blood pressure in the anesthetized patient. Anesthesiology, *50*:253, 1979.
43. Apple, H.P.: Automated noninvasive blood pressure monitors. In Essential Noninvasive Monitoring. Edited by J.S. Gravenstein, et al. New York, Grune & Stratton, 1980.
44. Gruen, W.: An assessment of present automated methods of indirect blood pressure measurements. Ann. N.Y. Acad. Sci., *147*:107, 1968.
45. Showman, A., and Betts, E.K.: Hazards of automatic noninvasive blood pressure monitoring. Anesthesiology, *55*:717, 1981.
46a. Bordley, J., et al.: Recommendations for human blood pressure determinations by sphygmomanometers. Circulation, *4*:503, 1951.
46b. Kirkendall, N.N., Feinleib, M., Allyn L.: Recommendations for human blood pressure determinations by sphygmomanometers. Circulation 62:1154A, 1980.
47. Brunner, J.M.R., et al.: Comparison of direct and indirect methods of measuring arterial blood pressure. III. Med. Instrum., *15*:182, 1981.
48. Van Bergen, F.H., et al.: Comparison of indirect and direct methods of measuring arterial blood pressure. Circulation, *10*:481, 1954.
49. Collins, V.J., and Magora, F.: Sphygmomanometry: The indirect measurement of blood pressure. Anesth. Analg., *42*:443, 1963.
50. Cushing, H: Some principles of cerebral surgery: Note on precordial stethoscope. JAMA, *52*:184, 1909.
51. Trout, K.W., Bertrand, C.A. and Williams, M.H.: Measurement of blood pressure in obese persons. JAMA, *162*:170, 1956.
52a. Rappaport, M.B., and Sprague, H.B.: Physiologic and physical laws that govern auscultation and their clinical application. Am. Heart J., *21*:257, 1941.
52b. Rappaport, M.B., and Sprague, H.B.: The effects of tubing bore on stethoscope efficiency. Am. Heart J., *42*:605, 1951.
53. Blitt, C.D.: Catherization techniques of invasive cardiovascular monitoring. Springfield, IL, Charles C Thomas, 1981.
54. Allen, E.V.: Thromboangitis obliterans: Methods of diagnosis of chronic occlusive arterial lesions distal to the wrist with illustrative cases. Am. J. Med. Sci. *178*:237, 1929.
55. Bedford, R.F.: Radial arterial function following percutaneous cannulation with 18 and 20 gauge catheters. Anesthesiology, *47*:37, 1977.
56. Barr, P.O.: Percutaneous puncture of the radial artery with a multipurpose teflon catheter for indwelling use. Acta Physiol. Scand., *51*:343, 1961.
57. Jones, R.M., et al.: The effect of method of radial artery cannulation on past cannulation blood flow and thrombus formation. Anesthesiology, *55*:76, 1981.
58. Pinella, J.C., et al.: Study of the incidence of intravascular catheter infection and associated septicemia in critically ill patients. Crit. Care Med., *11*:21, 1983.
59. Maki, P.G., and Band, J.D.: A comparative study of polyantibiotic ointments and iodophore ointments in the prevention of vascular catheter related infection. Am. J. Med., *70*:739, 1981.
60. Shinozaki, T., et al.: Bacterial contamination of arterial lines: A prospective study. JAMA, *249*:223, 1983.
61a. Hayes, M.F., et al.: Radial artery catheterization by cutdown technique. Crit. Care Med., *1*:151, 1973.
61b. Kroll, D.A., Caplan, R.A.: Nerve injury associated with anesthesia. Anesthesiology 73:202, 1990.
62. Wyatt, R., Glaves, I., and Cooper, D.J.: Proximal skin necrosis after radial artery cannulation. Lancet, *2*:1135, 1974.
63. Thomson, I.R.: Cardiovascular physiology: Venous return. Can. Anaesth. Soc. J., *31*:S31, 1984.
64. Guyton, A.C., Jones, C.E., and Coleman, T.G.: Circulatory physiology: cardiac output and its regulation, 2nd ed. Philadelphia, W.B. Saunders, 1973.
65. Mangano, D.T.: Monitoring pulmonary arterial pressure in coronary-artery disease. Anesthesiology, *53*:364, 1980.
66. Holt, H.M.: Central venous pressure via peripheral veins. Anesthesiology, *28*:1093, 1967.
67. Johnson, A.O.B., and Clark, R.G.: Malpositioning of central venous catheters. Lancet, *2*:1395, 1972.
68. Sorenson, T.I.A., and Sonne-Holm, S.: Central venous catheterization through the basilic vein or by infra clavicular puncture. Acta Chir. Scand., *141*:323, 1975.
69. Bridges, B.B., Carden, E., and Takacs, F.A.: Introduction of central venous pressure catheters through arm veins with a high success rate. Can. Anaesth. Soc. J., *26*:128, 1979.
70. Belani, K.G., et al.: Percutaneous cervical central venous line placement: A comparison of the internal and external jugular vein routes. Anesth. Analg., *59*:40, 1980.
71. Rao, T.L.K., Wong, A.Y., and Salem, M.R.: A new approach to percutaneous catheterization of the internal jugular vein. Anesthesiology, *46*:362, 1977.
72. Blitt, C.D., et al.: Central venous catheterization via the external jugular vein: A technique employing the J-wire. JAMA, *229*:817, 1974.
73. Blitt, C.D.: Catheterization techniques of invasive cardiovascular monitoring. Springfield, IL, Charles C Thomas, 1981.
74. Swan, H.J.C., and Shah, P.: The rationale for bedside hemodynamic monitoring. J. Crit. Care Med. IL., *11*:24, 1986.
75. Rao, T.L.K., Jacobs, K.M., and El-Etr, A.A.: Reinfarction following anesthesia in patients with myocardial infarction. Anesthesiology, *59*:499, 1983.

76. Nadeau, S, and Noble, W.M.: Misinterpretation of pressure measurements from the pulmonary artery catheter. Can. Anaesth. Soc. J., 33:352, 1986.
77. Stevens, J.H., et al.: Thermodilution cardiac output measurement. JAMA, 253:2240, 1985.
78. Guyton, R.A., et al.: The influence of positive end-expiratory pressure on intrapericardial pressure and cardiac function after coronary artery bypass surgery. J. Cardiothorac. Anesth., 1:98, 1987.
79. Jardin, F., et al.: Influence of position and end-expiratory pressure on left ventricular performance. New Engl. J. Med., 304:387, 1981.
80. Swan, H.J.C., et al.: Catheterization of the heart in man with use of a flow-directed balloon-tipped catheter. N. Engl. J. Med., 283:447, 1970.
81. Sprung, C.L., et al.: Ventricular arrhythmias during Swan-Ganz catheterization of the critically ill. Chest, 79:413, 1981.
82. Barash, P.G., et al.: Catheter-induced pulmonary artery perforation: mechanisms, management, and modifications. J. Thorac. Cardiovasc. Surg. 82:5, 1981.
83. Ehlers, K.C., et al.: Cardiac output measurements: A review of current techniques and research. Ann. Biomed. Eng., 14:219, 1986.
84. Runciman, W.B., Ilsley, A.H., and Roberts, J.G.: An evaluation of thermodilution measurements using the Swan-Ganz catheter. Anaesth. Intens. Care, 9:208, 1981.
85. Nadeau, S., and Noble, W.H.: Limitations of cardiac output measurements by thermodilution. Can. Anaesth. Soc. J., 33:780, 1986.
86. Jebson, P.J.R., and Karkow, W.S.: Pulsatile flow simulator for comparison of cardiac output measurements by electromagnetic flow meter and thermodilution. J. Clin. Monit., 2:6, 1986.
87. Bernstein, D.P.: Continuous noninvasive real time monitoring of cardiac output by thoracic electrical bioimpedance. Crit. Care Med., 13:355, 1985.
88. Huntsman, L., et al.: Noninvasive doppler determination of cardiac output in man. Circulation, 67:593, 1983.
89. Lavandier, B., et al.: Noninvasive aortic blood flow measurement using an intraesophageal probe. Ultrasound Med. Biol., 11:45, 1985.
90. Matsumoto, M., et al.: Application of transesophageal echocardiography to continuous intraoperative monitoring of left ventricular performance. Am. J. Cardiol., 46:95, 1980.
91. Clements, F.M., and de Bruijn, N.P.: Perioperative evaluation of regional wall motion by transesophageal two-dimensional echocardiography. Anesth. Analg., 66:249, 1987.
92. Roizen M.F., et al.: Monitoring with two-dimensional transesophageal echocardiography: comparison of myocardial function in patients undergoing supraceliac, suprarenal-infraceliac, or infrarenal aortic occlusion. J. Vasc. Surg., 1:300, 1984.
93. Smith, J.S., et al.: Intraoperative detection of myocardial ischemia in high-risk patients: electrocardiography versus two-dimensional transesophageal echocardiography. Circulation, 72:1015, 1085.
94. Furuya, M., et al.: Detection of air embolism by transesophageal echocardiography. Anesthesiology, 58:124, 1983.
95. Evans, J.M., Davies, W.L., and Wise, C.C.: Lowere oesophageal contractility: A new monitor of anesthesia. Lancet, 1:1151, 1984.
96. Cork, R.C., Vaughan, R.W., and Humphrey, L.S.: Precision and accuracy of intraoperative temperature monitoring. Anesth. Analg., 62:211, 1983.
97. Blitt, C.D. (ed.): Monitoring in anesthesia and critical care medicine. New York, Churchill Livingstone, 1985.
98. Smalhout, B., and Kalenda, Z.: Atlas of Capnography. ed. 2, vol. 1. Utrecht-Zeist, The Netherlands, 1982.
99. Fairley, H.B.: Respiratory monitoring. In Monitoring in Anesthesia and Critical Care Medicine. Edited by C.D. Blitt. New York, Churchill Livingstone, 1985.
100. Epstein, M.A., and Epstein, R.A.: Airway flow patterns during mechanical ventilation of infants: A mathematical model. IEEE Trans. Biomed. Eng., 26:299, 1979.
101. Waterson, C.K., et al.: Preventing anesthetic mishaps: Are we monitoring the right variables? Anesthesiology, 65:A536, 1986.
102. Byles, P.M.: Observations on some continuously-acting spirometers. Br. J. Anaes., 32:470, 1960.
103. Mushin, W.W., et al.: Automatic ventilation of the lungs, 2nd ed. Oxford, Blackwell, 1969.
104. Grenvik, A., and Hedstrand, U.: The reliability of pneumotachography in respirator ventilation: An experimental study. Acta Anaesthesiol. Scand., 10:195, 1966.
105. Kafer, E.R.: Errors in pneumotachography as a result of transducer design and function. Anesthesiology, 38:275, 1973.
106. Myerson, K.R., Ilsley, A.H., and Runciman, W.B.: An evaluation of ventilator monitoring alarms. Anaesth. Intens. Care, 14:174, 1986.
107. Nunn, J.F.: Applied Respiratory Physiology, 2nd ed. London, Butterworths, 1977.
108. Kennedy, S.K., and Wilson, R.S.: Oxygen measurement. Int. Anesth. Clin., 19: 1981
109. Hill, D.W.: Electrode systems for measurement of blood-gas tensions, content, and saturation. In Scientific Foundations of Anesthesia. Edited by C. Scurr and S. Feldman. Chicago, Yearbook Medical Publishers, 1974.
110. Severinghaus, J.W.: Measurements of blood gases: P_{O_2} and P_{CO_2}. Ann. N.Y. Acad. Sci., 148:115, 1968.
111. Shapiro, B.A., Harrison, R.A., and Walton, J.R.: Clinical Application of Blood Gases, 3rd Ed. Chicago, Yearbook Medical Publishers, 1982.
112. Burnett, R.W., and Noonan, D.C.: Calculations and correction factors used in determination of blood pH and blood gases. Clin. Chem., 20:1499, 1974.
113. Willford, D.C., Hill, E.P., and Morres, W.Y.: Theoretical analysis of oxygen transport during hypothermia. J. Clin. Monit., 2:30, 1986.
114. Sperinde, J.M., and Senelly, K.M.: The Opticath oximetrix system: Theory and development. In Continuous Measurement of Blood Oxygen Saturation in the High Risk Patient. Theory and practice in monitoring mixed venous oxygen saturation, Vol. 2. Edited by P.J. Fahey. San Diego, Beach International, 1985.
115. Yoshiya, I., Shimada, Y., and Tanaka, K.: Spectrophotometric monitoring of critical oxygen saturation in the fingertip. Med. Biol. Eng. Comput., 18:27, 1980.
116. Yelderman, M., and New, W.: Evaluation of pulse oximetry. Anesthesiology, 59: 349, 1983.
117. Norfleet, E.A., and Watson, C.B.: Continuous mixed venous oxygen saturation measurement: A significant advance in hemodynamic monitoring? J. Clin. Monit., 1:245, 1985.
118. Eberhand, P., et al.: Continuous P_{O_2} monitoring in the neonate by skin electrodes. Med. Biol. Eng. Comput., 13:436, 1975.
119. New, W., Barker, S.J., and Tremper, K.K.: Pulse oximetry

versus measurement of transcutaneous oxygen. J. Clin. Monit., 1:126, 1985.
120. Barker, S.J., Tremper, K.K., and Gamel, D.M.: A clinical comparison of transcutaneous P_{O2} and pulse oximetry in the operating room. Anesth. Analg., 65:805, 1986.
121. Shaw, P.J.: Neurological complications of cardiovascular surgery. II. Procedures involving the heart and thoracic aorta. Int. Anesthesiol. Clin., 24:159, 1986.
122. Arieff, A.I.: Hyponatremia, convulsions, respiratory arrest, and permanent brain damage after elective surgery in healthy women. N. Engl. J. Med., 314:1529, 1986.
123. Faulconer, A., and Bickford, R.G.: Electroencephalography in anesthesiology. American Lecture Series. Springfield, IL, Charles C Thomas, 1960.
124. Berger, H.: Über das Electrensephalogram des Menschen. Arth. F. Psychiatr. 94:16, 1931.
125. Adrian, E.D., and Matthews, B.M.C.: The interpretation of potential waves in the cortex. J. Physiol., 81:440, 1934.
126a. Gibbs, F., Gibbs, E., and Lennox, W.: Effect on EEG of certain drugs. Arch. Intern. Med., 60:154, 1937.
126b. Gibbs, F., Williams, D., and Gibbs, E.: Modification of the cortical frequency spectrum by changes in carbon dioxide, blood sugar and oxygen. J. Neurophysiol. 3:49, 1940.
127. Beecher, H.: Effects of BP on cortical potentials during anesthesia. J. Neurophysiol., 1:324, 1938.
128. Rubin, M.A., and Freeman, H.: Brain potential changes in man during cyclopropane anesthesia. J. Neurophysiol., 3:33, 1940.
129a. Schiller, F.: Consciousness Reconsidered. Arch. Neurol. Psychiat., 67:199, 1952.
129b. French, J.D., Verseans, M. and Magoun, H.W.: A neural basis of the anesthetic state. Arch. Neuro. Psychiat., 69:519, 1953.
130a. Brazier, M.B.: Blood sugar levels and EEG potentials. J. Clin. Invest. 23:319, 1944.
130b. Brazier, M.B.: The effect of drugs on the electroencephalogram of man. Clin. Pharmacol. Ther. 5:102, 1964.
131. Courtin, R.F., Bickford, R.G., and Faulconer, A.: Classification and significance of EEG patterns produced by nitrous oxide-ether anesthesia during surgical operations. Mayo Clinic Proc., 25:197, 1950.
132. Kiersey, D.K., Bickford, R.G., and Faulconer, A.: Electroencephalographic patterns produced by thiopental sodium during surgical operations: description and classification. Br. J. Anaesth., 23:141, 1951.
133. Faulconer A: Correlation of concentrations of ether in arterial blood with electroencephalographic patterns during ether-oxygen and during nitrous oxide, oxygen and ether anesthesia of human surgical patients. Anesthesiology, 13:361, 1952.
134. Possati, S., et al.: EEG patterns during anesthesia with cyclopropane. Curr. Res. Anesth. Analg., 32:130, 1953.
135a. Patrick, R.T., et al.: Analysis of gases in blood with mass spectrometer. Anesthesiology, 15:95, 1954.
135b. Patrick, R.T., Scientific exhibit. Annual Convention American Society of Anesthesiologists (Oct) 1958.
136. Lopes da Silva, F.: EEG analysis: Theory and practice. In Electroencephalography: Basic Principles, Clinical Applications, and Related Fields. Edited by E. Niedermeyer, and F. Lopes da Silvas Baltimore, Urban & Schwarzenberg, 1982.
137. Dawson G.D., and Walter, W.G.: The scope and limitations of visual and automatic analysis of the electroencephalogram. J. Neural. Neurosurg. Psychiat., 7:119, 1944.
138. Kiloh, L.G. et al.: Electroencephalography, 4th ed. London, Butterworths, 1981.

139. Dempsey, E.W., and Morrison, R.S.: The production of rhythmically recurrent cortical potentials after localized thalamic stimulation. Am. J. Physiol., 135:293, 1942.
140. Martin, J.W., Faulconer, A., and Bickford, R.G.: Electroencephalography in anesthesia. Anesthesiology, 26:359, 1959.
141. Stockard, J., and Bickford, R.: The neurophysiology of anaesthesia: a basis and practice of neuroanesthesia. Edited by E. Gordon. Amsterdam, Excerpta Medica, 1981.
142. Woodbury, S.M., et al.: Effects of carbon dioxide on brain excitability and electrolytes. Am. J. Physiol., 192:79, 1958.
143. Clowes, G.H.A., Kretschmer, H.E., and McBurney, Encephalogram in the evaluation of the effects of anesthesia agents and carbon dioxide accumulation during surgery. Ann. Surg., 138:558, 1953.
144. Reilly, E.L., Branberg, J.A., and Doty, D.B.: The effect of deep hypothermia and total circulatory arrest on the electroencephalogram in children. Electroencephalogr. Clin. Neurophysiol., 36:661, 1974.
145. Levy, W.J.: Automated EEG processing for intraoperative monitoring: A comparison of techniques. Anesthesiology, 53:223, 1980.
146a. Grundy, B.L.: Intraoperative monitoring of sensory-evoked potentials. Anesthesiology, 58:72, 1983.
146b. Desmedt, J.E., Brunko, E.: Functional organization of far-field and cortical components of somatosensory evoked potentials in normal adults. Clinical uses of cerebral, brainstem and spinal somatosensory evoked potentials. Progress in clinical neurophysiology, Vol. 7. Edited by Desmedt, J.E., Basel, S. Karger, 1980. pp 27–50.
147. Sebel, P.S., Flynn, P.J., and Ingram, D.A.: Effect of nitrous oxide on visual, auditory and somatosensory evoked potentials. Br. J. Anaesth., 56:1403, 1984.
148. Sebel, P.S., Heneghan, C.P., and Ingram, D.A.: Evoked responses—a neurophysiological indicator of depth of anaesthesia? Br. J. Anaesth., 57:841, 1985.
149. Howell, W.K.: Physiology and Biophysics, 20th ed. Philadelphia, W.B. Saunders, 1979.
150. Burke, D.L.: Intraoperative heat conservation using a reflective blanket. Anesthesiology, 60:151, 1984.
151. Larson, C.P., et al.: Effects of anesthetics on cerebral, renal, and splanchnic circulations. Anesthesiology, 41:169, 1974.
152. Forreger, R.: Surface temperatures during anesthesia. Anesthesiology, 4:392, 1943.
153. Morley-Forster, P.K.: Unintentional hypothermia in the operating room. Can. Anaesth. Soc. J., 33:576, 1986.
154. Vaughan, M.S., Vaughan, R.W., and Cork, R.C.: Postoperative hypothermia in adults: Relationship of age, anesthesia, and shivering to rewarming. Anesth. Analg., 60:746, 1981.
155. Britt, B.A.: Malignant hyperthermia. Can. Anaesth. Soc. J., 32:666, 1985.
156. Benzinger, T.M., Tympanic thermometry in surgery and anesthesia. JAMA, 209:1207, 1969.
157. Vaughan, M.S., Cork, R.C., and Vaughan, R.W.: Inaccuracy of liquid crystal thermography to identify core temperature trends in postoperative adults. Anesth. Analg., 61:284, 1982.
158. Schrier, R.W.: Acute renal failure. JAMA, 247:2518, 1982.
159. Wilson, R.F., Soullier, G., and Antonenko, D.: Creatinine clearance in critically ill surgical patients. Arch. Surg., 114:461, 1979.
160. Waterson, C.K., and Calkins, J.M.: Development directions for monitoring in anesthesia. Semin. Anesth., 5:225, 1986.
161. Cooper, J.B., Newbower, R.S., and Kitz, R.J.: An analysis of major errors and equipment failure in anesthetic management: considerations for prevention and detection. Anesthesiology, 60:34, 1984.

4

FUNDAMENTAL PHYSICS

... It is my intention to make known some new properties in gases, the effects of which are regular, by showing that these substances combine amongst themselves in very simple properties....
—Joseph L. Gay-Lussac 1802

THE MOLECULAR THEORY OF MATTER

It is well established that ordinary matter is not a uniform continuous mass but is made up of minute particles called molecules. They may exist in various states of aggregation, and these states or phases are solid, liquid, and gas (Fig. 4–1). All substances may exist naturally or may be made to exist (theoretically) in any or all phases. For example the homogeneous parts, ice, liquid water, and water vapor, are the states of aggregation common to water.

KINETICS OF MATTER

The molecules are in constant motion. This characteristic of molecules to be in constant motion is called the Kinetic Theory of Matter. When the molecules are close together there are mutual forces of attraction exerted on each other. In *solids*, these forces so limit the molecules that there is little freedom of motion. The molecules do not alter their relative position but merely oscillate about a fixed point. In *liquids* the binding force is less; there is greater freedom, less rigidity, and the molecules change relative positions. The oscillating molecules may escape from the cage of their neighbors and enter a new cage. The cohesive forces are sufficient to maintain volume but not to maintain shape and changes in shape occur.

In *gases* the cohesive tendency is nil and the substances expand indefinitely regardless of the space. The molecules are moving rapidly at high speeds and are far apart. The cohesive or attraction forces are insufficient to overcome the effect of their high speeds and the molecules move apart. Changes in volume brought about by pressure are due to de-

SOLID

Cohesive forces—binding
Freedom of motion—small
Molecular position—constant
Motion—oscillatory about fixed point
Shape—rigid
Volume—constant

GAS

Cohesive tendency—none
Freedom of motion—complete
Molecular position—not constant
Motion—completely haphazard
Shape—not kept
Volume—not kept; molecules move apart

LIQUID

Cohesive forces—strong
Freedom of motion—great
Molecular position—not constant
Motion—in all directions
Shape—not maintained
Volume—constant

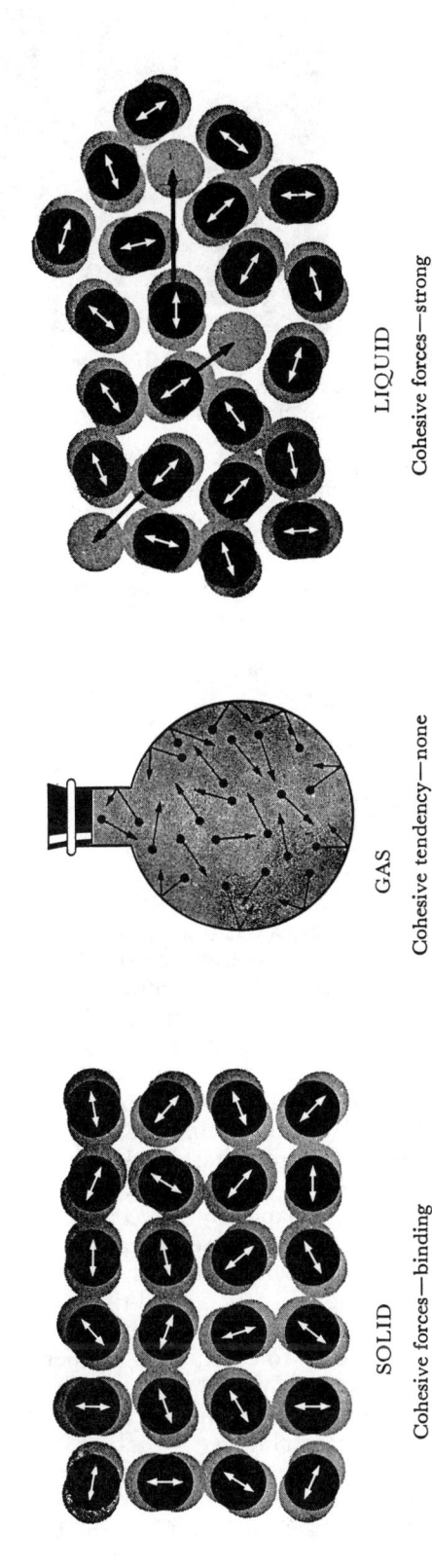

FIG. 4–1. Kinetic theory of matter. Composition of matter—Molecules. Physical property—Constant motion. Phases—solids, liquids, gases. From Chemical Bond Approach Project: Chemical Systems. New York, McGraw-Hill, 1964.[1]

101

creasing the space between molecules and not to change in size of molecules.

BEHAVIOR OF GASES

Since the molecules of a gas are moving about in space with huge velocity, they collide with each other frequently and strike the walls of the containing vessels. The path of each is absolutely hap-hazard. This bombardment gives rise to the pressure exerted by the gas. Furthermore the pressure exerted by a gas does not decrease with time; hence the average velocity is unaltered. If the volume or space in which a given quantity of gas is enclosed is increased, the number of molecular impacts on a given area is decreased, this is, a smaller number of molecules strikes any area of the wall in a given time and hence the pressure decreases. On the basis of the kinetic and molecular theories of matter, the behavior of gases can be predicted fairly accurately and laws expressing this behavior have been formulated.

Boyle's Law[2]

The relationship between the volume and pressure of a gas when temperature is constant was formulated by Boyle into a law in 1662. The law states that at any constant temperature the volume occupied by a quantity of gas is inversely proportional to the pressure exerted on it (Fig. 4–2).

Although all substances undergo some decrease in volume with increasing pressure, only gases undergo changes in volume that are inversely proportional. However, even under ideal conditions the gases show deviations and hence the law is not an exact one but a *limiting law*.

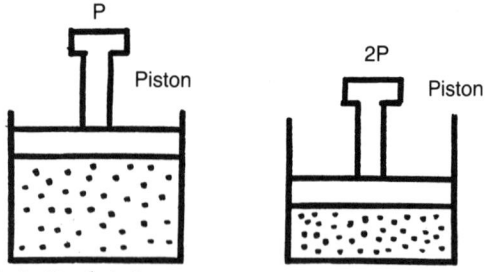

FIG. 4–2. Boyle's Law.

STATEMENT: The volume of a gas at constant temperature is inversely proportional to the pressure.

FORMULA: $V \propto \frac{1}{P}$ or $\frac{P}{P_o} = \frac{V_o}{V}$

EXAMPLE: If pressure P exerted on a volume gas V is doubled—2P—the volume is halved—$\frac{V}{2}$.

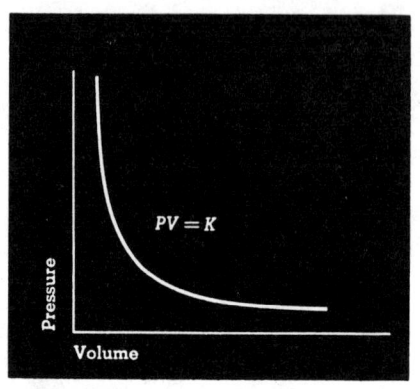

FIG. 4–3. The product of the pressure and volume of a gas sample is a constant provided that the total mass (g) and the temperature (T) of the sample are constant.

$$PV = K \ (T \text{ and } g \text{ constant})$$

From Chemical Bond Approach Project: Chemical Systems. New York, McGraw-Hill, 1964.

Generally it is expressed (as shown in Fig. 4–3) that the:

$$\text{Pressure} \propto \frac{1}{\text{Volume}} \text{ or}$$
$$\text{Pressure} \times \text{Volume} = K$$

Charles's Law[3]

Heating a substance increases molecular movement and in the case of gases there is a tendency to expand. Charles in 1787 found experimentally that equal volumes of all gases kept at *constant pressure* expand by equal increments of volume for each degree centigrade rise in temperature (Fig. 4–4).

The increment of increase for each degree is 1/273 of the volume of the gas at 0° C. On the other hand for each degree of cooling there is lessened molecular activity with contraction and a decrease of 1/273 of the volume at 0° C for each degree fall in temperature. Charles's Law may thus be restated as follows: A given quantity of gas, kept at constant pressure, expands by 1/273 of its volume at 0° C for each degree rise in temperature.

It is apparent from this that if a quantity of gas were progressively cooled there would be a progressive decrease in volume until at −273° C the gas would cease to exist. This temperature is called the absolute zero point below which it is impossible to go. From these conditions a gas scale of temperature has been established which is often called the absolute scale or the Kelvin temperature scale. On this scale 0° C is equal to 273° absolute and the boiling point of water of 100° C is equal to 373° absolute.

Charles's Law has been formulated likewise (Fig. 4–5) on the absolute scale

$$\frac{T}{T_1} = \frac{V}{V_1} \ (P \text{ constant})$$

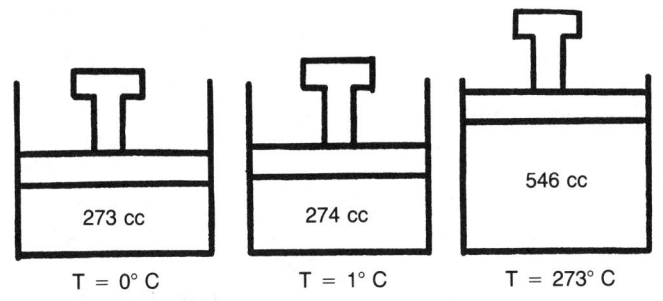

FIG. 4-4. Charles's Law.

STATEMENT: Equal volumes of all gases at constant pressure expand by equal increments of volume namely 1/273 of the volume of the gas at 0° C, for each degree centigrade rise in temperature.

FORMULA: $\frac{T}{T_o} = \frac{V}{V_o}$ (P is constant and T is absolute)

EXAMPLE: If the temperature of a 273 ml volume of gas at 0° C is raised 1° C, the volume becomes 274 ml. If T is raised to 273° C the resultant volume is doubled.

or if the progressive nature of the change is considered we may write for each increment change in volume denoted by (dv), an increment change in temperature denoted by (dt) and that the ratio is a constant dv/dt = k.

Gay-Lussac's Law[2]

In 1802 Gay-Lussac corroborated Charles's findings but he worked with a *constant volume*. He found that when a quantity of gas at 0° C is heated while the volume is kept constant, the pressure increases a definite fraction of its value at 0° C for each degree rise in temperature (Fig. 4–6). This fraction is 1/273 of the pressure at 0° C.

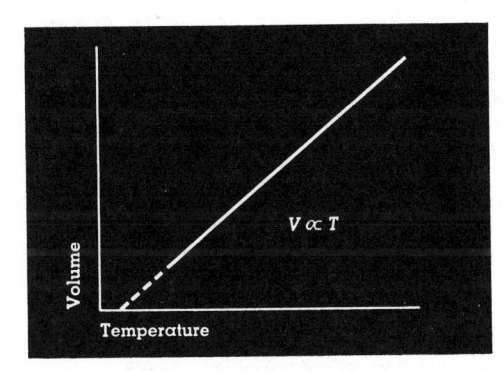

FIG. 4-5. The volume of a gas sample is proportional to the absolute temperature of the sample provided that the total mass (g) and pressure (P) of the sample are constant.

$V \propto T$ (P and g constant)

From Chemical Bond Approach Project: Chemical Systems. New York, McGraw-Hill, 1964.

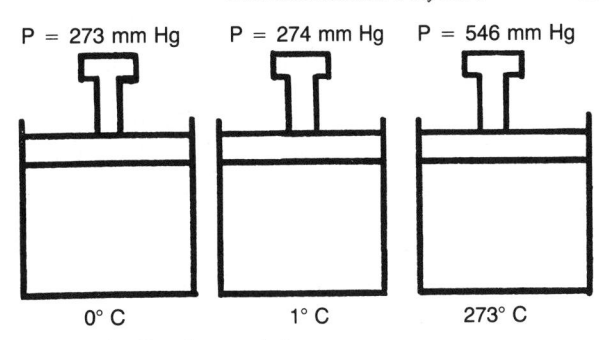

FIG. 4-6. Gay-Lussac's Law.

STATEMENT: When a quantity of gas kept at a constant volume is heated the pressure increases a definite fraction of its value at 0° C for each degree centigrade rise in temperature. The fraction is 1/273 of the pressure at 0° C. $P \propto T$.

FORMULA: $\frac{T}{T_o} = \frac{P}{P_o}$ (V is constant; T is absolute)

EXAMPLE: If the pressure of a volume of gas is 273 mm Hg at 0° C raising T 1° C increases P to 274 mm Hg. If T is raised to 273° C then P is doubled. V is constant.

Formulated on the absolute scale we may write (Fig. 4-7)

$$\frac{T}{T_1} = \frac{P}{P_1} \text{ (V = constant)}$$

or the ratio of each fraction change in pressure (dp) to each fraction change in temperature (dt) equals a constant or dp/dt = k.

By combining the three laws just given we can write the equation for the *ideal gas law* as

$$\frac{PV}{T} = k \text{ (constant)}$$

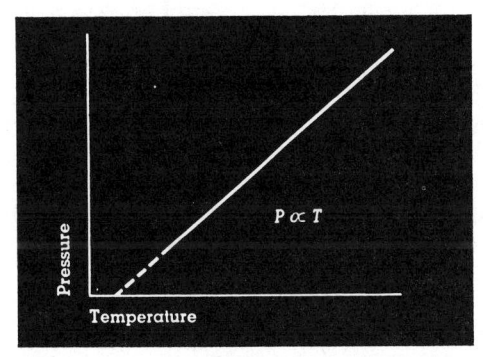

FIG. 4-7. The pressure of a gas sample is proportional to the absolute temperature of the sample provided that the total mass (g) and the volume (V) of the sample are constant.

$P \propto T$ (V and g constant)

From Chemical Bond Approach Project: Chemical Systems. New York, McGraw-Hill, 1964.

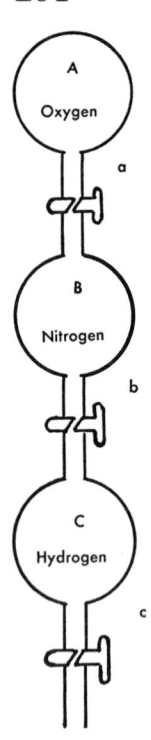

FIG. 4–8. Dalton's Law.

LAW: In a mixture of gases each exerts its own pressure independent of the other gases, or the total pressure (P) equals the sum of the pressures exerted by the parts (p).

FORMULA: $P = p_1 + p_2 + \ldots\ldots p_x$

EXAMPLE: Three bulbs of equal volume are filled with oxygen, nitrogen, and hydrogen each at a pressure of one atmosphere. If stopcock (b) is opened and the hydrogen forced into B by allowing mercury to flow into C through (c) then the pressure in B becomes 2 atmospheres or the sum of the pressures of the parts pH and pN. By forcing the contents of B into A the total pressure in A becomes 3 atmospheres, that is,
$P = pO + pN + pH$.

Dalton's Law[2]

This law states that in a mixture of gases each exerts its pressure independently of the others (Fig. 4–8). The pressure exerted by one gas is called the "partial pressure" and is that part of the total pressure due to the particular species of molecules under consideration. It follows that the total pressure in any gaseous mixture must be the sum of the partial pressures of all the gaseous substances present.

For example, the atmosphere (dry) exerts a pressure of 760 mm Hg at sea level. It is composed chiefly of oxygen, nitrogen, and carbon dioxide in the proportions of 20.96%, 79%, and 0.04%, respectively. Thus the partial pressure of oxygen is 20.96/100 of the total pressure or 159.2 mm Hg; that of nitrogen is 79/100 of 760 mm Hg or 596.45 mm Hg; and that of carbon dioxide is 0.04/100 of 760 mm Hg or 0.30 mm Hg. Dalton's Law may therefore be stated in another form, namely, the partial pressure of a gas is proportional to its percentage by volume in the mixture. Or, for instance atmospheric pressure (P) may be written as follows:

$$P = P_{O_2} + P_{N_2} + P_{CO_2}$$

Where P_{O_2} is partial pressure of oxygen, P_{N_2} the partial pressure of nitrogen, and P_{CO_2} the partial pressure of carbon dioxide.

Henry's Law[2]

The solubility of a gas in a liquid at a given temperature is proportional to the partial pressure of the gas above the liquid. This is Henry's Law. The same law may be expressed as a *vapor pressure law* for volatile solutes. Thus, the partial pressure of a volatile solute from a solution is porportional to its concentration in the solution:

P (partial pressure) ∝ C (concentration in solution).

Or the concentration of solute molecules above the solution is proportional to the concentration of solute molecules in the solution. For this law to apply there must be no chemical combination of the solute and the solvent. The law applies to oxygen, nitrogen, and inert gases but *not* to carbon dioxide.

For example if a gas lies in contact with the surface of a liquid, some of the gas molecules will penetrate the surface and become dissolved in it. Initially a few molecules of the gas will leave the liquid, but a greater number will be entering the liquid. This process continues until the tensions of the gas within and without the liquid are in equilibrium. At this point the number of molecules entering the solution is equal to the number leaving.

SOLUBILITY OF GASES IN LIQUIDS[3]

The amount dissolved depends on the nature of the liquid, the presence of solutes, and the temperature. The higher the temperature, the less the amount of gas dissolved. When a state of equilibrium is attained between the gas dissolved in a liquid and the overlying gas phase, the tensions will equalize. Techniques for the measurement of the dissolved gas or vapor utilize the basic tonometer method and the polarographic electrode.

In Table 4–1 of the solubilities of gases, the solubility coefficients are listed in terms of ml of gas measured at 38° C and 760 mm Hg that will dissolve in 100 ml of water.

At conditions of 0° C and barometric pressure of 1 atmosphere, the solubility of oxygen at a pressure of 760 mm Hg is 0.049 ml in 1 ml of water (or 4.9 ml in 1 dl).

At conditions of 20° C and 760 mm Hg, 0.03 ml of oxygen dissolves in 1 ml of water, which is 3 ml in 100 ml of water.

At 38° C, 2.38 ml of oxygen is dissolved in 100 ml of water.

In biologic systems,[4] the blood and tissues represent the liquid system, while the respiratory gases and the inhaled anesthetic agents represent the gases. The amount of oxygen dissolved in blood depends on the partial pressure of the gas and the temperature. At 20° C and 1 atmosphere, the solubility coefficient of O_2 at 760 mm Hg in blood is 0.034 ml O_2 per 1 ml of blood. At body temperature of 37° C (barometric pressure of 1 atmosphere) when the partial pressure of oxygen is 760 mm Hg, (less vapor pressure of water) the amount dissolved in 1 ml of blood is 0.023 ml of oxygen. Actually, oxygen is dissolved in the plasma.

Coefficients of Solubility[3]

The extent to which a gas dissolves in a liquid is expressed in solubility coefficients. Three such coefficients have been defined.

BUNSEN SOLUBILITY COEFFICIENT (α). This is defined as the volume of gas at standard conditions of 0° C and 1 atmosphere pressure dissolved in a unit volume of solvent, when the partial pressure of the gas is 760 mm Hg. Measured at standard conditions of 0° C (or 273° K) and barometric pressure of 1 atmosphere, the Bunsen coefficient for oxygen in water when partial pressure of oxygen is 760 mm Hg is 0.049, i.e., 4.9 ml O_2 dissolves in 100 ml water at 0° C. At 38° C, the Bunsen coefficient for oxygen at 1 atmosphere pressure is 0.0238 ml per 1 ml of water. For blood at 38° C, the Bunsen coefficient for oxygen is 0.0230. Bunsen coefficients (named for Robert von Bunsen) are usually given in the International Critical Tables. This coefficient can be obtained from the Ostwald coefficient when the value is corrected to standard temperature of 273K (= 0° C) i.e., Ostwald coefficient multiplied by 273° K over the absolute temperature (KT) at which solubility is obtained at body temperatures Kt = 310K by 273° K/TK = Bunsen Coefficient (T/273).

OSTWALD SOLUBILITY COEFFICIENT (λ). This coefficient is determined by application of the basic gas law equation and uses absolute temperatures KT (Kelvin) for calculations. It is defined as the volume of a gas taken up by a unit volume of liquid under conditions noted above. The measurement and calculation assume that the gas phase is always pure gas. In anesthesia studies this is the most convenient coefficient.[4] It is numerically equal to the simple tissue (blood)–gas partition coefficient.

PARTITION COEFFICIENT. A partition coefficient describes the relative capacity of a substance to be distributed between equal volumes of two phases. The amount in each phase is determined at equilibrium when partial pressure in each phase is equal. Conventionally in anesthesia practice the coefficient refers to the distribution between tissue phase (blood) and gas phase. "Blood solubility" means a blood/gas partition coefficient and "tissue solubility" is a tissue/blood partition coefficient.

This is a distribution coefficient. It is defined as the ratio of the amount of a substance present in equal volumes of two phases at a stated temperature. This is a volume–volume distribution.

VARIATIONS. Coefficients will vary somewhat among different subjects. These variations are related to hematocrit, degree of hydration, and the lipid and protein content of the blood.

Lowe reports a significant relationship between hematocrit and blood–gas partition coefficient.[5] The

TABLE 4–1. COEFFICIENTS OF SOLUBILITY (INTERNATIONAL CRITICAL TABLES) IN 100 ml OF WATER AT 38° C OF AGENTS USED IN ANESTHESIA (AT 1 ATM).

Agent	Solubility Coefficient (ml)
Oxygen	2.4
Carbon dioxide	55.0
Nitrous oxide	0.41
Ethylene	0.09
Cyclopropane	0.011
Ethyl chloride	0.25
Vinyl ether	5.2
Ether diethyl	15.4
Chloroform	0.014
Halothane	0.74
Isoflurane	0.61
Enflurane	0.78
Methoxyflurane	4.5

halothane partition coefficient for plasma is 1.37. There is also a partition coefficient for the red blood cells of 0.021 for each hematocrit unit. Thus, the whole blood–gas partition coefficient is calculated as follows:

Halothane coefficient = 1.37 + 0.021 × Hct

i.e., for a hematocrit of 45 the coefficient is 2.31.

An alteration in brain lipid content, which increases with age, increases the anesthetic brain tissue concentration and hence brain–blood partition coefficient.

After eating, a person's blood–gas solubility coefficient increases for several inhaled volatile anesthetic agents by 17 to 34% (except nitrous oxide). The rate of rise of the end tidal air, therefore the alveolar air, is below pre-eating control values by 8%, while the rate of blood uptake is increased 20%.[6]

BLOOD SOLUBILITY OF ANESTHETICS[4,7]

This is best expressed as a blood–gas partition coefficient and is determined at body temperature (Table 4–2). It represents the ratio of the anesthetic concentration in blood to the anesthetic concentration in the gas phase at equilibrium. An equilibrium is established when the partial pressure is equal in the two phases.

Gas tensions in arterial blood of anesthetic agents progressively increase with duration of administration and approach an equilibrium with inspired tension.

The solubility of the agent largely determines the shape of the curve of blood uptake. The increase in partial pressure in blood is rapid for the relatively insoluble agents and slow for those that are more soluble. This is evident in the sharp bend or "knee" of the curve for slightly soluble agents. For more

TABLE 4–2. BLOOD–GAS PARTITION COEFFICIENTS AT 37° C

Gas	Blood/Gas	Brain Gray/White	Liver	Kidney	Muscle	Heart	Fat
Ethylene	0.16	—	—	—	—	1.0	6
Cyclopropane	0.46	1.34/3.6	1.1	0.7	0.7	1.8	15.0
Nitrous oxide	0.47	1.10/1.1	0.9	0.9	0.9	1.1	2.3
Fluroxene	1.37	1.14/1.7	1.4	0.9	1.4	1.4	23.0
Isoflurane	1.43	2.6/?	2.5	—	4.0	—	48.0
Enflurane	1.91	1.45/?	2.1	—	1.7	—	37.0
Halothane	2.36	2.1/3.3	2.5	1.5	2.5	2.9	65.0
Oxygen (100%)	2.40	—	—	—	—	—	—
Divinyl ether	2.80	—	—	—	—	—	—
Trichlorethylene	9.5	—	—	—	—	—	—
Chloroform	10.3	1.0	—	—	—	1.0	—
Diethylether	12.1	1.1	0.9	0.8	0.9	1.0	4.2
Methoxyflurane	13.0	1.8/2.4	2.3	1.8	1.8	—	61.0

From Eger, E.I., II Anesthetic Uptake and Action. Baltimore, Williams & Wilkins Co. 1974 and Larson, 1964, and Steward A., et al.: Solubility coefficient for inhaled anesthetics for water, and oil biological media. Br. J. Anaesth., 45:282; 1973.

soluble agents, the knee is not sharp and blood tension approaches the inspired concentration slowly.

Avogadro's Law[2]

In 1811 Avogadro stated that equal volumes of all gases under the same conditions of temperature and pressure contain the same number of molecules; that is, the number of molecules contained in a given volume of (ideal) gas under fixed conditions is independent of the nature of the gas.

It is possible to calculate the number of molecules in a gram molecule of a gas. A gram molecule (mol) is the molecular weight of a substance expressed in grams. All calculations indicate the number to be of the order of 6×10^{23}, and this is called "Avogadro's number" or *Avogadro's constant*. Thus 32 grams of oxygen (which is a gram molecule of oxygen, the molecular weight being 32) contains 6×10^{23} number of molecules. Furthermore, under standard conditions the number of gas molecules in a gram molecular weight of a substance will occupy 22.4 liters. This is one *molal volume*.

STANDARD CONDITIONS

Comparison of properties of different substances of similar state must be done under similar conditions. These conditions particularly refer to temperature and pressure and have been arbitrarily chosen as 0° C and 760 mm Hg pressure (atmospheric pressure at sea level). These are the standard conditions.

WEIGHT OF GAS OR VAPOR

The weight of a gas or vapor may be expressed either as density or specific gravity. The first is in absolute values and the latter in relative values. The latter is more commonly used.

DENSITY

Density is defined as the mass per unit volume for any substance. It is the ratio of mass to volume. It depends on both temperature and pressure and these must be specified. The standard density of a substance is its density at the standard temperature and pressure (0° C and 764 mm Hg). In SI units it is kilograms per cubic meter ($kg \cdot m^{-3}$). In the CGS system, it is grams per cubic centimeter ($g \cdot cm^{-3}$).

For solids and liquids, density is expressed as grams per cubic centimeter, at a stated temperature and pressure, although pressure is negligible for solids. An important density consent is that for water. The maximum density (Q_{max}) of air-free and ion-free water at 764 mm Hg and 4° C is 0.999972 ($kg \cdot cm^{-3}$ or g/cm^3). It is usually stated as 1 g/ml. At 37° C and 764 mm Hg, the density of distilled water is 0.9934.

The relationship between density and temperature is inverse. Measurements of water show a *curvilinear* decrease in density with increasing temperatures:[9]

Temperature (% C)	Density (1 g/ml)
4	0.999972
20	0.9968
25	0.9958
30	0.9948
37	0.9934

For gases, it is the weight in g of 1 L of that gas under standard conditions. If the molecular weight of the gas is known, the density or weight of 1 L at standard conditions may be determined by the formula:

$$\frac{\text{Molecular Weight}}{22.4} = \text{g/Liter}$$

Air density is stated according to temperature and at 764 mm Hg. At 20° C, the weight of 1 L is 1.20 g.

At 0° C it is 1.29 g. At 37° C the density of air is approximately 1.00. Measurements of air densities at different temperatures and 764 mm Hg also show a curvilinear inverse relationship:

Temperature (° C)	Air Density (g/L)
0	1.29
20	1.20
25	1.18
30	1.11
37	1.00

Densities of Some Anesthetics[2]

On this basis the density of nitrous oxide is 2 gL, that of ether vapor (mol. wt. = 74) is 3.3 gL and that of air is 1.3 gL at standard conditions. For practical purposes the density of air is often taken as 1 gL at room conditions (T = 20°; 760 mm Hg).

The densities of the volatile anesthetics in the *liquid state* are as follows: ether = 0.72; vinethene = 0.77; chloroform = 1.5; halothane = 1.86; enflurane = 1.5; and isoflurane = 1.49.

SPECIFIC GRAVITY

Specific gravity is the ratio of the weight of a unit volume of one substance to a similar volume of water in the case of solids and liquids or of air in the case of gases but both substances compared must be under the same conditions of temperature and pressure. The value of the weight of water and air is taken as unity. Specific gravities are therefore relative expressions of weight. In the case of gases the specific gravity is the ratio of the weight of a unit volume of the gas to the weight of a similar volume of air under similar circumstances. (Table 4–3).

DIFFUSION OF GASES

The passage of a gas from one place to another depends on molecular movement. The passage or movement is called *diffusion*. The direction of diffusion is determined by differences in partial pressure and not by any difference in the amount of the gas. A gas diffuses from a place where it is at a high partial pressure to one where it is at a lower partial pressure. This occurs even though at the point of lower partial pressure there is a larger volume of the gas.

The rate or velocity of molecular movement at which diffusion of a gas occurs through a porous earthenware partition or certain semipermeable membranes is inversely proportional to the square root of the molecular weight or the density of the gas. This is *Graham's Law*.

For example (Fig. 4–9) 100 ml of oxygen (M_2 = 32 molecular weight) will flow under a small (constant)

TABLE 4–3. SPECIFIC GRAVITIES OF GASES AND VAPORS COMMONLY USED IN ANESTHESIA

Agent	Specific Gravity
Carbon Dioxide	1.5
Nitrous Oxide	1.53
Cyclopropane	1.46
Oxygen	1.10
Air	1.0
Nitrogen	0.96
Ethylene	0.97
Helium 80%; Oxygen 20%	0.34
Helium	0.13
Water Vapor	0.6
Ether Vapor	2.6
Vinethene Vapor	2.2
Ethyl Chloride Vapor	2.28
Chloroform Vapor	4.12
Enflurane	8.21
Isoflurane	8.20

decreasing pressure through a pinhole in a thin plate in 76 sec (t_1) and under the same conditions 100 ml of carbon dioxide (M_2 = 44 molecular weight) will escape in 92 sec (t_2). Since time and velocity have an inverse relationship this example may be formulated using time in the following proportionality:

$$\frac{t_1}{t_2} = \frac{M_1}{M_2}$$

The passage of a gas into a liquid or the diffusion velocity into the liquid (absorption) may be calculated using certain constants peculiar to the situation under consideration. The diffusion velocity is inversely proportional to the square root of the density but it is directly proportional to the pressure gradient and to the solubility of the gas in the liquid. The formula is expressed as follows:

Diffusion Velocity =

$$\frac{\text{Pressure Gradient} \times \text{Solubility of Gas}}{\sqrt{\text{Density}}} \times K$$

Since the vapor density of most anesthetic gases falls within a narrow range, the pressure gradient and solubility of the gas become of chief importance in determining velocity of diffusion into liquid of agents commonly used.

SURFACE TENSION

A fundamental cause of surface tension is the intermolecular force of cohesion. All the molecules within the bulk of a liquid, for example, attract each other with a cohesive force sufficient to maintain the liquid state. Cohesion, however, does not exert a measurable effect unless molecules are very close to each other at a distance of the order of 1 mm between their centers. Consideration of a liquid–gas interface such as the surface of water in contact with

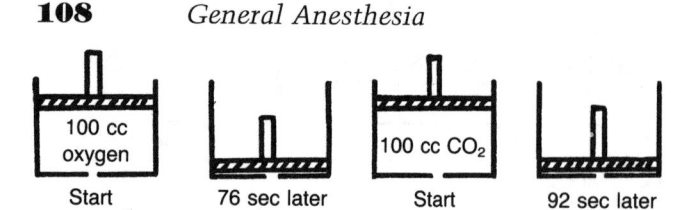

FIG. 4–9. Diffusion of Gases.

Depends on molecular activity.
Depends on pressure differences.
Direction of diffusion depends on differences in partial pressure of the gas and not on differences in volume.
Rate of diffusion depends on molecular weight.

GRAHAM'S LAW OF EFFUSION: The velocity (μ) of molecular movement through a porous earthenware partition is inversely proportional to the square root of the molecular weight or the density of the gas.

FORMULA: $\mu \propto \dfrac{1}{\sqrt{M}}$ or $\dfrac{\mu}{\mu_o} = \dfrac{\sqrt{M_o}}{\sqrt{M}}$

EXAMPLE: See text for explanation.

air shows the effects of cohesion at such a phase boundary.

The tension at any interface or surface, of a liquid in particular, follows the principles of minimal surfaces: due to the cohesive forces, substances assume a shape that affords the smallest area permitted by surrounding conditions. Those on the surface are not attracted equally and are pulled inward by the underlying molecules. The surface, therefore, shrinks, and the resultant inward force is designated as *surface* or *interfacial tension*. That is, the molecules in the surface layer are under a special strain of unbalanced forces. The surface, therefore, possesses free energy of which the intensity factor is the degree of tension and the capacity factor is the area. The work done in spreading or extending a surface by 1 cm against the spontaneous contracting surface force of T dynes per centimeter is T ergs per cm^2.

Measurement of Surface Tension

Surface tension may be defined as the force of contraction exerted across a line of unit length of the boundary edge of a membrane. It is stated in units of force per unit length and operates in the plane of the surface. Units of surface tension are expressed as dynes per centimeter. At 20° C, pure water has a surface tension of 73 dynes/cm, while plasma and tissue fluids at 37° C have a tension of 57 to 58 dynes/cm. It is estimated that the surface tension recoil of the lung is 20,000 dynes/cm, and would exert a pressure of 20 cm of water (1 cm of water = 980 dynes, the *gravitation constant*).

Surface tension is also measured in units of ergs per square centimeter. It is then represented by the symbol which is numerically equal to sigma (σ) or surface tension in dynes per centimeter since a weight of 1 g would be required to pull a film of 1 cm length and unit tension so as to make its area 1 sq cm, that is, *to do 1 erg of work on the film*.

Methods of measurement include: (1) capillary tube method; (2) stalagmometer or dripping device; and (3) torsion balance.

LA PLACE'S LAW. Considering spheres or bubbles it is evident that the tension in the wall of the surface tends to contract and that the pressure within tends to resist contraction or expansion. At the time there is no change in size an equilibrium will exist and the forces are equal. The relationship is expressed as

$$P \text{ (air pressure inside)} = \dfrac{2T}{r}$$

where T is tension and r is radius. If surface tension remains constant the air pressure required to inflate increases as radius decreases. Conversely as the radius increases less pressure is required to enlarge a bubble.

HEAT

This is a form of energy that can be given to or taken from matter. It is distinct from temperature, which is an expression of the thermal state, and indicates whether one substance will give or receive heat from another substance. The *calorie* is the unit of heat energy and is defined as the amount of heat required to raise the temperature of 1 g of water 1° C from 14.5 to 15.5° C.

PHYSICS OF VAPORIZATION

Molecules of water and other liquids are constantly in motion and some of these in the surface layer develop sufficient speed to overcome the attraction exerted by neighboring molecules. They thus escape from the liquid and enter the gaseous phase.

The change in state from a liquid to a gaseous phase is the process of vaporization. Cohesive forces of molecular attraction exist between the liquid molecules that are much greater than dispersive forces. The most important forces of molecular attraction are known as *van der Waals forces*. Such forces exist because of the following considerations: each molecule has a negative and positive pole; and two atoms or molecules when close together assume a dipolar relationship (Fig. 4–10). That is, there is attraction between areas of unlike charge and repulsion between areas of like charge. Large molecules of high molecular weight have strong van der Waals forces, accompanied by a decrease in volatility.

Dispersive forces depend on molecular motion

FIG. 4–10. Illustrates forces of molecular attraction (van der Waals forces) by virtue of dipolar orientation.

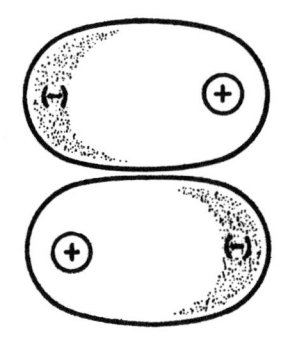

and the value of the kinetic energy of each molecule. The quantity of kinetic energy is proportional to the speed and molecular mass ($E = mv^2$). Addition of heat increases the speed and temperature, which reflects kinetic energy, provides an index to the dispersive force available.

Molecules move at different speeds in a different fluid. Collisions occur that impart more kinetic energy to some molecules and less to that of others. A frequency distribution curve exists of the molecules possessing various levels of energy. Those molecules that have sufficient kinetic energy to overcome van der Waals forces enter the gaseous phase and are in violent random motion (Fig. 4–11).

Vapor Pressure

Molecules of a substance existing above the liquid phase are collectively designated as a vapor and the process by which this vapor is formed is called *evaporation*. The molecules of a vapor are in violent

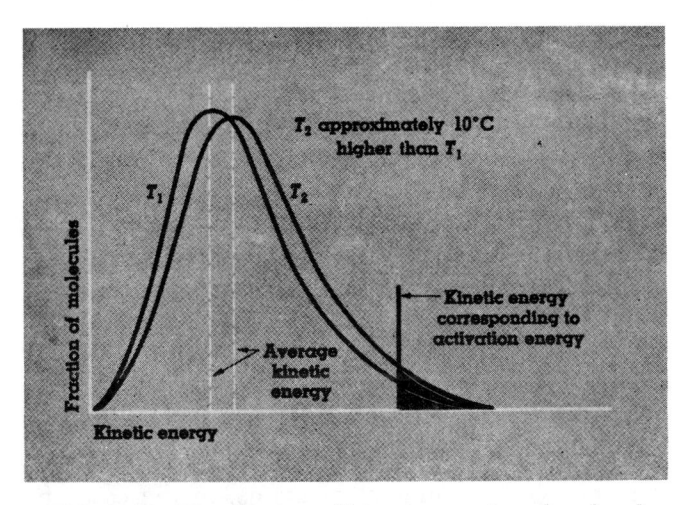

FIG. 4–11. Distribution of kinetic energies of molecules in a system at two different temperatures, T_1 and T_2. Shaded areas under curves at right show the relative fractions of molecules having kinetic energies greater than the activation energy for a reaction. From Chemical Bond Approach Project: Chemical Systems. New York, McGraw-Hill, 1964.

motion. As they strike the walls of the container they exert a pressure. At any definite temperature when a liquid and its vapor are in equilibrium the pressure exerted by the vapor is called the *vapor pressure* of the liquid. It must be clearly understood that vapor pressure is an equilibrium pressure and indeed is a saturation pressure. For example, water vapor in the absence of the liquid phase may exert a partial pressure that is anything less than the vapor pressure.

If the temperature of a liquid is raised by heating, molecular escape from the surface or vaporization is hastened. Finally a temperature is reached at which the vapor pressure of the liquid equals atmospheric pressure. This is the *boiling point*. Liquids whose vapors have anesthetic properties are usually considered useful and sufficiently volatile if the boiling point of the liquid is below 60° C.

The vapor pressure curves for the commonly used volatile agents are shown in Figure 4–12. From these curves one can calculate the percent saturation of an agent in the carrier gas.

Specific Heat

A definite quantity of heat is required by each substance for its temperature to be raised. The number of calories required to raise the temperature of 1 g of substance by 1° C is called specific heat. The specific heat of water is 1 since 1 calorie is necessary to raise the temperature of 1 g by 1° C. No other substance possesses such a high specific heat. The specific heats of some substances of importance to the anesthetist are noted in Table 4–4.

Latent Heat of Vaporization

At the boiling point a considerable amount of heat is required to change the liquid to a vapor without any rise in temperature. This heat is called the latent heat of vaporization and may be defined as the amount of heat in calories required to convert 1 g of a substance from the liquid to the vapor state without temperature change. It represents energy required to overcome the attractive forces acting between the molecules of a liquid. This latent heat of vaporization represents the energy of molecular separation.

For example, at barometric pressure of 760 mm Hg when a temperature of 100° C is attained by water, the continued addition of heat is needed to effect a change of state though there is no change in temperature. Each gram of water actually absorbs 537 calories before it changes to the vapor state. The latent heat of vaporization of ether is 83.9 calories per g or 63 calories per ml.

Measurements now are expressed as molar heat of vaporization (H_m) and defined as the amount of heat in joules required to change the state of 1 mol

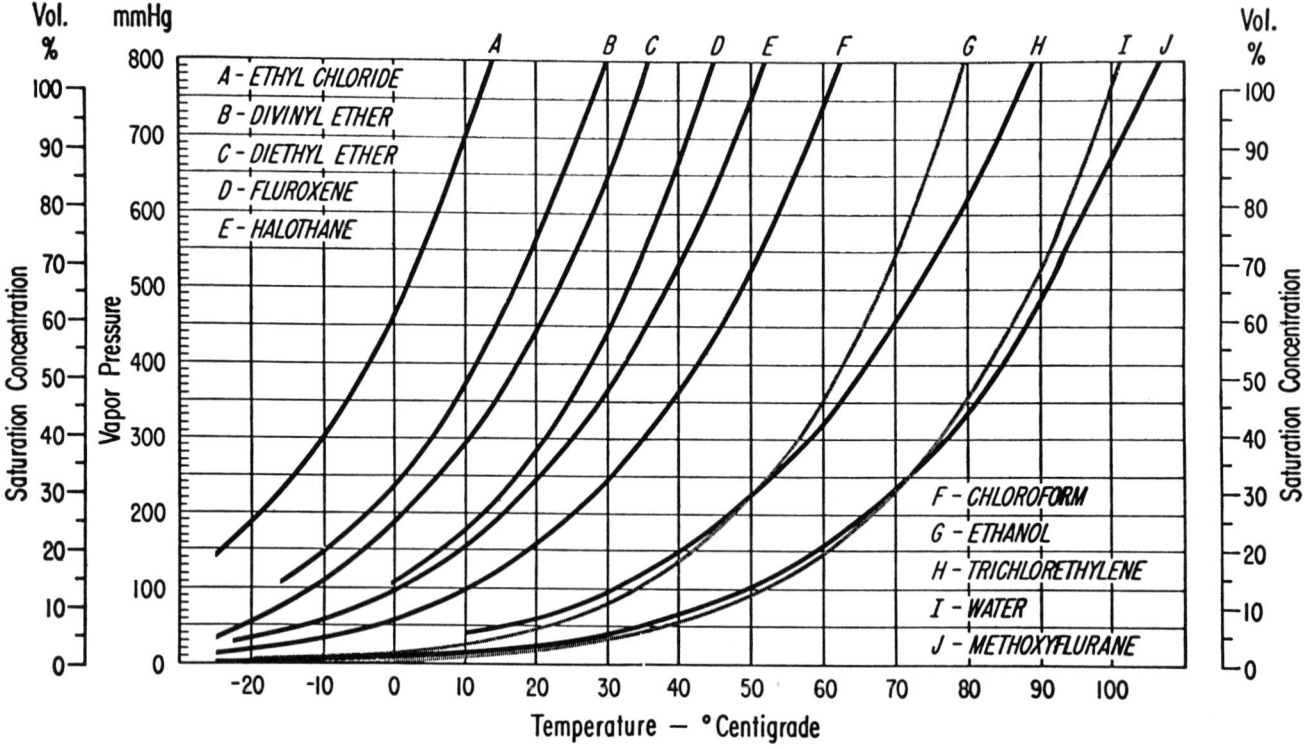

FIG. 4–12. The saturated vapor pressure curves of liquids commonly used in anesthesia. The curves give an indication of the comparative saturation pressures through the temperature range. They are *semidiagrammatic* and should not be used for obtaining accurate data. From: Macintosh, R.R., Mushin, W.W., Epstein, B.: Physics for the Anaesthetist, 4th ed. Revised by Mushin, W., and Jones, P.: Oxford, England, Blackwell Scientific Publications, 1987.

of the liquid into its vapour without a change in temperature. The unit is Joule mol^{-1}. Conversion units: one (1) joule = 0.239 cal; one (1) cal = 4.1875 J.

PROCESS OF VAPORIZATION

In this process of vaporization energy must be expended to overcome the natural cohesive tendency of the liquid. Such energy is obtained as heat from either an outside source or object or the liquid itself. Available heat depends on the specific heat of the source and is directed toward:

1. Raising the temperature of the liquid
2. Changing the physical state of the liquid (determined by latent heat of vaporization)

Thus, the chief requisites for vaporization are heat and a source of heat. To determine the amount of heat necessary to vaporize a substance one must first calculate the heat needed in calories to reach the boiling point and then add the heat in calories needed for the change of state.

One may apply the following formula:

1. Calories required for raising temperature = weight of substance × specific heat × temperature rise (C)
2. Calories required for change of state = the calories representing the latent heat of vaporization × weight of the substance

For example, if one wished to know the amount of heat necessary to vaporize 1 g of ether one would first determine the calories necessary to raise the temperature of the liquid ether from room temperature to the boiling point of ether. Thus, 1 g × 0.521 (specific heat of ether) × (34.5° C − 20.0° C) = 7.5 cal. A further quantity of heat is necessary for the change of state and here we must multiply the number of calories required as latent heat of vaporization per gram by the number of grams. In the case of ether this is 84.0 cal per g. The total caloric requirement then becomes 91.5 calories of heat to vaporize 1 g of ether.

Another method utilizes the heat of *adsorption*. The process of adsorption is characterized by surface tension and condensation. When substances are

TABLE 4–4. SPECIFIC HEATS AND LATENT HEATS OF VAPORIZATION OF SELECTED SUBSTANCES

Substance	Specific Heat (cal/g)	Specific Heat (cal/ml)	Latent Heat of Vaporization (cal/g)	Latent Heat of Vaporization (kJoule/g)
Water	1.0	1.0	537	4.19
Ether	0.52	0.36	83.9	0.37
Air (1 g = 770 ml)	0.14	0.0003	—	—
Copper	0.8	—	—	—
Vinethene	0.55	0.42	89	
Chloroform	0.23	0.34	64	247 0.28
Trichloroethylene	0.32	0.22	58	239 0.24
Ethyl chloride	0.36	0.33	92	—
Halothane	0.42	0.78	35	147 0.15
Isoflurane	0.28	0.42	44	151 0.15
Enflurane	0.29	0.35	42	157 0.16

brought in contact with a material of high adsorptive capacity (e.g., activated charcoal) the adsorptive surface tends to reduce its surface area and this is accompanied by evolution of large quantities of heat. It is an exothermic reaction. Thus, the simple contact of 1 g of ether with activated carbon will produce 30 calories of heat. This process is utilized in the Edison vaporizer.

Practical Aspects of Vaporization

Vaporization is accelerated (1) by increasing the surface from which vaporization may occur—hence, providing a greater contact area to furnish heat; and (2) by removing the molecules of vapor above a volatile substance there results a continuous low vapor pressure and a higher gradient of pressure from the liquid to the vapor. Air currents may pass over the surface or top of the volatile anesthetic and this is often called "topping" (see Chapter 5).

In practice, with open systems of anesthesia the mask provides a surface for evaporation and the air provides the heat. This is obviously an inefficient method since the specific heat of air is only .0003 calories per ml. Thus, to vaporize 1 g of ether (1.3 ml) over 300 L of air must pass over the evaporating surface.

More practical as a source of heat is the use of warm water baths and copper containers. Copper has a specific heat of only 0.093 cal/g but because of its great density, 1 ml has a heat capacity of 0.81 cal/g.

HUMIDITY

This is the term applied to the degree of moisture or water vapor in gases, especially in air. It varies with temperature. The *absolute humidity* is the actual mass of water vapor in a unit volume of air at a given temperature. It is usually expressed in grams of water per liter. The *relative humidity* is the ratio between the mass of vapor actually present in the air to that which it is capable of holding if saturated at the given temperature. It is expressed in terms of percent saturation. Indeed, humidity may be considered in terms of pressure of water vapor in relation to the saturation pressure at the given temperature. If air is saturated with water vapor, it has a relative humidity of 100%. The pressure at saturation is the vapor pressure. If the relative humidity is only 50%, then the partial pressure is half the vapor pressure.

CRITICAL CONDITIONS

All gases may be liquefied by compression under certain conditions. When pressure is exerted on a gas the molecules are forced closer together. This results in increased molecular motion as well as increased pressure. If the pressure is increased the energy of motion may be liberated in the form of heat. Cohesive forces may come into play and this gas may liquefy. However, this will not occur until the heat of the gas, that is its temperature, is below a certain critical level. This temperature, above which a substance cannot be liquefied regardless of the pressure exerted on it, is called the *critical temperature*. At any temperature below this critical one a substance becomes liquid when the applied pressure is greater than the vapor pressure of the substance at that temperature. The pressure that causes the liquid phase to form at the critical temperature is the *critical pressure*.

For example, the critical temperature of oxygen is −116° C. Therefore, at room temperature it cannot be compressed into the liquid state. At −116° C a pressure of 50 atmospheres is required to form the liquid phase. Actually, oxygen may be liquefied by decreasing its molecular action sufficiently by cooling. Thus if the temperature is reduced to −183° C gaseous oxygen will liquefy at a pressure of 1 atmosphere. This is the theoretical boiling point of oxygen.

On the other hand nitrous oxide has a critical

temperature of 36.15° C or 97° F. Above this temperature it can exist only as a true gas. At this temperature it can be liquefied by 51 atmospheres of pressure. Liquid nitrous oxide has a vapor and a vapor pressure which like any liquid, varies with temperature. For instance at −89° C the vapor pressure is below 1 atmosphere. Thus −89° C is the boiling point. At increasing temperatures up to the critical temperature the vapor pressure increases progressively until the material is entirely gaseous, i.e., it becomes a true gas (Fig. 4–13).

It follows, therefore, that the pressure within a cylinder of nitrous oxide is not always 750 lb per sq inch but depends on the vapor pressure at any temperature below 36° C and on Gay-Lussac's law above 36° C. Thus at 10° C the pressure may be 40 atmospheres; at 20° C, 51 atmospheres, and at any temperature above 36° C the pressure would increase 1/273 of the pressure at 0° C for each degree rise in temperature (Fig. 4–14).

Vapor and Gas

This discussion leads to the distinction between a vapor and a gas. The term vapor is used to designate the gaseous phase of a substance which at ordinary temperature and pressure exists as a liquid. Common examples are water vapor and ether vapor. A scientific definition of vapor, therefore, is a substance in the gaseous phase below its critical temperature;[3] above its critical temperature it is an ideal gas.

A gas on the other hand is a substance that does not exist as a liquid at ordinary temperature and pressure and thus may be defined as that phase of a substance when it exists at temperature above its

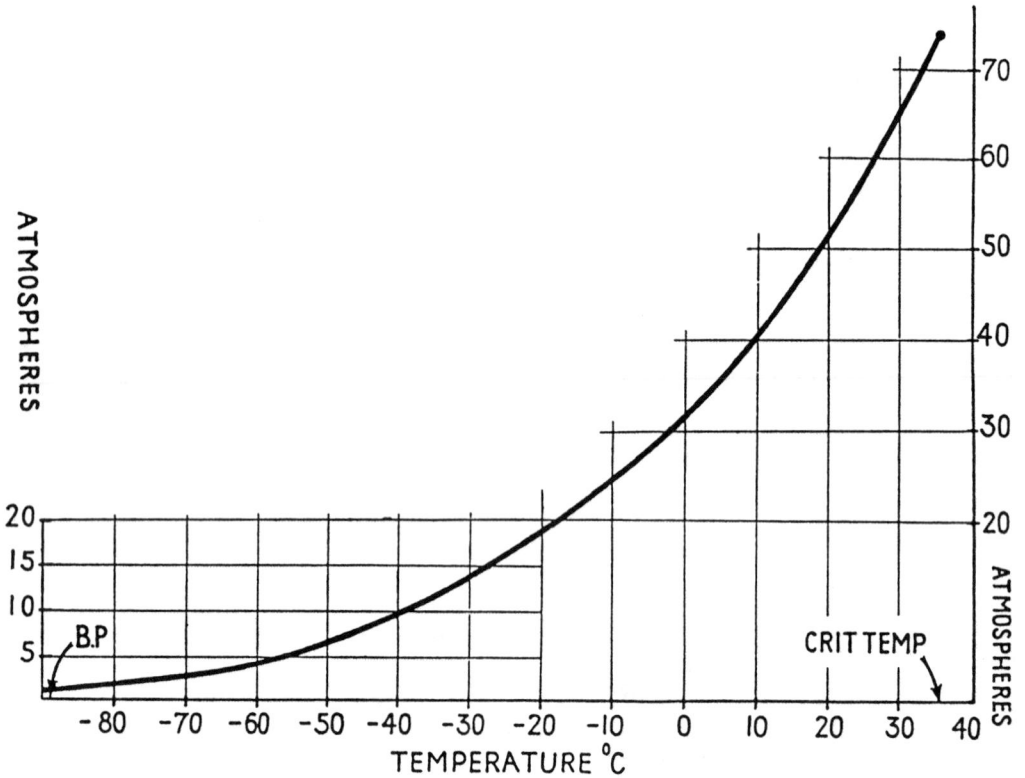

FIG. 4–13. Vapor pressure curve of nitrous oxide. Nitrous oxide is provided as a liquid inside cylinders when the temperature is below 36.15° C (97° F), which is the usual ambient temperature. At or just below this temperature the nitrous oxide is compressed at a pressure of 74 atm. Some of the nitrous oxide exists as a vapor above the liquid form. The pressure of the vapor above the liquid varies with the temperature. As the temperature of the liquid falls, the vapor pressure falls: at 20° C the vapor pressure in the cylinder will register 750 psi (50 atm); at 0° C the vapor pressure falls to 31 atm; at −89° C the vapor pressure falls to 1 atm. This is the boiling point (BP). From the BP to the critical temperature there is a progressive increase in pressure and more of the N_2O exists as a vapor until it is all vaporized; at the critical temperature, it becomes a true gas. It cannot be liquified by any amount of pressure. From Macintosh, Mushin, and Epstein: Physics for the Anesthetist, 1st ed. Springfield, IL, Charles C Thomas, 1958.

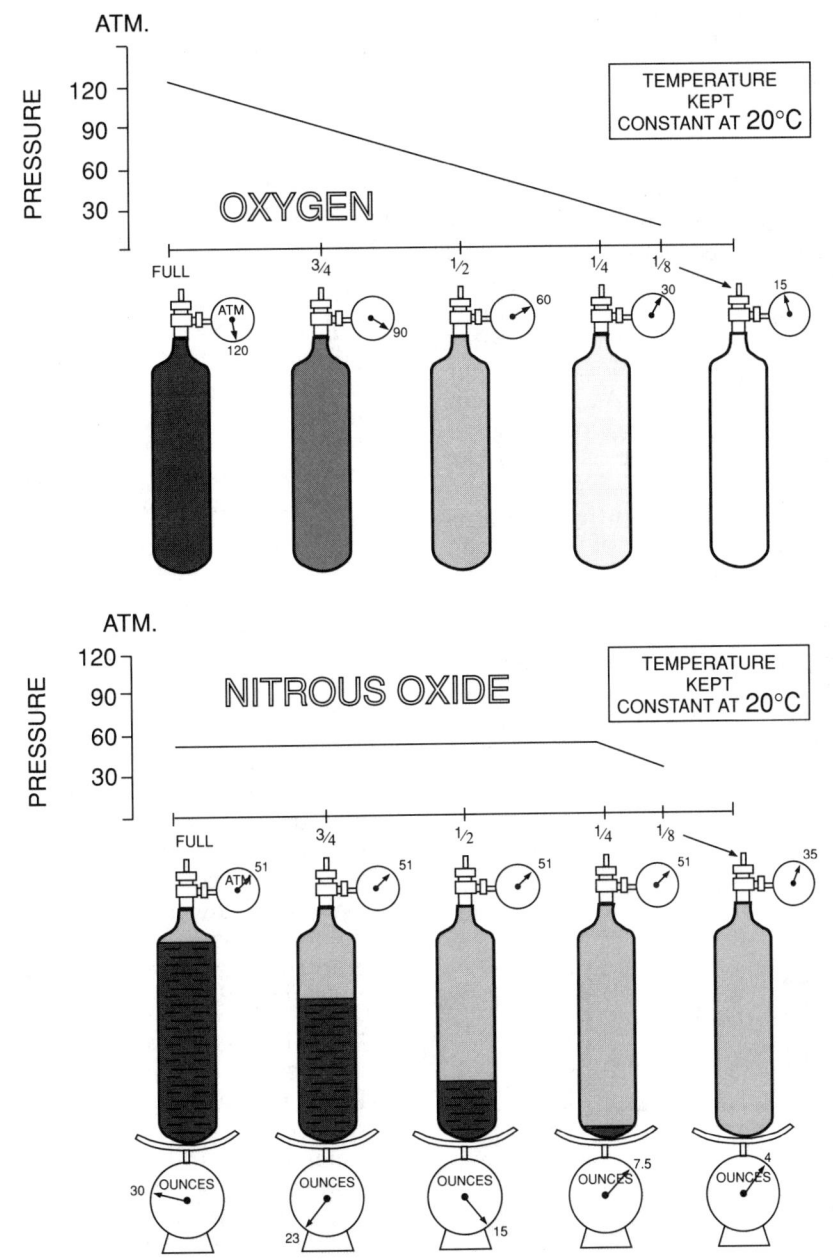

FIG. 4–14. Relationship between pressure in a cylinder and the amount of oxygen or nitrous oxide within it. *Upper.* A cylinder when 'full' contains oxygen under a pressure of 120 atmospheres. The valve is opened and the gas is allowed to escape; there is a progressive fall of pressure. When the pressure has fallen to 60 atmospheres the amount of gas within the cylinder has fallen, too, to half of what it was initially. A pressure reading at any stage gives an indication of the amount of oxygen remaining in the cylinder. As the density (represented by intensity of color) decreases there is a corresponding fall of pressure. *Lower.* The liquid nitrous oxide and the density of the vapor above it is represented by intensity of color. The temperature throughout the experiment is kept constant at 20° C, at which the pressure exerted by the saturated vapor over the liquid is 51 atmospheres. As the tap is opened gaseous nitrous oxide escapes, and is immediately replaced by further vapor from the liquid. When the cylinder is half full the density of the vapor, and therefore its pressure, are still the same. In fact these remain unaltered as long as any nitrous oxide exists in the liquid state. An accurate indication of the amount of nitrous oxide remaining in the cylinder can be obtained only by weighing the cylinder. The horizontal line shows that the pressure of the vapor within the cylinder remains uniform until it is just less than quarter full. When the liquid is all volatilized the pressure of the gas within the cylinder begins to fall. The relation between pressure and specific volume then gradually approximates to Boyle's Law. The Law applies only where the pressure of the nitrous oxide is considerably below its saturation pressure. From Macintosh, Mushin, and Epstein: Physics for the Anesthetist, 3rd ed. Springfield, IL, Charles C Thomas, 1963.

critical temperature. Hence liquefaction is impossible.[4] It is assumed that both vapors and gases at 1 atmosphere behave as ideal gases.

FLOW OF FLUIDS

The dynamics of the flow of fluids through any system of tubes are best studied by means of a model comprising a reservoir, a long horizontal outflow tube, and a series of upright tubes at strategic points. If such a system is closed and the reservoir filled with water, the water will rise to the same height in the reservoir and tubes (Fig. 4–15A). The height of the fluid represents potential energy or energy of position. The height in the reservoir is called the pressure head.

On opening the stopcock the potential energy is converted to kinetic energy or energy of motion and the fluid flows out the stopcock (Fig. 4–15B). The pressure decreases and this indicates that energy has been used. There is loss of energy in overcoming friction and in giving velocity to the fluid which is represented by a fall in lateral pressure. The difference in pressure between successive tubes is called the pressure gradient. As the stopcock is opened wider, the velocity of outflow is greater and the lateral pressure smaller.

Poiseuille's Law

If the diameter of the horizontal outflow tube is increased the volume outflow of a fluid increases greatly and if the diameter is reduced the volume outflow is also reduced. The exact relationship between the volume outflow of a fluid and the diameter of the tube was expressed by Poiseuille in 1841. He discovered that the volume of fluid flowing through a tube varies as the fourth power of the diameter of the tube. This is the fundamental basis of Poiseuille's Law (Fig. 4–15). For a nonviscous fluid a Newtonian series of relations may be expressed in the complete law as follows:

Volume flow per minute (Q) =
$$\frac{\text{Pressure Head } (P_1 - P_2) \times \text{area factors } (\pi r^4)}{\text{Viscosity } (\eta) \times 8 \text{ length of tube}}$$

For example an experiment may be set up with a 50 cm outflow tube of 6 mm internal diameter connected to a reservoir with a head of pressure of 16 cm of water kept constant. In 30 sec 100 ml of water will be collected from the outflow. If a 50 cm outflow tube with a diameter of 3 mm internal diameter is substituted only 6 ml of water will be collected in 30 sec. This represents $\frac{1}{16}$ of the first volume. In other words a reduction in the diameter of the tube by one-half reduces the outflow by one-half raised to the fourth power.

From these experiments a few rules may be summarized for fluids flowing smoothly through a tube.

1. Lateral pressure is inversely proportional to the velocity of the flow.
2. Resistance to flow is proportional to the frictional surface (length of tube) and to the velocity squared and inversely related to the cross sectional area.
3. Velocity of flow is proportional to: (a) the pressure gradient; (b) the fourth power of the diameter of the tube; (c) inversely to the viscosity; and (d) inversely to the sectional area of the tube.

Nature of Flow (Fig. 4–16)

When a fluid (also liquid or gas) streams through a tube, the particles comprising the fluid may move along two lines. If the movement of the molecules is in parallel layers it is termed *streamlined* or *laminar flow*. Under this circumstance the layers slip past one another and friction develops between adjacent layers. If some molecules slip from fast paths to slow paths the entire movement is slowed. This property of fluid friction is called *viscosity*.

On the other hand if the lines of flow are not parallel but irregular the movement is called *tur-*

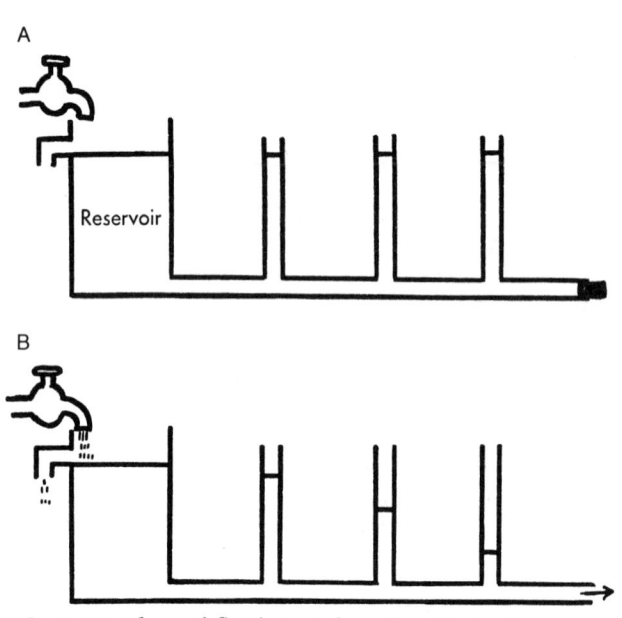

FIG. 4–15. Flow of fluids in tubes of uniform diameter. A. Outflow tube closed: Lateral pressure is inversely proportional to velocity of flow (V). B. Outflow tube opened:
1. Lateral pressure is inversely proportional to velocity of flow (V).
2. Resistance is proportional to $\frac{\text{length of tube}}{\text{sectional area}} \times V^2$.
3. Velocity is proportional to pressure gradient.
4. Volume of fluid flowing varies as fourth power of diameter. (Poiseuille's Law).

bulent flow. Thus, due to obstruction, branchings, and roughness of the conduit or fluid bed, changes in directions of the molecules are produced and eddy currents are formed.

Laminar flow is directly proportional to the volume flow and is dependent on viscosity of the substance. In contrast, turbulent flow is directly proportional to the volume flow *squared* and is dependent on the density of the gas.

Air flow tends to be laminar. In the respiratory system both types are seen. In the upper passages at the larynx and the carina or other branchings, turbulent flow predominates. In the trachea, bronchi, and other relatively straight conduits the flow is laminar.

Resistance to Flow

When fluids flow in any system there is opposition to this flow. Such opposition is due to the internal friction of fluid flow as a function of the velocity of flow and to the friction of the fluid against the walls of the system. This opposition to the flow of fluids is called *resistance*. It is measured by the pressure difference between the inlet and exit points of a given system for a given rate of flow (or volume flow). Based on this measurement the resistance of a system with a given volume flow of fluid is expressed in terms of the pressure gradient between any two points in the system. It may also be stated that this pressure represents the energy lost in overcoming the opposition to flow (or resistance) and in imparting velocity to the fluid.

It has become customary to express resistance in terms of the pressure differential measured in cm of water at a given rate of flow stated in liters per second, or

$$\text{Resistance} = \frac{\text{Difference in Pressure } (\Delta P)}{\text{Volume Flow/Second } (V)}$$

The amount of the pressure necessary to overcome resistance and to move fluid through a system depends on three variables. Together these provide a mathematical expression to Poiseuille's Law.

1. Volume of fluid flowing in a given time
2. The length of the tube
3. The internal diameter

VOLUME RATE OF FLOW. With the volume rate of flow the only variable, one may mathematically express the relationship of this with the pressure required:

$$\Delta p = k_1 V \text{ (laminar) or}$$
$$\Delta p = k_2 V^2 \text{ (turbulent flow)}$$

LENGTH OF TUBE. For a given flow rate and a fixed diameter of tube one may mathematically express the relationship between the pressure required to propel the fluid against the length of tube. This equation is as follows:

$$\Delta p = k_3 L \text{ (laminar flow)}$$
$$\Delta p = k_4 L \text{ (turbulent flow)}$$

DIAMETER OF TUBE. At constant volume flow rate and a fixed length of tube the pressure necessary to overcome resistance to flow is inversely related to the diameter or cross-sectional area. The relationship may be mathematically expressed as follows:

$$\Delta p = k_5 \frac{1}{d^4} \text{ (laminar flow)}$$
$$\Delta p = k_6 \frac{1}{d^5} \text{ (turbulent flow)}$$

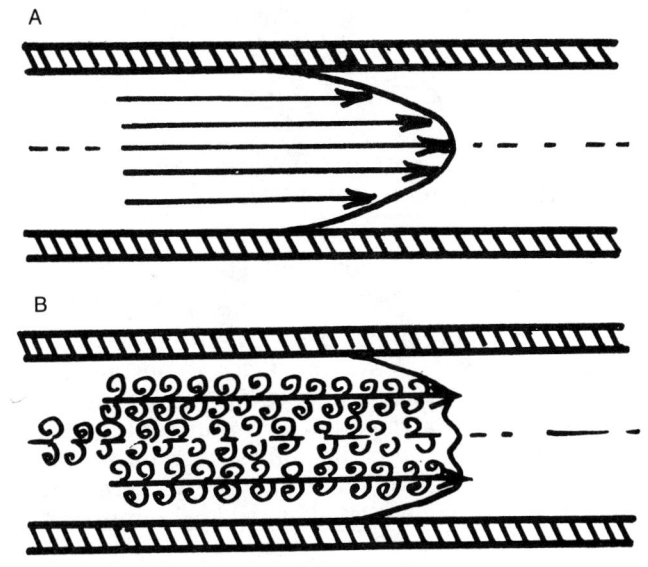

FIG. 4–16. Nature of air flow in tubes.

LAMINAR FLUID FLOW: Elements of the fluid move in essentially straight paths parallel to the axis of the tube. The greatest velocity is at the center and there is almost zero velocity for a thin layer near the walls. The shape of the flow head is parabolic. Pressure required to produce laminar flow is proportional to the volume flow × a constant.

$$\Delta P = K_1 \times V$$

TURBULENT FLUID FLOW: As velocity of flow increases or irregularities are encountered, the elements of the fluid acquire a radial component with the appearance of eddies. The velocity distribution tends to be uniform. Pressure required to produce turbulent flow is proportional to the square of the volume × a constant.

$$\Delta P = K_2 \times V^2$$

The empirically derived combined equation for approximate relationship is as follows:

$$\Delta p = K \frac{LV}{D^4}$$

when K is a constant including such factors as density, viscosity, and frictional forces.[10]

Flow in Tubes of Varying Diameter (Bernoulli's Theorem)

So far consideration has been given to tubes of uniform diameter. In a system under a constant pressure head and constant outflow the quantity of water passing a given point in a unit time must be the same at all points. It follows, therefore, that at a constricted area velocity must be greater. These observations may be stated by the law that in a tube of varying diameter the velocity is inversely proportional to the sectional area (Fig. 4–17A).

In 1738 Bernoulli formulated the relationship between changes in pressure and changes in speed. He demonstrated that in tubes of varying diameter the lateral pressure of a flowing fluid is least where the velocity is greatest (Fig. 4–17B). By increasing the volume flow rate, *i.e.*, by raising the pressure head, the lateral pressure in the side tube may be reduced to atmospheric pressure and even further. In this case air is drawn through the side tube into the flow tube; that is, air is "sucked in" or entrained. The pressure drop at constricted areas is due to the conversion of pressure energy to kinetic energy. An equivalent statement of this theory is as follows: As fluid flows from one place to another the velocity and pressure change in such a manner that kinetic energy (denoted by the expression $\frac{1}{2} dv^2$, *i.e.*, one-half the mass (d) times the velocity squared), plus potential energy (*i.e.*, pressure) remains constant.

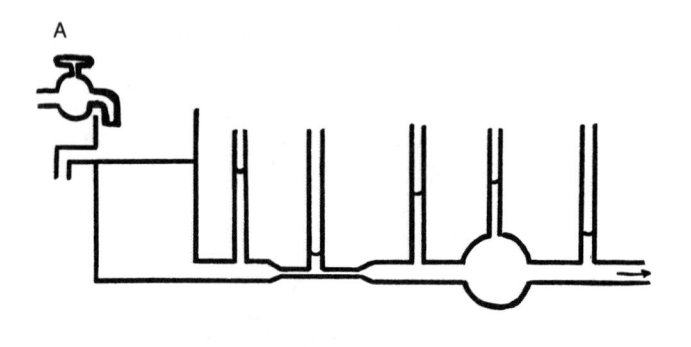

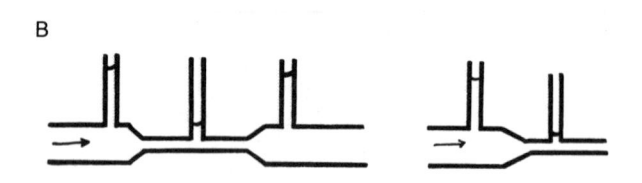

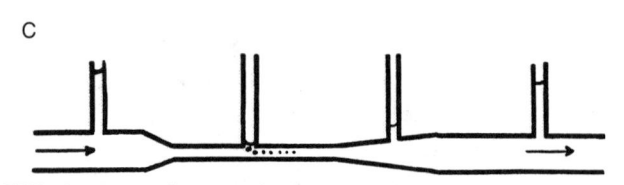

FIG. 4–17. Evolution of Venturi System.

A. FLOW PRINCIPLE: Velocity of flow is inversely proportional to sectional area.

B. BERNOULLI'S THEOREM: Lateral pressure is least where velocity is greatest or lateral pressure varies inversely with sectional area.

C. VENTURI PRINCIPLE: For pressure downstream to regain the value on the upstream side of a constriction the downstream tube must open gradually. If the angle of the cone exceeds 15° the pressure will not be regained maximally.

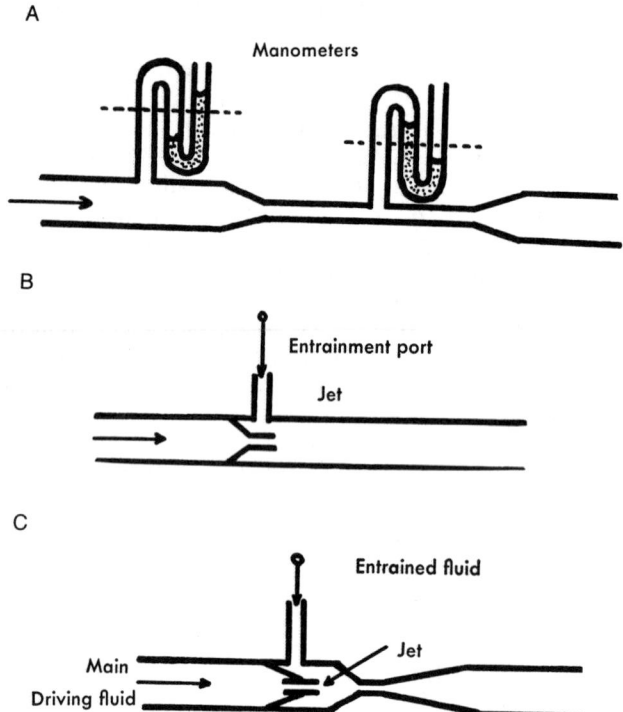

FIG. 4–18. Evolution of injector device. Based on a combination of Bernoulli's Theorem and the Venturi Principle.

A. A jet replaces constricted area of tube and a side entry tube or entrainment port replaces manometer.

B. Bernoulli's Theorem applied showing subatmospheric pressure created at a constriction because of rapid velocity of flow. This allows air to be sucked into flow tube and is called entrainment.

C. The entrainment port is moved closer to neck of jet and the downstream part of tube is modified into a Venturi tube now called a diffuser.

Fundamental Physics

TABLE 4-5. PHYSIOCHEMICAL PROPERTIES OF SOME VOLATILE ANESTHETIC AGENTS

Agent	Chloroform	Diethyl ether	Ethrane	Fluroxene	Forane	Halothane	Methoxy-flurane	Trichloro-ethylene
Formula	CHCl$_3$	C$_4$H$_{10}$O	C$_3$H$_2$OClF$_5$	C$_4$H$_5$OF$_3$	C$_3$H$_2$OClF$_5$	C$_2$HClBrF$_3$	C$_3$H$_4$OCl$_2$F$_2$	C$_2$HCl$_3$
Molecular weight	119.4	74.1	184.5	126.0	184.5	197.4	165.0	131.4
mg per ml of vapour at 760 mmHg 0° C	5.33	33.1	7.56	5.62	7.56	8.81	7.36	5.86
20° C	4.96	3.08	7.67	5.24	7.76	8.21	6.86	5.46
37° C	4.69	2.91	7.25	4.95	7.25	7.76	6.48	5.16
at 713 mmHg 37°C	4.40	2.73	6.80	4.64	6.80	7.28	6.08	4.84
Density g/ml at 20° C	1.47	0.72	1.52	1.13	1.49	1.86	1.42	1.46
ml vapour/ml liquid 20° C	296	234	198	216	194	227	207	267
Vapour pressure at 20° C in mm Hg	159	442	180	286	250	242	26	58
Latent heat of vaporization J g^{-1}	247	360	157	222	151	147	205	239

After Hill, D.W.: Physics Applied to Anaesthesia, 4th ed. London, Boston, Butterworth & Co. Ltd., 1980. With permission.

Observed pressures are somewhat different because no allowance is made for loss of pressure due to friction.

As a fluid passes from a constricted part to a wider area speed decreases and lateral pressure increases. In 1797 Venturi showed that for a fluid to regain a lateral pressure value similar to that before the constriction it was necessary that the tube distal to the constriction open up gradually. This is the principle underlying the design of the Venturi tube (Fig. 4-17C).

The combination of Bernoulli's theory, that lateral pressure is least where speed is greatest, and the principle of the Venturi tube results in the injector assembly. The evolution of this is illustrated (Fig. 4-18). Applications of the above principles are to be found in many modern engineering devices for measuring fluid volume flow; in the injector devices such as the atomizer and the Bunsen burner; and in the injector device used to obtain various air-oxygen mixtures during oxygen therapy.

SUMMARY OF PHYSIOCHEMICAL PROPERTIES. Physiochemical properties of some of the common volatile anesthetic agents are summarized in Table 4-5.

GENERAL REFERENCES

1. Adriani, J.: The Chemistry and Physics of Anesthesia, 2nd ed. Springfield, IL, Charles C Thomas Publishers, 1962.
2. Macintosh, R.R., Mushin, W.W., Epstein, B.: Physics for the Anaesthetist, 4th ed. Revised by Mushin W and Jones P: Oxford, Blackwell Scientific Publications, 1987.
3. Hill, D.W.: Physics Applied to Anaesthesia, 4th ed. London, Boston, Butterworths & Co. Ltd., 1980.

REFERENCES

1. Chemical Bond Approach Project: Chemical Systems. New York, McGraw-Hill, 1964.
2. Macintosh, R.R., Mushin, W.W., Epstein, B.: Physics for the Anaesthetist, 4th ed. Revised by Mushin, W. and Jones, P.: Oxford, England, Blackwell Scientific Publications, 1987.
3. Eger, E.I. (II): Anesthetic Uptake and Action. Baltimore, Williams & Wilkins Co., 1974.
4. Steward, A. et al.: Solubility coefficients for inhaled anesthetics for water, oil, and biological media. Brit. J. Anaesth., 45:282, 1973.
5. Lowe, H.J. and Ernst, E.A.: The Quantitative Practice of Anesthesia: Use of Closed Circuit. Baltimore, Williams & Wilkins, 1981.
6. Munson, E.S. et al.: Increase in anesthetic uptake excretion and blood solubility in man after eating. Anesth. Analg., 57:224, 1973.
7. Eger, E.I. (II), Larson, C.P. Jr.: Anaesthetic solubility in blood and tissues: values and significance. Brit. J. Anaesth., 36:140, 1964.
8. Eger, E.I. (II): Updated table. Personal Communication, 1988.
9. Weast, R.C.: Handbook of Chemistry and Physics, 57th Ed. Cleveland, CRC Press, 1976.
10. Orkin, L.R., Siegel, M., Rovenstine, E.A.: Resistance to breathing by apparatus used in Anesthesia I Endotracheal equipment. Anesth. Analg., 33:217, 1954.

Theodore C. Smith
Vincent J. Collins

ANESTHESIA MACHINES AND COMPONENTS

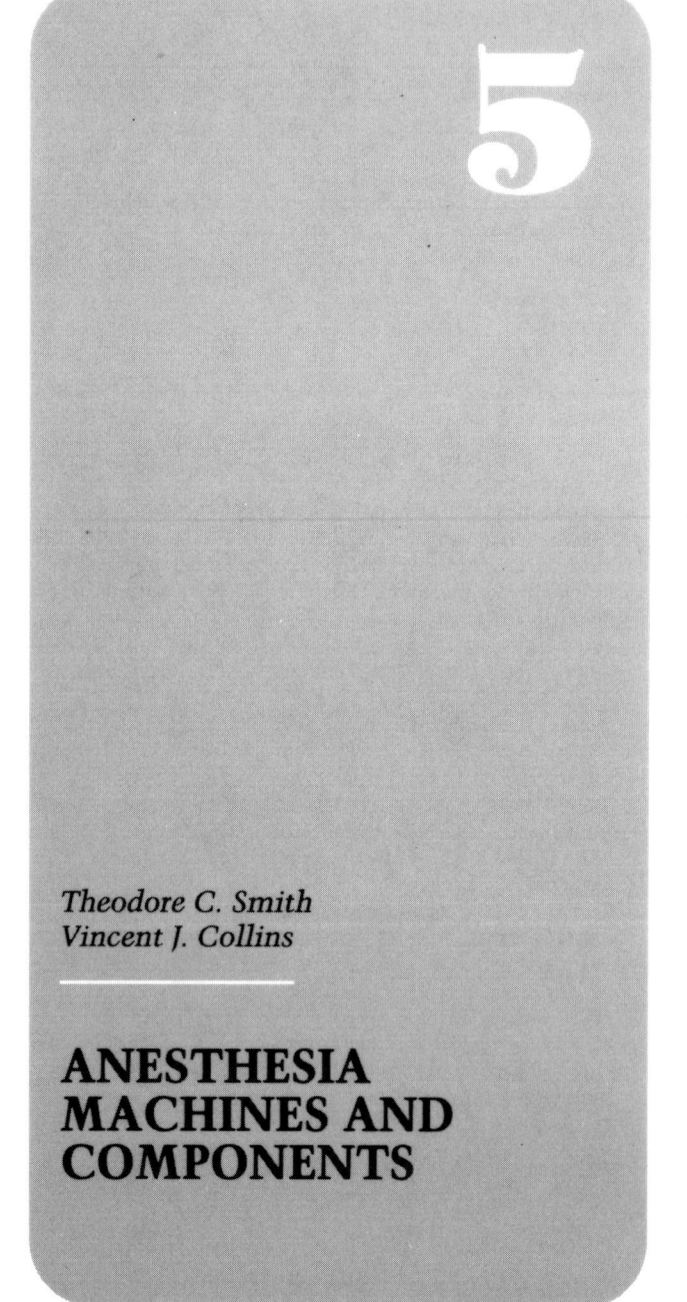

The Anesthesiologist is at once a physician, a scientist and an artist. As an artist he is judged by the condition of his equipment.

The anesthesia machine is a basic tool of the anesthetist and serves as the primary work station (Fig. 5–1). It allows the anesthetist to select and mix measured flows of gases, to vaporize known amounts of liquids, and thereby to administer safely controlled concentrations of oxygen and anesthetic gases and vapors to the patient via a breathing circuit. The anesthesia machine also provides a table top for placement of drugs and devices for immediate access and drawers for storage of small equipment, drugs, supplies, equipment instruction manuals, and Life Savers and chewing gum for use by the anesthetist during long procedures. Finally, the machine serves as a frame and source of pneumatic and electric power for various accessories such as ventilators and monitors.

One or more models of anesthesia machines are manufactured in more than half a dozen countries, and these models differ to varying degrees in design characteristics and component features. Their basic functional characteristics, however, are similar. This chapter provides the following: a description of these basic functional characteristics; a schema for classification of anesthesia machines and their attached equipment; simplified drawings of the major components of anesthesia machines; and references for more detailed descriptions of specific components. For determination of the operational characteristics of a specific machine or its components, the user should refer to the manufacturer's instructions, descriptions, and parts lists.

VISION CONSIDERATIONS

The anesthesiologist must be properly located to use the equipment and supplies, to "run" the machine, and to observe the patient as well as monitoring devices. His working position must allow for ready unobstructed vision of the anesthesia environment. Important displays of machine function such as

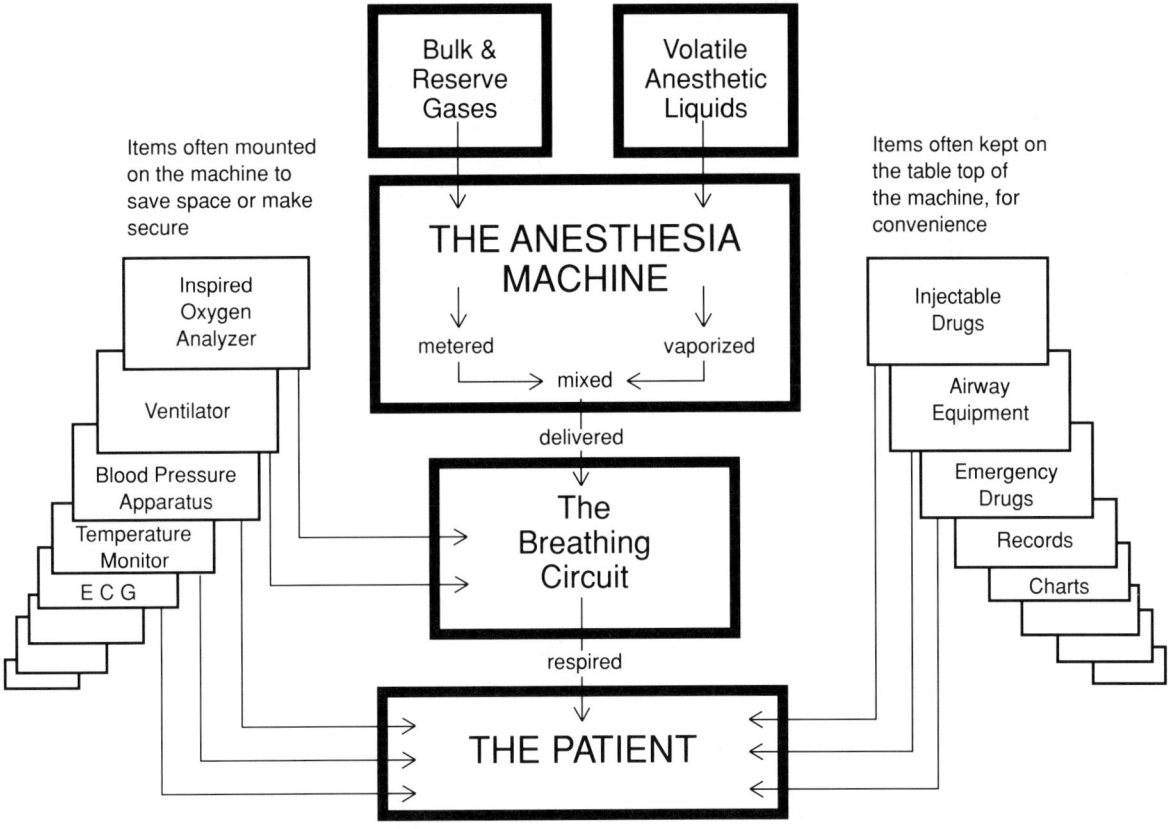

FIG. 5–1. Schematic diagram of the anesthetist's work station. The anesthesia machine permits the anesthetist to mix gases that are delivered via the breathing circuit to the patient. The machine is also used to store frequently used drugs and equipment and acts as a frame for the mounting of monitors and accessories.

flows of gases and of monitors should be primarily and readily observable. Cones of vision have been identified for the operator (Fig. 5–2).[1] The cone of vision is dynamic and changes with movement of the head. Visual information in the horizontal plane is most readily perceived if it is presented in a 30-degree critical zone of vision in front of the observer. The vertical plane, with the head stationary in the erect position, will be seen along a line 10 to 15 degrees above or below the horizontal plane of the eye level.[2]

For visual acuity, several recommendations are listed by Kendall:[1]

- Indirect or diffused lighting should be used.
- Glare and bright lights should be limited about the anesthetist's work station.
- The viewing distance should be about 20 in. while the operating distance should be about the length of the extended arm.
- Primary visual displays should center around the normal line of sight and not require great eye or head movement.
- All warning displays (those related to system failure or equipment hazard) should be within 30 degrees of the normal standing sight line or 45 degrees for a sit–stand position.
- Secondary displays may be placed to require eye movement but not head movement.
- Auxiliary displays—those not affecting the patient (on/off indicators)—may require head/eye movement.
- Know where the displays are located.[3]

HISTORICAL DEVELOPMENT

The first devices for administering anesthetics were glass or metal vessels that were partially filled with either diethyl ether or chloroform. The patient inhaled the vapor from the container. The requirement for large volumes of ether vapor to induce anesthesia was met by increasing the surface area available for vaporization with porous sponges, layers of cotton gauze, labyrinths of copper channels, or by the use of large tray-like vessels. With the introduction of more potent and dangerous chloroform, the problem became control of concentration, which was achieved by adding known liquid volumes to large bags of air, or by the use of hand bulbs that pumped a small controllable volume of air through liquid chloroform independent of the patient's respirations.[4] The less potent nitrous oxide was inhaled

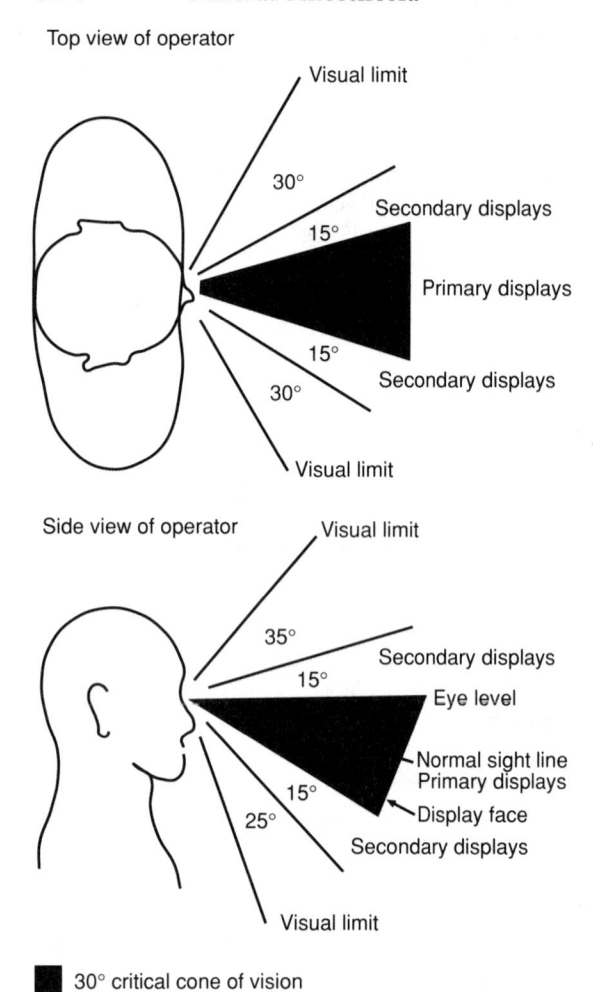

FIG. 5–2. *A.* Cones of vision. *B.* Many anesthesia machines do not present important displays (ECG monitor) in the human's critical cone of vision. From Kendall, J.: Visual considerations for the anesthesia machine operator. J. Assoc. Nurse Anesth., *54*:225, 1986.

directly from gasometers in which it was produced, or from impervious bags of gutta-percha or oiled silk.[4]

Technologic advances as well as escalating demand increased the complexity and sophistication of the various inhaler devices. The Harcourt chloroform inhaler of 1903 incorporated unidirectional valves, used a warming candle, and could alter inspired concentrations from 0.5 to 2%. The Ombrédanne ether inhaler of 1908 used a bovine urinary vesicle or caecum for the rebreathing bag and had air passages of low resistance.

Liquid nitrous oxide in cylinders was available from 1870 and was used by Clover as early as 1876. Compressed oxygen became available in the mid-1880s, produced first by the dentist and manufacturer, S. S. White of New England. Despite obvious advantages of compressed gases, acceptance was slow, due perhaps to an absence of reducing valves, pressure controls, and measuring or metering devices. Well into the twentieth century, anesthetic vapor-air mixtures were nearly universal. The collaborative experiences of the American anesthetist, James Gwathmey, with the English anesthetists, Sir Geoffrey Marshall and Edmund Boyle, during and after WWI;[5,6] the scientific studies of Ralph Waters; and the inventive contributions of physician-anesthetists such as Elmer McKesson, Jay Heidbrink, and Richard Forreger revolutionized the design of the anesthesia machine between 1910 and 1930.[7,8] In basic design and function, the anesthesia machine of the 1930s was similar to that used today. The major improvements between then and now have been in the development of important safety features, the use of better materials in the manufacturing process, the addition of useful convenience features, and the development of modern vaporizers. Modern vaporizers date from the copper kettle, developed in the late 1940s and the Fluotec, developed in the late 1950s.

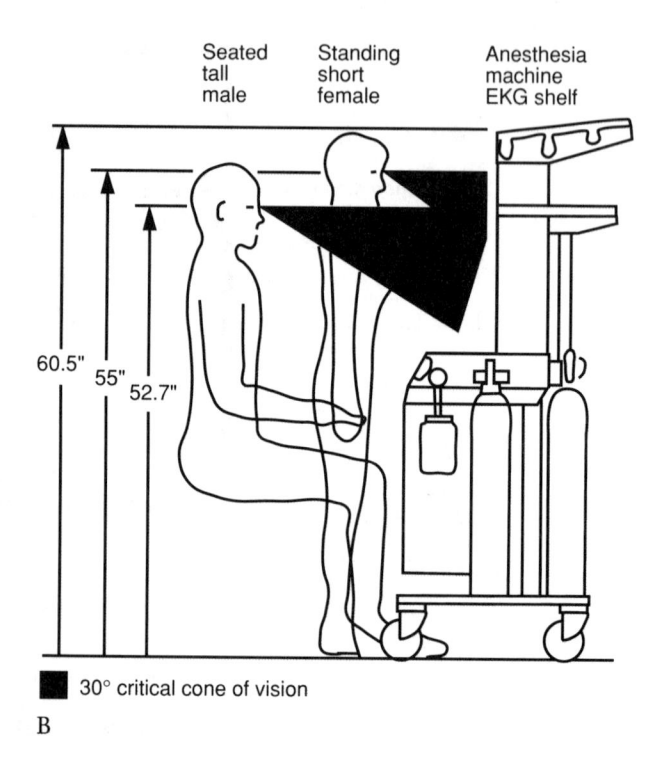

The vast majority of anesthesia machines in use today are continuous flow machines. On occasion, an intermittent or "demand" flow machine is used, usually in dental practice. However, radical departures from existing anesthesia machine design, in which many of the functions of the machine are under microprocessor control, are being evaluated.[9] In addition, there have been efforts to establish international standards for equipment design to enhance both equipment safety and compatibility.[10,11]

COMPONENTS OF CONTINUOUS-FLOW ANESTHESIA MACHINES

An anesthesia machine is an assembly of various components and devices: (1) gas cylinders with machine yokes; (2) pressure regulating and measuring devices; (3) valves; (4) flow controllers; (5) flowmeters; (6) vaporizers; (7) absorption canisters; and (8) breathing assembly (Figs. 5–3A and 5–3B).

Oxygen and nitrous oxide are generally delivered and stored in bulk form in the hospital and delivered to the operating rooms via pipelines. Because the piped systems can fail,[12] and because the machines may be used in areas of the hospital where piped gases are not available, all anesthesia machines are fitted with reserve cylinders of nitrous oxide and oxygen. The standard reserve cylinders of nitrous oxide and oxygen are of the E size (Table 5–1), although where piped gases are not available, the anesthesia machine may be fitted with G size cylinders in addition to the E cylinders. Both the bulk and cylinder sources of gas pass through backflow check valves. Bulk gases are delivered at a supply pressure of 45 to 60 psig* through quick disconnect couplings. Gases from cylinders, which may be at high pressures (750 to 2000 psig), pass through reducing valves set at 35 to 50 psig, thus permitting preferential use of the bulk supply if valves from both sources are open. Each bulk gas source has a separate pressure gauge, and each tank of compressed gas has a gauge that measures supply pressure and another that measures pressure after it has passed through reducing valves. Other than nitrous oxide and oxygen, machines upon which cylinders of cyclopropane, ethylene, helium, carbon dioxide, and air can be mounted and the gases delivered are available on special order from most manufacturers.

The gases are routed by copper or plastic tubing to failsafe devices. These devices are being increasingly used to shut off anesthetic gases if oxygen pressure becomes low. Some incorporate audible alarms. The gases then pass through needle valves and flowmeters for mixing and supply to vaporizers. At this point gas pressure has been reduced to near atmospheric pressure. The gases are then routed to the breathing circuit. A manual oxygen flush valve that permits rapid purging of the breathing circuit of anesthetic gases is also provided.

* Psig = pounds per square inch gauge, which is the difference between measured and atmospheric pressures.

FIG. 5–3A. The basic anesthesia machine with two gases. This is the teaching model selected for understanding the basics of machine operation. The design is traditional and lends itself to graphic representation. It incorporates all the components needed for learning the essentials. From Bowie, E., and Huffman, L.M.: Ohmeda, 1985.

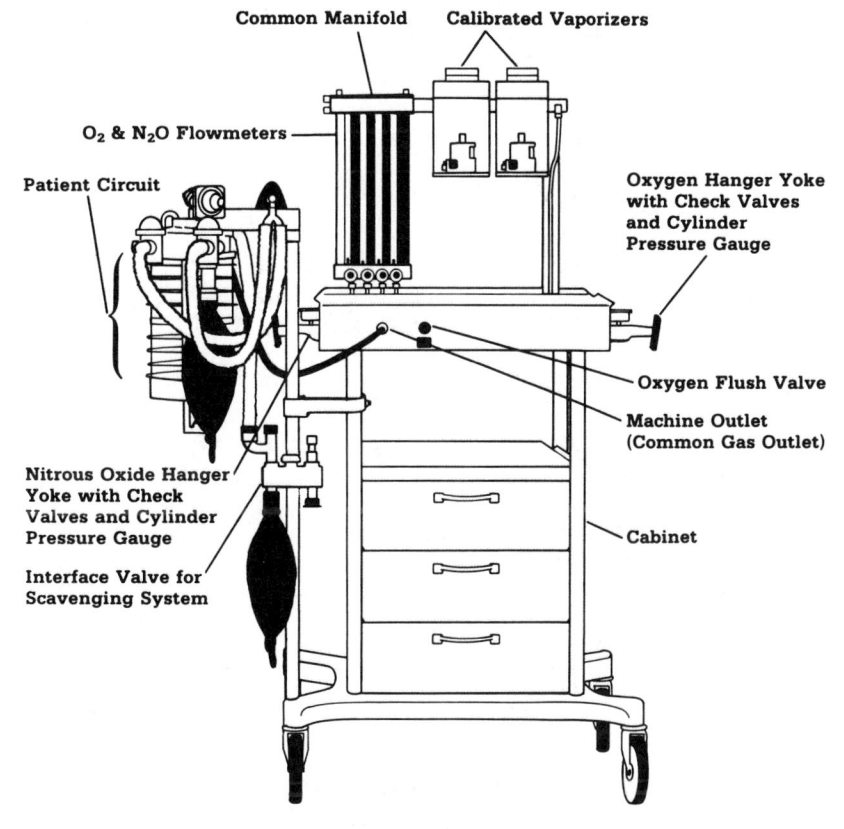

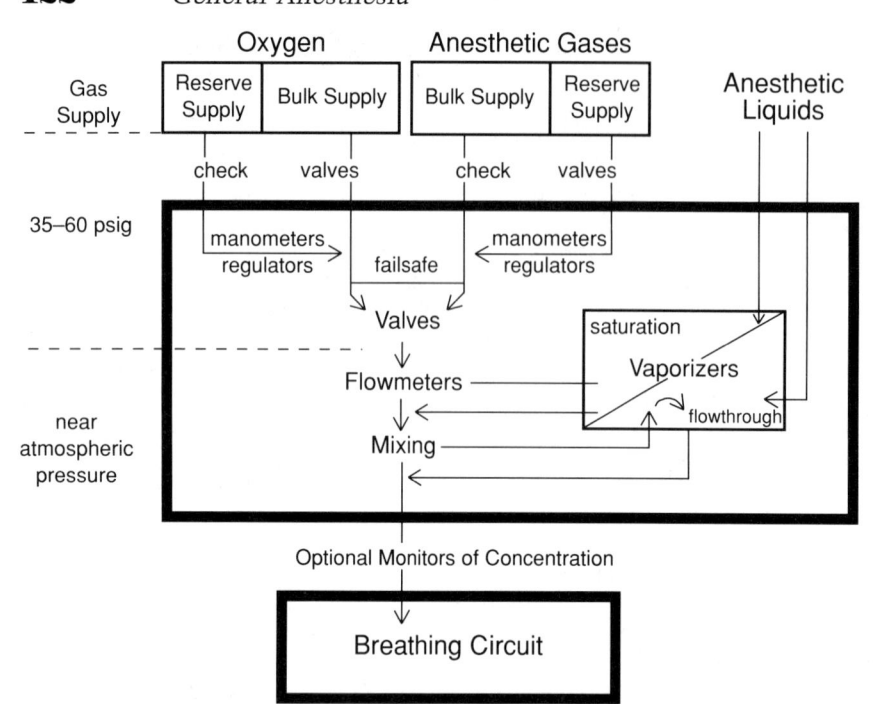

FIG. 5–3B. Schematic of the anesthesia machine. The essential elements of the anesthesia machine are contained in the large rectangular box. Oxygen and nitrous oxide are provided from central bulk stores or reserve tanks through internal plumbing and check valves, with the pipelines usually at working pressure of 35 to 60 pounds per square inch (psig). The flow of gases is controlled by needle valves and monitored by flow meters. Some or all of the gas may be diverted to vaporizers which are usually either saturation or flow-through type. The final gas mixture is then delivered through optional monitors (i.e., oxygen meter) to the breathing circuit.

The anesthesia machine should be sturdy, free of sharp corners and protrusions, and mounted on large-diameter wheels for ease of moving. The machine must have adequate shelf space for the various monitors and other accessories that are commonly used in anesthesia. The make and model of machine may be identical in each anesthetizing location of the hospital, to facilitate repair and preventive maintenance, or may be widely varied to suit individual preferences or teaching needs.

COMPRESSED GAS CYLINDERS[13]

A compressed gas is defined by the Department of Transportation (formerly the Interstate Commerce Commission) as *"any material or mixture having in the container either an absolute pressure exceeding 40 pounds per square inch at 70° F, or an absolute pressure exceeding 104 pounds per square inch at 130° F, or both; or any liquid flammable material having a vapor pressure exceeding 40 pounds per square inch absolute at 100° F."*[14]

A compressed gas may further be defined as any substance which exerts a gauge pressure exceeding 25 pounds per square inch at 70° F.

YOKES[15,16]

A yoke is the device used to attach gas cylinders to the apparatus or to a regulator. It consists of a metal "O" clamp with adjustable screw. The inside of the clamp is equipped with a nipple that fits snugly into the port of the cylinder valve (Fig. 5–4). In addition the Pin Index Safety System specifies that two small pins be located at designated positions (different for each gas) below the nipple to prevent cylinder yoke interchangeability (see below).

CONSTRUCTION OF CYLINDERS

All compressed gas cylinders are constructed according to Department of Transportation specifications (formerly Interstate Commerce Commission).[13]

For compressed medical and anesthetic gases the specification number is DOT followed by a letter indicating the cylinder size, with size A being the smallest and M and G being the largest. This marking and others must be placed on the shoulder of each cylinder.

Cylinders are constructed entirely of steel that meets certain chemical and physical requirements. The walls have a minimum thickness of $\frac{3}{8}$ of an inch. Some cylinders are constructed of a chrome molyb-

TABLE 5–1. CHARACTERISTICS OF STANDARD OXYGEN AND NITROUS OXIDE CYLINDERS

Cylinder	Weight Empty (lb)	Weight Full (lb)	Contents Liters	Contents Gallons
Oxygen				
E size	13	14.9	660	174
G size	110	125.5	5330	1408
Nitrous oxide				
E size	13	19.4	1590	420
G size	110	166	13,840	3655

denum alloy, which provides a cylinder approximately 20% lighter in weight. This fact is appropriately marked on the cylinder shoulder. Each cylinder is designed to contain a gas under a specified pressure. This pressure is called the authorized *service pressure*. If a cylinder is designed to withstand pressures exceeding 450 pounds per square inch, it must be able to resist pressure 1.66 (5/3) times the service pressure.

In addition to specific tensile strength a cylinder must possess some elasticity, but the expansion may not exceed 10%.

Each cylinder must be subjected to a test by interior hydrostatic pressure at least once every 5 years and this test must be recorded on the cylinder.

All cylinders have a precisely constructed valve to seal the contents, to provide an avenue for filling the cylinder, and to control the release of its contents.

Incorporated in each valve stem is a safety device which under hazardous circumstances of excessive heat or fire will allow the cylinder to become exhausted. The device is a simple plug or soft metal alloy called Wood's Metal; it is composed of bismuth, lead, tin and cadmium. This plug usually melts at 200° F.

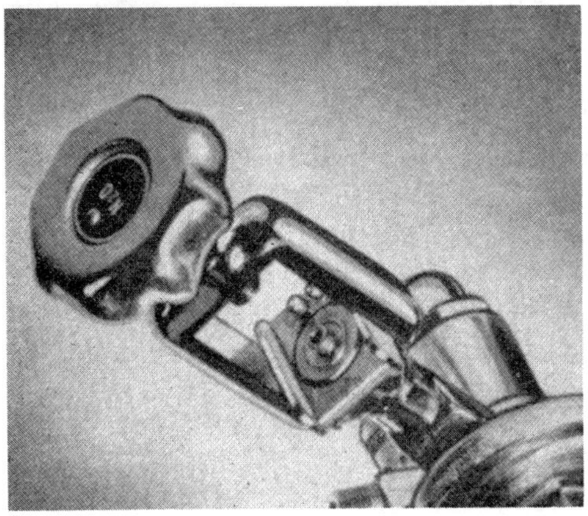

STANDARDS[19]

The Federal Food, Drug and Cosmetic Act also regulates the medical gases contained in cylinders. It is provided that the gases conform to the standards of the *United States Pharmacopeia*, and the purity and potency of the product are thereby assured. A label containing appropriate information is required. Besides identifying the product as well as the manufacturer an accurate statement of the quantity of the contents must be provided. The medical gas industry generally expresses the contents of full cylinders in terms of gallons measured at 70° F and normal atmospheric pressure; liquefied gases in cylinders are expressed also in terms of weight.

SIZE OF CYLINDERS

Cylinders designed for medical gas and anesthetic gas purposes are denoted not only by the specification number, DOT 3A, but also by a letter indicating the cylinder size. Sizes are designated by letters from A to M and the gas capacity increases as one advances in the alphabet. A chart of approximate dimensions and sizes is presented for reference (Table 5–2).

FILLING LIMITS

Since any gas in a closed container will increase in pressure with a rising temperature, the possibility

FIG. 5–4. Yoke assembly. Shows the essential "O"-type clamp and adjustable screw and nipple. Note the pins for the index safety system beneath the nipple. A fiber nonflammable-type washer is placed about the nipple to provide a leak-proof system. Courtesy Ohio Chemical and Surgical Equipment Company.

exists of dangerous pressures being attained. To prevent this occurrence regulations have been set for safe filling of cylinders. This applies whether the contents of the cylinders are in a gaseous or liquid state (see Table 5–3). In charging a cylinder the pressure in the cylinder at 70° F may not exceed service pressure for which it was designed. However, certain cylinders containing nonliquefied gases such as oxygen, helium, and carbon dioxide mixtures may be charged to a pressure 10% in excess of their marked service pressure (due to military emergency). Such cylinders are marked with a plus sign.

Further, a cylinder charged with medical gases (except CO_2 and N_2O) is limited to such amount that the pressure in the cylinder at 130° F does not exceed 1.25 times the serve pressure for which the cylinder was designed.

In the case of liquefied gases, the actual amount of gas in a given type of cylinder is limited by a maximum permissible *filling density* for each gas. This is determined from the water capacity of the cylinder expressed in pounds. Thus, the cylinders designed for the compressed liquefied gases are filled to a definite percentage of the water that the cylinder will hold.

LABELING AND MARKING

All cylinders must be marked according to DOT regulations. These markings are stamped permanently on the shoulder, top head or neck of the cylinder in letters or figures ¼" high as illustrated (Fig. 5–5). The following markings are required:

1. DOT specification number followed by service pressure in pounds per square inch at 70° F.

124 General Anesthesia

TABLE 5–2. STANDARD SIZES AND CAPACITIES OF MEDICAL GAS CYLINDERS

Style Cylinder and Appropriate Dimensions*		Carbon Dioxide	Cyclopropane	Ethylene	Helium	Nitrous Oxide	Oxygen†	Helium-Oxygen Mixtures	Carbon Dioxide-Oxygen Mixtures
A	gal	50	40	40	15	50	20	15	20
(3″ OD × 7″)	lb-oz	0–12.5	0–9.4	0–6.25	0–0.33	0–12.5	0–3.75	‡	‡
B	gal	100	100	100	28	100	40	29	40
(3½″ OD × 13″)	lb-oz	1–9.0	1–7.5	0–15.75	0–0.63	1–9.0	0–7.25	‡	‡
D	gal	250	230	200	80	250	95	82	95
(4¼″ OD × 17″)	lb-oz	3–14.5	3–5.5	1–15.5	0–1.8	3–14.5	1–1.0	‡	‡
E	gal	420		330	131	420	165	134	165
(4¼″ OD × 26″)	lb-oz	6–9.0		3–4.0	0–2.9	6–9.0	1–13.25	‡	‡
F	gal	1280		1100	425	1280	550	435	550
(5½″ OD × 51″)	lb-oz	20–0.0		10–12.0	0–9.4	20–0.0	6–2.0	‡	‡
M	gal	2000		1640	605	2000	800	620	800
(7⅛″ OD × 43″)	lb-oz	31–4		15–14.0	0–13.75	31–4	8–14.0	‡	‡
G	gal	3200		2800	1100	3200	1400	1126	1400
(8¼″ OD × 51″)	lb-oz	50–0.0		27–8.0	1–8.0	50–0.0	15–8.5	‡	‡

* The approximate dimensions given are for the cylinder less valve. Courtesy Ohio Chemical and Surgical Equipment Co.
† Oxygen is also supplied in styles "H" or "K" cylinders, 9″ OD × 51″ containing 220–244 cubic feet of gas.
‡ Varies with composition of the mixture.

2. Letter designating cylinder size followed by manufacturer's serial number. The identifying symbol and the serial number must be registered with the Bureau of Explosives. An ownership notation is allowed.
3. Inspector's official mark and date of original test.
4. Spun and plugged cylinders must be so marked.
5. The dates of all tests.

In addition, a label-tag is permitted; medical gas manufacturers use this on large cylinders, as well as small cylinders not packed in containers or cartons.

RECOMMENDED SAFE PRACTICES FOR HANDLING MEDICAL CASES

Special care must be exercised at all times in handling cylinders with compressed gases.[20] This is of such importance with regard to safety that the general rules recommended by the Compressed Gas Association are reprinted in full.[13,18,20]

1. Never permit oil, grease, or other readily combustible substance to come in contact with cylinders, valves, regulators, gauges, hoses, and fittings. Oil and certain gases such as oxygen or nitrous oxide may combine with explosive violence.
2. Never lubricate valves, regulators, gauges, or fittings with oil or any other combustible substance.
3. Do not handle cylinders or apparatus with oily hands or gloves.
4. Connections to piping, regulators, and other appliances should always be kept tight to prevent leakage. Where hose is used it should be kept in good condition.
5. Never use an open flame to detect gas leaks. Use soapy water.
6. Prevent sparks or flame from any source from coming in contact with cylinders and equipment.
7. Never interchange regulators or other appliances used with one gas with similar equipment intended for use with other gases.
8. All flowmeter valves should be closed.
9. Open cylinder valves slowly—only a half-turn first.
10. Cylinders must always be attached through the machine yoke to a pressure regulator.
11. Fully open the cylinder valve when cylinder is attached to machine and before connecting to the breathing apparatus to patient.

TABLE 5–3. PHYSICAL STATES OF COMPRESSED GASES IN THEIR CYLINDERS

Compressed Gases	Physical States in Cylinders
Nitrous oxide	Liquid (below 97.7° F)
Cyclopropane	Liquid (below 256° F)
Ethylene	Liquid (below 49.1° F)
Oxygen	Gas
Carbon dioxide	Liquid (below 88° F)
Carbon dioxide–oxygen	Gas
Helium	Gas
Helium–oxygen	Gas

FIG. 5–5. Labeling of cylinder shoulders. Labels now begin with the letters DOT rather than ICC.

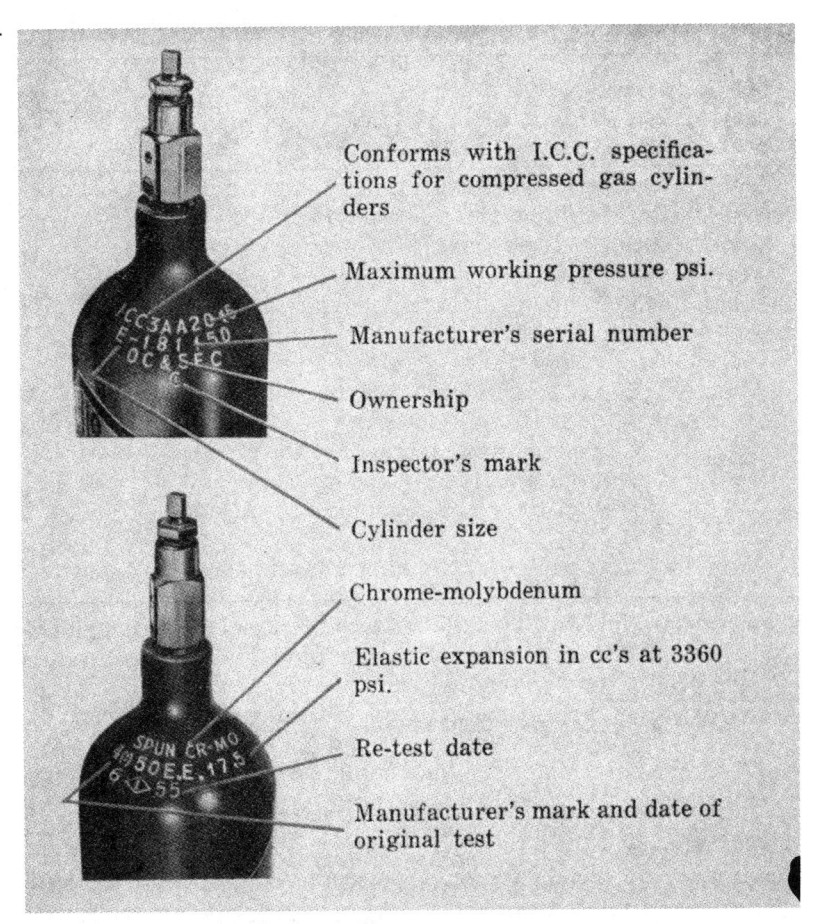

- Conforms with I.C.C. specifications for compressed gas cylinders
- Maximum working pressure psi.
- Manufacturer's serial number
- Ownership
- Inspector's mark
- Cylinder size
- Chrome-molybdenum
- Elastic expansion in cc's at 3360 psi.
- Re-test date
- Manufacturer's mark and date of original test

12. *Before placing cylinders in service,* any paper wrappings should be removed so that the cylinder label is clearly visible. Never drape a cylinder with sheets, hospital gown, or other items.
13. Do not deface or remove any markings that are used for identification of contents of cylinder. This applies to labels, decals, tags, stenciled marks, and upper half of shipping tag. Cylinders should not be refilled using label of previous filling.
14. Never attempt to mix gases in cylinders. (Mixtures should be obtained already prepared from recognized suppliers.) Never refill cylinders.
15. Store gases at temperatures below 72° F.
16. No part of any cylinder containing a compressed gas should be subjected to a temperature above 125° F. A direct flame should never be permitted to come in contact with any part of a compressed gas cylinder.
17. Never tamper with the safety relief devices in valves or cylinders.
18. Never attempt to repair or alter cylinders.
19. Never use cylinders for any purpose other than to contain gas.
20. Cylinder valves should be closed at all times except when gas is actually being used.
21. Notify supplier of cylinder if any condition has occurred which might permit any foreign substance to enter cylinder or valve, giving details and cylinder number.
22. Do not place cylinders where they might become part of an electric circuit.
23. Cylinders should be repainted only by the supplier.
24. Compressed gases should be handled only by experienced and properly instructed persons.

In addition, transfilling by the average hospital and medical personnel is considered an unsafe practice. Transfilling is the process of filling a small service cylinder from a large supply cylinder. During this process the gas coming from the reservoir or large cylinder must first expand; it is then rapidly recompressed and a large amount of heat is then evolved, which is a hazard even where conditions are controlled.

Closing cylinders requires care. During the transportation valves should be closed and protected; where caps are provided they should be kept on the cylinder head. Never drop a cylinder or permit one to strike another object or cylinder. It is recommended that large cylinders be moved by a hand truck and that all cylinders be well secured during movement.

USING CYLINDER CONTENTS. To use the contents of a gas cylinder the following steps should be followed:

1. The cylinder valve should be opened slightly for a moment to clear the outlet of possible dust. This procedure is called "cracking" the cylinder. The outlet should be pointed away from the operator and other personnel. This step is performed before attaching cylinder to a yoke.
2. A suitable pressure regulator device must be used and is attached to the outlet valve, of the cylinder. Generally, a pressure regulator is used, especially with large cylinders while a needle valve is frequently used in conjunction with small gas cylinders. All connections should be of the proper size with appropriate thread specifications and one should never force connections that do not fit.
3. After attaching the regulator determine that it is turned to the off position before cylinder valve is opened. In the case of needle valves of flowmeters these should be closed. When these precautions have been observed, the cylinder valve is opened slowly. Never permit gas to enter a regulator suddenly.
4. When the particular need for a compressed gas is completed, the cylinder valve should be closed. All pressure in the system should then be released by opening secondary valves or gauges. Finally, these valves and gauges should be closed.
5. Before a regulatory device is removed, close the cylinder valve and release all pressure in the system.
6. Valves on empty cylinders should remain closed.
7. Large cylinders are provided with a valve protection cap. These should not be removed until ready to withdraw contents of a cylinder or to connect to a manifold.

READING

In cylinders containing a liquefied compressed gas and vapor in equilibrium, the pressure in the container is determined almost solely by the vapor pressure on the liquid at the existing temperature, and bears no relation to the amount of liquid which remains in the cylinder. At a given temperature, the pressure in a cylinder containing a liquefied compressed gas such as nitrous oxide, cyclopropane, or carbon dioxide will remain approximately constant until all of the liquid has been withdrawn, at which time the pressure drops in relation to the rate at which the remaining gas is withdrawn. As long as liquid remains in the cylinder, the true contents can be determined only by weight.

In cylinders charged with a nonliquefied compressed gas, the pressure in the container is related both to temperature and the amount of gas in the container. For such gases whose physical state in the cylinder is gaseous, such as oxygen, ethylene, and helium and oxygen mixtures, cylinder content may be determined by pressure. At any given temperature the pressure will decrease proportionately as the cylinder contents are withdrawn. Thus, at a given temperature, when the pressure is reduced to half the given pressure, the cylinder will be half full.

For the various liquefied gases a table relating temperature and gas pressure will be presented when the pharmacology of a particular gas is discussed in subsequent chapters.

CONVERSION FACTORS

In dealing with compressed gases and the contents of anesthetic gas cylinders, it is necessary that the operator knows the volume of gas which he can expect will be delivered from a gas cylinder. This must depend on some of the factors presented above, considering whether the gas in question is liquefied or nonliquefied. However, certain factors are useful in making conversion volumes. These are as follows:

1 L	0.264 gal	or 0.035 cu ft
1 gal	3.785 L	or 0.132 cu ft
1 cu ft	28.3 L	or 7.48 gal

IDENTIFICATION STANDARDS[13–21]

Identification standards for medical gas containers have been set forth by the National Bureau of Standards in the Federal Register Vol. 37, No. 225, November 21, 1972. These standards are as follows:

1. American National Standards Institute (ANSI) Z 48.1–1954 (1970), "Methods for Marketing Portable Compressed Gas Containers to Identify the Material Contained."[13,20]
2. ANSI B 57.1–1965, "Compressed Gas Cylinder Valve Outlet and Inlet Connections (pin index safety system)."[15,16]
3. National Fire Protection Association (NF-PA) 56 A-1971, "Inhalation Anesthetics (Flammable and Nonflammable)"[22–24]
4. Military Standard 1018, December, 1970, "Color Code for Pipelines and Compressed Gas Cylinders."
5. Compressed Gas Association C-7, "Guide to the Preparation of Precautionary Labeling and Marketing of Compressed Gas Containers."[13]
6. Bureau of Standards SPR 176–41.[25,26]
7. Department of the Army Technical Bulletin TB 34–9–127, "Colors for Medical Gas Cylinders."
8. International Organization for Standardization (ISO) R 32, "Identification of Medical Gas Cylinders."[28,29]

9. Compressed Gas Association P–C9 1982 Color marking.[30]

COLOR CODE FOR CYLINDERS*

A color code to aid in identification of gas cylinders was adopted in 1949 by The Medical Gas Industry, The American Society of Anesthesiologists, and the American Hospital Association. The code was known as Simplified Practice Recommendation (R176–41) of the Bureau of Standards (Fig. 5–6).[25,26]

The current base for color code in the United States is contained in three principal standards: The SP Recommendation R–176–41;[25] Department of Army TB-34-9-127; and the Compressed Gas Association Pamphlet C-9 1982.[30]

The codes recommend that anesthetic gas cylinders approximately 4½ inches in diameter by 26 inches long and smaller, for use in anesthesia machines, be marked with the following colors or color combinations:

Oxygen	—Green (White in International Code)
Nitrous Oxide	—Light Blue
Cyclopropane	—Orange
Ethylene	—Red (Purple in International Code)
Carbon Dioxide	—Gray
Carbon Dioxide Oxygen	—Gray and Green
Helium	—Brown

The code for current practices in the United States differs from the International Standards Organization (ISO) color scheme with respect to the colors of oxygen and ethylene.[27,30] In the interests of standardization the various U.S. organizations concerned recommended that the ISO color code be adopted. Oxygen cylinders were to be identified by white and ethylene cylinders by purple.[29]

These colors are applied at least to the shoulders of the cylinders so as to be clearly visible. Where two colors are required the patterns must permit a sufficient amount of both colors to be seen together. In the case of chromium-plated cylinders (paint does not adhere) for cyclopropane, the labels shall bear the orange color.

PIN INDEX SYSTEM[31]

An ever-present hazard in anesthesia has been the possibility of error in attaching the flush-type valves of gas cylinders to gas apparatus with yoke connections. To eliminate this hazard of accidental substitution of the wrong gas, a combined cooperating group with representatives from the Compressed Gas Association, the American Society of Anesthesiologists and the American Hospital Association studied the problem and developed the Pin Index Safety System. The idea for this safety measure was first presented by Dr. Philip D. Woodbridge in a letter to Mr. J. G. Sholer of the Ohio Chemical and Manufacturing Company in 1939. This system was approved in 1952 by the three cooperating organizations as well as the military authority.[19]

The system consists of two pins projecting from the yoke assembly of the gas apparatus and positioned to fit into matching holes in the body of the cylinder valve. For any one gas there is only one combination of pins and holes. Unless the correct cylinder valve is attached the pins and holes will not match and parts will not fit.

There are six pin positions on the yoke and six holes on the gas cylinder. This allows ten different combinations using two position holes on the valve and two corresponding pins on the yoke. Eight medical gases or gas mixtures have been assigned combinations at present. With the system it is impossible for the cylinder of one type gas to be attached to a yoke pin indexed for another gas. The master index for the valve holes is illustrated as well as the eight assigned hole combinations (Fig. 5–7).

The central point of each position has been located as follows: A line drawn through the center of the valve outlet at an angle of 30 degrees to the right of the valve face passes through position number 1 while other positions are located at intervals of 12 degrees.

Attempts to mount the wrong cylinder will be met with frustration as the pins will not meet with the holes and the cylinder valve will not seal against the inlet washer. The pin indexing system can be defeated by force, ingenuity, and available adaptors but it is foolish and unsafe to do so.[32]

STORAGE OF CYLINDERS

In the storage of medical gas cylinders the recommendations of the Compressed Gas Association should be followed. These include:[13,17,18,20]

---

* In 1939, Dr. Paul Wood proposed that medical gas cylinders should be color-coded to help avoid accidental confusion of cylinders. As Chairman of the Committee of the Bureau of Standards, Dr. Wood prepared the Simplified Practice Recommendation that was adopted in 1941[25,26] as a Department of Commerce regulation.

This regulation formed the basis for the development of an international standard entitled "ISO Recommendation R 32, Identification of Medical Gas Cylinders," which was adopted in 1952. While in the formative stage, the British Standards Institution adopted the ISO proposal in 1955.

The ISO standard differs from the United States ICC (DOT) standard in that the color for oxygen is white while that of the SPR.41 is green. To update the Department of Commerce (DOT), the Standing Committee on Simplified Practice Recommendation revised the SPR 176-41 to conform to the ISO standard. A Standing Committee (V. J. Collins, Chairman) SPR 176-41 of the Department of Commerce proposed in 1951 that the color code for the United States should coincide with the ISO Code. This has not been implemented.

128 General Anesthesia

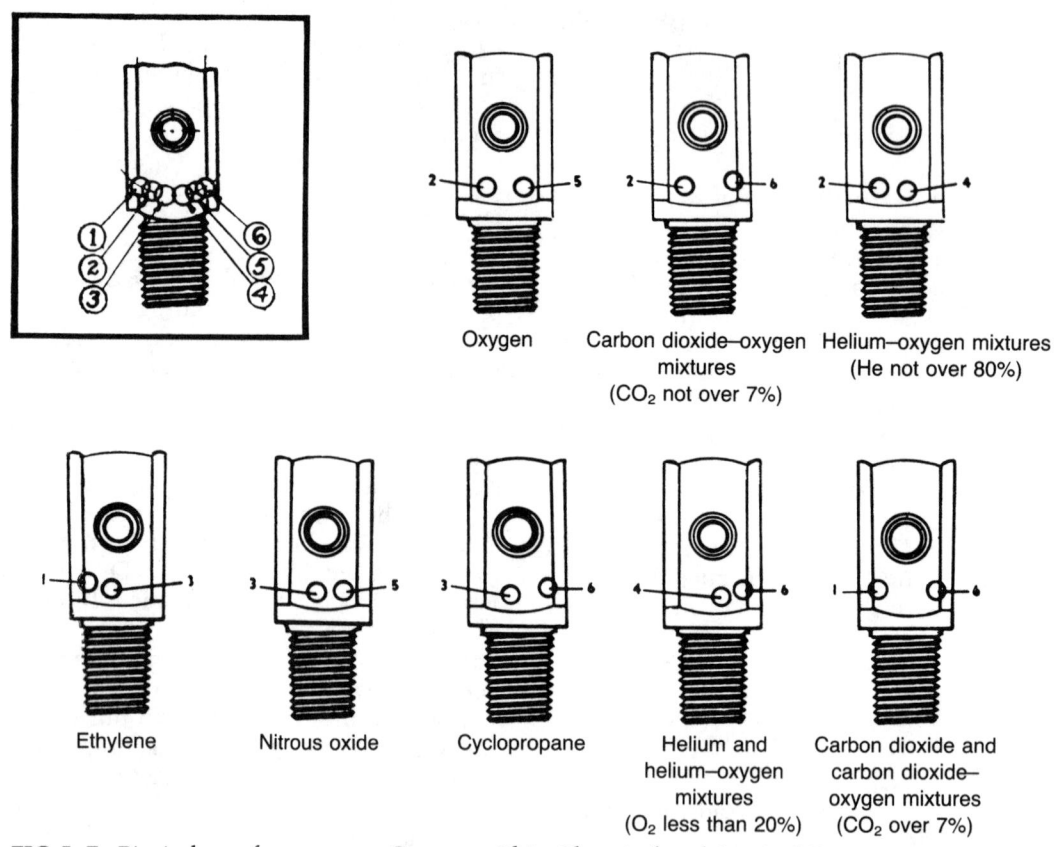

FIG 5–7. Pin index safety system. Courtesy Ohio Chemical and Surgical Equipment Company.

Oxygen

Carbon dioxide–oxygen mixtures (CO_2 not over 7%)

Helium–oxygen mixtures (He not over 80%)

Ethylene

Nitrous oxide

Cyclopropane

Helium and helium–oxygen mixtures (O_2 less than 20%)

Carbon dioxide and carbon dioxide–oxygen mixtures (CO_2 over 7%)

1. A definitely assigned location specific for cylinders. (No other products or items permitted.)
2. Storage rooms should be dry, cool, ventilated, and fireproof. Lighting fixtures should be shatterproof and electrical switches approved for hazardous locations used. Subsurface locations should be avoided.
3. Protect cylinders against the following hazards: excessive rise in temperatures; storage near radiators; highly inflammable substances as gasoline, oil, sparks, or flames; corrosive chemicals or fumes; dampness which promotes rust.
4. Storage of cylinders containing flammable gases must be separate from oxygen and nitrous oxide. Carbon dioxide cylinders should be with the flammable gases since this gas has a dampening effect on fires.
5. Full and empty cylinders should be separated. The storage layout should allow procurement of old stock with minimum handling of other cylinders. Small cylinders are satisfactorily stored in bins, while large cylinders should be placed against a wall, preferably with a chain fastening to prevent them from being knocked over.
6. Do not store in the operating room, in corridors, or in heavily trafficked areas. Unauthorized personnel should be prohibited from entering storage areas.
7. Valves must be kept closed at all times. In the case of large cylinders, covering caps must be in place.
8. Local, state, and municipal regulations should be fulfilled.

PRESSURE REGULATING AND MEASURING DEVICES

PRESSURE REGULATORS

Pressure regulators are used to convert a high source pressure (100 to 2000 psig) to a lower working pressure (35 to 60 psig). Using a lower working pressure offers two advantages: it decreases the chances for rupture of tubing or connections in the machine; and it permits finer adjustments and more constant settings of flowmeters than is possible when the pressure source is high. The principle of a regulator is that the force exerted by a high pressure on a surface of small cross-sectional area is equal to the force exerted by a lower (regulated) pressure acting on a diaphragm of larger area (Fig. 5–8). This is rather like two children of different weights on a teeter-totter. They can balance if they are at different distances from the fulcrum's center or if a weight is added to the side of the lighter child.

The reducing valve may be of the pneumatic balance demand type (Fig. 5–8) or, more commonly, of

—Net Contents of Cylinders for All Gases*

Size	CO₂	CO₂-O₂	(CH₂)₃	C₂H	He	He-O₂	N₂O	O₂	Cylinder Dimensions	Weight of Empty Cylinder (lbs.)
G	3200 gals.	1400 gals.		2800 gals.	1100 gals.	1126 gals.	3655 gals.	1400 gals.	8½ × 55"	100
M		800 gals.		1600 gals.			2000 gals.	800 gals.	7 × 47"	66
E		165 gals.		330 gals.			420 gals.	165 gals.	4¼ × 29¾"	15
D	250 gals.	95 gals.	230 gals.	200 gals.	80 gals.	82 gals.	250 gals.	95 gals.	4¼ × 20¼"	10¼
B	50 gals.	40 gals.		100 gals.	15 gals.	15 gals.	100 gals.	40 gals.	3¼ × 16½"	5¾
A		20 gals.		40 gals.			50 gals.	20 gals.	3 × 10¾"	2½
†DD			230 gals.						3¾ × 23¼"	8¾
†BB			100 gals.						2¾ × 19¾"	4
†AA			40 gals.						2¾ × 11"	3

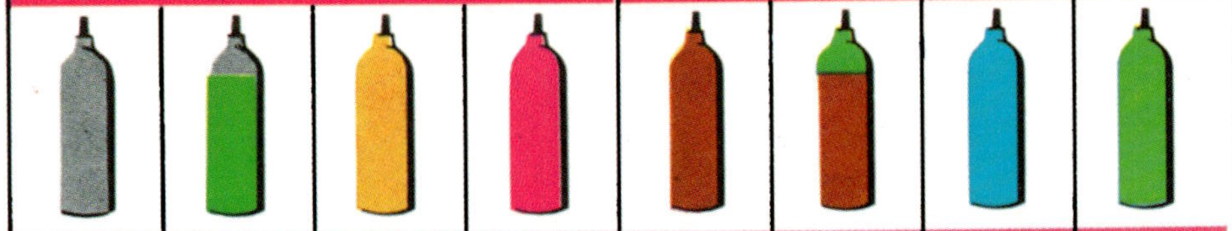

Cylinder Color Code

FIG. 5-6. Net contents of cylinders for all gases. Cyclopropane cylinders may be chrome plated and bear orange labels. Courtesy of Ohio Chemical and Surgical Equipment Company.

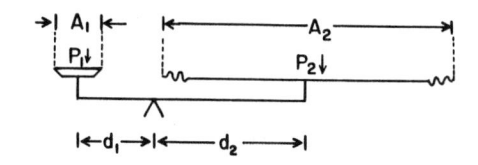

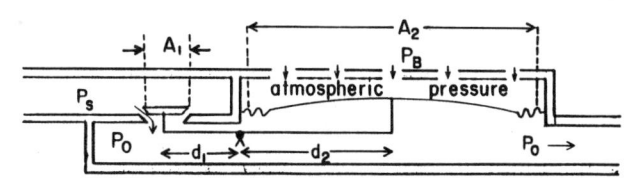

FIG. 5–8. The pneumatic balance and demand valve. A pneumatic balance is one in which the torque from a high pressure side is balanced against the torque from a low pressure side. The torque on the high pressure side is force times lever arm. Force is the product of pressure (P_1) and area (A_1). The lever arm is d_1. Thus, a high pressure acting over a small area and a short lever arm may be balanced by a lower pressure (P_2) operating on a large area (A_2) with a large lever arm (d_2). Mathematically the condition of balance in the upper diagram would be expressed as $P_1 \times A_1 \times d_1 = P_2 \times A_2 \times d_2$. The bottom panel shows a simplified demand valve based on the pneumatic balance. The regulator from a gas cylinder delivers gas at a supply pressure (P_s). When the patient inspires, the outlet pressure (P_o) is decreased below barometric pressure. The resulting pressure difference across the diaphragm (A_2) at the end of the lever arm (d_2) depresses the diaphragm, thus opening the supply valve of area A_1 via lever arm d_1. High pressure gas then enters the regulator chamber to restore P_o to atmospheric and close the valve again.

the reciprocal demand valve configuration (Fig. 5–9A), both of which reduce a high supply pressure to atmospheric pressure. The reciprocal demand valve becomes a regulator if a spring is added (Fig. 5–9B). This places tension on the output pressure side, resulting in an output pressure higher than atmospheric, but fixed by the force of the spring. If an adjustable spring is provided (Fig. 5–9C), it becomes an adjustable pressure regulator. With this device there may be some irregularities in output pressure if the supply pressure decreases, for instance as cylinders empty. Therefore, a two-stage regulator that employs two reducing valves in series (Fig. 5–10) is used to provide a more constant regulated pressure. Two-stage regulators are also less sensitive to back pressure or the effects of continued usage.

MANOMETERS

Manometers are pressure measuring devices and if carefully designed and manufactured, they will provide accurate measurements. Two types of manometers are commonly incorporated into anesthesia machines. One type is the Bourdon tube gauge, which is used in gas supply and other high pressure (over 15 psia*) lines. The Bourdon tube works like a long, empty balloon. As the inside is pressurized, it fills up, and just as it nears its nominal volume, it no longer hangs limply down but rises until it stands out horizontally. In the Bourdon tube gauge, the "balloon" is a small curved dead-end copper or bronze tube (Fig. 5–11). Increased pressure in the tube straightens the tube and moves an indicating needle. The range of motion of the needle may be augmented by one or more gears. The Bourdon gauge is usually linear within its design range and may be designed to indicate pressure changes of as little as 10 psi at 2000 psig.†

If a fixed resistance to gas flow is incorporated just downstream from a Bourdon tube gauge, the device becomes a flowmeter. The flowmeters on reducing valves used with cylinders for oxygen administration are usually of this type. The inlet pressure, which is essentially what the gauge measures, is approximately proportional to outflow through the resistance. In practice, the inlet pressure can be varied from atmospheric to about 50 psig to yield a flow from zero to about 20 L/min. The marks on the flowmeters are usually in liter gradations and are only approximate indicators of the actual flow. In addition, the Bourdon flowmeter assumes that the outflow pressure is essentially atmospheric pressure, as when oxygen is being supplied to an oxygen mask or nasal prongs. If the flowmeter is used with a Venturi mask, humidifier, or intermittent positive-pressure breathing (IPPB) apparatus, in which back pressure is generated, the indicated flow may overestimate the actual delivery rate.

The second type of manometer is the aneroid gauge, which is used to measure pressure in low pressure areas such as the outlet, breathing circuit, and ventilator locations. Aneroid gauges are also used in sphygmomanometers, oscillotonometers, and barometers. The aneroid manometer works like a concertina bellows, compressed by a spring. As gas under pressure enters the copper or stainless steel bellows, the bellows expands, compressing the spring and moving an indicating needle, the motion of which may be augmented by gears (Fig. 5–12). This type of manometer may also respond to decreased pressure, serving as well as a vacuum gauge. The linearity of the gauge depends on Hooke's law (within its elastic limit, strain is proportional to stress) and is usually ± 1%. With use, the needle may deviate from the zero point when no pressure is applied, but can be reset by altering the initial

---

* Psia stands for pounds per square inch absolute, which is the difference between the measured pressure and that at "absolute zero."

† As noted earlier in this chapter, psig stands for pounds per square inch gauge, which is the difference between measured and atmospheric pressures. Most gauges are set to read zero at 1 atmosphere (14.7 psia) pressure.

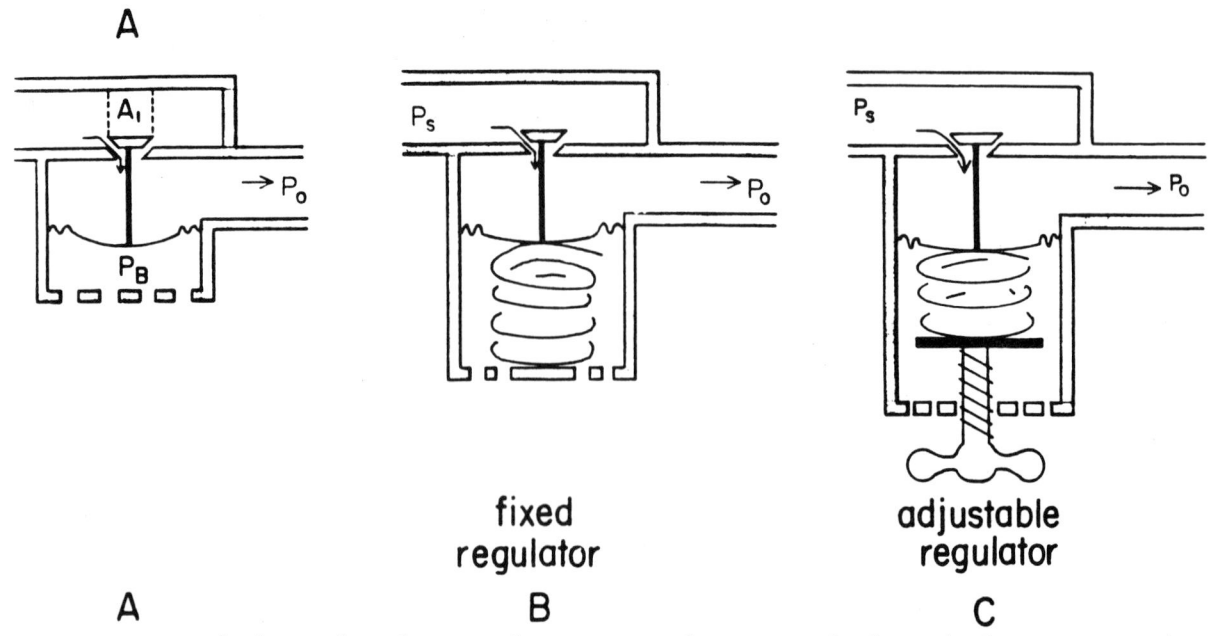

FIG. 5–9. Demand valves and regulators employing reciprocal action. *A.* The demand valve operates on the same principle as the pneumatic balance of Fig. 5–8. An attempt to inspire from the outlet of the valve lowers P_o below barometric pressure P_b. This pushes up the valve stem and opens the valve at A_1. Gas under pressure from the supply (P_s) flows in to restore the pressure P_o to atmospheric. If it is desirable to keep the outlet pressure above barometric pressure, as in the fixed regulator shown in *B.*, a spring can be inserted in the housing, pushing on the large diaphragm, thus augmenting the force opening the valve. The regulator may be made adjustable as in *C.* by a threaded screw which changes the compression on the spring. *C.* is a diagram of a typical one-stage adjustable regulator.

spring force with a screw adjustment. While some aneroid gauges can detect pressure changes of less than 0.1%, those used in anesthesia are less accurate and less expensive, but are usually accurate to 1% if properly maintained.

Other less common devices for pressure measurement include electronic displays of strain gauge imbalances, which are expensive; U-tube water or mercury manometers, which are fragile and messy if broken; and compression of a substance, usually air, in a dead-ended tube, which tends toward alinearity.

Fail-Safe Systems (Low-pressure Cut-off)[33]

Fail-safe devices for anesthetic gases are basically pressure manometers with mechanically coupled shut-off valves (Fig. 5–13). In addition to shutting off the nitrous oxide as the oxygen pressure decreases, the fail-safe device may also alert the user by means of a whistle alarm. The alarm comes from a small tank, about the size of an aerosol shave cream can, which fills with oxygen or nitrous oxide to operating pressure (usually 50 psig) when the oxygen side is first pressurized. If the pressure subsequently falls, the tank empties through a whistle (Fig. 5–14). Some fail-safe alarms whistle only if nitrous oxide is in use; others whistle even if only oxygen is in use and its pressure falls. As always, the user must be familiar with the equipment.

It is important to remember that fail-safe devices do not warn of low oxygen concentration. Oxygen monitors perform that function. Fail-safe devices merely warn of low oxygen pressure, for whatever reason.

THE DIAMETER INDEX SAFETY SYSTEM (DISS).[10] This system makes it impossible to interchange high-pressure gas lines at pressures of 200 psig (pipelines; large cylinder G) with the low-pressure medical gas connections. Each gas outlet (suction) is provided a threaded noninterchangeable connection; each outlet has its own special diameters and cannot be mated with connections for any other gas (Fig. 5–15).

DISS was developed by the Compressed Gas Association to help reduce the possibility of human error in the administration of inhalation anesthetics, oxygen therapy, resuscitation, and suction. The system is based on having two concentric and specific bores in the body and two concentric and specific shoulders on the connecting nipple. The small bore (BB) mates with the small shoulder (MM) and the large bore (CC) mates with the large shoulder (NN). Any attempt to match connections for dissimilar gases will fail because of interference. Oxygen retains its already established safe connection, which is quite different and apart from the other gases.

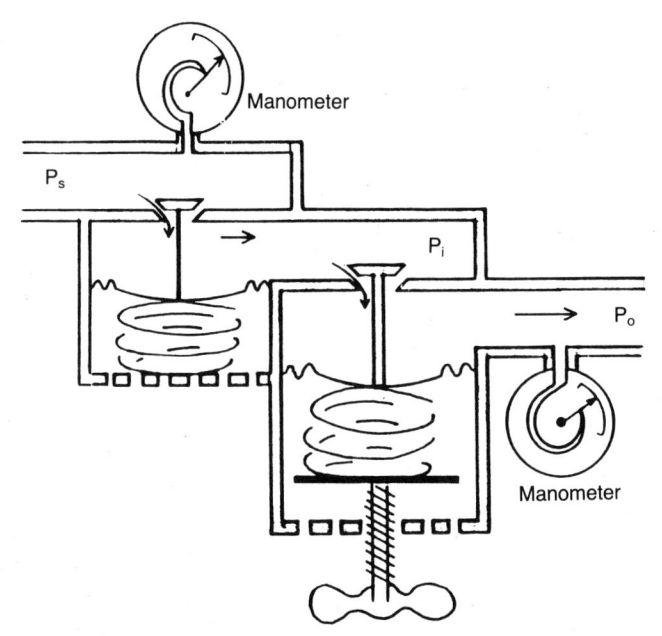

FIG. 5–10. Two-stage regulator. The two-stage regulator is essentially two one-stage regulators in a series. The advantage of an additional stage of regulation is that the output pressure is more constant than it is with a single-stage regulator. In this diagram, the supply (cylinder) pressure (P_s) is measured by the first manometer. Gas flows into the intermediate chamber whose pressure (P_i) is set at some value above atmospheric by the nonadjustable spring in the first stage. The output pressure (P_o) is set at the desired value by the adjustable spring in the second stage. When the output pressure (P_o) is lowered below that desired, the valve in the intermediate chamber opens and gas flows from the intermediate to the outlet chamber where the delivery pressure (P_o) is measured by the second manometer.

VALVES

Check Valves

When using gases under pressure, it is desirable to incorporate devices to prevent back flow (Fig. 5–16). For example, when one of a pair of cylinders on an anesthesia machine must be replaced, a check valve in the yoke prevents the loss of contents from the other tank and permits continued use of the full tank while the empty one is being replaced. Check valves also prevent transfilling from a full cylinder to a partially empty one. Check valves in the supply end of quick-disconnect gas lines and hoses prevent loss of gas when the line is not connected. Check valves in the delivery side of bypass vaporizers (see below) prevent changes in pressure due to the respiratory cycle from causing a backpressure into the vaporizer and possibly augmenting the vaporization of liquid anesthetics.[34]

Cylinder Valves[13,15]

Cylinder valves are used to seal the contents of a cylinder and to permit their controlled release when needed. There are two basic types of cylinder valves. First, valves of large cylinders (size F, G, H, or K) have a threaded valve outlet and a handle that, when turned, either displaces a seat (high-pressure oxygen type) or a diaphragm (low-pressure nitrous oxide type) upward, thereby allowing gas to flow. A single 360-degree turn counterclockwise changes the valve from off to full open. It is undesirable to turn this type of valve further as it may jam in the open position. Both the port that inserts into the cylinder and the delivery port of large cylinder valves have content-specific threading and diameters assigned by the Compressed Gas Association.

Second, valves of small cylinders (size A through E—"E" is most commonly used) have a "flush-type" surface for the cylinder valve outlet and a detachable handle that, when turned counterclockwise, displaces a seat or diaphragm upward, thereby allowing gas to flow.[15] In addition, the small cylinder valves are pin-indexed to fit specific yokes.[33-35]

Interlock and Switching Valves

Anesthesia machines may have one or more of a variety of interlock and switching valves. These valves may be stacked or mechanically ganged for convenience and flexibility in switching. For example, if an anesthesia machine has two or more vaporizers, the downstream vaporizer must not be supplied with output from the upstream vaporizer, because the contents of the downstream vaporizer will become contaminated and its subsequent output will be unknown. Simple two-way valves prevent this by putting the vaporizers in parallel.

Saturation vaporizers (see below) are supplied with oxygen from a dedicated flowmeter. A switch valve serves as a control, dumping any output of this flowmeter to room air when the control is "OFF." When the valve is turned to the "ON" position, it passes the flowmeter oxygen through the vaporizer and the combined oxygen-anesthetic is then mixed with the other gases.

FLUSH SWITCH VALVE

The flush valve is a common switch valve, whose purpose is to deliver a high flow of oxygen (usually 30 L/min or more) directly from the supply to the breathing circuit (Fig. 5–17). This valve is usually spring loaded so that it must be actively held in the ON position. In addition, it is usually mechanically ganged to the vaporizer control, turning it off when it is activated, thereby preventing the delivery of anesthetic at a time when only oxygen is desired. When the flush valve is released, oxygen flow to the

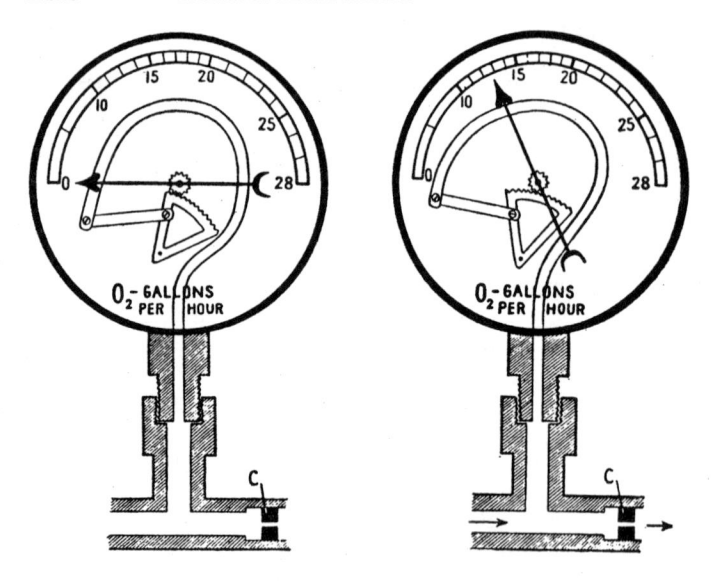

FIG. 5–11. Cross section of a Bourdon gauge type of flowmeter. A gas flowing from its source passes through the orifice (C) to a delivery tube. A pressure builds up proximal to (C) and is transmitted to the hollow spring tube which straightens. This movement operates a clockwork mechanism and the gas flow is indicated on a calibrated scale by a dial. Mushin, courtesy of Charles C. Thomas.

vaporizer is not reactivated until the valve is returned to the vaporizer output position. Because of this safety design, it is not desirable to utilize the oxygen flow through the vaporizer as the primary source of oxygen to meet the patient's needs.

When an anesthesia machine is equipped with two or more saturation vaporizers, the design of the combined selector/flush valve system is complex, and the manufacturer's brochure should be consulted. At one time, some anesthesia machines had flush valves for nitrous oxide, thereby permitting the administration of high concentrations of nitrous oxide.[8] This valve proved to be both unnecessary and unsafe.

FLOW CONTROLLERS

With the earliest anesthetic machines, patients were allowed to inspire through a liquid vaporizer and the diluent gas was usually air. As a result, the patient's minute volume determined the flow of gas through the vaporizer. When compressed gases became widely available, it became possible to control the flow of oxygen and anesthetic gases to a breathing circuit. The first controllers were simple shut-off valves, much like water faucets, where fractional turns of the handle admitted increasing amounts of gas. With these devices control was crude, and rates of flow changed with changing supply pressure. With the development of the needle valve, control of gas flow became easier, more stable, and more accurate.

NEEDLE VALVES

Needle valves deliver a selected gas flow from a regulated pressure source. They consist of a tapered or cylindrical rod moved into or out of a nearly complimentary seat by a threaded screw of fine pitch (i.e., many turns to the inch) (Fig. 5–18). As the area between the valve seat and the needle varies, the resistance to gas flow and hence the flow itself changes. The flow through the valve is extremely turbulent, hence the relationship between flow and revolution of the knob may not be linear. However, needle valves usually operate over a relatively small range of flows (rarely more than a 20-fold change) and thus the deviation from linearity is not great. Most needle valves may be opened much further than the amount necessary to cause

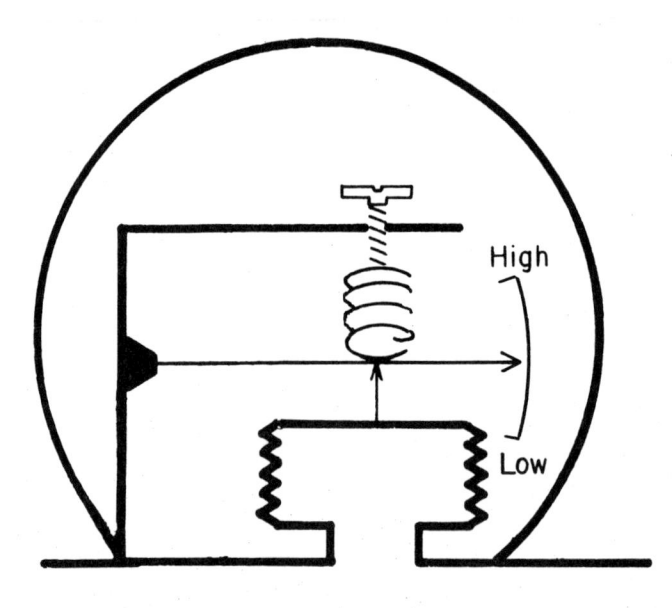

FIG. 5–12. The aneroid manometer. A concertina-like bellows that expands or contracts as the pressure within it changes is physically attached to a pointer that moves as the bellows opens and close. The set point of the aneroid is usually adjustable with a small control spring.

FIG. 5–13. Low-pressure cut-off system. Diagram illustrates the system used in the Foregger Guardian System. When oxygen pressure falls the pressure of the other gases being used also falls so that there is no further intermixing. Courtesy of Foregger Company.

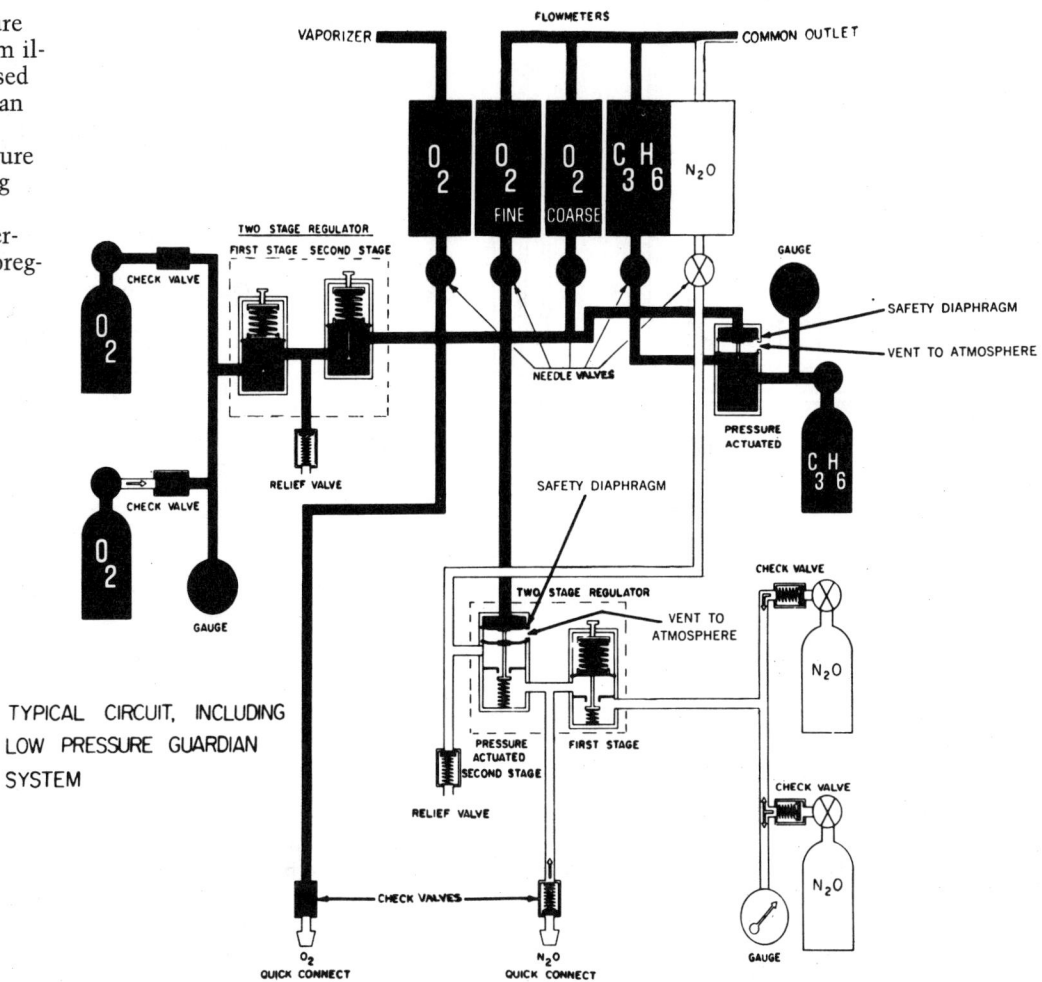

the associated flowmeter to reach the top of the calibrated scale. Use of the needle valve in this manner should be avoided because flow is then uncalibrated and may be overlooked because the flowmeter disappears off scale or becomes unobtrusive at the top of the scale.

Some needle valves may be damaged by grooving or bending if they are tightened beyond a gently closed position.[36] Others have a mechanical stop that prevents this. Either design may permit a small flow when the valve seems to be closed. The anesthetist should not try to correct this by overclosing the needle valve. Shut-off valves on tanks or bulk sources or ON–OFF switches on the machine serve this function. There is also the potential for gas to leak between the threads of the screw and the housing of a needle valve. With some valves this leak is prevented by compressing packing material over the end of the needle-valve stem threads. Maintenance involves tightening or repacking this fitting. Newer machines have tighter packless valves with negligible leaks.

The knobs of the various needle valves are arranged adjacent to, and usually below, their respective flowmeters. As a safety measure, the knobs are often of different shapes and are colored to match the compressed gas color code, but the shapes are not yet standardized.[37] Unusual shapes to these knobs, such as square or triangular, have been criticized as being prone to inadvertent movement by clipboards, laryngoscopes, suction catheters, or other pieces of equipment as they are used and returned to the table top.

FLOWMETERS

The first flowmeters were tubes immersed in water, so that the emerging bubbles of gas could be seen (Fig. 5–19). An improvement on this was the "sight tube" with a vertical row of small holes. With increasing flow, bubbles would issue from more and more holes. Thus one could give three bubbles of oxygen and six bubbles of nitrous oxide for a crude 1:2 mixture (Fig. 5–19). Dissatisfied with this semi-quantitative indicator, Professor Ralph Waters asked the Foregger Company to improve on the flowmeter and the "metric" flowmeter was born. The first

134 General Anesthesia

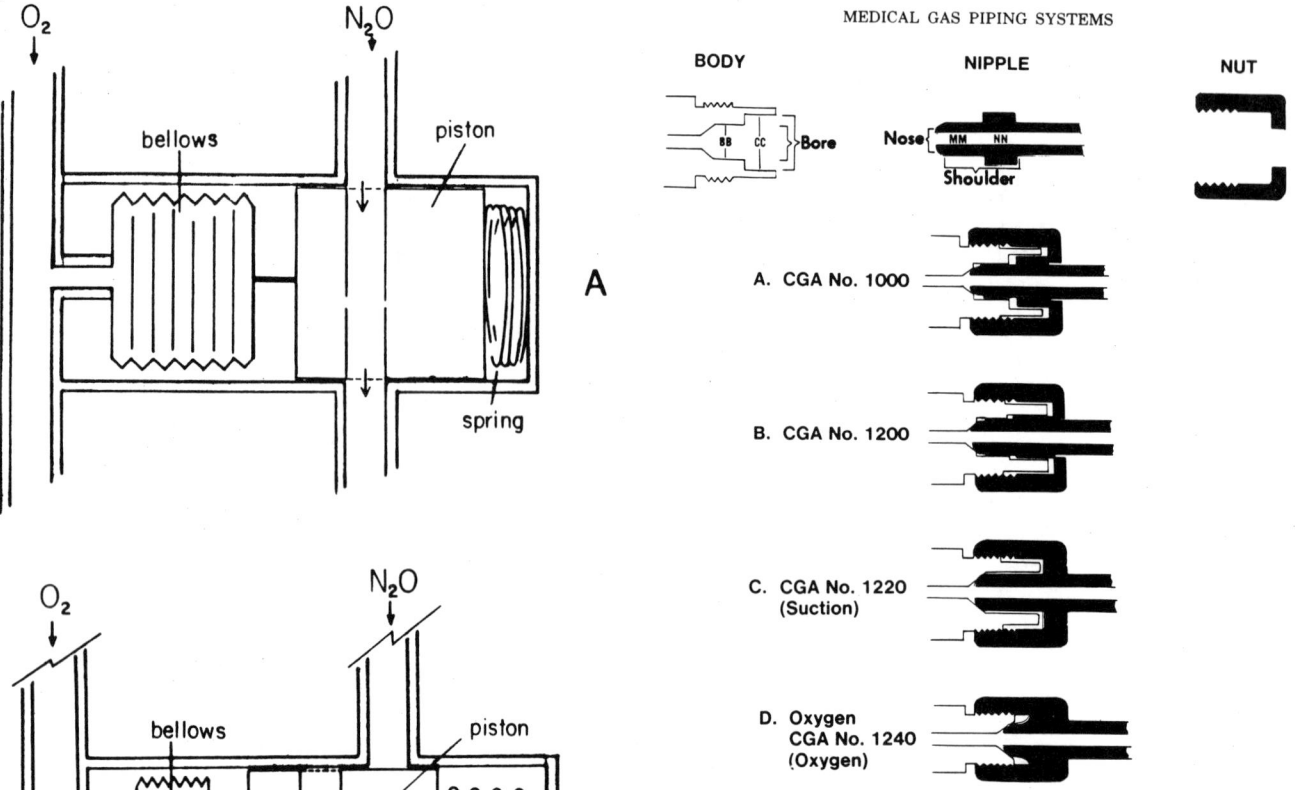

FIG. 5–14. A fail-safe device, which includes an audible alarm. *A.* shows the situation when oxygen pressure has opened the main nitrous oxide flow path. Also opened is a smaller flow path which permits nitrous oxide to fill a pressure tank, approximately the size of an aerosol shave can. Should the oxygen pressure fail, as in *B.*, the compressed spring expands, pushes the piston and collapses the bellows, occluding the nitrous oxide flow to the machine and to the pressure tank. In this position the tank is now vented to the outside through a whistle, and as the gas in the pressure tank discharges, the whistle sounds. This alarm, of course, can continue only for about 1 minute.

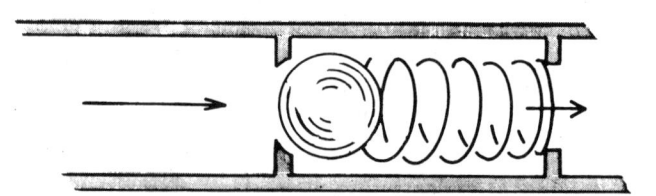

quantitative flowmeter was the inside water meter, an orifice device. It was based on the fact that the pressure drop across a perforated diaphragm in the gas line is roughly proportional to the square of the flow rate. This pressure drop is measured by an upstream glass tube immersed in a glass reservoir. The lower the water level in the tube is driven by the gas pressure, the higher the flow (Fig. 5–19). There was one tube for each gas. The reservoir was made of glass and was about 1 gal in size. Some of the problems with this flowmeter system were overcome by bringing the glass tube outside of the reservoir and making the reservoir of metal; hence, the "outside" water meter (Fig. 5–19). Still, the scale was compressed at low flows, dirt could clog the

FIG. 5–15. Diameter index safety system (1000 Series). With increasing CGA number, the small shoulder of the nipple becomes larger and the large diameter smaller. Noninterchangeability of connections is assured, since either *MM* will be too large for *BB* or *NN* will be too large for *CC* if assembly of a nonmating body and nipple is attempted. Redrawn from Compressed Gas Association; courtesy of Dorsch and Dorsch.

FIG. 5–16. A typical check valve. A ball of either plastic or metal is seated by the action of a compressed spring. However, when supply pressure produces a gas flow in the direction of the arrows, it pushes the ball away from the seat by compressing the spring. Should gas be pushed in the opposite direction, however, the ball would firmly seat itself and close the check valve, preventing back flow.

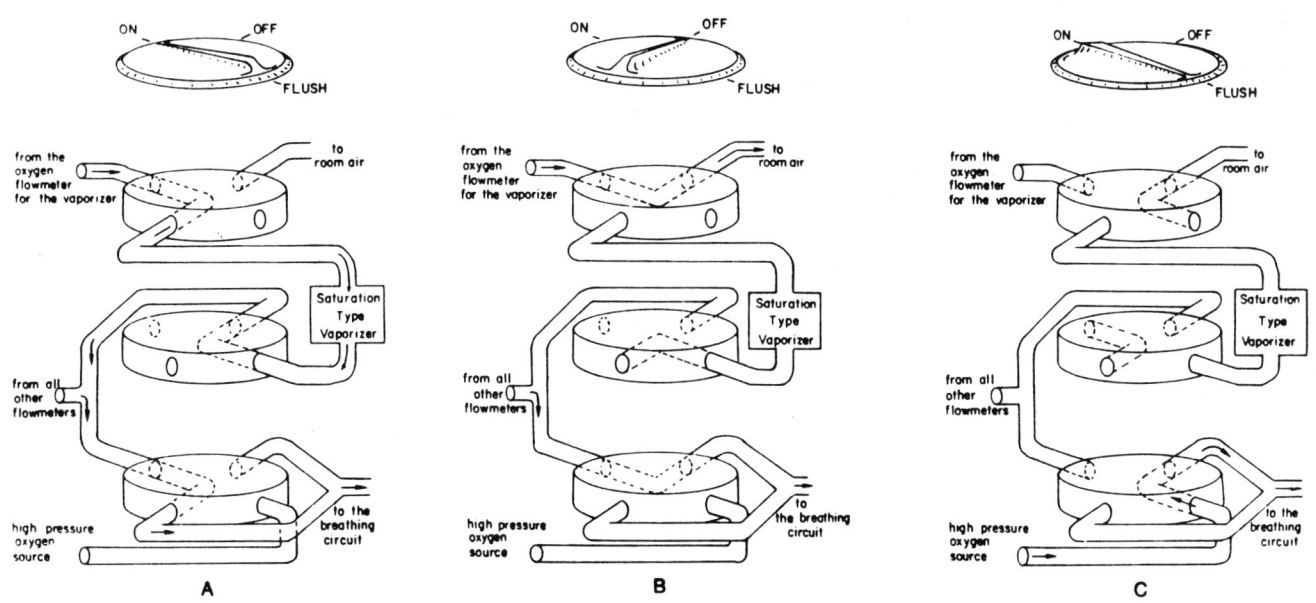

FIG. 5–17. A flush valve mechanically linked to the saturation vaporizer controls. This valve consists of three stopcock-like valves, stacked one on top of another. In the ON position (A.), gases are delivered to the flowmeters and to the saturation vaporizer and mixed before delivery to the breathing circuit. In the OFF position (B.), gases from the flowmeters are delivered to the breathing circuit, but no gas is delivered to the saturation vaporizer. In the FLUSH position (C.), the high pressure oxygen is supplied directly to the breathing circuit, bypassing the flowmeters and the vaporizer. Alternate schemes for flush valves may use push buttons or toggle switches without such mechanical linkage to flowmeters and vaporizer controls.

orifice, and pressure surges could convert the meter into a fountain.

THORPE TUBE FLOWMETERS

Modern anesthesia machines use flowmeters of the variable-orifice type based on the Thorpe tube, which is conically tapered.[38] In these flowmeters, a float is buoyed up by the flowing gas that passes between the float and the walls of the Thorpe tube (Fig. 5–20). The narrowing of the cross-sectional area at the float creates a resistance to gas flow and consequently a pressure drop across the float. The float settles in a position where the force represented by this pressure difference multiplied by the effective cross-sectional area of the float just equals the force of gravity on the mass of the float. Thus, as flow through the tube increases, the pressure differential increases and the float rises until the cross-sectional area between the float and the tube increases sufficiently to restore the pressure drop to its former value.

The float may be positioned in the center of the tube by a central guidewire, by three vertical ridges on the inside of the tube, or by small diagonal slots or vanes in the float causing it to spin and self-center. Recently, spherical floats have been used because they tend to be self-centering inside a vertical tube. Flowmeters are calibrated at ambient temperature and pressure. The flows are read at the top of bobbin floats and at the center of spherical floats. Individual tubes may be marked directly, or a card may be supplied with the tube for insertion behind it.

Extended range flowmeters are commonly used on machines (Fig. 5–21). One design uses a tube with two different tapers. Another uses two floats of different weights, e.g., glass and steel. A third uses two flowmeters in series, the second of which has either a heavier float or a wider tapered tube. However, most machines have two or more different flowmeters with individual needle valves, all in parallel. For example, a typical machine may have one oxygen flowmeter with a range of 50 to 600 ml/min for low-flow circuits; another of 20 to 400 ml/min for supply of a vaporizer containing easily volatilized agents such as halothane, enflurane, or isoflurane; a third of 200 to 2000 ml/min for supply of a vaporizer containing less easily volatilized agents such as methoxyflurane; and a fourth ranging from 0.5 to 10 L/min for providing a wide range of flows.

When more than one flowmeter is available for a particular gas, the anesthetist should choose the one in which the float will be closest to the top. The reason for this is that Thorpe tubes have two inherent errors in function. First, above the lower quarter of well-calibrated, clean vertical tubes, the errors are a constant fraction of the whole scale, not of indicated flow. Second, in the lower quarter or third,

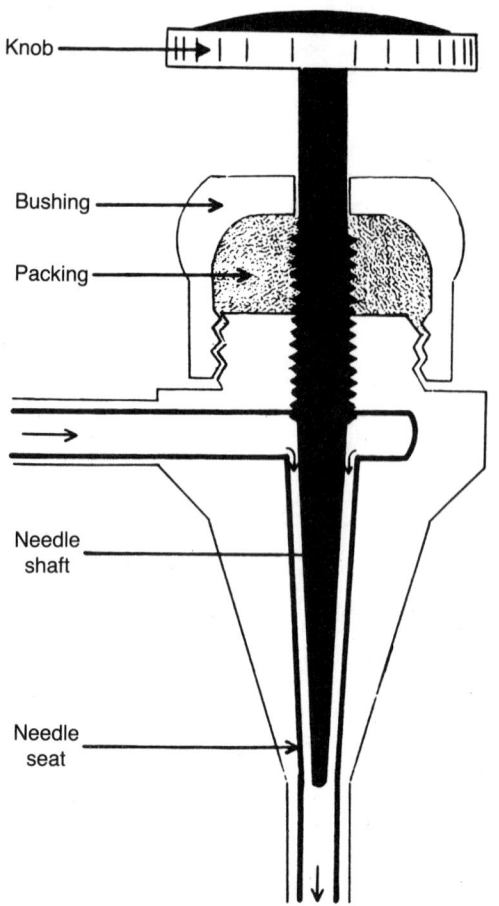

FIG. 5–18. A needle valve. A finely threaded rod with a tapered end fits into a cylindrical or conical tube permitting gas flow to occur between the shaft and the seat (*arrows*). When the rod is screwed fully down, it occludes the flow completely. Depending on the fineness of the threads and the taper of the needle, such valves can be made to control very small flows such as 0 to 100 ml/min, or very large flows such as 1 to 50 L/min.

friction between the float and tube, dirt in the tube, and turbulent eddy effects increase the absolute error somewhat, and the proportionate error greatly.[39] Thus, a 0.5 to 10 L/min flowmeter may be accurate within 100 ml/min at full scale (a 1% error), 100 ml/min at 2 L/min (a 5% error), and 200 ml/min at 0.5 L/min (a 40% error). This is a major reason for not interchanging agents in saturation vaporizers (see below). When the vaporizer is supplied with a flowmeter planned for an agent requiring relatively high flows (e.g., methoxyflurane), it can be grossly inaccurate when filled with an agent requiring lower flows (e.g., halothane), since the float will be riding extremely low in the tube.

OTHER TYPES OF FLOWMETERS

In most anesthesia machines the needle valve precedes the flowmeter and offers a high resistance to gas flow. The large pressure drop across the needle valve results in a flowmeter inlet pressure close to atmospheric and, hence, a small pressure drop across the float. This promotes accuracy and linearity of the flowmeter. However, a change in pressure downstream from the flowmeter, as when the anesthetist squeezes the reservoir bag or the ventilator cycles, produces a back pressure in the flowmeter, causing a relatively large change in the pressure drop across the float, and a tendency for the float to bob up and down. The flow tends to remain nearly constant during these bobbin excursions, at the valve indicated with no back pressure, but the movement of the float suggests loss of accuracy.

In "compensated" flowmeters the needle valve is placed downstream from the Thorpe tube. Since the pressure drop across the float is small, the inlet and outlet pressures are similar, close to the regulated line pressure, or about 50 psig. There is again a large pressure drop across the needle valve. In this situation, an increase in pressure of the magnitude found in breathing circuits (rarely over 50 mm Hg or about 1 psi) is small compared with the Thorpe tube pressure, so little movement of the float results. Compensated flowmeters are commonly found in conjunction with nebulizers and other respiratory therapy equipment, where large or variable back pressures may be expected, and where precision of the flowmeter reading is not important, since the output is not mixed with other gases.

Several novel flowmeter/controllers have been introduced. One mixes two gases, usually oxygen and nitrous oxide for use in anesthesia, or oxygen and air for use in intensive care units. It utilizes twin needle valves controlled by a single knob for mixing, and another needle valve and Thorpe tube flowmeter with a control knob to regulate flow rate. It can provide variable proportions from 30 to 100% oxygen. Another mechanically connects needle valves for oxygen and nitrous oxide in such a way that oxygen concentrations below 25% cannot be administered. Still another uses a manifold of constant flow nozzles or orifices. In this device, a tiny orifice in the path of gas flow produces a large pressure drop (½-half atm or more). The velocity of gas reaches the speed of sound at the orifice, setting up shock waves and back pressures resulting in a near constant flow despite small changes in either the upstream or downstream pressure. A series of seven such metering orifices, each double the capacity of the previous, with ON–OFF valves, can control and measure flows of 10 to 1270 ml/min ± 10 ml. The valves are solenoid-selected in combinations by an electromechanical switch or more recently, by a microprocessor chip.[9]

COMMON MANIFOLD

The outflow of the various flowmeters is collected by a manifold or mixing chamber so that it can be delivered as a mixture to the breathing circuit. The

Anesthesia Machines and Components

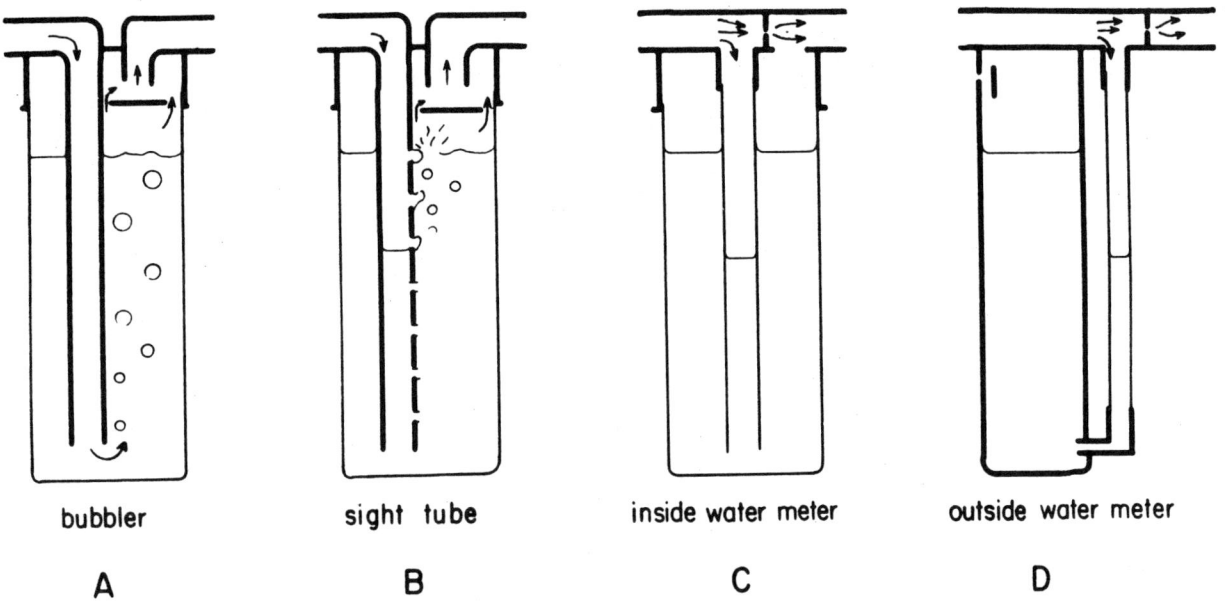

FIG. 5–19. Early flow meters. *A.* illustrates a tube under water. A rough estimate of gas flow is obtained from the vigor of the bubbling. Quantitation is improved in the sight tube (*B.*) where small holes emit bubbles at deeper and deeper levels as the gas flow increases. *C.* is a diagram of an "inside" water meter, a glass tube inside a glass reservoir. This device could be accurately calibrated so long as the orifice was not dirty or damaged. The fragility of the inside water meter was, in part, corrected in the "outside" water meter, where the glass tube is outside a reservoir made of metal (*D.*). However, both inside and outside water meters are inherently alinear, with the scale compressed at the low flow end where the anesthetist would most like the scale expanded.

order in which the flowmeters discharge into the manifold is of some importance. The safest arrangement is to have the oxygen flowmeter downstream from all other flowmeters, i.e., closest to the patient. If the oxygen flowmeter is not the most downstream flowmeter and a leak develops in the system proximal to the most downstream flowmeter, it is possible for the oxygen to leak to the atmosphere and only concentrated anesthetic gas or vapor be delivered to the patient. This cause for hypoxemia has been predicted, observed in practice, and corrected by placing the oxygen flowmeter in the most downstream location.[40–43] The location at which the oxygen-rich output from saturation vaporizers enters the common manifold is determined by its connections with the flush and vaporizer switch valves (see above).

DEMAND (INTERMITTENT-FLOW) MACHINES

Several machines used commonly in dental analgesia and occasionally in obstetric anesthesia provide intermittent flow of a desired nitrous oxide–oxygen mixture with each inspiration of the patient. In these demand flow machines, each inspiration opens both a nitrous oxide and an oxygen pneumatic balance (Figs. 5–8 and 5–9), providing gas flows of each at equal pressure. The concentration of the mixture is set by varying resistances in the outflow path of each gas. In one machine the accuracy of the delivered concentration of oxygen depends on careful balancing of pressure regulators, which are an integral part of the apparatus.[44] While the output

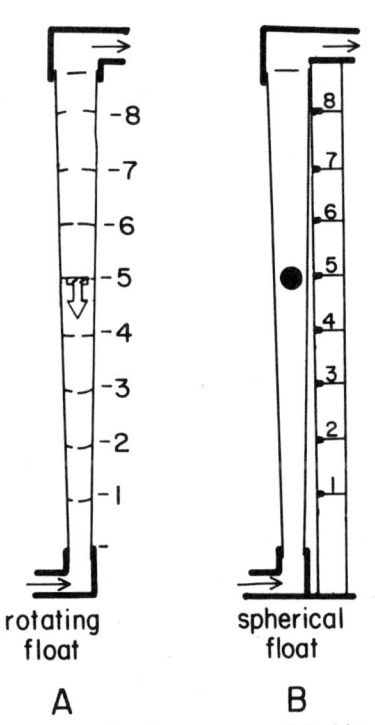

FIG. 5–20. Thorpe tube flow meters. A bobbin (*A.*) or a sphere (*B.*) is buoyed up by the flow of gas inside a conically tapered tube. A scale may be marked on the tube directly or mounted at its side.

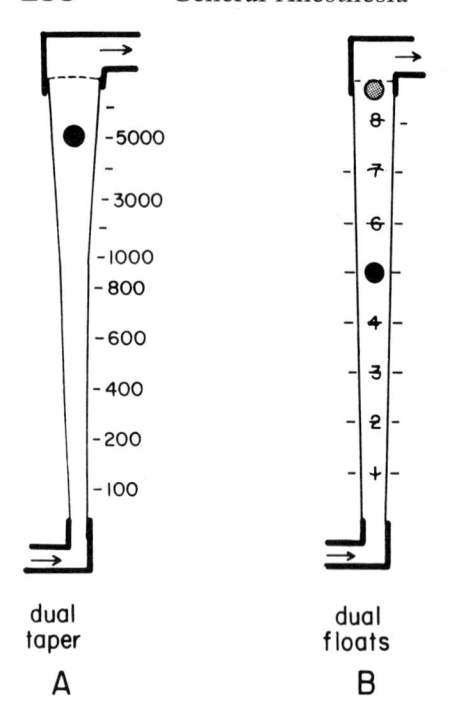

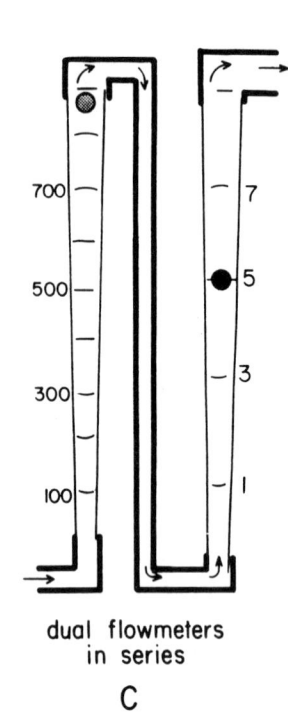

FIG. 5–21. Extended range flowmeters. In *A.*, a single float is utilized in a tube with dual tapers. In *B.*, two floats of different weights are used. In *C.*, dual flowmeters are used in series.

can be accurate to ± 1% oxygen, it is not uncommon to find machines of this type in use with inaccuracies in oxygen concentration of 10% or more. It is possible in principle to mix high-pressure gases in desired proportions, but the extant devices mix the gases after reduction to near ambient pressure.

When used in their intended fashion, demand machines deliver a mixture of nitrous oxide and oxygen when the pressure in the breathing circuit decreases just below atmospheric as a result of the patient's effort to inspire. The actual negative pressure at which flow is initiated depends on an independent and adjustable knob. The arrangement is similar in principle to that in Figure 5–9C. It is possible, by turning the adjustable knob, to provide a continuous delivery of anesthetic gases, although the flow rate may still increase with each inspiratory effort of the patient. If it is desired to use another agent as well, the mixture of nitrous oxide and oxygen may be passed through a low-resistance vaporizer before delivery to the patient. However, if the rebreathing feature is in use, this procedure can be extremely dangerous.[45]

MAINTENANCE AND SERVICE

Most manufacturers of anesthesia machines maintain regional service centers and supply depots in those countries where they sell their machines. Many independent firms offer service, supply, and maintenance in specific cities. Service contracts can provide preventive maintenance visits for two to six times a year. However, most machine service is simple and can be done in-house if necessary. Operating and maintenance manuals are supplied with new machines and are available for purchase for most of the older models. These provide necessary illustrations and parts lists so that with some simple equipment such as socket wrenches, screwdrivers, and Teflon tape, an anesthetist can accomplish routine preventive maintenance. Calibration of vaporizers, flowmeters, and gas analyzers is more equipment-intensive, but even these services can be done in-house or with mail-order laboratory help.

The basic operations in maintenance and service are periodic machine checkout, and written, collected and acted-on memos of deficiency. Many defects are not easily reproducible without details as to usage when the defect was noted. Some defects are intermittent, others obscure. Therefore, a big piece of tape labeled "BROKEN" is not sufficient. Once detected, defects should be corrected rather than allowed to persist and thus inconvenience or endanger others.

ACCESSORIES FOR THE ANESTHESIA MACHINE

Many accessories including a ventilator; spirometer; electrocardiographic and automated blood pressure monitors; oxygen, carbon dioxide, and anesthetic gas analyzers; thermometer; clock; timer; airway pressure meter; light; and telephone are commonly found on anesthesia machines. Some of these accessories increase the safety of anesthesia for patients while others are items that facilitate the work of the anesthetist and make him more effective and efficient. While the value of accessories ranges from essential to useful, their addition to the machine is not without problems. Most anesthesia machines manufactured today lack adequate shelf space to accommodate the large number and size of accessories that are commonly mounted on them. As a consequence, additional shelves must be added after delivery, which make the machine top heavy and hazardous to move. Furthermore, most accessories require electrical power, necessitating the instillation of auxillary electrical outlets on the machine. The electrical connections to the various accessories generate a maze of wires that, in some cases, may impair the anesthetist's full view of the monitors. Unfortunately, most accessories are not designed with the anesthesia machine in mind and most machines are not designed with the accessories in mind. Melding the accessories into the anesthesia machine in an efficient, safe manner may be the greatest challenge currently facing anesthesia machine and accessories manufacturers. The devices that require further description in this chapter are analyzers for oxygen, carbon dioxide, and anesthetic gases. See Chapter 15 for a discussion of ventilators and spirometers and Chapter 3 for a discussion of blood pressure and electrocardiographic monitors.

OXYGEN ANALYZERS

Three types of oxygen analyzers have been developed.[46] The earliest was invented by Linus Pauling and uses the unique paramagnetic property of oxygen.[47] No other respirable gas is paramagnetic and able to conduct magnatic lines of force, although some anesthetics are weakly diamagnetic and are able to disperse magnetic fields. The Pauling detector is a rotatable air-filled test body of dumbbell shape suspended from a string in a nonuniform magnetic field. When oxygen is introduced into the measuring chamber surrounding the dumbbell, the dumbbell is pushed out of the more intense field, into the weaker field. The higher the partial pressure of oxygen, the greater the rotation of the dumbbell. The degree of rotation of the dumbbell is detected by means of a light beam reflected from a small mirror attached to the suspension string. Since the unit detects partial pressure and not percentage of oxygen, atmospheric pressure must be known to obtain accurate oxygen values. The unit is simple in design and function and requires only a flashlight bulb and battery for recording; but owing to its sensitive suspension and the light weight of the dumbbell, it is fragile. The detecting chamber is also sensitive to moisture and a silica gel drying tube is provided to dry sample gas prior to its entry into the detecting chamber.

Another type of oxygen analyzer that is virtually indestructible is based on thermal conductivity. Two wires are heated in separate chambers, one of which contains air and the other of which contains the sample gas to be analyzed. The heated wires are connected in a Wheatstone bridge and balanced when both chambers contain air. When an oxygen-rich sample is sucked into the test chamber, the wire in that chamber cools, because of the slightly higher thermal conductivity of oxygen. The cooling changes the resistance of the wire, unbalancing the bridge and causing a meter to deflect. The device is quick-responding, reliable, and durable and for these reasons is widely used in newborn nurseries and intensive care units. However, it is intended only for air–oxygen mixtures. If gases other than air or oxygen are introduced into the mixture, the device yields spurious results. Normoxic oxygen–nitrous oxide mixtures would register as hypoxic mixtures and hence, the device is not useful where anesthetics are used.

The most recently developed and most widely used oxygen monitors are of the polarographic type. This type of monitor is based on the principle that oxygen in solution will conduct current at a rate proportional to the oxygen tension or concentration when an external field of 0.6 volts is applied. Other dissolved gases and anesthetics do so only at much higher potentials. These membrane-covered polarographs work like oxygen electrodes and are properly called Clark cells if they are externally polarized.[46,48] Those that are self-polarizing because the anode and cathode are made of metals, 0.6 volts apart in the electromotive series, have been called fuel cells. Calibration with air and pure oxygen is quick and convenient. However, the sensors require frequent replacement and do not function satisfactorily when the battery becomes weak or when the electrosurgical unit is active. Most new units have a battery check mode.

CARBON DIOXIDE ANALYZERS

Carbon dioxide in the gas phase can be analyzed either chemically or by infrared analysis.[49] Analysis using the Haldane or Scholander apparatus is based on chemical absorption of carbon dioxide and its attendent change in the volume of the sample. A change in pressure instead of volume can also be measured. In an early method, an end-tidal sample was trapped in a large bore tube between two valves. The tube was then shaken to break a small ampule containing sodium hydroxide with which the carbon dioxide reacted, thus lowering the total gas pressure. An attached aneroid gauge displayed the decrease in pressure. A newer device has entirely automated this process for end-tidal sample analysis.

Infrared analysis has become the most commonly used method in anesthesia for detecting carbon dioxide in airway or alveolar gas. This method of analysis is based on the Luft principle, in which a small volume of inhaled or exhaled gas is sampled continuously into a chamber where the absorption of infrared light by carbon dioxide is proportional to its concentration.[49] A second gas-filled detector chamber is heated by absorption of the infrared light that has passed through the gas sample. Thus there is less heating of the detector when there is more carbon dioxide in the sample chamber. The pressure change in the detector chamber owing to the change in temperature is measured by a capacitance manometer and displayed on a scale that registers in either concentration or partial pressure. Because the instrument is not linear, it must be calibrated with sample gases containing known concentrations or partial pressures of carbon dioxide. The operator can use his own exhaled breath when a rapid and only approximate calibration is desired. The newest infrared detectors are small and light enough to be placed directly in the airstream, sampling inhaled and exhaled gas, and obviating the need for a sample pump.

The major advantage of infrared analysis is the rapid response time, thereby allowing for breath-by-breath analysis of both inspired and expired carbon dioxide concentrations. Its major disadvantage is the fact that the instrument is affected by water vapor, nitrous oxide, and nitrogen. Carbon dioxide and nitrous oxide have a slight overlap in their infrared spectral bands, so that pure nitrous oxide will increase the carbon dioxide value by about 0.5%. This effect can be eliminated by filling the analyzer head with nitrous oxide, so the overlapping spectral waves are absorbed before they reach the detector chamber. Water vapor, nitrous oxide, and nitrogen broaden the infrared light spectrum absorbed by carbon dioxide, a phenomenon known as pressure broadening. The manufacturer of the infrared analyzer can lessen the pressure-broadening effect by keeping the carbon dioxide pressure in the detector cell low (10 mm Hg). Also, correction factors that minimize errors in analysis due to this effect are available.[50,51] Finally, the effect is less and greater accuracy is obtained by optically suppressing zero such that 4 or 5% carbon dioxide is at the zero position and full scale is somewhat above the highest value expected.

It is possible to measure carbon dioxide in gas by means of thermal conductivity, in which the differential cooling of a heated resistor on a Wheatstone bridge by a gas sample containing carbon dioxide is compared with the same sample after the carbon dioxide has been removed by soda lime. No commercially available carbon dioxide analyzers use this principle because a large gas sample is required, the response time is slow, and the analysis is greatly affected by the presence of anesthetic gases.

Both oxygen and carbon dioxide can be measured in inspired and expired gas by means of mass spectrometry.[52] A centrally located mass spectrometer can be programmed to sequentially sample airway gases from multiple patients. While a sample from one patient is being analyzed, samples from all other patients are stored in long nylon catheters and then sequentially analyzed. The results are reported on a terminal located at each sampling location. Although this form of gas analysis has a high initial cost, the analyses are rapid, accurate, and include the measurement of airway concentrations of volatile anesthetic gases as well as oxygen and carbon dioxide. It has been suggested that this method of analysis is cost-effective because it encourages the use of closed system anesthesia, increases patient safety, and monitors the effectiveness of gas scavenging systems.[52]

ANESTHETIC GAS ANALYZERS

Although a variety of anesthetic gas analyzers have been developed, none has been entirely satisfactory, and consequently they are not pieces of equipment that are commonly used in operating rooms. The simplest type of anesthetic gas analyzer that has been developed is the Narkotest, whose function is based on the elasticity of Silastic rubber.[53] The rubber is stretched by a spring at one end and a temperature-compensating bimetal strip at the other. Absorption of halothane alters the elasticity of the silastic so that a pointer, connected to the spring–Silastic junction, moves.

The device is calibrated for halothane at the factory. The lipid-like Silastic absorbs all anesthetics in proportion to their lipid solubility, however, so equipotent anesthetic mixtures tend to give equivalent Narkotest readings.[53] Although it was designed and calibrated for halothane, the device has been called a general Minimum Anesthetic Concentration meter. In addition to its nonspecificity for volatile agents, its readings are affected by water vapor and nitrous oxide, so correction factors must be used. Finally, the device has a slow response time (8 sec) and, consequently, only measures mean inspired or expired concentrations unless special efforts are taken to procure end-tidal samples.

The EMMA analyzer will measure any of the halogenated agents. It detects the presence of halogenated vapors by means of their effects on the oscillations of a lipid-coated quartz crystal. The frequency of oscillation changes as halogenated vapor is adsorbed onto the crystal. The analyzer must be calibrated for each anesthetic agent, but once done, it is stable and accurate. The major drawbacks to this analyzer are the lack of a self-calibrating system and a relatively slow response time.

Other analyzers that detect the refractive indices of halogenated drugs are accurate in the absence of nitrous oxide and water vapor and, hence, are used to calibrate vaporizers for halogenated anesthetics.[54]

Both infrared and ultraviolet spectrometers have been used for analysis of nitrous oxide and halogenated agents. The infrared devices work on principles similar to those for carbon dioxide. In the ultraviolet spectrometers, ultraviolet light is absorbed by a gas sample, and photoelectric detection measures the amount of absorption, which is proportional to the concentration.[55] The ultraviolet devices decompose halogenated vapors, producing toxic substances, and should not be used in a recirculating sample loop.[56,57] Both the infrared and ultraviolet spectrometers require regular recalibration with two known samples. Usually pure oxygen and the output of a reliable vaporizer suffice for daily calibration, but periodic checking with reference gases is advisable.

Finally, mass spectrometers are beginning to find application in critical care settings including the operating room.[58–60] These devices will measure anesthetic gas concentrations as well as oxygen and carbon dioxide concentrations (see above). The major drawbacks to mass spectrometry are the expertise and expense required to install and maintain it.

ALARM SYSTEMS

Alarms are an integral part of many pieces of equipment, particularly those that monitor vital functions or are critical to the safe administration of anesthetic gases. Alarms are either gas powered, as with fail-safe pressure-reducing valves for monitoring decreases in oxygen line pressure, or more commonly battery powered, as with electronic monitoring equipment. While alarms are extremely useful and may alert the anesthetist to an impending disaster, they are not without problems. Reports of alarms failing to function at critical times because of battery failure are not uncommon, and as a result, have fostered the recommendation that batteries be changed at frequent, regular intervals. Of equal concern is the fact that with multiple alarms on a machine, it becomes difficult for the anesthetist to determine from an auditory signal which alarm has been activated. Therefore, it is essential that auditory alarms be accompanied by a visual alarm, a flashing light being preferable to a continuously glowing one. The color of the flashing light can be used to indicate the urgency of the problem, with red being of immediate importance and yellow being more cautionary in nature. In general, it is not advisable for alarms to be optional devices or to be readily deactivated by a conveniently located switch. If an alarm is important enough to be installed on a piece of equipment, it should alarm when the equipment is malfunctioning and should not be deactivated permanently until the malfunction has been fixed or the equipment taken out of service. Alarms with delay intervals of 20 to 30 sec between signals are sometimes useful.

VAPORIZATION AND VAPORIZERS

PRACTICAL ASPECTS OF VAPORIZATION

In clinical anesthesia with volatile liquid anesthetics, the objective is to obtain controllable vaporization within an anesthetic range of concentration. Only with recently developed vaporizers have predictable and fairly accurate vapor concentrations become available.

Various principles have been applied to hasten vaporization. In all of these there exists one common requirement, namely, a source of heat. Generally, this is from outside, such as the environmental air interface, a contacting substance, and in part the substance itself. The latter is inefficient since vaporization decreases as the temperature of the liquid decreases, and there is a fall in the partial pressure of vapor above the liquid.

The main principles of increasing vaporization include:

1. Increase surface of evaporation
2. Decrease vapor pressure over the agent ("draw-over" principle)
3. Direct-heating of liquid container
4. Indirect source of heat for the agent

PROCESS OF VAPORIZATION

Most agents with a boiling point below 60° C can be vaporized relatively quickly under ambient conditions. For a substance to be vaporized, it must take up heat in two steps:

1. The liquid must be heated to its boiling point. This process depends on the specific heat of the particular substance. The liquid is raised from its ambient temperature to the boiling point by the specific heat value in calories per gram per degree centigrade.
2. Having reached the boiling point, it is necessary for the liquid phase to change to the gaseous phase by acquiring a substantial additional amount of heat in calories, designated as the latent heat of vaporization.

For halothane at a room temperature of 20° C, the liquid must acquire the following amounts of heat:

1. From 20° C to the boiling point of 50° C, the liquid must be heated such that its temperature is increased by 30° C; each gram requires 0.42 cal to reach the boiling point (the specific heat).
2. To pass into the vapor phase, each gram then requires 35.2 cal, which is the latent heat of vaporization.
3. The total caloric heat required for vaporization of 1 g halothane is

(Temperature to be raised × specific heat) + latent heat of vaporization = total.

In this case, it is (30 × .42) + 35.2 = 47.8.

CHARACTERISTICS OF VAPORIZERS

In the design of a vaporizer the method by which the carrier gas picks up the volatilized agent is an important consideration. From this viewpoint, vaporizers can be distinguished as the "draw over"

TABLE 5–4. CHARACTERISTICS OF VAPORIZERS

A. Method of vaporization
   1. Flow-over
      a. With wick
      b. Without wick
   2. Bubble-through (Pass through)
   3. Flow-over or bubble-through
B. Location
   1. Outside the breathing system
   2. Inside the breathing system
C. Method for regulating output concentration
   1. Variable bypass
   2. Measured flow
D. Temperature compensation
   1. None
   2. By supplied heat
   3. By flow alteration
E. Specificity
   1. Agent specific
   2. Multiple agent

From J. A. Dorsch, and S. E. Dorsch: *Understanding Anesthesia Equipment: Construction, Care, and Complications*, 2nd ed. Baltimore, Williams & Wilkins, 1984.

design where the carrier gas passes over the surface of the liquid and secondly, the design where the carrier gas passes through the liquid.

Clinically important characteristics (Table 5–4) of a vaporizer may be considered under several headings and further analyzed comparatively (Table 5–5):

1. *Complexity.* Increasing precision usually is accompanied by increasing complexity in design. The dangers of malfunction in an intricate device are evident. Simple devices, however, may be safe and satisfactory and sometimes more practical.
2. *Flow Resistance.* Draw over devices generally have lower resistance to gas flow. To obtain a large air-liquid interface, as in "bubble through" devices a break-down of the carrier gas into small particles is required and these must be forced through the liquid or through a baffle (wick type). This produces resistance and these devices are not suitable for "in-circuit" use.
3. *Temperature Stability.* Vaporization is an endothermic process. As a vapor is formed the kinetic energy and heat of the remaining liquid is reduced. This must be replenished from the surroundings. Vaporizers constructed of materials with a high heat capacitance and high heat conductivity are necessary for uniform vaporization. Thus, a chosen vapor concentration should be unaltered by temperature changes in the environment or in the liquid. Automatic compensation should be provided for changes in gas flow and variations in environmental temperature.
4. *Flow Stability.* With low flows of carrier gases equilibration of the gas with the vapor can occur in the time of passage and permits a higher concentration of vapor in the delivered gas. At high flow rates equilibration may be slowed and a low concentration of vapor will be delivered. Construction of a vaporizer to permit a relatively constant concentration at different flow rates of the carrier gas leads to stabilization. This is frequently attained when there is an extensive surface for evaporation. Thus, the chosen vapor concentration intended to reach the patient should be constant and unaltered by varied rates of gas flow through the vaporization chamber.
5. *Precision.* Volatile anesthetic agents like all potent drugs should be administered in precise doses. Vaporizers should permit controllable and predictable delivered concentrations so that inhaled anesthetics may be expressed in milligram doses. Provision for assuring delivery of a known accurate vapor concentration over the range of

TABLE 5–5. VAPORIZER CHARACTERISTICS COMPARED

Vaporizer	Complexity	Flow Resistance	Temperature Stability	Flow Stability	Precision
Draw-Over					
Open Drop	+	+ +	+	+ +	+
Drop-Type Ether	+ +	+	+ + +	+ + +	+
Heidbrink No. 8	+ + +	+	+ +	+ +	+ +
E.M.O.	+ + +	+	+ + + +	+ +	+ + +
F.N.S.	+ + +	+ + + +	+ +	+ +	+ +
Penlon	+ + +	+	+ + +	+ +	+ + +
Heidbrink Fluothane	+ + +	+ +	+ + +	+ +	+ +
Fluotec, Entec	+ + + +	+ + + +	+ + + +	+ + + +	+ + + +
Bubble-Through					
Copper Kettle	+ +	+ + + +	+ + +	+ + +	+ + + +
Vernitrol	+ +	+ + + +	+ + +	+ + +	+ + + +
Takaoka	+ + + +	+ + + +	+ + +	+ +	+ + + +
Mixed					
Richardson Bottle	+ + +	+ + + +	+	+	+
Heidbrink No. 10	+ + +	+ + + +	+	+	+
Boyle's Bottle	+ +	+ + +	+	+	+

(After Harp, Stephen and North.)

clinical usefulness of the agent is necessary. A control dial should indicate absolute concentrations preferably in fractional divisions.

CLASSIFICATION OF VAPORIZERS

Vaporizers may be classified into four groups distinguished by the practical methods used to hasten evaporation (Table 5–6).

Evaporative Surface Methods

Acceleration of vaporization by increasing the evaporative surface provides a greater contact area for the air–liquid interface and the transfer of heat from air to the liquid. This is referred to as the "ad plenum" principle. The heat is obtained from the surrounding air and from the liquid agent.

The simplest principle employed to aid the vaporization of volatile agents is that of providing a large free surface of contact. The open system of anesthesia by open drop mask with several layers of gauze (providing a free surface) is representative. The surrounding air is the source of heat. This is obviously inefficient since the specific heat of ether is 0.5 cal/g (0.36 cal/ml), and the specific heat of air is only .0003 cal/ml. Thus, to vaporize 1 g of ether, more than 300 L of air must pass over or through the evaporating surface. The warmer respiratory exhalations do help to vaporize, but usually the vapor is blown away.

This method is applied in the bubble-type vaporizer (Fig. 5–22). This is an inefficient system because a large volume of air must be available to provide heat, and the temperature of the liquid usually decreases, thereby decreasing the rate of vaporization and causing a fall in the partial pressure of the vapor

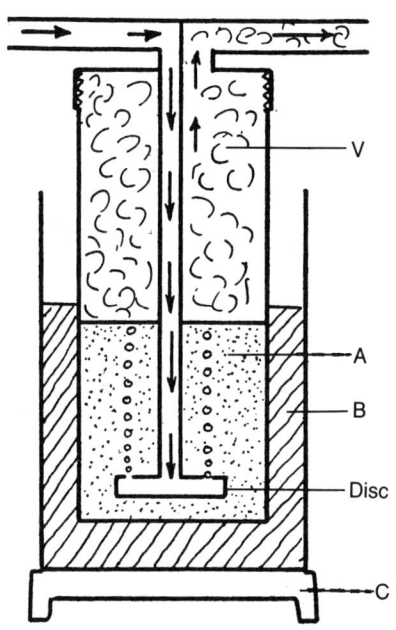

FIG. 5–22. Illustrates the bubble-type vaporizer. From Adriani, courtesy of Charles C Thomas. Gases flow from a cylinder source through a perforated disc (D) to be divided into fine bubbles which pass through the liquid anesthetic (A) to produce a vapor which passes off with the gas (V) in the direction of the arrows. (B) Represents a jacket containing warm water. (C) Represents a hot plate to warm the water. Adriani J.: Chemistry and Physics of Anesthesia 2nd ed. Charles C Thomas, 1972.

TABLE 5–6. TYPES OF VAPORIZERS ACCORDING TO VAPORIZATION METHOD

---

1. Units providing large free surfaces of evaporation—A variation portion of flow of anesthetic gases is directed over or through the liquid which is exposed on a large surface.
   - Gauze surfaces
   - Cotton wicks
   - Bubbling devices
   - Dropper; liquid ether drops on metal surfaces
2. Methods of decreasing vapor pressure—Utilizing "Draw-Over Principle" of currents of air or gas; depends on velocity of air currents.
   - Depending on air movement due to actual respiration.
   - Depending on independent currents of air.
3. Direct source of heat
   - Electrical hot plate
   - Water baths
4. Devices providing heat indirectly
   - Activated charcoal-heat of adsorption—Edison Etherizer
   - Heat of crystallization—chemical heat
     Crystals of low M.P.—hydrated CaCl$_2$; parachlorbenzine
   - Contact with material of high specific heat and conduction (Copper containers and other amalgams)

---

above the liquid. A further disadvantage is condensation of moisture in the air into the liquid anesthetics.

The simple bubble vaporizer has been improved by introducing a bronze sintered disc at the bottom of the delivery tube. As the oxygen passes through the disc it is broken up into multiple tiny globules which then bubble up to the surface. The disc provides a better heat source because it is of high specific heat. When the air or gas merely passes over the surface without going through the liquid, it is sometimes designated as "topping technique."

"Draw-Over" Methods

Removing molecules of the vapor from above a liquid anesthetic results in a continuous low vapor pressure. Thus, a high gradient of pressure from the liquid to vapor phase continues. This system is utilized in devices of the "draw-over" type (Fig. 5–23). It is also usually incorporated as part of many anesthesia vaporizing devices wherein a large evaporative surface is primarily employed. It depends on a given flow of gas over the agent's surface provided either by a metered flow from a gas source, or the active respiration of the patient.

In closed systems of anesthesia large areas of vaporization are provided by cotton wicks. This is an

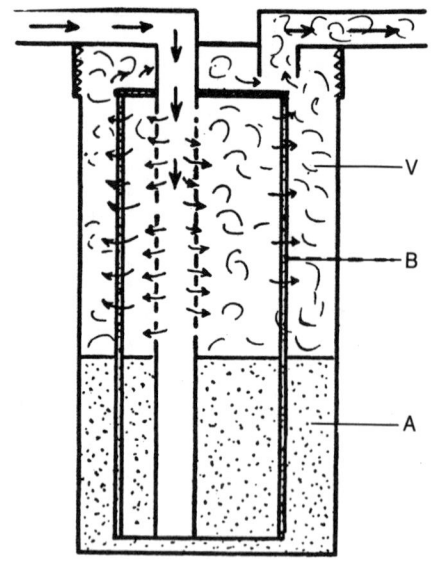

FIG. 5–23. Cross-section of a wick-type vaporizer illustrating the draw-over principle. From Adriani, *Chemistry of Anesthesia,* courtesy of Charles C Thomas. Springfield IL, 1972.
(A) Liquid anesthesia
(B) Wick assembly dipping into liquid
(V) Vapor and gas

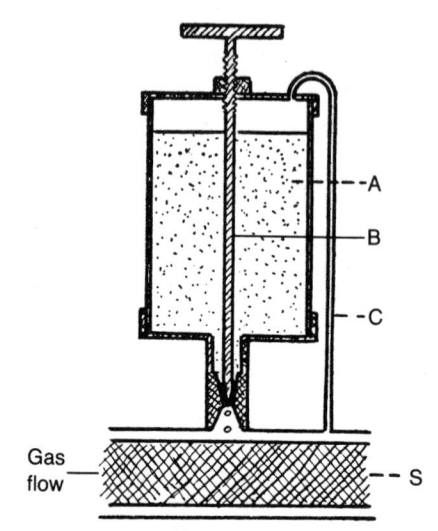

FIG. 5–24. Cross-section of dropper-type vaporizer. Illustrates the copper screen (S) with its high specific heat in the air stream delivered to patient. (Adriani, *Chemistry of Anesthesia,* courtesy of Charles C Thomas.)
(A) Liquid anesthetic in reservoir
(B) Pin valve which controls the number of drops contacting the copper screen in the air stream.
(C) A tube to equalize pressure between air stream and reservoir.

effective surface but again, heat is furnished directly by the moving respiratory atmosphere and the environmental air, which are limited.

Note should be taken of a classical controversy as to whether a vaporizer of the wick or dropper type should be on the inspiratory or expiratory side of a circle system. In a closed system, account must be taken of the carbon dioxide absorption chamber. If one is interested in the warmest atmosphere passing through or over the liquid anesthetic, one would prefer the mixture of gases *after* they pass through the canister where for each gram molecule of carbon dioxide absorbed, 14,000 calories of heat are produced as a heat source for vaporization of the anesthetic.

On the other hand, the dropper unit is a relatively satisfactory and efficient vaporizer. The liquid anesthetic drops on a metal gauze screen, usually copper or onto the soda lime of the canister. This screen is located in the stream of the breathing system (Fig. 5–24). This was modified by Adriani.[65]

Disadvantages of these methods include lack of vernier control of concentration and sudden gross changes in concentration, irritation, presence of liquid droplets.

Direct Heating

Direct heating of liquid anesthetic containers has been employed in several devices. These have obvious disadvantages including being cumbersome and possessing an explosion hazard. Also, the vaporization may be excessive and the concentrated vapors may condense in colder parts of the breathing system. Lastly, heating may favor decomposition.

As previously mentioned, direct heating of the anesthesia container is employed in two common devices. These are the hot water bath jackets surrounding the container of liquid anesthesia and hot plates, electrically operated. These are no longer used.

Indirect Sources of Heat

Methods employing indirect sources of heat have proved to be most efficient and subject to some control of concentration. There are three systems available. (1) The use of a copper container with its high specific heat acts as a physical means of furnishing heat by a rapid transfer. The heat capacity of copper is relatively low, 0.093 cal/g, but the density is high (9 g/ml), so that 1 ml of copper holds 0.81 cal, which is easily transferable. (2) The use of physiochemical heat of *adsorption* is utilized in the Edison Etherizer. (3) The chemical heat of crystallization of calcium chloride is used in the Oxford vaporizer.

HEAT OF ADSORPTION PRINCIPLE

The process of adsorption is characterized by increased surface tension and condensation. When substances are brought in contact with a substance of high-adsorptive capacity (inactivated charcoal), the adsorbing surface tends to reduce its surface area. This is accompanied by evolution of large quantities of heat, which is called an exothermic reaction. Thus, the simple contact of 1 g of ether with activated carbon will produce 30 cal of heat. This process is utilized in the Edison vaporizer.

In the Edison vaporizer liquid ether is introduced into the vaporizing unit from a funnel container. It passes through a sight glass downward onto a flared baffle and into a spreader tray. This results in an even distribution of the liquid ether on the underlying activated carbon. Dried air currents or oxygen passes downward to the bottom of the vaporizing chamber and mixes with the air–ether vapor, which then passes outward to an inhaler assembly.

CHEMICAL HEAT FOR VAPORIZATION

When a substance solidifies, heat is given up to the surrounding environment. Thus, when a pan of water has attained a temperature of 0° C, in order for ice to form, heat must be extracted from each gram. The amount of heat given off when 1 g of a substance is converted from the liquid to the solid state without alteration of temperature is called the *latent heat of crystallization* (Fig. 5–25).

Use is made of the large number of calories supplied by crystallization to aid in vaporization of volatile anesthetics. Substances of relatively low melting point are employed; one such substance is hydrated calcium chloride. Crystals of this substance are placed in a jacket surrounding a container of liquid ether or other volatile anesthetic. An outer jacket is provided as a water bath. When hot water is introduced into the outer jacket, the calcium chloride melts. Subsequently as the calcium chloride solidifies, heat is liberated that vaporizes the anesthetic. Approximately 40 cal of heat are liberated by each gram of calcium chloride that crystallizes. A fixed concentration of ether vapor is ensured for any particular setting of the control valve. This is the principle applied in the Oxford Vaporizer. (Used in Faulkland Islands War)

CONSIDERATION OF HEAT TRANSFER IN VAPORIZERS

On theoretical reasoning the vapor tension of an outflowing gas-vapor mixture can be determined in various systems if a steady state is established. The value of such depends on the stabilized temperature of the vaporizing liquid. With a given system and type of container a thermodynamic equilibrium equation can be established. Under these circumstances the efficiency of heat transfer between container and the gas-liquid is the crucial factor. Other variables include time required to achieve equilibrium and the ambient temperature. Based on physical constants and applicable thermodynamic laws, Faulconer[17a] has provided a functional and theoret-

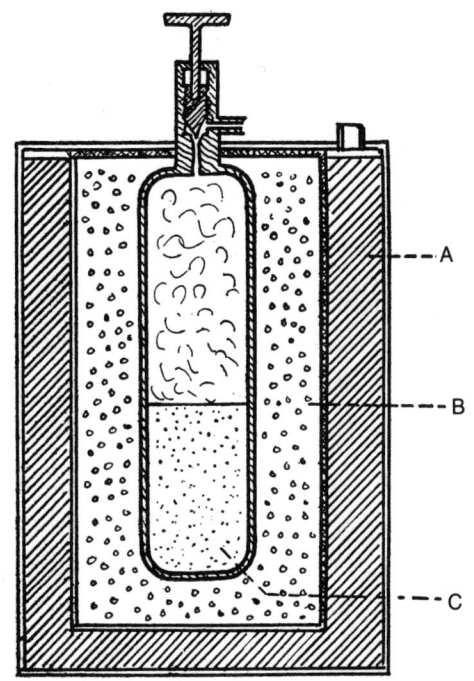

FIG. 5–25. Chemical heat of crystallization. This source of heat is utilized in the Oxford-type vaporizer. The outer container (A) is filled with hot water which melts the chemical in container (B). This chemical may be hydrated calcium chloride or paradichlorbenzene. As the melted chemical is cooled it crystallizes and releases the heat of crystallization. This heat is absorbed by the volatile anesthetic placed in the inner container (C). The pure vapor is delivered into the breathing circuit. The quantity delivered is controlled by a valve and measured by a flowmeter. From Adriani, *Physics and Chemistry of Anesthesia*, courtesy of Charles C Thomas.

ical classification of types of vaporizers. These are defined as follows:

I. LTE (Low Thermal-Transfer Efficiency Vaporizers)
   Container is an absolute insulator.
II. ITE (Intermediate Thermal-Transfer Efficiency Vaporizers)
   Most commercial vaporizers.
   "Open-Drop" Mask System.
   Least predictable vapor pressure output.
III. HTE (High Thermal-Transfer Efficiency Vaporizers)
   Physiochemical heat of adsorption
   Oxford Ether Vaporizers. Chemical heat
   Morris "Copper Kettle." (out of circuit)
   Out of Circuit—saturation vaporizers

VAPORIZERS

A variety of methods have been used to vaporize liquid anesthetics. These have included slow drip or injection into the breathing circuit, in-circuit devices using the patient's inspired gas to vaporize liquids, and accurate and complex out-of-circuit vaporizers of various designs.[60–62]

DIRECT ADDITION OF LIQUID ANESTHETIC

A number of methods, not commonly used today, have been devised to vaporize a volatile anesthetic by adding the liquid directly to the breathing circuit (Fig. 5–26).[63,64] Adriani incorporated a cup, needle valve drip chamber, and tube coiled within the soda lime canister of a breathing circuit to vaporize diethyl ether.[65] Up to 1 L/min of anesthetic vapor may be required early in induction of ether anesthesia in an adult. Since 1 ml of liquid ether yields about 250 ml of ether vapor, a liquid ether drip was an effective way of delivering these volumes, although not a good way of providing known concentrations. However, unlike for the halogenated agents used today, it was not important to know the exact concentration of ether being delivered and hence the usefulness of this device.

More recently, the injection of a measured amount of halogenated liquid into a breathing circuit has been proposed to produce precisely known amounts of vapor.[66,67] Injection directly onto the soda lime in the canister provides a large surface area and heat, which assures rapid and complete vaporization of the liquid. With a properly calibrated injection syringe, this is an extremely accurate way to administer volatile anesthetics and has particular application when closed-system anesthesia is being used. The major drawback to this form of vaporization is the lack of commercially manufactured machines that incorporate this type of device into the breathing circuit.

BREATHE-THROUGH OR IN-CIRCUIT VAPORIZERS

A variety of breathe-through vaporizers have been designed, but like direct injection, are not commonly used today. All vaporizers of this type work on the principle that as gas flows in the breathing circuit, it passes over a liquid anesthetic surface (where evaporation occurs) or bubbles through the liquid agent. Perhaps the most widely used of the in-circle vaporizers was the Heidbrink No. 8, a glass bottle that contained a cylinder of cotton string that was partially immersed in liquid ether (Fig. 5–27). The inspired gas passed through the interstices of nearly 10 in.^{2} of closely wound string moistened by ether. The effective surface area was several-fold greater than in bubble-type vaporizers available at the time, thus increasing the efficiency of vaporization. A variable bypass valve with 40 uncalibrated click-stop positions provided some controllability. The principal disadvantages of this type of vaporizer for delivery of halogenated anesthetics are the lack of calibration of the vaporizer and the dependency of vaporization on the patient's minute ventilation. As a result, the inspired concentration of anesthetic is unpredictable.

Other designs of these vaporizers focused on supplying heat. A particularly useful device for ether, developed by Epstein, a physicist at Oxford, in collaboration with MacIntosh, an anesthetist also at Oxford, is known as the EOM.[33] The base contains several liters of warmed water, which provides the heat of vaporization. Simple, rugged, portable, and accurate, this vaporizer is still in use in developing countries where more sophisticated apparatus is scarce and hard to maintain. An ingenious alternative is the use of crystals of calcium chloride, which,

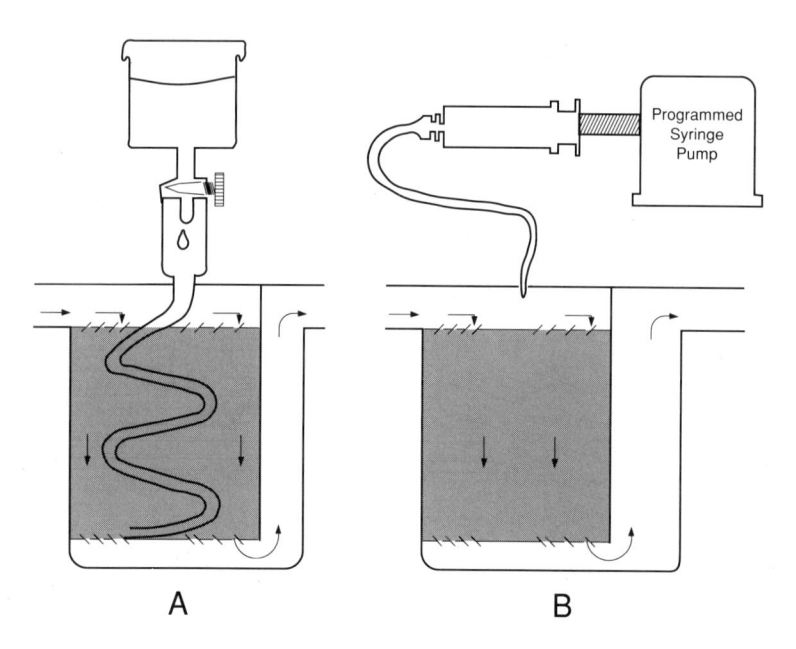

FIG. 5–26. Vaporization by direct addition by dropping or by injection. (Adaptation of dropper-type vaporizer) The soda lime canister of a circle breathing circuit provides heat and large surface area for vaporization of liquid anesthetics. *A.* shows Adriani's method for providing the large volumes of diethyl ether vapor necessary to induce anesthesia. Ether from a cup passes through a needle valve, drips past a sight chamber and into a coiled copper tube in the canister, from which ether vapor emerges to mix with the respired gases. *B.* illustrates Lowe's method of programmed injection where the syringe pump delivers liquid anesthetic at a precise rate designed to match calculated uptake of that agent by the patient. Many anesthetists are uncomfortable with these vaporizers because there is no simple indication of delivered concentration.

when exposed to a heat source, will melt at 29° C. When exposed to a cooler anesthetic solution, CaCl$_2$ recrystallizes and thus provides the heat of crystallization at constant temperature.[68] An electrically heated mantle is an obvious alternate idea that has been used but not widely accepted.

OUT-OF-CIRCUIT VAPORIZERS

Although there are a large variety of out-of-circuit vaporizers, they may be categorized into one of two types. One type saturates all of a small flow of oxygen supplied to it at measured or constant temperatures. The output of saturation vaporizers is then added to the main gas stream. The second type, or variable bypass vaporizer, achieves a reliable output concentration by passing a variable portion of all of the gas stream over or through the liquid anesthetic at measured or constant temperature. In some cases, a thermal compensating valve in the vaporizer obviates the need for temperature measurement or control.

SATURATION VAPORIZERS[68]

Saturation vaporizers were invented by Morris and Feldman at the suggestion of Ralph Waters and with the advice of Warren Gilson to provide for accurate vaporization of chloroform.[63,69–71] In the original copper kettle, heavy copper walls conducted heat from a copper table top to the liquid anesthetic. The gas, metered by a flowmeter with needle valves, passed through a "loving cup," which moderated pressure surges and helped equilibrate incoming gas temperature. The gas then passed through a sintered bronze disc that broke up the flow into myriads of tiny bubbles (Fig. 5–28). The high thermal conductivity of copper as well as the heat capacity of a thick-walled container and machine top assured a relatively constant temperature.

Several manufacturers produce similarly designed vaporizers made of brass or chrome plate. When the copper, brass, or chrome plating is polished, the vaporizer's radiation function is decreased, but the decrease is not of clinical importance when modern, potent agents are being used. The temperature of vaporizers that are descended from the copper kettle remains near that of the room, but thermometers are usually incorporated. The large surface of gas–liquid interface created by the fine bubbles assures complete saturation of the emerging gas at the temperature of the vaporizer.

The output of saturation vaporizers consists of the oxygen supplied to them plus the volume of the anesthetic vaporized, which depends on the vapor pressure of that agent at the vaporizer temperature (Table 5–7). As shown in the table, the vapor pressure of each agent at 20° C results in a particular

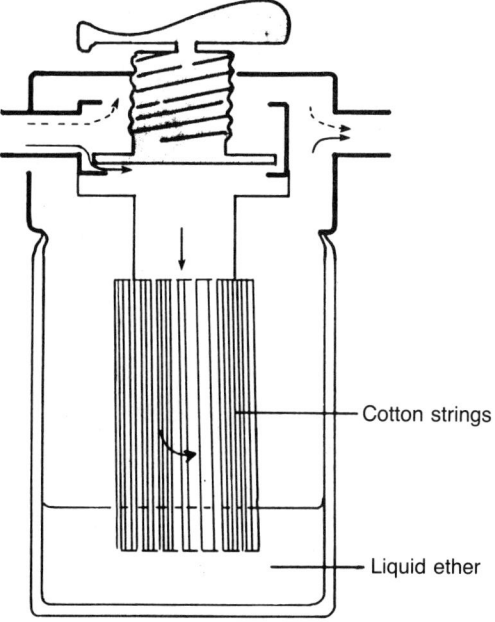

FIG. 5–27. A breathe-through vaporizer—wick type. Breathe-through vaporizers are incorporated within breathing circuits. They pass a variable portion of the entering gas stream through a vaporizing chamber (solid arrows). The fraction of gas which is shunted past the vaporizer and not exposed to ether (dotted arrows) is determined by rotating the lever at the top. This figure shows a cylinder of cotton string dipping into liquid ether, which wets the cotton and provides a large vaporization surface. The vaporizer can be on the expiratory side of the breathing circuit using the heat of expired gas and the dilution volume of the bag and canister to promote smooth increases to high concentration, or on the inspiratory side, to promote rapid changes in inspired concentration. The output of these vaporizers is not linearly related to rotation of the lever and varies greatly with respiratory minute volume and temperature.

concentration of that anesthetic in the outflow of a saturation vaporizer. Vapor pressure increases as temperature increases, and decreases as temperature decreases. Calculation of the concentration of anesthetic vapor delivered to the breathing circuit is made with the following equation:

$$C = \frac{F_{oxy}}{F_{tot}} \times \frac{P_V}{P_A - P_V} \times 100\%$$

where C = concentration (%) of anesthetic delivered to the breathing circuit; F_{oxy} = flow rate of oxygen through vaporizer (ml/min); F_{tot} = total flow rate of all gases (ml/min); P_V = vapor pressure of the anesthetic (mm Hg); and P_A = atmospheric pressure (mm Hg). This equation can be solved, provided the gas flows and the vapor pressure of the agent at the temperature of the vaporizer are known (Table 5–8). Atmospheric pressure may be assumed to be 760 mm Hg at or near sea level.

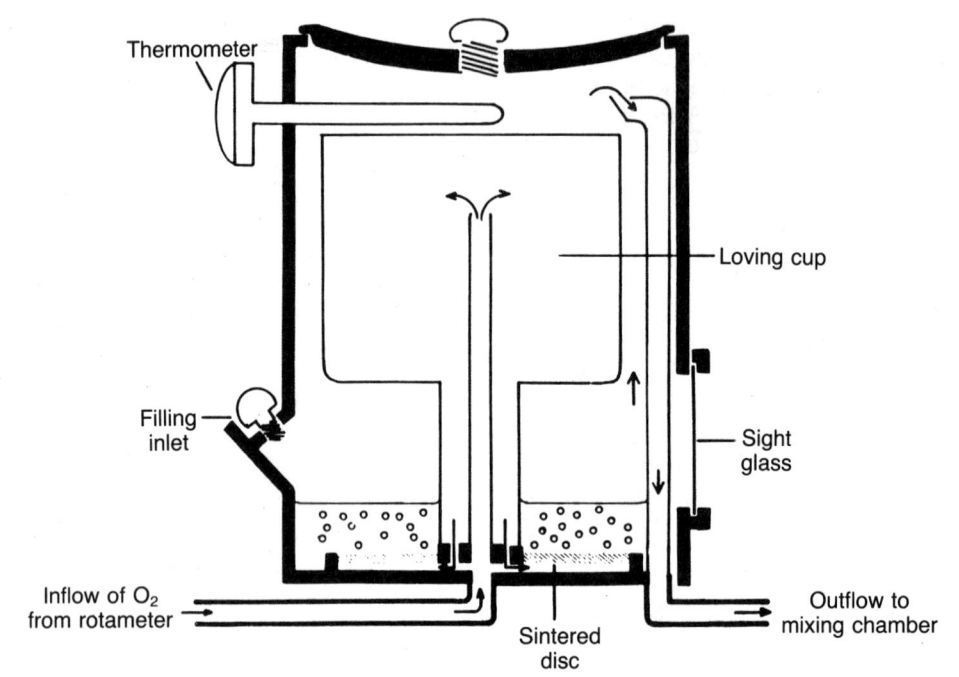

FIG. 5–28. A saturation vaporizer. The "kettle" type of vaporizer was designed to provide an output saturated with anesthetic vapor, which would then be diluted with other gases. The container is of copper, selected for its thermal conductivity, and is thermally well connected to the anesthesia machine frame so the whole unit acts as a radiator to provide the heat of vaporization to the liquid agent. The stream of oxygen (*arrows*) enters at the bottom and passes through a "loving cup." Its large volume buffers pressure surges when the gas inflow rate is changed and minimizes back-up by compression when the outlet pressure increases. The gas stream is then broken up into fine bubbles by a sintered disc, and these bubbles provide the large surface area that assures efficient vaporization of the anesthetic, whose level can be seen through the sight glass. The gas leaves through a covered outlet which prevents splashes of liquid from entering the output.

Many anesthetists find the previous equation cumbersome and confusing and prefer to calculate the concentration of anesthetic leaving the saturation vaporizer (Table 5–6). This is calculated as follows:

$$C = \frac{P_V}{P_A} \times 100\%$$

where C = concentration (%) of anesthetic leaving the saturation vaporizer; P_V = vapor pressure of the anesthetic (mm Hg); and P_A = atmospheric pressure. The concentration leaving the saturation vaporizer is then diluted to that which the anesthetist wishes to deliver to the breathing circuit by adding oxygen alone or with nitrous oxide via gas flows that bypass the vaporizer. Slide rules that simplify the calculation have been devised but are not popular.

Almost simultaneously, many anesthetists devised an even simpler method for establishing the desired concentration of volatile anesthetic. This method is based on the fact that a "magic number,"

TABLE 5–7. VAPOR PRESSURE AND TEMPERATURE CHANGE-EFFECT ON SATURATION VAPORIZER

Anesthetic	Vapor Pressure (mm Hg) At 20°C	Change per °C near 20° C	Concentration of Vapor Delivered by Saturation Vaporizer (%) At 20°C	Change per °C near 20° C
Diethyl ether	440	17	58	2.3
Fluroxene	285	13	38	1.7
Isoflurane	240	11	32	1.5
Halothane	244	11	32	1.4
Enflurane	172	8	23	1.1
Methoxyflurane	23	1	3	0.15

TABLE 5–8. CONCENTRATION OF ANESTHETIC DELIVERED TO CIRCUIT (%)

Anesthetic	Magic Number* (L/min)	Oxygen Flow Rate Through Vaporizer	
		(100 ml/min)	(200 ml/min)
Diethyl ether	14	1.01	2.00
Fluroxene	6	0.99	1.98
Isoflurane	5	0.95	1.87
Halothane	5	0.92	1.81
Enflurane	3	1.02	1.97
Methoxyflurane	0.2	1.05	1.58

*The magic number for each agent as described in the text is a total bypass flow of gases in L/min.

which represents the total bypass gas flow (in L/min) to be used, exists for each volatile anesthetic. At this total flow rate, when 100 ml/min of oxygen is passed through a saturation vaporizer, whose temperature is about 20° C, approximately 1% of the anesthetic agent is delivered to the breathing circuit. When 200 ml/min of oxygen is passed through the saturation vaporizer, approximately 2% of the anesthetic is delivered to the breathing circuit, except in the case of methoxyflurane, where low vapor pressure limits the concentrations that can be delivered.

When the operating room temperature is close to 20°C, the numbers are reasonably accurate (Table 5–7). The idea of magic numbers (5 L/min for halothane and isoflurane and 3 L/min for enflurane) has become so widespread that some anesthetists unthinkingly use 5 L/min total flow when using Fluotec for halothane and 3 L/min when using Vapor for enflurane, even though these devices deliver their indicated concentrations over wide ranges of inflow.

One modern machine incorporates a vaporizer of the saturation type with a thermostat and an electrical heating element controlled by a servo circuit set to 25° C. The oxygen flowmeter supplying the vaporizer is read in ml of anesthetic vapor produced, not oxygen flow rate to the vaporizer. Also of importance is the fact that the oxygen supplying the kettle is a portion of the "bypass" oxygen, not an independent supply. As always, it is essential that one be familiar with the peculiarities of the equipment being used, for the "magic numbers" are not useful in this situation.

VARIABLE BYPASS VAPORIZERS

A variable bypass vaporizer has a device that divides the total output of all of the flowmeters into two streams, one of which goes *through* the vaporizer and the other which goes *by* the vaporizer. A dial setting determines the proportion of total flow that is directed through the vaporizer. This gas becomes saturated or nearly so with the anesthetic agent, and it is diluted to the desired concentration by the bypass stream. When these vaporizers are used, no calculations of dosage are necessary. The concentration being delivered to the breathing circuit is read directly from the dial. When properly maintained, these vaporizers are reasonably accurate over flow ranges of 2 to 10 L/min.[72–77] In those vaporizers that are thermally compensated, at a given setting of the dial, the ratio of the two streams is affected by a bimetallic strip and plug (Fig. 5–29). Their accuracy can extend to flows as low as 0.5 L/min. Several manufacturers have produced a variety of vaporizers using this design, and they are distinguished by their name, which ends in "-tec," as in Fluotec, or in "-matic," as in Pentamatic. As a safety feature, these vaporizers are supplied with a filling device whose ends are specially shaped such that one will only accept a specific type of liquid anesthetic bottle and the other will only insert into a specific type of vaporizer. This keying is intended to prevent filling a vaporizer with the wrong agent.

The Vapor vaporizers are similar to the tec type in that they are agent-specific but different in that

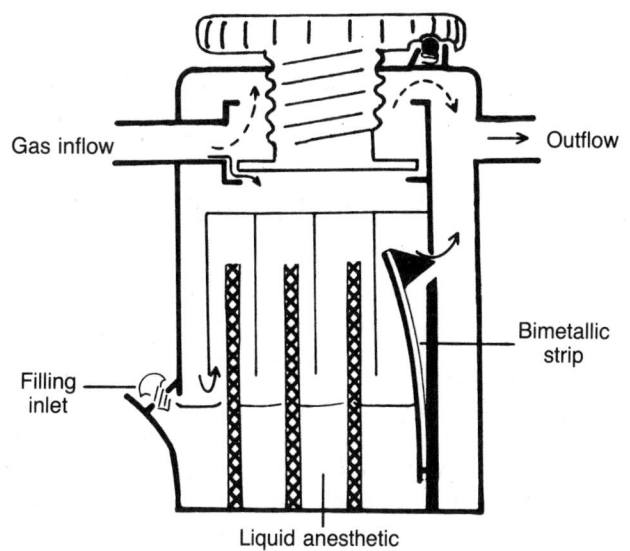

FIG. 5–29. Out-of-circuit–variable bypass vaporizer. These vaporizers are not much different in principle from many of the older breathe-through designs (Fig. 5–27). A portion of the gas stream (*solid arrows*) is passed over a liquid surface. The surface for vaporization is increased by wicks and a labyrinthine gas path. The remainder of the gas stream (*dotted arrows*) bypasses the anesthetic liquid. A large knob and indicator at the top control the bypass flow. The control has click-stops at quarter percents up to 3 or 4 MAC multiples. A temperature-sensitive bimetallic strip further modulates the flow, providing temperature compensation. Thick walls of high heat capacity promote reproducible function. These vaporizers are agent-specific and may be equipped with a shape-coded device to prevent filling with the wrong agent.

they do not have any thermally activated moving parts.[76,78] Instead, they are thermally calibrated. Heavy copper vessels, large liquid surface areas (using wicks when necessary), and precision-machined variable bypass valve mechanisms assure reproducible vaporization at any given temperature. The dial that sets concentration has a series of concentration lines, and a vertical index line on which a temperature scale from 15° to 25° C is inscribed. The output concentration of the vaporizer is read at the intersection of the desired concentration line with the appropriate vertical temperature index line, determined by reading an attached thermometer. The dial can easily be read to 0.1% concentration. This type of vaporizer is uniquely accurate at extremely low vaporizer flows and hence, is especially suited for use with closed system anesthesia. The volume of liquid anesthetic that this type of vaporizer holds is considerably smaller than that for the tec type, and the anesthetist must be alert to the need for regular refilling when standard (5 L/min) total gas flows are used.

THERMALLY CONFUSED VAPORIZERS

A myriad of thermally confused vaporizers, usually identified by eponyms, have been designed. They are similar in that they do not have any mechanism to compensate for temperature change, and hence their output is semiquantitative. The Boyle bottle is one such vaporizer. A supply of gas, usually the entire output of the machine, is split into two streams, one of which enters the vaporizer through a movable hooded tube. The hood can be raised well above the liquid level to produce a low concentration, or lowered nearer the liquid to increase the concentration, or placed below the liquid surface so that the gas bubbles through the liquid, greatly increasing the anesthetic output. These two controls, variable bypass and hood elevation, give considerable although uncalibrated control of the output. Even though they are functional, the Boyle and other similar types of vaporizers such as the Goldman, McKesson, Rowbottom, and FNS (Fabian, Newton and Stephens), to name a few, have mostly disappeared from use,[79,80] as anesthetists have emphasized the need for reliable delivery of accurately known concentrations of potent volatile anesthetics, whose margin of safety is narrow.

HAZARDS OF VAPORIZERS

Modern vaporizers are not hazard free, and several types of vaporizer accidents have been reported. Liquid anesthetic can be delivered to the breathing circuit, with the potential for massive overdose of anesthetic to the patient, if an insecurely fixed vaporizer is tipped or overturned, if a vaporizer is overfilled, or if a sudden large inflow of gas is permitted.[81-84] Less dramatic overdose can occur when a vaporizer is intermittently pressurized during assisted or controlled ventilation,[85-88] or when its temperature increases appreciably.[89] The pressure effects can be eliminated by a suitably placed valve.[34,90] Finally, when several vaporizers are set up in a series, contamination of those that are downstream can result in overdose.[91,92]

BREATHING ASSEMBLY

The gases and vapors mixed by the anesthesia machine are delivered to a breathing circuit, which in turn delivers them to the patient while providing for low resistance to inspiration and expiration, minimal rebreathing, absorption of carbon dioxide, humidification, and safe disposal of waste gases. The essential components of a breathing circuit include breathing tubing, respiratory valves, reservoir bag, carbon dioxde absorption cannister, a site for inflow of fresh gas, a pop-off valve for excess gas, a Y-piece, mask angle, and mask. This section is devoted to a functional analysis of the components used in common circuits.

BREATHING TUBING

The typical tubing used in breathing circuits has several characteristics. It is usually about 1 meter in length; has a large bore to make resistance negligible; and is corrugated or less commonly, reinforced to permit flexibility without kinking. For many years breathing tubing was made of conductive rubber, but since conductivity is rarely if ever necessary, plastic tubing has almost completely replaced rubber. Plastic has the advantages of being lighter in weight and disposable by design if not by use.[93] By convention, the ends of the tubing are 22 mm ID and identical in design. Future standards may specify a male–female configuration of the ends to prevent improper cross connecting of breathing circuit components. Tubing should be inspected before use as manufacturing difficulties can result in obstruction of the lumen.[94,95]

Distensibility of the tubing, which is not desirable, varies from nearly zero to over 5 ml/meter length/mm Hg of pressure applied, with plastic tubing having the lower values. Apparent distensibility is even greater because of compression of gas under pressure. This is of the order of 3% of the volume for typical inflation pressures (e.g., 20 mm Hg). The nominal volume of these tubes varies according to brand but is usually 400 to 500 ml/meter. Thus, positive pressure inflation of a patient's lungs to 20 mm Hg peak inspiratory pressure will store 30 to 150 ml of additional gas in the tubing.[96] This volume is not delivered to the patient's lungs but is measured by a ventilation meter within the circuit, thus adding a form of apparatus dead space to the system.

Resistance to gas flow in standard corrugated breathing tubes is exceedingly small (less than 1 cm $H_2O/L/min$).[97,98] When it is desirable to have the anesthesia machine at some distance from the patient's head, several tubings may be used in series connected by 22 mm OD nipples. These extensions do not increase the resistance of the system by any appreciable amount and affect the apparatus dead space only by their compliant volume.

The pattern of flow is almost always turbulent because of the corrugations in the tubing. This promotes radial mixing and plug-like flow patterns. Thus, a change in gas composition at one end, as when the delivered gas is altered at the machine, makes a distinct change in the inspired concentration within two to three breaths.

Tubing of smaller diameter is made for use in circle systems designed specifically for infants and children.

RESPIRATORY VALVES

Respiratory valves are incorporated into an anesthetic circuit to control gas flow. A circle system has two identical valves, one on the inspiratory limb and one on the expiratory limb. Their function is to maintain unidirectional flow of gases within the circle. That is, the inspiratory valve opens on inspiration but closes on expiration, thereby preventing the flow of exhaled gases back down the inspiratory limb of the circle. The expiratory valve works in a reciprocal manner. These valves can be mounted anywhere in the inspiratory and expiratory limbs of the circle, respectively, the only critical feature of their location being that they must be placed on opposite sides of the reservoir bag, the only easily collapsible structure in the circle system. So located and properly functioning, they prevent any part of the circle system from contributing to apparatus dead space. The respiratory valves on most modern anesthesia machines are located near or incorporated into the soda lime canister. Unidirectional valves have been incorporated into the housing of a Y-piece of a circle, but they have fallen into disfavor because of the weight they add to the mask, and more importantly, because they will cause an obstruction to respiration if they are inadvertently incorporated backward to the conventional valves in the circle system.[99] When valved Y-pieces were used, it was recommended that the circle system valves be removed, but failure to reinsert them when a nonvalved Y-piece was then used caused needless anesthetic complications.

The essential characteristics of respiratory valves in breathing circuits are low resistance and high competence.[100] That is, the valves must open widely with little pressure and close rapidly and completely with essentially no backflow. The common valves in anesthetic circuits are "dome" valves, consisting of a circular knife edge, occluded by a very light disc of slightly larger diameter (Fig. 5–30). When gas flow through the circle system is initiated, either by negative or positive pressure from the patient making an inspiratory or expiratory effort or from positive pressure being applied on the reservoir bag, the disc lifts off the knife edge, but is still contained by a small cage below the dome or by the dome itself. The disc must be hydrophobic so that water condensate does not cause the disc to stick to the knife edge and increase the resistance to opening. Most discs today are made of plastic and are thin and quite lightweight. They require vertical mounting so that the disc will fall properly into the closed position and seal the circuit from any backflow. Failure to seal converts the volume of the circle into apparatus dead space. The top of the valve is covered by a removable clear plastic dome so that the disc can be easily seen and periodically cleaned or replaced.

NONREBREATHING VALVES

Another type of respiratory valve is the nonrebreathing valve. Nonrebreathing valves permit the patient to inspire from a fresh gas reservoir other than a circle system and exhale into the room or into a scavenger exhaust. These usually consist of a pair of leaflets, one opening during inspiration and the other during expiration.

The early designs (e.g., Digby-Leigh or Stephen-Slater) required the anesthetist to occlude the expiratory valve with his finger if he wished to assist

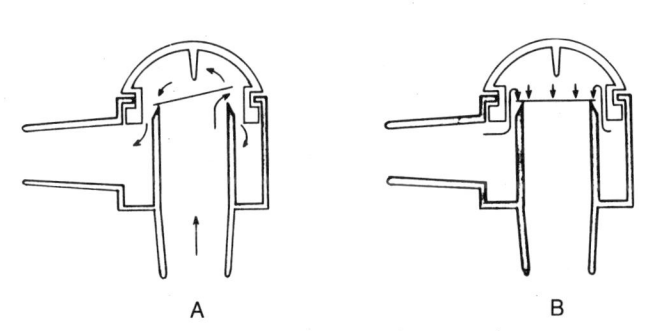

FIG. 5–30. Respiratory valves used in anesthesia machines. The figure is typical of the "dome" valves incorporated in circle absorber housings. In *A*., the valve is shown in the open position with gas flowing. In *B*., due to back pressure, the plastic disc seats on the knife edge and the valve is closed.

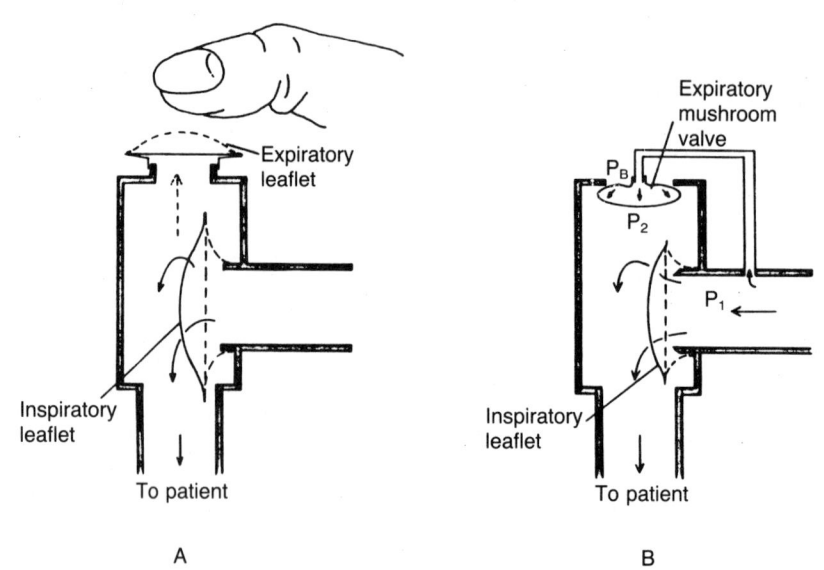

FIG. 5–31. Nonrebreathing valves shown during inspiration. These valves incorporate two leaflets which open alternately on inspiration or expiration. In the simplest form (*A.*), the valve functions well during spontaneous ventilation (*solid arrows*), but an attempt to inflate the patient's lungs manually would blow open both inspiratory and expiratory leaflets (*dotted arrow*) unless the anesthetist simultaneously occludes the expiratory valve with his finger. Several nonrebreathing valves have been designed to overcome the necessity for manual assistance of valve function. In *B.*, whenever gas flow opens the inspiratory leaflet, the pressure at point P_1 is greater than at point P_2. This pressure difference inflates the mushroom-shaped expiratory balloon, sealing the expiratory limb. But if no gas is supplied to the inspiratory limb, spontaneous effort on the part of the patient lowers both P_1 and P_2 well below atmospheric pressure, P_B, so that the mushroom valve collapses and the patient inspires room air.

or control ventilation (Fig. 5–31*A*).[101,102] Ingenious designs employing springs, magnets, flaps, etc. will provide a "semiautomatic finger" to close the expiratory valve when respiration is controlled (Fig. 5–31*B*).[103–106] Other designs use the pressure drop across the inspiratory valve to inflate a mushroom-shaped balloon valve (Frumin valve)[107] or depress a dome-shaped cover on the expiratory valve (Fink valve).[108] Resistance and backflow are negligible in both, but the former has the marked advantage of collapsing, permitting inspiration of room air or expirate if the inspiratory supply is inadequate (Fig. 5–31*B*). The Frumin valve is also lighter and more compact.[109,110] Some nonrebreathing valves are position sensitive and must be upright to function properly. Those that use flexible rubber leaflets or collapsible rubber tubing to provide the sealing function are nonpositional. Most nonrebreathing valves connect to masks and endotracheal tubes, but one is built into a mask.[111]

Self-inflating resuscitators for air or air–oxygen mixtures use valve pairs to control gas flow.[112,113] The Ruben valve has an inspiratory bobbin-shaped valve that, in opening, occludes the expiratory limb. Anesthetic vapors and secretions tend to expand the bobbin slightly, causing it to jam.[114]

BREATHING BAGS

Breathing bags, more commonly called reservoir bags, have three principal functions. They provide a reservoir of anesthetic gases or oxygen from which the patient can inspire; they permit a visual assessment of the existence and rough estimate of the volume of ventilation; and they provide a means for manual ventilation should that be necessary or desirable. The reservoir function is necessary because anesthesia machines cannot provide the instantaneous gas flows that are needed during the normal respiratory cycle. While the respiratory minute volume of an anesthetized adult is rarely more than 12 L/min, instantaneous gas flow rates at the peak of inspiration may reach 50 to 75 L/min, although for only 1 sec or less. Demand valves provide for such flows in intermittent flow systems, but in circuits supplied by continuous flow, such as a circle system, some compliant volume must be provided to supplement the delivered flow during inspiration.

The usefulness of a reservoir bag as a means of assessing the presence and volume of spontaneous ventilation is determined in large measure by the gas flowrate from the anesthesia machine. Certainly it is easier to see the reservoir move with inspiration and expiration than it is to see the chest expand and recede under the surgical drapes. The change in bag volume, however, is greatly affected by the inflow rate of gas from the machine. If a closed-circle system is used, virtually all of the gas inhaled by the patient comes from the reservoir bag and its excursion reflects tidal volume. If the inflow rate from the machine is in excess of 10 L/min, most of the gas inhaled by the patient comes from the inflow line and the reservoir bag shows little excursion. Assuming a respiratory minute volume of about 5 L/min in an anesthetized patient breathing spontaneously from a circle system, and a gas inflow rate from the machine to the circle of 5 L/min, approximately half of the tidal volume will come from the inflow line and half from the reservoir bag. Thus, the anesthetist can change the excursions of the reservoir bag during spontaneous breathing by changing the inflow rate.

Unlike reservoir bags in ventilators that are usually shaped like a concertina bellows, reservoir bags for anesthesia machines are usually elliptical to make them easy to grasp with one hand. They are made of nonslippery latex or rubber and are usually conductive, although this is rarely, if ever, necessary. Reservoir bags come in sizes ranging from 0.5 to 6 L. The optimal size is one that holds a volume between the patient's inspiratory capacity and vital capacity, so that a deep breath will not empty the bag. A 3-L bag meets these requirements for most adults and is of a size that is easy to grasp. Bags with a nipple at the bottom for use as an alternate pop-off are available but are rarely used.

The breathing bag may be attached to the machine at the gas outlet or at the soda lime canister housing, usually via a T-shaped fitting. Alternatively, the bag mount may be mechanically combined with the pop-off or respiratory valves, or the bag may be placed at the end of a corrugated tubing leading from the T connector. The latter arrangement provides the anesthetist with some freedom of movement. Since the reservoir bag is the only easily collapsible part of the anesthetic circuit, the only critical requirement is that the respiratory valves be positioned between the bag and the patient.

Because reservoir bags may have to function as pressure-limiting devices, it is essential that their pressure–volume characteristics permit large changes in volume with minimal or gradual changes in pressure (Fig. 5–32). This becomes important if the pop-off valve is inadvertently left in the closed

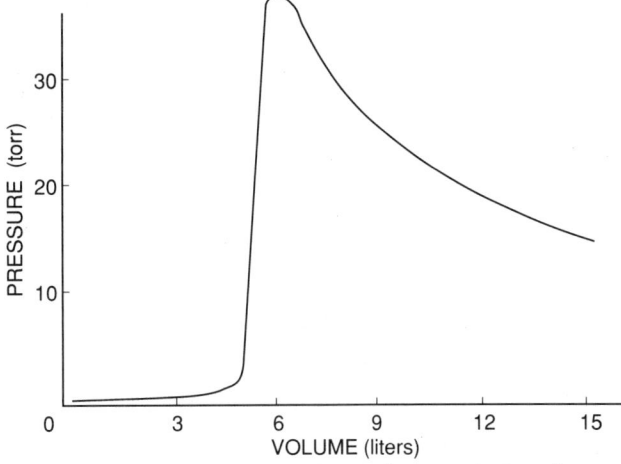

FIG. 5–32. The pressure–volume characteristics of a typical rubber reservoir bag. As the reservoir bag is filled from its evacuated volume to its nominal volume, the pressure increases little, but as the rubber is slightly stretched, a small increase in volume increases the pressure rapidly to some maximum, depending on bag shape and wall thickness. Further increase in bag volume causes a decrease in pressure. The decreasing pressure with increasing volume follows Pouiselle's law: $P = C/r$, where P is pressure, the constant C is a function of the bag thickness and material, and r is the radius.

position and gas inflow continues. Typical maximum pressures of 30 to 45 mm Hg are common with latex rubber bags, and prestretching may favorably lower the maximum pressure.[115–118] Plastic disposable bags may reach twice the pressure of rubber bags and then rupture abruptly.[93]

CARBON DIOXIDE ABSORPTION

In nonrebreathing systems, exhaled carbon dioxide is vented to room air. When a closed system is used, however, the exhaled carbon dioxide must be removed. Carbon dioxide in the presence of water hydrates to form carbonic acid. When carbonic acid reacts with a metal hydroxide, the reaction is one of neutralization, which results in the formation of water, a metal bicarbonate or carbonate, and the generation of heat. It is this reaction that is used in anesthesia for carbon dioxide absorption. Jackson is credited with developing the first method for bulk absorption of carbon dioxide. He passed respired gases over multiple trays containing sodium hydroxide solution to absorb carbon dioxide.[119] However, it was Waters who developed soda lime as it is used today and was the first anesthetist to use it in humans.[120,121]

"Wet" soda lime is composed of calcium hydroxide (about 80%), sodium and potassium hydroxide (about 5%), water (about 15%), and small amounts of inert substances, silica and kieselguhr, for hardness. The sodium and potassium hydroxide function as a catalyst to initiate the reaction of carbon dioxide with soda lime. The reaction of carbon dioxide with sodium and potassium hydroxide in the presence of moisture is an instantaneous one, forming sodium and potassium carbonate and bicarbonate. Subsequently, the sodium and potassium carbonate and bicarbonate react over the course of 1 min with the calcium hydroxide to form calcium carbonate and bicarbonate and water. In the process the sodium and potassium hydroxide catalyst is regenerated. When soda lime is exhausted, calcium carbonate is the principal end product. Soda lime absorbs 19% of its weight in carbon dioxide.[122]

The freshness of soda lime can be determined by feeling, tasting, and visually inspecting it. Fresh granules of soda lime crumble easily between the fingers and when placed on the tongue have a bitter taste and bite because of their alkaline nature (pH 9 to 10). In contrast, expended granules resemble chalk in that they are hard and have no taste. Finally, organic pH indicating dyes are added to soda lime to provide a visual check of its function. As carbonate and bicarbonate are formed from the hydroxide, the pH becomes less alkaline and the granules change color. The three most commonly used dyes are ethyl violet, which changes the granules from white to blue, ethyl orange, which changes the granules from orange to yellow, and clayton yellow, which changes the granules from red to yellow as the soda lime is expended. The regeneration of sodium hydroxide will cause a slight fading of color in the zone of active reaction when usage stops. If expended soda lime is allowed to remain in a canister for a prolonged period (weeks or months), the original color may return. However, upon first usage, the expended nature of the soda lime will quickly become evident because there is no regeneration of activity.

Soda lime is precisely made to maximize its absorption qualities and minimize resistance to gas flow through it, and for this reason is a relatively expensive compound. The granules are sized to 4 to 8 mesh (they will pass through a strainer having 4 to 8 holes/inch) and have a rough, irregular surface so as to maximize the surface to mass ratio, thus facilitating the rapid diffusion of carbon dioxide through pores into voids within the granules.[123–125] Soda lime is supplied in quart-size cartons that will just fill a canister, in disposable canisters, and in bulk containers ranging from 5 pounds to 5 gallons.

Alternates to soda lime are available. Lithium hydroxide offers more carbon dioxide absorption capacity per unit of volume and is used in submarines. Barium hydroxide (Baralyme) is a suitable alternative to soda lime, with the end product being barium carbonate instead of calcium carbonate.[126] It is initially pink and turns blue with exhaustion.

The initial clinical use of soda lime absorption by Waters was the result of careful and detailed experiments to delineate the optimal size and shape of to-and-fro canisters (Fig. 5–33).[121] Three reasons were advanced for preferring the to-and-fro canister:

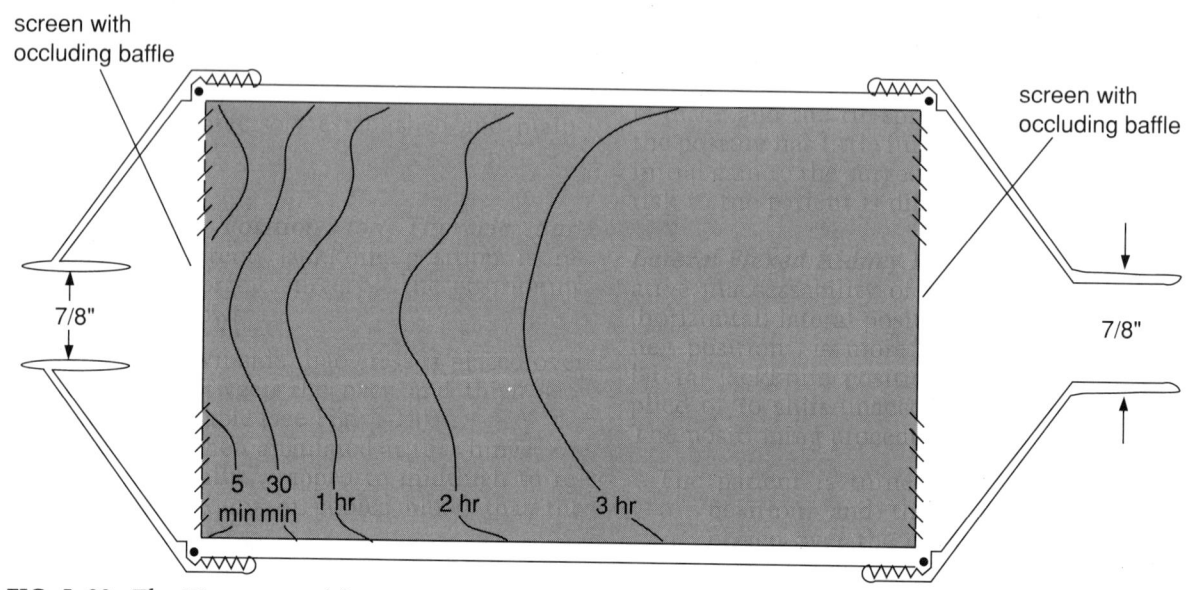

FIG. 5–33. The Waters to-and-fro canister. A screen with a central occluding baffle improves the pattern of soda lime exhaustion. A slip joint at either end permits end-to-end reversal in the breathing circuit with the use of a double male connector. With these two features, 6 to 8 h of closed circuit anesthesia are possible before inspired carbon dioxide concentration increases above 1%. Typical patterns of soda lime exhaustion are shown by the light lines.

the inspired gas was warmed and humidified by the soda lime; the small canister volume permitted rapid change of anesthetic concentration; and the absence of valves and tubes decreased resistance to breathing. These advantages were believed to be worth the awkwardness introduced by the necessity to balance several pounds of warm canister near the patient's face. As advances in equipment occurred, these advantages became less important. In time, the disadvantages of the to-and-fro canister, including the possibility of gas channeling in poorly packed canisters, and hence uncertain carbon dioxide absorption,[127] the possibility of dust inhalation,[128] the propensity to leaks and disconnects, and the required frequency of repacking with soda lime relegated this system to use only in pulmonary infections (for ease of sterilization) and then to history and museums.

With the addition of a pair of breathing tubes and respiratory valves, the to-and-fro canister was transformed by Sword in 1930 into a circle filter system.[129] The circle filter system offered several advantages, including the fact that the soda lime canister could be removed from the vicinity of the patient's head; it could be mounted upright to minimize channeling of gas flow; and it could be increased in size to lengthen its duration of useful function, thereby decreasing the frequency of servicing. The modern jumbo-size canisters used today were originally developed by Brown and Elam.[130] The canister contains two chambers for soda lime, separated by a wire screen (Fig. 5–34). Each chamber

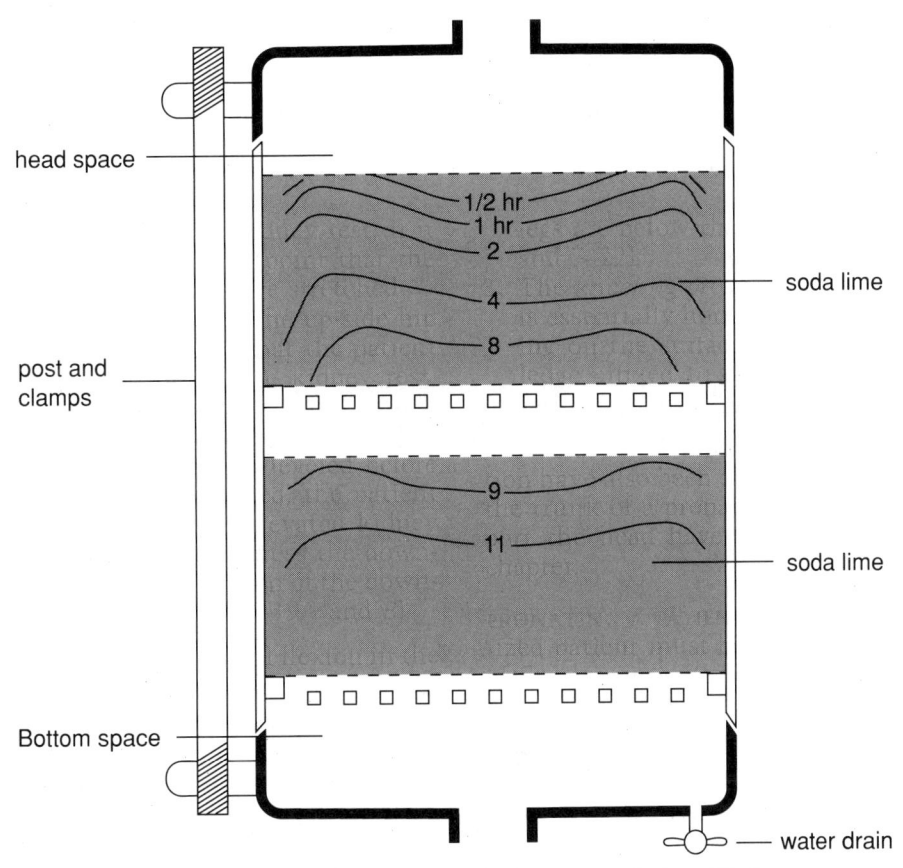

FIG. 5–34. The jumbo canister. Originated by Brown and Elam,[130] these transparent twin-chambered canisters are supplied by all manufacturers of anesthesia machines. Permanently mounted with a vertical gas flow axis, they eliminate dusting, channeling, and packing problems. Used as intended, changing the exhausted canister only when the second is partially exhausted, they utilize the absorptive capacity of soda lime fully, as shown by the lines illustrating patterns of exhaustion. Drop-in, prepacked containers add convenience. The nearly standard shape is 8 cm high, 15 cm in diameter. Since water of condensation may collect in the bottom forming a caustic lye solution with the dust, a drain valve is an important component. Convenience of opening, closing, and sealing varies with design but most now have a single screw-clamp mechanism. The casting for the top and bottom should be resistant to alkaline corrosion and may incorporate other components of the breathing circuit, e.g., bag mount, inflow site, and valve housings.

is large enough that when it is fully packed with soda lime, it will hold at least 500 ml gas volume, so that each exhaled breath remains in contact with soda lime for at least one respiratory cycle. This is sufficient time to assure the complete removal of carbon dioxide, provided the soda lime is functional. By using dual chambers in a series, the soda lime in the first chamber can be completely expended, thereby providing for maximum economy of use, and still have adequate absorption in the second chamber. When one chamber is expended, it is refilled with fresh soda lime and the canister remounted on the anesthesia machine in an inverted position so that the partially used second chamber is now the first to contact the exhaled gas. Canisters have a metal frame to dissipate heat, clear plastic sides to permit visualization of the color change of soda lime, and a reservoir at the bottom to collect excess water vapor from the exhaled gases. Originally, most canisters had a bypass or shunt valve on the top or side of the canister, so that exhaled gases from the patient could be directed around rather than through the soda lime, thereby permitting rebreathing of carbon dioxide as a ventilatory stimulus to speed induction of or emergence from anesthesia. Few canisters purchased today contain this shunt valve, in part because of the lack of perceived need in modern anesthesia for using carbon dioxide rebreathing to stimulate breathing, and in part because of the numerous unpleasant experiences of anesthetists with profound hypercarbia and its complications during the administration of an anesthetic from failure to recognize that the shunt valve was on.

GAS INFLOW AND POP-OFF

Gas is delivered from the machine to the breathing circuit via thick-walled tubing connected to a nipple incorporated into one of the respiratory valves or the canister housing. The site of fresh gas entry may be functionally in any portion of the circle, but the preferred site is between the carbon dioxide absorber and the inspiratory valve (see below).

Pop-off valves are designed to permit the exhaust of excess gas in sufficient quantities to match the inflow of fresh gas. There are many different designs but most are constructed like a dome valve, augmented by a spring and screw cap (Fig. 5–35). As the screw cap is tightened down, more and more pressure is required to open the valve. As it is loosened up, it should open at a pressure of less than 1 cm H_2O. The number of turns between fully open and fully closed should be one or two. If there are fewer than one, it becomes difficult to set a desired pressure accurately. If there are more than two, it is tedious to use and is usually fragile.

Special types of pop-off valves permit either spontaneous or assisted respiration without tedious read-

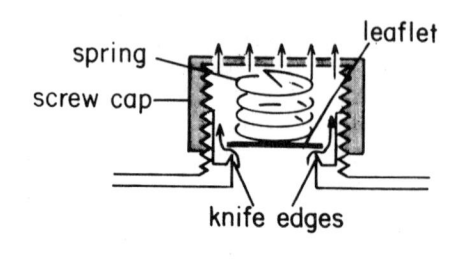

FIG. 5–35. A spring-loaded pop-off valve in the partially open position. When the cap is fully screwed down, the spring is compressed enough to prevent the valve leaflet from lifting at any airway pressure. When the top is loosened and the spring is not compressed at all, the valve opens at a pressure equal to the weight of the leaflet divided by its area, usually less than 1 mm Hg.

justment.[131,132] The simplest is the Steen valve (Fig. 5–36), which is essentially two knife-edge (dome-type) valves, one inverted over the other, sharing a common disc. The relatively slow flow of gas during the latter part of exhalation (up to 10 L/min) lifts the valve disc from one side only, so that the exhaled gas escapes around the disc. But if the anesthetist squeezes the bag, the abrupt increase in pressure lifts the valve disc vertically, seals it against the upper knife edge, and closes the circuit so that no gas is lost. The Georgia valve adds to the same design a light spring loading, which increases the range of gas flows with which it will exhaust, so that it can be used with mechanical ventilators.[133] The exhaust from any of the commonly used pop-off valves can be collected by a scavenging system.

CONNECTION OF THE PATIENT TO THE BREATHING CIRCUIT

The connection of the patient to the breathing circuit involves use of a Y- or T-shaped device, two ends of which are 22 mm OD to accept the breathing tubes and the third end of which has an OD of 22 mm and an ID of 15 mm so that it can accept a universal elbow or mask holder or an endotracheal tube connector. There may be a pop-off valve in the Y-piece, but this design is seldom used today because of the additional weight that it adds, the risk of serious hypoventilation that exists should the valve be left open inadvertently during controlled ventilation, and the satisfactory location of pop-off valves at the canister. Apparatus dead space begins distal to the bifurcation of the Y, but this volume is small (less than 5 ml) and if necessary, can be eliminated by using a Y-piece that has a septum distal to the bifurcation. The mask holder or elbow is a right-angle device that connects the Y-piece to the mask or endotracheal tube. The proximal (machine) end is 15 mm in OD and the distal (patient) end is

22 mm in OD and 15 mm in ID, so that it will accept either a mask or endotracheal tube connector. The mask holder is also apparatus dead space (less than 5 ml) but this too can be eliminated by using a holder that has a septum down its center. Flexible connectors that will provide extensions between an endotracheal tube connector and Y-piece are available, but they do add apparatus dead space as well as one more set of connections that can inadvertently become disconnected.

Masks are made of rubber, clear plastic (to make secretions or vomitus visible), or a combination of both. Most have an inflatable cuff that provides a pneumatic cushion that seals to the face. Masks come in a variety of sizes and styles to accommodate to the wide variety of facial contours. In general, it is desirable that masks be malleable so that they can be molded over the nasal bridge above, which is the most variable anatomic feature that prevents a tight mask fit, and between the mental process and alveolar ridge at each lower corner. Masks have prongs for attachment of a harness to aid the anesthetist in obtaining a tight seal of the mask to the face. The mask represents apparatus dead space, the volume of which varies according to how well it can be molded to the face.

Endotracheal tube connectors come in a variety of sizes and are usually straight, although those with 90 or 135 degree curves are available for use when it is desirable to minimize the intrusion of the tube and connector into the surgical field (See Endotracheal Anesthesia—Basic). Using a curved connector means that the tube must be cut to the proper length, that passage of a suction catheter through the tube will be difficult, and that use of a stylet is virtually impossible.

HAZARDS OF ANESTHESIA MACHINES

CONCENTRATION ERRORS FROM "OXYGEN FLUSHING"[134]

Free-standing "-tec" type vaporizers have been associated with hazards related to the position of the vaporizer "downstream" from the oxygen flush inlet. When vaporizers are in the OFF position, no vapor is delivered when there is an 8 L/min oxygen flow or when oxygen flushing is instituted; however, if the vaporizer is in the ON position and the dial set at zero, a vapor concentration is delivered. When oxygen flushing for 1 sec is employed, a vapor concentration is delivered, with peaks of 0.9% of enflurane.

Further studies indicate that when the vaporizer dial is set at 0.2%, often oxygen flushing of 1 sec duration will result in a peak delivered concentration of 1.4 to 1.8% of enflurane vapor. The highest peaks of anesthetic concentrations of enflurane in an enflurane-type vaporizer have been found to occur after a 5-sec flush with the vaporizer set at 0.2 vol% and the concentration actually delivered is of the order of 2.3%.

Oxygen flushing presents a high-system pressure at the vaporizer inlet. In the OFF position, this may be 100 mm Hg (13.6 kPa) but may rise to 300 mm Hg (38.5 kPa) when the vaporizer dial is set at 4.0%.

During flushing with the vaporizer in the ON position, it appears that gas is forced into the vaporizer and then escapes from the vaporizer after discontinuing the flush.

The hazards of flushing are thus evident with respect to the use of downstream vaporizers. There is an inadvertent delivery of higher concentrations of anesthetic vapors than are desired or safe.

Furthermore, the development of excessive pressure in the vaporizer may occur if the shunt valve to the vaporizer is open, resulting in breakage of the glass front of the vaporizer.

CONTAMINATION OF ANESTHETIC MIXTURES BY VAPORIZERS[135]

Contamination of inhaled anesthetic mixtures may occur as a result of exposure of the volatile anesthetic agents to components of the vaporizers used. It should be appreciated that this contamination is distinct from the occurrence of any impurities that may have existed in the volatile agents as prepared by the manufacturer and then used to fill the vaporizer reservoir chamber. Likewise, this mechanism is distinct from the breakdown of volatile anesthetics when they are exposed to soda lime, such as the breakdown of halothane, especially in closed-circuit systems.

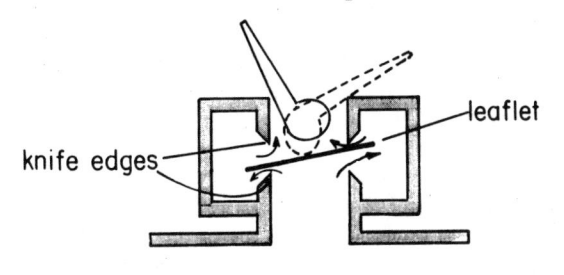

FIG. 5–36. The Steen valve during exhalation. This device permits gas to exit from a circuit under the slight pressure that occurs during exhalation. A sudden increase in pressure, such as occurs during an assisted or controlled inhalation, however, seals the leaflet against the upper circular knife edge. A lever-operated eccentric cam defeats this effect if desired and turns the valve into an ordinary pop-off that is not spring-loaded.

In 1981, Wald reported that enflurane could interact with wicks of the vaporizers and produce contaminants and impurities.[135] Wald determined that these impurities were not from the degradation of enflurane, but from an interaction with the sulfurous paper component in the vaporizer wick. The impact of this particular component, which produced a yellowish discoloration, as a toxic agent was not clearly established.

Utilizing the Ohio Calibrated Vaporizer for isoflurane vaporization, Welden has noted that a yellowish discoloration could also occur in the volatile agent isoflurane.[136] By both mass spectrometric and chromatographic techniques, three organic compounds were identified. One compound, designated as bis-phenol-(2,2-methylene-bis-[4-methyl, 6-tetrabutylphenol]) was found to be a contaminant in all vaporizers. Two other compounds could be detected routinely by gas chromatographic analysis but were not as concentrated as the first. These two additional substances in lesser quantity were identified as benzoresorcinol and diethyl hexyl-thalate (DEPH); however, none of these compounds could be considered to have produced the yellow discoloration of the volatile anesthetic. Only the vaporizers from the Ohio Medical Products were found to contain the yellow discoloration. The formation of these contaminants is apparently related to the extraction by the high solvent action of isoflurane, with respect to the plastic wick spacers and nylon bushings that are part of the vaporizer construction. Only when brass fittings and retainer nuts are involved in the construction of the vaporizer is there an absence of these particular contaminants.

COMPRESSED AIR: PIPELINES[137]

Compressed air is commonly used in operating rooms and intensive care units. This is usually available through a system of air storage tanks, air compressors, pipelines, and connectors to the source of use. Some studies indicate that there can be microbial contamination, so air samples collected in a specially constructed device have been analyzed for contamination. It was found that 70 to 80% of analyzed gas specimens contained a variety of bacteria. The most common organisms were Staphylococcus albus and Pseudomonas aeruginosa. It is indicated that air for medical use is rich in condensed water, and this together with the oil aerosol from compressors makes air storage tanks a favorable medium for proliferation of bacteria.

BACTERIAL INTERACTIONS[138]

Transmission of bacteria from infected patients to anesthesia practitioners and then to subsequent patients is always a concern. Of equal concern is the transmission of bacteria, viruses, or other pathogenic organisms from patients to anesthesiologists and patient to patient via the anesthesia circuit. A third source of cross-infection within the operating room is the anesthesiologist who only has a "little cold" but is coughing. Personnel in the operating room should be aware that they too pose a hazard to patients and then to colleagues. An important discussion of this subject is that by du Moulin and Hedley-Whyte.[138] Important facts are as follows:

- Speaking an average sentence results in over 100 bacteria-bearing droplets (0 to 250) being expelled from the airway.
- Coughing and sneezing release between 3000 and 1 million bacteria-laden droplets from healthy subjects at a high velocity of 300 m/s.
- Organisms expelled during sneezing or coughing originate largely from the anterior portion of the oropharynx, rarely from the nose or hypopharynx. Respiratory pathogens colonize in the nose and pharynx of their host. Only half of patients with streptococci expel the organism so as to be detected. In patients with open pulmonary tuberculosis, on coughing only 10% of droplets will contain bacilli.
- Many factors contribute to the risk of contaminating the anesthesia circuit and transmitting bacteria.
- Filters have not demonstrably minimized the contamination of anesthesia circuits or eliminated transmission of infection.
- The use of disposable circuits has not presented any significant difference in the development of postoperative respiratory infection.

Recommendations

Vigilant attention to interaction between patient–physician and environment, especially when acid-fast bacilli are considered includes:

1. Careful washing and sterilization or disinfection of nondisposable equipment after use
2. Use of disposable circle system may be helpful
3. Awareness of all operating room personnel of a "contaminated" case
4. Patients should wear masks
5. Appropriate disposition of gowns, masks, and covers
6. Minimal contact and traffic in the room of the contaminated case
7. Anesthesiologists should be gloved and intraoral manipulation kept to a minimum

Nosocomial Infections[139]

These are infections that occur in an institutional setting. Aerobic gram-negative bacilli cause 60% of such infections. Fungal infections and Staphylococcus aureus infections are also common. Routes of infection and outbreaks of septicemia have been related to careless intravenous delivery technique, to contaminated medications, and to sloppy management of hemodynamic monitoring systems.

Ventilators with humidifying cascades have been a source of patient contamination; however, careful studies by Craven demonstrate that the circuits need not be changed more frequently than 48 hours.

Intravenous infusion systems do not need to be changed more often than every 48 hours. Indeed, more frequent changes lead to unnecessary invasion and potential introduction of contaminants.

Multiple-dose vials may be easily contaminated. More important, particulate matter is introduced into the solution with the first puncture. For spinal, epidural, intramuscular, or nerve block injections, single vials of agents or ampules are recommended.

VAPORIZER OUTPUT AFFECTED BY COMPOSITION OF INPUT CARRIER GAS[140]

The output of a vaporizer varies with changes in composition of carrier gases. This is particularly evident in the variable bypass vaporizers. For example, in the ethrane vaporizer, when N_2O 70%/O_2 30% (3 L flow) is passed through the vaporizer, the output of ethrane is abruptly increased if the carrier gas is switched to air 70%/O_2 30% or to oxygen. The output of ethrane is almost tripled by the change. This aberrance is attributed to the differences in solubilities of the carrier gases in the liquid anesthetics. It is known that N_2O is highly soluble in the volatile liquids in contrast to nitrogen and/or oxygen. When a nonrebreathing system is used, the changing of carrier gas from nitrous oxide to oxygen may result in a clinically significant increase in the volatile anesthetic and represent an excessive dose.[140]

ANESTHESIA MACHINE CHECKLIST*

Prior to induction of anesthesia, the anesthesia machine and its contents should be made ready for use. All parts of the machine should be in good working order with all accessory equipment and necessary supplies on hand. The following checklist is a general guide to the inspection and testing procedures that should be carried out prior to administering an anesthetic. The exact procedures will vary according to the type of machine and monitors used. This checklist is based on guidelines developed by the Food and Drug Administration, as advised by anesthesiologists and manufacturers:

1. Inspect for condition and date of last servicing. Record machine serial number.

2. Inspect and turn on monitors and electrical equipment for warm-up.
3. Turn off flow control valves and vaporizers.
4. Check vaporizer filling, oxygen and nitrous oxide cylinder contents, and status of carbon dioxide absorbent.
5. Test flowmeters. Floats should move freely with flow and return to zero.
6. Test oxygen pressure failure system, oxygen ratio monitor/controller, and oxygen warning systems.
7. Check central gas supply pressures and alarm systems.
8. Calibrate oxygen monitor with air and oxygen. Set alarm limits.
9. Check breathing system valves.
10. Smell inspired gas; there should be no odor.
11. Test for leaks in machine and breathing system.
12. Check exhaust valve and scavenger system.
13. Test ventilator using a reservoir bag to simulate the patient's lungs.
14. Check, calibrate, and connect monitors and alarm devices.
15. Check final position of all controls. The machine is then ready for induction of anesthesia.

After anesthesia has been completed:
1. Turn off gas cylinders; allow pressure gauges to come to zero.
2. Allow flowmeter knobs to be open until float falls to bottom.
3. Close flowmeter knobs gently so that valve seats are not damaged.
4. Replace empty cylinders; disconnect central oxygen and nitrous oxide lines.
5. Remove face mask, breathing tubes, and reservoir bag for cleaning.
6. Turn off ventilator, monitors, and alarms; replace used supplies.
7. If machine, ventilator, monitors, or alarms are defective, remove machine from use and notify responsible individual.

RECOMMENDED READING

1. Boys, J.E., and Howells, T.H.: Humidification in anaesthesia. Br. J. Anaesth., 44:879, 1972.
2. Dorsch, J.A., and Dorsch, S.E.: Understanding Anesthesia Equipment: Construction, Care, and Complications, 2nd ed. Baltimore, Williams & Wilkins, 1984.
3. Eger, E.I., and Epstein, R.M.: Hazards of anesthetic equipment. Anesthesiology, 25:490, 1964.
4. Hill, D.W.: The design and calibration of vaporizers for volatile anaesthetic agents. Br. J. Anaesth., 40:648, 1968.
5. Lecky, J.H.: The mechanical aspects of anesthetic pollution control. Anesth. Analg., 56:769, 1977.
6. McPherson, S.P.: Respiratory Therapy Equipment, 2nd ed. St. Louis, C.V. Mosby, 1981.
7. Morris, L.E.: A new vaporizer for liquid anesthetic agents. Anesthesiology, 13:589, 1952.

* From Dripps, Eckenhoff, Vandam: Introduction to Anesthesia, 7th ed. Philadelphia, W.B. Saunders, 1988.

8. Pauling, L., Wood, R.E., and Sturdivant, J.H.: An instrument for determining the partial pressure of oxygen in a gas. J. Am. Chem. Soc., 68:795, 1946.
9. Schreiber, P.: Anaesthesia Equipment: Performance, Classification and Safety. New York, Springer-Verlag, 1972.
10. Thomas, K.: The Development of Anaesthetic Apparatus: A History Based on the Charles King Collection of the Association of Anaesthetists of Great Britain and Ireland. Philadelphia, J.B. Lippincott, 1975.
11. Ward, C.S.: Anaesthetic Equipment: Physical Principles and Maintenance. New York, Macmillan, 1975.
12. Waters, R.M.: Clinical scope and utility of carbon dioxide filtration in inhalation anesthesia. Anesth. Analg., 3:20, 1924.
13. Wyant, G.M.: Mechanical Misadventures in Anaesthesia. Toronto, University of Toronto Press, 1978.

REFERENCES

1. Kendall, J.: Visual considerations for the anesthesia machine operator. J. Assoc. Nurse Anesthetists, 54:225, 1986.
2. Diffrient, N.: Humanscale 1a. Cambridge, MA, MIT Press, 1981.
3. McIntyre, J.W.R.: Man–machine interface: The position of the anaesthesia machine in the operating room. Can. Anaesth. Soc. J., 29:74, 1982.
4. Keys, T.E.: A History of Surgical Anesthesia. New York, Krieger, 1978.
5. Foregger, R.: Gwathmey—Obituary. Anesthesiology, 5:296, 1944.
6. Thomas, K.B.: The Development of Anaesthetic Apparatus. Philadelphia, J.B. Lippincott, 1975.
7. Keys, T.E.: The development of anesthesia. Anesthesiology, 4:409, 1943.
8. McKesson, E.I.: Nitrous oxide–oxygen anesthesia with a description of a new apparatus. Surg. Gynecol. Obstet., 13:456, 1911.
9. Cooper, J.B., et al. A new anesthesia delivery system. Anesthesiology, 49:310, 1978.
10. Dornette, W.H.L.: Suggestions for standardization of anesthesia equipment. Anesthesiology, 16:1025, 1955.
11. Wyant, G.M.: Appendix B: Standards of interest to the anesthetist. In Mechanical Misadventures in Anesthesia. Toronto, University of Toronto Press, 1978.
12. Feeley, T.W., and Hedley-Whyte, J.: Bulk oxygen and nitrous oxide delivery systems: Design and dangers. Anesthesiology, 44:301, 1976.
13. Compressed Gas Association: Handbook of Compressed Gases, 2nd ed. New York, Reinhold Publishing, 1981.
14. Interstate Commerce Regulations, May 1954: Transportation of Explosive and Other Dangerous Articles.
15. Compressed Gas Association: Standard Compressed Gas Cylinder Valve Outlet and Inlet Connections. Pamphlet V1, 1977.
16. Compressed Gas Association: Diameter Intex-Safety System Non-Interchangeable Low Pressure Connections for Medical Gas Applications. Pamphlet V5, 1978.
17. Compressed Gas Association: Characteristics and Safe Handling of Medical Gases. Pamphlet P2, 1955.
18. Compressed Gas Association: Characteristics and Safe Handling of Medical Gases. Pamphlet P2, 1978.
19. American National Standards Institute: Minimizing Performance and Safety Requirements for Components and Systems of Continuous Flow Anesthesia. Machines for Human Use. ANSI 2:79.8. American National Standards Institute, Inc., 1430 Broadway, New York, NY 10036, 1979.
20. Compressed Gas Association: Safe Handling of Compressed Gases in Containers. Pamphlet P1; 3rd ed., 1956.
21. National Fire Protection Association: 470 Atlantic Ave., Boston, MA 02210, 1971.
22. NFPA N056A: Inhalation Anesthetics Flammable and Non-Flammable, 1971 (see Ref. 21).
23. NFPA N056A: Inhalation Anesthetics, 1978 (see Ref. 21).
24. NFPA N056F: Non-Flammable Medical Gases, 1983 (see Ref. 21).
25. Bureau of Standards (Department of Commerce) Simplified Practice Recommendation (R-176-41), 1941.
26. Standard Committee SPR 176-41. Department of Commerce, Chairman V.J. Collins. Federal Register Standards for Identification (November 16), 37:225, 1972.
27. I.S.O.: Recommendation International Standard Identification of Medical Gas Cylinders (Color Code), 1952.
28. Medical Gas Cylinders and Anaesthetic Apparatus. British Standard 1319 British Standards Institution, British Standards House, 2 Park St. London W, 1955 (I.S.O. 1957). Filed with ANSI, 1430 Broadway, New York, NY.
29. International Standards Organization (I.S.O.) Recommendation R-32. Identification of Medical Gas Cylinders. 1957.
30. Compressed Gas Association: Standard Color-Marking of Compressed Gas Cylinders Intended for Medical Use in the United States, Pamphlet C9. 1982.
31. Woodbridge, P.H.: Hazard of interchanging gas cylinders to wrong inlet—Pin Indexing Safety. Letter to J.G. Sholar, Ohio Chemical and Manufacturing Co., 1939. Archives A.S.A. Wood Library Museum.
32. Hogg, C.F.: Pin indexing failures. Anesthesiology, 38:85, 1973.
33. Epstein, R.M., et al.: Prevention of breathing of anoxic gas mixtures. Anesthesiology, 23:1, 1962.
34. Ohio Chemical Company: Safety in Hospitals. Form 2117, 1956.
35. Ohio Chemical Company: Medical Gases. Form No. 4662, 1956.
36. Eger, E.I., Epstein, R.M.: Hazards of anesthetic equipment. Anesthesiology, 24:490, 1964.
34. Keenan, R.L.: Prevention of increased pressure on anesthetic vaporizers with a unidirectional valve. Anesthesiology, 24:732, 1963.
37. Calverley, R.K.: A safety feature for anaesthetic machines—touch identification of oxygen flow control. Can. Anaesth. Soc. J., 18:225, 1971.
38. Foregger, R.: The rotameter in anesthesia. Anesthesiology, 7:549, 1946.
39. Waaben, J., Stokke, D.B., and Brinklov, M.M.: Accuracy of gas flowmeters determined by the bubble-water method. Br. J. Anaesth. 50:1251, 1978.
40. Bishop, C., Levick, C.H., Hodgson, C.: A design fault in the Boyle apparatus. Br. J. Anaesth., 39:908, 1967.
41. Eger, E.I., et al.: Anesthetic flow meter sequence—a cause for hypoxia. Anesthesiology, 24:396, 1963.
42. Katz, D.: Recurring cyanosis of intermittent mechanical origin in anesthetized patients. Anesth. Analg., 47:233, 1968.
43. Katz, D.: Increasing safety of anesthesia machines. Anesth. Analg., 48:242, 1969.
44. Gauert, W.B., and Husted, R.F.: Difference in metered and measured oxygen concentrations during nitrous oxide analgesia. Anesth. Analg., 47:441, 1968.
45. Everett, G., Hornbein, T.F., and Allen, G.D.: Hidden hazards

of the McKesson Narmatic anesthesia machine. Anesthesiology, 32:73, 1970.
46. Wilson, R.S., and Laver, M.B.: Oxygen analysis: Advances in methodology. Anesthesiology, 37:112, 1972.
47. Pauling, N.L., Wood, R.E., and Sturdivant, J.H.: An instrument for determining the partial pressure of oxygen in a gas. J. Am. Chem. Soc., 68:795, 1946.
48. Clark, L.C., et al.: Continuous recording of blood oxygen tension by polarography. J. Appl. Physiol., 6:189, 1953.
49. Severinghaus, J.W.: Methods of measurement of blood and gas carbon dioxide during anesthesia. Anesthesiology, 21:717, 1960.
50. Kennell, E.M., Andrews, R.W., and Wollman, H.: Correction factors for nitrous oxide in the infrared analysis of carbon dioxide. Anesthesiology, 39:441, 1973.
51. Severinghaus, J.W., Larson, C.P., and Eger, E.I.: Correction factors for infrared carbon dioxide pressure broadening by nitrogen, nitrous oxide and cyclopropane. Anesthesiology, 22:429, 1961.
52. Ozanne, G.M., et al.: Multipatient anesthetic mass spectrometry: Rapid analysis of data stored in long catheters. Anesthesiology, 55:62, 1981.
53. Lowe, H.J., and Hogler, K.: Clinical and laboratory evaluation of an expired anesthetic gas monitor (Narko-test). Anesthesiology, 34:378, 1971.
54. Hulands, G.H., Nunn, J.F.: Portable interference refractometers in anaesthesia. Br. J. Anaesth., 42:1051, 1970.
55. Wolfson, B.: Appraisal of the Hook and Tucker halothane meter. Anesthesiology, 29:157, 1968.
56. Robinson, H., Devison, J.S., and Summers, F.W.: Halothane analyzer. Anesthesiology, 23:391, 1962.
57. Tatnell, M.L., West, P.G., and Morris, P.: A rapid-response U.V. halothane meter. Br. J. Anaesth., 50:617, 1978.
58. Davies, N.J., Denison, D.M.: The uses of long sampling probes in respiratory mass spectrometry. Respir. Physiol., 37:335, 1979.
59. Yakulis, R., et al.: Mass spectrometry monitoring of respiratory variables in an intensive care unit. Resp. Care, 23:671, 1978.
60. Davison, M.H.A., Essex, L., and Pask, E.A.: Older methods of the vaporization of liquid anaesthetics. Anaesthesia, 18:302, 1963.
61. Faulconer, A. Jr.: Anesthetic vaporizers: A physical basis for functional classification. Anesthesiology, 18:372, 1957.
62. Hill, D.W.: The design and calibration of vaporizers for volatile anaesthetic agents. Br. J. Anaesth., 40:648, 1968.
63. Feldman, S.A., and Morris, L.E.: Vaporization of halothane and ether in the copper kettle. Anesthesiology, 19:650, 1958.
64. Hillmer, N.R., Kalandros, K., and Hummell, P.R.: A simple apparatus for administration of halothane. Anesthesiology, 22:1017, 1961.
65. Adriani, J.: Chemistry and Physics of Anesthesia. Springfield, IL, Charles C Thomas, 1970.
66. Hampton, L.J., and Flickinger, H.: Closed circuit anesthesia utilizing known increments of halothane. Anesthesiology, 22:413, 1961.
67. Weingarten, M., and Lowe, H.J.: A new circuit injection technique in syringe-measured administration of methoxyflurane: A new dimension in anesthesia. Anesth. Analg., 52:634, 1973.
68. Morris, L.E., and Feldman, S.A.: Considerations in the design and function of anesthetic vaporizers. Anesthesiology, 19:642, 1958.
69. Morris, L.E.: A new vaporizer for liquid anesthetic agents. Anesthesiology, 13:587, 1952.
70. Morris, L.E., and Feldman, S.A.: Evaluation of a new anesthetic vaporizer. Anaesthesia, 17:21, 1962.
71. Waters, R.M.: Chloroform. Madison, WI, University of Wisconsin Press, 1951.
72. Doblein, A.B., et al. Studies on the calibration of enflurane vaporizers. Anesth. Analg., 52:317, 1973.
73. Adner, M., and Hallen, B.: Reliability of halothane vaporizers. Acta Anaesthesiol. Scand., 9:233, 1965.
74. MacKay, I.M., and Kalow, W.: A clinical laboratory evaluation of four fluorothane vaporizers. Can. Anaesth. Soc. J., 5:248, 1958.
75. Massa, L.S., and Zauder, H.L.: Calibration of a new vaporizer. Anesthesiology, 25:708, 1964.
76. Noble, W.H.: Accuracy of halothane vaporizers in clinical use. Can. Anaesth. Soc. J., 17:135, 1970.
77. Paterson, G.M., Hulands, G.H., and Nunn, J.F.: Evaluation of a new halothane vaporizer: The cyprane fluotec mark 3. Br. J. Anaesth., 41:109, 1969.
78. Hill, D.W.: Halothane concentration obtained with a Drager "Vapor" vaporizer. Br. J. Anaesth., 35:285, 1963.
79. Hall, J.M., et al. A test of two types of halothane vaporizers. Br. J. Anaesth., 38:494, 1966.
80. Ward, C.S.: Anaesthetic Equipment. New York, Macmillan, 1975.
81. Greenhow, D.E., and Barth, R.L.: Oxygen flushing delivers anesthetic vapor—a hazard with a new machine. Anesthesiology, 38:409, 1973.
82. Kopriva, C.J., and Lowenstein, E.: An anesthetic accident: cardiovascular collapse from liquid halothane delivery. Anesthesiology, 30:246, 1969.
83. Munson, W.M.: Cardiac arrest: Hazard of tipping a vaporizer. Anesthesiology, 26:235, 1965.
84. Safar, P., and Galla, S.J.: Overdose with Ohio halothane vaporizer. Anesthesiology, 23:715–716, 1962.
85. Andreesen, I.H., and Bay, J.: Halothane concentrations obtained by the combined use of the Manley ventilator and the fluotec vaporizer. Br. J. Anaesth., 38:641, 1966.
86. Eger, E.I.: Pressure effect on the vernitrol vaporizer. Anesthesiology, 24:742, 1963.
87. Chatrath, R.R.: The effect of intermittent positive pressure on the output of halothane from a Blease thruway vaporizer. Br. J. Anaesth., 45:915, 1973.
88. Eger, E.I., and Ethans, C.T.: The effects of inflow, overflow and valve placement on economy of the circle system. Anesthesiology, 29:93, 1968.
89. Ngai, S.H.: Copper kettle. Anesthesiology, 19:559, 1958.
90. Keet, J.E., Valentine, G.W., and Riccio, J.S.: An arrangement to prevent pressure effect on the vernitrol vaporizer. Anesthesiology, 24:734, 1963.
91. Murray, W.J.: Zsigmond, E.K., and Fleming, P.: Contamination of in-series vaporizers with halothane-methoxyflurane. Anesthesiology, 38:487, 1973.
92. Wichett, R.E., Jenkins, L.C., and Root L.S.: Downstream contamination of in-series vaporizers. Can. Anaesth. Soc. J., 21:114, 1974.
93. Parmley, J.B., et al.: Disposable versus reusable rebreathing circuits: Advantages, disadvantages, hazards and bacteriologic studies. Anesth. Analg., 51:888, 1972.
94. Berry, F.A., and Eastwood, D.W.: Serious defects in "simple" equipment. Anesthesiology, 28:471, 1967.
95. Cozantis, O.A., and Tahkuman, O.: Aneurysm of ventilator tubing. Anaesthesia, 26:235, 1971.
96. Bushman, J.A., and Collis, J.M.: The estimation of gas losses in ventilator tubing. Anaesthesia, 22:664, 1967.
97. Nunn, J.F.: Ventilation and end-tidal carbon dioxide tension. Anaesthesia, 13:124, 1958.

98. Proctor, D.F.: Studies of respiratory air flow: Resistance to air flow through anesthetic apparatus. Bull. Johns Hopkins Hosp., 96:49, 1955.
99. Dogu, T.S., and Davis, H.S.: Hazards of inadvertently opposed valves. Anesthesiology, 33:122, 1970.
100. Hunt, K.H.: Resistance in respiratory valves and cannisters. Anesthesiology, 16:190, 1955.
101. Leigh, M.D., and Kester, H.A.: Endotracheal anesthesia for operations on cleft lip and cleft palate. Anesthesiology, 9:32, 1948.
102. Stephen, C.R., and Slater, H.M.: A nonresisting nonrebreathing valve. Anesthesiology, 9:550, 1948.
103. Hirano, T., and Saito, T.: A new automatic nonrebreathing valve. Anesthesiology, 31:84, 1969.
104. Lewis, G.: Nonrebreathing valve. Anesthesiology, 17:618, 1956.
105. Mitchell, J.V., and Epstein, H.G.: A pressure-operated inflating valve. Anaesthesia, 21:277, 1966.
106. Newton, G.W., Howill, W.K., and Stephen, C.R.: A piston-type nonrebreathing valve. Anesthesiology, 16:1037, 1955.
107. Frumin, M.J., Lee, A.S.J., and Papper, E.M.: New valve for nonrebreathing systems. Anesthesiology, 20:383, 1959.
108. Fink, B.R.: A non-rebreathing valve of new design. Anesthesiology, 15:471, 1954.
109. Loehning, R.W., Davis, G., and Safar, P.: Rebreathing with "nonrebreathing valves". Anesthesiology, 25:854, 1964.
110. Sten, S.N., and Chen, J.L.: Automatic non-rebreathing valve circuits: Some principles and modifications. Br. J. Anaesth., 35:379, 1963.
111. Stephen, C.R., and Slater, H.M.: A nonrebreathing mask. Anesthesiology, 13:226, 1952.
112. Redick, L.F., et al. An evaluation of hand-operated self-inflating resuscitation equipment. Anesth. Analg., 49:28, 1970.
113. Ruben, H.: A new nonrebreathing valve. Anesthesiology, 16:643, 1955.
114. Wisborg, K., and Jacobsen, E.: Functional disorders of Ruben and Ambu-E valves after dismantling and cleaning. Anesthesiology, 42:633, 1975.
115. Johnston, R.E., and Smith, T.C.: Rebreathing bags as pressure limiting devices. Anesthesiology, 38:192, 1973.
116. Linker, G.S., Holaday, D.A., and Waltuck, B.: A simply constructed automatic pressure relief valve. Anesthesiology, 32:563, 1970.
117. Stone, D.R., and Graves, S.A.: Compliance of pediatric rebreathing bags. Anesthesiology, 53:434, 1980.
118. Waters, D.J.: Use and misuse of a pressure-limited bag. Anaesthesia, 22:322, 1967.
119. Jackson, D.E.: A new method for the production of general analgesia and anaesthesia with a description of the apparatus used. J. Lab. Clin. Med., 1:, 1915.
120. Waters, R.M.: Clinical scope and utility of carbon dioxide filtration in inhalation anesthesia. Anesth. Analg., 3:20, 1924.
121. Waters, R.M.: Carbon dioxide absorption technic in anesthesia. Ann. Surg., 103:38, 1936.
122. Hale, D.E.: The rise and fall of soda lime. Anesth. Analg., 46:648, 1967.
123. Brown, E.S.: Voids, pores and total air space of carbon dioxide absorbents. Anesthesiology, 19:1, 1958.
124. Brown, E.S.: The activity and surface area of fresh soda lime. Anesthesiology, 19:208, 1958.
125. Brown, E.S., Bakamjian, V., and Seniff, A.M.: Performance of absorbents: Effects of moisture. Anesthesiology, 20:613, 1959.
126. Kitborn, M.G.: Preliminary clinical report on a new carbon dioxide absorbent—Baralyme. Anesthesiology, 2:621, 1941.
127. Adriani, J., Rovenstine, E.A.: Experimental studies in carbon dioxide absorbers for anesthesia. Anesthesiology, 2:1, 1941.
128. Tenpas, R.H., Brown, E.S., Elam, J.O.: Carbon dioxide absorption: The circle versus the to-and-fro. Anesthesiology, 19:231, 1958.
129. Sword, B.C.: The closed circle method of administration of gas anesthesia. Anesth. Analg., 9:198, 1930.
130. Brown, E.S., and Elam J.O.: Practical aspects of carbon dioxide absorption. N.Y. State J. Med., 55:3436, 1955.
131. Horn, B.: Valve for assisted or controlled ventilation. Anesthesiology, 21:83, 1960.
132. Lee, S.: A new pop-off valve. Anesthesiology, 25:240, 1964.
133. Smith, R.H., and Volpitto, P.P.: Volume ventilator valve. Anesthesiology, 20:885, 1959.
134. Kelly, D.A.: Free standing vaporizers: Another hazard. Anaesthesia, 40:661, 1985.
135. Wald, A.: Discoloration of enflurane. Anesth. Analg., 60:843, 1981.
136. Weldon, S.T., et al.: Production and characterization of impurities in isoflurane vaporizers. Anesth. Analg., 64:634, 1985.
137. Bjerring, P., and Oberg, V.: Bacterial contamination of compressed air for medical use. Anaesthesia, 41:148, 1986.
138. du Moulin, G.C., and Hedley-Whyte, J.: Bacterial interactions between anesthesiologists, their patients, and equipment. Anesthesiology, 57:37, 1982.
139. Eickhoff, T.C.: Nosocomial infections. New Engl. J. Med., 306:1545, 1982.
140. Scheller, M.S., and Drummond, J.C.: Solubility of N_2O in volatile anesthetics contributes to vaporizer aberrancy when changing carrier gases. Anesth. Analg., 65:88, 1986.

An intact human supports changes in body posture by complex, coordinated adjustments of many physiologic systems. Gravitational forces are potentially disruptive to effective body function in the new posture, and brisk organic reflexes must modify existing activity as sequential stresses occur. In the presence of disease, injury, starvation, prolonged physical inactivity, or anesthetic drugs, compensatory responses to postural changes are impaired or lost, and significant dysfunction of one or more organ systems may result. For the anesthesiologist the most important potential physiologic disruptions involve circulation, ventilation, and the central nervous system.

DEFINITION OF BODY POSTURES

In describing body positions we are forced to use jargon because of the inadequate definition of the term "decubitus." The most applicable of Dorland's definitions of *decubitus* states *"An act of lying down; also the position assumed in lying down"*;[1] neither of those usages fits our descriptive needs. Despite its appearance as semantic trivia, this issue becomes legally important when we attempt to describe a lateral position. The "left chest position" could mean either "the position that exposed the left chest to an incision," in which case the subject would be lying on his right side, or "the position in which the subject lies on the left side." For the purpose of the ensuing discussions, "decubitus" *will be used to indicate the body area that is in contact with the supporting surface of the operating table.* Thus "left lateral decubitus position" describes the position of a patient who is lying on his left side to permit surgery that involves structures on the right side of the body. The dorsal decubitus position is supine, and the ventral decubitus position is prone.

THE CARDIOVASCULAR SYSTEM

Restlessness appears in a supine, motionless, conscious human apparently for two reasons: (1) joints are extended into uncomfortable and nonneutral

John T. Martin

THE PHYSIOLOGY OF PATIENT POSTURE

positions[2]; and (2) normal spontaneous fluctuations of blood flow in the microcirculation fail after about 1 hour of immobility.[3] In a normothermic, normocarbic, and normovolemic subject, induction of anesthesia causes peripheral vasodilation; however, the resulting increase in tissue perfusion fades over time and spontaneous fluctuations in microcirculatory volume disappear until anesthesia ends and the patient begins to react.

GRAVITATION INFLUENCE ON VASCULAR PRESSURES

The forces of gravity play a major role in determining arterial pressures and the return of venous blood to the heart. Pressure gradients are determined by the vertical distance that separates two vascular beds. Pressures change by 2 mmHg each vertical 2.5 cm (1 inch).[4] In the standing position, the vascular axis is vertical and a person who is 6 feet tall, with a mean arterial blood pressure of about 90 mmHg at the level of the atria, will have mean arterial pressures of about 70 at the circle of Willis and 210 at the toes. In the supine position that vascular axis is in the same plane relative to gravity and hydrostatic differences in vascular pressures are minimized.

Distensible vessels tend to collapse at low or subatmospheric pressures and to engorge passively where the hydrostatic forces become significant. Because active changes in cardiac output and peripheral vascular resistance are frequent in the arterial tree, passive variations in hydrostatic pressure related to alterations in posture are more evident in the low-pressure venous circuit. Coonan and Hope[3] have reintroduced Wagner's 1886 concept[5] of a *hydrostatic indifferent point* (HIP) at which intravascular pressures and vessel caliber are independent of the hydrostatic forces in the circulation. Above that point, blood drains toward it; below it, the vessels are progressively more engorged as hydrostatic pressures increase. While the HIP may be specific for any given posture in a specific patient, it changes to some degree as the position is passively altered. The perception illuminates differences in cerebral perfusion and venous engorgement in the elevated head versus the head in the Trendelenberg position as well as shifts in distribution of pulmonary blood volume when the supine position is changed to a lateral position.

ZONES OF PULMONARY VASCULAR PRESSURE AND ALVEOLAR PRESSURE

West et al.[6] have defined three zones of varied relationships between alveoli and the pulmonary microcirculation (Fig. 6–1) in man. The basic zones are in the erect position.

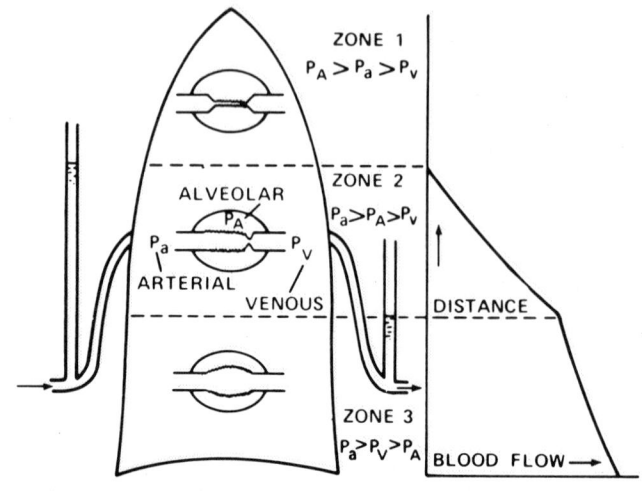

FIG. 6–1. Distribution of blood flow in the isolated lung. From West, J.B., Dollery, C.T., and Naimark, A.: Distribution of blood flow in isolated lung: Relationship to vascular and alveolar pressures. J. Appl. Physiol., *19:* 713, 1964.

In Zone 1, alveolar pressure exceeds either pulmonary arterial or pulmonary venous pressure and prevents pulmonary circulation. Pulmonary hypotension, exuberant positive end-expiratory pressure, or alveolar distension from large tidal volumes could create this relationship, which is normally not found in humans.

In Zone 2, pulmonary artery pressure exceeds alveolar pressure which, in turn, exceeds pulmonary venous pressure. This zone is found in the nondependent portions of the lung, and flow is a balance between arterial and alveolar pressures.

In Zone 3, hydrostatic pressures have raised venous pressure above alveolar pressure, and flow is determined by the difference between arterial pressure and venous pressure. Perfusion in Zone 3 is more homogenous than in Zone 2 and is less affected by the forces of gravity.

EFFECT OF DORSAL DECUBITUS POSITION (HORIZONTAL)

In the dorsal decubitus (supine) position, arterial pressures essentially are similar throughout the horizontal vascular axis, and perfusion of the head and lower extremities is not regionally compromised. Some degree of hydrostatic engorgement occurs in the dorsal portions of the pulmonary circulation, probably accounting for the volume of blood that is lost from the central circulation when posture is changed from supine to seated (Table 6–1).

A pillow beneath the occiput places the cerebral circulation somewhat above the level of the heart. A slight uphill gradient is established for arterial flow to the head, but rarely is this an important

TABLE 6–1. CARDIOVASCULAR EFFECTS OF CHANGE IN BODY POSITION OF CONSCIOUS AND ANESTHETIZED HUMANS FROM THE SUPINE TO THE SEATED POSITION*

	Conscious Supine to Seated	Anesthetized Supine to Seated
Blood pressure	+ 0%–20%	+ 0%–40%
Arterio–venous O$_2$ difference	+ 50%–60%	
Cardiac output	− 20%–40%	− 12%–20%
Heart rate	+ 15%–30%	0 or increased
Systemic vascular resistance	+ 30%–60%	+ 50%–80%
Pulmonary vascular resistance	Increased	
Stroke volume	− 40%–50%	
Central blood volume	− 400 ml	
Left and right atrial pressure	− Left and right	− (right < left)
Cerebral blood flow	− 20%	− 15%
Renal blood flow	− 30%	
Hepatic blood flow	− Slightly	

*Control baseline for Conscious Supine and Anesthetized Supine are separate and are not compared with each other.

Modified from Coonan, T.J., and Hope, C.E.: Cardiorespiratory effects of change of body position. Can. Anaesth. Soc. J., 30:424, 1983.

modification of cerebral perfusion. The downhill venous gradient, however, assists somewhat the venous outflow from the cerebral circulation.

Elevation of the legs (lithotomy position) produces an arterial perfusion gradient upward toward the feet, reduces vascular volume in the extremities, and augments venous return toward the central circulation. If mean arterial pressure is reduced significantly or if arterial flow to a leg is compromised either by luminal obstruction or by extramural pressure, arterial perfusion of the extremity may decrease enough to produce ischemia. Conversely, lowering legs rapidly from the lithotomy position to the supine may increase vascular capacitance so abruptly that perfusion cannot adjust and systemic hypotension results.[7]

Intra-abdominal masses can compress the great vessels along the spine of a supine patient. The most obvious example of this potential is the supine hypotensive syndrome, in which the enlarged gravid uterus rests on the aorta and inferior vena cava. It must be pushed laterally off of the vessels in order to restore circulation to the lower extremities and the uterine contents. Similar problems can occur with large tumor masses. Kaneko[8] has shown that the entire pulmonary circulation in the supine position acts as what West subsequently labeled a Zone 3, perhaps because of the ventral (substernal) location of the heart.

EFFECT OF SUPINE-HEAD DOWN TILT

As the supine patient is tilted head-down, hydraulic gradients increasingly alter the distribution of blood in the head and trunk.

An uphill gradient is established from the intracranial veins to the right atrium, favoring cerebral venous stasis. In the anesthetized and passively ventilated patient, the presence of an elevated inspiratory phase further disrupts venous return from the head.

With viscera forcing the diaphragm cephalad, lung bases are compressed and vascular congestion increases in the poorly expanding pulmonary apices. Considering both the effects of gravity and the zones described by West, one can conjecture that the lung bases tend to become Zone 2 as the head is tilted downward and the apices become Zone 3.

A conscious human usually finds the Trendelenburg position an unpleasant experience after a few minutes and may complain of a developing headache that subsides when the position is terminated. Kubal[9] has reported the development of chest pain in patients scheduled for coronary artery bypass grafting when they were placed in a head-down position to facilitate preanesthetic percutaneous introduction of pulmonary artery catheters via the internal jugular vein.

Several investigators[10-14] have each demonstrated the lack of value of the Trendelenburg position in the treatment of shock. Apparently the increased central blood volume, acquired from the lower extremities as a result of the head-down tilt, causes an initial increase in cardiac output that activates baroreceptors in the aortic arch and carotid bifurcation. The rapid result is peripheral vasodilation, reduced cardiac output, and decreased organ perfusion.[15] Because the head-down tilt also increases the hydrostatic pressure of cerebrospinal fluid within the closed cranial vault surrounding the brain, cerebral perfusion is at risk as cardiac output falls.

Kubal[9] found that the minor degree of Trendelenburg position used to distend neck vessels during introduction of catheters into the central circulation prior to anesthesia for cardiac bypass produced a measurable increase in myocardial oxygen demand. In patients with coronary artery disease this occurred at a time when myocardial oxygen supply was precarious, and one patient in their test series developed electrocardiographic changes of myocardial ischemia.

EFFECT OF SUPINE-HEAD-UP TILT

As a patient is changed from the horizontal dorsal recumbent position through various degrees of head elevation to reach a sitting position eventually (Table 6-1), the effects of gravity play a progressively more important role.

Blood pools in distensible vessels of the lower extremity and viscera, decreasing central venous volume and right heart filling to a degree that is modified by initial blood volume deficits, the intensity of drug-induced peripheral vasodilation, and the distance that the lower extremities are placed below the level of the heart.

As the HIP relocates from heart level to a point in the upper abdomen,[3] cardiac filling pressures are reduced, sympathetic tone increases, parasympathetic activity decreases, the renin-angiotensin-aldosterone system is activated, and the kidneys retain fluids and electrolytes.[16,17]

Intrathoracic blood volume decreases approximately 500 ml[18,19]; left atrial pressure, stroke volume, and cardiac output are reduced; pulse rate and peripheral resistance increase; and pulmonary vascular resistance increases.

Vascular tone changes only slightly in the systemic capacitance system, and right atrial pressure falls less than does left.

Because oxygen consumption does not change appreciably, the reduced cardiac output causes an increase in the arterio-venous difference in oxygen content as the patient becomes more erect.[18,20]

Cerebral blood flow can decrease by as much as 20%, although systemic mean arterial pressure may remain constant or actually increase. Cerebral venous pressure decreases 2 mm Hg per inch of elevation above the atria. At some point of head elevation it becomes subatmospheric throughout most of the respiratory cycle of a mechanically ventilated patient and permits air entrainment if a vein is incised or torn.

Kaneko's description of perfusion of the erect lung[8] resembles Zone 2 of West in the nondependent areas and Zone 3 in dependent.

All of these changes are usually of minor magnitude until the head of the patient is elevated more than 45 degrees; above that level they assume increasing significance and may continue to develop for as long as 1 hour after the final head-elevated position has been established. Differing anesthetic techniques and variations in the extent of systemic diseases between individual patients will influence the magnitude of these postural changes.

EFFECT OF POSTURAL CHANGES IN HYPOVOLEMIC PATIENTS

Dripps[15] showed that an injured individual who remained supine could compensate for about 1200 ml of blood loss without showing significant circulatory changes. Green and Metheny[21] introduced the use of the head-elevated position as a "tilt test" to provoke circulatory changes in the presence of blood loss and to determine from the magnitude of those changes approximately how much blood had been shed.

They maintained their subjects in 75 degrees of head-up tilt for 3 minutes. An increase in heart rate in excess of 25 bpm without concurrent hypotension or syncope indicated a blood volume deficit of 9 to 14 ml/kg and required a transfusion of about 1000 ml to correct. If syncope occurred with the pulse rate increase, the volume deficit was likely to be in the range of 14 to 20 ml/kg, requiring approximately 1500 ml of transfusion. If hypotension was evident without tilting, the deficit was estimated to be in excess of 20 ml/kg and needed more than 2000 ml of blood transfused to restore stability.

Because these data preceded our modern concepts of the proper fluid management of hemorrhagic hypovolemia, the exact values now may be more historic than therapeutic. The study emphasizes, however, the contention that movement of a hypovolemic patient can be an unsettling influence on cardiovascular compensation and tends to justify the inference that the effects of anesthesia may intensify the disruption.

VASCULAR PRESSURE CHANGES IN LATERAL DECUBITUS POSITIONS

When a patient is turned from the supine to a lateral decubitus position and maintained horizontally, the pressures at most locations along the vascular axis are almost identical. Exceptions are (1) the small gradients between the uppermost and the dependent arms; and (2) hydrostatic gradients occurring between the two lungs. If lateral flexion is added to the lateral decubitus position, vessels in the head and legs may be below heart level and obstructive angulation of the inferior vena cava may occur.

Because it is customary subsequently to adjust the operting table so that the uppermost chest wall of the laterally flexed patient is horizontal, the head is usually almost at heart level whereas the legs are angulated downward to a significant degree. Thus, intracranial congestion is less of a threat than is trapping of significant amounts of circulating blood volume in the dependent lower extremities.

EFFECT OF LATERAL POSITION ON PERFUSION OF EACH LUNG

Perfusion of the two lungs is dissimilar in the lateral decubitus position. Because the heart is more in the left hemithorax than right, dependent shifts in its position will occur differently in each lateral decubitus position. Nevertheless, it is generally true that the dependent lung lies below the level of the atrium whereas the uppermost lung lies above it. In the low-pressure pulmonary vascular circuit, gravitational forces tend to engorge the down-side lung, causing it to become a Zone 3 of West,[6] while the up-side lung is relatively hypoperfused and acts as Zone 2 and, perhaps, in some areas as Zone 1. Kaneko[8] identified the transition from Zone 3 to Zone 2 at a level 18 cm above the most dependent portion of the lung.

In a healthy, spontaneously ventilated lung this perfusion disparity may not be significant. It is magnified, however, by intermittent positive-pressure ventilation and diaphragmatic paralysis. Inflation volumes travel through the tracheobronchial tree along the line of least resistance and preferentially expand the more compliant uppermost lung unless larger tidal volumes are used than would be needed for adequate spontaneous ventilation.

EFFECT OF PRONE POSITION ON CIRCULATION

The ventral decubitus (prone) position offers several threats to circulation.[22] Usually the lower extremities are arranged so that the feet are below the level of the heart to a degree that varies from slight to that of the full kneeling position. Thus, pooling of blood in the legs is a common problem that can compromise adequate cardiac output.

Because the patient lies on the ventral surfaces of the thorax, intermittent positive-pressure ventilation must expand the lungs against the weight of the dorsal portions of the body. The resultant cyclic increases in intrathoracic pressure can further impede venous return from the lower extremities.

Unless the prone patient is supported so that the abdomen is relatively free from the surface of the operating table, pressure, caused by the weight of the trunk against the table surface, is transmitted to the abdominal viscera and great vessels. The result is additional obstruction to venous return from the dependent extremities or increased venous engorgement of an incision in the region of the spine.

Rotation of a supple neck permits a pronated patient to rest a cheek against the pillow. Forced rotation of the neck of a patient with arteriosclerosis and an arthritic cervical spine may compromise flow through the vertebral and internal carotid arteries[23] or obstruct venous return via the internal jugular vein.

Backofen[24] reviewed patients who were monitored with arterial and thermodilution pulmonary artery catheters before and after being turned prone during general anesthesia. Despite their careful use of measures to prevent venous pooling and abdominal compression, pronation caused: (1) a significant decrease in stroke volume and cardiac index; (2) increased vascular resistance in both the systemic and pulmonary circuits; and (3) no changes in mean arterial, right atrial, or pulmonary artery occlusion pressures.

When the circulatory status of the patient is precarious prior to the induction of anesthesia, Backofen recommends the use of invasive monitors to detect otherwise unrecognizable deterioration of cardiac function in the prone position. In the prone patient, the entire lung has been reported to conform to the Zone 3 described by West.[8]

EFFECT OF MORPHINE ON CARDIOVASCULAR POSITIONAL CHANGES. Drew and Dripps (1946) showed that both cardiac output and systolic pressure decreased on tilting to the 75° head-up position, but with quick compensation.[25] Morphine administration increased the incidence of significant falls in systolic pressure as well as their severity and the duration.

When normal human subjects change from the supine to a 70° head-up tilt, cardiac output decreases 15–30%.[25a] This is probably related to venous pooling in the lower extremities.

Studies of pregnant women in the third trimester show dramatic falls in maternal blood pressure on assuming the supine position from the erect position. However, changing from the supine to the left lateral position increased cardiac output up to 26%.[25b] The low pressure in the supine position is attributed to compression of the vena cava.

EFFECT OF ANESTHETICS

Hemodynamics on Sitting.[25c] Three anesthetic techniques have been investigated for changes in hemodynamics on assumption of the sitting position.

Both enflurane N_2O-O_2 and halothane N_2O-O_2 anesthesia caused significant changes in hemodynamics while patients were in the supine position. Decreases occurred in systemic arterial pressure, systemic vascular resistance, cardiac index (20%), and stroke volume index (30%). Only pulmonary vascular resistance increased slightly. Cardiovascular responses on placement of patients in the sitting position resulted in an exaggeration of all these changes.

A neurolept-narcotic technique (Innovar-fentanyl N_2O-O_2) resulted in greater impairment of cardiovascular dynamics, which was exaggerated in the sitting position. With this technique there was also a marked reduction in RAP and PCWP. Surgical stimulation resulted in increases in SAP, SVRI, and SVI, indicating autonomic stress.

Morphine-N_2O-O_2 anesthesia resulted in the least impairment of or change in hemodynamics, whether following induction, after placement in the sitting position, or on surgical stimulation.[25d] These changes differ from the tilt-table studies by Drew of low dose morphine, which showed marked hypotensive changes when volunteers were moved to the upright position from the supine.

Cardiovascular adjustments occur in the unanesthetized subjects on changing posture, so that postural hypotension does not occur when various sitting and upright postures are attained. Compensation occurs through at least three mechanisms: (1) the renin-angiotension system (Oparil),[25e] (2) the sympathetic nervous system, (3) and/or reflex baroreceptor mechanisms. It is concluded that the deleterious effects of general anesthesia and the sitting position are not fully compensated by the normal mechanisms in the unanesthetized state.

In the Marshall study plasma renin showed slight increases in the anesthetized patient on attainment of the seated position. Changes were noted from the awake resting supine value of 1.7 ng/ml/hour to 1.87 in the awake seated position and to 2.50 in the anesthetized seated subjects.

THE RESPIRATORY SYSTEM AND BODY POSITION

The various body positions inflicted upon anesthetized patients alter respiratory dynamics in numerous ways. Table 6–2 relates these changes to the lung of erect, conscious humans.

EFFECT OF ASSUMPTION OF SUPINE POSITION

When a conscious human changes from the erect to the supine position, abdominal viscera press against the diaphragm and stretch its dorsal portions cephalad.[26] The stretched part of the muscle becomes more efficient, permitting stronger contraction against the visceral load during spontaneous ventilation and producing more effective ventilation of the preferentially perfused posterior basal portions of the lung that are congested and compressed. The cephalad displacement of the dorsal diaphragm is increased somewhat by the induction of anesthesia and considerably more by the onset of muscle paralysis.[26a] Intermittent positive-pressure ventilation (IPPV) of the lung moves gas along the line of least resistance, so the less congested and more compliant ventral (substernal) lung units of the supine lung are inflated preferentially. Unless larger than normal tidal volumes are employed, the dorsal portions of the lung will be underventilated, and the ventilation/perfusion mismatch that results can be significant.

Changes in Subdivisions of Lung Air

Both total lung capacity (TLC) and functional residual capacity (FRC) are reduced in the supine position compared to erect posture. Nunn has stated that the normal FRC (adult subject, erect) of 3000 ml becomes 2200 ml when supine.[27] Sophisticated techniques to measure FRC, thoraco-abdominal dimensions (by computerized tomography), central blood volume (CBV), and extravascular lung water (EVLW), have shown[28] that the induction of halothane anes-

TABLE 6–2. EFFECTS OF CHANGE IN BODY POSITION OF CONSCIOUS OR ANESTHETIZED HUMANS RELATIVE TO THE ERECT POSITION WHILE CONSCIOUS

	Erect Alert	Erect Anesthetized/Paralyzed	Supine Alert	Supine Anesthetized/Paralyzed	Lateral or Prone Alert	Lateral or Prone Anesthetized/Paralyzed
FRC	Control	−3%	−24%	−DL +NDL	−44%	−12%
ICP	Control	—	Increased	—	—	—
ERV	Control	—	Decreased	—	—	—
CVP	Control	—	Variable	—	—	—
CPP	Control	—	Nil to slight increase	Nil to slight increase	—	—

FRC = functional residual capacity; ICP = intracranial pressure; ERV = expiratory reserve volume; CPP = cerebral perfusion pressure; CVP = central venous pressure; DL = dependent lung; NDL = nondependent lung.

Modified from Coonan, T.J., and Hope, C.E.: Cardiorespiratory effects of change of body position. Can. Anaesth. Soc. J., 30:424, 1983.

thesia, muscle paralysis, and mechanical ventilation caused a fall in FRC of 17% (500 ml), a reduction in thoracic volume of 800 ml (300 due to a reduction in thoracic cross sectional area and 500 due to craniad relocation of the diaphragm), a 300 ml shift of CBV from thorax to abdomen, and no change in EVLW. Rehder[29] obtained slightly different data using a more refined method of computerized imaging and noted an increase in thoracic fluid volume with induction of anesthesia. He found that the decrease in FRC accompanying induction of anesthesia occurred in the first few minutes and was not progressive. The causes of the loss in FRC supine remain elusive. A likely explanation involves decreased muscle tone in the chest wall and diaphragm that permits the elastic recoil of the lung, exerted through the pleuro-pleuro moisture seal, to reduce total thorax volume at the expense of FRC.

Closure of Airways

Studies of the closure of small airways in the dependent areas of the lung at low lung volumes, the closing capacity, have reached varied conclusions regarding the effects of posture and anesthesia.[3] Airway closure during spontaneous tidal breathing in the erect position has been demonstrated[30] in normal subjects over age 65 and in the supine position over age 45. Don[31] documented airway closure and gas trapping in anesthetized patients in the supine position. Preexisting lung disease would accentuate this finding.

Effect of Lithotomy Position

FRC decreases from supine values when the patient is placed in the lithotomy position, decreases still further in Trendelenburg position, and is reduced to the greatest extent when the lithotomy and Trendelenburg positions are used simultaneously.[32] Induction of anesthesia can be expected to worsen the FRC decrement and to facilitate airway closure and gas trapping.

EFFECT OF LATERAL POSITION

In the lateral position FRC is markedly lessened in the down-side lung. Redistribution of inspired gases toward nondependent and more compliant lung regions occurs in some subjects in the lateral position during spontaneous ventilation and in almost all patients who are anesthetized, paralyzed, placed in the lateral position, and mechanically ventilated.[33] Better distribution of inspired gases can be achieved during mechanical ventilation with larger tidal volumes or with the addition of positive end-expiratory pressure.[34]

POSITIONAL EFFECTS IN LUNG DISEASE. Gravity is the essential factor that affects both pulmonary circulation and ventilation. The rule is "down with the good lung."[34a] The mechanism is related to greater blood flow occurring in the dependent lung. With respect to ventilation, a remarkable matching to the increased circulation occurs related to the structural properties of the lung and to the vertical gradient of pleural pressure which enhances ventilation of lung bases and increases ventilation of the entire dependent lung. The design of the lungs alters the pressure-volume curve so that the smaller alveoli in the dependent areas have a greater compliance.

In the presence of unilateral lung disease, turning a patient so that the good lung is down results in an increase in both ventilation and perfusion of the dependent lung.[34b] Remolina[34c] has shown that this change in position results in improved oxygen uptake, with an average increase in arterial partial pressure of oxygen of 29 mm Hg. When a disease is equally distributed on both sides, arterial oxygen tension is higher when the right side is down.

Lying with a sick lung dependent is associated with dyspnea and cardiac arrhythmias.[34a]

EFFECT OF POSTURE POSTOPERATIVELY ON LUNG DIVISIONS. In normal individuals, changing from the supine to the sitting position will increase the FRC by 0.68 liter, or about 30% (Blair).[34d] On the first day following lower abdominal surgery (or extremity surgery) there is a 10% decrease in FRC; recovery to preoperative values occurs by the third day.[34e] After upper abdominal surgery the decrease in FRC is approximately 25% and recovery is delayed until the fifth day. These decreases are secondary to abdominal distention and pain that is increased by normal to deep inspiration.

After abdominal surgery assumption of the upright position produces a mean increase in FRC of 0.66 liter. This is roughly equated with the application of a 10 cm H_2O PEEP. Increases in FRC are consequent to both an increase in thoracic cage volume and a reduction in thoracic blood volume.[34f] Hence, position change and early ambulation have a physiologic basis for improving pulmonary function.

THE CENTRAL NERVOUS SYSTEM

Perfusion of the brain is a critical issue in positioning patients for a surgical procedure. By selective vasoconstriction or vasodilation, normal cerebral vasculature can, in the absence of anesthesia, autoregulate blood flow between mean arterial pressures (MAP) of roughly 50 and 150 mm Hg.[35] (To safeguard the patient, these MAP ranges should be read as values derived at the level of the circle of Willis.)

ROLE OF AUTOREGULATION

This autoregulatory capability affords the enclosed brain some degree of protection against either the battering effect of elevated systemic pressure or the ischemic results of systemic hypotension. In the presence of intracranial pathology or most anesthetic drugs, autoregulation is compromised or lost, and cerebral blood flow is affected directly by the pressures in the systemic circuit.

FACTORS IN CEREBRAL PERFUSION

A critical concept concerns cerebral perfusion pressure (CPP), the net result of the relationship between mean arterial pressure (the driving force of systemic blood pressure) and the resistance to flow within the bony encasement of the skull (intracranial pressure [ICP], or elevated central venous pressure [CVP]).

CPP = MAP − (the greater of either ICP or CVP)[36]

Raising or lowering MAP and ICP(CVP) simultaneously may have negligible effect on the balance between the driving force and the resistance to flow through the head; thus, global cerebral blood flow will be essentially unchanged. Altering either parameter alone, or each in opposite directions, can significantly change cerebral perfusion. As the values for ICP(CVP) approach MAP, cerebral ischemia results.

EFFECT OF ELEVATING THE HEAD

Elevating the head above the level of the heart, whether the patient is supine, lateral, or prone, establishes an uphill arterial gradient against perfusion, requires cerebral vasodilation to decrease resistance and maintain blood flow if MAP falls, and enhances drainage of venous blood via the jugular system to the superior vena cava and heart. With an arterial transducer placed at the level of the circle of Willis, an MAP in excess of 50 mm Hg ostensibly will maintain some degree of vascular autoregulation in the normal brain. In patients with arteriosclerosis, sclerotic plaques in the cerebral arteries may produce partially obstructed vascular segments that have high-pressure perfusion requirements and cannot tolerate lowered MAP. An orthostatic decrease in CPP may occur in a head-elevated position because of pooling of venous blood in the periphery and viscera with consequent decreases in preload, cardiac output, and MAP.[37] Add to this the effects of intermittently increased intrathoracic pressures needed to ventilate mechanically the patient who is placed in the lateral or prone position with the head elevated and the decrease in venous return from the periphery can become substantial. In the patient with an increased ICP, elevating the head may enhance other measures used to decrease ICP[38] unless orthostatic changes in MAP significantly compromise CPP.

EFFECT OF LOWERING THE HEAD

Placing the patient's head below the level of the heart produces an uphill gradient for venous return that increases ICP and promotes cerebral venous congestion. Increased jugular venous pressure, caused by gravity or reflected from elevated intrathoracic pressure produced by coughing, agitation, manipulation of the airway or mechanical ventilation, is transmitted as increased pressure in the acidotic, vasoparetic, and porous microvasculature that exists in areas containing intracranial pathology. The resulting extravasation of fluid accentuates local edema formation. This sequence is part of the reason that the Trendelenburg position is not useful for vascular resuscitation[14] and should be avoided in the presence of either intracranial pathology or a head injury.[39]

EFFECT OF NECK POSITIONS

Extremes of flexion or rotation of the neck can interfere with cerebral perfusion. Sherman[40] showed that excessive head turning can produce cerebral ischemia by compression of the carotid or vertebral arteries. Nornes and Magnaes[41] noted epidural pressure increases in patients when the neck was flexed; lessening the postural extreme resulted in restoration of cerebral blood flow. In these circumstances, a radial artery catheter connected to a transducer that is placed at level of the circle of Willis may not indicate cerebral MAP accurately, is not a reliable index of cerebral perfusion, and might permit the development of permanent sequelae.

ROLE OF CARBON DIOXIDE IN BRAIN PERFUSION

Cerebral blood flow is well known to be rapidly responsive to alterations of arterial carbon dioxide tensions. Increasing Pa_{CO_2} causes vasodilation; hyperventilative hypocarbia to a Pa_{CO_2} of about 20 mm Hg vasoconstricts normal cerebral vessels. Below a Pa_{CO_2} of about 20 mm Hg, vasoconstrictive hypoperfusion causes tissue ischemia and hypoxic vasodilation begins.[42] Hydrogen ion accumulation also leads to vasodilation. The vessels of the spinal cord behave in a manner similar to the cerebral vasculature regarding autoregulation and responsiveness to blood levels of oxygen, carbon dioxide, and hydrogen ions.[43] Evidence indicates that the blood supply to the spinal cord of certain people can be reduced by extremes of flexion or rotation of the neck, and ischemic changes in the cervical cord have been described.[34]

Changes in neural transmission have been recognized by monitoring somatosensory evoked potentials (SSEP) during positioning of patients.[44,45] Use of SSEP monitoring as a routine protective measure during patient positioning has been advocated, particularly in the presence of posterior fossa mass lesions that distort the brain stem.[45] Suggested causes of the altered neural transmission have included tissue compression, ischemia, and venous obstruction.

MOVING AN ANESTHETIZED PATIENT

Compensatory vascular reflexes are obtunded by general anesthesia, to a variable degree by spinal, epidural, and regional anesthesia, and significantly by acquired conditions such as serious illness, blood loss, spinal injury, starvation, or prolonged inanition.

When body posture is altered in the presence of one of the above, the circulatory system may not be able to adjust to the effects of either gravity or motion, and perfusion of vital organs can be threatened.

DURING GENERAL ANESTHESIA. The greatest challenge to moving an anesthetized patient ocurs during general anesthesia. When positioning is intended early after the induction of anesthesia, the patient should be depressed minimally by drugs, have perfusion stabilized (if possible by means other than vasopressors), be fully relaxed, and have a desensitized airway. Bucking on an endotracheal tube is disruptive to gentle positioning, can injure the airway, and is a frequent cause of reactive hypertension that may be severe.

REPOSITIONING DURING OPERATIONS

If the patient is to be repositioned during the course of a surgical procedure, adequate blood and fluid volume replacement must be assured, the intensity of anesthesia should be minimized as much as is permissible, and both analgesia and relaxation should be provided. The actual move requires slow, gentle manipulation and continuing monitoring of essential physiologic data. Enough personnel must be present to assist with the move so that neither they nor the patient is at risk of physical injury. One person, usually the anesthesiologist, should coordinate the move; however, when a part is at risk (e.g., an unstable neck), prudence requires that the responsible surgeon be actively involved in the process.

TRANSPORTATION TO INTENSIVE CARE UNIT

At the conclusion of the anesthetic, moving the patient to an intensive care unit may require that sedation and relaxation be continued along with artificial ventilation through a well-tolerated endotracheal tube. Vigorous motion of a bed over rough floors, or rapid lateral rotation of the patient as the bed rounds corners, can destabilize a precarious circulatory system. Adequate physiologic monitoring should be present and heeded during the move. Also present must be the necessary therapeutic agents in the event that circulatory distress becomes evident. It is folly to have conducted a meticulous and successful anesthetic procedure under life-threatening circumstances only to reach the critical care unit and find that the act of transportation has produced physiologic chaos.

PREPARATION FOR TRANSPORTATION. When the patient is to be transported to the postanesthesia recovery unit (PARU), the anesthetic should be terminated so that the patient's normal protective reflexes are as brisk as possible. The degree of monitoring needed during transport will vary with the condition of the patient and the distance to be travelled.

MOVING THE PATIENT UNDER REGIONAL ANESTHESIA. The stresses imposed by moving a patient during peridural, spinal, or regional anesthesia are usually less than during general anesthesia. Exceptions include postural changes that unmask an occult volume deficit that exceeds vascular compensation or changes that cause the level of spinal anesthesia to migrate cephalad.

ADDITIONAL READINGS

Coonan, T.J., and Hope, C.E.: Cardiorespiratory effects of change of body position. Can. Anaesth. Soc. J., 30:424, 1983.

Froese, A.B., and Bryan, A.C.: Effects of anesthesia and paralysis on diaphragmatic mechanics in man. Anesthesiology, 41:242, 1974.

Giffin, J.P.: Anesthesia for acute and chronic spinal cord injuries. In Refresher Courses in Anesthesiology, Vol. 13. Edited by P.G. Barash. Philadelphia, J.B. Lippincott, 1985.

Kaneko, K., et al.: Regional distribution of ventilation and perfusion as a function of body position. J. Appl. Physiol., 21:767, 1966.

Martin, J.T. (ed): Positioning in Anesthesia and Surgery, 2nd Ed. Philadelphia, W.B. Saunders, 1987.

Nunn, J.F.: Applied Respiratory Physiology, 2nd Ed., London, Butterworths, 1977.

Shapiro, H.: Anesthesia effects upon cerebral blood flow, cerebral metabolism, electroencephalogram and evoked potentials. In Anesthesia, 2nd Ed. Edited by R.D. Miller. New York, Churchill Livingstone, 1986.

Sibbald, W.J., et al.: The Trendelenburg position: Hemodynamic effects in hypotensive and normotensive patients. Crit. Care Med., 7:218, 1979.

West, J.B.: Ventilation, Blood Flow and Gas Exchange. Blackwell Scientific Publications, 1965.

REFERENCES

1. Dorland's Illustrated Medical Dictionary, 24th Ed. Philadelphia, W.B. Saunders, 1965.
2. Martin, J.T.: The lawn chair (contoured supine) position. In Positioning in Anesthesia and Surgery, 2nd Ed. Edited by J.T. Martin. Philadelphia, W.B. Saunders, 1987.
3. Coonan, T.J., and Hope, C.E.: Cardiorespiratory effects of change of body position. Can. Anaesth. Soc. J., 30:424, 1983.
4. Enderby, G.E.H.: Postural ischemia and blood pressure. Lancet, 1:185, 1954.
5. Wagner, E.: Fortgesetze Untersuchungen uber den Einfluss der Schwere auf den Kreislauf. Arch. Ges. Physiol., 39:371, 1886.
6. West, J.B., Dollery, C.T., and Naimark, A.: Distribution of blood flow in isolated lung: Relationship to vascular and alveolar pressures. J. Appl. Physiol., 19:713, 1964.
6a. West, J.B.: Ventilation, Blood Flow and Gas Exchange. Blackwell Scientific Publications, 1965.
7. Little, D.M.: Posture and anaesthesia. Can. Anaesth. Soc. J., 7:2, 1960.
8. Kaneko, K., et al.: Regional distribution of ventilation and perfusion as a function of body position. J. Appl. Physiol., 21:767, 1966.
9. Kubal, K., et al.: Trendelenburg position used during venous cannulation increases myocardial oxygen demands. Anes. Analg., 63:239, 1984.
10. Weil, M.H.: Current concepts on the management of shock. Circulation, 16:1097, 1957.
11. Weil, M.H., and Wigham, H.: Head-down (Trendelenburg) position for treatment of irreversible hemorrhagic shock. Ann. Surg., 162:905, 1965.
12. Guntheroth, W.G., Abel, F.L., and Mullins, G.L.: The effect of Trendelenburg's position on blood pressure and carotid flow. Surg. Gynecol. Obstet., 119:345, 1964.
13. Taylor, J., and Weil, M.H.: Failure of the Trendelenburg position to improve circulation during clinical shock. Surg. Gynecol. Obstet., 124:1005, 1967.
14. Sibbald, W.J., et al.: The Trendelenburg position: Hemodynamic effects in hypotensive and normotensive patients. Crit. Care Med., 7:218, 1979.
15. Dripps, R.D., and Comroe, J.H. Jr.: Circulatory physiology: The adjustment to blood loss and postural changes. Surg. Clin. North Am., p. 1368, Dec. 1946.
16. Railings, G.H., et al.: Studies on the control of plasma aldosterone concentration in normal man: Response to posture, acute and chronic volume depletion and sodium loading. J. Clin. Invest., 51:1731, 1972.
17. Sonkodi, S., et al.: Response of the renin-angiotensin-aldosterone system to upright tilting and to intravenous furosemide: Effect of prior metoprolol and propranolol. Br. J. Clin. Pharmacol., 13:341, 1982.
18. Gauer, O.H., and Thron, H.L.: Postural changes in the circulation. In Handbook of Physiology. Sect. 2, voila, Edited by W.F. Hamilton, and P. Dow. Washington, D.C., American Physiological Society, 1965.
19. Fourneir, P., et al.: Effect of sitting up on pulmonary blood pressure, flow, and volume in man. J. Appl. Physiol., 46:36, 1979.
20. Bevegard, S., Holmgren, A., and Johnson, B.: The effect of body position on the circulation at rest and during exercise, with special reference to the influence on stroke volume. Acta Physiol. Scand., 49:279, 1960.
21. Green, D.M., and Metheny, D.: Estimation of acute blood loss by tilt test. Surg. Gynecol. Obstet. 84:1045, 1947.
22. Martin, J.T.: The prone position: Anesthesiologic considerations. In Positioning in Anesthesia and Surgery, 2nd Ed. Edited by J.T. Martin. Philadelphia, W.B. Saunders, 1987.
23. Toole, J.F.: Effects of change of head, limb and body position on cephalic circulation, New Engl. J. Med., 279:307, 1968.
24. Backofen, J.E., and Schauble, J.F.: Hemodynamic changes with prone positioning during general anesthesia (abstract). Anes. Analg., 64:194, 1985.
25. Dripps, R.D., and Comroe, J.H.: Clinical studies on morphine. II. The effect of morphine upon the circulation of man and upon the circulatory and respiratory responses of tilting. Anesthesiology, 7:44, 1946.
25a. Smith, J.J., et al.: Application of impedance cardiography to study of postural stress. J. Appl. Physiol., 29:133, 1970.
25b. Ueland, K., et al.: Maternal cardiovascular dynamics: IV. The influence of gestational age on the maternal cardiovascular response to posture and exercise. Am. J. Obstet. Gynecol., 104:856, 1969.
25c. Marshall, W.K., Bedford, R.F., and Miller, E.D.: Cardiovascular responses in the seated position—Impact of four anesthetic techniques. Anesth. Analg., 61:648, 1983.
25d. Oparil, Z., et al.: Role of renin in acute postural homeostasis. Circulation, 41:89, 1970.
25e. Wong, K.C., et al.: The cardiovascular effects of morphine sulfate with oxygen and with nitrous oxide in man. Anesthesiology, 38:542, 1973.
26. Smith, B.L.: Physiologic changes in the normal conscious human subject on changing from the erect to the supine position. In Positioning in Anesthesia and Surgery, 2nd Ed. Edited by J.T. Martin. Philadelphia, W.B. Saunders, 1987.
26a. Froese, A.B., and Bryan, A.C.: Effects of anesthesia and paralysis on diaphragmatic mechanics in man. Anesthesiology, 41:242, 1974.
27. Nunn, J.F.: Applied Respiratory Physiology, 2nd Ed. London, Butterworths, 1977.
28. Hedenstierna, G., et al.: Functional residual capacity, thoraco-abdominal dimensions and central blood volume during general anesthesia with muscle paralysis and mechanical ventilation. Anesthesiology, 62:247, 1985.
29. Rehder, K., Cameron, P.D., and Krayer, S.: New dimensions of the respiratory system. Anesthesiology, 62:230, 1985.
30. LeBlanc, P., Ruff, F., and Milic-Emily, J.: Effects of age and body position on "airway closure" in man. J. Appl. Physiol., 28:448, 1970.
31. Don, H.F., Wahba, W.M., and Craig, D.B.: Airway closure, gas trapping and the functional residual capacity during anesthesia. Anesthesiology, 36:533, 1972.
32. Craig, D.B., Wahba, W.M., and Don, H.F.: Airway closure and lung volumes in surgical positions. Can. Anaesth. Soc. J., 18:92, 1971.
33. Rehder, K., and Sessler, A.D.: Function of each lung in spontaneously breathing man anesthetised with thiopental–meperidine. Anesthesiology, 38:320, 1973.
34. Rehder, K., Wenthe, F.M., and Sessler, A.D.: Function of each lung during mechanical ventilation with ZEEP and with PEEP in man anesthetised with thiopental–meperidine. Anesthesiology, 38:597, 1973.
34a. Fishman, A.P.: Down with the good lung (editorial). New Engl. J. Med., 204:537, 1981.

34b. Zack, M.B., Pontoppidan, H., and Kazemi, H.: The effect of lateral positions on gas exchange in pulmonary disease: A prospective evaluation. Am. Rev. Dis., *110:*49, 1974.

34c. Remolina, C., et al.: Positional hypoxemia in unilateral lung disease. New Engl. J. Med., *304:*523, 1982.

34d. Blair, E., and Hickam, J.B.: The effect of change in body position on lung volume and intrapulmonary gas mixing in normal subjects. J. Clin. Invest., *34:*383, 1955.

34e. Hsu, H.O., and Hickey, R.F.: Effect of posture on functional residual capacity postoperatively. Anesthesiology, *44:*520, 1976.

34f. Sjostrand, T.: Determination of changes in the intrathoracic blood volume in man. Acta Physiol. Scand., *22:*116, 1951.

35. Lassen, N.A.: Cerebral blood flow and oxygen consumption in man. Physiol. Rev., *39:*183, 1959.

36. Gravenstein, N., Grundy, B.L., and Reid, S.A.: Complications of positioning: The central nervous system. *In* Positioning in Anesthesia and Surgery, 2nd Ed. Edited by J.T. Martin. Philadelphia, W.B. Saunders, 1987.

37. Tindall, G.T., Craddock, A., and Greenfield, J.C.: Effects of the sitting position on blood flow in the internal carotid artery of man during general anesthesia. J. Neurosurg., *26:*383, 1967.

38. Kenning, J.A., Touting, S.M., and Saunders, R.L.: Upright patient positioning in the management of intracranial hypertension. Surg. Neurol., *15:*148, 1981.

39. Prentice, J.A., and Martin, J.T.: The Trendelenburg position: Anesthesiologic considerations. *In* Positioning in Anesthesia and Surgery, 2nd Ed. Edited by J.T. Martin. Philadelphia, W.B. Saunders, 1987.

40. Sherman, D.D., Hart, R.G., and Easton, J.D.: Abrupt changes in head position and cerebral infarction. Stroke, *12:*2, 1981.

41. Nornes, H., and Magnaes, B.: Supratentorial epidural pressure during posterior fossa surgery. J. Neurosurg., *35:*541, 1971.

42. Shapiro, H.: Anesthesia effects upon cerebral blood flow, cerebral metabolism, electroencephalogram and evoked potentials. *In* Anesthesia, 2nd Ed. Edited by R.D. Miller. New York, Churchill Livingstone, 1986.

43. Giffin, J.P.: Anesthesia for acute and chronic spinal cord injuries. *In* Refresher Courses in Anesthesiology, Vol. 13. Edited by P.G. Barash. Philadelphia, J.B. Lippincott, 1985.

44. Grundy, B.L., et al.: Evoked potential changes produced by positioning for retromastoid craniectomy. Neurosurgery, *10:*766, 1982.

45. McPherson, R.E., Szymanski, J., and Rogers, M.C.: Somatosensory evoked potential changes in position-related brain stem ischemia. Anesthesiology, *61:*88, 1984.

John T. Martin
Vincent J. Collins

TECHNICAL ASPECTS OF PATIENT POSITIONING

Positioning a patient for an operation is a persistent contest of varying degree between what the surgeon properly requires for access to the surgical pathology and what the patient can tolerate in the presence of the physiologic impairments produced by disease, injury, or the effects of anesthesia.

Many of the positions that must be inflicted on an anesthetized patient to permit an adequate surgical effort could not be tolerated awake. Each must be established gently, must include careful efforts to protect the patient, must be monitored attentively for signs of untoward physiologic responses that might be posture-related, and must be modified when patient intolerance is identified.

Collins[1] advised that proper positioning of a surgical patient on an operating table should offer minimal interference with ventilation; minimal interference with circulation; adequate padding to pressure areas to prevent nerve injury and provide good support; and comfort for the patient during regional anesthesia.

The techniques of positioning presented in this chapter are reliable for the neophyte and familiar to most experienced practitioners. Many acceptable alternatives exist; therefore, none of these comments can be construed as being an attempt to set standards or to restrict individual choices for physician or patient. Space limitations confine this presentation to essential important considerations. Readers interested in more details of patient positioning are referred to a dedicated text on the subject.[2]

THE OPERATING TABLE AND ITS ACCESSORIES

STANDARD TABLES

Most modern surgical tables rest on a wheeled base that can raise or lower the patient surface. Mechanical or hydraulic hoists and hinges interrelate the section of the table surface on which the torso of a supine patient rests with others that support the head, thighs, and legs.

Some tables have electric motors that give maximum mechanical advantage to adjusting the loads on their patient surfaces. When electrical controls are present, it is mandatory to have back-up mechanical controls with which to perform the same functions when the electrical systems fail. Many tables have surface tunnel attachments that are permeable to roentgen rays and permit intraoperative films to be taken. A recent innovation has been the ability to move the table surface horizontally with reference to its base, thereby permitting wider access of the portable radiologic image intensifier to the extremities or head of the patient.

While several makes and models of surgical tables are available, the most widely used, and most nearly "standard," is probably one of the AMSCO 2000 series made by the American Sterilizer Company of Erie, Pennsylvania. For the sake of convenience and clarity, all references to table controls made in this chapter will apply to the AMSCO table unless otherwise specified.

SPECIALIZED TABLES

Certain specialized surgical procedures and patient postures have required the development of surgical tables that have unique capabilities. Traction tables used to immobilize and align fractured extremities of traumatized patients, urologic and obstetric tables that permit procedures on the perineum, pediatric-sized tables, and the water-bath used in lithotripsy are examples. A series of detachable tops that serve specific patient postures has been a feature of one model.

Specialized tables that are used frequently are advantageous because their individual peculiarities are familiar and well understood. When they are used rarely, or are used by personnel who are new at the task, they need careful management to prevent misapplication and patient injury. These units require bulk floor space for storage as well as periodic inspection to assure the presence and proper function of their parts.

ARM SUPPORTS

Safe positioning of patients' arms is an issue that merits particular attention in order to avoid iatrogenic injury. The usual supportive device is an arm board that clamps to the side rail of the surgical table and allows adjustment cephalad or caudad as well as rotation about its point of attachment (Fig. 7–1A and B). A restless surgical assistant, searching for a comfortable stance during a long procedure, can inadvertently force the board cephalad enough, or rotate it enough, to hyperabduct the arm and stress the axillary neurovascular bundle of a supine patient (Fig. 7–1C). Unpadded elbows may allow compression of the ulnar nerve. An arm board that detaches unexpectedly can dislocate a shoulder or fracture an osteoporotic proximal humerus. The board should be well padded, attach easily to the table rail,

FIG. 7–1. Standard arm boards. *A* and *B*. Abduction of the supine arm up to 90 degrees will rarely stretch the axillary neurovascular bundle damagingly across the head of the humerus. *C*. Dangerous hyperabduction of the arm, threatening the axillary neurovascular bundle. *D*. Double-tiered arm board for the lateral position. Upper frame is covered with disposable stockingette. Its proximal end should be well padded if in contact with the thoracic wall (see also Fig. 7–15).

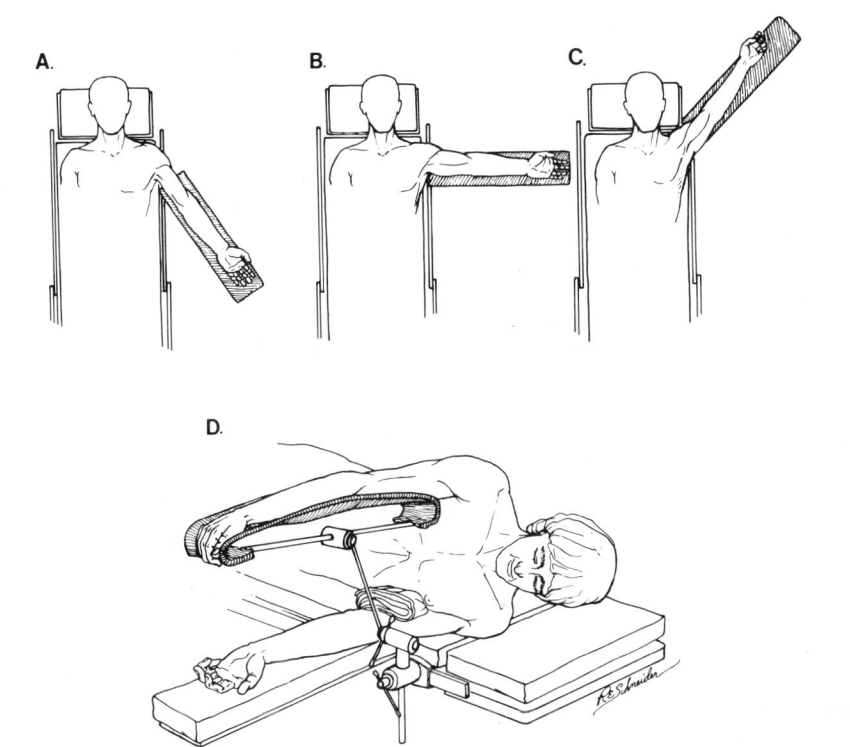

lock securely in place, and be adjustable only by deliberate intention.

Several versions of two-tiered arm boards[3] allow stable positioning of both upper extremities when the patient is in the lateral decubitus position (Fig. 7–1C). Padding should be arranged to prevent compression of the patient's chest wall by the axillary end of the upper board and to avoid inadvertent contact between metal and skin that could ground the patient and produce an electrical burn.

When an arm is supported above the patient's head on an "ether screen" (Fig. 7–2), the metal frame must be well padded, wrappings that restrain the arm should permit acceptable blood flow in the forearm and hand, and axillary structures should be relaxed. Careful torso support is needed so that neither the forces of gravity nor the pull of tissue retractors can reposition the patient sufficiently to stretch the restrained arm and cause the head of the humerus to injure the axillary neurovascular bundle.

TRUNK FRAMES

Several varieties of trunk supports ("ventral frames") are used to elevate a prone patient off of the ventral abdominal wall, remove compression from paraspinous vasculature, and separate spinous processes. When the vertebral column is fractured and unstable, ventral supports should be longitudinal to prevent a scissoring injury to the contents of the spinal canal; with an intact spine, a pedestal under each subclavicular hemithorax and each iliac crest can be effective.

The simplest trunk frame is a pair of identical cylinders, each made of a variable number of smooth folded sheets rolled tightly together (Fig. 7–3). Each roll must be even in diameter, free of wrinkles, relatively uncompressible, and long enough to reach from clavicle to groin of the patient in question. They are placed longitudinally in parallel on the table mattress, and each is tied to the contralateral rail. Although the rolls must be individually constructed for each patient, their major advantages are tailor-made thickness, minimal expense, and disposability.

Reusable soft ventral pads have been available from several manufacturers (Fig. 7–4). Although comfortable and easy to use, these devices tend to lose their already-limited thickness as they age. They must be cleaned carefully between uses.

Adjustable parallel metal frames with heavy padding are used effectively in many institutions (Fig. 7–5). As the patient's trunk is arched over the frame, the abdomen is suspended above the table surface and the head is below the level of the heart. A crank alters the contour of the frame to adjust the arch of the back according to the surgeon's need to enlarge the spaces between spinous processes.

Four pillars can be made of sandbags to elevate the trunk off of the table surface if the spine is intact. A similar reusable device is available as a Relton Frame (Fig. 7–6).

Kneeling frames attach to the depressed foot section of the operating table and allow the patient's knees to rest on a padded and adjustable ledge while the chest is supported by the major section of the table surface. The abdomen hangs free (Fig. 7–7).

HEAD HOLDERS

Stabilizing the head of a positioned patient can be a precarious maneuver unless suitable equipment is available.

1. *Padded face pieces* attach to the table by various frames and are useful unless they allow the head to be repositioned accidentally and the neck or eyes to be injured.
2. *Plastic foam rings*, or C-shaped cutouts (see Fig. 7–3A), can support the down-side cheek and pro-

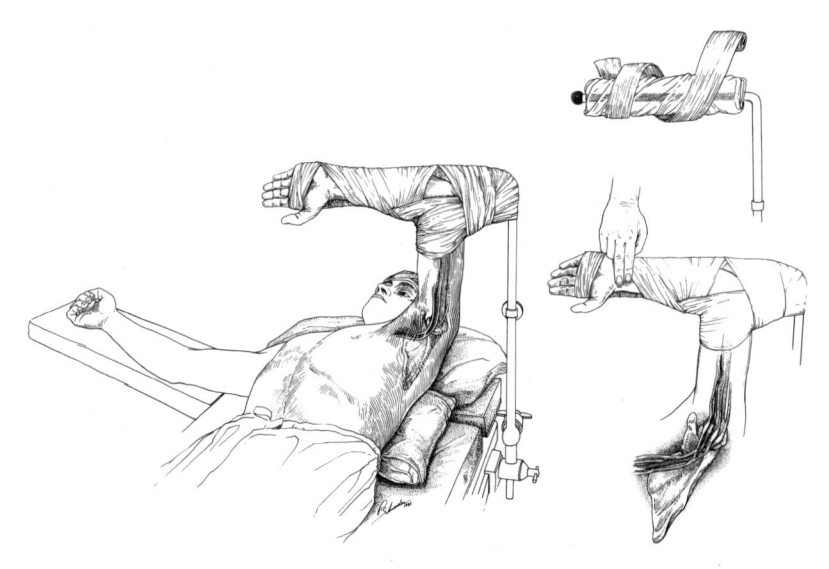

FIG. 7–2. Arm restrained on a well-padded (*upper insert*) adjustable overhead bar in the semisupine position, permitting a high anterolateral thoracic incision. Pads under the dorsal thorax keep torso from hanging from elevated arm and stretching axillary neurovascular bundle. Axillary contents (*lower insert*) not under tension from head of humerus and radial pulse not compromised.

FIG. 7–3. Plastic foam face rest (*A*) and ventral parallel supports for the prone position made of rolled sheeting and disposable plastic foam padding (*B*). Each roll can be sheathed in stockingette to avoid patient contact with plastic. Rolls are tiered to contralateral table rail. From Martin, J.T. (ed): Positioning in Anesthesia and Surgery. 2nd ed. Philadelphia, WB Saunders, 1987.

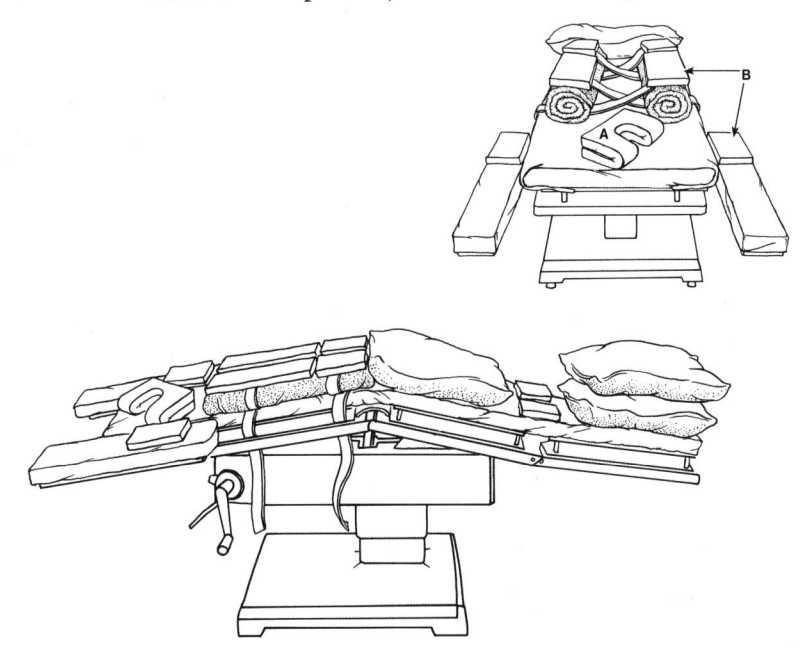

tect the eye and ear of a pronated patient whose head is turned.

3. A *rocker-based head holder* has been designed to allow the pronated face to be supported in the sagittal plane and avoid rotation of the neck.
4. An established method of firmly stabilizing the head is to use one of the several *three-pin head holders* that penetrate the outer table of the skull and attach to the operating table by a metal frame.

MOVING AND REPOSITIONING AN ANESTHETIZED PATIENT

Draw sheets, rollers, sliding boards, collapsible plastic tubes (large garbage bags), and sling hoists have all been used as assist devices to help move a patient between the bed or transport cart and the operating table. Physiologic consequences of moving an anesthetized patient are discussed in Chapter 6. The major mechanical risks involve injuries to members of the positioning team and trauma to the patient. Specifics are discussed in the chapter on Complications of Positioning.

ESTABLISHING SPECIFIC POSITIONS

THE TRADITIONAL SUPINE POSITION

The traditional supine position is the horizontal dorsal decubitus posture. The patient lies on his

FIG. 7–4. Soft reusable pads to support a patient in the prone position. *A.* Cloward surgical saddle. *B.* Bardeen pad. From Martin, J.T. (ed): Positioning in Anesthesia and Surgery, 2nd ed. Philadelphia, WB Saunders, 1987.

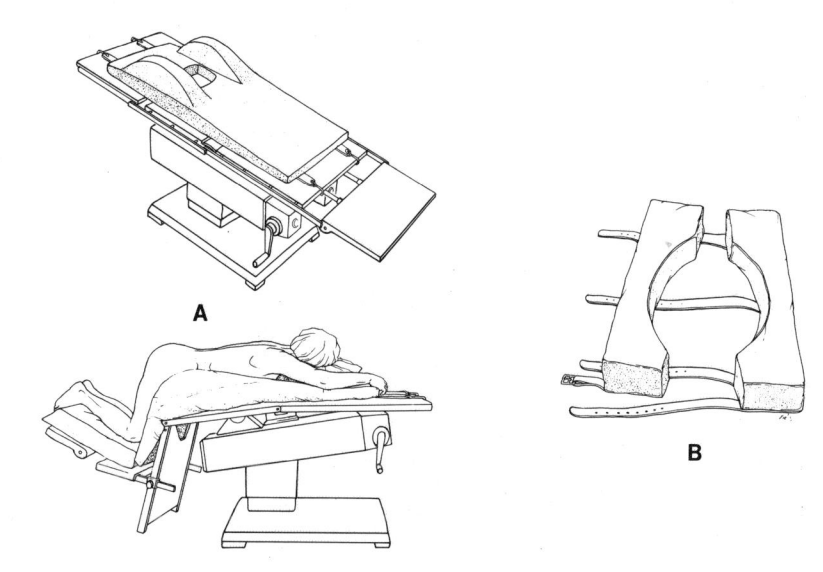

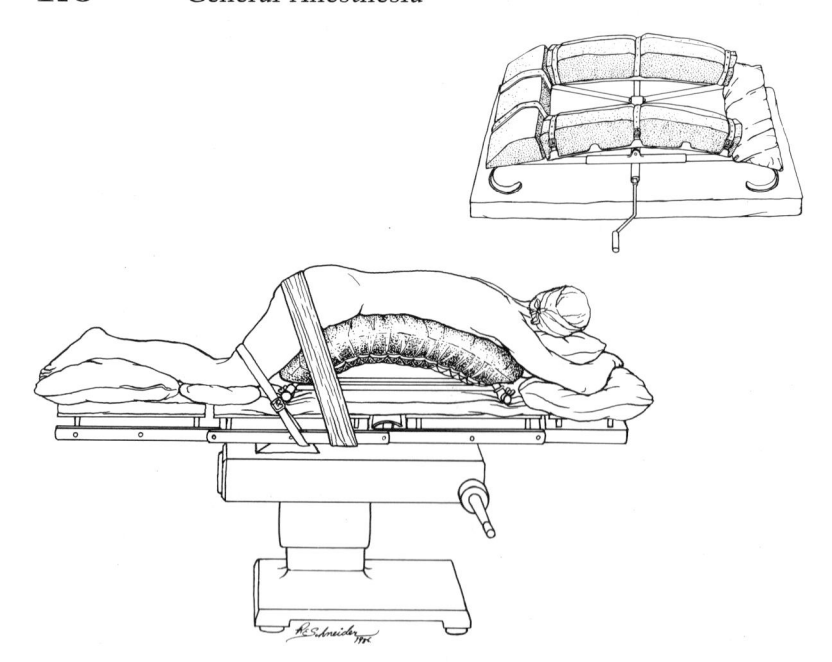

FIG. 7–5. Parallel metal frames for support in the prone position. From Martin, J.T. (ed): Positioning in Anesthesia and Surgery, 2nd ed. Philadelphia, WB Saunders, 1987.

than 90 degrees on armboards. A small pillow beneath the occiput eases stress on the neck and lumbar spine. Elbows and heels need to be padded for comfort. The posture is traditional, but for many patients it places joints in an uncomfortable, nonneutral position.

THE CONTOURED SUPINE POSITION

By slightly flexing the thighs on the trunk and the lower legs on the thighs (Fig. 7–8B), the lumbar spine can be relaxed and the supine lower extremities placed in a more comfortable position. This is accomplished either by placing pillows under the knees and legs or by manipulating the table-top positioning gears.

To contour the top of an American Sterilizer operating table, set the selector lever on "flex" and rotate the action handle three full turns so that the back and thigh sections each angle slightly upward and their mutual hinge. Then set the selector lever on "foot" and rotate the action handle three full turns in the reverse directions to gently depress the foot section.

The resulting contoured dorsal decubitus posture was called the *reflex abdominal position* by Miller many years ago,[1] and more recently has been termed the *lawn chair position*.[4,5] It places joints in a more neutral and comfortable arrangement than is the case with the traditional horizontal supine position, and it relaxes the abdomen somewhat by decreasing the distance between the xyphoid process and the symphysis pubis. It also serves to optimize perfusion and blood return from the lower extremities and head. Because it minimally congests the pulmonary apices, it is apt to be more effective in treating hypotension than is the Trendelenburg position.

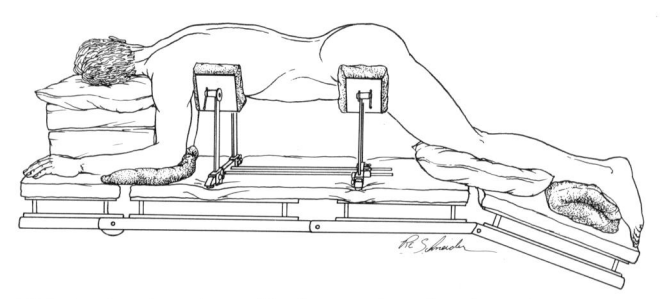

FIG. 7–6. The adjustable four-pedestal Relton frame. From Martin, J.T. (ed): Positioning in Anesthesia and Surgery, 2nd ed. Philadelphia, WB Saunders, 1987.

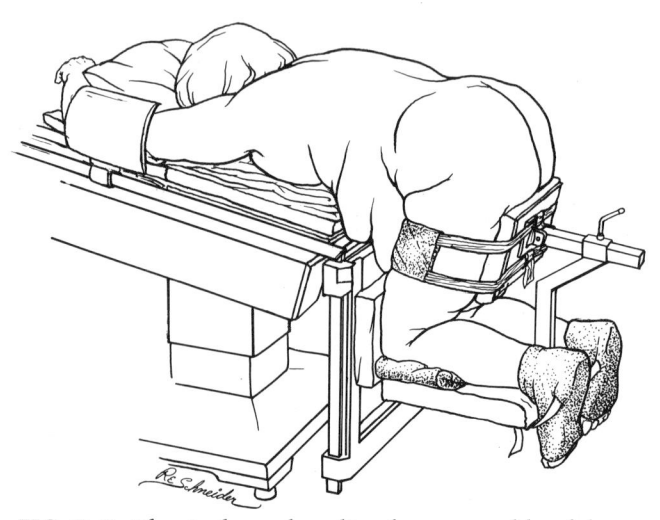

FIG. 7–7. The Andrews kneeling frame, capable of decompressing an obese abdomen. From Martin, J.T. (ed): Positioning in Anesthesia and Surgery, 2nd ed. Philadelphia, WB Saunders, 1987.

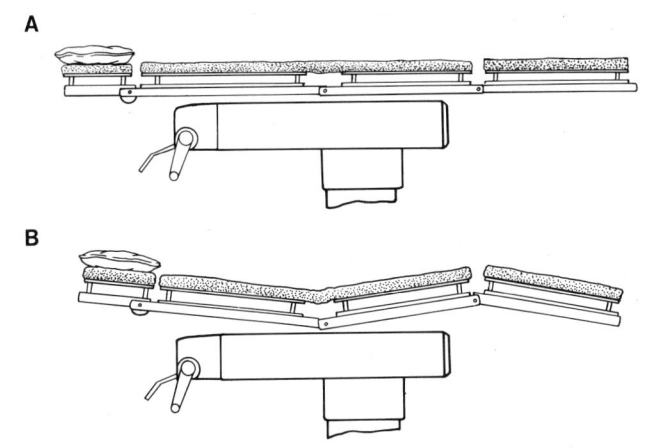

FIG. 7–8. The operating table arranged for a patient who is to be in the supine position. *A.* The horizontal (flat) supine position. *B.* The contoured supine position with the table angulated slightly at the thigh-back hinge and the leg section depressed. Redrawn from Martin, J.T. (ed): Positioning in Anesthesia and Surgery, 2nd ed. Philadelphia, WB Saunders, 1987.

THE LITHOTOMY POSITION

The lithotomy position (Fig. 7–9) is a dorsal decubitus posture in which the lower extremities are flexed at thigh and knee and held in place by vertical supports and ankle slings, by knee holders, or by leg crutches. The degree of leg elevation is minimal in urologic (cystoscopic) procedures and somewhat greater in gynecologic (uterine dilatation and curettage) or obstetric (delivery) usage. Some surgeons prefer to stand during a perineal procedure and often use a "high" lithotomy position in which the boot-clad feet of the patient are attached to a vertical pole that is elevated enough to have the lower leg almost fully extended upon the knee. When intra-abdominal and perineal procedures are accomplished simultaneously, the degree to which the legs are elevated and separated varies according to the build of the patient and the needs of the surgical team.

When establishing the lithotomy position, both lower extremities should be elevated together to avoid severe torsion stress on the pelvis and lumbar spine. When being lowered, the legs should be brought together in the midline and lowered slowly together in order to combat sudden increases in vascular capacitance that might disrupt preload and threaten systemic perfusion.

If low back pain exists preoperatively, the suitability of the lithotomy position can be tested before the induction of anesthesia by establishing it cautiously while the patient is still awake and able to indicate accentuated or new discomfort. A small support under the lumbar spine can maintain normal lordosis after the onset of anesthesia and minimize intensification of pain due to lumbar relaxation (a possibility with either general or spinal anesthesia).

In certain orthopedic procedures a restraining pole is placed against the perineum, the afflicted lower extremity is stretched in traction, and the nonsurgical lower extremity is placed in high lithotomy to permit access to the operative site for the roentgenologic camera on the C-shaped arm of the image intensifier.

When surgical access to the prostate must be gained via the perineum, the patient is placed in an exaggerated lithotomy position (Fig. 7–10) with the thighs flexed almost forcibly on the trunk at the hip, the knees flexed, and the lower legs high in the air. In an obese patient, thighs that compress the

FIG. 7–9. The standard lithotomy position. From Martin, J.T. (ed): Positioning in Anesthesia and Surgery, 2nd ed. Philadelphia, WB Saunders, 1987.

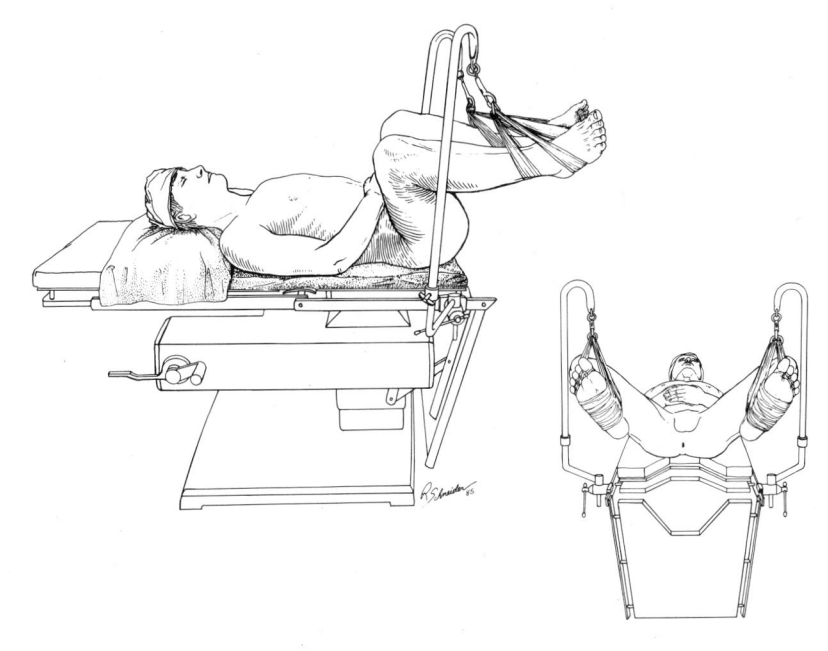

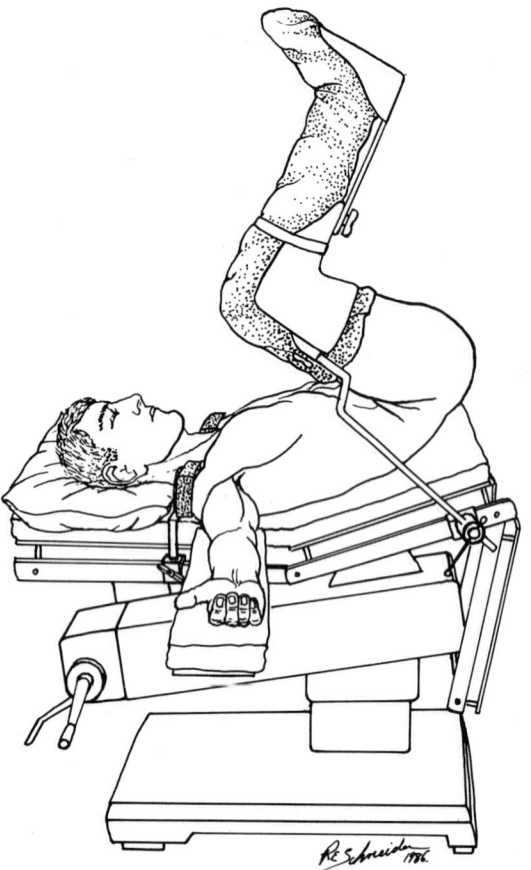

FIG. 7–10. Young's exaggerated lithotomy position, designed to provide maximum access to the perineum for prostatic surgery. From Martin, J.T. (ed): Positioning in Anesthesia and Surgery, 2nd ed. Philadelphia, WB Saunders, 1987.

back on a flat surface (Fig. 7–8A) with his arms either restrained alongside the torso or abducted less abdomen can impede ventilation by restricting the descent of the diaphragm. If blood pressure decreases, perfusion of the markedly elevated lower extremities may fall to ischemic levels.

Head-down tilt can be added to the exaggerated lithotomy position to improve perineal access to the retropubic space; in this instance the worst features of each position are combined, and carefully placed shoulder braces may be needed to stabilize the patient on the table.

THE TRENDELENBURG POSITION

Steep head-down tilt was apparently pioneered by Bardenhauer, a surgeon in Cologne, and popularized prior to 1870 by Friederich Trendelenburg, of Leipzig, as a means of improving transabdominal access to structures in the deep pelvis.[6] However, an 1885 description by Meyer, a New Yorker who had been his pupil, gave Trendelenburg credit for its origin.[7] For many years patients were placed in essentially 45 degrees of head-down tilt for best visceral exposure.

Walter Cannon, an eminent physiologist, advocated the head-down tilt during World War I as a means of improving venous return from the lower extremities in the management of shock. He also believed that the position improved cerebral perfusion.[8]

For almost 50 years, use of the Trendelenburg position to treat shock and expose viscera continued as an undisputed ritual until incriminating evidence accumulated to indicate that the head-down tilt altered blood pressure measurement in humans,[9] was lethal to bled laboratory animals,[10] and actually decreased cardiac output when applied to hypotensive, septic patients in a major intensive care unit.[11]

Subsequently, the degree of head-down tilt used during most surgical procedures has lessened and "shock blocks" have effectively disappeared from enlightened nursing units.

When the original steep Trendelenburg position is intended (Fig. 7–11, 30–45 degrees head-down tilt), the patient should be placed on the operating table so that the popliteal fossa is caudad of the hinge between the thigh and leg sections of the table top and the legs of the patient can be safely flexed at the knees. Using ankle straps to retain the feet and legs on the depressed foot section of the table, this placement of the popliteal fossa prevents the end of the thigh section of the table top from compressing the calf just below the knee and obstructing distal vessels. The arrangement also eliminates potential injury to the brachial plexus and vessels from shoulder braces that compress the root of the neck (or force the clavicle against the first rib) or from retaining wristlets that stretch the arm.

The slight amount of head-down tilt now employed during most procedures in the lower abdomen is referred to by some as a *scul60tus position*,[1,12] indicating that the head is lowered only between 10 and 15 degrees (Fig. 7–11, insert). It rarely requires leg or shoulder restraints; however, when some degree of the Trendelenburg position is added to the exaggerated lithotomy position, shifting of the patient is a potential problem and shoulder braces are helpful (see Fig. 7–10). If each brace is placed over the acromioclavicular joint rather than more medially at the root of the neck, they are rarely injurious to the brachial plexus or to the vasculature of the thoracic outlet.

As stated by Prentice,[13] and as was mentioned in the preceding chapter on the physiology of positioning, the Trendelenburg position is strongly contraindicated in patients with intracranial pathology, is not a useful adjunct to the treatment of shock, and should be used sparingly as a routine. If the tissue exposure produced by the position significantly shortens the duration of surgery and anesthesia, however, its use may be justified and the technical arrangements necessary to protect the patient should be assured.

FIG. 7–11. Trendelenburg's position, utilizing 30–45 degrees of head-down tilt and needing restraints on the angulated legs to prevent cephalad slippage, compared to the more usual scultetus position (*insert*), utilizing only 10–15 degrees of tilt and requiring minimal or no restraining devices. From Martin, J.T. (ed): Positioning in Anesthesia and Surgery, 2nd ed. Philadelphia, WB Saunders, 1987.

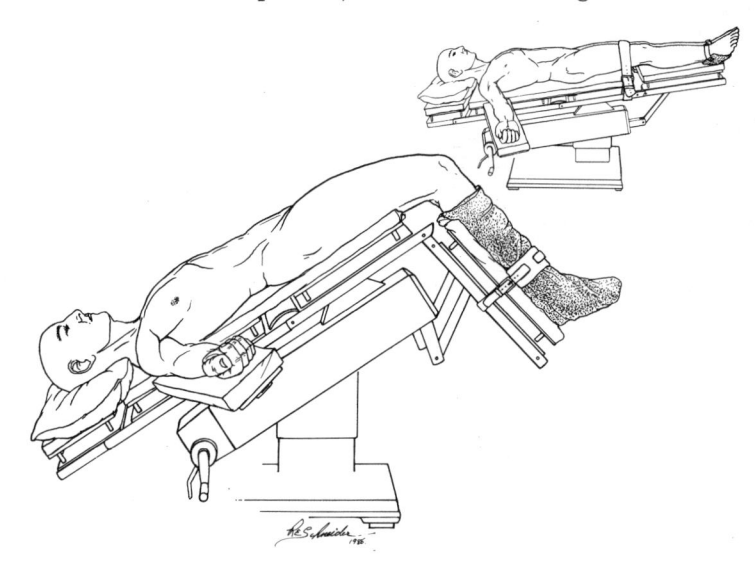

THE HEAD-ELEVATED POSITIONS

The head-elevated positions include the full sitting position, the "classic" sitting position, and head-elevated versions of the supine, lateral, and prone positions.[14]

The full sitting position, with the spine vertical and legs dependent, is a rarity in modern surgical and dental practice. As diagnostic pneumoencephalography has given way to sophisticated radiologic scanning devices, the full sitting position has become a curiosity even in neurosurgery.

The Full Sitting Position

This position is established by carefully placing the anesthetized patient in a chair-like arrangement that supports the head and neck, allows the arms to be retained on arm rests or in the patient's lap, maintains the spine vertical, supports the buttocks and thighs on a padded seat, and allows the legs to hang vertically from the knees. Some type of restraint that does not interfere with effective ventilation must be used to prevent the torso from slumping, and the extremities must be carefully restrained if postural change is contemplated. If a face rest is used to support the head, compression of the eyes must be avoided, and the head cannot be allowed to threaten the eyes as posture is changed.

For years such an arrangement was useful for introducing air into the lumbar subarachnoid space and allowing it to bubble cephalad into the cerebral ventricles for roentgenologic contrast studies. Several strong assistants were needed to manipulate the patient through the various positions required to help the contrast gas move around the components of the ventricular system during the filming process. More recently the development of multipositional chairs and wheels (e.g., the Garcia-Oller axioencephalographic wheel) that could rotate about vertical and horizontal axes made the procedure technically less complicated and safer for the patient.[15]

Classic Semi-Recumbent Dorsal Decubitus Position (Current "Sitting Position")

The term *sitting position* as it is now used describes a classic semirecumbent dorsal decubitus arrangement of a patient whose head and shoulders are elevated to about 60 degrees above the horizontal, whose legs are raised to the level of the atria, whose arms are folded across the lap, and whose neck may be gently flexed to render the cervical spine almost vertical. Often the head is rotated to facilitate exposure of structures in the cerebellopontine angle. It is a posture of controversy in neurosurgery and one that requires precise attention to the details of its establishment and management.[14]

The patient is placed supine with the cephalad edge of the back section of the operating table at the level of the first thoracic vertebra. (Fig. 7–12*A*). If the patient is thin or short of stature, one or more pillows can be placed beneath the buttocks to protect against pressure lesions and to elevate the shoulders toward the cephalad edge of the back section. Usually another pillow cushions the thighs.

Anesthesia and monitoring are established in the desired manner. While rapidly repeated measurements of systolic or mean arterial blood pressure are alertly observed to detect promptly the onset of postural hypotension, the thigh section of the table is flexed on the back section, the back and head sections are slowly elevated, and the foot section is depressed. The cephalad end of the table chassis is angulated downward so as to render the foot section parallel to the floor at the level of the patient's heart (Fig. 7–12*B* and *C*). In this intermediate position, the patient is semisitting with hips and knees flexed

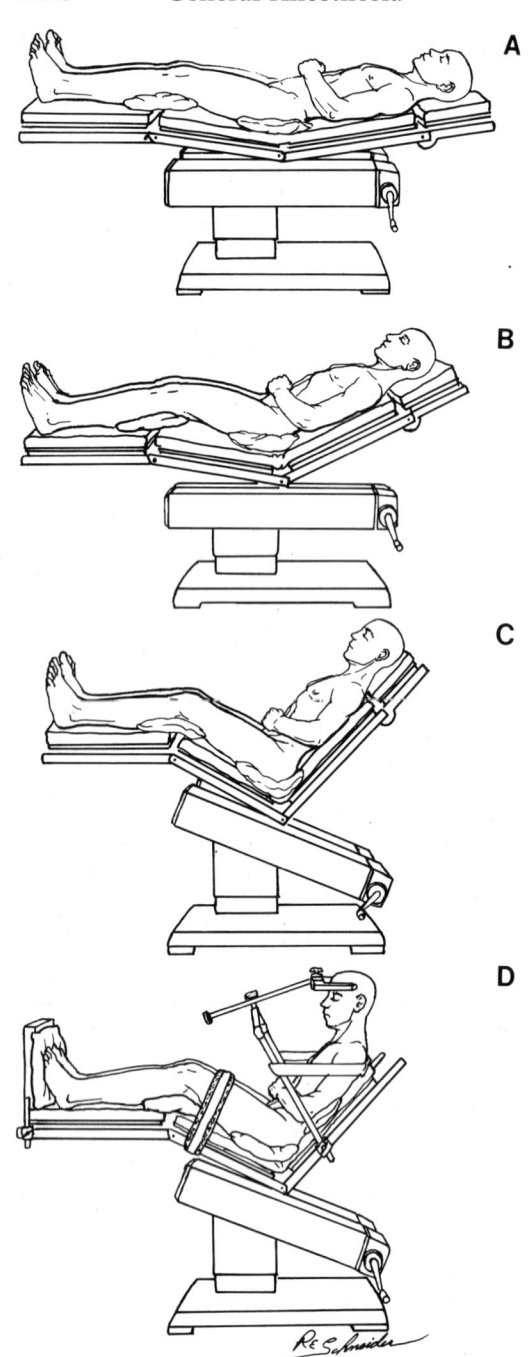

FIG. 7–12. Establishment of the standard ("classic") sitting position. See text for details. From Martin, J.T. (ed): Positioning in Anesthesia and Surgery, 2nd ed. Philadelphia, WB Saunders, 1987.

and the head still resting on the head section of the table (Fig. 7–12C). Should hypotension occur during these moves, the positioning sequence is delayed until adequate perfusion is restored.

The U-shaped supporting frame for the head holder is attached to each side rail of the back section of the table top (Fig. 7–12D). In this manner the frame will follow the back if the patient subsequently needs to be lowered toward the horizontal position because of the appearance of a venous air embolus. If the frame is attached to the thigh section, it cannot follow if the back is lowered and the patient will remain trapped unsupported in a partial sitting position, hanging dangerously from the head and neck.

If the three-pin head holder is to be used, at this point it is applied to the patient's head in the appropriate manner. The neck is gently flexed and the head rotated laterally if indicated, the holder is attached to the extension arm of the U-frame, the joints of the frame are locked, the head section of the table top is removed, and the final elevation of the back section is accomplished to attain the surgical posture (Fig. 7–12D).

If a padded head rest is used, rather than the three-pin head holder, it is first attached to the extension bar of the U-frame; then the patient is maneuvered into it so that it holds the head without compressing the eyes. Some type of retaining tape will be needed to stabilize the head of the "sitting" patient in the rest, and repeated checks will be needed during the surgical procedure to detect tape slipping and to assure that the position is correctly maintained. When the desired posture is assured, the head section of the table top is removed and any necessary final adjustments are made to the table sections or to the components of the frame holding the head.

In the final sitting position, the arms are folded in the patient's lap, are resting on the thighs, or are placed on arm board attachments to the table. The elbows should be supported and padded to assure that normal perfusion of the hands continues and that the ulnar nerve is not compressed. Heel pads should be applied and the feet held at right angles to the legs to prevent postoperative foot drop (Fig. 7–12D). The arterial transducer is positioned at the level of the circle of Willis and monitors on the ventral thorax are assured. Some surgeons tape the shoulders forward to the U-frame in order to add support to the torso and separate the medial borders of the scapulae (Fig. 7–12D).

Variations of Classical Sitting Position

Two important variations of the classical sitting position have been presented.

SIDESADDLE SITTING POSITION. Garcia-Bengochia et al.[16] have used a sidesaddle sitting position in which the patient is more upright than in the classic version and sits sideways on the operating table with legs supported in a special attachment (Fig. 7–13A). The back section of the table is raised against the side of the patient and the frame of the skull-pin head holder is attached to it (Fig. 7–13B); a padded

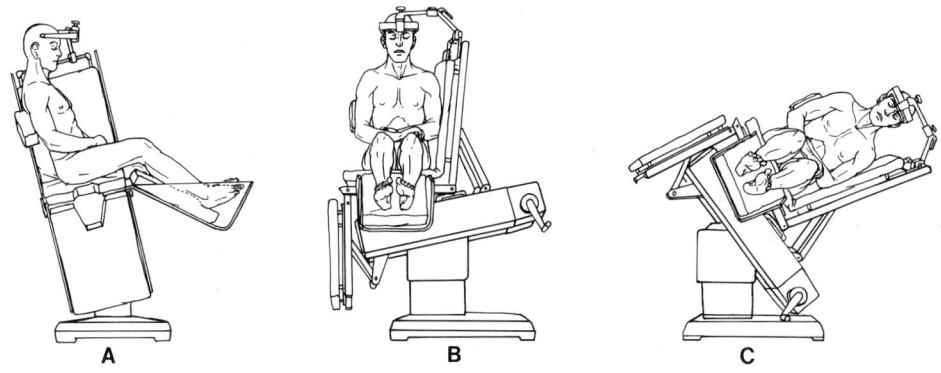

FIG. 7–13. The side-saddle sitting position of Garcia-Bengochia. Th surgeon operates behind the seated patient but at the side of the chassis of the operating table. The arrangement can be moved into Durant's position (C) without contaminating the surgical field should a venous air embolus occur. See text for discussion. From Martin, J.T. (ed): Positioning in Anesthesia and Surgery, 2nd ed. Philadelphia, WB Saunders, 1987.

attachment to the back section supports the patient's back (Figs. 7–13A and B). The chassis of the table is tilted so that the control end is high (Fig. 7–13B). If an air embolus is detected, the control end of the chassis is lowered (Fig. 7–13C) and the patient assumes a left lateral decubitus position without interference with the access to (and sterility of) the occipito–cervical operating field. This modification of the sitting position provides the surgeon with comfortable access to the field, but it requires special attachments to the table that have not become commercially available.

SHAPIRO'S MODIFICATION OF SITTING POSITION FOR AIR EMBOLISM. Shapiro[17] depicted a modification of the classic sitting position that elevates the control end of the table chassis with the patient otherwise in a customary semirecumbent posture (Fig. 7–14A). If an air embolus occurs, the control end of the chassis is lowered and the patient assumes a thorax-level and legs-high posture (Fig. 7–14B) that increases venous return to the chest, decreases the subatmospheric venous pressure gradient between operative site and heart, and preserves access to the surgical field. Special attachments for the standard operating table are not required for this arrangement.

The head may be elevated to varying degrees in the supine, lateral, or prone positions as well as in the sitting position. In most instances the posture is used to provide adequate access to the surgical site or because it is a more easily established alternative to the sitting position. Occasionally, however, it is chosen in the mistaken belief that air embolus is eliminated in the prone head-high or lateral head-high posture as opposed to the sitting position.

Head-Elevated Supine Position

The head-elevated supine position is used routinely by several surgical specialties for access to structures about the head and neck. In most instances the degree of elevation does not establish a gradient sufficient to allow air embolization, particularly in a patient who is being passively ventilated. Partial airway obstruction in a supine patient whose head is only mildly elevated, however, when combined with a vigorous spontaneous inspiratory effort, may transiently create sufficient subatmospheric pressure in the mediastinum for air to be entrained into a patulous vein in the surgical field.

Head-Elevation-Patient in Lateral Decubitus or Prone Position

Elevating the head of a patient who is either in the lateral decubitus position or in the prone position is usually employed as a means of decreasing venous congestion at the incision. In some instances the posture is chosen as an alternative to the sitting position in the belief that it eliminates the risk of air embolization. If the gradient established between the wound and the heart is low, the risk of venous air embolization is low, but present; if the gradient is relatively high, the risk is increased toward that of the sitting position. Either head-elevated posture adds the difficulties of head-up tilt to the problems inherent in its own positioning.

THE LATERAL POSITIONS

THE TERMINOLOGY TRAP. Describing a lateral position requires careful use of terminology. A surgeon may indicate that he wishes to operate on the right

184 General Anesthesia

lateral position, either with the chest horizontal and the legs dangling as for thoracic surgery, or with the kidney rest elevated as a lateral flexion fulcrum and chest and legs each angled somewhat downward.

THE CLASSIC LATERAL DECUBITUS POSITION. In the classic horizontal lateral decubitus position, the anesthetized patient is turned from the supine position onto one side (Figs. 7–15 and 7–16).

The down-side arm is extended parallel to the sagittal plane of the body and either placed on an arm board extending ventrally from the torso or flexed at the elbow to lie with the hand palm-up in front of the patient's face.

A small, firm roll or support is placed beneath the lateral rib cage just caudad to the down-side axilla to raise the thorax and shoulder off the table. This pad frees the shoulder from much of the direct lateral pressure of the position and minimizes ventral circumduction of the acromioclavicular joint that might stretch the supraclavicular nerve.

The down-side thigh is flexed on the trunk and the leg is flexed on the thigh to lie nearly perpendicular to the long axis of the torso (Fig. 7–16); in this position the down-side lower extremity acts to stabilize the patient's trunk against either ventral or dorsal displacement.

The up-side lower extremity is extended fully and supported on pillows in the long axis of the body.

One or two 3-inch-wide retaining tapes are placed across the up-side hip, located carefully in the space between the iliac crest and the head of the femur, and fixed at each end to the underside of the table top in front of and behind the patient (Fig. 7–15). The tapes assist the bent lower extremity in stabilizing the hips and reducing the chances for dorsal or ventral displacement of the torso.

The up-side upper extremity is placed either on the upper level of a two-tiered arm board[3] (see Figs. 7–1D and 7–15) or on pillows over the down-side

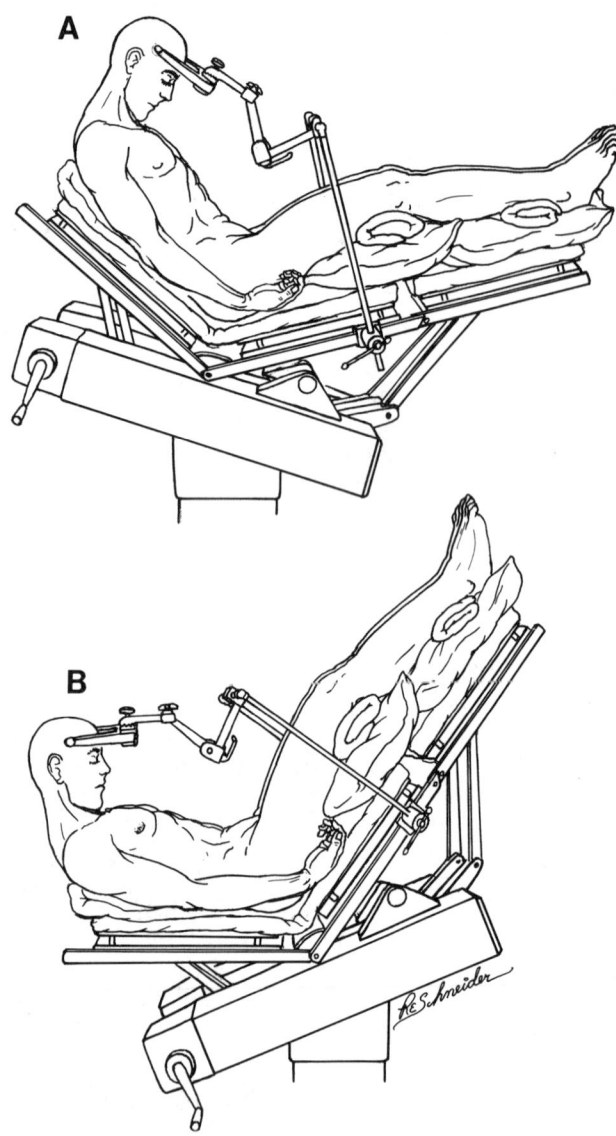

FIG. 7–14. Sitting position described by Shapiro. *A.* Position during operation. *B.* Resuscitative repositioning in the event of a venous air embolus. From Martin, J.T. (ed): Positioning in Anesthesia and Surgery, 2nd ed. Philadelphia, WB Saunders, 1987.

lung of the patient and have the patient placed in the "right lateral chest position." Actually, he has indicated the need for the *left lateral decubitus* position, which gives access to the right thorax. The terminology discussed in the chapters on patient positioning eschews obfuscation by using the decubitus description (defining *decubitus* as "that body part that rests upon the supporting surface of the operating table") synonymously with the simpler term *lateral position*.

The several versions of the lateral position to be discussed are: the classic horizontal lateral position with its variations, the Sims', spinal anesthesia, semisupine, and semiprone positions, and the flexed

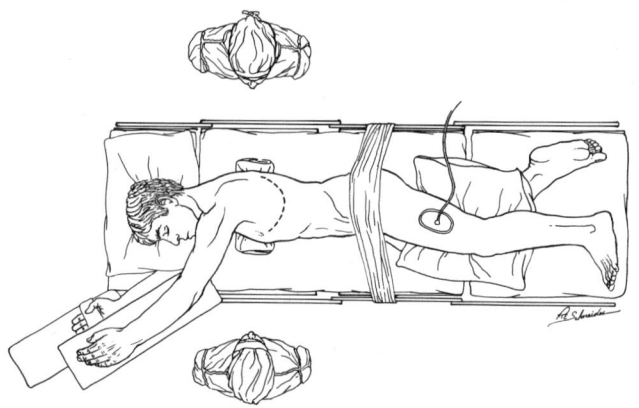

FIG. 7–15. The horizontal lateral position viewed from above. From Martin, J.T. (ed): Positioning in Anesthesia and Surgery, 2nd ed. Philadelphia, WB Saunders, 1987.

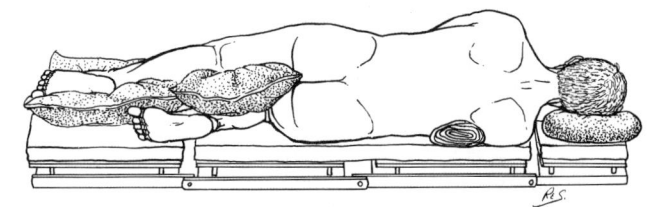

FIG. 7–16. The horizontal lateral position viewed from behind. From Martin, J.T. (ed): Positioning in Anesthesia and Surgery, 2nd ed. Philadelphia, WB Saunders, 1987.

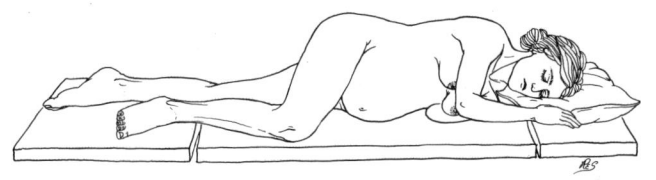

FIG. 7–17. The Sims' position. Note that up-side lower extremity is flexed at hip and knee while the down-side lower extremity is extended. The resulting semiprone posture exposes the perineum from behind to allow fetal delivery or operative surgery. See text for discussion. From Martin, J.T. (ed): Positioning in anesthesia and Surgery, 2nd ed. Philadelphia, WB Saunders, 1987.

arm on a single level arm board. An alternative choice is to flex it at the elbow and place its hand palm-down in front of the face of the patient, separated from the down-side palm by appropriate padding.

Careful attention must be paid to supporting the head of the patient in the lateral position (Fig. 7–16) so that no potentially injurious lateral angulation can occur in the cervical spine.

Occasionally a retaining tape is placed across the rib cage to prevent the patient from rolling out of the chosen lateral position. When this is done, it must be located as high as possible into the up-side axilla to avoid unduly restricting inspiratory expansion of the up-side hemithorax.

In some circumstances it is advisable to support the lumbar area by sliding a vertical rest onto the elevatable kidney bar at midtable and moving it against the patient. A similar rest against the abdomen may not be a wise choice if it compresses viscera to obstruct abdominal great vessels and restrict the descent of the diaphragm on inspiration.

THE SIMS' POSITION. The Sims'[18] modification of the lateral position, developed to permit the repair of vesicovaginal fistulas, has been useful for obstetric delivery and for surgical procedures about the perineum. It is achieved by placing the patient in a lateral position, extending the down-side lower extremity (with only slight flexion at the knee), and flexing the up-side hip and knee (each to about 90 degrees) (Fig. 7–17). The patient is allowed to roll ventrally until the up-side knee contacts the mattress and stabilizes the torso. In this position the perineum is well exposed from behind, and abdominal masses, such as a gravid uterus, usually do not compress the abdominal aorta or inferior vena cava. A pad under the down-side thorax can free the axilla if shoulder compression is troublesome, but the down-side upper extremity may need to be placed behind the patient to prevent uncomfortable ventral circumduction of the shoulder.

THE LATERAL POSITION FOR SPINAL ANESTHESIA. The lateral position used to facilitate the establishment of spinal or epidural anesthesia is rarely acceptable for a surgical procedure. It is accomplished by placing the patient on one side, flexing the neck, and drawing the flexed knees up as far as possible toward the chin. The sole purpose of the position is to arch the lumbar spine dorsally, separate the spinous processes, and improve access of the spinal needle to the ligamentum flavum and dura. A similar exposure can be gained with the patient bent forward while sitting. Excessive flexing of the back unduly stretches the ligaments and dura so that the spinal needle may produce greater tears in the dura and greater C.S.F. leakage.

SEMILATERAL POSITIONS. Semilateral positions can be established with the patient turned on one side and then allowed to roll dorsally (into a combination of lateral and supine positions—semisupine) or ventrally (into a combination of lateral and prone positions—semiprone). In each position, as well as in the classic lateral, the down-side axilla must be protected by a pad that elevates the thorax off of the table and avoids compressing the shoulder.

In the semisupine position the up-side arm becomes a concern. It cannot be used as a strap from which the torso hangs because a severe stretch injury can be inflicted on its brachial neurovascular bundle. Dorsal supports of some type should be placed beneath the shoulders and the pelvis to keep the patient from slipping fully supine (see Fig. 7–2). The down-side lower extremity should be straightened somewhat to allow it to lie flat on the table.

In the semiprone position the down-side arm is usually placed behind the patient, as it may be in the Sims position, to prevent problems with its shoulder. The legs are arranged as in the Sims position, and a soft support of some type is placed beneath the ventral thorax to keep the patient from rolling fully prone. This posture, often chosen for children who are awakening following a tonsillectomy, has been called a posttonsillectomy position.

THE FLEXED LATERAL POSITIONS. Bending a patient laterally at the waist increases the distance between the convex costal margin and its adjacent iliac crest. For surgical purposes, the maneuver is intended either to spread intercostal spaces and improve access

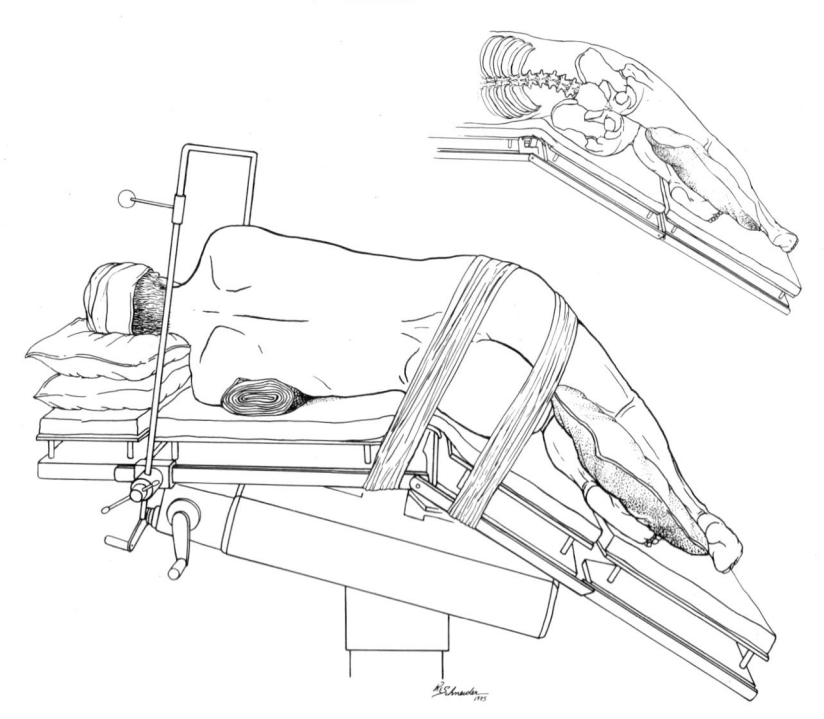

FIG. 7–18. The lateral jackknife position. The down-side iliac crest is properly placed over the flexion point of the table. Restraining straps thrust cephalad against the distracting weight of the legs. Head is supported to avoid injury to cervical spine. Leg wraps are not shown. Insert shows unrestrained slippage of the pelvis off the flexion point of the table, resulting in unacceptable compression of the down-side flank and respiratory embarrassment. From Martin, J.T. (ed): Positioning in Anesthesia and Surgery, 2nd ed. Philadelphia, WB Saunders, 1987.

to the lung (often referred to as the *lateral jackknife position*[19]) or to lengthen the flank enough to provide access to the up-side kidney (the "kidney position"). In neither instance is a patient likely to endure a flexed lateral posture when awake.

When the intention is to enhance intercostal space size and access to the thoracic cavity, the lateral jackknife position (Fig. 7–18) is of questionable value, and its physiologic risks of lumbar torsion and dangling legs are apt to be higher than acceptable for the patient.

When the intention is to enhance subcostal space size and renal exposure, the flexed lateral posture is acceptable if it is precisely established and maintained (Fig. 7–19).

Lateral Jackknife Position for Thoracic Surgery. When the lateral jackknife position is requested for intrathoracic surgery,[19] the positioning procedure is as follows:

- The patient's down-side iliac crest is placed over the hinge between the back and thigh sections of the table (see Fig. 7–18).
- The table top is then angulated at that hinge.
- The legs are usually wrapped to midthigh to reduce the amount of pooled blood that the posture produces.
- Restraining tapes and straps are arranged across the hips and legs (see Fig. 7–18) to keep the weight of the dangling legs from pulling the pelvis caudad and placing the angulation point of the table in the down-side flank (Fig. 7–18, *insert*).

The chassis is adjusted so that the patient lies in a lateral position with thorax horizontal and legs laterally flexed toward the floor.

While the lateral jackknife posture does tighten the up-side flank and widen intercostal spaces, it usually embarrasses circulation by pooling blood in the dependent extremities. It demonstrably reduces ventilatory motion of the up-side costal margin because of the taut flank muscles, and, if the patient slides caudad off of the flexion point of the table, excursions of the down-side lung are seriously threatened (See Fig. 7–18, *insert*). Once the incision is made and the rib-spreading retractor is in place, the posture has little further value. For the transient initial gain to the surgeon, the sustained physiologic risk to the patient is difficult to condone.[19]

Lateral Flexed Kidney Position. Because of the relative inaccessability of the kidney in the standard (horizontal) lateral position, the flexed lateral "kidney position" is more easily justified than is the lateral jackknife position. Its ability to be misapplied or to shift unacceptably, however, is greater. The positioning procedure follows.

- The patient is turned carefully into the lateral position, and the down-side iliac crest is placed over the elevatable kidney bar at the hinge between the trunk and thigh sections of the table top (Fig. 7–19C).
- The table top is then angulated downward at the hinge between the back and leg sections of its surface. As a result, the patient is flexed laterally and lies with head and feet below

FIG. 7–19. The flexed lateral kidney position. *A* and *B.* Show the flexion point of the table unacceptably positioned above the iliac crest and compressing the down-side flank. *C.* Shows proper position of the iliac crest over the elevated kidney rest at the flexion point of the table. Down-side flank is relatively free in *C.* Head is supported to avoid injury to the cervical spine. Leg wrappings and pelvic restraining tapes are not shown. Down-side hip and knee are flexed to stabilize the torso. From Martin, J.T. (ed): Positioning in Anesthesia and Surgery, 2nd ed. Philadelphia, WB Saunders, 1987.

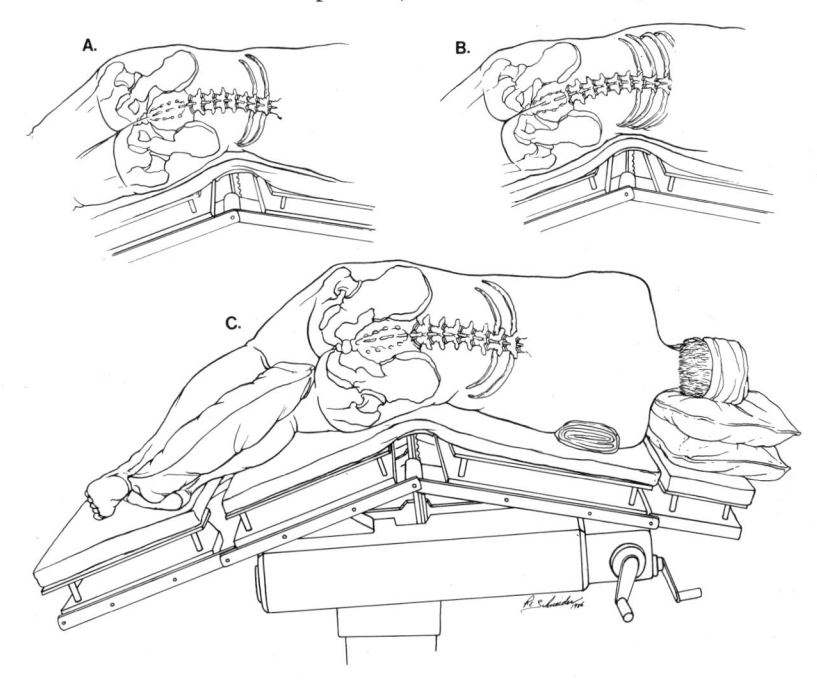

the level of the pelvis. The kidney rest, if it is to be used, is raised to the point that the muscles of the up-side flank are stretched.

Restraining tapes are placed over the up-side hip and thigh in such a manner that the patient cannot slide caudad off of the kidney rest. Then, and only then, the chassis of the table can be manipulated so that the thoracic spine is horizontal. If the thorax is leveled before the restraining tapes are placed, the patient will slide caudad off of the elevated kidney rest, causing the rest to compress the downside flank and impede expansion of the downside lung significantly (Figs. 7–19*A* and *B*).

While the resulting degree of lateral flexion in the kidney position offers at least the same amount of patient distress as that objected to in the earlier discussion of the thoracic flexed lateral position, the surgical advantage is sustained and greater for the urologist because the overhanging costal margin renders the target kidney almost inaccessible in the horizontal lateral position.

THE PRONE POSITIONS

Three versions of the prone position are generally employed:

1. The *extended prone position,* in which the thorax is horizontal and the lower extremities are almost in the same plane (Figs. 7–5, 7–6, and 7–20).
2. The *jackknife prone position,* in which the body is angulated ventrally at the hip and the head and legs are below the level of the pelvis (Figs. 7–21 and 7–22).
3. The *kneeling prone position,* in which the trunk is essentially horizontal and the patient is kneeling on the surface of the tilted table or upon a ledge affixed to the depressed foot section (see Figs. 7–4*A* and 7–7).

Several less-common versions of the prone position have also been described.[20,21] Frames to support the trunk of a pronated patient and devices to support the head have been discussed earlier in this chapter.

PRONATING A PATIENT—PRECAUTIONS. The anesthetized patient must be carefully turned into and out of the prone position. Sufficient personnel must be present so the anesthesiologist can attend to the management of ventilation and the airway as the turn progresses.

The arm over which the patient is pronated must be protected from injury, and the spine must not be twisted unnaturally during the turn. An acceptable final position for the arms must protect them from injury and not interfere with surgical access to a midline wound.

The head must be controlled at all times and never allowed to flop about because a damaging impact or severe injury can be inflicted on the cervical vertebrae and spinal cord.[22]

THE STANDARD PRONE POSITION. The extended (standard) prone position is accomplished by placing some type of supportive padding or frame (see previous section on Table Frames) beneath the pronated patient to assure that the abdominal viscera are free

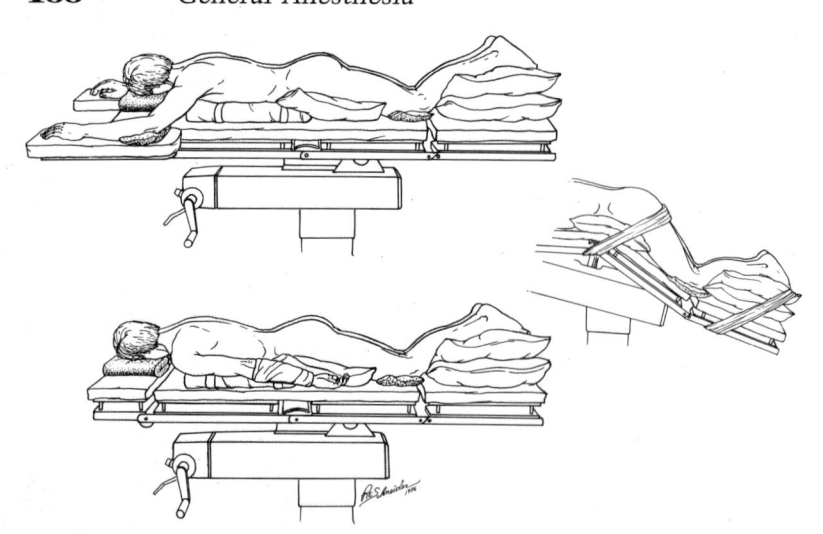

FIG. 7-20. The extended prone position utilizing parallel rolls of sheeting to free the abdomen. *Top.* Arms padded well on arm boards overhead. Pillow over caudad end of rolls prevents thighs from being gouged by roll ends. *Bottom.* Arms retained alongside of torso. *Insert.* Restraining straps under buttocks counteract caudad slippage from weight of legs after table is flexed to minimize lumbar lordosis and chassis is adjusted to level back. Feet are usually less extended than shown here. From Martin, J.T. (ed): Positioning in Anesthesia and Surgery, 2nd ed. Philadelphia, WB Saunders, 1987.

from compression by the weight of the trunk on the table (see Figs. 7-3, 7-4B, 7-5, 7-6, and 7-20).

The head is retained in the sagittal plane by an appropriate holder or gently turned laterally with the down-side eye and ear freed from pressure.

The arms are positioned alongside of the trunk or extended in a comfortable and well-padded position over the patient's head (Fig. 7-20).

If chest rolls are used, a pillow is placed across their caudad ends to prevent the rolls from digging into the ventral surfaces of the thighs (see Fig. 7-3). The patient's urinary drainage system is checked to assure freedom from obstruction.

Elbows are padded (Fig. 7-20), arms are checked to see that the contents of each axilla are neither compressed nor under tension, the knees are padded, the lower legs are flexed on the thighs by additional pillows under the shins, and padding at each ankle is arranged to allow the feet to remain approximately at right angles to the lower leg.

THE PRONE JACKKNIFE POSITION. The jackknife prone or flexed ventral decubitus position, used for surgery about the buttocks and within the anus and rectosigmoid, can be either minimally or markedly flexed.

In **the minimal jackknife position** (see Fig. 7-21), the iliac crest of the pronated patient is placed on a pillow over the flexion break of the table and the table top is flexed as much as possible. The result is a slight amount of ventral angulation of the thighs on the trunk and reasonably satisfactory exposure of the superficial sacrum and buttocks. Positioning is as follows:

The patient's head is turned gently toward one side, and the down-side eye and ear are protected by supportive padding.

Arms are usually placed alongside of the patient's head, although less neck torsion may occur if

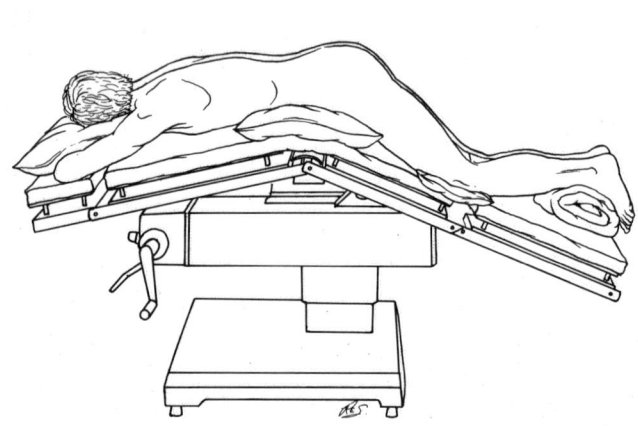

FIG. 7-21. Prone jackknife position with minimal flexion. Note that hip joints are over flexion point of the table. Hips, knees, and ankles are padded. Restraining tapes are usually not needed. Leg wraps not shown. From Martin, J.T. (ed): Positioning in Anesthesia and Surgery, 2nd ed. Philadelphia, WB Saunders, 1987.

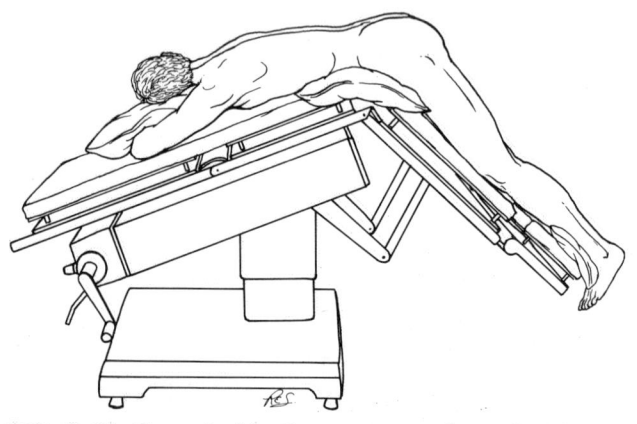

FIG. 7-22. Prone jackknife position with marked flexion. Note that head-piece of table has been added to the foot section as an extender. The hip joint of the patient is placed over the hinge between the thigh and foot sections. Flexion point becomes the thigh-foot section hinge, allowing greater flexion than in Figure 7-21. From Martin, J.T. (ed): Positioning in Anesthesia and Surgery, 2nd ed. Philadelphia, WB Saunders, 1987.

the arm toward which the patient's face is turned is alongside of the head and the other is along the side of the trunk.

Trunk frames and leg wrappings are rarely needed, although protective padding is helpful for arms, knees, and ankles.

For the *markedly flexed jackknife position* (Fig. 7–22), the flexion break of the table does not provide sufficient angulation. Therefore, the head section of the table is detached and transferred to the opposite end to extend the leg section. The table surface can then be angulated at the hinge between the thigh and leg sections and combined with chassis tilt to attain more effective flexion. Positioning is as follows:

The hips of the pronated patient are placed over the hinge between the thigh and leg sections, the extended leg section is depressed, and the chassis is tilted head-down. The patient is thereby arranged in an inverted "V." Lateral tapes are used to strap the buttocks apart and provide surgical access to the anus and rectum.

Legs may need to be wrapped to prevent pooling of blood in the dependent extremities, pads are needed under the lower shins to keep the feet at 90 degrees to the legs, the arms are usually placed alongside of the turned head, and padding should protect the down-side eye and ear.

Complication and Contraindication. In the markedly flexed jackknife position the patient's head is significantly below the level of the heart and conjunctival edema is commonly seen after all but the shortest of procedures. For this reason the posture should be avoided in patients with intracranial pathology and the risk of cerebral edema.

THE KNEELING PRONE POSITION. The kneeling prone position (see Figs. 7–4A and 7–7) is useful to provide surgical access to the dorsal trunk. Numerous variations exist according to the method used to stabilize the posture.[20] It is particularly useful when the patient is obese (see Fig. 7–7), and the extended prone position would probably not relieve visceral pressure on major abdominal blood vessels sufficiently to prevent venous congestion at the operative site.

With all of the usual precautions described above for the postural safety of the pronated patient fully activated, a ledge is placed on the foot section of the table top and the section is lowered so that the ledge becomes horizontal. With adequate padding and strapping, the patient is arranged to kneel on that ledge and the chassis of the table is tilted so that the abdomen hangs free.

Numerous mechanical hoists are available to vary the height of the kneeling ledge as are others, including simple stacks of sheets, that can elevate the ventral thorax off the table. The result should be a comfortable position for the patient's head and neck as well as freedom of the abdomen from pressure.

Arm position may be difficult with these table attachments unless the arms are crossed beneath the abdomen or held alongside of the patient. If the subject is massively obese, placing the large arms alongside of the trunk can add enough lateral body mass to make access to the dorsal midline difficult for the surgeon.

Extreme caution is advised when turning a supine patient with an unstable vertebral column into the prone position.[20,21] The responsible surgeon should be present and involved in the turn. Intubating the patient awake permits repeated neurologic assessments during and after the turn to assure no deterioration of the patient's condition or to return promptly to the safety of the original supine posture.

MOVING THE UNCONSCIOUS PATIENT. In moving unconscious patients, special care must be exercised to maintain the head and neck in a stable position. The head must not be allowed to "roll." Patients who have been paralyzed by relaxant drugs are vulnerable. The following is recommended:

1. Consider that a fractured cervical vertebra may already exist.
2. Place hands under shoulders.
3. Cradle the patient's head between the forearms.
4. Maintain the head and neck in the longitudinal axis of the vertebral column.

MANAGEMENT AND POSITIONING OF THE COMATOSE PATIENT (FOR CARE AND TRANSPORTATION)

Principles. The care and positioning of the comatose patient for *initial* first aid and transport the following basic principles must be observed.

1. *A free or patent airway* must be established and maintained.
2. A means of prevention of accumulation and/or removal of vomitus, regurgitation and/or oral pharyngeal secretions must be established.
3. *Ventilation* of an adequate volume must be maintained. If hyperventilation occurs, respirations must be assisted using such mechanical aids as a bag and mask (Air Viva Unit) with oxygen enrichment.
4. Patient must be protected from injury by objects or malposition. This includes pressure areas, thermal trauma, vascular occlusion, and protruded limbs.
5. Aggravation of the injury suffered must be prevented.
6. The patient must be comfortable (even when comatose). A patient lying flat on the back with arms and legs straight is not in a natural position.

7. Placing the patient on the transport vehicle and moving from one area to another should be gentle and as smooth as possible. Fast, jerky, uneven, and rough movements may cause deterioration of the patient's condition.
8. *Loss of body heat must be prevented.* Covering must be sufficient to protect the patient from loss of heat but at the same time not cause heat retention or be too heavy, causing unnecessary weight and restriction.

Procedure for Positioning a Comatose Patient. The following position is suited to the moving of a comatose patient. It should be used unless other factors prevent or modify it (some special considerations will be noted at the end of the memorandum).

1. The patient is placed on his *side* slightly rolled forward.
2. The head is placed in *extension* and *not* on a pillow (a slight lowering of the head by this means helps prevent aspiration and promotes drainage of secretions).
3. The *under arm* is placed in extension behind the back; it is not allowed to be under the patient's body or in a position that restricts abdominal or chest movements.
4. The *upper arm* is flexed in a manner to place the semiclosed fist under the jaw for support.
5. The *legs* are flexed as are the *knees* with the under leg and knee more flexed than the upper, thus using it for a support against the patient rolling onto his back or too far forward.
6. If *intravenous infusions* are established they should be in an upper limb, preferably in the forearm or on back of the hand.

In covering and strapping the patient, care must be taken to maintain control of the airway. Remember that a noisy airway (e.g., snoring) is an obstructed airway, but an airway that is completely obstructed is silent. Chest movements will be of help in determining if the airway is patent. If patient is strapped to stretcher, the band should be applied over the hip.

Transportation. During transportation, the portable suction apparatus must accompany the patient. The hand-bulb type is useful.

SPECIAL CONSIDERATIONS

Head Injuries. Patients with head injuries may be transported with the head and shoulders somewhat elevated. If this is done, the head must be extended (with a pillow or roll under the shoulder if the patient is on his back) and the jaw supported for a good airway. Watch for vomitus or other foreign material in the pharynx.

Orthopedic Injuries. Due to splinting or fixation these patients are often difficult or impossible to place in an ideal position. Extreme care must be taken to establish and maintain a good airway.

Delerium. Disoriented and delirious patients (alcoholics, etc.) should be restrained. This can be accomplished by anchoring wrist-straps on each wrist to the side rail proximal to the position of the hands noted in procedure.

Chest Injuries. When there is blood or fluid in the lungs or a collapsed lung, it is advisable to place the good lung uppermost to prevent restriction of its ventilation and contamination from the injured lung.

REMEMBER THE AIRWAY AND THE VENTILATION.

REFERENCES

1. Collins, V.J.: *In* Principles of Anesthesiology, 2nd ed. Edited by V.J. Collins. Philadelphia, Lea and Febiger, 1976.
2. Martin, J.T. (ed.): Positioning in Anesthesia and Surgery, 2nd ed. Philadelphia, WB Saunders, 1987.
3. Begenau, V.G.: Double tier arm support. Anesthesiology, 7:569, 1946.
4. Martin, J.T.: General requirements of safe positioning for the surgical patient. *In* Positioning in Anesthesia and Surgery, 1st ed. Edited by J.T. Martin. Philadelphia, WB Saunders, 1978.
5. Martin, J.T.: The lawn chair (contoured supine) position. *In* Positioning in Anesthesia and Surgery, 2nd ed. Edited by J.T. Martin. Philadelphia, WB Saunders, 1987.
6. Wilcox, S., and Vandam, L.D.: Alas, poor Trendelenburg and his position! A critique of its uses and effectiveness. Anesth. Analg., 67:574, 1988.
7. Meyer, W.: Uber die Nachbehandlung des hohen Steinschnittes sowie uber Verwendbarkeit desselben zur Operation von Blasenscheidenfisten. Arch. Klin. Clir., 31:494, 1885.
8. Porter, W.T.: Shock at the Front. Boston Med. Surg. J., 175:854, 1916.
9. Cole, F.: Head lowering in the treatment of hypotension. J.A.M.A., 150:273, 1952.
10. Weil, M.H., and Whigham, H.: Head-down (Trendelenburg) position for treatment of irreversible hemorrhagic shock: Experimental study in rats. Ann. Surg., 162:905, 1965.
11. Sibbald, W.J.: et al.: The Trendelenburg position: Hemodynamic effects in hypotensive and normotensive patients. Crit. Care Med., 7:218, 1979.
12. Dorland's Illustrated Medical Dictionary, 26th ed. Philadelphia, W.B. Saunders, 1965.
13. Prentice, J.A., and Martin, J.T.: The Trendelenburg position: Anesthesiologic considerations. *In* Positioning in Anesthesia and Surgery, 2nd ed. Edited by J.T. Martin. Philadelphia, WB Saunders, 1987.
14. Martin, J.T.: The head elevated positions: Anesthesiologic considerations. *In* Positioning in Anesthesia and Surgery, 2nd ed. Edited by J.T. Martin. Philadelphia, W.B. Saunders, 1987.
15. Wilson, R.D.: Abrupt postural changes in patients undergoing air contrast studies. Clinical and physiological evaluation. J.A.M.A., 198:970, 1966.
16. Garcia-Bengochea, F., Munson, E.S., and Freeman, J.V.: The

lateral sitting position for neurosurgery. Anesth. Analg., 55:326, 1976.
17. Shapiro, H.M.: Venous air embolism. *In* Anesthesia, 2nd ed. Edited by R.D. Miller. New York, Churchill Livingstone, 1986.
18. Sims, J.M.: Silver Suture in Surgery: The anniversary discourse before the New York Academy of Medicine, 18 November, 1857. New York, Samuel S. and William W. Wood, 1858.
19. Lawson, N.W.: The lateral decubitus position: Anesthesiologic considerations. *In* Positioning in Anesthesia and Surgery, 2nd ed. Edited by J.T. Martin. Philadelphia, W.B. Saunders, 1987.
20. Martin, J.T.: The prone position: Anesthesiologic considerations. *In* Positioning in Anesthesia and Surgery, 2nd ed. Edited by J.T. Martin. Philadelphia, W.B. Saunders, 1987.
21. Sing, I.: The prone position: Surgical aspects. *In* Positioning in Anesthesia and Surgery, 2nd ed. Edited by J.T. Martin. Philadelphia, W.B. Saunders, 1987.
22. Shellhas, K.P., et al.: Vertebrobasilar injuries following cervical manipulation. J.A.M.A., *244:*1450, 1986.

John T. Martin

COMPLICATIONS OF PATIENT POSITIONING

Complications associated with positioning a patient for surgery are, unfortunately, not rare. They may resolve rapidly and completely, resolve partially in a variable period of time, or become permanent. Almost always they are preventable; however, the occasional complication will occur despite deliberate preventive measures and meticulous technique. The opportunities for postural complications to occur persist and, perhaps, increase according to the number and complexity of procedures done in a given surgical suite. When the composite skill level of a surgical team is stable and attention is devoted to careful patient positioning, few problems should occur; when that skill level is altered by the inclusion of new team members, the opportunities for positioning complications may increase unless careful attention is paid to mundane details that provide patient safety.

Useful statistics regarding the occurrence of complications resulting from patient positioning are almost nonexistent. As a result, the discussions in this chapter are principally anecdotal and are based on personal communications, experience as an expert witness in litigation, or published data from many independent sources.

Because an injury or a complication can be associated with more than one surgical posture, this chapter is organized according to subjects and to regions of the body rather than by the positions involved.

COMPLICATIONS ASSOCIATED WITH PATIENT TRANSPORT

MONITORING LOSS. Vital sign monitors often are disconnected when critically ill patients are transferred from the emergency department or intensive care unit to the surgical suite or are returned from the operating room to an intensive care unit. Reattachment of the monitors on arrival at the destination may show that significant changes in vital signs have developed during transport and that resuscitative measures are overdue. Usually these alterations relate to hypoperfusion, but significant hypoxia and hypercarbia can result if appropriate oxygenation and ventilation are not continued during the trip. If these potentially catastrophic physiologic surprises are to be avoided, every surgical facility should possess some means of monitoring critical parameters during transport of an unstable patient to and from the operating suite, as well as the means to treat the incurred abnormality.

MOTION SICKNESS. Patients who are susceptible to nausea and vomiting may be provoked to vomit postoperatively by rapid directional changes as a transport cart rounds corners. Whether the occurrence is actually motion-oriented or is a sequel of the anesthetic is impossible to determine; however, the basic precept of gentle movement of the patient who is critically ill or who has just been anesthetized requires strict compliance.

MOTION-INDUCED HYPOTENSION. Occasionally patients who have compensated adequately on the operating table or in the emergency department for the loss of unrecognizedly large volumes of blood become hypotensive when they are moved to a transport cart and trundled through corridors and elevators to their next destination. The speculated cause is loss of effective splanchnic vascular resistance and resulting enlargement of the venous capacitance system. While the method of treatment is obvious, the possibility of motion-induced hypotension needs recognition and mandates appropriate monitoring.

COMPLICATIONS DURING PATIENT REPOSITIONING

POSTURAL HYPOTENSION. Changing the position of a patient can expose a failure of vascular adaptation that has been caused by underestimating and not replacing the fluid and blood volume deficit present at the start of the move. In some instances, a debilitated patient without a newly acquired volume deficit will compensate so slowly to a new posture that additional vascular volume and the temporary use of vasopressors may be needed to support perfusion.

Increases in effective vascular capacitance that exceed the ability of the available blood volume to perfuse the enlarged vascular space can occur when lithotomy is terminated and the legs are lowered to the horizontal supine posture, or when a patient is returned to the horizontal position from steep Trendelenburg. Similar hypotension may develop while the patient is being changed to one of the head-elevated positions. Less often it occurs during a turn from supine to prone.

Repositioning hypotension is usually readily correctable. Gentle use of vasopressors can temporarily reestablish effective perfusion, but correction of any existing volume deficit is the more durable therapeutic maneuver. The concentration of anesthetic drugs should be reduced until vasocompensation is achieved. Completion of the postural change may need to be delayed until appropriate vascular pressures have been restored.

EXTREMITY INJURIES. As a supine patient is turned into either the lateral or the prone positions, specific efforts must be made to protect the extremities from injury.

An arm that is alongside of the trunk may fall into a crevasse between the transport cart and the operating table, resulting in an injury to the capsule and articulations of the shoulder joint or causing a fracture of the humerus. This injury is more apt to occur and be serious as the pronated patient is returned to the supine position at the conclusion of a procedure.

The arm over which the patient is turned is apt to move from the dependent side to become lodged across the ventral surface of the torso as the turn progresses. In turning to the lateral position, this is not serious unless the capsule of the down-side shoulder is unduly stressed and damaged. When the patient is fully pronated, however, the arm may be trapped under the torso, causing monitor leads to be disconnected and intravascular lines to come apart in the process of its extrication.

The overgoing arm can also be a problem. Usually it flops dorsally to stress the capsule of the shoulder joint. Occasionally it can fall across the ventral torso and, as with the down-side arm, its recovery can threaten monitoring leads and vascular lines.

Each arm of the fully pronated patient can be allowed to dangle alongside the operating table while support of the torso is being completed or when lines are rearranged prior to supination at the end of the procedure. Final arm position, however, must be carefully achieved after pronation and the undergoing arm must be placed alongside of the torso before returning the patient to the supine position. If the undergoing arm is allowed to dangle or remains extended above the patient's head, the shoulder or humerus is at risk during supination.

A patient who is placed in the lateral position should have a small pad located just caudad of the down-side axilla to elevate the upper torso enough to take compressive weight off the down-side shoulder. It may also prevent significant ventral circumduction of the shoulder that can stretch and injure the suprascapular nerve.[1]

NECK INJURIES. When a patient is turned from the supine to a lateral or prone position, careful management of the head is essential. Sudden lateral motion of the unsupported head can injure osteoporotic cervical vertebrae or cause postoperative pain in the presence of an arthritic spine. Extreme or forced rotation of the pronated neck, needed to prevent compression of the down-side eye, may also cause new postoperative neck pain or exacerbate old distress.

When disease or trauma have rendered the cervical spine unstable, injury to the cervical spinal cord is a constant threat during any head movement. These patients are usually externally stabilized by traction devices or collars and may be nursed on turning beds such as Foster or Stryker frames. They benefit from being intubated awake,[2] perhaps with the help of a fiberoptic endoscope, and being carefully assisted as they turn themselves into the surgical position prior to anesthesia. With the cooperation of the patient, repeated neurologic checks are necessary to detect rapidly the presence of newly compromised spinal cord function. Where equipment and accurate interpretation are available, somatosensory evoked potential recordings may be helpful.

Enough personnel should be added to the turning team so that the risk of sudden shifting of the patient's weight and consequent loss of control of the unstable head and neck is minimized. A prudent precautionary arrangement is to have the responsible surgeon manually control the patient's head during the turn, thereby allowing the anesthesiologist to coordinate the move and protect the airway.

MISCELLANEOUS INJURIES. Corneal abrasions have occurred during the turning process when an attendant's hand or another rough object has brushed an uncovered eye. Eyes should always be lubricated and the lids gently taped shut before a turn.

Intravascular lines that disconnect during a turn may be a source of significant blood loss if not promptly discovered. Crystalloids lost during disconnection can cause enough dampening of mattress coverings to initiate maceration of fragile skin during a subsequent and lengthy surgical procedure.

Visceral drainage tubes and chest tubes can disconnect or be pulled out during a turn. Whereas a pneumothorax can be a damaging complication if not rapidly detected and treated, the loss of a visceral drainage tube may necessitate reopening the surgical wound and repeating much of the original operation. Careful attention to these lines and their connections is mandatory during any movement of the patient.

Male genitalia must be checked after a turn into the prone position to assure that they are not in contact with metal table parts or that sharp edges of supporting frames are not pressing against them.

INJURIES TO POSITIONING PERSONNEL. A bulky patient who needs to be repositioned can constitute a threat to attending personnel. Back injuries incurred by attendants while helping to lift a patient are well known to hospital administrators as compensatory issues. Having too few attendants to lift a massively obese patient effectively is an obvious risk factor to those who do assist. Footing for those who lift must be stable; back injuries occur when feet slip while a turn or lift is in progress.

COMPLICATIONS INVOLVING THE HEAD AND NECK

COMPRESSION ALOPECIA. Occipital alopecia has been reported to develop following prolonged use of a head strap to hold a face mask in place during anesthesia[3] and following lengthy operations with the patient in the dorsal decubitus position.[4] In the latter series, many patients were in some degree of Trendelenburg position for long periods and half had pain, swelling, exudation, and crusting in the area of the occiput where pressure had occurred. Alopecia occurred between the 3rd and 28th postanesthetic day, was temporary in all cases, and regrowth was complete in within 3 months.

Lawson[5] noted instances of both temporary and permanent alopecia following hypothermia and hypotension and thought that frequent changes in head position could reduce the risk of the complication. Patel[6] described temporary postanesthetic alopecia in a patient whose occiput had been protected by a foam ring, whose hair had been placed in a cap, and who had not been hypotensive. She also listed other causes of temporary alopecia unassociated with anesthesia.

Prudent protective measures would seem to include foam padding for the occiput and gentle periodic changes of the point of occipital pressure for a supine head. Contributory factors such as hypothermia and vasoconstrictive hypotension may not be completely avoidable.

EARS. Ear injuries are not frequent. Most are distortion or compression injuries of the external ear resulting from the ear being folded over or trapped between a firm surface and the skull. Occasionally the ear of a patient in the lateral position will rest on a misplaced foreign object such as intravenous tubing and be damaged by connectors or the sharp edges of control clamps. Occasionally a tape strap that circles the head to stabilize an endotracheal tube when the surgeon is working in the upper neck or mouth will compress the ear to produce a hematoma.

Careful attention to the details of ear placement on supportive head pieces, plus the use of foam padding or cut-outs, will usually be effective as preventive measures.

For the long-haired patient with multiple trauma, a careful examination should include inspection of the external ears to detect occult injuries that would affect the choice of head position during surgery.

Using somatosensory evoked potentials as a monitor, Grundy[7] has detected compromised function of the acoustic nerve during positioning for a retromastoid craniectomy. In most instances, the dysfunction is reversible and hearing recovers.

EYES. Injuries to the eyes consist mostly of corneal abrasions, although direct pressure on the globe by misplaced headrests can dislocate a crystalline lens or raise intraocular pressure sufficiently to restrict flow in the retinal artery, causing ischemia and blindness (Fig. 8–1).[8a]

In years past the sitting position, whether for pneumoencephalography or an occipito–cervical craniectomy, utilized a padded, horseshoe-shaped face rest to retain the head. An average-size rest fitted few faces properly. With a poorly fitting rest, or when a head moved during surgery, it was possible for pressure to relocate from the forehead and cheek to compress an eye. Recent use of a properly applied three-pin head clamp has eliminated most threats to the eyes in the sitting position.

In the lateral or prone position, the down-side eye must be protected from abrasion as well as from significant pressure resulting from contact with the mattress. Lubricating the conjunctivae and taping the lids shut prior to a turn in order to protect against abrasions of the cornea is a useful and widespread practice. When the pronated head is turned to one side and rests on the down-side cheek, a block of foam with a recess cut out of it can be placed under the forehead and jaw as cushioned support. The recess fits beneath the eye to remove pressure from the globe (a C-shaped face piece[8]). A new rocker-based face rest designed by Ray[8b] allows the pronated head to remain in the sagittal plane without threatening the eyes; however, initial models have allowed excessive pressure on the brows of some patients and the unit is being redesigned.

Patients who have been supine with head-down tilt, or in the lateral, flexed lateral, or prone positions may be noted, on arrival in the recovery facility, to have conjunctival edema of one or both eyes. While this may sometimes indicate excessive fluid replacement or a superior vena caval syndrome, it almost always is due to relative elevations in the venous drainage of the eyes in the posture used during anesthesia. Rarely is it either of significant duration or injurious to the eye itself.

NOSE. Positioning injuries to the nose are uncommon, and those that do occur are likely minor in nature and brief in duration. Abrasions of skin over the nose can occur during a turn. In the prone position, with the turned head initially resting on a cheek, it is possible for exogenous motion or a coughing spell to derotate the head toward the sagittal plane. This can develop lateral pressure on the cartilaginous nasal tip and distort it sideways. Almost never is this a prolonged or serious deformity.

FACE.[8b] The facial nerve leaves the skull by the stylomastoid foramen, whence it passes forward and outward to become superficial to the ramus of the mandible. It then enters the substance of the parotid gland and divides here into five major branches, the

FIG. 8–1. Improper position of head rest. Shows pressure being exerted on right eye with resultant retinal thrombosis (insert). From Slocum, H.C., O'Neal, K.C., and Allen, C.R.: Neurovascular complications from malposition on operating table. Surg. Gynecol. Obstet., 86:729, 1948.

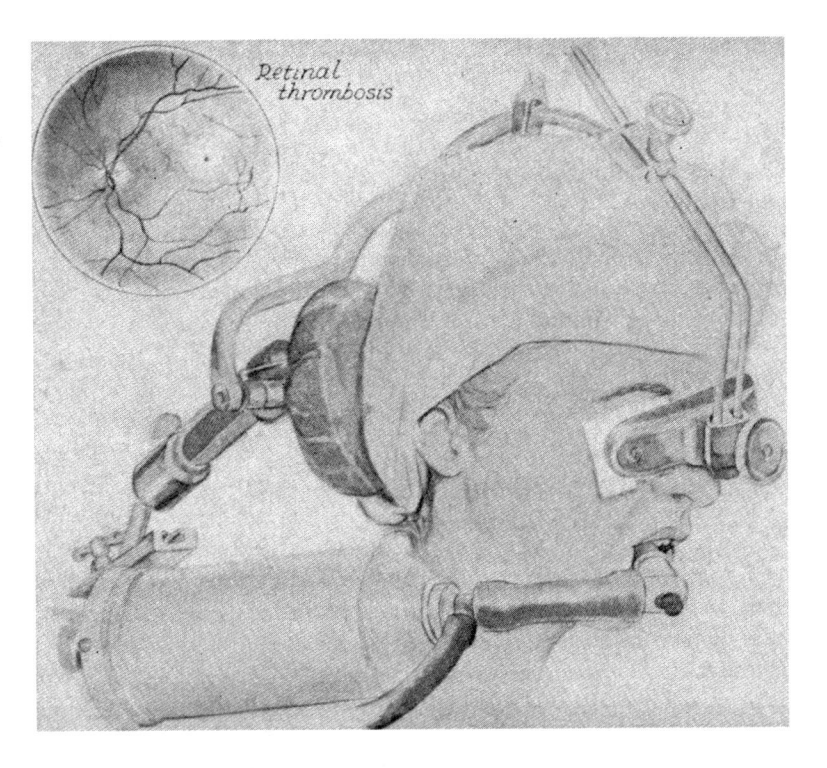

"crow's foot," which supply the facial muscles. The buccal and mandibular branches turn downward and are more superficial and more susceptible to injury. Injury may occur from (a) forward traction on jaw causing stretch of the nerves; (b) direct pressure applied to the nerves as they pass over the ramus of the jaw and cause interruption of conduction.

INTRACRANIAL INJURIES

PNEUMOCEPHALUS. Pneumocephalus indicates air inside of the cranium in the cerebrospinal fluid space. It occurs with every craniotomy and is usually of no functional consequence. An asymptomatic pneumocephalus may, however insulate the surface of the brain sufficiently to upset evoked potential monitoring.[9]

With a patient in the sitting position, a craniotomy incision made in the occiput has a significant volume of cranium above it. Cerebrospinal fluid can drain out of the incision and is usually replaced by air that bubbles upward over the surface of the brain. The air is then trapped in a functionally closed space. If it expands as it warms to body temperature, and if it expands further because nitrous oxide is present in adjacent capillaries to diffuse into and equilibrate in the newly formed gas pocket, it creates a tension pneumocephalus that is usually symptomatic and dangerous. Standefer[10] noted a 3% incidence of symptomatic pneumocephalus in a series of 275 patients operated on in the sitting position. Signs of delayed awakening and increased intracranial pressure should suggest the diagnosis. Skull radiographs are confirmatory, and decompression by twist drill holes made over the gas pocket is the usual treatment.

CEREBRAL EDEMA AND INCREASED INTRACRANIAL PRESSURE. Patients with existing increased intracranial pressure (ICP), or with intracranial pathology that has not yet elevated the ICP, are at risk of additional increases in ICP unless the anesthetic is carefully managed. If these patients are placed in a position in which the head is lower than the heart, gravity will increase intracranial pressure by increasing intracranial blood volume as well as by enlarging the edema space about the pathology. If steep head-down tilt is inflicted upon a head-injured patient in the mistaken notion that the posture is an effective resuscitative position for shock, the additional detriment to intracranial structures can be disastrous.

Flexing the neck of a patient can obstruct venous drainage from the skull and increase ICP[11] even in the sitting position. Unflexing the neck relieves the obstruction.

Head rotation can obstruct flow in the carotid and vertebral arteries.[12] Cerebral ischemia or stroke may occur despite a normal systemic mean arterial pressure. In a partially obstructed vessel that maintains low flow, thrombosis may occur, particularly in polycythemic patients.

Elevating the head above the level of the heart will reduce ICP and lessen the chance for edema formation.[13]

PARADOXICAL AIR EMBOLUS. An air embolus (see subsequent discussion) can cross from the venous to the arterial system via a probe-patent foramen ovale.[14] Variable patterns of neurologic damage occur because of air bubble obstruction of intracranial microvasculature and resultant ischemic foci in the brain.

The residual foramen ovale, present in 20 to 35% of the population[15,16] opens if pressure in the right atrium exceeds that in the left. Perkins-Pearson[17] found acute decreases in pulmonary capillary wedge pressures in half of newly seated anesthetized patients and believed that these patients were at risk for air emboli. She advocated that the patient whose right atrial pressure exceeded pulmonary capillary wedge pressure should not be operated upon in the sitting position. Lynch,[18] using echocardiographic screening, found right-to-left shunting at the atrial level in 18% of healthy volunteers who performed the Valsalva maneuver.

Based on the incidence of probe-patent foramen ovale (18–35%), venous air embolus (40%), and elevated right atrial pressure (50%), only about 1 sitting-position patient in 20 (5%) should be at risk for a paradoxical air embolus.

INJURIES TO THE NECK

An intact cervical spine can be injured by sudden lateral angulation, by the head becoming unsupported during a turn, or by prolonged lateral angulation if the head is improperly supported in the lateral position. While damage to the cervical spinal cord is unlikely to result, the patient may complain subsequently of a stiff, painful neck that can become a major therapeutic issue.

Protection of the neck during positioning becomes increasingly important when the preanesthetic evaluation reveals that a patient has a painful neck, a recognized herniated cervical disk, or has had previous surgery on the cervical vertebrae. While the patient is awake and cooperative, careful testing should establish the limits of painless head and neck motion. Once anesthesia is established, these limits should be strictly observed:

- Head rotation and neck flexion should be avoided during the turn.
- In the lateral position the head should be supported so that lateral angulation of the cervical spine is prevented.
- If the patient is to be pronated, the three-pin head

holder is a good choice for firm fixation of an intact adult skull in a position that will avoid stress on the neck.

Problems relating to an unstable cervical spine are discussed in the section on turning injuries earlier in this chapter.

CERVICAL VASCULAR (VERTEBROBASILAR ARTERY) INJURY. Hyperextension and rotation of the head cause stretch compression block and sometimes rupture of the contralateral (to rotation) vertebral artery.

The vertebral arteries are uniquely susceptible to mechanical injury. They ascend vertically in the foramina transversara of the first six cervical vertebrae. On exit from the foramina of the axis, they pass outward to reach the foramina or grooves in the atlas. The arteries then penetrate the strong atlantoccipital ligament, enter the spinal canal, and pass through the foramen magnum to enter the cranial cavity.

The arteries are vulnerable to mechanical injury at three sites: during ascent in the foramina of the cervical vertebrae, at the junction of the axis with the atlas, and as they pass over the atlas at the cervicocranial junction to enter the skull. The arteries are especially susceptible to stretching and to shearing forces. Thus, sudden rotation of the head, hyperextension, and sudden acceleration-deceleration movements are likely to cause injury. Greater vulnerability exists in the presence of cervical osteophytes and coexistent atherosclerosis.

Symptoms are more likely when the compromised artery is dominant or if the contralateral artery terminates in the posterior inferior cerebellar artery, instead of the basilar artery, without providing good collateral flow.

Vascular injury with diminished flow of the posterior inferior cerebellar artery produces the lateral medullary infarction syndrome (the stroke syndrome related to chiropractic manipulation). Physical findings include loss of ipsilateral cranial nerve function of V, IX, X, and XI; cerebellar ataxia; Horner's syndrome; and contralateral loss of pain and temperature sensation. Quadriplegia combined with loss of cranial nerve function may occur; this is known as "locked-in" syndrome.

Injuries to the Cervical Spinal Cord

Patients whose cervical spines are unstable are at risk of cord compression or transection with any motion of the head or neck, and particularly so when major body repositioning is undertaken. (See previous discussion of neck injuries during repositioning. See also Gravenstein.[19])

The presence of neck pain resulting from a protruded cervical disk also requires extreme caution and precision of neck stabilization during positioning, even though the threat of injury involves nerve roots more often than the cervical cord itself. The same degree of attention should be paid to neck stabilization when an asymptomatic cervical disk is present as when a cord injury is present. Particular caution should be applied during endotracheal intubation.

MIDCERVICAL TETRAPLEGIA. Within the past decade, midcervical tetraplegia has been recognized as a rare but devastating complication of the sitting position in which neck flexion and head rotation probably combine to stretch the spinal cord and compromise its vasculature.[10,20,21] The result is functional transection of the spinal cord at about the C5–6 level.

Levy[22] reported an adult male, left tied up for 12 hours in a position of extreme neck flexion by bandits, who developed signs of cervical spinal cord damage. In five of six anesthetized, seated monkeys, Cottrell[23] found that neck hyperflexion disrupted neural transmission through the cervical cord; the "normal" monkey, however, was quadriplegic on awakening. Midcervical tetraplegia has occurred in an infant who was operated on while in the supine position with the neck flexed but the chin still free of the chest and the head not rotated.[19] In adults, the role of spondylosis or a previously asymptomatic spondylitic bar in the causation of midcervical tetraplegia is speculated on but uncertain.[19]

While only a few instances of midcervical tetraplegia exist in the world literature, and an uncommon anomalous vasculature of the cervical spinal cord may need to be present if positioning is to produce tetraplegia, the complication is not restricted to the sitting position. Hyperflexing a patient's neck in any surgical posture should be considered dangerous.

CERVICAL SYMPATHETIC CHAIN INJURIES. Positioning injuries to cervical sympathetic nerves are either rare or are unrecognized as such. Jaffe[24] reported a patient who experienced a Horner's syndrome of 3 days' duration in the nondependent eye following an operation in the flexed lateral decubitus (kidney) position. He attributed the occurrence to a stretched cervical sympathetic chain.

CERVICAL PLEXUS PAIN. Except the first cervical nerve, the cervical plexus is predominantly sensory (C2, 3, 4, roots). The nerves emerge from the intervertebral foramina where they are held firmly in place by fibrous tunnels that are especially affixed at the tips of the transverse processes. The series of loops formed by the ascending and descending branches are intertwined in both a superficial and deep plexus. Although there is no peripheral point of fixation, under certain circumstances a stretch of these nerves may occur, causing annoying neck and shoulder pain. The circumstances are:

198 *General Anesthesia*

1. Trendelenburg position.
2. Shoulder brace at the acromio-clavicular point and the arm pulled down at patient's side.
3. Head turned to opposite side with cervical rotation.

The pain is rather constant, dull, and aching. It persists for an average of three weeks. The mechanism is simply that of stretch.[8a]

BRACHIAL PLEXUS INJURIES

Because the brachial plexus is long, anchored at its origin in the neck and in the axillary fascia,[25] and adjacent to mobile bony structures, it is easily susceptible to positioning injuries (Fig. 8–2). McAlpine[26] reviewed several reported series of peripheral nerve complications occurring following surgery and found that the most frequent damage was to the brachial plexus or its peripheral units. One of those series, constituting 421 consecutive thoracotomies for cardiac surgery, reported 63 neural complications, and 29 of the 63 involved components of the brachial plexus. McAlpine[26] also reemphasized a rapid method of identifying nerve injuries.

If the neck of a supine patient is allowed to flex laterally[27a] or if the head is unsupported when the patient is in the lateral position,[1] the plexus roots on the side of the obtuse neck–shoulder angle can be stretched and injured. A similar traction injury can be inflicted on the plexus of a patient who is anchored on the table by wrist restraints and who shifts cephalad while in a significant degree of head-down tilt.

Compression injuries to the brachial plexus can occur in several ways. A shoulder brace placed medially against the base of the neck can compress or stretch the roots of the plexus. Abduction of the arm may accentuate this risk.

If the acromioclavicular joint is pushed caudad, the clavicle can compress the brachial neurovascular bundle as it crosses the underlying first rib. When the arm is abducted and arranged in such a way that the head of the humerus is thrust into the axilla, the axillary neurovascular bundle can be stretched and compressed.

The Suprascapular Nerve

Schweiss[1] has identified diffuse shoulder pain caused by ventral circumduction of the shoulder sufficient to produce traction on the suprascapular nerve. The nerve is fixed at its origin and in the suprascapular notch that ventral circumduction of the scapula moves away from the spine. Blocking the nerve or freeing it by severing the ligament that closes the notch reportedly relieves the pain.

The Long Thoracic Nerve of Bell

The long thoracic nerve was described by Bell in 1825[28] and detailed in 100 cadavers by Horwitz and Tocantins[29] in 1938. It arises immediately from the anterior branches of spinal roots C5, 6, and 7 (and rarely C8), is long and unbranched, and is the sole supply to the serratus anterior muscle. C5 and 6 fibers are anchored by passage through the substance of the middle scalene muscle and join C7 fibers just beyond that muscle to complete the nerve trunk. The nerve is potentially subject to traction by con-

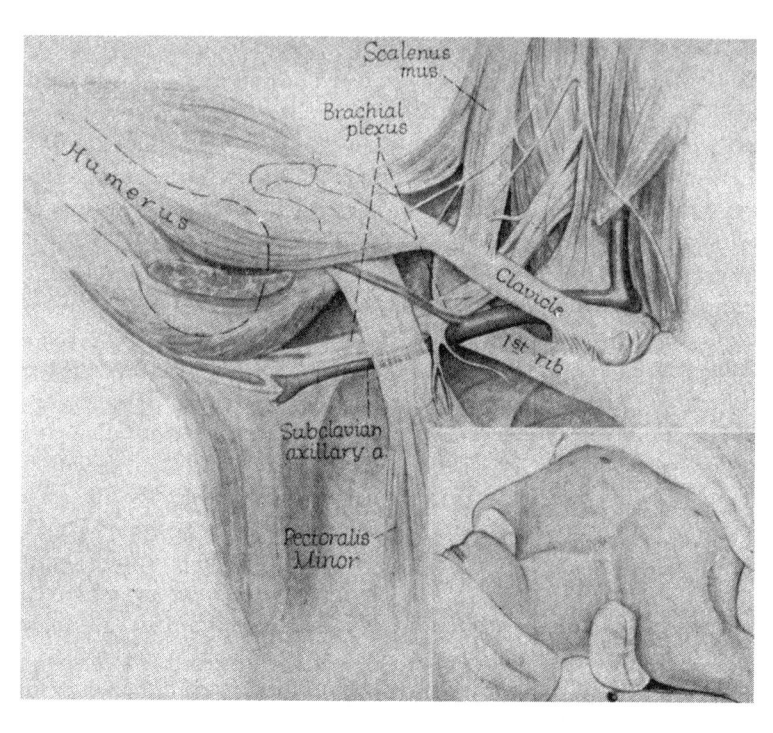

FIG. 8–2. Anatomic relationship of the brachial plexus. The four important structures that modify the course of the brachial plexus from the cervical transverse process to the axillary fascia are shown. From Slocum, H.C., O'Neal, K.C., and Allen, C.R.: Neurovascular complications from malposition on operating table. Surg. Gynecol. Obstet., 86:729, 1948.

tralateral tilt of the head and neck and to compression by adjacent structures that include the bursae and the clavicle.[29]

The serratus anterior muscle is a broad, flat muscle arising from the upper eight or nine ribs in the midaxillary line and inserting along the vertebral edge of the scapula. It helps to rotate the scapula ventrally, to elevate the abducted arm overhead, and to anchor the scapula to the chest wall. Also, it acts as an accessory muscle of inspiration when the scapula and upper extremity are fixed. When its function is impaired, the vertebral border of the scapula protrudes dorsally (the "winged" scapula), the shoulder droops caudad, and the arm cannot be raised beyond 90 degrees when abducted laterally.

Johnson[30a] reviewed 111 instances of long thoracic nerve palsy and found that 83% were right sided. In his series 45% were associated with acute (a blow to the neck) or chronic trauma (e.g., certain sports, knapsack straps); 31% were blamed upon causes that were quite doubtful; 12% were associated with recent obstetric deliveries or operations at remote body sites; and another 12% were considered idiopathic. Thus, 43% of the cases were of either doubtful or unknown cause. Foo[30b] presented 20 more cases and concluded that, in view of the uncertain causation in almost half of the cases, a likely cause was neuralgic amyotrophy (an entity of possible viral origin that causes pain followed by neural dysfunction).

The idea that postural trauma may affect the long thoracic nerve was recognized in 1947 by Lorhan,[30c] but the entity is unpublished in anesthesia literature until recently[30d] and is so rare that it is virtually unknown to the community of anesthesiologists.* An instance of pain in the upside shoulder and neck, experienced while the patient was unmedicated and in the lateral position for an epidural anesthetic, subsided when the supine position was resumed; surprisingly, that brief painful episode was followed in several days by the appearance of a winged scapula on the involved side.[30d] Nevertheless, routine care in patient handling and positioning should suffice to protect the patient from the rare appearance of such a neuropathy. A current report of a series of litigated occurrences of postoperative long thoracic nerve palsy,[30e] inferring from Foo's reasoning,[30b] contends that many instances of the dysfunction may represent an isolated and coincidental viral mononeuropathy and not an obligatory sequel of some type of positioning trauma.

The Thoracic Outlet Syndrome and Positioning

Patients who cannot elevate their arms over their heads during work or sleep without experiencing tingling, numbness, or pain in one or both arms should be considered at risk for serious damage to the brachial plexus if a similar posture is arranged during anesthesia. The affliction is apparently due to a restricted thoracic outlet or to an aberrant cervical rib and is frequently manifested by paresthesias or pain in the distribution of the ulnar nerve (C8–T1). Usually it is well recognized by the patient, who has learned what arm positions to avoid. A history of symptoms possibly due to a thoracic outlet syndrome should be deliberately inquired about in the preanesthetic interview of a candidate for surgery in the prone position,[8] and arm positions (extended overhead) that might activate it should not be utilized during anesthesia. When it occurs as a postoperative complication, brachial plexus pain from this cause is apt to be devastating, protracted, and very difficult to relieve.

PERIPHERAL NERVE INJURIES[27a]

Peripheral injuries to nerves derived from the cervical root are not uncommon. Because of their course and superficiality, the musculo-spiral, or radial, nerve and the ulnar nerve are especially vulnerable.

RADIAL NERVE PALSY.[27b] (Functional name: Extensor-Assistant Supinator Nerve.) All too frequently an improperly secured arm may sag during prolonged surgery and be compressed against the operating table. If the inner aspect of the upper arm rests against the table rail, the patient will awaken with a loss of hand control—the well-known wrist drop or "Saturday night palsy."

ULNAR NERVE PARALYSIS. During surgery the arm may be secure but allow a slight sag, enough that only the elbow rests on the table rail. The ulnar nerve may now be compressed at the "funny bone" site, and a paralysis of the flexor digitorum profundus muscle may result (Fig. 8–3). The functional name of the ulnar nerve is the "Finger Spreader—Approximator" (Fig. 8–3).

Diagnosis. Subsequent inability to spread or approximate the fingers results in a "claw" or "clergyman's" hand. The patient cannot form an "O" with thumb and index finger, scratch his palm, or hold a sheet of paper between his fingers.

MEDIAN NERVE PALSY. The median nerve, or flexor-pronator-thumb-finger-approximator, this nerve is not exempt from injury, as described by Pask.[27c] The median nerve lies superficially in the antecubital fossa just medial to the lacertus fibrosus tendon. Whenever infusions are administered via the medial antecubital vein, solutions can infiltrate to cause nerve ischemia or direct irritation; solutions containing thiopental or 10% dextrose have been im-

---

* Boals, D.C.: Personal communication, 1989.

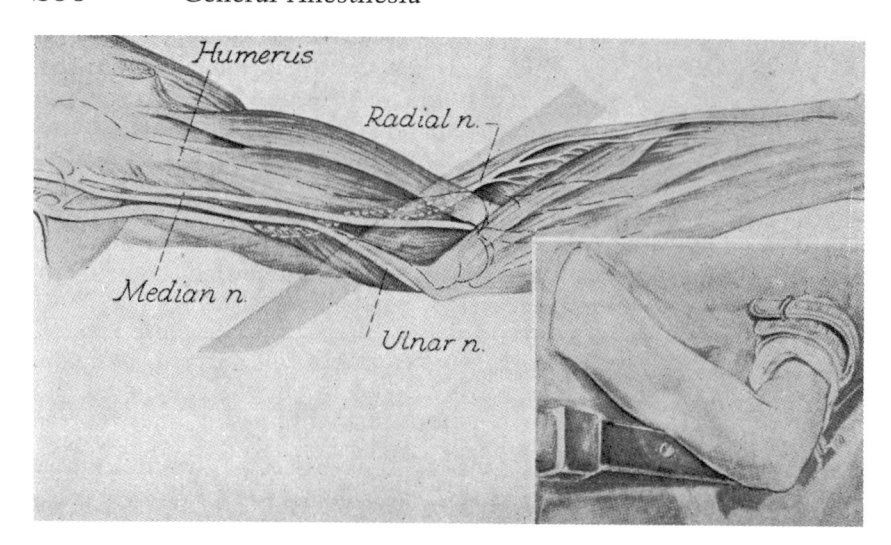

FIG. 8–3. Schema of nerves in the upper arm subject to injury. Insert shows pressure of operating room table guard-rail against inner aspect of arm. The ulnar nerve is particularly vulnerable. From Slocum, H.C., O'Neal, K.C., and Allen, C.R.: Neurovascular complications from malposition on operating table. Surg. Gynecol. Obstet., 86:729, 1948.

plicated. Demyelinization with subsequent paralysis occurs.

COMPLICATIONS INVOLVING THE THORAX

ASPIRATION PNEUMONITIS. With a patulous esophagus, a supine patient is at risk of aspiration of regurgitated gastric contents. Consequently, if an awake endotracheal intubation is not a useful choice, a rapid induction and cricoid pressure with either some degree of head elevation or significant head-down tilt should be considered as a protective maneuver prior to intubation.

THE TRAUMATIZED CHEST. An unstable or traumatized chest wall can seriously affect the choices of positioning for a surgical patient. In the lateral position, further compression of a down-side lung can be an atelectatic threat to its function. If ribs are newly broken or are incompletely healed, jagged ends may penetrate the lung to produce a pneumothorax. Shortening of the antero–posterior dimension of the chest in the prone position can be sufficient to obstruct grafted coronary arteries as the heart shifts ventrad due to gravity.[31]

The multiply traumatized patient with an unstable chest wall who requires an emergency decompressive laminectomy can be a difficult management problem.

BREASTS. The prone position is often a threat to a woman's breast and may be uncomfortable for the man with gynecomastia. Breast augmentation prostheses have been collapsed when the patient is placed in the prone position.[8] Stressed skin over the site of a mastectomy can be damaged by ventral supports when the patient is pronated and may require regrafting. Newly engorged lactating breasts may be tender and quite painful following surgery with the patient in the prone position.

True mammomegaly produces an unstable support for a pronated patient and may require an alternative position for spinal surgery. Longitudinal supporting frames can produce unequal pressure on large breasts and should be avoided. Supporting the thorax by folding bed sheets into a wide stack thick enough to raise the ventral chest wall off the table and free the abdomen[32] will distribute the patient's weight more evenly and less damagingly over large breasts. Recently available mechanical chest hoists may not extend laterally enough to encompass extremely large breasts and can produce uneven pressure that results in postoperative breast discomfort.

Because breasts that are thrust laterally under stress may tear and bleed in the upper inner quadrant, Martin[8] has advocated that breasts of a pronated patient be moved medially between chest rolls or pedestal-type ventral supports. Wrinkled sheets or sharp edges of supports should not contact breasts that are bearing the weight of the patient's thorax.

VENOUS AIR EMBOLUS. Venous air embolus occurs when the circulatory pressure in a vein falls below atmospheric, a hole appears in its wall, and the vessel is exposed to the atmosphere. Instead of pressure within the vein being sufficient to extrude blood through the leak, atmospheric pressure forces air into the lumen from whence it is disseminated systemically. When air reaches the heart it converts the normally noncompressible blood mass into compressible foam that absorbs and wastes the expulsive force of myocardial contraction. Foam that reaches the pulmonary microvasculature obstructs flow, reduces left atrial filling, and compromises cardiac output. (See also the previous discussion of paradoxical air embolism.)

A progressively widening pressure differential occurs as veins become raised above the level of the heart, the rate of pressure decrease being 2 mm Hg per vertical inch (2.5 centimeters) of elevation.[33] In the presence of a strong spontaneous inspiratory effort, or struggling inspiration because of partial airway obstruction, the gradient widens. Intermittent positive pressure with a significant increase in mean intrathoracic pressure throughout the respiratory cycle decreases the gradient. The degree of gradient needed to entrain air is uncertain.

Albin[34] believes that air has been embolized in prone patients with gradients of only 5 cm (4 mm Hg pressure differential). In the average patient who is placed in a classic sitting position, the circle of Willis is about 9 inches (22–23 cm) above the atria with an end expiratory venous pressure differential at an occipital wound of about 18 mm Hg. The head-elevated, prone, and lateral positions have similar pressure gradients, although each may be of lesser magnitude than the sitting gradient. Neither posture eliminates the opportunity for embolization of air.

For a more complete review of venous air embolism, the reader is referred to discussions by Shapiro[35] and by Glenski and colleagues.[36]

COMPLICATIONS INVOLVING THE ABDOMEN

USE OF THE TRENDELENBURG POSITION. Using the Trendelenburg position to improve exposure of pelvic viscera is a familiar technique in most surgical practices. Strictly speaking, the minimal degree of head-down tilt now in use in most surgical practices (10–15 degrees) should be termed a *Scultetus position*; Trendelenburg used much steeper tilt (30–45 degrees) as well as a break at knees to lower the foreleg.

Any degree of head dependency is hazardous in the presence of intracranial pathology and should be avoided. By increasing cerebral venous pressure and accelerating the formation of cerebral edema, the head-down tilt can intensify a neurologic defect or impair the postanesthetic level of consciousness of the patient.

As noted in Chapter 7, abundant evidence condemns the use of the Trendelenburg position as a resuscitative measure with which to treat shock.

VISCERAL STOMAS. Patients who have visceral stomata present on the abdominal wall are at risk of having a stoma injured if it is caught between a support and the body wall when placed in the prone position.

INTRA-ABDOMINAL MASSES. The presence of large intra-abdominal masses usually prevents use of the prone position. Not only is balance difficult, but the mass may cause pressure to be transmitted to the great vessels at the spine with resulting obstruction to flow in the aorta and vena cava. If the prone position must be used, a kneeling position with the chest elevated on some type of padded support may be tolerable. With the mass hanging relatively free from the dorsal abdominal wall, the potential for a venous air embolus should be seriously considered; appropriate monitoring and therapeutic modalities should be present.

In the supine position large abdominal masses can compress the aorta and vena cava. The supine hypotensive syndrome, due to aortocaval compression, is a familiar entity in obstetrics. It is relieved by elevating the right hip sufficiently to shift the uterine bulk into the left hemiabdomen and restore perfusion.

STABILIZATION BRACES. Not infrequently, a patient who is placed in a lateral position will have the down-side thigh properly flexed to almost a right angle on the trunk and then have a vertical rest shoved tightly against the abdominal wall. The intention of the rest is to help stabilize the torso when the more usual retaining strap across the hips would encroach on the operative site. Unfortunately, what it actually does is to impair diaphragmatic mobility and contribute to dysfunction of the down-side lung. Stability of the trunk should be sought by a less damaging method.

COMPLICATIONS INVOLVING THE SPINE

POSTOPERATIVE BACKACHE. Postoperative backache is not uncommon after operations done with the patient in one of the dorsal decubitus positions, as well as the lithotomy position particularly in females despite the fact that no injurious event has occurred during the anesthetic to create the problem. The probable cause is ligamentous stretch due to relaxation incidental to the anesthetic and paraspinous muscle relaxation that allows a change in the configuration of the lordotic lumbar spine. Neither regional nor general anesthesia is more apt to be associated with a postanesthetic backache. Brown[37a] showed that the duration of surgery was a more important issue than the type of anesthetic. Support placed under the lumbar spine prior to anesthesia can be used to maintain lordosis intraoperatively. If the patient has points about the lumbar spine that are tender to pressure, the lumbar support may not be tolerated and backache may be almost inevitable.

An important study by Donovan et al.[37b] has shown that a simple lumbar support using an inflatable bag or pillow (an inflatable 3-liter urological solution bag from Travenol Laboratories) will reduce the incidence and severity of backache. In a study by Hickmott et al.[37c] such an inflatable bag attached to a sphygmomanometer-aneroid gauge system was placed under the lumbosacral spine of volunteers to determine the bag pressure providing a maximum comfort pressure (MCP) for the subjects. A mean MCP was determined to be about 25 mm Hg or less for the supine position and about 35 mm Hg for the lithotomy position.

Among risk factors identified was that of the type

of table or surface. A hard table provided better comfort and lower pressures for MCP than did soft tables. Procedures lasting less than 40 minutes did not affect the occurrence of backache. Longer procedures by maintaining and prolonging ligamentour stretch was a major risk factor.

The use of the inflatable support applied to the individual's maximum comfort pressure reduced the incidence of backache from 46% to 21%. Patients with a preexisting back problem had an incidence of 56% backache if unsupported, but this was reduced to 22% when the lumbar support was used.

DISCOGENIC PAIN. The lack of postural reflexes and protective muscle spasm during anesthesia may allow muscular and ligamentous relaxation that worsens the status of a symptomatic herniated nucleus pulposis. If motion of the lower extremities is not carefully coordinated, or if torsion of the spine occurs during positioning, a partially extruded disc may become increasingly symptomatic.

In the dorsal decubitus position, the lawn chair variant usually offers more postural comfort than does the noncontoured, flat horizontal position.

When an operation requires the use of some version of the lithotomy position, prudence suggests that the patient's ability to tolerate the intended posture be tested by gently arranging the position prior to inducing the anesthetic. Increased distress strongly indicates that an alternative posture should be chosen.

The lateral lumbar flexion used in the flexed lateral position is particularly dangerous in the presence of a symptomatic lumbar disc.

IMPROPER DISENGAGEMENT FROM LITHOTOMY. In a stable back without a protruded lumbar disk, significant torsion of the lumbar spine can occur if the lower extremities are not raised and lowered simultaneously. Pain may result, arising either from the facets of lumbar vertebrae or from the joints of the sacrum and ilium. Putting one leg into lithotomy while the other is flat may be needed in an orthopedic procedure but it should be done carefully; its use in other specialties should require deliberate justification and the clear lack of a suitable alternative. Similarly, one leg should not be lowered from lithotomy while the other remains elevated.

To terminate the lithotomy position, both legs must be lowered slowly together. Rapid lowering enlarges vascular capacitance faster than it can be reflexly adjusted to available circulating blood volume. Hypotension results and may be marked if replacement of shed blood has been inadequate, the concentration of anesthesia is excessive, or vasomotor reflexes have been weakened by disease or debilitation.

THE UNSTABLE SPINE. The problem of the unstable cervical spine has been discussed in the section on problems encountered during turning a patient.

If instability exists in the thoracic or lumbar spine and the patient is to be turned from the supine to the lateral or prone position, the entire torso should be moved gently at one time without torsion or bending.

For the prone position, longitudinal supporting frames have a probable advantage over the four-pedestal type in that they have less chance of permitting movement at the point of instability that might have a scissoring action on elements of the spinal canal.

COMPLICATIONS INVOLVING THE EXTREMITIES

ARMS

Injuries to the arms during patient movement or positioning are discussed in the earlier sections of this chapter. Plexus injuries, concerns about the neurovascular bundle, and the problem of a cervical rib or the thoracic outlet syndrome are also discussed, as well as the principal peripheral nerve injuries to which the arms are susceptible (Fig. 8–3).

Lateral pressure on the outer surface of the upper arm, about at the junction of the middle and lower thirds of the humerus, can compress the radial nerve.

Whether the forearm is flexed or extended at the elbow, a pronated hand usually causes the notch (cubital tunnel) that contains the ulnar nerve on the medial dorsal surface of the elbow to rest against the surface of the operating table or arm board. Compression of the nerve at the notch may produce dysesthesias and anesthesia in its peripheral distribution that may be temporary and of variable duration or permanent.

Ulnar nerve dysfunction following a surgical procedure is a familiar issue for litigation. Deliberate and specific protection should be provided for the elbow of an arm that is either retained by the side of the patient or extended on a padded arm board. The anesthesia record should contain a notation to that effect.

Should a postoperative ulnar dysfunction occur, establishing its time of onset is an issue of maximum importance. If symptoms appear immediately following anesthesia (termination of regional anesthesia or arousal from general anesthesia), the cause of distress is likely to be associated with the time frame of the anesthetic. When the onset of symptoms is delayed beyond the stay of the patient in the recovery room, the cause of the distress is rarely associated with the events of the anesthetic; it is more logically associated with subsequent nursing care. Allegations commonly have been made that the recognition of ulnar dysfunction may be delayed by the presence of postoperative narcotic medications. While these drugs alleviate pain, they are not capable of reversing the hypesthesia or anesthesia that immediately accompanies ulnar injuries. Hence, the recovery room record is helpful if it regularly records the presence of sensation in ulnar distributions prior to the discharge of the patient.

Straps retaining arms on arm boards should be snug enough to retain the arm immobile but not tight enough to compress muscles on the volar surface of the forearm. The anterior interosseous nerve, a terminal branch of the median nerve, and its accompanying artery lie on or just superficial to the volar surface of the dense interosseous membrane. Compression of the volar muscle mass by a restraining strap, particularly if the perfusion pressure in that extremity is low, has been alleged to be the cause of a postoperative "anterior interosseous nerve syndrome," an ischemic injury similar to a compartment syndrome in the lower extremity (see following discussion). With the thousands of opportunities daily for such an event to occur, its astonishing rarity as a postoperative complication makes the alleged mechanism of its occurrence almost totally invalid. Nevertheless, the avoidance of undue constriction of the forearm by restraining devices is prudent. When the forearm in question has suffered recent trauma, the precaution is even more pertinent.

Acceptable arm positions vary according to the needs of the surgical team and the requirement for access to intravascular lines. Details are discussed in the chapter on the techniques of positioning.

In the dorsal decubitus position one or both arms can be placed on a well-padded arm board and abducted no more than 90 degrees from the sagittal plane of the torso. Additional abduction thrusts the head of the humerus into the axillary neurovascular bundle, threatening both a neural stretch injury and obstructive ischemia distally.

In the semiprone or posttonsillectomy position, the down-side arm should be placed just behind the torso to prevent: injury to the sternoclavicular joint; ventral circumduction of the shoulder that could stretch the suprascapular nerve; or neural compression and ischemic injury to the axillary neurovascular bundle.

When the patient who is placed in a full lateral position is allowed to rotate dorsally into the semisupine position, the arm on the side of the elevated shoulder can develop significant problems.

If the extremity is unsupported and extended dorsally, the shoulder joint is at risk of dislocation as the head of the humerus is forced against the ventral aspects of the joint capsule.

Dorsal shift of the acromioclavicular and glenohumeral joints may allow the clavicle to injure the brachial plexus and subclavian vessels by compressing them against the underlying first rib.

Useful solutions include strapping the arm to the side of the patient (although this is rarely used because the arm is almost always in the way of the surgical field) or restraining the arm on a well-padded overhead "ether screen" (see Fig. 7-2 in Chapter 7). If the arm is to be elevated on an ether screen, it must: remain well perfused, despite its wrappings; be protected from inadvertent contact with metal that could serve as a grounding path for the electrocautery unit; have firm support under the elevated shoulder to prevent dorsad displacement of the torso that could cause traction on the up-side humerus sufficient to produce a stretch injury of the brachial neurovascular bundle.

DIAGNOSIS OF PERIPHERAL NERVE INJURIES (ARM). Peripheral injuries to nerves derived from the cervical root are rather distressingly frequent. The musculo-spiral nerve or radial nerve and the ulnar nerve because of their course and superficial situation are quite vulnerable.

Radial Nerve Palsy. (Functional name: Extensor-Assistant Supinator Nerve.) All too frequently an improperly secured arm may sag during prolonged surgery and be compressed against the operating table. If the inner aspect of the upper arm rests against the table rail, the patient will awaken with a most distressing loss of hand control—the well-known wrist drop or "Saturday night palsy."

Ulnar Nerve Paralysis. The security of the arm may allow a slight sag, but enough so that only the elbow rests on the table rail. The ulnar nerve may now be compressed at the "funny bone site" and a paralysis of the flexor digitorum profundus muscle may result. The functional name of the ulnar nerve is the "Finger Spreader—Approximator" (Fig. 8-3).

Diagnosis. Inability to spread or approximate the fingers results in the claw hand or the clergyman's hand. The patient cannot form an "O" with thumb and index finger, scratch his palm, or hold a sheet of paper between fingers.

It is rather distressing for the patient and difficult for the doctor to explain to the patient why he, the patient, is going about his daily business with one hand ever in the position of a clergyman's benediction.

Median Nerve Palsy. The functional name of the median nerve is the flexor-pronator-thumb-finger-approximator. This nerve is not exempt from injury and such injury has been described by Pask.[27a] The mechanism of the compression and ischemia is somewhat different. The median nerve is rather superficial in the antecubital fossa just medial to the lacertus fibrosus tendon. Whenever infusions are administered through the medial antecubital vein, it is possible for infiltration of solutions to cause nerve ischemia or direct irritation; solutions containing thiopental or 10% dextrose have been implicated. Demyelinization with subsequent paralysis occurs.

FINGER HAZARDS

Fingers must be protected from contact with metal table edges that could provide low-resistance grounding pathways for current derived from the use of an electrocautery unit.

A less well-recognized hazard to fingers is the potential that they might protrude into the hinge mechanism of an operating table while the foot section was lowered to provide perineal access to a patient in the lithotomy position. When that foot section is subsequently raised to the horizontal level to accommodate the lowered legs of the patient at the conclusion of the need for lithotomy position, the protruding fingers can be scissored and amputated by the approximating edges of the foot and thigh surfaces of the table.[38] Welborn[39] has advocated wrapping each hand in a protective towel as a routine precaution against this injury when patients are placed in the lithotomy position.

LOWER EXTREMITIES

Lower extremities that are to be inactive and dependent during anesthesia have the potential of pooling a significant volume of blood and accentuating the significance of the amount of shed blood during an operation. Elastic wrappings that compress the lower legs, and possibly the thighs, without being tight enough to cause ischemia, can reduce the available vascular space in the extremities and minimize pooling of blood.

Padded protective heel cushions should be provided for the patient who is to spend hours in a dorsal decubitus position. Some type of supportive angulation should keep the foot at an approximately 90-degree angle with the lower leg in the supine, sitting, or prone positions in order to avoid postoperative foot drop.

If the lower extremities are flexed at the hip while the lower leg remains almost fully extended on the thigh, the sciatic nerve can be stretched and damaged. This mishap can occur either in the sitting position or, more infrequently, in the "high lithotomy position," an unusual version of lithotomy in which each leg is slung either from ankle straps or from a bootie on the foot to a high leg pole. Also at risk are the contents of the femoral canal when markedly angulated under the inguinal ligament by extreme flexion of the thigh on the trunk. Postoperative femoral neuropathies have been associated with use of the high lithotomy position.

A lower leg that is elevated and secured on a rest that supports the popliteal fossa is at risk of being hypoperfused if systemic blood pressure falls. The popliteal support can contribute to perfusion problems in the lower leg if it compresses muscle tissue of the upper calf either because of tight restraining straps or because of the added weight of an arm of a surgical assistant who must reach across the elevated leg to help with the operation. Hypoperfusion that causes ischemia initiates edema in the tight fascial compartment of the leg. As compartmental pressure increases, perfusion is further reduced and a compartment syndrome develops. Myonecrosis causes myoglobinuria and renal damage. Prompt decompression of the swollen compartments by fasciotomies is usually needed to treat the syndrome; protection of the kidneys from damage due to free myoglobin is also required. Assurance of adequate perfusion of the extremity plus a noncompressive arrangement for the leg are necessary preventive measures.

When the leg holder consists of a vertical bar and an ankle sling, the bar lateral to the leg requires padding to prevent it from compressing the common peroneal nerve just below the knee. That same bar medial to the leg also requires padding to protect the saphenous nerve.

When a patient is placed in the lateral position, the retaining tapes that are placed across the up-side hip should be located between the lateral iliac crest and the head of the femur. If placed across the head of the femur, pressure may occlude its nutrient vessel and lead to subsequent aseptic necrosis.

The common peroneal nerve courses laterally around the upper fibula about 2–3 cm distal to its head and bifurcates shortly thereafter. In many thin legs the nerve is palpable and susceptible to compressive trauma. When a patient is placed in the lateral position, the down-side knee should be padded to protect that nerve.

When a patient is placed in the kneeling prone position, padding on the knee rest should be sufficient so that the weight being borne on the distal end of the femur will not injure the flexed knee joint and its exposed articular surfaces.

THERMAL INSTABILITY

Concern about monitoring and regulating the body temperature of anesthetized patients is now common to every operating suite. The vast majority of anesthetized patients currently have some form of temperature monitoring throughout anesthesia. Inadvertent hypothermia is the most frequently encountered problem, but malignant hyperpyrexia is the most devastating.

Although an operating room is usually warmed to prevent heat loss in an anesthetized infant, most operating rooms are kept cool to prevent distracting discomfort for members of the surgical team who must wear layers of protective clothing and labor under hot lights. In these cool rooms the patient loses heat by exposure to atmospheres that are cooler than body temperature and that rapidly turn over the circulating air mass. Inadvertent hypothermia is frequent with small or frail bodies. Operating rooms with rapid air exchanges that attempt to provide laminar flow are particularly hazardous to the thermal stability of the patient and are frequently quite uncomfortable for the anesthesia team as well.

Warming the operating room is known to be the most effective method of preventing heat loss by the patient. When that is not practical, devices to combat inadvertent hypothermia in a cool environment include:

- Circulating water mattresses. The fluid in these units can be heated or cooled as needed to stabilize the patient's temperature. Not infrequently the patient surface in contact with the mattress will be too small for effective heat exchange (e.g., the lateral position or the prone position using a ventral supporting frame). The units have problems with kinked fluid paths if pressure of the patient on the table surface is uneven, and they rarely can stop a major fall in temperature in a heavy patient. Often the warming coils leave erythematous stripes on the skin of the patient surface that contacts the mattress; depending on the temperature gradient between skin and mattress, blisters may occur.
- Empty plastic bags that can swath the arms and head of a patient. These are useful to reduce opportunities for radiant heat loss and prevent access of convection currents.
- Heated airway humidification units. These insert into the patient's breathing circuit to warm inhaled gases and prevent heat loss from the respiratory system. Careful and continuing measurement must be made of the patient's airway temperature to prevent burning the tracheobronchial tree.
- An electrician's trouble light. With a 75-watt bulb, this is an astonishingly effective device that can be placed near the patient under a tent of drapes to radiate warmth to the exposed torso or head and shoulders. Properly arranged, it can halt thermal drift in even a bulky patient and can raise esophageal temperature in most patients. The bulb must be shatterproof and the unit must be approved by the safety engineers in the biomedical unit or the hospital. It must be kept carefully away from contact with the patient's skin to prevent burning.

REFERENCES

1. Lawson, N.W.: The lateral position: Anesthesiologic considerations. *In* Positioning in Anesthesia and Surgery, 2nd ed. Edited by J.T. Martin. Philadelphia, WB Saunders, 1987.
2. Lee, C., Blarneys, A., and Nagel, E.L.: Neuroleptoanalgesia for awake pronation of surgical patients. Anesth. Analg., *56*:276, 1977.
3. Gormley, T., and Sokoll, M.D.: Permanent alopecia from pressure of a head strap. J.A.M.A., *199*:157, 1967.
4. Abel, R.R., and Lewis, G.M.: Postoperative alopecia. Arch. Dermatol., *81*:72, 1960.
5. Lawson, N.W., Mills, N.L., and Ochsner, J.O.: Occipital alopecia following cardiopulmonary bypass. J. Thorac. Cardiovasc. Surg., *71*:342, 1976.
6. Patel, K.D., and Henschel, E.O.: Postoperative alopecia. Anesth. Analg., *59*:311, 1980.
7. Grundy, B.L., et al.: Evoked potential changes produced by positioning for retromastoid craniectomy. Neurosurgery. *10*:766, 1982.
8a. Slocum, H.C., O'Neal, K.C., and Allen, C.R.: Neurovascular complications from malposition on operating table. Surg. Gynecol. Obstet., *86*:729, 1948.
8b. Martin, J.T.: The prone position: Anesthesiologic considerations. *In* Positioning in Anesthesia and Surgery, 2nd ed. Edited by J.T. Martin. Philadelphia, WB Saunders, 1987.
8c. Fuller, J.E., and Thomas, D.V.: Facial nerve paralysis after general anesthesia. J.A.M.A., *162*:645, 1956.
9. McPherson, R.W., et al.: Intracranial subdural gas: A cause of false positive change of intraoperative somatosensory evoked potential. Anesthesiology, *62*:816, 1985.
10. Standefer, M., Bay, J.W., and Trusso, R.: The sitting position in neurosurgery: A retrospective analysis of 488 cases. Neurosurgery, *14*:649, 1984.
11. Nornes, H., and Magnaes, B.: Supratentorial epidural pressure during posterior fossa surgery. J. Neurosurg., *35*:541, 1971.
12. Sherman, D.D., Hart, R.D., and Easton, J.D.: Abrupt change in head position and cerebral infarction. Stroke, *12*:2, 1981.
13. Kenning, J.A., Touting, S.M., and Saunders, R.L.: Upright patient positioning in the management of intracranial hypertension. Surg. Neurol., *15*:148, 1981.
14. Gronert, G.A., et al.: Paradoxical air embolism from a patent foramen ovale. Anesthesiology, *50*:548, 1979.
15. Edwards, J.E.: Interatrial communications. *In* Pathology of the Heart. Edited by S.E. Gould. Springfield, Charles C Thomas, 1960.
16. Hagen, P.T., Scholz, D.G., and Edwards, W.D.: Incidence and size of patent foramen ovale during the first ten decades: A necropsy study of 965 normal hearts. Mayo Clin. Proc., *59*:17, 1984.
17. Perkins-Pearson, N., Marshall, N., and Bedford, R.: Atrial pressures in the seated position. Anesthesiology, *57*:493, 1982.
18. Lynch, J.J., et al.: Prevalence of right-to-left atrial shunting in a healthy population: Detection by Valsalva maneuver and contrast echocardiography. Am. J. Cardiol., *53*:1478, 1984.
19. Gravenstein, N., Grundy, B.L., and Reid, S.A.: Complications of positioning: The central nervous system. *In* Positioning in Anesthesia and Surgery, 2nd ed. Edited by J.T. Martin. Philadelphia, WB Saunders, 1987.
19a. Schellhas, K.P., et al.: Vertebrobasilar injuries following cervical manipulation. J.A.M.A., *244*:1450, 1987.
20. Hitselberger, W.E., and House, W.F.: A warning regarding the sitting position for acoustic tumor surgery. Arch. Otolaryngol., *106*:69, 1980.
21. Wilder, B.L.: Hypothesis: The etiology of midcervical quadriplegia after operation with the patient in the sitting position. Neurosurgery, *11*:530, 1982.
22. Levy, L.M.: An unusual case of flexion injury of the cervical spine. Surg. Neurol., *17*:491, 1982.
23. Cottrell, J.E., et al.: Hyperflexion and quadriplegia in the sitting position. Anesthesiol. Rev., *12*:34, 1985.
24. Jaffe, T.B., and McLeskey, C.H.: Position-related Horner's syndrome. Anesthesiology, *56*:49, 1982.

25. Westin, B.: Prevention of upper limb nerve injuries in the Trendelenburg position. Acta Chir. Scand., *108*:61, 1954.
26. McAlpine, F.S., and Seckel, B.R.: Peripheral nervous system complications. *In* Positioning in Anesthesia and Surgery, 2nd ed. Edited by J.T. Martin. Philadelphia, WB Saunders, 1987.
27a. Britt, B.A., and Gordon, R.A.: Peripheral nerve injuries associated with anesthesia. Can. Anaesth. Soc. J., *11*:514, 1964.
27b. Norman, J.E.: Nerve palsy following general anesthesia. Anaesthesia, *10*:87, 1955.
27c. Pask, E.A., and Robson, J.G.: Injury to the median nerve. Anaesthesia, *9*:94, 1954.
28. Bell, J., and Bell, C.: Anatomy and Physiology of the Human Body, vol. 1. 5th Am ed. New York, Collins, 1827.
29. Horwitz, M.T., and Tocantins, L.M.: An anatomic study of the role of the long thoracic nerve and the related scapular bursae in the pathogenesis of local paralysis of the serratus anterior muscle. Anat. Rec., *71*:375, 1938.
30a. Johnson, J.T.H., and Kendall, H.O.: Isolated paralysis of the serratus anterior muscle. J. Bone Joint Surg. (Am.), *37A*:567, 1955.
30b. Foo, C.L.: Isolated paralysis of the serratus anterior: A report of 20 cases. J. Bone Joint Surg. *65B*:552, 1983.
30c. Lorhan, P.H.: Isolated paralysis of the serratus magnus following surgical procedures. Arch. Surg., *54*:656, 1947.
30d. Hubbert, C.H.: Winged scapula associated with epidural anesthesia. Anesth. Analg., *67*:418, 1988.
30e. Martin, J.T.: Postoperative isolated dysfunction of the long thoracic nerve: A rare entity of uncertain etiology. Anesth. Analg., *69*:614, 1989.
31. Weinlander, C.M., Coombs, D.W., and Plume, S.K.: Myocardial ischemia due to obstruction of an aortocoronary bypass graft during intraoperative positioning. Anesth. Analg., *64*:933, 1985.
32. Smith, R.H., Gramling, Z.W., and Volpitto, P.P.: Problems related to the prone position for surgical operations. Anesthesiology, *22*:189, 1961.
33. Enderby, G.E.H.: Postural ischemia and blood pressure. Lancet, *1*:185, 1954.
34. Albin, M.S., et al.: Atrial catheter and lumbar disk surgery (correspondence). J.A.M.A., *239*:496, 1978.
35. Shapiro, H.M.: Venous air embolism. *In* Anesthesia, 2nd ed. Edited by R.D. Miller. New York, Churchill Livingstone, 1986.
36. Glenski, J.A., Cucchiara, R.F., and Michenfelder, J.D.: Transesophageal echocardiography and transcutaneous O_2 and CO_2 monitoring for detection of venous air embolism. Anesthesiology, *64*:541, 1986.
37a. Brown, E.M., and Elman, D.S.: Postoperative backache. Anesth. Analg., *40*:683, 1961.
37b. O'Donovan, M., et al.: A Postoperative backache: The use of an inflatable wedge. Br. J. Anaesth., *58*:280, 1986.
37c. Hicknott, K.C., et al.: Back pain following general anaesthesia and surgery: Evaluation of risk factors and the effect of an inflatable lumbar support. Br. J. Surg., *75*(5):571, 1990.
38. Courington, F.W., and Little, D.M. Jr.: The role of posture in anesthesia. Clin. Anesth., *3*:24, 1968.
39. Welborn, S.G.: The lithotomy position: Anesthesiologic considerations. *In* Positioning in Anesthesia and Surgery, 2nd ed. Edited by J.T. Martin. Philadelphia, WB Saunders, 1987.

"Moreover individual treatment is better than a common system in Education as in Medicine."
—ARISTOTLE: *The Nicomachean Ethics,* X, IX, 15

The role of the anesthesiologist is that of consultant to the surgeon in reference to pharmacology and physiology.[1] The anesthesiologist engages in the practice of medicine in its broadest sense when acting as the internist in the operating room, managing physiologic dysfunction, pharmacologic needs, and medical complications that arise during the course of anesthesia and surgery. The anesthesiologist's province and sphere of activity are thus clearly defined: to provide a stress free anesthetic surgical state and to care for the physiologic changes in the patient so the surgeon can concentrate his attention and skills to the correction of anatomic abnormalities. Thus, the surgeon's skills are directed toward anatomy, whereas the anesthesiologist's are directed more toward physiology.

PSYCHOLOGICAL CONSIDERATIONS

INFLUENCE OF FEAR. The psychological state of the patient scheduled for surgery has a profound influence on the outcome of an operation.[2,3]

Sheffer[3] has identified some of the fears related to anesthesia that are normally experienced by the patient prior to surgery. These include the fear that he "may tell secrets"; that "the operation will start too soon"; that he "may wake up during surgery"; that he "may not wake up after surgery"; of suffocation; of mutilation; of vomiting; and of cancer.

The influence of fear can be represented schematically as leading to apprehension and anxiety, then to irritability of the nervous system, and finally to resistance to anesthesia. Each stage can be increased or decreased by many factors (Table 9–1).

Emotional responses of surgical patients to anesthesia include:[3]

1. Defensive reactions—based on suspicion and manifested by resistance, withdrawal, and lack of cooperation
2. Conversion reactions—fear is expressed in two

PREANESTHETIC EVALUATION AND PREPARATION

TABLE 9–1. INFLUENCE OF FEAR
(After Nicholson)

Stages of Fear	Increased by	Decreased by
Apprehension ↓	Nontherapeutic approach	Therapeutic approach
Irritability of nervous system ↓	Excitement Stimulants	Rest and adequate sleep in hospital Sedatives
Resistance to anesthesia	Chronic alcoholism Smoking	Premedication

ways: by unusual motor behavior and by autonomic responses
3. Sleep disturbances—found in 40%
4. Mood disturbances—found in 38%; manifested by fatigue, fixations, feelings of guilt and unworthiness
5. Distortion of reality—panic reaction was evident in 11% of patients

PREOPERATIVE VISIT. In making a preoperative visit, the psychologic power of the anesthesiologist can be exerted; the extent of this power will be measured by the confidence of the patient and rapport achieved. It is important to realize that the hospital and surgical experience is new and strange for most patients and that they want information and wish to understand.

Some suggestions for a successful approach have been outlined by Buskirk:[4]

1. Treat all patients as human beings.
2. Be friendly; explain your visit and your plan.
3. Be attentive, sympathetic, and understanding.
4. Be patient.
5. Work at winning the patient; listen to his concerns.
6. Answer all questions in an understanding and warm manner.
7. Allay patient's fears.

In concluding the visit reassure the patient, calm anxieties, and explain the procedures of the operative day so that the experience will not be totally strange. *An informed patient is a tranquil patient.*[2] The value of a preoperative visit by the anesthetist has been shown to be at least equivalent to 100 mg of pentobarbital in its calming effect and is superior in allaying anxiety and providing emotional support.[5]

Occasionally a preoperative psychiatric consultation is helpful or even necessary to review suspected cases of psychosis and psychoneurosis so that postoperative reactions and psychotic episodes can be avoided. Sometimes an elective procedure may be cancelled if it is likely to result in psychiatric complications.[6]

TYPES OF ANXIETY. Patients should be assessed regarding their ability to deal with anxiety because anesthesia and surgery create a high-stress situation.[7] There is always an emotional reaction to the knowledge that there is both physical danger and pain to be confronted. The mentally stable person weighs these risks against the benefits.

Spielberger has delineated two types of anxiety:[8]

1. *Situational or state anxiety:* the immediate short-term fear that a person may experience in response to environmental or situational stresses that suddenly confront him. Situational anxiety is a transitory state that varies in intensity and fluctuates with time; however, it is not disproportionately intense and is nonpathologic, with reasonable adaptive behaviors and coping styles. These patients require only sedative hypnotic medication preoperatively.
2. *Trait anxiety:* a personality disposition that remains stable over time; it is a type of chronic anxiety that represents a state of continuous interpersonal treat. This maladaptive personality type is likely to be associated with pathologic and neurotic responses. Apprehension and hyperresponsiveness, panic attacks, neurotic depression, and avoidance behavior may occur. These patients usually require a tranquilizer (i.e., benzodiazepines).

PSYCHOLOGICAL RESPONSES.[9] Hospitalization is a psychologically upsetting experience for anyone. Janis has studied psychologic stress in surgical patients and demonstrated that "preoperative briefing," enabling patients to know what to expect, reduced the number and severity of postoperative emotional problems.[9a]

Behavior changes are seen postoperatively in patients, especially children poorly prepared for anesthesia. Vernon[10] has identified six types of responses, which provide a mood scale:

1. General anxiety and regression
2. Separation anxiety
3. Anxiety about sleep
4. Eating and bowel disturbances

5. Aggression to authority
6. Apathy—withdrawal

VARIABLES IN ANXIETY. Age, duration of hospitalization, and occupational status (of parents, for children) are significant variables.

Emergence phenomena in the absence of adequate preoperative briefing include delirium, postoperative confusion, and disorientation. Illusions are frequent and disturbing, whereas hallucinations are not often encountered. A distinction must be made between these terms based on definitions of the American Psychiatric Association:

Illusion—the misinterpretation of a real, external sensory experience; may be visual, auditory, or proprioceptive.
Hallucination—a false sensory perception in the absence of an external sensory experience.

PSYCHOLOGICAL EFFECTS IN CHILDREN.[10,11] General anesthesia effects have been evaluated in children 5 to 8 years of age in the absence of preanesthetic medication. It has been demonstrated that there is impairment of tests of reasoning, motor ability, and memory functions at 2 hours postanesthesia. At the end of 24 hours, no significant impairment was detected; however, some transient behavioral and sleep changes did occur.

INCIDENCE OF ANXIETY.[12] Some important aspects of preoperative anxiety have been recognized. In particular, the type of surgery has been associated with unusual anxiety.[13] Surgery of the genitourinary tract engenders great anxiety in over 80% of patients; possible cancer surgery excites intense anxiety in 85% of patients, as does potentially disabling or disfiguring surgery. Moderate anxiety, however, is typical for patients experiencing most elective surgery, wherein only about 50% of such patients are seriously concerned and disturbed. A night sedative is not as effective in patients who are extremely anxious and who do not have a preoperative visit from the anesthetist; a tranquilizer is needed. The combination of a visit and a sedative is more effective. Anxiety is higher in women than men; it is higher in asthenic women weighing less than 70 kg than in those of normal weight or heavier.[12]

PREANESTHETIC ANXIETY OF CANCER PATIENTS.[7] Cancer patients have intense psychological problems that affect physiologic function and disposition of drugs significantly. The following stresses should be considered in evaluation:

- Different emotional and situational anxiety
- Concern about death
- Concern about mutilation
- Anxiety about eventual survival and disability
- Less concern about present risk
- The long-term risk and outcome outweigh the short-term risk of the immediate anesthesia and surgery, as perceived by the patient

Hooper[7] has shown that cancer patients with high anxiety levels have a shorter survival than those with low anxiety levels.

PERSONALITY AND DRUG RESPONSES.[14] Some relationship is known to exist between personality and drug responses.

A personality study has been recommended prior to depressant drug use, especially analgesics. Caution should be exercised in such drug use for patients previously addicted or habituation-prone.

It is apparent to most physicians that there is great variability in the effects of a drug administered at the same dosage, for the same length of time, to similar groups of patients. Some of the factors that explain the variability are[15]:

1. The constitutionally determined responsiveness of the patient
2. The environmental conditions, e.g., hospital or home, presence of pain, acute or chronic illness
3. The personality of the patient

PREDICTORS OF PAIN AND BEHAVIORAL DISORDERS.[16] The patient's response to postoperative pain can be predicted based on the preoperative level of anxiety: the degree of anxiety and the amount and type of information about the surgery or anesthesia requested or provided significantly affect the perception of pain and the intensity of response after surgery. The *McGill Pain Questionnaire* (MPQ)* measures the level of pain intensity. In contrast to those with trait anxiety, patients with state anxiety usually seek more information and are therefore better informed to exert some control over their situation and request pain medication appropriately. Although the preoperative level of anxiety is high and emerges as part of the situation, the postoperative requirement for analgesia is less. The intensity of anxiety is elevated preoperatively and declines postoperatively in these patients.

Behavioral disorders seem to appear more commonly in patients with trait anxiety. Neurotic depression does occur, and sleep disorders such as insomnia, abnormal sleep latency, and difficulty in falling asleep, are prone to develop. Poor absorption of medication is a physiologic concomitant.

CONSTITUTION AND PERSONALITY.[14,17] Many constitutional factors are considered in determining medication dosage: age, weight, sex, and physiologic

---

* The MPQ is a self-report measure of pain that uses adjectives to describe sensory, affective, and evaluative components of pain. The Pain Rating Index (PRI) is a part of MPQ that divides the descriptors into three classes.

condition are a few of those factors. Attempts to classify patients on the basis of their physical makeup have not been too fruitful; however, certain generalizations may be made, so the classification of patients according to their physical constitution has been of some use. Kretschmer has recognized four types of body build together with their reaction patterns:[17a]

1. Asthenic—tall, thin person: generally tense; overresponsive to stress; sometimes referred to as the vagotonic individual
2. Pyknic—short, heavy person; tendency to obesity: rather jovial and outgoing; may be referred to as the sympathotonic individual
3. Athletic—good build, well proportioned; lean and muscular: adjusts well to most situations
4. Dysplastic—physically handicapped: these persons tend to withdraw; are shy; do not like to be disturbed; prefer a sheltered existence and environment.

Identifying the attitudes associated with body build makes it possible to predict to some extent the person's reaction pattern and response to drugs. The asthenic individual may require significant sedation and tranquilization. The pyknic person may more likely respond to suggestion, so only mild sedation is necessary. The athletic person requires reduction of metabolic activity. The dysplastic person needs support to deal with his fear and suspicion.

Another challenging concept relating drugs and personality is McDougall's *Chemical Theory of Temperament*.[17b] It is thought that the dimension of personality can be *scaled* on a continuum of temperament from extroversion to introversion: (1) the markedly extroverted personality is susceptible to depressant drugs, including alcohol; and (2) the introvert is resistant to depressant drugs.

This has been tested by Eysenk[18] using the sedation threshold as a measurement to relate personalities according to the ease of sedation.

In the personality inventory score, extroversion is associated with few perioperative complaints, whereas introversion or neuroticism is associated with frequent and more intense complaints.[19]

ROLE OF SYMPATHETIC NERVOUS SYSTEM. Emotions have been correlated with adrenal output.[20] In general, the anxious but passively reacting individual has an elevated epinephrine output and excretion. On the other hand, in subjects with an outgoing personality and aggressive tendency, there is an increased excretion of norepinephrine. These observations may provide some understanding of the varying responses to stress (Fig. 9-1).[21]

It is of interest to note that two members of the animal kingdom contrast sharply in their hormonal output when faced with threatening situations: the lion has a predominant release of norepinephrine,

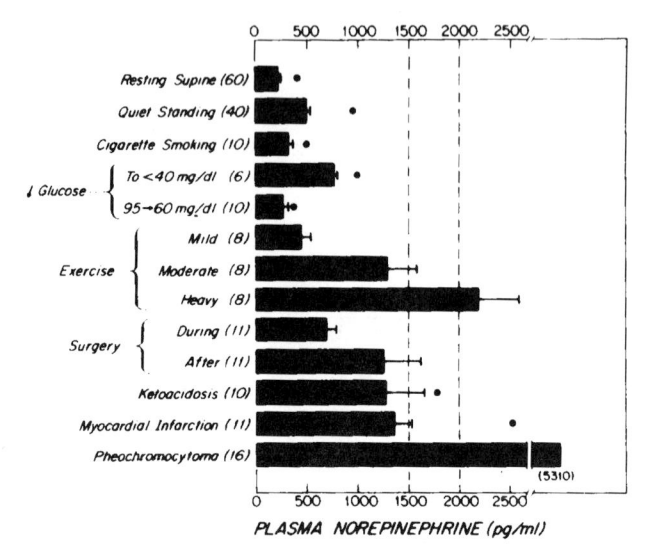

FIG. 9-1. Venous plasma levels of norepinephrine in various physiologic and pathophysiologic states in human beings (mean ± SEM). Numbers in parentheses indicate the number of persons studied; solid circles represent the highest value observed. Dashed lines encompass the range of concentrations required to produce measurable metabolic and hemodynamic changes in normal subjects. From Cryer, P.E. Plasma catecholamine levels in various physiologic and pathophysiologic states. N. Engl. J. Med., *303*:436, 1980.

whereas the rabbit, which usually flees, has a high output of epinephrine.

Psychological stress, as related to personality variables, can activate the sympathetic nervous system to the extent of precipitating life-threatening cardiac arrhythmias in the absence of underlying heart disease.[22] Ventricular tachyarrhythmias and sudden cardiac arrest have been reported. "Voodoo death," probably related to overactivity of the sympathoadrenal system, has been described during intense emotional stress by Cannon.[23] Many of these patients have been carefully evaluated, and some control of cardiac rhythm is accomplished by beta-blocker therapy. It is also of note that death from cardiac arrest due to *standstill* occurs more frequently in deeply depressed patients. Freud has described such instances as related to the psychology of the "death wish."[23b]

POSITIVE MEASURES TO REDUCE ANXIETY. Information about the possible reactions and experience of the anesthesia/surgery scenario results in significant reduction of anxiety. Reassurance and diversion are important approaches. Offering positive suggestions and assurance that there will be minimal but controlled pain and that medication will be available as needed greatly reduces anxiety about postoperative pain and its intensity. Poorly presented information may sensitize patients to preoperative stress and postoperative pain.[13]

PREANESTHETIC VISIT

Every surgical patient must be visited at the bedside by the anesthesiologist the day before an inhospital elective operation.[1,4,24] The visit should be both informative and supportive.[5] Egbert found that a beneficial 5-minute interview with a patient has the equivalent effect of 100 mg of pentobarbital in that anxiety is decreased and the degree of drowsiness is increased.[13] During the visit, there should be a complete assessment of the patient, including:

1. A pertinent personal and family history.
   a. Previous operations and anesthetics should be recorded and complications noted. Reactions of family members to anesthetics, especially hyperthermic reactions (malignant hyperthermia has a high associated mortality) should also be noted.
   b. Allergies: known drug reactions.
   c. Medications: many drugs prescribed by the patient's internist in the management of medical conditions may present significant interactions with anesthetic agents.
   d. Habits:
      (1) Use of alcohol
      (2) Drug addiction and use of drugs (inquire about "uppers" and "downers"; amphetamines, for example, when taken irregularly, increase the anesthetic requirement by 20% to 70%; if large doses are being taken, the anesthetic requirement may decrease by 20%)
      (3) Smoking (if excessive, postoperative pulmonary complications are increased sixfold[25]; smokers require more anesthetic and analgesic drugs than nonsmokers—a study of time/dose curves for pentazocine in anesthetized patients shows that there is more rapid metabolization of pentazocine in smokers[26]; oxidative enzymes are activated by smoking)[27]
2. Determination of physical condition by a pertinent physical examination and review of the patient's chart—pulse, blood pressure, and breathing patterns should be observed and recorded as part of the preanesthesia note; simple tests of pulmonary function and cardiovascular performance can be completed at the bedside.
   a. Physical habitus and weight: the patient's body build should be assessed. For this purpose, Kretschmer's classification is useful[17a]—four types of body build can be designated: asthenic, pyknic, athletic, and dysplastic (see "Constitution and Personality" in this chapter). Other qualifying adjectives such as obese, barrel-chested, or bull-necked may be included. The patient's weight should be recorded.
   b. General nutrition: dietary habits should be noted. Protein-calorie malnutrition can be judged by triceps skin fold and arm muscle circumference. (Standards have been prepared by the World Health Organization.[28,29])
   c. Facial characteristics: the contour of the face is assessed so that a properly fitting mask may be selected. Maxillary or mandibular deformities should be noted. Beards in men may represent a hazard because an adequate fit is difficult to obtain. Shaving of beards for surgery is required in some hospitals; that a spinal or epidural rather than general anesthetic may be given is not a compelling argument for not shaving the beard because these patients may require resuscitation.
   d. Dental hygiene: is evaluated and the presence of dentures noted. Full dentures may remain in situ when patients are transferred to the operating theater so a clear oral airway during induction can be maintained. This is especially important in emaciated and edentulous patients. When dentures are removed for any reason, such as during intubation, they should be carefully guarded.
   e. Airway check: the oral cavity should be checked for tongue size and deformities (e.g., cleft palate). The midline position of the trachea and any abnormal voice characteristics (such as hoarseness) should be noted. Patency of nares should be assessed for possible nasotracheal airway insertion or nasotracheal intubation.
3. Estimation of operative risk and designation of:
   a. ASA Physical Status grade
   b. American Heart Association functional class
   c. Goldman score
4. Choice of anesthetic technique and agent as well as informing the patient about the procedures to take place on the day of surgery.

ALCOHOLISM. Alcoholism is a psychosomatic disease that exists when the intake of alcohol produces a problem. An alcoholic is a human being escaping from intolerable stresses.[30,31]

Incidence. About 6% of men in the United States are problem drinkers, as is an almost equal percentage of women.

Definition.[32] The World Health Organization (WHO) Expert Committee on Drug Dependence defines alcoholism as any form of drinking that goes beyond traditional or customary use. Of practical importance is to consider the use of alcohol in quantitative terms; this serves a useful purpose in understanding pathophysiologic consequences.

Classification.[33] The extent of alcohol use and the corresponding effects provide a biologic gradient of alcoholism ranging from no effect to maximum effect. The entire population can thus be classified into five groups:[32,33]

1. Abstainers: A large percentage of the population abstains from alcohol
2. Social or cultural consumers: a second major part of the population consists of those who take alcohol customarily in diet or social use, but in limited amounts
3. Symptomatic alcoholics: those who consume alcohol to deal with a current problem, but not regularly or systematically
4. Addictive Alcoholics: those with an overpowering psychological craving and physiologic need for alcohol. Both tolerance and dependence phenomena are present.[34] Consumption approximates 1 pint of whiskey (80 proof) per day or about 150 g of alcohol over an extended but variable period. This amount is equivalent to 12 to 15 standard cocktails. Usually, no organic pathology is produced
5. Advanced alcoholics: those whose consumption of alcohol has produced organic or psychic deterioration. People who consume more than 1 pint and as much as 1 quart of whiskey per day, usually an intake of 250 g of alcohol, will invariably develop organ pathology.[35]

Rate of Metabolism.[36,37] Alcohol is almost completely metabolized in the liver to acetaldehyde and acetic acid. The latter is reduced by all tissues to carbon dioxide and water. Studies on alcohol labeled with radioactive carbon show that 90% appears as carbon dioxide, and less than 10% of alcohol is eliminated. The rate at which alcohol is metabolized is essentially slow. It has been estimated to vary between 100 and 200 mg/kg/h (200 mg is equivalent to 0.25 ml alcohol). It is expected that the average man weighing 70 kg can completely metabolize about 1 oz. whiskey per hour.[38]

Pharmacologic Effects on Central Nervous System.[39] A form of narcotic depression ensues, which is probably because of interference with synaptic transmission.[38]

As a CNS depressant, alcohol is similar to general anesthetic agents. The depression is a descending type, and the pattern of depression corresponds to the stages of anesthesia,[35,38] with progressive increases in blood alcohol levels from 0.05% to 0.1% in stage 1 to 0.15% to 0.2% in stage 2 to 0.3% to 0.5% in stage 3 ("dead drunk", unconsciousness or deep coma, often with vomiting).[40]

Heart and Circulation.[41] At a blood alcohol concentration of about 0.5%, an increase of 5% to 10% in pulse rate, blood pressure, and total blood flow occurs. This effect wanes in 30 minutes. No significant effect on coronary blood flow in humans has been established. In dogs, however, a marked augmentation of coronary flow occurs after intravenous injection. No significant electrocardiographic responses are to be seen after moderate or nonintoxicating doses.

Liver. Impairment of liver function does occur after drinking moderate to large amounts of alcohol.

Kidneys. Alcohol has a diuretic effect because it inhibits the production of antidiuretic hormone of the posterior pituitary.

Neuromuscular Junction. This effect includes a depolarization block, which is an anticurare effect.[42]

Catecholamine Effect. Ethanol causes a dose-dependent rise in plasma norepinephrine.

Metabolic Effect.[38] Both metabolic and respiratory acidosis occur from alcoholic intoxication.

Heart.

Cardiac Arrhythmias[43] Chronic alcoholics may experience arrhythmias only when drinking ("holiday heart"). Both atrial tachycardia and ventricular tachycardia are seen.[44,45] ECG shows prolonged PR, QRS, and QT intervals.[45] Cardiac contractility is considerably decreased and ventricular function curves are lowered.[46]

Cardiomyopathy[49] Cardiac muscle ultrastructural changes are similar to those in skeletal muscle.

Muscles. A so-called alcoholic myopathy, manifested by weakness and myoglobulinuria, occurs frequently,[47] and serum creatinine phosphokinase (CPK) activity may be increased after a long "binge."[48]

ACUTE ETHANOL INTOXICATION.[50a,50b] Occasionally, it is necessary to operate when these complications exist. If a life-saving surgical procedure is indicated in a wild, stuporous patient, the following is recommended:[34]

1. Tranquilization—IV midazolam (0.12 mg/kg) or promethazine (0.5 mg/hg) (H_1 blocker)
2. Gastric content control—H_1 and H_2 block with

IV promethazine (small doses), and ranitidine; gastric emptying: metoclopramide (5 mg IV)
3. Endotracheal intubation—awake, if possible
4. Rapid sequence induction—midazolam is preferred (0.25 mg/kg); avoid thiopental, if possible[51]
5. Inhalation agents for maintenance[52]

DOSAGE REQUIREMENTS IN THE ALCOHOLIC PATIENT.[53,54] Chronic alcohol consumption of one-half pint of whiskey per day (8 oz) or even less increases the anesthetic requirement of various drugs. For halothane, the MAC value increases from 0.76% to 1.10%.[55] Fentanyl supplementation is increased by 30% in the nitrous oxide–oxygen relaxant technique.[56] Impairment of liver function is well known. With greater daily consumption of alcohol, drug metabolism may be enhanced. Thiopental requirement is increased and may be doubled in patients scheduled for elective surgery who are poorly prepared or inadequately premedicated.[57,58]

Contrariwise, when alcohol is present in the body, the metabolism of many drugs is slowed, and the effect of alcohol on other CNS depressants is one of potentiation.[57] Chlorpromazine inhibits alcohol dehydrogenase and hence high blood levels of alcohol are attained; there is a simultaneous increase in the depressant effect of chlorpromazine. Diazepam is generally well tolerated in the noninebriated patient, even in large doses; however, in the presence of alcohol, this drug may become lethal.[59]

ABSTINENCE SYNDROMES OF CHRONIC ALCOHOLISM.[60,61]

SMOKING HISTORY AND SCORE.[62–64] A smoking history is reported by the numbers of "pack years."[65] For total smoking history, this is defined as the average packs per day *times* the years smoked. This should be modified by the period of current abstention. A habitual smoker is one who smokes 0.5 to 3.5 packs/day for more than 10 years. The average of one pack a day for 10 years has total smoking history of 1 × 10, or 10 "pack years."

A current smoking habit may also be graded according to a five-point score:[66]

1. —nonsmoker.
2. —ex-smoker
3. —smokes 1 to 14 g/day* (usually 1 to 14 cigarettes)
4. —smokes 15 to 24 g/day (usually 15 to 24 cigarettes)
5. —smokes more than 24 g/day (usually 24 cigarettes or more)

EFFECT OF SMOKING ON PHYSIOLOGIC FUNCTION. Respiratory function is significantly impaired in high-level smokers. The degree of impairment can be clinically classified on the basis of dyspnea.

Ciliary function is rapidly reduced and cilia destruction occurs.[67] Small airway conductance is decreased;[68] sputum becomes thicker, and production is increased.[69]

Acute respiratory tract illness is also more frequent in smokers, including young adults. The severity of the illness is greater with longer duration and intensity of coughs, as well as persistent abnormal auscultatory pulmonary findings.[70]

Cigarette smoking is a strong risk factor for coronary heart disease and occlusive peripheral arterial disease,[71] and systolic hypertension is potentiated.[72,73]

Chronic cigarette smoking also has an adverse effect on cerebral blood flow and is related to cerebral ischemic attacks.[74] Rogers measured cerebral gray matter blood flow in smokers and found significant reductions in both hemispheres; probably, as a result of enhanced cerebral arteriosclerosis. Cigarette smoking also relates to increased risk of stroke in those over 50 years of age.

Smokers have a higher gastric volume and higher gastric acidity than nonsmokers. Patients who smoke on the day of surgery have twice the gastric volume of nonsmokers and a greater acidity as well.[75]

SMOKING EFFECTS. A wide range of adverse effects is found on respiratory, cardiovascular, and immune systems, as well as on drug metabolism (Table 9–2), hemostasis, and patient psychology. Two factors contribute the most of the effect of smoking on physiology; carbon monoxide and nicotine.[64,76]

Carboxyhemoglobin COHb levels are increased in smokers. Because the affinity of hemoglobin for CO is 200 times that for oxygen, the consequence of smoking is a significant formation of COHb.[77] There

TABLE 9–2. INTERACTIONS BETWEEN SMOKING AND DRUGS BASED ON ALTERATIONS IN DRUG METABOLISM

Drug Class	Metabolic Response
Analgesics	
Propoxyphene	Higher rates of "ineffective" responses
Antipyrene	Increased hepatic metabolism
Phenacetin	Lower plasma levels
Pentazocine	Higher maintenance dose needed
Tricyclic Antidepressants	
Imipramine	Increased clearance rate
Xanthines	
Theophylline	Significantly accelerated metabolism
Tranquilizers	
Diazepam	CNS depression less frequent (probably due to increased rate of metabolism)
Chlorpromazine	Reduced drowsiness

From the Boston Collaborative Drug Surveillance Program: Clinical depression of the central nervous system due to diazepam and chlordiazepoxide in relation to cigarette smoking and age. N. Engl. J. Med., 288:277–280, 1973.

---
* One cigarette equals 1 g of tobacco; one cigarello equals 2 g of tobacco; one cigar equals 5 g of tobacco.

is some basic COHb of about 1% from endogenous CO metabolically produced, whereas cigarette smokers have levels ranging from 3% to 15%, directly related to the number of cigarettes inhaled. This increased COHb has two major effects: an absolute decrease in blood oxygen content and a shift in the oxygen dissociation curve to the left, and a decrease in oxygen delivery to tissues.[78]

The half-life of COHb is increased at low levels of activity, and during an 8-hour sleep the half-life doubles. Smoking at night and before sleep is a particular hazard.[79]

Nicotine Effect.[80] The blood levels of nicotine in smokers range between 15 and 50 ng/ml. The half-life after one cigarette is about 30 minutes.

The dominant pharmacologic effect is the ability of nicotine to stimulate the sympathoadrenal system.[81] The cardiovascular responses and oxygen requirements for both the cardiac and respiratory measurements are increased by this system. Hormonal levels of epinephrine, norepinephrine, growth factor, and cortisol are increased.[82]

Nicotine enhances drug disposition by inducing hepatic enzyme systems responsible for metabolism.[83] An accelerated rate of metabolism decreases the intensity and duration of effects of drugs metabolized in the liver.[84] The enhanced drug metabolism ranges from 10% to 15%.[85]

Respiratory Complications. The rate of respiratory complications is increased five to seven times.[86] Segmental atelectasis, bronchospasm, pleural effusion, as well as pneumothorax and postoperative "bronchitis" accompanied by cough, are noted. The incidence of these complications is increased with the number of cigarettes smoked.[87] The oxygen cost of breathing is increased 12% to 19%. Nonsmoking for 2 months reduces productive cough by at least 50% and decreases hyperirritability of the tracheobronchial tree;[88] however, the incidence of pulmonary complications remains two to three times greater than that in nonsmokers.

Mechanisms. Three major mechanisms are active in producing the adverse respiratory responses: (1) mucus hypersecretion; (2) impaired tracheobronchial clearance; and (3) narrowing of small bronchial airways.

There is hypersecretion of mucus. The mucus composition is increased. With mixed solids, there is a decrease in transport; the volume of sputum declines to a normal level over a 6-week period with cessation of smoking.[76]

Laurenco[89] demonstrated that clearance of particulate matter is delayed for up to 4 hours after smoking one cigarette and transport of mucus is slowed. Thus, even a normal mucus composition is poorly transported.

Many of the components of tobacco smoke are ciliostatic, and ciliary motion is markedly reduced.[90]

Gross spirometry: Forced expiratory volume at 1.0 second and Vital capacity (VC) may be normal in many smokers, but small airway disease may be present. FEV$_1$/VC and RV/TLC may be reduced, however, and closing capacity may reveal trapping of air.[91] There is also impaired diffusing capacity because of carbon monoxide.[92]

Hyperirritability.[65] A nonspecific bronchial reactivity, along with an increase in respiratory epithelial permeability, occurs in smokers. This is present even in those with normal lung function.[92]

Allergy Sensitization. Allergy sensitization has been demonstrated. Studies at Cornell indicate that a tobacco glycoprotein induces a variety of allergic reactions in smokers.[93,94]

Cardiovascular Response. An increase in blood pressure, both systolic and diastolic, and an increase in cardiac rate and peripheral vasoconstriction follow the smoking of one cigarette.[95] The sympathetic discharge is accompanied by an increased myocardial oxygen demand, whereas the carbon monoxide exerts a negative inotropic action on the myocardium.

A lowered threshold for ventricular fibrillation has been demonstrated experimentally, related to both nicotine and carbon monoxide.[96]

Recommendations[97,98]

1. Smoking should not be permitted within 24 hours of administration of anesthesia for surgery—nicotine levels, based on a half-life of 30 to 60 minutes, will fall appreciably but not completely.
2. For carbon monoxide levels to fall appreciably, a smoking-free period before anesthesia should be at least 3 half-lives, or 12 hours; however, a 48-hour smoking-free period will be sufficient time for COHb of most smokers to fall to a nonsmoker level. This will permit a significant rise in oxygen content and availability.
3. For reduction of sputum volume and postoperative respiratory complications, a smoking-free period of 4 to 8 weeks is required for maximum benefit. At that time the incidence of such complication is similar to that in nonsmokers.[97]
4. Improvement of airway function demonstrated by improved ratios (TV/VC and CV/TLC) occurs only after a minimum of 6 weeks of abstinence.

SURGICAL POSITION. Patients who are to be operated on in unusual operative positions, especially the lithotomy, lateral, and prone positions, should be placed in these positions the day before surgery so the physiologic responses and tolerances can be noted. In addition, a preliminary trial of positioning both in the supine and the planned surgical position should be conducted after premedication on the day of surgery to assess any physiologic changes.

GENERAL CONSIDERATIONS

AGE. The influence of age of the patient on the risks of anesthesia and surgery is determined by the type of associated diseases and dysfunction. In general, the very young and the very old do not tolerate much anesthesia or extensive surgery. Various stresses provoke significant strain and when any single system's function is disrupted, the breaking point is more quickly attained. Thus, one may say that an appreciable reduction in the margin of safety and diminished capacity for compensation occur at the extremes of life.

In the geriatric patient, the biologic effects of aging should be separated from actual degenerative disease processes with their impairment of functional reserve.[99] There are some physiologic changes that can be attributed to the aging process, including a decrease in cardiac output, an increase in cardiac size, and a decrease in efficiency of contractility and reserve.[100] A general reduction in oxygen requirement is accompanied by a diminished ventilatory capacity. There is a diminution in total body weight. Renal functional capacity is reduced; there is a progressive reduction in renal plasma flow and filtration rate and a decreased capacity of the tubules to perform osmotic work.[101]

Reflexes. Reflexes are progressively lost with age. For example, perception threshold is raised and reaction time is slowed. Older persons are less sensitive to pain. A given dose of narcotic provides progressively greater pain relief with advancing age from 40 to 80 years.[102] Deep reflexes are sluggish in the older patient but can be elicited and intensified by reenforcement.[103] The plantar flexor response and the superficial abdominal reflexes have an increased latent period.

The sensitivity of the protective reflexes of the airway are diminished or lost in humans.[104] There is a sixfold increase in the threshold to stimuli as one advances from the second to the eighth decade. Closure of the glottis to mechanical or chemical irritation is sluggish or lost and cough is impaired. The implication of more frequent pulmonary aspirations is a serious hazard.

Sensitivity to Drugs. Sensitivity to drugs as exemplified by β-adrenoreceptor responses in humans decreases with age.[105] In the studies by Vestal, the dose of isoproterenol needed to produce a given heart rate response progressively increases with age. Approximate increases were from 0.5 µg (single IV injection) at age 21 to 4 to 6 µg at age 60 to 70. An increasing resistance of these receptors to the blocking action of propranolol with age was also determined; larger doses are needed to block the β-receptor and produce a standard reduction in heart rate. Thus, there is a receptor insensitivity to both agonist and antagonist.

This appears to be a specific qualitative change in the condition of the receptor and not the result of a reduction in the number of receptors.

Geriatric Patient and Risk.[106] Age alone, however, with the expected changes in functional capacity associated with senescence is not a primary determinant of risk. Collected data for 1974 and 1975 showed the hospital mortality rate following anesthesia and surgery for patients over 65 to be 4.8%, compared to 0.75% for those under 65 years of age.[107] Nevertheless, most of the deaths in the over-65 age group were in patients with preexisting medical problems. Over the age of 80, the overall mortality rate at 1 month has been assessed at 6%. The mortality varied, however, with the Physical Status (PS) Classification and was significantly less in patients of PS I category. Thus, the PS system is a valid predictor of outcome. In a study by Denney and Denson[108] of patients over 90 years, the overall mortality was 29%. Again, those patients in PS I category, (without an identifiable preoperative disease or medical disability) had a mortality rate of only 5%.

WEIGHT LOSS.[109] Accurate determination of a patient's weight should be made because any changes are profoundly significant. Actual loss is usually the result of loss of body water. Chronic loss is due to depletion of body stores of protein and fat. In geriatric patients there is a decrease in total body water naturally. However, nutritional deficiencies may also occur and are associated with a reduction in intracellular water and a decrease in total potassium.

The correction of obvious protein, blood volume, and associated abnormalities cannot be carried out rapidly. If a patient loses 10% of his body weight, 5 to 7 days are required to prepare him for surgery; if he loses 20%, 10 to 12 days are necessary; and when weight losses are 25% or greater, 15 to 30 days may be needed.[110]

OBESITY.[111] This is a frequent condition only too often casually considered. The problems presented to the surgical team represent significant hazards. Recognition of these problems and their influence on the conduct of anesthesia and surgery is essential in evaluating and preparing the patient.

The anatomic factor profoundly affects anesthesia. Airway maintenance at best is difficult. Accommodation of the patient to the operating table is a challenge, and the surgical exposure is impeded.

Relaxation is always a problem: it is not a matter of muscular paralysis as much as a mechanical problem. Venipuncture is difficult and monitoring is uncertain. All of these enhance the *risk*.

Of greater importance are the physiologic derangements from associated diseases. Hypoventilation, emphysema and hypovolemia are frequently encountered.

Pharmacologically, the obese patient presents additional hazards. Fat tissue represents a storehouse for many agents including the volatile agents and many nonvolatile drugs such as the barbiturates. The employment of these results in prolonged depression.

Estimation of Overweight.[112] Determination of overweight should reflect the degree of fatness.

The body mass index (BMI) is an anthropometric measurement. It relates weight (W) to a power function of height (H) as W/H^2 to minimize influence of height in any correlation to fatness. BMI is one of the best indicators of obesity.[113,114] It is determined as a ratio of weight in kilograms to height in meters squared, or kg/m^2. Normal values are 10 to 20. Overweight values are 20 to 30. An index of 30 represents the cutoff point, and values above this number indicate varying degrees of obesity.

Classification of Obesity.[114,115] Obesity is classified as moderate (30 to 35), severe (36 to 40), and pathologic (40 to 50); values above 50 BMI are morbid and include the hypoventilation syndrome and the Pickwickian syndrome.

Clinical Estimation of Overweight. A practical and predictable determination of percent fat and estimation of overweight can be made at the bedside by measurement of skin fat folds.

Technique A skinfold caliper is employed.[116] Two sites for measurement may be used: (1) the *triceps*: an area midway between the shoulder and the elbow on the posterior aspect of the upper arm—this somewhat underestimates the percent of fat, and (2) the *scapula*: A point overlying the inferior (angle) aspect of the scapula.

The skin and subcutaneous tissues are lifted by pinching between the thumb and forefinger while the caliper is used to measure the thickness of the fold.

Skinfold measurement, percent fat, and percent overweight are summarized in Table 9–3. Correlation with height–weight tables (Table 9–4) is closest with scapular measurements. Accuracy is within 10% of the true fat value.[117]

Associated Diseases and Problems of Obesity.[114] Obesity is a disease entity. It imposes a physical burden on the victim and predisposes to other diseases. Among the diseases associated with obesity and concomitant dysfunction are the following.[118]

1. *Cardiovascular Disorders.* Hypertension is three times more frequent in obese people.[119a] In the Framingham heart disease study, hypertension occurred ten times more in persons 20% overweight than in the normal-weight population. Hypercholestcrolemia is usual. Ischemic heart disease occurs twice as often in the obese person.[119b] Cerebrovascular disease and cerebrovascular accidents are three times more frequent in obese subjects.[119a] As a result of increased pulmonary resistance, there is pulmonary hypertension and cor pulmonale.
2. *Cardiac Function.* Cardiac output is elevated and increases linearly with weight at rest.[120] A 100-kg increase above ideal weight doubles resting output. This is expected because of the general body demands that include increased preload; elevated Pulmonary artery pressure; cardiomegaly with left ventricular hypertrophy;[121,122] and electrocardiogram changes of prolonged QT interval, reduced QRS voltage, are first- and second-degree heart block.[123]
3. *Renal Disturbances.* Aluminumuria is frequent.
4. *Fat Storage.* Abnormal sites of fat storage include infiltration of the heart and the pancrease in morbid obesity. An excessive accumulation of fat occurs in the liver.

TABLE 9–3. SCAPULAR SKIN FOLD TEST

Skin Fold (mm)	Percent Fat	Percent Overweight	Classification of Obesity
4–5	9–10	Normal lean	Nonobese
10	16	10% overweight	Overweight
15	21	15% overweight	
20	27	20% overweight	Mild
35	33	25% overweight	Moderate
40	50	40% overweight	Severe
50 +	62	50% overweight	Pathologic to morbid

Adapted from Crook, G.H.: Evaluation of skin-fold measurements and weight chart to measure body fat. J.A.M.A., *198*:39, 1966.

TABLE 9–4. BODY MASS INDEX

(Weight in Kilograms)/(Height in Meters)² = BMI	
10 to 20	Normal
20 to 30	20% overweight
31 to 35	Moderate
36 to 40	Severe
40 to 50	Pathologic (double desired weight)
50+	

*Desirable weight according to current Metropolitan Life Insurance tables. 1983

5. *Diabetes Mellitus.* An elevated blood sugar and impaired glucose tolerance exist in the obese patient whether there is overt insulin-dependent diabetes or not.[124] Diabetes is prevalent in obese subjects with upper body obesity, and 20% of overweight subjects develop diabetes.[125,126] That is, the frequency of diabetes in the obese adult is 3 to 4 times the rate in comparable nonobese adults. Conversely, of patients with adult-onset diabetes, 85% are overweight.[124]
Many studies indicate the importance of an intact, functioning pancreas in maintaining normal weight. Involvement of the pancreas in obesity with fatty infiltration has been noted and demonstrated experimentally.
6. *Endocrine Disturbances.*[127] Abnormalities of 17 ketosteroid excretion have been reported in certain forms of juvenile adiposity. The thyroid, pituitary, and hypothalamus are all interrelated in an abnormal manner. Plasma norepinephrine (NE) concentrations are inversely related to the percentage of body fat.[128] NE decreases from about 400 pg/ml in people with 6% to 12% body fat to low levels of about 120 pg/ml in subjects with over 36% body fat.
7. *Hepatic Damage.* Abnormal liver function values are frequent. An enlarged liver and fatty infiltration occur in 25% of those 50% overweight. High-lipid-soluble agents such as halogenated volatile anesthetics tend to be retained in the body.
8. *Clotting Mechanisms.* Significant defects in blood clotting or coagulation are not pronounced, but thrombophlebitis and thromboembolism have a much higher incidence in the obese as a result, in part, to mechanical and positional factors.
9. *Respiratory Dysfunction.* Mechanical interference with ventilation occurs. There is specific diminished pulmonary compliance.
10. *Autonomic Nervous System.* Depression of both sympathetic and parasympathetic activity increases significantly with increasing percentage of body fat. As sympathetic activity decreases, there is an excessive storage of energy foodstuffs.[128]

Respiratory System. The ventilatory mechanical system is impaired by obesity in three ways:[129]

1. *A fixed thoracic cage* Compliance is reduced and elastic resistance greatly increased (Fig. 9–2).
2. *An elevated diaphragm.*[13] The diaphragm is restricted in its movements by the abdominal wall weight and the abdominal cavity contents so that a shallow bellows mechanism exists. Nonelastic resistance is sharply increased. A study by Vaughan showed that 88% of obese patients had gastric juice pH values below 2.5, whereas an equal percentage had resting gastric fluid volumes above 25 ml.[131]
3. *Parenchymal changes* lead to loss of compliance and compression of airways.

Changes in Respiratory Function Functional residual capacity (FRC) is reduced to 60% or less. Maximum voluntary ventilation (MVV) value is reduced as is maximum breathing capacity (MBC).[132] Ventilation perfusion ratios are low,[133,134] and Pa_{O_2} values result in the range of 60 to 70 mm Hg. A greater decline in Pa_{O_2} occurs with advancing age in the obese subject in the supine position.[135] Arterial oxygen saturation is reduced to 60%.[136]

Work of Breathing There is greater air flow resistance.[137] FEV_1 is less than 60% of predicted, and the work of breathing is increased. The amount of oxygen needed for the purpose of breathing increases greatly and progressively with the degree of obesity (Fig. 9–3). In mild to moderate obesity, the "oxygen cost" may be doubled or quadrupled.[138]

The actual oxygen cost of breathing needed in the

OBESITY: POSITION EFFECTS

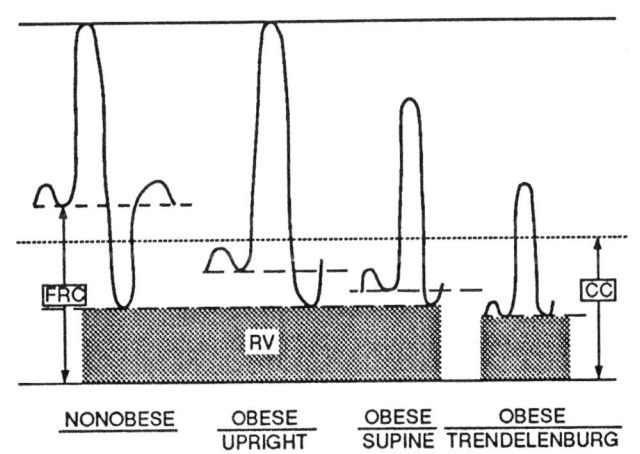

FIG. 9–2. In obesity, decreased chest wall compliance results in functional residual capacity (FRC) decreasing at the expense of expiratory reserve volume (RV). Closing capacity (CC) stays normal. Courtesy of Vaughan and Anesthesiology News, May 1987.

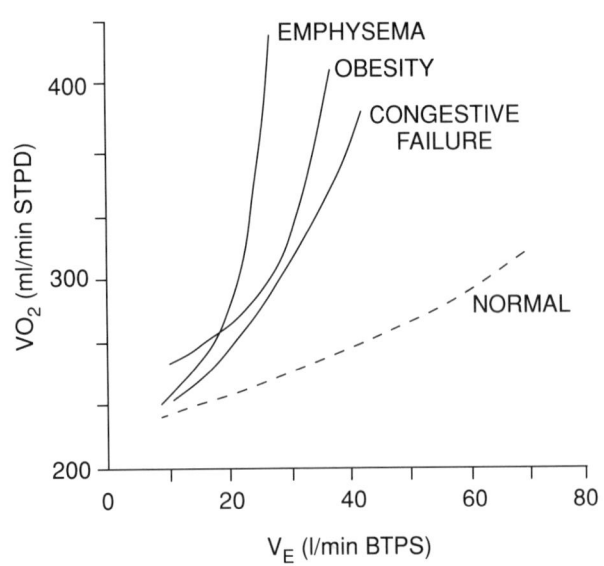

FIG. 9-3. The change in oxygen consumption associated with increases in ventilation in a normal subject and patients with respiratory insufficiency. From Cherniack, R.M.: Respiratory effects of obesity. Can. Med. Assoc. J., 80:613, 1959.

moderately obese subject is 4 ml of oxygen per liter of air moved. The normal requirement is 1 ml O_2 per liter of air moved.

Hypoventilation Syndrome [139] Hypoxemia is common, and Pa_{O_2} values of 50 to 60 mm Hg are observed.[140] The somnolence of marked obesity is often accompanied by sleep apnea.[141]

Blood Volume in Obese Patients. When blood volume is estimated on the basis of standard values (72 ml/kg), then obese subjects are hypovolemic. If the volume is calculated on the basis of lean mass and of circulatory capacity of fat tissue, however, the correct blood volume will be more closely approximated. The volume can be estimated by using a standard value of 65 ml/kg. Schwartz[111] has suggested that the ideal weight, plus one third of the difference between obese and ideal weight, will serve this purpose. If volume is actually reduced, it should be restored. The hematocrit is usually in normal range, but with advancing hypoxemia there is a polycythemia.

Hazards of Weight Reduction (Low-Calorie [18 K cal] Diets). The use of anorexiant drugs (fenfluramine—a sedative anorexiant with serotoninergic action; phentermine—a stimulant anorexiant with adrenergic action), metabolic stimulants of the amphetamine type, and water or starvation diets pose a hazard to anesthetic practice.[142]

Weight loss is related to an increase in α-adrenergic receptors[143] from a concentration in obese subjects of 85 f mol/mg of platelet binding sites to 113 f mol/mg. This up-regulation may be a response related to the concomitant decrease in circulating NE levels as obese patients lose weight. Among the consequences of weight reduction programs are:[144]

1. Increased sensitivity to catecholamines; sensitivity to foods and to catecholamine precursors, tyramine
2. Decreasing blood pressure and development of hypotension, along with a decrease in plasma renin. The decrease in blood pressure may be related to central α-adrenergic sensitivity (a clonidine-like effect)
3. Development of cardiac arrhythmias, spontaneous in obese subjects on extremely low caloric diets, especially liquid protein diets[144a]
4. Occurrence of sudden cardiac arrest, possibly related to increased sensitivity to β-adrenergic agents[144,145]

DEFORMITIES. Structural deformities encountered in patients, especially children, include lordosis, kyphosis, scoliosis, kyphoscoliosis and pectus excavatum as well as pectus carinatum. Of these, kyphoscoliosis or scoliosis alone and funnel chest cause sufficient changes as to impair pulmonary and cardiac function. The mechanism is apparent: the structural changes impose mechanical restrictions on thoracic viscera and these in turn are displaced and compressed. The etiological factors include, poliomyelitis as the most common cause today; congenital defects, vitamin D deficiency, and tuberculosis are still frequent. The tendency to pulmonary insufficiency and cardiac failure must be recognized.

UNUSUAL SYNDROMES AND ANESTHESIA.[145] Many rare syndromes, and some not so rare, are seen in patients who are candidates for anesthesia and surgery. These frequently are designated by eponyms and have been cataloged by Jones and Pelton in a remarkable index in which they have briefly commented on the anesthetic implications. This index can be found in the appendix to this chapter.

LABORATORY STUDIES[146]

Certain laboratory procedures may be necessary in the preoperative evaluation of the patient. These procedures should be considered as screening tests, and whenever a positive finding appears, it must be explored and further detailed examinations carried out. There are twelve tests that should be considered routinely (Table 9-5) and ordered according to indications. Normal limits for the laboratory tests are shown in Table 9-6. There are six others that are selective in nature (Table 9-7).[147]

TABLE 9–5. INDICATORS FOR COMMON LABORATORY PREOPERATIVE TEST ORDERING

Test	Indication
Type and screen	Potentially bloody operation, pregnancy, all major intracavitary surgery
Hemoglobin/hematocrit	Known anemia, hematologic disease, radiotherapy or chemotherapy, chronic renal failure, high prevalence of hemoglobinopathies, potentially bloody operation
Prothrombin time Partial thromboplastin time	Liver disease, biliary retention, malabsorption or poor nutrition, bleeding tendency, anticoagulant therapy, malignancy, alcoholism
Bleeding time Platelet count	Thrombopathy, bleeding tendency, hypersplenism
Serum electrolytes (Na^+, K^+, Cl^-, HCO_3, Proteins)	Acute metabolic situation, diuretics, steroids or any drug usage which action could lead to (or be modified by) fluid electrolyte disturbance, malabsorption or malnutrition, aged 70 years or older
Serum creatinine (or blood urea nitrogen)*	Renal disease, hypertension, diabetes mellitus or hyperuricemia, fluid and electrolyte disturbance, septic state, nephrotoxic drug usage, aged 70 years or older, high-risk surgery for renal function
Blood glucose	Diabetes mellitus, hypoglycemia, pancreatic disease, pituitary, hypothalamic or adrenal disease, steroid treatment, high risk for diabetes mellitus
Chest radiographs	Chronic lung disease, cardiovascular disease, high risk of asymptomatic disease
Electrocardiogram	Cardiovascular disease, chronic respiratory failure, aged 40 years or older, high risk of thromboembolic complication

*BUN when serum creatinine was not available (e.g., night service).
From Charpak, Y. et al. Usefulness of selectively ordered preoperative tests. Med. Care, 26:95–104, 1988.

The ordering of blood tests should be guided by the preoperative history and examination. In general, when no clinical indication exists, the chance of finding any abnormal test result that influences perioperative management is remote, whether the laboratory test,[148] the radiograph,[149] or the ECG is abnormal.

For specific medically compromised patients, there are several important tests that should be performed (Table 9–8).[150] These are in addition to the indicated routine tests and to selective tests.

STANDARD HEMOGRAM. To establish a proper blood profile, three basic laboratory studies are necessary: hemoglobin concentration; hematocrit; and the red blood cell (RBC) count. The normal hemoglobin value for white men is 15 g/dl ±2 g and for white women it is 14 g/dl ±2 g.[153] Patients with hemoglobin levels 8 g/dl or less should not undergo major surgery or surgery that might entail extensive blood loss. When an operation is contemplated, the anemia should be treated. When an operation is urgent, a patient should probably receive red blood

TABLE 9–6. NORMAL LIMITS FOR LABORATORY TESTS

			Normal Limits
Hemoglobin	♂	g/100 ml	14–17
	♀	g/100 ml	12–16
Prothrombin time*		%	>70
Partial thromboplastin time*		seconds	<10
Bleeding time		minutes	<8
Platelet count		$10^3/mm^3$	150–400
Serum electrolytes	Na	mmol/l	135–145
	K	mmol/l	3.5–5
	Cl	mmol/l	95–105
	CO_2	mmol/l	24–32
	Protein	g/l	60–75
Serum creatinine or		μmol/l	40–110
Blood urea nitrogen		mmol/l	<7.5
Blood glucose		mmol/l	3.5–5.5

* Patient versus control
From Charpak, Y., et al.: Usefulness of selectively ordering preoperative tests. Med. Care, 26:95, 1988.

TABLE 9–7. SELECTIVE TESTS BY GENERAL MEDICAL INDICATIONS

Laboratory Test	Period Valid For	Modifier
Creatinine phosphokinase	3 weeks	Only if deemed appropriate for anesthetic procedure or on basis of history
Sickle cell prep	Lifetime	Not necessary if documented by prior test
Sickle cell electrophoresis	Lifetime	On sickle cell prep positive patients; not necessary if documented by prior test
Pregnancy test	3 weeks	Physician discretion; recommend question and documentation
Syphilis serology	3 weeks	Over 11 years
Hepatitis antigen (HB$_s$Ag)	3 weeks	High-risk patients (see attachment); not necessary if previously positive

cell transfusions. This will furnish protein for maintenance of osmotic pressure as well as oxygen-carrying power.

Some racial differences exist for normal hemoglobin values. Blacks of a socioeconomic level similar to whites and black olympic athletes normally have a hemoglobin level 0.5–1 g/dl lower than whites. These should not be designated as anemic.[151,152]

Hematocrit Values. Hematocrit readings offer a rough index of red cell volume. Thus, a low reading indicates a red cell deficiency.[153] Hematocrit values of less than 2% are accompanied by a loss of oxygen-carrying power and decreased compensation to blood loss. Elective operations should probably be delayed or the patient actively treated according to clinical indications.

Acute blood loss is followed by a replenishment of the circulating volume with fluid from the "available fluid" compartments. This response is usually delayed for about 2 to 4 hours in the unanesthetized patient. Therefore, if no therapy is instituted, there is a steady fall in hematocrit for 3 days. The following are guides to these changes.

	24 Hours	72 Hours
Loss of 200 ml	2.5 mm ↓	4.5 mm ↓
Loss of 500–1000 ml	4–6 mm ↓	5.5–11 mm ↓

TABLE 9–8. TESTS FOR SPECIFIC MEDICALLY COMPROMISED PATIENTS

Medical Condition	Text	Valid For	Modifiers
Asthmatics—controlled on medication	Bronchodilator blood level, pulmonary function tests	3 weeks	None
Chronic obstructive lung disease	Pulmonary function test, chest radiograph, arterial blood gas	3 weeks	None
Diabetics	Blood glucose level	3 weeks and morning of surgery	None
Digitalis therapy	Digitalis level	3 weeks	None
History of liver disease within past year	Liver function tests (SPEP, protime, SGOT)	3 weeks	None
Hypertension or heart disease on diuretics	Chest radiograph, ECG Clin. Chem. I(Na$^+$ K$^+$ Cl$^-$ Ca^{++} Mg^{++})	3 weeks; potassium level 24 hr preop	None
Myocardial infarction (within the past 12 months) or frequent anginal attacks	Chest radiograph, ECG, cardiology or medicine consult	3 weeks	None
Thyroid disease, on medication	Blood T3 and T4 levels	3 weeks	None
Seizure disorder (epilepsy)	Phenobarbital and/or dilantin or other anticonvulsant drug level	3 weeks	None
Rheumatoid arthritis with cervical spine involvement	Cervical spine radiograph, anesthesia consult	3 weeks	None
Psychiatric disease on medication	None	—	Off MAO or tricyclics for 30 days
Steroid therapy	None	—	Continue medication regime, supplement Steroids day of surgery

Hematocrit values usually do not return to normal in uncompensated blood loss of 500 ml before the tenth day.

On the other hand, in the anesthetized patient microhematocrit values rapidly reflect acute blood loss and changes in circulating volume. There is a rapid increase in the circulating volume from the available fluid. Hence, the hematocrit does fall rather rapidly and will reflect changes in less than 30 minutes.[155a]

Elevated hematocrit values should also serve as a warning to the surgical team. With an increase of hematocrit of 50% above normal, there is a striking increase in total peripheral resistance due primarily to increased blood viscosity. This change is accompanied by a mean fall in cardiac output of almost 50%.

Blood Indices.[154] Using the three hemogram values, three blood indices can be calculated to establish types of anemia. These include[155]:

1. *Mean corpuscular hemoglobin concentration (MCHC).* This is the percentage of hemoglobin in each red blood cell. It is determined by the hemoglobin in g/dl of whole blood divided by the packed cell volume (the hematocrit) of 100 ml of whole blood, e.g., $(15 \div 45) \times 100 = 33\%$. Levels below 30% are considered to represent *hypochromic anemia.*
2. *Mean corpuscular hemoglobin (content) (MCH).* This is the actual amount (the mass) of hemoglobin per red cell expressed in picograms. This value is obtained by dividing the hemoglobin in 1000 ml of whole blood by the number of red blood cells in 1000 ml of blood, e.g., $150 \text{ g} \div 5.2 \times 10^{12}$. The normal MCH content is 29 picograms of hemoglobin in each erythrocyte (a 5 mM solution of hemoglobin; hemoglobin is 97.5% of cytoplasmic protein by weight)
3. *Mean corpuscular volume (MCV).* This is the volume of an individual red blood cell expressed in cubic micrometers or femtoliters. If the volume of packed red blood cells or the hematocrit expressed in milliliters per liter of whole blood is divided by the red cell count in millions per cubic millimeter or microliters, the MCV is derived, e.g., $450 \div (5 \times 10^{12}) = 90 \text{ }\mu m^3$. The normal MCV is 87 fl for men and 90 fl for women.

Hemogram in the Elderly.[156] Hematologic values in healthy patients (confirmed by long-term records) over the age of 80 have mean hemoglobin values of 14.8 ± 1.1 g/dl for men and 13.6 ± 1 g/dl for women. All other indices have also been calculated. When compared to young healthy adults, the values are similar. It can be concluded that abnormal values are the result of an underlying pathologic condition that can usually be identified by adequate investigation. It can also be stated that a hemoglobin level of 11 g/dl is abnormal, whether over 80 years of age or under 40 years of age.

USE OF ACTIVATED PARTIAL THROMBOPLASTIN TIME (PTT).[161a] This coagulation test is commonly used to screen patients before surgery to predict intraoperative and postoperative hemorrhage. The test is justified, however, only when there are indications of significant risk of bleeding. It has little or no ability to predict the occurrence of hemorrhage in the absence of indications.[161a] The test should be limited to a high-risk group of patients, including patients with active bleeding, known or suspected bleeding disorders, those on anticoagulants, liver disease, malabsorption, malnutrition, and conditions associated with acquired coagulopathies (Table 9-9). If prothrombin time and the PTT test are less than 1.5 times normal, fresh frozen plasma (FFP) is rarely indicated.

USE OF FRESH FROZEN PLASMA.[161b] The indications for the laboratory screening test are clearly defined. Consequent to information showing a deficiency of clotting factors, one should administer FFP.

Patients on the anticoagulant warfin sodium become deficient in vitamin K-dependent coagulation factors (II, VII, IX, and X). If the tests show prothrombin time (PT) and PTT values greater than 1.5 times normal and the patient is bleeding or requires emergency surgery, FFP plasma should be administered.[161c]

CROSSMATCH AND SCREEN PROTOCOL.[157] A major crossmatch has been a common practice when blood has been needed for surgery. A major crossmatch includes ABO grouping and Rh type determination,

TABLE 9-9. INDICATIONS FOR ACTIVATED PTT TEST

Risk Group	Criteria
Known coagulopathy	Diagnosis indicating coagulation disorder, or determination (chart audit for evaluation of hemorrhage, excessive transfusion requirement, or preoperative precoagulant administration) that patient was taking an anticoagulant before surgery
Potential factor deficiency	Any diagnosis code indicative of liver disease, malabsorption, or malnutrition
Trauma/hemorrhage	Diagnosis indicative of acute injury or hemorrhage at any site, or principal procedure of repair of laceration, surgical control of epistaxis, or suturing of gastric or duodenal ulcer site
Low risk	All others

Modified from Suchman, A.L., and Mushlin, A.I.: How well does the activated partial thromboplastin time predict postoperative hemorrhage? JAMA, 256:750, 1986.

as well as incubation at 37°C and an indirect antiglobulin test. This is both time consuming and costly and is not necessary in over two thirds of instances.

The present recommended practice is to perform an ABO and Rh type and a "screen" for unexpected antibodies. An immediate spin saline test is followed by 20-minute incubation and then an indirect antiglobulin test using antiIgG. If antibody status is negative, then as soon as blood is requested an "immediate spin crossmatch" is done (IS-Cx). This requires 3 to 4 minutes and provides blood in rapid order.

If a patient has a positive antibody test, a past record of unexpected antibodies or a positive direct antiglobulin test, a full crossmatch is performed (F-Cx).

PERIOPERATIVE RED BLOOD CELL TRANSFUSION. Recent surgical–anesthesia practice has been guided by the rule that a hemoglobin value of less than 10 g/dl, or a hematocrit less than 0.3 (33%), represents an oxygen-carrying deficit and a hazard.[212]

A study of patients who have refused blood transfusions for religious reasons has demonstrated that hemoglobin values much below 10 g/dl are not associated with increased morbidity or mortality. In patients with severe anemia, the hemoglobin level alone appears to be an inadequate index of risk.[158] Circulating volume was equally as important, and surgical blood loss was a strong predictor of complications independent of preoperative hemoglobin. No patients who had had a preanesthetic hemoglobin value of 8 g/dl and a blood loss of less than 500 ml died. The threshold value indicating a need for perioperative transfusion then appears to be values below 8 g/dl, and when surgical blood loss is anticipated to be greater than 500 ml.[159]

Because of the complications of whole blood transfusion, a change to component therapy has become the standard. The components are stored as frozen units until needed. The practice of autologous blood transfusions has also become a safe alternative. One must determine that the transfusion of blood components is clearly indicated.

The indication for transfusion of red blood cells to raise oxygen-carrying power resulting from moderate and even severe anemia has been greatly modified. Successful clinical anesthesia experience in managing patients with severe anemia from chronic renal failure and the administration of anesthesia to Jehovah's Witness patients with severe blood loss has not been accompanied by major morbidity or mortality. From this background, it has been concluded that:[160a]

1. Patients with 7 to 8 g or more of hemoglobin who are otherwise healthy do not require preoperative preparation with transfusions, providing that circulating volume is adequate
2. Patients with 7 g of hemoglobin or less (hematocrit less than 21%) because of acute anemia frequently require red blood cell transfusions, providing the intravascular volume is adequate for tissue perfusion. Transfusions of one unit of pooled red blood cells will increase the hemoglobin level about 1 g/dl and the hematocrit by 2.3% in an average 70-kg adult[160]
3. Patients with chronic anemia from chronic renal failure tolerate procedures with hemoglobin values less than 7 g/dl without perioperative transfusion. Usually, the oxygen-carrying capacity is adequate with this hemoglobin level if the circulating volume is adequate
4. If low hemoglobin levels are accompanied by hypovolemia (hematocrit below 21%), the combination represents a more serious condition, and volume replacement as well as red blood cell transfusion may be necessary. If volume expansion is indicated, crystalloid solutions or nonblood colloid solutions should be used

The decision to transfuse should be based on clinical evidence and laboratory data of arterial oxygenation, mixed venous oxygen content, oxygen extraction, cardiac output and blood volume. Cardiac output does not greatly increase until hemoglobin values decrease to 7 g/dl.[158] Hemoglobin values of 7 to 8 g/dl are not a necessary requirement for perioperative transfusion or cancellation of surgery, depending on clinical circumstances, i.e., if the patient is otherwise healthy, the surgery is minor without anticipated extensive blood loss, and the circulating volume is within normal limits.

BLEEDING TIME AND PLATELET COUNT. A patient presenting with a bleeding tendency, a known thrombopathy or coagulation defects, hypersplenism, sepsis, or platelet dysfunction resulting from medication such as recent aspirin intake, should have a bleeding time test; and a platelet count is indicated. If the platelet count is at least 50,000/μL even in the presence of thrombocytopenia purpura, prophylactic platelet transfusion is unlikely to be beneficial.[160c] If the platelet count is in the range of 10,000 to 20,000/μL in a clinically stable patient with an intact vascular system, prophylactic transfusions are indicated to prevent bleeding. One unit of platelet concentrate usually raises the platelet count by 5000 platelets per μL.

Polycythemia.[162] Recognition of polycythemia is as important as the recognition of anemia. First, there are physiologic dangers inherent in the condition, and second, the condition influences the type and amount of fluids to be administered.

Classification Two types of polycythemia are identified:

1. *Absolute* or *polycythemia vera* is characterized by a numerical increase in red blood cells per

unit volume of blood as well as an absolute increase in total circulating volume. Platelets also are increased.
2. *Relative polycythemia* is characterized by loss of circulating plasma and increased blood viscosity.

Although polycythemia vera is rare, the occurrence of relative polycythemia is common. It is especially to be noted in surgical patients with the following conditions: burns, shock, dehydration, peritonitis, or intestinal obstruction. Polycythemia vera (not idiopathic), however, may coexist or be consequent to such conditions as emphysema, pulmonary fibrosis, chronic bronchitis and bronchiectasis, mitral stenosis, asthma, congenital heart disease, and many other conditions associated with pulmonary hypertension.

Diagnosis Certain signs and symptoms characterize polycythemia: a ruddy complexion in a plethoric patient; conjunctival suffusion, venous engorgement, hypertension, and, in some relative types, severe degrees of dehydration. Cyanosis is often observed. These should make the anesthesiologist suspicious and stimulate further evaluation.

Pathologic Physiology In either type of polycythemia increased viscosity of the blood is the common denominator. The following pathologic changes result: stagnant peripheral circulation; tissue hypoxia and accumulation of metabolites and acidosis; increased permeability and edema; increased bleeding into surgical sites; and intravascular coagulation and occlusion. The formation of thrombus is the most dangerous complication.

Management For polycythemia vera, administration of any type of fluid is potentially dangerous and may lead to overload. Long-term therapeutic procedures such as spray irradiation or use of radioactive phosphorus is helpful. For rapid care in the surgical setting, "bleeding" is the procedure of choice.

Choice of Anesthesia Objectives should be to disturb circulation and respiration minimally. Relief of anxiety and blocking of stress responses are essential. In addition, measures to decrease the cardiac work load are instituted. Alpha-adrenergic blockade is important in both types, but in relative polycythemia rapid replenishment of volume at the time of blockade is necessary.

Inhalation anesthesia with ethrane is a good choice; an intravenous neuroleptic–narcotic relaxant technique with inhalation of nitrous oxide-oxygen is also acceptable. Ether, because of its tendency to increase prothrombin and clotting, is contraindicated. Regional anesthesia is preferred, but spinal anesthesia, whenever it can be used, is excellent, especially because the peripheral vasodilitation decreases cardiac work.

Monitoring Determination of total blood and total plasma volume is the most useful test in preoperative evaluation.[163] The hematocrit is of some use, and together these laboratory tests serve as a guide to fluid therapy.

During the course of extensive surgery in polycythemic patients a simple practical procedure to indicate changes in vicosity and polycythemia is the determination of blood and plasma specific gravity. This can be done by the falling plasma drop technique in copper sulfate solution.

In the absolute variety of polycythemia vera a sufficient volume of blood can be removed to reduce the hematocrit to normal. This blood can be preserved and used to replace surgical losses.

Conversely, in the face of relative polycythemia because of hemoconcentration related to surgical conditions (burns, dehydration, pancreatitis, or intestinal obstruction), the preparation must be vigorous with adequate and appropriate replenishment of water volume and electrolytes.

Effect Of Leukemia On Oxygen Requirements.[164]
In patients with leukemia, either myelocytic or chronic lymphatic, a degree of arterial hypoxemia may occur due to the tremendous uptake of oxygen by the leukocytes. This is a form of intravascular oxygen "steal" and has been termed "leukocyte larceny." Ordinarily, a sample of blood with a normal leukocyte count takes up oxygen at a rate depleting the oxygen supply by 0.2 mm Hg/min, whereas a count above 100,000 will take up oxygen at a rate depleting the supply by 12 to 70 mm Hg/min.

SCREEN FOR MALIGNANT HYPERTENSION (MH) SUSCEPTIBILITY.[165] In patients with predisposing conditions, it is recommended that a serum level be obtained to determine MH susceptibility. When a simple, inexpensive technique is available, this study should become routine. A preoperative serum CPK level will aid the practicing anesthesiologist in several ways, as stated by Zsigmond.[166]

1. Elevated serum CPK activity and abnormal MB/MM or BB/MM isoenzyme ratios will help to identify MH patients prior to induction. Note: These are isoenzymes of creatine kinase. BB is the brain and nerve type. MM is the muscle type. MB shows a mixed isoenzyme pattern.

    Normal plasma levels vary from 12–120 IU for men and 10 to 92 IU for women. The peak level is age related at 30–40 years. In MH susceptible subjects CPK values may exceed 400–800 IU.

    By electrophoresis CPK can be fractionated into two principal types. It has been proposed that the BB type predominates in MH.
2. Patients who developed myocardial infarction preoperatively would be recognized before induction.

3. Patients with myotonias who would develop muscle contracture following Sch could be recognized preoperatively.
4. In patients with central or peripherial neuropathies, the degree of muscle damage could be estimated and if indicated, the use of Sch avoided.
5. In traumatized patients, the degree of muscle trauma could be assessed before induction of anesthesia and Sch not used.
6. Properative baseline CPK values would be helpful in the assessment of the degree of skeletal muscle or cardiac muscle trauma that could have occurred during anesthesia and surgery, and the CPK isoenzymes would help differentiate between the two types of muscle damage.
7. Elevated serum CPK levels would call attention to the presence of unrecognized muscular dystrophies which may alter the response to anesthetic agents and muscle relaxants.
8. Routine serum CPK tests would lead to new discoveries of patients with MH, various muscular dystrophies, and cardiomyopathies. Based on this recognition, proper selection of anesthetics could be made.[166]

HYPOPROTEINEMIA. Plasma protein levels of 4.0 g or less represent a significant hazard. Low levels are usually part of the picture of chronic shock and hypovolemia. These patients are more likely to develop hypotension and clinical shock. In addition, Burstein[167] has demonstrated that the toxicity of many of the anesthetic agents, such as thiopental and especially the local agents, is enhanced in patients with low plasma protein levels.

Use of Routine Preoperative Urinalysis. In the absence of any clinical indication by history or by signs and symptoms, the urinalysis appears to be an unnecessary test. The detection of unsuspected disease is minimal, and only 1.8% of such tests lead to a new diagnosis.[168] Even in a study of patients with microhematuria, only 2.3% were found to have serious urologic disease.[169] In the ambulatory surgical setting, a routine screen by urinalysis affected diagnosis or altered anesthesia and surgical management in only 0.5% of patients.[170] It is apparent that the diagnosis and therapeutic yield of a urine test is low and does not merit the status of a routine test. Lawrence recommends that a urinalysis is appropriate preoperatively when there are medical indications or when bladder catheterization can be anticipated. It is remarked that abnormal results appear to be overlooked or ignored.[171] Medical indications for urinalysis include a history of renal disease; elevated serum urea nitrogen or creatinine; systemic diseases affecting kidneys; nephrotoxic drugs or Anticoagulants; metabolic acidosis; edema or hypoalbuminemia of unclear cause; or pregnancy.

BLOOD VOLUME. Estimation of any blood volume deficit is essential before major surgery. In many clinical situations a deficit can be expected. Blood loss effects are obvious. In nutritional deficiency, in debilitating disease and in elderly patients, hypovolemia is common. Determination of blood volume should be performed in these situations to complement hematocrit studies. The Evan's Blue Dye method and the radioiodine methods are satisfactory, but it must be realized that they measure so-called albumin space, which in part includes extravascular space. A more accurate determination is obtained by use of radioactive chromium (Cr^{51}) method.

When blood volume determinations are not possible and chronic weight loss exists, approximation of the blood volume deficit can be reached by using the following guides: (1) normal blood volume is set at 74 ml/kg of body weight (Table 9–10); (2) determine the weight loss in kilograms based on desirable weight for the patient's height according to life insurance tables. The indicated blood volume deficit is the product of these two figures. Thus, a 10-kg weight loss is closely associated with about 740 ml of blood volume deficit.

The chronic shock syndrome has been elucidated by Clark[173] and Randall.[174] It occurs in the debilitated patient, in geriatric patients, in nutritional deficiencies, and in chronic stress. It is denoted by the following triad:

1. Depleted plasma volume and/or total blood volume (hypovolemia)
2. Diminished circulating plasma protein (hypoproteinemia)
3. Decreased red cell mass (anemia)

In any situation where the hematocrit is low and the red blood cell count diminished, there is decreased compensation to blood loss; osmotic equilibrium is poor and there is decreased oxygen-carrying power. Tissue hypoxia is likely and adjustments to positional changes are poor. Correction by transfusion is reasonable.

Elevated hematocrit values should also serve as a warming to the surgical team. With an increase in hematocrit of 50% above normal there is a striking increase in total peripheral resistance due to increased blood viscosity. This change is accompanied by a mean fall in cardiac output of 51%.

CHEST ROENTGENOGRAM. A routine radiograph for every surgical patient is unnecessary. A careful clinical evaluation of the patient, considering history,

TABLE 9–10. NORMAL BLOOD VOLUMES
(As per cent of body weight in kilograms)
According to Body Build

	Athletic (or asthenic)	Normal Habitus	Pyknic Habitus (obese)
Male	7.5	7.0%	6.5
Female	7.0	6.5%	6.0

review of systems, and physical examination is first needed, and when positive risk factors are determined that offer a reasonable expectation that a radiograph will provide additional useful information, the procedure should be done.[175a]

In Sagel's review of "routine" preoperative chest radiographs (no clinical data on the radiology request form), only one of every six films revealed an abnormality.[175b] Of the patients with an abnormal radiologic report, a further review of the patients' records showed that in 70% of the instances, there was "a reasonable possibility of disease." In brief, clinical evidence alone will usually determine the need for chest radiographs. Routine films are unnecessary and expensive.

From the Rucker et al. study,[176] a list of risk factors has been identified that predicts whether a patient will have an abnormal preoperative chest film and provides useful information to confirm the existence of a pulmonary problem.

These risk factors are listed in Table 9–11. History factors include known cardiac or pulmonary disease; cancer at any body site; smoking habit; exposure to various fumes or dust; serious systemic disease and recent thoracic surgery; a review of systems *suggesting* cardiac, pulmonary or other systemic diseases, renal or hepatic; abnormal physical findings and age over 60 years. When any of these factors exist, the finding of an abnormal chest roentgenogram is usual.

Contrariwise, in patients with a negative profile and under 60 years of age (about 41% of preoperative chest examinations), only one patient in 360 has a positive insignificant finding, according to the Rucker study.

A study of routine preoperative chest radiographs in patients scheduled for vascular surgery showed that most of the abnormal radiographs were in those who had signs and symptoms of chest disease. Where an abnormality was found preoperatively, there was a 40% postoperative complication rate, which was anticipated. A normal chest radiograph in patients without clinical evidence of chest disease was associated with only a 9% postoperative complication rate and was not predictive. About 60% of routine radiographs were without impact on patient care. From this study, it was recommended that preoperative chest radiographs should be ordered only when signs or symptoms of chest disease are found or suspected, or when the patient is at risk for postoperative chest complications.[176]

Routine chest radiographs in patients admitted to medical services are also without benefit, except when signs and symptoms of chest disease are identifiable.[177]

ROUTINE CHEST RADIOGRAPH FOR CANCER PATIENTS. Preoperative chest radiographs should be ordered routinely for optimal care of cancer patients. About 23% of the patients under the age of 30 had chest abnormalities. Of cancer patients who had had a chest radiograph performed within the previous 6 months, 26% showed new significant abnormalities. Routine preoperative chest radiographs of cancer patients yielded a finding of 29% with clinically significant abnormalities, many of these previously undetected. Retrospectively, only 5% of the patients had standard cardiac or respiratory management altered during anesthesia. About 2% of the patients under the age of 40 had their care affected by preoperative radiographs. In older patients, however, there was a higher concordance between anticipated and actual management.[178]

TABLE 9–11. RISK FACTORS FOR ABNORMAL CHEST ROENTGENOGRAM

Medical History
Cancer at any site
Valvular heart disease
Stroke
Myocardial infarction
Angina
Asthma
Tuberculosis
Chronic obstructive pulmonary disease
Cigarettes
Occupational exposures: asbestos, fumes, or ores
Review of systems
General: fever, chills, sweats, or weight loss
Paroxysmal nocturnal dyspnea
Orthopnea
Class 3 or 4 dyspnea
Angina
Physical findings
Vital signs: fever, tachycardia, hypertension, or tachypnea
Chest: abnormal breath sounds, abnormal adventitial sounds, or dullness
Cardiovascular: severe murmurs, S_3, or displaced point of maximum impulse
Abdominal: tenderness, organomegaly, or ascites

From Rucker, L., et al.: Usefulness of screening chest roentgenograms in preoperative patients. J.A.M.A., *250*:3209–3211, 1983.

BEDSIDE TESTS OF FUNCTION

Simple bedside tests of pulmonary and cardiac function are helpful in identifying patient risk.[179,180] A standard history, observing the patient walk the corridor, and observing the patient's diaphragmatic chest respiratory movement are revealing.

BREATH-HOLDING TEST.[179] Sebarese's test is a simple test to screen for patients with cardiopulmonary problems. After two or three deep breaths the patient is asked to hold the next as long as possible. A holding time of 40 seconds or more is normal. A patient unable to hold his breath longer than 30 seconds has a diminished respiration reserve, and if the breath holding is less than 20 seconds function is severely compromised. (Severe pulmonary disease.)

VALSALVA TEST.[180-185] The Valsalva maneuver consists of taking a deep breath and then exerting a maximal expiratory effort or squeezing. Systolic pressure rises 40 mm Hg or more for 3 seconds; the blood pressure tapers off gradually over the next several seconds. On resumption of normal respiration there is a sudden fall to normal or slightly below and then a rebound rise or overshoot. These pressure changes may be divided into four phases (Fig. 9-4).

In carrying out the test certain simple items of equipment should be provided: (1) an aneroid sphygomomanometer with a short length of pressure tubing connected to a mouthpiece, and (2) an ordinary blood pressure apparatus and stethoscope.

While the patient is supine, a resting blood pressure is obtained. The mouthpiece is next inserted into the patient's mouth and the arm blood pressure cuff is inflated to 40 mm Hg above normal. The patient is now instructed to exhale vigorously so as to raise the aneroid pointer to 40 mm Hg. Meanwhile, the systemic pressure changes are followed. This is maintained for approximately 10 seconds.

An abnormal response is denoted by a sustained rise in pressure throughout the period of expiratory strain in contrast to the transient rise in the normal subject. In addition, on cessation of respiration no overshoot is seen.

This test has been found to provide reliable information about the presence of varying degrees of pulmonary congestion due to cardiac dysfunction. It is also useful in demonstrating incipient cardiac failure. Such conditions as left ventricular failure, mitral stenosis, aortic stenosis, myocardial failure, constrictive pericarditis, and others produce the abnormal response. If the test is negative in the presence of dyspnea, the dyspnea is due to pulmonary disease.[185]

RESPIRATORY FORCE TEST.[186] It is frequently desirable to assess whether significant airway obstruction exists while conducting a physical examination. Two simple tests of airway obstruction are: (1) the maximum breathing capacity and (2) the timed vital capacity. Both can be performed at the bedside, using an electronic digital recorder.

The ability of a patient to blow out a standard book match held 6 inches from the open mouth has been correlated with standard tests of pulmonary function. Eighty percent of patients who cannot blow out the match will have maximum breathing capacity below 60 L/min, while 80% of those who can blow out the match will have a maximum breathing capacity above 60 L/min. Eighty-five percent of the patients who cannot blow out the match will have a 1-sec vital capacity below 1.60 L, while 85% of patients who can blow out the match will have a 1-sec vital capacity above 1.6 L.

This simple bedside test is a fairly reliable guide to lower airway obstruction. It may fail in patients with greatly reduced total vital capacity due to interstitial fibrosis, without airway obstruction, because in these patients the 1-sec vital capacity may be a normal percentage of the reduced total vital capacity and still be inadequate to extinguish the match. Even in such cases the test may serve as an incentive to obtain further function studies.

COUGH TEST.[187] A vigorous cough induced in patients prior to surgery provides a screening test of patients susceptible to the development of atelectasis or pneumonia. It is a reliable method to detct the presence of disease such as bronchitis, abnormal quantities of mucus, or foreign material in the bronchial tree. The patient is requested to cough, then observed for (1) the ability to cough, (2) the strength, and (3) the effectiveness. A normal test is a "dry" response; in these patients major respiratory complications do not develop. A patient with a "wet" productive or a self-propagated paroxysm of coughing is a candidate for pulmonary complications.

PREANESTHETIC CARDIOVASCULAR EVALUATION

Two specific tests are available to estimate cardiovascular function;[188] these are the electrocardiogram (ECG) and the hemodynamic variables determined by cardiac catheterization.[189] Abnormalities of these tests have been shown to correlate closely with the development of complications.

An ECG serves as a screening test. It is not a measure of functional capacity, but it does serve to detect rhythm and conduction disturbances and premature contractions. One may be alerted to the presence of ischemic disease. In the older age group, it is a clue to many abnormalities, such as the diffuse myocardial disease. Preventive measures may be indicated and at least a baseline established for subsequent complications.

An exercise ECG test also reveals functional disease and the degree of cardiac reserve. It is useful to indicate possible coronary artery disease.[197]

Increased morbidity and mortality are found in the following circumstances, as revealed by the screening ECG: healed myocardial infarctions;[190] atrial premature contractions;[191] atrial fibrillation;[191] and bundle branch block.[192]

A high degree of postoperative complications is found when there is evidence of myocardial infarction and atrial premature contractions.

EVALUATION OF PATIENTS WITH CARDIAC DISEASE. The key to successful anesthesia and surgery in the cardiac patient is understanding that the cardiac reserve and any added risk is proportional to the decrease in this reserve. The cardiac reserve should be estimated by the cardiologist. Perhaps the best general index is a careful history. A patient's cardiac

FIG. 9–4. Valsalva maneuver showing effect on systolic blood pressure in normal subjects *(solid line)* and in patients with pulmonary congestion *(dotted line).*

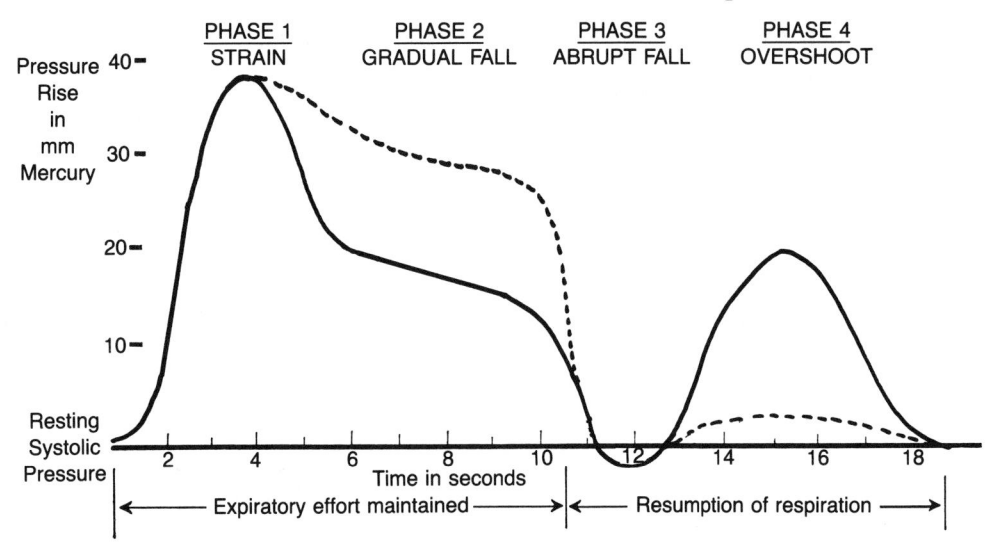

reserve is reflected in his ability to carry on work and in the extent and variety of everyday activities. This is a more accurate estimate of capacity than the mere description of the cardiac lesion.[194]

Diseases of the heart have been fairly well defined, and the New York Heart Association (NYHA) has established a classification of the elements of a complete cardiac diagnosis.[195] An outline of this classification is presented in Table 9–12 and should be familiar to all anesthesiologists. It represents the type of information that should be made available by medical consultants.

In practice, only the functional and therapeutic criteria are usually noted. The NYHA classification of great value in determining the degree of cardiovascular disability (Table 9–13). Supplementing this classification, Goldman et al have developed a specific activity scale based on the metabolic cost of activity.[196] Use of the Goldman Cardiac Risk Index has been presented, and its predictive value for complications and outcome has been amply confirmed.

SPECIFIC FACTORS.[191] Among the factors associated with underlying heart disease and contributing to increased complications and consequent increased mortality are the following:[191]

1. Inadequately digitalized patients
2. Recent congestive heart failure (within 2 months)
3. Severity of heart disease functionally
4. Cardiac enlargement
5. Atrial fibrillation
6. Arteriosclerosis and angina
7. Myocardial infarction within 1 year
8. Valvular disease

Physical Examination for Cardiac Performance. Among the conditions to be noted by the anesthesiologist are the following: presence of jugular vein distention (JVD); irregularity in pulse; abnormal heart sounds (S_3 and S_4); abnormal murmurs; peripheral edema; pulmonary rales and wheezes; and carotid bruits.

Clinical Cardiac Pump Performance. A classification of cardiac function indicative of pump performance has been proposed by Killip.[198] This is of value in the management of myocardial infarction and coronary ischemic disorders and provides clin-

TABLE 9–12. NYHA FUNCTIONAL CLASSIFICATION OF HEART DISEASE*

Class	Criteria
I	*No limitation:* ordinary physical activity does not cause undue fatigue, dyspnea, or palpitation
II	*Slight limitation of physical activity:* such patients are comfortable at rest; ordinary physical activity results in fatigue, palpitation, dyspnea, or angina
III	*Marked limitation of physical activity:* although patients are comfortable at rest, less than ordinary activity will lead to symptoms
IV	*Inability to carry on any physical activity without discomfort:* symptoms of congestive failure are present even at rest; With any physical activity, increased discomfort is experienced

* This element of the nomenclature of heart disease is based on the relation between symptoms and the amount of effort required to provoke them.

TABLE 9–13. NOMENCLATURE AND ALL CRITERIA FOR DIAGNOSIS OF DISEASE OF THE HEART

A. ETIOLOGIC
B. ANATOMIC
C. PHYSIOLOGIC
D. FUNCTIONAL
E. THERAPEUTIC
   a. No restriction of activity.
   b. No restriction of ordinary activity; but advised against strenuous activity.
   c. Moderate restriction of ordinary activity; discontinue strenuous activity.
   d. Extreme restriction of ordinary activity.
   e. Complete rest.

ical evidence of the degree of impairment of myocardial performance (Table 9–14).

Other Diagnostic Studies (as Indicated). The *dipyridamole-thallium stress test* is a noninvasive technique for detection of coronary artery disease (CAD).[199,200] Two-dimensional echocardiography with dipyridamole is also used to assess the presence of CAD.[201]

Coronary angiography is an invasive technique and is known as the "gold standard" for assessing the integrity of the coronary arteries.[202,203]

Preoperative Swan-Ganz evaluation, a system of preoperative invasive monitoring, has been recommended to assess operative risk, especially in the elderly patient.[204] In patients over 65, Swan-Ganz catheterization was routinely employed by Del Gurcico to obtain a cardiopulmonary profile. He reported that the Swan-Ganz evaluation was justified in over 80% of patients. The following measures or calculations were made, and they correlated with clinical assessment of ASA physical status (PS): preoperative oxygen tension, mean pulmonary artery pressures, mean pulmonary wedge pressure, pulmonary vascular resistance, mixed venous oxygen saturation, and shunt percent.

Preoperative oxygen tension in the elderly was below normal in 44% of patients, i.e., below 65 mm Hg. Mean pulmonary artery pressure showed relative pulmonary hypertension in about 60% of patients, whereas pulmonary vascular resistance was elevated over 250 dyne/sec/m^2 in 45% of patients. The mean pulmonary wedge pressure was above 8 mm Hg in 45% of patients. Left ventricular function plots of Sarnoff-type showed only 25% of patients with normal myocardial contractility, and 25% had poor ventricular function and contractility insufficiency. Shunts of 20% were found in 25% of patients. The arteriovenous oxygen difference was increased in 30% of patients.

Correlation of data with PS revealed that mixed venous oxygen showed an inverse trend in the estimation of PS. A decreasing venous oxygen saturation showed a worsening PS (Figs. 9–5 and 9–6). Mean pulmonary wedge pressure greater than 8 mm Hg corresponded to PS 4.

Another diagnostic study is *exercise ventriculography*.[205] Cardiac complications represent major causes of perioperative morbidity and mortality, especially in the elderly patient undergoing abdominal and nonthoracic surgery. To identify patients at high risk, Gerson and associates compared rest and exercise through the use of radionuclide ventriculog-

TABLE 9–14. CLASSIFICATION OF CARDIAC FUNCTION (PUMP PERFORMANCE)

Class	Criteria
1	No clinical signs of congestive heart failure
2	Pulmonary rales
3	Pulmonary edema
4	Cardiogenic shock

Adapted from Killip, T., and Kimball, J.T.: Treatment of myocardial infarction in a coronary care unit. Am. J. Cardiol., 20:457, 1967.

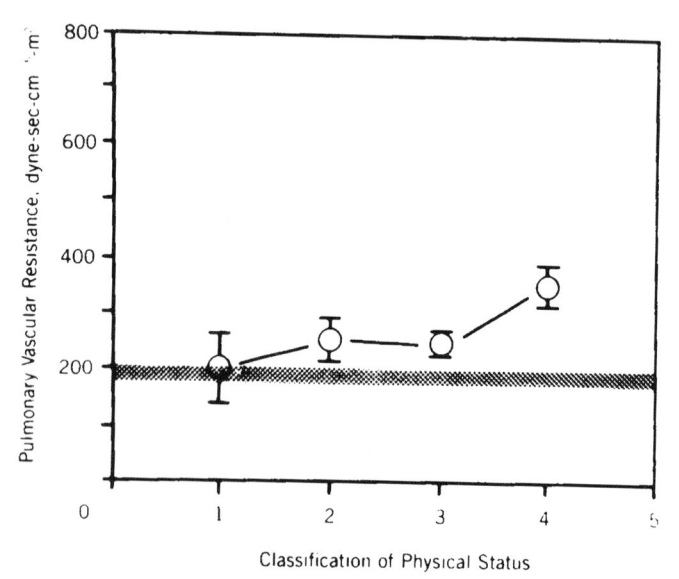

FIG. 9–5. Pulmonary vascular resistance and preoperative classification of physical status by anesthesiologists. Class 4 patients were found to have increased pulmonary vascular resistance. From Del Gurcico, L.R.M., and Cohn, D.J.: Monitoring operative risk in the elderly. J.A.M.A., 243:1350, 1980.

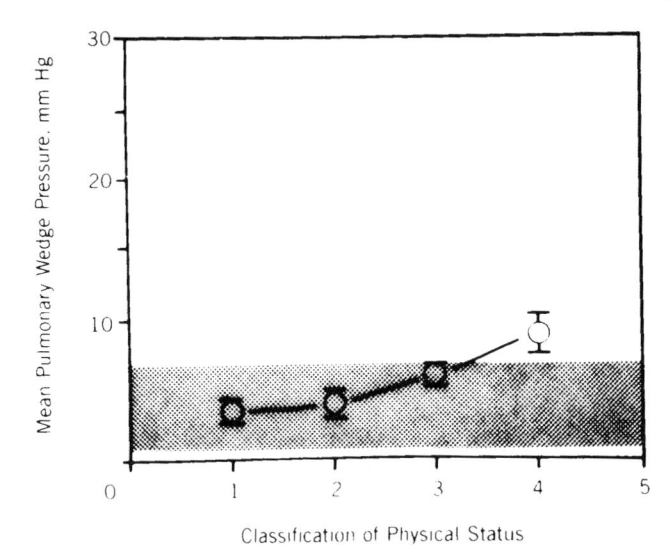

FIG. 9–6. Pulmonary artery wedge pressures in 148 preoperative patients compared with classification of physical status using American Society of Anesthesiologists criteria. Poor physical status generally predicted elevated wedge pressures. From Del Gurcico, L.R.M., and Cohn, J.D.: Monitoring operative risk in the elderly. J.A.M.A., 243:1350, 1980.

raphy. In an analysis of a group of patients, the only independent predictor of perioperative cardiac complications or death was the exercise testing procedure. It is noted that a larger study might identify other specific predictors of perioperative cardiac morbidity and mortality. The test had a significant sensitivity of about 80%, and it was specific for outcome in 53% of the patients studied.

Preoperative Assessment of Vagal Responsiveness.[206] Carotid sinus stimulation by massage is of value in detecting sinoatrial or atrioventricular node disease. Such disease may exist in the absence of abnormalities of the preoperative resting ECG. The test should be performed prior to surgical procedures of the head or neck or when excessive vagal stimulation is to be anticipated, as in upper abdominal surgery.

RESPIRATORY EVALUATION TESTS

The mechanics of breathing should be checked preoperatively; including the structural anatomy, the type of effort, and the pattern of movement. Patency of the nasal passages should be assessed. Hoarseness, stridor, or vocal abnormality should be checked. Indirect laryngoscopy will often reveal potential problems.

INDICATIONS. Table 9–15 summarizes the indications for preoperative pulmonary evaluation. Patients who show evidence of pulmonary disease or

TABLE 9–15. INDICATIONS FOR PREOPERATIVE PULMONARY EVALUATION

History	Physical
Smoking history	Cyanosis
Age >60 years	Tachypnea
Pulmonary symptoms	Upper airway anomaly
Known lung disease	Passive expiratory wheezing
Body weight >20% ideal	Forced expiration time >3 sec
Thoracic operation scheduled	Generalized weakness
Upper abdominal operation scheduled	Decreased mental status

respiratory dysfunction and who are scheduled for extensive intrathoracic or prolonged upper abdominal surgery should be carefully assessed clinically at the bedside and then by simple spirometric screening tests for FVC and FEV$_1$.[207] If the beside tests and the FEV$_1$ values are abnormal, more detailed and precise studies should be performed.

Three tests of pulmonary function are of predictive value in patients who have evidence of clinical disease.[208] These are:

1. *Spirometry:* for clinical capacity and "timed vital capacity" or forced expiratory volumes FEV(s). FEV$_1$ is the commonly used test with the most value.
2. *Ventilatory studies:* for maximum breathing capacity (MBC) and peak flow rate. Generally, peak flow rate and FEV$_1$ are closely correlated (Fig. 9–7a).
3. *Blood gas analysis:* Elevated PA$_{CO_2}$ has been associated with poor pulmonary function and has been of some predictive value and use in ventilatory management;[209] however, hypercapnea has not provided an absolute contraindication to surgery.[210] On the other hand, PA$_{O_2}$ has greater predictive value in determining the need for careful appropriate ventilatory management. (Fig 9–7b) It has been found to be one of the most important risk factors[208] and correlates with the degree of dyspnea.

VITAL CAPACITY AND FORCED VITAL CAPACITY MEASUREMENTS. Two specific and easily performed tests of pulmonary function are desirable in patients to be submitted to major surgery and in the geriatric patient. These are vital capacity measurements and a forced vital capacity (timed VC) test. A spirometer is used, and the calculations are easy. As a result, patients may be classified on a grid as having normal function or the following abnormal conditions:

1. A restrictive lesion—VC below 80% of predicted and a normal timed VC (above 60% of predicted).
2. An obstructive lesion—VC normal or above 80% of predicted and a timed FEV below 60% of predicted (0.5 to 1 L/sec is approximately 20% to 60% below predicted).
3. A combined lesion.

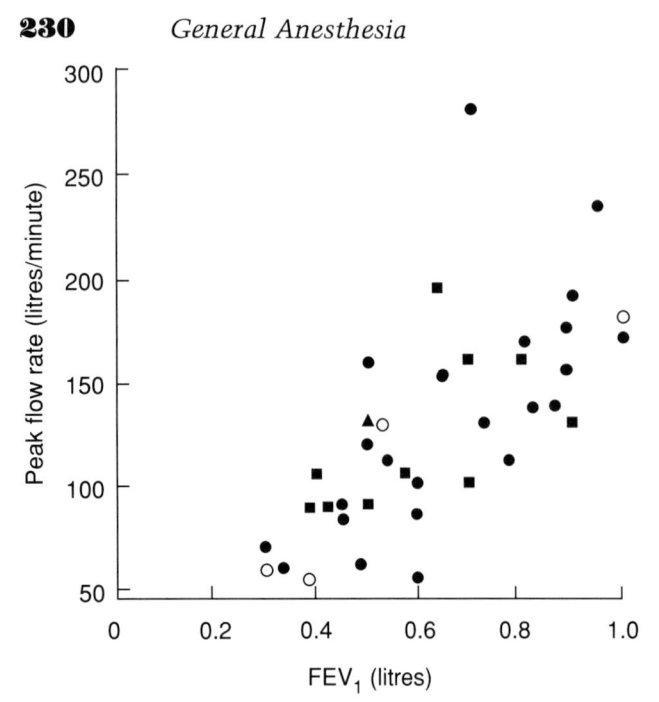

FIG. 9–7a. Preoperative values for FEV_1 and peak flow rate. ○ = ___; ● = ___; ▲ = ___; ■ = ___. From Nunn, J.F., et al.: Respiratory criteria of fitness for surgery and anaesthesia. Anaesthesia, 43:543, 1988.

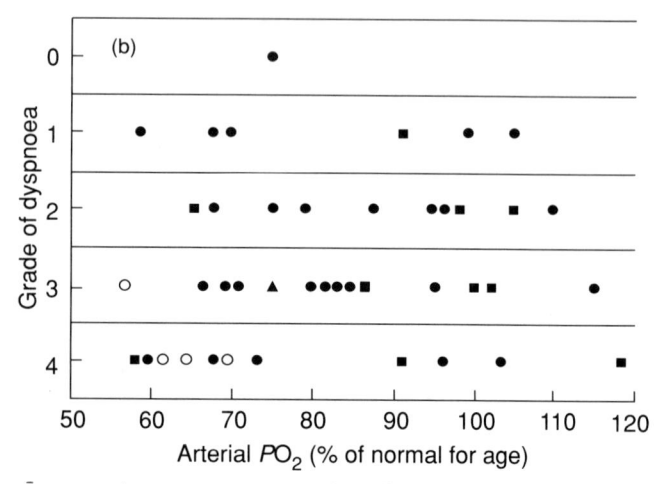

FIG. 9–7b. Pre-operative values for arterial P_{O_2}, as percentage of predicted and grades of dyspnoea. Note that all the patients whose lungs were ventilated postoperatively are clustered in the lower left hand corner. ●, general anaesthesia; ■, regional anaesthesia; ▲, combined regional and general anaesthesia; ○, artificial ventilation after the first operation (general anaesthesia).

As vital capacity may be decreased in both restrictive and obstructive pulmonary disease, a repetition of the test following the inhalation of 0.5% isoproterenol aerosol can differentiate obstruction due to contraction of smooth muscle from obstruction due to destructive or structural disease.

These studies enable the operative team to determine the extent of risk (Fig. 9–8), and they identify those patients who are in need of preoperative respiratory therapy. Thus, when an obstructive lesion is present the following regimen can be instituted: expectorants, antibiotics, liquefying agents, and postural drainage.

Howland[188] has found that any type of ventilatory defect increases the incidence of postoperative complications. Patients with emphysema are particularly vulnerable. In the geriatric patient, the mortality increases from about 2% in patients with normal pulmonary function to almost 10% in patients with combined lesions.

OTHER DIAGNOSTIC PULMONARY FUNCTION TESTS. Other relatively simple screening and diagnostic function tests that are more precise and detailed include:[211,212]

- Maximum breathing capacity by Wright respirometer (Turbine Type)*
- Peak flow rate (4 × MBC) by Wright respirometer correlates with FEV_1.
- Pulmonary diffusing capacity by single breath test of nontoxic carbon monoxide
- Measurements of pulmonary arterial and wedge pressure at rest and during exercise
- Bronchospirometry for estimation of regional lung function (especially for pulmonary surgery)
- Detection of regional disease, including presence, location, and extent, can be accomplished by presently available tests. These can show the distri-

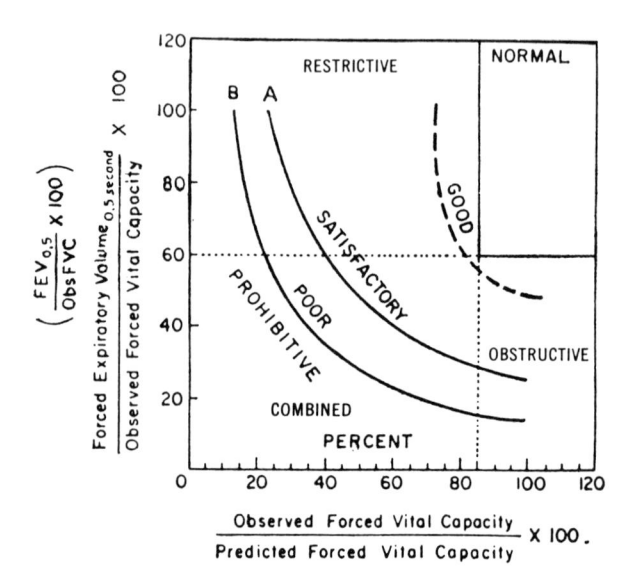

FIG. 9–8. Risk as related to ventilatory function. From Miller, W.F., et al.: Pulmonary function evaluation. Anesthesiology, 17:480, 1956.

---

* Richards Medical Equipment, Wheeling, Ill.

bution of air, the distribution of blood to pulmonary capillaries, and the matching of gas and blood to an alveolus.

- Single breath oxygen test—detects uneven distribution of air
- Single breath xenon test—shows the distribution of air to the lung fields
- Screening bronchograph test—shows structural abnormalities of airways
- Intravenous tagged albumin (also technetium)—shows perfusion at arteriolar and capillary levels; Abnormalities identify obstructed pulmonary arteries

APPLICATION IN THORACIC SURGERY. Pneumonectomy or lobectomy in the adult is well tolerated if FEV_1 is greater than 2 L (over 60% of predicted) and MBC is greater than 50%.[213] Stein[209] and Nunn,[208] however, have reported successful outcomes when the FEV_1 is less than 1 L, provided PA_{O_2} is monitored and maintained by adequate ventilatory care, especially postoperatively.[208] If calculated FEV_1 is greater than 800 ml, it is probable that the operation will be tolerated, but if it is less than 500 ml, the condition may be inoperable;[214] Nunn[208] and all but life-saving surgery should be avoided or delayed to optimize function.

DYSPNEA. This term has been concisely defined as "consciousness of the necessity for increased respiratory effort."[215] It is a subjective perception ("short of breath") by the patient of difficulty in breathing and connotes a symptom; hence, it cannot be directly measured.[216] But the severity of the difficulty can be graded according to the degree of exertion (Table 9–16).[217] The complaint is a sensitive indicator that the work of breathing has been changed and requires evaluation, particularly of the mechanics of ventilation. Undue awareness of breathing or breathlessness applies to the healthy person during severe exercise or work but is more usually applied in the medical context to the patient with impending respiratory or cardiac insufficiency during ordinary activity. There is usually clinical evidence of disease of either the lungs or the heart.

Among the multiple mechanisms producing dyspnea, the following have been presented:[211,212] (1) increased *work* of breathing; (2) a reduction in functional residual capacity (i.e., atelectasis, pulmonary edema); (3) increased sensory inflow from respiratory muscles or pulmonary stretch receptors (J); and (4) increased sensitivity to subjective phemonena (i.e., anxiety, airway obstruction).

Other Physiologic Studies of Dyspnea.

- Hypoxia and hypercapnea are often present but do not appear to be responsible for the sensation and are present when respiratory and cardiac disease are present.

TABLE 9–16. GRADES OF DYSPNEA ASSESSED BY THE EXERTION OF WALKING

Grade	Description
0	No history of dyspnea; no dyspnea on standard exercises or walking at a fast pace.
I	Mild dyspnea: fast walk on a level for a short distance; or a long distance at a slow pace.
II	Moderate dyspnea: "short of breath" walking at a normal pace on level ground for 2–3 blocks or climbing one flight of house stairs.
III	Severe dyspnea: "short of breath" at a slow walk on level ground with frequent pauses over a short distance, or unable to climb less than one flight of stairs.
IV	Incapacitating dyspnea: dyspnea at rest.

* Severity can be based on occurrence of the sensation (complaint) in response to physical exercise—walking is the usual exercise. The complaint of dyspnea is caused by respiratory and/or cardiac problems. Adapted from Boushy, S.F., et al.: Clinical course related to preoperative pulmonary function in patients with bronchogenic carcinoma. Chest, 59:383, 1971.

- Breath holding sheds some light on the causation of the sensation of "breathlessness." The sensation can be relieved by ventilation and a change in lung volume. The breath-holding time can be increased by such procedures as vagal and glossopharyngeal nerve block.[218a] These nerves carry pulmonary afferents that reflexly evoke involuntary contractions of the respiratory muscle.
- Breath-holding time is directly proportional to the lung volume at the beginning of breath holding. The time is usually limited in healthy subjects to 60 to 90 seconds. Some physiologic responses accompanying breath holding include vasoconstriction (skin, muscle, viscera, abdominal) and bradycardia. The "breaking point," or point of dyspnea, is in part related to the onset of hypoxia.[219]
- Breath holding can be greatly prolonged by administration of curare and blocking involuntary contraction of respiratory muscles.[220] Breath holding can also be prolonged by the diving reflex. In humans, this is due primarily to immersion of the face in water at a temperature of 10° to 20° C.[218b]

Role of Pulmonary and Respiratory Muscle Afferents Ordinary motor response consists of contraction of the respiratory muscles, especially the diaphragm, which is involuntary and driven by the ventilatory requirements of oxygen need and CO_2 elimination. When contraction of the respiratory muscles is impeded by breath holding, airway obstruction, or excessive work of breathing (cost of breathing itself), the failure of muscle shortening progressively excites the afferent component of the reflex from the diaphragm and intercostals.[221] This leads to the point where the need to breathe is no longer involuntary but becomes a conscious effort—a sensation. The afferent component is only modified reciprocally when the contractions are able to result in shortening of the respiratory muscles with movement of the chest and expansion of the lungs, thereby stimulating the MTJ (muscle-tendon-joint) proprioceptors in the chest wall and the pulmonary stretch receptors. This is the concept of "inappropriateness" between muscle activity and muscle movement as an explanation of the sensation of dyspnea.[219]

PULMONARY DISEASES. Respiratory diseases in surgical patients present real hazards and enhance the risk of complications and fatalities. The specific chest problem should be identified, the extent of interference with ventilation or gas exchange assessed by function studies, and attempts made to control the disease process or to correct the pathology. Rovenstine and Taylor[222] found that preoperative infection of the respiratory tract increased the frequency of postoperative chest complication *fourfold*.

Upper respiratory infections are frequent and often too casually viewed. The common cold and chronic sinusitis should be controlled. A safe decision can be reached by considering the urgency of the surgical situation. Elective surgery should be avoided in the presence of an acute cold. Urgent surgery requires vigorous treatment of a concurrent cold. Nasal inhaler therapy with aerosols and antibiotics; intravenous hydration; gargles for sore throat to decrease quantitatively the bacterial flora; and parenteral broad spectrum antibiotics are indicated preoperatively. Good oral hygiene is desirable. Beck[223] has shown that the use of a mouth wash preoperatively is effective in reducing bacterial counts and tracheal contamination, especially if endotracheal tubes are used.

Decreased ventilation can be caused by pleural effusions or ascitic fluid. This fluid should be removed. A pleural tap and removal of 1000 ml of fluid, such as may accumulate in elderly patients with heart failure as well as primary lung disease, will improve pulmonary function.

Asthmatic patients should be assessed carefully and attempts made to decrease bronchiolar constriction. It is equally important to decrease mucosal edema. Patients should not be exposed to offending allergens. Bronchodilator and bronchorrhea therapy should be instituted. Expectorants and potassium iodide are effective.

Patients with chronic lung disease such as chronic bronchitis, bronchiectasis, chronic obstructive pulmonary disease, emphysema and other conditions associated with increased secretions must be submitted to an "improvement regimen." Postural drainage, aerosol therapy to liquefy secretions,[224] and antibiotics are necessary. Surgery should be postponed to the afternoon; this allows the patient to spend the morning hours coughing and cleaning out his own respiratory tract. Tarhan et al have reported no mortality in a series of patients with chronic lung disease submitted to surgery under spinal or epidural anesthesia. This appears to be a safe choice when appropriate for the surgical site of operation.[225]

Emphysema. Emphysema is a serious complicating pulmonary problem encountered in surgical patients.[226] These patients have ineffective alveolar ventilation. It is usually due to both an interference with ventilation and secondarily to poor alveolar gas mixing with impaired alveolar–capillary diffusion. In truth, these patients are "respiratory disabled." Consequently carbon dioxide retention occurs and respiratory acidosis ensues. Superimposed on this functional inadequacy is invariably a secondary infection. In addition, the increased resistance to blood flow through the lungs produces corpulmonale and often right-sided failure.

The extent of the various functional deficiencies in emphysema must be assessed, and the pulmonary reserve must be evaluated. Not only should the pathophysiology be corrected, but a serious attempt made to improve function.

The first objective is attained by bronchodilators, pulmonary humidification, decongestants, postural drainage and expectorants.[227]

The second objective of improving pulmonary function can be attained by: (1) breathing exercises as advocated by Barach[228] and (2) by moderate general physical exercise and fitness programs.

Acute Respiratory Disease—Consensus Standard.[229] To persist with anything but emergency surgery in a patient with an upper respiratory infection (URI) is foolhardy. The incidence of complications is high, e.g., laryngeal spasm during induction or emergence, postoperative lower respiratory tract infections. Fitness for surgery is relative to the urgency, but pyrexia, nasal discharge, inflamed tonsils or ear drums, cough, and a raised white blood cell count are all indications for considering a delay before the surgery.[229]

Chronic URI or "Runny Nose" Syndrome.[230] The "runny nose" syndrome is frequently encountered, especially in children. This may be a benign condition or a serious condition imposing significant complications.

Such a subacute or chronic URI deserves careful evaluation. If the condition has existed or a cold has been present in the previous month, a preoperative chest radiograph (A–P and lateral) should be obtained. This is especially important in children. If the film is positive, surgery should be postponed.[231]

Preoperative chest films in a large series of pediatric patients without significant history or physical respiratory abnormalities showed 7.5% radiographic abnormalities. Pneumonia or atelectasis was present in 2.7% of these patients. Thus, without attention to chest physiology, significant pathology may be missed.[232] An additional study by Wood on asymptomatic children showed chest film abnormalities in 4.7%, and these abnormalities were significant in 1.2% of patients.

Hall has demonstrated abnormalities of pulmonary function after an uncomplicated flu bout persisting for at least 3 to 4 weeks.[233]

Children 1 to 4 years of age presenting symptoms of URI at the time of surgery, or who have had symptoms in the week prior to scheduled surgery, often show abnormally low saturation levels after general anesthesia on admission to the recovery room. These patients with preoperative URI symptoms should be monitored carefully and supplemental oxygen should be administered (Personal communication, R. Patel: Children's Hospital National Medical Center, Washington, D.C., 1989).

Clinical Aspects The causes of the benign "runny nose" are principally allergic rhinitis and vasomotor rhinitis. Clinically, the child is usually afebrile, eats well, plays well, and behaves normally. There is a degree of chronicity with a history of full-blown URI several times a year, especially in the winter and spring months. Anesthesia and surgery need not be cancelled under these circumstances.[234]

Acute URI.[235] A more serious situation is the "runny nose" developing acutely and representing the prodrome of an infectious process of the respiratory tract, with a reactive airway, excessive secretions, and infectious croup. Clinically, the history is that a child not behaving normally, usually cranky, not eating or sleeping well. The child may be slightly febrile and in the process of developing a productive cough. Anesthesia and surgery for such patients with an acute URI and nasopharyngitis, especially at the incipient stage, should be postponed for 4 to 6 weeks. With evidence of both upper and lower respiratory tract disease, one can be certain of a reactive airway and of excessive secretions. If a simple nasopharyngitis exists, without clinical evidence of a lower tract process, 2 to 3 weeks is usually sufficient.

Criteria for URI.[235] A person can be considered to have a URI if any three of the following signs and symptoms are present:[236]

1. Sore or scratchy throat
2. Rhinorrhea
3. Sneezing
4. Congestion of upper respiratory tract
5. Laryngitis
6. Nonproductive cough
7. Malaise
8. Fever less than 101°F

These symptoms may be acute or chronic, as in children with chronic otitis media. It is noted that a combination of these symptoms enables one to distinguish a URI from an allergic or vasomotor rhinitis. The latter are also seasonally related. The most prevalent symptoms in these children were rhinorrhea (80%), congestion (70%), nonproductive cough (60%), sneezing (40%), and sore throat (25%).

Subacute URI.[235] Tait has studied a large group of children with a history of chronic otitis media using the clinical criteria previously noted. Asymptomatic children with no recent history of a respiratory illness had perioperative complications presumed to be related to anesthesia in 1.25% of patients, consisting principally of laryngospasm and dysrhythmia. In symptomatic children, the incidence of complications was 1.28%. Children with symptoms of only one or two of the criteria, but with a history of a URI in the 2 weeks prior to their surgery, had an incidence of 2.38% of complications. These patients received halothane–N_2O–O_2 anesthesia by face mask. Noteworthy in this study is the significantly lesser prevalence and duration of respiratory symptoms in the anesthetized children compared with the matched nonanesthetized control group of children. It is evident that there is no increased morbidity related to anesthesia and surgery in these patients with otitis media. Indeed, it is suggested that either the anesthesia or the surgical procedure of myringotomy has a salutary effect on the URI.

Uncomplicated Chronic URI. Patients with uncomplicated URI infections may be safely anesthetized. Knight[237] has shown that asymptomatic children without a recent bout of a URI developed about 1.5% rate of respiratory complications, whereas children with an ongoing "runny nose" syndrome URI showed a 1.6% complication rate. In contrast, children with a history of a URI in the prior 2 weeks developed a 5.3% complication rate.[234]

In a comparison study, children presenting with a chronic URI infection, chiefly otitis media, symptomatic with rhinorrhea, congestion, sore throat but unproductive cough, when administered halothane anesthesia had a significantly shorter duration of old and new symptoms, such as malaise, fever and productive cough, than a nonanesthetized paired control group. In all instances, nasopharyngeal cultures revealed the presence of rhinovirus and respiratory syncytial virus.[237]

This clinical study complements both an in vitro and animal study of a number of viruses, wherein halothane exposure resulted in a reversible inhibition of viral replication. The extent of this inhibition was dose dependent.[238]

Anesthesia for Emergency Surgery in URI.[235] When anesthesia must be administered for emergency surgery to a patient with an infectious runny nose, two conditions complicate the administration of anesthesia and impose a perioperative and postoperative risk. First, the excess nasopharyngeal and tracheobronchial secretions must be managed because of the attendant airway obstruction. Second, the reactive airway is usually accompanied by a stormy induction, even with intravenous agents, and a stormy awakening and postoperative period. The increased sensitivity of the protective airway reflexes are particularly evident during induction. Coughing, breath holding, laryngospasm, and a "delirium" panic type of reaction is often encountered. The outpouring of secretions may be managed by an anticholinergic agent; a generous oral dose of 25 µg/kg of atropine may be given 30 minutes before or 10 µg/kg given IM 10 minutes before the induction of anesthesia. Induction may be accomplished by intramuscular midazolam or, if an intravenous line is in place, the anesthesia can be induced by the intravenous route with midazolam or ketamine. Thiopental and other shortacting barbiturates increase airway reactivity. Highly successful after an IM injection of midazolam is a gentle halothane–N_2O–oxygen mixture by inhalation. Postoperative coughing and excessive reacting to an airway can be controlled by the administration of lidocaine IV in doses of 1–1.5 mg/kg.

MEDICAL CONSULTATION[239]

When a medical condition coexists with a surgical disease, consultation with a general internist or a medical subspecialist is warranted. This defines the role and expertise of the medical consultant. The consultation request should be for medical evaluation (not a request for "clearance for surgery or anesthesia"). The selection of the patient for such consultation should be based on the judgment of the surgeon or anesthesiologist of the need for medical evaluation and benefit to the patient. The existence of a cardiac, pulmonary, renal, metabolic, or neurologic disease ("risk factors") represents general risks to the patient's health. The internist should define the disease and the degree of functional impairment. Therapy should be recommended and instituted and a statement entered into the medical evaluation note that the patient's condition has been stabilized and that he is optimally prepared medically. The anesthesiologist and surgeon, on this basis, are then in a position to estimate the operative risk of anesthesia and surgery and clear the patient for anesthesia for the planned procedure of the surgeon.[240a,240b]

For patients under 50 years of age, it is apparent that routine medical consultations have limited value and the benefits are infrequent. Consultations should be requested by the surgeon or anesthesiologist in limited circumstances, when some functional impairment exists, suggested from history and a review of systems.[240b]

For patients over 50 years of age, a routine general medical evaluation is indicated. In a study of preoperative examination by an internist, Levinson found that a significant medical risk condition existed in 20% of such consultations.

Some questions that should be answered by the internist include:

- What is the state of myocardial compensation? Reserve?
- Is the patient adequately digitalized?
- If patient is hypertensive, what has been done to control or stabilize the blood pressure? What is the medication regimen?
- What is the pulmonary status? What is the severity of dysfunction? Is an obstructive disorder under treatment? What medications?
- Is renal function or hepatic function within normal limits? If not, what is the problem and how is it managed?
- Are electrolytes within a normal range?
- Is there adequate metabolic reserve assessed by laboratory and blood gas analysis when indicated?
- Are all medications prescribed or being used by the patient, as well as doses, if determinable, noted?

The medical consultant should define the disease state, the degree of dysfunction, and the pathologic condition, and then treat the condition to an optimal level. It is appreciated when a patient's medical problems and organ functions are stabilized at a reasonable level of performance because it contributes to a successful outcome.[240c]

Statements often made in a medical "consultation," which are without any value (and may be legally compromising), are the following:[240c]

- "Okay for general anesthesia" (when regional anesthesia may be the safest)
- "No absolute contraindication to general anesthesia"
- "Cleared for spinal anesthesia" (in patient with a history of spinal cord dysfunction)
- "Avoid hypertension or hypotension" (Surgery is stressful, and blood is usually lost)
- "Avoid hypoxia (or hypercarbia)" (This is bringing coals to Newcastle)
- "Monitor electrocardiogram" (This is a standard of anesthesia practice since 1950)

CHOICE OF ANESTHESIA

PRINCIPLES IN CHOICE OF ANESTHESIA.[239] The choice of anesthesia should be based on an individualized plan for every patient who is presented for evaluation. In general, the goal of anesthesia is to provide a painless operation. Four factors must be considered in determining a technique and agent: (1) safety to the patient; (2) convenience for the surgeon; (3) comfort and preference of the patient; and (4) ability of the anesthesiologist.

Every patient plan should be individualized and

anesthetic technique and agent tailored to fit the situation. Each drug has its indications, its contraindications, and its field of usefulness. Whatever agents or techniques are used, they must be safe for the patient.

Either a general or a regional anesthesia may be most suitable for the patient, and one or the other may provide the greater margin of safety. Presently a wide armamentarium of drugs for general anesthesia is available, including intravenous agents, inhalation agents, and muscle relaxants. Similarly, there is a broad spectrum of local anesthetics with properties of onset and duration suitable for many surgical requirements and yet with a wide margin of safety.

All anesthetic drugs should be considered to cause some physiologic trespass. For the individual patient, the one producing the least disturbance should be chosen. When a medical disease is present in a patient, the drugs interacting with the least disturbance or alteration of function should be chosen. Choice is a matter based on physiologic and pharmacologic considerations as related to the type of disease and the pharmacologic effects of the agents.

Having provided a stress-free painless state and an anesthetic that is safe for the patient, the anesthesiologist should provide good working conditions for the surgeon. If such conditions are provided, the surgeon can complete the surgery expeditiously to the greater welfare and subsequent rapid convalescence of the patient. These conditions, however, must not be achieved at the price of safety.

It is also desirable to provide patient comfort, but this must not be achieved at the expense of favorable surgical conditions or safety to the patient. It may be necessary to sacrifice comfort or surgical convenience in the interest of safety.

Despite these important factors, it is often necessary to consider the ability of the anesthesiologist in determining the anesthetic technique or agent. It is preferable that an anesthesiologist use that technique with which he or she is most skilled and the agents with which he or she is most knowledgeable.

GENERAL ANESTHESIA VERSUS REGIONAL ANESTHESIA. For certain operative procedures, regional anesthesia reduces some intraoperative complications and postoperative morbidity. This is particularly true for epidural or spinal anesthesia.[241]

The endocrine and metabolic responses to trauma are reduced but not obliterated by epidural or spinal block. The antistress effect, however, is minimal in major abdominal or intrathoracic procedures, especially upper abdominal surgery.[242]

Intraoperative blood loss is reduced. In hip pinning, a reduction of 30% to 40% can be expected during extradural anesthesia.[243,244] Similar reductions of 30% or more are found during prostatectomy under subdural or epidural block.[245] Thromboembolic complications are reduced by 50% after hip surgery and prostatectomy managed by regional spinal techniques.[246]

For other complications, the evidence is not in favor of regional anesthesia. Indeed, postoperative mental dysfunction is equally as great with regional technics as with general anesthesia.

NEED FOR ANESTHESIA IN NEONATES.[247,248] The neonate has the anatomic equipment necessary to feel pain: cortex, thalamus, spinal cord, peripheral nerves and receptors, and developing neuronal connections to link them, they are functionally active.[247]

Many responses to painful stimuli in the newborn have been observed and studied. All are typical of those seen in the child or adult. Indeed, such responses are observed in utero and detailed as early as 5 months postconception.[249] Reactions to repeated pinprick in the lower limbs include an increase in heart rate, protective moments of upper and lower limbs, facial grimacing, and crying.[250] Changes in skin conductivity and transcutaneous P_{O_2} have also been noted.[251] Facial expressions associated with various emotional states, including pain, have been reliably differentiated by experienced observers. Cries are not acoustically unique, although they vary in intensity according to the amount of discomfort experienced by the neonate. Neonates who have been circumcised have shown that changes in behavior may persist for more than 22 hours postoperatively in babies who have received no analgesia.[252,253]

Behavioral changes and crying are responses that involve higher nervous system function and are not simple reflexes.[254]

Cortical activity in response to visual stimuli has been demonstrated in babies from the 25th week postconception.[255] Similarly, it has been shown that other stimuli, including auditory, olfactory, and tactile, result in cortical electroencephalographic activity in preterm neonates. Neonates[256] can distinguish voices over other sounds, and female over male voices. Motor cortical activity is also suggested in neonates with convulsions, as cortical convulsive potentials occur synchronously with peripheral massive muscle contractions.

The conclusion we must therefore make is that the neonate has the ability to perceive pain at a cortical level and does respond with typical efferent motor activity. Signs of distress such as crying, facial grimacing and tachycardia, when taken in the context of likely or actual tissue damage, are evidentiary. Other useful behavioral indicators include restlessness, being slow to settle after stimulation, and unusually long periods of wakefulness.[255]

The increasing use of local anesthesia in pediatric practice in general does not seem to have reached the neonate to a similar extent, partly because of technical difficulties and partly because of the reduced plasma protein binding and prolonged elimination of some agents in this age group. These problems, however, can be solved, and the use of anesthetic techniques, including local blockage, is advocated.[253,257]

Evidence of a stress response has also been provided by Stang[257] in a study of circumcision plasma levels. Presurgical baseline cortisol levels show a mean of 143 nmol/L (5.2 μg/ml). At 30 minutes after circumcision, without dorsal penile nerve block, the cortisol levels rise to levels of 475 nmol/L (17.2 μg/ml)[258] and remain high at 90 minutes at levels of about 350 nmol/L.[257] Return to baseline levels required 150 minutes. Saline injections also produce similar high levels of cortisol, which are prolonged as in patients without any injection.

In contrast, injections of lidocaine hydrochloride produced some elevation of plasma cortisol levels but significantly lower than when no anesthetic block was provided.[257] In Stang's studies, the neonates spent 70% of the time crying and manifesting behavioral distress. Again, in contrast, the neonates anesthetized with a penile nerve block exhibited distress and cried only 20% of the time. Injection of the penile nerve does not evoke behavioral distress any greater than that evoked by the restraint technic.

Other stress-related physiologic reactions in infants to surgical procedures have been well documented.[258] Dramatic changes in heart rate and respiratory rate have been reported; cyanosis related to crying is common, and transcutaneous P_{O_2} levels are greatly reduced.[259]

The American Academy of Pediatrics has published a policy statement endorsing the administration of local or systemic anesthesia to neonates undergoing surgical procedures.[260]

OTHER CONSIDERATIONS IN PREPARING PATIENTS

Gastrointestinal Tract

The gastrointestinal tract should be clear. It is axiomatic that the stomach devoid of foodstuff is less irritable and the likelihood of vomiting is minimized; also the possibility of aspiration of solid food particles is eliminated. A statement appropriate to this subject is that by Waters.[261]

> For each patient who has died from postoperative pneumonia due to the irritation of his lungs with the vapor of ether, dozens have died . . . following mechanical obstruction to their air passages. For each patient whose heart has stopped during anesthesia because of drug effect on the autonomic mechanism which controls it, the hearts of dozens of patients have stopped because the larynx was flooded with vomitus.

Patients scheduled for surgery in the afternoon should not be starved.[262] They should be allowed a light breakfast of grape, apple or prune juice, cream of wheat, a slice of toast (no butter), milk, and weak tea or coffee with sugar. Citrus juices such as orange and grapefruit remain in the stomach for long periods of time and should not be given.

THE EMPTY STOMACH. Solid foods pass through the stomach at unpredictable rates of up to 12 hours or more (e.g., in obstetric patients). Water and crystalloid fluids, however, have an emptying time of 12 minutes.[263] As stated by Maltby, it "appears illogical to have a single guideline for both preoperative solids and liquids." Several routine procedures are important in keeping the stomach empty prior to anesthesia and surgery.[264]

First, an essential procedure for elective surgery is the order *NPO* for solid foods for a minimum period of 6 to 8 hours in the absence of pain, trauma, apprehension, gastrointestinal disorders, or medications, and this is considered a reasonable time preoperatively. A complete fast has many drawbacks, and water or even clear fluids, if tolerated, should be allowed up to 2.5 to 3 hours pre-anesthetically.[264]

Second, the acidity of the basal gastric secretion should be reduced; this can be accomplished by neutralization of the secretions already present by antacids (1 hour preanesthetically) and by blocking of secretions. For the latter, an anticholinergic such as glycopyrrolate or atropine has been effective in raising the pH to above 2.5,[266] which is considered a critical value.[265]

Third, a reduction in the volume of gastric secretions is desirable. This can be accomplished, to some extent, by anticholinergic drugs. H_2 receptor blockers, however, are more effective either by mouth 2 hours or intravenously 1 hour preanesthetically. Ranitidine, about 1 mg/kg,[267] or famotidine, 0.5 mg/kg, are preferred. These have a duration of action for 12 hours; hence, only one dose has to be given in the late evening of the day before surgery.[268] The oral dose of ranitidine is 2 mg/kg. H_2 blockers simultaneously reduce the gastric volume to amounts below 25 ml,[269,270] and the pH is raised to reach a range of 5.0 to 6.0. The newer blocker famotidine is also effective in a dose of 0.5 mg/kg and is equal to that of ranitidine. An alternative is cimetidine at a dose of 3 mg/kg, resulting in a pH range of 5.0 to 6.0.[271]

Comparison of Cimetidine with Ranitidine and Famotidine.[272] Cimetidine has several adverse effects at other sites, which makes this drug less desirable than either ranitidine or famotidine.[237] These effects include: (1) prolongation of half-life of many drugs and inhibition of clearance of most oxidatively metabolized drugs (diazepam, theophylline, lidocaine, propanolol) by inhibition of hepatic microsomal enzymes; (2) reduction of hepatic blood flow;[274] (3) some altered CNS effects, causing confusion (long-term use);[275] (4) bone marrow effects; and (5) antiandrogenic effects.

Adverse effects of ranitidine are infrequent. There are also some further advantages of ranitidine in addition to the H_2 receptor block. An increase in lower esophageal tone occurs,[276] and there is a counteraction of the effects of anticholinergics at this site. Clearance of drugs is not prolonged because oxidative and conjugative mechanisms of metabolism are not impaired.[277]

Antacid Agents. Commonly prescribed antacids such as Mylanta, Maalox, Riopan, and other particulate agents have been used to neutralize gastric acidity in anesthesia practice.[278] These have been effective and have found patient acceptance.[279] It has been shown, however, that these particulate emulsified antacids, if aspirated, can have harmful physiologic and tissue effects.[280] It has also been shown that nonparticulate antacids such as sodium citrate (30 ml of 0.3 M sodium citrate) and bicitra are equally effective and safer. Alka-Seltzer, a mixture of bicarbonate (K and Na) and citric acid, administered within 20 minutes before anesthesia for emergency surgery, is also effective and raises gastric pH above 4.0.[281] Of similar activity is the oral intake of 2 to 3 ounces of Seven-Up, which has a citrate mixture.[282]

Metoclopramide. Another approach in the presence of a full stomach in a patient in urgent need of surgery is to empty the stomach actively by use of a benzamide derivative. To empty the stomach and limit aspiration, a cholinergic stimulant is useful. Metoclopramide (Reglan) (methoxychloroprocainamide) stimulates GI motility, and this appears to be a selective effect with little or no cardiac action. This cholinergic effect is largely restricted to the proximal gut. Gastrokinetic effects include an increase in resting muscle tension, notably at the lower esophageal valvular mechanism and the gastric fundus; an increase in amplitude of contractions of the peristaltic waves; and coordination of activity of gut tone and peristalsis with relaxation of the pylorus and duodenum. The result is greater esophageal clearance, accelerated gastric emptying, and hastening small bowel passage of contents.[283] This is the so-called "sweeping" effect. An additional effect of this drug is depression of the vomiting center. This antiemetic property of the drug is due to the antagonism of cerebral dopamine receptors.

Pharmacokinetics[283] The adult dose of metoclopramide intravenously is set at 10 to 20 mg, or 0.2 mg/kg of body weight. In children the dose is 0.1 mg/kg. It is also rapidly absorbed when taken orally. A therapeutic level is between 40 and 80 ng/ml. The plasma half-life is about 4 hours; most of the drug, i.e., 80%, is excreted unchanged in the urine or as a sulfate and glucuronide conjugate. Elimination is completed within 24 hours.

Side Effects Most of the side effects are related to central nervous system stimulation. These consist of nervousness, restlessness of the limbs, facial spasms, trismus, torticollis, and opisthotonus.

Uses[284]

1. As an antiemetic, this drug appears to be superior to the phenothiazines, especially in cancer patients where larger doses are employed
2. To empty the stomach, in anesthesia emergencies, and to minimize aspiration
3. For intubation of intestines in diagnostic radiography.
4. To decrease gastroesophageal reflux and esophagitis.
5. To relieve gastric motor failure from vagotomy.
6. To reduce gastric volume.[284]

PHYSIOLOGY OF GASTRIC EMPTYING. Gastric physiology and emptying of water or saline solutions is rapid. This has been known since 1824 and was first published in a classic paper by William Beaumont, an army surgeon, in 1833, from observations on Alexis St. Martin.[285]

In more recent times, Malagelada[286] clearly showed rapid emptying of a fluid meal (Fig. 9–9). On this basis, fasting prior to surgery, a traditional practice, has been reevaluated. Hester and Heath reported in 1977 that fasting from all intake for more than 4 hours before anesthesia did not influence the volume or acidity of gastric contents.[287] This report

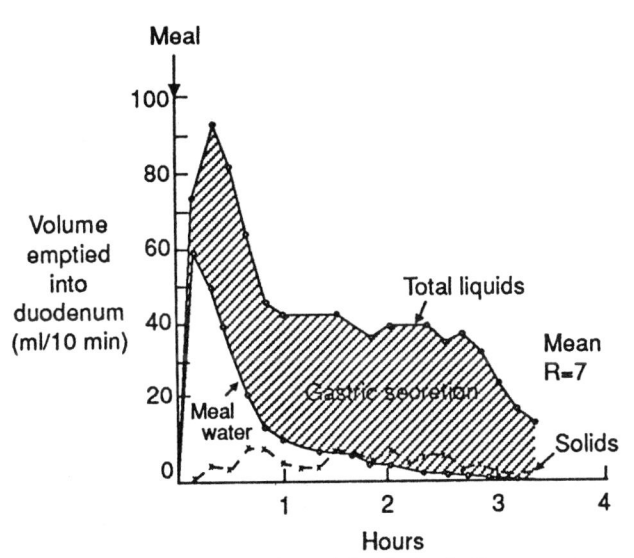

FIG. 9–9. Gastric emptying of fluids including gastric secretions after solid–liquid meals in normal human subjects. From Malagelada, J.R.: Quantitation of gastric solid–fluid discrimination during digestion of ordinary meals. Gastroenterology, 72:1264, 1977.

was further supported by Miller and colleagues, who found that fasting for more than 4 hours did not ensure an empty stomach or low acidity of the contents. Indeed, a light breakfast of tea and toast 2 to 3 hours preanesthesia did not affect the volume or acidity of gastric contents in the absence of narcotic premedication.[288]

Other studies have confirmed the concept that prolonged fasting, specifically from fluids, prior to anesthesia and surgery is not justified.[289] Inhospital children, adult, and geriatric patients scheduled for elective surgery, if placed on an "NPO after midnight" order do not have a significant change in gastric volume. Most children, outpatients, obese, or patients of normal habitus, if subject to overnight fasting, usually have a highly acid gastric aspirate (Table 9–17).[290]

VARIABLES TO GASTRIC VOLUME

- Fasting—the longer the fast, the higher the pH (Fig. 9–10);[289,291] after 4 hours, only small changes in pH or volume occur[287]
- Intravenous glucose 500 mg, i.e., 50 ml 50% glucose, inhibits gastric secretion[292]
- Narcotics paralyze gastric emptying for up to 2 hours (especially in patients in labor)[293]
- Anticholinergics increase gastric emptying
- Anesthetics decrease gastric secretion (halothane)[294,295]
- Age—gastric acidity and gastric volume both decrease with age[289]
- Smoking factor—smokers have a higher gastric volume and higher acidity than nonsmokers[296]

INFLUENCE OF AGE ON GASTRIC CONTENTS. A correlation exists between age and gastric contents. Generally, gastric acidity and volume both decrease with age.[273] Gastric pH varied from a mean of 1.99 in the pediatric group of patients to 2.40 in adults and to 3.32 in the geriatric patients. In the geriatric patients only 60% of patients had a pH of less than 2.5, whereas 92% of pediatric patients were below the critical pH of 2.5. Mean gastric volumes in the different age groups were found as follows: pediatric patients, 0.5 ml/kg; adult patients, 0.37 ml/kg; and geriatric patients (over 65 years), 0.25 ml/kg.

INFLUENCE OF DURATION OF FASTING ON GASTRIC CONTENTS. The duration of the fasting period as related to pH indicates an increasing alkalinity (increased pH) with the length of fasting.

The duration of fast has also been studied with respect to at-risk pH values below 2.5.[291] In those whom the duration of fast had a mean time of 12.5 hours, the mean pH was found to be 3.95. In contrast, for those who had a mean fast of 4.2 hours, the pH value was 2.93. Thus, it is apparent that a longer fast decreases the patients who are at risk.

INFLUENCE OF ANXIETY. Apprehension and anxiety have important effects on gastric juice, including increasing gastric volume, lowering pH, and delaying gastric emptying time.[302] In the pediatric patient,[302] adequate premedication with a sedative and narcotic plus an anticholinergic–glycopyrrolate reduce volume and raise pH well above the critical risk value of 2.5 units.[304]

TECHNIQUES FOR MEASURING GASTRIC EMPTYING. Common methods of measuring gastric emptying include the popular dye dilution, x-ray, and scintigraphic techniques. Noninvasive techniques involve real-time ultrasound and impedance techniques.[305]

The *epigastric impedance technique* is based on the increase in epigastric impedance after the ingestion of a nonionic fluid material.[305] In this technique, two electrodes are placed over the epigastrium in the midline below the xiphoid, and a second pair of electrodes is placed posteriorly about 6 cm apart in the midline. In the epigastrium, one electrode is placed below the xiphoid and is the input electrode (source) and the lower one just above the umbilicus is the recording electrode (the detector). Similarly, the electrodes posteriorly are placed about 6 cm apart in the midline and approximately at the same horizontal level as the anterior electrodes.

TABLE 9–17. CLINICAL CONDITIONS AFFECTING GASTRIC FLUID VOLUME AND ACIDITY IN PATIENTS PREOPERATIVELY

Condition	Reference Number	Gastric Volume* (ml)(%)	Percent With pH <2.5*
Emergency (no premedication)	287	>40 (30)	46
Obstetric patients	297,298	>40 (55)	40
Outpatients	299	Mean >10	Average 1.8
Morbidly obese patients	300	>25 (86)	38
Pediatric patients	301,302	—	100

* Shows percentage of subjects.

FIG. 9–10. Relationship of duration of fasting period to gastric pH, indicating increase in gastric pH as length of fasting period increased. From Manchikanti, L., et al.: Assessment of age-related acid aspiration risk factors in pediatric, adult, and geriatric patients. Anesth. Analg., 64:11, 1985.

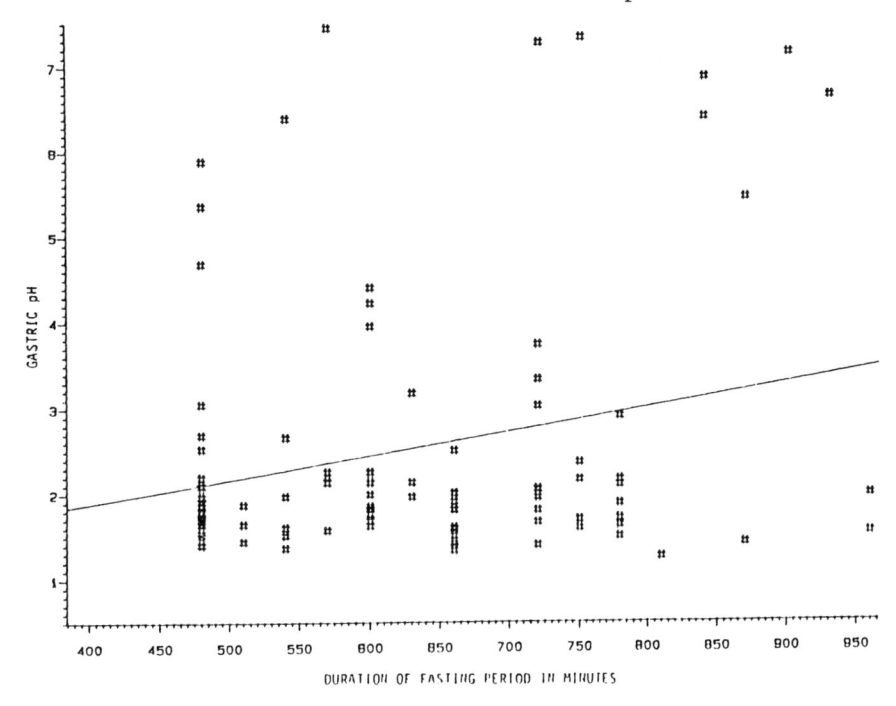

The resulting impedance on the ingestion of the fluid then declines over a period of time and represents a measure of the time for emptying of the stomach. The resulting record of impedance is the epigastrogram. It has been found to be a sensitive technique, equally as satisfactory as either the x-ray or the scintigraphic technique, and has even been available to measure gastric emptying in pregnancy.

GASTRIC EMPTYING IN PREGNANT PATIENTS. In O'Sullivan's study of pregnant women,[297,306] the time course of gastric emptying after drinking 500 ml of water or diluted orange concentrate over a 2-minute period is followed. The deflection heights above the baseline after gastric filling were then measured and followed for 15 to 30 minutes. The times to emptying from 100% impedance (full stomach) to 70%, 50%, and 30%, were about 4.5, 7, and 10 minutes, respectively. This was apparent in the third-trimester patients. In nonpregnant women, the times were 5, 8, and 11 minutes, respectively. These times, therefore, were somewhat similar.

This is a useful technique for assessing gastric emptying in the perioperative period. It is evident that water is rapidly propelled from the stomach. Hence, the intake of water does not need to be stopped, although it is emphasized that food itself should not be ingested. Labor was found to decrease emptying and was related to prior meperidine and promethazine premedication.

This study supports the position that fasting for more than 4 to 5 hours is not justified prior to elective surgery. On the other hand, fasting for less than 4 hours by allowing a light breakfast within 4 hours (2 to 3 hours prior to surgery) increases fluid volume, lowers the gastric pH significantly, and increases the risk of aspiration; therefore, this is not recommended.[306]

FASTING HAZARDS. Early warnings of the disadvantages of long fasts before elective surgery were expressed by Gwathmey in 1914:[307]

> While advantageous to have the stomach empty (preoperatively), it is not essential to starve the patient for 12 to 18 hours. Easily digested gruels of barley or rice can be given up to 2 to 3 hours of the operation with distinct advantage.

These hazards were also recognized by Booth in 1928:[308]

> The patient should be given a liquid diet for 18 hours prior to operation. Water should be freely given by mouth up to 3 hours of operation. This is to avoid mental distress.

An empty GI tract is essential preanesthetically, and the common practice to achieve this has been the order "NPO after midnight." This has been questioned, however.

It is also important to maintain good perioperative nutrition, because fasting for even 12 hours has its hazards.[309]

1. Hydration is compromised. Evidence indicates that renal function is depressed—oliguria is more likely, and renal hemodynamics are suppressed[310]
2. Fasting for 1 day may deplete liver glycogen;

Bruce has considered that these patients are at greater risk for hepatic toxicity from drugs[309]
3. Fasting for 24 hours or more increases free fatty acids (FFA) in humans;[311] but, generally, in patients who are designated "NPO-after-midnight," the increase is small;[312] however, halothane anesthesia may increase the FFA twofold to threefold[313]
4. Experimental evidence indicates that fasting, with an increase in FFA, lowers the threshold to epinephrine-induced arrythmias during halothane anesthesia;[314] this agent appears to interfere with the glycolytic process in the myocardium, and increased plasma FFA shifts metabolism from glycolytic to lipolytic paths.

To avoid such adverse effects, it is recommended that hydration and glucose administrations be started 2 hours before surgical time for an 8 A.M. surgery as a "parenteral breakfast." It is also important that the lipid infusions and hyperalimentation regimens be suspended in the immediate preoperative periods.

For patients who have recently eaten (i.e., within 2 hours) and are submitted for emergency operation, it should be appreciated that blood solubility coefficients are increased by 20% to 34%. This results in a more rapid uptake of anesthetic volatile agents by 20%[315] and a prolongation of elimination.[315]

Oral Fluids Preanesthesia.[317] In unpremedicated patients for ambulatory surgical care, an oral fluid intake of 150 ml water 2 to 3 hours preoperatively was permitted and then compared with patients restricted in all intake from the previous evening to the anesthetic period.[318] The residual gastric volume (RGV) in those receiving water was significantly lower, at a mean volume of 20.6 ± 14 ml, than in the fasting group. The RGV in the fasting group averaged 30 ml. The pH in those permitted water was also more alkaline, pH 6.7 versus pH 2.0. The critical values of RGV of 25 ml or more and pH less than 2.5 was found in 56% of patients who fasted; in those receiving water, the critical values of low pH and RGV over 25 ml were found in 28% (Table 9-18). In those receiving water and oral ranitidine (150 mg), only 2% had values outside the critical values.

It is evident that, at least for the type of patient treated in the ambulatory surgical setting, complete fasting to the time of operation is unnecessary. Second, the intake of 150 ml water plus 150 mg ranitidine reduces RGV and raises pH further, diminishing the risk of aspiration consequences. The volume of water recovered on suctioning the gastric contents was of the order of 8 ml (0 to 24 ml) and had a pH over 5.0.[317]

It is also evident from the study of Ong[299] that a light breakfast of tea and toast 2 to 3 hours preoperatively does not increase RGV and does not impose any additional risk. Also, one-third of patients who fast completely (no fluids) for more than 7 hours still have residual gastric fluid volumes of more than 25 ml and a pH of 2.5 or less.[318]

It is concluded that adult patients in the ambulatory setting may safely drink 4-5 ounces of water up to 2 to 3 hours preanesthetically. Not only is the residual gastric volume decreased as well as the acidity, but these patients have less thirst and are more comfortable.

Blood Glucose Levels in Infants and Young Children. Preoperative and perioperative glucose levels in children under 5 years of age vary with the development of the child and his or her percentile growth weight. Those below the third percentile of expected weight show remarkably low plasma glucose levels, representing significant hypoglycemia and posing serious operative risks.

For most purposes, a glucose level of less than 60 mg/dl (< 3 nmol/L) is defined as below normal for children.[319] In infants, a glucose level of 40 mg/dl (or less than 2.2 nmol/L) has been defined as hypoglycemic.[320]

Hypoglycemic levels have been found in children under the third percentile, even when children have received 5% dextrose by mouth up to 4 hours preinduction of anesthesia. Furthermore, Payne has

TABLE 9–18. INCIDENCE OF PATIENTS WITH RISK FACTORS IN EACH GROUP

Group	RGV > 25 ml No.	%	pH < 2.5 No.	%	Volume > 25 ml and pH < 2.5 No.	%
I (water & placebo)	9/25	36	20/22	91	7/25	28
II (water & ranitidine)	1/25	4	0/21	0	0/25	0
III (placebo only)	15/25	60	24/25	96	14/25	56
IV (ranitidine only)	2/25	8	1/19	5	1/25	4

Denominators in pH column represent patients in whom gastric aspirate was obtained.
P < 0.05 Group I vs. III.
P < 0.01 Groups II and IV vs. I and III.
Modified from Sutherland, A.D., et al.: The effect of preoperative oral fluid and ranitidine on gastric fluid, volume and pH. Can. J. Anaesth., 34:117, 1987.

demonstrated perioperative and postoperative hypoglycemia in healthy children in the 3rd to 25th percentile of growth.

1. Adequate preanesthesia feedings are recommended for children under 5 years of age, while the NPO order after midnight should be generally discontinued. Individualization of the pediatric patient is necessary.
2. Infant and those small for age need parenteral feedings preoperatively, and these should be continued through the operative period. If oral feedings are tolerated, the Alder-Hey guidelines are recommended (Table 9–19). It is also important to continue intravenous glucose postoperatively until oral intake is established. Discontinuing an intravenous glucose load prematurely can induce a serious rebound hypoglycemia.[321]

Fasting in Pediatric Patients. The occurrence of hypoglycemia as a result of fasting for surgery in pediatric patients is always a concern. The evidence shows, however, that hypoglycemia is not frequent in children *over* 5 years of age.[322]

A careful study of blood sugars can be rapidly carried out with a Glucometer technique. This has been found to be more useful and accurate as a bedside method for blood glucose monitoring. It is especially accurate when blood sugar levels are below 100 mg/dl. The results are readily available and correlate with a more precise glucose-oxidase method.

In Welborn's study, the following factors were clearly determined:[322]

1. Hypoglycemia is more likely in children less than 4 years of age and weighing less than 15 kg.[323]
2. Periods of fasting longer than 10 hours may be associated with perioperative low blood sugars, but not necessarily below 60 mg/dl.
3. When blood sugar levels were determined in infants after a 6-hour fast and in older children up to 6 years following a 10 to 12-hour fast, who received nonglucose-containing solutions (i.e., Ringer's lactate), all had preinduction blood sugar levels in a range of 80 to 90 mg/dl. Postoperatively, a slight increase in blood sugar was noted at an average of 110 mg/dl.
4. When 5% dextrose in Ringer's lactate was administered in the perioperative period, the preoperative blood sugar was also in the 80 to 90 mg/dl range, but at the conclusion of surgery, there was a greatly increased blood glucose level to a mean of 244 ± 60 mg/dl. This provides some concern because it may promote diuresis and result in some degree of dehydration. The significance of postoperative hyperglycemia is not yet fully assessed, but it is evidently physiologic trespass.[323] In healthy children, the administration of lower concentrations of dextrose or the avoidance of the use of dextrose completely for the first 12 hours postoperatively may be desirable.

To avoid hypoglycemia in children, Thomas has prepared a preoperative feeding regimen on the day of planned surgery. This Alder-Hey Children's Hospital Program considers whether patients are scheduled for morning or afternoon surgery. In general, children older than 1 year need not be fed if surgery is planned for the morning. After good sedation, parenteral fluids with dextrose will be sufficient. If surgery is planned for the afternoon period, however, some bland oral feedings are warranted in the early morning on awakening.[324]

DURATION OF FAST IN CHILDREN.[325] The appropriate length of time to withhold solid food from children over 5 years of age who are to undergo elective surgery is probably similar to that of adults. This is usually about 6 to 8 hours. For infants and children under 5 years of age, the Alder-Hey hospital regimen (see Table 9–19), involving a liquid diet, is safe and satisfactory.

For children older than 5 years, however, a simple regimen of clear fluids of a bland nature (such as apple or grape juice) has been found safe without retention. Such a regimen consists of a small drink 2 to 3 hours (or 2.5 hours) preanesthetically; the amount can be set at 3 ml/kg of the bland juices. This regimen provides several advantages:[325]

1. Hypoglycemia is allayed
2. Since clear fluids pass through the stomach rapidly, there is not retention after 10 to 12 minutes. There is actually a decreased gastric volume com-

TABLE 9–19. PREOPERATIVE FEEDING OF INPATIENT CHILDREN ON THE DAY OF PLANNED SURGERY*

Infants less than 1 yr	
Morning cases	No milk "feed" after midnight
	5% dextrose 10 ml/kg at 6 A.M. orally
Afternoon cases	Last milk feed at 7 A.M.
	5% dextrose 10 ml/kg at 10 A.M.
Children 1–5 yrs	
Morning cases	5% dextrose 10 ml/kg at 6 A.M.
	250 ml maximum for 8 A.M. surgery
	Milk 10 ml/kg at 6 A.M.
	250 ml maximum for 10 A.M. surgery
Afternoon cases	Light breakfast at 7 A.M.
	Milk 10 ml/kg at 10 A.M.
	250 ml maximum
Children more than 5 yrs	
Morning cases	Nothing by mouth in the morning
Afternoon cases	Light breakfast at 7 A.M.

* Modification of Alder Hey Children's Hospital Regimen
Adapted from Thomas, D.K.M.: Hypoglycemia in children before anesthesia. Br. J. Anaesth., 46:66, 1974, and Graham, I.F.M.: Preoperative starvation and plasmaglucose concentrations in children undergoing outpatient anesthesia. Br. J. Anaesth., 51:161, 1981.

pared to children who have not received the oral fluids
3. There is a decreased gastric acidity (overall pH is increased)
4. The children taking oral fluids are not hungry, nor do they complain of thirst
5. As a consequence, they are generally not as restless and are more cooperative than children who do not receive fluids.

RESPIRATORY TRACT

Before the preanesthetic medication is given, the patient should be instructed to cough several times and generally clear his upper respiratory passages. This procedure will minimize and decrease the incidence of postoperative pulmonary complications. Postural drainage is indicated for those patients with chronic pulmonary disease such as bronchitis and bronchiectasis.

MISCELLANEOUS

Before a patient leaves the unit to go to the operating room, watches, rings, and movable bridges should be removed and kept on the unit. Some anesthetists prefer that full dentures remain in place and feel that it is easier to get a better airway and mask-fit because of the more normal face contour which results. In addition, patient embarrassment is curtailed.

URINARY PROBLEM[326]

On the day preceding surgery and, if feasible, on several days preceding, the patient should be taught to urinate in bed into the urinal or bedpan. As a result, the incidence of postoperative urinary retention will be diminished.

It was found that among a large group of healthy Army personnel hospitalized for nondebilitating surgical conditions, 16% were unable to void either lying or sitting in bed preoperatively despite definite urgency. With practice and concentration, however, most men can learn to void easily in bed. By the simple expediency of preoperative training in one clinical series, a high incidence of 18% postoperative catheterizations was reduced to 3%.

POSTANESTHETIC RECOVERY SCORE.[327] A simple method of evaluation of postanesthetic patients applicable to all situations, regardless of the anesthetic and adjuvant agents administered, has been proposed by Aldrete (Fig. 9–11). The score is based on the observation of five signs. A score of 0, 1, or 2 is given to each sign, depending on whether it is present or absent. A score of 10 indicates a recovered patient in the best possible condition.

The following signs are described:[328]

1. *Activity:* The efficiency of muscle activity and coordination is assessed by observing the ability of the patient to move his limbs either spontaneously or on command. If able to move all four extremities, a score of 2 is given. When only two extremities are moved, this index is graded as 1, and if none of the extremities are moved, a score of 0 is recorded. This permits the evaluation of patients following subarachnoid or peridural blocks, and their total score increases when they regain muscle activity of the lower limbs.
2. *Respiration:* Respiratory efficiency is evaluated without the need for complicated gadgetry or sophisticated physical tests. A score of 2 indicates that patients are able to breathe deeply and cough. If respiratory effort is limited (i.e., splinting) or dyspnea is apparent, the score is 1. If no spontaneous respiratory activity is evident, the score is 0. To evaluate respiration, a patient has to recover sufficient central nervous system functional activity to understand to cough and to breathe deeply on command.
3. *Circulation:* Circulation is the most difficult vital function to evaluate by a single simple measurement or observation. Use changes of arterial blood pressure from the preanesthetic level to monitor this function. Blood pressure is monitored throughout the anesthetic state and is one of the first physical signs taken on arrival in the recovery room in virtually all hospitals. The grading system may be revised as further experience is gained with this score. When the systolic arterial blood pressure at recovery room arrival is between ± 20% of the preanesthetic level (as obtained by the Riva-Rocci method), the score is 2. If the same index ranges between ±20% and ±50% of the same control level, the score is 1. When blood pressure is ± 50% or more of the original reading, the score is 0.
4. *Consciousness:* Full alertness, demonstrated by the ability to answer questions clearly, is considered completely awake and is graded with 2 points. If patients are aroused only when called by their names, they receive 1 point. A score of 0 is given when there is no response to auditory stimulation. Painful stimulation is discarded for various reasons: (1) even decerebrate patients might respond to it; (2) it is not a desirable maneuver to repeat frequently; (3) it is difficult to develop a consistent and reliable method of painful stimulation that would be practical.
5. *Color:* In contrast to the evaluation of the newborn, this is an objective sign, relatively easy to judge. When the patients appear to have an obviously normal or "pink" color, a score of 2 is given. In those cases in which normal pigmentation of the skin prevents an accurate evaluation, the color of the oral mucosa is observed. When frank cyanosis is present, the score is 0. It

FIG. 9–11. The Postanesthesia recovery score. From Aldrete, J.A., and Kroulik, D.: A postanesthetic recovery score. Anesth. Analg., 49:924, 1970.

ASSESSMENT	ADM	15M	30M	1HR	1HR30M	2HR
ACTIVITY Purposeful - 2 Random - 1 None - 0						
RESPIRATION Regular Good Depth - 2 United - 1 APNEA or Assist - 0						
CONSCIOUSNESS Alert Awake - 2 Arousable - 1 Nonresponsive - 0						
COLOR Pink - 2 Pale, Duskey - 1 Cyanotic - 0						
CIRCULATION BP ± 20% - 2 ± 20-50% - 1 ± 50% - 0						
TOTAL						

should be noted, however, that this latter discoloration will be difficult to assess in dark-skinned or anemic, desaturated patients. Any alteration from the normal "pink" appearance that is not obviously cyanosis receives 1 point; this includes pale, congested, "dusky" or "blotchy" discolorations as well as jaundice.

The Aldrete score can be criticized on the basis of color assessment, which is dependent on many variables and difficult to interpret. Steward has proposed a simplified scoring system.[329] This also is deficient, in that circulation and reflexes are ignored.

EVALUATION OF UNCONSCIOUSNESS.[331] To aid the anesthesiologist in determining the depth of coma or the course of recovery from anesthesia, or to differentiate between clinically reversible or irreversible coma (clinical death) and biologic death, a viability scoring system is available.[332]

VIABILITY SCORE. This score system involves a continuous evaluation of five functions essential to total viability and human life, namely, cerebral, reflex, respiratory, circulatory, and cardiac. This scoring system serves a similar purpose to that of the Apgar score for evaluating the vitality of neonates.[330]

Accepting the basic premise that no single sign or function can or should be used to assess the capacity to live or to establish the certainty of absolute death, the five physiologic functions are assessed for presence, potential, or absence, using an arbitrary scoring system of 2, 1, or 0, respectively (Table 9–20).

A score of 5 or more points represents potential life; a score of less than 5 represents impending or presumptive death; and a score of 0 may be taken as showing absolute, irreversible death.

Serial determinations are made at least every 15 minutes over a period of from 1 to 6 hours; an increasing score indicates effective therapy and a prognosis of patient recovery, while a decreasing score indicates patient deterioration. To the five areas of clinical observation should be added such additional laboratory, pharmacologic, and monitoring tests of function and responsiveness as seem appropriate and feasible.

Commentary There are three objectives to this multiparameter scoring system.

1. The physician can employ it as a guide in deciding when efforts at resuscitation or attempts to prolong life are no longer justified and should be abandoned in the interest of humanitarianism[332,333]
2. It will protect potential donors from the risk of precipitous or premature removal of organs for transplantation, because it permits the establishment of irreversible biologic death beyond doubt.
3. It gives both the anesthesiologist and the surgeon a basis for quantitating the stages of recovery from anesthesia.

TOTAL PREPARATION

The challenge of the future is to reduce morbidity and mortality in the operating room to the infinitesimal. One unexploited aspect of this challenge is the preparation of the patient for elective surgery above and beyond the conventional treatment of disease and restoration of function. The concept of total physical preparation is presented as a newer approach.

The patient of the future should go through a process of physical conditioning. It is not enough simply to find that various organ systems are functioning adequately with or without therapy at rest and under ordinary circumstances of living. It is simply not sufficient to recognize that patients are up and about. Much more is necessary. They must be tuned to withstand stress and physical challenges. This process applied to patients may be compared to the physical training and conditioning of boxers and athletes for their entrance into a competitive event. In truth, the patient is pitting his physical stamina against the stress of anesthesia and surgery.

It is believed that the conditioning of the patient should begin weeks in advance of a major surgical event. The conditioning process is conceived as encompassing at least three areas. These are:

1. Regular living: This includes a properly balanced and regular diet; regularity of eating and sleeping.
2. Good habits: This includes the elimination or

TABLE 9–20. RECOVERY SCORE* FOR THE EVALUATION OF COMATOSE PATIENT RECOVERY POTENTIAL AND DYING PROCESS BASED ON FIVE FUNCTIONS

Function	Score 2 Present	Score 1 Abnormal	Score 0 Absent
I. CEREBRAL	NORMAL	DEPRESSED	ABSENT
1. Consciousness	Conscious		
Talking			
Response to command		EVOKED RESPONSE	NO EVOKED RESPONSE
Response to sound			
Response to light (pupil)			
Response to pain			
2. Movement—spontaneous			
3. EEG	Alpha	Spikes	Isoelectric
II. REFLEXIVE	PRESENT	DIMINISHED	ABSENT
1. Eyes	Constricted Pupils	Pupillary Response	Dilated
2. Laryngeal	Pharyngeal Reflex	Laryngeal–Carinal	
3. Tendon reflexes	Tracheal Buck		
4. Nerve stimulus		AN EVOKED RESPONSE	NO EVOKED RESPONSE
III. RESPIRATORY	NORMAL	ABNORMAL	ABSENT
1. Rate	Spontaneous	Assisted	Controlled
2. Depth	Adequate	Assisted	Controlled
3. Doxapram Test		EVOKED RESPONSE	NO EVOKED RESPONSE
IV. CIRCULATORY	NORMAL	DEPRESSED	ABSENT
1. Pulse	Spontaneous	Supported	
2. Pressure	Spontaneous	Supported	
3. Vasopressor test		EVOKED RESPONSE	NO EVOKED RESPONSE
V. CARDIAC	NORMAL	INEFFECTIVE	ABSENT
1. Auscultation	Heart sounds	Assisted	
2. ECG	Normal	Abnormal	Isoelectric
3. Pacemaker test	Not needed	EVOKED RESPONSE	NO EVOKED RESPONSE

* Guidelines:
1. Initial evaluation as soon as cardiopulmonary resuscitation has been instituted.
2. Serial determinations at least every 15 minutes.
3. A score of 10 indicates full function.
4. A score of 5 or more indicates *potential life*.
5. A score of < 5 indicates *impending* or *presumptive death*.
6. A score of 0 is *conclusive biologic death*.
7. An increasing score over a period of 1 hour represents effective therapy and patient recovery.
8. A decreasing score over a period of 1 hour represents failing therapy and patient deterioration.

modification of detrimental habits such as smoking and drinking.

  3. Physical activity: The patient should be placed on a program of regulated physical activity and exercise. The following seems to be both logical and reasonable.
    a. Daily walks of a prescribed and increasing amount.
    b. If appropriate and acceptable, swimming.
    c. Calisthenics and aerobic exercises (dynamic)

Final evaluation of the total physical state may then be tested by means of a variety of physical condition indices.[334]

The aerobic capacity or the oxygen requirement for a given amount of submaximal work or exercise appears to be the best index for physical fitness. The conditioning exercises or work are dynamic in nature (not static) and correlate with heart rate.[335] The primary change is an increase in stroke volume of the heart and an improvement in the oxygen delivery system to the body. The amount of oxygen one can deliver and utilize per kilogram of body weight per minute is called maximum oxygen consumption. It is recognized as the most reliable and useful measure of fitness.

Aerobic capacity is increased by regular, planned dynamic physical activity. By increasing capacity a person's physical condition is improved and general fitness is increased. Such persons are better prepared to cope with the stresses of anesthesia and surgery. Morbidity and mortality are thereby minimized.[336]

REFERENCES

1. Collins, V.J.: Preanesthetic evaluation and preparation. Iowa State Med. Soc., *58*:647, 1958.
2. Collins, V.J.: The anesthetist's second power (editorial). Anesthesiology, *9*:437, 1948.

3. Sheffer, M.B., and Greifenstein, F.E.: Emotional responses of surgical patients to anesthesia and surgery. Anesthesiology, 21:502, 1960.
4. Buskirk, J.H.: Report: American Society of Anesthesiologists, June 1956.
5. Egbert, L.D., et al.: The value of a preoperative visit by an anesthetist. J.A.M.A., 185:553, 1963.
6. Litin, E.M.: Preoperative psychiatric consultation. J.A.M.A., 170:1369, 1959.
7. Rardin, T.: Psychologic preparation of patients for surgery. Symposium AMA, June 14, 1960.
8. Spielberger, C.D., Gorsuch, R., and Lushene, R.: The State-Trait Anxiety Inventory. Palo Alto, CA, Consulting Psychologists Press, 1970.
9. Spielberger, C.D., et al.: Emotional reactions to surgery. J. Consult. Clin. Psychol., 40:33, 1973.
9a. Janis, I.L.: *Psychological Stress, Psychoanalytic and Behavioral Studies of Surgical Patients*, New York: John Wiley & Sons, Inc., 1958.
10. Vernon, D.T., Schulman, J.L., and Foley, J.M.: Changes in children's behavior after hospitalization. Am. J. Dis. Child., 111:581, 1966.
11. Morgan, S.F., Furman, E.D., and Dikmen, S.: Psychological effects of general anesthesia on five to eight year old children. Anesthesiology, 55:386, 1981.
12. Norris, W., and Baird, W.L.M.: Preoperative anxiety: Incidence and aetiology. Br. J. Anaesth., 39:503, 1967.
13. Egbert, L.D., et al.: Reduction of postoperative pain by encouragement and instruction of patients. N. Engl. J. Med., 270:825, 1964.
14. Eysenk, H.J.: Drugs and personality. J. Med. Sci., 57:372, 1957.
15. Woodrow, K.M., et al.: Pain tolerance: Differences according to age, sex and race. Psychosom. Med., 34:548, 1972.
16. Scott, L.E., Clum, G.A., and Peoples, J.B.: Preoperative predictors of postoperative pain. Pain, 15:283, 1983.
17. Schultz, J.H.: Psychotherapy and anesthesia. Anesthetist, 6:376, 1957.
17a. Kretschmer, Ernst. Der Körperbau der Gesunden und der Begriff der Affinität. Z. ges. Neur. Psychiat., 107:749–757, 1927.
17b. McDougall, W.: Outline of abnormal psychology 6th Ed New York, 1960.
17c. McDougall, W.B.: Body and Mind Greenwood Press, Westport CT, 1974.
18. Eysenck, H.J., and Eysenck, S.B.G.: Manual of Eysenck Personality Inventory. London, University of London Press, 1964.
19. Cronin, M., Redfern, P.A., and Utting, J.E.: Psychosometry and postoperative complaints in surgical patients. Br. J. Anaesth., 45:879, 1973.
20. Elmajian, F., Hope, J.M., and Lampson, E.T.: Excretion of epinephrine and norepinephrine in various emotional states. J. Clin. Endocrinol., 17:608, 1957.
21. Cryer, P.E.: Plasma catecholamine levels in various physiologic and pathophysiologic states. N. Engl. J. Med., 303:436, 1980.
22. Brodsky, M.A., et al.: Ventricular tachyarrhythmia associated with psychological stress: The role of the sympathetic nervous system. J.A.M.A., 257:2064, 1987.
23a. Cannon, S.B.: Voodoo death. Am. Anthropol., 44:169, 1942.
23b. Freud, S.: Thoughts For the Times on War and Death. *In* Collected Papers, Vol. 4. London, Hogarth Press, 1948, p. 288.
24. Collins, V.J.: Concepts in anesthesiology. J.A.M.A., 182:105, 1962.
25. Morton, H.J.V.: Smoking in surgical patients. Lancet, 1:368, 1944.
26. Hart, P., et al.: Enhanced drug metabolism in cigarette smokers. Br. Med. J., 2:147, 1976.
27. Kerri-Szanto, M., and Pomeroy, J.R.: Enzyme activation by smoking. Lancet, 1:947, 1971.
28. Jelliffe, D.D.: The Assessment of Nutritional Status of the Community. Geneva, World Health Organization, 1966.
29. Bistrian, B.R., et al.: Protein status of general surgical patients. J.A.M.A., 230:858, 1974.

ALCOHOLISM

30. Sellers, E.M., and Kalant, H.: Alcohol intoxication and withdrawal. N. Engl. J. Med., 294:757, 1976.
31. Block, M.A.: Alcoholism (editorial). J.A.M.A., 163:550, 1957.
32. World Health Organization Expert Committee on Drug Dependence. Twentieth Report. Technical Report No. 551; Geneva, World Health Organization, 1974.
33. Gordon, J.E.: The epidemiology of alcoholism. NY State J. Med., 58:1911, 1958.
34. Smith, J.A.: Psychiatric treatment of the alcoholic. N.Y. State J. Med., 58:3157, 1958.
35. Harger, R.N.: The pharmacology and toxicology of alcohol. J.A.M.A., 167:2199, 1958.
36. Westerfeld, W.W., and Schulman, M.P.: Metabolism and caloric value of alcohol. J.A.M.A., 170:197, 1959.
37. Greenberg, L.A.: Alcohol in the body. Sci. Am., 189:86, 1953.
38. Himwich, H.E.: The physiology of alcohol. J.A.M.A., 163:545, 1957.
39. Fazekas, J.: Influences of CP and alcohol on cerebral hemodynamics. Am. J. Med. Sci., 230:128, 1955.
40. Newman, H.W.: Emetic action of ethyl alcohol. AMA Arch. Intern. Med., 94:417, 1954.
41. Grollman, A.: Influence of alcohol on circulation. Q. J. Stud. Alcohol, 3:5, 1942.
42. Rummel, W., and Schmitz, J.: Die Anti-curare wirking des Alkahols. Arch. Exper. Pathol. Pharmacol., 222:257, 1954.
43. Regan, T.J.: Of beverages, cigarettes, and cardiac arrhythmias. N. Engl. J. Med., 301:1060, 1979.
44. Greenspan, A.J., et al.: Provocation of ventricular tachycardia after consumption of alcohol. N. Engl. J. Med., 301:1049, 1979.
45. Ettinger, P.O., et al.: Arrhythmias and the "holiday heart": alcohol-associated cardiac rhythm disorders. Am. Heart J., 95:555, 1978.
46. Bing, R.J., and Tillmanns, H.: The Effects of Alcohol on the Heart: Metabolic Aspects of Alcoholism. Baltimore, University Park Press, 1977, p. 117.
47. Spector, R., et al.: Alcoholic myopathy, diagnosis by alcohol challenge. J.A.M.A., 242:1648, 1979.
48. Rubin, E., et al.: Muscle damage produced by chronic alcohol consumption. Am. J. Pathol., 83:499, 1976.
49. Rubin, E.: Alcoholic myopathy in heart and skeletal muscle. N. Engl. J. Med., 301:28, 1979.
50a. Sellers, E.M., and Kalant H.: Alcohol intoxication and withdrawal. N. Engl. J. Med., 294:757, 1976.
50b. Sellers, E.M., et al.: Diazepam loading: Simplified treatment of alcohol withdrawal. Clin. Pharmacol. Ther., 34:822, 1983.
51. Editorial: Metabolic fate of thiopental. J.A.M.A., 147:875, 1958.
52. Zinn, S.E., Fairley, H.B., and Glenn, J.D.: Liver function in patients with mild alcoholic hepatitis, after enflurane, ni-

trous oxide-narcotic, and spinal anesthesia. Anesth. Analg., 64:487, 1985.
53. Adriani, J., and Morton, R.C.: Drug dependence: Important conclusions from the anesthesiologist's viewpoint. Anesth. Analg., 47:472, 1968.
54. Han, Y.M.: Why do chronic alcoholics require more anesthesia? Anesthesiology, 30:341, 1969.
55. Barber, R.E.: Anesthetic requirement in alcoholic patients. Abstracts of Scientific Papers. Presented at the October 1978 Annual Meeting of the American Society of Anesthesiologists, Chicago, IL, p. 623.
56. Tammisto, T., and Tigerstedt, I.: The need for fentanyl supplementation of N_2O–O_2 relaxant anaesthesia in chronic alcoholics. Acta Anaesth Scand., 21:216, 1977.
57. Mirsky, H., and Giarmian, N.J.: Studies on potentiation of pentothal. J. Pharm. Exper. Therap. and 114:240, 1955.
58a. Lee, P.K., Cho, M.H., and Dobkin, A.B.: Effects of alcoholism, morphinism, and barbiturate resistance on induction and maintenance of general anesthesia. Can. Anaesth. Soc. J., 11:354, 1964.
58b. Keilty, S.R.: Anesthesia for the alcoholic patient. Anesth. Analg., 68:659, 1968.
59. Boston Collaborative Drug Surveillance Program: Clinical depression of the central nervous system due to diazepam and chlordiazepoxide in relation to cigarette smoking and age. N. Engl. J. Med., 288:277–280, 1973.
60. Wilkins, A.J. et al.: Treatment of alcohol withdrawal symptoms. Psychopharmacol., 81:78, 1983.
61. Kraus, M.L., et al.: Effects of beta-adrenergic blockade in the treatment of alcohol withdrawal. N. Engl. J. Med., 313:905, 1985.

SMOKING

62. Morton, H.J.V.: Tobacco smoking and pulmonary complications after operation. Lancet, 1:368, 1944.
63. Kerri-Szanto, M., and Pomeroy, J.R.: Enzyme activation by smoking. Lancet, 1:947, 1971.
64. Conroy, J.P.: Smoking and the anesthetic risk. Anesth. Analg., 48:388, 1969.
65. Warner, M.A., et al.: Role of preoperative cessation of smoking and other factors in postoperative pulmonary complications: A blinded prospective study of coronary artery bypass patients. Mayo Clin. Proc., June 1989.
66. Samuelsson, O., et al.: Cardiovascular morbidity in relation to change in blood pressure and serum cholesterol levels in treated hypertension: Results from the primary prevention trial in Goteborg, Sweden. J.A.M.A., 258:1768, 1987.
67. Camner, P., and Philipson, K.: Some studies of tracheobronchial clearance in man. Chest, 63:235–240, 1973.
68a. Buist, A.S., et al.: The effect of smoking cessation and modification on lung function. Am. Rev. Respir. Dis., 114:115–122, 1976.
68b. Bode, F.R., et al.: Reversibility of pulmonary function abnormalities in smokers. Am. J. Med., 59:43–52, 1975.
68c. McCarthy, D.S., Craig, D.B., and Cherniack, R.M.: Effect of modification of the smoking habit on lung function. Am. Rev. Resp. Dis., 114:103, 1976.
69. Mitchell, C., Garrahy, P., and Peake, P.: Postoperative respiratory morbidity: Identification and risk factors. Aust. N.Z. J. Surg., 52:203–209, 1982.
70. Aronson, M.D., et al.: Association between cigarette smoking and acute respiratory tract illness in young adults. J.A.M.A., 248:2:181–183, 1982.
71. Warner, M.A., Divertie, M.B., and Tinker, J.H.: Preoperative cessation of smoking and pulmonary complications in coronary artery bypass patients. Anesthesiology, 60:380–383, 1984.
72. Public Health Service: The Health Consequences of Smoking. Dept. of Health, Education and Welfare Publication (CDC) 78–8351. Washington, DC, Government Printing Office, 1964, 1–120.
73. Wolf, P.A., and Kannel, W.B.: Controllable risk factors for stroke: Preventative implications of trends in stroke mortality. In Prognosis and Management of Stroke and TIAs. Edited by J.S. Meyer and T. Shaw. London, Addison Wesley, 1981, pp. 25–57.
74. Rogers, R.L., et al.: Cigarette smoking decreases cerebral blood flow suggesting increased risk for stroke. J.A.M.A., 250:20:2796–2800, 1983.
75. Wright, D.J., and Pandya, A.: Smoking and gastric juice volume in outpatients. Can. Anaesth. Soc. J., 26:328, 1979.
76. Pearce, A.C., and Jones, R.M.: Smoking and anesthesia: Preoperative abstinence and perioperative morbidity. Anesthesiology, 61:576, 1984.
77. Douglas, C.G., Haldane, J.S., and Haldane, J.B.S.: The laws of combination of haemoglobin with carbon monoxide and oxygen. J. Physiol. (Lond), 44:275, 1912.
78. Roughton, F.J.W., and Darling, R.C.: The effect of carbon monoxide on the oxyhemoglobin dissociation curve. Am. J. Physiol., 141:17, 1944.
79. Lawther, P.J., and Commins, B.T.: Cigarette smoking and exposure to carbon monoxide. Ann. N.Y. Acad. Sci., 174:135, 1970.
80. Comroe, J.H., Jr.: The pharmacological actions of nicotine. Ann. N.Y. Acad. Sci., 90:48, 1960.
81. Roth, G.M., and Schick, R.M.: The cardiovascular effects of smoking with special reference to hypertension. Ann. N.Y. Acad. Sci., 90:308, 1960.
82. Cryer, P.E., et al.: Norepinephrine and epinephrine release and adrenergic mediation of smoking associated hemodynamic and metabolic events. N. Engl. J. Med., 295:573, 1976.
83. Beckett, A.H., and Triggs, E.J.: Enzyme induction in man caused by smoking. Nature, 216:587, 1967.
84. Collaborative Drug Surveillance Program: Clinical depression of central nervous system in relation to cigarette smoking and age. N. Engl J. Med., 288:277, 1973.
85. Hart, P., et al.: Enhanced drug metabolism in cigarette smokers. Br. Med. J., 2:147, 1976.
86. Morton, H.J.V.: Tobacco smoking and pulmonary complications after operation. Lancet, 1:368, 1944.
87. Chalon, J., Tayyab, M.A., and Ramanathan, S.: Cytology of respiratory epithelium as a predictor of respiratory complications after operation. Chest, 67:321, 1975.
88. Warner, M.A., Divertie, M.B., and Tinker, J.H.: Preoperative cessation of smoking and pulmonary complications in coronary artery bypass patients. Anesthesiology, 60:380, 1984.
89. Laurenco, R.V., Klimek, M.F., and Borowski, C.J.: Deposition and clearance of 2μ particles in the tracheobronchial tree of normal subjects—smokers and non-smokers. J. Clin. Invest., 50:1141, 1971.
90. Dalhamn, T., and Rylander, R.: Ciliastatic action of cigarette smoke. Arch. Otolaryngol., 81:379, 1965.
91. Tockman, M., et al.: A comparison of pulmonary function in male smokers and nonsmokers. Am. Rev. Respir. Dis., 114:711, 1976.
92. Gerrard, J.W., et al.: Increased nonspecific bronchial reactivity in cigarette smokers with normal lung function. Am. Rev. Respir. Dis., 122:577, 1980.

93. Levi, R.: Induction of allergy in smokers by a glycoprotein component. Am. J. Pathol., 86:432, 1982.
94. Bierenbaum, M.D., et al.: Effect of cigarette smoking upon in vivo platelet function in man. Thromb. Res., 12:1051, 1978.
95. Roth, G.M., and Shick, R.M.: The cardiovascular effects of smoking with special reference to hypertension. Ann. N.Y. Acad. Sci., 90:308, 1960.
96. Greenspan, K., et al.: Some effects of nicotine on cardiac automaticity, conduction, and inotropy. Arch. Intern. Med., 123:707, 1969.
97. Gracey, D.R., Divertie, M.B., and Didier, E.P.: Preoperative pulmonary preparation of patients with chronic obstructive pulmonary disease: A prospective study. Chest, 76:123, 1979.
98. Kambam, J.R., Chen, L.H., and Hyman, S.A.: Effect of short-term smoking halt on carboxyhemoglobin levels and P_{50} values. Anesth. Analg., 65:1186, 1986.

AGING

99. Hayflick, L.: The cell biology of human aging. N. Engl. J. Med., 295:1302, 1976.
100. LaDue, J.S.: Evaluation and preparation of patients with degenerative cardiovascular disease for major surgery. Bull. N.Y. Acad. Med., 32:418, 1956.
101. Shock, N.W.: Some physiological aspects of aging in man. Bull. N.Y. Acad. Med., 32:208, 1956.
102. Bellville, J.W., et al.: Influence of age on pain relief from analgesics: A study of postoperative patients. J.A.M.A., 217:1835, 1971.
103. Ellenberg, M.: Reflexes—deep reflexes in old age. J.A.M.A., 174:468–469, 1960.
104. Pontoppidan, H., and Beecher, H.K.: Protective reflexes in the airway with aging. J.A.M.A., 174:2209, 1960.
105. Vestal, R.E., Wood, A.J.J., and Shand, D.G.: Reduced β-adrenoceptor sensitivity in the elderly. Clin. Pharmacol. Ther., 26:181–185, 1979.
106. Hospital Mortality: PAS Hospitals, United States 1974–1975. Ann Arbor, MI, Commission on Professional and Hospital Activities, 1977.
107. Djokovic, J.L., and Hedley-Whyte, J.: Prediction of outcome of surgery and anesthesia in patients over 80. J.A.M.A., 242:2301–2306, 1979.
108. Denney, J.L., and Denson, J.S.: Risk of surgery in patients over 90. Geriatrics, 27:115–118, 1972.
109. Beal, J.M.: Basic principles in the surgical management of the aged. Geriatrics, 14:269, 1959.
110. LaDue, J.S.: Evaluation of operative risk in patients with cancer. N.Y. State J. Med., 59:2942, 1959.

OBESITY

111. Schwartz, H.: The problem of obesity in anesthesia. N.Y. State J. Med., 55:3257, 1955.
112. Crook, G.H., et al.: Evaluation of skin-fold measurements and weight chart to measure body fat. J.A.M.A., 198:39, 1966.
113. Keys, A., et al.: Indices of relative weight and obesity. J. Chronic Dis., 25:329–343, 1972.
114. Mann, G.V.: The influence of obesity on health. N. Engl. J. Med., 291:I, 178–185; II, 226–232, 1974.
115. Fertman, M.B.: Etiology and severe obesity. J. Am. Geriatr. Soc., 7:38, 1959.
116. Lange, E.: The Slim Guide Skinfold Caliper. Plymouth, MI, Creative Health Products, 1976.
117. Entmacher, P.S.: Chief Medical Director, Metropolitan Life Insurance Company, 1983.
118. Abraham, S., et al.: Obese and Overweight Adults in the United States. U.S. Dept. of Health and Human Services Publication (PHS) 83-1680. Hyattsville, MD, National Center for Health Statistics, 1983.
119a. Hypertension Detection and Follow-Up Program: Five-year findings. 1. Reduction in mortality of persons with high blood pressure, including mild hypertension. Hypertension Detection and Follow-Up Program Cooperative Group. J.A.M.A., 242:2562–2571, 1979.
119b. Harris, T., et al.: Body mass index and mortality among nonsmoking older persons: The Framingham Heart Study. J.A.M.A., 259:1520–1524, 1988.
120. Alexander, J.F.: Obesity and cardiac performance. Am. J. Cardiol., 14:860, 1964.
121. MacMahon, S.W., Wilcken, D.E.L., and Macdonald, G.J.: The effect of weight reduction on left ventricular mass: A randomized controlled trial in young, overweight hypertensive patients. N. Engl. J. Med., 314:334–339, 1986.
122. Messerli, F.H.: Cardiomyopathy of obesity—a not-so-Victorian disease. N. Engl. J. Med., 314:378–380, 1986.
123. Alexander, J.K.: The cardiomyopathy of obesity. Prog. Cardiovasc. Dis., 27:325–334, 1985.
124. Joslin, E.P., Dublin, L.I., and Marks, H.H.: Studies on diabetes mellitus. III. Interpretation of variations in diabetes mellitus. Am. J. Med. Sci., 189:163, 1934.
125. Kissebah, A.H., et al.: Relation of body fat distribution to metabolic complications of obesity. J. Clin. Endocrinol. Metab., 54:254–260, 1982.
126. Krotkiewski, M., et al.: Regional adipose tissue cellularity in relation to metabolism in young and middle aged women. Metabolism, 24:703, 1975.
127. Tuck, M.L., and Sowers, J.: The effect of weight reduction on blood pressure, plasma renin activity, and plasma aldosterone levels in obese patients. N. Engl. J. Med., 304:930, 1981.
128. Peterson, H.R., et al.: Body fat and the activity of the autonomic nervous system. N. Engl. J. Med., 318:1077–1083, 1988.
129. Sharp, J.T., et al.: The total work of breathing in normal and obese men. J. Clin. Invest., 43:728–739, 1964.
130. Laurenco, R.V.: Diaphragm activity in obesity. J. Clin. Invest., 48:1609–1614, 1964.
131. Vaughan, R.W., Bauer, S., and Wise, L.: Volume and pH of gastric juice in obese patients. Anesthesiology, 43:686–689, 1975.
132. Cherniack, R.M.: Respiratory effects of obesity. Can. Med. Assoc. J., 80:613, 1959.
133. Dempsey, J.A., et al.: Alveolar–arterial gas exchange during muscular work in obesity. J. Appl. Physiol., 21:1807, 1966.
134. Barrera, F., et al.: Ventilation perfusion relationship in the obese patient. J. Appl. Physiol., 26:420, 1969.
135a. Vaughan, R.W., and Wise, L.: Postoperative arterial blood gas measurements in the obese patient: Effect of position on gas exchange. Ann. Surg., 182:705–709, 1975.
135b. Vaughan, R.W., and Wise, L.: Choice of abdominal operative incision in the obese patient: A study using blood gas measurements. Ann. Surg., 181:829–839, 1975.
135c. Tsueda, K., et al.: Obese supine death syndrome: Reports of two morbidly obese patients. Anesth. Analg., 58:345–347, 1979.

136. Wyner, J., Brodsky, J.B., and Merrell, R.C.: Massive obesity and arterial oxygenation. Anesth. Analg., 60:691–693, 1981.
137. Sharp, J.T., et al.: Effects of mass loading the respiratory system in man. J. Appl. Physiol., 19:959, 1964.
138. Kaufman, B.J., Ferguson, M.H., and Cherniack, R.M.: Hypoventilation in obesity. J. Clin. Invest., 38:500, 1959.
139. Burwell, C.S., et al.: Extreme obesity associated with alveolar hypoventilation—A Pickwickian syndrome. Am. J. Med., 21:811, 1956.
140. Andersen, J., Rasmussen, P.J., and Eriksen, J.: Pulmonary function in obese patients scheduled for jejuno-ileostomy. Acta Anaesth. Scand., 21:346–351, 1977.
141. Edelist, G.: Extreme obesity. Anesthesiology, 29:846, 1968.
142. DeHaven, J., et al.: Nitrogen and sodium balance and sympathetic nervous system activity in obese subjects treated with a low-calorie protein or mixed diet. N. Engl. J. Med., 302:477–482, 1980.
143. Sundaresan, P.R., et al.: Platelet alpha-adrenergic receptors in obesity: Alteration with weight loss. Clin. Pharmacol. Ther., 33:776–785, 1983.
144a. Lantigua, R.A., et al.: Cardiac arrhythmias associated with a liquid protein diet for the treatment of obesity. N. Engl. J. Med., 303:735–738, 1980.
144b. Sours, H.E., et al.: Sudden death associated with very low calorie weight reduction regimens. Am. J. Clin. Nutr., 34:453–461, 1981.
145. Jones, A.E.P., and Pelton, D.A.: An index of syndromes and their anaesthetic implications. Can. Anaesth. Soc. J., 23:207–226, 1976.

LABORATORY

146. Charpek Y, et al.: Usefulness of selectivity ordered preoperative tests. Med. Care, 26:95–104, 1988.
147. Blery C, et al.: Evaluation of a protocol for selective ordering of preoperative tests. Lancet, 1:139–141, 1986.
148. Kaplan, E.B., et al.: The usefulness of preoperative laboratory screening. J.A.M.A., 253:3576, 1985.
149. Rucker, L., Frye, E.B., and Staten, M.A.: Usefulness of screening chest roentgenograms in preoperative patients. J.A.M.A., 250:3209, 1983.
150. Johnson, P., Winnie, A.P., and Collins, V.J.: Special laboratory tests—indicators. Chicago, University of Illinois Hospital, Department of Anesthesiology Guidelines, 1988.
151. Garn, S.M., Smith, N.J., and Clark, D.C.: Lifelong differences in hemoglobin levels between blacks and whites. J. Nat. Med. Assoc., 67:91, 1975.
152. Dallman, P.R., et al.: Hemoglobin concentration in white, black and oriental children: Is there need for separate criteria in screening for anemia? Am. J. Clin. Nutr., 31:377–380, 1978.
153. Wintrobe, M.M., et al.: Clinical Hematology, 7th ed. Philadelphia, Lea & Febiger, 1974.
154. Crosby, W.H.: Red cell indices. Arch. Intern. Med., 139:23, 1979.
154a. Crosby, W.H.: Red cell mass: Its precursors and its perturbations. Hosp. Prac., 15:71–81, 1980.
155a. Howland, W.S., and Jacobs, R.: Serial microhematocrit determinations in evaluating blood replacement. Anesthesiology, 22:342, 1961.
155b. Barbour, H.G.: Water exchanges due to anesthetic drugs. Anesthesiology, 1:121, 1940.
155c. Lyon, R.P., et al.: Blood and "available fluid" volume studies in surgical patients. Surg. Gynecol. Obstet., 89:9, 1949.
155d. Gregersen, M.I.: A practical method for the determination of blood volume with the dye T-1824. J. Lab. Clin. Med., 29:1966, 1944.
155e. Albert, S.: I. Blood Volume Determinations with Radioactive Isotopes and Observations on Blood Volume Fluctuations. II. Index of Cardiac Clearance. AECU-361. Washington, DC, George Washington University for U.S. Atomic Energy Commission, 1958.
156. Zauber, N.P., and Zauber, A.G.: Hematologic data of healthy very old people. J.A.M.A., 257:2181, 1987.
157. Shulman, I.A., et al.: Experience with a cost-effective crossmatch protocol. J.A.M.A., 254:93, 1985.
158. Gillies, I.D.S.: Anaemia and anesthesia. Br. J. Anaesth., 46:589, 1974.
159. Carson, J.L., et al.: Severity of anaemia and operative morbidity and mortality. Lancet 1:727–729, 1988.
160a. Consensus Conference: Perioperative red blood cell transfusion. J.A.M.A., 260:2700, 1988.
160b. Office of Medical Appliances of Research. National Institutes of Health: Perioperative red cell transfusion. J.A.M.A., 260:2700–2703, 1988.
160c. Office of Medical Applications of Research. National Institutes of Health: Platelet transfusion therapy. J.A.M.A., 257:1777–1780, 1987.
161a. Suchman, A.L., and Mushlin, A.I.: How well does the activated partial thromboplastin time predict postoperative hemorrhage? J.A.M.A., 256:750, 1986.
161b. Office of Medical Applications of Research. National Institutes of Health: Fresh frozen plasma: Indications and risks. J.A.M.A., 253:551–553, 1985.
161c. Bove, J.R.: Fresh frozen plasma: Too few indications—too much use (editorial). Anesth. Analg., 64:849–850, 1985.
162. Barbour, C.M. Jr.: Polycythemia in relation to anesthesia and surgery. Presented at the Annual Meeting of the American Society of Anesthesiologists, St. Louis, MO, 1948.
163. Barbour, C.M.: Polycythemia in relation to anesthesia and surgery. Anesthesiology, 11:155, 1950.
164. Fox, M.J., et al.: Leukocyte larceny: A cause of spurious hypoxemia. Am. J. Med., 67:742, 1979.
165. Zsigmond, E.K., et al.: Abnormal creatine-phosphokinase isoenzyme pattern in families with malignant hyperpyrexia. Anesth. Analg., 51:827, 1972.
166. Zsigmond, E.K.: Creatine phosphokinase. In Enzymes in Anesthesiology. Edited by Foldes. New York, Springer-Verlag, 1978.
167. Burstein, C.L., Cotui, A.: Relationship between hypoproteinemia and toxicity of anesthetic agents. Anesth. Analg., 27:287, 1948.
168. Coogan, T.J., Turner, I.R., and Lashof, J.C.: Periodic evaluation of outpatients. Arch. Environ. Health, 21:192–199, 1970.
169. Mohr, D.N., et al.: Asymptomatic microhematuria and urologic disease: A population-based study. J.A.M.A., 256:224–229, 1986.
170. Fraser, C.G., Smith, B.C., and Peake, M.J.: Effectiveness of an outpatient urine screening program. Clin. Chem., 23:2216–2218, 1977.
171. Lawrence, VA, and Kroenke, K.: The unproven utility of preoperative urinalysis: Clinical use. Arch. Intern. Med., 148:1370–1373, 1988.
172. Entmacher, P.S.: Chief Medical Director, Metropolitan Life Insurance Company, 1983.
173. Clark, A.E.: Chronic shock syndrome. Ann. Surg., 125:626, 1947.
174. Roberts, K.E., DeCosse, J.J., Randall, H.T.: Fluid and electrolyte problems in surgery of the aged. Bull. N.Y. Acad. Med., 32:180, 1956.

175a. Sagel, S., et al.: Efficacy of routine screening and lateral chest radiographs in a hospital-based population. N. Engl. J. Med., 291:1001–1004, 1974.
175b. Rucker, L., Frye, E., Staten, M.: Usefulness of screening chest roentgenograms in preoperative patients. J.A.M.A., 250:3209–3211, 1983.
176. Tape, T.G., and Mushlin, A.I.: How useful are routine chest x-rays on preoperative patients at risk for postoperative chest disease? J. Gen. Intern. Med., 3:15–20, 1988.
177. Hubbell, F.A., et al.: The impact of routine admission chest x-ray films on patient care. N. Engl. J. Med., 312:209, 1985.
178. Weibman, M.: Routine chest x-rays for cancer patients. New York, Memorial Sloan-Kettering Cancer Center. ASA Annual Convention, 1988.
179. Kohn, R.M.: Breath-holding test for cardiac states. Circulation, 20:721, 1959.
180. Irvin, C.W.: Valsalva maneuver as a diagnostic aid. J.A.M.A., 170:787, 1959.
181. Valsalva, A.M.: De Aura Humana. *University of Utrecht, 1707* p. 84.
182. Sharpey-Schafer, E.P.: The effects of valsalva manoeuver on the normal and failing circulation. Br. Med. J., 1:693, 1955.
183. Knowles, J.H., Garlin, R., and Storey, C.F.: Clinical test for pulmonary congestion with use of valsalva maneuver. J.A.M.A., 160:44, 1956.
184. Garlin, R. Knowles, J.H., and Storey, C.F.: Valsalva maneuver as a test of cardiac function; pathologic physiology. Am. J. Med., 22:197, 1957.
185. Ard, R.W., and Twining, R.H.: Evaluation of valsalva test in bedside diagnosis of dyspnea. Am. J. Med. Sci., 234:403, 1957.
186. Snider, T.H., et al.: Simple bedside test of respiratory function. J.A.M.A., 170:1631, 1959.
187. Greene, B.A., and Berkowitz, S.: Preanesthetic induced cough as a method of diagnosis of preoperative bronchitis. Ann. Intern. Med., 37:723, 1952.
188. Howland, W.S., and Wang, K.C.: Preanesthesia clinic. N. Y. J. Med., 56:2497, 1956.
189. Mangano, D.T.: Monitoring pulmonary arterial pressure in coronary artery disease. Anesthesiology, 53:364–370, 1980.
190. Hannigan, C.A., et al.: Major surgery in patients with healed myocardial infarction. Am. J. Med. Sci., 222:628, 1951.
191. Finkbeiner, J.A., Wroblewski, F., and LaDue, J.S.: Major surgery in patient with chronic auricular fibrillation. N. Y. J. Med., 54:1175, 1954.
192. Pfeiffer, P.H., and LaDue, J.S.: Major surgical operations in presence of bundle branch block: Study of operative risk in 59 patients. Am. J. Med. Sci., 217:369, 1949.
193. Starr, I.: Present status of ballistocardiogram. Ann. Intern. Med., 37:839, 1952.
194. Wang, K.C., and Howland, W.S.: Cardiac and pulmonary evaluation in elderly patients before elective surgical operation. J.A.M.A., 166:993, 1958.
195. New York Heart Association, Criteria Committee: Nomenclature and Criteria for Diagnosis of Diseases of the Heart and Great Vessels, 8th ed. Boston, Little, Brown, 1981.
196. Goldman, L., et al.: Comparative reproducibility and validity of systems for assessing cardiovascular functional class: Advantages of a new specific activity scale. Circulation, 64:1227, 1981.
197. London, M.J., and Mangano, D.T.: Assessment of perioperative cardiac risk. Prob. Anesth., 1:337–358, 1987.
198. Killip, T., and Kimball, J.T.: Treatment of myocardial infarction in a coronary care unit. Am. J. Cardiol., 20:457, 1967.
199. Brewster, D.C., et al.: Selection of patients for preoperative coronary angiography: Use of dipyridamole-stress-thallium myocardial imaging. J. Vasc. Surg., 2:504, 1985.
200. Leppo, J., et al.: Serial thallium-201 myocardial imaging with dipyridamole infusion: Diagnostic utility in detecting coronary stenoses and relationship to regional wall motion. Circulation, 66:649, 1982.
201. Picano E., Lattanzi F., Masini M et al.: High dose dipyridamole-echocardiography test in effort angina. J. Am. Col. Cardiol., 8:84, 1986.
202. Foster E.D., Davis K.B., Carpenter J.A. et al.: Risk of noncardiac operation in patients with defined coronary disease: The Coronary Artery Surgery Study (CASS) Registry Experience. Ann. Thorac. Surg., 41:42–50, 1986.
203. Kleinman B., Henkin R.E., Glisson S.N. et al.: Qualitative evaluation of coronary flow during anesthetic induction using thallium-201 perfusion scans. Anesthesiology 64:157–164, 1986.
204. Del Gurcico L.R.M., Cohn D.J.: Monitoring operative risk in the elderly. J.A.M.A., 243:1350, 1980.
205. Gerson M.C., Hurst J.M., Hertzberg V.S., Doogan P.A. et al.: Cardiac prognosis in cardiac geriatric surgery. Ann. Intern. Med., 103:832, 1985.
206. McConachie I.: Value of pre-operative carotid sinus massage. Anaesthesia, 42:636, 1987.
207. Miller W.: Pulmonary function evaluation. Anesthesiology, 17:480, 1956.
208. Nunn J.F., Milledge J.S., Chen D., Dore C.: Respiratory criteria of fitness for surgery and anaesthesia. Anaesthesia, 43:543–551, 1988.
209. Stein M., Koota G.M., Simon M., Frank H.A.: Pulmonary evaluation of surgical patients. J.A.M.A., 181:765–70, 1962.
210. Tisi G.M.: Preoperative evaluation of pulmonary function. Validity, indications, and benefits. Amer. Rev. Resp. Dis., 119:293–310, 1979.
211. Comroe J.H.: Physiology of Respiration. 2nd Ed. Chicago, Year Book Medical Publishers, 1974.
212. Bendixen H. et al.: Respiratory Care. St. Louis, The C.V. Mosby Co., 1975.
213. Benumof J.L., Alfery D.D.: Pulmonary function testing. *In:* Anesthesia, Vol. 2 (Miller R.D., Ed.). New York, Churchill-Livingstone, pp. 1363–77, 1981.
214. Schwaber J.R.: Evaluation of respiratory status in surgical patients. Surg. Clin. North. Amer., 50:637–44, 1970.
215. Meakins J.C.: Dyspnea. J.A.M.A., 103:1442, 1934.
216. Shapiro B.A., Harrison R.A., Trout C.A.: Clinical Applications of Respiratory Care. Chicago, Year Book Medical Publishers Inc., 1975.
217. Boushy S.F., Billig D.M., North L.B., Helgason A.H.: Clinical course related to preoperative and postoperative pulmonary function in patients with bronchogenic carcinoma. Chest, 59(4):383–391, 1971.
218a. Guz A., Noble M.I.M., Widdicombe J.G., Trenchard D., Mushin W.W., Makey A.R.: The role of the vagal and glossopharyngeal afferent nerves in respiratory sensation, control of breathing and arterial pressure regulation in conscious man. Clin. Sci., 30:161, 1966b.
218b. Gooden B.A.: The diving response in clinical medicine. Anat Space Environ Med., 53:273, 1982.
219. Campbell, E.J.M., and Howell, J.B.L.: The sensation of breathlessness. Br. Med. Bull., 19:36, 1963.
220. Campbell, E.J.M., et al.: The effect of muscular paralysis induced by tubocurarine on the duration and sensation of breath-holding. Clin. Sci., 32:425, 1967.

221. Agostoni, E.: Diaphragm activity during breath-holding: Factors related to its onset. J. Appl. Physiol., 18:30, 1963.
222. Rovenstine, E.A., and Taylor, I.B.: Postoperative chest complications. Am. J. Med. Sci., 191:807, 1936.
223. Beck, H., and Preisler, O.: Laryngeal and tracheal flora before and after intubation. Der. Anaesthetist, 8:110, 1959.
224. Solomon, A., Herschfus, J.A., and Segal, M.S.: Aerosols of pancreatic dornase in broncho-pulmonary disease. Ann. Allergy, 12:71, 1959.
225. Tarhan, S., et al.: Risk of anesthesia and surgery in patients with chronic bronchitis and chronic obstructive lung disease. Surgery, 74:720, 1973.
226. Greene, N.M.: Anesthetic management of patients with respiratory disease. J.A.M.A., 162:1276, 1956.
227. Clifton, E.E.: Pancreatic dornase aerosol in pulmonary endotracheal and endobronchial disease. Dis. Chest, 30:373, 1956.
228. Barach, A.L., et al.: Physical methods simulating cough mechanism. J.A.M.A., 150:1300, 1952.
229. Patrick, M.: Preparation for Anaesthesia. Baltimore, University Park Press, 1980.
230. McGill, W.A., Coveler, L.A., and Epstein, B.S.: Subacute respiratory infections in small children. Anesth. Analg., 58:331, 1979.
231. Wood, R.A., and Hoekelman, R.A.: Value of the chest x-ray as a screening test for elective surgery in children. J. Pediatr., 67:447, 1981.
232. Sane, S.M., et al.: Value of preoperative chest x-ray examinations in children. J. Pediatr., 60:669, 1977.
233. Hall, W.J., et al.: Pulmonary mechanics after uncomplicated influenza. Am. Rev. Resp. Dis., 113:141, 1976.
234. Tait, A.R., and Knight, P.R.: The effect of general anesthesia on upper respiratory tract infections in children. Anesthesiology, 67:930–935, 1987.
235. Tait, A.R., McLear, A.S., and Knight, P.R.: Anesthesia and the common cold (abstract). Anesthesiology, 65:492, 1986.
236. Belshe, R.B.: Textbook of Human Virology. Littleton, PSE Publishing, 1984, p. 361.
237. Knight, P.R., et al.: Alterations in influenza virus pulmonary pathology induced by diethyl ether, halothane, enflurane, and phenobarbital in mice. Anesthesiology, 58:209, 1983.
238. Bedows, E., Davidson, B., and Knight, P.R.: Effect of halothane on the replication of animal viruses. Antimicrob. Agents Chemother., 25:719, 1984.
239. Collins, V.J.: Concepts in anesthesiology. J.A.M.A., 182:105, 1962.
240a. Collins, V.J.: Management of patients requiring operations. N.Y. State J. Med., 59:4359, 1959.
240b. Levinson, W.: Preoperative evaluations by an internist—are they worthwhile? Western Med., 141:395, 1984.
240c. Choi, J.J.: An anesthesiologists' philosophy on 'medical clearance' for surgical patients. Arch. Intern. Med., 147:2090, 1987.
241. Kehlet, H.: Does regional anesthesia reduce postoperative morbidity? Intens. Care Med., 10:165, 1984.
242. Kehlet, H.: The modifying effect of general and regional anesthesia on the endocrine-metabolic response to surgery. Reg. Anesth., 7:38, 1982.
243. Keith, I.: Anaesthesia and blood loss in total hip replacement. Anaesthesia, 32:444, 1977.
244. Chin, S.P., et al.: Blood loss in total hip replacement: Extradural vs. phenoperidine analgesia. Br. J. Anaesth., 54:491, 1982.
245. McGowan, S.W., and Smith, G.F.N.: Anaesthesia for transurethral prostatectomy: A comparison of spinal intradural analgesia with two methods of general anaesthesia. Anaesthesia, 35:847, 1980.
246. Modig, J., et al.: Thromboembolism after total hip replacement: Role of epidural and general anesthesia. Anesth. Analg., 62:174, 1983.
247. Owens, M.E.: Pain in infancy: Conceptual and methodological issues. Pain, 20:213, 1984.
248. Berry, F.A., and Gregory, G.A.: Do premature infants require anesthesia for surgery (editorial)? Anesthesiology, 67:291, 1987.
249. Gregory, G.A., et al.: Fetal anesthetic requirement (MAC) for halothane. Anesth. Analg., 62:9, 1983.
250. Anand, K.J.S., and Hickey, P.R.: Pain and its effects in the human neonate and fetus. N. Engl. J. Med., 317:1321, 1987.
251. Rawlings, D.J., Miller, P.A., and Engle, R.R.: The effect of circumcision on transcutaneous P_{O_2} in term infants. Am. J. Dis. Child., 134:676, 1980.
252. Booker, P.D.: Postoperative analgesia for neonates (editorial)? Anaesthesia, 42:343, 1987.
253. Marshall, R.E., et al.: Circumcision: Effects on newborn behavior. Infant Behavior. Devel. 3:1, 1980.
254. Fletcher, A.M.: Pain in the neonate (editorial). N. Engl. J. Med., 317:1347, 1987.
255. McGrath, P.A.: An assessment of children's pain: A review of behavioral, physiological and direct scaling techniques. Pain, 31:147, 1987.
256. Anand, K.J.S., Sippell, W.G., and Anysley-Green, A.: Randomized trial of fentanyl anaesthesia in preterm babies undergoing surgery: Effects on the stress response. Lancet, 1:243, 1987.
257. Stang, H.J., et al.: Local anesthesia for neonatal circumcision: Effects on distress and cortisol response. J.A.M.A., 259:1507, 1988.
258. Gunnar, M.R., et al.: The effects of circumcision on serum cortisol and behavior. Psychoneuroendocrinology, 6:269, 1981.
259. Talbert, L.M., Kraybill, E.N., and Potter, H.D.: Adrenal cortical response to circumcision in the neonate. Obstet. Gynecol., 48:208, 1976.
260. American Academy of Pediatrics Committee on Fetus and Newborn and Committee on Drugs: Neonatal anesthesia. Pediatrics, 80:446, 1987.
261. Waters, R.W.: Comments. Newsletter, American Society of Anesthesiology. 13:21, 1949.
262. Woodbridge, P.D.: Preanesthetic breakfast. Anesthesiology, 4:81, 1943.
263. Hunt, J.N.: Some properties of an alimentary osmoreceptor mechanism. J. Physiol., 132:267, 1956.
264. Maltby, J.R., et al.: Preoperative oral fluids: Is a 5-hour fast justified prior to elective surgery? Anesth. Analg., 65:1112, 1986.
265. Teabeaut, J.R.: Aspiration of gastric contents: Experimental study. Am. J. Pathol., 28:51–62, 1952.
266. Baraka, A., et al.: Control of gastric acidity by glycopyrrolate premedication in the parturient. Anesth. Analg., 56:642–645, 1977.
267. Strum, W.B.: Ranitidine. J.A.M.A., 250:1894, 1983.
268. Gallagher, E.G., et al.: Prophylaxis against acid aspiration syndrome: Single oral dose of H_2-antagonist on the evening before elective surgery. Anaesthesia, 43:1011–1014, 1988.
269. Coombs, D.W., Hooper, D., and Colton, T.: Pre-anesthetic cimetidine alteration of gastric fluid volume and pH. Anesth. Analg., 58:183–188, 1979.

270. Sutherland, T., Davies, J.M., and Stock, J.: The price and value of preoperative outpatient fasting—effects on gastric contents and outpatient morbidity. Can. Anaesth. Soc. J., 32:S100, 1985.
271. Stoelting, R.L.: Gastric fluid pH in patients receiving cimetidine. Anesth. Analg., 57:675–677, 1978.
272. Brater, D.C., Clinical comparison of cimetidine and ranitidine. Clin. Pharmacol. Ther., 32:484–489, 1982.
273. Manchikanti, L., Kraus, J.W., and Edds, S.P.: Cimetidine and related drugs in anesthesia. Anesth. Analg., 61:595–608, 1982.
274. Feely, J., Wilkinson, G.R., and Wood, A.J.J.: Reduction of liver blood flow and propranolol metabolism by cimetidine. N. Engl. J. Med., 304:692–695, 1981.
275. Lam, A.L., and Parkin, J.A.: Cimetidine and prolonged postoperative somnolence. Can. Anaesth. Soc. J., 28:450–452, 1981.
276. Brock-Utne, J.G., Downing, J.W., and Humphrey, D.: Effect of ranitidine given before atropine sulphate on lower oesophageal sphincter tone. Anaesth. Intens. Care, 12:140, 1984.
277. Abernethy, D.R., et al.: Ranitidine does not impair oxidative or conjugative metabolism. Clin. Pharmacol. Ther., 35:188, 1984.
278. Taylor, G., and Pryse-Davies, J.: The prophylactic use of antacids in the prevention of acid pulmonary aspiration syndrome. Lancet, 1:288–291, 1966.
279. Dewan, D.M., et al.: Patient acceptance of orally administered antacid therapy during labor. Anesthesiology, 52:526–527, 1980.
280. Gibbs, C.P., Spohr, L., and Schmidt, D.: The effectiveness of sodium citrate as an antacid. Anesthesiology, 57:44–46, 1982.
281. Chen, C.T., et al.: Evaluation of the efficacy of Alka-Seltzer effervescent in gastric acid neutralization. Anesth. Analg., 63:325, 1984.
282. Collins, V.J.: Use of a common popular citrate drink—Seven Up: A substitute for bicitra. Morbidity and Mortality Conference Report. University of Illinois Dep. of Anesthesiology, March 1988.
283. Schulze-Delrieu, J.: Metoclopramide. N. Engl. J. Med., 305:28, 1981.
284. Wyner, J., and Cohen, S.E.: Gastric volume in early pregnancy. Anesthesiology, 57:209, 1982.
285. Beaumont, W.: Experiments and observations on the gastric juice and the physiology of digestion. Plattsburg, NY, Allen 277:159, 1833.
286. Malagelada, J.R.: Quantitation of gastric solid-fluid discrimination during digestion of ordinary meals. Gastroenterology, 72:1264, 1977.
287. Hester, J.B., and Heath, M.L.: Pulmonary acid aspiration syndrome: Should prophylaxis be routine? Br. J. Anaesth., 49:595, 1977.
288. Miller, M., Wishart, H.Y., and Nimmo, W.S.: Gastric contents at induction of anaesthesia: Is a 4-hour fast necessary? Br. J. Anaesth., 55:1185, 1983.
289. Manchikanti, L., et al.: Assessment of age-related acid aspiration risk factors in pediatric, adult, and geriatric patients. Anesth. Analg., 64:11, 1985.
290. Maltby, J.R., et al.: Preoperative oral fluids: Is a 5-hour fast justified prior to elective surgery? Anesth. Analg., 65:1112, 1986.
291. Hutchinson, B.R., Merry, A.F., and Wild, C.J.: The relationship of duration of fast to the volume and pH of gastric contents. Anaesth. Intens. Care, 14:128, 1986.
292. Shay, H., et al.: The influence of glucose on response of human stomach to test meals. Am. J. Digest. Dis., 9:363, 1942.
293. Nimmo, W.S., Wilson, J., and Prescott, L.F.: Narcotic analgesics and delayed gastric emptying during labour. Lancet, 1:890, 1975.
294. Adelhoj, B., Petring, O.U., and Hagelsten, J.O.: Inaccuracy of preanesthetic gastric intubation for emptying liquid stomach contents. Acta Anaesthiol. Scand., 30:41, 1986.
295. Christensen, V., and Skovsted, P.: Effects of general anesthesia on pH of gastric contents in man during surgery: A survey of halothane, fluorexene and cyclopropane. Acta Anaesthiol. Scand., 19:49, 1975.
296. Wright, D.J., and Pandya, A.: Smoking and gastric juice volume in outpatients. Can. Anaesth. Soc. J., 26:328, 1979.
297. O'Sullivan, G.M., et al.: Noninvasive measurement of gastric emptying in obstetric patients. Anesth. Analg., 66:505, 1987.
298. Taylor, G.: Acid pulmonary aspiration syndrome after antacids. Br. J. Anaesth., 47:615–617, 1975.
299. Ong, B., Palahnuik, R.J., and Cummings, M.: Gastric volume and pH in outpatients. Can. Anaesth. Soc. J., 25:36, 1978.
300. Vaughan, R.W., Bauer, S., and Wise, L.: Volume and pH of gastric juice in obese patients. Anesthesiology, 43:686–689, 1975.
301. Coté, C.J., et al.: Assessment of risk factors related to the acid aspiration syndrome in pediatric patients—gastric pH and residual volume. Anesthesiology, 56:70–72, 1982.
302. Salem, M.R., et al.: Premedicant drugs and gastric juice pH and volume in pediatric patients. Anesthesiology, 44:216–219, 1976.
303. Salem, M.R., Wong, A.Y., and Collins, V.J.: The pediatric patient with a full stomach. Anesthesiology, 39:435–440, 1973.
304. Blom, H., Schmidt, J.F., and Rytlander, M.: Rectal diazepam compared to intramuscular pethidine/promethazine/chlorpromazine with regard to gastric contents in paediatric anaesthesia. Acta Anaesth. Scand., 28:652–653, 1984.
305. Sutton, J.A., Thompson, S., and Sobnack, R.: Measurement of gastric emptying rates by radioactive isotope scanning and epigastric impedance. Lancet, 1:898–900, 1985.
306. Lewis, M., and Crawford, J.S.: Can one risk fasting the obstetric patient for less than 4 hours? Br. J. Anaesth., 59:312–314, 1987.
307. Gwathmey, J.T.: Anesthesia. New York, Appleton, 1914, p. 365.
308. Booth, L.: A diet before surgery: American practice of surgery. Am. J. Surg., 4:131, 1928.
309. Bruce, D.L.: Anesthetic implications of fasting. Anesth. Analg., 50:612–619, 1971.
310. Barry, K.G., Mazze, R.I., and Schwartz, F.D.: Prevention of surgical oliguria and renal-hemodynamic suppression of sustained hydration. N. Engl. J. Med., 270:1371–1377, 1964.
311. Cahill, G.F.: Starvation in man. N. Engl. J. Med., 282:668–675, 1970.
312. Merin, R.G., Samuelson, P.N., and Schalch, D.S.: Major inhalation anesthetics and carbohydrate metabolism. Anesth. Analg., 59:625–632, 1971.
313. Merin, R.G.: Inhalation anesthetics and myocardial metabolism: Possible complications for functional effects. Anesthesiology, 39:216–255, 1973.
314. Miletich, D.J., Albrecht, R.F., and Seals, C.: Responses to fasting and lipid infusion of epinephrine-induced arrhythmias during halothane anesthesia. Anesthesiology, 48:245–248, 1978.

315. Munson, E.S., et al.: Increase in anesthetic uptake excretion and blood solubility in man after eating. Anesth. Analg., 57:224, 1978.
316. Sutherland, T., Davies, J.M., and Stock, J.: The price and value of preoperative outpatient fasting—effects on gastric contents and outpatient morbidity. Can. Anaesth. Soc. J., 32:S100, 1985.
317. Maltby, J.R., et al.: Preoperative oral fluids: Is a 5-hour fast justified prior to elective surgery? Anesth. Analg., 65:1112, 1986.
318. Sutherland, A.D., et al.: The effect of preoperative oral fluid and ranitidine on gastric fluid volume and pH. Can. J. Anaesth., 34:117, 1987.
319. Behrman, R.E., and Vaughan, V.S.: Nelson Textbook of Pediatrics. Philadelphia, WB Saunders, 1983, p. 1421.
320. Cornblath, M., and Schwartz, R.: Disorders of Carbohydrate Metabolism in Infancy 2nd ed. Philadelphia, WB Saunders, 1976, p. 345.
321. Bowie, M.D., Mulligan, P.B., and Schwartz, R.: Intravenous glucose tolerance in the normal newborn infant. Pediatrics, 31:590, 1963.
322. Welborn, L.G., et al.: Perioperative blood glucose concentrations in pediatric outpatients. Anesthesiology, 65:543, 1986.
323. Thomas, D.K.M.: Hypoglycemia in children before operation: Its incidence and prevention. Br. J. Anaesth., 46:66, 1974.
324. Jensen, B.H., Wernberg, M., and Andersen, M.: Preoperative starvation and blood glucose concentrations in children undergoing inpatient and outpatient anaesthesia. Br. J. Anaesth., 54:1071, 1982.
325. Splinter, W.M., Stewart, J.A., and Muir, J.G.: The effect of preoperative apple juice on gastric contents, thirst and hunger in children. Can. J. Anaesth., 36:55, 1989.
326. Collins, V.J.: Urinary retention in male patients following anesthesia and surgery. Unpublished data. U.S. Army, Glennan General Hosp., 1945.
327. Aldrete, J.A., and Kroulik, D.: A post-anesthetic recovery score. Anesth. Analg., 49:924, 1970.
328. Aldrete, J.A., and McDonald, J.S.: The post-anesthetic recovery score as a method of evaluation of anesthesia performance. Symposium Workshop, Proceed Demograph. Epidemiol., Washington, DC, December 2, 1977.
329. Steward, D.J.: A simplified scoring system for the postoperative recovery room. Can. Anaesth. Soc. J., 22:111, 1975.
330. Apgar, V., et al.: Evaluation of the newborn infant. Second report. J.A.M.A., 168:1985, 1958.
331. Beecher, H.K.: A definition of irreversible coma. J.A.M.A., 205:337, 1968.
332a. Collins, V.J.: Limits of medical responsibility in prolonging life—guides to decisions. J.A.M.A., 206:389, 1968.
332b. Collins, V.J.: Address at Special Program on Medicine and Religion Title as in 332a. Annual Convention AMA. San Francisco, June 16, 1968.
332c. Collins, V.J.: Concepts and ethics in defining death and a scoring system. J. Ill. State. Soc. Med., 148:43, 1975.
333. Sugar, O., and Gerald, R.W.: Anoxia and brain potentials. J. Neurophysiol., 1:558, 1938.
334. American College of Sports Medicine. *Guidelines for Graded Exercise Testing and Exercise Prescription,* ed. 2, pp. 45–48. Philadelphia, Lea & Febiger, 1980.
335. Astrand, P.O., Ryhming, I.: A normogram for calculation of aerobic capacity (physical fitness) from pulse rate during submaximal work. J. Appl. Physiol., 7:218, 1954.
336. Jette, M., et al.: The Canadian home fitness test. Can. Med. Assoc. J., 114:680, 1976.

DRUG INTERACTIONS

DRUG THERAPY UNRELATED TO ANESTHESIA AS A RISK[1,2]

The prevalence of drug therapy for medical diseases in patients scheduled for anesthesia and surgery poses a variety of problems and hazards. Approximately 10% of the population will receive an anesthesia and an operation in any single year. When it is recognized that half the adult population is taking some form of medication, the problem can be seen as a general one.[4] Most patients admitted to a hospital are frequent partakers of at least three drugs. In a hospital the average patient receives 6 to 10 drugs, and the incidence of adverse reactions is 7% to 10%. If 10 to 20 drugs are administered, the chances of an adverse reaction are 40%. Because the body mechanisms for reacting to drugs are limited, the intake of many drugs must result in some drug interaction.[3]

More important than the influence of an actual drug is the need for awareness on the part of the anesthesiologist of medication, of the extent of use and the extent of dependency. Upon recognizing a situation of drug use or abuse, two approaches may be pursued: (1) wait to see if symptoms of a disorder or drug deficiency occur and then treat, or (2) assume that undesirable effects exist or will occur and attempt to prevent. It is essential to consider some of the drugs commonly used.[6]

MECHANISMS OF ADVERSE DRUG INTERACTION

Adverse drug reactions can occur as a result of:

1. Immune or hypersensitivity responses
2. Idiosyncrasy—hyporeactions or hyperreactions
3. Defects in metabolism (genetic)
4. Overdosage or underdosage
5. Drug interaction

An important and expanding cause of *adverse reactions* is that of drug interaction.* Physical, chem-

---

* A table listing major adverse drug interactions has been prepared by the Editors of *Medical Letter*. The reader is referred to this detailed list in volume 123, March 6, 1981.

ical, and biologic drug interactions can occur at five sites: point of intake; transport and distribution points; action sites; metabolic stations; and portals of excretion.

Many specific mechanisms[5] may operate to alter the action of one drug in the presence of another: altered binding of a drug in the presence of a second drug; competition for receptors; preferential utilization of metabolic paths; chemical or pharmacologic antagonism; enhanced or inhibited uptake; interference with metabolism; genetic differences in metabolism; and changes in distribution or delay or enhancement of excretion of one drug by another (Table 10–1).

In many circumstances, altered metabolism is involved in drug disposition and action. One variable is the speed of metabolism which is dependent on availability of substrate, the chemical environment, and level of enzyme activity. Endogenous control of enzymes includes genetic, hormonal, nutritional, and physicochemical conditions.

PLASMA PROTEIN BINDING.[8] A principle of pharmacodynamics is that drugs bound to transport protein are inactive. Plasma proteins possess a variable number of anionic and cationic sites, depending on pH, to which many ionizable or polar drugs can bind avidly and extensively. Such protein can be considered an inactive or storage receptor, and different drugs compete for these binding receptors. Decreased drug binding may occur due to altered albumin composition. In uremia altered binding can be related to altered molecular structure due to increased alanine amino acid content.

Weakly bound drugs include oral hypoglycemics and coumarin anticoagulants.[7] The unbound plasma fraction of these can be increased two- to fivefold when displaced by strongly bound drugs. Strongly bound drugs include diphenylhydantoin, barbiturates, chloral hydrate, curare, salicylates, PABA (from hydrolysis of procaine), and ethacrynic acid. Curare is an important example: at pH of 7.4 about 30% to 35% is plasma protein-bound; the remaining free 65% to 70% participates in ionization balance. When pH is increased, the binding is enhanced and the free drug available for action is decreased. Conversely, acidosis increases the unbound fraction and enhances the action of curare.

Consideration must also be given to the effect of pH on the ionization of the effector *receptor* protein and its attraction for a drug. This variable influences the amount of drug uptake.

Drugs with a high protein-binding capacity may have their effect decreased by several means:

1. IV protein solution—to provide *more* binding power for competitive binding.
2. Enhanced binding by transport protein—to decrease availability of free drug.
3. To displace drug from effector sites by one or more highly bound and less active, or by decreasing occupancy of effector protein.
4. Enhance biotransformation.
5. Increase *urine* pH and urine ionization of drug (only nonionized fraction is reabsorbed) to decrease reabsorption. Ionized or polar drugs are excreted more rapidly.
6. Decrease nonionized fraction in plasma (only this fraction penetrates), *i.e.*, increase ionized fraction.

IONIZATION.[2] The effect of pH is twofold: to influence the degree of binding (see above) and to determine the ratio of ionized to nonionized drug of the unbound fraction.

The extent of ionization of the drug (unbound plasma fraction) is dependent on both the dissociation constant pK_a and the pH of the solution. The ionization constant pK_a is the pH or hydrogen ion concentration at which half of a drug is ionized and half is nonionized. For example, carbonic acid has a pK_a of 6.1 and this is the pH at which half of the acid exists as the bicarbonate. *Pharmacodynamically* only the nonionized fraction of a drug is lipoid soluble and capable of membrane penetration (Fig. 10–1).

The pK_a is a function of the nature of the drug. Thus, the following relationships exist: For those drugs that behave as acids, the stronger the acid, the lower its pK_a; for those drugs that behave as bases, the stronger the base, the higher its pK_a. Conversely, an acid with a high pK value is a weak acid; a base with a low pK value is a weak base. The relationshp

TABLE 10–1. DRUG INTERACTION MECHANISMS

I. PHYSICAL REACTIONS
　1. Competition for effector receptors:
　　—Occupancy level receptor
　　—Displacement capacity
　2. Competition for binding protein in plasma:
　　—Relative binding (avidity of one drug for another)
　　—Influence of pH on binding
　3. Ionization factors:
　　—Ratio of free to ionized drug
　　—Influence of different pK's
　　—Influence of pH
II. CHEMICAL REACTIONS
　1. Simple chemical neutralization; redox; hydrolysis
　2. Preferential use of metabolic pathways by one drug over another
　3. Differential metabolic rates and biotransformation
III. BIOLOGICAL REACTIONS
　1. Level of microsomal enzyme activity
　　—Enzyme control of factors of:
　　　(a) Genetic control
　　　(b) Quality and quantity of enzyme
　　　(c) Nutritional state
　　　(d) Physiocochemical conditions
　2. Stimulation or inhibition of enzyme levels by drugs (xenobiotic drugs):
　　　(a) Enzyme induction—increased synthesis
　　　(b) Enzyme depression—decreased synthesis
　　　(c) Enzyme utilization
　3. Differences in elimination

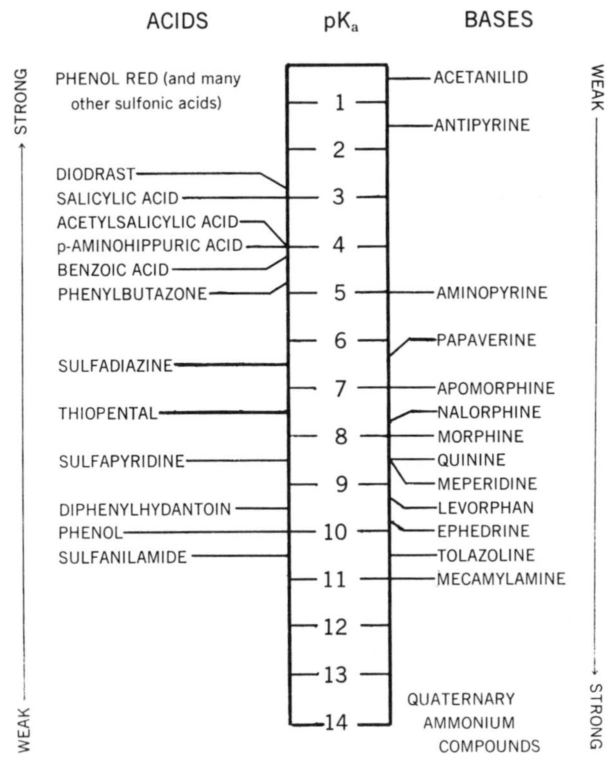
ACIDS
pKa
BASES
STRONG
WEAK
PHENOL RED (and many other sulfonic acids)
DIODRAST
SALICYLIC ACID
ACETYLSALICYLIC ACID
p-AMINOHIPPURIC ACID
BENZOIC ACID
PHENYLBUTAZONE
SULFADIAZINE
THIOPENTAL
SULFAPYRIDINE
DIPHENYLHYDANTOIN
PHENOL
SULFANILAMIDE
1
2
3
4
5
6
7
8
9
10
11
12
13
14
ACETANILID
ANTIPYRINE
AMINOPYRINE
PAPAVERINE
APOMORPHINE
NALORPHINE
MORPHINE
QUININE
MEPERIDINE
LEVORPHAN
EPHEDRINE
TOLAZOLINE
MECAMYLAMINE
QUATERNARY AMMONIUM COMPOUNDS
WEAK
STRONG

52

FIG. 10–1. Approximate pK_a values of some compounds of pharmacologic interest.

between pK_a and pH and the degree of ionization is expressed in the Henderson-Hasselbalch equation.

$$\text{For an acid: } pK_a - pH = \log \frac{[\text{Nonionized acid form}]}{[\text{Ionized acid}]}$$

$$\text{For a base: } pK_a - pH = \log \frac{[\text{Ionized base}]}{[\text{Nonionized base form}]}$$

Drugs that are weakly acid show an increasing ionization as the pH rises or the solution becomes alkaline. Conversely, acidosis decreases the dissociation so that more of the nonionized or active form is present.

Drugs that form weak bases (e.g., local anesthetics) show a decreasing ionization with more free base as the pH rises, whereas acidosis results in more ionized drug and diminished free drug.

Barbiturates form weak acids and are prepared as cationic salts. Thiopental is provided as the sodium salt. Once in plasma a portion is protein bound and inactive (some 75% is bound at a plasma pH of 7.4), whereas the remaining portion, some 25%, is free to ionize in accordance with the mass-action law. The free NaP ionizes into sodium ions and the conjugate base (P^-), which combines with hydrogen ions to form the nonionized acid (HP). The amount of non-ionized thiopental acid is dependent on the dissociation constant (K_a):

$$(H^+) + (P^-) \underset{\longleftarrow}{\overset{K_a}{\longrightarrow}} (HP)$$

TABLE 10–2. EFFECT OF DISSOCIATION CONSTANT ON FRACTION OF THIOPENTAL AND PENTOBARBITAL BOUND TO PROTEIN AND FRACTION NONIONIZED IN PLASMA

	Thiopental	Pentobarbital
pK_a	7.6	8.1
Fraction bound to protein at pH 7.4	0.75	0.40
Fraction nonionized at pH 7.4	0.61	0.83

At the pH of the dissociation constant of thiopental, i.e., pK_a of 7.6, half of the thiopental is in the acid nonionized form (HP) and half is in the ionized conjugate base form (P^-). At the normal plasma pH of 7.4 a larger absolute amount is unbound and available for dissociation reactions. At this pH a larger fraction, about 60%, is nonionized (Table 10–2). At lower pHs an increasing fraction is in the nonionized from. Conversely, at higher pHs (increasing alkalinity) more drug is ionized and becomes inactive.

Curare contrasts with the barbiturates. It is prepared as the chloride salt of a strong acid (hydrochloride) and behaves generally as a weak base, but more appropriately as an amphoteric electrolyte.* At the normal plasma pH of 7.4 only about 30% of curare is protein bound, leaving 70% free to obey the mass action law of dissociation. The free salt ionizes to form the poorly dissociated nonionized curare.

At lower pHs the fraction of curare bound (inactive) is decreased and the free active curare is increased. In turn the hydroxyls of this free curare at acid pHs are less ionized and more exist in the nonionized form, available for membrane penetration. Simultaneously, the amine group of the curare is more ionized as cations and more is available to combine with receptor-anionic sites.

ENZYME ACTIVITY. Introduction of a second drug, called a xenobiotic, may alter enzyme activity by two mechanisms: (1) increasing enzyme synthesis and raising the level of enzyme activity, which is designated as *enzyme induction* (an effective agent must be administered chronically, and the effect persists after discontinuing the agent); and (2) by interacting with the enzyme system one drug may permit inhibition or stimulation of the intensity of activity of a second drug (this effect persists only while the second agent is present).

ENZYME INDUCTION. Many drugs have the capacity to stimulate microsomal enzyme synthesis in the liver cells. Hypnotic drugs and large doses of steroids are effective in increasing enzyme levels, which has been interpreted as subtle evidence of hepatic toxicity.

* *D*-tubocurarine chloride pentohydrate is prepared as 1% solution at pH 4.6 to 4.8.

Other examples include:

1. *Phenobarbital* is a classic example: consequent to its chronic administration many other drugs are more rapidly degraded, e.g., warfarin, dicumarol, and other anticoagulants are readily destroyed, necessitating the use of larger doses for anticoagulant purposes. When the phenobarbital is discontinued, an excessive amount of anticoagulant may be present, causing hemorrhage; bilirubin conjugation is increased simultaneously; phenobarbital pretreatment increases the rate of uptake and transformation of methoxyflurane. Similarly, methoxyflurane breakdown is enhanced by tetrahydrocannabinol (THC).
2. Antipyrine is metabolized almost completely in the liver. It is also evenly distributed throughout body water and less than 10% is bound to plasma protein—the rate of antipyrine elimination has become a suitable method to assess liver microsomal drug metabolism.
3. Short-acting barbiturates such as amobarbital and secobarbital
4. DDT and similar organic pesticides increase microsomal enzymes—farm workers may have enhanced metabolism of hypnotic drugs and often show great tolerance
5. Steroids in *large doses* are enzyme inducers and drugs metabolized by liver enzymes are readily inactivated
6. Phenytoin
7. Alcoholism: Drugs dependent on hepatic metabolism are slowed in their degradation, and high plasma levels are achieved with the usual doses in the presence of alcohol. On the other hand, in the chronic alcoholic not inebriated, the same drugs undergo more rapid degradation, and higher doses are needed.
8. Smoking contributes to enzyme induction.[9]

ENZYME INHIBITION. Drugs dependent upon *liver* microsomal enzymes may not be readily metabolized if a chronically administered drug inhibits or "uses up" the available enzymes. Examples include antipyrine and steroids in *ordinary doses*, which do not promote enzyme synthesis but decrease the level of activity of liver enzymes by utilization. If administered, they are metabolized more slowly. Women taking oral contraceptive agents have a reduced metabolizing capacity and a concomitant increased activity of opiates and tranquilizers.

Alcohol diminishes the ability of enzymes to detoxify other liver-dependent drugs. Anticoagulant plasma levels are usually higher during alcohol intake. After periods of abstinence, intake of alcohol may raise anticoagulant levels to precipitate hemorrhage.

Many inhalation anesthetic drugs inhibit the metabolism of nonvolatile agents. Thus, diethyl ether inhibits barbiturate degradation. Halothane has a dual action on oxidative metabolism: (1) it depresses metabolism of certain barbiturates—amobarbital, hexobarbital, pentobarbital—this effect is dose dependent, reversible, and noncompetitive; in contrast, (2) it enhances the metabolism of aniline and similar substrates.

INTERACTION AT RECEPTOR SITES. The impact at the site of action of drugs administered by anesthetists is of special concern. Several circumstances are enumerated: atropine to counteract the bradycardia of narcotics and general anesthetics; protamine to eliminate the effects of heparin; vasopressors to counteract the hypotensive effect of a number of drugs; neostigmine to reverse curare; mylaxen to block cholinesterase and prolong succinylcholine; and naloxone to eliminate the respiratory depression of narcotics.

Other mechanisms by which one drug may enhance (or diminish) another are the increased synthesis of endogenous neuromediators, increased release of endogenous chemicals, prevention of binding to secondary receptors, sensitization receptors to drugs, and enhanced affinity between receptors and drugs.

Receptor binding capacity at the effector site can be considered as an additional compartment for distribution of drugs (Hull).[10]

SPECIFIC DRUG INTERACTIONS

ACRYLIC BONE CEMENT. Acrylic bone cement is now an established procedure in prosthetic hip surgery. The substance used is designated as methylmethacrylate (MM) and has been used extensively as dental prosthetic, as a bone substitute in cranioplasties, and extensively in hip replacement surgery. In 1960, Charnley introduced this cement in hip replacement surgery for the fixation of his prostheses.[1]

Composition and Preparation of Cement.

Methylmethacrylate is supplied as two components: a liquid and a powder, which are mixed shortly before use. The liquid is a monomer of methylmethacrylate. The monomer contains small quantities of dimethyl-p-toludine and hydroquinone. Hydroquinone prevents premature polymerization when mixed with the powder, and the toludine promotes what is known as "cold curing" of the finished compound. The powder consists basically of a polymer of methylmethacrylate. The mixing together of the liquid and the powder brings about polymerization of the liquid monomer, which then binds together the polymerized powder. The mixture forms a dough that sets within 5 to 10 minutes. In the course of this mixing, there is a marked exothermic reaction that produces a cement-like complex. The peak of the heat production is reached in about 6 minutes. Early in the mixing process, which is done in a dry shallow bowl and mixed with a metal spoon, the liquid being added to the powder, the mixture becomes liquid and should be mixed vigorously to promote evaporation of the monomer. This evaporation period allows a reduction in residual nonpolymerized monomer available that might enter into the circulation when the cement is inserted into the femoral shaft and into the acetabulum. Mixing should be done carefully so that bubbles in the cement are not increased, thereby allowing the material to become porous and weak. When the mixture assumes a doughy consistency, it can be then kneaded with the hands until it no longer sticks to the surgical gloves. At this point, it is ready for insertion manually into the acetabulum, after it ceases to stick to the gloves. The acetabulum should be dry and free of soft tissue and blood. The cement is also inserted into the femoral canal manually. It is recommended that a small suction tube be introduced into the femoral canal to remove blood and air when the cement is inserted.

This entire process is fraught with a number of hazards that present several intraoperative complications.

Absorption of MM into Circulation. MM has been demonstrated in the central venous circulation.[1] The peak level is noted at about 3 minutes after insertion of the prosthesis. By 5 to 10 minutes, the MM is not detected.

The acrylic monomer, in experimental studies, leaks into the venous circulation during the curing phase of the cement. Only the surface monomer is available for absorption. It is cleared principally by the lungs, and the odor can be detected in the expired air. It is recommended that the mixture should not be inserted until the monomer has had time to evaporate from the surface of the mix and the odor is not detectable.

Peripheral vasodilatation occurs when the monomer is absorbed into the circulation and can contribute to hypotension without histamine being released.[2,3]

Pulmonary Edema. Noncardiovascular pulmonary edema may occur following hip arthroplasty and the use of acrylic bone cement. It is often referred to as the "capillary leak syndrome." The clinical picture is that of hypotension, hypovolemia, low systemic vascular resistance, and a typical picture of pulmonary edema. The diagnosis may be confirmed by low pulmonary capillary wedge pressure (PCWP). Pulmonary emboli appear to be the cause arising from release of fat or cement substance from intramedullary vessels. These emboli block the small arterioles and pulmonary capillaries. Hydrolysis of the fat by lipase into free fatty acids can disrupt the alveolar–capillary membrane.

Hypoxemia.[4] A common consequence of fat embolism is hypoxemia. Significant falls in Pa_{O_2} are to be noted within 2 minutes of the application of bone cement. It is noted that this effect is transient and not associated with changes in cardiac rate or blood pressure. It is postulated that there is a sudden change in the pulmonary vasculature produced by the absorbed acrylic components[5] or by fat embolism and a fall in CVP.[4] Contributory to cardiac arrest is the presence of hypovolemia, dehydration, and the occurrence of hypotension.

Cardiac Arrest. Cardiac arrest as a risk is fully recognized. Most fatal cases are related to fat embolization and the risk is present for up to 48 hours after implantation of a prosthesis, after which the fat is finely dispersed and of little consequence.

Clinically, this event is more likely in the elderly, more in women, in fracture of the femoral neck, and in poorly hydrated patients.

Anesthetic Considerations. Awareness of the complications associated with the use of acrylic cement for prosthesis is essential. Early recognition is important. Intraarterial monitoring is probably justified.

Hydration of the patient must be accomplished before the start of anesthesia. Prophylactic administration of Ringer's salt solution in a volume of 500 ml to 1 L prior to the insertion of the cement substance is recommended.[1] Administration of a small dose of phenylephrine is also recommended prophylactically, and inhalation of 100% oxygen for the critical period seems reasonable.

Cadle has reported that the occurrence of hypotension is infrequent during neurolept–narcotic general anesthesia.

ASPIRIN AND ASPIRIN-LIKE DRUGS.[6] Aspirin is one of the most widely used drugs and possesses five important actions:

1. Analgesia: Analgesia of somatic type pain of the skeletal system and of the vascular system, such as headache. The mechanism is twofold: (a) interference in transmission of pain impulse between thalamus–hypothalamus and sensory cortex; and (b) peripherally by a reduction of local edema. An enhancement of the effect of narcotic and other analgesic drugs occurs.
2. Antipyresis: Fever is reduced by changing the hypothalamic thermostat with ensuing cutaneous vasodilatation and dissipation of heat. The posterior hypothalamic thermostat is set to a lower level.
3. Antiinflammatory: Useful in rheumatoid arthritis. This action is related in increased levels of corticoid and to inhibition of synthesis of those prostaglandins involved in the inflammatory process.
4. Respiratory and metabolic: (a) a central stimulatory effect, which causes a hyperventilation syndrome may occur with large doses. This results in a respiratory alkalosis and upset acid–base balance. (b) a hypoglycemic effect may occur

and is related to an action on the hypothalamus and pituitary axis.
5. Antithrombotic: This is one of the important actions that is employed to prevent postoperative vein thrombosis and thrombophlebitis.[6] A secondary area of usefulness is the low-dose intake regimen of acetylsalicylic acid in patients with cerebrovascular disease to limit stroke accidents.[7] Platelet aggregation is inhibited; bleeding time is prolonged.

Antithrombotic Action. Platelet aggregation is inhibited, and accompanying this effect is a prolongation of bleeding time. Even single doses of 365 mg (5 g) are effective, and bleeding time may be increased for 2 to 4 days after discontinuing the aspirin.[8] However, the platelet dysfunction appears to be irreversible and lasts for the life of the platelet. Several more days are required for a return to normal level of functional platelets, even when the bleeding time is within the normal range.[9]

Antiplatelet Importance. Two aspects of platelet dysfunction induced by aspirin are: (1) the usefulness in prophylaxis against venous thromboembolic disease postoperatively following certain orthopedic and vascular surgical procedures; and (2) the usefulness in prevention of strokes in patients with cerebrovascular disease.[7]

Harris[6] reported on the efficacy of low daily doses of aspirin of 1.2 g in men following total hip replacement, and McKenna the same, following total knee replacement. Women appear to have a better response to high-dose aspirin (daily dose 3.6 g), but bleeding difficulties are more likely. At the present time, the low-dose aspirin regimen is used only in men as prophylaxis.

Renal Effect of Antiinflammatory Drugs.[10] Aspirin and ibuprofen are commonly used antiinflammatory drugs in the management of rheumatoid arthritis. Both are inhibitors of prostaglandin synthesis and, thereby, may decrease renal function, which is dependent on intact renal prostaglandin synthesis. This may be revealed in elevations of BUN or serum creatinine levels.

Ibuprofen may produce occasional serious elevations of BUN or creatinine in about 1% of patients, whereas aspirin even in doses 2.6 to 3.9 does not.

Mechanism of Antiplatelet Action. Acetylsalicylic acid inhibits platelet aggregation and prolongs bleeding time. This is accomplished by the breakdown of aspirin to furnish the acetyl ion for acetylation and inactivation of the enzyme cyclooxygenase. The platelet enzyme (cyclooxygenase) system is essential in the metabolism of arachidonic acid to the precursors of thromboxane and prostaglandins. It is the thromboxanes that promote platelet aggregation and thrombosis formation. Inhibition of formation of thromboxin-A_2 is followed by a decrease in the levels of thromboxin-B_2, as well as a selective inhibition of prostaglandin synthesis.[11] Note that thromboxin-A_2 is a vasoconstrictor. It is emphasized that it is the acetyl ion that is important in this inhibitory action and that the salicylate moiety of aspirin, which is the main metabolite, is inactive on platelets. Oral intake of aspirin, insuring first-path deacetylation in the portal circulation, provides the acetyl ion for the acetylation of platelet enzymes and in their inactivation.

Vascular wall cyclooxygenase, however, is not inhibited in the small doses that are generally employed for an antithrombotic effect. With the low doses, the endothelial cells of the vascular wall continue to produce prostaglandin, a vasodilator, especially of cerebral vessels. Prostaglandin PGI_2 in the vessel wall is a potent inhibitor of platelet aggregation and attachment of platelets to the endothelial wall. With large doses, however, there is inhibition of prostaglandin (PGI_2) synthesis in vessel walls, which may be due to the salicylate moiety.[12] Thus, there is a dissociation between the two types of cyclooxygenase, depending on the dose. The platelet enzyme is more sensitive than the vascular wall cyclooxygenase to acetylsalicylic acid.

Other drugs affecting platelet function and bleeding time are numerous and include: ibuprofen; dipyridamole; propranolol; nitroglycerine; calcium channel blocking drugs; many antibiotics; other nonsteroidal antiinflammatory drugs; and some inhalation volatile agents, such as halothane.

Dextran is also capable of affecting platelet function *in vivo*. This branched-chain polysaccharide, of a molecular weight of 40 million average, is a partially hydrolyzed polymer of glucose derived from beet sugar. It has an oncotic pressure similar to albumin and is used as a plasma expander in small amounts. It does impair bleeding times and polymerizes fibrin. Dextran 40 and 70 induce rouleaux formation and interfere with typing and crossmatching. Dextran is also being studied and used in the prevention of postoperative thromboembolic phenomena with some success. The most serious defect, however, is that it is a potent antigen and does induce hypersensitivity reactions.

Dextran should not be used in patients who have chronic anemia, thrombocytopenia, or reduced fibrinogen. It has a long half-life.

Heta-starch has all the characteristics of dextran, but the large molecules are metabolized, and 40% of the small molecules are excreted within 24 hours.

Anesthetic Considerations.

1. Most bleeding during surgery is due to inadequate hemostasis. There may be dilution of coagulation factors (V–VIII) from administration of large volumes of fluid or blood components. Fibrinolytic activators may be released when trauma is extensive.
2. Patients on aspirin should have a bleeding time

and a platelet count. The prothrombin time (PT) and partial thromboplastin time (PTT) have little value, except if there is a suspected coagulation profile defect.
3. Alcohol potentiates the bleeding time of aspirin.
4. Bleeding times up to 10 minutes have not been associated with excess intraoperative blood loss. Mean bleeding times may be elevated, but 37% of individuals may be in the normal range.[9]
5. Caution must be exercised by the anesthesiologist in manipulations such as laryngoscopy to prevent trauma. The nasal route for intubation should be avoided. Preoperative bleeding times have not been predictive of intraoperative bleeding.[9]
6. Regional anesthesia should be avoided if the bleeding time is twice normal or over 10 minutes or the coagulation profile is markedly abnormal.
7. Spinal and epidural anesthesia may be administered, provided the bleeding time is less than 10 minutes and coagulation profile is not abnormal. There is a potential risk of hematoma formation in the spinal area; however, there is no evidence of its occurrence.[13]

ANTICANCER DRUGS. The objective of all cancer therapy is "total cell-kill," whether it is by surgery, chemotherapy, or radiation. Antineoplastic agents follow first-order kinetics, so that a constant percentage of the malignant cells are killed. To achieve this, several agents are employed. Most of the agents act on different phases of cell division. Cells with a high proliferative capacity are most susceptible, and normal cells, which ordinarily exhibit a high turnover, also are affected. This explains many of the undesirable effects, that is, hair follicles, bone marrow, intestinal and pulmonary epithelium, and many receptors are subject to destruction.

A comprehensive classification of chemotherapeutic agents is to be found in Goodman and Gilman.[14] Mechanisms and sites of action are summarized and concern molecular mechanisms in the cell cycle. Some drugs may affect the initial process of purine or pyrimidine formation; other drugs affect the sequence of the synthetic order on ribonucleotides (RNT) → desoxyribonucleotides (DNT) and the progression from DNA to RNA and protein synthesis and then cell mitosis.

Only some of the major and more commonly used drugs that have an important interaction affecting physiologic function and anesthetic management of complications are discussed here (and summarized in Table 10–3).

General Effects. Many systems are taxed by chemotherapeutic agents and a laboratory data base schedule should be established prior to forming an anesthetic plan.

Immunosuppression occurs with nearly all the antineoplastic drugs. This requires that meticulous aseptic technics be employed for all invasive monitoring procedures, as well as in the management of the airway and laryngoscopy. Extra caution is needed in laryngoscopy to avoid scratching and abrading the oropharyngeal and laryngeal tissues.

Myelosuppression is also a common and, to some extent, serious consequence of most of the anticancer agents. Anemia should be treated before major surgery. If the bleeding and coagulation profile is abnormal, especially if the platelet count is low, preparations should be made to correct the deficits.

Pulmonary toxicity and pneumonitis vary widely in severity, but appear to occur with nearly all of the anticancer agents. An enhanced oxygen toxicity occurs, causing dysplasia of the tracheobronchial mucosa and of the alveolar membrane. Interstitial pneumonitis is frequent. Fibrosis may be a late stage following long-term therapy. It is recommended that oxygen administration be kept to a value less than 0.33 FI_{O_2}. Chest radiographs and arterial blood gas studies are essential.

The alkylating agents are particularly associated with pulmonary toxicity and are listed in the order of decreasing severity:

- *Carmustine:* interstitial pneumonitis, dose related, with incidence of 2% to 20%; not reversible on discontinuing drug
- *Busulfan:* pneumonitis; 2% to 11%; may be progressive
- *Cyclophosphamide:* pneumonitis; pulmonary damage is rare and reversible; bronchopulmonary dysplasia from oxygen
- *Melphalan:* few pulmonary problems; some alveolar atypia

The antibiotic type drugs are also denoted by some pulmonary toxicity. *Bleomycin*, an extremely toxic agent, is the most toxic of all antineoplastic drugs on the pulmonary system.

Cardiac toxicity is an adverse effect of the anthracycline antibiotic drugs with antineoplastic action. In addition to a singular cardiomyopathy, arrhythmias, and congestive heart failure frequently may occur.

The *effect on plasma acetylcholinesterase (AChE) activity* is principally an effect of the alkylating agents. These agents are associated with a 35% to 70% reduction in the AChE activity.[15] This is demonstrable by the inhibition of benzylcholine technic (Kalow's ultraviolet spectrophotometric technique). This inhibition lasts for several days. The inhibition-50 factor (I_{50}) is greatest to least with these drugs in the following order: triethylene compounds > cyclophosphamides > mechlorethamine (nitrogen mustard).

Central nervous system malignancies respond poorly to peripherally administered therapeutic drugs. The reason for a poor response appears to be the existence of a blood–brain barrier.

One technique to provide efficacy of the anticancer drugs, specifically methotrexate, is the tech-

TABLE 10-3. CANCER CHEMOTHERAPEUTIC AGENTS

Agent	Action	Remarks
Alkylating	Most agents cross-link DNA	
Busulfan		Low plasma AChE; pulmonary toxicity 2–10%
Carmustine (nitrosurea)		Thrombocytopenia; myelosuppression; pneumonitis
Cyclophosphamide (cytotoxin)		Oxygen dysplasia; no CNS toxicity; alopecia
Melphalan (nitrogen mustard)		
Mechlorethamine		
Antimetabolites		
Methotrexate (folic acid analog)	Inhibits presynthetic phase and RNT	Immunosuppression; GI tract; bone marrow
Fluorouracil	Blocks thymidylate synthesis Inhibits RNT formation	Stomatitis; GI hemorrhage; myocardial ischemia; for breast and GI cancer
Cytarabine	Inhibits DNA formation and RNA synthesis	Pulmonary infiltrates; dyspnea; cough is common
Antibiotic-type		
Bleomycin	Damages DNA	A direct lung toxin 3%–5% oxygen toxicity; dermatologic; mucosa
Dactinomycin (actinomycin D)	Inhibits RNA synthesis	Cardiomyopathy
Daunorubicin (anthracyclene derivative)	Inhibits RNA synthesis	Arrhythmias; congestive heart failure
Doxorubicin (Adriamycin) (anthracyclene derivative)	Inhibits RNA synthesis	Normal rapidly proliferating tissues inhibited; includes hair follicles, epithelial cells, receptors
Mitomycin	Binds with helical DNA	Dermatitis; pneumonia
Mithramycin		Liver, kidney, bone; bleeding; CNS reactions; severe hemorrhagic disease
Vinca Alkaloids		
Vincristine	Interfere with mitosis	Leukopenia; hypoglycemia
Vinblastine		CNS paresthesias; autonomic NS
Colchicine		
Miscellaneous		
Cisplatin derivatives	Similar to alkylating agents	Nephrotoxicity; ototoxicity; hematologic; occasional anaphylaxis

nique of osmotic disruption of the blood–brain barrier, which allows the agents to enter the brain parenchyma. This disruption is accomplished with administration of 250 to 350 ml 25% mannitol injected over 20 to 30 seconds through a catheter in the internal carotid or vertebral artery. After 1 minute, a radionucleotide is injected intravenously and a brain scan performed to document the degree of disruption. When all is checked, methotrexate, 500 to 2500 mg, is then given through the catheter.

Seizures have been encountered with the injection of methotrexate, and these have been treated with diazepam or thiopental. Either pentobarbitol 200 mg or thiopental, 2 to 3 mg/kg of body weight, are injected intravenously.

One danger is that space-occupying intracranial lesions are frequently accompanied by increased intracranial pressure. The administration of the mannitol to cause disruption of the blood–brain barrier will increase the brain water, and mild to transient increases in intracranial pressure not exceeding 10 mm Hg may occur. Subsequently, an additional risk involves the marked diuresis that occurs at a rate of 2 to 3 L/hr produced by the mannitol. Thus, careful fluid monitoring is essential, and, re-establishment of corticosteroid therapy should be considered because most of these patients have a discontinuation of the steroids prior to disruption (corticosteroids stabilize the blood–brain barrier membranes). The problem of seizures can be controlled by the administration of both pentobarbital and phenytoin prior to the disruption procedure, and large doses of pentobarbital as well as thiopental and diazepam can be administered at the time of the seizures.[16]

Alkylating Agents. The molecular structure of these drugs contains many tertiary ammonium groups that undergo intramolecular cyclization, with the formation of quaternary ammonium groups. These can act directly at the neuromuscular junction (NMJ) in a curare-like manner. In addition, these agents significantly inhibit cholinesterase. Two consequences are to be noted: succinylcholine's effect is potentiated and prolonged; and a prolonged cholinergic-type crisis (as in myasthenia) may be induced, with prolonged apnea and a type II desensitization block. On the other hand, antidepolarizing relaxant drugs may be needed in larger doses to achieve a full NMJ block. Although a quaternary N blocking effect occurs at the NMJ receptor, the cholinesterase activity is reduced in greater proportion, requiring the larger doses of relaxant drugs. These are the preferred relaxants, and judicious doses of antagonists—usually smaller doses—are required. In every instance, a nerve block monitor is essential.

Pulmonary abnormalities are frequent. The incidence varies from 2% to 10%. Mucosal dysplasia, alveolitis, and interstitial pneumonitis occur. Ventilatory insufficiency may be identified, along with diffusion and gas exchange abnormalities. Adult respiratory distress syndrome (ARDS) may occur as a postoperative complication. Avoidance of concentrations of oxygen over 40% is recommended.

Thrombocytopenia and leukopenia occur, so aseptic precautions are necessary and platelet transfusions must be considered. Anemia does occur, and correction may be warranted by red blood cell infusion.

Antimetabolites. *Methotrexate* is a folic acid *antagonist* that inhibits dihydrofolate reductase necessary for the conversion of dihydrofolate to tetrahydrofolatic acid. The latter acid is involved in carbon transfer reactions necessary for DNA synthesis. Other physiologic processes dependent on reduced folates, such as the conversion of homocysteine to methionine, are also inhibited. This reaction is important in bone marrow processes. It is also catalyzed by a cobalamin-dependent methyltransferase.

Methotrexate is especially useful in acute lymphatic leukemia in children, choriocarcinoma, testicular carcinoma, and sarcoma. The drug causes significant bone marrow depression. To reduce the bone marrow side effects of large doses administered to treat acute cancers in children, a technique of "rescue therapy" using leucovorin (a tetrahydrofolate) is often employed. Anesthesia is usually necessary in the high-dose methotrexate–leucovorin sequence. Because nitrous oxide oxidizes vitamin B_{12} (cobalamine) irreversibly, the effect of methotrexate may be reduced and the rescue effect of leucovorin also reduced, thereby increasing side effects. Nitrous oxide should, therefore, be avoided.[17]

Pyrimidine analogs, especially the fluorinated compounds, are powerful metabolic poisons. They have been effective in carcinoma of breast, of the gastrointestinal tract, and of the genitourinary system. Carcinoma of the oropharyngeal area responds well to these compounds.

Major toxic effects are myelosuppression with leukopenia. Anemia and thrombocytopenia must be anticipated. Neurologic complications have been reported.

Cytarabine, a useful agent in acute leukemia, is a potent myelosuppressive agent and may produce all the pathologic features of bone marrow depression. Dermatologic and hepatic disturbances occur.

Antibiotic-type Drugs. Anticancer drugs of this type are derived from various species of Streptomyces. Five types of toxicity are associated with their use and present problems for anesthesia. These are:

- Pulmonary pathology
- Cardiomyopathy
- Dermatologic and mucosal
- CNS reactions, including convulsions
- Bleeding tendency

Bleomycin is one of the most toxic drugs to the pulmonary system. Pulmonary pathology is frequent, to the extent of 3% to 5%. It is a direct lung toxin and the degree of damage is dose related. Restrictive pulmonary dysfunction occurs, together with a decreased diffusion capacity and a lowered PA_{O_2}. Symptoms of cough and dyspnea precede radiologic changes in the lung. Mortality in patients developing a pulmonary lesion is about 10%.

Dactinomycin (Actinomycin-D) binds with double-helical DNA (intercalation) and interrupts the cell cycle in its progress to RNA (blocks synthesis of RNA). It inhibits rapidly proliferating cells and is one of the most potent antitumor agents. The rapidly proliferating cells (bone marrow, hair follicles, and intestinal mucosa), as noted above, are subject to damage and account in part for the toxic effects.

Pancytopenia occurs because of hematopoietic suppression and coagulation tests and platelet count are needed; inflammatory responses are seen in the mouth and gastrointestinal tract; alopecia is common.

Daunorubicin and doxorubicin are antibiotic drugs that also are Streptomyces derivatives and chemically are anthracyclines (they bind to helical DNA). They are effective against acute lymphocytic and granulocytic leukemias. Daunorubicin is effective against lymphomas in children but not in adults. Doxorubicin is effective against many solid tumors, especially sarcomas, metastatic breast adenocarcinomas, and carcinoma of bladder and metastatic thyroid tumors.

Toxic effects are those generally expected of the anticancer drugs: bone marrow depression; gastrointestinal disturbances; dermatologic changes: stomatitis; and alopecia. Cardiac toxicity is a peculiar toxic effect of these anthracycline antibiotics. There is avid binding of the drug to myocardial DNA. Tachycardia, arrhythmias and ST–T wave changes are often seen early. Hypotension can be expected in 6% of patients. Cardiomyopathy with left ventricular enlargement is to be found and severe progressive congestive heart failure may occur, but this complication occurs in patients with a clinical history of myocardial disease.[18]

Anesthetic precautions include avoiding depression of myocardium and treating arrhythmias carefully.

Mithramycin and mitomycin act by inhibiting RNA synthesis. They are extremely toxic and of limited value. Clinical use is largely confined to bone tumors, especially when these tumors are accompanied by hypercalcemia and hypercalcuria. *Mitotane* is principally used in the treatment of tumors of the adrenal cortex. The effect on plasma calcium is relatively specific. It is toxic to marrow, liver, and kidneys. CNS reactions and bleeding diathesis are seen.

Vinca Alkaloids. These are derived from the periwinkle plant. They are specific agents interfering with the cell cycle and, like colchicine, they block mitosis at the metaphase step. Good antineoplastic responses to these aklaloids are seen in a variety of tumors.

Vinblastine is used in the treatment of sarcomas; neuroblastomas; and carcinoma of breast, lung, oral cavity, urinary bladder, and testes. Good response is seen in treating Hodgkin's disease and in lymphocytic leukemia. Alopecia occurs in 20% of treated patients but is reversible.

The toxicity of these natural products is mostly neurologic. Central effects, including convulsions, are to be observed. Peripheral effects include paresthesias and loss of deep tendon reflexes.

Autonomic NS dysfunction occurs. Constipation, paralytic ileus, and urinary retention are noteworthy. An anticholinergic-type effect is apparent.

Anesthetic precautions include the avoidance of spinal and epidural anesthesia and of factors likely to contribute to convulsions.

Miscellaneous Agents. *Cisplatin* is an inorganic platinum-containing compound. It is used particularly in the treatment of testicular tumors and ovarian carcinoma. It has also been found useful in tumors of the bladder and is often combined with bleomycin or vinblastine for maximum effect.

Cisplatin is one isomer of the platinum compound; it enters tumor cells by diffusion; forming a covalent linkage and disrupting the helix formation of DNA. In this regard, it cross links both interstrand and intrastrand within the helix of DNA. It is thus similar as a bifunctional agent to the alkylating agents in its mechanism. The binding appears to be principally at the guanine base.

Of importance to the anesthesiologist is the fact that nephrotoxicity is seen with this drug, as is ototoxicity.

The nephrotoxicity consists of renal tubular dysfunction that appears in the second week of treatment. Persistent or repeated courses of therapy with cisplatin may then result in irreversible renal damage. Other adverse reactions include mild to moderate myelosuppression as well as occasional seizures, and anaphylaxis is to be anticipated.

The drug is also strongly bound (90%) to plasma proteins. This may be of consideration with respect to anesthetic drugs that are highly plasma protein-bound, including the relaxant drugs and other intravenous preparations.

ANTICOAGULANT THERAPY. Anticoagulant drugs are commonly used to prevent thromboembolic complications following surgery, especially in orthopedic and peripheral vascular types. The drugs employed are heparin and dicoumarin.

The issues are twofold: (1) to appreciate that bleeding may occur during surgery in patients on anticoagulant or antiplatelet therapy; and (2) to recognize the risk of spinal and epidural anesthesia and perhaps other regional techniques when patients are on anticoagulants or antiplatelets.

Heparin Techniques. Low-dose heparin in orthopedic surgery and in other selected procedures, such as lower extremity surgery: heparin 5000 IU is administered subcutaneously as an initial bolus injection 2 hours postoperatively and continued every 8 to 12 hours postoperatively. The objective with heparinization is to increase the partial thromboplastin time (PTT) period 2 to 2.5 times control. Note that heparin is a biologic preparation so it shows weight variability and must be assayed. USP heparin is lung derived, and 1 mg is approximately 120 IU. A low-molecular-weight heparin fraction has been found effective, with less subsequent bleeding and fewer side effects.[19]

High-dose heparin, 300 to 400 IU/kg, is employed in cardiac surgery. The anticoagulant effect is then reversed on discontinuing pump bypass.

Coumarin Derivatives (dicumarol and warfarin). Warfarin is considered to be the easiest derivative to control (dose 10 to 15 mg po/day, maintenance 2 to 15 mg).

These agents are chemical variations of vitamin K. They are active in vivo and act as vitamin K agonists. The mechanism of action is to prevent the reduction of vitamin K, which is necessary for the hepatic biosynthesis of prothrombin, plasma thromboplastin component, and other K dependent clotting factors.

Dosage and Technique Warfarin has been administered the night before surgery in an oral dose of 10 mg, and again in the evening after surgery. The objective is to obtain a prothrombin time 1.5 times the control value. In Harris' studies,[20] warfarin or aspirin prophylactic therapy was found superior to heparin, while fewer bleeding complications occurred with aspirin. Detection of thrombi was accomplished by phlebography. These patients were administered general anesthesia.

Pharmacodynamics After administration, about 24 hours is necessary before the available prothrombin is used up and the desired action of anticoagulation is delayed. Coumarin derivatives themselves are bound to plasma protein. They are metabolized in the liver slowly, requiring about 1 week.

Control Plasma prothrombin levels must be closely determined. A safe level, between 15% to 30% of normal activity, should be maintained. A level below 15% of control is dangerous and leads to bleeding. Reversal of a low level and of bleeding is accomplished by administration of 5 to 20 mg of vitamin K.[21]

Role of Regional Anesthesia. The administration of spinal or epidural anesthesia to patients on anticoagulant therapy is controversial. Owens[22] found that spinal subarachnoid lumbar puncture for diagnostic purposes, followed by systemic anticoagulation, was associated with an incidence of 1.6% spinal hematomas. Rao and El-Etr's[23] experience, however, in administering either continuous spinal or epidural anesthesia followed by intravenous heparinization in about 1 hour is impressive. In over 3000 patients, no patient developed signs of spinal, subarachnoid, or epidural hematoma. The risk, by statistical analysis, of 95% confidence limit of a hematoma with either approach is about 0.3%.

Matthews and Abrams[24] administered subarachnoid morphine for pain relief to patients undergoing open heart surgery after induction of general anesthesia. Heparinization was instituted about 50 minutes after the lumbar puncture. No spinal hematomas were reported.

Another situation where the benefit of regional anesthesia makes the procedure acceptable is in the management of intractable chronic pain of malignant origin. Regional anesthesia may be the choice in terms of overall safety. Patients with profound thrombocytopenia, suffering from severe pain of malignancy and fully anticoagulated have been provided caudal analgesia via a 25-gauge needle. In 56 patients so treated, the complication of excessive bleeding or hematoma was not encountered after 336 caudal blocks.[25] Other reports of safe use include those of Odoom[26] and of Mathews.[27]

Recommendations.

1. Avoid regional anesthesia when predisposing factors are present, such as blood dyscrasias, thrombocytopenia, hemophilia, leukemia, or anticipated difficult needle placement.
2. Low-dose heparin therapy has become common practice in many surgical procedures to prevent thromboembolic complications. The benefit of this therapy appears to outweigh the risk of bleeding during general anesthesia.
3. If spinal subarachnoid or epidural anesthesia is chosen for good reasons and the patient is provided perioperative anticoagulant therapy, the risk of hematoma should be recognized—perhaps about 1%.
4. Monitor patient frequently and closely during postoperative period.
5. A coagulation profile of PTT less than 2.5 times normal, a PT of less than twice normal, and a bleeding time less than 10 minutes may be acceptable when a regional anesthesia is strongly indicated but should be avoided otherwise.

Effectiveness of Anticoagulant Therapy. Six alternative methods customarily employed to present deep vein thrombosis (DVT) (Table 10–4) were studied. In a cost-effectiveness analysis, where it was estimated that the mortality rate in major orthopedic surgery from DVT and embolization is about 15 per 1000 operations. When a method of prophylaxis is used, this mortality is halved, while a heparin-dehydroergotamine method or warfarin and/or stocking method reduces DVT mortality by 75%. It is estimated that when pulmonary embolism occurs, about 11% of patients die within 1 hour of onset of symptoms.

Antiaggregation Effect of Anesthetics. Many anesthetic agents inhibit platelet aggregation. This has been demonstrated experimentally by Ueda[29] for the commonly used volatile agents as well as cyclopropane.

In human subjects, there have been varied reports, but generally there is an antiaggregation effect in vivo.

In vitro studies using an aggregating agent such as an adenosine diphosphate (ADP) mixture shows that any induced aggregation is inhibited by most of the inhaled agents:

Halothane Exposure to atmospheres of *halothane* used in clinical practice shows a decrease in platelet aggregation.[30] This is in contrast to some studies using liquid halothane, which causes an increase in platelet aggregation.

Enflurane Platelet aggregation appears not to change during anesthesia in patients anesthetized with *enflurane*.[31]

Isoflurane, at an atmospheric concentration of 1.5% in vitro, shows a small but significant inhibition of ADP-induced platelet aggregation.[32] In vivo studies reveal the same antiaggregation effect.

Nitrous Oxide At 80% concentration in oxygen, it has a small but significant antiaggregation effect.[32]

Inhibition of platelet function by the volatile and gas anesthetics is probably not clinically significant in most healthy patients. In those with congenital or acquired platelet disorders, however, the effect may be important, especially in the presence of antiplatelet drugs such as aspirin or ibuprofen.

Protamine Sulfate.[33,34] This drug is used principally to antagonize the effects of the anticoagulant, sodium heparin. It is a low-molecular-weight protein

TABLE 10–4. MINIMUM REGIMENS OF PROPHYLAXIS FOR INCLUSION OF REPORTS OF CLINICAL TRIALS

Method of Prophylaxis	Preoperative Administration	Postoperative Administration
Warfarin sodium	Loading dose of 15 mg	Adjusted to maintain prothrombin time at 10%–30% of normal
Heparin sodium	2500 IU	5000 IU every 12 h for 5 days
Intermittent pneumatic compression	Bilaterally applied prior to anesthesia and continued for 16 h	
Graduated compression stockings	Bilateral stockings applied	Stockings worn continuously until ambulation or discharge
Heparin and dihydroergotamine mesylate	Heparin sodium, 2500 IU, and dihydroergotamine mesylate, 0.5 mg	Heparin sodium, 2500 IU, and dihydroergotamine mesylate 0.5 mg every 12 h for 5 days
Heparin and stockings	Heparin sodium, 2500 IU, plus bilateral stockings applied	Heparin sodium, 5000 IU every 12 h for 5 days, plus bilateral stockings worn continuously until ambulation or discharge

From Oster, G., Tuden, R.L., and Colditz, G.A.: A cost-effectiveness analysis of prophylaxis against deep-vein thrombosis in major orthopedic surgery. JAMA, 257:203, 1987.

derived principally from fish sperm of the salmonid type. It is a strong base and has a high content of argenine amino acids. A dose of 1 mg antagonizes 100 IU of heparin. This dosage of protamine is related to the amount of nondepolarized heparin still present and to the half-life of sodium heparin, which is dose related.[35,36] For example, 100 IU/kg of body weight of heparin will last approximately 1 hour; 200 IU/kg is 1.5 hours; 400 IU/kg has a half-life of 2.5 hours.

When a dose of 100 IU/kg is administered, the amount of heparin in the plasma will be reduced by one-half in 30 minutes; therefore, the dose of protamine can be reduced to 0.5 mg/100 IU of the heparin dose. In contrast, with large doses of 300 to 400 IU/kg, the amount of plasma nondepolarized heparin remains high and a larger but precise protamine dose should be administered.[37] This can be accomplished by use of a linear dose–response curve relating activated clotting time (ACT) to heparin levels in a patient at a given time. Each laboratory must establish its curve data. The excretion of the sodium heparin is in the form of uroheparin.

Slow administration of protamine over a 30-minute period of the calculated dose is safer than a rapid intravenous bolus administered in 5 minutes or less.[40] This circumvents any negative inotropic effect of protamine. Other advantages include better, more rapid, and smooth decrease in heparin; normal postoperative coagulation develops without hypercoagulability. A normal antithrombin (AT III) activity returns in 24 hours, at a time when heparin levels are zero. Rebound heparinization is less likely to occur. Reactions are less likely to be seen.

When protamine is administered to a patient who has received heparin, the protamine, a strong basic substance, combines ionically in a typical acid–base fashion and forms a strong compound with the acid heparin. It is thus a straight, direct neutralization reaction. The compound that is formed is excreted in the urine.

Reactions are frequent and these include hypotension that may proceed to a shock state.[33] Bradycardia, however, is a common feature of the hypotension. Dyspnea, flushing, and peripheral vasodilatation may occur. It is apparent that there is some depression of the myocardium, as well as depression of the vascular smooth muscle.[38] Observations have shown episodes of right ventricular failure, but these occur infrequently.

Pulmonary artery vasoconstriction has been reported in patients with mitral valve disease. The mechanism of this is undetermined. In patients for coronary artery bypass surgery, protamine does not appear to alter right ventricular function.[39] It is considered that these reactions occur when protamine in high doses is rapidly administered in less than 5 minutes. When administered over a period of 10 to 20 minutes in patients with good left ventricular function, changes in cardiac output, systemic blood pressure, or vascular resistance are minimal.[38]

By itself, protamine, in the absence of heparin, interacts with platelets and many proteins, including fibrinogen. Excess protamine will also interact with other organic acids, such as d-tubocurarine. By itself, protamine sulfate acts as an anticoagulant.

In patients who are insulin-dependent diabetics receiving NPH insulin, there is an increased risk of reactions to protamine. In these patients, clinical reactions occur about 4% or twice as often as in nondiabetics.[40]

Consideration of regional anesthesia in patients on low-dose heparin often presents itself.[41] As long as the PT is less than 30 seconds and the PTT is less than 60 seconds, patients should not necessarily be deprived of regional anesthesia. In Rao's studies[42] of patients who have received continuous epidural and spinal anesthesia, anticoagulant therapy has been instituted after a period of absence of heparin administration.

Avoidance of Reactions Several recommendations for the safe administration of protamine include:

1. The dose of protamine should be appropriate to the dose of heparin administered. Excess of protamine leads to adverse reactions.
2. The amount of protamine needed to reverse residual heparin should be calculated according to the measurement of the activated clotting time. A dose–response curve has been provided by Bull (Fig. 10–2).
3. For low-dose heparin use (100 IU/kg), the dose of protamine be reduced after 30 minutes.
4. With high-dose heparin use (300 to 400 IU/kg), the full calculated dose of protamine be administered, but over a 20-minute period. In patients with good left ventricular function, a rate of 0.5 mg/kg/min has not caused adverse cardiovascular responses.[39]

ANTIHISTAMINIC AGENTS. The prototype of the H_1 blockers is diphenhydramine (Benadryl), but promethazine is equally potent. The main site of metabolic transformation of the H_1 blockers is the liver. Little if any of the drug is excreted unchanged. The products of metabolism are excreted in the urine. Most drugs that are metabolized by the liver are enhanced in their action and prolonged in the presence of H_1 blocker drugs.

The H_2 blocker drug, cimetidine, is also transformed in the liver and the products are excreted in the urine. This drug is dependent on liver-oxidative enzymes. Hence, those drugs dependent on hepatic degradation are inhibited and the effects are enhanced and prolonged. In addition, cimetidine diminishes liver blood flow and is a factor in increased toxicity. Some benzodiazepines, such as midazolam, are not completely dependent on liver metabolism and may be used simultaneously with cimetidine.

Ranitidine is an H_2 blocker that blocks basal acid secretion as well as histamine-induced secretion. Peak levels of ranitidine are evident after intravenous injection in 15 minutes. This drug is not dependent on oxidative enzymes, and only 4% is metabolized to the N-oxide and about 1% to the desmethyl metabolite. Most of the drug is excreted in the feces. Some serum protein binding, to the extent of 15%, occurs; however, no significant changes in half-life, distribution, or clearance of the drug in patients with liver disease have been observed. Furthermore, there is no reduction in liver blood flow.

Large doses of antihistaminic drugs are often needed in a variety of allergic and immune responses, including patients with mastocytosis (see below). It should be appreciated that the H_1 histaminergic blocking agents have central as well as peripheral anticholinergic activity. Large doses may produce symptoms that mimic atropine toxicity. In addition, there may be action on the cardiac mechanism that is related to the quinidine-like effect of these agents on the conduction system, a property that is shared by other anticholinergic agents in large doses. Although conduction disturbances and dysrhythmias may be noted as side effects, large doses may rarely produce clinically significant myocardial depression and pump failure producing cardiogenic shock.[43]

Mastocytosis is an abnormal proliferation and accumulation of mast cells commonly in the skin, but not limited to this area, and is likely to involve selectively multiple organs and sites such as the bone marrow, lymph nodes, and gastrointestinal tract. The dermal proliferation is manifested by macules, papules, or nodules with vesicle and bullae formation, particularly in infants and children. Manifestations are related to the release of stored mediators from the mast cells. These are largely vasodepressor products, including heparin, prostaglandin D, as well as serotonin, hyaluronic acid, and histamine.

Symptoms are protean: episodic flushing, tachycardia, hypotension, abdominal pain, headache, and cardiovascular collapse are representative. Provocative and aggravating conditions include such stress situations as emotional upset, cold, physical exertion, anxiety, and trauma. Certain foods, such as

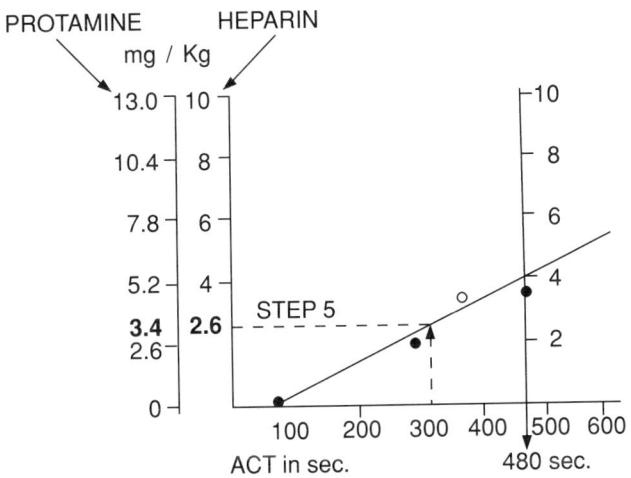

FIG. 10–2. To reverse anticoagulation, the circulating heparin level is determined. A rapid clotting time test is the celite activated coagulation time (ACT), which relates to heparin levels in a linear manner. (The partial thromboplastin time does not respond linearly.) The neutralizing dose of protamine is the heparin level in mg/kg multiplied by 1.3. The heparin level in mg can be converted to IU when multiplied by 120 (USP heparin is 120 IU/mg). From Bull, B., et al.: Heparin therapy during extracorporeal circulation: The use of dose–response curve to individualize heparin and protamine dosage. J. Thorac. Cardiovasc. Surg., 69:685, 1975.

beans, have also been implicated. Urine assay for prostaglandin D metabolites and histamine (which are usually elevated) is confirmatory. Treatment is generally symptomatic and includes antihistaminics, both H_1 and H_2 blockers, antimetabolites, steroids, and adrenocorticotropic hormone (ACTH). Ephedrine is an effective vasopressor agent, as are beta$_2$-adrenergic stimulants. Chlorpheniramine 25 mg is frequently used to avoid or attenuate a response.

Anesthesia considerations include careful preoperative evaluation, especially with intradermal testing of drugs intended to be used during the anesthetic state. Regional anesthesia with the amide local anesthetics has been recommended as safe, but lidocaine or bupivacaine should be skin tested. Analgesia with butorphanol 0.5 mg has been used without untoward effect and avoids the use of morphine and analogs. General anesthesia with ketamine induction and maintenance with nitrous oxide oxygen are recommended. Vecuronium is a safe relaxant, as are pancuronium and atracurium.

ANTIBIOTICS. Clinical hypersensitivity reactions to antibiotics are relatively frequent. Type I immune reaction, involving IgE antibodies and the release of mediators from mast cells and basophils, is seen especially from the penicillins. A full-blown classical systemic reaction readily occurs. Administration by the IM and IV route results in greater incidence than from oral intake. The incidence of penicillin anaphylaxis ranges from 0.015% to 0.04% in the general population, with a fatality rate of 0.002%.[44]

Cephalosporin drugs also may induce anaphylaxis. The incidence is less than for penicillin and is estimated at 0.02%. Skin and joint reactions to either the penicillin or cephalosporin, such as maculopapular or vesicular rash, erythema multiforme, serum sickness, joint swelling, and urticaria are more frequent. These forms range from 2% to 6%. For amoxicillin, it is reported at 3.7% and cefaclor 5.35%. Urticaria alone may be about 2.5% from cephalosporin and 0.7% for amoxicillin.[45]

Some evidence exists for cross-sensitizing to cephalosporins in patients allergic to penicillin.[46] The incidence, however, is probably less than 2%.

Patients with a history of penicillin reaction should probably be skin tested with cephalosporin agents; however, the tests at this time are crude.

The wisest course is to provide preventive and prophylactic measures. In anesthesia practice, avoidance of histamine and other mediator-releasing drugs is necessary. Thiopental, methohexital, and the curariform agents should not be used. Midazolam or ketamine are excellent, safe induction agents, whereas vecuronium or pancuronium are the relaxants of choice.

Many antibiotics, including penicillin, streptomycin, and nitrofurantoin, have produced anaphylactic reactions, dose-dependent cardiac depression, and venous dilitation.

Vancomycin is a potent antibiotic (Streptomyces derivative) employed in the management of severe resistant Staphylococcus infections. It is valuable in pneumonia, empyema, and osteomyelitis. It is also used in patients sensitive to penicillin and cephalosporins; however, it is accompanied occasionally by severe hypersensitivity reactions. Macular skin rashes, anaphylaxis, and a severe shock-like syndrome called the *red-neck syndrome* may follow intravenous administration. Hypotension and bradycardia may be seen. Administration through a central venous line is particularly hazardous, and cardiac arrest has been reported to follow.[47]

Procaine penicillin G is used for a variety of infections, especially gonorrhea. After the administration of 4 to 6 million units, plasma procaine levels range from 3.5 to 11.0 μg/ml. This appears to be an *in vivo* liberation of the procaine and can produce bizarre behavioral and neurologic reactions. These include auditory, visual, and taste disturbances; palpitation and dizziness are often encountered, and neuromuscular twitching may be a confusing disturbance in anesthesia practice.[47b]

ANTIHYPERTENSIVE AGENTS. In judging the role of these drugs in producing undesirable effects during anesthesia and the value of discontinuance, one must consider the risk of the disease state being unchecked against the risk of adverse drug interaction.[48]

The central-acting antihypertensive drugs are effective in reducing MAC values of inhalation agents. They are also capable of reducing the narcotic requirements for pain relief.[48,49]

Of the central-acting antihypertensive drugs reserpine, alphamethyldopa, and clonidine, it appears that clonidine is the most potent in this regard. It is an $α_2$-adrenergic receptor agonist and modulates the monoaminergic portion of the sympathetic central system. Gordh[50] has also demonstrated that clonidine itself has some analgesic action, and this may be, in part, the mechanism whereby narcotic dose requirements are reduced.

Rauwolfia Derivatives. Rauwolfia derivatives for the treatment of hypertension represent a significant hazard in patients scheduled for anesthesia. Agents such as reserpine block the sympathetic system both centrally at the hypothalamus and peripherally at ganglia and nerve endings. Anesthetic drugs are potentiated; therefore, the anesthetic dose should be reduced. It has been shown that reserpine liberates serotonin from brain tissues, which has a tranquilizing effect.[60a] Because serotonin is the central precursor to norepinephrine, it also follows that stores of norepinephrine are not replenished and a deficiency occurs. Peripherally, reserpine and guanethidine interfere with norepinephrine uptake and nerve ending stores are depleted. The net effect is to leave the autonomic nervous system with the parasympathetic component dominant.

Hypotension and bradycardia are prone to occur during reserpine therapy.[60b] These effects are enhanced by vagomimetic anesthetics such as thiopental and cyclopropane. Furthermore, the hypotension is resistant to therapy by vasopressors. Such a state of blockade may last for 10 days to 2 weeks. Patients on antihypertensive therapy should have the reserpine compounds withheld for at least 10 days prior to elective surgery. During the initial period of reserpine therapy the anesthetic requirement may be increased. Once maintenance is achieved the anesthetic requirement decreases by as much as 33%, as reflected in MAC values.

Guanethidine.[60c] This antihypertensive agent has been most valuable and widely used. It is representative of a class of agents that depress postganglionic adrenergic nerve activity. The major effect is blockade of effector response to sympathetic adrenergic nerve stimulation; there is also a reduction in the release of norepinephrine. In the early stages of action the inhibition of response develops rapidly without changes in catecholamine levels. Subsequently, the nerve stores of norepinephrine are depleted, but the content of the adrenal medulla is unaffected. Patients on this agent who are given sedative, analgesic, and anesthetic agents are prone to show a decrease in cardiac output, hypotension, and a sensitivity to position changes.

Other actions of concern include the sensitization of effector cells during chronic administration; this action is similar to that seen after sympathetic postganglionic denervation. Certain sympathomimetic effects also occur and include occasional hypertensive episodes, piloerection, and myocardial stimulation.

As an antihypertensive agent, guanethidine has been useful in the long-term treatment of severe hypertensive disease. The drug is initially combined with diuretic therapy; the initial dose of guanethidine is 10 mg. This is increased daily until an optimal maintenance dose is attained. Caution must be observed—any hypotension must be judged relative to the severity of the patient's disease. Because severe hypertension itself represents a substantial risk, discontinuance of therapy should be brief, perhaps only for the two preceding operative days and the day of operation.

Methyldopa (Aldomet). Methyldopa (chemically, *l*-methyl-3,4-dihydroxy-*l*-phenylalanine) serves as a "false" substrate in the synthetic process for norepinephrine. The enzymes dopa decarboxylase (*l*-aromatic amino acid decarboxylase) and dopamine *p*-oxidase act on the methyl form and produce methyl norepinephrine, probably in brain adrenergic neurons. This derivative replaces norepinephrine. It is direct-acting and similar to norepinephrine but less potent. It thus has become known as a false transmitter or a "mime" of norepinephrine. It is responsible for the hypotensive effect in hypertensive patients.[60d]

In antihypertensive therapy the oral dose of methyldopa is 0.25 to 0.5 grams orally. Because the duration of action is about 8 hours, it is taken two or three times a day.

Patients on methyldopa therapy given anesthetic agents may have enhanced undesirable hypotensive effects. Postural hypotension occurs.

Of greater concern are the following side effects:

1. Significant CNS action: the drug regularly produces sedation and drowsiness; vertigo; psychic depression. All these may emerge in the postoperative period.
2. Abnormal motor activity: subcortical and basal ganglia effects; parkinsonian reactions.
3. In patients with concomitant renal insufficiency there may be exaggerated CNS and other effects—the drug is in part eliminated by the kidney.
4. Hepatitis may be induced.
5. Cross-matching is rendered difficult. The Coomb's test may be unpredictable.
6. Retention of salt and water occurs. Edema and occasional congestive heart failure may ensue.

Management Discontinuance of some central-acting antihypertensive drugs may be advisable. Duration of withdrawal period depends on type of drug and extent to which sympathetic activity can recover. Rauwolfia compounds should be withheld for at least 5 days, and other agents for 3 days. Some deaths have occurred in fully reserpinized patients but not in those partially reserpinized.

For emergency surgery in such patients, generous doses of vagal blocking agent are required. Ordinary doses of belladonna are not sufficient, but a dose of 0.75 to 1.2 mg of atropine for the average adult has been found satisfactory. This should be given IV slowly if the pulse is below 72. As a substitute for belladonna alkaloids, it is recommended that *oxyphenonium bromide* (antrenyl) or glycopyrrolate be administered.[60b]

Additional effective measures to combat any antihypertensive drug-induced hypotension include wrapping the legs of the patient snugly from toes to upper thighs. Vasopressor agents with a direct action on vessels are indicated: methoxamine IM, 10 to 20 mg, or mephenteramine, 20 to 40 mg, slowly IV are effective.

Hydralazine and Minoxidil. These peripheral-acting antihypertensive agents have not been found to influence the course of anesthesia significantly. Mechanism of action is direct relaxation of arteriolar smooth muscle. The molecular mechanism is similar to that of organic nitrates.[33] A selective decrease in vascular resistance of cerebral, coronary, and renal circulation occurs. Preeclamptic patients undergoing necessary general surgical procedures have tolerated the anesthetic and the total stress well.

Adrenergic Blocking Drugs. Prazosin and labetalol are commonly used. The first selectively blocks post synaptic alpha-1 receptors. It is useful in reducing afterload. Labetalol is both a selective alpha-1 adrenergic antagonist and a nonselective beta-1 and beta-2 receptor antagonist. Bronchospasm is rarely seen, but orthostatic hypotension may occur.

DRUGS FOR TREATMENT OF ANGINA

Effect of Calcium Channel Blockers on Neuromuscular Blockers. In humans, increased neuromuscular blockade occurs when nondepolarizing muscle relaxants are administered to patients on calcium channel blockers (CCB). Verapamil particularly enhances the block of pancuronium and d-tubocurarine.[51] This is expected since calcium is part of the mechanism of transmitter release of acetylcholine at the presynaptic membrane.

Patients on chronic verapamil therapy who receive IV pancuronium have developed prolonged paralysis and ventilatory insufficiency. The administration of neostigmine failed to reverse the neuromuscular paralyis in some instances; however, edrophonium was promptly effective.[52]

Potentiation of vecuronium by verapamil has been reported. Neostigmine may fail to completely antagonize the paralysis.[53] It has been suggested that 4-aminopyridine, which facilitates the entry of calcium or the administration of calcium salts, should be used with the anticholinesterases for reversal of nondepolarizing block.

Interaction with calcium entry blockers such as verapamil and diltiazem with the administration of dantrolene in malignant-hyperthermia (MH)–susceptible or MH-treated patients may result in marked hyperkalemia and cardiovascular collapse.[54]

Calcium Channel Blockers and Inhalation Agents. These drugs interact with the commonly used volatile anesthetic agents. Halothane, enflurane, and isoflurane have calcium channel blocking properties that depress sinoatrial node conduction; this effect is similar to that of verapamil and diltiazem.[55]

Isoflurane has activity similar to the dehydroperidine blockers nifedipine and nicardopin; that is, the intracellular calcium kinetics are altered. Nifedipine has a predominant and potent peripheral vasodilator action and may be less depressant to ventricular muscle function.[56,57]

Verapamil and diltiazem apparently are more depressant to ventricular function than nifedipine, although experimental studies indicate that verapamil and isoflurane or verapamil and halothane produce dose-related depression of ventricular function. This is not supported by clinical experience.

Merin[58] states that the calcium channel blockers are useful dugs to combat or treat supraventricular tachycardias, hypertension, or coronary spasm during anesthesia with volatile agents. This is apparent when patients are on chronic therapy; however, caution should be exercised in administering the calcium channel blockers intravenously to treat arrhythmias developing during anesthesia. There is no evidence to indicate that patients on chronic therapy are at increased risk when given inhalation volatile agents.

High doses of either calcium channel blockers or high concentrations of the volatile agent (greater than 1.5 MAC) can produce clinically significant hemodynamic changes. Verapamil is a much greater depressant to myocardial ventricular function that is already compromised by disease.[59]

GOUT THERAPY.[60] Colchicine is useful in gout. It is one of the oldest therapies for this condition. However, colchicine has significant neuromuscular toxicity in humans. A myopathy may occur in patients with gout who take ordinary doses of the drug, but who may have elevated plasma drug levels because of altered renal function. An excessive action of the colchicine usually presents with proximal muscle weakness, and it is associated with an elevation of serum creatinine kinase. Electromyography demonstrates marked spontaneous activity. Pathologically, there is vacuolization of the skeletal muscle beds.

These patients usually show an enhanced response to the nondepolarizing drugs, and the doses of such should be reduced. On the other hand, succinylcholine administration may result in an abnormal degree of fasciculation and a further elevation of serum creatinine kinase. The latter drug is, therefore, not recommended.

DIURETIC THERAPY. Oral diuretics contributing to the control of the hypertensive patient can be safely taken up to 2 or 3 days before anesthesia. The longer acting diuretics (chlorthalidone, polythiazine, and cyclothiazide) should be discontinued at least 3 or 4 days before anesthesia.

Diuretic therapy over a long period may result in potassium loss and complicate the course of anesthesia by producing such responses as hypertension, cardiac arrhythmias, and respiratory paralysis. Patients who are receiving guanethidine and methyldopa and have hypertension should have these drugs discontinued at least 1 week prior to anesthesia. These patients should have a potassium determination and if hypokalemia exists, potassium should be administered. Central nervous system depressants are markedly potentiated by both of these agents. It is recommended that antihypertensive drugs be discontinued prior to anesthesia; in most instances bedrest and sedation are sufficient to maintain the patient in sound cardiovascular status.

ANTIDEPRESSANTS: MAO INHIBITORS.[61a] Affective disorders have been treated with monoamine oxidase (MAO) inhibitors. Although the treatment of such disorders has largely been replaced with the tricyclic antidepressants, nevertheless certain patients continue to be treated effectively with these agents. Elderly patients in particular who do not respond well to tricyclic antidepressants may respond to MAO inhibitors. Likewise, many patients receive MAO inhibitors for postelectroconvulsive maintenance therapy. Other conditions in which they appear to have advantages over tricyclic antidepressants include atypical and endogenous depression. These drugs may also be useful for regulation of weight and posttraumatic stress.

There are two classes of MAO inhibitors: the hydralazine and the nonhydralazine compounds. Among widely used hydralazines are phenelzine and isocarboxide. The only nonhydralazine in wide use is tranylcypromine (Parnate).

The mechanism whereby these drugs are effective relates to the increase in CNS biogenic amines in contrast to circulating catecholamines (dependent on COMT degradation). There is an irreversible inactivation of MAO followed by an increase of all endogenous catecholamines in peripheral tissues and the brain. Ordinarily, the sympathetic amines are degraded by monoamine oxidase, an intraneural enzyme. Two forms of the enzyme have been defined, MAO-A and MAO-B.[61b] Type A enzyme selectively deaminates serotonin, norepinephrine, and dopamine. A significant reduction of these neurotransmitters results in depression and mood changes. Type B enzyme preferentially deaminates phenylethylamine and tyramine.

Inhibition of Type A oxidase increases serotonin and norepinephrine in the CNS. This action is the most important because these transmitters are needed to elevate mood and manage affective disorders. If a type A selective inhibitor were available, it would be preferable. This would allow deamination of phenylethylamine and tyramine to proceed; such an action could minimize the hypertensive reaction consequent to tyramine's releasing effect of norepinephrine peripherally.

Nonselective drugs inhibit both forms, whereas selective MAO inhibitors inhibit either the A or the B form; however, only nonselective inhibitors are available in the United States and are chemically divisible into hydrazine and nonhydrazine drugs. In the course of treatment, it is estimated that at least 80% of the oxidase enzyme must be inhibited before an adequate therapeutic effect is observed. The nonhydrazine derivatives are reversible blockers, and their pharmacologic effects wane after 24 hours. The hydrazine class is an irreversible type of blocker, and the effects may persist for 2 to 3 weeks after therapy is stopped.

Adverse interactions include:

1. Interaction with sympathomimetic agents causes hypertensive crises. The drugs for which such crises have been reported include tyramine, ephedrine, metaraminol, and norepinephrine. Epinephrine in local anesthetic solutions carries a real danger. Cheese (containing tyramine, an indirect-acting amine), wine, and beer all seem to elevate blood pressure. If a vasopressor is required during anesthesia, small doses of a direct-acting agent such as neosynephrine should be used. If a hypertensive crisis does occur, a beta-blocking agent or a direct vasodilator (hydralazine; nitroprusside) is recommended.
2. These drugs interact with narcotic analgesics. Meperidine administration to patients taking MAO inhibitors may result in the development of severe agitation, excitement, hypertension, convulsions, hyperpyrexia, and coma.[62a] The mechanism whereby there is a marked CNS reaction is considered to be the result of marked increases in CNS serotonin.
3. The potentiation of narcotic effects has also been reported. This is likely with morphine and derivatives and is probably related to the inhibition of narcotic metabolism in the liver. Janowsky has recommended that one fourth of the usual dose of the narcotic should be used in patients on MAO-inhibitor drugs.[62b]
4. After 2 to 3 weeks of therapy, an antihypertensive effect may be seen. It is postural in nature and appears to be related to diminished venoconstriction. Hypotensive reactions may occur with narcotics, sedatives and alcohol.

A urinary antimicrobial, furazoladone, and an acute neoplastic drug, procarbazine, also inhibit MAO; hence, these two drugs may be responsible for overactivity to vasopressor therapy.

It has been the practice to discontinue the MAO inhibitors for at least 10 to 14 days prior to the administration of anesthetic agents in elective and planned surgery. This has not been necessarily possible for emergency surgery, especially in the elderly person, and there have been no significant increases in complication. Other reports indicate that anesthesia without undue complications has been successful in cardiac surgery in patients receiving MAO inhibitors. It is concluded that there is no need to discontinue long-term MAO inhibitor therapy in elective surgical procedures. No hard data have been adduced to discontinue therapy. In fact, discontinuing therapy presents hazards.[63,64]

ANTIDEPRESSANTS: TRICYCLICS.[65a,65b] These agents resemble the phenothiazines. Structurally, they differ by an absence of the sulfur ("S") moeity in the central ring. The principal mechanism of action is by blockade of the *amine pump*—the active transport system located in the presynaptic nerve endings. Amine neurotransmitters that have been released are not returned or taken up by the nerve in the presence of the tricyclics. In the CNS, this results in either a high serum concentration of norepinephrine or of serotonin, especially during the early period of therapy. It is curious that these drugs are not effective when norepinephrine stores are depleted. Thus, a deficiency of CNS biogenic amines has been proposed as the mechanism of depression (catecholamine hypothesis).[65c] Additional evidence indicates that depression results from increased sensitivity of the noradrenergic cyclic-AMP generating sytem in the limbic system, with an overabundance of cyclic-AMP. The tricyclic drugs decrease the ability of norepinephrine to stimulate cyclic-AMP formation in the brain. This desensitization requires 2 to 3 weeks; however, many of the side effects (antihistamine and anticholinergic) are seen within 24 hours.

Three major peripheral pharmacologic effects are evident: alpha-adrenergic blockade of norepinephrine amine uptake at nerve endings (presynaptic) (Fig. 10–3); anticholinergic activity (antimuscarinic)[65d]; and antihistaminic action (block of H_1 receptor) with mild sedation due to effect at the reticular activating system. Block of H_2 receptors also occurs; amitriptyline is 20 times as potent as cimetidine in this regard.

Interaction of tricyclics with other drugs includes the following: potentiation of CNS depressants; augmentation of pressor effects of sympathomimetic amines; and blockade of antihypertensive effects of such drugs as guanethidine by competition at the presynaptic membrane. After long-term therapy, with depletion of NE, the administration of anesthetic and sedative drugs may be followed by hypotension.

Many adverse reactions are principally related to the block of amine uptake, resulting in high plasma concentrations of norepinephrine. Tachycardia and other arrhythmias are frequent.

The tricyclics are divided into two groups: the tertiary amines (amitriptyline, imipramine, and doxepin) and the secondary amines (desipramine, nortriptyline, and protriptyline). Studies of depressed patients show that some have a lowered level of brain norepinephrine, as reflected in lower levels of the phenyloglycol metabolite (MHPG). These respond better to drugs, e.g., desipramine that block reuptake of norepinephrine. Other patients may have normal levels of MHPG but have a lowered level of 5-HIAA and a deficiency of brain serotonin. These patients respond better to agents that block reuptake of serotonin (amitriptyline). The relative effect on serotonin and norepinephrine of the commonly used agents shows the methylated drugs to be stronger blockers of serotonin reuptake, while the demethylated analogues are stronger blockers of norepinephrine uptake (Table 10–5). At high doses, these drugs act peripherally to block alpha-adrenergic receptors.

One important effect of action of the antidepressants is the alteration of cerebrovascular permeability with an increase in brain water uptake. Simultaneously, there is a reduction of 20% to 30% in cerebral metabolic rate and of blood flow.[66]

Pharmacokinetics. The elimination half-lives of these drugs may range from 10 to 20 hours for imipramine to 80 hours for protriptyline. The amelioration of states of depression is delayed for 1 to 3 weeks, but the plasma half-life is short, about 3 to 4 hours.

Metabolism of tricyclic drugs is primarily oxidation by hepatic microsomal enzymes, and, reciprocally, there is either potentiation or diminution in the effectiveness of each group. Steroids, neurolept drugs,[67] and phenothiazines potentiate tricyclic drugs, because these drugs are preferentially metabolized leaving the tricyclics intact. Prior barbiturate or sedative administration causes enzyme induction and thereby increases metabolism of tricyclic antidepressants, thereby hastening their elimination. Concurrent administration, however, will result in excessive effects, and the sedative drug dose should be reduced.

Imipramine (Tofranil) and amitriptyline hydrochloride (Elavil) are frequently used agents. Onset of effective action is prolonged and requires a latency period of 7 to 14 days. Excretion, however, is fairly rapid: about 40% of radioactive imipramine hydrochloride appears in urine in 24 hours and 70% is excreted in 72 hours. They have significant hypotensive effects and, although short acting, some clinicians believe they should be discontinued about 3 days before a general anesthetic is administered; however, more complications occur postanesthetically. Noncatecholamine vasopressors (oxymetazoline; methoxamine) should be available for treatment of hypotensive episodes. The hypotension is principally of orthostatic type and seen after chronic therapy, but it remains a risk factor.

Studies by Veith[68] reveal that there is no significant effect on left ventricular pump function. Evidence for depression of myocardial contractility is

		Serotonin	Norepinephrine	
Tertiary Amines	Amitriptyline	++++	—	Methylated
	Imipramine	+++	++	
	Doxepin	++	++	
Secondary Amines	Nortriptyline	++	++	Demethylated Analogues
	Protriptyline	++	+++	
	Desipramine	—	++++	

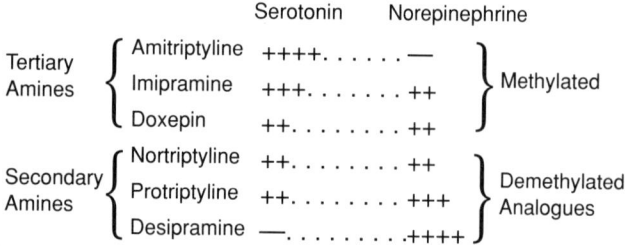

FIG. 10–3. Effects of various tricyclic antidepressants on blockade of biogenic amine reuptake. Adapted from Maas, J.W.: Biogenic amines: Biochemical and pharmacologic separation of two types of depression. Arch. Gen. Psychiatr., 32:1357, 1975.

TABLE 10–5. RELATIVE POTENCIES OF TRICYCLIC AGENTS AS ANTIHISTAMINES AND ANTICHOLINERGICS*

Compound	Antihistamine	Anticholinergic
Tertiary amines		
Amitriptyline	+++	++++
Doxepin	++++	+++
Imipramine	++	++
Secondary amines		
Nortriptyline	++	+
Protriptyline	+	++
Desipramine	+	+

*+ = least, ++++ = most.
Adapted from Snyder, S.H., and Yamamura, H.: Antidepressants and the muscarine-acetylcholine receptor. Arch. Gen. Psychiatr., 34:236, 1977.

based on animal work and on systolic time intervals.[69]

Two principal side effects of sedation and anticholinergic action of the different agents are presented in relation to one another with regard to potency (Fig. 10–4).

Overdoses of tricyclic drugs can cause hyperpyrexia or hypothermia, and hypertension or hypotension; most often, they cause hypotension and cardiac arrhythmias. Delirium, seizures and coma are central anticholinergic effects. Electroencephalographic seizure activity and the initiation of epileptic fits can occur.[70] These effects can be overcome by the administration of 1 to 2 mg of physostigmine, which, by antagonizing acetylcholinesterase and allowing cholinergic mechanisms to prevail, counteracts the central reactions.

Electrocardiographic (ECG) changes include prolonged PR intervals, intraventricular conduction delay, T-wave depression, and prolonged QRS.[71a,71b] Atrial arrhythmias are seen. Few changes are seen with doxepin, while imipramine has an antiarrhythmic effect.[68] Generally depressed patients with chronic heart disease can be safely and effectively treated with tricyclic drugs, when modest doses are given (avoid overdoses).

Cardiac complications and arrhythmias occur as a result of overdose. These are usually seen during the period of peak blood levels and during the first 24 hours following stoppage of drug administration. A careful study of overdose reveals that patients with a normal level of unconsciousness and a normal ECG for 24 hours do not develop arrhythmias.[72]

Anesthetic Considerations Include:

1. Tricyclics potentiate the effect of barbiturate and other sedative drugs by limiting their metabolism. Thiopental and brevital doses should be reduced; however, many patients exhibit rapid metabolism of the barbiturates, especially if the tricyclic is combined with a phenothiazine.
2. Anticholinergic effects are enhanced; caution should be exercised in determining doses of atropine or glycopyrrolate.
3. Sympathomimetic effects of amines (epinephrine and norepinephrine) are enhanced; acute hypertension and dysrhythmias are prone to occur.
    a. Ketamine, which also blocks norepinephrine uptake, may produce dangerous cardiovascular complications and should be avoided. Hypertensive crises may occur.

Sedation

High — Doxepin — Amitriptyline — Imipramine — Nortriptyline / Desipramine — Protriptyline — Isocarboxazid — Phenelzine — Tranylcypromine — Low

Anticholinergic Side Effects

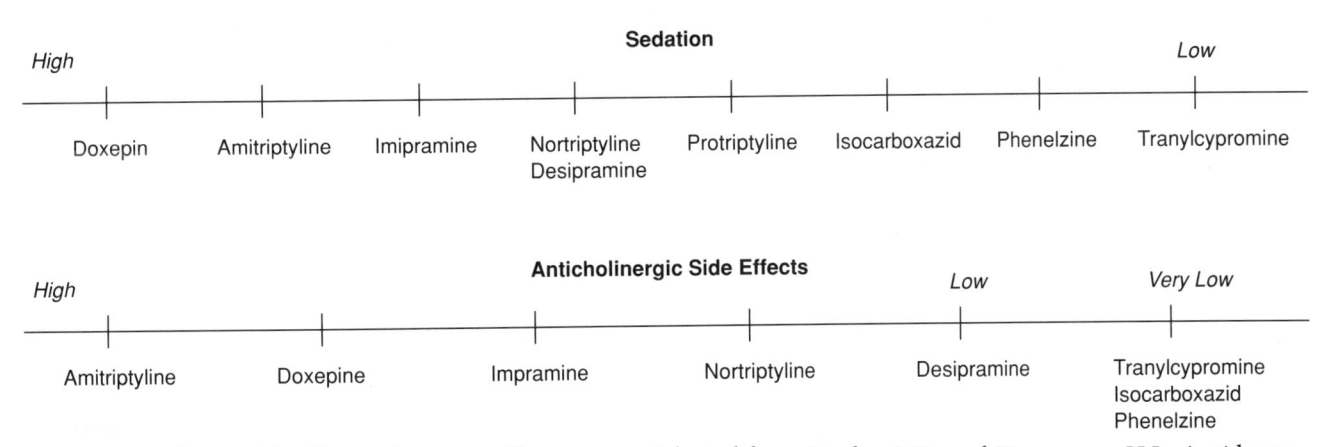

High — Amitriptyline — Doxepine — Impramine — Nortriptyline — Desipramine — Low — Tranylcypromine / Isocarboxazid / Phenelzine — Very Low

FIG. 10–4. Relative side effects of some antidepressants. Adapted from Snyder, S.H., and Yamamura, H.I.: Antidepressants and the acetylcholine receptor. Arch. Gen. Psychiatr., 34:236, 1977.

b. Halothane predisposes the myocardium to dysrhythmias and lowers the threshold for production of premature ventricular contractions by epinephrine and should be avoided.
c. Enflurane requires large amounts of epinephrine to produce dysrhythmias and is the anesthetic agent of choice.[73] The challenge dose of epinephrine to produce arrhythmias is least with enflurane. The ED_{50} for halothane is about 2 μg/kg; for isoflurane 6.7 μg/kg; and for enflurane 10.9 μg/kg. The administration of enflurane, however, may be accompanied by seizure activity in patients who are taking amitriptyline or other methylated analogues (tertiary amines).[73,74]
d. The cardiac risks of administration of local anesthetics with epinephrine exceed the benefit of low plasma levels of the local anesthetic.
e. Pancuronium blocks norepinephrine uptake, and dysrhythmias are more common. A similar effect is consequent to gallamine administration. The recommended relaxant is d-tubocurarine.[75a]
f. Reversal of d-tubocurarine should be cautious. Neostigmine can produce conduction defects and ST-T wave abnormalities.[75b] If tricyclic antidepressants are discontinued 24 to 48 hours prior to anesthesia, these cardiac effects are not seen. Either pyridostigmine or edrophonium are recommended as the choice of reversal agents because they have less muscarinic blocking effect[75c] than neostigmine. Of these, edrophonium has the least muscarinic effect, and newer studies indicate a duration of 60 minutes in doses of 0.5 mg/kg.[75d]

LITHIUM SALTS. In 1949, Cade[76] showed that lithium is effective in the management of manic-depressive psychoses and controls the manic episodes. It also corrects any associated sleep disorder. Since then, lithium has been used to manage other mental disorders, but this is the limit of approved therapeutic uses, although it has been useful in cluster headaches. The carbonate salts of lithium in doses of 900 to 1500 mg/day are taken by mouth and are readily absorbed. Larger doses are suggested for hospitalized patients. The drug is also rapidly excreted by the kidney. There is a low therapeutic index, however, and toxic symptoms are frequent.

Lithium decreases the availability of the neurotransmitter norepinephrine to the norepinephrine receptor. Like potassium, this cation shifts the sodium transport. Biochemically, as a monovalent cation, it has some of the characteristics of potassium.

Some clinical reports suggest an effect at the neuromuscular junction in which potentiation of pancuronium was considered and, curiously so, was potentiation of succinylcholine.

Waud[77] has studied the effect of lithium at the neuromuscular junction and found no strong evidence for a cellular effect. Negligible changes were observed on membrane behavior and on response to carbachol, and there was a failure to depolarize the end-plate. At high doses, not to be seen clinically, some slight reduction in ED_{50} to d-tubocurarine but not to pancuronium was observed. Even if the effect of chronic lithium exposure on response to d-tubocurarine is real, the effect may only indicate a slight dosage reduction for competitive blocking agents and, indeed, probably only for d-tubocurarine.

Two specific concerns of the anesthesiologist in managing patients on lithium are that the drug decreases pressor response to norepinephrine, and it causes diuresis.

Average doses may result in nausea, polyurea, diuresis, and diarrhea. Large doses may produce tremors, slurred speech, confusion, lethargy, and coma.

Renal clearance is decreased by furosemide, K-sparing thiazide, and ethacrinic acid. These drugs increase the levels of plasma lithium and increase toxicity. Renal clearance is increased by acetazolamide, aminophylline, sodium bicarbonate, sodium chloride, and mannitol. The sodium salts and mannitol may be used to reduce toxic levels of lithium.

DISULFIRAM. A thiuram disulfide derivative, disulfiram is used as an adjunct in the treatment of alcoholics. This substance blocks the dehydrogenase in the metabolism of alcohol at the second step of conversion from acetaldehyde to acetic acid, and an "acetaldehyde syndrome" develops. The toxic effects include throbbing headache, flushing of face and skin; marked diaphoresis; tachycardia and other arrhythmias; hypotension; and syncope occur. Respiratory depression, convulsions, and death have been reported. The antabuse–alcohol reaction occurs with blood alcohol concentrations of only 5 to 10 mg/dl.

If the drug is discontinued, the full syndrome may be precipitated during the ensuing 3 to 6 days with any alcohol intake. As a fat-soluble drug, disulfiram is stored in the body for several days. One fifth of a dose is present for 1 week.

Antabuse potentiates many CNS depressant drugs; after discontinuing the drug, sensitization to such drugs continues for 3 to 6 days. Hypotension occurs readily from sedatives, narcotics, and anesthetics.

Disulfiram inhibits dopamine β-hydroxylase so that there is reduction in norepinephrine synthesis. This explains, in part, the cardiovascular depressant effect of anesthetic and sedative drugs.

BARBITURATES. The barbiturates represent a widely used and abused group of drugs. Habituation and primary addiction occur; either a psychological reaction or a characteristic and dangerous abstinence syndrome may develop if adequate doses are not provided. Tolerance is a relatively frequent problem.

Patients who take over 1 g a day may be presumed to be addicted and the withdrawal syndrome is an occasional problem.

TRANQUILIZERS. A new era in medical therapy and especially in psychiatry has been introduced by the use of tranquilizers. The extent of use is extreme; many people give little thought to the fact that they are taking these drugs and it is often difficult to elicit the information.

Two types are popular, namely, the phenothiazines and the carbamates. Problems arise in the long-term use of these for anxiety or other psychologic disorders (Fig. 10–5). The phenothiazines are capable of producing hypotension and they potentiate barbiturates.[77a] It is presumed that they potentiate narcotic action and anesthetic agents. When chlorpromazine is combined with a regional anesthesia that blocks the thoracolumbar sympathetic outflow, such as epidural and spinal anesthesia, a more profound and prolonged hypotension may be encountered. This is resistant to vasopressor therapy (phenylephrine, ephedrine or norepinephrine). However, methoxamine and metaraminol have been found effective. On the other hand, some do not believe a real hazard exists when chlorpromazine is used with other agents; Lear's[77b] studies indicate that any hypotension is not serious.

Chlorpromazine potentiates the action of depolarizing muscle relaxants such as succinylcholine. Thus, the anesthesiologist should be more cautious in determining a dose of succinylcholine for patients on chlorpromazine therapy. It is probable that a similar situation exists with the other phenothiazines.

Meprobamate has not been found to influence greatly the effects of anesthesia. However, patients who have been on large doses have an exaggerated depressant effect when sedatives, narcotics, and anesthetics are used. Hypotension is not infrequent and seems to be pronounced in the postoperative period. Vasopressors such as metaraminol and methoxamine give a better therapeutic response than oxymetazoline. It is recommended that the drug be withheld from these patients for 5 days preoperative, or that the dose level be sharply curtailed.

Schizophrenic patients who have been on phenolthiazine therapy for more than 2 years also have a greater perioperative risk.[77c] There is an increased morbidity in the immediate postoperative period. The continued action of phenylthiazine should be appreciated and hypotensive episodes recognized and treated early. With recovery room care today, increased morbidity is not greater than that in nonschizophrenic patients. It is recommended that the patients be given adrenocorticotropic hormone (ACTH) or hydrocortisone as part of perioperative control.

PSYCHOTROPIC AGENTS IN THE ELDERLY. Most psychotropic drugs should be prescribed in doses one

FIG. 10–5. Side effects of antipsychotics. Courtesy of Dr. Oscar A. Cordoba.

Side Effects of Antipsychotics

Adverse Reactions	Phenothiazines Aliphatic	Piperidine	Piperazine	Thioxanthenes	Butyrophenones	Dihydroindolones	Dibenzoxazepines
Extrapyramidal							
Dystonic reaction	R	R	U	U	C	U	R
Parkinsonism	U	R	C	U	C		
Akathisia	U	U	C	U	C		
Anticholinergic	U	C	U	U	R		
Cardiovascular							
Hypotension	C	C	R	U	R	A	R
ECG abnormalities	R	U	R	U			
Endocrine	C	C	C	U	R		
Inhibition of ejaculation	U	C	U	A	A		
Skin							
Photosensitivity	U	U	R	R	R		
Skin pigmentation	U	A	A	A	A		
Allergic reaction	U	R	R	R	R		
Ophthalmologic							
Retinitis pigmentosa	A	U	A	A	A		
Lenticular pigmentation	U	A	R	R	R		
Cholestatic jaundice	U	R	R	R	R		
Blood dyscrasias	U	R	R	R	U		
Sedation	C	U	A	U	A	R	U

R = Rare U = Uncommon C = Common A = Absent

third to one half of that for those under 50 years of age. In addition, it is a basic rule in geriatric pharmacology to begin with a lower dose than calculated and increase the dose gradually until the desired effect is obtained without adverse effects.

Of the antianxiety agents, the benzodiazepines are quite effective and the most widely used. The indication is for the short-term relief of anxiety, not for prolonged antistress use.

The pharmacokinetic effect of antianxiety and sedative drugs on the CNS are related to the following:

- Increased organ sensitivity to benzodiazepines
- Impairment of drug disposition
- Increased apparent volume of disposition
- Reduced hepatic clearance

Duration of action in the elderly varies with the agent. The higher lipoid-soluble agents have a longer half-life. Diazepam has an elimination half-life of 20 hours in 20-year-olds, but 90 hours in 80-year-olds. In contrast, lorazepam and oxazepam show no major pharmacokinetic changes.[78]

Of the benzodiazepines with a significant sedative effect, flurazepam and temazepam are noted and considered undesirable in the elderly patient. The duration of action even in the younger subject of flurazepam is 48 or more hours and may be 100 hours in the elderly.[79] For sleep disturbances, these drugs are widely used; however, the alteration in sleep patterns is undesirable. There is a decrease in the amount of stage 3 and 4 sleep and a decrease in rapid eye movement (REM), which leads to hangover. Depression is also a problem with these drugs in older patients, and significant adverse effects are seen in 40% of this group.

Triazolam is an ultra rapidly eliminated congener of benzodiazepine. Doses of 0.125 to 0.25 mg are well tolerated in elderly or debilitated patients with minimal adverse effects.

THYROID PREPARATIONS. Several thyroid preparations, including thyroid extracts and thyroxine, are in popular use for weight reduction. Less frequent is the use of these agents to provide symptomatic relief from menopausal tension. Many such patients are potentially victims of induced hyperthyroidism. Appreciation of the hypermetabolism produced is necessary in determining sedative and narcotic doses and in selecting anesthesia. Also, any overactive subjects are not suitable for regional anesthesia. In general, it is desirable to taper off thyroid agents or to discontinue their use prior to anesthesia and surgery when they are not being used as substitutional therapy in primary thyroid deficiency.

On the other hand, one may encounter patients who are being treated for hyperthyroidism by antithyroid agents such as thiouracil or substitutes. These patients may have a significant reduction in thyroid activity to the extent that they are unduly sensitive to all depressant agents. Morphine is particularly poorly tolerated. Barbiturates in normal doses have an exaggerated effect. All dosages should be accordingly reduced.

CARDIOVASCULAR DRUGS. The overdigitalized patient may present some anesthesia problems. Vagomimetic drugs are potentiated and the use of cyclopropane and thiopental as well as chloroform and fluothane is likely to result in difficulties. Bradycardia, varying degrees of heart block, and hypotension are characteristic. Any patient who has been rapidly digitalized on the day of surgery by the medical department had best be cancelled—unless there is a surgical emergency—until digitalization is stable, or at least 24 hours have elapsed from the start of digitalization.

Anginal patients are often on significant doses of nitroglycerine or of one of the nitrites. These patients, when subjected to anesthesia, may develop a state of hypotension. If the hypotension is severe, i.e., more than 25% fall in systolic pressure, then a vasopressor is indicated.

Many patients have been placed on quinidine for the suppression of arrhythmias. This drug produces myocardial depression. For these patients it is preferable to employ agents which cause minimal depression of myocardial contractility such as nitrous oxide (with adequate oxygen), cyclopropane, or ethylene and to avoid the ethers and thiopental. Well-administered spinal and regional techniques are safe.

In addition to the cardiac effect, quinidine and quinine have a peripheral skeletal muscle blocking effect and tend to produce a myasthenic response; potentiation with blocking agents occurs. Thus, the use of curare is to be avoided. Succinylcholine in the lower dose range is acceptable, but when large doses are used, the phase II effect is manifest and potentiation of paralysis occurs. Postoperative hypoventilation and apnea are possible.

ANTIDIABETIC DRUGS. Loss of control of diabetes in patients taking insulin preparations is not unusual. Better control during the anesthesia and surgical period is possible if the patient is stabilized on regular insulin. Many patients who regulate their own diabetes are prone to increase their dosage when faced with any stress. They realize that such circumstances as anesthesia and surgery increase their requirements, and they automatically adjust without necessarily consulting their physician. Papper[30] refers to these patients, particularly the younger group, as sophisticated diabetics who wish to fortify themselves against the bad period of surgery by taking larger doses of insulin. A hypoglycemic reaction also may be encountered. During anesthesia this may be detected by the pounding pulse of "waterhammer" type with a falling diastolic pressure. Sweating is often profuse and subsequently a tachycardia is evident.

The increasing use of oral insulin preparations

must also be considered. These drugs (tolbutamide, etc.) depend upon residual pancreatic function for effect and are of most use in the milder diabetics. Preoperatively, these patients should be placed on parenteral regular insulin for more adequate control. Some evidence also exists that large doses of atropine are capable of suppressing to varying degrees pancreatic insular function. Thus, a mild case may be aggravated by this medication and care must be exercised in the determining of dosage of atropine.[80a]

Oral hypoglycemic agents also have positive inotropic effect. Patients on these drugs are more prone to arrhythmias. The frequency of ventricular fibrillation is greater in diabetics on these agents.[80b,80c]

ADRENAL CORTICOSTEROIDS. Medical conditions that benefit from the administration of corticosteroids include arthritis, asthma, nephrosis, allergies and others. Long-term use, therefore, of adrenal steroids is widespread. That these drugs may upset compensatory mechanisms and the reaction to stress was emphasized by Lundy[81] and Salessa.[82]

Withdrawal of these drugs at varying periods prior to surgery may lead to sudden circulatory collapse when anesthesia is induced or surgical stress imposed. The mechanism appears to be the following: prolonged therapy with corticosteroids leads to suppression of function and then atrophy of the adrenal gland. This is indirect by way of inhibition of the pituitary adrenotropic hormone. Thus, a patient may be completely dependent on substitution therapy and actually have incipient adrenal insufficiency. These patients respond poorly to stress.

All patients who have been on corticosteroid therapy within 4 to 6 months should be given supplementary corticoid hormone. Doses of at least 200 mg of cortisone on the preoperative day and 100 mg via intravenous infusion at the time of surgery are recommended.

Cortisone has a hyperglycemic effect. This should be appreciated in diabetics. In addition, epinephrine and other sympathomimetic amines potentiate this effect and raise the blood sugar.

Oral Contraceptives.[83a]
Patients who are receiving various "sex hormones" also have mild metabolic disturbances. Thus, the estrogenic preparations are known to increase tissue oxygen requirements. Stilbestrol has a similar action. Patients in the menopausal group and those with prostatic cancer should be treated carefully.

The estrogenic component (Wood) of oral[83b] contraceptives is a major factor affecting blood vessels, causing a "loss of tone" of vascular smooth muscle. Elastic tissue of large vessels is affected which results in a permanent loss of elasticity, while hyperplasia of the intima occurs. Peripheral veins also dilate during the period of medication but return to normal distensibility within a few weeks. Blood flow changes in extremities are intriguing. An increased flow in upper extremities with no change in lower extremities occurs, though the vessels are dilated. The velocity of flow in the lower extremities is reduced producing flow stasis.

Clotting changes occur and estrogen produces an increased platelet "stickiness."[83c] There is also an inhibition of natural anticoagulant factors so that clotting is favored. The combination of clotting tendency, intimal or vessel hyperplasia and increased stasis in veins favors intravascular thrombus formation (Classic Wessler Experiment). This is reproduced in humans on oral contraceptives.

In a comparison of young females the incidence of thrombophlebitis in the women on oral contraceptives is 12 times higher and thromboembolism is 8 times higher than nonusers.[83d]

Cerebrovascular accidents are observed in young women on oral contraceptives especially those with a migraine predisposition. Some degree of hypertension can be expected to occur within 1 to 6 months of start of therapy. This usually reverses itself in 3 to 6 months.[83d]

Oral contraceptives using the low dose of estrogen, as well as other drugs, inhibit the metabolism of those benzodiazepines managed by oxidation in the body, including triazolam and alprazolam, and increase the elimination time, which results in an increased duration of action. Those benzodiazepines that are conjugated, such as temazepam and lorazepam, have a decreased elimination time with an increased clearance and accelerated metabolism.[83]

ASTHMATIC THERAPY. The xanthenes are commonly used in the treatment of asthma. In the presence of beta agonists, there may be an enhancement of the xanthene effect, and there appears to be an increase in cardiac arrhythmias. In animal studies, ventricular fibrillation can be produced.[84]

ANGIOTENSIN CONVERTING ENZYME INHIBITORS.[84a] Inhibition of the angiotensin converting enzyme (ACE or kinanase II) in the lung endothelial cells reduces the plasma levels of angiotensin II and effectively controls hypertension. Captopril was the first clinically useful inhibitor. Presently enalapril and lisinapril are also available. These drugs are all effective in the treatment of hypertension and have a favorable profile with few side effects.

SYMPATHOMIMETIC DRUGS. Patients taking drugs of this class in small doses or infrequently may have an increased anesthetic need. Large doses may inhibit endogenous production of catecholamines, and the anesthetic requirement may be decreased.

Amphetamines taken for mood elevation or weight control significantly alter anesthetic dose requirements. In the acute user, or when small occasional doses are taken, the anesthetic need for halothane may increase from 20% to 70% as shown by studies of MAC.[84b] In these patients reserpine will block such effects; however, daily doses of 2.5 mg/kg deplete catecholamines and decrease halothane requirements.

Other catecholamine-blocking agents such as alphamethylparatyrosine (AMT) block synthesis and decrease halothane MAC by 30%.

LEVODOPA.[33] Considerable numbers of patients with Parkinson's disease are effectively treated by levodopa. Entrance into the basal ganglia is permitted, where the drug is apparently converted to dopamine, the neurotransmitter. Control of extrapyramidal activity is then provided.

The duration and intensity of action are enhanced by the simultaneous administration of carbidopa. This agent is an inhibitor of the decarboxylase, which ordinarily degrades levodopa in plasma. Usually, the combination is available for treatment (carbodopa, 25 mg, with levodopa, 250 mg). The simultaneous administration of an anticholinergic such as benztropine alleviates any side effects such as tremor.

Concomitant cardiovascular effects are due to the formation of dopamine as well as norepinephrine. Dopamine itself has complex actions: on myocardium there is direct β-stimulation and indirectly dopamine releases norepinephrine from sympathetic nerves. It also acts on specific dopaminergic receptors to produce renal and splanchnic vasodilatation.

With small doses of levodopa vasodilatation usually predominates and larger doses induce hypertensive actions. Such adverse actions, and more frequently hypotension, are seen in patients undergoing surgery. After oral administration peak plasma concentrations occur in 1 to 3 hours. The half life is about 0.5 hour. To avoid intraoperative complications it is recommended that treatment with levodopa be reduced on the day prior to anesthesia and the day of surgery.

Longer periods of withdrawal may reintroduce the dysphagia of parkinsonism and result in aspiration pneumonia.

Discontinuation of therapy ("drug holiday") for as short a time as 3 days may result in a neuroleptic malignant syndrome similar to malignant hyperthermia (MH). Successful treatment follows the same course as MH. It also has been demonstrated that pancuronium is effective in the management of neuroleptic malignant syndrome.[85]

PARASYMPATHETIC DRUGS. Certain eye preparations and many pesticides alter the action of the parasympathetic system. The organophosphates inhibit cholinesterase. Echothiophate (phospholine), an irreversible cholinesterase inhibitor used in the eye, is absorbed via the lachrymal duct and can antagonize the nondepolarizing muscle relaxants and greatly augment the action of depolarizing drugs such as succinylcholine.

EPINEPHRINE'S INTERACTION WITH VOLATILE ANESTHETICS. During halothane anesthesia, ventricular arrhythmias frequently occur in adults. The incidence varies from 3% to 7% and is increased when exogenous adrenaline is administered. The incidence also increases with increased PA_{CO_2}.

The interaction of adrenaline during anesthesia with the commonly used volatile agents shows significant differences in the arrhythmic potential (Fig. 10–6). The threshold concentration, that is, the lowest concentration at which any patient may develop an arrhythmia, shows that halothane sensitizes the heart significantly more than either enflurane or isoflurane. The ED_{50} for production of arrhythmias has been defined as the concentration of adrenaline administered submucosally that produces three or more ventricular extrasystoles in 50% of patients. Low doses of adrenaline are effective in the presence of halothane, while enflurane is the least provocative of ventricular arrhythmia, and requires a dose five times the ED_{50} of halothane and two times the ED_{50} of isoflurane (Table 10–6).[87-90]

It is further evident that lidocaine will raise the arrhythmia threshold and the provocative dose of epinephrine by twofold to threefold.[91]

PRESENCE OF GLAUCOMA. Glaucoma is defined by the presence of three main features: an increase in intraocular pressure (IOP), development of increased cupping with pallor of optic disc, and loss of visual field.

Normal IOP ranges from 10 to 22 mm Hg. It is about 12 to 15 mm Hg higher than intracranial pressure. Ocular hypertension is defined as ocular pressures between 21 and 30 mm Hg without loss of vision. Pressures greater than 21 mm Hg increase markedly with age; at 45 years, 5% of the population

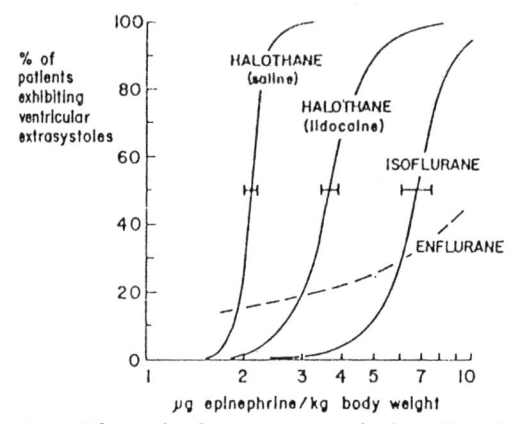

FIG. 10–6. The arrhythmogenicity of adrenaline determined in patients anaesthetized with 1.25 MAC of enflurane, halothane or isoflurane in oxygen. The effect of halothane was tested with or without lignocaine. From Johnston, R.R., Eger, E.I., and Wilson, C.: A comparative interaction of epinephrine with enflurane, isoflurane, and halothane in man. Anesth. Analg., 55:709, 1976.

TABLE 10–6. ADRENALINE DOSES ASSOCIATED WITH ARRHYTHMIAS

Agent	Arrhythmic Threshold Dose ($\mu g \cdot kg^{-1}$)	ED_{50} dose ($\mu g \cdot kg^{-1}$)
Halothane	1.8	2.1
Isoflurane	5.4	6.7
Enflurane	3.6	10.9

From Johnston, R., Eger, E.I., and Wilson C.: A comparative interaction of epinephrine with enflurane, isoflurane, and halothane in man. Anesth. Analg., 55:709, 1976.

have ocular hypertension; at 55 years, 10%; and at 75 years of age, 15%. About 3.5% of persons with ocular hypertension develop visual field loss within 5 years. A higher percentage of patients with pressures greater than 30 mm Hg develop visual field loss and open-angle glaucoma. The prevalance at large, of abnormal readings in the population is about 5%, while abnormal readings with visual loss is about 0.7% at age 65 and 1.3% at 75 years of age.

The essential basis of chronically elevated IOP is an obstruction to outflow of aqueous humor producing an increased IOP.

Formation of Aqueous Humor. Aqueous humor is formed from plasma by the ciliary body (supplied by choroidal vessels) at a rate of about 2.0 μl/min, and the humor is completely replaced every 2 hours. It enters the posterior chamber and passes through the pupil into the anterior chamber. From this chamber, the fluid leaves the eye at the angle between the iris and cornea through a trabecular meshwork (of Fontana) into Schlemm's canal and thence is absorbed into episcleral veins. These veins empty into superior and inferior ophthalmic veins.

Two-thirds of the aqueous is secreted by an active enzymatic process (carbonic anhydrase and cytochrome oxidase systems) and enters the posterior chamber; one-third filters through the anterior surface of the iris into the anterior chamber.

The volume of the anterior chamber is about 0.25 ml and that of the posterior chamber is about 0.06 ml.[92]

TABLE 10–7. CLASSIFICATION OF GLAUCOMA

PRIMARY GLAUCOMA
  Open-angle glaucoma
  Angle-closure glaucoma—acute, intermittent or subacute, chronic
SECONDARY GLAUCOMA
  Uveitis, trauma, intraocular tumor, corticosteroid-induced, and others

Classification. A primary and secondary group are recognized based on the type of obstruction (Table 10–7). The most common glaucoma is primary open or wide-angle glaucoma, representing about 80% of patients. In this condition, the obstruction exists on a microscopic level in the fine connective tissue meshwork through which the fluid in the anterior chamber drains into the canal of Schlemm (Fig. 10–7).

Primary angle closure glaucoma the result of which is the less common form representing about 15% to 20% of patients, is forward displacement of the iris (Fig. 10–7). This may be related to a higher posterior chamber pressure than anterior chamber or to overproduction of aqueous humor. There is usually a shallow anterior chamber, and the iris encroaches on the absorption meshwork at the angle. Commonly, obstruction of the pupillary opening by the lens also occurs, and the outflow of aqueous from posterior chamber to the anterior chamber is impeded.

Congenital or developmental glaucomas are rare, whereas secondary glaucomas are the result of a variety of causes corrected by other means.

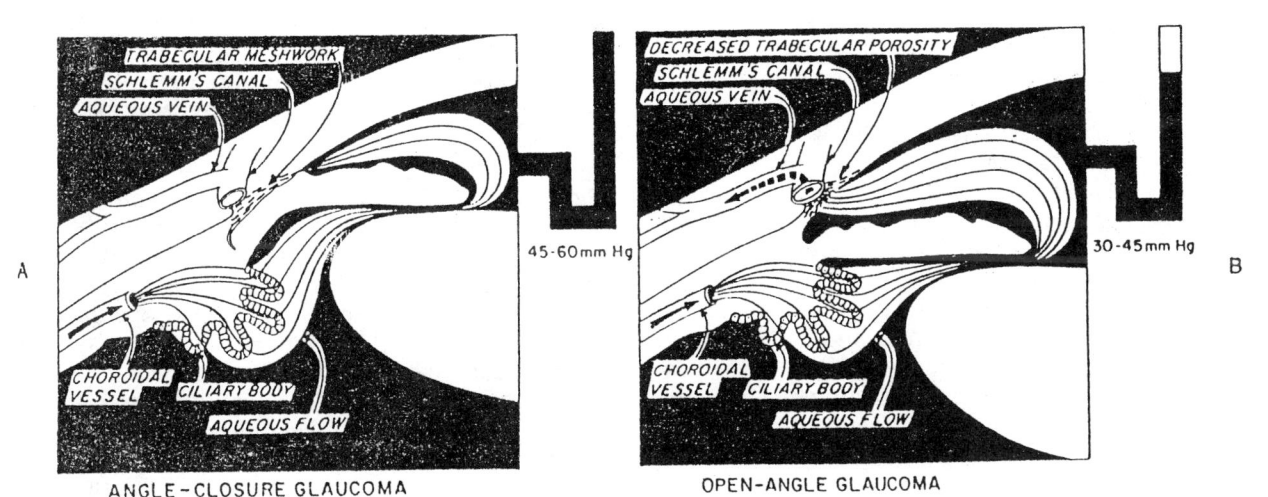

FIG. 10–7. Mechanism of the rise of intraocular pressure in angle-closure glaucoma (*left*) and in open-angle glaucoma due to trabecular obstruction preventing access to the canal of Schlemm (*right*). From Schwartz, B.: Current concepts in ophthalmology: The glaucomas. N. Engl. J. Med., 299:182, 1978.

Therapy. Open-angle glaucoma is treated primarily by medications that lower intraocular pressure to a safe level. The basic drugs are miotics, which induce contraction of the sphincter muscle of the iris. Realignment of the trabeculae occurs, allowing free outflow of aqueous. Three drug types are employed: (1) topical cholinomimetics—topical pilocarpine (0.5% to 4%) (a naturally occurring alkaloid) or carbachol (1.5%) (a synthetic cholinergic stimulant); (2) topical anticholinesterases, such as physostigmine (0.02% to 1%); demarcarium bromide—a bis compound with longer duration than simple anticholinesterase; echothiophate iodide (0.03% to 0.25%)—a long-lasting and widely used organic phosphate and anticholinesterase derivative; and (3) inhibitors of aqueous humor formation such as the systemic carbonic anhydrase inhibitors, i.e., acetazolamide (which inhibits the formation of carbonic acid from CO_2 and diminishes the subsequent formation of bicarbonate; Because aqueous humor has a high content of bicarbonate, the production of aqueous humor is greatly decreased by this drug) and blockers of beta adrenoreceptors, i.e., timilol eyedrop (0.25% to 0.5%) (1 drop twice a day; a non-specific beta-blocker; duration 7 to 12 hours).

Delta-tetrahydrocannabinol (THC), the active principle of marihuana, has been found to lower ocular hypertension in patients with wide-angle glaucoma. Administration of a solution of THC by eyedrops (nabilone) or a dose of 5 to 10 mg orally is effective. Intravenous urea (1 g) may be needed in acute narrow-angle glaucoma.

Sympathomimetic agents (epinephrine, 1%) paradoxically will reduce IOP by increasing outflow (in open-angle chronic glaucoma) and by vasoconstriction of choroidal vessels, thereby decreasing the rate of secretion. These must not be used in closed-angle glaucoma.

Formation of aqueous humor may be dependent on beta-adrenergic receptors, and recent studies demonstrate that beta-adrenergic blocking drugs (timolol) are effective topically in reducing formation of aqueous humor.

In open-angle glaucoma, drugs may not always be effective and disease may progress. When changes in the optic disc appear, the visual field narrows, and ocular pressure remains high, surgery is needed. The procedure consists of creating a drain route from the anterior chamber into the subconjunctival or intrascleral space.

Angle-closure glaucoma and congenital glaucoma are treated best by operation. A small opening in the iris is created, permitting easy flow from posterior chamber into anterior chamber. This decreases pressure in posterior chamber and allows the iris to fall away from absorption trabeculae.

Drug Interactions. *Corticosteroids* administered both topically and systemically can raise ocular pressure, produce optic disc change, and cause visual field loss.

Anticholinergic agents, such as belladonna derivatives, drugs used in gastrointestinal disorders, and agents used in parkinsonism, may greatly elevate IOP in patients predisposed to angle-closure (narrow-angle) glaucoma. This is the less prevalent form of glaucoma, however.

Other drugs that elevate IOP in angle-closure glaucoma include tranquilizers and nitrites. Precipitation of narrow-angle glaucoma by tricyclic drugs may occur. Depolarizing muscle relaxants, such as succinylcholine, also elevate IOP significantly in angle-closure glaucoma.

Note that these drugs have not been found to elevate intraocular pressure in *open-angle type* glaucoma.[93]

Complications of Drugs Used in Therapy. Most of the adverse responses of the principal drugs used in glaucoma are exaggerated parasympathomimetic effects due to systemic absorption. These include:

1. Sinus bradycardia
2. Occasional cardiac arrest[94]
3. Vasodepression followed by hypertension; both depressor and pressor responses are blocked by atropine
4. Bronchospasm
5. Sweating and salivation
6. Increased gastric secretion with low pH
7. Arousal effects
8. Hallucinogenesis

That the topical instillation of miotic drugs has systemic consequences should be appreciated.

A 1% pilocarpine solution has 10 mg/ml. Thus, 2 drops in the eye may result in 1.5 to 2 mg of the agent being absorbed. Similarly, 2 drops of an 0.5% physostigmine solution may quickly introduce 0.5 to 1 mg of this agent into the blood stream.

Anticholinesterases used as eye drops are absorbed systemically and depress both red blood cells and plasma cholinesterase. Depolarizing (succinylcholine) muscle relaxants administered to patients on this therapy may be prolonged in action and produce concomitant prolonged respiratory depression.

Echothiophate (Phospholine) is a potent organophosphorous compound. It is useful in chronic, simple wide-angle glaucoma and is a potent miotic. The topical application of 1 to 2 drops of 0.25% solution may be administered 1 to 2 times a day. As with the other topical agents instilled into the eye, it is readily absorbed and after a few weeks of therapy pseudocholinesterase activity may be reduced by 60% to 80%. The combination of this compound with the esterase is virtually irreversible. Recovery of levels depends on synthesis of the enzyme. In the absence of inhibitors, this process requires 7 to 14 days. If therapy is discontinued, the excretion of the inhibitor requires 2 to 3 weeks. Thus, a significant reduction of enzyme continues for 4 to 6 weeks. After 1 week of therapy, plasma enzyme levels are 50%

of normal. After 2 weeks of therapy, plasma enzyme levels are reduced to 30% of normal and by 1 month, levels are less than 10% of normal. Thereafter, there is a decline slowly for a year to levels of 5%. Red blood cell activity is reduced to below 50% by 6 weeks of therapy. Because this drug taken daily is cumulative, other system adverse reactions of anticholinesterase action may be manifested.

Beta blockers and, specifically, timolol, as an eyedrop solution are frequently used in glaucoma and decreases humor formation. It has minimal effects on vision and does not cause conjunctivitis. However, there are systemic effects at cardiac and pulmonary receptors. Sinus bradycardia and reduction in cardiac output may be seen; cardiac arrest as well as bronchospasm have been reported.[95] Sensitivity to insulin occurs from systemic nonspecific beta blockers and glycogenolysis in muscle is decreased. Hence, hypoglycemia may ensue. It has been reported that its central effect may produce respiratory depression and apnea in infants.[96]

Anesthetic Effect on IOP. Most inhalation anesthetic agents decrease IOP. The decrease is nonspecific for these agents, but Magora[97] has indicated that the decrease is proportional to the depth of anesthesia and that the pressure reaches a common value or "floor" for all agents during deep anesthesia (EEG level III). The following inhalation agents have been studied and confirm this general principle:

- Diethylether and cyclopropane[98]
- Chloroform and trichlorethylene[97]
- Carbon dioxide[97,99]
- Halothane[97,100]
- Methoxyflurane[101]
- Enflurane[102]

A "floor" level of IOP is often produced without regard to dosage or anesthetic depth. Enflurane appears to have this effect and produces a 40% decrease in IOP in light anesthesia with little or no further decline.

Most IV agents also lower IOP, including:

- Thiopental[98]
- Hydroxydione[97]
- Fentanyl–droperidol[101]
- Diazepam[103]

With neurolept-narcotics there is little or no IOP change in light levels of anesthesia techniques, but a uniform drop to a stable IOP level with deeper levels at EEG level II or III.

Ketamine is the one exception of the commonly used intravenous agents and produces a slight increase[104] in IOP or a clinically insignificant rise.[105] Shivering and muscular activity increase IOP.[106]

Relaxant Drugs. With d-tubocurarine,[107] a significant fall occurs probably as a result of paralysis of extraocular striated muscles and intraocular ciliary muscles; however, d-tubocurarine decreases the coefficient of facility of outflow. Pretreatment with d-tubocurarine before succinylcholine fails to inhibit succinylcholineinduced elevations of IOP.[108]

Pancuronium produces no change or transient decreases in intraocular pressure.[109] The reduction amounts to about 20% in unanesthetized patients

TABLE 10–8. DRUGS—MIXING COMPATIBILITIES

	Amobarbital	Atropine	Chlorpromazine	Diazepam	Diphenhydramine	Glycopyrrolate	Hydroxyzine	Meperidine	Morphine	Pentobarbital	Promethazine	Scopolamine	Secobarbital
Amobarbital		N	N	N	N	N	N	N	N	N	N	N	N
Atropine	N		Y	N	Y	Y	Y	Y	Y	N	Y	Y	N
Chlorpromazine	N	Y		N	?	Y	Y	Y	Y	N	Y	Y	N
Diazepam	N	N	N		N	N	N	N	N	N	N	N	N
Diphenhydramine	N	Y	?	N		?	Y	Y	Y	N	Y	?	N
Glycopyrrolate	N	Y	Y	N	Y		Y	Y	Y	N	Y	Y	N
Hydroxyzine	N	Y	Y	N	Y	Y		Y	Y	N	Y	Y	N
Meperidine	N	Y	Y	N	Y	Y	Y		Y	N	Y	Y	N
Morphine	N	Y	Y	N	Y	Y	Y	Y		N	Y	Y	N
Pentobarbital	N	N	N	N	N	N	N	N	N		N	N	N
Promethazine	N	Y	Y	N	Y	Y	Y	Y	Y	N		Y	N
Scopolamine	N	Y	Y	N	?	Y	Y	Y	Y	N	Y		N
Secobarbital	N	N	N	N	N	N	N	N	N	N	N	N	

Source: Trissel, Lawrence J.: Handbook of Injectable Drugs, 2nd ed., 1980.

and about 30% after induction with thiopental–oxygen–nitrous oxide. The reduction remains for 3 to 8 minutes and continues lower, even after intubation.

The depolarizing muscle relaxants and, specifically, succinylcholine, produce a marked increase in IOP, approximately doubling IOP and lasting 10 minutes or more.[110] This is due principally to the contraction of the extraocular striated muscles. Pretreatment with an antidepolarizing agent (d-tubocurarine) does not significantly alter the rise, nor does a large dose of thiopental immediately preceding the succinylcholine.[110]

Mechanisms of Anesthetic Action on IOP. The usual decreases in IOP noted for most of the anesthetic agents may be related to several mechanisms:

- Depression of central control at ocular centers in hypothalamus, diencephalon, and midbrain[111]
- An increased coefficient in facility of outflow of aqueous humor by general anesthetics[98]
- Paralysis of extraocular striated muscles
- Paralysis of intraocular smooth muscles

MANAGEMENT METHODS

For the prevention of adverse drug interactions, several positive measures are in order.

1. Take a careful drug history on each patient; when in doubt, send urine and blood samples to a laboratory for screening
2. Know what drugs are hidden in drug combination preparations. Be aware of mixing compatibilities (Table 10–8)
3. Provide drug "washout" time; discontinue long-term therapy with oral drugs in sufficient time to restore normal reactivity
4. Use supportive drugs cautiously; titrate for the desired effect
5. Limit the number of drugs given; use a drug only when there is a positive indication; be more critical of indication
6. Be prepared for possible reactions, with a special drug tray (glucose or glucagon for diabetics who have been on oral hypoglycemics; alpha-blockers for hypertensive patients who have been treated with MAO inhibitors or tricyclics.)

REFERENCES

GENERAL REFERENCES (pp. 253–256)

1. Medical Letter. Adverse Interactions of Drugs. 23:No. 5 (Issue 578) March 6, 1981.
2. Smith, N.T., Miller, R.D., Corbascio, A.N.: Drug Interactions in Anesthesia. Lea & Febiger, 1981, Philadelphia.
3. Martin, E.W.: Hazards of Medication. Philadelphia, J.P. Lippincott Co., 1971.
4. Medical News: Risk of drug interaction may exist in 1 of 13 prescriptions. J.A.M.A., 220:1287, 1972.
5. Solomon, H.M., Barakat, M.J. and Ashley, C.J.: Mechanisms of drug interaction. J.A.M.A., 216:1997, 1971.
6. Melmon, K.L.: Preventable drug reactions—causes and cures. New Engl. J. Med., 284:1361, 1971.
7. Sellers, E.M., Koch-Weser, J.: Displacement of warfarin from human albumin by diazoxide and ethacrynic, mefenamic and nalidrixic acids. Clin. Pharm. & Therap., 11:524, 1970.
8. Crawford, J.S.: Drug binding by serum albumin. Brit. J. Anaesth., 41:543, 1969.
9. Editorial: Smoking and anesthesia. Arch. Int. Med., 126:397, 1970.
10. Hull, C.J.: Pharmacokinetics and pharmacodynamics. Br. J. Anaesth. 51:579, 1979.

SPECIFIC REFERENCES (pp. 256–280)

1. Kim, R.C., and Ritter, M.A.: Hypotension associated with methylmethacrylate in total hip arthroplastics. Clin. Orthopaed. Rel. Res., 88:154, 1972.
2. Peebles, D.J., et al.: Cardiovascular effects of methylmethacrylate cement. Br. Med. J., 1:349, 1972.
3. Homsy, C.A., et al.: Some physiological aspects of prosthesis stabilization with acrylic polymer. Clin. Orthopaed. Rel. Res., 83:317, 1972.
4. Kallos, T., et al.: Intramedullary pressure and pulmonary embolism of femoral medullary contents in dogs during insertion of bone cement and a prosthesis. J. Bone Joint Surg., 56A:1363, 1974.
5. Park, W.Y., et al.: Changes in arterial oxygen tension during total hip replacement. Anesthesiology, 39:642, 1973.
6. Harris, W. H., et al.: High and low dose aspirin prophylaxis against venous thrombolic disease in total hip replacement. J. Bone Joint Surg., 64(A):63, 1982.
7. Boysen, G., et al.: Prolongation of bleeding time and inhibition of platelet aggregation by low dose acetysalicylic acid in patients with cerebrovascular disease. Stroke, 15:241, 1984.
8. Ferraris, V.A., and Swanson, E.: Bleeding times with respect to aspirin intake. Surg. Gynecol. Obstet., 156:439, 1983.
9. Hindman, B.J., and Kobu, B.V.: Usefulness of post-aspirin bleeding time. Anesthesiology, 64:368, 1986.
10. Bonney, S.L., et al.: Renal safety of two analgesics used over the counter: Ibuprofen and aspirin. Clin. Pharmacol. Ther., 40:373, 1986.
11. Smith, J.B., and Willis, A.L.: Aspirin selectively inhibits prostaglandin production in platelets. Nature, 231:235, 1971.
12. De Gaetano, G., et al.: Pharmacology of platelet inhibition in humans: Implications of the salicylate–aspirin interaction. Circulation, 72:1185, 1985.
13. Benzon, H.T., Brunner, E.A., ad Vaisrub, N.: Bleeding time and nerve blocks after aspirin. Region. Anesth., 9:86, 1984.
14. Calabresi, P., and Parks, R.E. Jr.: Chemotherapy of neoplastic diseases. The Pharmacological Basis of Therapeutics. Edited by L. Goodman and A. Gilman. New York, Macmillan, 1980.
15. Zsigmond, E.K., and Robius, G.: The effect of a series of anti-cancer drugs on plasma cholinesterase activity. Can. Anaesth. Soc. J., 19:75, 1972.
16. Williams, W.T., Lowry, L., and Eggers, G.W.N. Jr.: Anesthetic management during therapeutic disruption of the blood–brain barrier. Anesth. Analg., 65:188, 1986.
17. Ueland, P.M., Refsum, H., and Wesenberg, F.: Methotrexate

therapy and nitrous oxide anesthesia. N. Engl. J. Med., 314:1514, 1986.
18. Burrows, F.A., Hickey, P.R., and Colan, S.: Perioperative complications in patients with anthracycline chemotherapeutic agents. Can. Anaesth. Soc. J., 32:149, 1985.
19. Turpie, A.G.G., et al.: A randomized controlled trial of a low-molecular-weight heparin (enoxaparin) to prevent deep-vein thrombosis in patients undergoing elective hip surgery. N. Engl. J. Med., 315:925, 1986.
20. Harris, W.H., et al.: Comparison of warfarin, low-molecular-weight dextran, aspirin, and subcutaneous heparin in prevention of venous thromboembolism following total hip replacement. J. Bone Joint Surg., 56A:1552, 1974.
21. Cutting, W.C.: Handbook of Pharmacology, 7th ed. Norwalk, CT, Appleton-Century, 1984.
22. Owens, E.L., Kasten, G.W., and Hessel, E.A.: Spinal subarachnoid hematoma after lumbar puncture and heparinization: A case report, review of the literature, and discussion of anesthetic implications. Anesth. Analg., 65:1201, 1986.
23. Rao, T.L.K., and El-Etr, A.A.: Anticoagulation following placement of epidural and subarachnoid catheters: An evaluation of neurologic sequelae. Anesthesiology, 55:618, 1981.
24. Matthews, E.T., and Abrams, L.S.: Intrathecal morphine in open heart surgery. Lancet, 2:543, 1980.
25. Waldman, S.D., et al.: Caudal administration of morphine sulfate in anticoagulated and thrombocytopenic patients. Anesth. Analg., 66:367, 1987.
26. Odoom, J.A., and Sih, I.L.: Epidural analgesia and anticoagulant therapy: Experience with one thousand cases of continuous epidurals. Anesthesiology, 38:254, 1983.
27. Mathews, E.T., and Abrams, L.D.: Intrathecal morphine in open heart surgery. Lancet, 2:543, 1980.
28. Oster, G., Tuden, R.L., and Colditz, G.A.: A cost-effectiveness analysis of prophylaxis against deep-vein thrombosis in major orthopedic surgery. J.A.M.A., 257:203, 1987.
29. Ueda, I.: The effects of volatile general anesthetics on adenosine diphosphate-induced platelet aggregation. *Anesthesiology, 34:405, 1971.*
30. Dalsgaard-Nielsen, J., and Gormsen, J.: Effects of halothane on platelet function. Thromb. Haemost., 44:143, 1980.
31. Gotta, A.W., et al.: The effect of enflurane and fentanyl anesthesia on human platelet aggregation in vivo. Can. Anaesth. Soc. J., 27:319, 1980.
32. Fauss, B.G., et al.: The in vitro and in vivo effects of isoflurane and nitrous oxide on platelet aggregation. Anesth. Analg., 65:1170, 1986.
33. Gilman, A.G., et al.: The Pharmacologic Basis of Therapeutics 7th Ed. New York, Macmillan, 1985.
34. Horrow, J.: Protamine: A review of its toxicity. Anesth. Analg., 64:348, 1985.
35. McAvoy, T.J.: Pharmacokinetic modeling of heparin and its clinical implications. J. Pharmacokinet. Biopharm., 7:331, 1979.
36. Whitfield, L.R., Schentag, J.J., and Levy, G.: Relationship between concentration and anticoagulant effect of heparin in plasma of hospitalized patients: Magnitude and predictability of interindividual differences. Clin. Pharmacol. Ther., 32:503, 1982.
37. Bull, B., et al.: Heparin therapy during extracorporeal circulation: The use of dose–response curve to individualize heparin and protamine dosage. J. Thorac. Cardiovasc. Surg., 69:685, 1975.
38. Michaels, I., and Barash, G.: Hemodynamic changes during protamine administration. Anesth. Analg., 62:831, 1983.
39. Hines, R.L., and Barash, G.: Protamine: Does it alter right ventricular function? Anesth. Analg., 65:1271, 1986.
40. Levy, H.A., Zaidan, J.R., and Faraj, B.: Prospective evaluation of risk of protamine reactions in patients with NPH insulin-dependent diabetes. Anesth. Analg., 65:739, 1986.
41. Houle, G.: Practical considerations in regional anaesthesia. Can. Anaesth. Soc. J., 32:S47, 1985.
42. Rao, T.L.K.: Anticoagulation following placement of epidural and subarachnoid catheters: An evaluation of neurologic sequelae. Anesthesiology, 55:618, 1981.
43. Freedberg, R.S., et al.: Cardiogenic shock due to antihistamine overdose: Reversal with intra-aortic balloon counterpulsation. J.A.M.A., 257:660, 1987.
44. Iduoe, O., et al.: Nature and extent of penicillin side-reactions with particular reference to fatalities from anaphylactic shock. Bull WHO, 38:159, 1968.
45. Levine, L.R.: Quantitative comparison of adverse reactions to cefaclor vs. amoxicillin in a surveillance study. Pediatr. Infect. Dis., 4:358, 1985.
46. Anderson, J.A.: Cross-sensitivity to cephalosporins in patients allergic to penicillin. Pediatr. Infect. Dis., 5:557, 1986.
47a. Mayhew, J.F., and Deutsch, S.: Cardiac arrest following administration of vancomycin. Can. Anaesth. Soc. J., 32:65, 1985.
47b. Green, R.L., Frederickson, E.C.: Elevated plasma procaine concentration after administration of procaine penicillin G. N. Engl. J. Med., 291:223, 1974.
48. Prys-Roberts, C., Meloehe, R., and Foëx, P.: Studies of anesthesia in relation to hypertension I. Cardiovascular responses of treated and untreated patients. Br. J. Anaesth., 43:122, 1971.
48a. Bloor, B.C., and Flacke, W.E.: Reduction in halothane anesthetic requirement by clonidine, an alpha-adrenergic agonist. Anesth. Analg., 61:741, 1982.
49. Ghignone, M., et al.: Effects of clonidine on narcotic requirements and hemodynamic response during induction of fentanyl anesthesia and endotracheal intubation. Anesthesiology, 64:36, 1986.
50. Gordh, T.E., and Tamsen, A.: A study of the analgesic effect of clonidine in man (abstract). Acta Anaesthesiol. Scand. (suppl)2:78, 983.
51. Verapamil for hypertension. Medical Letter, 29(737):37–38, April 10, 1987.
52. Jones, R.M., et al.: Verapamil potentiation of neuromuscular blockade: Failure of reversal with neostigmine but prompt reversal with edrophonium. Anesth. Analg., 64:1021, 1985.
53. Van Poorten, J.F., et al.: Verapamil and reversal of vecuronium neuromuscular blockade. Anesth. Analg., 63:155, 1984.
54. Rubin, A.S., and Zablocki, A.D.: Hyperkalemia, verapamil, and dantrolene. Anesthesiology, 66:246, 1987.
55. Bosnyak, Z.J., and Kampine, J.P.: Effects of halothane, enflurane and isoflurane on the SA node. Anesthesiology, 58:314, 1983.
56. Chelly, J.E., et al.: Cardiovascular effects of and interaction between calcium blocking drugs and anesthetics in chronically instrumented dogs. I. Verapamil and halothane. Anesthesiology, 64:560, 1986.
57. Rogers, K., et al.: Cardiovascular effects of and interaction between calcium blocking drugs and anesthetics in chronically instrumented dogs. II. Verapamil, enflurane and isoflurane. Anesthesiology, 64:568, 1986.
58. Merin, R.G.: Calcium channel blocking drugs and anesthetics: Is the drug interaction beneficial or detrimental? Anesthesiology, 66:111, 1987.
59. Chew, C.Y.C., et al.: Influence of severity of ventricular dysfunction on hemodynamic responses to intravenously

administered verapamil in ischemic heart disease. Am. J. Cardiol., *47*:917,. 1981.
60. Kuncl, R.W., et al.: Colchicine myopathy and neuropathy. N. Engl. J. Med., *316*:1562, 1987.
60a. Hess, S.M., et al.: Effects of α-methylamino acids on catecholamines and serotonin. Fed. Proc., *20*:344, 1961.
60b. Coakley, C.S., et al.: Anesthesia during rauwolfian therapy. J.A.M.A., *161*:1143, 1956.
60c. Woosley, R.L., and Nies, A.S.: Guanethedine. N. Engl. J. Med., *295*:1053, 1976.
60d. Bobik, A., et al.: Evidence for a predominantly central hypotensive action of alpha-methyldopa in humans. Hypertension, *8*:16, 1986.
61. Roth, J.A.: Multiple forms of monoamine oxidase and their interaction with tricyclic psychomimetic drugs. Gen. Pharmacol., *7*:381, 1976.
62. Palmer, H.: Potentiation of pethidine. Br. Med. J., *2*:944, 1960.
63. El-Ganzouri, A.R., et al.: Monoamine oxidase inhibitors: Should they be discontinued preoperatively? Anesth. Analg., *64*:592, 1985.
64. Wong, K.C.: Preoperative discontinuation of monoamine oxidase inhibitor therapy: An old wives' tale? Sem. Anesth., *5*:145, 1986.
65. Maas, J.W.: Biogenic amines: Biochemical and pharmacologic separation of two types of depression. Arch. Gen. Psychiatr., *32*:1357, 1975.
66. Preskorn, S.H., Raichle, M.E., and Hartman, B.: Antidepressants alter cerebrovascular permeability and metabolic rate in primates. Science, *217*:250, 1982.
67. Domenech, J.S., et al.: Pancuronium bromide: An indirect sympathomimetic agent. Br. J. Anaesth., *48*:1143–1148, 1976.
68. Veith, R.C., et al.: Cardiovascular effects of tricyclic antidepressants in depressed patients with chronic heart disease. N. Engl. J. Med., *306*:954, 1984.
69. Burckhard, D., et al.: Cardiovascular effects of tricyclic and tetracyclic antidepressants. J.A.M.A., *239*:213, 1978.
70. Dallos, S.V., and Heathfield, J.: Iatrogenic epilepsy due to antidepressant drugs. Br. Med. J., *4*:80, 1969.
71. Spiker, D.G., et al.: Tricyclic antidepressant overdose: Clinical presentation and plasma levels. Clin. Pharmacol. Ther., *18*:539–546, 1975.
72. Goldberg, R.J., Capone, R.J., and Hunt, J.D.: Cardiac complications following tricyclic antidepressant overdose. J.A.M.A., *254*:1772, 1985.
73. Johnston, R.R., et al.: A comparative interaction of epinephrine with enflurane, isoflurane and halothane in man. Anesth. Analg., *55*:709, 1976.
74. Sprague, D.H., and Wolf, S.: Enflurane seizures in patients taking amitriptyline. Anesth. Analg., *61*:67, 1982.
75a. Ivankovich, A.D., et al.: The effect of pancuronium on myocardial contraction and catecholamine metabolism. J. Pharm. Pharmacol., *27*:837, 1976.
75b. Glisson, S.N., Fajardo, L., and El-Etr, A.A.: Amitriptyline therapy increases electrocardiographic changes during reversal of neuromuscular blockade. Anesth. Analg., *57*:77–83, 1978.
75c. Osserman, K.E.: Critical reappraisal of the use of Edrophonium tests in myasthenia gravis and significance of clinical classification. Annals of the New York Academy of Science, *135*:312, 1966.
75d. Cronnelly, R., Morris, R.B., and Miller, R.D.: Edrophonium: Duration of action and atropine requirement in humans during halothane anesthesia. Anesthesiology, *57*:261, 1982.
76. Cade, J.F.J.: Lithium salts in the treatment of psychotic excitement. Med. J. Aust., *2*:349, 1949.

77. Waud, B.E., Farrell, B.A., and Waud, D.R.: Lithium and neuromuscular transmission. Anesth. Analg., *61*:399, 1982.
77a. Berger, F.M.: Use of antianxiety drugs. Clin. Pharmacol. and Ther., *29*:291, 1981.
77b. Lear, E., et al.: A clinical study of mechanisms of action of chlorpromazine. J.A.M.A., *163*:30, 1957.
77c. Matsuki, A., and Oyama, T.: Excessive mortality in schizophrenic patients on chronic phenothiazine treatment. Travail Recu le 28 August: 407–415, 1972.
78. Thompson, T.L. II, Moran, M.G., and Nies, A.S.: Psychotropic drug use in the elderly. I and II. N. Engl. J. Med., *308*:134, 1983.
79. Greenblatt, D.J., et al.: Benzodiazepine hypnotics. Sleep, *5* (suppl)1:18, 1982.
80a. Papper, E.M.: Problems of commonly used drugs on patients who require surgery. N.Y. State J. Med., *59*:4368, 1959.
80b. Soler, N.G., et al.: Coronary care for myocardial infarction in diabetics. Lancet, *1*:475, 1974.
80c. Committee N.I.H.: Assessment of biometric aspects of controlled trials of hypoglycemic agents. J.A.M.A., *231*:583, 1975.
81. Lundy, J.S.: Cortisone problems involving anesthesia. Anesthesiology, *14*:377, 1953.
82. Salessa, R.M., et al.: Postoperative adrenal cortical insufficiency. J.A.M.A., *152*:1509, 1953.
83a. Stadel, B.V.: Oral contraceptives and cardiovascular disease. N. Engl. J. Med., *305*:672, 1981.
83b. Wood, J.E.: The cardiovascular effects of oral contraceptives. Concepts Cardiovas. Dis., *41*:37, 1972.
83c. Leff, B, Henriksen, R.A., Owen, W.G.: Effect of oral contraceptive use on platelet prothrombin converting (platelet factor 3) activity. Thromb. Res., *15*:631, 1979.
83d. Kannel, W.B.: Oral contraceptive hypertension and thromboembolism. Int. J. Gynaecol. Obstet., *16*:466, 1979.
83e. Heyman, A. (collaborative study): Oral contraception and increased risk of cerebral ischemia or thrombosis. N. Engl. J. Med., *288*:871, 1973.
83f. Stoehr, G.P., et al.: Effect of oral contraceptives on triazolam, temazepam, alprazolam, and lorazepam kinetics. Clin. Pharmacol. Ther., *36*:683, 1984.
84. Wilson, J.D., Sutherland, D.C., and Thomas, A.C.: Has the change to beta-agonists combined with oral theophylline increased cases of fatal asthma? Lancet, *1*:235, 1981.
84a. Garrison, J.C., and Peach, M.J.: Renin and angiotensin. In Goodman and Gilman's The Pharmacological Basis of Therapeutics. 8th Ed. Edited by A.G. Gilman, T.W. Rall, A.S. Nies, and P. Taylor. New York, Pergamon Press, 1990.
84b. Johnston, R.R., Way, W.W., and Miller, R.D.: Effect of CNS catecholamine-depleting drugs on dextroamphetamine induced elevation of halothane MAC. Anesthesiology, *41*:57, 1974.
85. Friedman, J.H., Feinberg, S.S., and Feldman, R.G.: A neuroleptic malignantlike syndrome due to levodopa therapy withdrawal. J.A.M.A., *254*:2792, 1985.
86. Katz, R.L., Matteo, R.S., and Paper, E.M.: The injection of epinephrine during general anesthesia with halogenated hydrocarbons and cyclopropane in man. Anesthesiology, *23*:597, 1962.
87. Reisner, L.S., and Lippman, M.: Ventricular arrhythmias after epinephrine injection in enflurane and in halothane anesthesia. Anesth. Analg., *54*:468, 1975.
88. Johnston, R.R., Eger, E.I., and Wilson, C.: A comparative interaction of epinephrine with enflurane, isoflurane and halothane in man. Anesth. Analg., *55*:709, 1976.
89. Konchigeri, H.N., Shaker, M.H., and Winnie, A.P.: Effect of epinephrine during enflurane anesthesia. Anesth. Analg., *53*:894, 1974.

90. Halsey, M.: Drug interactions in anaesthesia. Br. J. Anaesth., 59:112, 1987.
91. Horrigan, R.W., Eger, E.I., and Wilson, C.: Epinephrine-induced arrhythmias during enflurane anaesthesia in man: A nonlinear dose–response relationship and dose-dependent protection from lidocaine. Anesth. Analg., 57:547, 1978.
92. Adler, F.H.: Physiology of the Eye, 5th ed. St. Louis, C.V. Mosby, 1970.
93. Grant, W.M.: Systemic drugs and adverse influence on ocular pressure. In Symposium on Ocular Therapy. Edited by I.H. Leopold, vol. 3. St. Louis, C.V. Mosby, 1968, pp. 57–87.
94. Hiscox, P.E.A., and McCulloch, C.: Cardiac arrest occurring in a patient on echothiophate iodide therapy. Am. J. Ophthalmol., 60:425, 1965.
95. Britman, N.A.: Cardiac effects of topical timolol. N. Engl. J. Med., 300:566, 1979.
96. Bailey, P.L.: Timolol postoperative apnea in neonates and young infants. Anesthesiology, 61:622, 1984.
97. Magora, F., and Collins, V.: The influence of anesthetic agents on intraocular pressure. Arch. Ophthalmol., 66:806, 1965.
98. Kornbleuth, W., et al.: Influence of general anesthesia on intraocular pressure in man. Arch. Ophthalmol., 61:84, 1959.
99. Duncalf, D., and Weitzner, S.W.: The influence of ventilation and hypercapnea on intraocular pressure during anesthesia. Anesth. Analg., 42:232, 1963.
100. Esposito, A.C.: The role of general anesthesia (halothane) in cataract surgery. South. Med. J., 58:922, 1965.
101. Ivankovic, A.D., and Lowe, J.H.: Influence of methoxyflurane and neurolept anesthesia on intraocular pressure in man. Anesth. Analg., 48:933, 1969.
102. Presbitero, J.V., et al.: Intraocular pressure during enflurane and neurolept anesthesia in adult patients undergoing ophthalmic surgery. Anesth. Analg., 59:50, 1980.
103. Cunningham, A.J., et al.: The effect of intravenous diazepam on rise of intraocular pressure following succinylcholine. Can. Anaesth. Soc. J., 28:581, 1981.
104. Corssen, G., and Hay, J.E.: A new parenteral anesthetic CL-581: Its effect on intraocular pressure J. Pediatr. Ophthalmol., 3:20, 1967.
105. Peuler, M., Glass, D.D., and Arens, J.F.: Ketamine and intraocular pressure. Anesthesiology, 43:575, 1975.
106. Mahajan, B.P., et al.: Intraocular pressure changes during muscular hyperactivity after general anesthesia. Anesthesiology, 66:419, 1987.
107. Al-Abrak, M.H., Samuel, J.R.: Effects of general anesthesia on the intraocular pressure in man: Comparison of tubocurarine and pancuronium with nitrous oxide and oxygen. Br. J. Ophthalmol., 58:806, 1974.
108. Myers, E.F., et al.: Failure of non-depolarizing neuromuscular blockers to inhibit succinylcholine-induced increases in intraocular pressure. Anesthesiology, 48:149, 1978.
109. Smith, R.B., and Leano, N.: Intraocular pressure following pancuronium. Can. Anaesth. Soc. J., 20:742, 1974.
110. Cook, J.H.: The effect of succinylcholine on intraocular pressure. Anaesthesia, 36:359, 1981.
111. Schmerl, E., and Steinberg, B.: The role of the diencephalon in regulating ocular tension. Am. J. Ophthalmol., 31:155, 1948.

11

PRINCIPLES OF PREANESTHETIC MEDICATION

Preanesthetic medication has a twofold purpose: (1) it serves to prepare a patient for anesthesia by providing a state of acquiescence to the induction of anesthesia and by obtunding nervous system activity; and (2) it serves to contribute to the anesthetic state and reduce the anesthetic drug requirements.

OBJECTIVES

Four general objectives are the following:

1. Promotion of mental and emotional relaxation
    a. Cortical sedation, subcortical tranquilization, and amnesia.
    b. Reduced limbic system activity (emotional centers).
2. Reduction of sensory input
    a. Analgesia for actual or anticipatory pain.
    b. Reduction of thalamic center activity.
    c. Depression of reticular activating system (RAS).
3. Reduction of metabolic rate
    a. Reduction of oxygen needs.
    b. Decrease in amount of anesthetic drugs required.
4. Antagonizing of adverse autonomic nervous system stresses
    a. Blockade of parasympathetic activity.
    b. Blockade of sympathetic (adrenergic) activity.

REDUCTION OF CENTRAL NERVOUS SYSTEM (CNS) ACTIVITY. The objective of the clinician is to produce mental and emotional relaxation with sedatives, tranquilizers, and psychological support to provide anxiolysis, sedation, amnesia, antiemesis, antihistaminic action, and reduced need for the patient to think (history, physical, and admission paperwork the day before surgery).

REDUCTION OF SENSORY INPUT. The clinician should reduce visual and auditory stimuli (by providing a quiet room and less talk). Analgesia should be administered as needed. Simple manipulations, e.g., applying blood pressure cuffs, setting up monitors, evoke more than an interest and may be uncomfortable or interpreted as unpleasant or painful (anticipatory pain). Invasive procedures should be performed when the patient is under anesthesia. The number of staff in contact with the patient should be minimized as much as possible.

REDUCTION OF METABOLISM WITH OPIOIDS. The advantages of using opioids for preanesthetics include: Analgesia for both anticipated and actual pain; reduced oxygen requirement (20%); reduced MAC for inhalation agents (15% to 25%); and reduced induction dose of intravenous drug to produce unconsciousness (the UD_{95}).[1] Also, priming opiate receptors by premedication with a narcotic (morphine) enhances the effect of subsequent opioids in control of postoperative pain (the shadow effect).[2]

CONTROL OF AUTONOMIC NERVOUS SYSTEM RESPONSES (ANTICHOLINERGICS; NEUROLEPTS). Parasympathetic blockade lowers vagal tone; reduces mucus and salivary secretion (antisialagogic), gastric fluid volume, and gastric acidity; decreases gastrointestinal (GI) tone and motility; provides prophylaxis against hypersensitivity reactions; and decreases nausea and vomiting (H_1 and H_2 block).

Sympathetic blockade (alpha-adrenergic sympathetic block) decreases catecholamine release (tranquilizers, droperidol); decreases nausea and emesis; blocks dopaminergic Chemoreceptor Trigger Zone; and suppresses central noradrenergic outflow (clonidine).

ANXIETY FACTORS.[3] The incidence and degree of anxiety and apprehension are proportionate to the type and magnitude of the surgery (Table 11–1).[4]

Many factors contribute to preoperative anxiety.[3,4] A restless sleep the night before surgery increases the anxiety level the following day. Thus, a "good night's sleep" is a cliche, but a sound one that should be assured. For the patient with a trait anxiety, a tranquilizer is indicated; for simple situational anxiety, a sedative may be sufficient.

A night sedative is not as effective in anxious patients who do not have a visit by an anesthesiologist; a tranquilizer is preferred. The combination of a visit and a sedative, however, is more effective.

Anxiety is higher in women than men; it is higher in women under 70 kg.[3]

Most inhospital patients have a high degree of anxiety because of their medical problems or more serious illness. Ambulatory patients have a milder degree of apprehension, but this may be more related to the arrangements and activity. Preanesthetic medication dosage may be reduced. Patients undergoing regional anesthesia are likely to be concerned about "being awake" and should be adequately sedated or tranquilized preanesthetically. Infants may experience psychological trauma (parental separation) and fear of pain, with long-lasting untoward psychological effects or personality changes (see later discussion).[5] The process of obtaining informed consent can sometimes create anxiety for the patient.[6]

ANXIETY AND THE ENDOCRINE SYSTEM. Anxiety and stress activate the sympathoadrenal axis[8,9] as well as the pituitary-hypothalamic-adrenal cortical system.[10] Some psychological and physiologic stresses have been quantified with regard to catecholamine response (Table 11–2).[11]

Using the *Linear Analogue Anxiety Scale*, Fell demonstrated that this scale correlates the degree of anxiety and the percentage change in plasma adrenaline concentration, but not noradrenaline. Adrenaline increased significantly by 40% before induction of anesthesia and correlated with the increased anxiety.[12]

HORMONAL ASSESSMENT OF PREANESTHETIC MEDICATION.[12] Control of anxiety, both situational and trait, is essential for stress-free anesthesia. Assessment can be *qualitatively* reported by observation and questioning of the patient. Assessment also can

TABLE 11–1. ANXIETY FACTORS

Type of Surgery	Incidence of Anxiety (%)
Genitourinary	80
Other elective	57
Possible cancer	85
Cardiac	60

TABLE 11–2. QUANTITATION OF STRESS AND ARTERIAL BLOOD CATECHOLAMINE LEVELS

Normal plasma catecholamine levels in arterial blood:

	Mean	Range
Epinephrine	50 pg/ml (5.0 ng/dl) (0.27 nMol)	20–120 pg/ml
Norepinephrine	250 pg/ml (25 ng/dl) (1.7 nMol)	120–500 pg/ml (12–50 ng/dl)

Production rate of:	Epinephrine	Norepinephrine*
State	Rate/min (nanograms)	Rate/min (nanograms)
Normal	5	25 (12–50)†
Rest (recumbent)	2–3	10
Upright posture[7]	6.7	30
Excitement (anger or fear)	18–30	—
Cold	12–14	—
Mental stress (exam, etc.)	18.6	—

* Epinephrine is more affected by emotions than norepinephrine. Norepinephrine is affected by physical and mental stress.
† Range in parentheses.
Data from vonEuler, U.S.: Quantitation of stress by catecholamine analysis. Clin. Pharmacol. Exp. Ther., 5:398, 1964.

be *quantified* by measurements of plasma cortisol and plasma catecholamines. Utting[13] has shown that a poor night's sleep is associated with high morning levels of cortisol. In patients who have a restful sleep, plasma levels approximate 16 μg/100 ml, whereas those who sleep poorly have levels of 20 μg/100 ml or more. Similarly, higher levels of norepinephrine are found in the morning in anxious preoperative patients when sleep has been fitful and interrupted.

EFFECT OF ANXIETY ON GI FUNCTION. Apprehension and anxiety have important effects on gastric juice, including increasing gastric volume and acidity and delaying gastric emptying time.[14] In the pediatric patient,[15] adequate premedication with a sedative and narcotic plus an anticholinergic, glycopyrrolate, reduces volume to below 50 ml and raises the gastric pH well above the critical risk value of 2.5 units. A similar study found that a "lytic cocktail" of meperidine/promethazine/chlorpromazine is effective in allaying apprehension (and reducing catecholamines) and in reducing gastric volume and raising pH. Promethazine has an antiemetic effect, whereas chlorpromazine (atropine-like action) affects alimentary tract secretion.[16] The cocktail used is a mixture of meperidine 30 mg, promethazine 8.0 mg, and chlorpromazine 8.0 mg in 1 ml of saline. The intramuscular dose for children is 0.05 mg/kg (see later discussion and Table 11-7).

APPROACHES TO PREANESTHETIC MEDICATION

THE CLASSIC APPROACH. Medication of a patient prior to anesthesia according to the traditional concept is concerned with reducing metabolic activity and rate. It is presumed that this is accomplished by the sedation of the patient and by direct metabolic depression through the effects of narcotic drugs. Historically, the use of morphine to provide a calm patient prior to anesthesia was suggested by Lorenzo Bruno in 1850.[17] Subsequently, Claude Bernard gave the practice his support.[18]

Beecher[19a] disputed this approach and contended that the narcotics do not achieve a reduction in basal metabolism. Because the chief drugs, morphine and meperidine, are primarily pain relievers, they should be used only under circumstances of pain.[19b] It is claimed that little effective sedation or a state of well being can be provided with the narcotics while the opposite effect—a state of dysphoria—may result.[19a] These contentions need assessment. In fact, the test of long clinical experience indicates a salutary effect and definite ease in the production of the anesthetic state as well as some contribution to the anesthetic process.[20a,20b]

Indeed, because all surgical patients have at least one standardized feature of the pain complex, namely a *wound*—a standard pain stimulus—it seems logical to change both the perception to this eventual pain and the reaction pattern. Keats[21a] has demonstrated that patients premedicated with narcotics are more comfortable postoperatively; they also recover more rapidly.[21b] Furthermore, there is a significant and interesting type of anxiety that develops and is associated with the mere anticipation of pain.[22a,22b] No drug compares with morphine and similar agents in reducing this anxiety.[23a,b]

OPIOID PREMEDICATION OR INTRAVENOUS INDUCTION PRETREATMENT.[23] Nearly all opioids are capable of reducing MAC values and the amount of inhalation anesthetic needed[24a] when administered as part of preanesthetic medication or when administered intravenously prior to induction. They are able to decrease the dose of intravenous induction drugs such as thiopental, methohexital, and midazolam.[24b] Opioids also reduce the incidence of excitatory effects of methohexital and shorten the onset time of midazolam.[24c]

Fentanyl and alfentanil administered prior to induction reduce MAC values and also the UD_{95} (ED_{95}) doses of intravenous induction agents.[24b]

Sufentanil has a more rapid onset of action than fentanyl, if administered shortly before induction, in reducing the UD of thiopental, methohexital, and midazolam. It also has a shorter duration of action and is more potent.[24d]

PRIMARY CORTICAL SEDATION. One may recognize *simple cortical sedation* without the use of narcotics as second and distinct approach to preanesthetic medication. The available drugs recommended are chiefly sedative drugs exemplified by the barbiturates. The consequences of lessened mental activity are calmness and lessened physical activity, which lead to a basal state.

In brief *cortical depression* is the keystone of this second approach. By itself, this approach is inadequate. Stress responses usually are enhanced. Larger doses of induction drugs are needed, and MAC values of inhalation agents are not reduced. In the presence of pain, a disoriented state may be produced.

SUBCORTICAL SUPPRESSION. A third distinct approach, *subcortical depression*, is available. By subduing the arousal mechanisms, the alertness and sensitivity of the patient are diminished. The locus of action is placed chiefly at the RAS.[25] In addition, the drugs capable of this effect also depress the hypothalamus and the thalamus.[26] Hence, a degree of diminished autonomic sensitivity results, and the deleterious effects of stress are obtunded. Tranquilizers are key agents in achieving these goals.[26,27]

BALANCED MEDICATION. A balanced or selective approach seems more logical, where each of the above modes are used. According to circumstances and indications, a specific mode is emphasized but combined with other approaches. Medication is directed at specific targets, represented by segments of the CNS that are evidently overactive. Thus, if cortical depression is needed, the barbiturates are indicated for sedation; if the needs are for tranquility, a state of acquiescence, or the suppression of agitated and anxiety states, tranquilizers are employed. In other words, medication is directed specifically at that segment or segments of the nervous system that are evidently most overactive. Inherent in using any medication is the danger of reactions because of the chemical nature of the drug and individual sensitivity and response.

For a generalized depression of the CNS, the narcotics are of inestimable value. They provide analgesia for the traumatic experiences of preparing a patient for anesthesia, and they will potentiate anesthetics, thereby lessening the dose; furthermore, the effect carries into the postoperative period and diminishes the early need for analgesics as well as the emergence delirium due to pain.

In conclusion, the approach to premedication is a matter of understanding the particular objectives in a given case and selecting that drug which is most appropriate. Whether the emphasis in medication is on depression of the cortex or depression of the subcortical centers determines the approach.

PARASYMPATHETIC BLOCKADE. An anticholinergic, such as scopolamine, atropine, or glycopyrrolate, should be given to every patient before anesthesia; atropine is the reference anticholinergic and the optimal dose for preanesthetic medication is about 6.0 μg/kg. Thus an optimal dose of 10 mg of morphine is accompanied by a dose of 0.4 mg of atropine. A dose of 15 mg of morphine is optimally accompanied by a 0.6 mg dose of atropine. This is known as the 25 to 1 ratio, or Waters ratio of morphine to atropine. The dose of scopolamine with 15 mg of morphine is 0.3 mg or about one third less than that of atropine. The dose of glycopyrrolate is one half that of atropine.

The use of parasympathetic blockade in regional anesthesia is controversial; however, when spinal or epidural anesthesia is chosen, or regional blocks of head, neck, and arms are planned, it is essential to avoid complications as follows:

1. An anticholinergic prevents GI cramping sensations and discomfort by decreasing motility and propulsive movements of the gut.
2. A sensory level above the umbilicus (T9) results in vagal dominance when the vagus is likely to dominate (sympathetic block may be up to T6).
3. An anticholinergic will obtund adverse cardiovascular responses during head and neck anesthesia.
4. An anticholinergic with a narcotic decreases the incidence of postoperative nausea and vomiting.[24d]

STATE OF AWARENESS. To understand the problem of sleep and depression, it is desirable to understand the state of wakefulness and, hence, acuity of perception. The physiology of arousal is discussed here.[25]

Consciousness or the waking state is thought to depend on a stream of impulses radiated to the central hemispheres from an area in the brain stem and hypothalamic region termed the *reticular activating system*.[25] This system has a multisynaptic structure similar to the cortex.

Afferent stimuli capable of arousing a patient may take the following two routes to the brain:

1. Through the classical sensory system of the medial and lateral leminisci via the thalamus to the appropriate part of the sensory cortex.
2. Through the central part of the brain stem in a neuronal mesh or network called the reticular system. The input to this system is via collaterals from the main sensory tracts, and the output is to the cortex.

The main function of the secondary system is to alert the brain to receive and appreciate stimuli from the classical pathways so they may enter more completely into the field of consciousness. To produce unconsciousness, therefore, two activities must be obtunded. That is, the cortical integration of sensation over classical paths must be abolished, and the effectiveness of the arousal system must be blocked. It is evident that to diminish the background sensitivity of the cortex or the alertness of the cortex, it is fundamental that the RAS be inhibited. A major consequence of such depression is the production of a favorable mental state.

DEFINITIONS. It is suggested that the cortex, the RAS, and the subcortical centers are the areas largely affected in producing sedation and the anesthetic state.[26] In achieving a depression of consciousness (to relieve mental and physical distress) there is a progression from complete awareness to unconsciousness and anesthesia. By the use of silver electrodes placed at various levels in the brain, it has been shown that the electrical changes of normal sleep and the effects of pharmacologic depressants first appear in the subcortical zone when the patient feels drowsy. With onset of sleep electrical changes spread into the overlying cortex.[27]

King[28] states that barbiturates, in general, alter the state of consciousness by preventing the stimulation of the RAS via the collaterals from the classical somatic pathways. Ether, on the other hand, depresses both reticular formation and the diffuse thalamic projection system to the cortex.[29] Thus, this drug, in small doses, may produce sedation and analgesia; as greater doses are administered, further electrical activity of the CNS is altered until unconsciousness occurs.

Depending on extent of CNS depression, one recognizes arbitrary *clinical states* of awareness merging into unconsciousness[26] (Table 11–3.)[30a]

TABLE 11-3. STATES OF AWARENESS FROM FULL CONSCIOUSNESS TO COMPLETE UNCONSCIOUSNESS DEPENDING ON DEGREE OF CNS DEPRESSION

	Conscious		Unconscious	
Degree of Depression	Awake but Calm and Tranquil	Asleep Responsive to Verbal Commands Coordinate	Arousable to Pain Stimulus Somatic Response Incoordinate	Autonomic Responses Only to Pain Stimulus
SEDATION Cortical Depression	Barbiturates			
HYPNOSIS Subcortical depression		Large doses of barbiturates Tranquilizers		
NARCOSIS Subcortical depression		Narcotics		
STAGE—ANALGESIA Cortical and subcortical depression		Large doses of narcotics Light doses of anesthetics		
BASAL ANESTHESIA Cortical–subcortical, midbrain, and medullary depression			Large doses of aliphatic depressants: barbiturates, avertin, light anesthesia	
ANESTHESIA				Anesthetics

From Goodman, L., and Gilman, A.: The Pharmacological Basis of Therapeutics. New York, Macmillan, 1970.

Amnesia. Amnesia is defined as the inability to remember experiences. The loss of memory may be of recent events or of long-past events. Anterograde amnesia is that form for events occurring after a trauma, onset of a disease, or administration of a drug. Retrograde amnesia refers to loss of memory of events that occurred before a new condition. Anterograde amnesia is of particular importance in anesthesia practice because amnesia of events relating to the perioperative and anesthesia experiences can be obtained. Studies of the neuroanatomy of amnesia indicate that damage to the medial temporal region of the human brain causes a profound amnesic syndrome. Careful experimental studies indicate that the conjoint injury of the hippocampus-amygdala produces a severe memory defect.[30]

Drugs of value to produce amnesia include the benzodiazepines, especially diazepam. The classical drug producing anterograde amnesia is scopolamine.

Sedation. This is a mild state of cortical depression in which the patient is calm and tranquil but awake. Barbiturates are the classic drugs that provide this degree of depression.

Hypnosis. This is the condition of mild sleep or semiconsciousness brought about by the use of sedatives and nonnarcotic drugs from which the patient may be aroused by noxious or painful stimuli. Cortical and subcortical depression can be accomplished by larger doses of barbiturates, but the tranquilizers are the reference drugs. The major tranquilizers of the phenothiazine and the benzodiazepine groups are used for this purpose.

Narcosis. This is the condition of sleep or stupor similar to hypnosis. It is brought about by the use of narcotics. These drugs differ from other central depressants in that they relieve pain before unconsciousness occurs. In contrast, most sedative or nonanalgesic drugs do not relieve pain until complete unconsciousness is attained. The locus of action is both cortical and subcortical.

Analgesia. Analgesia is defined as the absence of sensibility to pain. The agents used depress pain without causing loss of consciousness. The agents act by blocking central pain perception and, in varying measures, the pattern of response to the sensation.

State of Analgesia. This is a state of profound sleep from which the patient can be aroused to respond in an appropriate coordinate fashion. Amnesia and loss of pain sense designates the state. It is readily produced by minimal concentrations of anesthetic drugs. It can also be produced by larger doses of narcotics and barbiturates.

Basal Anesthesia. This is a state of unconsciousness short of surgical anesthesia. The patient will respond with somatic reflex responses to painful stimuli but not respond to the spoken word. The responses are uncoordinate, generally.

State of Anesthesia. This is a state of unconsciousness in which intense noxious stimulation evokes only autonomic-type reflex responses. Thus, there are no protective reflex reactions involving the voluntary movements; however, changes in respiration and cardiocirculatory dynamics are evident.

SPECIFIC OBJECTIVES IN PREMEDICATION. Among the specific objects attained by adequate medication are:

amnesia lessened *apprehension*; reduction in the *amount of anesthetic required*, and hence, lessening the toxicity of the agent; the counteracting of untoward or *undesirable effects*, such as respiratory irregularities, excitement, and the excessive flow of mucous or saliva. By depressing *reflex excitability*, agents that are not potent, such as nitrous oxide and ethylene, can be used. Finally, the proper selection of drugs will *lower basal metabolism*. This is the term used to indicate the rate of heat production in the postabsorptive state with the patient supine and motionless. Much lowering of metabolism is accomplished through lessened muscular activity.

FACTORS DETERMINING DOSAGE

From his anesthetic experience, Guedel[31] early enunciated the conditions and factors influencing metabolism and the size of dose, as discussed here.

AGE. Basal metabolism varies distinctly with different ages.[32] Expressed in calories per square meter of body surface per hour (cal/m^2/hr), an approximate curve of metabolic rate may be established (Fig. 11-1). At birth and in early infancy it is low and may be given a value of 35 to 40 cal/m^2/hr, but it rises rapidly during the first few months of life to 45 to 50 cal/m^2/hr. This rise continues to reach a maximum at about the second year of life of 55 cal/m^2/hr. From this maximum, there is a gradual decline to about 41 cal/m^2/hr at the age of 12 years.[32]

With pubescence there is a rise in basal metabolism out of proportion to size, and between the ages of 12 to 14, with variations, the rate is about 45 cal/m^2/hr. This is followed by a decline to 40 cal/m^2/hr at age 20. Between the ages of 20 and 40, basal metabolism maintains a fairly constant level, with values between 38 and 40 cal/m^2/hr. Thereafter there is a gradual decline to about 35 cal/m^2/hr at the age of 70 years. It is obvious that the times at which the greatest amount of morphine or other depressing agents can be given per pound of body weight are those periods when caloric consumption is at its highest: at about the age of 2; again at the age of puberty. These are mean ages, so it is preferred that one be guided not by chronologic age but by physiologic age.

Age is a most important variable in determining the action of drugs.[33] After the age of 40 years there is *increasing* effect of narcotic and sedative drugs. A striking increased pain relief with increasing age is evident, and for the decades 50 through 80, there is approximately a 10 to 15% increased effect for each decade. The phenomenon of decreased sensitivity to sensory modalities with age is not only evident by decreased pain perception but by decreased activity of airway reflexes (laryngeal). Conversely, progressively smaller doses of these drugs are needed to achieve a given response. The decreased sensitivity is related to decreased responsiveness of the receptors.

The sensitivity of beta-adrenergic receptors is also age dependent. These receptors become less sensitive with age, i.e., resistance of the receptor to combining with either agonists or antagonists increases with age.[34] A positive correlation between age and receptor resistance for propranolol has been demonstrated;[35] i.e., propranolol does not readily combine with receptors in older subjects.[34]

Generally, an age-related decrease in enzyme induction of drug-metabolizing enzymes occurs. This is consistent with the concept of aging as a reduced ability to adapt or respond to stimuli and is a biochemical expression of the aging process. Conversely, a marked increase in oxidative–reductive drug-metabolizing enzymes occurs in young mature animals.

STHENICITY. Closely related to basal metabolic rate is the body habitus or build. This is essentially a matter of size and weight. Thus large, heavy-set people will require more of a given drug. Pyknic-type individuals are usually somewhat phlegmatic, not apprehensive, and their metabolic processes are relatively sluggish. At the other extreme is the as-

FIG. 11-1. Basal metabolism expressed in cal/m^2/hr as related to age and sex. Adapted from AMA Fundamentals of Anesthesia, 3rd ed. Philadelphia, W.B. Saunders, 1954. Based on Tables of Dubois[38] and Dubois[39].

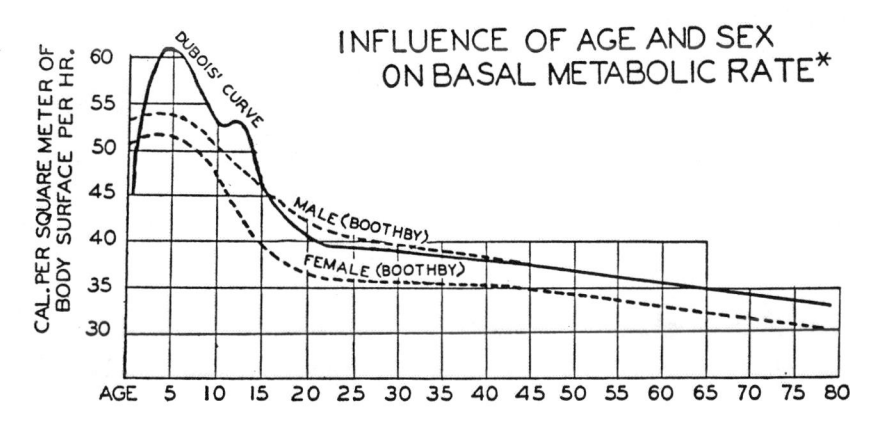

thenic individual—tall, emotional, whose metabolic processes are usually overactive.

SEX.[31] The basal metabolism of women is distinctly lower than men of the same size and age. This discrepancy is noticeable from the age of 2, when the difference is about 4%; the difference increases to about 9% at 13 years, and during adult life is 7% to 10%.

TEMPERATURE. There is about a 7% increase in the basal metabolic rate for each degree Farenheit rise in temperature.[36]

EMOTIONS. This is probably the most frequent cause of preanesthetic rise in basal metabolic rate. Fear and excitement are the principal factors. Both increase the sensitivity to pain, and it is well to estimate emotional excitability with some degree of accuracy. This can be done after a short conversation with your patient. Mental activity such as a mathematical exercise alone has little influence on metabolism, but excitement may raise the metabolism 20%.[39]

ENDOCRINE EFFECTS. The thyroid hormone is a key determinant of basal metabolism. There can be increases or decreases of 50% from normal, depending on the level of hormone. The thyroid effect is mediated via increases in ion flux and the associated increase in activity of membrane-bound sodium-potassium-adenosine triphosphatase.[37]

Ingestion of food is associated with an increase in energy production (diet-induced thermogenesis). The specific dynamic action can raise heat production by 20% over the normal caloric value of the foodstuff. Overnight fasting is thus an important factor in preparing patients for surgery and to reduce preoperative metabolism.[38,39]

Catecholamines increase basal metabolic rate. Stress is the important factor in releasing both epinephrine and norepinephrine as well as cortisol.

Psychosocial stimuli (anxiety) and physical trauma (pain) can elicit a stress-strain response on either or both neuroendocrine systems:[40a] (1) the sympathetic-adrenal medullary system[40b] and (2) arousal of the pituitary-adrenal cortical system.[40c] Such stimulation adversely affect homeostasis and increases metabolism. Opiates are capable of obtunding the stimuli and the responses.[40d]

EFFECT OF DIURNAL RHYTHM (TIME OF DAY). Diurnal rhythm affects the analgesic activity of morphine and the hypothalamic control of neuroendocrine activity (endogenous opiates). Morphine has an increasing analgesic effect in the late afternoon and evening and throughout most of the hours of darkness; during the early morning and daylight hours from 4:30 AM to 12:00 noon, there is decreased effect.[41a] Conversely, there is diurnal rhythm to be observed in response to painful stimuli. Some hyperalgesia occurs during the morning hours from 4:30 AM to 12:00 noon and a decreasing response to any stimuli during the period of 12:00 noon to 12:00 midnight. Naloxone effects show a diurnal pattern; i.e., enhancement of the hypersensitivity to pain during the morning hours, and this drug lessens the ability to tolerate pain in the evening and dark hours.[41b]

TOXEMIAS. The function of the thyroid markedly influences metabolic rate, and hence larger doses of depressing drugs can be used. In hyperthyroidism, for instance, the basal metabolic rate usually is markedly elevated, and the pain threshold is lowered.

PAIN. The increase in basal metabolic rate due to pain is a well-known physiologic phenomenon and the increase is directly proportional to the intensity of the pain.

DISEASES. Patients should be evaluated regarding their illnesses and treatment. A patient with a severe chronic infection, as an osteomyelitis, may be rated toxic, in poor nutrition, and with a liver not capable of handling large doses of morphine. Anemic patients fare better when given small doses of opiates or other depressant drugs. In contrast, many patients with chronic diseases, such as tuberculosis or empyema, have often been on extended courses of opium derivatives for sedative purposes; because of this they tolerate morphine and related agents extremely well.

AGENTS. Potency of the anesthetic agent also is a modifying factor. It should be emphasized that the degree of sedation should vary inversely with the potency of the anesthetic agent. One must remember that atropine is a cortical stimulant and raises metabolism somewhat, whereas scopolamine depresses cortical activity.

Adequate premedication is perhaps one of the most important factors in smooth anesthesia, especially for inhalation techniques. Too much will depress respiration and prevent the anesthesia from getting into the blood stream, whereas too little may cause copious secretions and result in an apprehensive patient. It is perhaps better to err on the side of too little. Waters[42] recommends almost no morphine, especially with cyclopropane, and believed that better anesthesia is attained.

GUIDE FOR PREANESTHETIC MEDICATION (ADULTS)

Preanesthetic medication begins with a night sedative. This has a sufficient carry-over time effect to contribute to the morning premedication.

Suggested preanesthetic medications for adults and the dosages are discussed. These should be modified under special circumstances. A variety of agents is available to satisfy most patients' mental and emotional states and avoid undesirable side effects.

As a general rule, increase the dosage for pain, thyrotoxicosis, inappropriate anxiety, and for muscular patients (not for mere fat). Precautions dictating a lowered dose are presented (Table 11–4).

EVENING BEFORE SURGERY. A patient should receive an oral sedative, such as secobarbital or pentobarbital, 50 to 100 mg or amobarbital (125 mg), for a patient in good physical condition under 50 years. Chloral hydrate for patients in fair condition or over 65 years provides physiologic sleep.

A tranquilizer is needed for patients with trait anxiety or extreme apprehension. Of the phenothiazines, promethazine (Phenergan), 25 to 50 mg, is one of the preferred agents with many additional advantages. The benzodiazepines are particularly effective: temazepam (15 to 30 mg); diazepam (Valium) (10 to 50 mg); triazolam is not recommended because of its short period of action and hangover effects. Avoid fluorinated tranquilizers (i.e., fluphenazine; flurazepam) when a fluorinated inhalation anesthetic agent is planned.

MORNING OF SURGERY (PREANESTHETIC). *Time of Administration.* The timing is important in order to obtain full benefit of preanesthetic medication, which should be scheduled as follows:

1. *Sedative or tranquilizer:* 2 hours preoperative IM
2. *Opiate:* 1 hour preoperative IM
3. *Anticholinergic:* 1 hour preoperative IM with the opiate

For emergency or urgent procedures, use IV medication, which should be adjusted intravenously in half dose and slowly, initially, to achieve a satisfactory end point.

SEDATIVES AND TRANQUILIZERS. All patients scheduled for regional or general anesthesia (spinal, caudal, local or nerve blocks) should receive one of the following:

1. A sedative, barbiturate such as sodium amytal (60 to 125 mg), pentobarbital, 50 to 100 mg, (under 60 years of age), or secobarbital, 50 to 100 mg, to provide a state of calmness; or amobarbital, 125 mg *or*
2. A tranquilizer, such as promethazine, 25 to 75 mg, or chlorpromazine, 0.2 mg/kg, 2 hours prior to surgery when patient shows inappropriate anxiety; *or*
3. A benzodiazepine, which is recommended for emotional states, such as lorazepam (2 to 4 mg), midazolam (0.1 mg/kg), tremazepam (15 to 30 mg, single dose), triazolam (0.25 mg, single dose), or diazepam 0.2 mg/kg.

NARCOTIC MORPHINE SULFATE. This may be used for most cases as a preanesthetic agent. In pulmonary disease, however, meperidine is preferred. Doses for patients under 60 years of age, if preceded by a sedative/tranquilizer (halve the dose in patients over 60 years of age) are as follows:

Morphine sulfate: 0.1 mg for each kg up to 25 kg; 0.1 to 0.2 mg/kg over 25 kg
Meperidine: 1 mg/kg; 1 to 1.5 mg for each kg over 25 kg

OUTPATIENT ANESTHESIA AND SURGERY. The use of premedication for anesthesia in patients in the ambulatory surgical setting as opposed to no premedication presents a dilemma. Premedication may prolong recovery and introduce side effects, but anesthesia and surgery without preliminary sedation may be unpleasant for the patient. Raeder[43] has compared the effects of two premedication routines, morphine–scopolamine or intramuscular midazolam, with placebo. Only 3% of patients preferred no premedication, but 80% preferred a combination of an anxiolytic or a tranquilizer. Over 60% of patients preferred premedication by injection. The morphine–scopolamine combination, as well as midazolam injection, were equally effective. More amnesia was noted with midazolam than with morphine–scopolamine. Midazolam was also a more reliable premedicant than diazepam. Recovery of daily functions at home was better than in those patients given a placebo. Additionally, premedication with either midazolam or morphine–scopolamine lessened the amount of anesthesia needed for the surgery.

Unpremedicated patients in an ambulatory surgical center present with anxiety greater than similar inhospital patients and are at considerable risk for aspiration pneumonitis. Gastric pH is less than the critical value of 2.5 in 88% of patients. In many patients, there are levels of 1.5 to 1.8 pH. The volume of gastric contents is also more than 25 ml in 56% of patients. In Manchikanti's studies,[44] premedication with meperidine and phenothiazine was associated with a significant decrease in volume and pH.

The use of a narcotic has been noted to provide significant advantages in preanesthetic medication

TABLE 11–4. PRECAUTIONS IN NARCOTIC PREOPERATIVE MEDICATION

- Infants and elderly
- Debilitated patients
- Presence of intracranial pathology
- Reduced level of consciousness (drug induced or injury)
- Hypovolemia or shock (administer fractional doses intravenously)
- Obstructive lung disease (avoid morphinan derivatives)
- Outpatients (ambulatory surgery)
- When in doubt, reduce dose or do not use a drug

TABLE 11-5. AMBULATORY SURGERY NARCOTIC USE

Controls anxiety
Lowers induction doses
Lowers maintenance doses
Smooth awakening
No prolongation of recovery
Dosage:
    Morphine 50 µg/kg
    Meperidine 0.35 mg/kg
    Fentanyl 0.75 µg/kg
    Sufentanil 0.15 µg/kg
Time:
    Administer IV 30 minutes preinduction

Adapted from Pandit, S.K., and Kothary, S.P.: Should we premedicate ambulatory surgical patients. Anesthesiology, *52*:A352, 1986.

of patients in outpatient surgical anesthesia (Table 11–5).

CLONIDINE IN PREANESTHETIC MEDICATION. Clonidine in oral doses of 5 µg/kg has been shown to be a safe and effective drug to achieve preoperative blood pressure control in mild to moderate hypertension.

The drug also may be administered as part of preanesthetic medication in normotensive patients or given intravenously a few minutes prior to induction. As a preanesthetic medication, it provides many anesthetic advantages:

- The doses of commonly used intravenous induction agents are reduced. The UD_{95} is decreased 15% to 30%. This has been shown by Dundee for thiopental, methohexital, and midazolam.[1,19]
- Reduction of MAC values of inhalation agents occurs.
- About a 40% reduction in isoflurane concentrations has been demonstrated.[45]
- Halothane requirements are lessened experimentally to 40% or more.[46]
- Improved perioperative cardiovascular stability is assured.[45]
- Diminished cardiovascular response to laryngoscopy and intubation, which appears to be superior to either lidocaine[45] or fentanyl pretreatment.
- Reduction in peripheral sympathetic tone is effected.[47]
- A significant reduction in catecholamines occurs, either during rest or exercise.[48]
- Potent analgesic properties have been demonstrated in humans and have been used to produce spinal and epidural analgesia.[49,50]
- In narcotic-based anesthetic techniques, the dose requirements are reduced, as in patients undergoing coronary artery bypass surgery. A total dose of either 200 or 300 µg orally 90 minutes before arrival in the operating room is effective.[51]
- Shivering in the operative and postoperative period is significantly curtailed.[51]
- Bronchospastic responses to noxious stimuli are inhibited.[52]
- Nicotine addiction (smokers): The role of clonidine in heavy smokers for reducing their nicotine dependence and craving has been reported.[53] Thus, smokers who are scheduled for surgery may have an amelioration of their urges when a small oral dose of clonidine is provided preanesthetically or the evening before surgery.
- Sympathoadrenal stress responses are readily obtunded. This is especially advantageous in patients with coronary artery disease. Adrenaline and noradrenaline plasma levels are lowered throughout surgery and for 3 hours postoperatively. On the other hand, growth hormone vasopressin and cortisol levels are not changed.[54]
- A base is provided for producing smooth controlled hypotension, as with isoflurane-induced hypotension, at lower inspired concentrations (2% versus 3%).[55]

Mechanism of Action. Clonidine is a central-acting alpha$_2$-adrenergic agonist, which induces an inhibitory action on central dopaminergic systems. There is suppression of central noradrenergic action with a reduced sympathetic outflow to the peripheral system. In addition, there is a balanced central control of the cardiovascular system, modulation of sleep/wake cycle, diminished cortical arousal, and decreased nociception.

PARENTERAL DRUG ADMINISTRATION METHODOLOGY

The parenteral administration of medications rests on the use of a syringe and a needle. The development of these two tools is of historical interest.

The syringe was born in the concept of the piston and cylinder, which originated with a Greek, Ktesibios, in Alexandria, Egypt, about 200 B.C. He was a barber's son and was acknowledged as one of the greatest engineers of antiquity. The first application of this concept to a syringe is noted in Heron's "pneumatics" about 100 B.C.[56] The instrument was used primarily for sucking pus out of wounds and, hence, named *pyulkos* (Greek) or *pyulcus* (Latin), or pus puller, but it was also used for injecting liquids. It is noted that the Egyptians were giving themselves enemas before the Alexandrian syringe was invented. Their clyster kit probably consisted of a tube, an animal bladder, and a string, an assembly which did its job well into the 19th century.[57] In 1851, Charles Pravez developed a modern type syringe, which he described in 1853.[58] In 1845, however, F. Rynd of Dublin had already developed a similar syringe.[59]

Needles have a separate story. The first hollow needles were quills and were used in 1656 by Sir Christopher Wren to inject fluids intravenously into animals. In 1836, Lafargue successfully deadened pain by pressing morphine paste subcutaneously through a vaccination lance cut. Thereafter, others found new ways of introducing morphine and other drugs into the body. Taylor and Washington, in New York, practiced hypodermic medications by first puncturing the skin with a lancet and then forcing a solution of morphine under the skin with an eye syringe.

HYPODERMIC INJECTION. The major advance came when the Scottish physician, Alexander Wood,[60] in 1853 devised a metallic, hollow needle and introduced the technique of hypodermic medication. About this time, Pravez attached the hollow needle to his syringe. Wood intended his procedure as a means to relieve pain of neuralgia by injecting morphine at the site of pain, presumably to anesthetize the peripheral nerves. However, Charles Hunter, a London surgeon, had already realized in 1856 that it was not necessary to inject into the painful area. His conclusion that the effect of hypodermic injection was general and not local seems obvious today but was revolutionary in the 19th century.[61]

ROUTES OF ADMINISTRATION. In the parenteral administration of drugs, it is important to consider the route of administration of the drug, the site of injection, and the timing of optimal effects.

In the healthy patient with good circulation, the subcutaneous or intramuscular route is satisfactory and can be accomplished by nursing personnel.

Suitable sites for relatively safe intramuscular injection include the gluteal muscles, the vastus lateralis, and the deltoid muscle. These are recommended to avoid injury to nerves and to muscles.

INTRAMUSCULAR INJECTION TECHNIQUE. The intramuscular route for injection of drugs is the most important and frequently used route for administering drugs next to the intravenous route. By this route, a drug is exposed to a rich capillary bed, and absorption is rapid and dependable in the normal patient (not vasoconstricted). Improper technique, however, involves the risk of neural damage to the sciatic nerve, especially in infants.[62] Skin fragments may be introduced into deeper tissue, or muscle damage may occur.[63] Therefore, the site of injection is important.[64]

Fundamental Principles. The point of injection should be as far from major nerves and vessels as possible. In addition, the muscular bed selected should have a mass large enough to accommodate significant volumes of fluid. The needle used should be of sufficient length to deposit the solution into the muscle bed; and the needle should be sharp, without burrs, and introduced quickly to make the procedure as painless as possible.[65]

Sites for Intramuscular Injection. Considering the above factors, three suitable muscular areas are available: the gluteal muscle mass, the vastus lateralis, and the deltoid.

Gluteal Area (Fig. 11–2). This is the most frequently used site for intramuscular injection. Topographically, the gluteal area takes in the entire space overlying the three glutei muscles. It extends from the entire iliac crest downward to the crease of the buttocks (lower margin of gluteus maximus). The entire area can be divided into quadrants by a perpendicular line from the peak of the iliac crest and a horizontal line through the greater trochanter. Only the upper outer quadrant, with the anterior superior iliac spine representing the upper outer landmark, should be used. This is the correct classic site. Neither the "buttock" nor the "cheek" should be equated with the gluteal muscle mass used for injection. The lateral or Sims position with the patient relaxed is desirable.

Hanson* recommends that needles should be inserted anterior and superior to a line drawn from the posterosuperior iliac spine to the greater trochanter (Fig. 11-3). This line is parallel to and lateral to the course to the sciatic nerve.

Hochstetter† recommends that the ventrogluteal area overlying the gluteus medius muscle be used. It is located just below the iliac crest and extends from the midpoint forward to the anterior superior iliac spine (Fig. 11–4). It is farthest from both major nerves and large vessels. The skin is thinner than over the remainder of the gluteal area and appears to be less sensitive. The subcutaneous fat is less and the muscle bed is thick. Special positioning of the patient is not required, and the muscle is easily relaxed.

Vastus Lateralis Muscle Site The midline of the lateral thigh is the preferred site for intramuscular injection of infants and children. The area is a narrow band extending a few fingerbreadths below the greater trochanter to a line a similar distance above the knee. This overlies the vastus lateralis muscle, which is a thick muscle. There are no major vessels or nerves in this region, and the skin is minimally sensitive. A significant volume of fluid can be accommodated at each injection, and the area can be used several times. The midanterior site over the quadriceps also has been used effectively.

Deltoid Muscle The midportion of this muscle is readily accessible. The topographical site is a small, bulging area on the lateral surface of the upper third of the arm located below the acromion and above the insertion of the deltoid muscle in the tuberosity of the humerus (2 fingerbreadths).

---

* Hanson, D.J.: Personal communication, 1976.

† Hochstetter, H.: Personal communication, 1970.

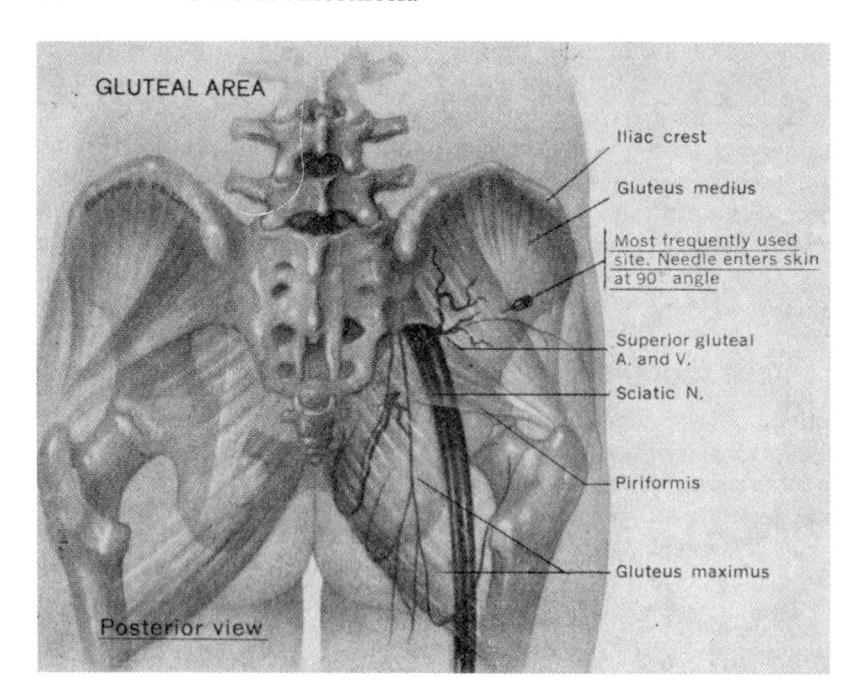

FIG. 11–2. Gluteal area used for intramuscular injections. Courtesy of Abbott Laboratories.

Complications of Intramuscular Injection. Intramuscular injections produce various local effects and complications. These include sterile abscess formation, infection, pain and, in certain sites, nerve damage. Hematomas are not infrequent.

Muscle injury usually occurs and the activity of serum creatine phosphokinase (CPK) increases. In a human study of intramuscular injection, increases are directly related to the concentration of a drug, osmolality of the injected solution, and volume of the diluent solution.[66] CPK activity may increase maximally by 60 to 120 mU/ml of serum over the normal range of 82 mU/ml.

THE INTRAVENOUS ROUTE. The intravenous route provides significant advantages for the administration of medications prior to anesthesia. It is recommended when the patient is in a state of vasoconstriction or circulation is impaired. The medication can be administered intravenously by the anesthesiologist in the operating theater or in an adjacent holding area. This procedure provides assurance that the drugs enter the circulation.

Careful venipuncture technique is important.

FIG. 11–3. *A* and *A'*: Lines representing boundaries used in classic method. *B*: Line demonstrating ease with which misplacement of boundary can expose sciatic nerve to injection. *C*: Recommended modification: any injection lateral and superior to this line will be well away from the sciatic nerve. Courtesy of D.J. Hanson, M.D.

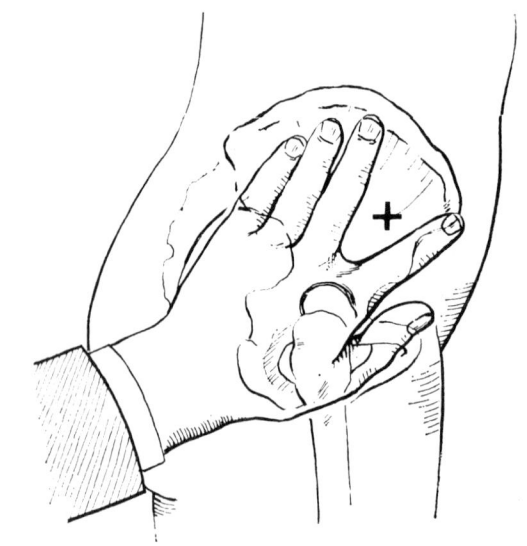

FIG. 11–4. The injection is made between the index and middle fingers, spread as far as possible, forming a "V." Courtesy of H. Hochstetter, Abbott Laboratories.

Large hollow needles (no stylet) may biopsy skin fragments (69%) or core portions of a vessel wall.[67] When the usual veins are inaccessible, the intraglossal or subglossal site is an alternative route and provides rapid induction of drug solutions into the circulation.

Technique of Venipuncture. *Selection of Suitable Veins*[68] The procedure should be carried out using a suitable vein away from the area of surgery and away from infections.

Evaluate all the veins available and select the best. To some extent, suitable veins depend on age and habitus of the patient. Usually the veins of the antecubital fossa and on the forearm are easily accessible: these are the median basilic and the median cephalic. A vein that is to be used repeatedly may be outlined with a dye.

Other veins that should be investigated include the following:

1. Veins on dorsum of hand
2. Radial vein of wrist—large and invariably present
3. Saphenous vein
4. Scalp veins in infants

For occasional single intravenous injections of drugs or the obtaining of blood one may use the external jugular, the internal jugular, the femoral, and the superficial temporal vein. The sagittal sinus and veins of the scalp are also useful and are particularly adaptable in infants and children. An apparatus for immobilization of head for scalp transfusions and an efficient method of immobilizing the leg for saphenous vein transfusions have been described.[69]

Developing Veins Gentle friction or slapping the area of a vein will often dilate the vein. Hot compresses are helpful in causing venous dilatation; these should be applied so as to include the entire extremity below the site of venipuncture and well above. Mere application to site of puncture is unphysiologic.

Small veins may be punctured with a large needle by first introducing a small hypodermic needle into the vein and then distending the vein with normal saline solution; then a 19- or 18-gauge needle may be introduced into the vein. The tourniquet remains applied throughout the procedure of introducing the small needle, the injection of saline, and the introduction of the large neede.

Introduction of Needle[70] Select vein. Prepare skin with alcohol or other antiseptic. (If a colored antiseptic such as povidone-iodine is used, remove excess after completion of procedure.)

Apply tourniquet.

Select needle of a size as large as vein will accept and insert needle as follows:

Principles of Preanesthetic Medication **295**

1. Pierce the skin to the side of the vein.
2. Immobilize the vein by drawing the skin taut below the site of penetration of vein. With bevel of needle toward vein, pick up the superficial adventitia of vein.
3. Introduce needle through the wall. When bevel of needle is facing away from vein, hematomas are prone to occur as shown in Figure 11–5A. Correct position of needle is seen in Figure 11–5B. Insert nearly two thirds of needle shaft for better security.

Cut-down A cut-down may be done when veins are thrombosed, collapsed, or inaccessible. The technique consists in making a transverse incision across the area where a vein is usually found. The tissues around the vein are dissected away bluntly and the vein mobilized over an area of about 1 inch. Silk ligatures are placed above and below the area in the vein to be entered. The vein is then nicked, a cannula inserted, and the superior ligature tightened around the cannula; the lower ligature is tightened about the vein.

Increasing Fluid Flow of Intravenous Systems[71] The rate of flow through standard guage needles depends on the bore of the needle and the "head of fluid pressure." The actual flow rate can be mathematically expressed in Poiseuille's Law (see below).

1. *Size of needle*—In practice the following observations have been made: when the increment in bore of a needle is 2 times, i.e., an 18-gauge needle compared to a 22-gauge needle, increment in flow is 7 times; when the increment in bore is 3.4 times, i.e., a 15-guage needle compared to a 22-gauge needle, the increment in flow is 16 times. An increment in bore of 4.4 times, as when a 13-gauge needle is compared to a 22-gauge needle, the increment in blood flow is 18 times. It is readily apparent from these few observations that a gauge 15, 16, or 17 will give optimum results.
2. *Positive pressure*—According to Poiseuille's Law, and from experimental observations, pressure on a fluid system increases the flow linearly and roughly in proportion to the increment in pressure.[72] Using a 20-gauge needle, blood will flow at a rate of about 14 ml/min at 50 mm Hg pressure; if pressure is increased to 200 mm Hg or quadrupled, the flow is only about 30 ml/min.
3. *Increase gravity effect*—Raising the distance of fluid container above level of arm will increase flow rate. If a transfusion is set up with a 17-gauge needle at a height of 4.5 feet, 600 ml of blood will be administered in approximately 10 minutes, while at a height of 7 feet it will take 6 minutes.[72]
4. *Several sites* of introduction of fluids.[73]
5. Use of tubing roller or *stripper*.[68]

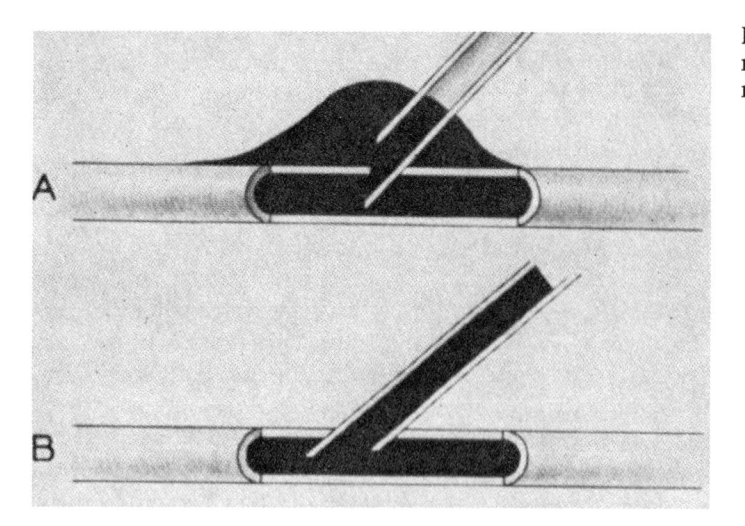

FIG. 11–5. *A.* The incorrect introduction of a needle into a vein and hematoma formation. *B.* Correct introduction. From Lundy[68] and Adams[70].

6. The *introduction of saline solution* into the circulation also has a dilatory effect and helps to release spasm. Hence, an initial administration of normal saline solution may facilitate the administration of whole blood. A Y-shaped glass connector may be used: through one arm, balanced Ringer's solution is introduced and through the other, blood is allowed to flow.
7. *Procaine infiltration* about the site of needle placement will relieve vessel spasm.

INTRAVENOUS INFUSION PRACTICES. Infusion therapy, or access infusions, required for monitoring may be complicated by a local infection about the needle or catheter wound. Phlebitis, bacteremia, and septicemia have been reported.[74]

Because bacteremia and septicemia most often begin as a local infection about a catheter (contaminated infusion solutions, when properly used, are a rare source of bacteremia) they are related to the cutaneous flora of the patient.[75] Therefore, it becomes important to provide effective antisepsis before insertion of a needle or catheter intravenously.[76]

Risk factors associated with catheter-related infections, and particularly predictive of septicemia, are as follows:[76,77]

- Colonization at the site of intravascular puncture
- Contamination of the needle or catheter hub
- Moisture or blood that accumulates beneath the dressing
- Duration of catheter placement

Recommendation for Infection Control.[78] The following guidelines are from the Centers for Disease Control (CDC):

1. The operator should perform a short scrub before handling intravascular catheter sets and proceeding with the venous invasion.
2. Careful and thorough skin antisepsis should be practiced.
3. Administration sets and catheters together should be changed every 48 hours.[77] This is accompanied by a low rate of fluid contamination of only 0.8%. A 72-hour change schedule has a rate of 1.5% contamination; however, the contaminant concentration is low. Coagulase-negative staphylococci have been found exclusively. Because a 72-hour schedule is cost effective, it appears that this interval can be safely followed.[77]
4. A 24-hour and up to 48-hour schedule is recommended for therapy with blood products or lipid emulsions. This schedule is also recommended for arterial catheters used for monitoring.
5. The use of Teflon catheters is much safer than polyvinylchloride or polyethylene catheters. The latter have been associated with a 2% to 5% risk of bacteremia when in place for 48 hours. It is noted that Teflon catheters are resistant to microbial adherence.[79]
6. Contamination at the needle and catheter hub occurs in 20% to 25% of patients when the access wound is examined.
7. The dressing over the catheter and puncture site may either be a sterile gauze covering or a transparent polyurethane dressing.[77] The dressing should provide an inclusive coverage. Less moisture has been noted to accumulate under a simple sterile gauze dressing.

Inflammation at the site of intravenous access is relatively high. Swelling, tenderness, and erythema are noted. This occurs in approximately half of the intravenous sites. Phlebitis is likewise high and is defined as the existence of one or more of the inflammatory signs mentioned. The incidence is approximately 10% of patients. Under the procedure recommended, the inflammation did not progress and was relatively mild. Most wounds can be treated by simple measures of local cleansing and antiseptic care. In the study by Maki, only 5 patients in more than 2000 showed bacteremia.[77]

ALTERNATIVE ROUTES OF DRUG ADMINISTRATION FOR PREMEDICATION

Alternative routes of administration that can be used effectively are Transbuccal instillation; Nasal instillation; Transdermal application; Rectal instillation; and Alternative Intravascular techniques.

TRANSBUCCAL MUCOSAL ABSORPTION

- Morphine[80,81]
  - Tablet of 10 mg in an absorbable packet;[80] peak effect between 1 and 2 hours
  - *Location:* May be sublingual, in upper buccal sulcus. On mucosa of gum, above the gingival margin, not a good site for solubilization.
  - Comparison with IM:[81] IM more profound, more rapid onset; level of anxiety less; variability and slower plasma decay.[82]
- Sublingual buprenorphine:[83,84] Increases salivation.
- Lollipop sucking
  - Morphine sulfate lollipop[85]
  - Fentanyl lollipop[86]

Buccal absorption shows significant variability. Patients experience a bitter taste and experience interference with taste postoperatively.

Lollipop Preparations. Morphine sulfate has been successfully used in lollipops. The drug was suspended in a candy mixture and then formed into lollipops. The lollipops were flavored as peppermint 5 mg (green color) or 10 mg in a lemon-flavored (yellow) pop (1-inch diameter) or lemon flavored with a red coloring. Children were provided with the lollipop when readied for the operating room suite. Children under 4 years usually received the 5 mg pop and older children received the 10 mg pop.[85a] It is considered that the children swallowed a variable portion of the lollipop. In most instances, only half of the pop was used. Most of the children were allowed to finish the lollipop before the start of anesthesia.

Fentanyl has been incorporated in a candy matrix, in amounts ranging from 200 to 1000 μg fentanyl citrate.[86b] Children were provided a lollipop in a holding area and allowed sufficient time to consume the lollipop. The effects were dose related. The optimal sedative dose was determined to be in children consuming 15 to 20 μg/kg. This dose also had minimal side effects.[86b] Onset of sedation was rapid, occurring in 5 to 20 minutes and was accompanied by an itchy nose or eye. Some increased gastric volume occurs, but nausea and vomiting are infrequent.

NASAL INSTILLATION. The nasal mucosa is a rich vascular area and provides the following advantages for drug administration:[89]

- Rapid absorption directly into the systemic circulation.
- The absorbed drugs do not pass through the portal circulation and, hence, are not immediately subject to hepatic clearance.
- The route is particularly agreeable to preschool children.
- Absorption and action are dependable.

In contrast, the oral and rectal routes are denoted by slow onset, some unpredictability, and delayed recovery.

Medication can be administered via a 1- or 3-ml syringe without the presence of a needle, by a nasal spray, or by drops. Children can be held in the parent's or nurse's arms during the instillation.

Preanesthetic Sedation. Midazolam has been found to be an excellent sedative medication for children when administered by the intramuscular route but is accompanied by discomfort.[90] As a water-soluble agent it lends itself to rapid absorption from the nasal mucosa with an onset of action within 5 minutes. The drug is prepared in a concentration of 1 mg/ml and administered in doses of 0.2 mg/5 kg (a volume of 0.2 ml/5 kg. Larger doses do not offer any improved sedation and result in more sneezing and coughing. Administration of midazolam by this route not only has great acceptability by children but has been found to be an effective anxiolytic and sedative. Few instances of agitation occur on inhalation induction in contrast with over 60% excitement in unpremedicated children.[91] There is less retching and vomiting (17%) than with other sedative medications. Recovery is rapid.

Preanesthetic Opiates. Opiate solutions may be instilled nasally. A sufentanil solution when instilled by a syringe, nasal spray, or nose drops is effective. A spray solution containing 50 μg/ml is an effective preparation; one puff provides 0.1 ml or 5 μg from a standard spray unit. The nose-drop preparation contains 2.5 μg/drop. In the spray technique the patient should be upright or sitting, whereas in the nose-drop administration the patient should have the head tilted back or be in the supine position. Two puffs of a spray provides 10 μg and is effective, with a rapid onset of sedation, which continues for 50 minutes after administration. The effect decreases after 60 minutes. A larger dose (4 puffs equals 20 μg) appears not to improve the effect. The drop-dose selected is 1 drop (2.5 μg) per 10 kg; 6 drops, 3 in each nostril, provides a dose of 15 μg.

The onset of action has been found to be more rapid than an IM injection. There is relative freedom from the side effects of opioids.

Infants and children scheduled for elective surgery have been premedicated in a preoperative holding area with intranasal sufentanil before induction of anesthesia.[88] The dose recommended is 1.5 to 3 μg/kg (0.03 to 0.06 μg/ml/kg) of an undiluted solution of 50 μg/ml. The lower dose enables the anesthesiologist to separate infants from parents, usually at the end of 4 minutes, but by 10 minutes at the latest.

TRANSDERMAL INSTILLATION.[92,93] Many drugs can be administered by dermal application with local effect on absorption into the circulation for a systemic effect. Dermal application in various ointments and pastes of local anesthetic is used to provide local anesthesia, without needle injection, to prepare a site for venipuncture, especially in children.[94] A cream containing a combination of lidocaine and prilocaine has been successfully applied to the forearm of children prior to venipuncture. Mucosal application of local anesthetic is widely used in dentistry at the site of insertion of needle for subsequent alveolar block (mandibular/maxillary block) to produce surface anesthesia. Mucosal application of local anesthetic to the anorectal area can provide analgesia, i.e., hemorrhoids. Application of local anesthetic in gels or lubricants is used to provide mucosal anesthesia of the urethra.

For systemic absorption, the following drugs have been successfully used in transdermal preparations: scopolamine,[95] fentanyl,[96] nitroglycerine,[97] clonidine,[98] estrogens.[99]

These drugs are usually incorporated into an impermeable plastic adhesive skin patch containing the drug in a sealed reservoir from which the drug seeps out gradually. Such patches are applied to a hair-free skin area on the upper chest. With fentanyl (TTS System, Alza Corp., Sheffield, England), the absorption rate is slow, and at least 2 hours are necessary for a significant blood level to be attained.

RECTAL ADMINISTRATION

- Seconal or pentobarbital capsules have provided rectal sedation in children. Piercing the ends of 100 to 200-mg capsules and inserting rectally will provide sedation.[100]
- Methohexitone is used rectally to provide a basal state of unconsciousness. The dose for this purpose is 25 mg/kg prepared as a 10% solution in sterile distilled water.[101] The time to sleep is between 6 and 12 minutes. Half of this dose will provide good sedation without sleep in the same period.
- Diazepam 1 hour preanesthesia, in doses of 0.75 mg/kg of body weight, has been used and provides anxiolysis and freedom from agitation.[102] Compared to an intramuscular lytic cocktail, however, it is less effective in reducing gastric acidity or gastric volume or providing an antiemetic effect.[103,104]
- Morphine in a polyethylene oxide hydrogel has been formulated as a suppository to provide an initial burst of 6 to 10 mg, followed by sustained release over 12 hours.[105] This has been useful for postoperative pain but inadequate and too slow in onset for preanesthetic medication.

Rectal administration of medication is not accepted well by most children.

BONE MARROW INFUSIONS. The bone marrow route is just another portal of entry for parenteral fluids. Tocantins, a hematologist in Philadelphia, after obtaining marrow for study, injected the saline and could not retrieve the saline.[106] Experimentally, dyes injected into the marrow cavity could be found in systemic circulation within minutes. He proceeded to demonstrate that the bone marrow is a good route for parenteral fluids in human patients and published his first paper in 1940.[107] In 1941 Tocantins and O'Neill[108] reported on 52 administrations of various fluids via bone marrow. Papper[108] studied the rate of absorption of material from sternal marrow into general circulation. The tests indicated that absorption may be more rapid than by vein.

Indications.[109,110] Bone marrow infusions should be considered for situations in which the veins are simply inaccessible because of burns, profound shock, anasarca, or thrombosis. This route is useful in excited and delirious patients; it is indicated for patients who are to be transported and require parenteral fluids. It is an excellent route for the administration of fluids to infants and children who are to undergo extensive surgery.[111]

Pertinent Anatomy. The site of choice for marrow injection is the sternum for adult and tibia for infants and children. Near the junction of the manubrium and the gladiolus (corpus sterni), the thickness of the sternum from anterior periosteum to posterior periosteum is 3 cm. This junction is at the level of the second costal cartilage. One should be aware of the profusion of veins beside the sternum as well as the internal mammary artery.

The requirements of a good portal of entry for the injection of fluid are accessibility, rapid absorption, and no untoward effects. The sternum is subcutaneous; the anterior plate is thin, compact, and relatively easy to pierce with a needle. Because of an ample spongy marrow and rich venous drainage, absorption into general circulation is rapid.

Technique of Needle Placement. Introduction of a needle for marrow infusions is accomplished at the lower end of the manubrium or upper portion of the body (gladiolus or corpus sterni). The skin and the anterior periosteum are infiltrated with 1% procaine and an 18-gauge needle 1 inch long with stylet is inserted at a 30-degree angle cephalad using a *rotary, pushing motion*. A sudden "give" indicates entrance into the marrow cavity. Marrow can be aspirated and usually the patient will complain. The needle is secured with proper placement of gauze squares and packs. Fluids are administered by gravity—any greater force is uncomfortable.

Introduction of the needle into the tibia is usually accomplished on the anteromedial aspect of the tibia. One should direct the needle away from the knee joint.

Errors and Complications.[112] A common error is to insufficiently insert the needle into the marrow cavity with the result that the fluids are injected subcutaneously.

Introduction of the needle too vigorously may result in perforation of posterior plate and entering the great veins on the heart. This is of little consequence if recognized; however, one may also enter the mediastinum or the pleural cavity, which is serious.

Osteomyelitis occasionally occurs and is dangerous.

In tibial marrow infusions, one must not introduce the needle too close to the knee joint nor should the needle be directed toward the knee joint. Injury to the epiphysis may result.

Materials Injected. Any fluids or solutions that can be given by vein may be given via the marrow cavity. Such fluids as crystalloid solutions (saline, dextrose), and plasma are easily infused. Blood enters but more slowly. Drugs such as pentothal in solution may be so administered. It is generally best to avoid the injection of irritating solutions.

TECHNIQUES FOR MISCELLANEOUS ROUTES. ***Internal Jugular Vein.*** Puncture of this vein is performed by selecting the midpoint between tip of mastoid and angle of mandible. Needle is inserted perpendicular to the skin at this point while withdrawing on plunger to exert a negative pressure.

Intracardiac.[113] This route has been utilized as a desperate route. The technique as described consists in the insertion of a 7- to 8-cm needle into the lower part of the fourth intercostal space approximately 2.5 to 3 cm to the left of the left sternal margin. This results in placement of needle in the left ventricle. Blood is then injected by syringe or by pressure transfusion apparatus.

Intraaortic.[114–117] Administration of blood into the aorta is feasible during intrathoracic surgery. With the chest open, the aorta is readily exposed and the surgeon merely inserts a sterile, large-gauge (18) needle into the vessel. In a sense this is a modified intra-arterial transfusion. The blood is given under pressure.

Corpora Cavernosa.[118,119] The extensive venous spaces of the penile corpora have been used as an avenue for transfusion as well as regional penile anesthesia. A needle is inserted by quick stab just lateral to midline of shaft. Blood is administered under pressure.

Femoral Vein.[120,121] Administration is accomplished as follows: The skin of the groin adjacent to the inguinal ligament is prepared with an antiseptic solution. The area of the groin is palpated for the pulsation of the femoral artery and the large common femoral vein is located adjacent to the artery on the medial side at or just above the inguinal ligament. A two and one-half inch long 20 gauge needle with a short bevel with an attached syringe is introduced through the skin and perpendicular to the leg just medial to the artery. The needle is advanced until dark venous blood is observed usually at a depth of 2.0–3.5 cm. The needle is then secured usually with a Kelly forceps applied to the needle at the skin level. A catheter can be introduced if a larger needle is employed.

Cord Transfusions.[122,123] These can be given through the umbilical vein and may be accomplished in utero or at the time of delivery. The reader is referred to the articles cited for details of the procedure.

PREANESTHETIC MEDICATION IN PEDIATRICS

That infants and children are without significant apprehension or fear and that they can be quickly anesthetized with an inhalation agent without prior sedation (or needle stick) is a fallacious and unreasonable concept.[124–128]

Coté has shown that unpremedicated children are at significant risk of vomiting and aspiration of gastric juice of hazardous composition. In 95% of the children, the pH values were below 2.5, and in 76% of the children the gastric volumes exceeded 0.4 ml/kg. Premedication has been shown to minimize this risk.[104,129,130]

Catecholamines are significantly increased in children. On entering a hospital, the levels are usually elevated (often used as the control levels) and are further elevated on being taken into the operating theater[131] unless properly managed by psychologic measures or premedication.[131]

The principles and objectives of premedication in pediatric patients are the same as those for adults:

1. Reduce apprehension and fear, anxiety, agitation; increase cooperation; and permit easy separation from parents.
2. Control catecholamines and stress response.
3. Control gastric acidity and volume.
4. Reduce metabolic requirements.
5. Reduce the anesthetic dose requirements.
6. Achieve rapid recovery by avoiding overdose.
7. Monitor throughout the period of drug action (especially newborns and infants).

MEDICATION PROGRAMS.[127] Three general approaches to the preanesthetic management of children have emerged: (1) basal hypnosis; (2) moderate sedation and narcosis; and (3) no medication.

Basal Hypnosis. Basal hypnosis is defined as the production of sleep equivalent to the second stage of general anesthesia. This can be accomplished either by rectal instillation of drugs or by intramuscular injection. Several drugs are used rectally (this route avoids the use of needles or mask):

1. Barbiturates: Thiopental (20 to 30 mg/kg), methohexital (10 to 15 mg/kg), and secobarbital (seconal) (5 to 10 mg/kg) have been employed.
2. Classically, rectal tribromethanol (Avertin) was used for basal hypnosis.
3. Diazepam: 0.75 mg/kg of body weight.

The major disadvantages of this method include: (1) the rectal instillation is distasteful and uncomfortable and is resisted by children; (2) it is essentially the induction stage of anesthesia and should be carried out by the anesthesiologist; (3) absorption of the drugs is variable; (4) the administration is usually made 10–15 minutes before the establishment of the anesthetic state. Hence, a child may be waiting a considerable period of time after awakening, held NPO and without any sedation, thus permitting thirst and apprehension to develop.

Basal hypnosis can also be achieved more satisfactorily and effectively by intramuscular injection. Two drugs have been employed: (1) midazolam—dosage 0.1 mg/kg (diazepam has been used, but the pain and burning are unacceptable); and (2) ketamine—dosage 3 to 5 mg/kg of body weight. When sleep is obtained, a dose of an anticholinergic should be given. Scopolamine or glycopyrrolate may be mixed with the ketamine and a single injection of the two drugs achieved. These intramuscular injections are best administered 10 to 15 minutes before induction of anesthesia.

Moderate Medication. [124,125] This has been the standard approach since Waters' classic report in 1936 on pediatric medication and the tabulation of medication by Leigh and Belton in 1946. It is a widely used and effective approach for allaying emotional turmoil and fear responses in children. Crying is controlled and a postoperative psychic trauma minimized. The stress responses of the autonomic nervous system are reduced. The objective is to achieve a calmness and acquiescence and a state of somnolence without depression.[126,127]

Medication is usually accomplished in two time stages, with a sedative or tranquilizer administered first, followed by a narcotic 30 minutes later. The barbiturates are the foundation of sedative medication in children. Most children do not manifest a trait or neurotic anxiety. Their apprehension and fear stems from the medical hospital situation and the strangeness of their environment. This hospital environment for most, including adults, is a strange one and a strange experience. In general, the apprehension of children can be designated as situational anxiety and can be alleviated by sedatives. Occasionally, tranquilizers are necessary, as when a neurotic type of anxiety is identified or extreme agitation is manifest.

Hypnotics A sedative, such as secobarbital or pentobarbital, may be administered to healthy, normal children after 6 months of age to control restlessness and fear. The rectal route is a common avenue of pentobarbital or secobarbital administration in children up to the age of 5 years.[104,132] The oral administration is acceptable by children and preferable thereafter. The dosage of these barbiturates must be individualized and based on a lean body mass.

Oral pentobarbital or secobarbital in capsules at doses of 1 mg/kg or promethazine in doses of 1 mg/kg in a syrup form have been singularly satisfactory. Elixir of phenobarbital provides excellent sedation in infants.

The nonbarbiturate tranquilizers for oral use have not been found satisfactory in general for children. The drugs that have been studied include most of the phenothiazines, hydroxyzine, meprobamate, and benzodiazepines.

Sedatives are usually given approximately 60 minutes before the time of administration of anesthesia. The narcotic is then administered 30 to 45 minutes before the time of operation or on call, if there is any question of delay. It is important that at least a 30- to 60-minute interval occur between the administration of the sedative and the administration of any narcotics.

For children who are scheduled to be operated on late in the morning or early afternoon, the sedative should be administered early in the morning at about 9:00 A.M., or when considered optimal, but a narcotic is administered on call at approximately 30 minutes before the time of induction of anesthesia.

Narcotics[133] The advantages of adequate preanesthetic medication using the narcotics, with or without a prior sedative, far outweigh any advantages. It is also probably the most predictable and dependable technique of preanesthetic medication for children, based on widespread experience. A single needlestick in the nursery or in the presence of a cuddling parent is less traumatic than transportation of an unsedated child to an operating theatre and the application of the mask or the surreptitious gravity administration of a flow of inhalation agents over the face.

In addition to producing a calm, sleepy child, the narcotic drug also enhances the ease of induction and lowers the MAC value of the potent inhalation volatile agents. Narcotic premedication obtunds crying and agitation and reduces apprehension and reflex excitability. There is a checking of the rapid, exhaustive respiratory rates seen in anxious children.

Hypnotic–Narcotic Dosage Dosage must be guided by physiologic age and lean body mass. The dosages presented in Table 11–6 are for the average well-developed child. Increases or reductions are necessary by medical modifying factors, notably debility, obesity, mental retardation, physical anomalies, hyperactivity, and various disease states.[127]

Tranquilizers With the exception of midazolam, nonbarbiturate drugs have not provided the type of calmness or control of apprehension that is desired. Most children do not manifest a trait or neurotic anxiety, where the tranquilizers have their benefits in the adult. The apprehension and fear exhibited by children stems from the medical and hospital situation. Hence, it is noted as situational anxiety because of the strange environment or experience. In general, the apprehension of children can be alleviated by the sedatives, and only rarely are tranquilizers necessary. Both major and minor tranquilizers have been disappointing. Among the drugs that have proven to be less than effective include meprobamate, glutethimide, hydroxyzine, and most of the phenothiazines.[127,134]

Of singular value has been the use of intramuscular ketamine to produce a moderate state of somnolence. In doses of 4 mg/kg of body weight, ketamine is capable of producing an excellent state of sleep without depression and at the same time provide significant analgesia. As a result, invasive techniques may be carried out, including intravenous, without the occurrence of struggling or withdrawal movements.

MIDAZOLAM PREANESTHETIC MEDICATIONS.[135] Intramuscular midazolam is an excellent sedative–tranquilizer agent for pediatric preanesthetic medication. It has been found effective at all age levels, especially young children in the 1 to 5-year age group, who are usually more apprehensive and less cooperative.[136] With midazolam premedication, there is an increasing level of sedation as the age of patients increases; in this regard, children can be divided into three age groups: (1) 1 to 5 years; (2) 6 to 10 years; and (3) 10 to 15 years. All patients are more drowsy than with other sedative agents.[137] Midazolam, however, is a sedative tranquilizer, not a narcotic, and does not provide pain obtundation.

The recommended intramuscular dose has been determined to be between 50 and 100 μg/kg of body weight in children,[135] with an average of approximately 80 μg/kg. This average dose has been associated with the following advantages: a smoother inhalation induction of anesthesia, a lower concentration of halothane and other volatile agents, and

TABLE 11–6. PREANESTHESIA MEDICATION SCHEDULE*

Age	Average Weight (kg)	Pentobarbital†‡ (mg)	Morphine§ (mg)	Atropine (mg)	Glycopyrrolate (mg)	Demerol (mg)
Newborn	3	—	—	0.15	0.1	—
6 mo	8.1	30 Rectal	0.5	0.15	0.1	5
1 yr	10.6	45 Rectal	1	0.2	0.1	10
2 yr	14	60 Rectal	1.5	0.3	0.15	15
3 yr	15	60 Rectal	2	0.3	0.15	15
4 yr	17	90 Rectal	3	0.3	0.15	20
5 yr	19	90 Rectal	3	0.3	0.15	20
6 yr	22	90 Rectal	4	0.4	0.2	20
7 yr	25	90 Rectal	5	0.4	0.2	25
8 yr	28	100 Oral	5	0.4	0.2	25
9 yr	31	100 Oral	5	0.4	0.2	30
10 yr	35	100 Oral	6	0.4	0.2	40
11 yr	40	100 Oral	6	0.4	0.2	40
12 yr	45	100 Oral	6	0.4	0.2	50
13 yr	50	100 Oral	8	0.4	0.25	50
14 yr	55	100 Oral	8	0.4	0.25	60
15 yr	58	100 Oral	8	0.4	0.25	60
16 yr	60	100 Oral	8	0.4	0.25	70

* This table is a guide to be followed for average, well-developed patients. Increases or reductions in medication must be made for patients who do not fall in this category, i.e., hyperactive, obese, or poor-risk patients.

† Pentobarbital (Nembutal) should be given at least 60 minutes before surgery.

‡ Suggested guide for pentobarbital when followed by morphine is 4 mg/kg for rectal use (maximum 120 mg) and 3 mg/kg for oral use (maximum 100 mg).

§ Morphine should be given 30 to 45 minutes (IM or SC) before anesthetic induction. Suggested guide for morphine is 0.75 mg/yr of age.

Adapted from Smith, R.M.: Anesthesia for Infants and Children, 4th ed. St. Louis, C.V. Mosby, 1980.

a shorter length of stay in the recovery room than in control subjects. When midazolam was compared to morphine in Rita's study,[135] there was a lower incidence of postoperative nausea and vomiting.

ADVANTAGES OF ADEQUATE PEDIATRIC PREMEDICATION. Proper premedication achieves the following:

- Fear is absent.
- Relaxation and comfort—the pharmacologic "mother."
- Pain is obtunded—both physical and anticipatory.
- Agitation (struggling and crying)—absent during induction.
- Stress response—minimized (less catecholamine, cortisol and hormonal disturbance).[138a,138b]
- Amnesia occurs.
- Premedication contributes to the anesthesia process:[138c]
  - Reduction in doses of volatile agents (MAC decreases).
  - Reduction in doses of intravenous anesthetic agents or adjuncts.
- Minimizes tachyarrhythmias associated with psychological stress by obtunding the sympathetic nervous system.[138d]
- Smoother emergence—preanesthetic narcotics provide opiate-receptor occupancy into the early postoperative period. Pain is already partially obtunded, and smaller postoperative doses of analgesics are effective (the *pharmacologic shadow*).

In addition, Coté[129] and Salem[130] have shown:

- Reduced volume of gastric juice.
- Increased gastric fluid pH to levels within the "safe range," i.e., pH is greater than 2.5 and volume is less than 25 ml or 0.4 ml/kg (average 0.18 ml/kg; mean pH = 3.5).

NO MEDICATION. Except under special environmental circumstances and parental presence, this approach is not an acceptable practice.[127,131] The circumstances mentioned require homelike surroundings, a colorful nursery play area with toys, and several diversionary techniques. Movies, music, and television are helpful. Nursing personnel should be in casual dress.

For most infants and children, parting from parents is a frightening occasion. It is possible at times for those under 2 years of age to remain with hand held by parents during an inhalation induction. Even then, a struggle is frequent. Above all, intravenous infusions and other invasive monitoring approaches should await the establishment of anesthesia.

The *parental–separation syndrome* is a psychological trauma, accompanied by more than the emotional reactions of crying, yelling and struggling, and nightmares.[127] There are endocrine stress responses that set the stage for cardiorespiratory complications.

Even the anesthesiologist possessed of a great capacity for administering tender, loving care (TLC) is, at best, a stranger. There are hyperkinetic children, those at all ages who are retarded, and those with language difficulties who cannot cooperate and require pharmacologic intervention.

In brief, even a large dose of psychology needs the supporting doses of pharmacologic agents. In Cook County Children's Hospital in Chicago, where anesthesiologists were involved with the concept of psychological preparation, TLC and the "singing" technique, preanesthetic preparation almost always involved adequate premedication. Interest in the alternative preparation of children began 40 years ago with an analysis of the psychology of children and the emphasis of this as the "second power of the anesthesiologist"—the first being pharmacology.[128]

ANTICHOLINERGICS IN PEDIATRIC PATIENTS. The anticholinergic drugs are a valuable part of preanesthetic medication.

The objectives of anticholinergic use and advantages are as follows: (1) to prevent vagal/cardiovascular responses; (2) to diminish gastric acidity and volume;[130] (3) to provide amnesia (with scopolamine) and potentiate sedation (with narcotics); (4) to diminish respiratory tract (i.e., bronchoconstriction) responses to drugs or to endoscopic procedures; (5) to antagonize respiratory depressant effect of narcotics by atropine;[133] (6) to diminish respiratory and salivary secretion; and (7) to diminish excessive GI motility.

The mechanism for effectiveness of anticholinergics is basically related to the vagolytic action. In the recommended doses, especially in the pediatric patient, few unfavorable responses are to be noted. Most adverse effects can be related to an excessive dose and not necessarily to a peculiarity of the agent. The central anticholinergic action is likewise to be encountered when excessive doses are used. In this regard, the synthetic agent glycopyrrolate, which does not penetrate the blood–brain barrier, is devoid of any unusual CNS adverse response.

The belladonna derivatives have been the classic agents in combination with a narcotic or a hypnotic drug. Atropine itself has been the favorite in pediatric practice, especially in the infant. Scopolamine, on the other hand, has been preferred in children over 2 years of age.[125,133] Its singular advantage is that it provides additional sedation and reinforces narcotic and sedative effects of other drugs and, at the same time, provides a significant valuable amnesia that is hardly duplicated by any of the newer agents, such as the benzodiazepines.

In today's practice, one does not seek a drying effect on the salivary and other glands of the mouth and upper airway. Other objectives achieved by anticholinergic medication have been and are sought. Thus, Salem and coworkers have demonstrated that glycopyrrolate in particular is capable of reducing gastric acidity and gastric volume.[130,138]

In children, the cardiovascular stability achieved

prevents adverse effects such as bradycardia when drugs such as halothane or succinylcholine are employed. Likewise, endoscopic procedures are not accompanied by unusual arrhythmias if an anticholinergic has been used in the preanesthetic period. It is important to realize that the priming of the vagal receptors by an appropriate dose is able to fortify the subsequent dose that might be needed when a severe adverse reaction of vagal stimulation occurs.

The timing of the anticholinergic drug is approximately 30 to 45 minutes before the induction of anesthesia. The drug is usually given in a mixture simultaneously with the narcotic. An intramuscular injection is a more predictable route. In general, this drug and the narcotics should not be given subcutaneously inasmuch as this route results in great variability in drug response.

The conclusion is that a small dose of the anticholinergic should be given at the time of the narcotic premedication. Do not wait until an adverse reaction occurs.

SOME PREMEDICATION REGIMENS. See Table 11-7.

EFFECT OF OPIATE PREMEDICATION ON RESPIRATORY DEPRESSION AND HYPOXEMIA. The use of narcotics in the pediatric patient has often been questioned because of possible respiratory depression that may occur. Experience with modest doses of morphine in healthy pediatric patients does not support this concern.[139,140]

Concomitant with a decrease in respiratory activity is a decrease in metabolism. A reduction in the MAC values of different induction and inhalation agents is achieved, and emergence from anesthesia is smoother.

A study of postoperative hypoxemia in children, when meperidine (1.5 mg/kg) has been used as premedication with a benzodiazepine (diazepam 0.1 mg/kg), showed better oxygen saturation than nonmedicated subjects. The Sa_{O_2} of those asleep on arrival in recovery, but unpremedicated, was 93.6% and in those premedicated the Sa_{O_2} was 96.3%; of those awake on arrival in recovery, the Sa_{O_2} was 94.6% in those unpremedicated and 96.4% in those premedicated.

Of patients not receiving oxygen in the recovery room, the administration of morphine sulfate in doses of 0.05 mg (50 µg/kg) for comfort and pain relief, no adverse effect of the morphine sulfate was observed on saturation, but an actual improvement—before morphine the Sa_{O_2} was 97.1% and 10 minutes after morphine, the Sa_{O_2} was 97.6%.

Mayhew[141] reported an average Sa_{O_2} of children admitted to Post Anesthesia Recovery; Glazener[139] has reported an average Sa_{O_2} of 93.3%. Such levels of saturation are below a desirable level of 97.9% and are, in part, attributable to the reduced functional residual capacity in infants and children following general anesthesia. Both investigators recommend that oxygen supplementation is needed for the first 15 to 30 minutes postoperatively.

Although premedication increases the number of patients asleep on entering the PAR, there is an associated increase in oxygen saturation by 30 minutes and most patients are awake.

EVALUATION OF DRUGS

DEFINITIONS. "Pharmacology is a science of natural phenomena dealing with the measurable, predictable and therefore reproducible effects of drugs on function and cellular structure of animals and humans."[142] It borrows its methodology from physics, chemistry, and physiology. It may be, for practical purposes, divided into *fundamental pharmacology* and *clinical pharmacology*. In fundamental pharmacology and the pharmacology of screening new drugs, the various actions of the drug are primary. All drugs are first tested in animals in whom assumptions of drug action are put to the experimental test. The suggestion to test drug action in animals (by intravenous route) probably came from Sir Christopher Wren and was applied by Robert Boyle to dogs in 1660 using opium.

Clinical pharmacology may be defined as the application of pharmacologic tests to obtain objective evidence of the value of drugs in patients.[143,144] It is a team effort usually, and the drugs used have already been evaluated in animals. The services of

TABLE 11-7. PEDIATRIC PREMEDICATION REGIMENS

Drug	Dose	Comments
Sedative–Narcotic Combination[130]		
Pentobarbital	2.2 mg/kg oral	Reduce volume of gastric juice and increase pH levels within the "safe range" (58%); i.e., pH above 2.5 and volume < 0.4 ml/kg (mean vol. = 0.18 ml/kg)
Morphine	0.18 mg/kg IM	
Glycopyrrolate	7 µg/kg IM	
Premedication by Lytic Cocktail[104]		
Promethazine	8 mg	0.5 ml/kg IM
Meperidine	30 mg	
Chlorpromazine	8 mg	

three scientists are necessary: the clinician, the pharmacologist, and the statistician.

PRINCIPLES. In recent years, investigators have found that drugs that alter subjective feelings and patient mood can be appraised with acceptable precision. Factors that determine the sensitivity and the reliability of methods of clinical drug evaluation are as follows:[145]

1. *Inherent pharmacodynamic activity* of the drug.
2. *Dosage:* Neither token nor toxic doses are useful in drug assessment. A series of graded doses provide a more substantial basis for evaluation than a single dose.
3. *Choice of subject:*[146] This depends on the purpose of the investigation, whether it is (1) *a therapeutic evaluation*, in which it is desired to predict the value of a drug in the treatment of a particular disease; or (2) *pharmacological evaluation*, in which it is desired to define the actions of a drug in man.

    In humans, the investigation of pharmacologic actions of a drug is necessary preliminary to its therapeutic evaluation. Subsequently, the therapeutic potential of a drug must be carried out on patients with the particular disease state or clinical situation in which it is supposed to be effective. Thus, the choice of subject differs according to the *aim* of the investigation. Next, it is necessary to have an adequate size of the group to be tested. Then, the *composition* of the control group as well as the experimental group must be representative of the general population. The subjects must also be able to discriminate between active and inert agents. In many instances, "volunteers" are desirable; however, these may not be representative. Finally, the constitutionally determined responsiveness of the subject is significant.

    The selection of the subject population for whom the investigation is to be conducted may be procured by various artificial means, including *random sampling* and *purposive* or *selective sampling*. Randomization incurs the uncertainty of chance fluctuations, whereas purposive sampling is influenced by investigator bias.
4. *Use of controls.* A control is a basis of comparison. It must be decided by the investigator whether the selected control is sound and valid. Several types of control are recognized. The simplest method is to study the effects against a passive placebo or an active placebo or a reference standard (Yardstick placebo: Experience). The *historical control* is one in which previous personal or recorded experience is the basis of comparison. This is fraught with chance, error and poor judgement.

    Paired controls or the classic control method employs two separate groups; one is nontreated and the other is treated. This requires large homogeneous groups. Proper matching of the two groups is essential. Such matching is preferably achieved by alternating patients to be treated and not treated. One may assign all patients meeting the experimental specifications to the treated group for a time and then assigning all patients to the nontreated control group for a similar period or until an equal number is observed. This last method introduces errors of weather, season, and changing conditions. An alternate method is to give each patient the medicaments and placebo so that each patient serves as his own control.
5. *Collection of data.* As long as objective measurements are possible, there is little difficulty when subjective responses must be determined. A scale of effectiveness must be established and the patient must be able to communicate his reactions. Further in the interest of accuracy, recording should be done immediately and not delayed. If reliance is made on patient's memory, outside influences will operate.
6. *Sensitivity of method.* A scale of sensitivity must be established. The method employed must first indicate that drug effect is present, *i.e.*, it should enable the subject and investigator to detect a drug action. Second, the method should allow one to discriminate degrees of action or increments in effects.
7. *Placebo actions.* See later discussion.
8. *Bias.* This introduces many variables from multiple sources. The symbolic nature of the physician as a helper will color the results. Knowledge of the nature of a drug is prejudicial. Thus, the identity of the drug should be concealed from both the investigator and the subject. The double-blind technique serves partially to remove this variable as well as to offer a control.
9. *Extraneous forces.* The subject's psychic state and the investigator's mood will influence observations. The situation in which the drug is administered and the personality of the subject are important determinants.[147]

DOUBLE-BLIND TECHNIQUE.[146,148] This is a basic method of study evolved by Denton and Beecher. A score of subjective responses have been studied, and pain has served as a prototype of the stimulus and sensation. Special methods have been developed for other sensations and for the hypnotic and antitussive drugs. In general, this method requires the following:

1. Use of a group of cooperative people who report on the sensation under study.
2. Arbitrary criteria of change in or relief of a symptom are set up.
3. Controls are the "double unknown," *i.e.*, neither subject nor observer knows when test agents are employed.
4. Placebos are inserted as unknowns.

5. The order of administration of drugs and placebo is randomized.
6. Correlated data are used; all agents are employed on all subjects.

PERSONALITY AND DRUG REACTIONS.[149] The correlation between personality and response to drugs has been attempted by a number of investigators. Lasagna[147] has done this in terms of typical and atypical effects of drugs on mood and wakefulness. Thus, to morphine and heroin, dysphoria and sedation were typical; to barbiturates, euphoria and sedation were characteristic. Two chief personality types are suggested: *First* is the impulsive, egocentric, anxious person. His personality is not well balanced and *atypical* reactions are prone to appear. *Second*, is the well-integrated balanced personality; in him *typical* reactions are expected.

Mood changes can be induced in humans by many drugs. The nature of the drug is, of course, primary and it is desirable to rate a drug according to whether it produces a state of pleasantness or unpleasantness. Thus, the opiates and, to some extent, the barbiturates may produce a state of dysphoria or unpleasantness that has a bearing on the effectiveness of the drug.

It should be appreciated that therapeutic doses of sedative drugs may have profound effects. Thus, after a hypnotic dose of a barbiturate, physiologic performance is significantly diminished, and mental impairment may persist for several hours beyond the time of so-called drug effect.[150,151]

THE PLACEBO[152]

DEFINITION. A placebo may be defined as any inert substance that, by virtue of its chemical composition, does not enter into or influence directly any physiologic process. In addition, such substances cannot be divorced from having a psychological efect and therefore, "please the patient." The derivation of the word is from the Latin for *"I shall please."*

Dorland's defines placebo as "an inactive substance or preparation given to satisfy the patient's symbolic need for drug therapy and used in controlled studies to determine efficacy of medicinal substances."

An expanded definition is that of Arthur K. Shapiro:[153]

> Any therapy (or component of therapy) that is deliberately or knowingly used for its nonspecific, psychologic or psychophysiologic effect, or that is without specific activity for the condition being treated.

TYPES OF PLACEBO

- *Impure placebo (or active placebo).* This is a placebo that contains a substance with some inherent pharmacologic activity not relevant to the immediate problem being treated.
- *Placebo effect.* The effect of any therapeutic procedure or component which objectively does not have any specific activity for the condition being treated.[153]
- *Placebo reactors.* Subjects who obtain either an exaggerated therapeutic response or experience an adverse effect.
- *Adverse placebo effects.* Placebo addiction occurs; it is manifested chiefly by dependence.

FUNCTION OF A PLACEBO.[142] Two main functions of placebo use are recognized: (1) to distinguish pharmacologic effects from the effects of suggestion; and (2) to obtain an unbiased assessment of the result of experiment.

The reasons for the use of the placebo have been summarized by Beecher and in reviewing these uses one also gains insight into the function of the placebo.[146,152]

- As a psychological instrument in the therapy of certain ailments arising out of mental illness.
- As a resource to the harassed doctor in dealing with neurotic patients.
- To determine the true effect of drugs apart from suggestion in experimental work.
- As a device for eliminating bias on part of patient and when used as an unknown on part of observer.
- As a tool for study of mechanism of drug action.

In a study of postoperative wound pain,[141] it was determined that patients could be divided into placebo reactors and nonreactors. Differences in backgrounds, education, and personalities determined the response. Almost 30% of patients obtained a positive therapeutic response in terms of pain relief after placebo administration. Furthermore, the magnitude of the therapeutic effect was significant because the degree of relief of pain was 35%. Thus, the placebo is capable of altering subjective responses and symptoms by affecting the reaction component of pain.

In addition to remarkable psychotherapeutic effects, placebos also have toxic effects. A wide range of complaints have been recorded, ranging from nausea and fatigue to drowsiness and headache; toxic rashes, collapse and angioneurotic edema have been reported.[154] Placebo dependency can occur, and reliance may be placed by a subject on the placebo when some specific therapy is needed. Many objective signs of effect have also been reported following use of placebos. Thus, gastric acidity has been known to fall, and the typical adrenal responses to stress noted in anxiety states are obtunded.

ETHICS OF PLACEBO USE.[155] In view of the above aspects, the ethics of placebo use must be reviewed in every situation. The use of placebo is intentionally deceptive.

This ethical dimension must be assessed on the basis of a risk–benefit ratio. There are many situations in which the use of a placebo is beneficial and promotes the welfare of the patient. A basic requirement is that the placebo therapy be part of a careful clinical plan. It must help physician–patient communication and must be intended to achieve optimal health of the patient.[155]

Some requirements include the following:

1. No pharmacologic harm.
2. No psychologic harm. Recognize that a subject's feeling of well being may lead to harmful acts in some circumstances.
3. Informed consent. Pharmacologic deception is involved, but the placebo may benefit the patient psychologically.
4. Recognize risks and potential for above.
5. Recognize indirect physiologic and toxic effects.
6. Selection of subjects. They should have right of free choice.
7. Recognition that the duplicity involved may damage the profession of medicine.

When and in what situations should placebos be used?

1. Only after careful diagnosis.
2. No active pharmacologic agents (use inert placebo).
3. Right of patient to information. Answer questions honestly.
4. Never use if patient objects or is not informed (right of consent).
5. Never use when other therapy is clearly indicated.

INDICATIONS. Some specific indications include:

1. Weaning patient from narcotics and sedatives.
2. A drug substitute when a complex clinical picture related to drugs exists.
3. In a careful plan to establish a diagnosis, especially in chronic pain states.
4. To reduce pain medication in terminal states when the active medication dosage is producing adverse effects (constipation, nausea).

The role of inert substances when subjective responses are being assessed must be recognized. The effect of suggestion in relief must be separated from a true pharmacologic response induced by an active agent.

MEASUREMENT OF PAIN.[156] Pain is a complete reflex with both afferent and efferent components; this duality is often designated as *pain perception* and *pain reaction*. Because pain reaction is modified by innumerable variables, it is necessary to attempt evaluation of only the first component. The lowest perceptible intensity of pain caused by a pain stimulus is called the *pain threshold*. Obviously, this threshold value is best identified by the subject and his recognition of when a stimulus is just painful or not is critical.

Many methods have been introduced based on the use of a particular type of stimulus to measure pain. The stimuli used have been mechanical, chemical, electrical, and thermal. Most methods have attempted to evaluate cutaneous pain, although deep somatic and visceral pain have also been subjected to analysis.

The oldest technique is that of Von Frey, a mechanical method. Stiff hairs were used, and pain was elicited by graduated pressure on the skin surface or on the cornea. It was assumed that the amount of pressure could be correlated with the pain threshold and the intensity of pain. Chemical methods have not been completely investigated, but various irritants have been proposed. Lewis has used an ischemia-producing technique by occlusion of vessels to a subject's arm. According to Lewis, ischemia produces a metabolite called the "P" factor which will produce pain. Electrical methods of physiologic stimulation were introduced by Helmholtz. The voltage is correlated with the intensity of the pain. Recently, Harris[157] used electrical stimuli applied to tooth pulp.

Perhaps the most useful and informative method for measuring pain is that introduced by Wolff.[158] The technique uses a thermal stimulus. It involves the application of a measurable amount of heat to a 3.5 cm area of skin on the forehead of the test subject. The heat intensity is raised in graduated amounts until pain is evoked. This is the threshold stimulus. The amount of applied heat is further increased to the point where the subject states that it is maximal and no further increase in stimulus intensity evokes a further increase in the value of the pain sensation. The actual average heat value necessary to have the subject recognize the stimulus as painful was 218 mcal/sec/cm^2, and the ceiling level was reached with a heat value of 680 mcal/sec/cm^2.

Between these two values, an arbitrary division into ten levels is made, and these are called *dols*. The instrument is called the *dolometer*. Although the technique has its limitations and is open to criticism, nevertheless many characteristics of pain have been elucidated.

The following physiologic characteristics of pain are summarized:

1. There is a narrow range between the threshold stimulus and the maximal pain stimulus.
2. Lack of spatial summation differs from other sense modalities—threshold pain is dependent on the strength of stimulus and not on the number of end organs stimulated.
3. Lack of adaptation.

It has been further determined that many factors influence pain perception, these include:

Neurologic factors—injury, irradiation, inflammation.
Pharmacologic agents—local anesthetics; analgesics.

Psychological factors—distraction, suggestion; mood.

Constitutional factors—age, sex, emotional status, racial and cultural characteristics; fatigue.

It should be appreciated that the pain threshold is not constant from day to day in a given individual. Beecher[159] has pointed out that a pain sensation is already subject to "psychic processing" before awareness is achieved. Furthermore, pain sensations probably "reverberate in the internuncial neurons, before arriving at the level of consciousness." Changes in mood also alter the threshold to pain. Thus, amphetamine, which tends to elate, is capable of raising the pain threshold and making pain more tolerable.

INTRODUCTION TO DRUG DEPENDENCE

DEFINITIONS.[160] Drug dependence is a developed state of reliance on a psychoactive agent, developed by the individual to maintain psychophysical well being in the environment.

The word *drug* is widely used to identify active substances taken for pleasurable nontherapeutic purposes, whereas therapeutic agents are referred to as *medicines*.

Drug dependence includes habituation and addiction. These terms were originally introduced by Seevers.[161] *Habituation* is that type of drug dependence that specifies the continuing aspect of the drug taking and implies psychological rather than physiologic dependence.

Addiction implies tissue dependence, tolerance, and withdrawal symptoms. This is the phenomenon of physical dependence that plays a significant role in drug-seeking behavior. Without the withdrawal syndrome, there would be a minimal urge to obtain more drug. The reward of more drug is no abstinence reaction—a negative reinforcement. In a sense, there is secondary essential psychological dependence.

Susceptibility is the term used to identify those individuals who inherently, or because of environment, are unable to use potent psychoactive agents without compulsion to continue drug taking with ensuing personal harm or harm to society.[161]

PATHOGENESIS. Inherent in this descriptive definition of drug-dependence is that the state is complex, that it is a developed state, that a sequence of events is present, and that a number of promotional factors can be recognized.

1. Drug dependence can occur only when a person has an experience with a psychoactive drug. No drug experience—no dependency. Susceptibility is only relative. If conditions are optimal, almost any individual can be made drug dependent.[162]
2. The first drug trial must be rewarding. By a few more drug trials, positive reinforcement occurs and a conditioned pattern of behavior results.
3. This leads to primary psychological dependence.
4. Uncontrollable compulsive use (abuse) may now occur in susceptible individuals.

Drug dependence thus is related to the nature of the agent and the pharmacologic effects on the individual (stimulant or depressant); the quantity used; the character of the individual; the environment and the pathogenetic sequence.

CAUSES. Although there are many complexities, it is useful to classify drug dependence into three categories based on the chief underlying cause.[163] These are social, neurotic, and psychotic (Table 11–8). In each type any of the available drugs may be used. The degree of dependence may be mild or intense; may be intermittent or continuous and may or may not lead to severe habituation or to addiction.

Social Drug Dependence.[164] Many drugs such as opium, alcohol, coffee, tobacco and the hallucinogens, have been taken socially by many persons over the years. All produce varying stages of psychic and physical intoxication, and all are potentially dangerous. To take these drugs is usually the "in thing." They are taken "where the action is." Abuse in taking of these drugs develops out of continued dissatisfaction with things as they are, a degree of immaturity and confusion, and the desire for status or identity. Users of alcohol and of the hallucinogens belong to this group.

Neurotic Drug Dependence. A neurosis is a disorder of the emotions. Unconscious conflicts exist between instinctual impulses and total personality. Expression of this conflict may be in psychological symptoms (phobias, obsessions); psychopathologic symptoms (hypochondriasis, headaches, indiges-

TABLE 11–8. TYPES OF DRUG DEPENDENCE AND THEIR CHARACTERISTICS

Type	Basic Symptoms Subserved by Drug Taking	Patient's Fear	Goal of Drug Taking	Chief Treatment	Danger
Social	Dissatisfaction	Unfulfillment, rejection	Identity, status, pleasure	Educational	Waste, crime
Neurotic	Anxiety	Suffering	Relief	Psychological	Addiction
Psychotic	Horror	Annihilation	Escape	Medical	Suicide, murder

tion, palpitation); character traits (compulsive, anxious, fearful, aggressive) or abnormal behavior (overeating, gambling, delinquency).

Many alcoholics as well as barbiturate, and narcotic drug takers belong to this class. The motivating force is to escape from reality. Inferiority feelings are often involved, and the use of the drugs may, in the young, express defiance and rebellion against authority.

Psychotic Drug Dependence.[165] Psychotic people are those who, in part or on the whole (major psychosis) live in a world of unreality. There are many persons who live a quiet, apparently normal life, yet frequently have periods during which they feel inadequate. These are periods of depersonalization, persecution, and delusions, and these people have suicidal or homicidal impulses. Such personalities are prey to drug "pushers."

PHARMACOLOGIC CONSIDERATIONS. All psychoactive agents may be divided for simplicity into two broad pharmacological groups.

Stimulants. These drugs enhance and excite psychic functions and increase motor activity. Included are the psychomotor stimulants (amphetamines) and the hallucinogens, when initially used. Characteristic of these drugs is the inducement of psychotoxicity, with distortion of perception, illusions, hallucinations, and disordered behavior. The difference between the hallucinogens and the other stimulants is the magnitude of the dose. With hallucinogens, distortion occurs early in to the dose–response curve, whereas large doses of amphetamines are required to achieve the same effect.

Abnormal and antisocial behavior is induced as a direct action to these drugs. There is no impairment in performance and often increased capacity to perform. Physical dependence does not occur, but on withdrawal there is commonly a state of fatigue and depression. Compulsion for the drug is not related to any physical need but to desire for reward.

Depressants. These drugs reduce both mental and physical functions, as their predominant pharmacologic action. The depressants can cause loss of consciousness and loss of motor function and thus their intake is self-limited. The spree use of drugs such as alcohol, barbiturates, or narcotics may cause personal injury and abnormal behavior.

The chronic use of depressant drugs is associated with the phenomenon of tolerance and physical dependence. These are mutually independent. *Tolerance* is the state that exists when increasing doses are required to achieve the original pharmacologic effect. The development of this state involves a modification of drug action, especially by reducing the effect on vital mechanisms. All parts of the CNS do not become tolerant to these drugs at the same rate. A single dose of morphine may produce acute tolerance recognized after 7 days and persisting for as long as 180 days.[162]

Physical dependence is the state of latent CNS hyperexcitability brought about by uninterrupted exposure of the CNS to large doses of depressant drugs. It becomes manifest when administration of the drug is stopped. The signs and symptoms of increased nervous system activity that appears is designated as the *abstinence syndrome*, and two distinct types are recognized.

Morphine-Abstinence Syndrome. This is produced by all narcotic drugs and appears on cessation of drug use. It is a unique clinical syndrome of hyperactivity of all responsive tissues and characterized by a marked *increase* in all somatic and autonomic nervous system activity. Changes in behavior result.

1. All morphine-like drugs can be used interchangeably to create the state or to prevent the withdrawal syndrome.
2. The rate of development of physical dependence with narcotics is according to the classical dose–response curve. With increasing doses and frequency of administration, there is increasing intensity of dependence until a peak dose effect is achieved. Doses beyond this level do not further the intensity of dependence.
3. The withdrawal syndrome is distressing but is infrequently life threatening. The syndrome is characterized by two types of symptoms: (1) *purposive symptoms*, which are goal oriented, behavioral, and directed at getting more drug; and (2) *nonpurposive symptoms* that are involuntary and not directed.

The latter appear 8 to 12 hours after the last dose with lacrimation, rhinorrhea, perspiration, and yawning. Then, the addict falls into a tossing, restless sleep known as the "yen." In 24 hours, additional signs of restlessness, instability, tremors, dilated pupils, gooseflesh, and anorexia appear. By 72 hours the syndrome reaches peak intensity with greater irritability, insomnia, violent yawning, sneezing, and coryza. Nausea and vomiting along with cramps and diarrhea are common. Flushing, sweating, and chilliness alternate. The prominent pilomotor response is the basis for the expression "cold turkey." Blood pressure and pulse are elevated.

Signs of CNS hyperexcitability are prominent. Skeletal muscle spasms, pain in muscles and bones, and wild, kicking movements are characteristics. Ejaculations and orgasms occur. Leukocytosis is common, and 17-ketosteroids rise in the urine. The syndrome runs its course in 7 to 10 days for morphinelike drugs.

Meperidine abstinence appears in 3 to 4 hours, reaches a peak in 12 hours, and declines by 4 to 5 days.

Alcohol-Barbiturate Abstinence Syndrome

1. The rate of development of physical dependence does not follow a classic dose–response curve.
   Prolonged administration of large, almost incapacitating doses is necessary to produce dependence. Moderate or intermittent does are not effective. A critical dose level is needed (about 500 ml/day of alcohol; about 500 mg/day of barbiturates).
2. Abstinence is characterized by delirium, hallucinations, tremors, hyperthermia, and grand mal seizures. It is life threatening.
3. Induction is achieved with most CNS depressants including alcohol, barbiturates, hydrocarbons, and the minor tranquilizers but not the phenothiazines. All these may be used interchangeably. Morphine-like drugs do not suppress withdrawal from these sedative classes of drugs.

CONCLUSIONS. All drug dependence has a basic psychological conditioning to the pharmacologic effects of drugs. The primary psychological dependence results from the situational reward to the user. Further use provides positive reinforcement through the continued reward effect. Secondary psychologic dependence results from the negative reinforcement by the fear of actual or anticipated withdrawal.

REFERENCES

1. Dundee, J.W.: Some effects of premedication on the induction characteristics of intravenous anaesthetics. Anaesthesia, 20:299, 1965.
2. Lasagna, L., Von Felsinger, J.M., and Beecher, H.K.: Drug-induced mood changes in man. J.A.M.A., 157:1006, 1955.
3. Norris, W., and Baird, W.L.M.: Preoperative anxiety: Incidence and aetiology. Br. J. Anaesth., 39:503, 1967.
4. Egbert, L.D., et al.: The value of preoperative visit by an anesthetist. J.A.M.A., 185:553, 1963.
5. Eckenhoff, J.E.: Relationship of anesthesia to postoperative personality changes in children. Am. J. Dis. Child., 86:587, 1953.
6. Antrobus, J.H.L.: Anxiety and informed consent: Does anxiety influence consent for inclusion in a study of anxiolytic premedication? Anaesthesia, 43:267, 1988.
7. Johnson, G.A., Peuler, J.D., and Baker, C.A.: Plasma catecholamine concentrations in normal subjects. Curr. Ther. Res., 21:898, 1977.
8. Cannon, W.B.: Emergency function of the adrenal medulla in pain and the major emotions. Am. J. Physiol., 33:356, 1914.
9. Cannon, W.B.: Stresses and strains of homeostasis. Am. J. Med. Sci., 189:1, 1935.
10. Selye, H.: The general adaptation syndrome and the diseases of adaptation. J. Clin. Endocrinol., 6:117, 1946.
11. von Euler, U.S.: Quantitation of stress by catecholamine analysis. Clin. Pharmacol. Exper. Therap., 5:398, 1964.
12. Fell, D., et al.: Measurement of plasma catecholamine concentrations: An assessment of anxiety. Br. J. Anaesth., 57:770, 1985.
13. Utting, J.E., and Whitford, J.H.W.: Assessment of premedicant drugs using measurements of plasma cortisol. Br. J. Anaesth., 44:43, 1972.
14. Coté, C.J., et al.: Assessment of risk factors related to the acid aspiration syndrome in pediatric patients: Gastric pH and residual volume. Anesthesiology, 56:70, 1982.
15. Salem, M.R., et al.: Premedicant drugs and gastric juice pH and volume in pediatric patients. Anesthesiology, 44:216, 1976.
16. Blom, H., Schmidt, J.F., and Rytlander, M.: Rectal diazepam compared to intramuscular pethidine/promethazine/chlorpromazine with regard to gastric contents in pediatric anaesthesia. Acta Anaesthesiol. Scand., 28:652, 1984.
17. Bruno, L.: (Referenced) Dogliotti, A.M. Anesthesia: Narcosis, Local, Regional, Spinal. Chicago, S.B. Debour, Publishers, 1939, p. 20; p. 63.
18. Bernard, C.: Des effets physiologiques de la morphine et de leur combinaison avec leux du chloroforme. Bull. Gen. de Therap., 77:241, 1869.
19a. Beecher, H.K.: Preanesthetic medication (editorial). J.A.M.A., 157:242, 1955.
19b. Beecher, H.K., and Cohen, B.D.: The routine use of opiates questioned. J.A.M.A., 147:1664, 1951.
20a. Lasagne, L., and Beecher, H.K.: The optimal dose of morphine. J.A.M.A., 156:230, 1954.
20b. Connor, J.T., Belleville, J.W., et al.: Morphine, scopolamine and atropine as intravenous surgical premedicants. Anesth. Analg., 56:606, 1977.
21a. Keats, A.S.: Postoperative pain, research and treatment. J. Chron. Dis., 4:72, 1956.
21b. Gravenstein, J., and Beecher, H.K.: The effect of preoperative medication with morphine on postoperative analgesia with morphine. J. Pharmacol. and Exper. Ther., 119:506, 1954.
21c. Epstein, B.S., et al.: Evaluation of fentanyl as an adjunct to thiopental-nitrous oxide-oxygen anesthesia. Anesth. Rev. 2(3):24, 1975.
22a. Hill, H.E., Belleville, R.E., and Wikler, A.: Studies on anxiety, associated with anticipation of pain: Effect of pentothal. Arch. Neurol. Psychiatr., 73:602, 1955.
22b. Hill, H.E., et al.: Studies on anxiety associated with anticipation of pain. I. Effects of morphine. A.M.A. Arch. Neurol. Psychiatr., 67:612, 1952.
23a. Saidman, L.J., and Eger, E.I. II: Effect on nitrous oxide and of narcotic premedication on the alveolar concentration of halothane required for anesthesia. Anesthesiology, 25:302, 1964.
23b. Hoffman, J.C., and Di Fazio, C.A.: The anesthetic sparing effect of pentazocine, meperidine and morphine. Arch. Int. Pharmacodynam. Ther., 186:261, 1970.
24a. Traynor, C., and Hall, G.M.: Endocrine and changes during surgery: Anesthetic implications. Br. J. Anaesth., 53:153, 1981.
24b. Dundee, J.W., et al.: Effect of opioid pretreatment on thiopentone induction requirements and the onset of action of midazolam. Anaesthesia, 41:159, 1986.
24c. Dundee, J.W., et al.: Some factors influencing the induction characteristics of methohexitone anaesthesia. Br. J. Anaesth., 33:296, 1961.
24d. Furness, G., Dundee, J.W., and Milligan, K.R.: Low dose sufentanil pretreatment. Anaesthesia, 42:1264, 1987.
24e. Riding, J.E.: Postoperative vomiting. Proc. R. Soc. Med., 53:671, 1960.
25. Magoun, H.W.: Caudal and cephalic influences of the brain stem reticular formation. Physiol. Rev., 30:459, 1950.
26. French, J.D., Verzeano, M., and Magoun, J.W.: Neural basis

of the anesthetic state. Arch. Neural. Psychiatr., *69*:519, 1953.
27. Heath, R.G.: Symposium on Sedative and Hypnotic Drugs. Baltimore, Williams & Wilkins, 1954.
28. King, E.E.: Differential action of anesthetics and intravenous depressants upon EEG arousal and recruitment responses. J. Pharmacol., *116*:404, 1956.
29. Belleville, J., and Artusio, J.: Electro-encephalographic pattern and frequency spectrum analysis during diethyl ether analgesia. Anesthesiology, *16*:379, 1955.
30a. Goodman, L., and Gilman, A.: The pharmacological basis of therapeutics. 4th ed. New York: The Macmillan Company, 1970.
30b. Zolan-Morgan, S., Squire, L.R., and Mishkin, M.: The neuroanatomy of amnesia amygdala-hippocampus versus temporal stem. Science, *218*:1337, 1982.
31. Guedel, A.E.: Inhalation Anesthesia, 2nd ed. New York, Macmillan, 1937.
32. Peters, J.P., and Van Slyke, D.D.: Quantitative Clinical Chemistry, vol. 1, 2nd ed. Baltimore, Williams & Wilkins, 1946.
33. Belleville, J.W., et al.: Influence of age on pain relief from analgesics. J.A.M.A., *217*:1835, 1971.
34. Vestel, R.E., Wood, A.J.J., and Chand, D.J.: Reduced beta-adrenoreceptor sensitivity in the elderly. Clin. Pharmacol. Therap., *26*:181, 1979.
35. Vestel, R.E., et al.: Effect of age and cigarette smoking on propranolol disposition. Clin. Pharmacol. Therap., *26*:8, 1979.
36. DuBois, E.F.: The basal metabolism in fever. J.A.M.A., *77*:352, 1921.
37. Smith, T.J., and Edelman, I.S.: The role of sodium transport in thyroid thermogenesis. Fed. Proc., *38*:2150, 1979.
38. DuBois, D., and DuBois, E.F.: Clinical calorimetry: A formula to estimate the approximate surface area if height and weight are known. Arch. Intern. Med., *17*:863, 1916.
39. DuBois, E.F.: Basal Metabolism in Health and Disease, 3rd ed. Philadelphia, Lea & Febiger, 1936.
40a. Mason, J.W.: A historical view of the stress field. Part 2. J. Hum. Stress, *1*:22, 1975.
40b. Cannon, W.B.: Stresses and strains of homeostasis. Am. J. Med. Sci., *189*:1, 1935.
40c. Seyle, H.: The general adaptation syndrome and diseases of adaptation. J. Clin. Endocrin., *6*:117, 1946.
40d. Savege, T.: Reduction or obliteration of reflex responses to surgery. In Stress-Free Anaesthesia. Analgesia and the suppression of stress responses. Internal Congress Royal Society of Medicine Series Number 3. Published by Royal Society of Medicine London. New York, Grune & Stratton, 1978.
41a. Morris, R.W., and Lutche, F.: Diurnal rhythm in analgesic effect of morphine. J. Pharm. Sci., *58*:374, 1969.
41b. Frederickson, R.C.A., Burgis, V., and Edwards, J.D.: Hyperalgesia induced by naloxone follows diurnal rhythm on responsivity to painful stimuli. Science, *198*:756, 1977.
42a. Waters, R.M.: Pain relief for children. Am. J. Surg., *39*:470, 1938.
42b. Waters, R.M.: A study of morphine, scopolamine, and atropine and their relation to preoperative medication and pain relief. Texas State J. Med., *34*:304, 1936.
42c. Wangeman, C.R., and Hawk, M.H.: The effects of morphine, atropine, and scopolamine. Anesthesiology, *3*:24, 1942.
43. Raeder, J.C., and Breivik, H.: Premedication with midazolam in out-patient general anaesthesia: A comparison with morphine-scopolamine and placebo. Acta Anaesthesiol. Scand., *31*:509, 1987.
44. Manchikanti, L., et al.: Assessment of effect of various models of premedication on acid aspiration risk factors in outpatient surgery. Anesth. Analg., *66*:81, 1987.
45. Ghigone, M., Calvillo, O., and Quintin, L.: Anesthesia and hypertension: The effect of clonidine on perioperative hemodynamics and isoflurane requirements. Anesthesiology, *67*:3, 1987.
46. Bloor, B.C., and Flacke, W.E.: Reduction in halothane anesthetic requirement by clonidine, an alpha-adrenergic agonist. Anesth. Analg., *61*:741, 1982.
47. Cavero, I., and Roach, A.G.: Effects of clonidine on canine cardiac neuroeffector structures controlling heart rate. Br. J. Pharmacol., *70*:269, 1980.
48. Maurer, W., et al.: Effect of the centrally acting agent clonidine on circulating catecholamines at rest and during exercise: Comparison with the effects of beta-blocking agents. Chest, *2*(Suppl):366, 1983.
49. Gordh, T.E., and Tamsen, A.: A study of the analgesic effect of clonidine in man (abstract). Acta Anaesthesiol. Scand. *2*(Suppl):78, 1983.
50. Tamsen, A., and Gordh, T.E.: Epidural clonidine produces analgesia. Lancet, *2*:231, 1984.
51. Flacke, J.W., et al.: Reduced narcotic requirement by clonidine with improved hemodynamic and adrenergic stability in patients undergoing coronary bypass surgery. Anesthesiology, *67*:11, 1987.
52. Anderson, R.G.G., et al.: Inhibitory effects of an alpha$_2$-adrenoceptor agonist, clonidine, on bronchospastic response in guinea-pig and man. Acta Physiol. Scand., *124*(Suppl):378, 1985.
53. Glassman, A.H., et al.: Heavy smokers, smoking cessation, and clonidine. J.A.M.A., *259*:2863, 1988.
54. Pouttu, J., et al.: Oral premedication with clonidine: Effects on stress responses during general anaesthesia. Acta Anaesthesiol. Scand., *31*:730, 1987.
55. Woodcock, T.E., et al.: Clonidine premedication for isoflurane-induced hypotension. Br. J. Anaesth., *60*:388, 1988.

PARENTERAL DRUG ADMINISTRATION METHODOLOGY

56. Drachmann, A.G.: Ktesibios, Philon and Heron. A Study in Ancient Pneumatics. Copenhagen, Munskgaard, Swets and Zeitlinger, 1948.
57. Majno, G.: The Healing Hand. Cambridge, Harvard University Press, 1975.
58. Pravez, C.G.: Sur un nouveau moyen d'opérér la coagulation du sang dans les arteries. Applicable à la guérison des aneurismes. C.R. Seances. Acad. Sci. [III], *36*:88, 1853.
59. Rynd, F.: Treatment of Neuralgia. Dublin Med. Press, 1845; Description of an instrument for the subcutaneous introduction of fluids in affections of the nerves. Dublin Q. J. Med. Sci., *32*:13, 1861.
60. Wood, A.: New method of treating neuralgia by the direct application of opiates to the painful joints. Edin. Med. J., *82*:265, 1855.
61. Howard-Jones, N.: The origins of hypodermic medication. Sci. Am., *224*:94, 1969.
62. Combes, M.A., et al.: Sciatic nerve injury in infants: Recognition and prevention of impairment resulting from intragluteal injections. J.A.M.A., *173*:1336, 1960.
63. Crawford, L.D.: Skin fragments in end-opening needles. Can. Med. Assoc. J., *72*:374, 1955.
64. Rees, R.M.: The importance of site selection in intramuscular injection. Pfizer Lab. Spectrum, 1960.

65. Travell, J.: Factors affecting pain of injection. J.A.M.A., *158*:367, 1955.
66. Sidell, F.R., Culver, D.L., and Kaminskis, A.: Serum creatine phosphokinase activity after intramuscular injection: The effect of dose, concentration and volume. J.A.M.A., *229*:1894, 1974.
67. Norris, B.: Skin fragments removed by intravenous needles. Lancet, *2*:983, 1958.
68. Lundy, J.S., and Osterberg, A.E.: Technic of venipuncture. Surgery, *2*:590, 1937.
69. Spohn, P.H., and Statten, T.: Apparatus for scalp and lower limb transfusions in pediatrics. J. Pediatr., *31*:207, 1947.
70. Adams, R.: Venipuncture—A neglected subject. Surg. Clin. North Am., *24*:792, 1945.
71. Brew, J.D., and Dill, L.V.: Rate of blood flow through standard gauge needles under pressure. J.A.M.A., *140*:1145, 1949.
72. Ginsberg, V., and Marsh, M.R.: Rapid administration of blood by use of gravity and large-bore needles. N.Y. St. J. Med., *50*:2302, 1950.
73. Peirce, V.K., Robbins, G.F., and Brunschweig, A.: Ultrarapid blood transfusion: Clinical and experimental observations. Surg. Gynecol. Obstet., *89*:442, 1949.
74a. Maki, D.G., et al.: Nationwide epidemic of septicemia caused by contaminated intravenous products. I. Epidemiologic and clinical features. Am. J. Med., *60*:471, 1976.
74b. Maki, D.G.: Skin as a source of nosocomial infection. Infect. Control., *7*(Suppl):113, 1986.
75. Curry, C.R., and Quie, P.G.: Fungal septicemia in patients receiving parenteral hyperalimentation. N. Engl. J. Med., *285*:1221, 1971.
76. Maki, D.G., and Ringer, M.: Evaluation of dressing regimens for prevention of infection with peripheral intravenous catheters: Gauze, a transparent polyurethane dressing, and an iodophor-transparent dressing. J.A.M.A., *258*:2396, 1987.
77. Maki, D.G., et al.: Prospective study of replacing administration sets for intravenous therapy at 48- vs. 72-hour intervals: 72 hours is safe and cost-effective. J.A.M.A., *258*:1777, 1987.
78a. Goldmann, D.A., et al.: Guidelines for infection control in intravenous therapy. Ann. Intern. Med., *79*:848, 1973.
78b. Centers for Disease Control Working Group: Guidelines for prevention of intravenous therapy-related infections. Infect. Control, *3*:62, 1981.
79a. Sheth, N.K., et al.: Colonization of bacteria on polyvinyl chloride and teflon intravenous catheters in hospitalized patients. J. Clin. Microbiol., *18*:1061, 1983.
79b. Band, J.D., and Maki, D.C.: Infections caused by arterial catheters used for hemodynamic monitoring. Am J. Med., *67*:735, 1979.
80. Stanley, T.H.: New routes of administration and new delivery systems of anesthetics. Anesthesiology, *68*:665, 1988.

ALTERNATE ROUTES OF ADMINISTRATION

81a. Bardgett, D., et al.: Plasma concentration and bioavailability of a buccal preparation of morphine sulphate. Br. J. Clin. Pharmacol., *17*:198P, 1984.
81b. Bell, M.D.D., et al.: Buccal morphine—a new route for analgesia? Lancet, *1*:71, 1985.
82. Fisher, A.P., et al.: Buccal morphine premedication: A double-blind comparison with intramuscular morphine. Anaesthesia, *41*:1104, 1986.
83. Barry, P., and Kay, B.: Post-operative sublingual buprenorphine for peri-operative analgesia. In Buprenorphine and Anaesthesiology. Edited by Bevan, P.L.T., and Firth, M. London, Royal Society of Medicine, International Congress and Symposium Series, Number 65;5–10, 1984.
84. Risbo, A., et al.: Sublingual buprenorphine for premedication and postoperative pain relief in orthopaedic surgery. Acta Anaesthesiol. Scand., *29*:180, 1985.
85. Collins, V.J.: The anesthetist's second power (editorial). Anesthesiology, *9*:437, 1948.
86a. Streisand, J.B., et al.: Oral transmucosal fentanyl premedication in children (abstract). Anesth. Analg., *66*:S170, 1987.
86b. Nelson, P.S., et al.: Premedication in children: A comparison of oral transmural fentanyl citrate (fentanyl lollipop) and an oral solution of meperidine, diazepam and atropine (abstract). Anesthesiology, *67*:A490, 1987.
87. Vercauteren, M., et al.: Intranasal sufentanil for pre-operative sedation. Anaesthesia, *43*:270, 1988.
88. Henderson, J.M., et al.: Pre-induction of anesthesia in pediatric patients with nasally administered sufentanil. Anesthesiology, *68*:671, 1988.
89. Boer, A.G., DeLeede, L.G.J., and Breimer, D.D.: Drug absorption by sublingual and rectal routes. Br. J. Anaesth., *56*:69, 1984.
90. Rita, L., et al.: Intramuscular midazolam for pediatric preanesthetic sedation: A double blind controlled study with morphine. Anesthesiology, *63*:528, 1985.
91. Wilton, N.C.T., et al.: Preanesthetic sedation of preschool children using intranasal midazolam. Anesthesiology, *69*:972, 1988.
92. Adriani, J., and Dalili, H.: Penetration of local anesthetics through epithelial barriers. Anesth. Analg., *50*:834, 1971.
93. Adriani, J., Savoie, A., and Naraghi, M.: Scope and limitations of topical anesthetics in anesthesiology practice. Anesth. Rev., *10*:10, 1983.
94. Shaw, J.E., and Urquhart, J.: Transdermal drug administration—a nuisance becomes an opportunity. Br. Med. J., *283*:875, 1981.
95. Uppington, J., Dunnet, J., and Blogg, C.E.: Transdermal hyoscine and postoperative nausea and vomiting. Anaesthesia, *41*:16, 1986.
96. Duthie, D.J.R., et al.: Plasma fentanyl concentrations during transdermal delivery of fentanyl to surgical patients. Br. J. Anaesth., *60*:614, 1988.
97. Bogaert, M.G.: Clinical pharmacokinetics of glyceryl trinitrate following the use of systemic and topical preparations. Clin. Pharmacokinet., *12*:1, 1987.
98. Mroczek, W.J., Ulrych, M., and Yoder, S.: Weekly transdermal clonidine administration in hypertensive patients. Clin. Pharmacol. Therap., *31*:352, 1982.
99. Laufer, L.R., et al.: Estrogen replacement therapy by transdermal estradiol administration. Am. J. Obstet. Gynecol., *146*:533, 1983.
100. Poe, M.F., and Karp, M.: Seconal as a basal anesthetic for children. Anesth. Analg., *27*:88, 1948.
101. Goresky, C.V., and Steward, B.J.: Rectal methohexitone for induction of anesthesia in children. Can. Anaesth. Soc. J., *26*:213, 1979.
102. Lindahl, S., Olsson, A.K., and Thomson, D.: Rectal premedication in childhood: Use of diazepam, morphine and hyosine. Anesthesiology, *36*:376, 1981.
103. Haagensen, R.E.: Rectal premedication in children: Comparison of diazepam with a mixture of morphine, scopolamine and diazepam. Anaesthesia, *40*:956, 1985.
104. Blom, H., Schmidt, J.F., and Rytlander, M.: Rectal diazepam compared to intramuscular pethidine/promethazine/

chlorpromazine with regard to gastric contents in paediatric anaesthesia. Acta Anaesthesiol. Scand., 28:652, 1984.
105. Hanning, C.D., et al.: Further development of a sustained release morphine suppository. Br. J. Anaesth., 56:802P, 1984.
106. Tocantins, L.M.: Rapid absorption of substances injected into bone marrow. Proc. Soc. Exp. Biol. Med., 45:292, 1940.
107. Tocantins, L.M.: Infusions of blood and other fluids via the bone marrow. J.A.M.A., 117:1229, 1941.
108. Tocantins, L.M., and O'Neill, J.F.: Infusion of blood and other fluids into the circulation via the bone marrow. Proc. Soc. Exp. Biol. Med. 45:782, 1940.
109. Papper, E.M.: The bone marrow route for injecting fluids and drugs into the general circulation. Anesthesiology, 3:307, 1942.
110. Tocantins, L.M., and O'Neill, J.F.: Infusions of blood and other fluids into circulation via bone marrow. Surg. Gynec. Obst., 73:287, 1941.
111. Tocantins, L.M., Price, A.H., and O'Neill, J.F.: Infusions via the bone marrow in children. Penn. Med. J. (Sept.), 1943.
112. Tocantins, L.M., and O'Neill, J.F.: Complications of intraosseous therapy. Ann. Surg., 122:266, 1945.
113. Iokhveds, B.I.: Intracardiac blood transfusion: Amer. Rev. Soviet Med., 3:97, 1945.
114. Kay, E.B., and Hacker, V.D.: The treatment of shock by aortic transfusion during thoracic operations. J.A.M.A., 134:604, 1947.
115. Jones, P.G., et al.: Physiologic mechanisms of intraarterial transfusion. Surg., 27:189, 1950.
116. Keet, J., and Collins, V.J.: Unpublished, 1950.
117. Ciliberti, B.J.: Intraarterial transfusion in hemorrhagic emergencies. J.A.M.A., 144:382, 1950.
118a. Shaw, E.C.: The venous spaces of the penis as an avenue for transfusion. J.A.M.A., 90:446, 1928.
118b. Strain, R.E.: The corpus cavernosa as a receptor of blood. Lancet, 1:61, 1942.
119. Magid, M.A., and Culp, A.S.: Ideal penile anesthesia obtained by injection of corpus cavernosa. J. Urol., 50:508, 1943.
120. Stove, Douglas H.: Femoral transfusion in shock. Bull. U.S. Army Med. Dept., 7:492, 1947.
121. Schaffer, J.O.: A method of rapid transfusion into femoral vessels in patients without adequate superficial veins. Surg., 21:659, 1947.
122a. Harville, C.H.: Cord transfusions in management of prematurely delivered infants with erythroblastosis fetalis. J.A.M.A., 129:801, 1945.
122b. Liley, A.W.: Intrauterine transfusion of foetus in hemolytic disease. Br. Med. J., 2:1107, 1963.
122c. Spielman, F.J., Seeds, J.W., and Corke, B.C.: Anaesthesia for fetal surgery. Anaesthesia, 39:756, 1983.
123. Arnold, D.P., and Alford, K.M.: A new technique for replacement-transfusion in newborn infants. J. Pediatr., 32:113, 1948.

PEDIATRIC PREMEDICATION

124. Waters, R.M.: Pain relief for children. Am. J. Surg., 39:470, 1938.
125. Leigh, D., and Belton, M.K.: Premedication in infants or children. Anesthesiology, 7:611, 1946.
126. Downes, J.J., and Nicodemus, H.: Preparation for and recovery from anesthesia. Pediatr. Clin. North Am., 16:601, 1969.
127. Smith, R.M.: Anesthesia for Infants and Children, 4th ed. St. Louis, C.V. Mosby, 1980.
128. Collins, V.J.: The anesthetist's second power (editorial). Anesthesiology, 9:437, 1948.
129. Coté, C.J., et al.: Assessment of risk factors related to the acid aspiration syndrome in pediatric patients—gastric pH and residual volume. Anesthesiology, 56:70, 1982.
130. Salem, M.R., et al.: Premedicant drugs and gastric juice pH and volume in pediatric patients. Anesthesiology, 44:216, 1976.
131. Epstein, B.: In Anesthesia for Infants and Children, 4th ed. Edited by R.M. Smith. St. Louis, C.V. Mosby, 1980.
132. Haagensen, R.E.: Rectal premedication in children: Comparison of diazepam with a mixture of morphine, scopolamine and diazepam. Anaesthesia, 40:956, 1985.
133. Waters, R.M., Bennett, J.H., and Leigh, D.M.: Effects upon human subject of morphine and scopolamine alone and combined. J. Pharmacol. Exper. Therap., 63:38, 1939.
134. Smith, M.J., and Miller, M.M.: Severe extrapyramidal reaction to perphenazine treated with diphenhydramine. N. Engl. J. Med., 264:396, 1961.
135. Rita, L., et al.: Intramuscular midazolam for pediatric preanesthetic sedation: A double-blind controlled study with morphine. Anesthesiology, 63:528, 1985.
136. Goulding, R.R., Helliwell, P.J., and Jerr, A.C.: Sedation of children as outpatients for dental operations under general anesthesia. Br. Med. J., 1:855, 1957.
137a. Fragen, R.J., et al.: Midazolam versus hydroxyzine as intramuscular premedicant. Can. Anaesth. Soc. J., 30:136, 1983.
137b. Reves, J.G., Fragen, R.J.: Midazolam pharmacology and uses. Anesthesiology, 62:310, 1985.
138. Manchikanti, L., et al.: Assessment of effect of various modes of premedication on acid aspiration risk factors in outpatient surgery. Anesth. Analg., 66:81, 1987.
138a. Oyama, T.: Endocrine responses to anaesthetic agents. Br. J. Anaesth., 45:276, 1973.
138b. George, J.M., et al.: Morphine anaesthesia blocks cortisol and growth-hormone response. J. Clin. Endocrin. Metab., 38:736, 1974.
138c. Cullen, S.C.: Anesthesia in General Practice, 3rd ed. Chicago, Year Book Publishers, Inc., 1948.
138d. Brodsky, J.B., Brose, W.G., and Vivenzo, K.: A postoperative pain management service. Anesthesiology, 70:719, 1989.
138e. Cahalan, M.K., Lurz, F.W., Eger, E.I. II: Narcotics decrease heart rate during anesthesia. Anesth. Analg., 66:166, 1987.
139. Glazener, C., and Motoyama, E.K.: Hypoxemia in children following general anesthesia. Anesthesiology, 61:A416, 1984.
140. Motoyama, E.K., et al.: Reduced FRC in anesthetized infants: Effect of PEEP. Anesthesiology, 57:A418, 1982.
141. Mayhew, J.F., Seifen, A.B., and Guinee, W.S.: Postoperative hypoxemia in children. Anesthesiol. Rev., p. 33, 1987.

EVALUATION OF DRUGS

142. Koppanyi, T.: From animal to human: Some basic principles of comparative pharmacology. Clin. Pharmacol. Therap., 1:7, 1960.
143. Gold, H.: The proper study of mankind is man. Am. J. Med., 12:619, 1952.
144. Gaddum, J.H.: Clinical pharmacology. Proc. Roy. Soc. Med., 47:195, 1954.
145. Modell, W., and Houde, R.W.: Factors influencing clinical evaluation of drugs (with special reference to the double blind technique). J.A.M.A., 167:2190, 1950.

146. Beecher, H.K.: Experimentation in Man. Springfield, Charles C. Thomas, 1959.
147. Lasagna, L., Von Felsinger, J.M., and Beecher, H.K.: Drug-induced mood changes in man. J.A.M.A., *157*:1006, 1955.
148. Denton, J.E., and Beecher, H.K.: New analgesics: Report to the Council on Pharmacy and Chemistry. J.A.M.A., *141*:1051, 1146, 1148, 1949.
149. Eysenck, H.J.: Methodology of drug research. J. Med. Sci., *57*:372, 1957.
150. Goodnow, E.R., et al.: Physiological performance following a hypnotic dose of a barbiturate. J. Pharmacol. Exp. Ther., *102*:55, 1951.
151. Von Felsinger, M., Lasagna, L., and Beecher, H.K.: The persistence of mental impairment following a hypnotic dose of a barbiturate. J. Pharmacol. Exp. Ther., *109*:284, 1953.
152. Beecher, H.K.: The powerful placebo. J.A.M.A., *159*:1602, 1955.
153. Shapiro, A.K.: Factors contributing to the placebo effect. Am. J. Psychiatr., *18*:72, 1964.
155. Silber, T.J.: Placebo therapy: The ethical dimension. J.A.M.A., *242*:245, 1979.
154. Wolf, S., and Pinsky, R.H.: Toxic reactions to placebos. J.A.M.A., *155*:339, 1954.
156. Bonica, J.J.: The Management of Pain. Philadelphia, Lea & Febiger, 1956.
157. Harris, S.C., and Worley, R.C.: Human analgesic action of d-amphetamine, amobarbital, acetylsalicylic acid, and acetophenetid in combination. Proc. Soc. Exp. Biol. Med., *83*:515, 1953.
158. Wolff, H.G., Hardy, J.D., and Goodell, H.: Studies on pain. J. Pharmacol. Exp. Ther., *75*:38, 1942.
159. Beecher, H.K.: Appraisal of drugs intended to alter subjective responses, symptoms. J.A.M.A., *158*:399, 1955.

DRUG DEPENDENCE

160. Jaffe, J.H.: Drug addiction and drug abuse. *In* Goodman and Gilman, The Pharmacological Basis of Therapeutics, 8th ed. Gilman, Rall, Nies, Taylor, eds. Chapter 22. New York, Pergamon Press, 1990.
161. Seevers, M.H.: Psychopharmacological elements of drug dependence. J.A.M.A., *206*:1263, 1968.
162. Konetsky, C., and Bain, G.: Morphine-single dose tolerance. Science, *162*:1011, 1968.
163. Solomon, P.: Medical management of drug dependence. J.A.M.A., *206*:1521, 1968.
164. De Quincey, T.: Confessions of an English Opium Eater. London, Oxford University Press, 1966.
165. Taylor, N.: Narcotics—Nature's Dangerous Gifts. New York, Delta, 1963.

12
GENERAL ANESTHESIA—FUNDAMENTAL CONSIDERATONS

DEFINITION.[1-3] General anesthesia may be defined as an irregular descending depression of the nervous system. It may be further defined as a state in which certain physiologic systems of the body are brought under a condition of external regulation by the action of various chemical agents. It is brought about by supplying to the brain by way of the circulatory system a sufficient concentration of an agent to cause unconsciousness. Such an agent may be introduced by the following routes:

1. Oral administration
   a. Buccal and transmucosal absorption
   b. Gastric absorption
2. Nasal administration
3. Subcutaneous injection
4. Rectal instillation
5. Intravenous injection
6. Inhalation administration
7. Transdermal administration

The descending central depression is irregular because the medullary centers are skipped and the spinal axis is depressed preferentially. The order of descending depression is (1) the cortical and psychic centers; (2) the basal ganglia and the cerebellum; (3) the spinal cord; and (4) the medullary centers. The signs of anesthesia are based on the time at which various reflexes and responses referable to these major divisions of the central nervous system (CNS) are obtunded.

COMPONENTS OF GENERAL ANESTHESIA. With the advent of new anesthetic agents, it has become apparent that a redefinition of general anesthesia is warranted and that it is not simply a "descending depression of the nervous system." The ability to provide a sleep state separate from sensory deprivation and to control reflexes or muscular activity independently of one another indicates that general anesthesia is broader than originally conceived. That it is a state in which physiologic systems of the body are under a condition of external regulation by the action of chemical agents is evident.

The elements of general anesthesia include four components:[4]

1. Sensory Block. During general anesthesia stimuli applied to end organs are blocked centrally and do not enter into consciousness or cortical appreciation. They may reach the cortex and, indeed, bombard the cortex. The degree of this effect ranges from light depth or analgesia (stage I) to true anesthesia or absence of all sensation (stage III). When there is complete sensory loss, the following areas of the brain are considered to be depressed: (a) cortex, hypothalamus, cortical relay, and associated nuclei; (b) subcortical thalamic nuclei; (c) all cranial sensory nuclei; and (d) motor nuclei of the extrinsic muscles of the eye. It should be noted that regional anesthesia blocks stimuli applied to end organs peripherally. Hence, the impulses do not reach the cortex.

2. Motor Block. A blood-borne anesthetic can eventually depress motor areas of the brain and block efferent impulses. The areas include the premotor and motor cortex. The anesthetic can progressively affect subcortical and extrapyramidal centers controlling muscle tone and function. An increasing effect is denoted by progressive muscular relaxation of skeletal muscles—the muscles of respiration are the last to be affected. The order of paralysis is the lower thoracic intercostal muscles → upper thoracic intercostal muscles → diaphragm. However, Fink[5] indicates that all the intercostal muscles may be paralyzed simultaneously.

At this stage of motor cortex block there is only proprioceptive activity with globus pallidus function, and the patient may show decorticate signs (slight flexor tone). With progressive anesthetic depression, there is depression of motor nuclei integrating proprioceptive information at the pallidus, pons, and brain stem. There follows progressive depression of the globus pallidus and red nucleus with the development of decerebrate rigidity. This is intensified with further depression until the vestibular nucleus (Dieters nucleus) is inactivated, when rigidity is abolished.

3. Block of Reflexes. Undesirable effects of a reflex must also be blocked. Among the reflexes involved and requiring consideration are the following:

- Respiratory: mucus formation; laryngeal and bronchiolar spasm
- Circulatory: altered homeostasis of vasopressor mechanisms; changes in vascular tone; arrhythmias
- Gastrointestinal: salivation, vomiting, ileus

4. Mental Block. The eventual production of sleep or unconsciousness may progress through several steps or degrees, each of which overlaps the other, as noted in the following:

- Calmness, ataraxia (lack of tension)
- Sedation or drowsiness (lack of alertness)
- Light sleep or hypnosis (lack of consciousness but arousable)
- Deep sleep or narcosis (lack of consciousness but arousable, responsive to primitive sensory stimulation)
- Complete anesthesia
- Medullary depression

The above considerations have led Woodbridge to suggest the term *nothria* to describe the combined state rather than *anesthesia*. The latter term applies by derivation to "loss of sensibility," whereas nothria implies mental and motor inactivity with insensibility.

BASIS OF THE ANESTHETIC STATE

NEURAL BASIS.[6] *Anesthetic state* is a progressive condition from complete consciousness through imperfect consciousness through unconsciousness to complete loss of reflex excitability and, finally, to alteration of vital functions. It is the logical consequence of the absorption of an effective concentration of an anesthetic by specific areas of the brain. These areas are depressed in a standard biologic sequence, reflected by findings based on consideration of the following:

1. Clinical manifestations (signs of anesthesia).
2. Changes in bioelectric activity (as measured by an electroencephalogram [EEG]).
3. Neural structures and their responsiveness.
4. Metabolic function of the areas.

This analysis shows that the CNS is depressed in a standard manner (Fig. 12–1). Evidence from clinical signs first shows impairment of the most highly integrated centers. The electrical activity of the different parts of the brain is similarly depressed. The order of depression is also related to the phylogenetic development of the brain.[7] Thus, the most recently acquired cerebral functions are the first to be depressed. These newer areas are also the more sensitive to oxygen deprivation.[8] A relationship also appears to exist between enzyme activity in the different brain areas and the ease of inhibiting these systems in the higher centers.

SPINAL CORD CONTROL OF SENSORY INPUT.[9] Anatomic and physiologic evidence exists that sensory information is initially processed at the first dorsal horn relay. The microanatomy of the dorsal horn reveals six cell layers, and, as first described by Rexed,[10] the spinal gray matter in all mammals resembles a multilaminated cerebral cortex. The cells in each layer show differences in size, number, and compactness, which permits differentiation of layers. These are designated *Rexed laminae* (Fig. 12–2), after the Swedish anatomist.

Physiologic differences exist at the different layers (Table 12–1), and control over afferent impulses is exerted.[11] For example, gentle tactile stimulation

STAGE	ANESTHESIA	CHARACTERISTICS	SITE of DEPRESSION	BRAIN
I	CLOUDING	EUPHORIA LOSS of DISCRIMINATION TO IMPAIRMENT of ENVIRONMENTAL CONTACT	SLIGHT DEPRESSION of CORTEX TO MODERATE DEPRESSION of CORTEX	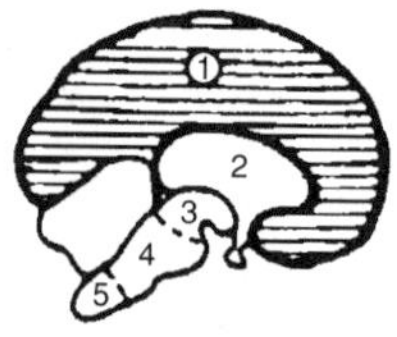 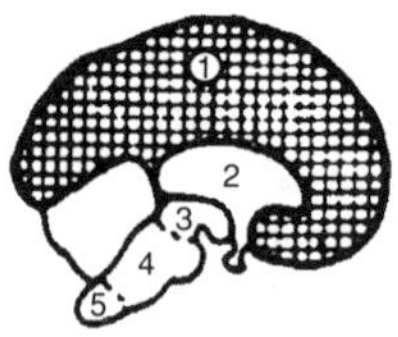
II	HYPER-SENSITIVITY	LOSS of CONSCIOUSNESS	PREDOMINANT CONTROL by SUBCORTEX	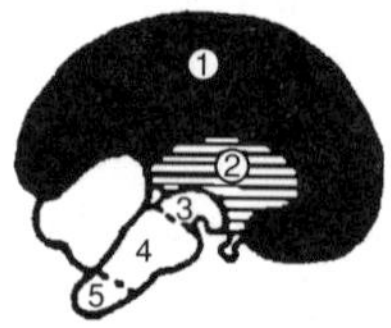
III Plane I	LIGHT SURGICAL	HYPOACTIVITY to PAINFUL STIMULUS	MODERATE DEPRESSION of SUBCORTEX	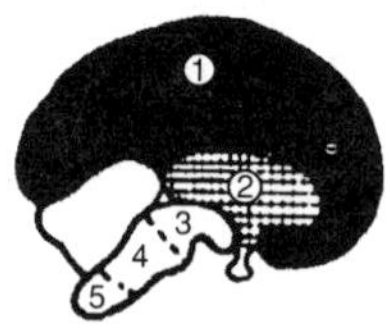
Plane II	MODERATE SURGICAL	LOSS of SOMATIC RESPONSE to PAIN	PREDOMINANT CONTROL by MIDBRAIN	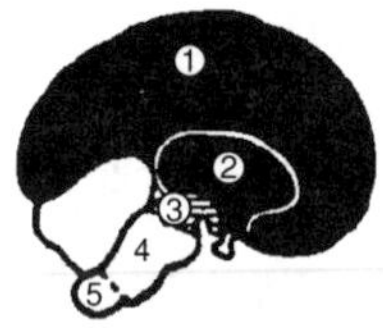
Plane III	DEEP SURGICAL	LOSS of VISCERAL RESPONSE to PAIN	MODERATE DEPRESSION of MIDBRAIN	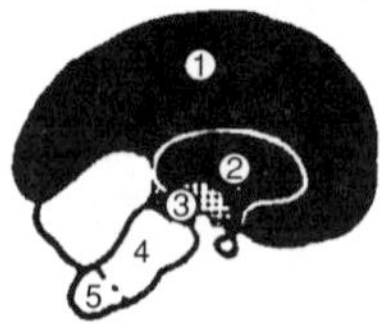
IV	IMPENDING FAILURE	FALL in PULSE PRESSURE	MODERATE DEPRESSION of PONS	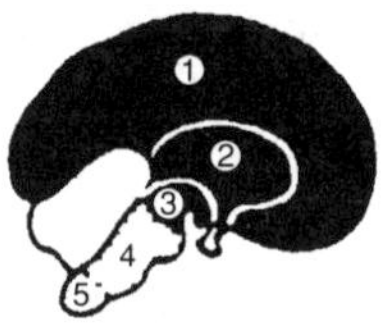

FIG. 12–1. Effects of thiopental on the order of depression of the central nervous system. A correlation is shown between the stages of thiopental anesthesia and the outstanding clinical signs and their neuroanatomic locations. From Etsten, B., and Himwich, H.E.: Stages and signs of pentothal anesthesia: Physiologic Basis. Anesthesiology, 7:536, 1946.

causes laminae II and III (substantia gelatinosa) neurons to depolarize the terminals of small nerve fibers that transmit pain. When depolarized these fibers cannot relay impulses to the CNS, i.e., access (the gate) to the brain is closed. Anesthetics alter the functional state of the dorsal horn cells. All agents tested—halothane, ether, N_2O, thiopental—depress both spontaneous and evoked discharges of the neurons in laminae IV, V, and VI. Most general anesthetic agents tend to keep pain signals from the CNS by diffusely shutting down primary relays. Ketamine suppresses the transmission of sensory impulses at both lamina I and V. The most profound effect of most anesthetic agents is on lamina V cells, which respond principally to noxious stimuli.

NATURE OF THE WAKING STATE.[12] The waking state is a person's awareness of environment and appreciation of stimulation. Integrating the sensory information and establishing a state of awareness ob-

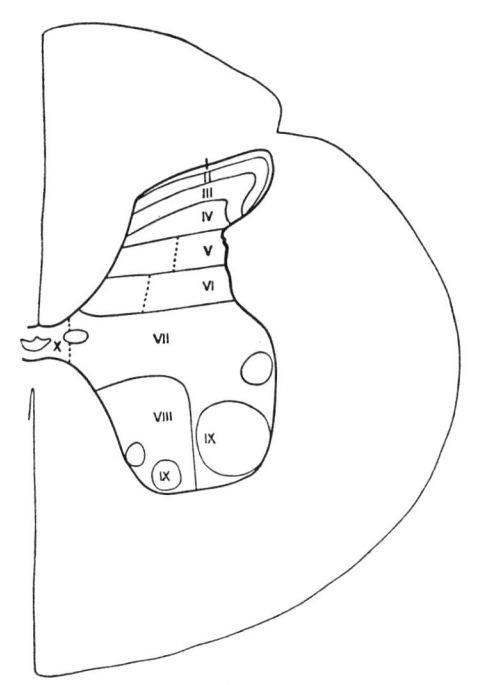

FIG. 12–2. Lamination of the spinal cord gray matter of L-5 of the adult cat. (VII–X indicate Rexed laminae outside the dorsal horn. These laminae mostly subserve association and motor functions.) From Rexed, B.: The cytoarchitectonic organization of the spinal cord in the cat. Neurol., 96:415, 1952.

viously depend on the CNS. A structural basis for such a function has been postulated. In 1942, Morrison[13] described a nonspecific thalamocortical projection system that mediates various stimulation response patterns. In 1949, the classic work of Moruzzi[14] defined the functions of the subcortical reticular activating system. The relationship between these systems and the cortex were established by Jasper.[15] This definable system (RAS) is capable of screening and modulating an infinite variety of sensory impulses and funneling them into the cortex.

The maintenance of the ". . . waking state may be attributed to a tonic barrage of impulses from the ascending reticular system."[16] Study of the waking state using the EEG to analyze the electrical activity of the brain reveals various patterns.[17]

Awake patterns are desynchronized and composed of waves of low voltage and fast activity. This contrasts with the sleep pattern, which is synchronous and consists of high-voltage slow activity. Arousal from sleep can be induced by stimulation of specific subcortical areas.[14] The excitable areas are composed of a collection of reticular relays in the midbrain ascending to the diencephalon and then distributed to cortical hemispheres.[18] Included are the medial reticular formation, the tegmentum of the lower brain stem, and the hypothalamus. Together these have been termed the *reticuar activating system* (RAS).[14] The pathways in and from this system are multineuronal. Characteristics of the action potentials in these neurons include a longer latency for discharge, a slower rise to a peak, and a gradual fall that contrasts with classic direct somatic pathway potentials (Fig. 12–3).

Destruction of this area in monkeys results in a profound state of sleep or of deep anesthesia. The EEG pattern is synchronous and is similar to the patterns of humans in coma or stupor.[16]

Every sensory modality is thus regulated by the subcortical reticular system. The functions of the system are listed as follows:[12]

1. To set background activity of mesencephalic, diencephalic, and cortical structures (to provide a scanning mechanism).
2. To moderate activity beyond the first neuronal sensory relay.
3. To monitor incoming information.

NATURE OF SLEEP

Natural sleep is associated with electrical changes in the neuraxis.[20] The electrical findings in sleep first appear in the subcortical structures and then shortly, if the subject is not aroused, in the cortex.

TABLE 12–1. PHYSIOLOGIC LAMINATION OF THE DORSAL HORN OF THE FELINE LUMBAR SPINAL CORD*

Lamina	Spontaneous Activity	Receptive Field	Modality
1	Slow	Large	High-threshold cutaneous; thermal
2	None		
3	None (brief bursts)	Small	Low-threshold cutaneous
4	Bursts and relative silence	Small-large	Low-threshold cutaneous; pressure; pinch; ethyl chloride
5	Bursts and steady firing	Large	High-threshold cutaneous; thermal; visceral
6	Maintained bursts		Proprioceptive

* Summary of characteristics of Rexed laminae. From Kitahata, L.M., Taub, A., and Kosaka, Y.: Lamina-specific suppression of dorsal-horn unit activity by ketamine hydrochloride. Anesthesiology, 38:4, 1973.

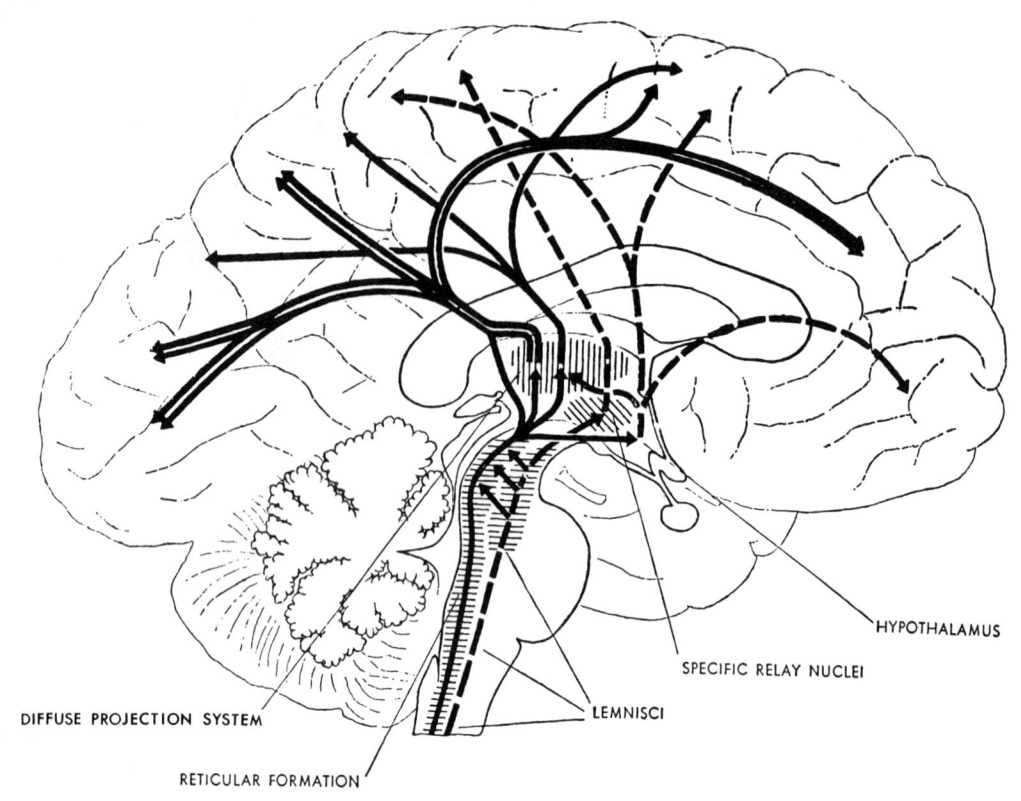

FIG. 12-3. Two pathways of stimulation in the human brain are shown. Sensory impulses pass through the lemnisci to the specific relay nuclei of the thalamus in the center of the brain. From there they are relayed to the parts of the cerebral cortex concerned with the analysis of specific sensations. This system is shown by the dashed black arrows. The other set of pathways, called the activating system, begins with branches from the lemnisci. They carry impulses to the midbrain reticular formation, which in turn relays these impulses to the thalamus. From there the activating impulses are carried to the cerebral cortex by way of the diffuse projection system. These paths are indicated by black lines. The reticular formation also sends impulses to the hypothalamus. Secondary impulses from the hypothalamus are suggested by dashed black lines; from the thalamus, by solid black lines, paralleling the black. From Himwich, H.E.: New psychiatric drugs. Sci. Am., *193*:38, 1955.

When the first changes occur, the subject may be drowsy or dull but not clinically asleep until the cortical electrical changes appear. When reduction in the state of awareness is produced (in monkeys by lesions of appropriate subcortical circuits) to a point resembling the induction of sleep, there is an associated reduction in the output of urinary 1-ketosteroids. It is noteworthy that sodium amytal affects subcortical structures first, whereas phenobarbital affects the cortex first.

CLASSIC CONCEPT OF SLEEP.[16,21] Sleep is considered to be a unique passive state opposed to waking. The discovery of the ascending RAS offered a simple explanation that waking is an increase in the activity of the RAS, and sleep a passive dampening of the system.[22] This is an attractive theory requiring only one system to explain two phenomena and thus subscribing to the law of biologic economy. Sleep, however, is a complex phenomenon, and major advances in neurophysiology now provide information that leads to the general theory that sleep is an active phenomenon. It is not to be regarded as the absence of wakefulness, and its genesis is not entirely based on changes in sensory input.

TYPES OF SLEEP (Table 12-2). In the *presleep—awake period*, drifting off to sleep requires about 10 minutes, during which subjects relax and may reflect on their experiences. Body temperature, pulse, and respiration decline. Both beta and alpha EEG activity is present; there is a fast pattern with low voltage. Subjects close their eyes, which show a slow nystagmus (not rapid-eye-movement [REM]), and alpha activity is more evident.[23]

In the process of going to sleep, the brain passes through two states, which can easily be identified as slow-wave sleep and paradoxic sleep.

Slow-wave Sleep. Slow-wave sleep (SWS) (nondreaming; non-REM [NREM]) is probably "ordinary" sleep. Within this state, four stages of intensity may be identified by EEG tracings.

In the first stage of NREM, the subject dozes and a decline in alpha activity occurs. Asynchronous

TABLE 12–2. EEG ACTIVITY AND OTHER CHARACTERISTICS OF THE STAGES OF SLEEP

Stage*	EEG Wave Activity†	Eyeball Activity	Effect of Deprivation	Other Observations

0 Awake
  Eyes open
  Eyes closed
	Beta
	Alpha
		Irregular, except slowing rolling when drowsy	—	Insomniacs have longer stages 0 and 1 than normal subjects

1 "Descending" sleep; dozing	Alpha Beta Theta	Slight, but bursts of rolling movement	Prevents all following sleep stages; no selective deprivation	
2 Unequivocal sleep	Theta Spindles K complexes	Slight rolling movements; occasional REM‡	Prevents following stages	Subject easily aroused; sensory stimuli evoke K complexes
Slow-wave sleep (SWS, deep sleep) 3 Deep-sleep transition	Theta Delta Spindles K complexes	Slight	Prevents stage 4	Subject hard to arouse; K complexes are hard to evoke
4 Cerebral sleep	Delta	Slight	Suicidal ideation and day terrors Rebound excessive; SWS begins on first night of restored sleep and may last for weeks	Subject very hard to arouse; K complexes cannot be evoked Night terrors and somnambulism occur in this stage Insomniacs have normal SWS
REM sleep‡ (REMS)	Mixed frequency but no spindles or K complexes Theta frequency	Considerable; darting, irregular, in bursts (REM)‡§	Anxiety, overeating, behavioral disturbances, decreased concentration and learning, hypersexuality, decreased seizure threshold	Stage of recallable dreaming; 74% of dreams occur in REMS Dreams are more vivid, sexual, and bizarre than in non-REMS; nightmares usually occur during REMS In men, REMS frequently begins with an erection

* Order of sleep stages is 0, 1, 2, 3, 4, REMS, 1, 2, 3, 4, REMS, etc.; stage 0 may also be repeated, especially in subjects with insomnia. A complete cycle takes approximately 90 minutes. Narcoleptics may bypass any or all of stages 1 to 4. In young adults, the percentage of total sleep time spent in the various stages is as follows: stage 0, 1% to 2%; stage 1, 3% to 6%; stage 2, 40% to 52%; stage 3, 5% to 8%; stage 4, 10% to 19%; REMS 23% to 34%.

† Alpha is high-amplitude, sinusoidal activity of 8 to 14 cycles per second (cps); beta is low amplitude, 15 to 35 cps; delta is high amplitude (>75 μvolt), 0.5 to 3 cps; theta is low amplitude, 4 to 7 cps; spindles are bursts (each, 0.5-second duration) of high amplitude, 12 to 15 cps; K complex is a high-amplitude negative wave followed by a positive wave, with spindles sometimes superimposed.

‡ REM stands for rapid eyeball movement.

§ REM activity is expressed as "density," ie, number of movements per epoch.

From Harvey, S.C.: *Sedatives and Hypnotics* Chap. 17. In Goodman and Gilman's The Pharmacologic Basis of Therapeutics, 7th ed. Edited by A.G. Goodman, T.W. Rall, F. Murad and A. Gilman. New York, Macmillan, 1985.

theta waves are present. This phase accounts for about 5% of sleep time.

In the second stage of NREM, which lasts about 30 minutes, a slow-wave pattern with spindles and theta wave activity is seen. This is classic unequivocal sleep, but the subject is arousable.

In the third stage of NREM, the subject enters into an EEG-determined high-voltage, slow-wave period and, in addition, theta activity and spindles are present. Heart rate and temperature decline slightly, and muscular relaxation is good. The subject, however, may change position; there is little recall, and the subject is hard to arouse. Respiratory rate decreases; pupils are constricted; and brain blood flow is reduced.

In the fourth stage of NREM, deep S and delta waves are dominant; the EEG waves are about five times higher at stage 4 than waking rhythms. This is designated as *cerebral sleep*. The physiologic changes seen in stage 3 become greater in stage 4.

NREM is clinically characterized by a low level of activity, sleep posture, closed eyes, myotic pupils that react readily, sphincters that contract strongly, postural tonus of neck muscles, and minimal muscle relaxation.

After 90 minutes, sleep patterns begin to reverse, and the sleeper enters the first REM period (10 to 30 minutes).

Paradoxic Sleep.[17,24] The REM state follows SWS after a varying period of time. There is cortical activity with low-voltage fast activity similar to that of waking but with absence of electromyographic (EMG) activity in various muscle groups, especially the neck. Brief movements of the face and the extremities are seen.

REM sleep depends on the integrity of areas in the pontine reticular formation. It is characterized by REMs that are conjugate and resemble purposeful waking movements. Autonomic irregular activity is present. Heart rate increases, blood pressure rises, and respiration accelerates with frequent periods of apnea lasting as long as 10 seconds. Cerebral blood flow increases, and thermoregulation is suspended. *Dreaming* is related to this phase. Men experience erections and women clitoral engorgement; but certain abnormal phenomena such as enuresis, nightmares, and sleep-walking are not related.[25]

This REM type of sleep interrupts NREM sleep about once every 90 minutes and lasts approximately 20 minutes. It thus accounts for 20% to 25% of total sleep time in normal young adults.[21]

Two different phenomena appear in this state:[17,23]

1. *Tonic Activity.* A fast, low-voltage cortical activity (as in waking) associated with theta rhythm in the hippocampus is found, and there is total disappearance of muscular activity; although muscles may twitch, the sleeper seems paralyzed. This persists for several minutes and may be accompanied by superimposed EMG phasic behavior.
2. *Phasic Activity.* REMs (50 to 60 per minute) associated with deep sleep waves are termed *pontogeniculo-occipital activity*. These are high-voltage waves and are similar to those recorded during visual attention.

Lower forms of animals do not exhibit paradoxic sleep, but it is present in every mammalian form studied. In the newborn mammalian animal slow-wave sleep appears only in mammals whose CNS is well developed, while the general pattern is an alternation between waking and paradoxic sleep.

CYCLIC ASPECT OF NREM-REM.[26,27] Normal adult subjects show several cycles (commonly three to four) during natural sleep (Fig. 12-4). The duration of NREM is longest usually after the first occurrence of the REM stage. The REM stages become longer with each successive cycle. It appears that the periodicity of the NREM-REM cycle is controlled by reciprocal activity of aminergic and cholinergic cell groups. The need for sleep varies, as do the rhythms, according to individual activities. The need for sleep also decreases with age. In the infant, the sleep period occupies two thirds of the wake-sleep cycle. REM occupies about 40% of the sleep period. At maturity, two thirds of the wake-sleep cycle is the awake phase. The REM state of sleep is sharply reduced to 20% of the sleep stages. After 70 years of age, total sleep time decreases to about 6 hours, while REM remains at about 20% of the sleep cycle.

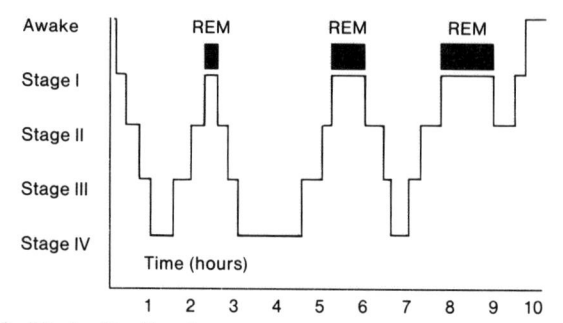

FIG. 12-4. Cyclic alternation of NREM and REM sleep. Normal patients progress through several cycles of NREM and REM sleep during the night. From Zsigmond, E.K.: Hypnotic therapy. Upjohn, 1981.

SLEEP AS AN ACTIVE PHENOMENON. Sleep can be induced by stimulation of many different parts of the brain. Electrical induction is accomplished by impulses of low frequency corresponding to the frequency of sleep spindles, applied to synchronizing or "hypnogenic" structures located in the lower brain stem. Destruction of certain pontine areas produces insomnia, while a midpontine transection produces a definite increase in waking behavior and EEG trances of the waking state. Lesions ventral to the locus coeruleus at the level of the nucleus reticulaus pontis-caudalis suppresses paradoxic sleep.

PACEMAKER FOR SLEEP.[28] Sleep is part of the biologic circadian rhythms; as such, it has a neuroanatomic correlate.[29] This is located in the area of the ventral-lateral hypothalamus.[30] Investigation identified a monosynaptic retinohypothalamic projection that terminates specifically in the suprachiasmatic nuclei of the hypothalamus. These nuclei play an important role in the coordination of circadian rhythms and are an internal master clock that proceeds almost independently on a 24.5-hour solar cycle in the absence of light or other environmental clues (A monthly cycle of a 29.5-day lunar month also exists). The pacemaker, however, is exquisitely sensitive to light.[26] Most rhythms are set by the diurnal alternation of light and darkness.[31]

In the absence or reduction of light stimulation, a secretion of the pineal gland, i.e., melatonin, greatly increases and has sedative effects. This effect may account for feelings of depression seen in subjects in temperate climates during the winter season.

Sleep episodes correlate with temperature changes, and temperature appears to be a determinant of the length of sleep. Higher temperatures relate to longer sleep, whereas reduced temperatures shorten the length of sleep.

NEUROANATOMIC MECHANISMS.[31] Two neuroanatomic complexes are involved in the control of the awake-sleep cycle.

For the *awake period*, the control is by the tegmentum (pons) of the brain stem.

For the *sleep period*, the control is by the lateral hypothalamus.

These anatomic sites are characterized by different neurohumoral mechanisms. Dopamine is the neurotransmitter for the waking phase. Serotonin is the principal transmitter for the sleep phase. An inverse reciprocal relationship exists between these two neurotransmitters. The sleep phase is modified by cyclic release of norepinephrine, which induces the REM state.[32]

The hippocampus is also a possible site for sleep control because it involves the release of the neurotransmitter serotonin during sleep. The metabolism and concentration of serotonin (5-hydroxytryptamine) (5-HT) and 5-HIAA (5-hydroxy-indole acetic acid) increase in the hippocampus during sleep. In animal studies, the increase is 40 times for HT and 3 times for HIAA over wakefulness. On the other hand, the metabolism of dopamine decreases in the striatum and the thalamus in SWS, but its concentration increases as a prelude to REM or paradoxic sleep.[33] In general, dopamine induces alertness and sets conditions for the waking state.

QUANTITATIVE ASPECTS. The sleep state can be measured quantitatively. Studies indicate that sleep is a biologic constant. Circadian variations of the sleep states can be correlated with circadian biochemical variations in the brain.

NEUROTRANSMITTER CORRELATES.[34,35a] Biogenic amines (serotonin, dopamine, norepinephrine) are the controllers of sleep. Cerebral serotonergic elements play an important role in producing sleep and appear related to quiet, slow-wave sleep. Noradrenergic systems are involved for active (REM) sleep.

The onset of sleep into the slow-wave stages, according to Hobson,[35b] is first related to decreasing activity of amine-containing cells of the locus ceruleus, especially decreasing dopamine activity. This is accompanied by an increasing level of serotonin. The onset of each REM, or paradoxic sleep period, is accompanied by the accumulation and increasing activity of norepinephrine and decreasing activity of serotonin. The norepinephrine activates the cortex.

Meanwhile, acetylcholine-containing cells reach a high level of activity during REM. Pharmacologic and biochemical evidence support the concept that awakening is a cholinergic process and is related to reticular activity. Stimulation of the RAS causes a marked increase in acetylcholine release in the cerebral cortex.[36]

Inhibition of synthesis of serotonin at the tryptophan hydroxylase step (by P-chlorophenylalanine) leads to insomnia. This can be reversed and sleep produced by the injection of 5-hydroxytryptophan, the immediate precursor of serotonin. In addition, total destruction of serotonin-containing neurons in the raphe system also leads to a persistent waking state.

Noradrenaline plays a role in paradoxic (REM) sleep. Cells containing this amine are located in the locus coeruleus. Thus, paradoxic sleep may depend on priming by serotonin mechanisms and triggering of the state by noradrenergic mechanisms.

BIOCHEMICAL CORRELATES.[31,37] (Fig. 12-5) Plasma potassium concentration varies as little as 10%, but this variation may be much larger. The rate of urinary potassium excretion varies fivefold in normal subjects in the course of a 24-hour day.[38]

Plasma cortisol[39] shows great normal differences between the levels just before awakening and the levels before going to sleep (Fig. 12-6). Cortisol levels are higher in the early morning; they are slightly reduced at midmorning and rise again at noon, then decrease in the late afternoon and evening. During sleep, there is a progressive increase in cortisol levels from about 5 μg/dL at midnight to more than 15 μg/dL before awakening. The cortisol rhythm is a result of a circadian rhythm in cortisol production and secretion.[40]

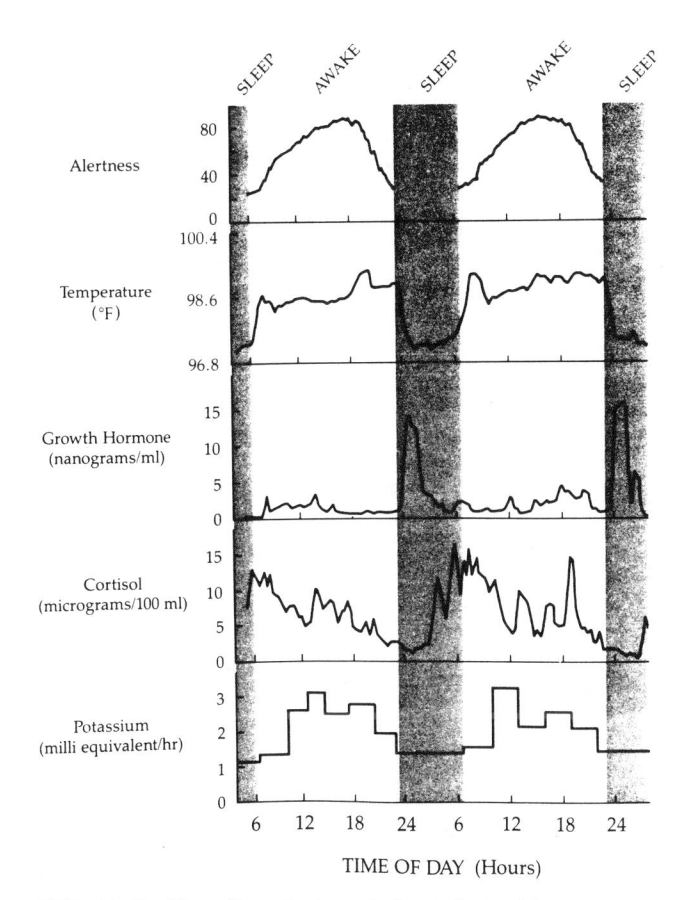

FIG. 12-5. Circadian timing of physiological functions over two days. From C. Czeisler: PhD Thesis, Stanford University, 1978, and R.C. Coleman: Wide Awake at 3:00 A.M.: By Choice or by Chance? New York, W.H. Freeman & Co., 1968. With permission.

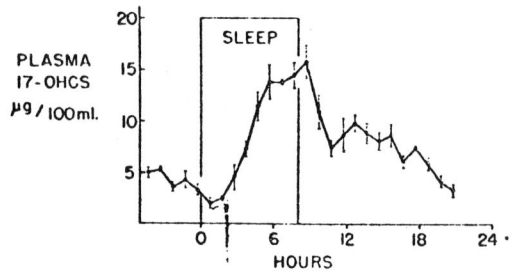

FIG. 12–6. Plasma cortisol (17-OHCS) concentrations in eight normal subjects confined to a metabolic ward. They slept regularly from 10 P.M. until 6 A.M. for several days before and during the period when blood was sampled hourly via indwelling venous catheters. The mean 17-OHCS and the standard error of the means are shown. From Best, C.H., and Taylor, N.B., Physiologic Basis of Medical Practice, 10th ed. Edited by J. R. Brobeck. Baltimore, Williams & Wilkins, 1979, pp. 7–13.

Growth hormone secretion is generally increased during SWS and is accompanied by a high net protein synthesis. This may be important for wound healing. During REM sleep, when skeletal muscle tone is low, there is a net skeletal muscle synthesis.

EFFECT OF CNS DEPRESSANTS.[41–44] Almost all CNS-depressant drugs in soporific doses induce some suppression of REM sleep. Many drugs of the nonbarbiturate type (glutethimide, quinozolone) as well as barbiturates suppress REM sleep time, but a pronounced rebound increase occurs in REM time after withdrawal. Chloral hydrate in 1000 mg doses, however, does not appreciably suppress REM time.

Sleep latency and insomnia are frequent after the use of sedative and cerebral-depressant drugs. Treatment of these abnormalities may be partially accomplished by tranquilizers and other agents, which are effective in the following order: flurazepam > perphenazine-amytriptaline combination > chloral hydrate > chlorpromazine > diphenylhydramine.[27]

Benzodiazepines and other tranquilizers do not suppress REM, but they do eliminate stage 4 SWS. They are also useful in preventing night terrors.

Monoamine oxidase inhibitors, or 5-hydroxytryptophan, suppress REM sleep, and a state of catatonia may be induced.

In classic experiments on dream deprivation, suppression of REM sleep in normal subjects by awakening them causes irritability and anxiety.[45] This does not occur if subjects are awakened during NREM sleep. Drug suppression may produce the same results.[22]

METABOLISM IN SLEEP. Metabolism slows during sleep and oxygen consumption is reduced. During SWS stages 3 and 4 delta-wave (deep) sleep, metabolism is lowest.[46] Synthetic and anabolic processes are activated, and growth hormone secretion is increased.

PHYSIOLOGIC CHANGES. Changes in blood gas constituents are a secondary effect. Since the basic changes are rapidly reversible, they are best explained by the neurogenic mechanism. Sleep is not a static state and there are frequent changes in depth, movements, alveolar gas tensions, blood pH, and EEG patterns. Biochemical changes are of the nature of a respiratory acidosis. Despite the well-recognized decrease in production of CO_2, there is an increase in alveolar and blood P_{CO_2}. It is considered that this is due to a decreased sensitivity of the respiratory center to carbon dioxide. Such decreased sensitivity appears to depend on a decrease in the number of afferent impulses reaching the medullary chemoreceptors. The production of hypoxemia or the administration of carbon dioxide may stimulate the REM phase.

A mean decrease in alveolar oxygen tension is also to be noted but it is not significant and does not produce arterial oxygen desaturation.[47]

Block has determined that, in normal healthy adults, there is a mean maximal sleep desaturation of 10%, which corresponds to a fall in oxygen tension of about 6 mm Hg.[48] There may be a 50% fall in saturation in subjects with sickle cell disease.[49]

NATURE OF ANESTHETIC STATE

Anesthesia is a state of altered cerebral and nervous system function; it is a depression of the CNS and a depression of the brain stem reticular formation. There are three assumptions to this concept:[50]

- *That* consciousness resides in the cerebral cortex
- *That* the RAS has an excitable action on the part or parts of the brain where conscious processes are developed
- *That* removal of the tonic reticular action results in loss of consciousness; when certain alerting nervous system processes are lost, the anesthetic state results

Much of this theory describes the anatomic locus of action of the anesthetic agent. Analysis of the details provides more specific information. The reticular formation is composed of a rich, complex multisynaptic network through which sensory information is relayed to the brain. These synapses may be weak or vulnerable points in the transfer of information and can be altered or blocked.[51] This is an oversimplification, for no simple relationship exists between consciousness and the amount of cortical activity. Fast EEG activity can be associated either with waking state or deep sleep; arousal is often associated only with temporary increases in neuronal excitability, while stimulation of the reticular system may inhibit some cortical neurons.

Different synapses vary widely in their vulnerability.[52] Some are weak with a low safety factor.

Monosynaptic dorsal-ventral root connections transmit at low frequency and are readily blocked by anesthesia. The first central synapses in direct afferent paths (dorsal column) conduct impulses at high frequency and are resistant to depressants.[22] Another variant is the thalamic relay in the primary somatosensory pathway that transmits at low frequency but is insensitive to anesthesia; the frequency limiting factor is caused by a negative feedback.

In general, anesthetics depress spontaneous and repetitive activity before there is any marked effect on transmission of primary short-latency responses. Some anesthetics may facilitate inhibitory control and thus may alter the excitatory-inhibitory balance. Evidence indicates that conscious processes depend on a high degree of central spontaneous repetitive activity. This is mediated by acetylcholine, which is liberated by an ascending cholinergic system. In the central areas this chemical appears to reduce permeability to potassium.[52]

DIFFERENCES IN ANESTHETICS. Anesthetic agents do not all act alike. Most agents produce a variable but reversible chemical (pharmacologic) lesion of the reticular formation, that depresses all of the listed functions of the RAS and produces electrical sleep patterns.[19,50–52]

A contrast in site of action is noted between the barbiturates, the tranquilizers, and anesthetics. Administration of barbiturates blocks the arousing influence of reticular stimulation.[53] The electrical activity of the RAS is depressed by pentobarbital and thiopental. Simultaneously, the cortex exhibits diminished responsiveness.

Tranquilizers such as chlorpromazine, however, allow cortical arousal and appear to increase the ability of the reticular formation to be more selective of sensory information that reaches the cortex. Indeed, sensory information is regulated without altering cortical function.

On the other hand, the anesthetics differ from the barbiturates and have a greater effect on the afferent lemniscothalamic system. Ether has a pronounced depressant action on this system but also causes an early marked depression of the cortex. Davis[54,55] has shown that cyclopropane, ethylene, and nitrous oxide depress the afferent lemniscothalamic and thalamocortical projection systems. The extent parallels the anesthetic potency.

Atropine and related drugs affect cortical activity. Wikler[56] found that after administration of atropine the EEG is characteristically one of a sleeping animal; yet, the animal is behaviorally awake.

GENERAL METABOLISM.[50] Altered cerebral function or metabolism is not the determinant of general body metabolism. Reduction of body metabolism is a reflection of the direct reduction of metabolism in the individual organs and the total body reduction is the cumulative effect. Depression of active organs contributes extensively to the decreased body $\dot{V}_{O_2}$. For example, halothane produces a dose-related progressive reduction of body metabolism of 27% to 60%. The myocardial contribution represents over 47% of this value, whereas cerebral effects account for only 2%.

Because thiopental produces a general reduction of body oxygen consumption, it is capable of a dose-related reduction of cerebral oxygen consumption. Ether and cyclopropane show a diphasic effect. Although they cause reduced body $\dot{V}_{O_2}$, they may produce an increase in cerebral $\dot{V}_{O_2}$.

The overall effect of inhalation anesthesia may be related to the state of the cardiocirculatory system. As seen with halothane, the activity of the myocardium plays a prominent role in its effect on body oxygen consumption.

Reduction in myocardial $\dot{V}_{O_2}$ is a major component in decreasing whole body $\dot{V}_{O_2}$. Such changes can be duplicated by measures that reduce arterial pressure and cardiac output.[58]

SUMMARY. From the above observation, the initial stages of anesthesia with loss of awareness may be considered to be a reversible pharmacologic block of the subcortical arousal system. Induction of anesthesia thus prevents arousal. Special sensory (auditory) and somatic stimuli, however, may still evoke a primary cortical response by transmission over classic paths. This is not reduced until large doses of ether or barbiturate are administered, when the cortex is depressed.

THE GENERAL ANESTHESIA PROCESS

The objective in administering a general anesthetic is to attain a proper concentration of agent in the brain tissues.[59] In inhalation methods, a concentration must be first established in the anesthesia circuit and then delivered to the body and its separate tissues. Thus, a downward gradient in concentration exists between the anesthetic machine reservoir and the body cells. Agents introduced into the body by other routes must eventually be absorbed into the circulation and delivered to the brain and other tissues. A gradient, therefore, is established from the point of administration to the brain and other tissues. Tissues and cells may be divided into separate compartments that vary in their ability to take up anesthetic drugs. The gradient of anesthetic agents in the body is a continuum and not a step-wise process, although consideration will be given to separate stations along the gradient. Similarly, a gradient exists until equilibrium is established. An end point will thus be the time when concentration at any one point is in balance (not equal) to other points.

ABSORPTION OF INHALATION AGENTS.[51,52] Absorption of an anesthetic may be defined as the intake of an agent by the body and the uptake of the agent by tissues with the assumption of an equilibrium between the anesthetic and the cells of the entire body.

Absorption of anesthetic agents by inhalation is a sequence of events that may be described in five phases (Table 12–3):[59]

Phase 1 consists of the mass movement of gases and vapors from the anesthetic atmosphere to the lung alveoli. The process is largely mechanical. An atmosphere containing a determined concentration of anesthesia is moved into the lungs by ventilation.

Phase 2 consists of distribution of atmospheric gases and anesthetic agents with the alveolar air. It is then mixed with the alveolar air and is changed by dilution with the gases already present. Water vapor is added to decrease the partial pressure of the inspired anesthetic mixture. It is also heated rapidly (less than 1/100 second). Furthermore, a portion is lost to the capillary blood by uptake and tends to limit the build-up of alveolar concentration. This mixing process in the alveoli is relatively rapid so that equilibrium between alveolar air and the atmospheric mixture occurs in about 2 minutes. In the diseased or emphysematous lungs this may require 11 minutes or longer.

Phase 3 is divisible into two parts: (1) the diffusion of the alveolar gases through the respiratory alveolar-capillary membrane to the blood; and (2) the flow of the solution of anesthetics in the blood through the pulmonary capillaries. This depends on concentration of agent in alveoli, the pulmonary perfusion, and the anesthetic agent solubility in blood.

Phase 4 is the transportation by the circulation of the anesthetic agents dissolved in the blood of the pulmonary capillaries to the capillary beds of body tissues and cells.

Phase 5 is the process of diffusion from the tissue capillaries into the interstitial and extracellular fluid followed by passage across the cell membranes into the intracellular fluid. The extent of this process again depends on tissue circulation, blood concentration of agent, and anesthetic agent solubility in tissues as shown by the blood-tissue partition coefficient.

When an equilibrium between the partial pressure of the anesthetic in the breathing atmosphere and the cells is established, the absorption process is complete. The total amount of anesthetic agent dissolved in the cells plus all other volumes dissolved in the intermediate stages is defined as the absorption capacity of the body for the particular agent under conditions of administration.

Total uptake by the body is dependent on three primary factors: (U):

1. The solubility coefficient of the anesthetic agent, (λ) which is the main feature of the drug profile.
2. The cardiac output ($\dot{Q}$) as the determinant of circulation through the lung and to the tissues.
3. The alveolar air partial pressure of the anesthetic agent minus the venous blood partial pressure of the agent.

$$(U) = \lambda \times (\dot{Q}) \times (P_A - P_V)$$

Fundamentally, inhalation anesthesia depends on the laws of diffusion of gases and vapors, and an anesthetist's problem is to deliver an anesthetic agent to the various tissues of the body with a minimal disturbance of the body's physiology. Five conditions must be kept in mind constantly.[52]

I. PARTIAL PRESSURE OF ANESTHETIC AGENT INSPIRED

In administering inhalation anesthesia, time is required to establish a proper mixture in the anesthesia system and to deliver this to the patient. Thus, a delay results from the difference between gas flowing into the system and the gas inspired.[60,61]

Fundamental to this is a consideration of partial pressure and of the washout effect on the anesthetic system, the pulmonary system, and the blood and tissues.[62]

Diffusion is always in the direction of lessening partial pressure. Thus, at the beginning the partial pressure of the anesthetic agent will be greatest at

TABLE 12–3. THE FIVE-PHASE CONTINUUM OF THE GENERAL ANESTHESIA PROCESS

Phase	Action
1	Gas from anesthetic atmosphere → lung • Moved by ventilation and pressure gradient
2	Distribution of atmospheric gases and anesthetic agent with alveolar air • Mixing with alveolar air • Brownian dispersion • Molecular diffusion
3	Distribution of alveolar gases through respiratory alveolar-capillary membrane to blood Solution of anesthetic in blood flowing through pulmonary capillary
4	Circulation of anesthetic agents in pulmonary capillary blood to capillary bed of tissue
5	Diffusion from tissue capillaries → interstitial extracellular followed by passage across the cell membrane into intracellular fluid

the point of administration, and the patient's pulmonary system and will be least in the tissues and cells of the body. The gradient, is therefore, downward. Stations along this gradient are the upper respiratory tract, the alveolar air, the alveolar membrane, the blood, and the tissue cells. During recovery the anesthetic gradient is reversed.

Washout is a mass dilution effect.[63] For example, if an anesthetic circle system has a volume of 8 L filled with nitrogen and another gas is allowed to flow into the system at a rate of 4 L/min, the concentration of the new gas in the circuit rises exponentially (Fig. 12–7) and represents a washout curve. Thus, when a total of 8 L has flowed into the system, there will be a concentration of 63% of the new or inflowing gas in the system. This per cent is the point on a simple exponential curve at which the time is equal to one time constant. In such a system, a time constant equals the volume of the system divided by the flow.

When a proper anesthetic mixture in the anesthesia machine is established, the mixture may then be administered to a patient and the agent introduced into the lungs. If the lungs are continuously ventilated with a constant flow of gas, the curve would represent the lung washout, provided no other factor affects the simple relation. The rate at which the alveolar concentration of different anesthetic agents approaches that of the inspired concentration follows a pattern (Fig. 12–8).

The *effect of different anesthetic systems* in establishing a proper inspired partial pressure and the related alveolar partial pressure is illustrated in Figure 12–9.

II. ESTABLISHMENT OF AN ALVEOLAR CONCENTRATION OF ANESTHETIC

Attainment of atmospheric and alveolar gas equilibrium depends on *effective* alveolar ventilation. Thus, hyperventilation hastens the process. When there is respiratory depression, there is a decrease in the area of alveolar membrane exposed to the inhaled gases; likewise, the amount of anesthetic agent brought in contact with the blood stream through the pulmonary alveoli is lessened.

NATURE OF CURVES. The curves of alveolar concentration of agents follow a similar pattern in relation to the inspired concentration. Ventilation is the primary determinant of the curve, but it is modified by other factors such as: (1) the anesthetic agent and its anesthetic character; (2) differences in inspired concentration; (3) type of anesthetic system; (4) the circulation; (5) the coefficient of solubility; and (6) the tissue uptake. Examination of the curves (Fig. 12–8) for different agents shows the following:[64]

A rapid initial rise followed by a "knee," which then tapers off into a gradually ascending curve until eventually it reaches 100% of the inspired concentration.

FIG. 12–7. A well-mixed gas or fluid system washes out exponentially, where the time constant is the ratio of volume to flow. Concentration may be replaced by voltage across an equivalent capacitor in an electrical analog. (From Severinghaus, J.W.: The role of lung factors. In Uptake and Distribution of Anesthetic Agents. Edited by E.M. Papper and R.J. Kitz. New York, McGraw-Hill, 1963.

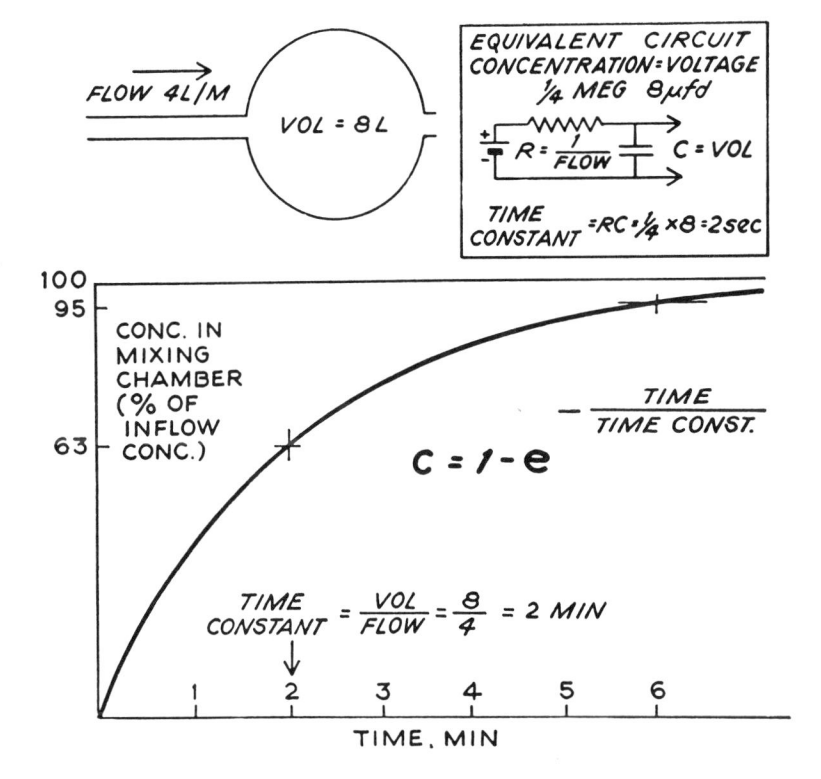

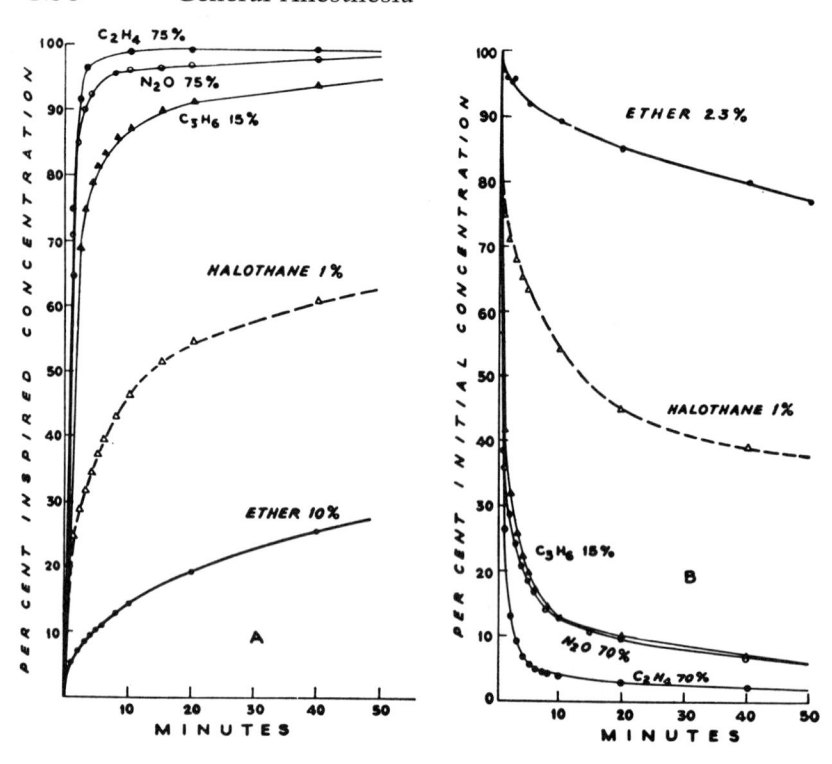

FIG. 12–8. The effect of change in inert gas on the rate at which alveolar concentration approaches that inspired. The curves on the left represent induction, and those on the right, recovery. The actual inspired concentration during induction is noted on the respective curves. Alveolar concentrations at the start of recovery are noted on the respective curves. The curves for recovery assume complete tissue equilibration. (From Eger, E.I.: Applications of a mathematical model of gas intake. *In* Uptake and Distribution of Anesthetic Agents. Edited by E.M. Papper and R.J. Kitz. New York, McGraw-Hill, 1963.

Analysis of a curve indicates that the initial rise is the result of lung washout. The knee represents the time at which a balance is achieved between the gas flow into the lungs and the uptake by the blood. Beyond the knee, the gradual rise is related to equilibrium of the agent with the tissues.

EFFECT OF ALVEOLAR VENTILATION ON THE ALVEOLAR CONCENTRATION CURVE. Alteration of the alveolar ventilation affects the concentration of agent in the alveoli as well as the washout previously discussed. With an increase in minute volume, there is a more rapid increase in alveolar concentration because of

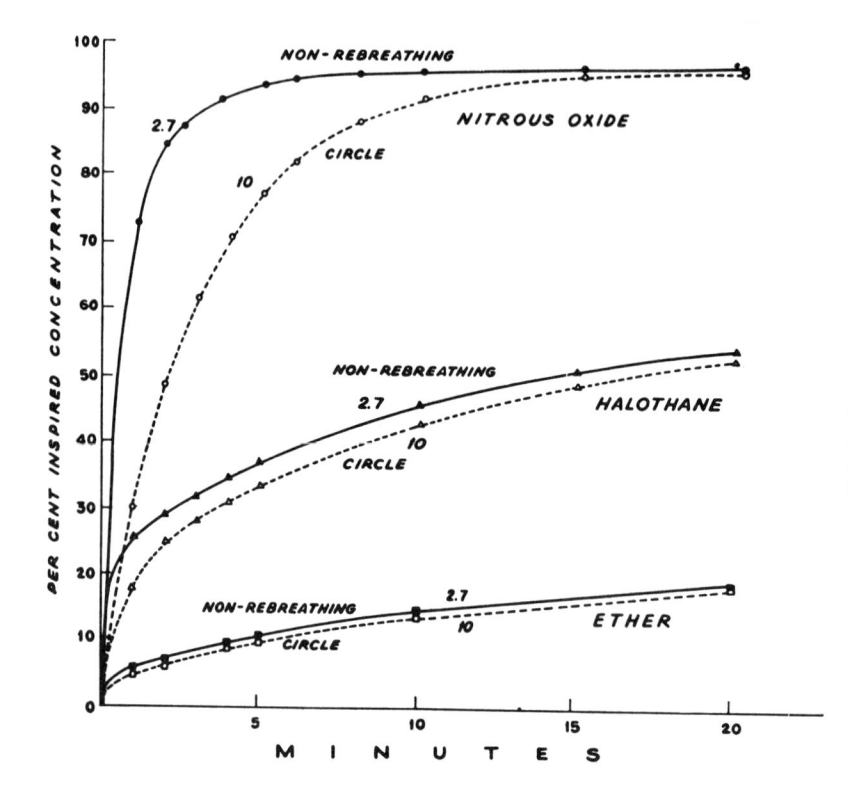

FIG. 12–9. The effect on alveolar concentration of interposing an anesthetic circle system between the patient and the gas source. This opposes a 10-L total gas phase (circle system + functional residual capacity (FRC) to a 2.7-L gas phase (nonrebreathing system, that is, FRC). Gas is flowing into the circle at 4 L/min. Inspired alveolar ventilation is 4 L/min plus whatever is drawn into the lungs by uptake. Nitrous oxide, 75% inspired (*top two graphs*), halothane, 1% (*middle two*), and ether, 10% (*lower two*) are compared. From Eger, E.I.: Applications of a mathematical model of gas uptake. *In* Uptake and Distribution of Anesthetic Agents. Edited by E.M. Papper and R.J. Kitz. New York, McGraw-Hill, 1963.

FIG. 12–10. The left side shows the effect on alveolar concentration of varying cardiac output from 2 to 6 to 18 L/min as indicated on each graph. Relative distribution of output is unchanged. The top three graphs are those of nitrous oxide, the middle three those of halothane, and the lower three those of ether. The right side similarly illustrates the effect of alteration of alveolar ventilation from 2 to 4 to 8 L/min. From Eger, E.I.: Applications of a mathematical model of gas uptake. *In* Uptake and Distribution of Anesthetic Agents. Edited by E.M. Papper and R.J. Kitz. New York, McGraw-Hill, 1963.

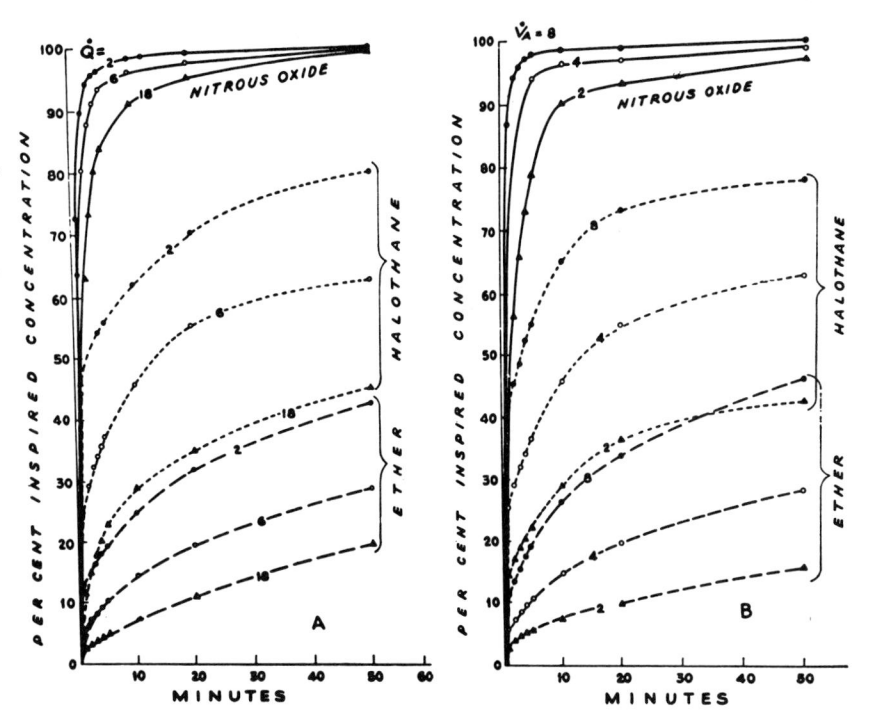

a more rapid washout. The increased input of anesthetic agent into the lungs also compensates for uptake by the blood. Washout is rapid with all of the agents. Blood uptake of soluble agents, however, affects the alveolar concentration. Ventilation has a limited effect on the alveolar concentration of nitrous oxide but a pronounced effect on the concentration of ether. Halothane is intermediate (Fig. 12–10).

Tidal volume must be an optimal volume. Too small a tidal volume will not effectively bring the anesthetic mixture into the alveoli. On the other hand, too large a tidal volume will raise the mean volume of the total gas phase, and this will dilute the rise in alveolar concentrations. This is a small factor but, on occasion, may be important.

DISTRIBUTION OF PULMONARY GASES. Inert gases within an alveolus are rapidly mixed and uniformly distributed. The mixing occurs at all times by diffusion and within hundredths of a second.

Uneven distribution between alveoli or pulmonary segments with some parts poorly ventilated will have a delaying effect on equilibrium between inspired agents and arterial concentration. This dead-space effect will also diminish the excretion of carbon dioxide and the oxygenation.

EFFECT OF PULMONARY CAPILLARY FLOW. Alveolar concentration of anesthetic agent varies with the perfusion of the pulmonary segment, which in turn depends on cardiac output. The effect of the pulmonary capillary flow as determined by cardiac output is shown for several agents (Fig. 12–10).

With nitrous oxide administered in the usual high concentration, this capillary flow effect on alveolar concentration is negligible. It is likewise of lesser importance with other insoluble agents. With highly soluble agents, however, blood uptake and the circulation are important. With halothane an increase in pulmonary segment perfusion results in a considerable reduction of alveolar concentration; with ether an increased perfusion or increased cardiac output results in the greatest reduction of alveolar concentration.

Another manner of expressing the effect of pulmonary capillary perfusion on the alveolar concentration is that of clearance fractions.[63] Briefly, it is the percent clearance of a unit of blood of its anesthetic agent in one passage through the lung during the elimination process. Conversely, it is the percentage approach to equilibrium of the blood with alveolar gas during one passage through the lung.

The elimination process is selected for discussion. The venous anesthetic content reaching the lung must equal the arterial content *plus* that lost to the alveoli (assuming a zero alveolar or inspired concentration). Thus, anesthetic inflow or venous content must equal arterial content plus the amount expired (Eq. 1)

$$\text{(Eq. 1)} \quad \begin{matrix} \text{ANESTHETIC INFLOW} \\ \text{OR} \\ \text{VENOUS ANESTHETIC} \\ \text{CONTENT} \end{matrix} = \text{Expired Anesthetic Volume} + \text{Arterial Anesthetic Volume}$$

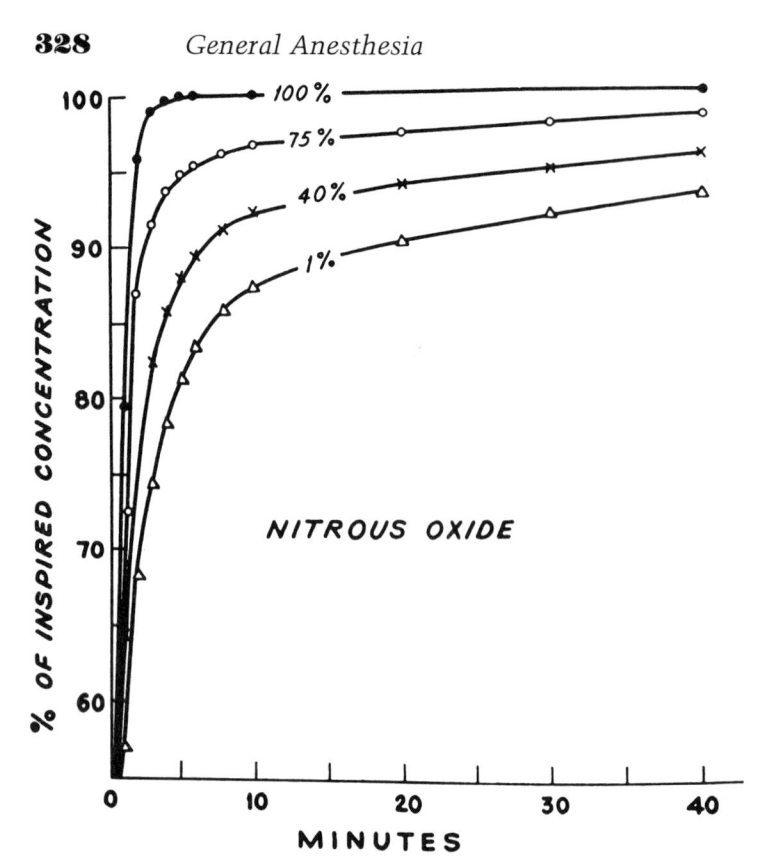

FIG. 12–11. Approach of alveolar nitrous oxide concentration to that inspired. Inspired concentrations are noted on the respective curves. From Eger, E.I.: Applications of a mathematical model of gas uptake. *In* Uptake and Distribution of Anesthetic Agents. Edited by E.M. Papper and R.J. Kitz. New York, McGraw-Hill, 1963.

Clearances can be calculated for different agents using the blood-gas partition coefficient. Thus, the clearance for ethylene is 85%; that is, 85% of the blood is cleared of its anesthetic content in one passage through the lung. Diethyl ether has a clearance of only 5% (Eq. 2).

EFFECT OF TISSUE UPTAKE ON CURVE OF ALVEOLAR CONCENTRATION.[65] The shape of the last part of the curve of alveolar concentration shows the effect of tissue uptake on alveolar concentration. Equilibration occurs first in tissues with a rich circulation and more slowly in tissues with a poor circulation. As tissues become saturated, the venous blood concentrations leaving the tissues show a rising concentration of agent so that the venous-alveolar gradient falls, alveolar-capillary uptake falls, and, consequently, alveolar concentrations rise. The influence of the vessel-rich group of tissues with a large relative blood flow is dominant with nitrous oxide and ether during the first 4 to 8 minutes. Halothane has a high tissue-blood partition coefficient with a high tissue uptake so that this effect on alveolar concentration lasts for 12 minutes or more before it is limited and a sharp break (or knee) appears in the alveolar concentration. After saturation of highly vascular tissues, the uptake by muscle and fat then becomes important.

In general, alveolar concentration approaches the inspired concentrations most rapidly with the insoluble agents such as ethylene, nitrous oxide, and cyclopropane. With the most soluble group of drugs the tissue uptake continues for a longer period and, during this time, influences alveolar concentrations.

For the two insoluble agents nitrous oxide and cyclopropane, each with a similar blood-gas partition coefficient, there is a noticeable difference in the attainment of alveolar equilibration with inspired gas. This is related to the *concentration effect*. With higher concentrations of agents in the inspired mixtures, there is a more rapid increase in alveolar concentration (Fig. 12–11). This effect is seen in the curves of different inspired nitrous oxide and ether-inspired concentrations (Fig. 12–12).

Attainment of an alveolar concentration is thus limited when inspired concentration is low and when uptake by the blood is high. This is exemplified by ether. If high concentrations of ether (such as 100%) are employed, however, the washout of the lung can be as fast as when other gases are breathed at 100% concentration.

THE SECOND GAS EFFECT.[66] In 1964, Epstein and colleagues suggested that the "uptake of large volumes of a first or primary gas (usually nitrous oxide) accelerates the alveolar rate of rise of a second gas given concomitantly."[66] This is known as the *second gas effect* (Table 12–4). Because the uptake of the first gas requires that there be an increase in subsequent inspiratory volumes to maintain a

$$\text{(Eq. 2)} \quad \text{PER CENT CLEARANCE} = \frac{\text{Expired Anesthetic Volume}}{\text{Venous Volume (Inflow Concentration)}} \times 100$$

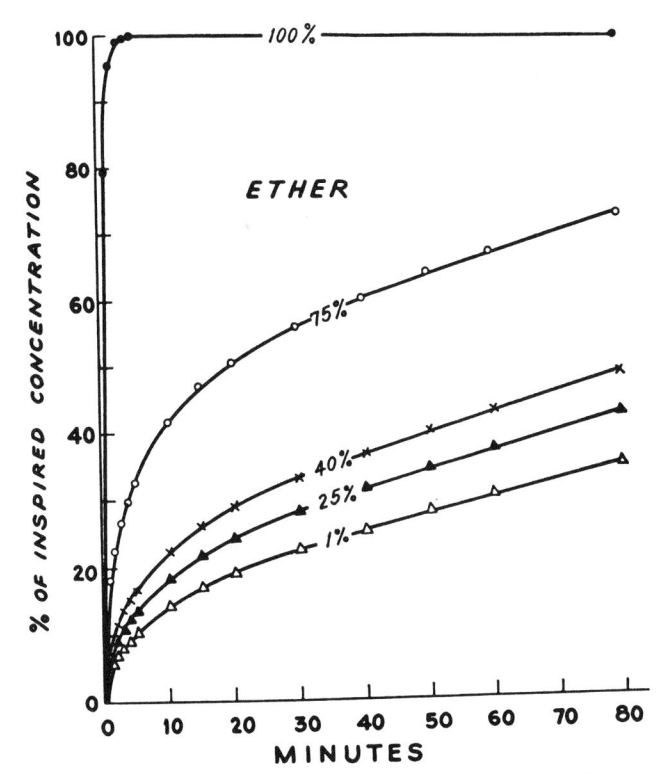

General Anesthesia—Fundamental Considerations **329**

FIG. 12–12. Approach of alveolar ether concentration to that inspired. Inspired concentrations are noted on the respective curves. From Eger, E.I.: Applications of a mathematical model of gas uptake. *In* Uptake and Distribution of Anesthetic Agents. Edited by E.M. Papper and R.J. Kitz. New York, McGraw-Hill, 1963.

proper pulmonary volume, Epstein concluded that the increase in ventilation should increase the alveolar concentration of all concomitantly inspired gases. Using a dog model, 0.5% halothane was administered under two conditions, (1) with 70% nitrous oxide and 30% oxygen, and (2) with 10% nitrous oxide and 90% oxygen. The alveolar rate of rise of both nitrous oxide and halothane were more rapid with higher nitrous oxide concentrations (Fig. 12–13). Not only did nitrous oxide concentration at 70% become higher at the higher inspired concentration, but at the same time, the alveolar halothane concentration rose more rapidly when mixed with 70% nitrous oxide and 30% oxygen as opposed to a mixture of 0.5% halothane in 10% nitrous oxide with 90% oxygen. With nitrous oxide, a poorly soluble agent, the uptake relies on the high concentration.

Stoelting, however, has suggested that the uptake of the primary gas in fact reduces the total lung gas volume and thereby concentrates any gas that has a different uptake rate when given concomitantly.[67]

III. ALVEOLAR-CAPILLARY MEMBRANE EQUILIBRIUM

The alveolar-capillary membrane may be regarded as a major dividing point in the progress of inhaled anesthetics from the atmosphere to the nervous system. An equilibrium of the anesthetic agent must be established between the alveolar air and the blood flowing in pulmonary capillaries. On the alveolar side, the anesthetics are in the gaseous state; on the capillary side these same agents are in solution. It is assumed that inert-gas exchange in the human body takes place only by diffusion (there is no significant contrary evidence).[68a] Diffusion velocity depends on properties of the membrane and characteristics of the agent.

TABLE 12–4. SECOND GAS EFFECT

- The uptake of large volumes of a first or primary gas (usually N_2O) is greater when the concentration of agent is increased.
- As uptake increases, there is increased alveolar ventilation and mixing with fresh mixture.
- The alveolar rate of rise of a second gas or vapor administered concomitantly is accelerated.
- Highly soluble agents cause a fractional increase in remaining agents in the alveoli and an increased fresh-gas-flow FGF inspiratory input (ventilation).
- Poorly soluble agents rely on the concentration effect of the inspired mixtures.

Adapted from Epstein, R.M., Racknow, H., Salanitre, E., and Wolf, G.L.: Influence of the concentration effect on the uptake of anesthetic mixtures: The second gas effect. Anesthesiology, 25:364–371, 1964.

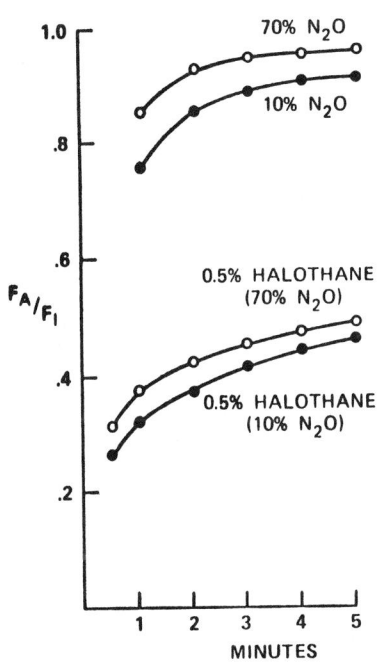

FIG. 12–13. Half percent halothane was administered to dogs under two conditions: (1) with 70% nitrous oxide; and (2) with 10% nitrous oxide. The alveolar rate of rise of both nitrous oxide and of halothane were more rapid with the higher nitrous oxide concentration. Adapted from Epstein, R.M., Rackow, H., Salanitre, E., and Wolf, G.L.: Influence of the concentration effect on the uptake of anesthetic mixtures: The second gas effect. Anesthesiology, 25:364, 1964.

ALVEOLAR-CAPILLARY INTERFACE.[69] Epithelium of the alveoli is separated from capillary endothelium by an interstitial space (ISS). This ISS measures about 1 μm and contains loose alveolar connective tissue and a lymphatic system.

The alveolar surface is composed of 95% alveolar type I cells—thin flat sheets 0.1 to 0.3 μm thick. The remaining surface cells are type II and are concerned with production of surfactant.

Electron microscopic studies indicate that the edges of capillary cells generally overlap, but there are some intercellular gaps about 2 to 6 nm in width through which particulate matter such as lipid droplets and leucocytes can pass. Of greater importance is the evidence for functional pores or fenestrations in the cell membrane through which water electrolytes and proteins may pass.

The endothelial cells of the capillary act as a semipermeable membrane and serve to process angiotension 1, bradykinin, prostacyclin, and factor VIII.

From the physiochemical standpoint, the membrane may be considered a thin film of a watery solution of protein. The membrane factors include the thickness and the total respiratory alveolar area. Tissue membranes (and cell boundaries) appear to present little resistance to the diffusion of chemically inert gases. Such membranes are thin, and the passage of gases is not restricted to the hydrophilic portion of the membrane. (Surface films of solution on the membrane may offer considerable resistance). In the passage of gases across the biologic membranes, a number of mechanisms and transport systems are available.[70]

PASSIVE TRANSPORT SYSTEM. This system is related to lipid solubility of diffusing molecules in the membrane. To some degree, permeability to lipid-soluble substances is increased as the molecules become more soluble in fatty oils and ether.* Molecular size also is important with respect to the time of penetration. With short chains, penetration time is not greatly different, although lipid solubility may increase with each carbon atom by a factor of 6 until the length of a carbon chain increases to 7 or 8 carbons, when the time for penetration gets longer. Thus, large lipid-soluble molecules are a factor of importance in the rate of diffusion. It must be stressed that the solubility of anesthetic gases in human lipids is not identical to the solubility in olive oil.

PHYSICAL TRANSPORT SYSTEM. Pores in a cell membrane offer a route for lipid-insoluble agents to enter a cell. Investigations indicate that a pore radius of 4 Å is representative of a number of cell membranes. Thus, 3-carbon chains of nonlipid substances may pass but larger molecules may not. Obviously, the shape of a molecule is a factor. Thus, the substitution of a hydroxyl group for a hydrogen atom as represented by tartrate versus the maleate molecule increases penetration time by a factor of 7. Hormones as well as pharmacologic agents influence the pore size. The antidiuretic hormone increases the pore radius in Necturus kidney slices.

The process of solvent drag is an example of a passive transport system that also can carry agents through membranes. It describes the carriage of a solute by a stream of water that is flowing through a pore.

ACTIVE TRANSPORT SYSTEM. Such systems cause a *net* movement of ions and molecules against a concentration gradient. Energy is needed, and an unequal transmembrane distribution of ions results.

The rate of diffusion of an agent follows laws described by Fick.[60b] Pertinent characteristics of diffusion of agents are four: (A) partial pressure of the gas (pressure gradient) (a reasonable substitute for concentration of an agent); (B) blood flow; (C) membrane property; and (D) drug profile. In a normal individual, there is a controlled movement of gas determined by and directly proportional to the pressure gradient and the solubility of the gas in water (the membrane is a film of water); the movement also is inversely proportional to the square root of the molecular weight of the gas.

Two of these factors, solubility and molecular weight, are constant for a particular agent. The membrane factor consists of two parts: the area, and thickness of the membrane. The quantity or rate of diffusion of an agent that goes across a membrane is directly proportional to the area and inversely to the thickness. In general, the membrane factor is also a constant for a given person.

Hence, with these factors the following formula (Eq. 3) may be established:

---

* The Classical Theory.
Overton, E.: Studien uber die Narkose Zugleich ein Beitrag zur Allgemeinen Pharmakologie, Jena, G. Fischer, 1901

(Eq. 3)

$$\text{DIFFUSION VELOCITY} \atop \text{(Quantity Transferred Per Unit Time Across a Membrane)} = \underbrace{\text{Concentration Gradient} \atop \text{(Partial Pressure)}}_{[A]} \times \underbrace{\text{Blood Flow}}_{[B]} \times \underbrace{K_1 \text{(Membrane Property)}}_{[C]} \times \underbrace{\text{Drug Profile } K_2 \; \frac{\text{Solubility of Gas in Blood}}{\sqrt{\text{Molecular Weight}}}}_{[D]}$$

Only the partial pressure is a variable. Passage across the membrane, therefore, depends on two factors: (1) partial pressure of the gas in the alveoli; and (2) the solubility of the agent in the membrane and in water.

The entry into solution in the blood similarly depends on partial pressure (Law of Partial Pressure) and blood solubility (Henry's Law). From the mathematic and experimental evidence, it appears that equilibrium always exists between alveolar gas and blood leaving the capillaries.

TIME FOR ALVEOLAR-CAPILLARY EQUILIBRIUM. The time required for an inert gas in an alveolus to cross the alveolar membrane and to equilibrate with a segment of flowing capillary blood has been calculated from studies using carbon monoxide. According to these studies blood will be 99% equilibrated in less than 0.01 second. Since blood spends a little less than 1 second in the capillaries, equilibration can easily take place.[69]

Intracapillary blood will have a uniform gas tension. Even for gases of high molecular weight whose diffusion might be slower, equilibrium will rapidly occur and no significant inert gas tension gradient will exist in capillary blood. Therefore, equilibrium always exists between alveolar gas and blood leaving the capillaries of the lung.

BLOOD SOLUBILITY OF ANESTHETICS.[71-73, 76-78] Blood solubility is best expressed as a blood-gas partition coefficient and is determined at body temperature. This coefficient represents the ratio of the anesthetic concentration in blood to the anesthetic concentration in the gas phase at equilibrium. An equilibrium is established when the partial pressure is equal in the two phases. With gases, this is the same as the Ostwald coefficient (Table 12–5).[72-80]

TABLE 12–5. PARTITION COEFFICIENTS OF SOME ANESTHETIC GASES AT 37° C. ± 0.5° C.

Anesthetic Gas	Water/Gas	Blood/Gas	Oil/Gas	Tissue/Blood
Ethylene	0.081*	0.140	1.28	1.0 (Heart)
				1.2 (Brain)
Xenon	0.102	0.20	1.90	1.25 (Brain-White)
	0.097*		1.93*	0.7 (Brain-Grey)
Cyclopropane	0.204	0.415	11.2*	0.81 (Muscle)†
				1.36 (Liver)†
Nitrous Oxide	0.435*	0.468*	1.4	1.13 (Heart)
				1.06 (Brain)
Servoflurane		0.59	55.0	1.0 (Lung)
Fluroxene	0.84	1.37	47.7	1.43 (Brain)
				1.37 (Liver)
				2.27 (Muscle)
Halothane	0.74	2.3	224	2.6 (Brain)
		2.36		2.6 (Liver)
		2.4		1.6 (Kidney)
				3.5 (Muscle)
				60.0 (Fat)
Enflurane	0.8	1.9	98.5	2.6 (Brain)
				3.0 (Muscle)
				3.8 (Liver)
Isoflurane	0.61	1.4	98.0	3.6 (Brain)
				3.5 (Liver)
				4.6 (Muscle)
				94.5 (Fat)
Oxygen (100%)	1.33	2.40	—	—
Divinyl Ether	1.40	2.8	58†	—
Ethyl Chloride	—	3.0	4.05	—
Trichloroethylene	1.55	9.15	960	
		9.85		
Chloroform	3.8	10.3	265	1.0 (Heart)
		8.4		1.0 (Brain)
Methoxyflurane	4.5	13.0	825	2.34 (Brain-White)
		11–12		1.70 (Brain-Grey)
				1.34 (Muscle)
Diethyl Ether	13.1	12.1	65	1.14 (Brain)
	15.61	15.2	50.2	1.2 (Lung)

* Bunsen coefficient corrected to 37° C.
† Calculated from published data.
Source: Larson, C.P., Jr., Eger E.I., Severinghaus, J.W.: Ostwald solubility coefficients for anesthetic gases in various fluids and tissues. Anesthesiology, 23:868, 1962, and communication of E.I. Eger, 1974.[71-76]

Gas tensions of anesthetic agents in arterial blood progressively increase with the duration of administration and approach an equilibrium with inspired tension.

The solubility of the agent largely determines the shape of the curve of blood uptake.[71] The increase in partial pressure in blood is rapid for the relatively insoluble agents and slow for those that are more soluble. This is evident in the sharp bend or knee of the curve for slightly soluble agents. For more soluble agents, the knee is not sharp and blood tension approaches the inspired concentration more slowly.

Difference in clinical behavior or the establishment of anesthesia by different agents is based essentially on the alveolar concentration and the factor of solubility. The more lipid soluble an anesthetic agent, the lower the arterial concentration required to produce anesthesia. It is also clear that the more lipid soluble an anesthetic agent, the longer it takes to establish an alveolar concentration in equilibrium with the capillary blood.

Three groups of agents may be recognized on the basis of solubility.

1. Low Coefficient of Solubility. Agents in this group include nitrous oxide, ethylene, and cyclopropane. These drugs are poorly soluble in whole blood (37° C). The first equilibrium between anesthetic atmosphere and alveolar air is relatively rapid and is achieved in about 5 minutes. As soon as this occurs, the tension of the agent in the blood stream quickly equals that in the alveoli because of the high alveolar concentration. Therefore, the attainment of an anesthetic tissue concentration is rapid.

2. Intermediate Coefficient of Solubility. Agents included in this group are halothane, fluroxene, ethyl chloride, and divinyl ether. The first equilibrium between atmospheric mixture and alveolar air is established somewhat slowly compared with ethylene or nitrous oxide. Because of an intermediate solubility ratio, the uptake of these agents by the blood and tissues is relatively rapid. Thus, attainment of an alveolar partial pressure of the agent is delayed. Attainment of anesthesia is thus intermediate between the other two groups of agents.

3. High Coefficient of Solubility. This group includes such substances as diethyl ether, trichloroethylene, chloroform, and methoxyflurane. These agents pass across the alveolar membrane and are quickly taken up by the blood. This rapid absorption by the blood also rapidly depletes the anesthetic concentration in the alveolar air. Because the mass of anesthetic brought to the alveoli is relatively small, an adequate concentration in the alveoli and the first stage of the equilibrium between inhaled atmosphere and the alveolar air are delayed. An adequate alveolar concentration depends on ventilation. In view of this, Haggard stated that absorption ether is for practical purposes "proportional with volume of lung ventilation."[79]

FACTORS MODIFYING SOLUBILITY. The commonly used values for blood-gas partition coefficients of various inhalation agents show variations with respect to weight, age, and hemoglobin levels.

Age significantly affects blood solubility coefficients (Table 12–6). The greatest coefficient is in adults and the least in infants. The coefficient in infants is lower by about 18% than in adults. Children show intermediate values, and the coefficient is about 12% lower than in adults. Elderly subjects show values similar to children.[81]

Blood-gas partition coefficients depend to some extent on the concentration of several serum lipid and protein constituents. At least two constituents are needed to predict the partition coefficient.[82] The coefficients of isoflurane and enflurane correlate directly with serum albumin and triglyceride concentrations. Halothane's coefficient correlates with cholesterol and triglycerides and less so with albumin and globulin. Methoxyflurane correlates with cholesterol and both albumin and globulin.[82,83]

The lower coefficient in infants and children explains the more rapid rate of rise in alveolar partial pressure of these volatile agents. Consequently, the rate of induction of anesthesia is more rapid in infants and children than in adults, because the induction rate is proportional to the rate of rise of alveolar partial pressures with respect to the inspired anesthetic partial pressure. A stable alveolar partial pressure presents the establishment of a uniform alveolar-blood equilibrium.

There is a negative correlation for weight that is approximately linear. Obese subjects have a lowered coefficient.[84]

Blood solubility coefficients of anesthetic drugs may be modified by factors altering the composition of blood.[85] For example, a decreased concentration of red blood cells from hemorrhage or anemia reduces blood solubility. A hematocrit of 30 reduces the solubility of halothane by 24% and of methoxyflurane by 22%.[85] As hematocrit increases, the coefficient increases.[85]

One important implication of the above is that the blood-gas coefficients for patients with anemia are significantly less than those with a normal hematocrit. Simultaneously, the equilibrium between inspired concentration and alveolar concentration is more rapidly established, and both induction and recovery are more rapid.

Eating significantly increases blood solubility of all volatile anesthetic agents.[86] The increase varies from 17% to 24%. The mechanism involves both carbohydrate and protein metabolism. In the process of digestion, a release of insulin occurs and a reduction in free fatty acids in the blood ensues. Because the fatty acids are transported bound to plasma al-

TABLE 12–6. INFLUENCE OF AGE ON BLOOD SOLUBILITY COEFFICIENTS OF SELECTED ANESTHETIC AGENTS

	Newborns/Infants	Children (3–7 yr)	Adults (26–40 yr)	Elderly (75–85 yr)
Isoflurane	1.19	1.28	1.46	1.29
Ethrane	1.78	1.78	2.07	1.79
Halothane	2.14	2.39	2.65	2.41
Methoxyflurane	13.30	15.0	16.0	15.0

bumin, a decrease in free fatty acids will allow more albumin binding sites for inhalation anesthetic agents and an increase in solubility (inhalation anesthetics are bound loosely to plasma albumin).

Because there is an increased blood uptake and binding in the postprandial state for as long as 6 hours, there is a slowing in the rate of rise of end-tidal alveolar concentration of the anesthetics and a prolongation of induction.

Excretion rates are also changed. There is a relatively slower initial rate during the first 15 minutes that is followed by a more rapid excretion. Also, a greater biodegradation may occur as a result of increased liver perfusion consequent to eating.[86]

Some evidence shows a correlation between the increase in blood cholesterol and triglyceride and an increased solubility of agents, but this has not been found by Munson.[86]

ANESTHETIC POTENCY

DEVELOPMENT OF CONCEPTS. Quantification of depth of general anesthesia was proposed by John Snow in 1858 as a patient's varying response to a painful stimulus. A minimal stimulus might not evoke signs of pain during light anesthesia, but a more intense stimulus would do so and require more anesthesia. Thus, responses of patients during anesthesia enabled one to assess the depth of anesthesia and estimate the potency of agents used, which at that time included ether and chloroform.[87]

In 1946 Robbins defined potency as the AD_{50}.[88] This was determined as the inspired concentration of an anesthetic at which 50% of mice failed to right themselves in 15 seconds after tumbling in a bottle. A lethal dose (LD_{50}) was considered as the anesthetic concentration that produced apnea in 50% of mice. These indices obviously had little clinical merit.

Guedel defined general anesthesia as a descending depression of the entire CNS and outlined the signs and reflexes as obtundation progressed with increasing concentrations of inspired anesthetic.[89] Haggard showed that blood levels of ether correlated with progressive obtundation and related these to Guedel's stages.[89a] At the clinical level, these signs remain of practical value, and variations can be related to different anesthetic agents.

Other approaches to depth of anesthesia include Faulconer's EEG signs,[89b] which correlate with progressive obtundation of nervous system phenomena (see Chapter 13).

Because of the development of balanced anesthetic technique, Woodbridge introduced the valuable concept of components of general anesthesia, each of which should be appropriately blocked if an adequate stress-free state is to be produced.[91]

All of these concepts have proved clinically satisfactory. Precision was given to potency, however, with the development of the concept of (MAC) by Eger in 1963.[92] Such potency is based on the alveolar concentrations of inhaled anesthetic drugs.

Minimum Alveolar Concentration

DEFINITION. Minimum alveolar concentration[92] (MAC) is defined as that alveolar concentration necessary to prevent a gross skeletal muscle response to a standard painful stimulus (skin incision) in 50% of patients. This is known as 1.0 MAC for an agent at 1.0 atmosphere. Potency is considered as the reciprocal of the partial pressure of an agent that is required to achieve the stated anesthetic effect. Thus, an inverse relationship exists between MAC and potency.[61,93]

At equilibrium, the partial pressures of an anesthetic are equal in all tissues; the actual concentrations of an agent in different tissues, however, are not equal, because concentration is a function of the solubility of the agent in the different tissues. Yet, at equilibrium, the partial pressure in the gray matter of the brain is almost equal to that in the alveoli because the gray brain matter is richly profused. The end-tidal anesthetic partial pressure thus corresponds to (reflects) the brain anesthetic partial pressure more accurately than the inspired or venous percentage concentrations. It is also important in administration of anesthesia at higher altitudes, because partial pressures and not concentrations are the effective pharmacologic factors.

MAC thus defines one point on a hypothetical dose-response curve. Such a curve is a plot of anesthetic dose against an index of depth of anesthesia. It is a useful biologic unit of anesthetic-induced CNS depression.

Two important features relate the value of MAC to oil-gas solubility. Because the potency of any an-

334 General Anesthesia

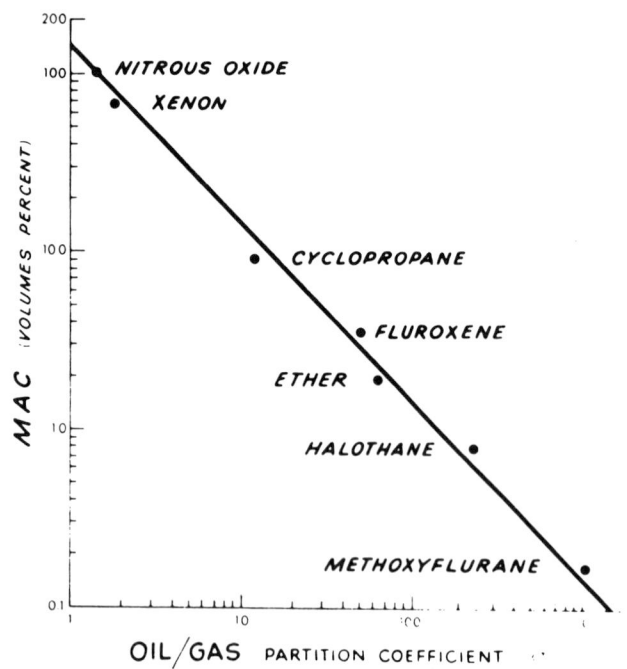

FIG. 12–14. The relation between MAC and oil-gas partition coefficient. The correlation is shown for several general anesthetic agents and some inert gases not used for anesthesia. The log scales show the correlation over a wide range of fat solubilities and potencies. The line through the points satisfies the equation MAC × oil/gas partition coefficient = 143. This value is the average of all multiplications of MAC × the Partition Coefficient from experimental data. (Modified from Saidman et al., 1967; Eger, 1969; Miller, 1972.) From Goodman and Gilman's The Pharmacological Basis of Therapeutics (Gilman, A.G., Goodman, L.S., Rall, T.W., Murad, F. Eds.) in Chapter 13: 7th ed. History and Principles of Anesthesiology, T.C. Smith and H. Wollman, pp. 260–275, New York, Macmillan Publishing Co., 1985. With permission.

esthetic agent may be related directly to its oil-gas solubility coefficient (lipid solubility), the value of MAC multiplied by the oil-gas partition coefficient should be approximately the same for all agents. (Fig. 12–14).[93]

Work on dogs has substantiated this concept: an inverse relationship between MAC and the oil-gas partition coefficient has been demonstrated, and the multiplication of these two factors results in essentially the same product. From the MAC value, a parameter known as the *minimum alveolar tension* of the agent may also be derived when the barometric pressure is known.

MAC MEASURE OF ANESTHETIC DOSE.[94] MAC provides a clinical yardstick for determining an anesthetic dose. It allows a comparison of anesthetizing equipotency with respect to its anesthetic effect on CNS depression, which is a clinical sign of anesthesia.

Because MAC defines only the dose of an inhaled anesthetic agent that produces a CNS depression to eliminate movement in response to a skin incision in only 50% of patients, it is necessary to determine the MAC value for ED_{95}, i.e., a clinically practical anesthetic dose that will immobilize 100% of patients.[95,96] An ED_{95} can be ascertained from clinical practice. To this extent, it has been demonstrated that there is a 5% to 40% increase in the value of MAC for most common inhalation anesthetic agents. In brief, the available data indicate that at 1.4 MAC for any inhalational anesthetic, at least 95% of all patients will be anesthetized in surgical planes of anesthesia.

RELATIONSHIP OF MAC TO TOXICITY. MAC provides a means of expressing a total dose of inhalation anesthetic. This is expressed as MAC hours, i.e., the dose multiplied by time. For the moderately to highly lipid-soluble anesthetics, MAC hours provides a relatively accurate estimation of the amount of anesthetic delivered and metabolized. It thus provides a means of comparing different anesthetics with regard to side effects on other systems, such as respiratory, cardiac, and renal, at equipotency levels. It also provides a tool to compare toxicities.[94]

TABLE 12–7. ANESTHETIC DOSE, PATIENT NOREPINEPHRINE RESPONSES, AND CALCULATED DOSES BLOCKING ADRENERGIC RESPONSE

	MAC Multiple/Morphine dose (mg/kg)*				MAC BAR$_{50}$†	MAC BAR$_{95}$
	1.0	1.3/0.4	1.6/0.9	1.9/1.4		
Enflurane	—	34 (9)‡	43 (14)	73 (11)	1.60 ± 0.13 MAC	2.57 MAC
Halothane	0 (6)	42 (12)	56 (9)	87 (15)	1.45 ± 0.08 MAC	2.10 MAC
Morphine	—	0 (8)	13 (8)	87 (8)	1.13 ± 0.09 mg/kg plus 60% N$_2$O	1.45 mg/kg plus 60% N$_2$O

* Sixty percent nitrous oxide was administered as a background to all general anesthetics. MAC doses for enflurane and halothane include calculated MAC contribution of nitrous oxide.
† Dose for blocking adrenergic response ± 1 SD.
‡ Results are given as percentages of patient population whose plasma level of norepinephrine did not increase by 10% or more following skin incision; the number of patients studied is given in parentheses.
From Roizen, M.F., Horrigan, R.W., and Frazer, B.M.: Anesthetic doses blocking adrenergic (stress) and cardiovascular responses to incision: MAC BAR. Anesthesiology, 54:390, 1981.

General Anesthesia—Fundamental Considerations

TABLE 12–8. COMPARISON OF MAC WITH MAC EI AND MAC BAR*

	MAC$_{50}$[†]	MAC$_{95}$	MAC EI$_{50}$[‡]	MAC EI$_{95}$	MAC BAR$_{50}$[§]	MAC BAR$_{95}$
Halothane	1.0 MAC 0.74 ± 0.03%	1.2 MAC	1.3 MAC	1.7 MAC	1.5 ± 0.1 MAC	2.1 MAC
Enflurane	1.0 MAC 1.68 ± 0.04%	1.1 MAC	1.4 MAC	1.9 MAC	1.6 ± 0.1 MAC	2.6 MAC
Morphine sulfate	—	—	—	—	1.13 ± 0.1 mg/kg plus 60% N_2O	1.5 mg/kg plus 60% N_2O

* Decimals for MAC equivalents have been rounded off to first order.
† Minimum alveolar concentration that inhibits movement in response to a noxious stimulus in 50% of individuals.
‡ Minimum alveolar concentration that inhibits movement and coughing to endotracheal intubation in 50% of individuals.
§ Minimum alveolar concentration that inhibits adrenergic response to skin incision in 50% of individuals.
From Roizen, M.F., Horrigan, R.W., and Frazer, B.M.: Anesthetic doses blocking adrenergic (stress) and cardiovascular responses to incision: MAC BAR. Anesthesiology, 54:390, 1981.

For example, subclinical nephrotoxicity of methoxyflurane occurs at about 2.5 MAC hours. In contrast, as much as 2.7 MAC hours of enflurane will not result in any renal impairment.

MAC-BAR.[97] To access the stress-ablating capacity of different inhalation agents, the concept of MAC-BAR has been proposed. MAC-BAR has been defined as "the minimum alveolar concentration that inhibits adrenergic response to skin incision in 50% of individuals (MAC-BAR$_{50}$). The MAC-BAR$_{95}$ is that alveolar concentration which inhibits the adrenergic responses in 95% of individuals."

A refined MAC value has also been considered applicable at the time of intubation and has been designated as MAC-EI$_{50}$. This is essentially the anesthetic concentration value in MAC units that prevents a sympathetic response to endotracheal intubation (EI) in 50% of patients.

In the study by Roizen,[97] the age-adjusted values for anesthetic agents that block the neuroendocrine adrenergic response to a skin incision for different inhalation agents is presented in Tables 12–7 and 12–8 and Fig. 12–15.

The MAC values for different anesthetic objectives are essentially *multiples* of the basic MAC value (Table 12–8):

- The MAC-EI$_{95}$, which inhibits movement and coughing to endotracheal intubation in 95% of subjects, shows multiples of 1.7 MAC for halothane and 1.9 MAC for enflurane.
- The MAC-BAR$_{95}$, which inhibits adrenergic responses in 95% of subjects, shows multiples of 2.1 MAC for halothane and 2.6 MAC for enflurane in terms of plasma norepinephrine (Table 12–8).
- The dose of morphine preventing various responses during 60% of nitrous oxide is stated as 1.5 mg/kg to inhibit an adrenergic response in terms of increased plasma norepinephrine.

FACTORS MODIFYING MAC (Tables 12–9A and 9B).[87] A knowledge of MAC values permits useful clinical applications and enables the clinician to modify the inspired concentrations. Variations in MAC val-

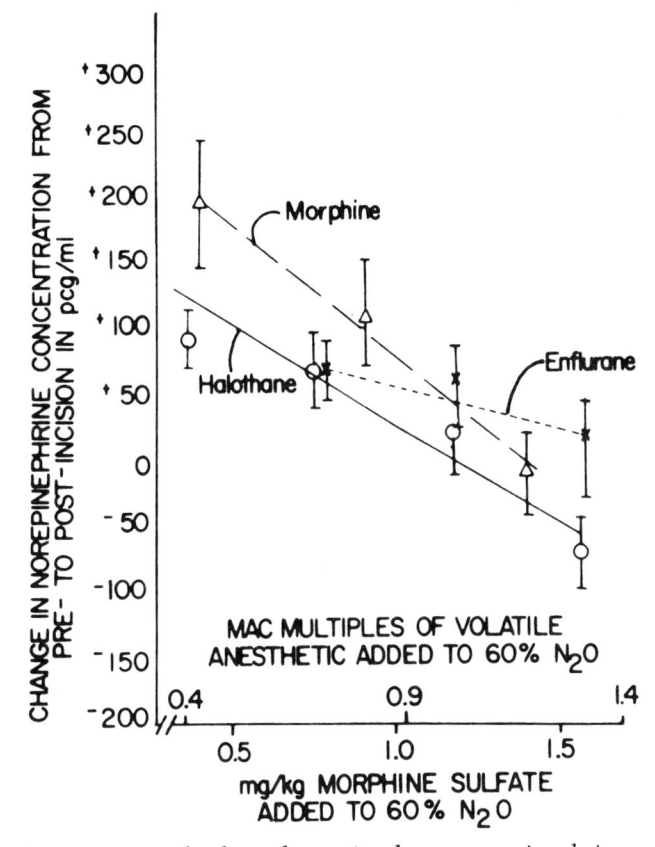

FIG. 12–15. Absolute change in plasma norepinephrine levels (pg/ml) after incision *vs.* the end-tidal dose of anesthesia the patient was receiving. The lines are described as follows: for morphine, the change in norepinephrine = (−207) (mg/kg dose of morphine) + 292 (r = 0.60); for halothane, the change in norepinephrine = (−199) (MAC dose of halothane including 60% N_2O) + 326 (r = 0.60); for enflurane, the change in norepinephrine = (−80) (MAC dose of enflurane including 60% N_2O) + 179 (r = 0.56). *Note:* These equations represent an alternate method of depicting data presented in the text. The x-axis MAC values in the figure do not include the 0.57 MAC contribution of nitrous oxide that is included in the text and tables. From Roizen, M.F., Horrigan, R.W., and Frazer, B.M.: Anesthetic doses blocking adrenergic (stress) and cardiovascular responses to incision: MAC BAR. Anesthesiology, 54:390, 1981.

TABLE 12-9A. FACTORS DECREASING MAC OF VOLATILE AGENTS

Advancing age
Sex (no known change)
Diurnal variation parallels metabolic activity[103]
Electrolytes
   Magnesium elevation
   Hyponatremia
Narcotics
   Morphine > fentanyl > nalbuphine
Intravenous anesthetics
   Diazepam[104]
   Ketamine[105]
Relaxants
   Pancuronium Reduces MAC of halothane 0.75 to 0.55[106]
Drugs decreasing CNS
   Catecholamines
Antihypertensive drugs (central acting)
   Clonidine
   Reserpine
   Methyldopa
Intravenous lidocaine[107,108]
Increased uptake after *eating*
   increases blood solubility[103]
Alcohol ingestion[109,110]
   (not chronic alcoholism)
Deliberate hypotension with pentolinum, trimethaphan, or nitroprusside
    MAC reduction by 20%
    parallels MAP[111]
Hypothermia
   8% reduction/°C[112,113]
Chronic sympathomimetic amine intake
$Pa_{CO_2} > 70$ mm Hg[85]
Metabolic Acidosis
   Hypoxemia ($Pa_{O_2} < 38$ mm Hg

Adapted from Quasha, A.L., Eger, E.I., and Tinker, J.H.: Determination and applications of MAC: Review. Anesthesiology, 53:315, 1980.

ues may result from many physiologic and pharmacologic factors.

Age. The effect of age is significant. There is an inverse relationship of age to MAC values (Table 12–9A).[65] For example, the MAC value for halothane decreases with advancing years from a high of 1.08 in infants to a low of 0.64 in the eighth decade.[98] Another example is that of enflurane. The usual MAC value for enflurane is 1.68 in the age group of 20 to 40; the MAC value in infants is 2.4; in children, the value is 2.0. The MAC value for those at 60 years of age is 1.4.[99] Isoflurane shows a continuous decrease in MAC from birth to 80 years or older (Fig. 12–16). Only at puberty is there a slight leveling in value.[100–102]

Sex. Sex has not been shown to produce any changes in MAC values.

Diurnal Variations. These are recognized, and they parallel metabolic activity (Fig. 12–17).[103] Thus, in the daytime period between 3:00 A.M. and 10:00 A.M., when catecholamines are at their lowest, the MAC values are also decreased. Ordinarily, epinephrine increases during the morning and peaks at about 4:00 P.M.[114] Any action or stress that increases metabolic activity will also increase the MAC value for a given anesthetic state.

Body Temperature. Values for MAC also vary directly with body temperature.[115,116] As temperature increases, MAC also increases. Febrile patients may require more agent over the duration of anesthesia. Altered physiology due to fever, however, enhances toxicity.

CNS Catecholamines. Anesthetic requirements and MAC values are altered by the level of CNS catecholamines.[117] The release, by any stress, of nor-

TABLE 12-9B. FACTORS INCREASING MAC[122A]

Young age—Newborn and infants[130A]
Temperature elevation—Increases in proportion to increased metabolism (8% increase for each °C on halothane)[115]
Increased central catecholamines
Drug effects
   Amphetamines (acute administration)[119]
   Only ephedrine of common vasopressors[116]
   Cocaine[161]
   Monoamine oxidase inhibitors[118]
   Other antidepressants
   Atracurium (laudanosine)[145]
Alcoholism (chronic)[109,156]—Isoflurane: 30% to 45% increase;[157] halothane 30% increase[110]

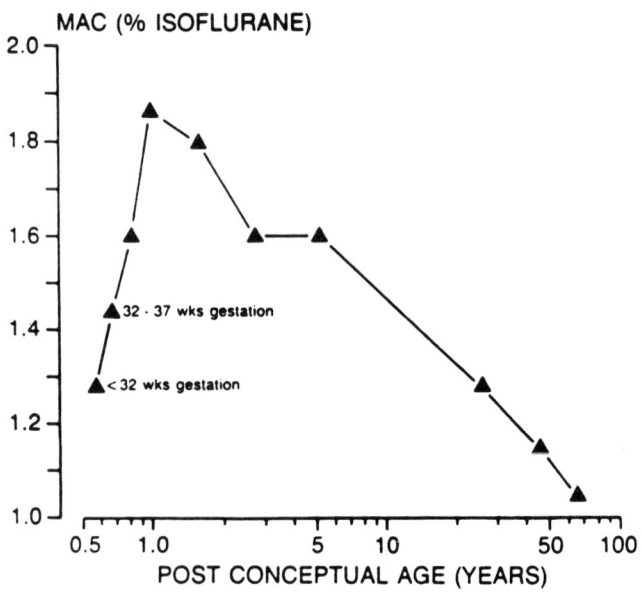

FIG. 12–16. The MAC of isoflurane as related to all ages. Values for postconceptual age were obtained by adding 40 weeks to the mean postnatal age for each age group. A similar curve for ages postpartum has been determined for halothane. A slight increase has been noted at puberty. From LeDez, K.M., and Lerman, J.: The minimum alveolar concentration (MAC) of isoflurane in preterm neonates. Anesthesiology, 67:301, 1987.

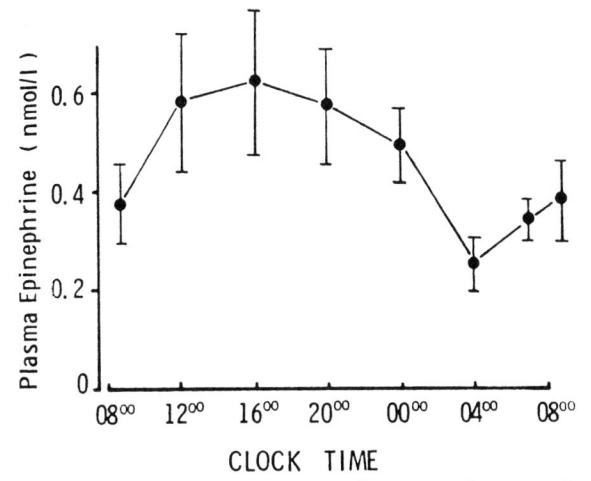

FIG. 12–17. Circadian variation of venous plasma epinephrine. To convert nmol/L to μg/L, multiply by 0.18. From Barnes, P.: Nocturnal asthma and changes in circulating epinephrine, histamine, and cortisol. N. Engl. J. Med., 303:263, 1980.

epinephrine in the CNS increases the anesthetic need and raises MAC values. Intake of certain sympathomimetic amines, such as amphetamines, releases norepinephrine centrally; amphetamines cause a dose-dependent increase in MAC values.[118] Chronic sympathomimetic amine intake, however, reduces the CNS levels of norepinephrine and thereby reduces the MAC value. Chronic intake of such agents decreases MAC of halothane by 21% ± 5%. Chronic amphetamine abusers also respond poorly to indirectly acting sympathomimetic agents such as ephedrine.[117] Most drugs that act by depleting CNS catecholamines reduce the MAC values.[119,120]

Levodopa is the precursor to dopamine synthesis and does not directly affect norepinephrine and epinephrine concentrations. Thus, ordinary doses may reduce MAC, but acutely administered large doses may increase MAC requirement.[121]

Because circulating catecholamines do not readily cross the blood-brain barrier, the peripheral release of such catecholamines does not contribute to CNS stimulation.

Mixtures of Inhalation Anesthetics. Each component is reduced so that the sum is equal to the whole MAC value for the anesthetic requirement.[108] Thus, halothane (when administered in a 70% nitrous oxide atmosphere) has a MAC value of 0.29 (equal to a concentration of 0.29%); in contrast, halothane in air or oxygen has a MAC of 0.71 (equal to a concentration of 0.71%)—that is, the requirement for halothane is reduced by 61%.[122] Simply stated, 0.5 MAC of one agent plus 0.5 MAC of a second is equal to the effect of 1.0 MAC of either agent.

Most inhalation anesthetics show a similar synergistic effect, which is in accordance with the gas-hydrate theory of anesthesia.[123] One exception is the combination or mixing of cyclopropane with either nitrous oxide or ethylene; these agents are antagonistic when given together. The effect is explained by the competition between these agents for the spaces in the hydrate structure.[108]

Hypotension and Anemia. Hypotension from any cause will reduce MAC values.[111] Hemorrhage and severe chronic anemia (hemoglobin level less than 7.0 g) both will decrease the values for MAC.[85]

Respiratory Gases. MAC is not altered by elevated Pa_{CO_2} within the range of 20 to 80 mm Hg, nor by hypocapnea,[124] but Pa_{CO_2} values above 80 mm Hg are associated with a decreased value.[85] Metabolic acidosis decreases MAC value by 10% to 20%. Hypoxia has no effect until Pa_{O_2} reaches values below 30 mm Hg, when MAC is decreased by 20%; when Pa_{O_2} is reduced to 18 mm Hg, the MAC value is reduced by 50%. Hyperoxia does not influence MAC.

Relationship of MAC to Solubility. Eating prior to anesthesia appears to alter MAC. One might expect this, because an increased relation exists between MAC values and blood-gas coefficient of solubility.[86]

The validity of these values is corroborated by the fact that the product of the MAC and the oil-gas partition coefficient is approximately the same for each agent and represents a constant. Thus, if the MAC 1 value of halothane (0.74%) is multiplied by the oil-gas partition coefficient of this agent (224), a value of 165 is obtained. Fluroxene's MAC 1 is 3.45% and, if multiplied by its oil-gas partition coefficient of 47.7, a value of 162 is obtained. Nitrous oxide, with an estimated MAC 1 of 115%, also gives a value of 162 when multiplied by its oil-gas partition coefficient of 1.4. Additional study of this approach to potency may provide a practical clinical guide in anesthesia practice.

Electrolytes. Of the body electrolytes, only a sodium imbalance significantly affects MAC values. Thus, hyponatremia is associated with a reduced need for an inhalation anesthetic. The MAC values are reduced.[125]

Hypothermia. In 1924, Guedel reported the finding that body metabolism and drug requirements parallel each other. A reduction in body temperature is known to decrease metabolism and oxygen demands as well as the doses of anesthetic drugs required.[126]

Deliberate or accidental production of hypothermia is associated with decreased MAC values.[112] Other investigations confirm this effect.[113,127] A reduction in core temperature produces about 8% per

°C reduction in metabolism and a similar reduction in MAC.

Thyroid Function. Thyroid hormone activity significantly affects anesthetic requirements, probably through its influence on metabolism. Hyperthyroidism increases metabolism and oxygen requirements. Anesthetic requirements are greatly increased, and this increase is accompanied by increased MAC values. Conversely, hypothyroidism reduces anesthetic requirements and MAC values. Experimental studies confirm the changes in MAC.[128,129]

Effect of Adjunctive Drugs on MAC Values

OPIOID PREMEDICATION OR IV INDUCTION.[130] Nearly all opioids are capable of reducing MAC values when administered as part of preanesthetic medication or when administered intravenously prior to induction. They are also able to decrease the dose of intravenous induction drugs, such as thiopental, methohexital, and midazolam.*[131]

Preanesthetic medication with narcotics reduces the requirement of inhalation anesthetics and lowers MAC values by 7% to 15% (Table 12–10). Morphine is capable of the greatest reduction, followed by meperidine, fentanyl, alfentanil, sulfentanil, nalbuphine, and pentazocine in that order.[130–132] The doses of intravenous induction drugs are also lowered by opioid premedication. Note that intrathecal morphine also lowers the minimum alveolar concentration.[133]

Fentanyl and alfentanil, administered prior to induction, reduce MAC values and also the unconscious doses (UD_{95}) (ED_{95}) doses of intravenous induction agents.[134,135]

Compared with fentanyl, sulfentanil has a more rapid onset of action, if administered shortly before induction, in reducing the UD of thiopental, methohexital, and midazolam. It also has a shorter duration of action and is more potent.[136]

Intravenous anesthetics for induction are also capable of reducing MAC values. Thiopental without narcotic premedication administered to unconsciousness reduces MAC of halothane, enflurane, and isoflurane by about 15% to 20%. Diazepam

---

* Opioids also reduce the incidence of excitatory effects of methohexital and shorten midazolam's time of onset.

induction intravenously lowers the MAC values of halothane in oxygen.[137] In doses of 0.2 mg/kg intravenously, the MAC values of halothane–O_2 are reduced from 0.75 to 0.48.[104]

INCREASING FENTANYL PLASMA LEVELS. Increasing fentanyl plasma levels produces a proportional decrease in MAC values for enflurane. At high plasma concentrations of fentanyl, the reduction in enflurane MAC may be more than 50%. (In dogs, a concentration of fentanyl of 30 ng/ml causes a reduction of 65% in MAC enflurane.)[135]

Increasing levels of agonist-antagonist narcotic analgesics (butorphanol, nalbuphine) produce a significant reduction in MAC values for enflurane. Experimentally, this occurs at low-dose levels and only results in a MAC reduction of 11% and 8%, respectively. This is in contrast to morphine, which produces a progressive reduction of MAC enflurane up to a maximum decrease of two thirds.[132]

INTRAVENOUS LIDOCAINE. This local anesthetic agent reduces anesthetic requirements for inhalation agents. Plasma concentrations of 3 to 6 µg/ml decrease halothane or nitrous oxide requirements by 15% to 28%.[107] Such concentrations of lidocaine are not unusual in humans after epidural anesthesia or the injection of lidocaine for antiarrythmic purposes. Thus, plasma lidocaine contributes to the total MAC values of general anesthetic agents that are simultaneously administered. Conversely, increasing plasma levels of lidocaine from 1 to 6 µg/ml reduces the MAC values of inhalation agents in a linear fashion from 5% to 45%.[138]

The primary metabolite of lidocaine is monoethylglycinexylidide, which represents less than 20% of the total amide concentration in the plasma and appears not to have an anesthetic effect.[138]

ROLE OF RELAXANT DRUGS. Relaxant drugs were once considered to contribute to CNS depression. Pick demonstrated in animals that large doses (2.5 times the paralyzing dose) of curare abolished EEG activity.[139] Doses of 10 times the paralyzing dose block synaptic nerve conduction and abolish cortical activity in the cat.[140] Small amounts of *d*-tubocurarine enter the cerebrospinal fluid (CSF) at a rate of 4 mg/ml/5 min and 15 mg/ml/h,[141] but these levels do not affect CNS activity. In the monkey, intravenous *d*-tubocurarine and gallamine have been found to

---

TABLE 12–10. ALTERED MAC VALUES

	Unpremedicated	Morphine	Nitrous Oxide
Halothane	0.74%	0.69%	0.29%
Fluroxene	3.45%	2.70%	0.82%
Nitrous oxide	115%	—	—

In volumes percent at 1 atmosphere.

elevate the seizure threshold to lidocaine, whereas decamethonium and succinylcholine do not.[142] More drug enters the CSF in the presence of hypokalemia.

The elegant and definitive studies on humans by Whitacre, however, did not demonstrate any effect of curare.[143]

In humans, pancuronium is the only relaxant that has been demonstrated to reduce the halothane MAC requirement. In Eger's studies, 0.1 mg/kg of pancuronium reduced the MAC of halothane from a control value of 0.75% to 0.55%.[106] The mechanism appears to be a block of muscarinic receptors in the RAS ie, pancuronium acts as a specific antagonist in the cholinergic pathways of the RAS.[144] Vecuronium, a chemical analog, has not been found to affect MAC.

MAC values may be increased by laudanosine, a metabolite of atracurine. As a result of animal studies, there is an increase in cerebral irritability, and this may account for the increased MAC value for halothane.[145]

ANTIHYPERTENSIVE DRUGS AFFECTING MAC. Among the drugs that are effective in reducing MAC values are the central-acting antihypertension drugs.[120] These central-acting drugs include reserpine, methyldopa, and clonidine. Each of these, in turn, significantly affects the alpha$_2$-adrenergic receptor in the CNS. These are agonists that modulate central monoaminergic pathways involved in the sympathetic response to noxious stimuli as well as to the mechanisms involved in essential hypertension. Each of these drugs is capable of reducing MAC values of the inhalation agents.

Prior administration over a period of 1 week to 10 days of alpha-methyldopa, reserpine, clonidine, and other agents that deplete CNS brain norepinephrine is associated with a reduction of MAC, which is dose related.[120]

Guanethedine and other peripheral-acting sympathomimetic blocks have no effect on MAC.[120]

EFFECT OF CLONIDINE. Of the drugs that are used in the management of hypertension, clonidine appears to be the most effective in reducing MAC values. Reduction of MAC values of inhalation anesthetic agents occurs when clonidine has been part of preoperative preparation in hypertensive patients. The administration of 5 µg/kg orally 90 minutes prior to anesthetic induction also reduces the MAC values when administered orally in normotensive subjects. Reductions range from 25% to 40%. Halothane MAC is reduced about 25%;[146] enflurane MAC is reduced about 30%; and isoflurane MAC is reduced about 40%.[147]

Additional effects contributing to this action are the reduction in central sympathetic tone and reduction of circulating catecholamines.[148] It is considered that inhibition of central monoadrenergic systems is the responsible mechanism.[149,150]

DELIBERATE HYPOTENSION. Deliberate hypotension achieved with either pentolinium, trimethaphan, or nitroprusside during anesthesia reduces MAC values. In animal studies by Rao, there is about a 30% reduction in MAC for halothane. The change in MAC appears to be related to the decrease in mean arterial pressure. The lessened need for the anesthetic persists, even when normotension is established.[111,151]

EFFECT OF ANTICHOLINERGIC AGENTS. Both atropine and scopolamine pass the blood-brain barrier into the human brain cells.[152] The result is often the appearance of the "central anticholinergic syndrome."[153] Atropine is particularly effective, especially in excessive cases, by producing excitatory signs that are often accompanied by elevation of temperature. This is reversed by physostigmine.[154] Scopolamine in usual doses appears to decrease MAC values, probably because of its amnesic sedative effects. Large doses produce the central anticholinergic syndrome, which is reversed by physostigmine.

CHOLINESTERASE INHIBITORS. Physostigmine does penetrate the blood-brain barrier and has an "awakening action" on sleepy subjects, as well as EEG arousal, by increasing acetylcholine. It usually increases anesthetic requirements and MAC values.[155] Neostigmine does not readily penetrate into the brain and does not affect MAC.

ALCOHOLISM.[156a] Alcohol significantly influences anesthetic requirements. Clinical reports and experience support this statement.[156b] Chronic alcohol ingestion causes an increased requirement for anesthetic agents. This has been demonstrated for MAC values. Han showed that human halothane MAC is significantly increased.[109] For alcoholics, the MAC value for halothane increases from 0.75% to 1.1%, which is about 44% greater than normal.[110] Animal studies confirm this influence.[157] Ethanol increases fluidity of membranes, and chronic exposure causes resistance to fluidization. Such tolerance may be a cause of increased requirement.[158]

Acute alcoholism reduces the MAC requirement.[110] Most studies demonstrate an additive effect of ethanol and volatile anesthetics. For isoflurane or halothane, the MAC requirement in the presence of alcohol is reduced 15% to 20%.

MISCELLANEOUS DRUGS. The following have been shown experimentally to reduce MAC values: propranolol[159] and tetrahydrocannibol and derivatives.[160] In contrast, isoproterenol[159] and ketamine increase anesthetic needs and MAC values.[105] Cocaine increases MAC values.[161]

INFLUENCE OF OBESITY. Obese patients metabolize many anesthetic agents to a greater extent than those of normal weight. Enflurane and isoflurane are metabolized at a faster rate to reactive metabolites and to free fluoride.[162] Enflurane biodegradation occurs at a faster rate—twice that for patients of normal weight. The serum peak levels are significantly higher and continue for a longer period of time. The serum level of fluoride occurs at about 2 to 4 hours postanesthesia. Peak levels for enflurane have been reported to reach 31.5 μmol/L, compared with 7.9 μmol/L for isoflurane. The mean peak levels at 2 hours are 22.7 μmol/L for enflurane and 6.5 μmol/L for isoflurane.[163] The isoflurane levels are not significantly different from the levels seen after anesthesia in the nonobese subject. Considering organ toxicity and renal function impairment, isoflurane should be considered to be the anesthetic choice in morbidly obese patients.[163]

CNS ELECTRICAL STIMULATION–REDUCTION OF MAC.[164] A reduced anesthetic requirement after electrical stimulation of periaqueductal gray matter has been reported. Electrical stimulation of the periaqueductal gray has been employed in the treatment of chronic intractable pain. Relief of such pain is accompanied by an increase in beta-endorphin levels in the ventricular CSF. The analgesic effect is unique in that no other changes in sensorium or motor activity are noted. Likewise, the high specificity noted is not for acute pain related to somatic stimulation. With regard to the interaction with anesthetic agents, Roizen[164] has demonstrated that there is a marked reduction in the overall MAC value, if an anesthetic is administered following preoperative stimulation of the periaqueductal gray. The mean anesthetic requirement of halothane mixed with 60% nitrous oxide in unstimulated patients was determined as 0.75 ± 0.10 MAC. For the stimulated patient, the anesthetic requirement was assessed at 1.26 ± 0.03 MAC. In terms of the end-tidal halothane concentration, a decrease in the end-tidal halothane is quite significant. In the unstimulated patient, halothane in a concentration of 0.51 was necessary to maintain a nonmoving state. With the stimulated patient, however, the end-tidal concentration of halothane was reduced to 0.15%.

MINIMUM ALVEOLAR CONCENTRATION AWAKE.[165] The alveolar concentration of anesthetic agents at which awakening from inhalation anesthesia occurs has been determined. Consciousness is defined as when patients make a proper response to a verbal request, so when patients first open their eyes on request (verbal command), the concentration of the agent is measured. The concentration of agent preventing the response during recovery has similarly been measured. The concentration midway between the value *permitting,* and the value *preventing* a response has been defined as *MAC awake.* Such a value is approximately half the standard MAC value.

The MAC awake values are listed in Table 12–

TABLE 12–11. MAC AWAKE VALUES

Agent	Value
Methoxyflurane	0.81 (±0.021)
Halothane	0.41 (±0.05)
Ether	1.41 (±0.22)
Fluroxene	2.20 (±0.49)

11. These values were obtained when alveolar concentration was constant for 15 minutes (an equilibration with cerebral anesthetic concentration is assumed).

MAC AWAKE–MAC ASLEEP RATIO. When alveolar concentrations are determined at equilibrium states, the ratios are relatively consistent. The MAC awake to MAC asleep ratios were found to average about 0.58 for the various agents studied. Thus, for methoxyflurane the value is 0.53, for halothane 0.52, for ether 0.67, and 0.60 for fluroxene (Fig. 12–18).

On this basis certain predictions for other agents are possible. If MAC for cyclopropane is 9.2%, then MAC awake for this agent would be about 5.3% (MAC awake equals MAC times 0.58). Nitrous oxide MAC awake may be calculated at 59% (101 times 0.57).

The consistency of the ratios also indicates that differences in awakening time may be caused by differences in rates of elimination; this agrees with the experience that a slow recovery is seen with highly soluble agents, and a rapid recovery with poorly soluble agents.

MEDIAN ANESTHETIC DOSE.[166] A logical extension of the MAC concept is the term AD_{50}, which represents the median anesthetic dose. The AD_{50}, anal-

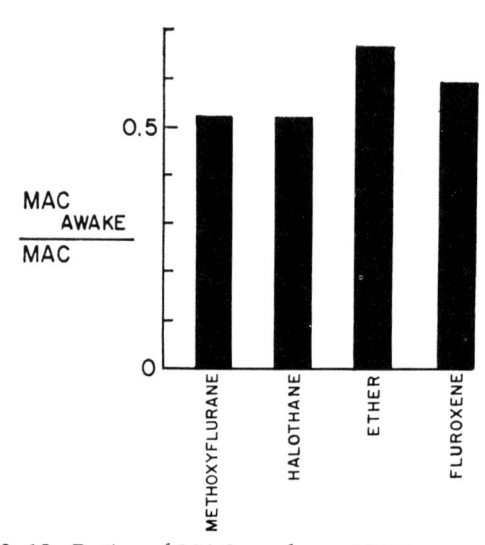

FIG. 12–18. Ratios of MAC awake to MAC at constant alveolar concentrations. From Stoelting, R.K., et al.: MAC awake. Anesthesiology, 33:5, 1970.

ogous to the ED$_{50}$ in pharmacology, is defined as the drug dose (or concentration) that produces anesthesia in half the subjects. The AD$_{50}$ is identical to MAC in concept and generally is numerically identical to MAC. (The standard error furnishes confidence limits.) Advantages include compatibility with statistical and pharmacologic practices and derivation of log dose-response equations. The latter permits calculation of other points such as AD$_{95}$, the dose that anesthetizes 95% of subjects. Computed AD$_{95}$ is shown in Table 12-12; on the average this value exceeds AD$_{50}$ by about 20%. The relationship of AD$_{95}$ to AD$_{50}$ is also presented.[166]

IV. TRANSPORTATION OF AGENTS[60,61]

The establishment of a proper tissue concentration or tissue saturation of agent emphasizes the role of the circulation. Tissue saturation depends on: (1) the adequacy of circulatory system, including the blood volume; (2) the blood flow or perfusion of organs as seen in the capillary circulation; and (3) the tissue uptake of agents as evidenced by blood-tissue partition coefficients and the solubility of agents in intercellular and intracellular fluids.

CIRCULATORY CAPACITY. The volume of blood is an obvious factor in transport of anesthetic agents from the lung to the tissues. A decreased volume may cause peripheral vasoconstriction and limit the exposure of tissues to anesthetic concentrations.

Exposure of all the blood in the circulatory system to an effective alveolar concentration is necessary to have uniform distribution and equilibrium. The time for the circulation of all the blood in an adult that is, the cardiac output, is estimated to be approximately a few seconds over 1 minute. This has been termed the *round of blood* by Haldane.[61b] It represents the time taken by the total blood volume to pass from the pulmonary capillaries, through the systemic circulation, and back to the pulmonary capillaries. This is of importance with fast-acting agents such as ethylene, nitrous oxide, and cyclopropane to which the blood must be exposed two or three times to obtain an adequate blood concentration. It is also important with agents of high blood solubility and relatively low alveolar concentration because the alveolar source may be exhausted by passage of units of blood, leaving none for immediate succeeding units.

BLOOD SUPPLY TO TISSUES. Because the brain has a more abundant blood supply than any other organ in the body as well as an avidity for lipoid-soluble substances, it will take up an anesthetic agent more quickly than other body tissues. Other tissues, particularly the fat of the body, having a poor circulation, will become saturated only after considerable time. Because of the great avidity by fats for lipoid-soluble drugs, they will become concentrated in the fat compartment and will remain there for long periods. This means that there is a further gradient in the partial pressures of the anesthetic gases in the body between the various organs of the body. Thus, there will be a downward gradient from the brain to general body fat and to total body water.

Obesity. Pharmacokinetic differences exist between overweight and underweight patients. Overweight patients of 45% adiposity have about three times the rate of halothane uptake as do underweight patients (15% adiposity). The rate of uptake per per cent of inspired concentration increases with increased adiposity. Recovery time increases with adiposity and can be twice as long as 45% adiposity (as compared with 15% adiposity).[167]

V. ESTABLISHMENT OF TISSUE CONCENTRATION OF AGENT

FACTORS IN TISSUE UPTAKE OF DRUGS.[168] The diffusion of drugs across biologic membranes occurs at

TABLE 12-12. MINIMUM ALVEOLAR CONCENTRATIONS

Agent	MAC Atm.	MAC %	AD$_{50}$	AD$_{95}$	AD$_{95}$/AD$_{60}$
Nitrous Oxide	1.0	100	—	—	—
Xenon	0.71	71	69.4	87.16	1.26
Ethylene*	0.67	67	67.2	74.47	1.11
Cyclopropane	0.10	9.2	9.1	10.07	1.10
Fluroxene	0.034	3.4	3.4	3.57	1.05
Diethyl ether	0.019	1.9	1.9	2.22	1.16
Enflurane	0.016	1.68	1.69	1.88	1.11
Isoflurane	0.011	1.15	1.16	1.63	1.41
Halothane	0.0074	0.74	0.74	.90	1.22
Chloroform†	0.0067	—	—	—	—
Methoxyflurane	0.0016	0.16	0.16	0.22	1.38

* Personal communication from Eric Wahrenbrock, M.D.
† Chloroform—for dog

From de Jong, R.H., and Eger, E.I. II: MAC expanded: AD$_{50}$ and AD$_{95}$ values of common inhalation anesthetics in man. Anesthesiology, *42*:384–389, 1975.

TABLE 12-13. REGIONAL BLOOD FLOW AND OXYGEN CONSUMPTION

Region	Weight (kg)	Percentage of Total Weight	Organ Blood Flow (ml/min)	Cardiac Output (%)	Organ Oxygen Uptake (ml/min)	Total Oxygen Uptake (%)
Brain	1.4	2.2	750	13.9	46.2	22.9
Heart	0.3	0.5	255	4.7	29.1	11.6
Hepatic-portal	2.6	4.1	1500	27.7	51.0	20.4
Kidney	0.3	0.5	1260	23.3	17.6	5.0
Skeletal muscle	31.0	49.2	840	15.6	49.6	20.0
Skin	3.6	5.7	460	8.4	10.9	4.8
Residual tissue	23.8	37.8	380	6.4	50.0	15.3

Adapted from Bazett, H.C.: *Medical Physiology.* St. Louis, C.V. Mosby, 1966.

speeds governed by physiologic and physiochemical factors. These factors are expressed in the general Fick principle, which relates the quantity (Q) of a drug taken up by a tissue per unit time (speed of transfer) to four groups of factors, as follows:

1. Regional blood flow and the microcirculation.
2. Concentration gradient between the blood and the tissue.
3. Membrane characteristics of the tissue and its cells.
4. Drug profile: molecular size; stereoisomerism; ionizability.

These factors are formulated as follows:

$$Q/t = (\text{Blood Flow}) \times \begin{pmatrix} \text{Concentration} \\ \text{Gradient} \\ C_{blood} - C_{tissue} \end{pmatrix}$$
$$\times \begin{pmatrix} \text{Membrane} \\ \text{Characteristics} \\ (K_1) \end{pmatrix} \times \begin{pmatrix} \text{Drug} \\ \text{Profile} \\ (K_2) \end{pmatrix}$$

REGIONAL BLOOD FLOW–TISSUE GROUPS. Great variations exists between different tissues of the body and their blood flow per unit volume. Regional blood flow and oxygen consumption has been summarized by Bazett[169] (Tables 12–13 and 12–14). The body tissues can conveniently be divided into four compartments[170,171] (Fig. 12–19).[171,172] (1) The vessel-rich group (VRG) includes the brain, heart, hepatoportal system, kidney, and endocrine glands. (2) The muscle group (MG) is composed of muscle and skin and has an intermediate circulatory flow rate. (3) The fat group (FG) is composed of adipose tissue and marrow. (4) The vessel-poor group (VPG), with a poor circulation, is composed of tendons, ligaments, connective tissue, teeth, bone, and other relatively avascular tissues.

It should be emphasized that 75% of the cardiac output goes to the VRG of tissues. Hence, after this tissue group becomes saturated, there will be a rapid rise in venous anesthetic concentrations and consequently a diminished blood uptake of agents from the lung.

CONCENTRATION GRADIENT. In the presence of an adequate circulatory pattern, the uptake of drugs by a tissue from the blood is first a function of the blood concentration of the drug in the two compartments. The difference in concentration provides a gradient for molecular diffusion.

TISSUE-BLOOD PARTITION COEFFICIENT. Solubility of anesthetic agents in tissues is expressed as a ratio of the amount of the anesthetic agent in equal volumes of the two phases of tissue and of blood. This is a partition coefficient or distribution ratio. When gases are involved, this partition coefficient is numerically equal to the Ostwald solubility coefficient which is a distribution ratio. The coefficients for several anesthetic agents is given in the following table (Table 12–15).

TABLE 12-14. COMPARISON OF REGIONAL BLOOD FLOW AND OXYGEN CONSUMPTION OF VITAL ORGANS AND OTHER TISSUES

Region	Weight (kg)	Percentage of Total Weight	Organ Blood Flow (ml/min)	Cardiac Output (%)	Organ Oxygen Uptake (ml/min)	Total Oxygen Uptake (%)
Vital organs (brain, heart, hepatoportal, kidneys)	4.6	7.3	3765	69.6	143.9	59.9
Other tissues	58.4	92.7	1680	30.4	110.5	40

From Papper, E.M., and Kitz, R.J.: *Uptake and Distribution of Anesthetic Agents.* New York, McGraw-Hill, 1963.

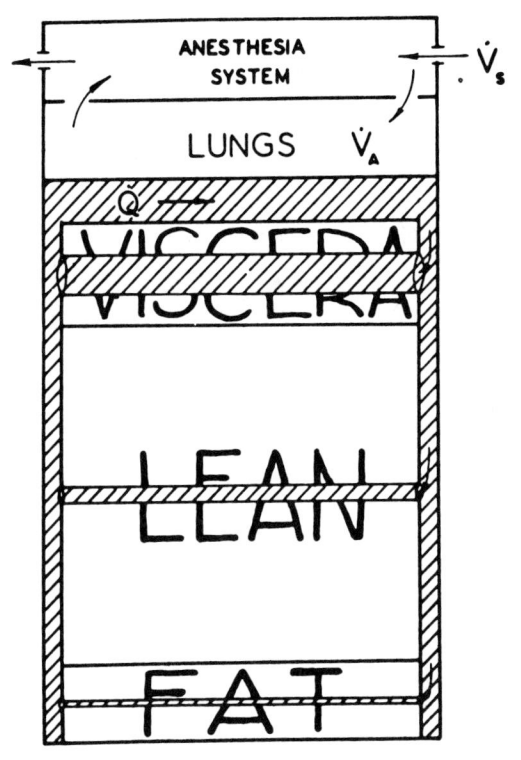

FIG. 12–19. Arbitrary compartments of the anesthesia body system. From Papper, E.M., and Kitz, R.J.: Uptake and Distribution of Anesthetic Agents. New York, McGraw-Hill, 1963.

It is to be noted that the tissue-blood solubility coefficients approach unity for most anesthetic agents regardless of the tissue. Halothane is an exception. It is two to three times as soluble in tissue compartments as in whole blood. This may be related to its high-lipoid solubility.

EQUILIBRIUM BETWEEN TISSUES AND VENOUS BLOOD. A diffusion equilibrium exists between tissue groups and the effluent or venous blood. This equilibrium can be reasonably assumed to occur in hundredths of a second or within the capillary transit time, which is about 1 second. It would be true

TABLE 12–15. PARTITION COEFFICIENTS FOR VARIOUS GASES AT 37° C

Gas	Blood/Gas	Tissue-Blood			
		VRG	MG	FG	VPG
Ethylene	0.14	1.0	1.0	5.9	1.0
Nitrous Oxide	0.468	1.06	1.13	2.3	1.0
Cyclopropane	0.47	1.34	0.92	14.7	1.0
Halothane	2.3	2.5	3.5	60.0	1.0
Ether	15.0	1.14	1.0	2.0	1.0

See text for abbreviations.
From Papper, E.M., and Kitz, R.J.: Uptake and Distribution of Anesthetic Agents. New York, McGraw-Hill, 1963.

of highly perfused tissues but not of vessel-poor tissues (Fig. 12–20). Comparison of three different agents as to their uptake rate shows a general similarity of the curves (Fig. 12–21).

NATURE OF MEMBRANE BOUNDARIES (K_1). Most biologic membranes are bilipid layers of molecules interspersed with small aqueous pores. Agents with molecular weights of 100 or less may pass through these pores, but other drugs largely depend on the solubility in the lipid layer. Thus, the degree of lipoid solubility of a drug is of prime importance.

The geometry of any membrane also plays a role. Two features are evident: the surface area of the membrane that is exposed to the microcirculation and the thickness of the membrane.

TRANSFER SYSTEMS INTO CELLS. For the passage of substances from the circulation into tissues and cells, the following four principal mechanisms of transfer are defined:[168]

1. Simple diffusion
2. Facilitated diffusion (carrier systems)
3. Active transport (enzymatic)
4. Special processes (pinocytosis). Surface vesicles on endothelium take up substances into the cell.

Membrane boundaries possess a dual function by (1) acting as a simple boundary through which many substances may diffuse passively; and (2) providing active transport mechanisms for special substances. A number of compounds (some gases) enter at a similar rate by simple diffusion. Natural substrates, such as some sugars, amino acids, and inorganic ions, have a low solubility but pass readily by active transport.

DRUG DIFFUSION PROFILE. With the development of accurate techniques for estimating the presence of drugs in biologic material, the ability of drugs to penetrate blood-tissue boundaries has been measured. A variety of drugs enter the tissues and cells at rates roughly parallel to their physiologic properties, often expressed as a constant (K_2). Six principal properties of drugs affect this process, as follows:

1. Molecular size
2. Steric configuration
3. Lipoid solubility
4. Protein binding
5. Ionization constant
6. Receptor-drug binding

Molecular size is of significance, because diffusion is inversely related to the square root of the molecular weight. The physical nature of a drug modifies its mobility. The higher the molecular weight, the lower the mobility and diffusion. Generally, compounds of less than 600 molecular weight diffuse relatively easily. Those under 200 molecular weight

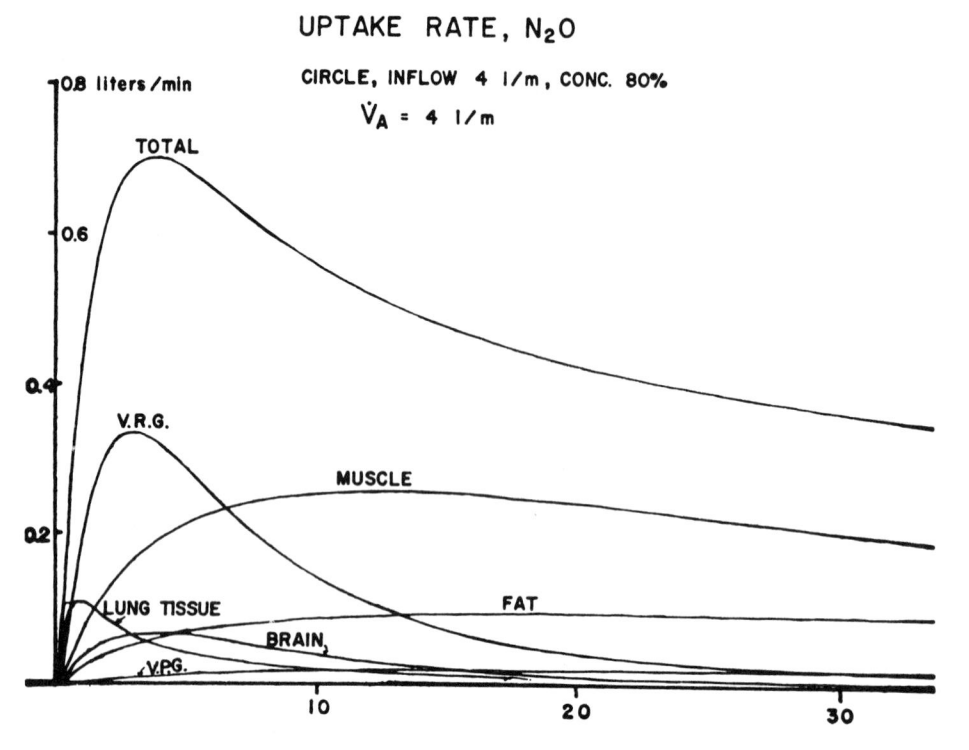

FIG. 12–20. The uptake rate of individual tissues was computed by inserting a very small resistance in series with one tissue analog capacitor at a time and recording the voltage drop across it. It is evident that the vessel-poor group contributes a negligible part of the total body uptake. From Papper, E.M., and Kitz, R.J.: Uptake and Distribution of Anesthetic Agents. New York, McGraw-Hill, 1963.

diffuse rapidly, whereas those over 1000 molecular weight are impermeable. Even with large molecules, however, the size factor may be offset by increased lipoid solubility or by unusually large concentrations. Simple chain compounds usually diffuse more readily through membranes than do bulky molecules.

A number of compounds (some gases) enter at a similar rate, and it appears that the transfer process is one of simple diffusion. Most drugs pass by virtue of their lipoid solubility and, more precisely, a lipid-water partition coefficient at a pH of 7.4. High-lipid–soluble substances, such as barbiturates, have a rapid rate of entry, and the only limiting factor appears to be the blood flow.[173]

Binding of Drugs. The binding of drugs, nonspecifically by plasma and other body proteins, diminishes the amount of free drug active and available for ionization.

Drugs penetrate the boundary mainly in their nonionized form. The ionization capacity of the free fraction is a limiting factor and is related to the drug's dissociation constant, or pKa. The degree of ionization for highly ionized substances is a limiting factor; these compounds enter the various tissues and the brain at rates roughly parallel to the proportion of drug nonionized at pH 7.4. Again, the property of the nonionized portion that determines entry is the lipid solubility. A given drug, however, does not penetrate all regions of the tissue with the same speed. Thus, phenobarbital penetrates white matter more slowly than gray matter, and the tissue microconstruction is a limiting factor.

Substances that ionize distribute themselves unevenly across the boundary between blood and the cells. This is the result of the preferential permeability to the nonionized form and the difference in hydrogen ion concentrations of fluids on either side. Acidic drugs attain a tissue-plasma concentration ratio of less than 1.00, whereas basic drugs attain a ratio somewhat greater than 1.00. By affecting the concentration of the unionized form, acidity limits transfer of many substances.

UPTAKE OF DRUGS BY THE BRAIN

The factors that determine drug uptake by tissues and cells in general also apply specifically to brain uptake of drugs.[174] A number of limiting factors operate to control the passage of drugs and natural substances into the brain, including:

1. Anatomic construction and variations in circulation
2. Differences in metabolism and vascularity between gray and white matter
3. The pH of extracellular fluid and effect of CO_2 and circulation

BRAIN PERFUSION. A profusion of vessels and capillaries denotes the brain circulation. Two anatomic features are important, namely, that no arteriovenous shunts exist and that capillaries are randomly distributed and are not oriented along a particular axis. The latter makes it possible for diffusion of substances to be in an outward and not a longitu-

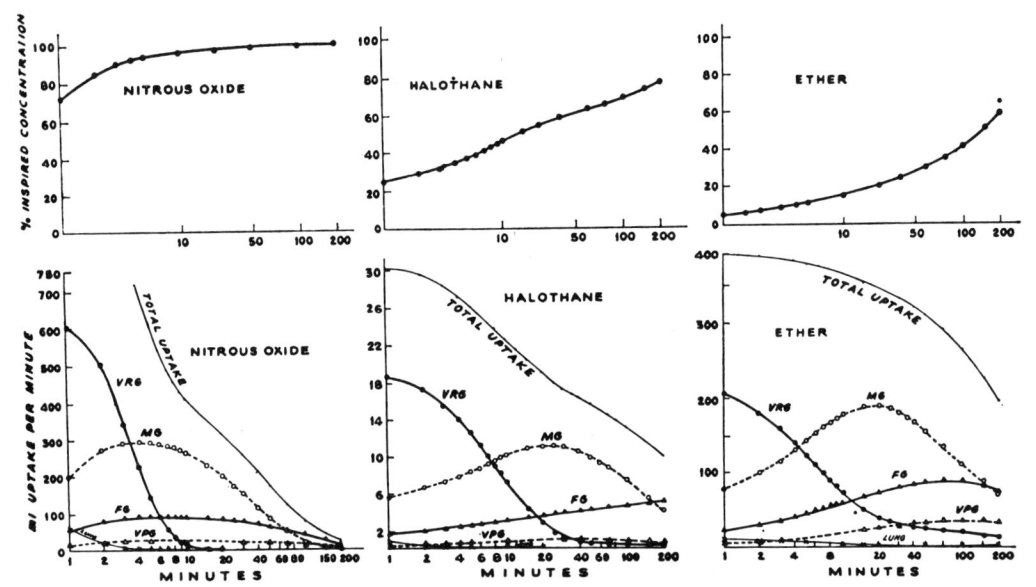

General Anesthesia—Fundamental Considerations **345**

FIG. 12–21. Concentration changes with three gases. From left to right: nitrous oxide, 75% inspired; halothane, 1% inspired; ether, 10% inspired. The three top graphs are percent of inspired concentration found within the alveoli plotted against time. They are the same as those seen in Fig. 12–8, but appear different since they are plotted on a log-base abscissa. The three bottom graphs describe the milliliter uptake of gas per minute by each tissue group. Within these the uppermost graph is total uptake. Uptake by each tissue group is indicated by the curves under total uptake. Uptake by the lung is of consequence in the first minute only. Uptake by the VPG is insignificant. The VRG, MG, and FG are the main determinants of uptake. The VRG uptake dominates the first 5 to 10 min; the MG is then dominant for 70 to 170 min, after which the FG is the principal determinant of uptake. From Papper, E.M., and Kitz, R.J.: Uptake and Distribution of Anesthetic Agents. New York, McGraw-Hill, 1969.

dinal pattern and, hence, to expose all cells uniformly to a diffusing material. If the radius of a capillary is about 4 μ and the radius of a surrounding tissue cylinder is 18 μ,[175] then, with the range of diffusion coefficients commonly encountered with inert gases, the equilibrium of an element of blood with brain tissue will be complete when the blood is about one tenth of the way along a capillary. In brief, diffusion in brain tissue is not limited by anatomic factors.

From studies by Kety,[175] using a nitrous oxide-brain uptake technique, the mean cerebral blood flow in humans is set at 54 ml/100 g of tissue per minute. Blood flows in various regions of the brain have also been determined by Landau.[174] The cerebral cortex has a generally high flow but exhibits a certain degree of differentiation, with primary sensory and motor areas having a significantly higher perfusion rate than other areas. The auditory and visual areas have a slightly smaller perfusion. Of all areas, the inferior colliculus in the midbrain shows the highest blood flow. At the other extreme, white matter has a low value and is generally about one fifth that of gray matter.

It is considered that brain structures that have the greatest functional activity have the highest blood flow. This is consistent with regard to the sensorimotor cortex. Sokoloff[176] has shown by photic stimulation of cats that there results a significant increase in blood flow, probably reflecting an increased metabolic and functional activity. That the inferior colliculus has the highest flow is curious, but it is of further interest that this area has the highest concentration of certain enzymes of the Krebs cycle to further suggest a high metabolic rate.

Factors controlling and altering basic regional cerebral blood flow (rCBF) will be dealt with elsewhere.

BRAIN TISSUE UPTAKE. In general, the distribution and uptake of diffusible and unmetabolized substances, especially the inhalation anesthetics, by different regions of the brain tissue are determined by the factor of lipid solubility or the tissue-blood partition ratio and by the rate of blood flow to the specific areas.

REGIONAL CEREBRAL BLOOD FLOW. Comparative values of blood flow during consciousness and in a lightly anesthetized state are revealing. Under well-controlled, light thiopental anesthesia, significant reductions in flow occur in structures composed of gray matter. Flow in white matter is essentially unchanged. Greatest reductions in flow are observed primarily in the visual, auditory, and somatosensory areas, which reflect precisely the more profound effects of anesthesia on these highly active and sensitive areas. It is of further interest that, 1 minute after the injection of thiopental in cats, the level of the drug in the cortex is twice that in the plasma.

PENETRATION OF DRUGS INTO THE CNS.[177] The boundary between the blood stream and the brain is a characteristic watery membrane with lipid-like layers, behaving like other body membranes. This boundary has been usually designated as a barrier, but this is an inaccurate term for what is truly an active passageway for the transport of natural substances as well as drugs from the blood to the brain (Bradbury).[178]

Anatomically, the blood-brain boundary consists of the capillary endothelium, the perivascular and the perineural glial tissue (the supporting tissue), and an extracellular brain space. The brain capillaries generally differ from other tissue capillaries in having endothelial cells which have tight functions or merging of the outer layer with that of adjoining endothelial cells.[179] In addition, the myelin sheaths offer a barrier, especially with regard to penetration of white matter. It is known that many drugs enter white matter more slowly than gray matter structures.[178] Until recently, the brain was considered to be a uniformly compact cellular organ with only an insignificant extracellular space. Studies[180] by electron microscopy reveal this space to be about 4% in volume, while observations of insulin and dextran diffusion in the brain show values of 10% for the extracellular brain space. There is a 20 nm gap between cell surfaces (Davson).[181]

Penetration is defined as the rate at which the final concentration in the cell or tissue is approached. It is not balance of concentrations within or without a cell or tissue but due to selective transport mechanisms.[180]

The brain capillary endothelium provides the active transport mechanisms for special substances.[182] Some of the transporter systems through the membranes of the endothelial cells merely facilitate osmotic diffusion by a concentration gradient. D-glucose and large neutral amino acids (phenylalanine) reach the brain by this means and exit similarly. A special sodium-ion channel has been demonstrated and the movement of sodium is often accompanied by glycine, a potent inhibitory neurotransmitter but at a low level.

As with the cells of other tissues, drugs penetrate into the brain cells in the non-ionized form. This is a function of lipid solubility (Fig. 12–22). Certain molecules needed for brain metabolism cross the endothelial blood-brain barrier more readily than expected from their lipid coefficient of solubility. These are carried by the above-mentioned endothelial transport systems.[183]

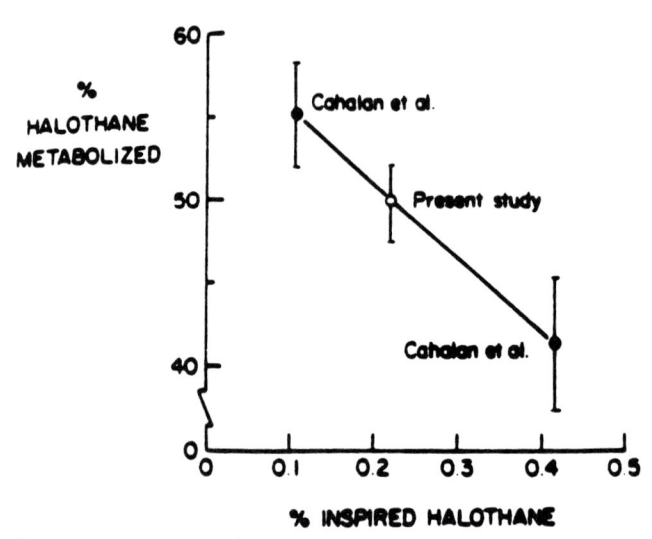

FIG. 12–22. Lipid solubility has the greatest effect on a substance's capacity to pierce the blood-brain barrier. The lipid solubility of a compound is measured according to how it distributes itself in a mixture of oil and water (*horizontal axis*). The ability to cross the barrier is measured in terms of how freely a molecule enters the brain compared with molecules known to do so most freely (*vertical axis*). For most substances ease of passage is determined largely by lipid solubility (*solid points*). Certain molecules needed for brain metabolism are carried across the barrier by a transport system. Most of the data on the graph are from William H. Oldendorf of the University of California at Los Angeles School of Medicine. From Goldstein, G.W., Betz, A.L.: The blood-brain barrier. Sci. American, 255:74, 1986.

A study of the influence of carbon dioxide on brain drug penetration indicates that hypercarbia exerts a profound effect on the penetration of ionizable substances into brain matter. There is a marked increase in the rate of entry. There is also a more marked effect on white matter, into which drugs like phenobarbital and salicyclic acid penetrate more extensively.

EXIT OF DRUGS FROM THE CNS. Three routes are available for the exit of drugs from the CNS. Physiochemical properties of a drug largely determine the route. (1) All drugs, regardless of molecular size or lipoid solubility, can leave the CSF by simple filtration across the arachnoid villi. The rate of this process is determined by the rate of CSF drainage into the villous area. (2) Drugs can leave cerebral tissue by diffusion across either the blood-brain boundary or the blood-CSF boundary. Such depends on lipoid solubility and the extent to which the drug is nonionized. This is the route extensively used by lipid-soluble drugs. The drugs either enter the capillary beds draining the cellular portions of the brain or enter the venous drainage of the CSF ventricular drainage system. (3) A third exit is across the brain-blood boundary by active transport mechanisms, wherein energy is required.

ELIMINATION OF INHALED ANESTHETICS*

Three principal pathways are recognized for the elimination of volatile inhaled anesthetic agents. These are as follows:

1. Pulmonary exhalation—The major route.
2. Renal excretion—A route for removal of only minimal amounts of parent volatile agents from the body but a major route for detoxified bodies or metabolic produce.
3. Biotransformation—Metabolites may be excreted by either the pulmonary or renal system.

There is minimal excretion of anesthetic agents through the skin.[1]

PULMONARY EXHALATION

The respiratory system is the primary route of elimination of inhaled gas and volatile agents. The process is dependent on gas laws and solubility factors and is essentially the reverse of uptake and distribution factors. A variable percentage of the original total drug introduced is excreted by this route. The gas agents nitrous oxide, ethylene, and cyclopropane are essentially eliminated entirely by ventilation. Theoretically, N_2O can be biotransformed and converted to nitrates and nitrite products, which could be excreted by the kidney into urine or by the liver into the bile. Ether and vinethrene are almost completely eliminated by the lungs, but a small fraction may be excreted via the gastrointestinal and renal tracts and through the skin. The volatile halogenated agents also are almost entirely eliminated by pulmonary exhalation, but a significant percentage is metabolized. The volatile products are eliminated by the lungs, whereas the nonvolatile products are eliminated by the kidneys and bile.

BIOTRANSFORMATION. The objective of drug metabolism is to increase the water solubility of drugs or to form polar units and, thereby, enhance elimination. Many of the inhaled anesthetic agents once considered to be metabolically inert have been found to be broken down in the body. The degree of metabolic change is related to many factors:

- The chemical nature and structural formula. The more stable the molecular structure and inert a drug, the less the breakdown.
- The solubility in lipids; i.e., the lipophilic or the hydrophilic nature of a drug. Anesthetic agents with low lipid solubility are less likely to be metabolized and hence have a lower toxicity.
- The concentration and duration of stay in the body. Trace amounts may be retained in the body lipids for days or weeks.
- The efficiency of required chemical reaction processes and pathways, both enzymatic and nonenzymatic.

The integrity of the chief organs involved in the chemical reactions—primarily the liver, kidney, and, to some extent, the lungs—is essential. Breakdown of drugs by enzymes in the other tissues and the blood depends on the liver as the principal source of enzymes. Simple alkaline hydrolysis may occur at a slow rate for many days.

FACTORS IN METABOLISM. Metabolites may be increased or decreased in accordance with different mechanisms of metabolism. Enzyme induction by other drugs will enhance transformation, while enzyme inhibition can diminish metabolism in some circumstances. Factors affecting the rate of breakdown and the degree of toxicity include the concentration of agent and duration in the body; accumulation of metabolites to toxic concentrations; the production of reactive versus inert products; the presence of intermediates, which form bonds with tissue macromolecules; and the formation of haptenes to produce a hypersensitive state. An important objective of drug metabolism is to detoxify, that is, to render exogenous substances inert and nontoxic. This is achieved not only by converting lipid-soluble substances and nonpolar drugs into water-soluble derivatives that can be excreted, but by conjugation. In general, the ordinary end products are low in concentration and nontoxic. Altered metabolism to undesirable products and high concentrations of some metabolites, however, can be toxic.

Depending on the duration of stay and the concentration in the plasma and the body, the volatile agents can exert acute physiologic dysfunction and initiate chronic pathologic processes. The intact agent is more important in the acute physiologic reactions, and the metabolites are important in chronic cytotoxic processes.

PATHWAYS OF DRUG METABOLISM. Two general phases of metabolism are the phase 1 and phase 2 reactions.[2]

Phase 1 Reactions. Transformation occurs not only in lipid-rich membranes, especially endoplasmic reticulum where enzymes are concentrated, but also in plasma and nuclear membranes. The liver has the highest level of activity followed by the kidneys and lungs. The phase 1 enzyme system depends on cytochromes or hemoproteins. The key enzyme is cytochrome P-450, described as a mixed-function oxidase system. Three types of reactions occur, as follows:

- *Oxidation Reactions*—All volatile anesthetics undergo phase 1 transformation. Oxidation is the common route and may be by dehalogenation or O-dealkylation (ether cleavage). Other types of oxidation reactions include aromatic hydroxylation, aliphatic hydroxylation, N-dealkylation, sufoxi-

---

* This section has been prepared with the assistance of Duncan A. Holaday, M.D.

dation desulfuration, epoxidation, and N-oxidation. Since this is the common and important mechanism, it will be discussed further.
- *Reduction Reactions*—These use the cytochrome P-450 system. Azo and nitro compounds undergo reductive changes. It appears that drugs of this nature accept electrons directly from cytochrome. Halothane also is a substrate for reductive reaction.
- *Hydrolysis*—Local anesthetics, both esters and amides, undergo this type of change. It may be simple alkaline hydrolysis or it may use nonmicrosomal enzymes, ie, esterases.

Phase 2 Reactions. Addition reactions are by conjugation pathways and occur in aqueous solution of the cytoplasm. The process is synthetic in nature. The enzymes involved have no specificity to substrates but do have specificity to chemical groups. The specific chemical groups are -NH$_2$; -SH; -OH; and -COOH.

Some types of conjugation are glucuronic acid conjugation; sulfate conjugation; amide synthesis; and mercapturic acid formation.

Glucuronic Acid Conjugation This is the most common path and is the only one discussed. Glucose is the precursor to glucuronic acid. When the glucuronic acid is activated a condensation with a specific chemical group is catalyzed by glucuronyl transferase. Glucuronides have a high water solubility, and small molecular conjugates are excreted by the kidney while large molecular conjugates are excreted in the bile.

OXIDATIVE METABOLISM

The primary chemical mechanism for transformation of most drugs and of the volatile inhalation agents is the oxidative pathway. The rate of electron transfer in the oxidative chain is determined by an enzyme system involving the cytochrome P-450 reductase. This is a nonspecific enzyme system for a variety of substrates and can attack a wide variety of chemicals, not only barbiturates, phenothiazines, benzodiazepines, meperidine congeners, and acetaminophens, but also the inhalation anesthetics. Thus, it serves as the enzyme for transformation of most drugs.

The extent and rate of transformation are altered by several factors. Sex differences are recognized—males metabolize greater amounts of volatile inhaled agents than females. Androgens are probably responsible for this effect. Age is an important factor—infants and children before puberty have an immature enzyme system, so substantially less of the inhaled anesthetic agents are metabolized. There is a low incidence of hepatotoxicity in the teenaged group.

With prolonged exposure and at high MAC values, the degree of biodegradation is enhanced. Repeated exposure to the fluorinated agents results in increased breakdown. Norgate[3] however, has demonstrated that this does not occur with enflurane.

THE ENZYME SYSTEM. Microsomal enzyme systems in the liver, kidney, and brain are responsible for degradation of inhalation agents. The liver is the principal organ involved. The site of enzymatic transformation and the source of the oxidative enzymes are the rough endoplasmic reticulum in the liver. Oxidative, reductive, and conjugative enzymes are present in this locus. In biochemical preparations (homogenized and centrifuged), the reticulum is concentrated into small spheres called *microsomes*, in which the enzymes are located.

Enzyme Induction. Enzyme activity may be increased by the process of induction. The chronic administration of certain drugs in small doses stimulates both the synthesis of more enzymes and the activity of enzymes in other pathways. Decreasing the rate of enzyme degradation also increases the enzyme level.

Exposure to certain chemicals, environmental or industrial, such as the polychlorbiphenyls, which are potent enzyme inducers, can result in increased rate of degradation and stimulate abnormal pathways of metabolism. This usually results in a shortened plasma half-life and decreased pharmacologic activity of the subsequent administered drugs.

Many agents and drugs are capable of enzyme induction (Table 12–16). Phenobarbitol and diphenylhydantoin are especially to be noted. After enzyme induction, the rate of degradation of other drugs is enhanced. Thus, the administration of methoxyflurane is accompanied by a marked increase in the break-off of fluoride; the administration of halothane is also accompanied by increased biodegradation with an enhanced break-off of fluoride. Isoflurane is not accompanied by significant increases in biodegradation, but enflurane biodegradation is increased, although to a lesser extent than halothane. Enflurane is also an enzyme inducer.

In the case of volatile anesthetics, the enhanced biotransformation to certain metabolites is adverse. For example, administration of enzyme inducers to animals prior to halothane administration produces centrolobular hepatic necrosis. Accompanying the damage is an increase in serum glutamic pyruvic transaminase (SPGT) and a decrease in hepatic microsomal cytochrome P-450. Regarding most highly potent nonvolatile drugs, enhanced breakdown and conjugation are protective mechanisms whereby the formation of toxic metabolites is suppressed.

Enzyme Inhibition. On the other hand, the enzyme system attacking volatile agents may be inhibited by certain drugs. Antioxidants protect the liver from damage by some agents. Disulfuram is a potent enzyme inhibitor. Pretreatment with this antimetab-

TABLE 12–16. DRUGS NOTED AS ENZYME INDUCERS

Hypnotics
  Barbiturates
  Glutethimide (Doriden)
  Ethanol
  Chloral hydrate
Tranquilizers
  Chlorpromazine (Thorazine)
  Promazine (Sparine)
  Meprobamate (Equanil)
  Chlordiazepoxide (Librium)
Anticonvulsants
  Diphenylhydantoin (Dilantin)
  Methyphenylethylhydantoin (Mesantoin)
Antihistaminics
  Diphenhydramine (Benadryl)
Steroids
  Cortisone
  Prednisolone
  Norethynodrel (Enovid)
  Methylestosterone
Anesthetics
  Diethyl ether
  Halothane (Fluothane)
  Methoxyflurane (Penthrane)
Insecticides
  DDT
  Chlordane
  o,p'-DDD

olite prevents the hepatotoxicity of chloroform. In contrast, phenobarbitol pretreatment enhances chloroform hepatotoxicity.

Glutathione may play a role as a conjugating agent for intermediate products. This is evident in chloroform or fluroxene anesthesia, wherein the products of degradation are rendered inert by glutathione.[4]

REDUCTIVE METABOLISM. Under aerobic conditions, metabolism of halothane is largely an oxidative process and preferentially leads to bromide and trifluoracetic acid and to some fluoride. Under anaerobic conditions,[5] reduction reactions may be more prevalent and dehalogenation with marked increase in fluoride occurs. This is accompanied by a threefold increase in covalent bonding of metabolites to microsomal lipids.

Two reductive metabolites have been identified: CDF (1,1 difluoro-2-chlorethylene) and CTF (1,1,1, trifluoro-2-chlorethane). These are present in exhaled air of humans under aerobic conditions. However, there is a four- to eightfold increase resulting from enzyme induction and moderate hypoxia.

The concentrations rapidly increase from the start of anesthesia, reach a plateau after 1 hour and then rapidly decline. The metabolites CDF and CTF have been designated as markers of reductive metabolism and of human hepatic toxicity.[6]

EXTRAHEPATIC BIOTRANSFORMATION. Some experimental studies indicate extrahepatic metabolism of volatile anesthetics, eg, methoxyflurane by rabbit pulmonary microsomal enzymes, trichlorethylene by lungs. Transformation of halothane and enflurane has been studied using three microsomal preparations: pulmonary, renal, and hepatic. All three enzyme preparations are capable of oxidative demethylation and epoxidation. Halothane undergoes reductive biotransformation by all three preparations, but the liver enzyme preparation produces three times as much product. Enflurane is defluorinated at an appreciable rate only by liver microenzymes.[7]

TYPE OF METABOLITES (TABLE 12–17)

A number of demonstrated and theoretical metabolites of halogenated anesthetics may be considered, as follows:

1. Trifluoroacetic acid—A major oxidative metabolite of halothane, fluroxene, and isoflurane. It is largely an ionized substance that does not penetrate membranes and has a low level of toxicity.
2. Trifluoroethanol—Produced from fluroxene in humans in small amounts. It has not been demonstrated after halothane administration.
3. Trifluoroacetaldehyde—Has not been isolated after halothane or other agents in humans but may be an intermediate.
4. Oxalic acid—Produced after methoxyflurane administration in humans. Crystalline oxalate deposits are seen in the renal tubules. Ordinarily, urinary oxalate concentrations are insufficient to cause obstruction, and toxicity occurs at concentration 10 times greater. But, in the presence of other agents such as the tetracyclines, high concentrations do occur.
5. Inorganic fluoride—A toxic metabolite. Release in large amounts occurs following methoxyflurane; release in small amounts occurs after halothane, enflurane, and isoflurane. Nephrotoxicity may appear at the minimal plasma range of 40 to 50 μmol/L and invariably at levels of 80 μmol/liter.[6] However, Mazze subsequently considered that serum levels of 20 μmol/L may cause renal damage.[8] The urinary excretion for 1 MAC hour of enflurane anesthesia is below 800 μmol/day. It is considered that nephrotoxicity occurs when the urinary excretion of inorganic fluoride exceeds 2500 μmol/day.[3,6]

Of the total amount of fluorinated agents absorbed by patients, a significant portion of the biotransformed products appears as the fluoride ion (Table 12–18). For methoxyflurane, 70% is degraded and, of the products, 46% is inorganic fluoride; for halothane, 20% of the total absorbed is degraded, representing principally trifluoroacetic acid, while about 0.6% to 1.2% appears as free fluoride; for enflurane, 2.4% of the total administered is recovered as metabolites, representing both inorganic

TABLE 12–17. PRIMARY PRODUCTS OF BIOTRANSFORMATION OF COMMON INHALATION ANESTHETICS

Anesthetic	Primary Products of Biotransformation	Approximate Amount of "Absorbed" Anesthetic Metabolized
Methoxyflurane (Penthrane) $CHCl_2CF_2OCH_3$	Difluoromethoxyacetic acid Fluoride ion Dichloracetic acid Oxalic acid Conjugates	70%
Halothane (Fluothane) $CF_3CHBrCl$	Trifluoroacetic acid Bromide ion Conjugates	20%
Trichloroethylene (Trilene) CCl_2CClH	Chloral hydrate Trichloroethanol Trichloroacetic acid Conjugates	80%
Enflurane (Ethrane) $CHCl_2F_2OCHF_2$	Difluoromethoxydifluoroacetic acid Fluoride ion Oxalic acid (?) Conjugates (?)	2–5%
Fluroxene (Fluoromar) $CF_3CH_2OCHCH_2$	Trifluoroacetic acid Ethanol (?) Trifluoroethanol (?) Conjugates	20%
Chloroform $CHCl_3$	CO_2 Chloride ion Mono- and dichloromethyl derivatives Glutathione conjugates	?
Isoflurane $CF_3CHClOCF_2H$	Trifluoromethanol Trifluoroacetic acid Formic acid Fluoride ion	0.17–1%

fluoride and organic metabolites. Of the total enflurane, about 0.5% appears as degraded inorganic fluoride.[9]

The mean peak serum concentrations in the intraanesthetic period of the fluoride ion metabolite of the commonly used fluorinated agents has been determined: halothane, 2 to 6 µmol/L;[10] isoflurane, 4.4 ± 0.4 µmol/L;[8] enflurane, 18 to 22 µmol/L;[6,10] and methoxyflurane, 50 to 80 µmol/L.[4]

MECHANISMS OF NEPHROTOXICITY. Renal toxicity is due to the fluoride ion, which interferes with the transport of sodium in the proximal convoluted tubule. There is inhibition of adenyl cyclase and of the action of antidiuretic hormone. Ordinarily, vasopressin increases the permeability to water of both the distal convoluted tubules and the collecting tubes. This allows more water to be reabsorbed.

Also, experimental evidence in rats indicates that free water reabsorption is markedly reduced. It is hypothesized that the inhibition occurs in the medullary portion of the ascending loop of Henle. Perhaps at this site, there is inhibition of the chloride pump.[11]

Urine concentrating ability of the kidney is altered by the administration of volatile fluorinated agents. With enflurane, reabsorption of water is inhibited; there is approximately a 25% decrease in maximum urinary osmolality after a vasopressin concentrating test. With halothane, there is an in-

TABLE 12-18. BIODEGRADATION OF HALOTHANE, ENFLURANE, AND METHOXYFLURANE[9,23]

Anesthetic Mean ± SD	Anesthetic Concentration (%)	Anesthetic Absorbed (g)	Per Cent Recovery of Anesthetic in Expired Gas	Fluoride Excretion in Urine (mmol)	Inorganic Fluoride % of Amount Degraded	Biodegradation (%)
Halothane	0.93 ± 0.12	6.64 ± 1.93	72.8 ± 9.2	18.2 ± 8.2	0.6 ± 0.6	17.7 ± 4.4
Enflurane	1.30 ± 0.09	5.62 ± 2.53	79.3 ± 14.6	3.7 ± 2.9	19.0 ± 4.1	2.3 ± 0.9
Methoxyflurane	0.31 ± 0.02	4.18 ± 0.89	34.8 ± 12.5	22.7 ± 4.1	21.2 ± 5.1	46.3 ± 11.7
Isoflurane	1.0 ± 0.1	18.0 ± 6.0	95.0 ± 7.0		4.2	<1.0

crease in urine concentrating ability on the second postanesthetic day after vasopressin testing of about 10%.[10] Normally, after vasopressin, there is a marked increase in urine osmolality from ordinary values of 1000 mOsm/kg of water.

DEFLUORINATION INDEX. Because nephrotoxicity is related to the levels of inorganic fluoride at the time of exposure, Mazze has proposed a defluorination index to reflect a nephrotoxic potential.[12] This index is the product of in vitro fluoride formation and the oil/gas partition coefficient of the anesthetic agent. Methoxyflurane has been assigned a potential of 1, and other agents are relative (Table 12-19).

REACTIVE INTERMEDIATES.[13] The demonstrated metabolites are stable and are excreted. Under certain circumstances, however, some intermediate compounds may exist for an appreciable time and then combine with cellular constituents. These intermediates are known as free radicals and are quite reactive. It is postulated that hepatotoxic intermediates are produced from halothane (and other agents probably) by a reductive pathway—nonoxygen dependent—involving cytochrome P-450 enzyme dependency. Some free radicals that theoretically can be produced from halothane are reactive acylhalides by hydroxylation and reactive carbanion.[13] Under anaerobic conditions, reduction reactions are enhanced.

Free radicals may readily react with unsaturated fatty acids and nucleic acids. Covalent binding with macromolecules of lipids and phospholipids is enhanced at lower oxygen tensions.[2] Peroxidative decomposition of the membranes of liver endoplasmic reticulum and mitochondria may ensue. In conditions of low concentration of antioxidants, such as glutathione, liver cell necrosis can occur after some anesthetics such as chloroform or halothane administration.

ALTERING BIOTRANSFORMATION (DEUTERATION). It would appear beneficial to decrease the metabolism of the volatile anesthetics and, thereby, reduce the metabolic products that are related to adverse effects.[14a] The replacement of hydrogen by deuterium in these anesthetics has been proposed on the basis that the carbon-deuterium (C-D) bond is less reactive than the carbon-hydrogen (C-H) bond. Total replacement of the hydrogen of methoxyflurane by deuterium results in a 29% decrease in the amount of fluoride produced. Deuteration of only the methoxyl group produces a 33% decrease in fluoride production. Deuteration of halothane resulted in a 15% to 26% decrease in sodium bromide. If the ethyl portion of enflurane is deuterated, there follows a 65% decrease in urinary fluoride. It is interesting that deuterated chloroform, when administered to experimental animals at a concentration of 0.35%, decreases the amount of SGPT. It was concluded from McCarty's study that deuteration of volatile anesthetics changes their rate of metabolism and in most instances produces a decrease.[14c] Although deuteration decreases the amount and rate of the metabolism, it may channel anesthetic biotransformation to other pathways and more undesirable products. As Holaday has demonstrated with regard to the metabolism of methoxyflurane, the metabolism can proceed by two pathways.[4] The deuteration of the methoxyl group limits the metabolic attack on methoxyflurane so that there is a marked decrease in the formation of fluoride, but biotransformation continues by the second pathway. Cohen has proposed three pathways for the metabolism of halothane.[15] Deuteration may decrease the path breaking off bromide but may permit other paths to be used preferentially.

NITRO COMPOUNDS. Some evidence exists that nitrous oxide may be metabolized. Nitrous oxide has some biologic activity and is a mild enzyme inducer.[16] It is possible that N_2O could be metabolized to nitric oxide or to nitrate ions,[17] and this can occur in the intestine.[15]

Some studies indicate that N_2 is the major metabolite. It is possible that other gaseous products, such as NO, NO_2, and NH_3, or water-soluble non-

TABLE 12-19. NEPHROTOXIC POTENTIAL OF FLUORINATED ANESTHETIC AGENTS

Agent	F− (nmol 30 min⁻¹ per mg protein)	×	λ (oil: gas)	=	Defluorination Index	Nephrotoxic Potential
Methoxyflurane	2.00		930		1860	1.00
Dioxychlorane	1.41		275		387	0.23
Enflurane	1.31		99		129	0.07
Senoflurane	1.82		56		101	0.05
Isoflurane	0.51		94		48	0.03
Halothane	0		230		0	0.00
Synthane	0		95		0	0.00

From Mazze, R.I., Beppu, W.J., and Hitt, B.A.: Metabolism of synthane: Comparison with in vivo and in vitro defluorination of other halogenated hydrocarbon anaesthetics. Br. J. Anaesth., 51:839, 1979.

volatile agents (NO_3^-, NO_2^-, NH_4^+) may be formed; the evidence using ^{15}N gas indicates that N_2 is the only significant derivative.[18]

OBESITY FACTOR. Obese patients metabolize volatile anesthetics to a greater extent than the nonobese.[19] Storage of the lipoid-soluble agents is greater and provides a continuing perianesthetic source of agent for biotransformation. The higher the oil-gas solubility coefficient, the greater the amount present for metabolism and the longer it will be available to be more completely changed. The enhanced breakdown may also be related to an increase in liver fat, because fatty infiltration of the liver occurs in 75% of people who are 50% to 100% overweight.

Methoxyflurane. Methoxyflurane metabolism after 3 hours of anesthesia (3 MAC hours) is at least doubled in the obese patient. Serum inorganic fluoride in nonobese subjects reaches a peak of 24 μmol/L 2 hours after anesthesia, compared to a peak of 55 μmol/L in obese subjects.

Halothane. Halothane breakdown is significantly greater in obese subjects; serum inorganic fluoride 1 hour after anesthesia (3 MAC hours) in nonobese subjects peaked at 2 to 4 μmol/L, but in obese subjects rises to 10 μmol/L.[20]

Enflurane. Enflurane metabolism is enhanced in the obese patient. Biotransformation in the morbidly obese subject may be 65% greater than in the nonobese. With this increased degradation, there is a greater increase in formation of free serum inorganic fluoride. In normal patients, the mean serum fluoride level is about 20 μmol/L but increases to over 28 μmol/L in obese subjects.[21] The metabolism occurs mostly in the period of 4 to 12 hours postanesthesia.

Isoflurane. Isoflurane metabolism is relatively small, ie, one tenth to one hundredth that of other commonly used halogenated agents. Obesity does not greatly enhance the metabolism. The mean peak serum fluoride concentration of 6.5 μmol/L in the obese patient is not significantly increased over the mean of 4.4 μmol/L in subjects of normal weight (Fig. 12–23).[22]

EFFECT OF BLOOD SOLUBILITY. Inhaled agents with a high blood or lipid solubility are retained in the blood and fat tissues of the body longer than agents of low solubility. Therefore, capillary blood-alveolar exchange is limited, and elimination by alveolar ventilation is low. Similarly, a high lipid solubility results in retention and slow release, so that hepatic and other mechanisms of biotransformation have a longer time to metabolize the agent and produce higher amounts of metabolites.[23]

PULMONARY RECOVERY OF UNCHANGED ANESTHETIC

In general, the primary route of elimination of most inhaled gas and volatile anesthetics is via ventilation. Studies of elimination of inhaled anesthetics have emphasized the role of metabolism. The recovery of metabolites, however, is probably incomplete, and the role of metabolism of inhaled anesthetic agents may be greater than the current evidence would indicate. In the past, most of the estimates of metabolism have been based on fluoride and fluorine compounds.

MASS BALANCE METHOD. In an elegant study using a technique of measurement of mass balance of administered anesthetics, Carpenter and associates have studied the total anesthetic recovered in exhaled gases.[24] This has been compared to the total uptake during administration. The difference is assumed to be the result of metabolism of the agent.

A mixture of four volatile agents—isoflurane, enflurane, halothane, and methoxyflurane—was administered simultaneously into a 60% nitrous-oxygen carrier stream. The inspired concentrations resulted in an additive alveolar concentration of 0.6 MAC. The total uptake over a period of 2 hours was measured, and, thereafter, the exhaled gases were measured for a period of 5 to 9 days. The per cent of the recovered gases over the total administered was calculated. Isoflurane recovery amounted to

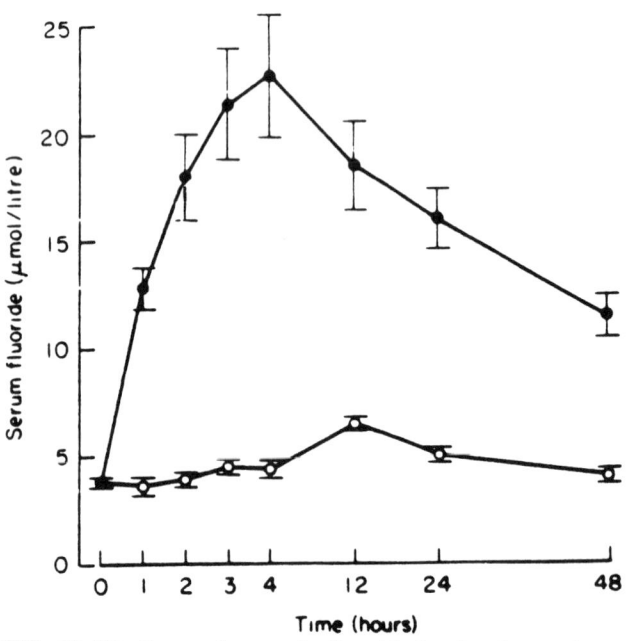

FIG. 12–23. Serum inorganic fluoride levels after enflurane anaesthesia (●) and isoflurane anaesthesia (○) (mean, SE). From Strube, P.J., et al.: Serum fluoride levels in morbidly obese patients: Enflurane compared with isoflurane anaesthesia. Anaesthesia, 42:685, 1987.

TABLE 12-20. UPTAKE AND METABOLISM OF ANESTHETICS AS ASSESSED BY MASS BALANCE IN NINE PATIENTS COMPARED WITH THE RESULTS OF PREVIOUS MASS BALANCE AND METABOLITE RECOVERY STUDIES

Anesthetic	Total Uptake (ml)	Total Recovery (ml)	Per Cent Recovery	Recovery Normalized to Isoflurane (%)	Normalized Metabolism (%)	Per Cent Recovery	Metabolism as a Per Cent of Total Uptake
Isoflurane	381 ± 25	354 ± 28	92.8 ± 4.0	100	0*	95	0.2
Enflurane	682 ± 43	379 ± 48	84.9 ± 3.8	91.5 ± 1.0	8.5 ± 1.0	85 90-91	2.4
Halothane	356 ± 22	179 ± 13	50.2 ± 3.8	53.9 ± 0.9	46.1 ± 0.9	7 41-45	11-25 17-20
Methoxyflurane	127 ± 12	29 ± 2	23.1 ± 1.9	24.7 ± 1.6	75.3 ± 1.6	29-35	48

Values are mean ± SE.
* Metabolism of isoflurane was assumed to be 0 for this calculation.
From Carpenter, R.L., Eger, E.I., and Johnson, B.H.: The extent of metabolism of inhaled anesthetics in humans. Anesthesiology, 65:201, 1986.

93%, and, because an insignificant amount of this agent has been identified in the form of metabolites, it was assumed that the 7% difference was related to losses from other sites. Isoflurane recovery from ventilation was normalized to 100%. The per cent recovery of the other anesthetic agents was then normalized to the isoflurane value.

Analysis by mass balance shows that ventilation is the primary route for isoflurane and enflurane; pulmonary clearance is about 93% of isoflurane and 85% of enflurane. For halothane, however, both metabolism and ventilation are equally important, hepatic and extrahepatic (kidney) routes for metabolism both being employed.[25]

For methoxyflurane, metabolism by liver, kidneys, and lungs is most important and exhalation relatively unimportant.

On this basis, the results indicate that a larger percentage of inhaled agents is metabolized than is evident by the amount of metabolites that have been recovered. It is estimated that enflurane is metabolized to the extent of 8%, halothane 46%, and methoxyflurane 75%.

OTHER ROUTES OF LOSS

Inhaled anesthetic agents are also lost intact by several other routes. Losses through the skin;[26] dissolved in urine and sweat; and in the feces[27] are minimal. Loss from surgical wounds and exposed body cavities may be appreciable. The loss depends on the area of exposure, the blood flow to the area, and the tissue-gas partition coefficient. Thus, an agent with a small coefficient will have a greater loss through the wound (isoflurane); an agent with a high tissue-gas coefficient will be retained by that tissue.

EFFECT OF INSPIRED CONCENTRATION ON METABOLISM.[26,28] The inspired concentration is an important determinant of the fraction of agent metabolized (Fig. 12-24). It is considered that with higher concentrations and exposure to degradation mechanisms, metabolism is limited by saturation of enzyme systems responsible for metabolism. This reduces the fraction of drug metabolized.[29]

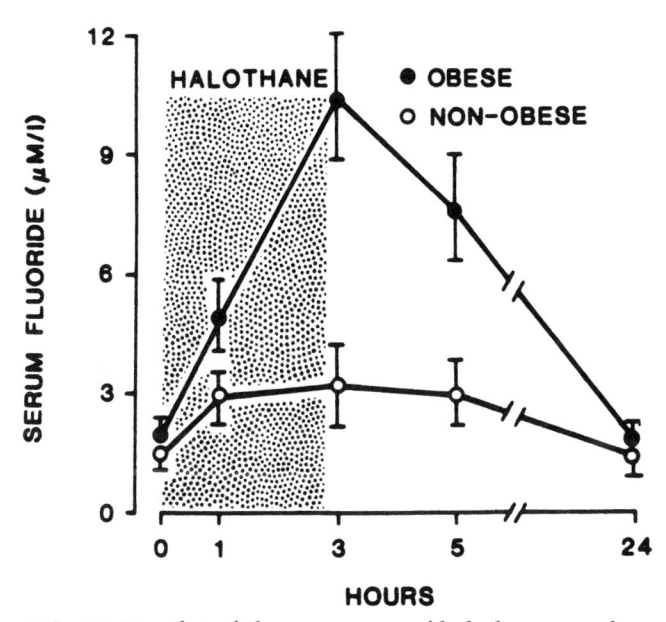

FIG. 12-24. Plot of the percentage of halothane metabolized against the inspired concentration in humans. The value measured in this study is plotted with those determined by Cahalan et al.[29] Values are mean ± SE. From Carpenter, R.L., Eger, E.I., and Johnson, B.H.: The extent of metabolism of inhaled anesthetics in humans. Anesthesiology, 65:201, 1986.

EFFECT OF DURATION OF ANESTHESIA ON PHARMACOKINETICS AND METABOLISM OF INHALED AGENTS.[30] By using the mass balance elimination technique, the percentage of anesthetic metabolized from total uptake and recovery of anesthetic was estimated. For short periods of anesthetic administration, the alveolar wash-out is more rapid. The duration of administration of anesthesia, however, does not affect the time constants determined for each drug, nor is there any change in the number of compartments into which the anesthetic agent is distributed or from which the anesthetic is metabolized. Further, the percentage of anesthetic metabolized does not change with the duration of administration.

REFERENCES

1. Guedel, A.L.: Inhalation Anesthesia, 2nd ed. New York, Macmillan, 1937.
2. Goodman, L., and Gilman, A.: The Pharmacological Basis of Therapeutics, 6th ed. New York, Macmillan, 1980.
2a. Smith, T.C., and Wollman, H.: History and Principles of Anesthesiology. In Goodman and Gilmans' The Pharmacological Basis of Therapeutics. Edited by A.G. Gilman, L.S. Goodman, T.W. Rall, and F. Murad. 7th ed. New York, Macmillan, 1985, pp. 260–275.
3. Stanley, T.H.: New routes of administration and new delivery systems of anesthesia. Anesthesiology, 68:665, 1988.
4. Woodbridge, P.D.: Changing concepts concerning depth of anesthesia. Anesthesiology, 18:536, 1957.
5. Fink, B.R.: Electromyography in general anesthesia. Brit. J. Anaesth., 33:555, 1961.
6. French, J.D., Verzeano, M., and Magoun, H.W.: A neural basis of the anesthetic state. Arch. Neurol. Psychiatr., 69:519, 1953.
7. Etsten, B., and Himwich, H.E.: Stages and signs of pentothal anesthesia: Physiologic basis. Anesthesiology, 7:536, 1946.
8. Himwich, W.A., et al.: Brain metabolism in man: In anesthesia and in pentothal narcosis. Am. J. Psychiatr., 103:689, 1947.
9. Heavner, J.E.: The spinal cord dorsal horn. Anesthesiology, 38:1, 1973.
10. Rexed, B.: The cytoarchitectonic organization of the spinal cord in the cat. J. Comp. Neurol., 96:415, 1952.
11. Kitahata, L.M., Taub, A., and Kosaka, Y.: Lamina-specific suppression of dorsal-horn unit activity by ketamine hydrochloride. Anesthesiology, 38:4, 1973.
12. Magoun, H.W.: The Waking Brain, 2nd ed. Springfield, Charles C. Thomas, 1969.
13. Morrison, R.S., and Dempsey, E.W.: Study of thalamocortical relations. Am. J. Physiol., 135:281, 1942.
14. Moruzzi, G., and Magoun, H.W.: Brain stem reticular formation and activation of EEG. Electroencephalogr. Clin. Neurophysiol., 1:455, 1949.
15. Jasper, H.: Thalamocortical relationship. Electroencephalogr. Clin. Neurophysiol., 1:405, 1949.
16. Dement, W.: Nature of sleep. Science, 131:1705, 1960.
17. Jouvet, M.: Neurophysiology of the states of sleep. Physiol. Rev., 47:117, 1967.
18a. Brazier, M.A.B.: Role of the limbic system in maintenance of consciousness. Anesth. Analg., 42:748, 1963.
18b. Himwich, H.E.: New psychiatric drugs. Scientif. Amer., 193:38, 1955.
18c. Himwich, H.E.: Psychopharmacologic drugs. Science, 27:59, 1958.
19. French, J.D., and Magoun, H.W.: Effects of chronic lesions in central cephalic brain stem of monkeys. Arch. Neurol. Psychiatr., 68:391, 1952.
20. Heath, R.G.: Symposium on Sedative and Hypnotic Drugs. Baltimore, Williams & Wilkins, 1954.
21. Kleitman, N.: Sleep and Wakefulness. Chicago, University of Chicago Press, 1939, pp. 131–147, 166.
22. Arduini, A., and Arduini, M.G.: Effects of drugs and metabolic alterations on brain stem arousal mechanism. J. Pharmacol. Reper. Therap., 110:76, 1954.
23. Harvey, S.C.: Sedatives and hypnotics. In The Pharmacologic Basis of Therapeutics, 6th ed. Edited by A.G. Goodman and A. Gilman. New York, Macmillan, 1980.
24. Jouvet, M.: Biogenic amines and the states of sleep. Science, 163:32, 1969.
25. Hartman, E.: The Biology of Dreaming. Springfield, Charles C. Thomas, 1967.
26. Czeisler, C.A., et al.: Human sleep: Its duration and organization dependent on its circadian phase. Science, 210:1264, 1980.
27. Zsigmond, E.: Hypnotic therapy. Upjohn Company, Kalamazoo, MI, 1981.
28. Moore-Ede, M.C., Czeisler, C.A., and Richardson, G.S.: Circadian timekeeping in health and disease. I. Basic properties of circadian pacemakers. N. Engl. J. Med., 309:469, 1983.
29. Richter, C.P.: Biological Clocks in Medicine and Psychiatry. Springfield, Charles C. Thomas, 1965.
30. Richter, C.P.: Sleep and activity: Their relation to the 24-hour clock. Res. Publ. Assoc. Res. Nerv. Ment. Dis., 45:8, 1967.
31. Moore-Ede, M.C., Czeisler, C.A., and Richardson, G.S.: Circadian timekeeping in health and disease. 2. Clinical implications of circadian rhythmicity. N. Engl. J. Med., 309:530, 1983.
32. Jouvet, M.: A possible role of the catecholamine-containing neurons of the brain stem of the cat in the sleep-waking cycle. Acta Physiol. Pol., 24:5, 1973.
33. Koračevič, R., and Radulovacki, M.: Monoamine changes in brain of cats during slow-wave sleep. Science, 193:1025, 1976.
34. Hornykiewicz, O.: Dopamine (3-hydroxytyramine) and brain function. Pharmacol. Rev., 18:925, 1966.
35a. Everett, G.M., and Borcherding, J.W.: L-dopa: Effect on concentrations of dopamine, norepinephrine, and serotonin in brains of mice. Science, 168:849, 1970.
35b. Hobson, J.A.: Sleep: Physiologic aspects. N. Engl. J. Med., 281:1343, 1969.
36. Kanai, T., and Szerk, J.: The mesencephalic reticular activating system and cortical acetylcholine output. Nature, 205:80, 1965.
37a. Czeisler, C.: Internal organization of temperature, sleep-wake, and neuroendocrine rhythms monitored in an environment free of time cues. PhD Thesis, Stanford University, 1978.
37b. Czeisler, C., et al.: Human sleep: Its duration and organization depend on its circadian phase. Science, 210:1264, 1980.
38. Moore-Ede, M.C., Brennan, M.F., and Ball, M.R.: Circadian variation of intercompartmental potassium fluxes in man. J. Appl. Physiol., 38:163, 1975.
39. Weitzman, E.D., et al.: Twenty-four hour pattern of the episodic secretion of cortisol in normal subjects. J. Clin. Endocrinol. Metab., 33:14, 1971.

40. Best, C.H., and Taylor, N.B.: Physiologic Basis of Medical Practice, 10th ed. Edited by J.R. Brobeik. Baltimore, Williams & Wilkins, 1979, Chap. 6, Function of Adrenal Glands, pp. 54–72.
41. Roizen, M.F., et al.: The effect of two anesthetic agents on norepinephrine and dopamine in discrete brain nuclei, fiber tracts, and terminal regions of the rat. Brain Res., 110:515, 1976.
42. Roizen, M.F., et al.: The effect of two diverse inhalation anesthetic agents on serotonin in discrete regions of the rat brain. Exp. Brain Res., 24:203, 1975.
43. Roizen, M.F., et al.: Effects of ablation of serotonin or norepinephrine brain-stem areas on halothane and cyclopropane MACs in rats. Anesthesiology, 49:252, 1978.
44. Hetzel, M.R., and Clark, T.J.H.: The clinical importance of circadian factors in severe asthma. In Chronopharmacology. Edited by A. Reinberg and F. Halberg. New York, Pergamon Press, 1979, pp. 213–221.
45. Coleman, R.M.: Wide Awake at 3:00 A.M.: By Choice or by Chance? New York, W.H. Freeman, 1986.
46. Adam, K.: Sleep is for tissue restoration. J. Coll. Physicians Lond., 11:376, 1977.
47. Robin, E.D., et al.: Alveolar gas tensions, pulmonary ventilation and blood pH during physiologic sleep. J. Clin. Invest., 37:98, 1958.
48. Block, A.J., et al.: Sleep apnea, hypapnea and oxygen desaturation in normal subjects. N. Engl. J. Med., 300:513, 1979.
49. Scharf, M.B., et al.: Nocturnal oxygen desaturation in patients with sickle cell anemia. J.A.M.A., 249:1753, 1983.
50. Krnjevic, K.: The mechanism of general anesthesia: Editorial views. Anesthesiology, 34:215, 1971.
51. Krnjevic, K., Pumain, R., and Renaud, L.: Excitation of cortical cells by barium. J. Physiol. Lond., 211:43P, 1970.
52. Darbinjan, T.M., Golovchinsky, V.B., and Plehotkina, S.I.: Effects of anesthetics on reticular and cortical activity. Anesthesiology, 34:219, 1971.
53. King, E.E.: Differential action of anesthetics and interneuronal depressants upon EEG arousal and recruiting responses. J. Pharmacol. Exper. Therap., 116:404, 1957.
54. Davis, H.S., et al.: Effect of anesthetic agents on evoked central nervous system responses: Gaseous agents. Anesthesiology, 18:634, 1957.
55. Davis, H.S., et al.: The effect of anesthetic agents on evoked central nervous system responses: Muscle relaxants and volatile agents. Anesthesiology, 19:441, 1958.
56. Wikler, A.: Pharmacologic dissociation of behavior and EEG "sleep patterns" in dogs: Morphine, n-allyl normorphine, and atropine. Proc. Soc. Exper. Biol. Med., 79:261, 1952.
57. Oswald, I., and Clemente, C.D.: Drug effects in sleep. Pharmacol. Rev., 20:273, 1968.
58. Theye, R.A., and Michenfelder, J.D.: Individual organ contributions to the decrease in whole-body VO$_2$ with isoflurane. Anesthesiology, 42:35, 1975.
59. Harris, T.A.B.: The Mode of Action of Anesthetics. Baltimore, Williams & Wilkins, 1954.
60. Papper, E.M., and Kitz, R.J.: Conference report. In Uptake and Distribution of Anesthetic Agents. 1st ed. New York, McGraw-Hill, 1963.
61a. Eger, E.I. II: Anesthetic Uptake and Action, 1st ed. Baltimore, Williams & Wilkins, 1974.
61b. Christiansen, J., Douglas, C.G., and Haldane, J.S.: The absorption and dissociation of carbon dioxide by human blood. J. Physiol. (Lond.) 48:244, 1914.
61c. Haldane, J.S., and Priestley, J.G.: Respiration. New Haven, Yale Univ. Press, 1935.
61d. Comroe, J.H., et al.: The Lung, 2nd ed. Chicago, Year Book Medical Publishers, Inc., 1962, pp. 140–161.
61e. Bohr, C., Hasselbalch, K.A., and Krogh, A.: Uhereinen in biologischer Beziehung wichtigen. Einfluss, dendie Kohlensauerspannung des Blutes auf dessen. Sauerstoffbinding übt. Sk and Arch. Physiol., 16:402, 1904.
62. Kety, S.S.: Theory and applications of exchange of inert gas at lungs and tissues. Pharmacol. Rev., 3:1, 1951.
63. Severinghaus, J.W.: Role of lung factors. In Uptake and Distribution of Anesthetic Agents. Edited by E.M. Papper and R.J. Kitz. New York, McGraw-Hill, 1963.
64. Eger, E.I.: Applications of a mathematical model of gas uptake. In Uptake and Distribution of Anesthetic Agents. Edited by E.M. Papper and R.J. Kitz. New York, McGraw-Hill, 1963.
65. Eger, E.I. II: Anesthetic Uptake and Action, 2nd ed. Baltimore, Williams & Wilkins, 1979, pp. 77–96.
66. Epstein, R.M., et al.: Influence of the concentration effect on the uptake of anesthetic mixtures: The second gas effect. Anesthesiology, 25:364, 1964.
67. Stoelting, R.K., and Eger, E.I. II: An additional explanation for the second gas effect. Anesthesiology, 30:273, 1969.
68a. Forster, R.E.: Diffusion factors in gases and liquids. In Uptake and Distribution of Anesthetic Agents. Edited by E.M. Papper and R.J. Kitz. New York, McGraw-Hill, 1963.
68b. Fick, A.E.: Uber diffusion. Ann. d. Phys. v. Chem. 94:59, 1855.
69. Forster, R.E.: Exchange of gases between alveolar air and pulmonary capillary blood: Pulmonary diffusing capacity. Physiol. Rev., 37:391, 1952.
70. Solomon, A.K.: Transport of solutes across biologic membranes. In Uptake and Distribution of Anesthetic Agents. Edited by E.M. Papper and R.J. Kitz. New York, McGraw-Hill, 1963.
71. Eger, E.I. II, and Larson, C.P. Jr.: Anesthetic solubility in blood and tissues: Values and significance. Br. J. Anaesth., 36:140, 1964.
72. Steward, A., et al.: Solubility coefficients for inhaled anesthetics for water, and oil biological media. Br. J. Anaesth., 45:282, 1973.
73. Wade, J.G., and Stevens, W.C.: Isoflurane: An anesthetic for the eighties? Anesth. Analg., 60:666, 1981.
74. Holaday, D.A., and Smith, F.R.: Clinical characteristics and biotransformation of sevoflurane in healthy human volunteers. Anesthesiology, 54:100, 1981.
75. Wallin, A.F., et al.: Sevoflurane: A new inhalation anesthetic agent. Anesth. Analg., 54:758, 1975.
76. Larson, C.P. Jr., Eger, E.I. II, and Severinghaus, J.W.: Ostwald solubility coefficients for anesthetic gases in various fluids and tissues. Anesthesiology, 23:868, 1962.
77. Eger, E.I. II: Personal communication, 1964.
78. Eger, E.I. II, et al.: Anesthetic potencies of sulfur hexafluride, carbon tetrafluoride, chloroform and ethane in dogs: Correlation with hydrate and lipid theories of anesthetic action. Anesthesiology, 30:129, 1969.
79. Haggard, H.W.: The absorption, distribution and elimination of ethyl ether. J. Biol. Chem., 59:737, 1924.
80. Katoh, T., and Ikeda, K.: The minimum alveolar concentration (MAC) of sevoflurane in humans. Anesthesiology, 66:301, 1987.
81. Lerman, J.: Age and solubility of volatile anesthetics in blood. Anesthesiology, 61:139, 1984.
82. Laasberg, L.H., and Hedley-Whyte, J.: Halothane solubility in blood and solutions of plasma proteins. Anesthesiology, 32:351, 1970.

83. Wagner, P.D., Nauman, P.F., and Laravuso, R.B.: Simultaneous measurement of eight foreign gases in blood by gas chromatography. J. Appl. Physiol., 36:600, 1974.
84. Borel, J.D., et al.: Enflurane blood-gas solubility: Influence of weight and hemoglobin. Anesth. Analg., 61:1006, 1982.
85. Ellis, D.E., and Stoelting, R.K.: Individual variations in fluroxene, halothane and methoxyflurane blood-gas partition coefficients, and the effect of anemia. Anesthesiology, 42:748, 1975.
86. Munson, E.S., et al.: Increase in anesthetic uptake, excretion, and blood solubility in man after eating. Anesth. Analg., 57:224, 1978.
87. Quasha, A.L., Eger, E.I. II, and Tinker, J.H.: Determination and applications of MAC: Review. Anesthesiology, 53:315, 1980.
88. Robbins, B.H.: Preliminary studies of the anesthetic activity of fluorinated hydrocarbons. J. Pharmacol. Exp. Ther., 86:197, 1946.
89a. Guedel, A.E.: Inhalation Anesthesia: A Fundamental Guide. New York, Macmillan, 1937, pp. 14–60.
89b. Faulconer, A. Sr., Pender, J.W., and Bickford, R.G.: The influence of partial pressure of nitrous oxide on the depth of anesthesia and the electroencephalogram in man. Anesthesiology, 10:601, 1949.
90. Haggard, H.W.: The absorption, distribution and elimination of ethyl ether. IV. The anesthetic tension. J. Biol. Chem. 59:783, 1924.
91. Woodbridge, P.D.: Changing concepts concerning depth of anesthesia. Anesthesiology, 18:536, 1957.
92. Eger, E.I. II, Saidman, L.J., and Brandstater, B.: Minimum alveolar anesthetic concentration: A standard of anesthetic potency. Anesthesiology, 26:756, 1965.
93a. Saidman, L.J., et al.: Minimum alveolar concentrations of methoxyflurane, halothane, ether and cyclopropane in man: Correlation with theories of anesthesia. Anesthesiology, 28:994, 1967.
93b. Eger, E.I. II, et al.: Anesthetic potencies of sulfur hexafluoride, carbon tetrafluoride, chloroform and ethrane in dogs: Correlation with the hydrate and lipid theories of anesthetic action. Anesthesiology, 30:129, 1969.
93c. Miller, K.W., et al.: Physicochemical approaches to the mode of action of general anesthetics. Anesthesiology, 36:339, 1972.
94. Quasha, A.L.: Why do we need to know the MAC of an anesthetic? In ASA Refresher Course. Edited by S. Hershey. 9:131, 1981.
95. Nicodemus, H.F., et al.: Median effective doses (ED_{50}) of halothane in adults and children. Anesthesiology, 31:344, 1969.
96. Eger, E.I. II: MAC and dose-response curves. Anesthesiology, 34:202, 1971.
97. Roizen, M.F., Horrigan, R.W., and Frazer, B.M.: Anesthetic doses blocking adrenergic (stress) and cardiovascular responses to incision: MAC BAR. Anesthesiology, 54:390, 1981.
98. Gregory, G.A., Eger, E.I. II, and Munson, E.S.: The relationship between age and halothane requirements in man. Anesthesiology, 30:488, 1969.
99. Gion, H., and Saidman, L.J.: The minimum alveolar concentration of enflurane in man. Anesthesiology, 35:361, 1971.
100. LeDez, K.M., and Lerman, J.: The minimum alveolar concentration (MAC) of isoflurane in preterm neonates. Anesthesiology, 67:301, 1987.
101. Cameron, C.B., Robinson, S., and Gregory, G.A.: The minimum alveolar concentration of isoflurane in children. Anesth. Analg., 63:418, 1984.
102. Stevens, W.C., et al.: Minimum alveolar concentrations (MAC) of isoflurane with and without nitrous oxide in patients of various ages. Anesthesiology, 42:197, 1975.
103. Munson, E.S., Martucci, R.W., and Smith, R.E.: Circadian variations in anesthetic requirement and toxicity in rats. Anesthesiology, 32:507, 1970.
104. Perisho, J.A., Beuchel, D.R., and Miller, R.D.: The effect of diazepam on minimum alveolar anesthetic requirements (MAC) in man. Can. Anaesth. Soc. J., 18:536, 1971.
105. White, P.F., Johnston, R.R., and Pudwill, C.R.: Interaction of ketamine and halothane in rats. Anesthesiology, 42:179, 1975.
106. Forbes, A.R., Cohen, N.H., and Eger, E.I.: Pancuronium reduces halothane requirement in man. Anesth. Analg., 58:497, 1979.
107. Himes, R.S. Jr, Di Fazio, A., and Burney, R.G.: Effects of lidocaine on the anesthetic requirements for nitrous oxide and halothane. Anesthesiology, 47:437, 1977.
108. Di Fazio, C.A., et al.: Additive effects of anesthetics and theories of anesthesia. Anesthesiology, 36:57, 1972.
109. Han, Y.J.: Why do chronic alcoholics require more anesthesia? Anesthesiology, 30:341, 1969.
110. Barber, R.E.: Anesthetic requirement in alcoholic patients. Abstracts of Scientific Papers. Annual Meeting of the American Society of Anesthesiologists, 1978, p. 623.
111. Tanifuji, Y., and Eger, E.I. II: Effect of arterial hypotension on anesthetic requirement in dogs. Br. J. Anaesth., 48:947, 1976.
112. Vitez, T.S., White, P.F., and Eger, E.I. II: Effects of hypothermia on halothane MAC and isoflurane MAC in the rat. Anesthesiology, 41:80, 1974.
113. Regan, M.J., and Eger, E.I. II: Effect of hypothermia in dogs on anesthetizing and apneic doses of inhalation agents: Determination of the anesthetic index (apnea/MAC). Anesthesiology, 28:689, 1967.
114. Barnes, P., et al.: Nocturnal asthma and changes in circulating epinephrine, histamine, and cortisol. N. Engl. J. Med., 303:263, 1980.
115. Eger, E.I. II, Saidman, L.J., and Brandstater, B.: Temperature dependence of halothane and cyclopropane anesthesia in dogs: Correlation with some theories of anesthetic action. Anesthesiology, 26:764, 1965.
116. Steffey, E.P., and Eger, E.I. II: Hyperthermia and halothane MAC in the dog. Anesthesiology, 41:392, 1974.
117. Johnston, R.R., Way, W.W., and Miller, R.P.: Alteration of anesthetic requirement by amphetamine. Anesthesiology, 36:357, 1972.
118. Mueller, R.A., et al.: Central monoaminergic neuronal effects on minimum alveolar concentrations (MAC) of halothane and cyclopropane in rats. Anesthesiology, 41:143, 1975.
119. Johnston, R.R., Way, W.L., and Miller, R.D.: The effect of CNS catecholamine-depleting drugs on dextroamphetamine induced elevation of halothane MAC. Anesthesiology, 41:57, 1974.
120. Miller, R.D., Way, W.L., and Eger, E.I., II: The effects of alpha-methyl dopa, reserpine, guanethedine, and iproniazid on minimum alveolar anesthetic requirement (MAC). Anesthesiology, 29:1153, 1968.
121. Johnston, R.R., et al.: The effect of levo-dopa on halothane dose requirements. Anesth. Analg., 54:178, 1975.
122. Saidman, L.J., and Eger, E.I. II: Effect of nitrous oxide and of narcotic premedication on the alveolar concentrations

of halothane required for anesthesia. Anesthesiology, 25:302, 1964.
122a. Lee, P.K., Cho, M.H., and Dobkin, A.B.: Effects of alcoholism, morphinism, and barbiturate resistance on induction and maintenance of general anesthesia. Can. Anaesth. Soc. J., 11:354, 1964.
123. Pauling, L.: A molecular theory of anesthesia. Science, 134:15, 1967.
124. Bridges, B.E., and Eger, E.I. II: The effect of hypocapnia on level of halothane anesthesia in man. Anesthesiology, 27:634, 1966.
125. Tanifuji, Y., and Eger, E.I. II: Brain sodium, potassium and osmolality: Effects on anesthetic requirement. Anesth. Analg. (Cleve.), 57:404, 1978.
126. Guedel, A.E.: Metabolism and reflex irritability in anesthesia. J.A.M.A., 83:1736, 1924.
127. Munson, E.S.: Effect of hypothermia on anesthetic requirement in rats. Lab. Anim. Care, 20:1109, 1970.
128. Babad, A.A., and Eger, E.I. II: The effects of hyperthyroidism and hypothyroidism on halothane and oxygen requirements in dogs. Anesthesiology, 29:1087, 1958.
129. Munson, E.S., Hoffman, J.C., and DiFazio, C.A.: The effects of acute hypothyroidism and hyperthyroidism on cyclopropane requirement (MAC) in rats. Anesthesiology, 29:1094, 1968.
130. Hoffman, J.C., and DiFazio, C.A.: The anesthesia sparing effect of pentazocine, meperidine, and morphine. Arch. Int. Pharmacodyn. Ther., 186:261, 1970.
130a. Deming, M.N.: Agents and techniques for induction of anesthesia in infants and young children. Anesth. Analg. 31:113, 1952.
131. Dundee, J.W., et al.: Effect of opioid pretreatment on thiopentone induction requirements and the onset of action of midazolam. Anaesthesia, 41:159, 1986.
132. Murphy, M.R., and Hug, C.C. Jr: The enflurane sparing effect of morphine, butorphanol, and nalbuphine. Anesthesiology, 57:489, 1982.
133. Drasner, K., Bernards, C.M., and Ozanne, G.M.: Intrathecal morphine reduces the minimum alveolar concentration of halothane in humans. Anesthesiology, 69:310, 1988.
134. Dundee, J.W., et al.: Some factors influencing the induction characteristics of methohexitone anaesthesia. Br. J. Anaesth., 33:296, 1961.
135. Murphy, M.R., and Hug, C.C. Jr: The anesthetic potency of fentanyl in terms of its reduction of enflurane MAC. Anesthesiology, 57:485, 1982.
136. Furness, G., Dundee, J.W., and Milligan, K.R.: Low dose sulfentanil pretreatment. Anaesthesia, 42:1264, 1987.
137. Tsunoda, Y., et al.: Effects of hydroxyzine, diazepam and pentazocine on halothane: Minimum alveolar anesthetic requirements. Anesth. Analg., 53:390, 1973.
138. Di Fazio, C.A., Niederlehner, J.R., and Burney, R.G.: The anesthetic potency of lidocaine in the rat. Anesth. Analg., 55:818, 1976.
139. Pick, E.P., and Unna, K.: The effect of curare and curare-like substances on the central nervous system. J. Pharmacol. Exp. Therap., 83:59, 1945.
140. Ostow, M., and Garcia, F.: Effect of curare on cortical responses evoked by afferent stimulation. J. Neurophysiol., 12:225, 1949.
141. Matteo, R.S., et al.: Cerebrospinal fluid levels of d-tubocurarine in man. Anesthesiology, 46:396, 1977.
142. Munson, E.S., and Wagman, T.H.: Elevation of lidocaine seizure threshold by gallamine. Arch. Neurol., 28:329, 1973.
143. Whitacre, R.J., and Fisher, A.J.: Clinical observations on the case of curare in anesthesia. Anesthesiology, 6:124, 1945.
144. Savarese, J.J.: How many neuromuscular blocking drugs affect the state of general anesthesia? (Editorial) Anesth. Analg., 58:449, 1979.
145. Shi, W., et al.: Laudanosine (a metabolite of atracurium) increases the minimal alveolar concentration of halothane in rabbits. Anesthesiology, 63:584, 1985.
146. Bloor, B.C., and Flacke, W.E.: Reduction in halothane anesthetic requirement by clonidine, an alpha-adrenergic agonist. Anesth. Analg., 61:741, 1982.
147. Ghigone, M., Calvillo, O., and Quintin, L.: Anesthesia and hypertension: The effect of clonidine on perioperative hemodynamics and isoflurane requirements. Anesthesiology, 67:3, 1987.
148. Maurer, W., et al.: Effect of the centrally acting agent clonidine on circulating catecholamines at rest and during exercise: Comparison with the effects of beta-blocking agents. Chest, 2(suppl):366, 1983.
149. Kobinger, W., and Pichler, L.: Localization in the CNS of adrenoreceptors which facilitate a cardioinhibitory reflex. Naunyn Schmiedebergs. Arch. Pharmacol., 286:371, 1975.
150. Cavero, I., and Roach, A.G.: Effects of clonidine on canine cardiac neuroeffector structures controlling heart rate. Br. J. Pharmacol., 70:269, 1980.
151. Rao, T.L.K., et al.: Deliberate hypotension and anesthetic requirements of halothane. Anesth. Analg., 60:513, 1981.
152. Kalser, S.C., et al.: Further studies of the excretion of atropine-alpha-C. J. Pharmacol. Exp. Therap., 121:449, 1957.
153. Ostfeld, M., and Unna, K.: Effects of atropine on EEG and behavior in man. J. Pharmacol. Exp. Therap., 128:265, 1960.
154. Duvaisin, R.C., and Katz, R.: Reversal of central anticholinergic syndrome in man by physostigmine. J.A.M.A., 206:1963, 1968.
155. Horrigan, R.W.: Physostigmine and anesthetic requirements for halothane in dogs. Anesth. Analg., 57:180, 1978.
156a. Orkin, L.R., and Chien-Hsu, C.: Addiction, alcoholism and anesthesia. South. Med. J., 70:1172, 1977.
156b. Lee, P.K., Cho, M.H., and Dobkin, A.B.: Effects of alcoholism, morphinism, and barbiturate resistance on induction and maintenance of general anesthesia. Can Anaesth. Soc. J. 11:354, 1964.
157. Johnstone, R.E., Kulp, R.A, and Smith, T.C.: Effects of acute and chronic ethanol administration on isoflurane requirement in mice. Anesth. Analg., 54:277, 1975.
158. Chin, J.H., and Goldstein, D.B.: Drug tolerance in biomembranes: A spin label study of effects of ethanol. Science, 196:684, 1977.
159. Tanifuji, Y., and Eger, E.I. II: Effect of isoproterenol and propranolol on halothane MAC in dogs. Anesth. Analg. (Cleve.), 55:383, 1976.
160. Vitez, T.S., et al.: Effects of delta-9-tetrahydrocannabinol on cyclopropane MAC in the rat. Anesthesiology, 38:525, 1973.
161. Stoelting, R.K., Creasser, C.W., and Martz, R.C.: Effect of cocaine administration on halothane MAC in dogs. Anesth. Analg. (Cleve.), 54:422, 1975.
162. Bentley, J.B., et al.: Hepatorenal indices among general anesthetics in obesity. Anesthesiology, 53:S259, 1980.
163. Strube, P.J., Hulands, G.H., and Halsey, M.J.: Serum fluoride levels in morbidly obese patients: enflurane compared with isoflurane anaesthesia. Anaesthesia, 42:685, 1987.
164. Roizen, M.F., et al.: Reduced anesthetic requirement after

electrical stimulation of periaqueductal gray matter. Anesthesiology, 62:120, 1985.
165. Stoelting, R.K.: MAC awake. Anesthesiology, 33:5, 1970.
166. de Jong, R.H., and Eger, E.I. II: MAC expanded: AD$_{50}$ and AD$_{95}$ values of common inhalation anesthetics in man. Anesthesiology, 42:384, 1975.
167. Saraiva, R.A., et al.: Adiposity and the pharmacokinetics of halothane. Anaesthesia, 32:240, 1977.
168. Papper, E.M., and Kitz, R.J.: Uptake and distribution of anesthetic agents. New York, McGraw-Hill, 1963.
169. Bazett, H.C.: Medical physiology. St Louis, C.V. Mosby, 1966.
170. Eger, E.I.: Applications of a mathematical model of gas uptake. In Uptake and distribution of anesthetic agents. New York, McGraw-Hill, 1963.
171. Hunter, A.R.: The group of pharmacology of anesthetic agents and the absorption-elimination of inhaled drugs. Br. J. Anaesth., 28:244, 1956.
172a. MacKree, G.: In Uptake and distribution of anesthetic agents. Edited by E.M. Papper and R.J. Kitz. New York, McGraw-Hill Book, 1963.
172b. Severinghaus J.W.: Role of lung factors. In Uptake and distribution of anesthetic agents. New York, McGraw-Hill Book Co., Chapter 6, 1963.
172c. Mellander S, Johansson B: Control of resistance, exchanges and capacitance functions in the peripheral circulation. Pharmacol. Rev. 20:117, 1968.
173. Brodie, B.B., and Hogben, C.A.M.: Some physio-chemical factors in drug action. J. Pharm. Pharmacol., 9:345, 1957.
174. Landau, W.M., et al.: The local circulation of the living brain. Trans. Am. Neurol. A., 80:125, 1955.
175. Kety, S.S.: Concepts of blood-flow distribution in the brain. In Uptake and distribution of anesthetic agents. Edited by E.M. Papper and R.J. Kitz. New York, McGraw-Hill, 1963.
176. Sokoloff, L.: Control of cerebral blood flow: The effects of anesthetics agents. In Uptake and distribution of anesthetic agents. Edited by E.M. Papper and R.J. Kitz. New York, McGraw-Hill, 1963.
177. Schauker, L.S.: Penetration of drugs into the central nervous system. In Uptake and distribution of anesthetic agents. Edited by E.M. Papper and R.J. Kitz. New York, McGraw-Hill, 1963.
178. Bradbury, M.: The concept of a blood-brain barrier. New York, John Wiley & Sons, Inc., 1979.
179. Brightman, M.W., Reese, T.S.: Junctions between intimately apposed cell membranes in the vertebrate brain. J. Cell Biol., 40:648, 1969.
180. Betz, A.L., Firth, J.A., Goldstein, G.W.: Polarity of the blood-brain barrier: Distribution of enzymes between the luminal and antiluminal membranes of brain capillary endothelial cells. Brain Res., 192(1):17, 1980.
181. Davson, H.: Physiology of cerebro-spinal fluid. London, Churchill, 1970.
182. Betz, A.L., Goldstein, G.W.: Specialized properties and solute transport in brain capillaries. Ann. Rev. Physiol., 48:241, 1986.
183. Goldstein, G.W., Retz, A.L.: The blood-brain barrier. Sci. American, 255(3):74, 1986.

ELIMINATION OF INHALED ANESTHETICS

1. Cullen, B.F., and Eger, E.I. II: Diffusion of nitrous oxide, cyclopropane, and halothane through human skin and amniotic membrane. Anesthesiology, 36:168, 1972.
2. Van Dyke, R.A.: Metabolism of volatile anesthetics: Implications for toxicity. Menlo Park, CA, Addison Wesley, 1977.
3. Norgate, C.E., Sharp, J.H., and Cousins, M.J.: Metabolism of enflurane in man following a second exposure. Anaesth. Intensive Care, 4:186, 1976.
4. Holaday, D.A., Rudofsky, S., and Treuhaft, P.S.: The metabolic degradation of methoxyflurane in man. Anesthesiology, 33:579, 1970.
5. Widger, L.A., Gandolfi, A.J., and Van Dyke, R.A.: Hypoxia and halothane metabolism in vivo: Release of inorganic fluoride and halothane metabolite binding to cellular constituents. Anesthesiology, 40:197, 1976.
6a. Chase, R.E., Holaday, D.A., Saidman, L.J., et al.: The biotransformation of ethrane in man. Anesthesiology, 35:262, 1971.
6b. Cousins, M.J., et al.: Metabolism and renal effects of enflurane in man. Anesthesiology, 44:44, 1976.
7. Blitt, C.D., et al.: Extrahepatic biotransformation of halothane and enflurane. Anesth. Analg., 60:129, 1981.
8. Mazze, R.I., Cousins, M.J., and Barr, G.A.: Renal effects and metabolism of isoflurane in man. Anesthesiology, 40:536, 1974.
9. Sakai, T., and Takaori, M.: Biodegradation of halothane, enflurane, and methoxyflurane. Br. J. Anaesth., 50:785, 1978.
10. Mazze, R.I., Calverley, R.K., and Smith, N.T.: Inorganic fluoride nephrotoxicity: Prolonged enflurane and halothane anesthesia in volunteers. Anesthesiology, 46:265, 1977.
11. Roman, R.J., et al.: Renal tubular site of action of fluoride in Fischer's 344 rats. Anesthesiology, 46:260, 1977.
12. Mazze, R.I., Beppu, W.J., and Hitt, B.A.: Metabolism of synthane: Comparison with in vivo and in vitro defluorination of other halogenated hydrocortion anesthetics. Br. J. Anaesth., 51:839, 1979.
13. Brown, B.R., and Sagalyn, A.M.: Reactive intermediates of anesthetic biotransformation and hepatotoxicity. In Molecular Mechanisms of Anesthesia. Edited by B.R. Fink. New York, Raven Press, 1975.
14a. Mazze, R.E., and Denson, D.D.: Deuteration of anesthetics. Anesthesiology, 51:101, 1979.
14b. McCarty, L.P., Malek, R.S., and Larsen, E.R.: The effects of deuteration on the metabolism of halogenated anesthetics in the rat. Anesthesiology, 51:106, 1979.
15. Cohen, E.N., and Trudell, J.R.: Biodegradation of inhalation anesthetics. In Metabolic Aspects of Anesthesia, Clinical Anesthesia Series. Edited by P.J. Cohen. Philadephia, F.A. Davis, 1975.
16. Eastwood, D.W., et al.: Effect of nitrous oxide on the white-cell count in leukemia. N. Engl. J. Med., 268:297, 1963.
17. Matsubara, T., and Mori, T.: Studies on denitrification. IX: Nitrous oxide, its production and reduction of nitrogen. J. Biochem., 64:871, 1968.
18. Hong, K., et al.: Metabolism of nitrous oxide by human and rat intestinal contents. Anesthesiology, 52:16, 1980.
19. Bentley, J.B., et al.: Serum inorganic fluoride levels in obese patients during and after enflurane anesthesia. Anesth. Analg., 58:409, 1979.
20. Young, S.R., et al.: Anesthetic biotransformation and renal function in obese patients during and after methoxyflurane or halothane anesthesia. Anesthesiology, 42:451, 1975.
21. Bentley, J.B., et al.: Hepatorenal indices among general anesthetics in obesity. Anesthesiology, 53:S259, 1980.
22. Strube, P.J., Hulands, G.H., and Halsey, M.J.: Serum fluoride levels in morbidly obese patients: Enflurane compared with isoflurane anaesthesia. Anaesthesia, 42:685, 1987.

23. Holaday, D.A., et al.: Resistance of isoflurane to biotransformation in man. Anesthesiology, *43:*325, 1975.
24. Carpenter, R.L., et al.: The extent of metabolism of inhaled anesthetics in humans. Anesthesiology, *65:*201, 1986.
25. Blitt, C.D., et al.: Extrahepatic biotransformation of halothane and enflurane. Anesth. Analg., *60:*129, 1981.
26. Stoelting, R.K., and Eger, E.I. II: Percutaneous loss of nitrous oxide, cyclopropane, ether and halothane in man. Anesthesiology, *30:*278, 1969.
27. Cascorbi, H.F., Blake, D.A., and Helrich, M.: Differences in the biotransformation of halothane in man. Anesthesiology, *32:*119, 1970.
28. Van Dyke, R.A., and Chenowith, M.B.: The metabolism of volatile anesthetics. II. In vitro metabolism of methoxyflurane and halothane in rat liver slices and cell fractions. Biochem. Pharmacol., *14:*603, 1965.
29. Cahalan, M.K., Johnson, B.H., and Eger, E.I. II: Relationship of concentrations of halothane and enflurane to their metabolism and elimination in man. Anesthesiology, *54:*3, 1981.
30. Carpenter, R.L., et al.: Does the duration of anesthetic administration affect the pharmacokinetics or metabolism of inhaled anesthetics in humans? Anesth. Analg., *66:*1, 1987.

13

GENERAL ANESTHESIA—CLINICAL SIGNS

HISTORY OF STAGES AND SIGNS IN ANESTHESIA

1847—Francis Plomley[1] (January 1847)—Separated stages of anesthesia into three parts.

1847—P. Jean Marie Flourens.[2]—Experiments demonstrating successive action on the central nervous system.

1847—John Snow[3] (September 1847)—Divided the anesthesia into five degrees of narcotism.

1918—Joseph T. Gwathmey and H. T. Karsner[4a]—Reported analgesia for short surgical procedures.

1920—Arthur E. Guedel[5a,5b]—Published his well-known classification of stages and signs in anesthesia (divided into four parts).

1925—A. H. Miller[6]—Called attention to the intercostal paralysis as a sign of anesthesia.

1925—Ralph M. Waters[7]—Placed the intercostal paralysis in Plane 3, Stage III.

1933—Hans Berger[8]—Demonstrated the effect of chloroform anesthesia on the brain potentials of humans.

1950—R. F. Courtin, R. G. Bickford, and A. Faulconer, Jr.[9]—Reported the first clinical use of the encephalogram (EEG) in estimating the depth of anesthesia.

1954—Joseph F. Artusio[10]—Reported a detailed description of stage I of ether anesthesia in humans.

1957—Philip D. Woodbridge[11]—Divided general anesthesia into sensory, motor, reflex, and mental block. (designated as Nothria)

HISTORY OF CLINICAL SIGNS. In March 1847, Flourens[2], the French physiologist, recognized three degrees of depression when the agents ether or chloroform were administered. Under ether the nervous centers lose their power in regular succession: (1) cerebral lobes, (2) cerebellum, and (3) spinal areas.

Flourens pointed out that under anesthesia the medulla oblongata still retains its functions and the animal continues to live, but, with loss of action of medulla, life is lost.

Snow's pioneer monograph on ether appeared in

September 1847,[3] when he published his observations on the stages or degrees of anesthesia. Anesthesia was divided into the four well-known stages that continue to be recognized.

Snow emphasized that the chief requisite in administering anesthesia was the skill of determining when anesthesia had progressed to the operative stage. He stated that the divisions were arbitrary.

CLASSIFICATION OF SIGNS.[5c] The clinical signs of anesthesia have been classified and carefully charted in relation to the four stages of Guedel. The clinical signs are the consequence of the *absorption* of an anesthetic by specific areas of the brain. This process of anesthesia must be examined carefully.

In 1952,[10] Artusio clarified the first stage of Anesthesia and *described* the clinical signs or events occurring at this time (Table 13-1). As a result of his investigations, the first stage has been termed the *analgesic stage*. He demonstrated conclusively that major surgery could be performed during this period.

The signs of anesthesia are thus a description of patients and their biologic responses. They are produced by all agents that are depressant and blood borne to the nervous system regardless of the method of introduction into the circulation.

CLINICAL SIGNS OF ANESTHESIA

Under optimal conditions and with a favorable pressure gradient as well as a continued supply of an anesthetic agent, a patient may be taken from the state of complete consciousness to that of respiratory arrest and death. In doing so the patient passes through four well-defined stages. These stages are demarcated, one from another by the absence of particular responses but merge, one with another. The classic "ether stages" and planes are noted in Figure 13–1 and form a base for discussion.

Variations and modifications of these basic stages are seen with different agents (Fig. 13–2).

STAGE I: INDUCTION PERIOD

During the induction stage, volitional reactions are gradually depressed. There is usually a sensation of floating, followed by sinking and a sense of suffocation. Thoughts are blurred, and amnesia soon develops. In the latter part of this stage, 85% of the patients have analgesia. During this stage one may observe slight stiffening of the body and some dilatation of the pupils. Pulse is usually accelerated, mostly due to apprehension. Respiration usually slows and blood pressure usually falls. The special senses of smell and taste may be heightened.

STAGE II: THE STAGE OF UNCONSCIOUSNESS

Stage II is often erroneously called the *excitement stage*. It corresponds to the time when all volitional reactions are lost. It should be pleasant in the psychologically prepared patient and not disturbed or nightmarish.

The stage may be conveniently divided into two

TABLE 13–1. SUMMARY OF STAGE I OF ANESTHESIA

Characteristics	Plane 1	Plane 2	Plane 3
State	Preanalgesia Preamnesia Sedation	Partial analgesia Total amnesia	Total analgesia Total amnesia Loss of consciousness
Clinical signs			
Amnesia	0	XXXX	XXXX
Memory for recent events	XXXX	XXXX	XX⟶0
Memory for past events	XXXX	XXXX	XXXX→0
Response to spoken voice	XXXX	XXXX	XXXX→0
Cerebration	XXXX	XXXX	XXXX→0
Ability to focus eyes	XXXX	XXXX	XX⟶0
Ability to distingish color	XXXX	XXXX	XXXX⟶0
Analgesia	0	XX	XXXX

0 indicates *absence of* or *none*; X indicates *degree of*, i.e., XX is partial, XXXX is complete.

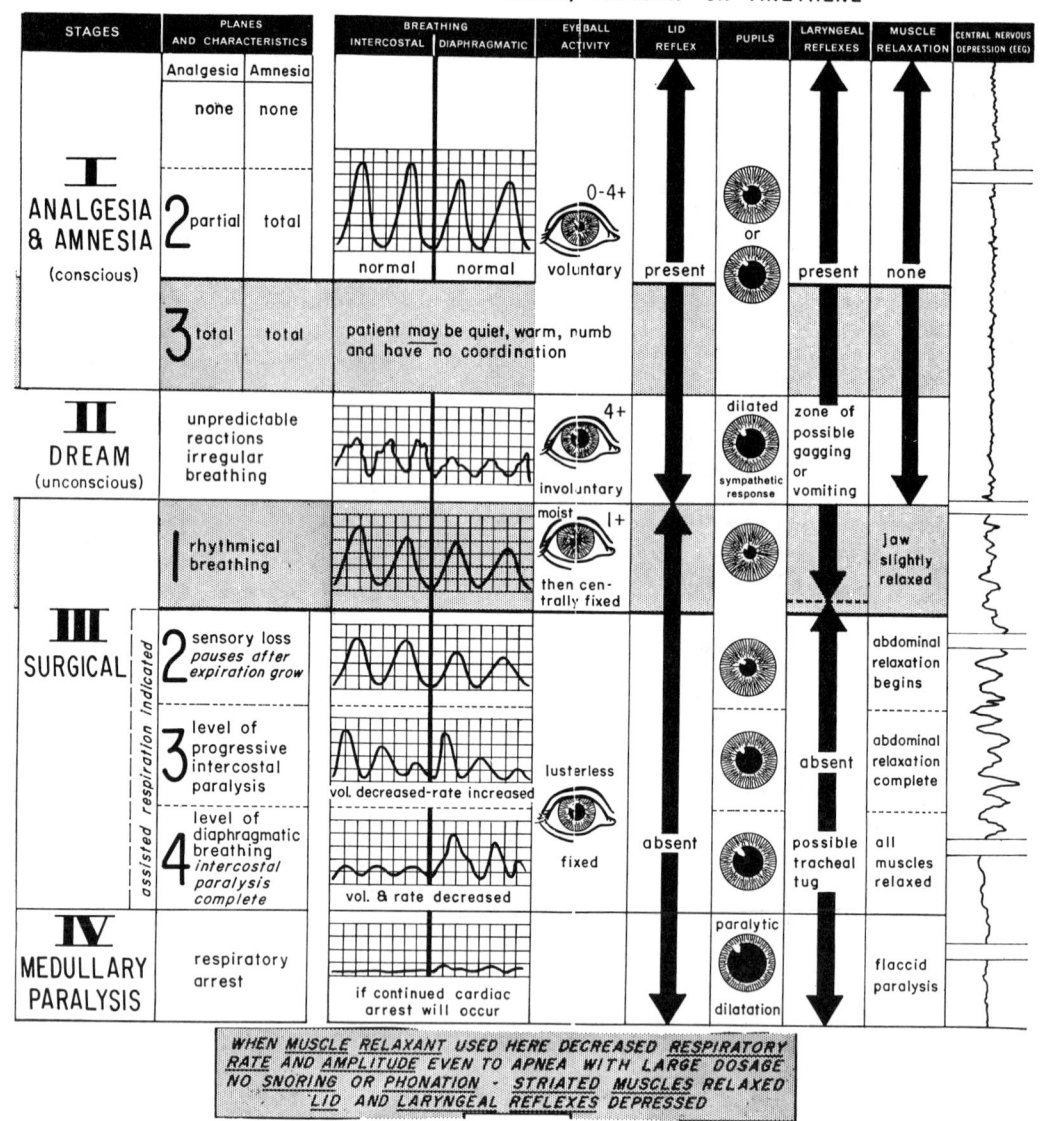

FIG. 13–1. Stages and signs of anesthesia with inhalation of volatile ethers enflurane and isoflurane. *Shaded areas* show planes when muscle relaxant administration results in decreased respiratory rate and amplitude, even to apnea, with large dosage; no snoring or phonation; relaxed striated muscles; and depressed lid and pharyngeal reflexes. Modified from Thomas G.J., et al.: Summary of stages and signs in anesthesia. Anesth. Analg., 40:42, 1961.

parts: (1) the decorticate plane of depression, and (2) the decerebrate plane, which follows.

DIVISION OF STAGE II

The manifestations of stage II usually depend on various external stimuli and are usually exaggerated when basal metabolism is high. If the stimuli are unpleasant, there may be a great deal of struggling. During this stage the special senses (cranial) are obtunded. Usually smell, taste, and sight are the first to go while the sense of hearing may be initially heightened and is the last to be depressed. It is thus important that noises be excluded from a room in which a patient is being inducted into anesthesia. As consciousness is lost, involuntary but rhythmic muscular movements are usually noted accompanied by cerebral release in which the patient may sing or swear. During this stage the swallowing re-

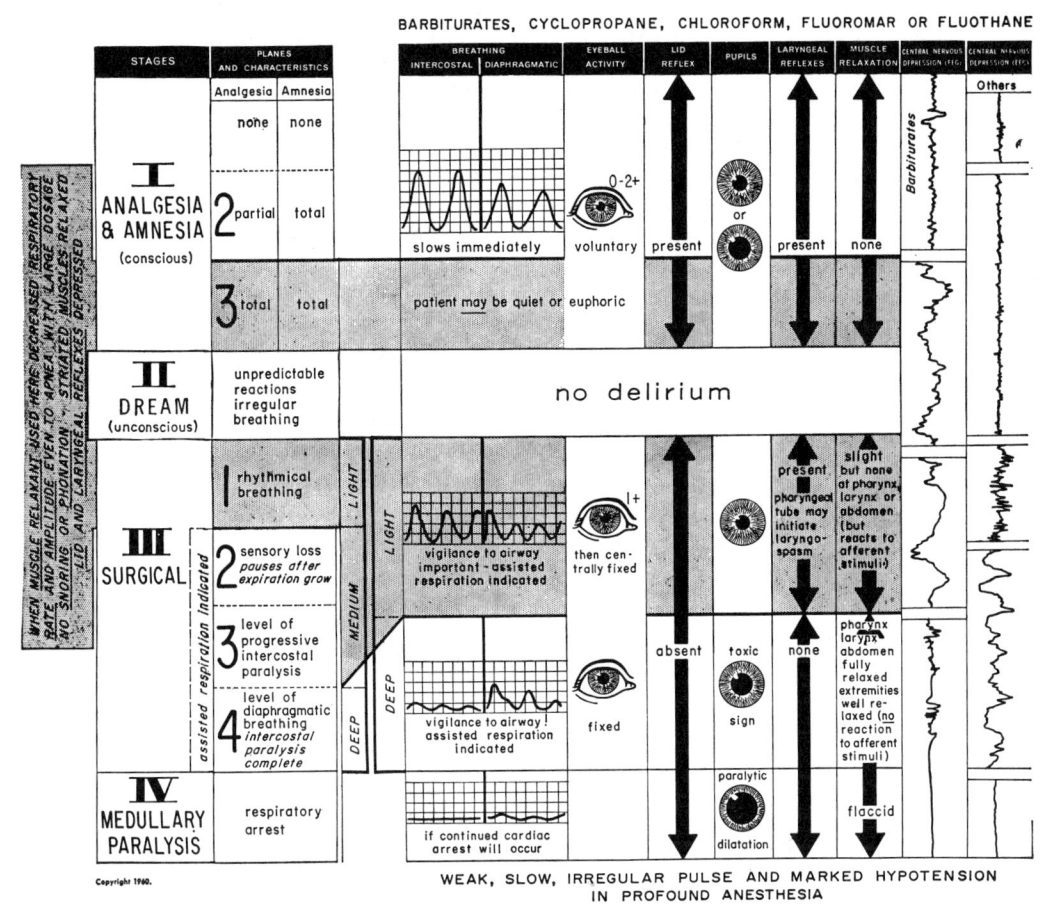

FIG. 13–2. Stages and signs of anesthesia with barbiturate or intravenous induction and halothane, enflurane, or isoflurane maintenance. See Figure 13–1 legend for definition of shaded areas. Modified from Thomas, G.J., et al.: Summary of stages and signs in anesthesia. Anesth. Analg., 40:42, 1961.

flex is quite active, and the corneal reflex is present. Often vomiting will occur because of direct action on the medulla; however, this may also be due to gastric irritation. The pulse is fast and respiration is irregular. Characteristic of this stage is the roving eyeball, due to an imbalance in tone of the ocular muscles. Pupils are widely dilated.

It is during this stage that ventricular fibrillation is likely to occur, especially when the patient is at an age when physiologic activity is greatest, namely, between 5 and 30 years. Its occurrence depends on a greatly increased activity of the sympathetic nervous system. This overactivity is apparently the result of adrenalin release, particularly with ether, and to the stimulus of emotional excitement. One other danger of this stage is that of physical violence. This, as has been previously mentioned, usually results from external stimuli, which tend to increase the apprehension of the patient. Nursing personnel should control any violent movements and restrain the extremities to prevent possible injury.

STAGE III: THE STAGE OF ANESTHESIA

The stage III planes 1 and 2 (surgical anesthesia) are achieved by MAC multples of 1.4 to 2.0 × MAC. At this MAC level producing surgical anesthesia, a rough correlation exists with increased plasma concentrations of the anesthetic agent over the concentration at 1.0 MAC. Thus, for the different anesthetic agents, the plasma concentration for surgical anesthesia is approximately as follows:

- Diethyl ether: 100 to 120 mg%
- Enflurane: 15 to 25 mg%
- Halothane: 10 to 20 mg%
- Methoxyflurane: 0.5 to 2.0 mg%

Stage III is divided into four planes. There is a progressive obtundation of protective reflexes in this stage, and there is also a gradual paralysis of all muscles of the body. Small muscle groups are the first to be paralyzed. In the fourth plane, or plane of greatest depth, respiratory arrest occurs (with ether). If the anesthetic medication is discontinued or its concentration is decreased to allow a reversal of the anesthetic gradient, respiration will be resumed by the patient spontaneously, in the absence of muscle relaxants.

PRINCIPLE OF CURRENT PRACTICE. In current practice it is no longer necessary to deepen the level of surgical anesthesia by high inhalation anesthetic concentrations to achieve muscle paralysis and surgical relaxation. This is accomplished by muscle relaxants. Hence, deep planes 3 and 4 of stage III are avoided to prevent toxic effects. Nevertheless, the effects of deep anesthesia are noted on the functions of the various body systems.

OBSERVATIONS AT DIFFERENT PLANES

Plane 1

Respiration—regular and deep, similar to that of normal sleep.

Circulation—pulse and blood pressure attain a normal level after the effects of Stage II diminish.

Pupils are constricted; corneal reflex is present but the blink reflex is absent.

Roving eyeballs may be present but usually are absent.

Reflexes—response to skin stimulation depressed; gag or pharyngeal reflex obtunded in lower half of plane.

Plane 2

Respiration—a pause between inspiration and expiration appears, and inspiration becomes shorter than expiration.

Circulation—pulse and blood pressure normal.

Eyeball is centered and up; no roving.

Pupils show slight dilatation; corneal reflex sluggish.

Rigidity of skeletal muscle begins to disappear, and reflex contraction of abdominal wall muscles is abolished at lower border of this plane.

Reflexes—cough and skin reflexes lost.

Plane 3

Respiration—intercostal paralysis begins; breathing gradually becomes diaphragmatic; inspiration definitely shorter than expiration and jerky.

Circulation—with the progressive muscular relaxation there is progressive pooling of blood and an increase in pulse rate; a fall in blood pressure and a fall in pulse pressure at expense of systolic pressure occurs.

Pupils show greater dilatation, corneal reflex obtunded.

Large skeletal muscle groups relax, and smooth muscle tone is lost.

Reflexes—visceral and traction reflexes obtunded.

Plane 4

Respiration—completely diaphragmatic; there is paradoxic respiration, namely, the thoracic cage collapses when inspiration occurs and the abdomen protrudes. This becomes marked until central respiratory paralysis occurs; jerky character of respiration prominent.

Circulation—pulse faster and blood pressure continues to drop.

Pupils are greatly dilated.

Muscular relaxation is cadaveric.

Reflexes—response to corneal reflex obtunded.

STAGE IV: STAGE OF VITAL ARREST

Stage IV has been termed that of medullary paralysis; however, it is more properly related to cardiac depression.

CLINICAL ASSESSMENT OF DEPTH OF GENERAL ANESTHESIA.[5c,11,12] The state of anesthesia has been defined as a descending central nervous system (CNS) depression. One can observe the presence or absence of nervous system faculties and functions by applying the principle of stimulus–response. Various stimuli are applied and responses are noted. A neurologic examination corresponding to Woodbridge's components is usually followed.[11]

1. *Cortical depression*—This can be determined by observing the following:
    a. Levels of orientation
    b. Consciousness
        (1) Response to conversation—alertness
        (2) Response to commands
        (3) Response to a loud sound, eg, a bell (startle reaction)
2. *Sensory stimulus*—Voluntary Motor Reactions
    a. Somatosensory stimuli of a noxious nature such as a pin prick or a skin incision ordinarily evokes a withdrawal phenomenon employing voluntary muscles.
    b. When these sensory impulses do not produce a response, somatosensory block has occurred.
    c. In plane 2 eye and pharyngeal reflex responses are obtunded.
3. *Visceral Response*
    a. Viscerosensory stimuli are more potent than somatosensory stimuli. They can evoke skeletal motor activity (tightening of muscles) as well as some sympathetic responses.
    b. In plane 2, the pharyngeal reflex is absent and laryngeal-tracheal reflexes are obtunded.
4. *Autonomic Viscerosympathetic Reflexes*
    a. There are no responses in stage III, planes 2 and 3, when MAC-BAR levels are at-

tained. This occurs at multiples of MAC.[13,14]

(1) Laryngeal reflexes are absent.
(2) Tracheal reflexes are obtunded, and intubation responses are minimized.
(3) Catecholamine (norepinephrine) release is obtunded.

CONFOUNDING FACTORS. Many factors may alter the appearance or modify stimulus–response testing. The graded intensity of a stimulus will produce graded responses: a mild stimulus may produce a negligible response, whereas a strong stimulus will produce an extensive physiologic reaction. It is evident that the CNS stimulus–response principle is not an all-or-none phenomenon, as with many peripheral reactions. Important modifiers include the following:

1. Adjunctive CNS depressants
2. Muscle relaxants
3. Supplementary narcotics
4. Local anesthetics
5. Automonic nervous system blockade
   a. Alpha and beta blockers
   b. Topical anesthetics
   c. Regional epidural anesthesia
   d. IV local anesthetics
6. Pharmacologic Differences of Inhalation Agents on Brain Physiology—The various inhalation agents have significant differences in their effect on cerebral blood flow (CBF), global cerebral metabolic rate (CMR), and regional CMR (gray matter).

EFFECT OF ANESTHETIC DRUGS. Most anesthetic drugs depress electrical activity to an isoelectric state. Metabolic activity is simultaneously depressed, and cell activity is subdivided into the oxygen requirements for the performance of function and the basal lower requirement for the simple maintenance of cell life. To depress the latter requires greater concentrations of anesthetic agents. Metabolic activity also varies with the type of brain tissue: gray matter has an oxygen requirement three times that of the white matter. For the cerebral metabolic rate of oxygen (CMR_{O_2}) the depression is nonlinear at anesthetic concentrations less than 1.0 MAC.[15]

On the anesthetic dose-response at the transition of the EEG, there is a rapid decrease in the CMR_{O_2}; thereafter, there is a linear decrease in CMR_{O_2}. Some examples are as follows:

- Halothane[16,17]—Increases CBF from 40% at 1% inhaled concentration to 140% at 3% concentration; global CMR_{O_2} shows a dose-related depression. At 1% the CMR_{O_2} decreases 40%, whereas at 3% there is a 70% decrease.
- Nitrous oxide 70%[16]—CBF increases 200% or more; CMR_{O_2} increases 160%; global CMR_{O_2} increases 120% (Gray matter)
- Enflurane[15,17]—CBF is not affected at 0.6 MAC but increases at 1.2 MAC; CMR_{O_2} is not affected at 0.6 MAC but is reduced at 1.2 MAC.
- Isoflurane[18,19]—CBF is little affected below 1.0 MAC; at 1.0% CBF increases 10% to 12% and increases further at 2.3% inhaled concentration; CMR_{O_2} decreases in a dose-related manner; at 2.5 MAC the EEG reaches an isoelectric level. Increased concentrations do not further affect the EEG level.
- Hypothermia[20,21]—CMR_{O_2} is progressively and continuously reduced.
- Ketamine[22]—CBF increases by 60% to 80% but returns to normal in 20 to 30 minutes; CMR increases 15% to 20%; visual pathways show increased metabolic activity and the limbic system remains active. The auditory paths are depressed.

ANALYSIS OF SPECIAL REFLEXES

BLINK REFLEX.[23] This is a reflex that is commonly evaluated early in the induction period of anesthesia to provide evidence of the occurrence of unconsciousness. This eyelid or blink reflex in patients is obtunded at the end of the second stage of unconsciousness and at the beginning of the third stage, the stage of anesthesia. This is a brain stem reflex that was originally described by Kugelberg and has been extensively investigated.[24] A stimulus applied to the eyelid or conjunctiva (also the cornea) produces afferent impulses that travel over the ophthalmic division of the trigeminal nerve.[25] Such stimulation evokes a double-component reflex response in the ipsilateral orbicularis oculi muscle.[26] The first part of the reflex has a short latency (9 to 11 mec) and is transmitted through an oligosynaptic reflex arc involving the nucleus caudalis of the trigeminal nerve and projecting to the motoneuronal pool of the facial nerve. The second part of the response is of longer latency (25 to 35 msec) and is a multisynaptic central relay system that includes numerous brain stem structures of the mesencephalic reticular formation. It is clear that the second component of the blink reflex serves a nociceptive function and produces eyelid closure, which protects the eyeball against the noxious stimulus. The afferent arc is over the facial nerve.[24] This reflex can also be elicited by stimulation of the supraorbital nerve branch of the ophthalmic division.

Pupillary Light Reflex. Observation of this reflex has been a traditional stimulus–response test of the effects of anesthetics on the brain and a test of the depth of anesthesia.[25,26] As anesthesia is deepened, the pupil dilates and fails to actively respond in a normal manner.[28,29] Because volatile anesthetics depress the reflex, it has been considered that sluggish response or its absence indicates deep surgical anesthesia. The technique of eliciting the reflex, however, has not been standardized, and different agents appear to have variable responses.

An elegant study by Larson using an infrared pupillometer provides the following:[30]

Thiopental, used for induction and for short procedures, causes an initial reduction in the degree of reflex response but does not produce a sustained response or abolition of the response. The reflex is abolished only when a volatile anesthetic is introduced.[31]

The *volatile inhalation anesthetics* (eg, isoflurane) depress the response, and this is profound. It is abolished when MAC-BAR levels of anesthesia are attained. A response may be noted on skin incision.[30]

Succinylcholine was not found to block the pupillary response even when patients were only under light thiopental sedation.[30] Because the iris contains only smooth muscle, it would be expected that the skeletal muscle relaxants would not block the contraction of the sphincter muscle of the iris. The claim that this relaxant blocks the reflex and hence could be used to assess the depth of coma is invalid.[32]

Age modifies the reflex. In elderly patients a reduced response reflex is already present even when they are awake (senile miosis).

Mechanism.[30] The pupillary light response is a parasympathetic reflex. The reduction in the response by anesthetics appears to occur in the afferent pathway of the reflex. The efferent path is not significantly obtunded; direct stimulation of this pathway can evoke pupillary contraction. Intense surgical stimulation will often cause pupillary constriction, but this is the result of sympathetic activation.

LOWER ESOPHAGEAL CONTRACTILITY.[33] Lower esophagus contractility (LEC) is denoted by two forms of muscular activity consisting of *peristaltic* and *nonperistaltic* (nonpropulsive) movements.[34] Nonpropulsive contractility as well as contractions provoked by an inflation of a balloon are of interest because it is reported that they are stress related.[35] In the nonanesthetized subject there are spontaneous contractions of the lower esophagus characterized by isolated contractions at a rate of 4 to 10 per minute, lasting about 5 seconds, at an amplitude with a mean of 30 mm Hg. With the onset of anesthesia, there is a suppression of frequency of activity, but amplitude of the remaining contractions is not greatly altered.

As anesthesia is deepened, there is progressive suppression of both frequency and amplitude until there is no intrinsic esophageal activity at 2 MAC for inhalation agents. Suppression is also evident with large doses of fentanyl. As anesthesia is lightened, there is progressive return of LEC with a particular rise in the frequency of spontaneous contractions. The provoked LEC also shows a rise in frequency and amplitude.

It is evident that the measurement of LEC could be a useful guide and monitor of the adequacy and depth of general anesthesia.

RECOVERY.[11,36] The neurologic changes occurring during the recovery are the reverse of those seen during progressive deepening of anesthesia. The more primitive brain-stem centers are the earliest to recover, whereas cortical functions manifested by the return of consciousness and intellectual functions recover later. Although patients may respond to noise (bellringing), painful stimuli, and verbal commands, and may be able to speak and be oriented, nevertheless, some degree of mental impairment may continue for 2 to 4 days. Performance can be studied with refined and sophisticated psychological methods. Impairment is more evident in the elderly patient. It is evident from various studies that this postoperative impairment may occur following either general or regional (epidural) anesthesia. Because epidural anesthesia inhibits some of the stress response to anesthesia and surgery (ie, cortisol and glucose levels do not significantly change), it is concluded that factors other than stress evoke the transient mental impairment.[36]

AWARENESS DURING ANESTHESIA

The phenomenon of perioperative awareness during anesthesia has been recognized since 1844.[37] As stated by Waterman, it is still a mystery, but certain negative aspects are definable.[38] Intraoperative awareness with recall must be distinguished from dreams and hallucinations. The word *hallucination* means to wonder in mind. It is defined as a subjective perception of what does not exist and evoked without a peripheral sensory stimulus. The description of an hallucination is a description of a vision, sound, or sensation that is unreal.

Awareness is defined as one's ability to consciously integrate actual events of reality into the memory system.[39] Experiences are recorded first as a temporary imprint, but if important or vivid, may be consolidated for long-term memory subject to indeterminant time recall.

Recall is the ability to take actual experiences, either abstract concepts or physical events, from memory stores and to recount the sequence as a scenario. It is important to recognize that recall is memory of actual events without pain. A painful experience may not be consolidated in the memory system.[40]

It appears that anesthetic agents impair memory consolidation and impair registration of events in long-term memory.[41] Both RNA brain and protein synthesis are inhibited. Amnesia is essentially the impairment of consolidation of events into memory.

On the other hand, even under the influence of anesthetic agents, sensory input from potent stimuli may be perceived. Intraoperative awareness occurs when auditory or tactile stimuli are intense. Unconsciousness alone does not preclude awareness.

INCIDENCE.[39,41] Recall of intraoperative events by patients who have been anesthetized occurs in about 1% of patients, but the incidence of recall may be as high as 10%. The higher incidence is particularly likely after balanced anesthesia and when depth of inhalation anesthesia is inadequate—at levels lighter than stage III, planes 1 and 2, ie, at MAC less than 1.3 to 1.5 MAC.[40,41] The timing of recall is usually associated with the induction period and the onset of surgery; recall awareness is also frequent during the emergence period.

The injudicious use of relaxants without an adequate state of unconsciousness or stage of anesthesia is the most common condition in which awareness develops.

CAUSES.[42] The causes of recall of intraoperative events are related to the following:

1. Poor or inadequate preanesthetic medications
2. Lack of amnesic agents
3. Balanced anesthetic techniques[43]
4. Use of muscle relaxants[42,44]
5. Light levels of anesthesia (unconsciousness only) ie, stages I and II[39]

PERIODS OF AWARENESS.[39,44] Induction is often performed in an atmosphere of activity and conversation that is both disturbing and frightening. The unpleasantness of the surgical theater is often recalled. Even when the patient is unconscious, recall is frequent—especially when life-threatening statements are made and such statements and unusual sounds can penetrate to the subconscious. It should be emphasized that hearing is the last of the central special senses to be obtunded.

Intubation is frequently performed in an unconscious but unanesthetized patient—one only under a sedative hypnotic such as thiopental or a benzodiazepine but paralyzed. This circumstance is too frequently remembered.[45]

Intraoperative recall with or without pain occurs and is related to "dissociative" phenomenon.[40,41] Dreams may be unpleasant especially after a disturbing preanesthetic operating room experience. A frequent condition for recall is the trend toward light anesthesia and muscular paralysis presumably to minimize depression of respiratory and cardiovascular function. The designation of this state as the stage of anesthesia is inaccurate. It is clearly the second stage of the anesthesia process[10] and is only the dream stage. Certain procedures, however, may dictate a period of awakening for diagnostic purposes. During Harrington rod procedures, this is often desired, but if explained adequately preoperatively, it is not unpleasant nor painful. In neurosurgery, a relative state of consciousness is often desirable but is acceptable and not disturbing when patients are fully instructed and prepared.

ROLE OF MUSCLE RELAXANTS. With the advent of muscle relaxants, many of the signs of the depth of unconsciousness and of the planes of anesthesia have been lost.[44] In 1950, Winterbottom noted that patients can awaken during insufficient anesthesia.[37] Others reported that consciousness and pain can exist during apparent anesthesia.[40,43] Intraoperative awareness was more frequently evident during balanced type anesthesia and especially with intravenous narcotic technics.[43] Distressing experiences of patients undergoing heart surgery, who awakened during narcotic "anesthesia" (analgesia) while paralyzed by succinylcholine, have been described.[42] These patients suffered postoperative traumatic neurosis, denoted by persistent anxiety, nightmares, and preoccupation with death.[40,45] Most patients are unwilling to discuss their experience.

POSTOPERATIVE AWARENESS.[40,46] This is a frequent experience. It is unpleasant if a patient becomes conscious before muscle control returns or pain relief is provided. After long procedures of more than 3 to 4 hours, any narcotic, premedication or anesthetic, may have been dissipated and pain rapidly returns. Such a circumstance is conducive to agitation and delirium. Consideration of respiratory depression from analgesic drugs needs to be weighed against the respiratory depressant effect of pain and the enhanced metabolism from stress and fear.[46,47] The administration of a small dose of a narcotic intravenously, such as 2 mg morphine, 20 mg meperidine, or 20 μg fentanyl, prior to discontinuing nitrous oxide and/or volatile anesthetic mixtures has been found satisfactory and safe.

RECALL.[45,48] Suggestions made during anesthesia are often followed postoperatively without patient knowledge of the suggestion. Sentence recognition is frequent but does not reach significance. Recall of perioperative events, however, has been recorded in 23% of patients, all men, some recall being achieved with the aid of hypnosis. These memories were both kinesthetic and auditory. Postoperative psychosis and dreaming with or without nightmares are observed.[49]

It is evident that the inability of patients to recall operative events does not mean they were not aware. Postoperative anxiety and light premedication are predictors of postoperative recall. If the anesthetic technique is based primarily on inhalation agents and small doses of intravenous analgesics, then when the inhalation agent is withdrawn at particular parts of the surgery, information and events may be registered. Recall more often occurs in the absence of narcotic supplementation or when inhalation agents are not being administered or are withdrawn, as during bypass.

TESTS OF AWARENESS. During general anesthesia with relaxants, some recognition of wakefulness may be determined by the method of Tunstall.[50] He describes the isolated forearm technique in which the arm and hand are spared from neuromuscular blockade by a pneumatic tourniquet. This provides an opportunity for the patient to signal to the anesthetist when he is aware or awake.[50]

Nonverbal Response. Nonverbal response postoperatively to intraoperative conversation has been demonstrated (Bennett).[51] A double-blind study under known clinical levels of nitrous oxide–enflurane or halothane anesthesia was conducted in which patients were exposed to a repetitive suggestion. The importance of touching their ear during a postoperative interview was emphasized. All patients were amnesic to the intraoperative suggestion but did touch their ear at the time of the postoperative interview. Thus, deep-seated psychomotor actions can be suggested and carried out without a conscious awareness. This suggestion technique may have value in prevention of nausea, vomiting, and headache and in minimizing pain.

USE OF POSITIVE SUGGESTIONS.[49–52] A clinical study of unconscious perception during general anesthesia shows the merit of positive suggestions on posoperative recovery. In the experimental group, suggestions from a cassette recorder were made over earphones attached to the patients. In a reassuring voice, suggestions were made of relaxation, well being, comfort, lack of nausea and vomiting, no difficulty with bladder or bowel function, and rapid recovery. In comparison, other patients were exposed to either ordinary operating room sounds or a continuous monotonous low-frequency noise.

In older patients, over 55 years of age, the positive suggestions contribute to a rapid recovery and shorter hospital stay (at least following gall bladder surgery).[52]

PREVENTION OF AWARENESS. Scopalamine as an amnesic agent remains a prototype and should be employed more frequently. Contrary to some reports, it does not produce postoperative delirium unless pain is present and pain centers have not been obtunded.

Benzodiazepines provide excellent prograde amnesia. Diazepam effect is short lived, but lorazepam lasts for 12 to 24 hours;[53,54] midazolam appears to offer greater advantages over the other agents for its amnesic effect.[55]

Quiet in the operating room and recovery area is essential; unnecessary conversation must be avoided and noise excluded.

Adequate general anesthesia at least to first plane stage III should be provided. Pain must be controlled throughout any surgical procedure and into the postoperative period.

Narcotic supplementation and at least 1.5 MAC levels of volatile anesthetics reduces the amount of relaxants needed and minimizes awareness. At the end of surgery and during recovery from general anesthesia, the judicious use of small doses of analgesics is useful in blunting the immediate postoperative pain experience.

Ear plugs have been recommended, especially for regional anesthesia. Music in the operating room situations is an excellent supplementation for many cases.

Clinical signs presumptive of intraoperative awareness have been proposed for the totally paralyzed patient.[56] The signs are principally sympathetic responses to surgical stimulation but may be activated by auditory stimuli when patients are not completely anesthetized to the third stage of depth (Table 13–2).

SUMMARY OF RECOMMENDATIONS.[41]

1. Provide surgical anesthesia with an inhalation agent to a depth of stage III, planes 1 and 2.
2. Remember that the special sense of hearing is the last to be obtunded and the first to recover.
3. Assume that the patient may be awake in any case and provide words of comfort and reassurance during maintenance.
4. Use a benzodiazepine or scopolamine preanesthetically to achieve some amnesia.
5. Patients for emergency surgery (especially trauma patients) are at high risk for awareness.
6. Avoid discussions that would be disturbing or unsuitable to the patient or derogatory of the patient. Judicious conversation in the operating room is necessary.
7. Patients should have an opportunity to discuss postoperatively any awareness they experienced during surgery and then be helped to gain an understanding of why it occurred.

Recall of events during surgery from major trauma has been studied by Bogetz and Katz.[48] Concern was expressed over the tendency to reduce MAC requirements because of such conditions as hypotension, shock, acidemia, hypothermia, or intoxication in the interest of safety. Some patients were provided a steady state of light surgical anesthesia, yet 11% had recall. Of those more seriously injured and managed by rapid sequence (ketamine or thiopental plus relaxant SCH), 43% recalled their surgery. In either instance, the patients considered the awareness their worst hospital experience. Pain during surgery was the most distressing feature of their experiences (despite presumed adequate doses of narcotics), whereas hearing voices and knowing that they were being operated on were secondarily distressing.[40]

TABLE 13–2. PRESUMPTIVE SIGNS OF AWARENESS
Sympathetically Activated Responses

	1st Stage	2nd Stage	3rd Stage
Lacrimation	Active	Passive	Absent
Salivation	Active	Passive	Absent
Perspiration	Active	Passive	Absent
Peristalsis (borborygmus)	Active	Passive	Absent
Piloerector reflex	Active	Passive	Absent
Areola reflex	Active	Passive	Absent
Consciousness	Yes	Perhaps	No

From Massa, D.J.: Presumptive signs of intraoperative awareness. Anesthesiol. Rev., 9:33, 1982.

EEG SIGNS OF ANESTHESIA

Changes in the brain wave pattern have been found to parallel changes in consciousness in humans.[57] The EEG has been found to be a reliable index of the depth of anesthesia. Because the EEG can be readily recorded from the surface of the scalp, this technique has provided a useful monitoring method in the operating room.

EEG techniques have been worked out for the study of cortical activity during anesthesia by the Mayo Clinic group, and patterns of activity have been correlated with various anesthetic depths.[7]

TECHNIQUE.[9a-9c] The EEG technique employs a frontal to occipital bipolar derivation on one side. This simplification of the EEG channels has been found satisfactory, because investigation revealed that characteristic rhythms of anesthesia were present in all parts of the cortex but maximal precentrally. Second, fast frequencies have been removed by use of a filter to increase the legibility of the slow waves that characterize anesthesia.

GENERAL PATTERN. As the cortex is depressed by increasing amounts of anesthetic agents, a characteristic EEG pattern is obtained. A general pattern is recognized and can be graphically illustrated as a continuum of progressive cerebral depression. Although there are minor differences between the patterns if obtained with different agents, there is sufficient similarity to form a composite pattern (Fig. 13–3).[58]

The results have been striking and consistent with nitrous oxide-ether anesthesia. The first noticeable effect is a disappearance of the resting alpha

FIG. 13–3. Pattern classification in the continuum of progressing cerebral depression. 1. Fast-frequency, low-voltage activity. 2. Rhythmic waves of slower frequency and higher voltage. 3. Pattern of mixed waves—low-voltage, faster frequency superimposed on high-voltage, slower frequency. 4. Periods of cortical inactivity separating periods of activity (burst suppression). As depression progresses, cortical activity decreases in voltage and frequency and appears at more infrequent intervals. From Brechner, V.L.[58] *The Electroencephalogram in Anesthesia.* Worcester, MA, Edin, 1962.

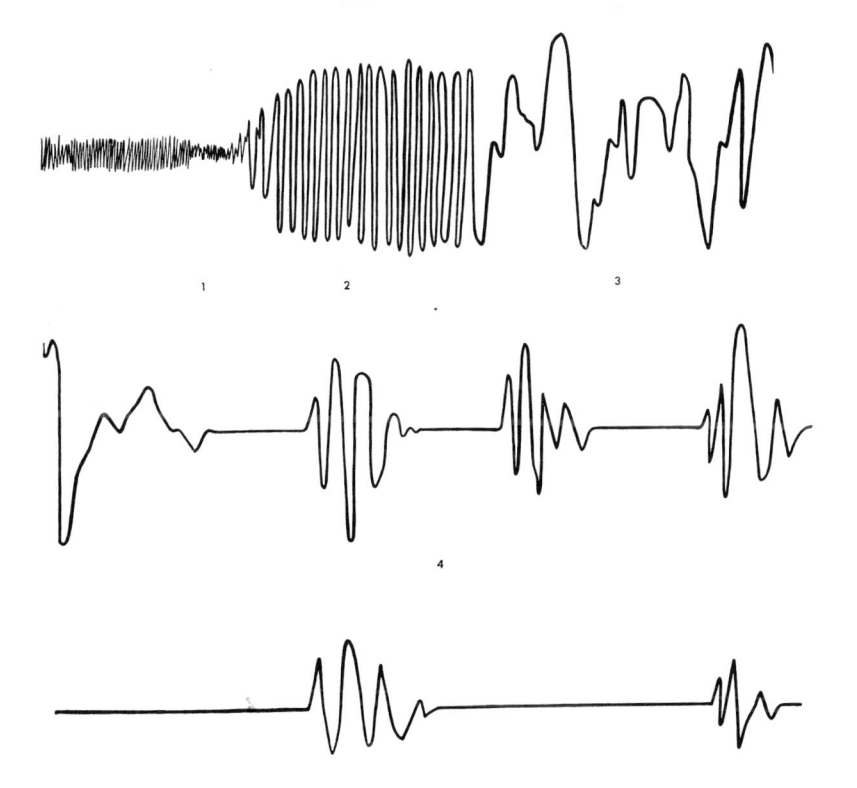

rhythm with flattening of the record alpha rhythm with flattening of the record that persists into the dream stage. As the stage of surgical anesthesia is approached, a high-amplitude rhythmic discharge appears, which lasts approximately 1 minute and is rapidly replaced by a complex type of discharge. As anesthesia deepens, an inhibition of electrical activity takes place until the cortex is completely inactive at the stage of respiratory paralysis.[59]

CLASSIFICATION. Because the changes described above were reproducible and consistent, they have been classified into seven levels. These are illustrated in Figure 13–4 and Table 13–3.[9a]

First Level. The first level has a flat pattern. The alpha frequencies present during consciousness have disappeared. Occasional fast discharges of low amplitude (30 μV) are seen. This pattern lasts for the duration of induction, usually 7 minutes. It apparently corresponds to the clinical first stage,[51] or the stage of imperfect consciousness and analgesia. Excitement may be seen in the latter part of this level.[59]

Second Level. The second level is characterized by a rhythmic pattern that consists of high-amplitude, regular discharges that appear abruptly. The amplitude varies between 200 and 300 μV with a frequency of 2.8 cps. This pattern rarely lasts longer than 1 minute and abruptly changes to the pattern of the third level. Excitement may be seen during this level.

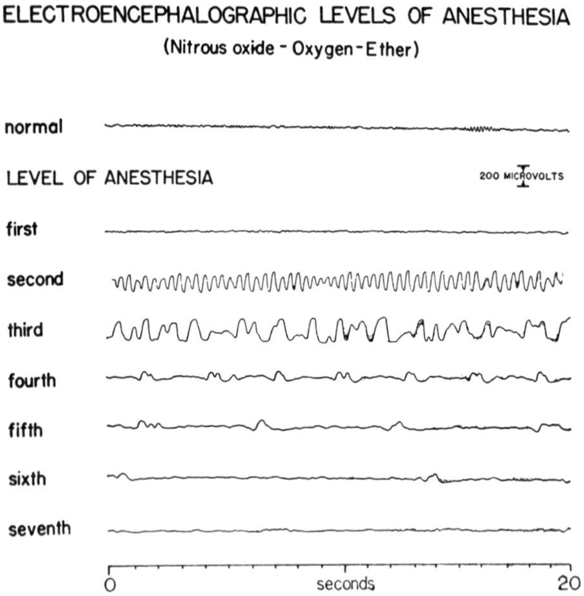

TABLE 13–3. EEG LEVELS RELATED TO ARTERIAL ETHER CONCENTRATIONS[9a]

Clinical Stage	EEG Level	Ether Concentration (mg %)
I	I	60
II	II	78
III	III	98
III plane 1	IV	116
III plane 2	V	125
III plane 3	VI	135
IV	VII	135

Third Level. There is a complex pattern in the third level. This level is characterized by little rhythmicity or repetition of wave forms. Waves of slower frequency predominate with some faster components. The amplitude begins to fall. At this level minor surgical operations are possible, and it therefore corresponds to first plane (light surgical anesthesia).

Fourth Level. Beginning at the fourth level, there is suppression of cortical activity that is progressive. There are small groups of high-voltage waves separated by short periods of relative cortical inactivity with waves of amplitude no greater than 20 μV. Such sequences of inactivity are fairly constant in length. The wave groups have a frequency of 2 to 4 cps with an average amplitude of 150 μV. The intervals of inactivity do not exceed 3 seconds in length. This conforms to the second plane, and there is beginning muscular relaxation. Abdominal surgery may be performed at this level.

Fifth Level. In the fifth level, there is moderate suppression, with periods of cortical inactivity lasting between 3 and 10 seconds. The amplitude of the wave groups is less. This level corresponds to third plane anesthesia, and muscular relaxation is nearly flaccid. Intubation of the trachea is easily performed at this time.

Sixth Level. Severe suppression is present in the sixth level. The wave groups do not appear more than once every 10 seconds. The average amplitude is about 76 μV. This level is unnecessarily deep and corresponds to fourth plane anesthesia or a period of diaphragmatic muscular paralysis.

Seventh Level. Complete suppression is seen in the seventh level. Absence of measurable waves characterize this level. Such waves that occasionally appear have an amplitude of 20 μV or less. This level corresponds to fourth stage, or stage of respiratory

FIG. 13–4. EEG patterns during nitrous oxide–oxygen–ether anesthesia at varying depths. From Courtin, R.F., Bickford, R.G., and Faulconer, A., Jr.: The classification and significance of Electro-encephalographic patterns produced by nitrous oxide-ether anesthesia during surgical operations. Proc. Staff Meet. Mayo Clin., 35:197, 1950.

arrest. It is also seen under conditions of anesthetic difficulty.

There are many transitional patterns of the EEG tracings. Composite EEG patterns representative of the different common general anesthetic agents are presented. It is to be noted that the seven levels originally presented for nitrous-oxide oxygen-ether have been slightly modified. The fourth through the seventh levels, depending on the degree of suppression show electrical burst activity of high-voltage, slow frequency irregular waves of delta pattern.

INFLUENCE OF DIFFERENT ANESTHETIC DRUGS

Nitrous Oxide.[9c] A gradual and progressive diminution of amplitude of alpha waves occurs during administration of nitrous oxide. A random delta rhythm with waves of frequency between 4 and 6 cps appears. These increase in amplitude. The anesthetic level does not depend on hypoxemia, and good first-plane nitrous oxide anesthesia is directly proportional to the partial pressure of the anesthetic gas.

Sodium Pentothal.[59] The flattening of the first level is rarely seen. There is usually a pattern containing slow waves of low amplitude with superimposed frequencies. When ether is added, the pattern sequence is picked up at the second level.

Cyclopropane. Possati[60] correlated EEG patterns with blood levels of this drug. Six levels of cortical electrical activity were defined. The first five are similar to ether, but amplitude is less throughout. The last two levels could probably be broken into three parts, depending on how suppression of the small wave group is divided.[61]

Intravenous Thiobarbiturates. Kiersey[62-63] has classified thiopental EEG patterns into five levels.

Halothane–Nitrous Oxide. Observations have been made on humans by Gain.[64] They have identified seven levels in the pattern of the EEG waves from induction to complete cortical suppression. With occurence of a mixed-wave pattern as a level three, one can subsequently recognize varying degrees of suppression conveniently separated into four levels.

Hypothermia and Occluded Circulation. Effect of decreasing temperature on the EEG has been studied by Quasha.[65] There is a progressive decrease in potential during cooling to 28° C. and less thiopental is needed to produce burst suppression.

Chloroform. The patterns of electrocortical activity obtained under chloroform anesthesia have been studied by Pearcy.[66] He defined six distinct levels. One can divide the sixth level into two degrees of suppression before complete suppression or inactivity greater than 30 seconds is attained.

Fluoromar. Changes produced by this drug in humans were studied by Brechner,[67] who classified six levels of cortical activity. Greater suppression of the waves was not achieved because of the circulatory depression.

Other Drugs.[68] See Table 13-4 for a summary of other commonly used drugs that produce EEG changes.

OTHER INFLUENCES. Progressive depression of electrical cortical activity is produced by a number of nonanesthetic influences. A normal EEG depends on adequate cerebral perfusion. Thus, ischemia, hypoxia, deep anesthesia, hypotension, or sudden temperature falls will result in an abnormal pattern.

Hypoxia.[69] Any fall in blood oxygen saturation diminishes cerebral activity. It is especially marked with severe burst suppression when saturation reaches 60% or less.[70]

Hypercarbia.[71] The accumulation of carbon dioxide hastens the onset of deeper levels of anesthesia and makes slow rhythms pronounced. This was noted by Rubin[61] during cyclopropane anesthesia. An increase in carbon dioxide appears to increase the average frequency of brain potentials. It is also recognized that the inhalation of carbon dioxide will prevent the changes in frequency seen when hypoxic mixtures are inhaled.

Automatic Regulation.[72] With the demonstration that reliable patterns of depth of anesthesia can be produced and that there generally is a progressive decrease in the total bioelectric potential, the possibility of using these values to determine the administration of agents appeared. To this end, the total brain electric potential is determined and converted into a simple numeric measure.[73] This is then integrated with the anesthesia input. Thus, a self-regulatory system called *servo-anesthesia*, is established.[74]

EFFECTS OF EXTREME ETHER ANESTHESIA.[75] Dogs deeply anesthetized with ether (and artificially ventilated) beyond the point when complete suppression is observed in the EEG show reactivation of the EEG. This return of cortical reactivity follows a fairly consistent pattern. Beyond Courtin's standard EEG seven levels, four additional levels before complete quiescence have been recognized by Pearcy.[59] These changes are noted as the circulation begins to fail, and it is hypothesized that this reactivation is due to cerebral ischemia.

TABLE 13–14. COMMONLY USED DRUGS PRODUCING CHANGES IN EEG WAVE PATTERNS AND FREQUENCIES

Drugs producing 18–30 cps high-voltage waves—CNS depressants (basal narcotics).
Barbiturates
    Amobarbital (Amytal)
    Phenobarbital
    Secobarbital (Second)
    Pentobarbital (Nembutal)

Nonbarbiturate sedatives
    Methylparafynol (Somnesin)
    Ethchlorvynol (Placidyl)
    Methylpentynol (Oblivon)
    Meprobamate
    Diphenhydramine HCl (Benadryl)
    Sodium bromide.

May obscure spike discharges and slow-wave foci or generalized slow-wave activity from other causes.

Drugs producing 5–8 cps high-voltage wave activity in paroxysms.
CNS depressants in high and prolonged dosages abruptly withdrawn.
Barbiturates
Meprobamate
Ethyl alcohol
Meperidine HCl (Demerol)

May produce convulsive seizures.

Drugs producing 1.2–7 cps moderate voltage slow-wave activity, focally and generally.
Modern tranquilizers
Reserpine
Phenothiazines
    Chlorpromazine (Thorazine)
    Thioridazine (Mellaril)
    Others
CNS depressants (analgesics)
    Morphine
    Meperidine HCl (Demerol)

After high dosage and prolonged administration: May obscure slow wave foci (lesions) or generalized slow wave activity from other causes.

Drugs that may eliminate focal and bisynchronous spike discharges.
CNS depressants
Anticonvulsants
    Phenytoin
    Mesantoin
    Milontin
    Thiantoin
    Mysoline
    Phenurone
    Phenobarbital
    Mebaral
    Gemonil

May obscure evidence of epileptogenic activity.

Drugs that increase the convulsive threshold for spike-and-wave activity accompanying clinical petit mal attacks.
CNS stimulants
    Amphetamines
    Caffeine
Anticonvulsants
    Tridione
    Paradione
    Celontin
    Phenurone
    Barbiturates

May obscure spike and 3 cps slow-wave activity or generalized slow-wave activity from other causes.

Drugs producing random 5–7 cps waves (theta frequencies).
Thymelephic
True antidepressant
    Imipramine HCl (Tofranil)

Not likely to be seen in the usual therapeutic dosage

From Towler, U.L., Beall, B.D., and King, J.B.: Drug effects on electroencephalographic pattern. J South. Med. Assoc., 55:832, 1962.

REFERENCES

1. Plomley F.: Stages of anesthesia. Lancet *1*:134, 1847.
2. Flourens P.J.M.: Note touchant les effets de l'inhalation etherée sur la moelle épinière. Comp. Rend. Acad. Sci. (Paris) *24*:161; 253; 340 (March), 1947.
   idem: Note touchant l'action de l'éther sur les centres nerveux. Comp. Rend. Acad. Sci. (Paris) *24*:340, 1947.
3a. Snow J.: Stages of anesthesia. Lancet *1*(March):228, 1847.
3b. Snow J.: A lecture on the inhalation of vapour of ether in surgical operations. Lancet *1*:551, 1847.
3c. Snow J.: *On Inhalation of Vapour of Ether in Surgical Operations*. London, John Churchill, September, 1847.
4a. Gwathmey J.T., Karsner H.T.: General *analgesia* by oral or rectal administration. Brit. Med. J *2*:312, 1918.
4b. Gwathmey J.T.: *Anesthesia*, 2nd Edition (Textbook). New York, The Macmillan Co., 1924.
5a. Guedel A.E.: Anesthesiology Supplement. Am. J. Surg. *24*:53, 1920.
5b. Guedel A.E.: Signs. Internat. Anesth. Research Soc. Bull. No. 3(May), 1920.
5c. Guedel A.E.: *Inhalation Anesthesia—A Fundamental Guide*, 2nd Edition. New York, The Macmillan Co., 1951.
6. Miller A.H.: Ascending respiratory paralysis under general anesthesia. J.A.M.A. *84*:202, 1925.
7. Waters R.: Quoted by Guedel in: *Inhalation Anesthesia*, p. 28. New York, The Macmillan Co, 1937.
8. Berger H.: Über das Elektrenkephalogramm des Menschen. Arch. Psychiatr. *99*:555, 1933.
9a. Courtin R.F., Bickford R.G., Faulconer A. Jr.: The classification and significance of electro-encephalographic patterns produced by nitrous oxide-ether anesthesia during surgical operations. Proc. Staff. Meet., Mayo Clinic *25*:197, 1950.
9b. Mayo C.W., Bickford R.G., Faulconer A. Jr.: Electroencephalographically controlled anesthesia in abdominal surgery, J.A.M.A. *144*:1081, 1950.
9c. Faulconer A. Jr., Pender J.W., Bickford R.G.: The influence of partial pressure of nitrous oxide on the depth of anesthesia and the electroencephalogram in man. Anesthesiology *10*:601, 1949.
10. Artusio J.F. Jr.: Di-ethyl ether analgesia: A detailed description of the first stage of ether anesthesia in man. J. Pharmacol. Exp. Therap. *3*:343, 1954.
11. Woodbridge P.D.: Changing concepts concerning depth of anesthesia. Anesthesiology *18*:536, 1957.
12. Thomas G.J. et al: Summary of stages and signs in anesthesia. Anesth. Analg. *40*:42, 1961.
13. Eger, E.I. II, Saidman, L.J., and Brandstater, B.: Minimum alveolar anesthetic concentration: A standard of anesthetic potency. Anesthesiology, *26*:756, 1965.
14. Roizen, M.F., Horrigan, R.W., and Frazer, B.M.: Anesthetic doses blocking adrenergic (stress) and cardiovascular responses to incision MAC-BAR. Anesthesiology, *54*:390, 1981.
15. Sullken, E.H., Jr., et al. The non-linear responses of cerebral metabolism to low concentrations of halothane, enflurane, isoflurane, and thiopental. Anesthesiology, *46*:28, 1977.
16. Smith, A.L., and Wollman, H.: Cerebral blood flow and metabolism: Effects of anesthetic drugs and techniques. Anesthesiology, *36*:378, 1972.
17. Mitchenfelder, J.D., and Milde, J.H.: Influence of anesthetics on metabolic functional and pathological response to regional cerebral ischemia. Stroke, *6*:405, 1975.
18. Newburg, L.A., Milde, J.H., and Mitchenfelder, J.D.: The cerebral metabolic effects of isoflurane at and above concentrations that surpass cortical electrical activity. Anesthesiology, *59*:23, 1983.
19. Newman, B., Gelb, A.W., and Lam, A.M.: The effect of isoflurane-induced hypotension on cerebral blood flow and cerebral metabolic rate for oxygen in humans. Anesthesiology, *64*:307, 1986.
20. Bigelow, W.G.: Oxygen transport and utilization of oxygen in dogs. Am. J. Physiol., *160*:125, 1950.
21. Bigelow, W.G.: and Callaghan, J. C.: General hypothermia for experimental intracardiac surgery. Ann. Surg., *132*:531, 1950.
22. Dawson, E.V.: *In* Intravenous Anesthesia and Analgesia. Edited by G. Corssen, J.G. Reves, and T.H. Stanley. Philadelphia, Lea & Febiger, 1988.
23. Willer, J.-C., et al.: Failure of naloxone to reverse the nitrous oxide-induced depression of a brain stem reflex: An electrophysiologic and double-blind study in humans. Anesthesiology, *63*:467, 1985.
24. Kugelberg, E.: Facial reflexes. Brain, *75*:385, 1952.
25. Olzewski, J.: On the anatomical and functional organization of the spinal trigeminal nucleus. J. Comp. Neurol., *92*:401, 1950.
26. Hiraoka, M., and Shimamura, M.: Neural mechanisms of the corneal blinking reflex in cats. Brain Res., *125*:265, 1977.
27. Flagg, P.J.: The Art of Anesthesia. Philadelphia, J.B. Lippincott, 1916, pp. 108–113.
28. Guedel, A.E.: Inhalation Anesthesia. New York, Macmillan, 1937, pp. 25–36.
29. Larson, M.D.: Pupillary effects of general anesthesia. Anesth. Rev., *13*:25–31, 1986.
30. Larson, M.D.: Alteration of the human pupillary light reflex by general anesthesia. Anesth. Rev., *16*:25–29, 1989.
31. Larson, M.D.: Dilation of the pupil in human subjects after intravenous thiopental. Anesthesiology, *54*:246–249, 1981.
32. Plum, F., and Posner, J.B.: The Diagnosis of Stupor and Coma, 3rd ed. Philadelphia, F.A. Davis, 1980, pp. 320–321.
33. Evans, J.M., Davies, W.L., and Wise, C.C.: Lower oesogeal contractility: A new monitor of anaesthesia. Lancet, *1*:1151–1153, 1984.
34. Ingelfinger, F.J.: Esophageal motility. Physiol. Rev., *38*:533–584, 1958.
35. Faulkner, W.B.: Objective esophageal changes due to psychic factors. Am. J. Med. Sci., *200*:796–803, 1940.
36. Riis, J., et al. Immediate and long-term mental recovery from general versus epidural anesthesia in elderly patients. Acta Anaesthiol Scand., *27*:44, 1983.
37. Winterbottom, E.H.: Insufficient anesthesia. Br. Med. J. *1*:247, 1950.
38. Waterman, P.: Postop recall by patients after general anesthesia. Surgical Rounds, *2*:27–29 (August) 1979.
39. Scott, D.H.: Awareness during general anesthesia. Can. Anaesth. Soc. J., *19*:173, 1972.
40. Graff, T.D., and Phillips, O.C.: Consciousness and pain during apparent surgical anesthesia. J.A.M.A., *170*:2069, 1959.
41. Blacher, R.S.: Awareness during surgery. Anesthesiology, *61*:1, 1984.
42. Meyer, B.C., and Blacher, R.S.: A traumatic neurotic reaction induced by succinylcholine chloride. N.Y. State J. Med., *61*:1255, 1961.
43. Hilgenberg, J.C.: Intraoperative awareness during high-dose fentanyl-oxygen anesthesia. Anesthesiology, *54*:341, 1981.
44. Mainzer, J., Jr.: Awareness, muscle relaxants and balanced anaesthesia. Can. Anaesth. Soc. J., *6*:386, 1979.
44a. Mainzer, J., Jr.: Muscle relaxants and problems of surgical awareness. Anesthesiol. Rev., *8*:30, 1981.

45. Blacher, R.S.: On awakening paralyzed during surgery. A syndrome of traumatic neurosis. J.A.M.A., 234:67, 1975.
46. Editorial: On being aware. Br. J. Anaesth., 51:711, 1979; 53:1, 1981.
47. Van Valen, L.: Baroreceptor activation reduces reactivity to noxious stimulation: Implications for hypertension. Science, 205:1299, 1979.
48. Bogetz, M.S., and Katz, J.A.: Recall of surgery for major trauma. Anesthesiology, 61:6, 1984.
49. Goldmann, L., Shah, M.V., and Hebden, M.H.: Memory of cardiac anaesthesia: Psychological sequelae in cardiac patients of intraoperative suggestion and operating room conversation. Anaesthesia, 42:596, 1987.
50. Tunstall, M.E.: Detecting wakefulness during anesthesia for caesarean section. Br. Med. J., 1:1321, 1977.
51. Bennett, H.L., Davis, H.S., and Giannini, J.A.: Non-verbal response to intraoperative conversation. Br. J. Anaesth., 57:174, 1985.
52. Bonke, B., et al. Clinical study of so-called unconscious perception during general anaesthesia. Br. J. Anaesth., 58:957, 1986.
53. Knapp, R.: Evaluation of the cardiopulmonary safety and effects of lorazepam as a premedicant. Anesth. Analg., 53:122, 1974.
54. Gale, G., Galloon, S.: Lorazepam as a premedication. Can. Anaesth. Soc. J., 23:22, 1976.
55. Reeves, J.G., Fragen, R.J., and Vinik, H.R.: Midzolam: Pharmacology and uses. Anesthesiology, 63:310, 1985.
56. Massa, D.J.: Presumptive signs of intraoperative awareness. Anesthesiol. Rev., 9:33, 1982.
57. Gibbs, F.A., Gibbs, E.L., and Lennox, W.G.: Effect on the electroencephalogram of certain drugs which influence nervous activity. Arch. Int. Med., 60:154, 1937.
57a. Brechner, V.L., and Dornette, W.H.L.: Electroencephalographic patterns during nitrous oxide trifluoethylvinyl ether anesthesia. Anesthesiology, 18:321, 1957.
58. Brechner, V.L., Walter, R.D., and Dillon, J.B.: Practical Electroencephalography for the Anesthesiologist. Springfield, IL, Charles C. Thomas, 1962.
59. Galla, S.J., Rocco, A.G., and Vandam, L.D.: Evaluation of the traditional signs and stages of anesthesia: An electroencephalographic and clinical study. Anesthesiology, 19:328, 1958.
60. Possati, S. et al. Electroencephalographic patterns during anesthesia with cyclopropane: Correlation with concentration of cyclopropane in arterial blood. Anesth. Analg., 32:130, 1953.
61. Rubin, M.A., and Freeman, H.: Brain potential changes in man during cyclopropane anesthesia. J. Neurophysiol., 3:33, 1940.
62. Kiersey, D.K., Bickford, R.G., and Faulconer, A., Jr.: Electroencephalographic patterns produced by thiopental sodium during surgical operations: Description and classification. Br. J. Anaesth., 23:141, 1951.
63. Kiersey, D.K., Faulconer, A., Jr., and Bickford, R.G.: Automatic electro-encephalographic control of thiopental anesthesia. Anesthesiology, 15:356, 1954.
64. Gain, E.A., and Paletz, S.G.: An attempt to correlate the clinical signs of fluothane with electroencephalographic levels. Can. Anesth. Soc. J., 4:289, 1957.
65. Quasha, A.L., Tinker, J.H., and Sharbrough, F.W.: Hypothermia plus thiopental: Prolonged electroencephalographic suppression. Anesthesiology, 55:636, 1981.
66. Pearcy, W.C., et al.: Electroencephalographic and circulatory effects of chloroform anesthesia in dogs. Anesthesiology, 18:88, 1957.
67. Brechner, V.L., and Dornette, W.H.L.: Electroencephalographic patterns during nitrous oxide-trifluoroethylvinyl ether anesthesia. Anesthesiology, 18:321, 1957.
68. Towler, U.L., Beall, B.D., and King, J.B.: Drug effects on electroencephalographic pattern. J. of So. Med. Assoc., 55:832, 1962.
69. Gronqvist, Y.K.J., Seldon, T.H., and Faulconer, Albert, Jr.: Cerebral anoxia during anesthesia: Prognostic significance of electroencephalographic changes. Ann. chir. et gynaec. Fenniae, 41:149, 1952.
70. Siegar, O. and Gerard, R.W.: Anoxia and train potentials. J. Neurophysiol., 1:558, 1938.
71. Clowes, G.H.A., Jr., Kretchmer, H.E., McBurney, R.W., and Simeone, F.A.: The electro-encephalogram in the evaluation of the effects of anesthetic agents and carbon dioxide accumulation during surgery. Ann. Surg., 138:558, 1953.
72. Bickford, R.: Use of frequency discrimination in the automatic electroencephalographic control of anesthesia. Anesthesiology, 13:83, 1951.
73. Faulconer, A., and Bickford, R.G.: Electroencephalography in Anesthesiology. Springfield, IL. Charles C Thomas, 1960.
74. Findeiss, J.C., et al.: Power spectral density of the electroencephalogram during halothane and cyclopropane anesthesia. Anesth. Analg., 48:1018, 1969.
75. Pearcy, W.C.: Circulatory and electroencephalographic effects of extreme ether anesthesia in dogs. Anesthesiology, 23:605, 1962.

14

GENERAL ANESTHESIA—SPECIAL CONSIDERATIONS

RESPIRATION

INTRODUCTION. Perhaps the most important clinical signs of depth of anesthesia are the changes in respiration. These are modified to some extent by the anesthetic agent and are confounded by the administration of muscle relaxants.

To appreciate the effects of anesthesia on the mechanisms of respiration, it is essential to review the muscles of respiration and their function.

MUSCLES OF RESPIRATION. (Table 14–1). In the unanesthetized normal subject at rest, the diaphragm is the primary muscle of respiration. There is also a significant contribution from intercostals (Campbell[1]). It is estimated that, at rest, the diaphragm contributes approximately 60% to tidal exchange and the intercostals about 40%.[2] As activity and demands increase, there is increasing diaphragmatic action, and there is progressive downward recruitment of the external intercostals and the intercartilaginous portion of the internal intercostals. The diaphragm contracts a fraction of a second before the flow of air.[3] The first intercostal also contracts, and if there are greater respiratory demands, there is recruitment of successively lower intercostal muscles. The external intercostals are the ones involved.[4,5]

As the effort increases, abdominal muscles become active, raise intraabdominal pressure, and lower the ribs to assist in expiration.[2] With maximum effort, the accessory inspiratory muscles are brought into play.[6]

The diaphragm has been studied by electromyography.[4] During resting conscious breathing, there is initially a gradual rise in electrical activity during inspiration that wanes during normal expiration (Petit[7]). During forced exhaling, straining, or coughing, the electrical activity recorded from the diaphragm is strong.[8a,8b]

The diaphragm is not only resistant to fatigue but exhibits resistance to anesthetic depression.

MUSCLE FIBER TYPES. The capacity to generate ventilatory force by the respiratory muscle depends on

TABLE 14–1. MUSCLES OF RESPIRATION

PRIMARY[2]
  Diaphragm   60% of normal tidal exchange
  Intercostals   40% of normal tidal exchange
    Inspiration: All external intercostals and intercartilaginous portion of internal intercostal
    Expiration: Remainder of internal intercostals[5]
SECONDARY
1. Abdominal wall muscles
  The power muscles for expiration and coughing[6]
  —"Splint" the abdomen and raising intraabdominal pressure.
  —Contribute to rib depression—an expiratory function.
2. Cervical strap muscles of the neck
  Most important accessory inspiratory muscles.
  —Elevate and fix the first two ribs and enlarge the upper thoracic cavity—active even in normal resting breathing.
3. Sternocleidomastoid
  Elevates the sternum and increases anterior-posterior diameter of chest cavity.
4. Back muscles
  —Augment inspiration.
  —Enlarge rib cage.
  —Used at demanding activity levels requiring maximal respiratory effort.

the mass of the muscle and the muscle fiber type. The latter is related to the number of motor units and their contraction frequency.[9] Two types of fibers can be distinguished:[10]

1. Fatigue-resistant fibers (50% of diaphragmatic fibers) characterized by slow twitch response, high oxidative capacity, and endurance.
2. Fatigue-susceptible fibers[11] characterized by rapid twitch response, development of great force, maximum energy requirements, significant shortening, and limited endurance

EFFECTS OF ANESTHETICS. Anesthesia causes profound changes in respiratory function. Nunn has stated that there is "an overall depression of every facet of the . . . functions which contribute to oxygenation of blood".[13]

In 1857,[14] Snow observed that deepening anesthesia decreased thoracic ventilatory excursion. Guedel[15] emphasized the role of respiration as a clinical guide to depth of anesthesia, while Miller[16] described the pattern of respiration as first an ascending depression of the intercostal muscles followed by diaphragmatic paralysis.[17]

At first, the volatile agents, ether, euflurane, isoflurane ethyl chloride, vinethene, and chloroform appear to stimulate in the order named. Then, in plane 2 of stage III anesthesia, these are respiratory depressants in the reverse order.[12] On the other hand, nitrous oxide and ethylene are stimulants throughout anesthesia and do not depress respiration directly. With cyclopropane and halothane, respiration is generally quiet and depression is continuous and gradual.[13] It is not noticeable until the patient is well into third plane anesthesia, and often there is abrupt change with complete paralysis of intercostal respiration that is rapidly followed by diaphragmatic paralysis and apnea.

PATTERN OF BREATHING DURING ANESTHESIA. All anesthetics produce a progressive dose-related depression of the central nervous system, accompanied by a progressive depression of the respiratory system. This respiratory depression can be correlated with the stages of anesthesia.

In *stage I*, respirations are at first normal, but in the lower limits of this stage there is some increase in rate. This increase may be readily related to the degree of apprehension or excitement of the patient preceding induction. Hyperpnea and breath holding are two other changes that are frequently seen. The latter is entirely voluntary.

In *stage II*, respiration is completely irregular, and any abnormality can occur.

In *stage III*, the respiratory changes noted will be considered according to the plane in which they occur. Refer to Figure 14–1 for a diagrammatic representation of respiratory changes during general anesthesia.

Plane 1. Respiratory exchange is similar to that of normal sleep. Respiration is full and rhythmic. Usually there is an increase of volume. If the first two stages have been smooth the increase is roughly 25%, and in closed-system anesthesia this increase is undoubtedly the result of some accumulation of carbon dioxide. This pattern is particularly evident with ether anesthesia.[12] In the unmedicated patient given cyclopropane, the increase is hardly detectable.[18a,18b] There is also some reflex stimulation, particularly in trauma surgery. There may be a decrease in respiration and minute volume, however, which usually develops as a result of the hyperpnea of stages I and II.

Plane 2. Respiration is very similar to that of Plane 1. A longer pause between inspiration and expiration may be detected. The time for inspiratory effort is shorter than for expiration.

Plane 3. This is the plane of intercostal paralysis. Until this depth of anesthesia is obtained, both components of respiration are synchronous, that is, the diaphragm and the intercostal muscles contract simultaneously to produce a coordinated inspiratory effort.[3] However, with the advent of the third plane there is a delay in thoracic effort.[17] Because the respiratory demand is not lessened, the diaphragmatic component of respiration must compensate for the diminished intercostal component, and because of this it will be noted that the abdomen usually bulges on inspiration.[13a–20]

If anesthetists place their hand on the thoracic cage during this plane, they will detect the delayed thoracic effort in the early phases. There is an ascending paralysis of the intercostal muscles of res-

FIG. 14–1. Respiratory changes during general anesthesia. Shows relationship between thoracic and diaphragmatic components at different anesthetic levels. Courtesy D.E. Brace, Dept. of Anesthesia, New York Medical College, New York.

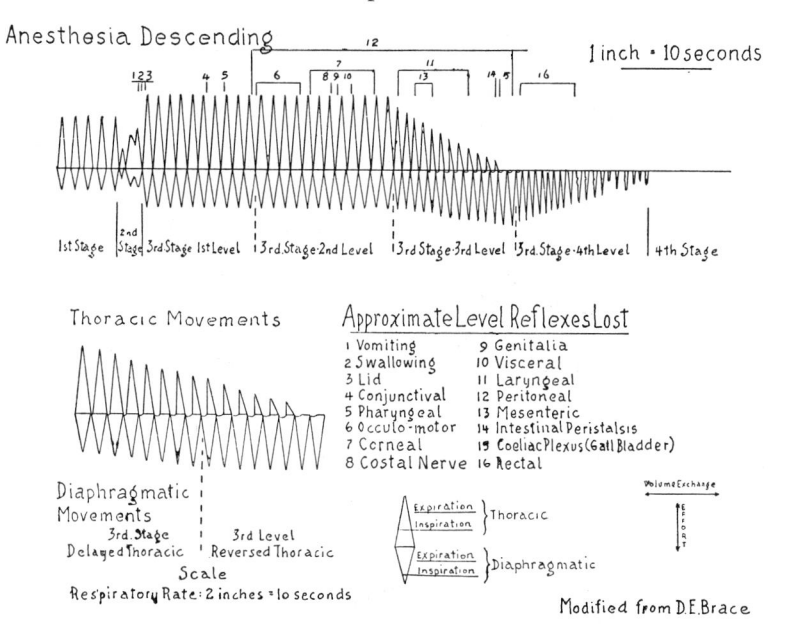

piration. The lower intercostal series is paralyzed first, followed by relaxation of the upper series.[17] Somewhat later no effort will be noted, and in the lower limits of this plane there may be actual caving in or retraction of the chest. Respiration in deep anesthesia can be described as gasping in type. All of these observations are related to the differential paralysis of the various muscle groups.[21]

Plane 4. In this level of anesthesia, the diaphragmatic component of respiration is gradually depressed. The sternocostal portion is paralyzed first, followed by the crural portion.[21] Toward the lower limits there is an irregularity in the diaphragmatic respiration, and finally complete cessation. The cessation of the diaphragmatic portion of respiration denotes the beginning of the fourth stage of anesthesia, or the stage of respiratory arrest.

RESPIRATORY PATTERNS. Generally two patterns of a normal respiratory cycle may be distinguished, depending upon anesthetic agents used. The variations are not too distinct in the first plane of anesthesia but are more evident in the second plane.

Apneustic Pattern.[22] With diethyl ether and vinethene there is a shift of the respiratory pattern to the inspiratory side. Inspiration tends to be sharp, strong, and brief in duration, and there is an *end-inspiratory pause.* This is similar to the pattern of respiration found after vagotomy in the unanesthetized animal and more dramatically when this is accompanied by low-pontile transection. Such conditions remove most inhibitory effects on the respiratory center with the production of "respiratory cramp."[23]

During ether anesthesia, all respiratory vagal effects are apparently removed or overcome (Fig. 14–2). Neither cutting the vagi nor stimulating the vagi by tilting the head up 30 degrees produces any respiratory effects.[17] As far as the vagal system is concerned, ether anesthesia may be considered as causing a functional central vagotomy.

Expiratory Pattern. An expiratory pattern of respiration indicative of enhanced vagal activity may be seen with thiopental anesthesia. Other agents that shift the level of respiratory action to the expiratory side include morphine, tribromoethanol and halothane (Avertin) and cyclopropane. These drugs potentiate the vagal expiratory drive,[24] and during their administration an expiratory or vagal apnea is readily produced. Thus, in various experiments conducted by Gordh,[12] tilting the head of an animal or human up to 30 degrees produces prolonged expiration or apnea in the expiratory position (Fig. 14–3). The same result occurs if the vagus is stimulated with a single shock of mild intensity. However, these responses are prevented when bilateral vagotomy is performed. It is of note that the respiratory pattern is similar to that seen in brain stem section when the pontile center's influence on the medullary center is removed, thereby leaving the vagal influence dominant. Thus, further evidence is available to indicate that at least thiopental causes a functional decerebration.

TRACHEAL TUG.[25] A sharp downward movement of the trachea may be seen on inspiration during anesthesia. This is an exaggeration of the normal downward movement seen on inspiration in the unanesthetized subject. It is pronounced with deep anesthesia—stage III planes 3 or 4. It is also seen in

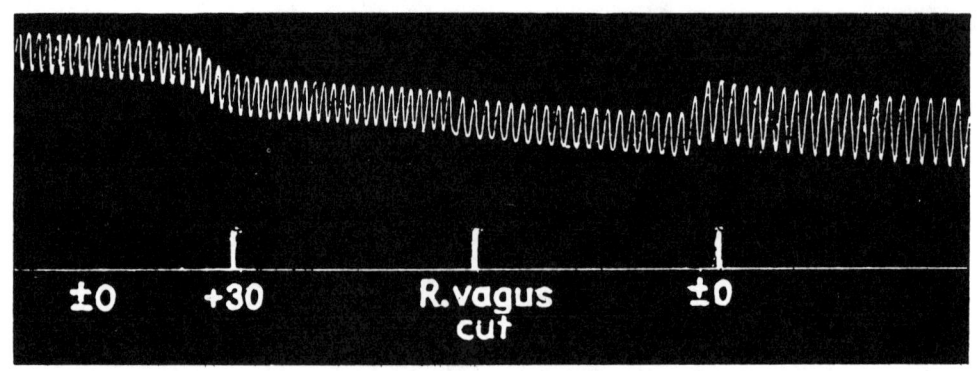

FIG. 14–2. Vagotomy during deep ether anesthesia. Demonstrates that vagus exerts little of its inhibitory influence on respiration with this agent and that a functional vagotomy is probably produced. Actually there is a shift to the inspiratory side. From Gordh, T.: Postural circulatory and respiratory changes during ether and intravenous anesthesia. Acta Chir. Scand., *92*(Suppl):102, 1945.

partially curarized subjects breathing spontaneously and in the presence of respiratory obstruction.

The mechanism is mechanical. Two muscular situations exist that can account for the phenomenon. One[26] explanation relates to the dual origin of the muscles of the diaphragm, namely the sternocostal fibers and the crural fibers. Because the sternocostals are paralyzed first, the crural component is allowed to exert a more direct force on the central tendon. There results a sharper contraction transmitted to the entire mediastinum pulling the lung root down.

A more valid explanation relates to the extrinsic muscles of the larynx.[1] These consist of the sternothyroid and sternohyoid muscles, which are depressors of larynx and are opposed by the mylohyoid, stylohyoid, styloglossus and posterior belly of digastric, which are elevators of the larynx. Ordinarily, the larynx is stabilized by these two sets and remains stationary. With increasing depth of anesthesia the elevator muscles are paralyzed first, leaving the depressors relatively active.

SIGH.[27] A sigh is a single deep inspiration seen in conscious subjects. It has been further defined as an inspiration that is *three times* the normal tidal volume. Its purpose appears to be that of expanding poorly aerated alveoli and to prevent segmental atelectasis.

Sighing is often associated with anesthetic agents that produce apneustic respiration, especially diethyl ether. It must be distinguished from gasping

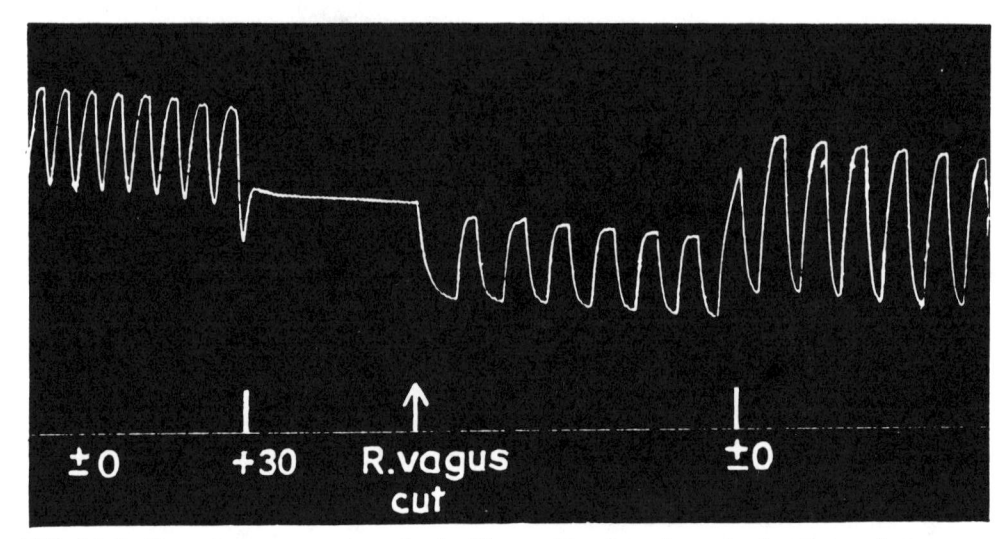

FIG. 14–3. Deep intravenous anesthesia. The application of vagal stimulus such as a 30-degree head-up posture produces apnea. Cutting the vagus at this time restores respiratory activity and removes the potentiated inhibitory influence of the vagus. From Gordh, T.: Postural circulatory and respiratory changes during ether and intravenous anesthesia. Acta Chir. Scand., *92*(Suppl.):102, 1945.

respiration or breath-holding. Although seen in the anesthetized subject it is greatly obtunded; it is also suppressed during physiologic sleep and by both sedative and narcotic drugs.

Of great importance in anesthesia is the fact that sighing is abolished during assisted and controlled respiration. Therefore, it is imperative during general anesthesia with respiratory control that artificial sighing be provided either mechanically (or manually) or pharmacologically.

Mechanical sighing is produced by occasional deep sustained positive pressure applications during anesthesia (single pressures of 40 cm of H_2O for 20 seconds or several applied pressures to provide volumes three times the maintenance tidal volume).[28] In addition, pharmacologic sighing may be produced by respirogenic drugs. This is especially applicable in the postoperative period by intermittent injections of a drug such as doxapram HCl (Dopram).[29]

MUSCULAR RELAXATION AND DEPTHS OF ANESTHESIA FOR VARIOUS TYPES OF SURGERY

The grading of anesthetic depth introduces the two major problems to be overcome if surgery is to proceed smoothly. These are (1) reflexes and (2) relaxation. Which reflexes must be obtunded and degrees of relaxation obtained depend on the type of surgery (Table 14–1). If good working conditions are to be provided, the recognition of anesthesia depth is required of the anesthetist. Working conditions are provided best by anticipating surgical needs and obtaining adequate anesthesia before it is required. The problem of reflexes will be dealt with separately, but a brief note will be made here concerning relaxation.[26]

Furnishing good muscular relaxation requires an understanding of simple muscle physiology. Living muscle is in a state of semicontraction. This is called muscle tone and is dependent first on intrinsic irritability and contractility and second on nervous impulses arising from higher neurologic centers and modifying the intrinsic contracted state of the muscle.

Intrinsic irritability refers to the property of living tissue to respond to a directly applied stimulus, and in the case of muscle the response is one of shortening or contraction. This property is possessed by living muscle independent of any neurologic connection.

The modifying impulses from higher centers arrive at a muscle through the motor neuron after being coordinated in the cell body of these neurons which are situated in the anterior horns of the spinal cord. This motor neuron actually possesses a great deal of independence. As the efferent path of the simple spinal reflex arc, it furnishes basic tone to a muscle. The afferent path carries proprioceptive impulses arising in the muscle itself as a result of stretching; the interplay between muscle stretching and muscle contraction carried over the single afferent and efferent path is called the myotatic reflex.

The basic myotatic reflex is also modified by stimulating and suppressing impulses from higher centers, which are both pyramidal and extrapyramidal. Such impulses impinge upon the cell body of the spinal motor neuron and are coordinated into a final integrated impulse. These impulses are thus both facilitatory and inhibitory. Sherrington[30] termed the motor neuron carrying an integrated impulse to an effector organ the *final common pathway* (Fig. 14–4). Among the centers originating impulses which impinge upon the anterior horn cells, several are well defined:[26]

CORTEX. Impulses originating here pass in the corticospinal or pyramidal tracts to the motor cells for voluntary control of muscle activity. Removal of the motor area or area four of the cortex or cutting the pyramidal tracts results in flaccidity.

Decortication, leaving the optic thalami intact (ie, producing the thalamic animal) results in little departure from normal muscle tone. However, subcortical centers (diencephalic or hypothalamic) are released from certain central inhibitory influences, and manifestations of sympathetic overactivity appear. There is also a slight increase in extensor tone.

TECTAL NUCLEI. Retinal impulses are correlated by cell groups in the superior colliculi with body movements. This results in visuospinal reflexes carried by fibers of the tectospinal tract to anterior horn cells.

TABLE 14–2. ANESTHETIC DEPTH (MAINTENANCE) REQUIRED FOR REPRESENTATIVE OPERATIONS

Lower part of plane 1
  Most operations on integumental structures
  Extrapleural thoracic surgery
  Most surgery about the head and neck, including thyroidectomy and tonsillectomy
  Herniorrhaphy
  Amputation, fracture, and tendon repairs
  Caesarean section and most obstetric surgery
  Intracranial neurosurgery
Upper plane 2
  Perineal operations, including most rectal and genital surgery
  Laryngeal surgery
Lower plane 2
  Intrauterine operation
  Most abdominal procedures may be carried in this plane
  Intrapleural thoracic surgery
Plane 3
  Introduction of endotracheal tube
  Gastric operations
  Other intraabdominal procedures in which reflexes are too active to be performed in lower plane 2, such as splenectomy and ventral hernia repair
  Versions

380 *General Anesthesia*

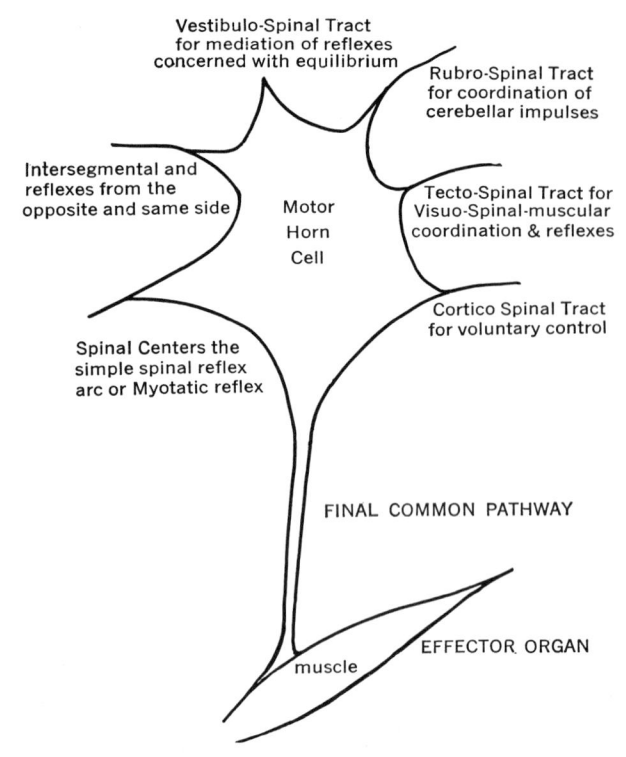

FIG. 14–4. The final common pathway. The effector side of the reflex arc concerned with muscle action and hence surgical relaxation.

RED NUCLEUS. This nucleus lies in the tegmentum of the midbrain beneath the thalamus. It functions to maintain tone or postural background, against which voluntary movements are executed. Phylogenetically, this nucleus conditions muscle behavior and coordinates involuntary influences from the cerebellum and striate body. The outflowing fiber tract forms part of the extrapyramidal system and is called the rubrospinal tract. The so-called reticulospinal tracts arising in scattered cells of the reticular formation of the midbrain also transmit impulses arising in the cerebellum and striate bodies for regulating postural tone.

VESTIBULAR NUCLEUS. Equilibrium impulses from labyrinthine and cerebellar areas are mediated by this nucleus and transmitted through the vestibulospinal tracts to motor neurons for reflex controls of muscles. When the brain stem is transected between the anterior colliculus and the vestibular nucleus, extensor muscle spasm results, which is called decerebrate rigidity. It is due to the uninhibited action of the vestibular nucleus—it represents a release of lower centers from the suppressive influence of the extrapyramidal cortical (strip region and area 6) projection system (corticopontocerebellar, corticostriatonigral, and corticothalamic projections). Decerebrate rigidity is abolished on destruction of vestibular nuclei.

INTERSEGMENTAL NEURONS. These neurons channel reflexes from the opposite and same side of a body segment as well as from higher and lower spinal segments into the anterior horn cells. Mediation of these impulses is through the spinospinal tracts. This results in intersegmental correlation.

SPINAL CENTER. This is simply the cell bodies of the motor neurons. When combined with a single afferent proprioceptive path the myotatic reflex arc is formed.

DISCUSSION. These centrally originated impulses all mediate influences that can modify tone and hence must be blocked to obtain relaxation. This block can be accomplished by regional anesthetization of the peripheral nerve to eliminate all the reflexes from the anterior horn cells; or the block may be accomplished by general anesthesia which obtunds the central origins of the impulses. Curare as an adjunct to anesthesia achieves its relaxing effect by blocking the impulses of the final common pathway at the myoneural junction. However, neither regional anesthesia nor general anesthesia with or without curare will interfere with intrinsic irritability, and a muscle can be made to contract by direct stimulation. Such a stimulation is frequently seen during surgery when strong retraction stretches a muscle excessively and suddenly.[31–34]

THE GAMMA SYSTEM. The classic innervation of voluntary muscle consists of large motor nerve fibers, cholinergic in action, known as the alpha fiber system. The diaphragm, for example, is richly supplied by alpha motoneurons, which show phasic activity. In addition, it has been recognized that in the ventral roots there are small nerve fibers known as the gamma fibers, which innervate the contractile substance of the muscle spindles (Fig. 14–5). This system provides tonic postural activity. For example, the muscles of locomotion have a rich gamma and fusiomotor system. The intercostal and respiratory muscles have a rich gamma system, which modulates the phasic muscle activity.

The role of these fibers has been studied and may be described briefly. First, the synapse between the small motor fibers and the spindle contractile substance is cholinergic in nature. Parasympathetic substances such as acetylcholine or succinylcholine excite the endings, while *d*-tubocurarine reduce activity. Secondly, an impulse over the gamma fibers causes contraction of the spindle and thereby stimulates the spindle afferent fiber. Activation of these afferents then increases the discharge over the primary motor nerve fiber. Thus, the ordinary stretch reflex is modulated by the magnitude of incoming afferent impulses from muscle spindles.

Muscular movement may be initiated or augmented in two ways: (1) There may be a direct discharge down the large motor nerves to elicit muscle contraction of varying grade, depending on the dis-

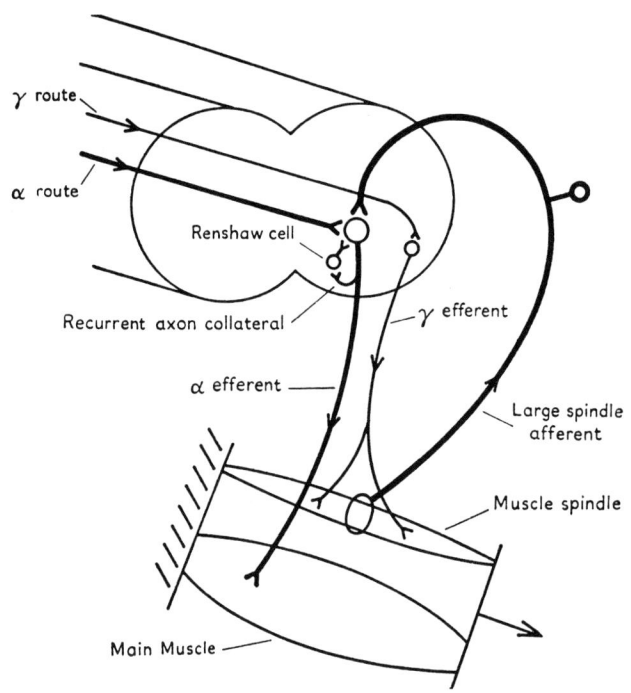

FIG. 14-5. The stretch reflex and related mechanisms. The muscle spindle lies parallel with the main muscle and its fast-conducting afferent is in synaptic connection with the large α motor neuron supplying the main muscle fibers. A slow-conducting γ synaptic efferent (*thin line*) supplies the contractile poles of the spindle and thus can alter the bias on the spindle sensory ending. The muscle can be made to contract, either by impulses from higher centers exciting the α motor neuron direct (the α route) or by impulses in the γ efferents (the γ route), which activate the muscle indirectly through the stretch-reflex arc (the "follow-up" servo). A subsidiary feedback loop through the recurrent axon collateral and an inhibitory Renshaw interneurone may be concerned in stabilizing the response of the α motor neuron to its excitatory input. From Hammond, P.H., Merton, P.A., and Sutton, G.G.: Nervous gradation of muscular contraction. Br. Med. Bull., *12*:214, 1956.

charge; and (2) muscular activity may be initiated by small motor nerve fibers which cause a change in the length of the spindle. The general muscle bed will then change its length to match that of the spindle. The latter offers a finer gradation in muscle contraction.[32]

THE "H" REFLEX.[35] In studies of muscle activity as related to mixed nerve stimulation, the initial response is the action potential, designated as the *M response*, resulting form the impulse traveling orthodromically. This is followed by a second action potential, resulting from the same stimulus, which produces an impulse that travels by sensory paths centrally and then is relayed from the spinal cord back to the muscle. This is called the "H" response.

The H-reflex was first described by Hoffman in 1918 and is analagous to the monosynaptic muscle stretch reflex.[36] The afferent impulses arise from stimuli originating in the muscle spindles; they pass centrally to the dorsal roots and then reach the anterior horn nuclei. These cells are activated, and the efferent path is over the motoneuron. The testing of this reflex is considered to assess motoneuronal function, as well as the integrity of the afferent arc.

BALANCED ANESTHESIA

HISTORY.[37] When the first anesthetic agent was administered that embodied a rudimentary concept of what is now termed '*balanced anesthesia*' is difficult to identify. The use of morphine prior to ether and chloroform anesthesia in 1850 represented premedication, but the morphine contributed to the anesthetic process and may be considered a combination of anesthetic drugs. In 1858, Benjamin Bell of Edinburgh showed that belladonna drugs antagonized morphine effects and contributed to the anesthesia.

The concept of using several agents each with a specific purpose was proposed and applied by Crile[38] between 1900 and 1911. His theory of "anoci-association" resulted from observations on patients exposed to nontoxic concentrations of general anesthesia. He noted that noxious auditory, visual, and olfactory impulses were obtunded but not the traumatic impulses arising from the surgical site. The latter, he observed, could be blocked by local anesthesia. Therefore, he recommended selecting and combining anesthetic agents in such a way that all noxious stimuli could be excluded from the brain, thereby attaining complete dissociation of these stimuli without cost to the patient in terms of deranged metabolism resulting from the use of very deep anesthesia produced by only one agent.

This theory of anoci-association was the immediate precursor of the term balanced anesthesia coined by Lundy[39] in 1926. It designates the use of a combination of anesthetic agents and methods so balanced that part of the burden of relief of pain is borne by preliminary medication, part by local anesthesia, and part by one or more general anesthetic agents. The method was believed to increase patient safety by minimizing immediate and remote untoward effects of any single agent.

Subsequently, the introduction of cyclopropane in 1930, thiopental (Pentothal)[39] in 1934, and curare as an adjunct to anesthesia by Griffith in 1942, as well as the development of neuroleptic techniques by Laborit in 1950 for protection against shock, led to the term *combined anesthesia*. According to Little,[40] this referred to the combination of hypnosis by thiopental analgesia by nitrous oxide, and relaxation by curare. For the sake of simplicity, this latter concept can be included in Lundy's version of balanced anesthesia.

DEFINITION. Balanced anesthesia is thus a coined term, a descriptive term, and may be defined as anesthesia produced by a combination of drugs and techniques, each with a primary purpose and specific effect but with overlapping secondary effects. The following is implied: Surgical anesthetic conditions are produced by several agents often administerd by different routes; the amount of any one agent used is diminished if the administrator does not need to rely for all effects on any one drug (deep levels of general anesthesia); the drugs may be detoxified and excreted in several different ways and thus not burden any one path. Thus, the components of general anesthesia as noted by Woodbridge[41] are each achieved by a specific drug and these drugs may interact and be interdependent in part: *Mental block* by sedatives, hypnotics, and small concentrations of anesthetic agents; *sensory block*, including pain relief, by large doses of sedatives, hypnotics, large doses of opiates and/or low concentrations of potent volatile inhalation anesthetics, or nitrous oxide analgesia; *relaxation* by peripheral relaxants and secondarily by the anesthetic agents; and *autonomic block* by some anesthetic and sympathetic blocking agents. An ideal agent would be one which achieves all these objectives but with limited toxicity. However, the state of balanced anesthesia achieved has no basis in fact, pharmacologically or biochemically. A state of physiologic balance is assumed.

The techniques of administration of widely accepted anesthetic agents in combination fall into four main categories:

1. General anesthesia administered by combinations of inhalation, parenteral, or rectal anesthesia
2. General anesthesia combined with regional anesthesia, including spinal anesthesia
3. General anesthesia combined with relaxants
4. General anesthesia combined with neurolepsis[42] and relaxants

APPLICATION OF WOODBRIDGE COMPONENTS. Pertinent to balanced anesthesia and the recognition of the depth of anesthesia is the application of the Woodbridge components.[41] It is evident from prior discussions that all of these components can be successfully and safely blocked by single potent inhalation volatile and gaseous anesthetic agents. In balanced anesthesia techniques, it is relatively easy to provide unconsciousness, analgesia, and skeletal muscle relaxation by using several pharmacologic agents.

However, block of the autonomic nervous system is essential to provide a stress-strain free state for surgery and, in lieu of high doses of opiates, usually requires sympathetic blocking agents (alpha and beta). Eidence of sympathetic stimulation should be sought, and then the system should be obtunded. Observation of skeletal muscle movement can indicate light depths of anesthesia, because pain will evoke a somatosensory or viscerosensory voluntary motor response. This is not possible in the unconscious paralyzed patient. Block of the autonomic nervous system is essential to provide a stress-strain free state for surgery. Evidence of an active sympathetic system and, consequently, light anesthesia is collected by the observation of cardiovascular changes. In light stage III or stage II anesthesia, blood pressure elevations and tachycardia or bradycardia (intense noxious stimulation) may be observed. Catecholamines are elevated and can be measured, but at present this is not a practical, immediate monitoring technique.

MONITORING OF RELAXATION (LEC). One monitoring technique proposed to assess the adequacy of a state of autonomic nervous system blockade is the measurement of lower esophageal contractility (LEC) (see Chapter 13). The muscles of the lower half of the esophagus are nonstriated and not affected by skeletal muscle relaxants. Esophageal activity can be described as being of two types: primary peristaltic and secondary nonpropulsive. The rate of spontaneous LEC and the magnitude of LEC, especially provoked secondary peristalsis, can be measured.[4] The measurement of LEC is simple. A probe is used simultaneously with an esophageal stethoscope, and changes in lower esophageal tone and movement are observed. Initially, the probe is used to measure changes in contractility as well as in over-all peristaltic movement. Deepening anesthesia will result in a progressive suppression of LEC. It should be emphasized that the smooth muscles of the lower esophagus will remain active despite skeletal muscle paralysis. Drugs or conditions that increase the activity of the sympathetic nervous system will enhance LEC. On the other hand, ganglionic blocking drugs and large doses of anticholinergics can reduce the activity. Smooth muscle relaxants, such as nitroprusside, are capable of paralyzing the lower esophageal muscles.

This probe technique of the lower esophageal tone and contractility offers some objective guide to the depth of anesthesia depending on the anesthetic agent. Thus, it has been found significant during halothane anesthesia but not during nitrous oxide alfentanil anesthesia.[43] It has not been found to be predictable of depth during isoflurane anesthesia.

COMBINATIONS OF ANESTHETIC TECHNIQUES AND AGENTS

INTRAVENOUS–INHALATION. Combining inhalation, parenteral, and rectal anesthesia to provide balanced anesthesia, Barton[47] found that when a 50–50 mixture of nitrous oxide–oxygen was administered with thiopental, the amount of thiopental required to maintain a given plane of anesthesia was only one fourth that previously necessary when thiopental was used alone or with oxygen. This observation stressed the importance of adding oxygen or nitrous oxide-oxygen to thiopental anesthesia in order to maintain blood arterial oxygen values, especially in the poorer risk patients.

Paulson[48] noted that the disadvantages of thiopental could be obviated or minimized by the use of small amounts of ether as a supplement, finding that the total dose of thiopental was thus markedly reduced. Laryngeal spasm was not encountered during several hundred anesthetic administrations with this technique. Endotracheal intubation could be accomplished more easily and safely. Studies of respiratory minute volume revealed greater minute volume while the patient was under anesthesia with thiopental and ether than before anesthesia when the patient was conscious and had not received any medication. Most patients awoke or reacted at the time they left the operating room with no postanesthetic depression, and nausea and vomiting was minimal.

Faulconer[49] found that a lower concentration of ether was required to produce each of the electroencephalographic levels studied when nitrous oxide was present in the arterial blood in excess of 10 mg/100 mL than when no nitrous oxide was present. This difference was shown to be statistically significant to a high degree for the observations made during the electroencephalographic levels 4 and 5, corresponding to moderate an deep surgical anesthesia.

OPIATE–BARBITURATE–GAS COMBINATION.[50] Regarding the use of opiates in combination with thiopental and nitrous oxide–oxygen, Widdowson[51] found that the average recovery time following repeated doses of morphine and thiopental (107 minutes) was longer than after repeated doses of meperidine (43.5 minutes) when meperidine was used as a supplement to anesthesia induced with thiopental, nitrous oxide–oxygen. They concluded that meperidine has a transient effect while the barbiturates have a cumulative effect, contributing to postoperative depression.

Hamilton,[52] commenting on the need to reinforce the potency of the analgesic property of nitrous oxide without having to resort to undue depression of vital functions as a result of excessive doses of thiopental alone, suggested supplementation of these agents with opiates, observing that the respiratory depression associated with opiates can be successfully antagonized by levallorphan or n-allylnormorphine.

The work by Eger[52a] on *minimum anesthetic concentrations* (MAC) of various agents has shown that an opiate reduces the amount of anesthetic agent necessary to produce a given state of anesthesia.[53,54]

Antagonist Addition. Ausherman,[55] by using n-allylnormorphine to antagonize the respiratory depression of meperidine administered by continuous drip technique prior to administration of thiopental and nitrous oxide–oxygen, were able to obtain satisfactory anesthesia with 48% less thiopental than was required in a control group anesthetized with thiopental and nitrous oxide–oxygen but without meperidine. In this study, meperidine was found to have a short duration of effect when administered by the continuous drip technique; the only evidence of allergic phenomena was the appearance of urticarial wheals and redness along the course of the vein through which meperidine was flowing. It is possible but not substantiated that with the judicious use of the opiate antagonists one might achieve maximal analgesia with minimal respiratory depression.

In 1949, Marsh[58] reported on the use of rectal thiopental as a basal hypnotic in pediatric surgery. Rectal thiopental for children as a preoperative hypnotic in all types of surgery was found to lessen apprehension, to permit smoother administration of anesthetic agents, and to diminish the amount of primary anesthesia required. Local anesthesia, combined with this sequence, proved satisfactory in children who have recently eaten and are admitted for minor procedures.

LARGE-DOSE INTRAVENOUS OPIATE TECHNIQUES.[56] Morphine or fentanyl have been administered intravenously in 5 to 10 times the usual amount to provide the analgesic component of general balanced anesthesia. Doses of morphine of 1 to 3 mg/kg of body weight[56] or fentanyl (and its analogues) in doses of 10 to 100 μg/kg have been recommended.[57] It is noted that fentanyl and its analogues are structurally related to meperidine. These techniques are discussed in the chapter on Intravenous Narcotic Techniques.

COMBINATION OF GENERAL AND REGIONAL ANESTHESIA. Wiggin[59] made the following claims regarding balanced spinal anesthesia before the days of curare:

1. The patient is more completely under the control of the anesthetist.
2. The psychic factors of apprehension, restlessness, and undue stimulation are completely allayed.
3. Respirations can be controlled by the administration of oxygen.
4. Blood pressure and pulse remain more stable than they do with any other method of anesthesia.
5. Complete relaxation can be obtained without the administration of large doses of spinal anesthetic agents.

Cognizant of these observations and realizing the shortcomings of spinal anesthesia, Lorhan[60] advocated combining spinal anesthesia with inhalation anesthesia, cyclopropane being the unanimous choice because it was a potent agent permitting easy induction, and could be used with a high concentration of oxygen.

Keyes[61] was the first to use intravenous anesthesia in conjunction with spinal anesthesia by using hexobarbital or thiopental in 50 patients for the following purposes:

1. To quiet the apprehensive patient for spinal induction and during the operation
2. To supplement the inadequate spinal
3. To prolong anesthesia

Grady[62] used a balanced anesthetic technique consisting of spinal anesthesia, intravenous thiopental, and an inhalation agent. Nitrous oxide–oxygen was the most frequent agent used, while cyclopropane was used chiefly to prevent hiccough, coughing, or laryngospasm produced by thiopental; ether was used in few cases wherein the surgical procedure outlasted the spinal anesthesia. Pentobarbital (Nembutal) and secobarbital (Seconal) were used intravenously as supplementary agents primarily in hysterectomies and appendectomies but were not advised for long upper abdominal operations because they produce excessive postoperative depression.

Herbert[63] advocated a combination of agents and techniques to provide anesthesia for thoracoplasty. After adequate premedication, paravertebral block of the appropriate spinal nerves is performed followed by intravenous thiopental and nitrous oxide–oxygen. Such a balanced anesthesia provides a safe and satisfactory method of anesthesia to meet the special requirements of poor risk patients undergoing thoracoplasty. It is nonexplosive and suitable for use of electrocautery. Concurrent use of paravertebral nerve block with general anesthesia has the advantage of abolishing undesirable respiratory reflexes and reducing the dose of thiopental required. The incidence of postanesthetic complications appears to be no greater with this type than with other agents and methods.

The use of fractional segmental spinal anesthesia supplemented by intravenous and inhalation agents advocated by Brown[64] represents another method of providing good surgical operating conditions with minimal deleterious physiologic effects in the poor risk surgical patient. Johnson[65] recommended the establishment of a continuous spinal system, beginning the operation under local infiltration anesthesia and subsequently injecting intrathecal procaine in small divided doses when relaxation is required.

COMBINATION OF GENERAL AGENTS AND RELAXANTS. The third major classification of the techniques of balanced anesthesia consists of the use of general anesthesia in combination with muscle relaxants. The advantages of obtaining muscular relaxation by means of peripherally acting drugs rather than by the effects of profound central narcosis are obvious. The muscle relaxants have been successfully employed in reducing the amount of an inhalation agent required for a given procedure.

Morris[66] found a combination of nitrous oxide, curare, and edrophonium (Tensilon) to be satisfactory and useful in the management of poor risk patients, craniotomies, thoracotomies, and cesarean sections. They observed that Tensilon usually reduces the effects of curare but does not terminate them. They also observed that the increased respiratory exchange observed after the administration of Tensilon is frequently followed within 5 to 10 minutes by a return to a state of partial curarization that was not so severe as had been present before the injection of Tensilon.

Espinosa[67] reported on the use of succinylcholine in combination with analgesic drugs and general inhalation anesthesia. It was found that when critical dose of 50 µg/kg/min of succinylcholine is exceeded, profound respiratory depression results.

MISCELLANEOUS COMBINATIONS. The use of neurolept analgesic agents and general anesthesia is considered elsewhere. Reference is made to hypothermia, the antihistaminic drugs, and the so-called steroid anesthetic agents.

REFERENCES

1. Campbell, E.J.M.: The Respiratory Muscles and the Mechanics of Breathing. Chicago, Year Book Publishers, Inc., 1958.
2. Tusiewicz, K., Bryan, A.C., Froese, A.B.: Contributions of changing ribcage-diaphragm interactions to the ventilatory depression of halothane anesthesia. Anesthesiology 47:327, 1977.
3. Koepke, G.H., Smith, E.M., Murphy, A.J., et al.: Sequence of action of diaphragm and intercostal muscles during respiration. Part I. Arch. Phys. Med., 39:426, 1958.
4. Murphy, A.J., Koepke, G.H., Smith, E.M., et al.: Sequence of action of diaphragm and intercostal muscles during respiration. II. Expiration. Arch. Phys. Med., 40:337, 1959.
5. Campbell, E.J.M.: An electromyographic examination of the role of the intercostal muscles in breathing in man. J. Physiol. (Lond.), 129:12, 1955.
6. Campbell, E.J.M., Green, J.H.: The behavior of the abdominal muscles and the intraabdominal pressure during quiet breathing and increased pulmonary ventilation. A study in man. J. Physiol. (Lond.), 127:423, 1955.
7. Petit, J.M., Milic-Emili, G., Delhez, L.: Role of the diaphragm in breathing in coscious normal man: An electromyographic study. J. Appl. Physiol. 15:1101, 1960.
8a. Coryllos, P.N.: Action of the diaphragm in cough. Experimental and clinical study on the human. Am. J. Med. Sci., 194:523, 1937.
8b. Huizunga, E.: The tussic squeeze and bechic blast. Ann. Oto. Rhino. Laryngol., 76:923, 1967.
9. Bigland, B., Lippold, D.O.: Motor unit activity in the voluntary contraction of human muscle. J. Physiol. (Lond.), 125:322, 1954.
10. Lieberman, D.A., Falkner, J.A., Craig, A.B. Jr., et al.: Performance of histochemical composition of guinea pig and human diaphragm. J. Appl. Physiol., 34:233, 1973.

11. Roussos, C., and Macklin, P.T.: Diaphragmatic fatigue in man. J. Appl. Physiol., 43:189, 1977.
12. Gordh, T.: Postural circulatory and respiratory changes during ether and intravenous anesthesia. Acta. Chirurgica. Scand., 92(Suppl):102, 1945.
13a. Nunn, J.F.: Effects of anaesthesia on respiration. Br. J. Anaesth., 65:54–62, 1990.
13b. Hedenstierna, G., et al.: Functional residual capacity thoracoabdominal dimensions and central blood volume during general anesthesia with muscle paralysis. Anesthesiology, 62:247, 1985.
14. Snow, J.: On Chloroform and Other Anaesthetics. London, John Churchill, 1857.
15. Guedel, A.E.: Inhalation Anesthesia, 2nd ed. New York, Macmillan, 1951.
16. Miller, A.H.: Ascending respiratory paralysis under general anesthesia. J.A.M.A., 84:201, 1925.
17. Miller, A.H.: The role of diaphragmatic breathing in anesthesia and a pneumographic method of recording. Anesth. Analg., 17:38, 1939.
18a. Munson, E.S., Larson, C.P., Jr., Babad, A.A., et al.: The effect of halothane, fluroxene and cyclopropane on ventilation: A comparative study in man. Anesthesiology, 27:716, 1966.
18b. Rehder, K., Mallow, J.E., Fibuch, E.E., et al.: Effects of isoflurane anesthesia and muscle paralysis on respiratory mechanics in normal man. Anesthesiology, 41:477, 1974.
19. Nishino, T., Shirahata, M., Yonezawa, T., et al.: Comparison of changes in the hypoglossal and the phrenic nerve activity in response to increasing depth of anesthesia in cats. Anesthesiology, 60:19, 1984.
20. Behrakis, P.K., Higgs, B.D., Baydur, A., et al.: Active inspiratory impedance in halothane-anesthetized humans. J. Appl. Physiol., 54:1477, 1983.
21. Westbrook, P.R., Stubbs, S.E., Sessler, A.D., et al.: Effect of anesthesia and muscle paralysis on respiratory mechanics in man. J. Appl. Physiol., 34:81, 1973.
22. Stella, G.: On the mechanism of production and physiologic significance of "apneusis." J. Physiol. (Lond.), 93:10, 1938.
23. Comroe, J.: Physiology of Respiration. Chicago, Year Book Publishers, 1970.
24. Gesell, R.: Respiration and its adjustments. Am. Rev. Physiol., 1:185, 1939.
25. Hunan, J.V.: Chin retraction: A new sign of anaesthesia. Br. J. Anaesth., 15:66, 1938.
26. Harris, T.A.B.: The Mode of Action of Anesthetics. Baltimore, Williams & Wilkins, 1951.
27. Bendixen, H.H., Smith, G.M., Mead, J.: Pattern of ventilation in young adults. J. Appl. Physiol., 19:195, 1964.
28. Shapiro, B.: Clinical Application of Respiratory Care. Chicago, Year Book Publishers, Inc., 1975.
29. Winnie, A.P., Collins, V.J.: The doxapran test: A new technique for differential diagnosis of apnea. Anesthesiology, 26:27, 1965.
30. Sherrington, C.: The Integrative Action of the Nervous System. New Haven, Yale University Press, 1947.
31. Smith, C.M.: Neuromuscular pharmacology: Drugs and muscle spindles. Ann. Rev. Pharm., 3:223, 1963.
32. Hammond, P.H., Merton, P.A., Sutton, G.G.: Nervous gradation of muscular contraction. Br. Med. Bull., 12:214, 1956.
33. Hutter, O.F.: Effect of choline on neuromuscular transmission in the cat. J. Physiol., 117:241, 1952.
34. Paton, W.D.M.: Possible causes of apnea. Anaesthesia, 13:253, 1958.
35. Mayer, R.F., Mawdsley, C.: Studies in man and cat on the significance of the H wave. J. Neurol. Neurosurg. Psychiat., 28:201, 1965.
36. Grossi, P., and Arner, S.: Effect of epidural morphine on the Hoffman-Reflex in man. Acta. Anaesth. Scand., 28:152, 1984.
37. Keyes, T.E.: The History of Surgical Anesthesia. New York, Schuman's, 1945.
38. Crile, G.W., and Lower, W.E.: Surgical Shock and the Shockless Operation Through Anoci-Association. Philadelphia, W.B. Saunders Co., 1921.
39. Lundy, J.S.: Clinical Anesthesia. Philadelphia, W.B. Saunders Co., 1942.
40. Little, D.M., Jr., Stephen, C.R.: Modern balanced anesthesia: A concept. Anesthesiology, 15:246, 1954.
41. Woodbridge, P.: Changing concepts concerning depth of anesthesia. Anesthesiology, 18:536, 1957.
42. DeCastro, J., and Mundeleer, P.: Die neuroleptanalgesie. Auswahl der praeparate, bedeutung der analgesie und de neurolepsia. Anaesthetist, 11:10, 962.
43. Evans, J.M., Davies, W.L., Wise, C.C.: Lower esophageal contractility. A new monitor of anaesthesia. Lancet 1:1151, 1984.
44. Sessler, D.I., Olofsson, C.I., Chow, F.: Lower esophageal contractility predicts movement during skin incision in patients anesthetized with halothane but not with nitrous oxide and alfentanil. Anesthesiology, 70:42, 1989.
45. Erickson, P., Foss, J., Kuni, D.R.: A controlled trial of efficacy of lower esophageal contractility as a measure of depth of anesthesia (abstract). Anesthesiology, 67:A672, 1987.
46. Sebel, P.S., Heneghan, C.P., Ingram, D.A.: Evoked responses—a neurophysiological indicator of the depth of anesthesia? Br. J. Anaesth., 57:841, 1985.
47. Barton, G.D., Wicks, W.R., Livingston, H.M.: The effect of pentothal alone and in combination with oxygen on arterial blood gases. Anesthesiology, 7:505, 1946.
48. Paulson, J.A.: Thiopental sodium and ether anesthesia. J.A.M.A., 150:983, 1952.
49. Faulconer, A., Jr.: Correlation of concentrations of ether in arterial blood with electroencephalographic patterns occurring during ether-oxygen and during nitrous oxide-oxygen and ether anesthesia of human surgical patients. Anesthesiology, 13:361, 1952.
50. Corssen, G., Reves, J.G., Stanley, T.H.: Intravenous Anesthesia and Analgesia. Philadelphia, Lea & Febiger, 1988.
51. Widdowson, H.R., Aquino, T.D., Virtue, R.W.: Recovery time following demerol or pentothal supplementation of nitrous oxide anesthesia. Anesthesiology, 16:747, 1955.
52. Hamilton, W.K., and Cullen, S.C.: Supplementation of nitrous oxide anesthesia with opiates and a new opiate antagonist. Anesthesiology, 16:22, 1955.
52a. Quasha, A.L., Eger, E.I. II and Tinker, J.H.: Determination and applications of MAC. Anesthesiology 53:315, 1980.
53. Hoffman, J.C., and DiFazio, C.A.: The anesthesia sparing effect of pentazocine, meperidine, and morphine. Arch. Int. Pharmacodyn. Ther., 186:261, 1970.
54. Quasha, A.L.: Why do we need to know the MAC of an anesthetic? ASA Refresher Course. Ed. S. Hershey, 9:131, 1981.
55. Ausherman, H.M., Nowill, N.C., Stephen, C.R.: Controlled analgesia with continuous drip meperidine. J.A.M.A., 160:175, 1956.
56. Lowenstein, E., et al.: Cardiovascular responses to large dose of intravenous morphine in man. N. Engl. J. Med., 281:1389, 1969.
57. Stanley, T.H., Webster, L.R.: Anesthetic requirements and cardiovascular effects of fentanyl-oxygen and fentanyl-diazepam-oxygen anesthesia in man. Anesth. Analg., 56:836, 1977.
58. Marsh, L.C., Fox, J.L., Burstein, C.L.: Preanesthetic hypno-

sis with rectal pentothal in children. Anesthesiology, *10:*401, 1949.
59. Wiggin, S.C.: Balanced spinal anesthesia. Anesth. Analg. (Curr. Res.), *18:*193, 1939.
60. Lorhan, P.H., Orr, T.G.: Combined spinal anesthesia and light inhalation cyclopropane anesthesia for abdominal surgical relaxation. Kansas Med. Soc. J., *41:*13, 1940.
61. Keyes, P.A.: Combined intravenous spinal anesthesia. Anesth. Analg. (Curr. Res.), *20:*24, 1941.
62. Grady, R.W., Stough, J.A., Robinson, E.B.: A survey of spinal anesthesia from 1949 through 1952. Anesthesiology, *15:*310, 1954.
63. Herbert, C.L.: Balanced anesthesia for thoracoplasty. Anesthesiology, *9:*537, 1948.
64. Brown, S.: Fractional segmental spinal anesthesia in poor risk surgical patients. Report of 600 cases. Anesthesiology, *13:*540, 1952.
65. Johnson, N.P., Livingstone, H.M.: Anesthesia for urgent intra-abdominal surgical procedures in patients with cardiovascular disease. Anesthesiology, *15:*150, 1954.
66. Morris, L.E., Schilling, E.A., Frederickson, E.L.: The use of tensilon with curare and nitrous oxide anesthesia. Anesthesiology, *14:*117, 1963.
67. Espinosa, A.M., Artusio, J.F.: The dose response relationship and duration of action of succinylcholine in anesthetized man. Anesthesiology, *15:*239, 1954.

15

INHALATION ANESTHESIA— BREATHING SYSTEMS

INTRODUCTION. The modern anesthesiologist is offered a choice of various anesthetic circuits. This chapter focuses on the functional characteristics of these circuits to help the clinician select the most suitable system for a given situation. The essential features common to all anesthetic circuits are (1) accurate delivery of anesthetic gases, (2) accurate delivery of desired FIO_2, (3) prevention of CO_2 accumulation in the circuit, and (4) low resistance and dead space in the apparatus, especially when it is used for infants and young children. Other desirable features in these circuits include (1) ease of scavenging, (2) humidification of gases, (3) simplicity in design, (4) light in weight, and (5) cost-effectiveness.

A major objective in the design of breathing systems is the removal of carbon dioxide and the prevention of its accumulation. This can be accomplished by (1) by chemical neutralization using absorbents for the carbon dioxide, and (2) by a circuit permitting large volume inflow of fresh gases to dilute and "wash out" the carbon dioxide from the circuit into the atmosphere (Table 15–1).

CLASSIFICATION OF SYSTEMS. Breathing circuits may be classified according to the technical method (chemical or physical) by which exhaled carbon dioxide is removed. Four methods of carbon dioxide removal are available:

1. Absorption of carbon dioxide using soda lime: Closed systems such as a closed circle system or to-and-fro system rely on this technique, because exhaled carbon dioxide is absorbed and all other expired gas is rebreathed while only those quantities of fresh oxygen and anesthetic agent that are needed to replace uptake, metabolic losses, and circuit leaks are added.
2. Addition of fresh gas to dilute carbon dioxide to insignificant levels: Because of the intermittent nature of carbon dioxide excretion (during exhalation only) and the continuous inflow of fresh gas, the choice of location of the inflow site, reservoir bag, and popoff valve and the choice of

This chapter has been written with the assistance of Theodore C. Smith of Loyola University School of Medicine, Maywood, IL.

TABLE 15–1. CLASSIFICATION OF ANESTHESIA CIRCUITS

CO_2 absorption circuits (circle and to-and-fro systems)
  Semiclosed (FGF greater than uptake; partial rebreathing)
  Closed   (FGF = uptake)
CO_2 washout circuits
  Open (no reservoir bag)
    Open mask (open drop)
    Insufflation
    T-piece
  Semiopen (with reservoir bag)
    Nonbreathing valve systems
    Mapelson A (Magill circuit)
    Mapelson D
    Rees and Bain circuits

inflow rate may all contribute to carbon dioxide removal. Semiclosed systems, such as a circle system in which flow is in excess of uptake, metabolic losses, and leaks use this method in part for carbon dioxide removal. When flow rates into a circle system approach 10 L/min, dilution alone is sufficient to remove carbon dioxide. At lesser flow rates, both absorption and dilution account for its removal.

3. Use of valves to exclude exhaled from inhaled gases: Nonrebreathing circuits and systems using nonrebreathing valves use this method of carbon dioxide removal.
4. Dilution of exhaled carbon dioxide in room air: Open systems, such as the open drop technique or a T-piece without a reservoir, in which the expired gases, including carbon dioxide, are exhausted to the room are examples of this form of carbon dioxide elimination. This method has similarities to method 2, and anesthetic systems such as a T-piece with a reservoir may rely on dilution of carbon dioxide by both fresh gas and room air for its removal.

Other methods for classifying anesthetic circuits exist. Moyers proposed classifying them according to whether a reservoir was used and whether rebreathing occurred.[1a] By his classification, an open system has no reservoir and no rebreathing; a semiopen system has a reservoir but no rebreathing; a semiclosed system has a reservoir and partial rebreathing; and a closed system has a reservoir and complete rebreathing.[1b] Others have proposed variations to this classification based on the use of carbon dioxide absorption and unidirectional valves. Because of the needless confusion that the traditional nomenclature of open, semiopen, semiclosed, and closed systems has caused, Hamilton[2] has recommended its abandonment in favor of a description of the design of the system (eg, circle filter system, coaxial circuit, T-tube, and so on) and flow rates being used. Anesthetists have tended to adopt this recommendation because of its simplicity and greater accuracy and utility in describing what system is being used and how. However, the traditional nomenclature provides a conceptual basis for the

TABLE 15–2. CHARACTERISTICS OF VARIOUS INHALATION SYSTEMS

System	Reservoir Bag	Rebreathing of Exhaled Gases	Chemical Absorption of Exhaled Carbon Dioxide	Access to Atmosphere Inspir.	Access to Atmosphere Expir.	Unidirectional Valves	FGI Rate[†]
Open							
Open drop (gravity)	No	No	No	Yes	Yes	None	Unknown
Insufflation	No	No	No	Yes	Yes	None	Unknown
Modified Ayre-T	No	No	No[†]	Yes	Yes	None	High ($2^{-3} \times$ RMV)
Semiopen-nonrebreathing							
Valvular	Yes	No*	No	No	Yes	Two in one housing	High
Leigh, Fink, Ruben, Stephen-Slater, or Frumin valve							
Semiclosed							
Mapelson class A, B, C, D	Yes	Partial*	No	No	Yes	One	Intermediate
Jackson-Rees	Yes	Partial*	No	No	Yes	One	Intermediate
Coaxial							
Bain	Yes	Partial*	No	No	Yes	One	Intermediate
Circle	Yes	Partial	Yes	No	Yes	Three	Moderate
Closed							
Circle	Yes	Yes	Yes	No	No	Three	Low
To-and-fro	Yes	Yes	Yes	No	No	None	Low

* No breathing of exhaled gases only when FGI is adequate.
† High = greater than 6 L/min; intermediate = 3 to 6 L/min; low = 0.3 to 0.5 L/min.
Modified from Collins, V. J.: Principles of Anesthesiology. Philadelphia, Lea & Febiger, 1977; Stoelting, R., and Miller, R.: Basics of Anesthesia. 1984; Aldrete, J.A.: Acta Anaesth. Belg. *34*:251, 1984.

multiplicity of systems and also provides a base for conveniently tabulating general and functional characteristics of different systems (Table 15–2). Because the removal of carbon dioxide from a breathing circuit is a key feature, one may further identify the method as either the result of chemical neutralization or physical washout (Table 15–1).

CIRCLE BREATHING SYSTEMS

COMPONENTS. The circle system of administering inhalation anesthetics was introduced into anesthesia practice in 1928 by Brian Sword in consultation with the physiologist Yandell Henderson of Yale.

The basic components of a circle breathing system are an inspiratory and expiratory limb (corrugated tubes, each with a unidirectional valve, a Y-shaped airway adapter, and a rebreathing bag or spirometer moving reciprocally with the patient's lungs (and thus known as a counterlung). The system may be divided into quadrants (Fig. 15–1). The patient and the counterlung separate the inspiratory and expiratory limbs of the system, while the valves separate the patient from the bag side of the system. The position of the valves within the limbs is not necessarily fixed. They may be anywhere between the patient and the bag with little practical difference in function. They are usually incorporated with the bag mount and canister for manufacturing ease and durability. Even if the valves are moved to other locations, it is convenient to think of four quadrants when analyzing circle systems.

To make the circle system functional, it is necessary to add three other components: a carbon dioxide absorber, a fresh gas inflow (FGI) site, and a valve for exhaust of excess gas. Each of the three may be placed in any of the four quadrants. In theory, there are many ways that these three components might be located in the circle, but only a few are encountered in practice because most are impractical. Different manufacturers use different arrangements, and some designs allow the user to change the configuration with resulting changes in function. Disposable circuits may also vary the arrangement of components. Finally, the optimal configurations for spontaneous and controlled respiration are different.[3]

PLACEMENT OF ADDITIONAL COMPONENTS. The carbon dioxide absorber may be placed in any of the four quadrants but is almost invariably placed in the inspiratory limb on the bag side (Fig. 15–2). Since gravity-sensitive valves need a firm mounting site for optimal function, the inspiratory valve is often mechanically attached to the absorber.

The inflow site for fresh gases may also be placed in any of the four quadrants,[3] but convenience dictates that it be as close as possible to the other components (ie, absorber, bag mount, and valves). There is nearly universal acceptance for its placement on the bag side of the inspiratory limb, functionally downstream from the absorber (quadrant A, Fig. 15–2). In this location, during inspiration, fresh gas provides most or all of the respired gas with high-flow techniques or enriches the oxygen and anesthetic-depleted expiratory gas with low-flow techniques. During exhalation, a mixture of fresh and exhaled gases fills the bag or exits through the popoff valve, with the composition of the vented gas depending somewhat on the site of the popoff valve. Furthermore, if the absorber housing has appreciable head space, as is common, this inflow site serves to store the continuously delivered fresh gas during exhalation and preferentially exhaust exhaled gas. Finally, with the inflow site on the bag side of the inspiratory limb, gas flows down the inspiratory

FIG. 15–1. The basic circle breathing system. Two corrugated breathing tubes connect the patient and the counterlung (a reservoir bag or spirometer). A one-way valve is located in the inspiratory limb and another in the expiratory limb. The circle system can thus be bisected twice, dividing it into four quadrants: A, B, and D. To make a practical circuit for anesthesia, three more essential components must be added: an inflow site, a popoff valve, and a carbon dioxide absorber (See Fig. 15–2).

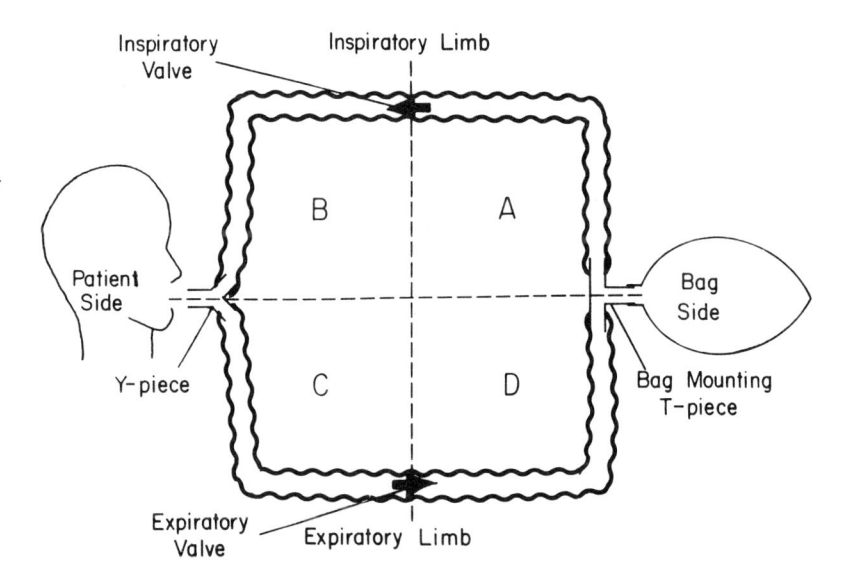

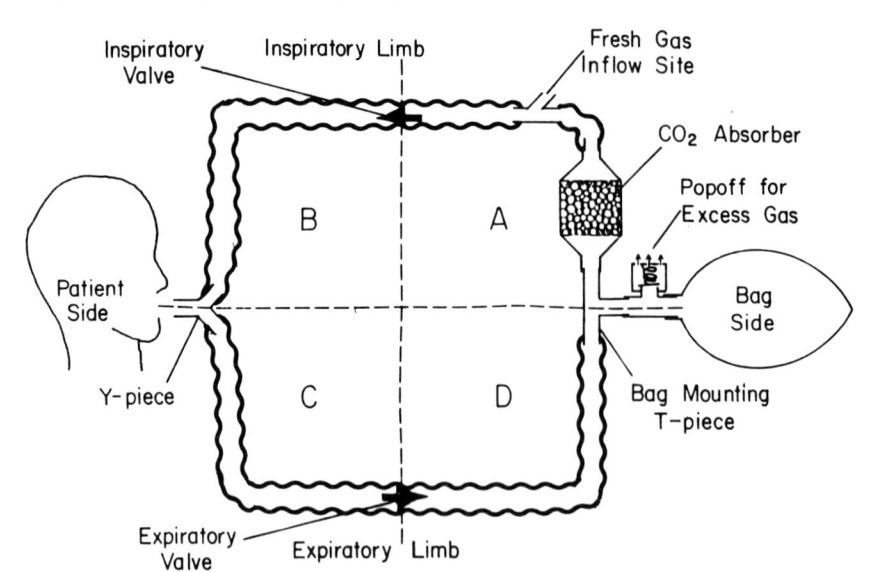

FIG. 15–2. Placement of the carbon dioxide absorber, fresh gas inflow, and popoff valve. The usual site for the absorber is in the inspiratory limb on the bag side, i.e., in quadrant A. The respiratory valves are usually mechanically attached to the canister but are shown here as they were in Fig. 15–1 for ease of functional analysis. FGI is usually on the bag side in the inspiratory limb (quadrant A), downstream from the soda lime absorber. The popoff valve is usually downstream from the expiratory valve near the bag. It is shown here in quadrant D but could be in A, before the soda lime absorber, or at the Y-piece between B and C.

limb only during inspiration, while during the remainder of the respiratory cycle it goes backwards toward the absorber, bag, and popoff valve. If the inflow site is located on the patient side of the inspiratory valve (quadrant B, Fig. 15–2), gas flows continuously around the circle throughout the respiratory cycle, making measurement of exhaled volumes with a spirometer located in the expiratory limb inaccurate unless total gas flow is shut off.[4]

The popoff valve may be placed anywhere in the circle, but some locations are more rational than others. Most locations in the inspiratory limb would tend to vent fresh anesthetic and carbon-dioxide-free gas, and this is clearly undesirable. It is usually found convenient to place the popoff valve between the expiratory valve and bag mount, or just opposite the bag mount, or just downstream from the bag but before the absorber (ie, in quadrants D or A but close to the bag mount). Incorporating the popoff valve into a one-piece, absorber-bag mount-expiratory valve-popoff-valve assembly gives convenience and durability.

There is at least theoretical value to locating the popoff valve on the patient side at the Y-piece or next to it (quadrant C, Fig. 15–2). During spontaneous inspiration, the pressure at this site is below atmospheric, and the popoff valve is closed. During exhalation, the pressure is just slightly above atmospheric, and gas flows to the reservoir bag until it is distended to its nominal volume. Then the pressure in the entire circuit increases as FGI and exhalation from the patient continue, thereby opening the popoff valve. What is then exhausted is primarily carbon-dioxide–rich and oxygen-anesthetic–depleted end-tidal gas that has been minimally diluted with fresh gas. However, the situation is reversed during assisted or controlled ventilation when, during inspiration, the pressure in the circuit at the Y-piece is positive with respect to atmosphere. In this situation, a popoff valve located at the Y-piece would dump fresh gas, while one near the bag would dump mostly a mixture of dead space and end-tidal gas.

MIXING DEVICES. Most of the resistance to gas flow in a circle system is located in the respiratory valves. While exact values for resistance are not known, most modern, properly functioning anesthesia machines have a resistance of less than 1 cm H_2O/L/min of gas flow.[5] Because this value is extremely low (less than one third to one half of the normal resistance to gas flow in the human lungs), it is safe to allow patients, including infants and children, to breathe spontaneously from a circle system for prolonged periods. However, before circuit design permitted such low resistances, attempts were made to decrease resistance to breathing in a circle system by providing a continuous flow of gas around the circle, thereby causing the inspiratory and expiratory valves to float rather than open and close with respiration. Both pumps and venturi devices driven by fresh gas flow (FGF) were designed, the most prominent of which was the Revell circulator.[6,7] While these devices will decrease apparatus dead space and may decrease resistance, the latter effect is small and may backfire under some circumstances, and actually increase resistance. Because resistance with modern equipment is so low (and can be eliminated by controlled ventilation), these mixing devices are of little practical value. Devices to reduce the mean airway pressure during controlled ventilation have been suggested but are not commonly used.[8]

FLOWS AND CONCENTRATIONS.[9] The gas mixture inspired by a patient breathing from a circle system is determined by the FGI, the configuration of the circle, the respiratory pattern and the uptake of oxygen and anesthetic agents by the patient. At inflow rates of 7 L/min or more, the circle behaves like a semi-open nonrebreathing system, and the concentration of inspired gas approaches that being delivered by the flowmeters. As flow progressively decreases below 7 L/min, the disparity between inflow and inspired concentration of anesthetic agents increases, and the system behaves more like a semiclosed rebreathing system.

FUNCTION OF THE CIRCLE SYSTEM.[10] The circle system functions similarly during spontaneous and controlled ventilation (Fig. 15–3). Opening of the inspiratory valve is initiated by the negative pressure created during spontaneous ventilation or by compression of the reservoir bag during controlled ventilation. With the opening of the inspiratory valve, fresh gas enters the inspiratory limb. Since the inspiratory flow rate exceeds the FGF, gases that have passed through the canister to the reservoir bag follow the FGF into the inspiratory limb. On exhalation, the increase in pressure in the system closes the inspiratory valve and opens the expiratory valve. Exhaled gases are therefore directed down the expiratory limb towards the overflow valve and canister while fresh gas flows through the canister toward the reservoir bag. During the expiratory pause, both valves are closed, and fresh gas continues to flow toward the reservoir bag.

DEAD SPACE

Any space occupied by respiratory gases in which no gas exchange takes place is termed *dead space.* Such space functions merely as a conduit or passageway. Anatomically, the mouth, pharynx, and tracheobronchial tree are dead space. In inhalation anesthestic systems, various appliances and masks are used to produce mechanical dead space. This is space within the inhalation system occupied by respiratory gases that do not come in contact with an absorbent and are rebreathed without losing their content of carbon dioxide.

CIRCLE FILTER SYSTEM. The dead space is the volume of air in the mask and the connectors up to the outlet tube or exhalation tube. In a circle system, the apparatus dead space extends only from the partition of the Y-piece to the patient's airway. Provided the unidirectional valves are competent and the soda lime is functioning, all gas entering the inspiratory limb will be free of carbon dioxide. However, if the inspiratory valve does not close immediately during exhalation, exhaled gases may enter the inspiratory limb, resulting in inspiration of some of the expired gases (rebreathing). Valves can leak as much as 150 mL of gas, resulting in significant rebreathing.[10] This can be detected easily by capnography or massspectrometry as a rise of inspired carbon dioxide to a level higher than 0%.

TO-AND-FRO FILTER SYSTEM. In this system, the dead space is the volume of air in the mask and the connectors up to the wire mesh of the canister. When absorbent in the forepart of the canister becomes exhausted, this becomes dead space.

SEMICLOSED SYSTEM. The dead space in this system consists of the volume of air in the mask and up to and including the exhalation valve cage.

OPEN SYSTEM. The volume of air contained under the mask constitutes the dead space in this system. Face pieces vary considerably in the intramask volume, and the amount of potential or actual dead

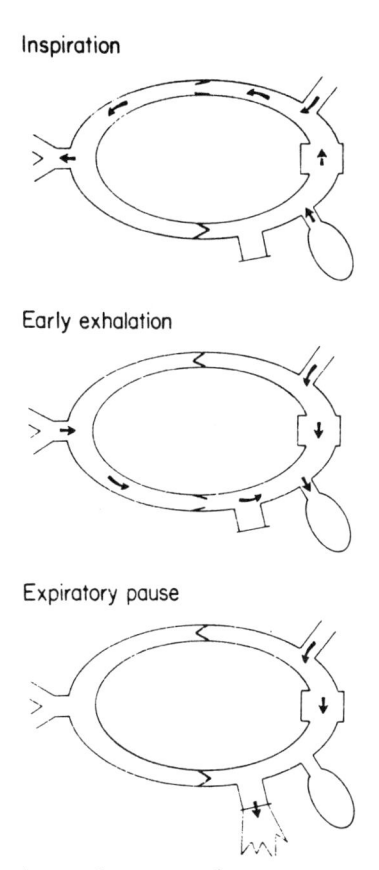

FIG. 15–3. The circle system during spontaneous ventilation. During inspiration the inspiratory valve is open. During exhalation, the inspiratory valve closes, expired gas is directed through the expiratory valve, and fresh gas flows toward the reservoir bag. During the expiratory pause, both valves are closed and fresh gas continues to flow toward the reservoir bag. From Fisher, D.: Anesthesia equipment for pediatrics. *In* Pediatric Anesthesia. G.A. Gregory. New York, Churchill Livingstone, 1983.

space depends on the mask size relative to the patient's face and the proper application of the mask. The average will-fitting and properly applied mask for adults provides a dead space of approximately 25 to 60 mL of air. A large face piece, improperly applied, may provide a dead space of 200 mL of air.

Endotracheal tubes reduce both the anatomic and mechanical dead space. The tube eliminates the air space of the nasal and pharyngeal passages as well as that of the mask. The air space of these passages in an adult (including the mouth, nose, and pharynx) measures between 60 and 75 mL.

Adjustments to respiratory activity occur in response to increases in external dead space.[11] In normal unmedicated subjects, even small increases in external dead space are of significance. An increase of 125 mL can produce appreciable increases in tidal and minute volumes and may be considered a critical additional volume of dead space for adults.

When a critical mechanical dead space volume is added to an anesthesia system, the minute volume increase in respiration does not equal the calculated dead space minute volume. That is, the minute volume increase is less than could be expected from simply adding the dead space to tidal volume value times rate. This indicates that compensation to increased dead space of even this small amount is not complete. Moreover, the end expiratory PE_{CO_2} will be significantly elevated over the controls.[12] Therefore, in using anesthetic equipment one must be careful to avoid increasing dead space and ever alert to compensate respirations.

CLOSED CIRCLE SYSTEMS

DEFINITION. The closed system of inhalation anesthesia allows no escape of anesthetic mixtures. It involves complete rebreathing and a reservoir is required. There is no access to the atmosphere, either on inspiration or expiration. In order for the system to be safe, enough oxygen must be delivered to supply the patient's needs each minute and the carbon dioxide produced by metabolism removed. Hence, closed systems are carbon dioxide absorption circuits. Simultaneously, an anesthetic vapor or gas must be added to the system according to the demands and tissue uptake. Larger amounts are needed for induction and lesser amounts for maintenance.[13,14]

HISTORY. John Snow introduced the concept of carbon dioxide absorption into clinical practice in 1850, using potassium hydroxide to absorb CO_2 during chloroform anesthesia.[15] Jackson revived Snow's concept by using sodium hydroxide as the absorbent.[16] More efficient and less caustic mixtures followed the development of granular forms of gas absorbents containing silicate as a binder for use in gas masks during World War I.[17] During the 1920s, the to-and-fro system was described by Waters,[13] and the circle system was introduced by Sword in 1928.[18] The introduction of cyclopropane in the early 1930s led to the widespread use of low-flow CO_2 absorption circuits. With the introduction of muscle relaxants and newer, nonflammable anesthetics in the 1950s and 1960s, the popularity of cyclopropane fell, but CO_2 absorption circuits became widely used.

REQUIREMENTS. It should be noted that an absorbent for carbon dioxide should be available and should be fresh; dead space must be minimized; all fittings must be tight, and the masks must be snugly applied to the patient's face to avoid leaks. An endotracheal system should be leak-proof. Apertures connecting various parts of the system must be at least 2-½ cm in diameter. This diameter was determined after experimentation and corresponds to the diameter of the adult trachea. Carbon dioxide is a waste product and in high concentrations is a depressant that possesses narcotic properties. Its use to stimulate respiration is unjustified. This by-product of tissue metabolism should be considered dangerous and removed at all times.

ADVANTAGES. The closed system provides maximal humidification, warming of inhaled gases, reuse of agents, minimalization of pollution, and reduction of costs.

RESISTANCE.[19,20] In any closed system, resistance is encountered to the passage of gases through the conduits. In the anesthetized, spontaneously breathing patient, the resistance to breathing is the sum of the resistance of the natural air passages and the anesthetic apparatus to the flow of gases. Most of the resistance to air flow is in the upper respiratory tract. Proctor has shown that simply changing from oral to nasal respiration may cause a fivefold increase in the atmospheric-alveolar pressure gradient.[21]

The resistance to flow of gases is a function of (1), the density and viscosity of the gases; (2), the caliber, length, shape, and internal smoothness of the tube; and (3) the velocity of flow (volume rate of flow).[19]

During closed system anesthesia, the resistance to spontaneous normal respiration is influenced by fit of the mask; size of the aperture (between masks, canisters, tubes, and bags); shape and size of canisters; length of tubing; constrictions; valves; and size of granules of the absorbent.[20]

In the face mask of a circle system, a positive pressure of 8 mm of water occurs on expiration and hence represents resistance, while on inspiration a negative pressure of 5 mm develops.

Furthermore, beyond the canister, the pressure in the circle system varies from 2.5 mm water during expiration to zero during inspiration, while in the breathing bag the pressure is nearly always positive.[20] Thus, it is recognized that the absorbent canister divides the apparatus into the two separate compartments: one on the patient's side (inspiratory limb) where the pressure is alternately positive and negative, and one on the expiratory limb, where the pressure is never negative (Table 15–3).

In experiments measuring pressures in the mask, conditions were optimal and the rebreathing reservoirs used were limitless so that the pressures reflected the influence of the system itself, exclusive of the breathing bag. When, however, a standard breathing bag of 5 L is inserted into the system, there is a further increase in the pressures depending upon how much the bag is filled. Thus, with a rebreathing bag that is completely filled but not overdistended at the end of expiration, a positive intrabronchial pressure occurs of +12 to 18 mm Hg. If the bag is half-filled at the end of expiration, a positive intrabronchial pressure of 2 to 14 mm Hg is produced.[23]

Resistance of Other Components. Resistance of various connectors, tubing, and endotracheal equipment may be summarized as follows:[19,20]

1. Higher resistance is encountered when there is a sudden change in direction of air flow. Curved connectors exhibit considerably higher resistance, so sharp corners and changing diameters of the passageway are to be avoided.
2. The internal diameter of equipment is the most critical dimension influencing resistance. Adapters should be wide-bored. Connection with rubber tubes should be smooth, ie, the tube should be stretched. All airways, connectors, and tubing should be as large in internal diameter as possible.

Obviously, to overcome resistance the spontaneously breathing patient must exert a greater effort to maintain proper gas exchange. It is usually difficult to measure the effect on ventilation of changes in resistance because the patient usually adapts his effort to the varying situation. One method depicts changes in air flow by a pneumotachograph when resistance factors are varied in anesthetic appliances; it uses a phrenic nerve stimulator to provide a constant respiratory effort.[24] This technique graphically illustrates the reduction in ventilation occurring with the to-and-fro absorber introduced into the airway and the much greater reduction occurring when circle absorbers of adult type are used (Fig. 15–4). The impact of dirty valves on ventilation is also clearly depicted, and it is apparent that such valves may reduce ventilation by at least 50%; to maintain adequate ventilation the patient must increase respiratory effort by a like amount (see Equipment—Valves) (Fig. 15–5).

Comment on Resistance Most anesthetists at present control respiration; hence the impact of breathing circuit resistances as seen during spontaneous breathing is irrelevant.

WATER VAPOR. The relative humidity in a closed system of anesthesia is approximately 100%. The water comes from two sources: the water vapor ordinarily found in exhaled gases (normal level 6.20%, water content of air about 1%); and the water of neutralization produced in the absorption of carbon dioxide. Such a heavy saturation with water of the anesthetic breathing mixture gradually reduces the amount of water vaporized in the alveoli and thereby reduces heat loss. As a consequence, body temperatures tend to rise. The increased temperature then increases the capacity of the respiratory atmosphere to hold more water and a vicious cycle develops. High water vapor content diminishes the oxygen content and dilutes the anesthetic mixture. Further, it *binds water-miscible* anesthetic agents and *may* interfere with anesthetization. Cole[25] describes a condition of water intoxication occurring during deep inhalation anesthesia. Edema of the brain with failure to regain consciousness may exist; water retention with oliguria and "extrarenal uremia" are to be expected.

TEMPERATURE OF INSPIRED GASES. After the establishment of closed system anesthesia, the average

TABLE 15–3. PRESSURE CHANGES IN SOME ANESTHESIA SYSTEMS DURING RESPIRATORY CYCLE

	Inhalation	Exhalation
Ayre T' system	0	1.0 mm H_2O
D–L valvular system (15 L/min)	17.5 mm H_2O	10 mm H_2O
Infant circle (10 L flow/min)	−1.3 mm H_2O	+2.5 mm H_2O
Adult to-and-fro mask	−2.3 mm H_2O	+3.0 mm H_2O
Adult circle		
Mask	−5.0 mm H_2O	+8.0 mm H_2O
Tube inhalation	0	+2.5 mm H_2O
Bag	+25 mm H_2O	—
Intrabronchial		
Full bag	—	120–180 mm H_2O
Part full	—	20–140 mm H_2O

394 *General Anesthesia*

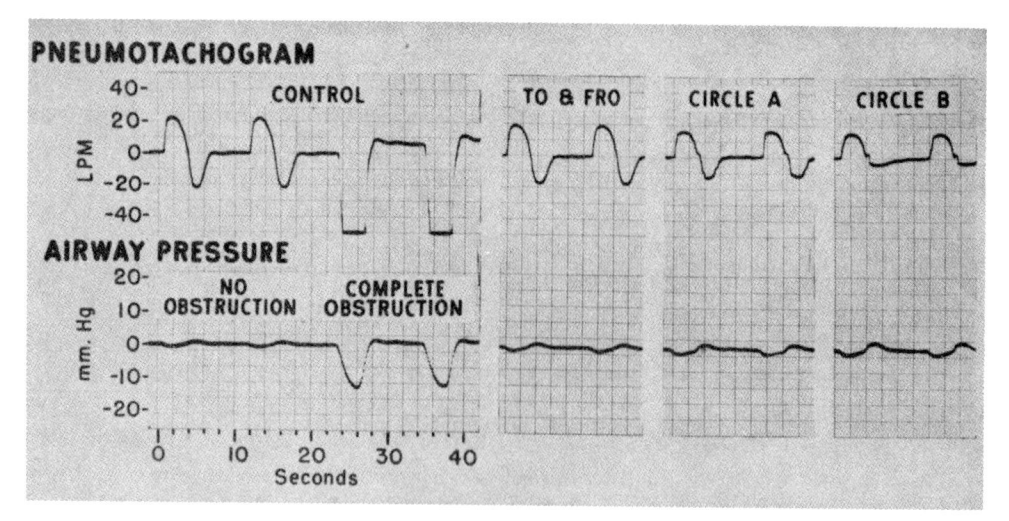

FIG. 15–4. Effect of obstruction on air flow and thus on resistance and respiratory effort. From Hamilton, W.K., and Eastwood, D.W.: A new method of depicting resistance of inhalation anesthetic equipment. Anesthesiology *17*:222, 1956.

temperature at the face piece is 32 to 33° C in the circle filter method and from 39 to 41° C in the to-and-fro method.[22] Two mechanisms operate to raise the temperature of the anesthetic atmosphere. First, the absorption of carbon dioxide liberates heat; secondly, closed systems maintain the heat regulatory function of the lungs. Ordinarily, the lungs help to lower the body temperature by warming inspired tidal air and by vaporizing water in the alveoli and furnishing the heat of vaporization. Thus a closed circuit humidifies and warms inspired anesthetic gases.

CARBON DIOXIDE CONTENT. In closed systems the carbon dioxide content of the atmosphere is elevated. The degree depends on the efficiency of the absorption but occurs even under optimal conditions. A fresh change of absorbent will effectively reduce the carbon dioxide content of an atmosphere to 0.1 or 0.2%. (Atmospheric carbon dioxide concentration is 0.04%.) However, in a matter of minutes, the concentration exceeds 0.15% and mounts progressively to 2.0%. Simultaneously the blood CO_2 tension increases. Furthermore, it is difficult to detect clinically percentages of carbon dioxide of

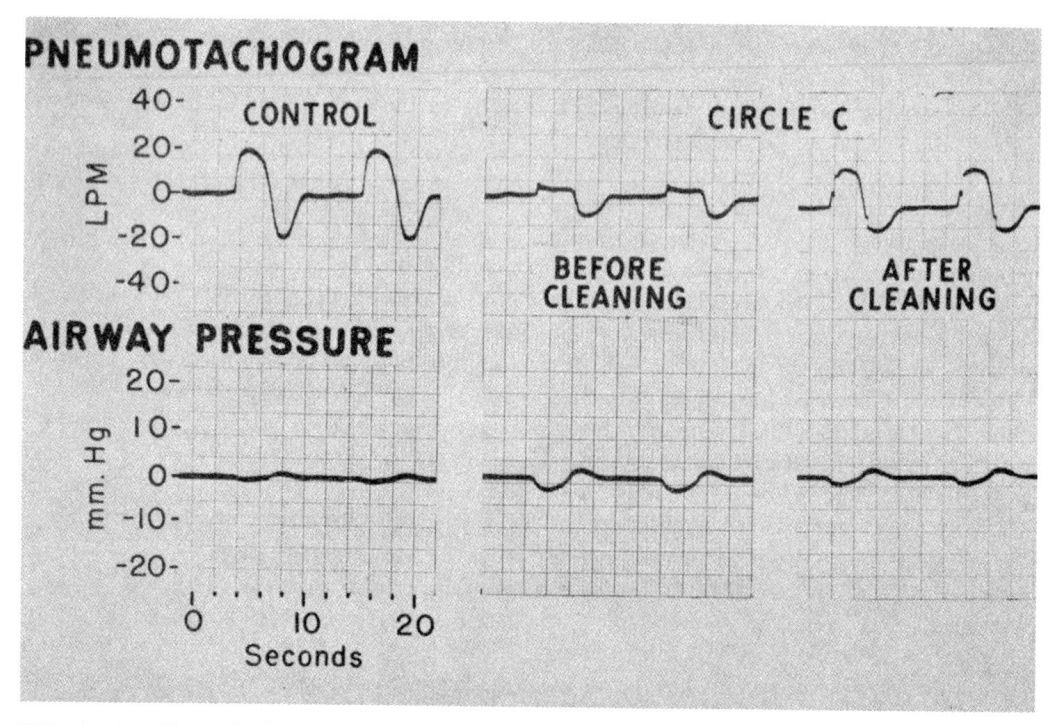

FIG. 15–5. Effect of valves on air flow and resistance and thus on respiratory effort. Dirty valves show great effort requirements. Cleaning the valves permits easy air flow. From Hamilton, W.K., and Eastwood, D.W.: A new method of depicting resistance of inhalation anesthetic equipment. Anesthesiology *17*:222, 1956.

2% during administration of inhalation anesthesia.[26] Factors such as depth of anesthesia, type of agent, and reflex stimuli detract from ability to judge carbon dioxide accumulation.

DILUTION OF ANESTHETIC GASES. The anesthetic contents of a closed system of anesthesia are altered by (1) the presence in the pulmonary tract of atmospheric gases, and (2) air entry through leaks in the apparatus. In order to obviate the influence of the inert nitrogen particularly, a procedure of flushing must be carried out. The procedure of using large volume flows of gases is called "washout technique," and the use of direct flows is called "flushing." The combined process is called denitrogenation. It is mandatory to use this procedure when weak inhalation agents such as nitrous oxide or ethylene are administered.

Loss of Gases Through Diffusion. Apart from leaks that may occur in overt openings in the anesthetic equipment (ie, poor mask fit, holes in bags and tubing), a loss of gas from the system results from the diffusion of anesthetic gases through the skin and through the structure of new rubber bags and tubing.

Wineland has demonstrated the extremely rapid diffusibility through rubber of N_2O as compared to other gases.[27] Carbon dioxide also diffuses rapidly and approaches N_2O in its ability to pass through rubber sheeting (common breathing bags) (Table 15-4).

Loss of inert gases through the skin also occurs and influences total body equilibration. Orcutt reported nitrous oxide loss through the skin to be about 230 mL/hr/m^2 after 1 hour of anesthesia.[28] Studies with better controls established a loss rate of 3.6 mL/min/m^2 and confirmed this value. Cutaneous blood flow of 150 mL/min was assumed and a steady alveolar concentration. During the first hour percutaneous loss increased and reached a plateau by 100 minutes. At the same time the body uptake of nitrous oxide decreased. After 100 minutes the nitrous oxide loss amounted to about 6.4% of the steady body uptake of nitrous oxide of 100 mL/min.[29]

The loss of other anesthetic gases through the skin is shown in Table 15-5). Factors in the amount of gas lost include the following:[30]

1. Simple diffusion is the principal determinant.
2. Skin temperature—a rectilinear increase with increasing skin temperature over range of 20 to 40° C. Over this range there is a fivefold increase in N_2O loss.
3. Fat solubility—an inverse relationship of percutaneous loss with fat solubility and therefore the influence of subcutaneous fat.
4. The effective body surface area.
5. The cutaneous blood flow. Stoelting's[29] studies suggest that nitrous oxide transfer across the skin is limited more by diffusion than by flow.

Leaks in System. In describing the closed system, Waters[13,28] emphasized the importance of leaks, stressing the need to eliminate leaks in the apparatus itself and at the contact of mask with the face and prevent air from leaking in and diluting the anesthetic mixture.

If a leak exists in a system three effects are possible:[31]

1. *Loss of gas.* When a hole in the breathing bag exists on the far side of the canister, away from the patient (ie, expiratory side in circle method) or the part of the system as mentioned above where the pressure is *always* positive), gas can be lost to atmosphere without any air entering the system during spontaneous breathing. During positive pressure inflations, gas will be lost from an aperture in any part of the system.
2. *Alternate loss of gas and entry of air.* When an aperture exists between the canister and the patient (inspiratory side of circle setup), it will be subjected to alternate positive and negative pressure. Gas will be lost during *positive* phase, while during *negative* phase air will be drawn into the system. Such a situation exists when a poorly fitted face piece leaves an opening between the mask and the face. Usually more gas is lost than is gained. However, it is apparent that as little as 1 L/min of air entering a system can greatly reduce the concentration of agents. Mathematical

TABLE 15-4. DIFFUSION OF N$_2$O THROUGH HUMAN SKIN DURING ANESTHESIA

Case Illustration	
Total body surface (cm^2)	19,500–17,100
Surface enclosed in pletysomograph	937–1,128
Time of anesthesia in minutes	50–80
Percent N$_2$O found	1.2–23
Mg N$_2$O/hr from surface in pletysmograph	37.75–45.2
ML (N$_2$O/hr from body surface 27° C, 740 mm	450–394
Mg N$_2$O/hr/cm$_2$ body surface	0.0403–0.0401

From Wineland A.J., and Waters, R.M.: The diffusion of anesthetic gases through rubber. Anesth. Analg. 8:322, 1929.

TABLE 15–5. CHARACTERISTICS OF PERCUTANEOUS LOSSES OF ANESTHETICS AT PLATEAU LEVELS

	Nitrous Oxide	Ether	Halothane
1. Alveolar percent	70	4	0.9
2. Percutaneous loss (mL/min/m²)*	3.57 ± 0.97 mL	0.15 ± 0.16	0.0076 ± 0.0031
3. mL anesthetic carried in 150 mL blood†	49.4 mL	72.6	3.1
4. Percent of (3) lost through the skin	7.2	0.21	0.25
5. mL percutaneous loss/min/1.8 m²*	6.43 mL	0.27	0.014
6. Calculated total body uptake (mL/min)*	100	300	13
7. Percent percutaneous loss/uptake* (5)/(6) × 100	6.43	0.09	0.10

* After 60 (ether and halothane) or 100 (nitrous oxide and cyclopropane) minutes of anesthesia.
† Calculated as alveolar percent times 150 mL/min times the blood/gas partition coefficient.
From Stoelting, R.K., and Eger, E.I., II: Percutaneous loss of nitrogen oxide, cyclopropane, ether and halothane in man. Anesthesiology 30:280, 1969.

analysis of actual conditions of administration of agents indicates that nitrous oxide concentrations can be greatly reduced, cyclopropane can be diluted drastically, and oxygen content can be lowered, even to subatmospheric levels.

3. *Loss of incoming anesthetic gases.* When openings exist at any joint or connection between the fine adjustment valves and the site of entry into the breathing system, loss of gas can occur. The gas loss is proportionately greater when small rates of flow are employed. Conditions may exist in which a patient can be suboxygenated.

INCOMPATIBILITY OF ABSORPTION TECHNIQUE WITH CERTAIN AGENTS. Certain inhalation agents cannot be administered in a closed carbon dioxide absorption system because of decomposition. The decomposition results from reaction to the chemical absorbents and from breakdown by the heat developed.

In 1943, cranial nerve palsy was reported by McCauley following administration of trichlorethylene.[32] Other reports followed.[33] It was determined that trichlorethylene reacted with the sodium hydroxide of soda lime in the formation of a toxic product, dichloracetylene.[33]

Decomposition of the trichlorethylene occurs in the presence of alkalies and is enhanced by heat. Both conditions exist in the soda lime cannister.[34] Dichloracetylene can cause paralysis of other cranial nerves and some peripheral nerve paresthesias. Servoflurane is incompatible.

Halothane interaction with soda lime was first reported by Reventos in 1965.[35] Sharp has detected that 2-bromo-2-chloro-1,1-difluoro-ethylene is formed when halothane contacts soda lime during routine anesthesia in semiclosed and closed system anesthesia.[36] It was not found in nonrebreathing systems.

Enflurane and isoflurane are retained by the soda lime.[37,38] However, the quantities of degraded products are relatively small.

CONTAMINANTS FROM VAPORIZERS. Volatile agents such as enflurane and isoflurane may interact with such vaporizer components as wicks, screens, and plastic connectors to produce contaminants in the inhaled mixtures.[39] Leaching of chemicals from the vaporizer parts may occur with isoflurane. This aspect of contamination is distinguished from impurities that may be present in the commercial product supplied.

WASTE GASES-HUMAN METABOLITES. Several gases produced as "waste" metabolites may accumulate during closed system general anesthesia. These include methane, acetone, and nitrogen largely the result of intestinal bacterial action and although absorbed into the circulation are released into the lungs. They then accumulate in the breathing circuit and are rebreathed.[40]

CLOSED SYSTEM—TO-AND-FRO

The closed to-and-fro system of administration of inhalation anesthetic agents was developed by Waters and Jackson and introduced in 1924.[13,16] This was the first widely adopted closed-absorption system. It is a nonrebreathing system and is distinct from the circle system in having a single channel for both inspiration and expiration. The assembly consists of a metal connector between the face mask and a breathing bag; this connector is provided with an inlet port for anesthetic gases, oxygen, and vapors. A carbon dioxide absorption canister open at both ends is interposed between the connector and the breathing bag. It is thus a single-line breathing channel and eliminates the two corrugated tubes of the circle system. It is a prototype of the Mapelson C configuration with the interposition of the CO_2 absorption canister (Fig. 15–6).

COMMENT. The to-and-fro system is simple and requires a minimum of breathing components. The resistance of the system to spontaneous breathing is also minimal and is less than that of the circle system. In the face mask, a positive pressure of 8 mm water may be measured on exhalation, and a negative pressure of 2.5 mm water develops on inhalation. However, in current practice using ventilators, this is not of concern. Further, the equipment is cumbersome because it is all assembled near the patient's head and is difficult to manage, especially the carbon dioxide absorber. There is a progressive increase in the dead space of the apparatus as soda lime is exhausted. There also exists the possibility of inhalation of soda lime dust and excessive heat production close to the patient's airway. Hence, it has fallen into disuse.

LOW-FLOW AND INJECTION OF LIQUID AGENT TECHNIQUE (Lowe–Aldrete Technique).

INTRODUCTION.[41,42] A low-flow liquid anesthetic injection technique has as its principle an FGI equal to uptake and losses of anesthetic and oxygen. The objectives of this closed system injection anesthetic technique are

- An oxygen inflow equal to or slightly in excess of oxygen consumption, based on Brody's equation and sufficient to meet metabolic demands.
- Elimination of carbon dioxide by standard circuit absorption.
- A calculated dose of volatile anesthetic to more closely approximate the anesthetic requirements. The vapor dose is converted to a liquid volume equivalent.

The inhalation anesthetic agent is introduced in liquid form into the circuit by syringe injection of precisely calculated unit-doses in milliliters of the liquid anesthetic (volatile agent), which is then vaporized in the circuit to produce a vapor concentration sufficient to produce the anesthetic state. Larger amounts of vapor are required initially, and so a greater number of units in a given time period is injected. As anesthesia progresses and uptake and saturation of body tissues occurs, the amount of vapor required is less and units are injected less frequently.

The uptake of inhalation anesthetics towards a saturation end point decreases with time. This was shown in 1924 by Haggard for diethylether.[43] Eger determined exponential equations for uptake and saturation of body tissue.[44] Lowe demonstrated that the exponential saturation equation predicts that the *rate* of whole body uptake of anesthetic vapors at the 4th, 9th, 16th, 25th . . . minute is one half, one third, one fourth, one fifth of the initial one-minute uptake rate. The rate of whole body uptake of an agent shows a linear decrease with the square root of time:[41,44]

$$\text{Rate of uptake at } t \text{ minutes} = \frac{\text{rate of uptake at 1 minute}}{\sqrt{t}}$$

A corollary of this equation is that the total cumulative dose over any given *interval* of time is the same as the initial dose.

BASIC PHYSIOLOGIC CONCEPTS. In 1942 Brody empirically discovered that oxygen consumption of all mammals is related as an exponential function of body weight. When expressed in milliliters per minute, the oxygen consumption is related to body weight in kilograms in a linear logarithmic manner.[45]

Oxygen consumption (mL/min) = weight $(kg)^{3/4} \times 10$.

Other physiologic parameters are similarly related. Cardiac output, in accordance with Fick's equation, establishes a direct correlation with oxygen consumption $\dot{V}O_2$. Therefore, the Brody index of weight in kilograms to the exponent $3/4$ has been found to be a more accurate index of cardiac output;[46] the equation for cardiac output is Brody number $(kg^{3/4}) \times 2 = dL/min$. Carbon dioxide production is also related to Brody's number. Thus, $(kg^{3/4})$ mul-

FIG. 15–6. To-and-fro rebreathing system. From National Research Council. Subcommittee on Anesthesia: **Fundamentals of Anesthesia.** American Medical Association, Editorial Direction 3rd Ed. Philadelphia, W. B. Saunders Company, 1954.

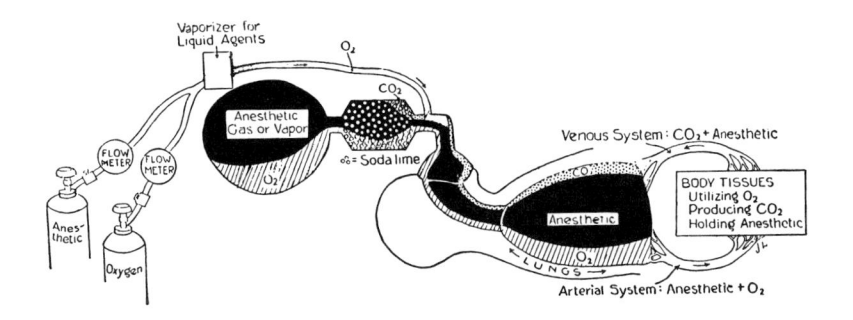

TABLE 15–6. CONVERSION OF VAPOR TO LIQUID VOLATILE ANESTHETICS

To convert milliliters of vapor to milliliters of liquid, the vapor volume must be divided by
240 for halothane
212 for enflurane
212 for isoflurane
Conversion is based on Avogadro's Law: The number of gas molecules in a gram-molecular weight of a substance is the same for each substance and each occupies a volume of 22.4 L.

---

tiplied by a factor of 8 will give the amount of milliliters produced per minute.[47] Clinical conditions may alter these basic values.

CALCULATION OF UNIT DOSE.[41] Anesthetic arterial concentration (Ca) and cardiac output per minute ($\dot{Q}$) determine the rate at which tissues become saturated with anesthetic molecules. Their product is the amount of anesthetic delivered to the tissues each and every minute (Ca × $\dot{Q}$ = mL vapor). The anesthetic arterial concentration is a function of anesthetic potency in MAC values and the blood gas solubility coefficient. In most patients, anesthesia is achieved at 1.3 MAC, and the amount of anesthetic gas delivered each minute in milliliters of vapor is predicted by the equation:

$$1.3 \,(f) \times MAC \times \lambda B/G \times \dot{Q} = mL \text{ vapor/min}$$

To attain the desired arterial concentration, one must also consider the alveolar concentration. Hence, the prime dose equals the minute arterial delivery *plus* the amount to fill the ventilatory delivery system, which is approximately the same volume. From these facts, the unit dose (mL vapor) to fill the ventilatory and arterial systems when $t = 1$ minute is as follows:

$$\text{Volume of vapor} = 2 \,(fMAC \times \lambda B/G \times \dot{Q})$$

where $\dot{Q}$ or cardiac output is determined by Brody's number or two times weight in kilograms to the exponent ¾. To determine the amount of the anesthetic unit dose in liquid form, the milliliters of vapor are converted (Table 15–6).

Tables have been constructed of unit doses. The vapor unit is converted to the milliliters of unit liquid dose for each of the currently available volatile inhalation agents that is injected into the system (Table 15–7).

DOSING INTERVALS.[41,48] The timing of administration of unit doses of liquid in practice is in accordance with the exponential saturation curve of tissue uptake. The intervals at which a unit dose is repeated correlates with the numbered sequence of the dose. The timing is the square of the sequence number. Thus, the second dose after prime dose is administered at 4 minutes, the third dose at 9 minutes . . . and ad seriatim. Doses 4, 5, 6, 7, 8 . . . N are administered at 16, 25, 36, 49, 64 . . . N^2 minutes.

The calculated unit amount of liquid agent that is injected after prescribed *intervals* of time is sufficient to provide a concentration for maintenance of the anesthetic during the time interval.

CLOSED CIRCUIT INJECTION DOSE TECHNIQUE FOR CHILDREN.[49] The closed circuit low-flow injection technique with the volatile agents has been used in infants and children,[49] employing a modified Bloomquist circle system[50] or a modified pediatric breath-

TABLE 15–7. UNIT LIQUID ANESTHETIC DOSES AND OXYGEN CONSUMPTION WITH 100% OXYGEN FOR ADULTS

Weight (kg)	Brody's Number ($kg^{3/4}$)	$\dot{V}O_2$ (10 × $kg^{3/4}$) (mL/min)	$\dot{Q}$ (2 × $kg^{3/4}$) (dL)	Halothane (mL)	Enflurane (mL)	Isoflurane (mL)
10	5.6	56	11.2	0.21	0.44	0.27
20	9.5	95	20.0	0.36	0.76	0.46
30	12.8	128	25	0.48	1.02	0.62
40	15.9	159	30	0.61	1.28	0.78
50	18.8	188	36	0.72	1.52	0.92
60	21.6	216	43	0.81	1.72	1.04
70	24.2	242	48	0.91	1.92	1.16
80	26.8	268	54	1.00	2.12	1.29
90	29.2	292	58	1.10	2.32	1.41
100	31.6	316	62	1.20	2.52	1.53

* Divide doses in half if 65% N_2O is used.
$\dot{V}O_2$ = oxygen consumption; $kg^{3/4}$ = weight in kilograms to three-fourths power.
$\dot{Q}$ = cardiac output.
Modified from Aldrete, J.A., Lowe, H.J., and Virtue, R.M.: Low Flow and Closed System Anesthesia. New York, Grune and Stratton, 1979.
Courtesy of Paul O'Leary, MD, Detroit, MI, and Lowe, H.J. and Ernst, C.A.: The Quantitative Practice of Anesthesia Use of Closed System, Baltimore, Mount Sinai Hosp Procedures Anesthesia, Williams and Wilkins, 1981.
Courtesy of Paul O'Leary, Detroit MI, 1988.

ing assembly adapted to a standard anesthesia machine.[51] The breathing pediatric assembly consists of short plastic breathing tubes, plastic Y-adapter with endotracheal tube connector, and an appropriately sized infant or child's mask. The breathing tubes are attached to the inflow and outflow parts of a standard adult circle anesthesia machine. The assembly is usually disposable.[51] Graff has shown that the adult circle system does not impose significant strain on infants breathing spontaneously.[52] Reynolds confirmed this, but advises that assisted or controlled respiration should be used.[53]

After preoxygenation and denitrogenation for 3 minutes, the gas flow of oxygen into the system is decreased to a level of approximately 100 mL·min^{-1} in infants; for older children, approximately 150 mL·min^{-1} is administered. The calculated priming dose of liquid anesthetic is injected into the exhalation arm of the breathing system (Table 15–8). For induction, several unit doses at 15, 30, 60, and 90 seconds are administered after the prime dose. Maintenance is achieved by supplemental unit doses in a time sequence. The first and second supplements are given at 2 minutes and 4 minutes, the third at 9 minutes, and the fourth at 16 minutes; the time of subsequent injections is the square of the numbered injections. For a duration of anesthesia of 40 to 50 minutes, the average for enflurane is 3.7 ± 1.1 mL, while for halothane and isoflurane, it is 3.0 ± 0.9 mL.

PRECAUTIONS

In a closed circle system, in which inflow just matches loss from the system and the popoff or overflow valve is closed, the composition of inspired gas is not predictable from the inflow concentration of gases.[9] Furthermore, expired and inspired gases will differ because of uptake of oxygen and anesthetic and excretion of carbon dioxide. Oxygen concentration in the expiratory limb is usually about 4 or 5% lower than in the inspiratory limb. Although oxygen uptake remains relatively constant during an anesthetic procedure (about 200 to 250 mL/min in the average adult) provided body temperature does not change appreciably, anesthetic uptake will vary, being greatest at the start of anesthesia and then decreasing with time. If oxygen concentration (or partial pressure) is maintained constant during closed system anesthesia, the flowmeter values reflect oxygen consumption and anesthetic uptake by the patient, rather than inspired concentrations.

When nitrous oxide is used in closed system anesthesia, the oxygen tension or concentration in the circle must be monitored continuously, because nitrous oxide uptake declines rapidly while oxygen uptake does not, thus making the inspired gas mixture progressively more hypoxic if the nitrous oxide inflow is not gradually decreased. Whether it is necessary to measure the concentration of potential volatile anesthetics during closed system anesthesia remains controversial. Some believe that it is necessary, while others prefer to monitor anesthetic depth and patient responses. Further, when nitrous oxide is part of the carrier gas–oxygen–anesthetic mixture, the inflow is usually in excess of the patient's needs and the popoff valve must be open. This is now a semiclosed partial rebreathing circle system.

Other concerns include dangerous increases in carbon dioxide, the accumulation of toxic metabolites from biotransformation of volatile anesthetics or build-up of excretory metabolic gases (methane), and the difficulty in administering correct doses.[41] With a properly functioning absorber of the Jumbo type with replacement of the absorbent after 8 to 10 hours, this has not been a problem, assuming the ventilation is adequate. The accumulation of anesthetic agent metabolites or of changes in respiratory gases resulting from normal metabolism is discussed under biotransformation, but they have not

TABLE 15–8. LIQUID ANESTHETIC DOSES AND OXYGEN CONSUMPTION FOR INFANTS AND CHILDREN (Couto da Silva)

Weight (kg)	Brody's Number (kg$^{3/4}$)	$\dot{V}O_2$ (10 × kg$^{3/4}$)	$\dot{Q}$ (2 × kg$^{3/4}$)	Doses Halothane	Doses Isoflurane	Doses Enflurane
9	5.1	51	10.2	0.21	0.21	0.42
8	4.7	47	9.4	0.19	0.19	0.39
7	4.3	43	8.6	0.17	0.17	0.35
6	3.8	38	7.6	0.15	0.15	0.31
5	3.3	33	6.6	0.13	0.13	0.27
4	2.8	28	5.6	0.11	0.11	0.23
3	2.3	23	4.6	0.09	0.09	0.18
2	1.6	16	3.2	0.06	0.06	0.13

This table is used to predict the doses and consumption of liquid anesthetic. Oxygen consumption ($\dot{V}_{O_2}$) and cardiac output ($\dot{Q}$) were calculated according to Brody[4,5]. Doses of liquid anesthetic were injected in the expiratory limb of the system according to the square root of time sequence, except during induction of anesthesia, when higher concentrations of anesthetic vapors are needed. From Couto da Silva, J.M., Tubino, P.J., Vieira, Z.E.G., and Saraiva, R.A.: Closed circuit anesthesia in infants and children. Anesth. Analg., 63:765, 1984.

clearly caused a greater problem than with other systems. Dosage with volatile agents depends largely on the vigilance of the anesthesiologist and his observation of the patient.

With proper precautions, closed systems are safe. Witness the 30-year (1930–1960) use and popularity of closed-system cyclopropane. A closed system in which FGI equals uptake is mandatory. In the hands of physicians properly trained in the use of cyclopropane in either the to-and-fro or circle system, the safety record has been unparalleled.*[41]

SEMICLOSED CIRCLE–PARTIAL REBREATHING METHOD

DEFINITION. In the partial rebreathing system, part of the expired gases escape through an exhalation valve into the air or are scavenged, and part passes into a breathing bag. There is no admixture with atmospheric air on inspiration.

FGI is always greater than the uptake, ie, FGF > uptake. Unless the FGF is greater than two to two and one half times the respiratory minute volume, carbon dioxide washout will only be partial. Therefore, the excess inflow is exhaled through the popoff valve, carrying some CO_2, but the remaining CO_2 requires the presence of a CO_2 absorber canister.

The inspired concentration will be variable, depending on the volume-rate of FGF into the system. It will approach uniformity or approximate the mixture calculated from the volumes of gases set by the flowmeters after varying periods of time.

The inspired nitrogen percentage with different FGF is illustrated in (Figure 15–7).[24] Note that with a nonrebreathing system, no expired gas is returned to the reservoir and nitrogen "washout" of the lung is rapid, no nitrogen is rebreathed, and the inspired gases are entirely fresh and constant in percentage. On the other hand, in a semiclosed partial rebreathing system, the attainment of a constant inspired concentration of fresh gas is more rapid with high gas flow, but a low gas inflow may take an indefinite time to become constant or to wash out nitrogen.

This technique is applicable in the use of nitrous oxide. An adequate supply of oxygen must be available at all times to the patient. The first physician to use oxygen with nitrous oxide was Andrews (1868).† When combining these gases, he described the fundamental principles underlying the use of nitrous oxide, which included the removal of nitrogen from the lungs and the circuit. High flows of gas mixture were used, and oxygen in concentrations greater than 25% were recommended. Because

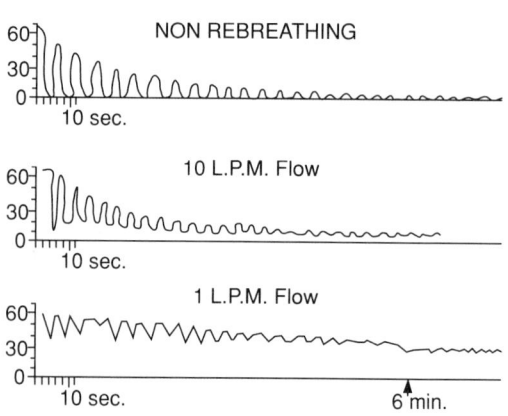

FIG. 15–7. Airway nitrogen concentrations occurring when subjects previously breathing air inhale from anesthesia apparatus to which oxygen is added in amounts indicated. The ordinate is percentage nitrogen. The "valleys" in the tracing represent inspiration. Hamilton, W.F., Eastwood, D.W.: A new method of depicting resistance of inhalation anesthetic equipment. Anesthesiology, 17:222, 1956.

an escape valve was needed, the first valve was developed by Boothby from his observations of the valves on kegs in local breweries. Later, the technique and equipment for the administration of gases, particularly by a semiclosed system, was perfected by McKesson.

PRINCIPLES. The flow of gases must be continuous and at anesthetic concentrations. The volume of gases flowing should equal or exceed the respiratory volume. With low rates of flow, the oxygen actually available to the patient is less than the mixture delivered, even though the original mixture may contain an amount of oxygen in excess of minimal requirements. It is recommended that with mixtures delivered and containing at least 50% oxygen the total rates of flow be kept in excess of 8 L/min, or approximately the minute respiratory volume. Under these circumstances, the oxygen available to the patient will reasonably approach the original tension of 152 to 158 mm Hg. Otherwise, at the end of 3 minutes, there may be some hypoxia. In addition, the volume of gases flowing per unit time must equal the respiratory minute volume in order to effectively eliminate carbon dioxide.

Preliminary flushing out of air or residual gases from the anesthetic circuit with oxygen is essential, followed by denitrogenation of the pulmonary and circulatory system. This is mandatory if concentrations of nitrous oxide greater than 50% are to be employed.

NITROUS OXIDE TECHNIQUES. In the application of nitrous oxide–oxygen mixtures using 50–50% as a supplement to intravenous or balanced anesthesia or as a carrier for potent anesthetic vapors, it is

---

* Robbins, B.H.: Cyclopropane anesthesia (closed system) 2nd ed., Baltimore, The Williams and Wilkins Co., 1958.

† Heironimus, T.W. History of nitrous oxide. Clin. Anes. 1:1, 1964.

important to preoxygenate and denitrogenate the patient. It is recommended that a relatively high total flow rate be continued by allowing 3 to 4 L each per minute of nitrous oxide and oxygen to flow into the anesthesia system. One may use smaller flow rates such as 2 L/min if a carbon dioxide absorber is in the circuit.

INFLUENCE OF LEAKS.[31] Leaks are as important in semiclosed as in closed system anesthesia. Even if flow rates are ideal for a given patient, the achievement of good results is negated by both loss of gases and dilution from the atmosphere. In general, nitrogen elimination is difficult, and concentrations of anesthetic nitrous oxide greater than 50% are rarely obtained in the anesthetic system.

SUMMARY. The following conditions must be satisfied to provide a proper semiclosed partial rebreathing method of anesthesia:

1. A minimal resistance exhalation valve
2. Continuous flow of gases at anesthetic concentrations
3. Total flow of gases at least equal to respiratory minute volume
4. Oxygen concentration calculated at 20% of mixture admitted to system
5. No leaks in the system
6. CO_2 absorption unit

It is important to realize that the nitrous oxide carrier agent used in semiclosed anesthesia is weak. The anesthetic system and the respiratory tract must be flushed thoroughly in order to diminish the concentration of nitrogen, which otherwise would dilute the anesthetic gas and the oxygen.

NONREBREATHING VALVULAR SYSTEMS

Unidirectional nonrebreathing valves have been used as a method of administering anesthesia. During the 1950s, a number of flap and mushroom valves were introduced. Later, valves of the disk or spring-loaded type became available.[54,59]

Externally, these systems resemble a semiclosed system of the Mapleson A type, differing only in that a second valve is inserted somewhere between the reservoir bag and the patient. This becomes an inspiratory valve that opens on inhalation, allowing fresh gas from the reservoir bag to be inspired, and closes on exhalation. The popoff is the expiratory valve that opens on exhalation, allowing exhaled gases to pass to the atmosphere, but closes on inspiration. There is no rebreathing. Only the FGF can fill the reservoir bag. Therefore, FGF must be at least equal to respiratory minute volume. Generally, the two valves are incorporated into one housing.

Several such valves were developed for administering anesthesia (Fig. 15-8). The first valve (the DL) was introduced by Digby Leigh in 1946.[54] The Stephen-Slater valve, an improvement, was introduced in 1948.[55,56] Fink modified the DL valve so as to permit easy positive pressure ventilation.[57] These modifications employed flap and mushroom valves.[58,59] Frumin introduced a valve modification in which the expiratory valve is opened if the delivered flow from the reservoir bag decreases below the inspiratory flow, thereby allowing an atmospheric inflow and preventing asphyxia.[60]

The Ruben valve[61] deserves special comment. This is an ingeniously designed valve in which the FGI changes direction, going either toward the bag or toward the patient on the different phases of the respiratory cycle. The inflow goes toward the patient on inspiration, along with gas from the reservoir, and goes toward the bag and a popoff component on exhalation. This valve can be used in low-flow spontaneous breathing techniques but does not lend itself to a true closed system anesthesia.

With any of these valves, the expiratory valve closes upon inspiration whether it is spontaneous, assisted, or controlled. Resistance is negligible and is balanced by the natural tendency of the reservoir bag to collapse. Generally, valves constructed of rubber flaps are more efficient and have less resistance. The resistance with gas flow rates up to 15 L/min has been shown to be only 1.75 cm water on the inspiratory side and 1 cm water on the expiratory side.[58,62]

The technique has been employed in infants of 2 or 3 months of age for 2 or more hours, as well as in children. The valve is placed in juxtaposition to the endotracheal tube or special mask so that the dead space of the upper respiratory or pharyngeal portion of the respiratory tract is reduced to about 9 mL. At the other end of the valve, a reservoir bag is placed (2.5 L for children up to 10 years of age). The distal end of the bag is connected to the source of inflow of fresh gases.[59,63]

Advantages of valvular systems include

Excellent carbon dioxide elimination
Dissipation of heat and prevention of hyperthermia
Elimination of respiratory water vapor
Minimal intrapulmonic pressure
Facilitation of respiratory assistance, possible by placing the hand over the exhalation valve on inspiration
Possibility of deep anesthesia minimized by high-flow gases

Other advantages include ease of use during transport and resuscitation and fresh gas economy, because the required fresh gas equals the patient's minute volume.

FIG. 15–8. Types of nonrebreathing valves.

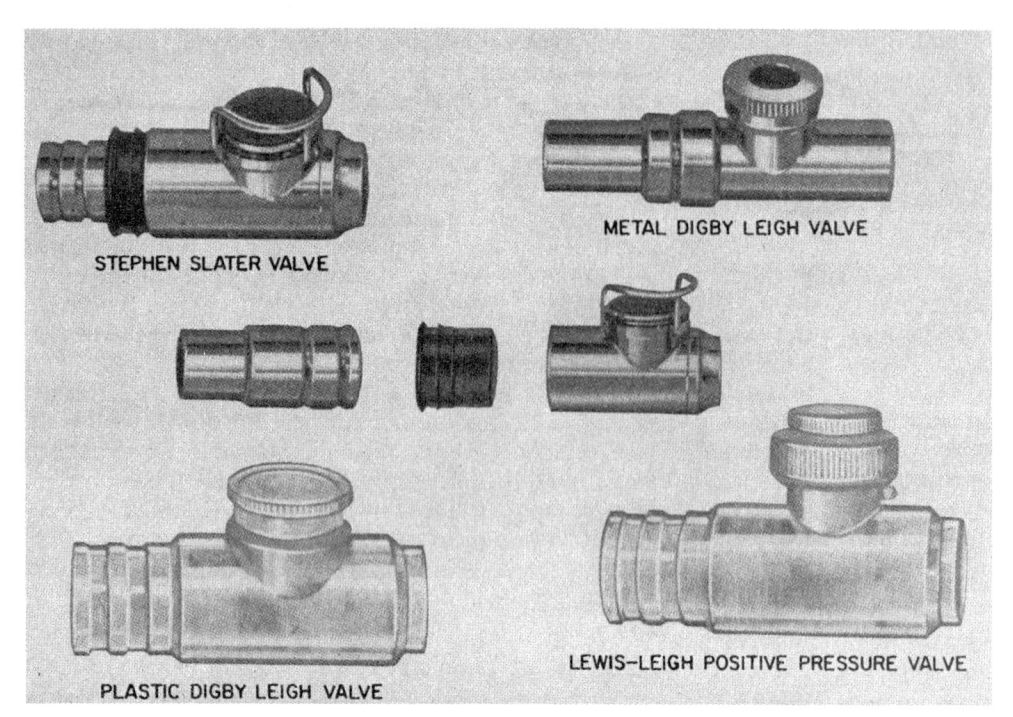

Disadvantages include malfunction of valves (increased apparatus resistance and rebreathing); cumbersomeness when used in certain surgical procedures; operating room pollution (no scavenging); inability to be set up for ventilator use; and problems with humidification. Because of these problems, these systems have been abandoned in administration of anesthesia. They are used in gas masks, scuba gear, self-inflating bags, and pneumatic ventilators. The self-inflating bags with nonrebreathing valves are used in patient transport and resuscitation.

SEMICLOSED SINGLE-LIMB SYSTEMS: MAPLESON CONFIGURATIONS

Mapleson configurations are single-limb systems and partial rebreathing systems, unless the FGI into the system is large enough to wash out the exhaled gas volume.[63] Nearly all involve a corrugated, widebore (2.5 cm) extension from the patient's airway.[64–66] Variations depend on the location of the gas flow inlet, the placement of an exhalation port, and the inclusion of a reservoir bag. These semiclosed breathing systems have several advantages: simplicity, single tube design, no absorption canister, no absorbent, and easy sterilization. These have been classified by Mapleson.[64]

The Magill circuit was one of the first semiclosed systems to be designed. The original Magill apparatus consisted of a simple breathing elbow connector attached to a mask and to an expiratory valve close to the patient's face. From the valve an extension connects to a breathing bag. An inlet for fresh gas, is located either through a nipple located at the extension or at the tail of the bag.[67] The bag ideally contains a volume equal to the inspiratory capacity of the patient (about 3 L in an adult) to permit spontaneous deep breaths without the feeling of suffocation. Gas flows of one to two times per minute volume are used.[68] In Mapleson's analysis, this became known as the Mapleson C configuration (Fig. 15–9).[64] To remove the reservoir bag from the area of the face, as for head and neck operations, a breathing tube is interposed between the bag and the mask. This is known as the Mapleson A configuration (Fig. 15–9). Reversing the location of the inflow and popoff valve sites yields the Mapleson D configuration (Fig. 15–9).

Each of these breathing systems may be thought of as lying somewhere along the following continuum:

Maximum CO$_2$ Excretion		Maximum CO$_2$ Retention
No mixing of fresh and alveolar gas	Complete mixing of alveolar and fresh gas	No mixing of fresh and alveolar gas
Fresh gas goes to patient	Mixture is inhaled and popped off simultaneously	Fresh gas goes to popoff
Alveolar gas goes to popoff		Alveolar gas is rebreathed

The far right situation represents rebreathing and is of use only in the study of respiratory control and as one treatment for hiccups. The original Mapleson

patient side   bag side

Mapleson C
Original Magill System

Mapleson A
Magill attachment (extension)

Mapleson D
Modified by Rees.

Bain Circuit
Coaxial

Modified Ayre T-Tube
An open system often designated as Mapleson E

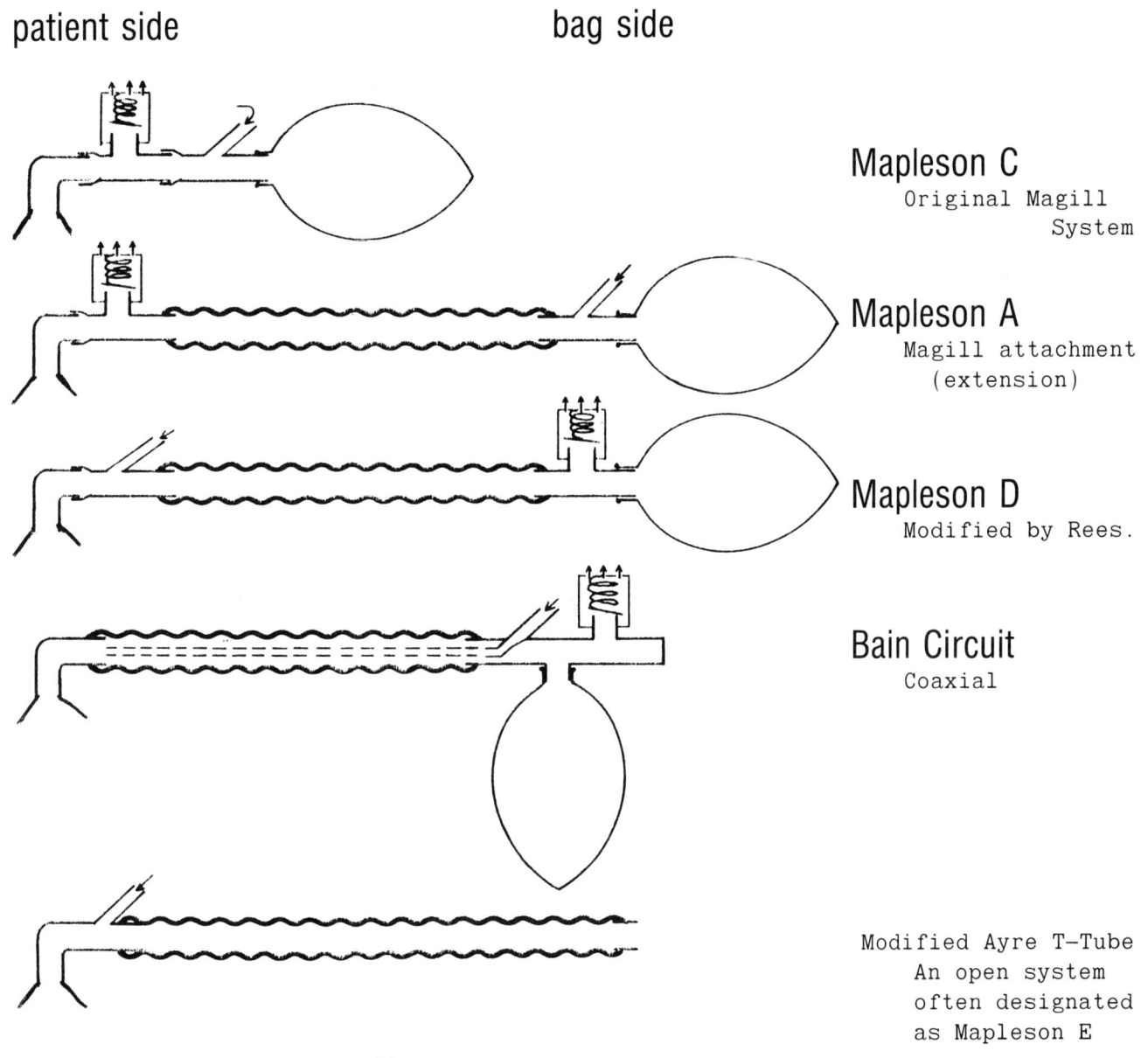

FIG. 15–9. The Mapleson configurations. The semiclosed or Magill circuits (*top four*) contain most of the components of a circle system: tubing, connectors, bag, FGI, and popoff site. They lack carbon dioxide absorbers because carbon dioxide is lowered by addition of fresh gas. They also lack separate inspiratory and expiratory limbs. One tubing serves both purposes. Thus no inspiratory or expiratory valves are required and are thus single-limb systems.

The Mapleson C system is a simple bag and mask. Because it permits more mixing of fresh and exhaled gas, it is less efficient than the Mapleson A, D, or E. The A and D are similar except that the inflow and popoff sites have been exchanged. A is optimal for spontaneous breathing, D for controlled breathing.

The coaxial (Bain) circuit, which has a gas delivery tube inside of a corrugated exhaust tube, behaves functionally like the Mapleson D. Its fresh gas delivery is effectively deposited at the patient connector, having been delivered there through a small tubing (*dotted lines*) whose connector is near the bag for convenience. This system differs from the Mapleson D in three ways: It can be rigidly mounted, it can be conveniently scavenged, and a pressure gauge is included with the circuitry.

The Mapleson E system (modified Ayre system) is essentially an Ayre Y-piece (or T-piece) to which has been added a corrugated reservoir tube. It is an open, not a semiclosed system. It is simple but lacks the convenience of a bag for ventilatory assistance or control. A bag can be added to it, but the system still lacks an adjustable popoff valve, and thus assistance or control of respiration is not convenient.

All of these circuits share a common advantage. Vigorous hyperventilation cannot decrease the patient's carbon dioxide tension much below normal if the FGF are kept between one and two times the patient's normal respiratory minute volume. Of course, they all share the same disadvantage, the wasting of large volumes of anesthetic gases and vapors. The Mapleson B system, with the inflow site and the exhalation popoff site positioned together near the patient's face at the mask or endotracheal tube, is an unsound design on the basis of physical principles of gas flow and is physiologically unsatisfactory. It is devoid of merit and is not illustrated.

B configuration lies midway on this continuum and is judged to have no particular merit, as other configurations are more efficient. None of the Mapleson systems meet the requirements on the far left, which are essentially a description of nonrebreathing systems. There is always a partial pressure difference for carbon dioxide such that

| Alveolar gas CO_2 concentration | > | Mixed expired CO_2 concentration | > | Dead space CO_2 concentration | > | Fresh gas CO_2 concentration |

The efficient breathing circuit configurations place the popoff valve where the highest carbon dioxide concentration is to be found during the phase of breathing when the circuit pressure is above atmospheric. This occurs at end expiration during spontaneous breathing and with inspiration during controlled breathing. Since the Mapleson A, D, and Jackson Rees systems each permit the fresh gas to mix well with exhaled air, they are more efficient than the C system. Complete mixing and/or proper placement of the popoff valve site contribute to the efficiency of the A, D, Jackson Rees, and Bain systems.

THE JACKSON REES SYSTEM.[69] This system was designed by Jackson Rees for pediatric use in 1950. It is classified as a modification of the Mapleson D configuration. It provides an inlet at the patient end or proximal end near the patient's airway for FGI and a corrugated tube extension from the patient to a breathing bag with an open tail. The popoff valve of the Mapleson D configuration is eliminated and, thereby, a potential device failure is removed and valve resistance is eliminated. Exhalation of excess gas and of carbon dioxide occurs through the partially occluded tail of the breathing bag (Fig. 15–10).

This arrangement is designed primarily for controlled respiration. In this system, FGF is close to the patient, while the outlet is remote. If a bag tail is used and partially occluded by a clamp, the exhalation valve may be eliminated and exhalation permitted through the tail.[70] FGF should be between one and one half to two times the patient's calculated minute ventilation to prevent CO_2 accumulation during controlled breathing. A simple calculation to achieve this requirement is to deliver a FGF equal to 7 mL/kg body weight × respiratory rate with a minimum FGF of 3 L/min and a maximum FGF of 8 L/min.[71]

COAXIAL BAIN CIRCUIT. A streamlined type of Mapleson D semiclosed circuit in which a FGF tube is positioned inside a corrugated expiratory tube (coaxial circuit) was proposed by Bushman and Robinson[72] and developed in detail by Bain and Spoerel.[73] A lightweight, disposable model of the Bain circuit is popular for use in circumstances where it is desirable to minimize the bulk of the apparatus located at the patient's mouth or head and provide less drag at the face. With this system, the ratio of ventilation to FGF determines the arterial P_{CO_2}. If ventilation is controlled at a minute volume equal to that at rest, a FGI of 70 mL/kg will maintain a normal arterial P_{CO_2} in most patients.[74,75]

The construction of the system is as follows: a corrugated tube attachment with a uniform diameter of 22 mm, about 150 to 180 cm in length, with an internal volume of about 500 mL (about 85 mL/30 cm of tubing). The patient end of the attachment has an internal diameter of 15 mm adaptable to a mask angle or directly to an endotracheal tube.

Exhalation is accomplished either by a popoff valve on a special bag mount with a close reservoir bag or by an open-tailed reservoir bag. Assisted or controlled ventilation can be accomplished by manual compression of the breathing bag or by attaching a respirator directly to the end of the system at the site of the reservoir bag.

In adult patients, a FGI of 7 L/min appears sufficient to prevent CO_2 retention.[76] Nightingale has determined that for most modified Ayre T-system and single tube systems that a FGI of 220 mL/kg/min is needed.[71]

There are advantages to this system in that it is lightweight and requires minimal apparatus at the patient's airway because of the elimination of the delivery tube and valves. Elimination of valves reduces breathing resistance. The system can be used in all age groups, although a smaller attachment is designed for children under 10 years of age. It is ideal for head and neck procedures.

LACK CIRCUIT.[77] This is a coaxial circuit in which fresh gas flows down the main or outer tube, while exhalation occurs through an inner tube of larger diameter than the delivery tube of the Bain cir-

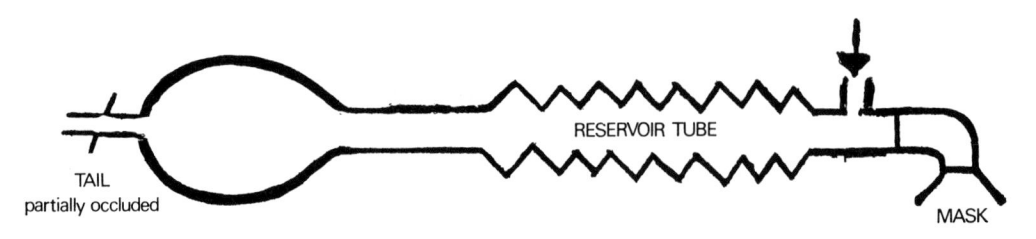

FIG. 15–10. Rees System (T-piece modification). Similar to Mapelson D-arrangement without the exhalation valve.

cuit.[78,79] It is claimed that it is suitable for spontaneous respiration and that it requires a lower FGI.[79]

SEMIOPEN SYSTEMS

DEFINITION.[86] A semiopen system of anesthesia is one in which the patient's respiratory system is open to the atmosphere both on inspiration and expiration. A reservoir is created that is open to the atmosphere but is sufficiently flushed with oxygen or air to dilute and wash out carbon dioxide. Rebreathing of an atmosphere with carbon dioxide is technically absent; atmospheric air either carries or dilutes the anesthetic agent.

SEMIOPEN METHOD.[81] Whenever a towel is folded so as to encircle an open drop mask and form a moat about the mask for the purpose of preventing the escape of anesthetic vapor and gas, a semiopen system is created. In such a method higher concentrations of anesthetic vapor or gas result but the ingress of oxygen diminishes and carbon dioxide increases. One must, therefore, be cautious in the use of towels as well as in the use of extra layers of gauze because hypoxia may result if too many are used.

AYRE T-TUBE SYSTEM

Although Ayre is credited with establishing the basic T-piece system for infants and children, the concept had been introduced during World War I by Sir Ivan Magill.[67,68] The Ayre T-piece and its modifications can also be considered as the prototype of the various single-limb constructions. These have been reviewed by Harrison and classified by Mapleson, combining reservoir bags and exhalation and inhalation ports, as well as their relative placement, in a given system.[82]

The Ayre apparatus consists of a light metal tube, or T-piece, with one end connected to the patient's airway at a face mask or at an endotracheal tube through a rubber connector or through a metal modification of the patient's end of the T-piece (the Bissonnette modification).[83,84] The other end is an open exhalation limb that may be extended by rubber tubes. The interior diameter of the T-piece is not less than 1 cm. Between the two metal ends is a small metal inlet nipple for attachment of the gas–anesthetic hose. This inlet port was "placed at a right angle to the main tube" in the original arrangement,[83,84] but subsequently has been directed toward the patient to form a "Y."

Surgical procedures about the head and neck require an anesthetic breathing system with the following features:[85] equipment and anesthetists removed from the surgical field, no interference or distortion of the surgical field, simple design, and lightweight equipment without excessive drag on the endotracheal tube. It should provide system security and permit control of ventilation without CO_2 retention.

The Ayre T-tube system satisfies many of these requirements.[82,86]

FUNCTION OF THE AYRE T-SYSTEM.[86] The Ayre T-tube technique is an example of either an open or a semiopen system. In the classic technique, the expiratory arm of the T-piece is short and has a rubber extension, which in the usual situations of employment (children, with low tidal air and minute volume), represents a small but definite reservoir. Rebreathing is precluded by the volume of anesthetic gases and oxygen flowing into the system. During inspiration, however, atmospheric air may be drawn into the lung and dilute the anesthetic mixture. It thus functions as an open system. If the expiratory arm is now extended, a larger volume of reservoir air will be available in the extension and be inhaled, so that the system may be considered technically more as a semiopen system. Detailed description of the technique is considered in the ensuing section (Fig. 15–11).

PRACTICAL APPLICATION. The Ayre T-system technique is one of the simplest in inhalation anesthesia. It is safe and essentially free of resistance. There are no bulky appliances or special apparatus. It can be considered the forerunner of the valvular nonrebreathing technique. In the past, the expiratory side arm has been used on an empirical basis to provide a reservoir and diminish breathing of room air. Two basic questions must be answered for the effective use of the system:

1. What is the flow rate of the anesthetic mixture?
2. What is the correct length of reservoir or exhalation tubing?

The flow rate must be sufficiently high to minimize inspiration of atmospheric air and thus preserve the anesthetic mixture.[86] Too low a flow rate will result in air dilution, diminished washout, and rebreathing. Too high a flow rate creates positive pressure in the airway and on the alveoli. A minute flow volume of anesthetic gases of at least two to three times the patient's respiratory minute volume minimizes both rebreathing and air dilution.[87]

Extending the expiratory arm sufficiently to provide a reservoir permits a reduction in the FGF rate appreciably without dilution by air of the anesthetic mixture. Such reservoir arms should be at least 12 mm in diameter to eliminate inspiratory and expiratory resistance. The inflow nipple should be 6 mm in diameter and enter perpendicular to the main lumen of the T-piece; otherwise, an elevated pressure will occur at the point of gas inflow and cause resistance to expiration. If the expiratory arm is too

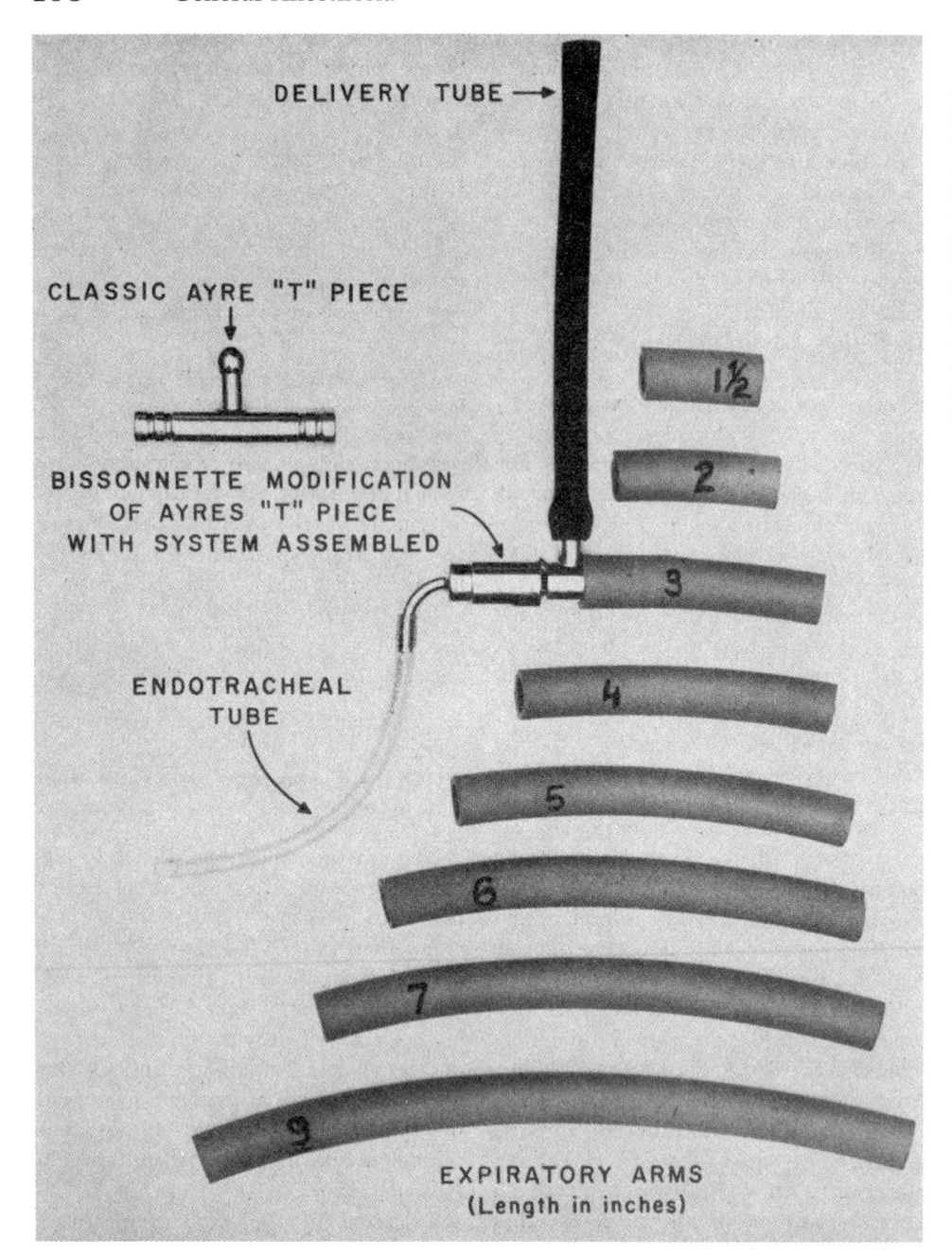

FIG. 15–11. Anesthesia system showing Ayre T-tube assembly. The arm connected to the endotracheal tube is usually designated as the inspiratory arm or patient end; the continuation of this arm beyond the point of delivery of anesthetic gases is designated the expiratory arm. This is extended by varying lengths of rubber tubing according to the principles outlined and the table of specifications.

long, a large unflushed reservoir may exist, and carbon dioxide retention with rebreathing may occur.

ANALYSIS OF SYSTEM. It has been stated that the percentage of air dilution is dependent on the ratio

$$\frac{\text{Volume flow rate of anesthetic mixture}}{\text{Respiratory minute volume (patient)}}$$

It is also assumed that the sine-wave pattern of inspiratory flow rate pertains (Fig. 15–12).

Mathematical studies of the system and of this general principle by Onchi[88] have provided the following information:

1. If the flow rate of gases is three times larger than the respiratory minute volume, air dilution will not occur, even if the length of reservoir tube is zero or very short. Also, with this flow rate, even with long reservoir tubes, dead space and rebreathing is not increased.
2. If the flow rate of gases is two times the respiratory minute volume and the reservoir tube is zero or very short, then air dilution will occur, and the concentration of anesthetic mixture inspired will be 78% with 22% air.

To avoid appreciable air dilution with this flow rate of anesthetic gases, an expiratory arm having

FIG. 15–12. Relation of inspiratory gas demands of a sine-wave pattern of inspiration to available FGF.

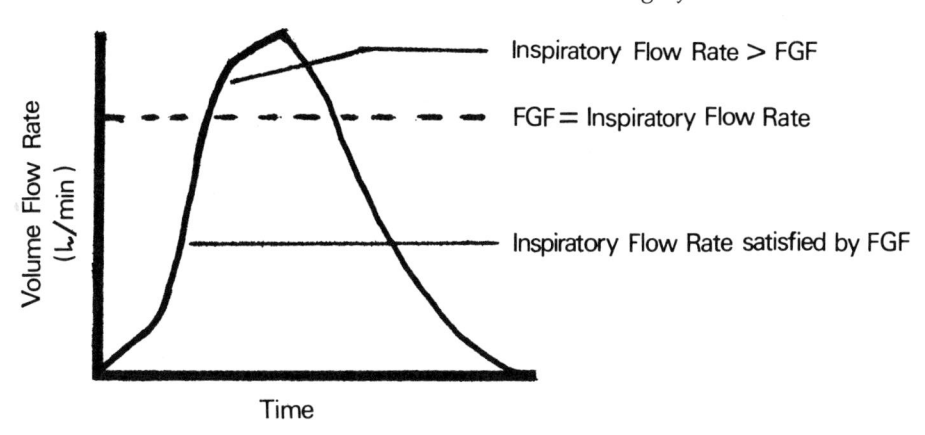

an air capacity of at least 12.5% of the tidal volume is necessary. In practice, with a flow rate of twice the respiratory minute volume, an expiratory arm with an air capacity of 20% of the tidal volume is desired.
3. If the flow rate of gases is equal to the respiratory minute volume, air dilution occurs, and the concentration of the inspired anesthetic mixture is 50% of that delivered.
4. Regarding the development of pressure, flow rates of 5 L/min raise pressure toward the lung less than 5 mm water.

In summary, the following practices are recommended for the simple open Ayre T-system:

1. Classic simple Ayre T-piece and *no* expiratory arm (for infants only): Because the sine-wave pattern of flow rate is characteristic of infants, an FGF three times the minute ventilation will satisfy the respiratory flow rate demands and prevent air from being pulled into the system during inspiration.
2. In infants and children using the Ayre T-piece with an expiratory arm (reservoir): If reservoir has an air capacity of 20% of tidal volume, a flow rate of the breathing mixture of twice the respiratory minute volume is needed to minimize air dilution. These conditions allow only 2% of the expired air to be rebreathed.
3. In the adult breathing pattern of older children: Higher peak flow rates are achieved during respiration and therefore the FGF must be three to five times the minute volume ventilation to avoid air being pulled into the system—but this produces high airway pressure.

If a reservoir arm is added amounting to one third the tidal volume, then FGF only three times the minute ventilation need be provided.

CLINICAL APPLICATION.[89] It is essential to determine respiratory tidal volume and respiratory minute volume in children and to calculate the flow rates and expiratory arm length. Using the medium-sized T-tube having a diameter of 10 to 12 mm and rubber tubes as arms having a similar diameter, the accompanying table of arm lengths and gas flows has been devised (Table 15–9). These arm lengths provide an air capacity of approximately 20% of the tidal respiratory volume. The mathematical value has been calculated and then corroborated by actual volume measurements.

BISSONNETTE MODIFICATION OF AYRE T-TUBE. This modification of the Ayre T-tube consists essentially

TABLE 15–9. AYRE T-TUBE SPECIFICATIONS FOR PRACTICE

Age of Patient	Weight (lb)	Respiratory (rate/min)	Tidal Volume (mL)	Arm Length* (in)	Total Gas Flow (mL)
Newborn	6	50	20	1.5	1800
3 months	12	45	30	2	2700
6 months	16	45	40	3	3200
1 year	20	40	50	4	4000
2 years	30	35	65	5	4500
3 years	35	30	80	6	4800
4 years	40	25	100	7	5500
5 years	45	25	125	9	6250

* The tube lengths are calculated to provide an air capacity of approximately 20% of the tidal air. (Minimal capacity recommended: 12.5% of tidal air.[88] From Collins, V.J., Brehner, B., and Rovenstein, E.A.: The Ayre T-tube technique. Practical applications. Anesth. Analg. 40:392, 1961.

of molding the patient arm of the main metal tube and incorporating a female connector whose internal circumference is tapered. This permits easy insertion of a slip joint or other fitting from an endotracheal tube or breathing mask and eliminates the use of rubber tubing to make connections within the circuit.[90]

MODIFICATION OF AYRE SYSTEM. Modification of the Ayre T-system by the addition of a corrugated reservoir tube to the expiratory arm overcomes some of the original's disadvantages, which include a lack of a reservoir, the occurrence of air-breathing and the dilution of the anesthetic mixture, a high-flow gas anesthetic delivery, and poor control of ventilation. The modification is often designated as a Mapleson E configuration. A tidal reservoir is provided, air dilution of the anesthetic mixture is prevented, and rebreathing is minimized by an appropriate anesthetic–diluent inflow volume. In most T-piece systems, an inflow of two and one half to three times the respiratory minute volume prevents CO_2 retention.[82,88] Spontaneous breathing is required, but ventilation can be assisted or even controlled by intermittent occlusion of the exhalation port (see Fig. 15–9).

BARAKA DOUBLE-T-SYSTEM.[91] A system using two T-pieces has been designed by Baraka to permit a flexible system for both spontaneous breathing and controlled respiration. This is a practical combination of the Magill and Rees design. A T-piece is attached to either side of the reservoir tubing (60 mL capacity) and allows an easy change of the point of gas inflow. The anesthetist may introduce his breathing mixture either near the patient for controlled respiration or remote for spontaneous respiration, and exhalation occurs conversely.

During spontaneous respiration, rebreathing is negligible in the Magill type of arrangement *if* FGI equals the minute volume of the child; however, in the Rees system, at least double the minute volume is required to eliminate rebreathing. During controlled ventilation, rebreathing is approximately the same with both arrangements.

OPEN INHALATION SYSTEMS (CARBON DIOXIDE WASHOUT METHODS)

DEFINITION. An open anesthesia system is one in which there is no reservoir bag or valves and that allows the patient to have ready access to the atmosphere both on inhalation and exhalation. Exhaled carbon dioxide is diluted and "washed" away into the room air.[76–81]

"Open drop" anesthesia is one type of open system, as are gravity and insufflation methods. The simple Ayre T-tube is also an open system. A slightly more complex Ayre T-tube modification with an extended exhalation arm, a direct patient connection, and an FGI is a semiopen system often referred to as a Mapleson E configuration. A classification of open-inhalation system appears in Table 15–10. With open systems and their simple equipment, malfunctions are unlikely.

These systems were used commonly up to 1960. The patients breathe spontaneously. The anesthetic gases or vapors are delivered from the anesthesia machine by a tube that is inserted under the mask. The anesthetic liquid is dropped onto layers of gauze stretched over a frame shaped like a face mask.

Rebreathing usually does not occur when open systems are used. The inhaled anesthetics are diluted by room air, unless high flows are used from the anesthesia machine. An increase in minute ventilation further dilutes inhaled anesthetics with atmospheric air, resulting in lighter levels of anesthesia, while a decrease in minute ventilation may result in a deeper anesthetic level. Thus, it is difficult to predict the anesthetic depth from the anesthetic concentrations delivered from the anesthesia machine, and reliance on clinical signs is essential. Since exhaled gases are spilled to atmospheric air, operating room pollution is an undesirable feature of open systems. Another problem is the difficulty or inability of the system (depending on the method used) to permit assisted or controlled ventilation if required.

OPEN DROP INHALATION METHOD[80–81]

In this technique, a liquid anesthetic agent is dropped onto a gauze surface in order to be vaporized, and the vapor is then drawn into the lungs mixed with atmospheric air inhaled through the mask. This technique was popularized for the use of the volatile anesthetics ether, ethyl chloride, divinyl ether, and chloroform. Although it can be used for newer volatile anesthetics, the development of superior systems of anesthetic administration has made open drop inhalation chiefly of historical interest. However, its historical importance warrants

TABLE 15–10. CLASSIFICATION OF OPEN INHALATION SYSTEMS

OPEN SYSTEMS
Open drop method
Gravity method
Insufflation method
Ayre T-tube without expiratory arm; Slocum hook (cheiloplasty)
SEMIOPEN SYSTEMS
Semiopen drop (with moat)
Ayre T-tube with expiratory arm.
T-tube modifications
Baraka double-T-piece
Magill original system

brief review of the technique, which may still be used in some developing countries.

A sponge was first used by Morton as a means to confine the anesthetic agent.[92] This sponge was actually placed over the nose and mouth of the patient, and asphyxia invariably accompanied the anesthetic procedure. Warren also employed a sponge but later shifted to a truncated cone. At Bellevue Hospital, a newspaper folded into the form of a cone open at both ends was used and called the Bellevue mask. In 1857, John Snow constructed a mask that was connected to a small cylindrical container resting in an evaporating pan. The anesthetic agents were placed in the container, and warm water was placed in the pan. Thus, a good concentration of vapor was obtainable. A similar ether inhaler was developed in 1872 by Morgan of Dublin. Later, Prince developed a gauze evaporating surface over a wire, which has been designated the Ochsner (or Ferguson) mask.[93,94] At about the same time, Yankhauer developed a gauze evaporating surface over a screen. This has been referred to as the Yankhauer–Gwathmey mask.[95]

PROCEDURE. Equipment is simple and consists of three items: a mask, a container of liquid anesthetic, and a dripper.[80,81]

The mask is designed to provide a surface for volatilizing liquid agents and a means for confining the anesthetic agent. The Yankhauer or Ochsner mask is most suitable and was widely used. It consists of 6 to 12 layers of gauze covering a wire or screen. The most effective number of gauze layers is 8 in temperate climates. In warm climates, one usually increased the layers of gauze to 12; and in cold climates, one decreased the number of layers to 6. This rule enabled one to better contain an anesthetic concentration of agent beneath the mask.

The dripper may be prepared by using a safety pin stuck through the cap of the ether can. This allows air to enter the can at one point of puncture and the ether to drop out of the other. However, the dropping rate and drip size is quite uneven. Another simple arrangement and the preferred method is a dripper arrangement made by cutting two notches into a suitable cork opposite each other, one notch being larger than the other; into the larger of the notches a wick of either gauze or cotton is set (Fig. 15–13). The wick should be long enough to reach to the bottom of the container and the other end should come to a fine point beyond the cork. The liquid rises to the tip of the wick by capillary action and, indeed, provides a steady smooth drop. The mask selected should be appropriate to cover the face and nose but as small as possible to minimize dead space.

TECHNIQUE OF OPEN DROP.[78–81] Administration should begin slowly and the agent given smoothly. The entire vaporizing area should be used. Altering the rate of drip rapidly, suddenly, increasing concen-

THE DRIPPER
(A simple type)

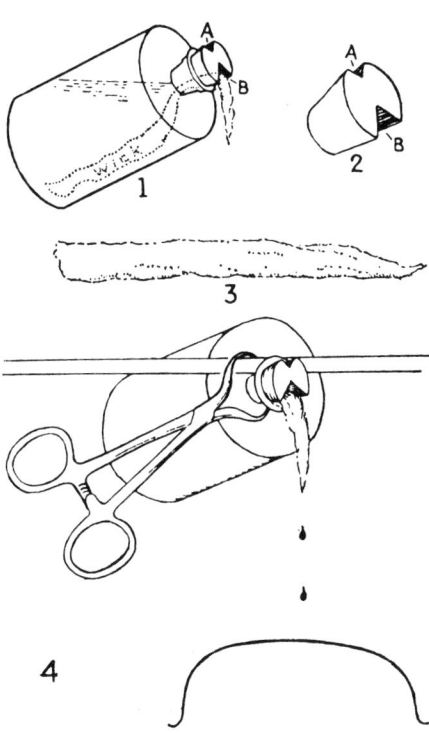

FIG. 15–13. *1*, the container of the anesthetic liquid; *2*, the cork with two notches—one small (*A*) and one large (*B*); *3*, the wick—a strip of gauze or cotton long enough to reach to the bottom of the container and coming to a fine point at the outer end; *4*, arrangement for convenience in maintaining a constant drip—the dripper may be fixed above the mask to a gooseneck support or to a screen by means of a bull's horn forceps. From AMA Committee on Anesthesia. Council on Pharmacy and Chemistry: *Fundamentals of Anesthesia*, 1st ed. Chicago, AMA Press, 1942.

trations of drug, or any irregularity is unpleasant. Do not pour ether! An initial ether vapor concentration of 3% is irrespirable for a conscious patient.

An approximate dropping rate with the percentage concentrations of ether under the mask is as follows:

	Drops	Percent Concentration
First minute	12	1
Second minute	25	3
Third minute	50	6
Fourth minute	100	10–12

The last is approximately total saturation of the usual Yankhauer mask. Once surgical anesthesia is established, a concentration of 6% is needed for maintenance of anesthesia. As for the dropping rate, it should be remembered that the object is to produce narcosis, and whether this is done with 20 or 200 drops is unimportant.

In humid atmosphere, water vapor in the exhaled air may condense on the mask and saturate the gauze because of the cooling effects of vaporized agents. This water slows vaporization of the agent and impedes respiration. It is recommended that additional masks be prepared before anesthesia and that several changes be made during conduct of anesthesia. A saturated mask should be changed for a dry one.

Induction should be started with the mask held a few inches above the face after a word of explanation and instruction to the patient to breathe naturally. A slow rate of drip is begun, about one for each breath, as the mask is gradually lowered. Thereafter, the rate of administration is increased.

The agent is administered as long as the patient continues to breathe naturally. Administration is immediately discontinued if breath-holding, laryngospasm, or coughing occurs. It is resumed when breathing is in order.

Maintenance is achieved by a dropping rate of one half that is required for induction. With each successive hour of anesthesia, the dropping rate should again be drastically curtailed; a rule of thumb is that the dropping rate should be halved with each hour.

PHYSIOLOGY. Safety and practicality of open drop administration of anesthesia is dependent upon the freedom with which air is able to pass into and out of the mask (Fig. 15–14). It is quite possible to have oxygen lack and an accumulation of carbon dioxide if there is an impedance. Though the method is called "open," it is open only as long as atmospheric air is truly accessible to the space beneath the mask. The administrator should not wrap the mask in towels. It is well to remember that air is the source of the oxygen supply to the patient. Under the mask during open administration of anesthetic agents is a constantly changing mixture of the following:[97] room air, anesthetic vapors, and exhaled gases with reduced amount of oxygen, carbon dioxide, and water vapor. As ether administration by open system progresses, there is a steady reduction of the oxygen tension (Fig. 15–15). The ether vapor has a diluting effect on atmospheric gases, especially oxygen. Therefore, supplementary oxygen should be provided. Oxygen may be flowed under a mask by means of a beveled delivery tube or a nasal catheter; as little as 500 mL/min flow under the mask will elevate the PaO_2. As ether vapor is added, the constituents of the air and of the exhaled gases are changed in their concentrations as shown:[98]

	Preanesthetic	Induction	Stage III
Nitrogen	80%	76%	72%
Oxygen	20%	19%	18%
Ether	0%	5%	10%

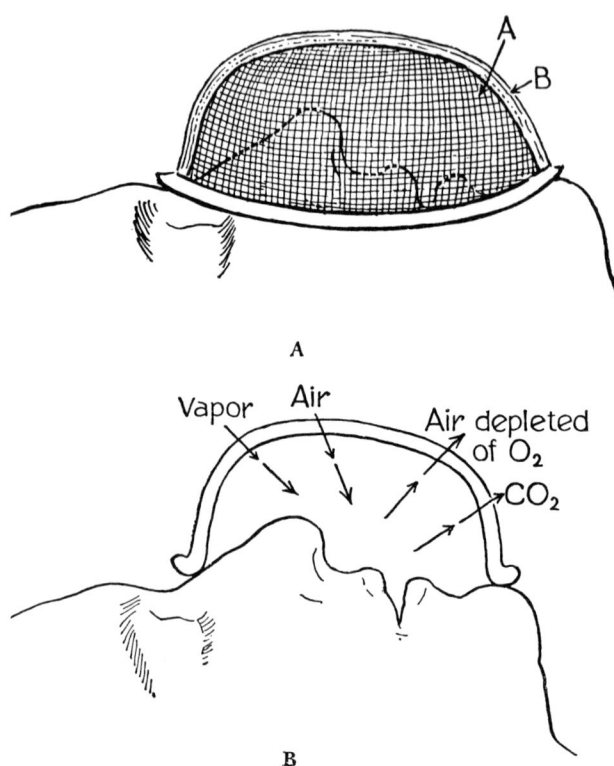

FIG. 15–14. (Top), Open drop anesthesia. A, Wire frame; B, 6 to 12 layers of gauze. (Bottom), Exchange of gases in open method. Composition of inhaled atmosphere depends on size and fit of mask, thickness of gauze, position of head, tidal and minute respiratory volumes, temperature, humidity, moisture, movement of room air, and amount and distribution of liquid anesthetic agent on the gauze. From AMA Committee on Anesthesia. Council on Pharmacy and Chemistry: *Fundamentals of Anesthesia*, 3rd ed. Philadelphia, W. B. Saunders Co, 1954.

As the concentration of ether rises in the inhaled atmosphere, a gradient is established with the blood stream and eventually the brain. The lipids in the brain tissue are the first to become saturated.[99] This is followed by saturation of the lipids in other organ tissues. To achieve satisfactory saturation of the brain and also achieve the various planes of anesthesia, a certain degree of ether concentration in the blood stream must be attained. When plane 1 of stage III is attained, there is about 100 mg/dL ether in the blood stream. In plane 2, approximately 110 mg/dL ether is present. In plane 3, 130 mg/dL ether and in plane 4, about 140 mg/dL is found in the blood stream.[100]

ADVANTAGES AND DISADVANTAGES OF OPEN SYSTEMS. Simplicity of equipment and technique is paramount. It is generally difficult to administer an overdose of anesthetic agent by the open system in contrast to closed system techniques. Hence, there is a wide margin of safety. Adaptability to primitive operating situations is obvious.

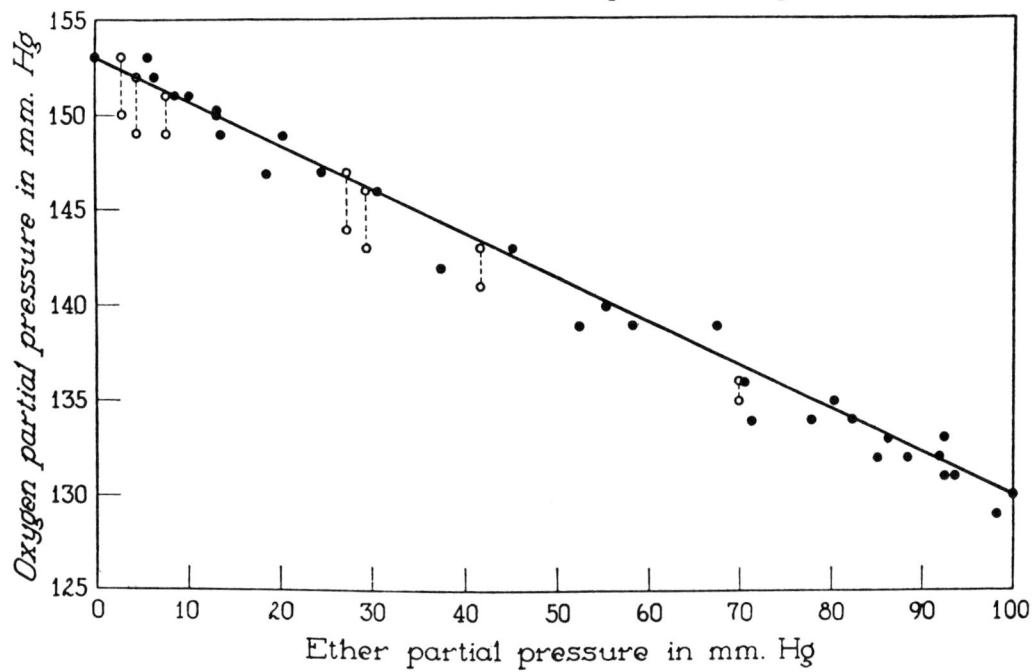

FIG. 15–15. Oxygen-diluting effect of ether vapor. Solid black line represents calculated dilution of ether vapor with oxygen. Dots are observations. From Faulconer, courtesy of Anesthesiology.

On the other hand, the composition of inhaled vapors is quite variable. It is relatively difficult to maintain a smooth and even concentration of anesthetic agent. There is a great deal of waste, and in warm operating rooms, the vapor concentration needed for anesthesia may not be attainable. Of major importance is the fact that the oxygen supply is dependent upon the atmosphere, and by improper application of the equipment, the oxygen concentration is readily compromised. Thus, vapor concentration and oxygen tension are not controlled, and carbon dioxide excess is prone to develop. There is much waste, and the fire hazard is ever present. Skin irritation or erythema of the face and burns of the face and eyes (sometimes referred to as ether burns) may occur. Eye protection can be achieved by placing a towel over the eyes or by use of an ophthalmic solution.* Despite protective measures an irritative conjunctivitis is frequent. The technique allows the patient to inhale gases that are both cold and irritating. Lastly, anesthetic pollution of the operating room is a problem.

GRAVITY ADMINISTRATION[80,81,101]

Anesthetic gases and/or vapors can be delivered from an anesthesia machine to a mask held above the patient's face or by the delivery tube so held. This allows the mixture to flow over the face and diffuse into the atmosphere above the face, whereupon it is then inhaled by the patient. As the patient becomes sleepy, the mask is lowered until it rests on the face and a proper fit is then secured. This is a commonly performed inhalation induction technique in pediatric practice.

Because anesthetic gases and vapors and oxygen are heavier than air (ethylene is an exception but is no longer used), they gravitate to the patient's face and are then inhaled.

INSUFFLATION

Insufflation is defined as the delivery of a directed stream of an anesthetic gas mixture (or oxygen for inhalation therapy) directly into the mouth by a metal hook (Slocum) or into the pharynx by an oropharyngeal or nasopharyngeal catheter.[80,81,103]

The anesthetic is vaporized in air or oxygen from a gas machine and the flow is directed by the hook or catheter in a stream into the mouth or pharynx. The mixture is delivered under varying degrees of pressure related to the portion of the compressed gas cylinder pressure permitted by the size of the opening of the flowmeter valve. The unit pressure beyond the flowmeter forcing a unit volume flow is approximately the square of the volume flow rate,

---
* Methyl or isopropyl cellulose (no ointments)

that is, the volume flow rate of gas is approximately the square root of the applied pressure at the orifice of the flowmeter.

Low-flow rates of 2 to 4 L/min are under pressures of 5 to 10 mm Hg; high-flow rates of 6 to 8 L/min are under pressures of 20 to 25 mm Hg. Flow rates above 10 L/min are not used in catheter techniques.[102]

The pressure beyond the flowmeter is modified by the catheter size. The delivery is confined to the tip of the mouth hook or catheter tip and hence is physically gas *infusion* or insufflation.

The catheter sizes vary: No. 4F to No. 6F for children, No. 6F to No. 12F for adults.

An extended catheter may be placed in the trachea and enable the delivered gas mixture to mix more completely with trochopulmonary gases. In these methods, there is lessened dilution by atmospheric air than in the open drop or gravity technique and, if the catheter is placed near the carina, there is minimal rebreathing. The inflow of the anesthetic mixture should be about 8L of gas per minute.[103]

During insufflation, the insufflated anesthetic gas mixture is diluted with varying amounts of room air and the final mixture is inhaled to reach the alveolar system. If the Slocum mouth hook is used, there is significant dilution with air; with the pharyngeal catheter, dilution is moderate; with the tracheal catheter, dilution is least. With the pharyngeal or tracheal placement of the catheter, the dilution is related to the dead space of the pharynx or the minimal volume of the trachea.

Exhalation occurs around the insufflation device and is spilled directly into the atmosphere. The expired air does not pass through the catheter tube or hook.

Although not commonly used at present, the method offers the advantage of simple equipment and minimal resistance to breathing.

Insufflation techniques are still used in conjunction with topical anesthesia for laryngoscopy, bronchoscopy, or similar endoscopic techniques.

If a small endotracheal tube is in place and anesthetic gases are allowed to flow continuously through the tube into the trachea, a system of endotracheal insufflation is created. The endotracheal tube should only partially fill the glottic chink, and there must be adequate free space for exhalation to occur around the tube and through the glottis.[104] The patient should be breathing spontaneously. If dependence is placed on diffusion respiration in apneic subjects, it will be found that oxygenation will be adequate but also that carbon dioxide will accumulate.

The ventilating bronchoscope follows the principles of insufflation in which a small side arm nipple and delivery tube attached to the bronchoscope carry oxygen and/or anesthetic mixture into the trachea. The fiberoptic bronchoscope is equipped with an incorporated delivery channel for oxygen.

This technique represents an early application of Jet Ventilation. By intermittent opening and closing of the delivery tube, pressure surges are created with surges of gas flow—a jet effect. High frequencies of these surges cause extensive mixing of fresh gas with pulmonary gas, causing dilution and washout.

Disadvantages include the waste of anesthetic gases and the variable composition of the inhaled mixtures. There is inability to assist respiration in the absence of a reservoir bay, but some ventilation and oxygenation can be accomplished by a higher inflow rate and the intermittent occlusion of the delivery tube to produce a jet effect.

The method contrasts with the open drop of liquid anesthetic technique or the flow of anesthetic gases above the face representing the gravity technique. By these methods, the anesthetics *diffuse* into the atmosphere and are highly diluted.

HUMIDITY AND HEAT EXCHANGE IN BREATHING SYSTEMS

INTRODUCTION. Exhaled alveolar gas is saturated with water vapor, which at body temperature (37°C) has a partial pressure of 47 mm Hg. The specific heat of gases is so low that they cool nearly to room temperature almost immediately upon exhalation. In a circle system, the exhaled gases are rewarmed as they pass through the soda lime in the absorber and again cool to near room temperature before being inhaled.[105] If the cooled gas remains saturated with water vapor at 20°C, its partial pressure of water can be only 17.5 mm Hg, with the rest having been lost by condensation. It may literally "rain out" within the circle. When this gas is then rewarmed, it will contain water at a vapor pressure of only 17.5 mm Hg unless additional water and the energy to vaporize it are supplied. This is accomplished during normal breathing by an exchange of heat and water in the nose and upper pharynx. Inspired dry gas is humidified and warmed by the mucosa, which itself is partially dried and cooled. The mucosa then serves as a condenser for the next expiration. As water condenses on the mucosa of the nasopharynx, the mucosa is warmed and moistened, preparing it for the next inspiration. About two thirds of the alveolar water is conserved by this exchange process. Mouth breathing, and especially tracheal intubation, bypass the natural exchanger, putting the burden of humidification on the tracheobronchial tree.

WATER AND HEAT LOSS. In anesthetic systems in which fresh dry gas is inhaled, humidity is lost with each breath, the loss averaging about 10 mL/hr.[107] The heat lost with evaporation of this water is about 5 kcal/hr, or less than 10% of the basal metabolic rate.[106] Heat and water losses are decreased in those systems in which some gas is rebreathed and therefore some moisture is inhaled. To-and-fro systems provide the highest inspired moisture content and nonrebreathing systems the lowest. Closed or low-inflow (<2.5 L/min) circle systems retain some moisture (about 18 mm Hg) in the inspired gas, but additional warmth and humidity must be provided by the patient breathing from the system. Heat loss in low-flow or closed circle systems can be as low as 1 kcal/hr and water loss as low as 3 mL/hr.[107–109] These values increase as the total flow through a circle filter system is increased.

While adult man is able to breathe fresh dry gases for many hours without evidence of serious injury, infants and small children may develop dehydration and hypothermia rather quickly, especially if high-flow semiclosed systems are used.[110] Therefore humidification is necessary for infants and children, and even for adults if prolonged respiration of dry gases is contemplated. A wide variety of devices are available for providing humidity, with or without heating the humidified gas. They may be grouped into two broad classes: those providing water vapor and properly called humidifiers, and those providing aerosols (droplets), usually with specified or controlled particle diameter. Either type can be adapted to most anesthetic systems.

HUMIDIFIERS. The simplest type of humidifier is the "artificial nose," which consists of wetted low-resistance metal, felt, or plastic screens added to the breathing circuit. Its value as a humidifier for anesthetic gases has been difficult to document.[111,112] Humidifiers used in anesthetic circuits are similar in design to anesthetic vaporizers. The gas to be humidified passes over a large water surface or bubbles through the water. The humidifier may or may not be heated. In heated humidifiers, it is customary to warm the gas to about 40°C to allow for some loss of heat and water in the breathing circuit between the humidifier and the patient. The current to the humidifier is usually cut off if the reservoir goes dry, and thermostats are necessary to prevent overheating. The optimal design would sense the temperature at the Y-piece, and several units have this capability. Heated water baths are important sources of bacterial contamination and nosocomial infections and hence must be sterile initially and then replaced frequently. Inexpensive disposable humidifiers are available and have been shown to be satisfactory for routine use.[113,114]

AEROSOL DEVICES. Several types of devices will generate aerosols or droplets. The perfume atomizer, sprayer for topical anesthetics, and aerosol dispenser for paint, hair spray, or deodorant are functionally similar. Water is broken into myriads or droplets by a blast of gas through a nozzle. Usually the larger droplets are filtered by impaction on a deflector, while the rest travel with the gas. In another device, water is flowed over a sphere with a pin hole in it. Gas under pressure leaves the pinhole, blowing bubbles in the film of water flowing over the sphere. When the bubbles break up, droplets are formed. Anyone who has blown soap bubbles has felt the little droplets hit his face when the bubbles pop. The effect is the same but more rapid without the use of soap to lower the surface tension of water. Another aerosol generator uses a film of water flowing over a screen. Gas passing through the screen blows small, short-lived bubbles that burst, forming droplets. Still other generators use piezoelectric crystals vibrated at ultrasonic frequencies. This creates a microtempest on the surface of a water cup above the crystal, and the air is filled with spray.

Aerosols of water may increase the water content of inhaled gases above 43.3 mg/L, which is the weight of saturated water vapor at 37°C. If the droplet size is of the range of 10 to 100 µm in diameter, the droplets will, in large part, impact on the turbinates and pharyngeal wall. Particles 1 to 10 µm will penetrate into the bronchioles and alveolar ducts, while those 0.5 µm will be inhaled and exhaled with little loss by tissue deposition. The surface area of aerosols may be immense, contributing to rapid evaporation and increase of dry gas humidity toward saturation. However, as the particle diameter decreases, surface tension at the air–water interface creates an increasingly large force opposing evaporation so that the droplets become quite stable. Because not much evaporative loss occurs with small particle size, when isotonic salt solutions are used, the droplets formed remain isotonic.

BACTERIAL CONTAMINATION IN BREATHING SYSTEMS

In view of the possibilities for bacterial contamination of components of anesthetic systems that are reused, the use of sterile, disposable systems whenever possible has become popular. Another approach has been the use of bacterial filters in reusable systems. However, the value of disposable systems and bacterial filters to improving patient care remains to be documented. While it is clear that bacterial counts are lower distal to a bacterial filter and in a presterilized disposable system, the use of these devices does not decrease the incidence of postoperative respiratory infections.[114–116] Washing of circuits with soap and water and drying before use appear to be satisfactory precautions. Bacterial filters will remove particulate matter such as soda lime dust if that should be of concern.

VENTILATION MONITORS

The measurement of tidal volume or minute ventilation is useful during anesthesia and can be accomplished with ventilation monitors in the breathing circuit. Two types of ventilation monitors are available: anemometers and volume displacement meters.

ANEMOMETERS. The most common anemometers use rotating vanes in turbine designs. The measured flow through a fixed cross section is mechanically converted to accumulated volume by clockwork type of gear trains. Flow through the meter is possible in either direction but is measured in only one direction. Turbine anemometers, such as the Wright or Boehringer models, are conveniently sized, reasonably durable, and relatively inexpensive. Though scale readings to 10 mL are possible, there is potential for up to 30 to 40% error in measurements of intermittent flow such as occurs during breathing. Causes of error include inertial delays at the start and stop of flow and from water condensation. Measurement errors may also occur if fresh gas flows continuously around the circle system,[4] if leaks to or from the atmosphere occur, or if the anesthetic system becomes overdistended.

VOLUME DISPLACEMENT METERS. Volume displacement meters are affected by flow in either direction and will not work usefully unless they are properly placed in a circle system or cycled by a ventilator bellows. The Drager volumeter employs a pair of gears that rotate with gas flow (North American Drager, Telford, PA). The rotation is mechanically added by clockwork gears and indicated on a dial. Other volumetric gas meters using bellows, slide valves, and gear chains to measure volume are bulky, hard to clean, and not especially accurate with intermittent flow. They can, however, be very accurate when flow is constant and are useful in respiratory research.

The most common volume displacement device is the collapsible concertina bag incorporated into most anesthesia ventilators. The concertina bag become the counterlung in most anesthesia circuits. During exhalation, it fills, providing a measure of tidal volume. Its performance is predictable, but volumes may not be easily readable to less than 50 mL per breath. Volume displacement devices are subject to the same errors from circuit distensibility and leaks as are other devices.

SCAVENGING OF EXCESS GAS

The general use of flow rates of fresh gases into anesthetic systems in excess of those required to compensate for uptake, metabolism, leaks, or removal of exhaled carbon dioxide results in variable volumes of anesthetic gases and vapors exiting from the breathing circuit. There has been considerable concern that prolonged exposure of operating room and perhaps recovery room personnel to trace concentrations of anesthetic agents may increase their incidence of spontaneous abortion or leukemia or developmental anomalies in their offspring.[117] In a typical operating room ventilated with an air flow 15 times its volume per hour, the excess gases may not be diluted to currently proposed safe levels of nitrous oxide of 25 ppm and halogenated anesthetics of 0.5 ppm.[118] This problem is overcome by collecting the excess gas and absorbing it onto charcoal or, more commonly, by venting it safely.

Methods for collecting the excess gases have been devised for all anesthetic systems except the open system.[119,120] For anesthetic systems having a popoff valve, the typical collection system consists of an airtight hood or cap that encloses the valve but still permits regulation of popoff pressure. For anesthetic systems with no valves or with nonrebreathing valves, special collecting devices have been designed. Methods have also been designed to collect the exhaust from ventilators.

Once collected, excess gases are disposed of by one of three methods. One method is to absorb the gases onto activated charcoal filters. Unfortunately, charcoal will not remove nitrous oxide, so its use does not obviate the need for other scavenging systems. For this reason, charcoal absorption is not widely used for scavenging.

Another method for disposal involves directing the excess gases, through large-bore tubing, to the ventilator grille where the room air is removed.[121] If the air supply to the operating rooms is not recirculated, or only partially recirculated, this method may be sufficient. However, nitrous oxide, 5 L/min, vented into a typical room of 210 m^3 that is ventilated with 15 changes of air per hour would result in average air level of nitrous oxide of 100 ppm. If more than 1/10th of the mixed exhaust were recirculated, the 25 ppm standard for nitrous oxide would be exceeded.

The third method involves continuous aspiration of the collection site by operating room suction. Because the excess gases popoff only during part of the respiratory cycle, popoff flow rate may transiently be very high, up to 50 L/min. This much inflow to most operating room suction systems will transiently degrade the vacuum available for surgical suction or aspiration of secretions. A switch or valve that diverts the suction line to the surgeon's or anesthetist's use on demand has been suggested, but this is clumsy and not often used in practice. A dedicated vacuum line just for the scavenger can be provided. Alternatively, a suction flow of 8 to 10 L/min for each anesthetizing location can de dedicated to scavenging and a number of rooms scavenged with the same vacuum line. If this is done, the excess gases flow into a partially open interface volume, ie, a reservoir, which must be greater than the volume of gas that is popped off with each breath (Fig. 15–16). The interface volume is emptied by the constant suction of 8 to 10 L/min, a flow rate that exceeds the average popoff flow rate.

The scavenged gases must ultimately be returned to the atmosphere. If this occurs within the hospital,

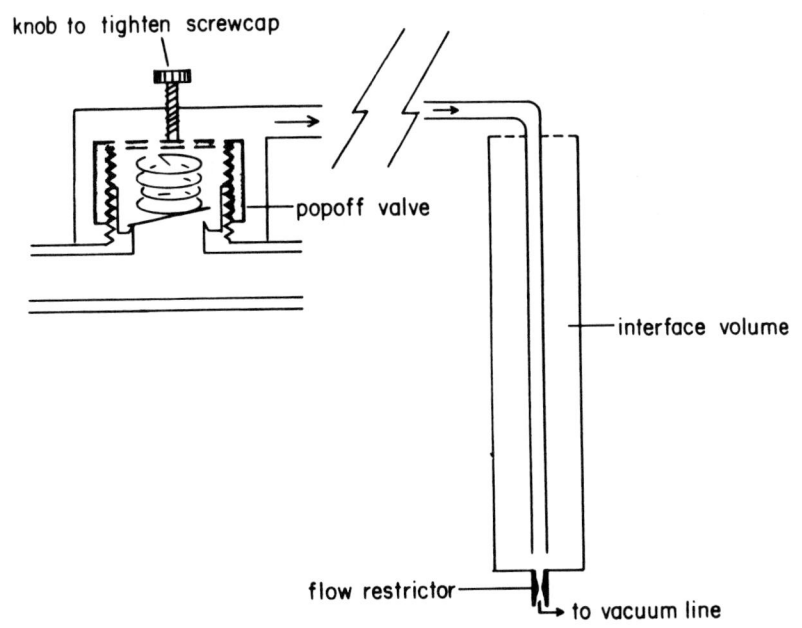

FIG. 15–16. Gas scavenging. Scavenged gas enters an interface volume that is open to the atmosphere at the top so that pressure does not build up in it during the popoff of excess gases. The interface volume is emptied at a flow rate of 8 to 10 L/min into a suction line through a flow restrictor, which permits use of one suction line for the efficient scavenging of many operating rooms. Similar gas collection and scavenging devices have been described for essentially all anesthetic circuits and ventilators. From Lecky, J.H.: The mechanical aspects of Anesthetic pollution control. Anesth. Analg. 56:769, 1977; Whitcher, C., Piziali, R., and Sher, R.: Development and evaluation of methods for the elimination of waste anesthetic gases and vapors in hospitals. Publication No. 75–137. Cincinnati, U.S. Department of Health, Education, and Welfare, Public Health Service, Center for Disease Control, National Institute for Occupational Safety & Health, 1975.

the risks are merely transferred from one group of hospital personnel to another. It is far preferable to exhaust the scavenged gases on the hospital roof.

IATROGENIC CONSIDERATION

Despite continual improvement in the design and function of anesthesia machines and related equipment, patient mishaps resulting from their misuse or malfunction continue to occur. One analysis of preventable anesthesia mishaps occurring in one hospital indicates that most were due to either equipment failures or human errors committed while using equipment.[122] While some of the problems identified were not of a serious nature, many others had the potential for being so. For example, the two most common occurrences were breathing circuit disconnections and inadvertent gas flow changes, either of which has the potential for serious or lethal consequences for the patients involved. From this and other similar analyses come several important recommendations that anesthetists and manufacturers of anesthesia equipment should heed.[123] <u>First</u>, it is essential that the anesthetist be thoroughly familiar with the equipment that he is using so he understands what it is supposed to do and how it is supposed to function. <u>Second</u>, it is equally essential that the anesthetist have a routine for establishing that equipment is functioning properly. <u>Third</u>, it is important that faulty equipment be removed from service and appropriate repairs made before the item is used again. <u>Fourth</u>, anesthetists are well advised to employ monitoring devices that enhance their ability to detect important malfunctions of anesthesia equipment. Such devices might include an oxygen monitor, a ventilator disconnect alarm, and perhaps an end tidal carbon dioxide analyzer or other ventilation monitor to detect circuit disconnections. <u>Fifth</u>, manufacturers should design a piece of equipment as simply as possible to do the job for which it is intended. Needless elaboration or detail may only serve to confuse the user and detract from the basic utility of the device. <u>Finally</u>, all po-

416 *General Anesthesia*

tential equipment malfunctions or errors in their use cannot be anticipated, so anesthetists must be constantly vigilant to their occurrence and be prepared to manage their consequences.[124]

PRINCIPLES AND PHYSICS OF HUMIDITY AND HUMIDIFICATION*

The amount of water vapor an atmosphere can hold depends on temperature. This is because the evaporation of water is related solely to its vapor pressure, which is entirely thermally regulated (Table 15-11). Thus, the humidity of a gas can be expressed as its percent saturation with water vapor at a given temperature (relative humidity) or the actual weight of water vapor held per unit volume of gas (absolute humidity). Absolute humidity can also be expressed in terms of actual water vapor pressure.

Instruments that measure humidity are called hygrometers, and as a rule, indicate relative humidity at a given temperature. The moisture content of a gas or gas mixture can also be measured gravimetrically (by condensation of the water vapor held by a known volume of gas) or by gas chromatography or mass spectrometry.

When the relative humidity of a gas at a given temperature is known, it is possible to calculate its absolute humidity. For instance, a relative humidity of 67% at 23° C can be expressed as 67% of the vapor pressure of water at 23° C. Because Table 15-10 indicates that this vapor pressure is 21 mm Hg, absolute humidity becomes $(21 \times 67) \div 100 = 15.4$ mm Hg. To calculate the weight of water vapor held by a unit volume of gas (usually milligrams of water per liter of gas), use Avogadro's Law, which states that 1 g molecule of water (18 g) will occupy 22.4 L at 0°C and 760 mm Hg (or 18 mg will occupy 22.4 mL). Because water vapor expands by 1/273 of its volume for each 1° C rise in temperature (Law of Charles), 18 mg of water will occupy 24.3 mL at 23° C:

$$22.4 + \frac{22.4 \times 23}{273} = 24.3$$

Because the vapor pressure of water at 23° C is 21 mm Hg (Table 15-11), the percentage of water vapor an atmosphere could hold if it were saturated with moisture at sea level would be $\frac{21 \times 100}{760} = 2.76$ ml/100 mL or 27.6 mL/L. We have shown that 18 mg of water will vaporize to 24.3 mL at 23° C. Thus, 1 mL of water vapor will weigh $18 \div 24.3 = 0.74$ mg at that temperature. The weight of water held in 1 L of an atmosphere saturated with moisture at 23° C will therefore be $27.6 \times 0.74 = 20.4$ mg H$_2$O. And because the humidity is only 67%, absolute humidity becomes $\frac{20.4 \times 67}{100} = 13.7$ mg H$_2$O/L.

Because it is tedious to repeat these calculations, use the curve depicted in Figure 15-17 to convert

* This section prepared by Jack Chalon, Professor, New York University Medical Center.

TABLE 15-11. VAPOR PRESSURE OF WATER IN RELATION TO TEMPERATURE

Temperature °C	Vapor Pressure	Temperture °C	Vapor Pressure
15	12.788	28	28.349
15.5	13.206	28.5	29.185
16	13.634	29	30.043
16.5	14.077	29.5	30.924
17	14.530	30	31.824
17.5	14.998	30.5	32.748
18	15.477	31	33.695
18.5	15.971	31.5	34.668
19	16.477	32	35.663
19.5	17.0	32.5	36.684
20	17.535	33	37.729
20.5	18.086	33.5	38.801
21	18.650	34	39.898
21.5	19.231	34.5	41.024
22	19.827	35	42.175
22.5	20.441	35.5	43.356
23	21.068	36	44.563
23.5	21.714	36.5	45.800
24	22.377	37	47.067
24.5	23.06	37.5	48.365
25	23.756	38	49.692
25.5	24.472	38.5	51.049
26	25.209	39	52.442
26.5	25.965	39.5	53.868
27	26.739	40	55.324
27.5	27.535	40.5	56.81

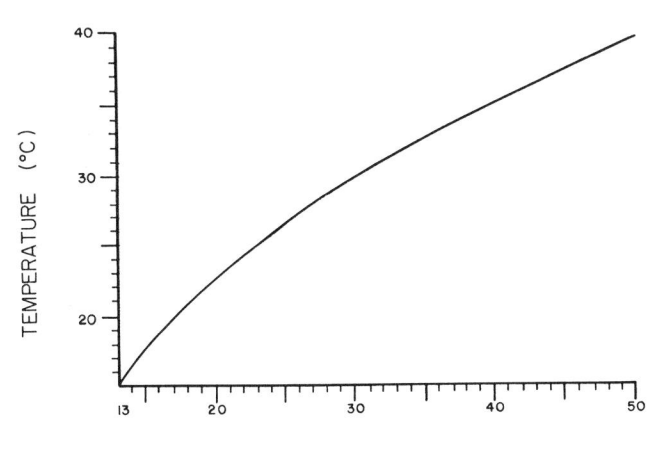

Inhalation Anesthesia—Breathing Systems **417**

FIG. 15–17. Saturated absolute humidity as function of temperature.

relative humidity into absolute humidity expressed as milligrams of water per liter of gas. Alternatively, tables giving saturated absolute humidity in relation to temperature can be drawn.

When an atmosphere is found to have an 80% relative humidity at 30° C, it is easy to calculate from Figure 15–17 that its absolute humidity is 80% of 30 mg H$_2$O/L, or 24 mg H$_2$O/L. If it is cooled to 15° C, its water content drops to 13 mg H$_2$O/L because of a condensation of (24 − 13 mg H$_2$O/L) 11 mg H$_2$O/L. Conversely, if a second atmosphere saturated with 5 mg H$_2$O/L is warmed to 40° C, its relative humidity becomes a fraction of the saturated humidity at 40° C seen as 50 mg H$_2$O/L in Figure 15–17, or (5 × 100) ÷ 50 = a 10% relative humidity at 40° C.

Because vaporization of water depends only on ambient temperature, variations in ambient atmospheric pressure will not affect the amount of water vaporized at the same temperature, but the percentage of water vapor in the gas mixture will vary. For instance, at 20° C, water vapor pressure is 17.5 mm Hg. At sea level the percentage of saturated water vapor would be (17.5 × 100) ÷ 760, or 2.3%. However, if ambient atmospheric pressure falls to 500 mm Hg (eg, in an operating room warmed to 20° C at an altitude of 5000 meters) the saturated water vapor content of the atmosphere would rise to (17.5 × 100) ÷ 500, or 3.5%.

The principles governing the evaporation and condensation of water according to temperature also apply to the minienvironment of anesthetic systems. Anesthetic gases are dried intentionally to prevent clogging of valves and regulators. Therefore, they reduce the amount of water vapor available to the patient. Humidity in anesthetic circuitry depends on (1) ambient temperature, (2) exhalation of water vapor by the patient into the system (32 mg H$_2$O/L), and (3) respiratory minute volume (V̇). The humidity output of systems that recycle anesthetic gases by the neutralization of lime mixtures by carbon dioxide (an exothermic reaction that generates water vapor) is affected by the amount of exhaled carbon dioxide or V̇CO$_2$. In addition, because water is intentionally added to lime granules (5–20% weight for weight), it contributes to the initial humidity output of these systems.

Finally, previous use of all systems will cause water vapor to condense in the circuitry and anesthesia bag or ventilator, thus raising initial humidity output during subsequent use.

TUBE BAG SYSTEMS. Tube bag systems include semiopen and nonrebreathing circuits. Nonrebreathing systems have an extremely poor humidity output because most of the moisture exhaled by the patient is lost through the nonrebreathing valve. The only source of humidity from these circuits is derived from their mechanical dead space, which acts as a heat and moisture exchanger. They are used rarely and should be humidified by either wetting the corrugated breathing tube[123] or adding vaporizers to the circuitry.

Semiopen circuits in use in this country include the Bain circuit, a coaxial version of the Mapleson D system, and the Jackson Rees pediatric system (Fig. 15–18).

The Bain circuit has coaxial breathing and fresh gas delivery tubes. According to Bain,[73] the system should be used solely during mechanical ventilation, provided minute ventilation exceeds the fresh gas inflow (FGI) estimated at 70 mL/kg/min. According to Ramanathan,[124] the circuit used in this

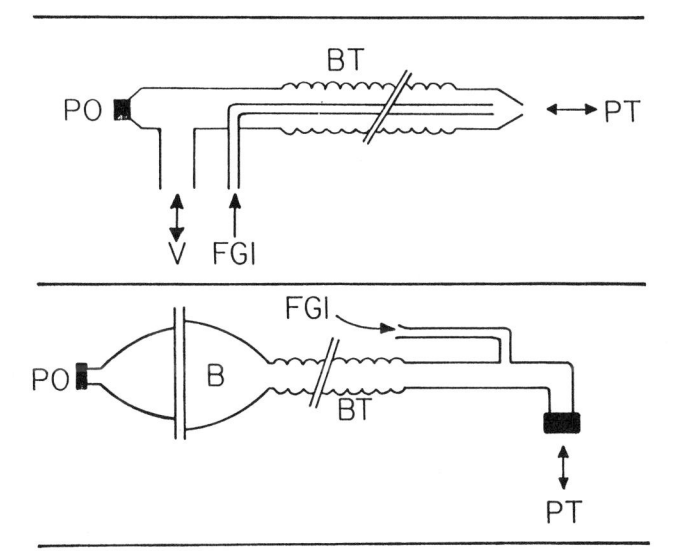

FIG. 15–18. Bain circuit (*top*) and Jackson Rees circuit (*bottom*). PO = pressure release valve, v = ventilator connector, B = anesthesia bag, PT = patient end of system, FGI = fresh gas inflow delivery tube, BT = breathing tube.

fashion delivers an initial absolute humidity of 14 mg H_2O/L, reaching 21 mg H_2O/L after 80 minutes. Rayburn[125] estimated the humidity output of the circuit at 24 to 26 mg H_2O/L after 30 minutes of use with a FGI of 2500 mL/m^2/min and a ventilatory minute volume three times this value. We repeated the experiments both in the laboratory and during clinical anesthesia but were unable to obtain a humidity output exceeding 21 ± 1 mg H_2O/L. It is possible that the difference in measurements were due to insufficient drying of the ventilator used by Rayburn. A previously used ventilator containing approximately 10 mL of water, when placed on a nonrebreathing system with a FGI of 10 L/min, delivers 7 mg H_2O/L, decreasing exponentially to 0.5 mg H_2O/L after 10 hours. It can thus act as a water vaporizer and inadvertently increase experimental figures.

The Jackson-Rees pediatric system (Fig. 15–18) is also a modified Mapleson D system, but the FGI is delivered by a T-piece at the patient end of the circuit and the pressure release valve is inserted at the tail end of the anesthesia bag. In order to ensure adequate venting of expired carbon dioxide, the FGI is usually set at two or three times the ° of the child anesthetized on it. This high FGI vents most of the water vapor exhaled by the patient, causing a low humidity output, especially during spontaneous ventilation when it reaches 3 ± 0.5 mg H_2O/L.[126] Controlling ventilation increases inspired humidity to 8 ± 1 mg H_2O/L, presumably because the resistance of the endotracheal tube is less than that of the pressure release valve, thus increasing rebreathing.

CIRCLE SYSTEMS. Circle systems are anesthetic circuits that recycle anesthetic gases by passing them through a carbon dioxide absorber canister (containing hydroxide mixtures) placed between an inspiratory and an expiratory valve (Fig. 15–19). They can be used as semiclosed or closed systems according to the amount of FGI used.

Semiclosed circle systems have a low humidity output, ranging from 6 mg H_2O/L at the onset of anesthesia to 12 mg H_2O/L within 90 minutes (with a FGI of 5 L/min and a ° of 6 L/min).[107] Closing the system will raise initial humidity to 7.5 mg H_2O/L, reaching 19 mg H_2O/L within 120 minutes.

Variations in the construction of the system will affect its humidity output. Placing the pressure release valve on the expiratory side of the circuit will economize lime, because it will vent some of the expired carbon dioxide, but it will reduce the heat and moisture produced by the quantitative reaction of neutralization of the lime. On the other hand, introducing the FGI into the expiratory end of the circuit, as recommended by Berry,[127] will prevent the dilution of humidified gases reaching the inspiratory valve by the FGI and considerably raise inspired humidity.

A glance at Figure 15–19 will show that builders of circle systems were more preoccupied with ensuring adequate absorption of carbon dioxide than in providing the patient with sufficient inhaled moisture. Gases reaching the bottom of the canister being warmed and humidified by the reaction of neutralization of the lime lose most of their water vapor content in the cool external conduits leading to the inspiratory dome valve. The use of coaxial inspiratory and expiratory limbs, together with the insertion of all external conduits through the center of the lime and the insertion of the FGI into the lid of the canister, will raise inspired moisture.[128] Gases leaving the bottom of the canister will reach the inspiratory dome valve through a conduit heated by the reaction of neutralization of the lime, and the inspiratory limb will be warmed by the surrounding expiratory limb containing warm, moist gases expired by the patient. These modifications will produce an initial inspired humidity to 14 mg H_2O/L and a stabilized humidity to 29 mg H_2O/L within 2 hours (oversaturation by 9 mg H_2O/L at an ambient temperature of 23° C), using a ° of 6 L/min and a FGI of 5 L/min.

Infant circle systems available in this country include the Bloomquist and the Columbia pediatric circuits. The humidity output of the Bloomquist circuit is very low. This is because the dry FGI is delivered on line with gases emerging from the absorber and thus reduce inspired humidity.[129] Thus an infant exhaling 15 mL CO_2/min and anesthetized on a Bloomquist circle system receiving a FGI of 5 L/min will inspire less than 1 mg H_2O/L, while a larger infant exhaling 60 mL CO_2/min will inhale anesthetic gases containing 11 mg H_2O/L if the FGI is reduced to 1 L/min. Reversing the bag and FGI attachments, as recommended by Berry,[127] raises the humidity output of the system. An infant exhaling 15 mL CO_2/min in a system receiving FGI of 5 L/min will now inhale anesthetic gases containing 5 mg H_2O/L, and a child exhaling 60 mL CO_2/min into a Bloomquist circle receiving a FGI of 1 L/min will inhale anesthetic gases containing 26 mg H_2O/L. These figures were obtained only after a 3-hour period of stabilization. At the onset of anesthesia the humidity output of the circuit attained only one third the values quoted above.

Children anesthetized on the Columbia circle system inhale better humidified anesthetic gases. An infant with a $\dot{V}CO_2$ of 15 mL/min on a Columbia circuit receiving an FGI of 1 L/min will inhale 6 mg H_2O/L after a 2-hour stabilization period, while a child with a $\dot{V}CO_2$ of 60 L/min will inhale 20 mg H_2O/L with the same FGI. At the onset of anesthesia inhaled moisture attains only half these values.

Both the Bloomquist and the Columbia pediatric circles provide very little humidity for children with a $\dot{V}CO_2$ of less than 30 mL/min. Applying modifications used on adult systems to raise inspired moisture[128] will effectively humidify infant cir-

FIG. 15–19. A circle absorber system. EDV and IDV = expiratory and inspiratory dome valves, EXPIR. and INSPIR. = expiratory and inspiratory limbs, FGI = fresh gas inflow, PO = pressure release valve, B/V = bag or ventilator, PT = patient attachment.

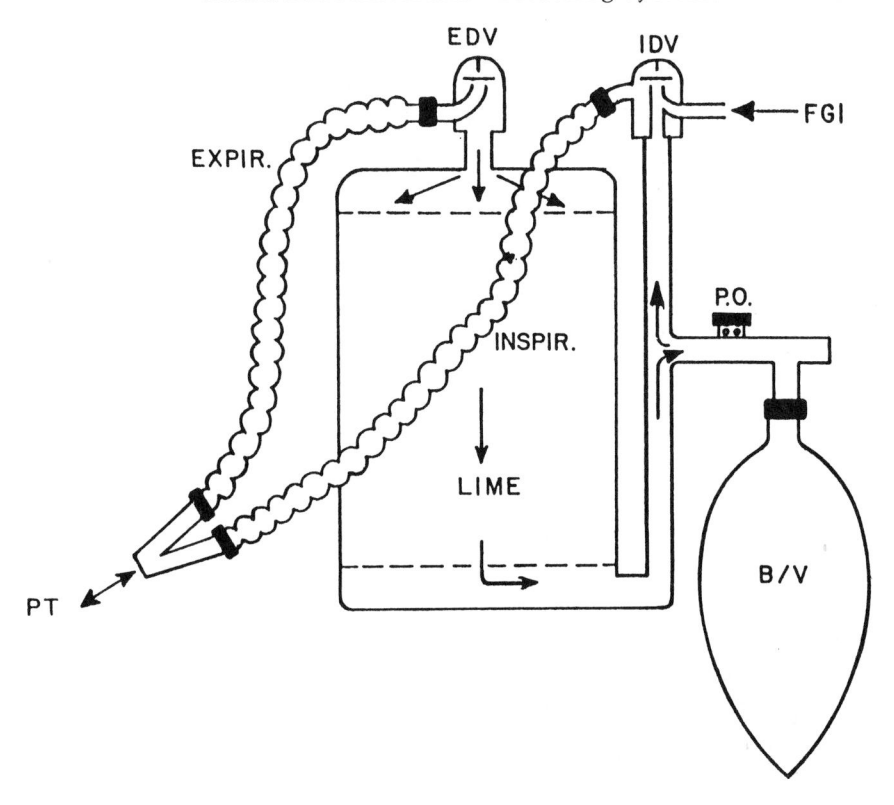

cles.[130] Thus an infant circuit with coaxial breathing tubes receiving FGI into the lid of the canister (in which the inferior compartment is connected to the inspiratory valve by a tube passing through the center of the lime) will provide anesthetic gases containing 14 to 24 mg H_2O/L. It will thus satisfy the needs of small infants and premature babies. The humidity output of the aforementioned systems is summarized in Table 15–12.

The question of the use of high inhaled humidity has been the subject of numerous publications. In an early article, Toremalm showed that poorly humidified gases arrested the tracheal ciliary activity of rats.[132] Chalon[133] later showed that dry anesthetic gases injured the ciliated cells of the tracheal mucosa if anesthesia lasted over 1 hour and recommended a minimum humidity of 12 mg H_2O/L. Marfatia[134] confirmed these findings in histologic sections of the lower airway of rabbits that had breathed dry anesthetic gases.

Knudsen[135] failed to find statistically significant postoperative pulmonary complication rate differences in 82 patients who breathed either dry anesthetic gases or gases saturated with water vapor at 32° C. Chalon[136] compared tracheobronchial cytologic damage and postoperative complication rate in 202 patients who breathed either dry anesthetic gases or gases containing 12 and 33.5 mg H_2O/L. It

TABLE 15–12. HUMIDITY OUTPUT OF THE SYSTEMS DISCUSSED

Type of System	Ventilation (mL/min)	$\dot{V}CO_2$ (mL/min)	FGI (L/min)	$\dot{V}$ (L/min)	Absolute Humidity (mg H_2O/L)
Bain circuit[124]	Controlled	Irrelevant	5	6	21 ± 1
Jackson Rees[126]	Spontaneous	Irrelevant	5	2.5	3 ± 0.5
	Controlled	Irrelevant	5	2.5	8 ± 1
Regular circle system[107]	Controlled	300	1–12.5	5–16	20–10
		200	1–12.5	5–16	19.5–9.5
		100	1–12.5	2.9–6.6	6–16
Modified circle system[128] (adult)	Controlled	200	5	6	28 ± 3
	Controlled	200	1–5	6	29 ± 1.5
Bloomquist[129]					
Unmodified	Controlled	15–60	1–5	1.2–3.6	0.5–11
Modified according to Berry[127]	Controlled	15–60	1–5	1–5	5–26
Columbia[131]					
Pediatric system	Controlled	15–60	1–5	1.2–3.6	3–20
Modified infant circle[130]	Controlled	15–60	1–5	1.2–3.6	14–23

was found that both factors studied diminished exponentially as humidification of inhaled gases increased toward 33 mg H$_2$O/L. In addition, because 12–15% of body heat is lost through the lung, the patient group that inhaled the highest degree of moisture lost the least amount of heat during surgery.[136] It is my personal opinion that the use of humidified anesthetic gases is beneficial to the patient. It prevents mucosal damage, reduces postoperative complication rate, and inhibits postoperative shivering because of reduced heat loss during surgery.

REFERENCES

1a. Moyers, J.: A nomenclature for methods of inhalation anesthesia. Anesthesiology, 14:609, 1953.
1b. Ernst, E.A.: Selection of the Anesthesia Delivery System: From Open Drop to Closed Circuit. Lecture 119: Annual Refresher Courses, A.S.A., Atlanta, GA, Oct. 7–10, 1983.
2. Hamilton, W.K.: Nomenclature of inhalation anesthetic systems. Anesthesiology, 25:3, 1964.
3. Eger, E.I., and Ethans, C.T.: The effects of inflow, overflow and valve placement on economy of the circle system. Anesthesiology, 29:93, 1968.
4. Briere, C., Patoine, J.G., and Audet, R.: Inaccurate ventimetry by fresh gas inlet position. Can. Anaesth. J., 21:117, 1974.
5. Foregger, R.: The classification and performance of respiratory valves. Anesthesiology, 20:296, 1959.
6. Neff, W.B., Burke, S.F., and Thompson, R.: A venturi circulator for anesthetic systems. Anesthesiology, 29:838, 1968.
7. Revell, D.G.: An improved circulator for closed circle anaesthesia. Can. J. Anaesth., 6:104, 1959.
8. Eger, E.I., and Hamilton, W.K.: Positive-negative pressure ventilation with a modified Ayre T-piece. Anesthesiology, 19:611, 1958.
9. Smith, T.C.: Nitrous oxide and low inflow circle system. Anesthesiology, 27:266, 1966.
10. Fisher, D.: Anesthesia equipment for pediatrics. In Pediatric Anesthesia. Edited by G.A. Gregory. New York, Churchill Livingstone, 1983.
11. Stannard, J.N., and Russ, E.M.: Estimation of critical dead space in respiratory protective devices. J. Appl. Physiol., 1:326, 1948.
12. Clappison, G.B., and Hamilton, W.K.: Respiratory adjustments to increases in external dead space. Anesthesiology, 17:643, 1956.
13a. Waters, R.M.: Clinical scope and utility of carbon dioxide filtration in inhalation anesthesia. Anesth. Analg. Curr. Res., 3:20, 1924.
13b. Waters, R.M.: Advantages and technique of carbon dioxide filtration with inhalation anesthesia. Anesth. Analg., Curr. Res., 5:160, 1926.
14. AMA Subcommittee on Anesthesia. In Fundamentals of Anesthesia, 3rd ed. Philadelphia, W.B. Saunders, 1954.
15a. Snow, J.: Inhalation of Vapour of Ether. London, John Churchill, 1947.
15b. Snow, J.: On Chloroform and Other Anesthetics. London, B.W. Richardson, 1958.
15c. Snow, J.: Inhalation of Vapour of Ether. Reprinted from original in Churchillian type. Philadelphia, Lea & Febiger, 1956.
16. Jackson, D.: A new method for the production of general anesthesia with a description of the apparatus used. J. Lab. Clin. Med., 1:1, 1915.
17a. Wilson, R.E.: Preparation of soda lime. J. Ind. Eng. Chem., 12:1000, 1920.
17b. Wilson, R.E., Lamb, C., and Cheney, R.B.: Chemical Warfare IV, 3, 4, 5. Edgewood, MD, U.S. Government Printing Office, 1920.
18. Sword, B.C.: Closed circle method of administration of gas anesthesia. Anesth. Analg., 9:198, 1930.
19. Orkin, L.R., Siegel, M., and Rovenstine, E.A.: Resistance to breathing by apparatus used in anesthesia: I. Endotracheal equipment. Anesth. Analg., 33:217, 1954.
20. Orkin, L.R., Siegel, M., and Rovenstine, E.A.: Resistance to breathing: II. Valves and machines. Anesth. Analg., 36:19, 1957.
21. Proctor, D.F., Hardy, J.B., and McLean, R.: Studies of respiratory air flow. Bull. Johns Hopkins Hosp., 87:255, 1950.
22. Adriani, J., and Rovenstine, E.A.: Experimental studies on carbon dioxide absorption for anesthesia. Anesthesiology, 2:1, 1941.
23. Wilhelm, R., Gilson, W.E., and Orth, O.S.: Pressures produced in the respiratory tract of anesthetized patients during spontaneous, controlled or artificial respiration. Fed. Proc., 67:227, 1947.
24. Hamilton, W.K., and Eastwood, D.W.: A new method of depicting resistance of inhalation anesthetic equipment. Anesthesiology, 17:222, 1956.
25. Cole, F.: Water accumulation as a hazard of rebreathing in anesthesia. J.A.M.A., 151:910, 1953.
26. Mousel L.: Personal communication of unpublished data. Concentrations of carbon dioxide—clinical detection. Mayo Clin. Proc., Department of Anesthesia, 1942.
27a. Wineland, A.J., and Waters, R.M.: The diffusion of anesthetic gases through rubber. Anesth. Analg., 8:322, 1929.
27b. Lowe, H.J., Titel, J.H., and Hagler, K.J.: Absorption of anesthetics by conductive rubber in breathing circuits. Anesthesiology, 34:283, 1971.
28. Orcutt, F.S., and Waters, R.M.: The diffusion of nitrous oxide, ethylene and carbon dioxide through human skin during anesthesia. Anesth. Analg. Current Researches, 12:45, 1933.
29. Stoelting, R.K., and Eger, E.I., II: Percutaneous loss of nitrogen oxide, cyclopropane, ether and halothane in man. Anesthesiology, 30:279, 1969.
30. Cullen, B.F., and Eger, E.I., II: Diffusion of nitrous oxide, cyclopropane and halothane through the human skin and amniotic membrane. Anesthesiology, 36:168, 1972.
31. Cole, W.H.J.: Gas loss and air entry in closed circuit technique anaesthesia. Anaesthesia, 10:46, 1955.
32. McCauley, J.: Trichloroethylene and trigeminal anaesthesia. Brit. Med. J., 2:713, 1943.
33. Firth, J.B., and Stuckey, R.E.: Decomposition of Trilene in closed circuit anaesthesia. Lancet, 1:814, 1945.
34. Carden, S.: Hazards in the use of closed circuit technique for Trilene anaesthesia. Brit. Med. J., 1:319, 1944.
35. Reventos, J., and Lemon, P.G.: The impurities of flurothane. Brit. J. Anaesth., 37:716, 1965.
36. Sharp, J.H., Trudell, J.R., and Cohen, E.N.: Volatile metabolites and decomposition products of halothane in man. Anesthesiology, 50:2, 1978.
37. Grodin, W.K., and Epstein, R.A.: Halothane absorption complicating the use of soda-lime to humidify anaesthetic gases. Brit. J. Anaesth., 54:555, 1982.

38. Eger, E.I., and Strum, D.P.: The absorption and degradation of isoflurane and I-653 by dry soda lime at various temperatures. Anesth. Analg., 66:1312, 1987.
39. Waldon, D.T., et al.: Production and characterization of impurities in isoflurane vaporizers. Anesth. Analg., 64:634, 1985.
40. Morita, S., et al.: Accumulation of methane, acetone, and nitrogen in the inspired gas during closed-circuit anesthesia. Anesth. Analg., 64:343, 1985.
41. Lowe, H.J., and Ernst, E.A.: Quantitative Practice of Anesthesia. Baltimore, Williams & Wilkins, 1981, pp. 11–14.
42. Aldrete, J.A., Lowe, H.J., and Virtue, R.M.: Low Flow and Closed System Anesthesia. New York, Grune and Stratton, 1979.
43. Haggard, H.W.: The absorption, distribution and elimination of ethyl ether. J. Biol. Chem., 59:737, 1924.
44. Eger, E.I.: Applications of a mathematical model of gas uptake. In Uptake and Distribution of Anesthetic Agents, Chaps. 7,8. New York, McGraw-Hill, 1963.
45. Brody, S.: Bioenergetics and Growth. New York, Reinhold, 1945.
46. Guyton, A.C., et al.: Evidence of tissue oxygen demand as a major factor causing auto regulation. Circ. Res. (Suppl.)15:60, 1964.
47. Kleiber, M.: Body size and metabolic rate. Physiol. Rev., 27:511, 1947.
48. O'Leary, P.: Personal communication. Report of procedure at Sinai Hospital of Detroit, 1988.
49. Couto da Silva, J.M., et al.: Closed circuit anesthesia in infants and children. Anesth. Analg., 63:765, 1984.
50. Bloomquist, E.R.: Pediatric circle absorber. Anesthesiology, 18:787, 1957.
51. Smith, R.M.: Anesthesia for Infants and Children, 4th ed. St. Louis, C.V. Mosby, 1980.
52. Graff, T.D., Holzman, R.S., and Benson, D.W.: Acid–base balance in infants during halothane anesthesia with the use of an adult circle absorption system. Anesth. Analg., 43:583, 1964.
53. Reynolds, G.J.: Acid–base equilibrium during C_3H_6 anesthesia and surgery in infants. Anesthesiology, 27:127, 1966.
54. Leigh, M.P., and Belton, M.K.: Pediatric Anesthesia. New York, Macmillan, 1948.
55. Stephen, C.R., and Slater, H.M.: Nonresisting nonrebreathing valve. Anesthesiology, 9:550, 1948.
56. Slater, H.M., and Stephen, C.R.: Anesthesia for infants and children: Nonrebreathing technique. Arch. Surg., 62:251, 1951.
57. Fink, B.R.: A nonrebreathing valve of a new design. Anesthesiology, 15:471, 1954.
58. Lewis, G.: Nonrebreathing valves. Anesthesiology, 17:618, 1956.
59. Stephen, C.R., Ahlgren, E.W., and Bennett, E.J.: Elements of Pediatric Anesthesia. Springfield, IL, Charles C. Thomas, 1970.
60. Frumin, M.J., Lee, A.S.J., and Papper, E.M.: New valve for nonrebreathing systems. Anesthesiology, 20:383, 1959.
61. Reuben, H.: A new nonrebreathing valve. Anesthesiology, 16:643, 1955.
62. Molyneux, L., Pask, E.A.: The flow of gases in a semiclosed anaesthetic system. Brit. J. Anaesth., 23:81, 1951.
63. Woolmer, R., and Lind, B.: Rebreathing with a semiclosed system. Brit. J. Anaesth., 26:316, 1954.
64. Mapleson, W.W.: The elimination of rebreathing in various semiclosed anaesthetic systems. Brit. J. Anaesth., 26:323, 1954.
65. Waters, D.J.: A composite semi-closed anaesthetic system suitable for controlled or spontaneous respiration. Brit. J. Anaesth., 33:417, 1961.
66. Waters, D.J., and Mapleson, W.: Rebreathing during controlled respiration with semi-closed system. Brit. J. Anaesth., 33:374, 1961.
67. Magill, I.: Endotracheal anaesthesia. Proc. R. Soc. Lond., 22:83, 1928.
68. Magill, I.: Endotracheal anaesthesia discussion. Proc. R. Soc. Lond., 60:749, 1967.
69. Rees, G.J.: Anaesthesia in the newborn. Brit. Med. J., 2:1419, 1950.
70. Rees, G.J.: Pediatric anaesthesia. Brit. J. Anaesth., 32:132, 1960.
71. Nightingale, D.A., Richards, C.R., and Glass, A.: An evaluation of rebreathing in a modified T-piece system during controlled ventilation of anaesthetized children. Brit. J. Anaesth., 37:762, 1965.
72. Bushman, J.A., and Robinson, J.S.: A "single" ventilator hose. Brit. J. Anaesth., 40:796, 1968.
73. Bain, J.A., and Spoerel, W.E.: A streamlined anaesthetic system. Can. J. Anaesth,. 19:426, 1972.
74. Bain, J.A., and Spoerel, W.E.: Flow requirements for modified Mapleson D system. Can. J. Anaesth., 20:629, 1973.
75. Bain, J.A., and Spoerel, W.E.: Carbon dioxide output and elimination in children under anaesthesia. Can. J. Anaesth., 24:533, 1977.
76. Bain, J.A., and Spoerel, W.E.: Low flow anesthesia utilizing a single limb circuit. In Low Flow and Closed System Anesthesia. Edited by J.A. Aldrete, H.J. Lowe, and R.M. Virtue. New York, Grune and Stratton, 1979, pp. 151–164.
77. Lack, J.A.: Theatre pollution control. Anaesthesia 31:259, 1976.
78. Humphrey, D.: The Lack Magill and Bain circuits anaesthetic breathing system: A direct comparison in spontaneously breathing anaesthetized adults. J. R. Soc. Med., 75:513, 1982.
79. Humphrey, D.: A new anaesthetic breathing system combining Mapleson A, D, and E principles. Anaesthesia, 38:361, 1983.
80. Guedel, A.E.: Inhalation Anesthesia, 2nd ed. New York, Macmillan, 1951.
81a. AMA Committee on Anesthesia. Council on Pharmacy and Chemistry: Fundamentals of Anesthesia, 3rd ed. Philadelphia, W.B. Saunders Co., 1954.
81b. AMA Committee on Anesthesia. R.M. Waters, Chairman. 1st ed. Chicago, AMA Press, 1942.
82. Harrison, G.A.: Ayre's T-piece: A review of its modifications. Brit. J. Anaesth., 36:115, 1964.
83. Ayre, P.: Endotracheal anesthesia for babies with special reference to hare-lip and cleft palate operations. Anesth. Analg., 16:330, 1937.
84. Ayre, P.: Anaesthesia for hare-lip and cleft palate in babies. Brit. J. Surg., 25:131, 1937.
85. Ayre, P.: Endotracheal anaesthesia with the T tube. Brit. J. Anaesth., 28:520, 1956.
86. Mapleson, W.W.: Ayre-T piece breathing system. Brit. J. Anaesth., 26:323, 1954.
87. Inkster, J.S.: Volume flow of gases in T-piece systems. Brit. J. Anaesth., 28:512, 1956.
88. Onchi, Y., Hayashi, T., and Ueyama, H.: Studies on the Ayre-T piece techniques. Far East J. Anesth., 1:30, 1957.
89. Collins, V.J., Brenner, B., and Rovenstine, E.A.: The Ayre T-Tube technic. Practical application. Anesth. Analg., 40:392, 1961.

90. Bissonnette, B.: T-piece connection. *In* Foregger Catalogue. 1956.
91. Baraka, A., and Brandstater, B.: Rebreathing in a double T-piece system. Brit. J. Anaesth., *41*:47, 1969.
92. Keys, T.E.: The History of Surgical Anesthesia. New York, Schuman's, 1945.
93. Prince, L.H.: An ether mask with an evaporating surface. Chicago Med. Rec., *12*:232, 1897.
94. Tovell, R.M.: Useful agents and methods for gynecological and obstetrics. *In* Obstetrics and Gynecology, Vol. 3. Edited by A.H. Curtis. Philadelphia, W.B. Saunders Co., 1935, p. 989.
95. Gwathmey, J.J.: Anesthesia, 1st ed. New York, Appleton, 1914.
96. Faulconer, A.: A study of physical methods for the determination of the tension of ether vapor in air-ether mixtures. Anesthesiology, *10*:1, 1949.
97. Faulconer, A., and Latterell, K.E.: Tensions of oxygen and ether vapor during use of semi-open, air-ether method of anesthesia. Anesthesiology, *10*:247, 1949.
98. Branch, D.: Ether anesthesia—A true gas technic. Anesth. Analg., *32*:217, 1953.
99. Draper, W.B., Whitehead, R.W., and Spencer, J.N.: Studies on diffusion respiration, III. Alveolar gases and venous blood pH of dogs during diffusion respiration. Anesthesiology, *8*:524, 1947.
100. Haggard, H.W.: Absorption fate and elimination of di-ethyl ether. J. Biol. Chem., *59*:737, 1924.
101. Stephen, C.R.: Technics in pediatric anesthesia. Anesthesiology, *13*:77, 1952.
102. Adriani, J.: The Chemistry and Physics of Anesthesia, 2nd ed. Springfield, IL, Charles C. Thomas, 1962.
103. Rovenstine, E.A., Taylor, I.B., and Lemmer, K.E.: Oropharyngeal insufflation of oxygen: Gas tensions in bronchus. Anesth. Analg., *15*:10, 1936.
104. Reiman, J.: Personal communication. Report—Section on Anesthesia. AMA convention, 1956.
105. Déry, R., et al.: Humidity in anesthesiology, II. Evolution of heat and moisture in the large CO_2 absorbers. Can. J. Anaesth., *14*:205, 1967.
106. Burch, J.E.: Rate of water and heat loss from respiratory tract of normal subjects in a subtropical climate. Arch. Intern. Med., *76*:315, 1945.
107. Chalon, J., et al.: Humidity output of the circle absorber system. Anesthesiology, *38*:458, 1973.
108. Chase, H.F., Kilmore, M.A., and Trotta, R.: Respiratory water loss via anesthesia systems: Mask breathing. Anesthesiology, *22*:205, 1961.
109. Clark, R.E., Orkin, L.R., and Rovenstine, E.A.: Body temperatures in anesthetized man. J.A.M.A., *154*:311, 1954.
110. MacKvanying, N., and Chalon, J.: Humidification of anesthetic gases for children. Anesth. Analg., *53*:387, 1974.
111. Déry, R., et al.: Humidity in anesthesiology, III. Heat and moisture patterns in the respiratory tract during anesthesia with the semi-closed system. Can. J. Anaesth., *14*:287, 1967.
112a. Bissonnette, B., and Sessler, D.: Passive and active inspired gas humidification increases thermal steady-state temperatures in anesthetized infants. Anesth. Analg., *69*:783, 1989.
112b. Bissonnette, B., and Sessler, D.: Passive and active inspired gas humidification in infants and children. Anesthesiology, *71*:381, 1989.
113. Weeks, D.B.: Evaluation of a disposable humidifier for use during anesthesia. Anesthesiology, *54*:337, 1981.
114. Feeley, T.W., et al.: Sterile anesthesia breathing circuits do not prevent postoperative pulmonary infection. Anesthesiology, *54*:369, 1981.
115. Garibaldi, R.A., et al.: Failure of bacterial filters to reduce the incidence of pneumonia after inhalation anesthesia. Anesthesiology, *54*:364, 1981.
116. Mazze, R.I.: Bacterial air filters. Anesthesiology, *54*:359, 1981.
117. Cohen, E.N., et al.: Occupational disease among operating room personnel: A national study. Report of an ad hoc Committee on the Effect of Trace Anesthetics on the Health of Operating Room Personnel, American Society of Anesthesiologists. Anesthesiology, *41*:321, 1974.
118. Mazze, R.I.: Waste anesthetic gases and the regulatory agencies. Anesthesiology, *52*:248, 1980.
119. Lecky, J.H.: The mechanical aspects of anesthetic pollution control. Anesth. Analg., *56*:769, 1977.
120. Whitcher, C., Piziali, R., and Sher, R.: Development and evaluation of methods for the elimination of waste anesthetic gases and vapors in hospitals. Publication No. 75-137. Cincinnati, US Department of Health, Education, and Welfare, Public Health Service, Center for Disease Control, National Institute for Occupational Safety and Health, 1975.
121. Bruce, D.L.: A simple way to vent anesthetic gases. Anesth. Analg., *52*:595, 1973.
122a. Cooper, J.B., et al.: Preventable anesthesia mishaps: A study of human factors. Anesthesiology, *49*:399, 1978.
122b. Goldman, H.S.: Anesthetic mistakes, mishaps, and misadventures. Curr. Rev. Clin. Anesth., *8*:115, 1988.
122c. Orkin, F.K.: Practice standards: The Midas touch of the emperor's new clothes. Anesthesiology, *70*:567, 1989.
123. Chase, H., Trotta, R., and Kilmore, M.A.: A simple method for humidifying nonrebreathing anesthesia gas systems. Anesth. Analg. *4*:249, 1962.
124. Ramanathan, S., et al.: Rebreathing characteristics of the Bain anesthesia circuit. Anesth. Analg. *56*:822, 1977.
125. Rayburn, R.L., and Watson, R.L.: Humidity in children and adults using the controlled partial rebreathing anesthesia method. Anesthesiology *52*:291, 1980.
126. Ramanathan, S.: Personal communication.
127. Berry, F.A., Jr., and Hughes-Davies, D.I.: Methods of increasing the humidity and temperature of inspired gases in the infant circle system. Anesthesiology *37*:456, 1972.
128. Chalon, J., et al.: Humidification of the circle absorber system. Anesthesiology *48*:142, 1978.
129. Ramanathan, S., Chalon, J., and Turndorf, H.: Humidity output of the Bloomquist infant circle. Anesthesiology *43*:679, 1975.
130. Chalon, J., et al.: A high humidity circle system for infants and children. Anesthesiology *49*:205, 1978.
131. Ramanathan, S., et al.: Humidity output of the Columbia pediatric circle. Anesth. Analg. *55*:877, 1976.
132. Toremalm, N.G.: Airflow patterns and ciliary activity in the trachea after tracheotomy. Acta Otolaryngol (Stockh) *53*:442, 1961.
133. Chalon, J., Lowe, D.A.Y., and Malebranche, J.: Effect of dry anesthetic gases on tracheobronchial epithelium Anesthesiology *37*:338, 1972.
134. Marfatia, S., Donahoe, P.K., and Hendrin, W.H.: Effect of dry and humidified gases on the respiratory epithelium in rabbits. J. Pediatr. Surg. *10*:583, 1975.
135. Knudsen, J., Lomholt, N., and Wisborg, K.: Postoperative pulmonary complications using dry and humidified anaesthetic gases. Br. J. Anaesth. *45*:636, 1973.
136. Chalon, J., et al.: Humidity and the anesthetized patient. Anesthesiology *50*:195, 1979.

16

INHALATION ANESTHESIA—PROCEDURAL CONSIDERATIONS

PRELIMINARY CONSIDERATIONS

Inhalation anesthesia may be defined as the production of general anesthesia by the inhalation of anesthetic agents into the pulmonary system for uptake into the circulation and thence to the brain.[1,2]

With the administration of agents into a breathing system, the proportions and partial pressure of the various constituents of the air are changed as the anesthetic agent is added. All inhalation techniques possess four common features:[2]

1. Source of oxygen
2. Means of carbon dioxide elimination
3. Breathing system for confining anesthetic gas or vapor
4. Vaporizer for liquid (volatile) anesthetics

CLASSIFICATION OF BREATHING SYSTEMS. Classification of the techniques for administration of anesthetic agents by inhalation is determined by three factors:[3-9]

1. The utilization or not of a reservoir
2. The provision or preclusion of rebreathing
    - using chemical CO_2 absorption
    - using CO_2 washout by fresh gas flow (FGF)
3. The access of the pulmonary system to the atmosphere, either on inspiration, expiration, or both

On this basis, four inhalation techniques may be classified as seen in Table 15–2.

In describing or labeling any system, two features must be stated: (1) an accurate description of the equipment used and how it is used, and (2) the volume flow rates of fresh gas with any vaporized agents introduced into the system.[4,10]

CHOICE OF BREATHING SYSTEM.[5-8] The design and function of breathing systems have been described, and the characteristics are summarized in Table 15–2. The choice depends on surgical conditions such as the position of the patient, the surgical "field," environmental hazards, the age of the patient, and the monitoring needs and preferences of the anesthesiologist.

The open systems are not commonly used, although they are simple and practical for short procedures in infants and children. They carry the hazard of operating room contamination and the associated occupational hazard; the systems are not readily adaptable to scavenging methods.

The semiopen nonrebreathing systems are commonly chosen for procedures in infants and children. The breathing tube can be extended away from the surgical field and hence is suitable for neurosurgery and for many extensive head and facial procedures. Scavenging methods are feasible and should be employed.

Semiclosed partial rebreathing techniques with a circle system are commonly used and are adaptable to most surgical conditions and to most patients. Scavenging is an essential feature.

A closed system with low gas flow and CO_2 absorption with the circle breathing system has the advantages of minimal environmental hazard (no scavenging needed) and the conservation of agents with resulting minimal cost. An efficient absorption canister for the chemical neutralization of CO_2 is absolutely necessary. The method of injecting by syringe a calculated amount of volatile agents into the system has been proposed and used during maintenance and elevates, to some extent, the concentration produced by vaporizers.

INDUCTION DEFINED.[9] *Induction* is defined as the production of a deep state of unconsciousness and the progressive depression of the central nervous system. In the process, the subject passes from the awake conscious state to the state of anesthesia, or the stage III, equivalent to the classic Guedel Stage III, wherein there is not only a complete lack of cortical and subcortical activity but obtundation of major reflexes, including blockade of the autonomic nervous system.

Two main approaches to induction are practiced: (1) inhalation induction with adequate and the appropriate premedication; and (2) the intravenous approach, which should also be preceded by appropriate premedication to allay anxiety and promote an acquiescent state in the patient.

PREOXYGENATION[11]

In either method, induction is immediately preceded by the technique of preoxygenation. The purpose of having a patient breathe oxygen for a period of 1 to 5 minutes is to increase the oxygen stores in the body and to eliminate a significant portion of the nitrogen that is in the lungs of a person who has been breathing air. This will increase the saturation of the hemoglobin and also increase the dissolved oxygen in the blood. Further, a high pulmonary-alveolar oxygen content in the FRC (Functional Residual Capacity) of about 2.5 L in adults will be provided as an oxygen reserve.

Preoxygenation can be accomplished by one of two approaches: (1) having the patient breath at a normal tidal volume 100% oxygen for 3 minutes, or (2) having the patient breathe full volumes up to and including vital capacity volumes for 1 to 2 minutes. The latter more rapidly eliminates the nitrogen and provides a more rapid hemoglobin saturation (see also preoxygenation under Intravenous Induction).

One aspect of the preoxygenation technique concerns the need to first eliminate the air and gas from the breathing circuits and fill the circuits with fresh oxygen. This is done *before* placing the mask on the patient by flushing the system with oxygen.

BASIS OF PREOXYGENATION. The introduction of preoxygenation is related to the basic work carried out by McClure[11] and subsequently by Medrado.[12] In the absence of preoxygenation, oxyhemographic studies show that blood oxygen saturation drops to levels of about 60 to 70%[11] on induction with thiopental in healthy patients breathing room air.[13,14]

Preoxygenation consists essentially of having the patient breathe 100% oxygen for periods of time from 2 to 8 minutes and with varying ventilatory volumes. In a circle system, a fresh gas inflow of 4 L oxygen per minute was recommended for 3 or more minutes. This results in elimination of pulmonary nitrogen and maintenance of blood oxygenation. Preoxygenation raises arterial oxygen tension to values above 400 mm Hg. On induction and after 2 minutes of apnea, the arterial oxygen tension will be maintained at values around 200 mm Hg. Failure to oxygenate before induction permits fall of arterial oxygen tension below 100 mm Hg (Pa_{O_2} levels of 80), considered a critical level during anesthesia.[12]

TECHNIQUES OF PREOXYGENATION. Oxygenation of blood and nitrogen washout varies with the duration of oxygen administration and the type of breathing. Using a semiclosed circle system, a FGF of 4 L oxygen per minute for 3 to 4 minutes produces saturation of the blood and results in the elimination of 80% of pulmonary nitrogen.[15] A more rapid pulmonary nitrogen washout with effective oxygenation can be obtained if a nonrebreathing system is used and the patient is allowed to breathe normally for 2 to 3 minutes.[16] However, shorter periods of preoxygenation have been suggested, as these will be effective if deep breaths are taken by the patient,[17,18] although denitrogenation may be incomplete.[15] To this end, an assessment of oxygenation techniques has been carried out by Drummond and Park.[19]

The preliminary administration of 100% oxygen for 2 to 3 minutes while the patient is breathing at a normal depth and rate will produce Pa_{O_2} values that will remain satisfactory in most patients for as long as 4 minutes after preoxygenation.[20] During the period after preoxygenation, induction with anesthetic drugs and intubation is accomplished. It is necessary, of course, that tracheal intubation be carried out promptly.[21]

In the study by Drummond,[19] the breathing pattern for the inhalation of 100% oxygen involved maximal breaths. It was demonstrated that only three or four vital capacity breaths in 30 seconds will wash in oxygen more effectively than breaths involving the inspiratory reserve volume only, that is, normal tidal volume breathing.

Recommendations. Preoxygenation can be accomplished by one of two procedures using a well-fitted and comfortable mask (minimal leaks):

1. Have the patient breathe 100% oxygen at normal tidal volumes for 3 minutes. This will raise the Pa_{O_2} values to 300 mm Hg or more. This approach is satisfactory in elective surgical procedures.
2. Use the "four-deep-breaths-technique." There is a rapid removal of nitrogen from the lungs and adequate oxygen saturation of the blood, resulting in Pa_{O_2} values of 300 mm Hg or more, by vital capacity breathing (maximal) with only four respiratory efforts within 30 seconds. This is the recommended technique in emergency circumstances and for rapid sequence induction.

The four-deep-breaths technique is also useful and recommended in the pregnant patient undergoing emergency delivery or cesarean section, especially when fetal distress is present. It has been shown that arterial oxygen tension is reduced to a greater extent in the pregnant patient than in the nonpregnant patient on rapid induction of anesthesia with intravenous agents.[22] In addition, pregnant patients have decreased FRC, airway closure occurs more readily, and in the supine position there are underventilated alveoli. All these changes lead to hypoxemia. Maximal deep breathing for four breaths significantly raises blood saturation and oxygen tension and is recommended in these circumstances.[18]

When these techniques are carried out, there is a persistence of oxygen saturation for 3 to 5 minutes, even if patients become apneic.[18,22] If small leaks about the mask are allowed to exist, oxygenation may not be adequate.[23]

Comparison of the Two Techniques.[24] Arterial saturation to 99 to 100% (Sa_{O_2}) is accomplished by either technique. The shortest time to beginning desaturation is between 6 and 8 minutes. However, when patients are rendered apneic, desaturation to 97% and to 95% occur earlier with the four-deep-breaths-technique at 5 to 6 minutes, while the 3-minute preoxygenation technique takes 8 minutes. This time difference is clinically insignificant. One can make a case if prolonged apnea of more than 6 to 8 minutes is expected to occur during induction, but this reflects unskilled care or poor anesthetic preparation, resulting in failure to establish an airway and ventilate the patient.

DENITROGENATION[23-27]

The process of eliminating nitrogen from the pulmonary system, and to some extent the circulation, by the administration of high concentrations of fresh oxygen is called *denitrogenation* or *nitrogen desaturation*. Denitrogenation accompanies the technique of preoxygenation and is a dividend of that process. As with preoxygenation, the breathing system is flushed with oxygen before application of the mask to the patient, and this step is again stated. The patient then breathes from the anesthesia circuit continuously or deeply while a FGF continues to flow into the circuit (Fig. 16–1).

Two phases can be distinguished: The first is the

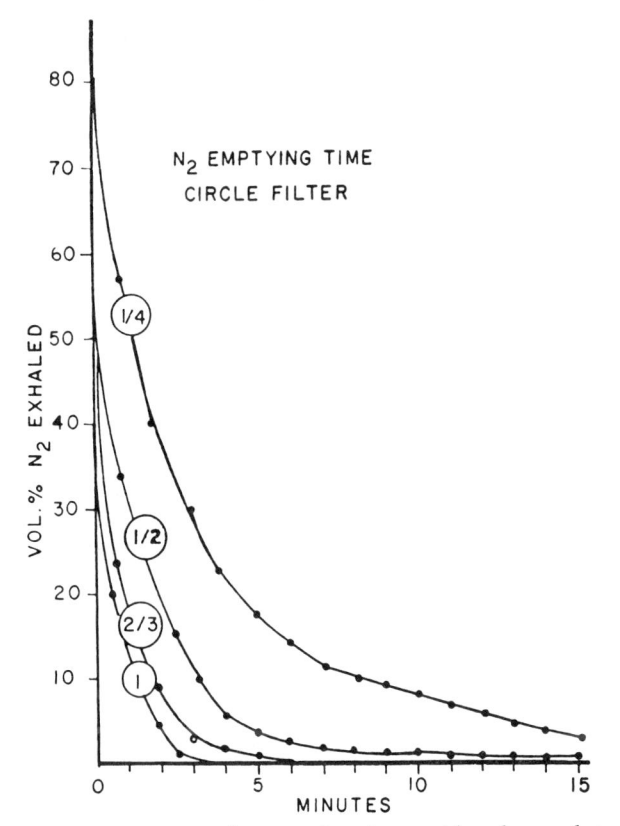

FIG. 16–1. Typical curve showing rapid and complete elimination of nitrogen from the lungs of a healthy young volunteer breathing pure oxygen from a circle filter at his minute volume exchange and with no rebreathing and at one quarter, one half, and two thirds of the minute volume exchange with rebreathing. From Miles, G.G., Martin, N.T., and Adriani, J.: Factors influencing the elimination of nitrogen using semi-closed inhalers. Anesthesiology, *17*:213, 1956.

elimination of nitrogen from the pulmonary system, and the second is the elimination of nitrogen from the tissues. The alveolar rate of nitrogen washout from the pulmonary system depends on gas mixing and gas displacement. This is influenced by[28]

- Variations in ventilation
- Functional residual air volume, dead space
- Alveolar gas mixing
- Capacity of anesthesia circuit
- Volume flow of gases introduced

If respiratory function is within normal limits, then the elimination of nitrogen depends upon volume flow of gases into the combined machine-lung system. When the flow equals the respiratory minute volume, the pulmonary nitrogen is eliminated in 2 to 3 minutes. It may be stated that the quantity of nitrogen elimination is a constant percentage of the amount present at any given time.

The following analysis illustrates the importance of removing nitrogen from an anesthetic system:[25,27]

1. Apparatus was flushed (10 seconds) with pure nitrous oxide. The concentrations of gases were found to be as follows: Oxygen—2.3%; nitrogen—3.1%, and nitrous oxide—95.6%.

    With flowmeters regulated at 4000 cc nitrous oxide and 1000 cc oxygen (80–20 mixture) and the pop-off valve open, the anesthetic mask was applied to the face; after several breaths (1 minute), analysis revealed oxygen—15%, nitrogen—40.0%, and nitrous oxide—40.6%.

2. Without flushing and the flowmeters maintained as above, at the end of 3 minutes with the pop-off valve open, analysis showed the following approximate concentrations: Oxygen—15%, nitrogen—21.1%, and nitrous oxide—66.1%. At the end of 8 minutes, analysis revealed oxygen—15%, nitrogen—17.2%, and nitrous oxide—71.7%.

3. With the administration of a 90–10 mixture after the mask has been applied to the patient's face for 3 minutes, the following analysis resulted: Oxygen—10.1%, nitrogen—9.5%, and nitrous oxide—81.0%.

4. With the constant administration of an 80–20 mixture after the mask has been applied to the patient's face and following at least three flushings with pure nitrous oxide, at the end of 3 minutes the following concentrations were found: Oxygen—13.5%, nitrogen—5.5%, and nitrous oxide—81%.

These analyses are presented to show primarily the percentage of nitrogen remaining in the respiratory system even after vigorous flushing maneuvers. It is evident that at the total volume flow of 5 L/min a significant percentage of nitrogen remains in the respiratory tract. Similarly, achieving an anesthetic concentration of nitrous oxide is delayed. When gases are admitted at the respiratory minute volume of the patient, the nitrogen tension falls rapidly. One significant investigation provides the following information:[25,26]

When an anesthetic gas mixture was admitted into an inhaler at the minute volume exchange of the subject, with no rebreathing, the nitrogen tension fell to the zero level in an average of 2.5 minutes. If the flow rate of gases admitted was two thirds of the minute volume, elimination of nitrogen was prolonged to 4 to 6 minutes. At one half the minute volume, elimination required 8 to 10 minutes, and at one fourth the minute volume, elimination required 15 to 18 minutes.

This time period for desaturation is essentially the same for normal patients regardless of individual minute volume if gases are supplied at the individual demand rate. The rate of elimination of nitrogen from the pulmonary system with different gas flows is represented in Figure 16–1. The reverse phenomenon, namely pulmonary nitrogen refill, follows a similar curve to that for pulmonary desaturation.

TISSUE NITROGEN DESATURATION. The elimination of nitrogen from the tissues represents a secondary phase of the process of nitrogen desaturation. Total body tissue nitrogen amounts to 700 to 1200 cc.[29] Because the tension of pulmonary gases is in equilibrium with the same gases in the plasma, it is to be expected that there is a nitrogen equilibrium with all extracellular water compartments of the body. The process of tissue desaturation occurs after the alveolar nitrogen has been replaced by another gas. This occurs rapidly, and therefore there is a gradient of nitrogen partial pressure from tissues to alveoli.

The depletion of tissue nitrogen is gradual; an average of 0.5 L volume of nitrogen may be excreted in 30 minutes. At the end of this time one may expect to find in the breathing circuits a concentration of nitrogen of about 9 vol %.

UPTAKE OF INERT GASES.[30,31] Having eliminated the nitrogen to an insignificant value, the next phase of the anesthetic process must consider the uptake of the inert anesthetic gas, nitrous oxide, which is commonly used as part of the inhaled anesthetic gas mixture.

Absorption of a gas may be defined as the uptake of the gas or agent by the blood stream and body tissues. In inhalation administration of agents, it is the transfer of the gas from the pulmonary alveoli into the liquid blood and subsequently into tissues and cells. The rate of uptake is determined by (1) the gradient in gas tension and (2) by Henry's Law of solubility of gases in liquids.

In general, the uptake of any inert gas continues for many hours at a decreasing rate until saturation occurs. Saturation involves two processes: (1) arterial saturation and (2) tissue saturation.

The rate of uptake, although progressive, shows three time phases: The first is very rapid and represents initial blood saturation. About 5 minutes is required. The second is the period of relative complete arterial saturation and requires another 20 to 30 minutes. The last time phase is that of tissue saturation and requires about 5 hours.

It is believed that the rate of uptake or the amount absorbed in a given period of time is proportional to the amount necessary to reach saturation. One may express the process of rate of absorption:

$$\frac{dx}{dt} = k(A - X)$$

In this expression, t is time, x is the amount of gas absorbed in time t, A is the amount of saturation, and k a constant.

Behnke has studied nitrogen elimination and nitrogen uptake.[29] One process is essentially the converse of the other. Approximately 5 hours is required for complete nitrogen desaturation and an equivalent period of time for nitrogen saturation.

SUMMARY. It is evident that with low total flow rates the percentage of oxygen as actually available to patients is less than the proportion delivered.[32] Secondly, the amount of nitrous oxide available to the patient is seen to be much less than the concentration delivered to the breathing system as indicated by flow-meters. This is related to a persistent residual low nitrogen value. Lastly, with low flow rates and nonabsorption technique, there is accumulation of carbon dioxide.

EFFECT OF PREOXYGENATION ON ALVEOLAR GASES

In the process of preoxygenation and resulting pulmonary denitrogenation, the nitrogen concentration in a semiclosed circle system is reduced to an average of 16% (15–20%) within 10 minutes because of alveolar washout.[25,26]

Further pulmonary ventilation with a continuous inflow of fresh gas (oxygen or helium oxygen)[28] will further reduce the nitrogen to levels of about 5%, but this requires about 33 minutes. This reduction is related to the slow transfer of blood nitrogen into the pulmonary system and hence into the anesthesia circuit. At this level, there still remains a store of 650 mL of nitrogen in body tissues. To reduce the nitrogen content of exhaled air further may require 30 hours of fresh air breathing.[29] Nitrogen elimination may be hastened by breathing a mixture of helium and oxygen.[28]

Simultaneously, with the reduction of nitrogen in a closed circuit, certain trace gases are detectable and accumulate in the gas mixture of the closed circle system.[33] Besides small amounts of residual nitrogen, the other gases that are detectable (after 30 minutes) and accumulate as metabolic contaminants in the inspired inhalation gas mixture of a closed circle system are as follows:[34,35]

Methane may increase from an average of 0.30 ppm to 17 ppm (4.3–22.5 ppm)
Acetone may increase from a base level of 0.3 ppm to 2.2 ppm (1.3–6 ppm)
Hydrogen may increase from 10 pp to 100 ppm
Carbon monoxide may increase from 300 ppm to 600 ppm

SOURCES OF EXTRANEOUS GASES. Nitrogen may also be introduced into the circuit, as well as other gases, from trace amounts present in cylinders or piped USP medical grade oxygen. Liquid oxygen sources may have 1900 ppm of nitrogen. Other gases include argon at 3000 to 5000 ppm and methane at 50 ppm.

Methane is derived from the ambient atmosphere, where it is present to the extent of 1.2 ppm. It also accumulates in the circuit from trace amounts in medical gas stores and from bowel gas, which is produced by intestinal digestion of foodstuffs, transferred into the circulation, and then passed into the pulmonary gas. The flammable level is about 5% and represents a hazard during the use of cautery.[33]

Acetone is produced largely in the liver from metabolism of free fatty acids in the liver and is partially excreted through the lungs.[34] In the fasting subject or the diabetic there may be an increased production and accumulation of greater amounts in a closed circuit breathing system. In a closed system with high humidity and condensation, acetone may be trapped in the water.

Ethanol may also be excreted in the lungs. With a water–gas coefficient of 1200, it may also be trapped in pulmonary water; "flushing" does not readily remove it from the circuit.

Hydrogen also enters the pulmonary system.[35] This is a product of tissue metabolism and bacterial action in the bowel and is ordinarily excreted by the lungs. Hydrogen up to 0.6 mL/min can be readily excreted. In a prolonged closed system (anesthesia), it is possible that concentrations of hydrogen might reach 4 to 5%—a possible flammable hazard.[36]

Carbon monoxide accumulates in the closed circle system of anesthesia.* The source is both exogenous from polluted air and endogenous, produced by metabolism and the destruction of red blood cells. In nonsmokers, levels that are first perceptible but nonlethal have been found in alveolar air at 300 to 600 ppm. Although not productive of symptoms,[37] these levels are sufficient to bind to hemoglobin. An alveolar concentration of 0.01% or 100 ppm will bind to about 3–6% of the body hemoglobin as COHb.[38] In heavy smokers (two packs of cigarettes per day), a median carboxyhemoglobin (COHb) level of 5.6% is to be found.[37a]

Continuous inflow of fresh gas mixtures and flushing of the system with oxygen will reduce the

---

* The average concentration of CO in the atmosphere is about 0.1 ppm.

nitrogen in the system, as well as the other extraneous gases.

INDUCTION

INHALATION INDUCTION. A state of general anesthesia can be readily accomplished by inhalation of potent volatile agents through a face mask in adequately premedicated patients assessed as well-sedated and tranquilized. It is emphasized that mask induction is preceded by preoxygenation. After preoxygenation, a mixture of anesthetic gases and agents is provided to the patient for inhalation. Usually, nitrous oxide–oxygen in a 50:50 mixture is the common carrier and diluent. To this is added a percentage of one of the potent volatile agents such as halothane, enflurane, or isoflurane. These agents are administered in concentrations of approximately 1 to 1.5 MAC and are adjusted as clinically indicated to provide surgical levels of anesthesia. This is continued for maintenance of the surgical anesthetic state. In most instances, an intravenous induction supplement is necessary for adults.

Some anesthesiologists have used halothane in high concentrations of 3 to 4% in nitrous oxide–oxygen for induction of children as well as adults.[39] Recent reports using a single-breath induction of anesthesia with a vital capacity breath of halothane 4% in a carrier mixture of nitrous oxide 66% and oxygen 34% have found the technique effective, safe, and acceptable.[40,41] The patient is instructed to inhale fully and hold his breath as long as is comfortable. The reports indicate that in patients who are unpremedicated the mean induction time is approximately 83 seconds. It was also noted that there is relative cardiovascular stability with only insignificant decreases in blood pressure if the heart rate is maintained by atropine premedication.[41]

A single breath of a high concentration of 2% isoflurane in nitrous oxide 66%–oxygen 34% has been advocated by Lamberty.[42] Some patients have found the method more acceptable than conventional inhalation induction, but the incidence of moderate-to-poor patient compliance was greater than with the halothane single-breath technique. Isoflurane is offered as an alternative to halothane by this technique in adults.[43]

INTRAVENOUS INDUCTION.[44,45] Although the potent inhalation anesthetic agents are used for induction to produce a state of unconsciousness, there are drawbacks—largely psychological—that have resulted in the use of intravenous agents to produce sleep. These do not create the feeling of suffocation often experienced by patients when breathing anesthetic gases. Since the uptake into the circulation is immediate with intravenous agents, they are rapidly distributed to the brain and suffuse the cortex and subcortical centers to produce an easy sleep. Again, *preoxygenation* is mandatory before the sleep dose of an intravenous agent is administered and before an anesthetic mixture is introduced for inhalation by the patient.

The intravenous agents used are discussed in detail in the chapters on intravenous barbiturates and nonbarbiturates. For the present purpose, the commonly used intravenous agents and the dose requirements to produce a state of unconsciousness (ie, the second stage of anesthesia) are listed in Table 16–1.

Intravenous Induction Drug Potencies.[46] In the unmedicated subject, the dose potency required to produce unconsciousness is termed the UD_{50}, or the dose producing unconsciousness in 50% of subjects. This is a pharmacologic index of potency and is the minimum amount necessary to produce sleep (not anesthesia). The dose producing unconsciousness in 95% of subjects is the UD_{95} and is generally twice the UD_{50}; this dose represents a clinical index of potency and approaches a state of "anesthesia".[46–49]

Table 16–1 lists the various drugs and their UD_{50}, as well as their UD_{95}, which is the dose that is generally used in unpremedicated patients.

In a recent comparative study of several commonly used intravenous induction drugs, thiopental was found to be superior to propofol, methohexital, and etomidate in outpatient surgery. The side effects of methohexitone and etidomate made them unacceptable. Propofol produced a higher incidence of sequelae on induction than thiopental but provided a high-quality and more rapid recovery[49] (Table 16–2).

CLINICAL MONITORING OF SLEEP INDUCTION. During the administration of an induction drug, the following neurologic observations should be made sequentially to monitor the developing depth of sleep:

1. Loss of verbalization by the patient (ie, ask the patient to count)
2. Loss of response to a command ("open your eyes"), usually considered a sleep level

TABLE 16–1. TABLE OF DOSES FOR INTRAVENOUS INDUCTION DRUGS

	UD_{50} (mg/kg)	UD_{95} (mg/kg)
Thiopental	2.2 –2.5	4.0 –5.0
Methohexital[47]	0.6 –1.0	1.5 –2.5
Diazepam	0.33–0.35	0.40–0.5
Midazolam[48]	0.15–0.18	0.20–0.25
Ketamine	0.14	1.0 –2.0
Propanidid	2.0	3.0
Althesin (alphaxalone)	0.25	0.30
Propofol[49]	1.5 –2.0	2.5

Data derived from references 44–48.

TABLE 16–2. COMPARATIVE EFFECTS OF 4 INDUCTION AGENTS, INJECTED OVER 20 S TO GROUPS OF 50 FIT PATIENTS (McCollum et al, 1986)

Agent	Dose mg kg⁻¹	Anaesthesia Induced+	SBP Fall 20+ mmHg	Apnoea 30+ s++	Excitatory Effects	Respiratory Disturbances	Induction Acceptable to Anaesthetist
Thiopentone	4.0	45(6)	3	11(1)	4	4	38
	5.0	50(5)	10	19(1)	4	4	43
Methohexitone	1.5	48(2)	1*	10(1)	18	10	37
Etomidate	0.3	50(0)	4	0	35	5	36
Propofol	2.0	45(5)	10	12(5)	16ˣ	2	35
	2.5	50(0)	19	22(6)	12ˣ	3	43

+ Figures in brackets: rapid lightening of anaesthesia
++ Figures in brackets; apnoea lasting over 1 min
* Average of 25% increase in heart rate (3–9% with other agents)
ˣ Very minor in nature, compared with methohexitone and etomidate
From Dundee, J.W., and Wyant, G.M.: *Intravenous Anesthesia*, 2nd ed. Edinburgh, Churchill Livingstone, 1988.

3. Lack of eyelash stimulus response and lack of eyelid touch response
4. Loss of eyeball movement and centering of eyeball
5. Loss of oropharyngeal responses
6. Depression of respiration; need to assist breathing

INHALATION INDUCTION IN CHILDREN. Children generally prefer an inhalation induction to an intravenous stick injection. Infusion should not be started in resistant and fearful children and infants, especially if the availability of veins is limited.[50]

Use of nitrous oxide–oxygen in a 50:50 concentration with an admixture of one of the volatile agents is a common procedure. The gaseous mixture can be allowed to flow over the child's face from above without direct application of a mask. The choice of agent may, in part, be dictated by the child. The ethers such as enflurane or isoflurane are thought to be pungent. However, Tierney[51] allowed children to sniff enflurane and halothane at the time of a preop visit and asked them which they preferred. No general trend was evident, but the preferred agent was administered.

Inhalation induction using halothane is a common practice in the management of pediatric patients. Halothane may be used at 3% concentrations in oxygen. However, the induction time is more rapid if the 3% halothane is carried by a mixture of 60% nitrous oxide and 40% oxygen. Cardiovascular stability is good and is well maintained if heart rate is kept high by atropine premedication.

Inhalation induction using isoflurane in infants is associated with significant depression of both blood pressure and heart rate.[52] Premedication with atropine has little effect on blood pressure, which stays depressed (unlike in halothane induction).

Effect of Mask Induction on Oxygen Saturation. Children receiving sedative opioid procedures show limited or no agitation during gravity and mask induction. Similarly, none of these patients showed arterial desaturation below 90% SaO₂ during inhalation induction with nitrous oxide–oxygen–halothane or isoflurane. Negligible decreases occurred with halothane.[53]

Phillips found appreciable desaturation, however. Preoxygenation as such was not attempted in children, but a mixture of nitrous oxide/6 L/min and oxygen (3 L/min) was allowed to flow over the patient's face. Induction was carried out by adding a volatile agent.[54]

Arterial desaturation below 85% occurred in about 10% of subjects. More frequent coughing, laryngospasm, and sinus tachycardia occurred with isoflurane, and induction required a longer time.

Comparison of Agents for Inhalation Induction. The method of direct mask inhalation induction is an established one for pediatric patients with many advantages and relatively few disadvantages.[50] A tranquil and mildly sedated child is desired. Halothane and enflurane appear to have few complications. Induction time is faster with halothane than with enflurane or isoflurane, but all are about 3 minutes (Table 16–3). Laryngospasm is greatest and most frequent with isoflurane and least with enflurane.[55] On recovery, coughing almost always occurs following isoflurane and is least common with enflurane.[50]

Emergence following enflurane is rapid, and most children have spontaneous eye opening within 2 minutes. Halothane is also associated with a significant incidence of headache, amounting to 9%. The incidence of nausea with all these agents is low (7%).[56]

Summary of Pharmacodynamics of Inhalation Agents. The overall acceptability of each agent without premedication or aid of intravenous agents has been studied and compared as follows:[50]

TABLE 16–3. INDUCTION CHARACTERISTICS WITH VOLATILE ANESTHETIC

	Induction Time (min)	Induction Excitement	Induction Laryngospasm	Emergence Time (min)	Total Duration
Halothane	2.7 ± (1.0)	13	4	6.2	22.3 ± 7.6
Enflurane	3.2 ± (0.8)	33	2	4.7	21.5 ± 8.6
Isoflurane	3.3 ± 1.2	34	23	6.4	25.1 ± 6.8

From Fisher, D.M., et al.: Comparison of enflurane, halothane, and isoflurane for diagnostic and therapeutic procedures in children with malignancies. Anesthesiology, 63:647, 1985.

Halothane. Faster induction than enflurane or isoflurane (2.7 min); least excitement. However, emergence is slower, and a significant incidence of postanesthetic hangover and headache occurs.

Enflurane. Induction is slightly longer than that of halothane (3.2 min), with the least amount of laryngospasm. Emergence is the most rapid of all the agents, and a hangover is not seen.

Isoflurane. Induction is slower than with the other agents and is accompanied by a high percentage of laryngospasm; excitement is about the same as with enflurane. Coughing is also frequent, and emergence is slower.

In infants, induction of anesthesia by mask inhalation of halothane or enflurane has been the most satisfactory method. In contrast, isoflurane is accompanied by a high frequency of laryngospasm and coughing, which is often severe.[57] It is generally considered a poor agent for mask inhalation induction.

Mask Induction Psychology.[58,59] Induction of anesthesia by mask in children can be made more acceptable by either a modification of the type of mask or by applying a pleasant scent to the rim of the standard commercial mask. Modified masks include a balloon mask and a Mickey Mouse face mask with a wide mouth.

The use of scented masks has been a time-honored technique used to diguise the odors of the inhalational agents. Its origins have been lost because of failure to report technical features in the early days of anesthesia practice when open drop ether anesthesia was the common practice. Paluel Flagg, in *The Art of Anaesthesia* (1911) noted the practice:

One may sometimes render the induction more pleasant by dropping upon the mask a little essence of orange, wintergreen or some essential oil before the ether is given. This serves to mask the disagreeable odor.[58]

The application of drops of fruit extract on masks makes inhalation induction for children, as well as adults, more pleasant. It was common practice by such attending anesthesiologists as Wood and Burdick at Doctors' Hospital in the 1940s to place a small dab of fruit extracts or oil of peppermint or oil of spearmint on the rim of the mask. At least one public report of the use of spearmint fragrance was presented in the *Saturday Evening Post* in January 1949, in an article entitled "Sing Them to Sleep, Doctor."[60] The smell of rubber of the commonly used masks in the early days was also disguised by a dab or drop of one of these agents.

A modification of the use of pleasant scents consists of vaporizing volatile fruit flavors into the anesthetic gas mixtures.[61] Aerosolizing fruit-flavored materials into an inhalational gas mixture, however, has been considered to have disadvantages. These fruit extracts may manifest both toxicologic and allergic responses and may be potential airway irritants.[62] It has been suggested that rather than introduce the various extracts into the breathing mixture, only a small quantity should be applied either to the face mask in the traditional manner or to use an especially designed face mask that already has a scent-release polymer base in its construction.[62]

The odor of isoflurane has been disguised by applying a small amount of a liquid strawberry extract on the face mask for induction of children.[63] Though induction complications are not significantly different from a group induced by a nonscented mask, Lewis found that patients in the scented-mask group were more cooperative and were quieter on induction. It is important not to place too much scented extract on masks because this may cause gagging or coughing.

APPLICATION OF MASK.[9] Because in inhalation techniques, the operator must use some type of mask, consideration should be given to the selection of the mask and the application of the mask. A mask should be selected that fits the face of the patient and is comfortable. This means it follows the facial contour and, when applied, is snug. Connecting apertures should be at least 2.5 cm in diameter for the average adult. The mask should be easily held by the anesthetist.

In applying the mask to the patient's face, the operator should explain what is about to happen and what the patient might expect to feel. The patient should be told to breathe naturally and quietly as if in bed going to sleep. The mask should be applied gently but firmly so that leaks are minimal. After the patient is asleep, straps may be used.

The mask should not be permitted to creep up above the bridge of the nose and cause pressure on the corners of the eye or directly on the eyeball. The former may cause edema and the latter either corneal injury or oculo-cardiac reflex responses.

Head straps for securing the mask must be used carefully. Excessive pressure has produced reversible and, on occasion, permanent alopecia.[64]

DIFFUSION HYPEROXIA DURING INDUCTION. It is recognized that when a patient breathes a 50% nitrous oxide–oxygen mixture there is an increase in the Pa_{O_2} of the blood. During the uptake of the nitrous oxide, whose coefficient of solubility is approximately 0.4 versus 0.0025 for oxygen, it is evident that with the rapid uptake of the nitrous oxide there would be an increase in the oxygen partial pressure in the alveoli and, simultaneously, an increase in the oxygen uptake by the blood.[31] This has been designated as diffusion hyperoxia[31,65] and is related to the "concentrating effect" on alveolar oxygen by the rapid uptake of the nitrous oxide.[66]

This diffusion hyperoxia during the administration of nitrous oxide is maximally obtained when a mixture of 79% nitrous oxide and 21% oxygen is inhaled by the patient.[66] Markello has studied this process and has shown that the mean rise in Pa_{O_2} of the blood approximates 27 mm Hg, with a range from a few millimeters of mercury to as high as 43 mm Hg. This increase is above that of the actual available inspired oxygen concentration. In subsequent studies, the same group determined that there was consistently a higher Pa_{O_2} value if the patient had breathed 100% oxygen for several minutes or if deep breathing of vital capacity volumes preceded the administration of the nitrous oxide–oxygen mixture, in contrast to the value in a patient who had not been preoxygenated.

The development of *diffusion hyperoxia* during induction with concentrations of oxygen over 50% has been suggested but has not represented a problem.[65,66]

DIFFUSION HYPOXIA DURING EMERGENCE. Essentially, the process of diffusion hyperoxia is the reverse of the process during emergence when diffusion hypoxia is prone to occur.[67,68] The nitrous oxide–oxygen washout with room air, as originally described by Fink, is recognized, and oxygenation during at least the first 5 minutes after discontinuing anesthesia is essential in preventing diffusion hypoxia.

OCULAR INJURY DURING ANESTHESIA

INCIDENCE. Eye exposure during general anesthesia or mask inhalation of gases should be avoided. A trauma incidence of 44% has been reported.[69]

TYPES OF INJURY. Eye injury can be mechanical and/or chemical. The types of injury and their causes are as follows:

- Face mask pressure on bulb and orbit
  Abrasion of cornea[70]
  Occlusion of retinal artery flow—blindness
  Detachment of retina
  Periorbital edema
  Numbness resulting from supraorbital nerve compression
  Masks with poorly inflated cushions producing tissue pressure.[71]
- Direct trauma to cornea
  Abrasion from instruments, drapes, tubes[69]
  Laceration of cornea by fingers of anesthesiologist during manipulations
  Drying of open eyes by flow of gases or by simple exposure to atmosphere for long periods
  Conjunctivitis from irritation by volatile agents and antiseptic solutions
  Head and neck surgery risk
  Prone position
  Great risk in patients with exophthalmas and patients with Bell's palsy
- Drying of open eyes[72]
  Exposure to flowing anesthetic gases and vapors
  Simple exposure to the atmosphere
  Anesthetic inhibition of basal tear production[73]

EXAMINATION. Preanesthetic evaluation of eyes for complaints or disorders should be routine. At the conclusion of every general anesthetic procedure, the eyes should be inspected. Complaints should be noted and care rendered. An ophthalmic consultation is good practice when indicated.

After an abrasion, the pain is similar to that of a foreign body. A laceration or abrasion appears as a dull, lusterless area. (In acute glaucoma, the eye is red with a steamy dull appearance of the cornea and a dilated pupil.)

Examination should be performed with a good light. A topical anesthetic agent should be applied, followed by fluorescin stain. A corneal laceration or abrasion is green.

DRUG EFFECTS.[74] Succinylcholine increases intraocular pressure and is contraindicated in eye trauma, penetrating eye injury, weakened cornea or sclera, or extraocular surgery if the sclera is incised. Pretreatment with antidepolarizing agents fails to prevent the increase.

PROTECTION OF THE EYE. Careful application of masks is important. When they are placed over the bridge of the nose, pressure on the eyeball can occur. This has a mechanical effect but also may elicit an ocular reflex. Frequently check the position of head pieces, of tubes, and of all paraphernalia about the head, including connections and methods of security.

An eye lubricant should be placed in the eyes of the patient, especially if the duration of surgery is to be more than an hour. After the drops are instilled, the eyes should be closed and ophthalmic eye pads placed over the orbits and secured with nonallergenic tape such as Dermaclear Tape or cellophane to the patient's temples. If a skin infection is present about the eyes and face, an antibiotic ophthalmic solution is instilled. Neosporin ophthalmic solution is effective against the majority of ocular bacteria but remains controversial because a fungus invasion may occur.[77]

For short procedures (anesthesia under 60 minutes) away from the head and neck, with the patient supine and not intubated, closing of the eyes alone without use of a lubricant and careful covering with eyepads taped in place is an effective preventive measure. Patients in coma, paralyzed, or those requiring ventilator care should have an opthalmic solution and eye patches. This care should be repeated every 12 hours or more often as needed.

Eye Lubricants.[75] A methylcellulose-based viscous artificial tear solution is recommended. Two solutions that have been used with highly favorable outcomes are Lubrifair solution and Tears Naturale.* They are the most bland and effective in minimizing the common complications; they are also accompanied by the least number of associated complications.

The petrolatum-based or mineral-oil–based ophthalmic ointments are not recommended. The common complications of these ointments are blurred vision and foreign body sensation, the incidence of which following Lacri-Lube (Allergan) is 75% and 62% respectively (Table 16–4). After Duratears (Alcon), also a petrolatum-based ointment, blurred vision is noted in 55% of patients and foreign body sensation in over 40%. The duration of these undesirable effects is of the order of 4 to 7 hours. Visual acuity is also significantly decreased by the Snellen eye chart test with these ointments. Additionally, scleral erythema occurred in a frequency ranging from 6% to 18%. Lacri-Lube is also associated with significant tearing. More serious complications observed are blockage of the meibomian glands with severe blepharitis and inflammation of the entire eyelids. A comparison study

---

* Lubrifair® solution (artificial tears/isopto-alkaline) contains dextran 70 (0.1%); hydroxypropyl methylcellulose (0.3%); 0.01 benzalkonium chloride (preservative); EDTA (preservative); sodium chloride; potassium chloride (pH adjustment); purified water (vehicle) (pH adjustment). ®Pharmafair Inc., Hauppauge, New York.

Tears Naturale II® solution contains dextran 70 (0.1%); a polymeric formulation with hydroxypropyl methylcellulose (0.3%); polyquaternium^{-1} (0.001%) (preservative); Edetate disodium (preservative); potassium chloride; sodium chloride (pH adjustment); purified water (vehicle) (pH adjustment). ®Alcon Laboratories, Fort Worth, Texas.

TABLE 16–4. EYE COMPLICATIONS ASSOCIATED WITH PETROLATUM-BASED OPHTHALMIC OINTMENTS

- Blurred vision
- Tearing
- Foreign body sensation
- Dryness
- Scleral erythema
- Corneal abrasion
- Visual acuity change
- Itching
- Meibomian gland blockade
- Blepharitis

has revealed that Tears Naturale or Lubrifair solution was the superior and most effective agent.[76]

The simple direct taping of the eyelids without an eye pad or lubricant was associated with significant dryness of the eyes, and tearing was also to be noted, along with foreign body sensation. Taping only has been associated with the development of erythema about the eye, as well as conjunctivitis. This has been noted even with use of nonallergenic tape.

TREATMENT. Pain must be relieved. This is accomplished by a topical ophthalmic anesthetic. Tetracaine 0.5% ophthalmic solution is effective and relieves pain in about 30 seconds.[78] Some burning is usually noted by the patient for the first ten seconds, but this agent minimally interferes with the healing process and is needed for only 1 to 2 days. Partial re-epithelialization occurs in 24 hours. Long-term use may cause some softening of the globe.

Steroids should be avoided.[79] Healing is retarded and inflammatory processes may be exacerbated. After long use, glaucoma or subcapsular cataracts may occur.

An antibiotic topical preparation should be used to treat infections. Neosporin is effective against most ocular bacteria,[77] and broad-spectrum antibiotic preparations of either erythromycin or tetracycline in petrolatum base are also available and effective for therapeutic purposes.[71] An eye patch and rest are the most effective therapeutic measures.

Atropine sulfate 1% ophthalmic ointment is useful when there is severe pain associated with spasm of iris or ciliary muscle but should be avoided in glaucoma.

SUMMARY. The recommended eye protection procedure is to use the methylcellulose-based ophthalmic solutions and standard ophthalmic eye pads over the closed eyes, secured by nonallergenic tape to the temples.

FACIAL NERVE PARALYSIS

Management of the airway during mask anesthesia may be associated with facial nerve paralysis.[80] Usually hard pressure on the nerve behind the angle of the mandible to relieve respiratory obstruction is the cause. This may be coupled with stretching of the nerve by forward traction on the mandible at the chin. A tight-fitting mask held by a head strap crossing the face and pressing on the parotid gland may contribute to nerve pressure.

The facial nerve leaves the skull through the stylomastoid foramen and passes superficially over the ascending ramus of the mandible to enter the parotid gland. At this point, the nerve divides into several branches—the "crow's foot" distribution. When the branches to the buccinator, masseter, and orbicularis oris muscles are in the superficial layer of the parotid gland, they are more vulnerable to pressure. Patients may have difficulty chewing, they may experience weakness and asymmetry of the face, or they may be unable to pucker the lips (whistle).[80]

PRECAUTIONS. Hold the mandible forward by placing the fingers at the chin and along the horizontal ramus. Use pressure at the angle of the mandible only for short periods and only with enough pressure to maintain the airway. Use head straps properly: one strap well forward of the area of the parotid and the other behind the ear.

UPPER AIRWAY OBSTRUCTION

An axiom in breathing is that "noisy respiration is obstructed respiration."[1,2] Upper airway obstruction in the unconscious patient may be due to loss of muscle tone of the upper air passage with mechanical obstruction from the tongue. Mechanical obstruction may also occur from foreign bodies, such as teeth, blood, secretions, dentures, or tumors present in the airway.[81]

Loss of skeletal muscle tone of upper airway passages occurs during normal sleep and is related to inhibition of gamma motor neuron system, which results in relaxation of tongue muscles and pharyngeal constrictor muscles. Increased tone of intrinsic muscles of larynx produces physiologic obstruction due to stridor and/or laryngospasm.

Infants have a shallow pharynx, a cephalad epiglottis and tongue, and a mobile mandible.[81a] These conditions are conducive to obstruction of the air passage, increase the effort of breathing, and lead to hypoxia. In addition there is failure of glottic closure at end of respiration, causing a reduction of FRC; a lowered reservoir of alveolar oxygen then results in hypoxemia. This set of physiologic changes is the probable mechanism in SIDS and in the postanesthetic period in some infants.

MECHANISMS IN OBSTRUCTION OF UPPER AIRWAY. At the level of the oral passageway, in the supine position, obstruction is usually a result of the tongue "falling back," causing obstruction at the level of the soft palate by making contact with the soft palate and partially to the hard palate. Because the tongue is attached to the mandible, simply lifting the chin will relieve the obstruction.[82] In these instances the nasopharyngeal passage is patent. Rarely does the tongue fall into the pharynx. However, the tongue can be forcibly pushed deeply into the mouth and the soft palate pushed into the nasopharynx, occluding the nasopharyngeal passage. A pharyngeal airway improperly placed or too large may be the cause of obstruction at the oronasopharyngeal level.[83]

At the level of the pharyngeal passage two mechanisms of obstruction may operate, both independent of position or movement of the tongue.[83] By fiberoptic visualization, it has been noted that the base of the epiglottis can close over the rima glottidis and the lateral parts of the epiglottis or rims can come in contact with the posterior pharyngeal wall; at the same time, the pars glottic of the epiglottis can occlude the esophagus (Fig. 16–2).

POSITION OF THE HEAD.[82,83] The position of the head in the supine unconscious patient greatly influences the patency of the upper airway.[84] In the neutral

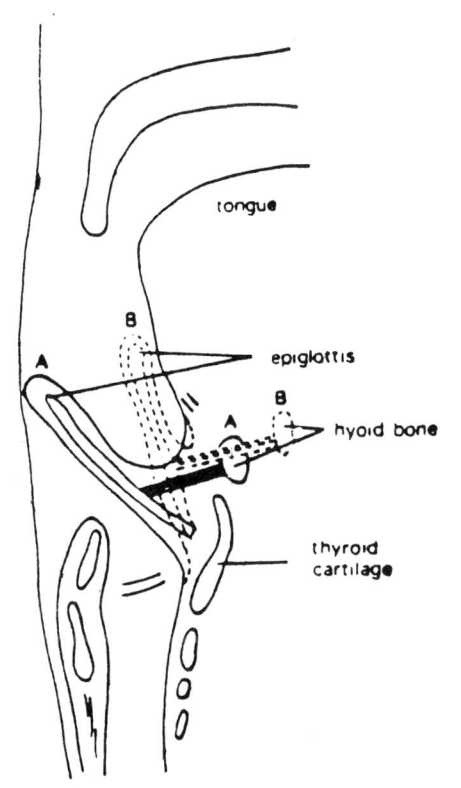

FIG. 16–2. Cross-section of the larynx in the neutral position showing obstruction of the upper airway by the epiglottis, A. Anterior displacement of the hyoid bone, B, by strong retroflexion of the head and stretching of the extra pharyngeal muscles clears the airway. From Boidin, M.P.: Anesthesia and Its Interactions With the Components of Critical Care Medicine [thesis]. Rotterdam, Erasmus University, October 1985.

position, with the head resting on the horizontal plane of the table, the oral axis makes an angle of about 105 degrees with the horizontal and is restrictive (Fig. 16–3). If the head of an adult is elevated by a pillow under the occiput from the neutral position the passageway is greatly improved. The forward position should be 2 to 4 in. above the horizontal. This achieves the sniffing position (Fig. 16–4).[82]

In an elegant study by Boidin using a flexible fiberoptic bronchoscope, the occiput was elevated to various heights and the patency of the upper airway observed.

To secure a patent airway in the neutral head position, the head needs to be greatly extended to an angle of retroflexion of approximately 115 degrees. As the occiput is elevated, the angle of retroflexion needed to obtain a clear airway lessens. When the occiput is elevated between 3 to 4 in., only a small tilt of the head at the atlanto-occipital junction is necessary.

Obstruction at the Hypopharynx.[82] It is evident from both lateral radiographic studies of the airway[89] and fiberoptic observations that the position of the epiglottis is a major determinant in the provision of a clear air passageway into the trachea. When the head is in a neutral position in the unconscious patient, the passageway is usually narrow or closed and the epiglottis lies in a horizontal position. Elevating the head so that the oral axis approximates a 90-degree angle with the horizontal then permits easy tilting of the head. This maneuver decreases the degree of retroflexion necessary to open the upper airway. Anterior displacement of the hyoid bone by lifting the chin advances the epiglottis anteriorly away from the laryngeal opening (Fig. 16–5).

MAINTENANCE OF AIRWAY.[82] Patency of airways is perhaps the most important necessity in induction and maintenance of general anesthesia. The anatomy of the upper airway is fundamental to the problem. The oropharyngeal passage has a rigid posterior wall formed by the cervical vertebrae and a collapsible anterolateral wall consisting of the soft tissues of the oral cavity enclosing the tongue and the epiglottis. The tongue is kept forward naturally by

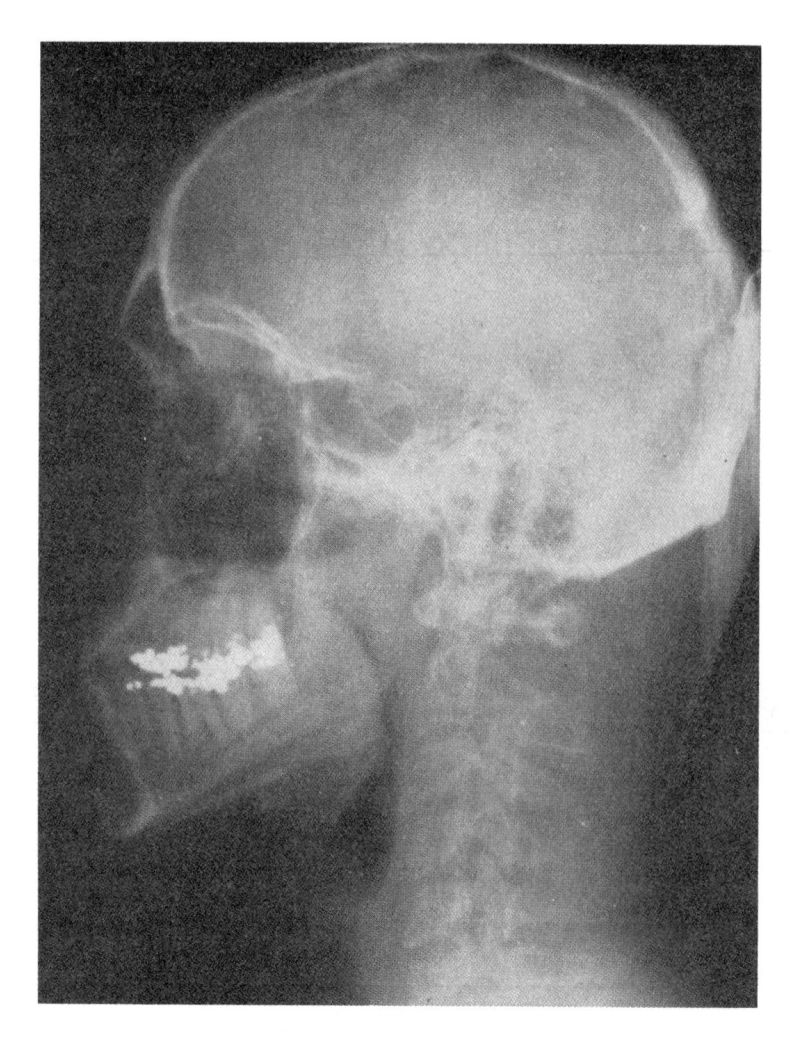

FIG. 16–3. Natural head position. The head is slightly forward with relation to the trunk. The passageway is clear but not large. As long as pharyngeal reflexes are present there will be no obstruction. (Courtesy J. Elam.)

Inhalation Anesthesia—Procedural Considerations **435**

FIG. 16–4. Raising the head to exaggerate the forward position of the head to a true sniffing position greatly improves the passageway. This is accomplished by placing a pillow under the head. This maneuver not only enlarges the pharyngeal passage but helps to move the tongue forward. (Courtesy J. Elam.)

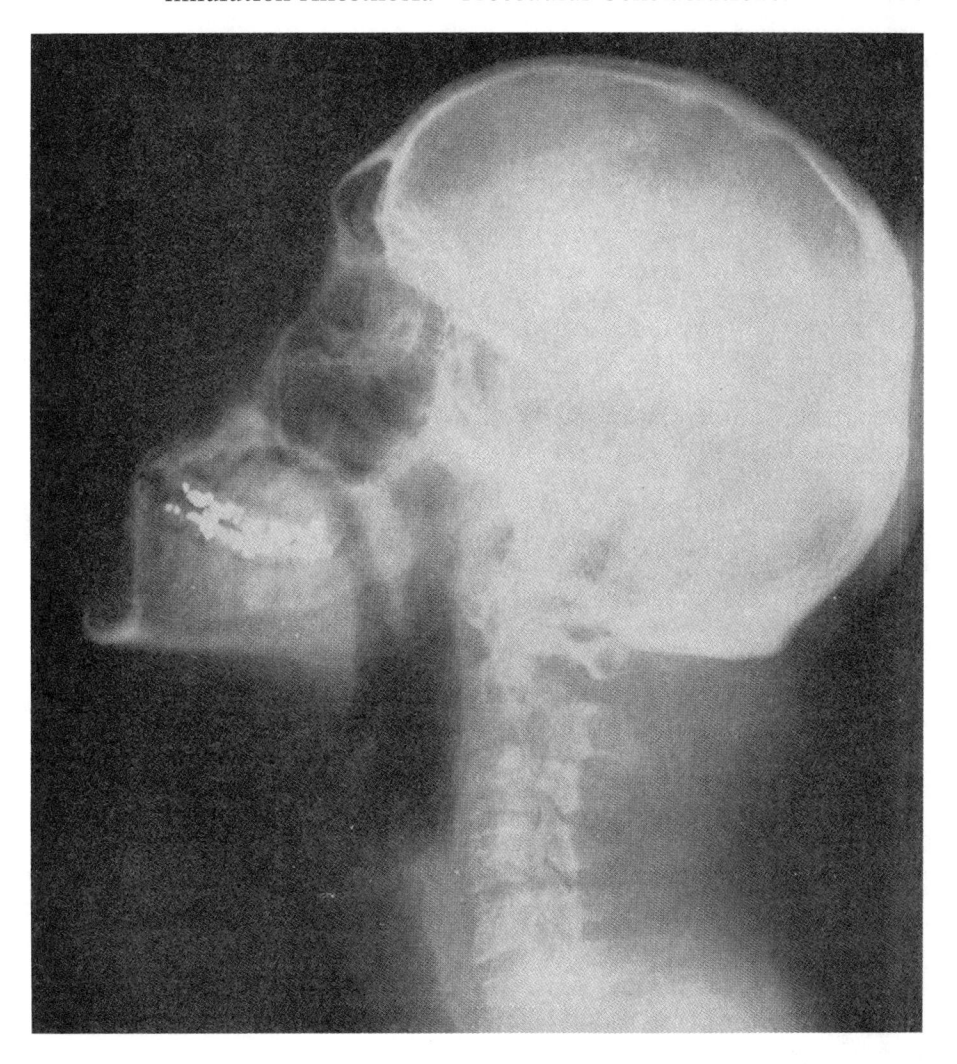

FIG. 16–5. The position of the hyoid bone determines which of two funnels is opened/closed. Note that the tongue is pushed away by the pressure of the epiglottis in position (B). From Boidin, M.P.: Anesthesia and Its Interactions With the Components of Critical Care Medicine [thesis]. Rotterdam, Erasmus University, October 1985.

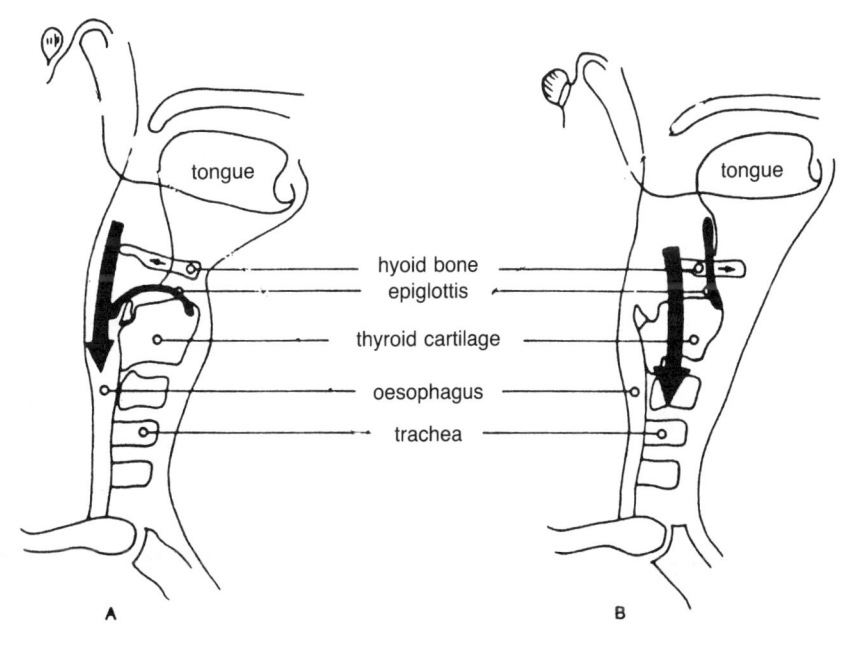

436 *General Anesthesia*

muscles attached forward to the mandible and hyoid bone. When tone of these muscles is lost, the tongue falls back into the oropharyngeal passage and the epiglottis may partially occlude the laryngeal entrance.

Often it is possible to secure a clear airway by simple measures that bring the tongue forward.

1. *Position of Head.* Most people naturally carry the head a little forward (see Fig. 16–3). If the head is brought into normal relation with the trunk, a clear passage may result. This is accomplished by placing a small pillow under the occiput to effect the "sniffing position" (Fig. 16–4).
2. *Tilting the Head* (Fig. 16–6). If one simply tilts the head backward, improvement in the airway is achieved, although the extent of this improvement is not as great as the maneuver of raising the head on a pillow. It should be emphasized that the tilt must be obtained at the atlanto-occipital junction. Hyperextending the entire head, causing a bowing of the cervical vertebrae, will actually obstruct the air passage.

A combination of raising the head about 1 to 3 inches on a pillow and tilting the head at the atlanto-occipital junction provides the maximum in a patent anatomic airway (Fig. 16–7).

3. *Supporting the Jaw.* Simply supporting the jaw forward by pressure at the angle of the mandibles is effective. Also, lifting by a force applied under the chin is oftentimes sufficient. Turning the head to one side will often result in clearing the airway. Remember that extending the head sharply backward is unnatural and that steep Trendelenburg position results in the tongue falling against the palate and posterior pharyngeal wall, resulting in obstructed breathing.
4. *Pulling Out the Tongue.* This is an obvious method of creating a clear passageway. It can be accomplished by placing a towel clip or a suture in the tip of the tongue. Various tongue clamps have been devised in the past but are little used today.

ARTIFICIAL AIRWAYS.[83] It is usually necessary to employ some artificial device when the pharyngeal re-

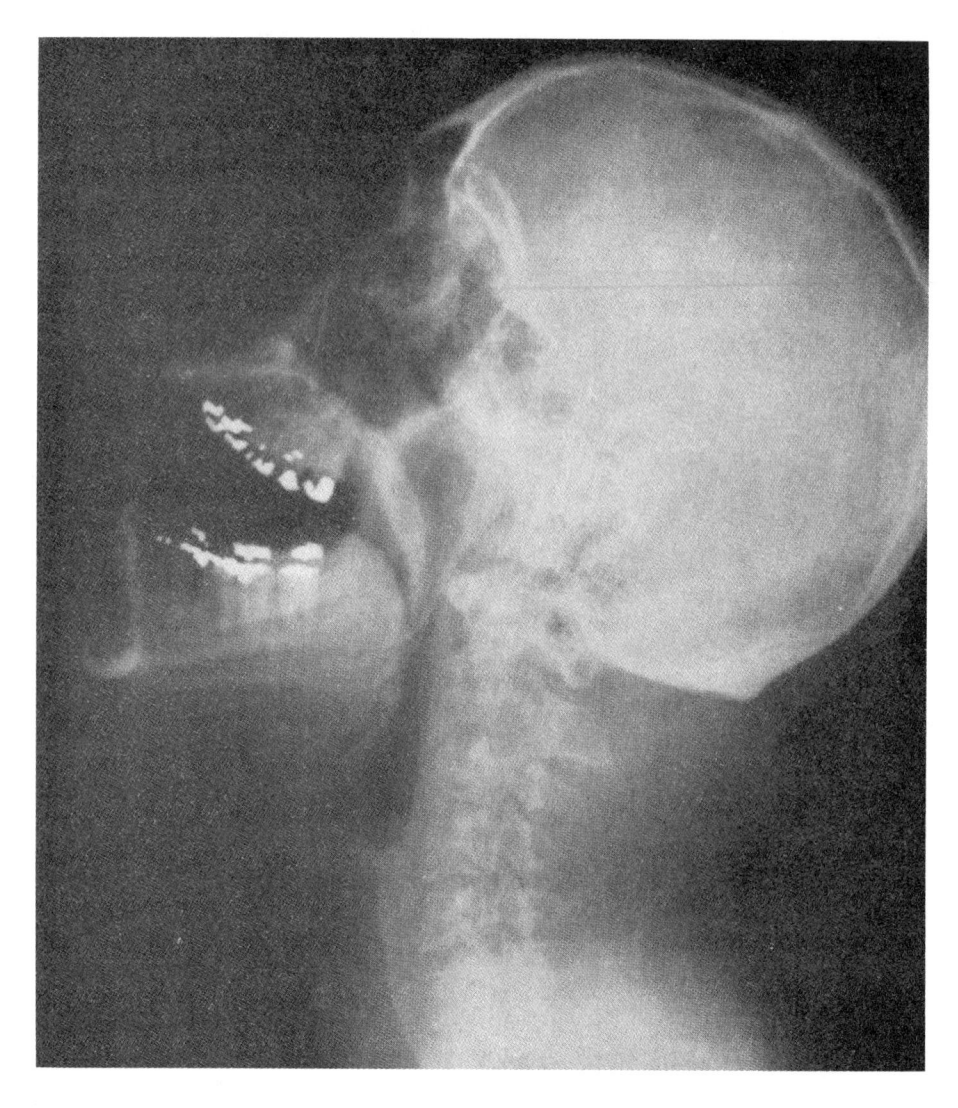

FIG. 16–6. Tilting the head. This maneuver especially aids in enlarging the pharyngeal passage and to some extent helps to move the tongue forward. (Courtesy J. Elam.)

FIG. 16–7. Combination. Head is raised on a pillow to a good sniffing position, and when the head is tilted at the atlanto-occipital junction, an optimum airway is provided. The tongue may be further moved forward by *chin lift*. (Courtesy J. Elam.)

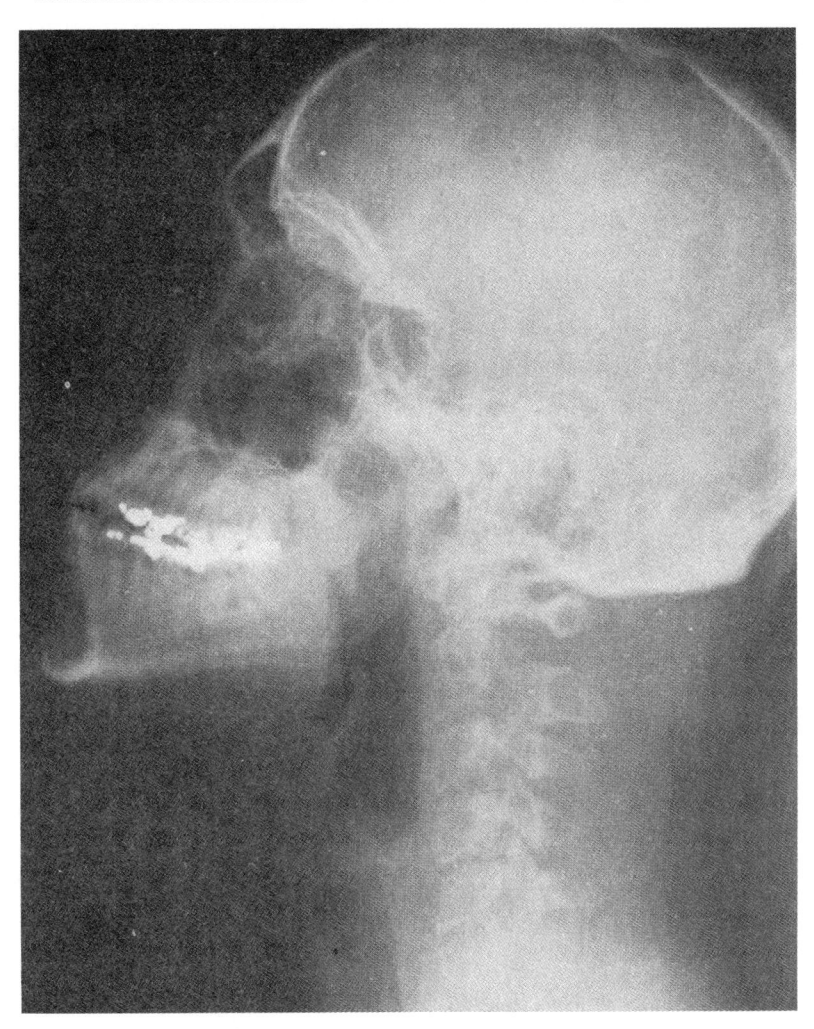

flexes are depressed and the tongue muscles relaxed. Many devices have been developed as upper respiratory tract airways and can be classified into three groups.

Oropharyngeal Airways (Fig. 16–8). These airways are designed to keep the base of the tongue forward; they function to provide a reliable clear pharyngeal air passage. They extend from the lips to the pharynx and are constructed so that there is a flange outside the lips, a portion between the lips that is straight, and then a curved portion extending upward and backward to correspond to the shape of the tongue and palate (see Fig. 16–9). The standard pharyngeal airway exemplified by the Guedel type has several limitations. Unless the size is appropriate, either the tongue can be pressed down and posterior into the pharynx, thus causing partial obstruction, or the tip of the long airway can press the epiglottis against the posterior pharyngeal wall and cover the laryngeal aperture.

To correct these difficulties, the vallecular airway has been developed by Fink.[83] This is a standard pharyngeal airway with a forward extension that fits into the vallecula of the tongue and presses the tongue forward at its base from the point of the linguoepiglottic junction.

Nasopharyngeal Airways. These airways are passed through the nose and extend from the nares to the pharynx just below the base of the tongue. They can be constructed by cutting down Magill endotracheal tubes to the proper length. Also, ordinary rubber tubing about 30 cm long (1 ft) with a moderate curve may be beveled at each end on the same side, while a window is made in the middle on the opposite side. Such an airway provides bilateral breathing through the nose. The diameter varies from No. 26 to 32 F. The length needed for each patient is estimated by the distance from the tragus of the ear to the tip of the nose plus 1 in.

Endotracheal Airways. These airways are designed to pass through the mouth or nose into the pharynx and through the glottic opening into the trachea. They are further described under endotracheal technique. Reusable tubes should be cleaned with a brush and soapy water, then rinsed in water and

FIG. 16–8. Pharyngeal airways.

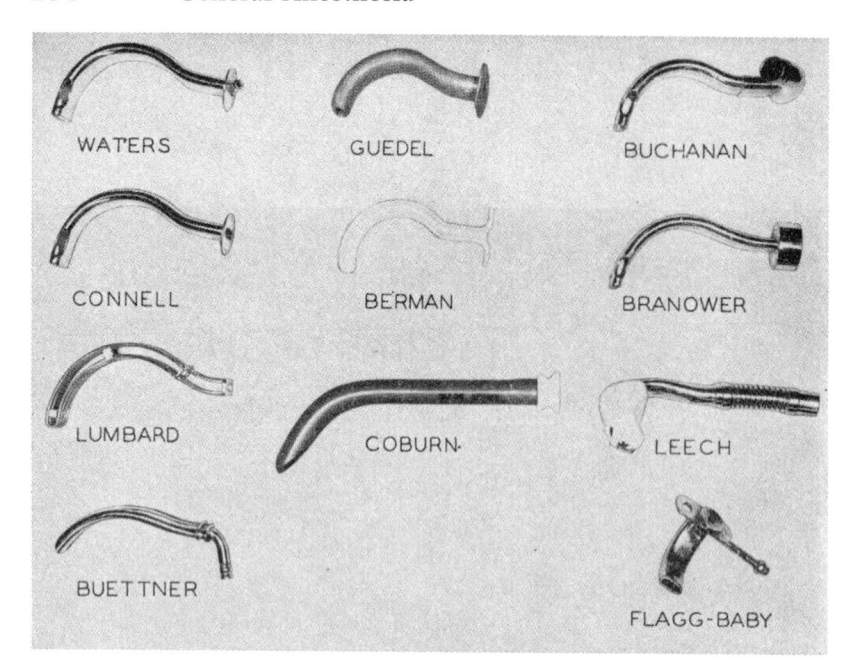

alcohol; at intervals they should be cleaned chemically with 70% alcohol by soaking for 30 minutes. At present disposable tubes are widely used.

MANAGEMENT OF THE PATIENT WITH A FULL STOMACH

A patient with a full stomach is at great risk for regurgitation and aspiration. To secure the airway against pulmonary aspiration becomes a primary objective for safe general anesthesia. It is usually accomplished by a rapid sequence technique, and endotracheal intubation with cuff inflation to seal off the trachea-bronchial passages from the oroesophageal passages. Intravenous agents are used for rapid induction at fairly large doses, with the simultaneous production of full paralysis by the use of muscle relaxants. A priming technique with nondepolarizing drugs is recommended; succinylcholine is also commonly used but is attended by a number of hazards, such as an increase in intragastric pressure and cardiac arrhythmias. Full paralysis will, of course, prevent vomiting but will not prevent regurgitation or passive gastroesophageal reflux.

PROTECTION OF AIRWAY—SELLICK MANEUVER.[87] To contribute to the safety of the rapid sequence induction and to minimize regurgitation of gastric material reaching the pharynx and upper airway, Sellick in 1961 demonstrated the effectiveness of cricoid compression. The maneuver consists of temporary occlusion of the upper esophagus by firm backward pressure on the cricoid ring against the bodies of the cervical vertebrae, usually the 5th to 7th vertebrae.

The compression force should be slightly off center to the left but uniform.

Efficacy of Sellick Technique. The efficacy of the Sellick maneuver has been demonstrated in adults

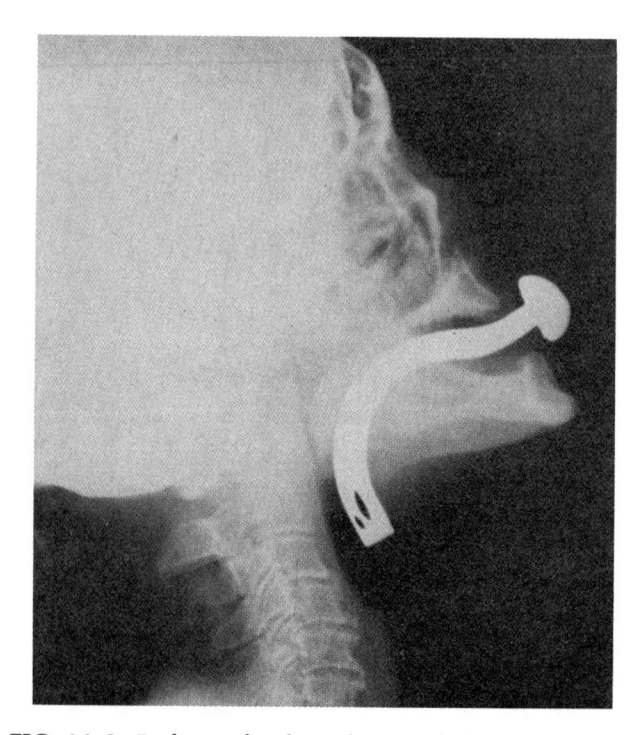

FIG. 16–9. Radiographic lateral view of pharyngeal airway properly placed. From Fink, B.R.: Roentgenographic studies of oropharyngeal airway. Anesthesiology, *18:*711, 1957.

by Fanning[88] and in children by Salem.[89] Significant complication arising from the technique itself has not been observed,[90] but the technique may be performed poorly, and incomplete occlusion may result. Two factors are important in correct application:

1. *The direction of the force* must be uniformly and completely against the vertebral bodies of the 6th and 7th cervical vertebrae. In children, the cricoid is slightly higher in topographical location to the vertebral bodies.
2. *The amount of pressure* needed to occlude the esophagus is approximately 4.5 kg (weight). This is considered to be sufficient weight to produce the desired effect in the majority of patients.[91]

To facilitate a uniform pressure, a cricoid yoke device has been introduced.[92] This is designed to produce consistent and reproducible cricoid pressure.

Frequently, a nasogastric tube is present in these patients, and the competence of the esophagogastric valvular mechanism (esophageal sphincter) may be compromised, allowing a greater volume of regurgitant material. Under these circumstances, one is concerned about the ability of the Sellick maneuver to prevent gastric contents from reaching the pharynx. Salem[93] has demonstrated that cricoid compression will seal off the esophagus from the pharynx and upper airway. Further, a standard nasogastric tube inserted prior to the beginning of anesthesia in patients with an overdistended stomach clearly fails to reduce intragastric pressure. Emptying the full stomach of those who have eaten recently by an oropharyngeal large-bore tube prior to anesthesia may be advisable, particularly in onset of labor.[94]

It should be noted that plastic nasogastric tubes are not occluded by cricoid pressure. These tubes are quite firm, in contrast to the soft latex nasogastric tubes, which can be readily occluded by slight pressure. It is recommended, therefore, that because there is no leakage from the esophagus along the course of the nasogastric tubes into the pharynx the nasogastric tubes be left unclamped.[93]

To further assure that leakage around a nasogastric tube would not occur, Salem designed a nasogastric tube with an anti-reflux valve: the Salem Sump.* The one-way design of this valve allows atmospheric air to enter the vent lumen of a double-lumen nasogastric tube while preventing gastric fluids from being expelled around the tube. This valve protects patients and hospital personnel from contact with potentially hazardous body fluids.

Problems of regurgitation, vomiting, and aspiration are discussed in greater length in a subsequent chapter.

* Argyle® Salem Sump®, marketed by Sherwood Medical, St. Louis.

RAPID SEQUENCE INDUCTION[95]

A rapid induction with a state of general anesthesia is best accomplished by the intravenous administration of appropriate drugs. It represents the "balanced anesthesia technique." The drugs are usually administered in sequence. When the goals of induction are attained, the anesthetic state may be maintained by inhalation of volatile agents by continued use, by neurolepts and higher dose narcotic agents, and by appropriate doses of muscle relaxants.

Three techniques have been used for rapid sequence induction, depending on the drugs used. They include use of an intravenous hypnotic, an opioid or analgesic, and a muscle relaxant.

The most frequently used technique utilizes thiopental-succinylcholine. Prior to induction, 1 mg pancuronium is administered, followed by oxygenation for 2 minutes. Thiopental 2.5% in doses of 4 to 5 mg/kg (smaller doses for patients in shock or debilitated) is administered intravenously and rapidly within 30 seconds, accompanied by 1.5 mg/kg succinylcholine. Intubation can be accomplished usually within 1 minute after completion of injection. The Sellick maneuver should be employed during laryngoscopy and intubation.

A second technique employs a combination of midazolam–ketamine–succinylcholine, preceded by 1 mg pancuronium and oxygenation.[94] This has been designated the "one–five technique." A combination of midazolam 0.15 mg/kg is administered intravenously and rapidly, followed immediately by ketamine 1.5 mg/kg. This is accompanied by succinylcholine in doses of 1.5 mg/kg. The midazolam effectively attenuates the dreaming and adverse behavioral responses often seen after ketamine and also provides some amnesia.

Ketamine has been found advantageous over thiopental when cardiovascular stability is needed. The dose for abolition of eyelid reflex and painful response is between 2 and 4 mg/kg.[96]

The sequence midazolam—succinylcholine without ketamine has been used, but larger doses of midazolam (3 mg/kg) are needed, the induction is slower, and recovery is delayed.

The third technique may be called the U of I sequence.[97] It consists of midazolam pretreatment—ketamine induction—vecuronium relaxation. The midazolam pretreatment may be accompanied by a priming dose of the nondepolarizing agent. The sequence and doses for the induction are the same as previously noted, but instead of succinylcholine, vecuronium is administered in doses of 0.10 mg/kg (pancuronium 0.15 mg/kg). Conditions of relaxation for intubation will develop as rapidly as with succinylcholine.

Thus, for induction, either midazolam alone in ED_{95} doses of 0.3 to 0.4 mg/kg or ketamine in ED_{95} doses of 2 to 4 mg, preceded by a small sedative dose of intravenous midazolam 0.1 mg/kg, are the choices and doses. These have been used safely in high-risk patients in ASA PS III and PS IV categories.[96]

CHOICE AND USE OF RELAXANTS. The availability of vecuronium is a consideration when a short surgical procedure is proposed. The dose is set at 0.10 mg/kg, which is the ED_{95} (effective dose) dose and two to three times the ED_{50}. The drug provides excellent hemodynamic conditions at even larger doses of 0.28 mg/kg. Cardiac output increases about 10%, and SVR (systemic vascular resistance) decreases 12%. Heart rate and MAP do not change.[98] Thus, cardiac performance improves. This relaxant is recommended over pancuronium.

More rapid relaxation and excellent intubation conditions can be achieved by the priming technique. The administration of vecuronium in a partial dose of 10 μg/kg while preliminary preparations are still ongoing will provide a 25% receptor occupancy without discomfort or risk. This will then enable the full dose of the vecuronium to be effective in about 60 seconds. Vecuronium can also be administered for longer surgical procedures by supplementary injections.

A comparative study of relaxants in the rapid sequence technique has been conducted.[99] Differences in cardiovascular effects are consistent in most studies.[100] Pancuronium generally increases cardiac rate, and in doses needed for rapid sequence, prolongs paralysis. Atracurium, in doses suitable for rapid relaxation (1 to 1.5 mg/kg), increases the heart rate by 30 ± 17 beats per minute, with a decrease in arterial blood pressure of about 22 mm Hg systolic. Thus, atracurium is associated with moderate hypotension and tachycardia, neither of which is desirable, in many situations requiring rapid sequence. In contrast, vecuronium in doses of 0.25 mg/kg causes only a slight increase in heart rate of about 15 beats per minute. There is no hypotension and usually a simultaneous slight increase in arterial pressure of about 15 mm Hg. Thus, there are minimal cardiovascular changes following large doses of vecuronium.[101]

It can be concluded that of currently available nondepolarizing relaxants, vecuronium is the choice for rapid sequence and can be used in place of succinylcholine, especially when the latter drug is contraindicated.

RAPID INDUCTION BY SINGLE SYRINGE INJECTION.[102] Ketamine and vecuronium can be combined in one syringe. These two drugs are miscible in all proportions. Vecuronium bromide is supplied as a sterile, nonpyrogenic, freeze-dried, buffered cake of very fine microscopic crystalline particles. The cake contains citric acid, dibasic sodium phosphate, sodium hydroxide, and/or phosphoric acid. When reconstituted with solvent water, the resultant solution is isotonic and has a pH of 4. The reconstituted preparation contains 2 mg/mL. Ketamine is a cyclohexane hydrochloride. It is formulated as a slightly acid sterile solution with a pH of 3.5 to 5.5 for intravenous or intramuscular injection. The commercial preparation contains benzethonium chloride as a preservative. The 100 mg/mL concentration is in isotonic sodium chloride.

Solutions of ketamine and vecuronium can be mixed in a single 10-mL syringe in various miscible proportions. One preparation consists of ketamine 2 mL (200 mg) of the concentrated ketamine base solution aspirated into a 10-mL syringe with vecuronium 5 mL (100 mg) aspirated into the same syringe. The resultant solution has 20 mg ketamine and 1 mg vecuronium per milliliter. This full volume contains the dose for the average healthy adult male of 60 to 80 kg. A portion of this mixture (8 mL or less) may be administered to females and the elderly patient.

A higher dose solution can be mixed in a single 10-mL syringe for younger patients and for robust males: 2.5 mL (250 mg) of the concentrated ketamine base solution (100 mg/mL) is aspirated into a 10-mL syringe (total 250 mg), to which is added 7.5 mL of the vecuronium solution (total 15 mg). The resultant solution has 25 mg and 1.5 mg/mL ketamine and vecuronium, respectively.

CARDIOVASCULAR EFFECTS OF RAPID INDUCTION. Thiopental is a common induction agent with the principal end-point of producing unconsciousness. It is usually accompanied by varying degrees of hypotension. A study of cardiac rate and left ventricular ejection fraction (LVEF) shows some impairment of cardiac function. In a comparison of rapid sequence induction and elective induction with thiopental and succinylcholine, the following observations have been made:[103]

- Rapid sequence—simultaneous administration of thiopental (5 mg/kg) and succinylcholine (1.5 mg/kg): A small decrease in LVEF of 6% was observed. On laryngoscopy and intubation, the LVEF decreased 30%, the heart rate increased by about 30%, and the MAP by 38%.
- Elective induction—(thiopental followed in 1 minute by succinylcholine): A fall in LVEF of 18% was observed after thiopental but returned to normal levels after succinylcholine. After laryngoscopy and intubation, LVEF decreased by 32%, accompanied by a heart rate increase of 12% and an increase in MAP of 30%.

Comment. A depression of left ventricular performance is evident with both induction regimens. However, hypertensive and tachycardic responses were more pronounced in the rapid sequence technique. It is believed that this imposes a higher oxygen demand.

REFERENCES

1. Guedel, A.E.: Inhalation Anesthesia. New York, The Macmillan Co, 1951.
2. AMA Commitee on Anesthesia, Council on Pharmacy and Chemistry, T. Sollnanz Chairman of Council. (Originally chaired by R.M. Waters for National Research Council WWII Program, 1942.) *Fundamentals of Anesthesia*, 3rd ed. Philadelphia, W.B. Saunders, 1954.
3. Moyers, J.: A nomenclature for methods of inhalation anesthesia. Anesthesiology, *14*:609, 1953.
4. Adriani, J.: The Chemistry and Physics of Anesthesia, 2nd ed. Springfield, Charles C. Thomas, 1962.
5. Ernst, E.A.: Selection of the anesthesia delivery system: From open drop to closed circuit [Lecture 119]. Annual Refresher Courses, American Society of Anesthesiologists Annual Meeting, 1983.
6. Aldrete, J.A.: A practical perspective of low, minimal and closed system anesthesia. Acta. Anaesthesiol. Belg., *34*:251, 1984.
7. Stoelting, R., and Miller, R.: Basics of Anesthesia. New York, Churchill Livingstone, 1984.
8. Dripps, R.D., Eckenhoff, J.A., and Vandam, L.: Introduction of Anesthesia, 7th ed. Philadelphia, W.B. Saunders, 1988.
9. Collins, V.J.: Chapter 15. *In* Inhalation Anesthesia: Principles of Anesthesiology, 2nd ed. Philadelphia, Lea & Febiger, 1977.
10. Hamilton, W.K.: Nomenclature of inhalation anesthetic systems. Anesthesiology, *25*:3, 1964.
11. McClure, R.D., Behrmann, V.G., and Hartman, F.W.: The control of anoxemia during surgery anesthesia with the aid of the oxyhemograph. Ann. Surg., *128*:685, 1948.
12. Medrado, V., and Stephen, C.R.: Arterial blood gas studies during induction of anesthesia and endotracheal intubation. Surg. Gynecol. Obstet., *123*:1275, 1966.
13. Chen, K.K.: Symposium on Sedative and Hypnotic Drugs. Baltimore, Williams & Wilkins, 1954.
14. Werner, H.W., Pratt, T.W., and Tatum, A.L.: A comparative study of several ultra-short acting barbiturates. J. Pharmacol. Exp. Ther., *60*:189, 1937.
15. Hamilton, W.K., and Eastwood, D.W.: Study of denitrogenation with some inhalation anesthetic systems. Anesthesiology, *16*:861, 1955.
16. Berthoud, M., Read, D.H., and Norman, J.: Preoxygenation: How long? Anaesthesia, *38*:96, 1983.
17. Gold, M.I., Duarte, I., and Muravchick, S.: Arterial oxygenation in conscious patients after 5 minutes and 30 seconds of oxygen breathing. Anesth. Analg., *60*:313, 1981.
18. Bone, M.E., and May, K.E.: Preoxygenation techniques in obstetric patient. Anesth. Rev., *15*(3):37, 1988.
19. Drummond, G.B., and Park, G.R.: Arterial oxygen saturation before intubation of the trachea: An assessment of oxygenation techniques. Br. J. Anaesth., *56*:987, 1984.
20. Heller, M.L., and Watson, T.R.: Polarographic study of arterial oxygenation during apnea in man. N. Engl. J. Med., *264*:326, 1961.
21. Heller, M.L., and Watson, T.R.: The role of preliminary oxygenation prior to inhalation with high nitrous oxide mixtures: Polarographic Pa_{O_2} study. Anesthesiology, *23*:219, 1962.
22. Archer, G.W., and Marx, G.F.: Arterial oxygen tension during apnea in parturient women. Brit. J. Anaesth., *46*:358, 1974.
23. Norris, M.C., and Dewan, D.M.: Preoxygenation for cesarean section: A comparison of two techniques. Anesthesiology, *62*:827, 1985.
24. Gambee, A.M., Hertzka, R.E., and Fisher, D.M.: Preoxygenation techniques: Comparison of three minutes and four breaths. Anesth. Analg., *66*:468, 1987.
25. Miles, G.G., Martin, N.T., and Adriani, J.: Factors influencing the elimination of nitrogen using semi-closed inhalers. Anesthesiology, *17*:213, 1956.
26. Swartz, C.H., Adriani, J., and Mih, A.: Semi-closed inhalers: Studies of oxygen and carbon dioxide tensions during various conditions of use. Anesthesiology, *14*:437, 1953.
27. Mousel, L.: Unpublished data courtesy of Dr. Mousel from Mayo Clinic Studies, 1942.
28. Behnke, A.R., and Willmon, T.L.: Gaseous nitrogen and helium elimination from the body during rest and exercise. Am. J. Physiol., *131*:619, 1941.
29. Behnke, A.R.: The absorption and elimination of gases of body in relation to fat and water content. Medicine, *24*:359, 1945.
30. Kety, S.S.: Uptake and distribution of gases. Pharmacol. Rev., *3*:1, 1951.
31. Severinghaus, J.W.: Rate of uptake of nitrous oxide in man. J. Clin. Invest., *33*:1183, 1954.
32. Proctor, D.F., Hardy, J.B., and McLean, R.: Studies of respiratory air flow. Bull. Johns Hopkins Hosp., *87*:255, 1950.
33. Morita, S., et al.: Accumulation of methane, acetone, and nitrogen in the inspired gas during closed-circuit anesthesia. Anesth. Analg., *64*:343, 1985.
34. Crofford, O.B., et al.: Acetone in breath and blood. Trans. Am. Clin. Climatol. Assoc., *88*:128, 1977.
35. Levitt, M.D.: Production and excretion of hydrogen gas in man. N. Engl. J. Med., *281*:122, 1969.
36. MacIntosh, R., Mushin, W.W., and Epstein, H.G.: Physics for the Anaesthetist. Oxford, Blackwell, 1958, p. 284.
37. Henderson, L.J., and Haggard, H.W., quoted by von-Oettingen, W.F.: Carbon monoxide: Its hazards and the mechanism of its action. Public Health Bulletin #290.
37a. Goldsmith, J.R., and Landaw, S.A.: Carbon monoxide and human health. Science, *162*:1352, 1968.
38. Middleton, V., et al.: Carbon monoxide accumulation in closed circle anesthesia system. Anesthesiology, *26*:715, 1965.
39. Bennett, E.J.: *In* Elements of Pediatric Anesthesia. Edited by S.A. Bennett. Springfield, IL, Charles C. Thomas, 1970.
40. Ruffle, J.M., et al.: Rapid induction of halothane in man. Br. J. Anaesth., *57*:607, 1985.
41. Wilton, N.C.T., and Thomas, V.L.: Single breath induction of anaesthesia, using a vital capacity breath of halothane, nitrous oxide and oxygen. Anaesthesia, *41*:472, 1986.
42. Lamberty, J.M., and Wilson, I.H.: Single breath induction of anaesthesia with isoflurane. Br. J. Anaesth., *59*:1214, 1987.
43. Loper, K., et al.: Comparison of halothane and isoflurane for rapid anesthetic induction. Anesth. Analg., *66*:766, 1987.
44. Dundee, J.W.: Clinical studies of induction agents, VII. A comparison of eight intravenous anaesthetics as main agents for a standard operation. Brit. J. Anaesth., *35*:784, 1963.
45. Clarke, R.S., et al.: Clinical studies of induction agents, XXVI. The relative potencies of thiopentone, methohexitone and propanidid. Brit. J. Anaesth., *40*:593, 1968.
46. Stella, L., Torri, G., and Castiglioni, C.L.: The relative potencies of thiopentone, ketamine, propanidid, alphaxalone and diazepam: A statistical study in man. Brit. J. Anaesth., *51*:119, 1979.
47a. Dundee, J.W., and Wyant, G.M.: Intravenous Anesthesia 2nd ed. Edinburgh, Churchill Livingstone, 1988.
47. Stoelting, V.K.: The use of a new intravenous oxygen bar-

biturate 25398 for intravenous anesthesia (a preliminary report). Anesth. Analg., 36:49, 1957.
48. Reeves, J.G., et al.: Midazolam compared with thiopentone as a hypnotic component in balanced anesthesia: randomized, double-blind study. Can. J. Anaesth., 26:42, 1979.
49. Heath, P.J., et al.: Which intravenous induction agent for day surgery? Anaesthesia, 43:365, 1988.
50. Fisher, D.M., et al.: Comparison of enflurane, halothane, and isoflurane for diagnostic and therapeutic procedures in children with malignancies. Anesthesiology, 63:647, 1985.
51. Tierney, E., et al.: Halothane or enflurane for inhalation induction. Anesth. Analg., 64:77, 1985.
52. Friesen, R.H., and Lichtor, J.L.: Cardiovascular depression during halothane anesthesia in infants: A study of three induction technics. Anesth. Analg., 51:S313, 1979.
53. Laycock, G.J.A., and McNicol, L.R.: Hypoxaemia during induction of anaesthesia—an audit of children who underwent general anaesthesia for routine elective surgery. Anaesthesia, 43:981, 1988.
54. Phillips, A.J., Brimacombe, J.R., and Simpson, D.L.: Anaesthetic induction with isoflurane or halothane. Anaesthesia, 43:927, 1988.
55. Lindgren, L.: Comparison of halothane and enflurane anaesthesia for otolaryngological surgery in children. Br. J. Anaesth., 53:537, 1981.
56. Davidson, S.H.: A comparative study of halothane and enflurane in paediatric outpatient anaesthesia. Acta. Anaesthesiol. Scand., 22:58, 1978.
57. Friesen, R.H., and Lichtor, J.L.: Cardiovascular effects of inhalation induction with isoflurane in infants. Anesth. Analg., 62:411, 1983.
58. Flagg, P.: The Art of Anaesthesia. Philadelphia, J.B. Lippincott, 1911.
59. Collins, V.J.: The anesthetist's second power (editorial). Anesthesiology, 9:437, 1948.
60. Collins, V.J.: Sing them to sleep, doctor. Saturday Evening Post, August 29, 1949.
61. Yamashita, M., and Motokawa, K.: 'Fruit-flavored' mask induction for children. Anesthesiology, 64:837, 1986.
62. Hinkle, A.J.: Scented masks in pediatric anesthesia (editorial). Anesthesiology, 66:104, 1987.
63. Lewis, R.P., et al.: Fruit-flavored mask for isoflurane induction in children. Anaesthesia, 43:1052, 1988.
64. Gormley, T.P., and Sokoll, M.D.: Permanent alopecia from pressure of a head strap. J.A.M.A., 199:747, 1967.
65. Rackow, H., Salanitre, E., and Frumin, M.J.: Dilution of alveolar gases during nitrous oxide excretion in man. J. Appl. Physiol., 16:723, 1961.
66. Markello, R., Maceda, L., and Goplerud, D.: Diffusion hyperoxia, a "concentrating" effect. Anesth. Analg., 53:233, 1974.
67. Fink, B.R.: Diffusion anoxia. Anesthesiology, 16:511, 1955.
68. Frumin, M.J., and Edelist, G.: Diffusion anoxia: A critical reappraisal. Anesthesiology, 31:243, 1969.
69. Batra, Y.K., and Bali, I.M.: Corneal abrasions during general anesthesia. Anesth. Analg., 56:363, 1977.
70. Snow, J.C., et al.: Corneal injuries during general anesthesia. Anesth. Analg., 54:465, 1975.
71. Durkan, W., and Fleming, N.: Potential eye damage from reusable masks. Anesthesiology, 67:444, 1987.
72. Krupin, T., Cross, D.A., and Becker, B.: Decreased basal tear production associated with general anesthesia. Arch. Ophthalmol., 95:107, 1977.
73. Cross, D.A., and Krupin, T.: Implications of the effects of general anesthesia on basal tear production. Anesth. Analg., 56:35, 1977.
74. Meyers, E.F., et al.: Failure of non-depolarizing neuromuscular blockers to inhibit succinylcholine-induced increased intraocular pressure. Anesthesiology, 48:149, 1978.
75. Bøggild-Madsen, N.B., et al.: Comparison of eye protection with methyl cellulose and paraffin ointments during general anesthesia. Can. J. Anaesth., 28:575, 1981.
76. Siffring, P.A., and Poulton, T.J.: Prevention of ophthalmic complications during general anesthesia. Anesthesiology, 66:569, 1987.
77. Hallett, J.W., Wolkowicz, M.I., and Leopold, I.H.: Ophthalmic use of Neosporin. Am. J. Ophthalmol., 41:850, 1956.
78. Marr, W.G., et al.: Effect of topical anesthetics on regeneration of corneal epithelium. Am. J. Ophthalmol., 43:606, 1957.
79. Aquevella, J.V., Gasset, A.R., and Dohlman, C.H.: Corticosteroids in wound healing. Am. J. Ophthalmol., 58:621, 1964.
80. Glauber, D.T.: Facial paralysis after general anesthesia. Anesthesiology, 65:516, 1986.
81. Safar, P., Escarraga, L.A., and Chang, F.: Upper airway obstruction in unconscious patients. J. Appl. Physiol., 14:760, 1959.
81a. Thach, B.T.: Sudden infant death: Old causes rediscovered. N. Engl. J. Med., 315:126, 1986.
82. Elam, J.O., et al.: Head-tilt method of oral resuscitation. J.A.M.A., 172:812, 1960.
83. Fink, B.R.: Roentgenographic studies of oropharyngeal airway. Anesthesiology, 18:711, 1957.
84. Morikawa, S., Safar, P., and DeCarlo, J.: Influence of the head-jaw position upon airway patency. Anesthesiology, 22:265, 1961.
85. Boidin, M.P.: Anesthesia and Its Interactions With the Components of Critical Care Medicine (thesis). Rotterdam, Erasmus University, October 1985.
86. Boidin, M.P.: Airway patency in the unconscious patient. Br. J. Anaesth., 57:306, 1985.
87. Sellick, B.A.: Cricoid pressure to control regurgitation of stomach contents during induction of anaesthesia. Lancet, 2:404, 1961.
88. Fanning, G.L.: The efficacy of cricoid pressure in preventing regurgitation of gastric contents. Anesthesiology, 32:553, 1970.
89. Salem, M.R., Wong, A.Y., and Fizzoti, G.F.: Efficacy of cricoid pressure in preventing aspiration of gastric contents in paediatric patients. Br. J. Anaesth., 44:401, 1972.
90. Sellick, B.A.: Rupture of the aesophagus following cricoid pressure? Anaesthesia, 37:213, 1982.
91. Lawes, E.G.: Cricoid pressure with or without the "cricoid yoke." Br. J. Anaesth., 58:1376, 1986.
92. Lawes, E.G., et al.: The cricoid yoke—a device producing consistent and reproducible cricoid pressure. Br. J. Anaesth., 58:925, 1986.
93. Salem, M.R., et al.: Cricoid compression is effective in obliterating the esophageal lumen in the presence of a nasogastric tube. Anesthesiology, 63:443, 1985.
94. Cohen, S.E.: Aspiration syndromes in pregnancy. Anesthesiology, 51:375, 1979.
95. White, P.F.: Comparative evaluation of intravenous agents for rapid sequence induction—thiopental, ketamine, and midazolam. Anesthesiology, 57:279, 1982.
96. Gross, J.B., Caldwell, C.B., and Edwards, M.W.: Induction dose-response curves for midazolam and ketamine in premedicated ASA Class III and IV patients. Anesth. Analg., 64:795, 1985.
97 Vieira, Z., et al.: Mistura de quetamina con vecuronio para

induçaô anestesica e intubaçào traqueal em sequencia rapida. Rev. Bras. Anest., *39*:Sup 11 CBA 32, 1989.
98. Morris, R.B., et al.: The cardiovascular effects of vecuronium (ORG NC 45) and pancuronium in patients undergoing coronary artery bypass grafting. Anesthesiology, *58*:438, 1983.
99. Miller, R.D., et al.: Clinical pharmacology of vecuronium and atracurium. Anesthesiology, *61*:444, 1984.
100. Lennon, R.L., Olson, R.A., and Gronert, G.A.: Atracurium or vecuronium for rapid sequence endotracheal intubation. Anesthesiology, *64*:510, 1986.
101. Kunjappan, V.E., Brown, E.M., and Alexander, G.D.: Rapid sequence induction using vecuronium. Anesth. Analg., *65*:503, 1986.
102. Mahisekar, U., et al.: Ketamine and vecuronium mixture for rapid induction intubation. *In* Book of Abstracts. Proceedings of 25th Anniversary Symposium on Ketamine, Ann Arbor, Michigan, June 19–21, 1989. Edited by Domino.
103. Chaemmer-Jørgensen, B., Høilund-Carlsen, P., and Marving, J.: Left ventricular ejection fraction during anesthetic induction: Comparison of rapid-sequence and elective induction. Can. J. Anaesth., *33*:754, 1986.

17

M.F.M. James

CLIMATE, ALTITUDE, AND ANESTHESIA

Although it is well known that altitude may affect anesthetic systems and pose special problems for anesthetists, it is generally assumed that levels of altitude of less than 10,000 ft have negligible effects because there is little alteration in basic physiology at moderate altitude.[1,2] Consequently, anesthetic problems at such altitudes have received relatively little attention.

ALTERED PARTIAL PRESSURES OF GASES

At 5000 ft, the partial pressure of oxygen in *air* is reduced from the sea level value of 21 kPa (158 mm Hg) to 17 kPa (128 mm Hg). Consequently, the maximum *arterial* Pa_{O_2} that can be achieved in normal subjects is in the region of 11 kPa (83 mm Hg). At 10,000 ft, the inspired oxygen pressure (Pi_{O_2}) decreases to 14.8 kPa (111 mm Hg), and arterial oxygen tension (Pa_{O_2}) is in the order of 8.6 kPa (65 mm Hg). As a result of the hypoxia, the carbon dioxide response curve is shifted to the left, and there is a progressive increase in minute volume as the barometric pressure decreases. This results in a reduction in the arterial P_{CO_2} to 4.8 kPa (36 mm Hg) at 5000 ft[3] and 4.5 kPa (34 mm Hg) at 10,000 ft. To compensate for the reduced arterial oxygen content during anesthesia, Powell[4] recommended that a minimum of 40% oxygen be administered during anesthesia at altitudes of 1 mile. Perhaps more rationally, Aldrete[5] recommended a minimum inhaled partial pressure of oxygen of 215 mm Hg (28.3 kPa) at altitude, which represents 33% oxygen at 5000 ft and 40% oxygen at 10,000 ft. For patients with normal pulmonary function, this figure provides adequate oxygenation for routine anesthesia at altitude.

The partial pressure and hence the effectiveness of nitrous oxide is also reduced progressively as the barometric pressure decreases. James[6] studied the analgesic effect of 50% nitrous oxide in oxygen on conscious volunteers at barometric pressures of 760 mm Hg, 640 mm Hg and 524 mm Hg. Nitrous oxide 50% was found to be a highly effective analgesic at sea level pressures, but the analgesic effectiveness of this concentration of nitrous oxide was reduced by nearly 50% at 5000 ft and to insignificant levels of 10,000 ft (Fig. 17–1). Reliance on nitrous oxide to provide anesthesia at an altitude of 1 mile has been questioned,[4] and its use at altitudes of 10,000 ft or more condemned.[1] While similar considerations should apply to any gas such as cyclopropane, the potency of this agent is such that the changes in partial pressure are of minor importance.

GAS ANALYZERS

Anesthetic gas mixtures are usually described in terms of the concentration of the individual gases in the mixture. This is probably a consequence of volumetric devices such as the Haldane apparatus being the only type of equipment available for gas analysis in early studies. However, virtually all of the devices currently used by anesthetists for the determination of gas composition are based on one or other physical property of the agent being measured. These devices respond to the number and activity of molecules present unrelated to the presence of other substances unless there is some degree of interference. Such instruments, therefore, measure partial pressure, not concentration, but because of the trend to think in terms of concentration, these devices are almost universally calibrated in percentages. This may introduce important errors with changes in barometric pressure, and, because it is partial pressure and not concentration that is of primary importance, errors in clinical management may ensue.

OXYGEN ANALYZERS. There are four main types of analyzers currently in common use for measurement of the oxygen content of gas mixtures. They are paramagnetic, fuel cell, oxygen electrode, and mass spectrometer devices. All respond to partial pressure of oxygen alone, and the output changes as the barometric pressure changes. At an altitude of 5000 ft an oxygen analyzer set to measure 21% oxygen at sea level will give a reading of 17.4% unless it is recalibrated to read 21% in air at the new pressure (Table 17–1). If the device were to be calibrated in terms of partial pressure the scale readings would reflect the true state of oxygen availability to the patient. This effect is of relatively minor importance unless accurate research work is being performed or the changes in barometric pressure are extreme. At altitudes of 10,000 ft and above, 21% oxygen becomes a relatively hypoxic mixture, and measurements of partial pressure are the only sensible ones to follow. It is worth noting that breathing air at this altitude is equivalent to breathing 14% oxygen at sea level. As a practical point, the gain controls on some models of oxygen analyzers do not permit resetting of the scale to read 21% in air at such low partial pressures of oxygen. These devices will, however, continue to reflect the reduced partial pressure. Under hyperbaric conditions, it is again important to know the partial pressure of oxygen in the mixture inhaled, because 21% oxygen at 5 atmospheres pressure will exert a partial pressure greater than that of 100% oxygen at sea level, with the consequent risks of oxygen toxicity.

CARBON DIOXIDE ANALYZER. Carbon dioxide is most commonly measured by absorption of infrared radiation by the gas. Such instruments are often produced commecially with an internal calibration device that is supposed to read in percentages. Because the instrument actually responds to partial pressure, this is misleading, and reliance on the internal calibration device will introduce errors of clinical importance when such equipment is used at altitude. A device with internal calibration nominally set at 7% will, in fact, be calibrated to 7 kPa (53 mm Hg), which is actually 8.2% of barometric pressure at 5000 ft altitude. For such equipment to function correctly, it must be either recalibrated against known concentrations of carbon dioxide at the correct barometric pressure or the scale converted to read partial pressure. If kilopascals are used, this conversion is simple because sea level percentages and kilopascals are, for practical purposes, the same. Fortunately, many CO_2 analyzers now available display the transducer output in pressure units and not as percentages. The effect of varying barometric pressures on the output of an infrared analyzer using

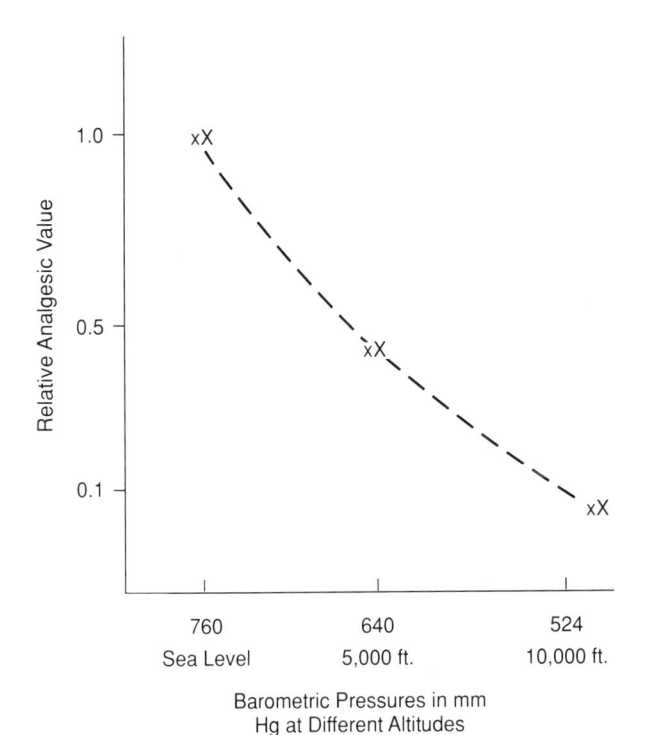

FIG. 17–1. The analgesic effect of 50% nitrous oxide in oxygen at barometric pressures of 760 mm Hg (101.3 kPa), 643 mm Hg (84 kPa), and 512 mm Hg (69 kPa).

TABLE 17–1. INFLUENCE OF BAROMETRIC PRESSURE ON OXYGEN CONTENT OF AIR AS MEASURED BY PARAMAGNETIC OXYGEN ANALYZER

Altitude (ft)	Barometric Pressure (kPa)	Barometric Pressure (mm Hg)	Scale Reading (% oxygen)	Partial Pressure of Oxygen (kPa)	Partial Pressure of Oxygen (mm Hg)
0	101.5	760	21.0	20.9	165
5000	83.2	624	17.4	17.4	122
10000	69.0	518	14.2	14.2	110

a fixed concentration of carbon dioxide is shown in Table 17–2. At an altitude of 5000 ft, the concentration of carbon dioxide in alveolar gas is 5.5%. If a device calibrated in percentages is used to monitor end tidal CO_2 to maintain normocapnia, the use of the percentage figure will result in the patient being rendered significantly hypercapnic, because the partial pressure of expired CO_2 will be 5.5 kPa (42 mm Hg), the normal at this altitude being 4.6 kPa (35 mm Hg).

A more subtle error may also be introduced if a machine of this nature is used to monitor a patient being ventilated inside a one-man hyperbaric chamber in, for example, the management of carbon monoxide poisoning. If the analyzer is placed outside the chamber and the patient's expired gas led outside the chamber before measurement, the gas will expand. The concentration of carbon dioxide in the mixture will remain unchanged, but the partial pressure will decrease, thus giving a falsely low reading.

VAPOR ANALYZERS. Similar arguments apply to the use of vapor analyzers, all of which in modern practice respond to partial pressure, although they are invariably calibrated in percentages. This situation can be confirmed by producing a gas mixture of known composition by vaporizing a known mass of a volatile anesthetic liquid into a closed vessel of known volume. Reduction of the ambient pressure to which the flask and its contents are subjected will result in a fall in the partial pressure of the vapor in the flask, with a consequent reduction in the reading of the analyzer, even though the concentration of the vapor is unchanged.

Alternatively, a fresh vapor mixture can be prepared at different ambient pressures by adding the same mass of liquid to the cleaned flask after the pressure had been altered. In this way, a constant mass of anesthetic vapor would be contained within the flask and the partial pressure of the vapor should be the same at each level of pressure, although the concentration would be different. The output of the analyzer remains constant despite the altered concentration. These effects are illustrated in Tables 17–3 and 17–4.

From this discussion, it is clear that most modern methods of analyzing gases and vapors depend on the partial pressure of the gas, not its concentration, despite the fact that the output of these devices is usually calibrated in percentages. One important exception to this rule is the gas chromatograph, in which the composition of gases in a mixture is described by the area under the curve of the output of a katharometer. Once the instrument is calibrated, the gas mixture is analyzed by the proportion of each gas in the mixture, thus giving a true percentage figure for composition.

VAPORIZERS

The saturated vapor pressure of a volatile anesthetic is, for practical purposes, dependent only on temperature.[7] Consequently, at any given temperature, the concentration of a given mass of vapor increases as the barometric pressure decreases but the partial pressure of the agent remains unchanged. Since the effect of an inhaled vapor depends on the mass of agent delivered per unit time and not on its concentration, the anesthetic effectiveness of a given partial pressure of vapor will remain unchanged. Similarly, the output of calibrated vaporizers will be

TABLE 17–2. INFLUENCE OF BAROMETRIC PRESSURE ON 4.5% MIXTURE OF CO_2 AS MEASURED BY INFRARED ANALYZER

Altitude (ft)	Barometric Pressure (kPa)	Barometric Pressure (mm Hg)	Scale Reading (% CO_2)	Partial Pressure of Oxygen (kPa)	Partial Pressure of Oxygen (mm Hg)
0	101.5	760	4.5	4.5	34.2
5000	83.2	624	3.7	3.74	28.5
10000	69.0	518	3.1	3.18	24.3

TABLE 17–3. RESULTS OF MEASURING FIXED CONCENTRATION OF HALOTHANE VAPOR AT DIFFERENT BAROMETRIC PRESSURES

Barometric Pressure		Halothane Concentration	Scale Reading	Partial Pressure of Halothane	
(kPa)	(mm Hg)	(%)	(%)	(kPa)	(mm Hg)
101.5	760	1.6	1.5	1.6	12.2
83.2	624	1.6	1.2	1.33	10.1
69.0	518	1.6	1.0	1.11	8.5

altered with changes in barometric pressure only as far as the concentration of vapor is concerned. The partial pressure of the vapor should, in theory, remain unchanged, and so the patient response at any given setting should be the same as that expected at sea level. This, of course, assumes that the characteristics of the vaporizer do not change as a result of the altered density and viscosity of the carrier gases. In his experiments under conditions of increased barometric pressures, McDowell[8] found that small alterations in the output of Fluotec Mk II occurred, which were attributed to altered flow characteristics within the vaporizer. Safar[1] studied the performance of the Foregger vaporizer at 10,000 ft and found that the vaporizer produced a higher partial pressure at increased altitude. James[9] tested the Fluotec Mk II and Drager Vapor halothane vaporizers[14] at three altitude levels: sea level (101.5 kPa), 5000 ft (83.2 kPa), and 10,000 ft (69 kPa). At each level of pressure, three flow rates were used (3, 5, and 8L/min), and the output from the vaporizer was measured at each flow rate. The vaporizers were also tested in a circuit driving a Manley ventilator to determine whether or not back pressure from the ventilator produced any additional change in the vaporizer output with changes in barometric pressure. No change greater than 0.1 kPa compared to sea level values was demonstrated, whether or not a ventilator was included in the circuit. Speer[10] produced a mathematical model of the copper kettle in which he calculated that the mass output of the vaporizer would increase with decreasing barometric pressure but did not verify the model experimentally. The overall conclusion would seem to be that the output of vaporizers is little changed by alterations in barometric pressure.

GAS DENSITY AND FLOW

Changes in barometric pressure produce changes in the density of gases. As a result, an apparatus whose function is partly or wholly dependent on gas density will not behave as it would at the altitude at which the device was calibrated (almost invariably sea level). Consequently, equipment used by anesthesiologists in the operating room, critical care area, and laboratory may not function in the expected manner.

FLOWMETERS. Most flowmeters use the decrease in pressure that occurs when a gas passes through a resistance as a measure of gas movement. The magnitude of the decrease in pressure depends on the density and viscosity of the gas. In situations where the resistance represents an orifice, resistance depends primarily on the density of the gas. Where the resistance is tubular, viscosity becomes the prime determinant of the magnitude of the decrease in pressure provided that the flow remains laminar. Most flowmeters use a floating ball or bobbin supported by the stream of gas in a tapered tube. At low levels of flow, the device depends primarily on tubular flow, and as the float moves up the tube, the resistance behaves progressively more like an orifice. The density of a gas changes, of course, with changes in barometric pressure, but the viscosity changes relatively little, as it is primarily dependent on temperature.[11] Safar reported an error of 1% for every 1000 ft of altitude in the Foregger flowmeter and recommended that with this minor correction, flowmeters could be safely used at any altitude.[1] Collins supported this view.[2] Halsey,[12] on the other hand, stated that as the accuracy of a flowmeter

TABLE 17–4. RESULTS OF ADDING FIXED MASS OF HALOTHANE VAPOR TO A KNOWN VOLUME OF GAS AT DIFFERENT BAROMETRIC PRESSURES

Barometric Pressure		Halothane Concentration	Scale Reading	Partial Pressure of Halothane	
(kPa)	(mm Hg)	(%)	(%)	(kPa)	(mm Hg)
101.5	760	1.2	1.1	1.2	8.8
83.2	624	1.4	1.0	1.2	8.8
69.0	518	1.7	1.1	1.2	8.8

changes with the ambient pressure, recalibration becomes necessary if the ambient pressure differs significantly from 1 atmosphere. Coleman[13] concurred. Gas flow through an orifice is inversely proportional to the square root of the density of the gas. As the density of the gas falls, therefore, the flow through an orifice of given size will increase. Thus at altitude the actual flow delivered by a flowmeter will be greater than that indicated by the position of the float. It has been suggested that the actual flow delivered by a flowmeter under conditions of altered barometric pressure can be described by Equation 1:

EQUATION 1. $F_1 = F_0 \sqrt{\dfrac{\rho_0}{\rho_1}}$

where F_1 is the flow delivered at the new pressure, F_0 is the flow delivered at the original pressure, ρ_0 is the original density of the gas, ρ_1 is the density of the gas at the new pressure.

As density is directly proportional to pressure, values for barometric pressure may be substituted for density.[13,14]

The relative contributions of density and viscosity to the behavior of a flowmeter are unpredictable, as each flowmeter has its own characteristics determined by the relationship between the shape of the bobbin and the taper of the tube. Thus, the exact role of viscosity in the determination of the position of the float has not been well established. Viscosity has been shown to exert an important effect in clinically used flows,[15] and at flow rates at which viscosity is the predominant factor, Equation 1 will not apply. Little if any error in measured flow will occur with changes in altitude at the lower settings of the flowmeter where viscosity is the main determinant of the pressure drop. Friedman[16] studied a Fischer and Porter flowmeter, which is not specific for any one gas, and showed that at flow rates of less than 3 L/min there was virtually no error induced by changes in barometric pressure. Other flowmeters that are custom built for an individual agent have their own particular characteristics as regards the relative contributions of density and viscosity, and the degree of error predicted by changes in density do not apply accurately at low gas flows. James[9] studied nitrous oxide and oxygen flowmeters of the floating bobbin or floating ball type over a range of flows from 0.5 L/min to 8 L/min and at barometric pressures of 760 mm Hg, 640 mm Hg, and 512 mm Hg. The accuracy of the flowmeters was also checked under loaded conditions in which the gas stream was used to drive a Manley ventilater. The error in flow rate for the two types of flowmeter are shown in Figures 17–2 and 17–3.

It can be seen that the error is not constant but gradually increases with flow rate and reaches a

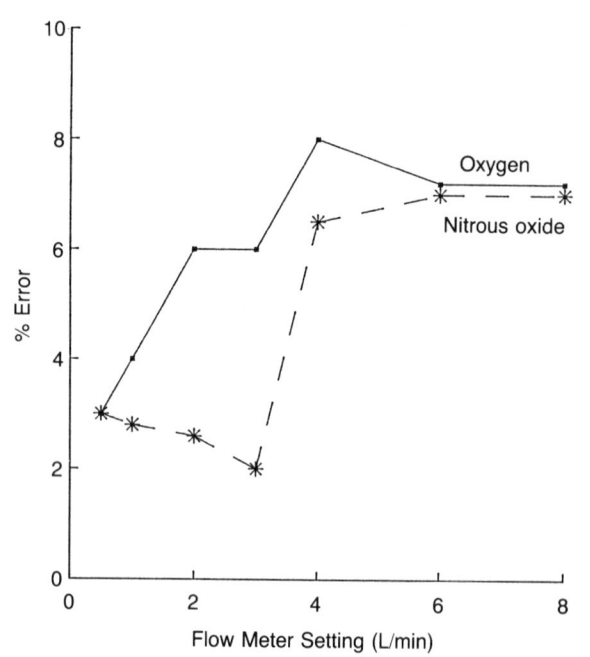

FIG. 17–2. The percentage error in an oxygen and a nitrous oxide rotameter-type flow meter at an altitude of 4800 ft. Barometric pressure = 643 mm Hg, 84 kPa.

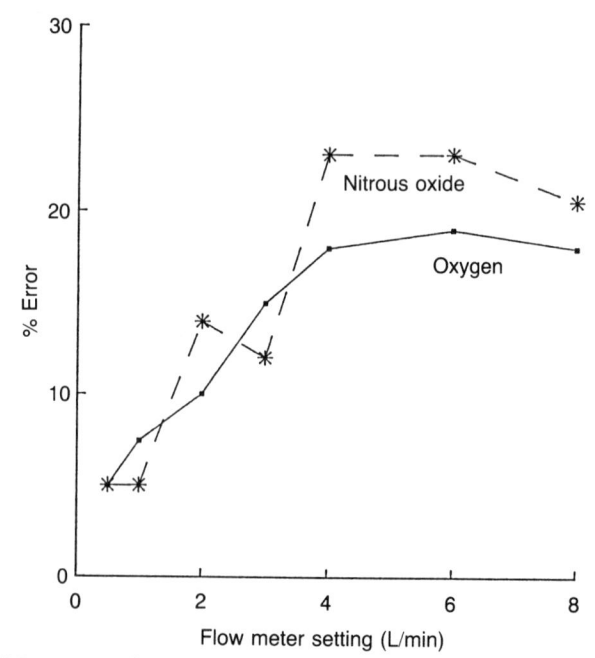

FIG. 17–3. The percentage error in an oxygen and a nitrous oxide rotameter-type flow meter at an altitude of 10,000 ft. Barometric pressure = 512 mm Hg, 69 kPa.

relatively steady level at flows above 4 L/min. This presumably reflects the changing contribution of viscosity and density as the flow rate increases. The relatively constant error at flows greater than 4 L/min suggests that density is the major determinant of the pressure drop at flow rates of this magnitude or greater, and this impression is supported by the fact that the measured and calculated errors using Equation 1 are in good agreement. At low flows, where the error is much smaller (presumably because viscosity is playing a more important role than density in determining the position of the bobbin), Equation 1 does not apply. Low-reading flowmeters were not tested, and it is possible that these comments may not apply to these devices because the orifice characteristics may be different. The contention that the error in flow is approximately 1%/1000 ft change in altitude is not supported by these findings.[1] It is clear, therefore, that the common attitude that flowmeters may be safely used at altitude because they underread is not wholly reliable if low flows are being used, and anesthesiologists using low-flow techniques should be aware of this possible hazard. Errors may arise when low flows of oxygen are mixed with higher flows of nitrous oxide in an attempt to administer a 30% oxygen mixture. If, for example, 1.5 L/min oxygen and 3 L/min nitrous oxide are administered at 10,000 ft, it is possible the mixture could contain as little as 25% oxygen, which has been shown to pose a serious risk of hypoxemia during anesthesia at altitude.[4] Under such circumstances, the use of an oxygen analyzer is advisable, although a cheaper alternative, expecially in the Third World, would be to dispense with nitrous oxide altogether. If accurate measurements are to be made, the only practical approach is to recalibrate the flowmeter at the altitude at which it is to be used. These comments do not apply to fixed orifice flowmeters, in which turbulent flow is probable at all flow rates, and the error should be accurately described by Equation 1 at any flow.

Various other flow-measuring devices will also perform inaccurately at altitude. The manufacturers of the Wright respirometer include a guide to the inaccuracy of the instrument at altitude.* Devices that depend on other physical properties of the gas, such as katharometers, will also tend to underread, because the number of gas molecules per unit volume, and hence the thermal capacity, will be reduced. Consequently, when such devices are used to adjust ventilator settings, there will be a tendency towards hyperventilation. Minute volume dividers, driven by the flows delivered from flowmeters, will also tend to overventilate if the same settings are used as those adopted at sea level. Pneumotachographs, on the other hand, use laminar flow to generate a pressure drop, and therefore viscosity, not density, will be the prime determinant of the measurement obtained. These devices should, therefore, continue to perform well regardless of changes in barometric pressure but may be sensitive to temperature fluctuations. Ventilators that use a bellows to measure expired volumes will obviously perform accurately, but it should be remembered that patients at altitude normally hyperventilate, and this should be allowed for when setting the ventilator.

HIGH AIR FLOW OXYGEN ENRICHMENT DEVICES

The importance of administering known concentrations of oxygen at flows exceeding peak inspiratory flow in the management of patients with respiratory disease has often been stressed. High air flow oxygen enrichment equipment usually consist of a fixed orifice Venturi device for which a specified minimum gas flow must be provided in order to produce adequate flow rates. Changes in barometric pressure might be expected to exert profound effects on such devices, because the driving force that accelerates air along the breathing pathway is the pressure gradient between the atmosphere and the negative pressure area created by the jet of oxygen emerging from the nozzle. Under conditions of reduced barometric pressure, these devices might be expected to "run rich," that is, to produce higher oxygen concentrations than those set but at a lower flow rate than that delivered at sea level. When tested, however, these devices performed better than might have been anticipated.[9] In virtually every case, there was a small but consistent increase in the oxygen percentage and a similar decrease in the total flow produced by the device. The magnitude of these errors, however, was smaller than had been anticipated when a standard flowmeter, not corrected for altitude, was used. When a fresh gas flow is set on a standard flowmeter, it appears that the increased flow delivered by the flowmeter at altitude largely offsets the errors in delivered flow and oxygen concentration that would otherwise occur with decreases in barometric pressure.

When flows corrected for altitude are used, the performance of the device deteriorates to the point where the flow delivered by the mask may well decrease below the patient's peak inspiratory flow, and higher than expected percentages of oxygen are produced. This is unlikely to be of major importance at altitudes of 5000 ft or less. It should be noted that although the oxygen percentage may have remained more or less constant, there is a reduction in its partial pressure, and this effect must be allowed for when prescribing such a device for patient use.

---

* Wright Peak Flow Meter designed by B.M. Wright of Medical Research Council. Bay Medical Inc., 16001 Bay Vista Dr., Clearwater FL 34620.

TABLE 17–5. VARIATIONS IN MAC AT VARIOUS ALTITUDE LEVELS AS COMPARED TO VALUES FOR MAPP.

Agent	MAC Sea Level	MAC 5000 ft	MAC 10,000 ft	MAPP kPa	MAPP mm Hg
Nitrous Oxide	105.0	126.5	152.2	106.1	798.0
Ethyl ether	1.92	2.31	2.78	1.94	14.6
Halothane	0.75	0.90	1.09	0.76	5.7
Enflurane	1.68	2.02	2.43	1.70	12.8
Isoflurane	1.20	1.45	1.73	1.22	9.1

CONCLUSIONS

Reduced barometric pressures exert considerable influence on the delivery and utilization of anesthetic gases and vapors as a result of changes in the partial pressures and densities of these agents. There is a serious risk that patients anesthetized at high altitudes using unmodified sea-level techniques may be made hypoxic, despite the fact that apparently adequate concentrations of oxygen are being administered. For example, at an altitude of 10,000 ft, 30% oxygen has the same partial pressure as 20% oxygen at sea level. As a result of the reduction in partial pressure of nitrous oxide that occurs, the effectiveness of this agent will be seriously impaired to the point that little if any benefit is derived from its use. The increased concentrations of oxygen needed to maintain adequate inspired partial pressures will further reduce the partial pressure of nitrous oxide.

This problem may be compounded by inaccuracies in flow measurement. It is clear that the commonly held views on the performance of flowmeters at altitude are excessively simplistic and that errors in patient management may follow if such assumptions are applied. By far the most logical approach for anesthetists working at altitude is to have flowmeters that are calibrated for the appropriate barometric pressure. This, however, would create problems with the use of such equipment as high air flow oxygen enrichment devices and is excessively expensive. It would seem that the errors are relatively small at altitudes of 5000 ft but steadily increase thereafter. In view of the potential risks of error arising at altitudes higher than this, the value of nitrous oxide in such situations remains questionable.

Errors in measurement of gas concentrations may occur with potentially serious consequences for patients. Such errors can be avoided by thinking in terms of partial pressures, rather than concentration, and consideration should be given to the recalibration of measuring devices in units that reflect partial pressure, not concentration. This is of particular importance in the case of oxygen. The minimum Pi_{O_2} that should be administered is of the order of 220 mm Hg (approximately 30 kPa), which represents 35% oxygen at 5000 ft and 42% oxygen at 10,000 ft.

Although the output of calibrated vaporizers is little affected by changes in barometric pressure, it is important to realize that there is an increase in the concentration of vapor with no change in partial pressure, so the anesthetic potency expected for any given vaporizer setting is effectively unchanged, even though the concentration of vapor will be increased. Small deviations in performance may be expected as a result of alterations in the flow-splitting ratios, but they are unlikely to be of major importance.

Oxygen entrainment devices can obviously be used with relative safety if recalibrated flowmeters are not used, but it behooves clinicians working at altitude to be fully conversant with the effects of reduced barometric pressure on partial pressures of inspired gases.

MINIMAL ALVEOLAR PARTIAL PRESSURE. Partial pressure is the factor determining the effectiveness of the volatile agents as well as of the inhaled gases. Consequently, because the concentration of an agent required to produce a given effect increases with reductions in barometric pressure, the concept of MAC does not apply accurately at altitude and should be converted to minimal alveolar partial pressure (MAPP).[17] The idea has much to recommend it; using this concept would eliminate many of the problems described herein. For ease of reference, the MAC and MAPP values of the commonly used anesthetic agents are listed in Table 17–5.

REFERENCES

1. Safar, P., and Tenicela, R.: High altitude physiology in relation to anesthesia and inhalation therapy. Anesthesiology 25:515, 1964.
2. Collins, V.J.: Principles of Anesthesiology, 2nd ed. Philadelphia, Lea & Febiger, 1976, pp. 1312–1313.
3. Kanarak, D.J., Goldman, H.I., and Zwi S.: Arterial O_2 tension values in normal adults at an altitude of 1763 m. S Afr. Med J. 46:315, 1972.
4. Powell, J.N., and Gingrich, T.F.: Some aspects of nitrous

oxide analgesia at an altitude of one mile. Anesth. Analg. *48*:680, 1969.
5. Aldrete, J.A., and Romo-Salas, F.: Oxygenation with high, intermediate, and low gas flows during thoracic and abdominal surgery: Studies at an altitude of one mile. *In* Low Flow and Closed System Anesthesia. Edited by J.A. Aldrete, H.J. Lowe, and R.W. Virtue. New York, Grune & Stratton, 1979.
6. James, M.F.M., Manson, E.D.M., and Dennett J.E.: Nitrous oxide analgesia and altitude. Anaesthesia *37*:285, 1982.
7. Hill, D.W.: Physics Applied to Anesthesia, 4th ed. Boston, Butterworths, 1980, pp. 336–337.
8. McDowall, R.G.: Anaesthesia in a pressure chamber. Anaesthesia *19*:321, 1964.
9. James, M.F.M., and White, J.F.: Anesthetic considerations at moderate altitude. Anesth. Analg. *63*:1097, 1984.
10. Speer, D.L.: Vaporization of anesthetic agents at high altitude. *In* Low Flow and Closed System Anesthesia. Edited by J.A. Aldrete, H.J. Lowe, and R.W. Virtue. New York, Grune & Stratton, 1979.
11. Van Wazer, J.R., et al: Viscosity and Flow Measurement. New York, John Wiley & Sons, 1975, p. 31.
12. Halsey, M.J., and White, D.C.: Gas and vapour supply. *In* General Anaesthesia, 4th ed. Edited by T.C. Gray, J.F., Nunn, and J.E. Utting. London, Butterworth, 1980.
13. Coleman, A.J.: Hyperbaric physiology and medicine. *In* A Practice of Anaesthesia, 4th ed. Edited by H.C. Churchill-Davidson. London, LloydLuke Ltd., 1978, p. 235.
14. Dorsch, J.A., and Dorsch, S.E.: *In* Understanding Anesthesia Equipment. Baltimore, Williams & Wilkins, 1975, p. 46.
15. McIntosh, R.R., Mushin, W.W., and Epstein, H.G.: In Physics for the Anaesthetist, 3rd ed. Oxford, Blackwell, 1963, pp. 192–208.
16. Friedman, M.D., and Lightstone, P.J.: The effect of high altitude on flowmeter performance. Anesthesiology *55*:17, 1981.
17. Fink, B.R.: How much anesthetic? Anesthesiology *34*:403, 1971.

18

CARBON DIOXIDE ABSORBPTION TECHNIQUE

INTRODUCTION. The closed-system technique of anesthetic administration involves complete rebreathing of anesthetic mixtures. The technique permits no escape of gases. Because the patient consumes oxygen and produces carbon dioxide, the exhaled gas has had part of its oxygen extracted and replaced by carbon dioxide. The latter is a waste product and will accumulate in the system. Therefore, oxygen must be added and carbon dioxide removed from the gas mixture before it is rebreathed. Similarly, in semiclosed systems there is partial rebreathing, and if the total amount of gas admitted to the system is less than the respiratory minute volume ($\dot{V}$), there will be accumulation of carbon dioxide.

Snow introduced the closed system of anesthesia in clinical anesthesia in 1850, using potassium hydroxide as an absorbent for the exhaled carbon dioxide during chloroform anesthesia. The concept that carbon dioxide was an acid when exposed to water and that it could be neutralized or absorbed by alkalies during rebreathing was established. However, the use of potassium hydroxide proved to be too caustic and presented significant hazards.[1]

To overcome these hazards, Jackson in 1915 introduced an absorption technique using alkalies investigated in laboratory experiments on animals. During World War I, Wilson,[2] working in conjunction with the Chemical Warfare Service, found that sodium hydroxide alone gave off too much heat and devised a soda lime mixture. In 1923, Waters applied the absorption technique to humans and published the first clinical report in 1926.[3,4]

For the application of the absorption technique certain equipment is needed:

1. Compressed gases and regulators
2. Needle valves and flowmeters
3. Vaporizers for liquid agents
4. Delivery tube to breathing circuit
5. Absorber and unidirectional valves
6. Reservoir (bag and bellows)
7. Relief valve for excess gas
8. Inhaler assembly with minimal dead space
9. A free airway with minimal resistance
10. A tight system free from leaks

PROCESS OF ABSORPTION

CHEMICAL NATURE. Absorption of CO_2 is essentially a chemical reaction, that of neutralization.[5] It is a reaction between an acid and a base. The acid is carbonic acid, formed by the combination of CO_2 with water; when the carbonic acid ionizes, H-ions result. The base is the absorbent, and at the present time the only satisfactory absorbents are the hydroxides of the alkali metals (potassium, sodium, lithium) and of the alkaline earths (barium, strontium, calcium, and magnesium). The hydroxides of the alkali metals are more active chemically than the alkaline earths but are very caustic and highly hygroscopic. For clinical purposes, mixtures have been found practical and cheap.

MOISTURE FACTOR. Absorption is a surface phenomenon.[6] The outer surface of the absorbent granule is relatively small and contributes only minimally to absorption, while the surface area of the pores is about 100 times greater.[7] Filling of the pores with water to about 85% of their volume provides sufficient moisture to dissipate by vaporization the heat of reaction and facilitates the chemical reaction. Moisture is needed to facilitate the formation of carbonic acid.

The moisture content of granular lime amounts to 20 to 25% water on a dry basis, and the absorbent is called wet soda lime. More moisture fills the pores and reduces the surface area for absorption. Less moisture shortens absorbent life because the lime dries out before its reactants are completely used.[8] To obtain the desired moisture content, water is added physically to soda lime during its preparation and, to be retained, lime is packaged in air tight containers.

Moisture can also be chemically associated with the absorbent by using barium hydroxide octahydrate, $Ba(OH)_2 \cdot 8H_2O$ (Baralyme). On reacting with carbon dioxide, this compound yields 45 mL of water of crystallization per 100 grams. Because Baralyme granules contain only 5% water of crystallization, the manufacturer increases the moisture content to 10 to 15% to improve the absorption capacity.

In both the to-and-fro and circle systems, all specimens of lime with moisture content below 10% are equally inefficient. The optimum water content for both soda lime and Baralyme is between 10 and 22%.

GRANULES. Granules of 4 × 8 mesh are used in anesthesia. Mesh refers to the number of wires per inch in a sieve screen. A 4 × 8 mesh granule size can be sieved through a screen with 4 wires per inch, but only a small specified amount can go through a screen with 8 wires per inch. Carbon dioxide absorption techniques must provide minimal breathing resistance through the absorbent bed and efficient removal of expired carbon dioxide with each passage through the absorber. Since the activity increases as granule diameter decreases, while resistance to air flow increases, this mesh specification represents a compromise.

Resistance to air flow through an absorbent can be estimated by the following relationship:

$$R = \frac{KLV}{A}$$

In this equation (R) is the resistance, (V) is velocity of air flow, (L) is the length of the canister, and (A) is the effective cross-sectional area of the absorber. (K) is the specific resistance of 4 × 8 mesh absorbent and is of the order of 1 mm of water per liter flow per minute.[9]

In larger absorbers, resistance through the absorbent does not exceed 1 cm of water at 100 L/min, or the maximum respiratory flow rates expected in anesthetized adults. This resistance valve does not include the effect of the breathing tubes, unidirectional valves, and fittings.

ABSORBENTS

SODA LIME. Soda lime is basically porous limestone granules that are activated for carbon dioxide absorption by the addition of the caustics, ie, the alkali metals. Potassium hydroxide is a better activator than sodium hydroxide.[10a,10b]

Thus, soda lime is a mixture of sodium, potassium, and calcium hydroxides, which by ionization furnish OH-ions. Sodium hydroxide and potassium hydroxide make up about 4.5% of the mixture and calcium hydroxide about 95%.[11a,11b] The calcium hydroxide decreases the tendency to deliquescence. Small amounts of silica are added to make the mixture hard and to minimize fragmentation and alkaline dust formation. In soda lime silica amounts to about 0.2%.

$$\begin{aligned} 2CO_2 + 2H_2O &\rightarrow 2H_2CO_3 \rightarrow 4H^+ + 2CO_3^- \\ 2NaOH &\rightarrow 2OH^- + 2Na^+ \\ Ca(OH)_2 &\rightarrow OH^- + Ca^{++} \\ &\qquad \downarrow \\ &\quad 4H_2O + Na_2CO_3 + CaCO_3 \end{aligned}$$

Equation 1. Reaction of carbon dioxide with soda lime.

(1) $Ba(OH)_2 \cdot 8H_2O + CO_2 \rightarrow BaCO_3 + 9H_2O$
(2) $9H_2O + 9CO_2 \rightarrow 9H_2CO_3$
(3) $9H_2CO_3 + 9Ca(OH)_2 \rightarrow CaCO_3 + 18H_2O$

Equation 2. Reaction of carbon dioxide with Baralyme.

BARALYME. As noted previously, another absorbent of CO_2 that is as efficient as soda lime is a mixture of barium and calcium hydroxide.[12a,12b] Baralyme consists of 20% barium hydroxide and 80% calcium hydroxide. The barium hydroxide is a chemical hydrate with eight molecules of water bound as water of crystallization. This water acts as the bonding agent for the entire granule so that no inert material is necessary. The same water is used for dissolving carbon dioxide. Because absorbents containing such hydrates have an inherent stability of water content, they are more dependable and efficient under varying circumstances of use.[12] Baralyme also possesses a greater degree of hardness and is less subject to fragmentation and dust formation.

THE REACTION. Carbon dioxide dissolves in the moisture film on the surface of the lime granule. Carbonic acid is formed and dissociates into hydrogen ions and bicarbonate ions.

$$CO_2 + H_2O \rightarrow H_2CO_3 \rightarrow H^+ + HCO_3^-$$

The very soluble activators of the absorbent provide a high concentration of hydroxyl ions for neutralizing the hydrogen ions produced.[13] Calcium hydroxide also ionizes into calcium ions and hydroxide ions. The hydroxide ion maintains a concentration necessary for the acid H-ion, while the calcium ions react to form calcium carbonate, which precipitates from the solution. In this reaction (Equation 1) the heat of neutralization released with the absorption of each gram molecular weight (44 grams = 22.4 L) of carbon dioxide amounts to 13,500 calories.

The reaction with Baralyme is shown in equation 2. The heat of neutralization is the same as with soda lime. Hence for each gram molecular weight of carbon dioxide absorbed about 13,500 calories of heat are produced.

ABSORPTIVE CAPACITY. The "break point" in absorption of carbon dioxide is the time at which unabsorbed traces of the gas begin to pass through the absorbents. A standard test procedure is to pass through a 150-m canister an air mixture containing 2% → of CO_2 and moisture equivalent to 85% humidity at 20° C. The rate of flow of air mixture is 3.5 L/min. The capacity for CO_2 absorption by granular Baralyme and soda lime is essentially identical and, in single-chamber absorbers, is 10 to 15 L CO_2 per 100 grams absorbent. In two-chamber absorbers, these absorbents yield a capacity of 18 to 20 L CO_2 per 100 grams.

INDICATORS.[14] Chemical indicators have been incorporated into the granules of absorbents. These are dyes that change color when exposed to different acidities or basicities. Usually, they are acids or bases themselves and in the reaction process are converted from or to a salt. The acid form has one color and the base form another. Indicators added to the absorbent denote the exhaustion of absorbing activity. Indictors such as ethyl violet or Clayton yellow are dyes that change color at a pH below 12. As carbonic acid accumulates, the indicator on the absorbent granules changes as follows:

1. Ethyl violet is a colorless base and reacts with carbonic acid to form a colored carbonate. Changes to violet color occur at pH below 10.3.
2. Clayton yellow is pink in color at high pH ranges and changes to yellow (acid form) at low pH ranges (below 6.5).

Baralyme contains two indicators, Mimosa Z (pink at pH above 7.8) and ethyl violet. When this absorbent is inefficient it changes from pink to blue, and when it is completely exhausted it will be gray.

Absorbents must be observed for such indicator change during active use because they subsequently revert to their original color on standing. At this point, the remaining capacity of absorption is negligible because the hydroxide ion is no longer maintained at concentrations useful for absorption. With re-use, the indicator changes color again quickly. Other evidences of exhaustion in an absorber are the decreased heat in the reaction zone and a zone of moisture condensation slightly downstream from this reaction zone. This ring of moisture, along with the color change of the indicator, travels through the absorbent bed. Hence, observation of both indicator and the moisture ring reveal the exhaustion status in the transparent circle absorber.

With opaque-walled canisters, incomplete CO_2 removal is suspected if the patient develops hyperpnea or hypertension.[8] A more reliable practice is noting the color of the indicator in a transparent-walled two-chamber absorber. If no change has occurred in the lower compartment, CO_2 absorption is complete. However, the adequacy of ventilation and competence of the unidirectional valves must also be assessed.

ABSORBER SYSTEMS

BREATHING CIRCUITS. The to-and-fro system of absorption employs only a canister and a breathing bag. The canister is attached to the patient's airway with a minimum of fittings to minimize dead air space. The activity of absorbent at the patient end of the canister is exhausted at a rate that adds 50 to 75 mL of dead space per hour. Increasing the tidal volume can compensate for this increased dead space for about 90 minutes.[15] Alternating canisters at frequent intervals allows cooling. Regeneration of absorbent activity during rest periods is negligible.[16,17] Each canister should be recharged after 90 minutes use. Packed to-and-fro absorbers can lose absorbing life within several days when left unsealed in warm, dry areas. Heat loss through respiration is small with this technique because exhaled gas is kept warm by the heat of reaction. Water vapor content is also high.

The circle system is more efficient than the to-and-fro.[15] In the circle absorption system, valves direct exhaled gas one way through the canister and then back to the patient.[18] Flow through this system is intermittent and in sequential segments corresponding to the patient's successive tidal volumes. Depending upon the position of the absorber in relation to the reservoir bag, flow through the canister stops either during expiration or inspiration.

ABSORBER SIZE. The optimal size of an absorber's lime compartment depends upon the patient's carbon dioxide production rate, his tidal volume, the presence of channeling, and the anticipated period of use before the absorbent can be conveniently changed. A 1-L lime compartment packed with lime accommodates a tidal volume of 470 mL. Note, however, that during use this relationship changes as the activity of lime is exhausted.[9]

The air space of an absorber is the total volume of voids (spaces between granules) and the pores (spaces within granules). If the air space in the canister is equal to or larger than the tidal volume, all the exhaled gas will be in contact with the absorbent for at least one respiratory cycle.[19] If the tidal volume is larger than the air space, part of the exhaled gas passes through the canister without a pause and adequate contact with absorbent. Because gas does not flow through the pores of absorbent, only the air spaces between granules (the voids) in the absorbent bed accommodate the exhaled gas. The effective air space is about 47% of the compartment volume of a filled absorber[20] (Table 18–1). This effective air space decreases at a rate of approximately 60 mL/hr with the exhaustion of absorbent.[9]

Each compartment of jumbo or similar canisters holds 1 to 1.5 kg of lime and accommodates tidal volumes of 500 to 775 mL in the void space. Therefore, in a closed system, when this void space in the upper lime compartment is exhausted over a period of 9 to 15 hours, the void space of the lower lime compartment still accommodates tidal volumes of 500 to 775 mL and provides complete CO_2 absorption.

If the tidal volume does not grossly exceed the effective air space, the absorbent efficiency is 60 to 80%.[19] The theoretical capacity of high-moisture soda lime is about 250 mL CO_2 absorbed per gram of lime or 25 L/100 grams. Many absorbers permit channeling, however, which reduces their performance to 15 L CO_2 per 100 grams. Adult patients produce 200 to 300 mL CO_2 per minute or 12 to 18 L/hr.[21] In a closed circuit, each 100 grams of soda lime should last an hour. In a semiclosed system in which gas inflow is equal to the minute volume, this time is doubled because half the exhaled carbon dioxide is discarded, provided the pop-off valve is placed in the expiratory system ahead of the absorber.

With the large absorbers (jumbo) in which two chambers for lime are arranged in series, an absorbent efficiency of 80% for soda lime is obtained or 200 mL per gram or 20 L per 100 grams. The reserve or lower chamber removes the carbon dioxide passed by the active upper chamber as its exhaustion nears completion. Because moisture condenses in the reserve chamber, lime that has partially dried out is hydrated to useful levels. This condensation of moisture evaporated by the heat of reaction rehydrates lime ahead of the reaction zone in circle absorbers and permits use of absorbents with any moisture content in these two-chambered absorbers.[8] On the other hand, in single-chambered absorbers, the moisture content of lime should be above 12%.

Proper closure of the unidirectional valves in a circle system is necessary for removal of carbon dioxide. Incompetent valves may permit rebreathing of carbon dioxide concentrations of over 6%.[22]

PREPARATION OF CANISTER. Packing of the canister must be done carefully or channeling will result. In

TABLE 18–1. CHARACTERISTICS AND PERFORMANCE OF ABSORBERS

	Manufacturer and Designation	Lime Compartment (mL)	Soda Lime (g)	Void Space (mL)	Time Efficiency (hr)
Single Lime Compartment	Foregger To-and-Fro	635	570	300	1.5†
		445	400	205	1.5†
		285	260	135	1.5†
		112	100	53	1.5†
	Foregger Morris	635	570	300	3.5†
	McKesson 1200	1380	1250	650	12.0†
	Ohio 9B	865	780	405	5.5†
	Ohio 19	1220	1100	575	11.0†
Double Lime Compartments*	Anesthesia Associates RPA	1060	960	500	9.5‡
	Foregger Jumbo	1000	910	470	9.0‡
	Ohio 20	1500	960	705	14.0‡
	Quantiflex	1650	1500	775	15.5‡

* All data for upper lime compartment only
† To 1% exit CO_2 concentration
‡ To complete color change of indicator in upper lime compartment
From Brown, E.S.: Factors affecting the performance of absorbents. Anesthesiology 20:613, 1959.

to-and-fro absorbers, underpacking can leave an open path along the top of a canister used in a horizontal position. Improper design of baffles or packing lime in any absorber may reduce efficiency considerably.[23] The following rules have been formulated by Neff.[24]

1. Remove lime from stock by hand or by strainer. Do not pour lime through small orifices; this causes fragmentation.
2. Reseal stock securely to assure moderate air tightness.
3. Avoid filling canister with dusty absorbents and avoid fragmentation.
4. After introduction of every two to three handfuls of soda lime, tap side of canister gently. This aids in completely filling canister.
5. Test canister after each filling by blowing or breathing through it.

Careful packing of the absorbent, as required in small absorbers, is of less consequence in absorbers of this size although the fine alkaline dust, which tends to accumulate in large bulk containers with handling, should never be placed in any absorber. Not only is the dust harmful if inhaled from a to-and-fro canister, it can find its way into the water trap of circle absorbers and can burn the hands of the person servicing the absorber. Dust may be eliminated by sifting lime in a kitchen strainer as it is taken from bulk container to absorber. Packing of the absorbent has been further simplified for the user by manufacturers who supply a disposable clear plastic cartridge of absorbent which fits directly into the two-chamber absorber.

SUMMARY OF CANISTER FACTORS IN OPTIMAL CO_2 ABSORPTION. During the decade 1955 to 1965, the design and performance of absorbers were vastly improved. For optimal performance, an absorber should have transparent walls and should include the following (Fig. 18–1):

1. A distributor space above the absorbent bed to prevent channeling
2. Two lime compartments, each with a volume of 1 L or more (diameter of 5–6 in. and height of 3 in.)
3. Baffle rings to prevent channeling
4. A water trap arranged below the level of the inspiratory tube

Expired air should enter the top of the absorber to help carry the water formed in the reaction into the trap.

If these simple principles are observed, CO_2 absorption is efficient, reliable, continuously evaluated by inspection, and relatively inexpensive. In contrast, the storage of lime in open containers in warm, dry areas and its use in undersized, unbaffled canisters that permit channeling in breathing systems with leaky unidirectional valves renders CO_2 absorption unpredictably incomplete and creates nuisance, inconvenience, and, occasionally, hazard for the patient.

PERFORMANCE

The performance of various absorbers in closed system is given in Table 18–1. The upper chamber of a large two-chamber absorber provides absorption for 9 to 15 hours in a closed system, thereby neutralizing 160 to 270 L CO_2, depending upon the size of the absorber.

In semiclosed systems with fresh gas inflow equal to the patient's minute volume, this time efficiency is extended to 60 to 90 hours.[25] This remarkably increased period in the semiclosed usage, however, is not attained in circle systems with the overflow or pop-off valve placed in the inspiratory part of the circuit.

If channeling through the absorbent is negligible, the change in indicator is as informative of complete

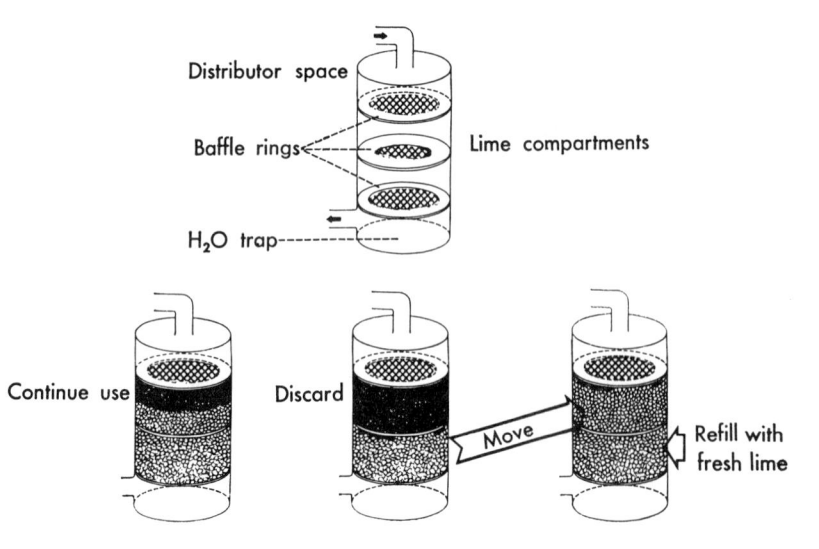

FIG. 18–1. Essential design features and sequence of usage and service of the two-chamber absorber.

removal as CO$_2$ analysis of the gas leaving the absorber. When this color change has occurred throughout the upper lime compartment, adding fresh lime is timely but can be postponed for the duration of an anesthetic procedure because without the prospect of CO$_2$ rebreathing the lower compartment will continue to remove all expired CO$_2$ for several hours. There is seldom need to change absorbent during an anesthetic procedure.

The color of indicator will fade after the absorber has rested several hours because of migration of hydroxyl ions from the interior of the lime granules to the surface. Therefore, assessment of the need to service an absorber should always be made toward the end of the period of active use.

Because the lime in the lower compartment may be partially exhausted, it is moved at the time of servicing to the upper position and fresh absorbent is placed in the lower compartment (Fig. 18–1).

The resistance of the absorbent to respiratory flow of 30 L/min is less than 0.5 cm H$_2$O. Overpacking of lime and fragmentation of granules increase the resistance of the absorbent bed.

TEMPERATURE CHANGE. The temperature in the absorbent bed may reach 65° C. The circle system yields inspired gas temperatures 8° C cooler than the to-and-fro (Fig. 18–2).

ADSORPTION OF ANESTHETICS. Chemical breakdown of certain anesthetics occurs when these agents are exposed to the alkaline absorbents. Common principles involved in the adsorption and degradation of volatile agents are tabulated. Table 18–2.

In addition, many inhalation volatile agents are trapped in the pure air space or *adsorbed*.[27] Adsorption is a physiochemical process. There is a reversible bonding between the agent and the surface of the absorbent, which is related to the molecular dimensions of the agent. Calculation of interatomic distances and bond angles of the anesthetics provides a base for determining two important dimensions of the anesthetics: chain length and kinetic diameter.[27] These characteristics determine the extent of vapor phase adsorption of small organic molecules by molecular sieves.

The process of adsorption is biphasic with respect to soda lime, which acts as a molecular sieve.[27] With dry soda lime, the pores of the absorbent are saturated in the initial phase—a sieve-like process. During this period the uptake is extensive, and little or no vapor is detectable above the absorbent. A critical volume is held in the interstices of the soda lime and may be retained for considerable time. Once the sieve is saturated, the second phase ensues in which an equilibrium is established between the surface and the overlying vapor, and this equilibrium is governed by Henry's Law.

Halothane is adsorbed by soda lime, and when exposed to dry lime,[26,28] clinically significant quantities are reversibly retained.[29] Subsequent use may expose another patient to larger than expected concentrations of anesthetic agent.

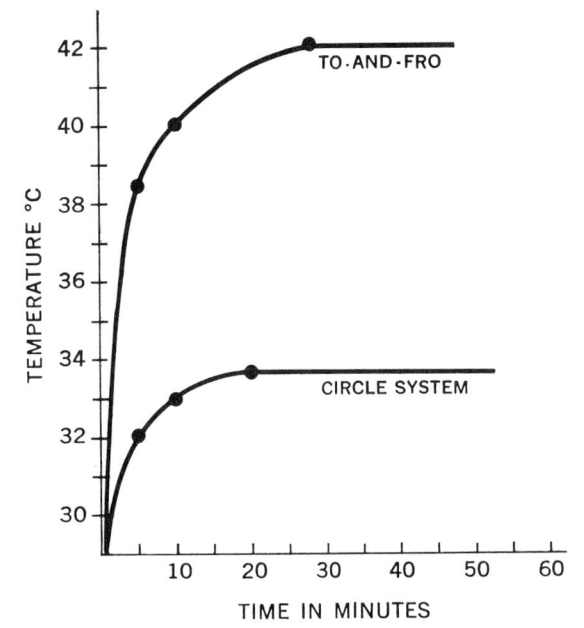

FIG. 18–2. Temperature changes in mask air during closed system inhalation anesthesia. Comparison is made under identical ventilating conditions. In the circle system the Foregger unit with corrugated tubing 30 × 1-¼ in. was used. In the to-and-fro system a 13 × 8 cm brass canister was used. The time to reach temperature equilibrium is shown. In the circle system a temperature equilibrium is reached in 10 minutes at 31° C. In the to-and-fro-system a rapid rise in temperature to 40° occurs in 10 minutes and an equilibrium is reached in 30 minutes at 42° C. (After Adriani. The Chemistry and Physics of Anesthesia 2nd Ed. p 175. Springfield IL. Courtesy of Charles C Thomas, 1962.)

Enflurane and isoflurane are also adsorbed but in lesser amounts.[30] (Table 18–3). The magnitude of adsorption is evident from the slopes for equilibrium of the agents with dry lime: Halothane is the steepest, followed by enflurane, followed by insoflurane (Fig. 18–3). Adsorption of isoflurane is significantly greater than the newer substitute I-653 (desflurane) by about 30% at 40° C.[31]

When fresh soda lime (water-containing) is used, the slope of adsorption is similar for each agent and follows Henry's Law with an overlying vapor phase.[32]

CHEMICAL DEGRADATION.[27] All potent inhaled volatile anesthetic agents are adsorbed to soda lime and degraded to varying degrees. The breakdown of the anesthetic agents is due to an interaction with the alkalies of the soda lime. More specific is the reaction with the highly active sodium hydroxide and potassium hydroxide. These together form 4.5% of the absorbed mixture. Experimentally, if the con-

TABLE 18–2. COMMON PRINCIPLES FOR ALL AGENTS

Adsorption to soda lime occurs with all volatile agents
- Adsorption is markedly greater in dry soda lime; moist soda lime reduces capacity of agents to be adsorbed.
- Adsorption occurs at all temperatures, from 0° to 60° C.
- Adsorption decreases with increasing temperature.
- The reaction of exhaled CO_2 with soda lime liberates heat and water; this then decreases the amount adsorbed.
- Moist soda lime may become dry with high-flow nonrebreathing techniques and adsorption thus increased.

Degradation in soda lime
- All potent inhaled agents are degraded.
- Degradation is slow and limited in moist soda lime.
- Moist soda lime is maintained moist by the chemical reaction of CO_2 with soda lime
- Rate of degradation at high moisture levels of 14.5% is less than at 6.5%. An inverse relation exists between amount degraded and the moisture level.
- In moist soda lime containing 6.2% water, the degradation rate of isoflurane approaches zero.

Data from Sharp, J.H., Trudell, J.R. and Cohen, E.N.: Volatile metabolites and decomposition products of halothane in man. Anesthesiology 50:2, 1978; Breck, D.: Zeolite Molecular Sieves: Structure, Chemistry and Use. New York, Wiley Interscience, 1974, pp. 634–637; Cohen, E.N., and Van Dyke, P.A.: Metabolism of volatile anesthetics: Implications for toxicity. Reading, MA, Addison-Wesley, 1977; and Eger, E.I., II, and Strum, D.P.: The adsorption and degradation of isoflurane and I-653 by dry soda lime at various temperatures. Anesth. Analg. 66:1312, 1987.

centration of sodium hydroxide is reduced, the degree of degradation is diminished. The presence of silicates also retards chemical breakdown. Some factors in adsorption and degradation are tabulated in Table 18–2. It should be noted that retained parent drug in soda lime may alter subsequent anesthetic agents when the same machine and canister are used.

Dry soda lime adsorbs much more anesthetic vapor than moist soda lime.[32] Such an action will enhance degradation. Degradation of agents in moist soda lime is much slower than in dry soda lime. In soda lime containing 6.2% water, the rate of degradation approaches zero for isoflurane and I-653.

TABLE 18–3. SODA LIME ADSORPTION OF VOLATILE ANESTHETICS

Agent	r	g	V* ul	Q
FRESH SODA LIME				
Halothane	0.99	0.038 ± 0.0002	1.5 ± 0.4	1.12
Enflurane	0.99	0.033 ± 0.0004	1.8 ± 0.4	0.79
Isoflurane	0.99	0.034 ± 0.0004	1.2 ± 0.4	0.77
DRY SODA LIME				
Halothane	0.97	0.0174 ± 0.0008	318 ± 6	17.7
Enflurane	0.70	0.0048 ± 0.0006	229 ± 7	78.6
Isoflurane	0.86	0.0028 ± 0.0002	12.7 ± 3	146.0

N = number of studies; r = correlation coefficient; g = slope; V* = microliters x intercept; and Q = quasipartition coefficient. Vaues ± for the slope g represent standard deviations. Values ± for V* represent 95% confidence levels.
From Grodin, W.K., Epstein, M.A.F., and Epstein, R.A.: Soda lime adsorption of isoflurane and enflurane. Anesthesiology 62:60, 1985.

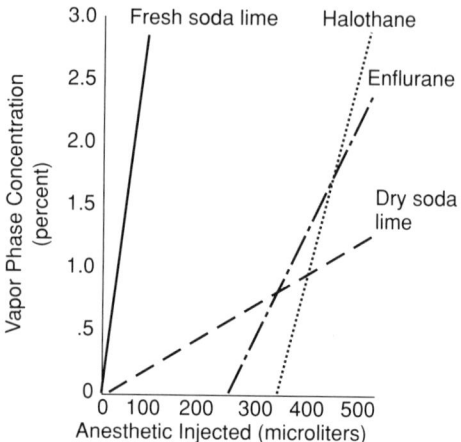

FIG. 18–3. Plot of linear regression of vapor phase concentration as a function of liquid anesthetic injected. Using fresh soda lime (solid line on left, r = 0.99) adsorption follows Henry's law. Using dry soda lime (broken lines) adsorption by a sieve-like process precedes the adsorption following Henry's law. Halothane adsorption is represented by the dotted line (r = 0.97), enflurane by the dash–dot line (r = 0.74), and isoflurane by the dashed line (r = 0.87). From Grodin, W.K., and Epstein, M.F., and Epstein, W.F.: Anesthesiology 62:60–64, 1985.

In 1943, cranial nerve palsy of the trigeminal nerve following trichloroethylene anesthesia was reported by McCauley.[33] Other reports followed, and it was determined that trichloroethylene reacted with the soda lime, principally with very reactive sodium hydroxide, in the formation of several products, of which dichloracetylene was the main toxic substance.[34] Trichloroethylene is rapidly degraded and must not be used in systems with absorbents.

Trichloroethylene + sodium hydroxide → dichloracetylene

$$\begin{array}{c} C = HCl \\ \| \\ C = Cl_2 \end{array} + NaOH \rightarrow \begin{array}{c} C - Cl \\ \||| \\ C - Cl \end{array} + NaCl + H_2O$$

Dichloracetylene is a toxic product, that can cause palsy of cranial nerves. Trigeminal (V) neuralgias were first reported. Other nerves have been involved, including palsy of the eye muscle nerves (III, IV, VI), the facial nerve, and sometimes, the vagus.

Halothane adsorption and degradation were first reported by Reventos in 1965[28] and have been demonstrated by Sharp and Grodin.[26,32] When halothane contacts soda lime during routine anesthesia in closed and semiclosed systems, one potentially toxic product of degradation detected by Sharp is 2-bromo-2-chloro-1,1-difluorethylene. Enflurane chemical degradation has been determined in the presence of soda lime.[31]

Rates of Degradation. Rates of degradation of isoflurane and the newer ether desflurane have been found to be roughly equivalent at any given temperature and starting concentration in dry soda lime.[31] Degradation rates of both drugs increase with increased temperature, but the fractional degradation is inversely related to the starting concentration.

REFERENCES

1. Snow, J.: On Chloroform and Other Anesthetics. London, Churchill, 1858.
2. Wilson, R.E.: Soda lime as absorbent for industrial purposes. Ind. Eng. Chem., 12:1000, 1920.
3. Waters, R.M.: Clinical scope and utility of carbon dioxide filtration in inhalation anesthesia. Anesth. Anal. 3:20, 1924.
4. Waters, R.M.: Advantages and technique of carbon dioxide filtration with inhalation anesthesia. Anesth. Analg. 5:160, 1926.
5. Adriani, J., and Rovenstine, E.A.: Experimental studies on carbon dioxide absorption for anesthesia. Anesthesiology 2:1, 1941.
6. Adriani, J.: The effect of varying the moisture content of soda lime upon the efficiency of carbon dioxide absorption. Anesthesiology 6:163, 1945.
7. Brown, E.S.: The activity and surface area of fresh soda lime. Anesthesiology 19:208, 1958.
8. Brown, E.S., Bakamjian, V., and Seniff, A.M.: Performance of absorbents: Effects of moisture. Anesthesiology 20:613, 1959; Performance of absorbents: Continuous flow. Anesthesiology 20:41, 1959.
9. Elam, J.O.: The design of circle absorbers. Anesthesiology 19:99, 1958.
10a. Letts, H.R.J.: Preparation and Properties of Granular Carbon Dioxide Absorbents. Part I: Soda Lime Granules. Porton Technical Paper No. 101, May 1949.
10b. Grant, W.J.: Medical Gases: Their Properties and Uses. Chicago, Year Book Medical Publishers, pp 133–134, 1978.
11a. Isom, L.W.: Dewey and Almy Chemical Company. Personal communication, 1946.
11b. The Sodasorb Manual of Carbon Dioxide Adsorption in inhalation anesthetic apparatus. New York, Dewey and Almy Chemical Division of W.R. Grace & Company, 1962.
12a. Adriani, J., and Batten, D.H.: The efficiency of mixtures of barium and calcium hydroxides in the absorption of CO_2 in rebreathing appliances. Anesthesiology 3:1, 1942.
12b. Hale, D.E.: The rise and fall of soda lime. Anesth. Analg. 46:648, 1967.
13. Weber, H.C., and Nilsson, K.T.: Absorption of gases in milk of lime. Ind. Eng. Chem. 18:1070, 1926.
14. Adriani, J.: Soda lime containing indicators. Anesthesiology 5:45, 1944.
15. Ten Pas, R.H., Brown, E.S., and Elam, J.O.: Carbon dioxide absorption. The circle versus the to-and-fro. Anesthesiology 19:231, 1958.
16. Brown, E.S., and Elam, J.O.: Practical aspects of carbon dioxide absorption. N.Y. State J. Med. 55:3436, 1955.
17. Mousel, J.H., Weiss, W.A., and Gilliom, L.A.: A clinical study of carbon dioxide during anesthesia. Anesthesiology 7:375, 1946.
18. Sword, B.C.: Closed circle method of administration of gas anesthesia. Anesth. Anal. 9:198, 1930.
19. Conroy, W.A., and Seevers, M.H.: Studies in carbon dioxide absorption. Anesthesiology 4:160, 1943.
20. Brown, E.S.: Factors affecting the performance of absorbents. Anesthesiology 20:613, 1959.
21. Petersen, P.N., and Elam, J.O.: Elimination of carbon dioxide. Anesth. Analg. Current Researches 37:91, 1958.
22. Kerr, J.H., and Evers, J.L.: Carbon dioxide accumulation: Valve leaks and inadequate absorption. Can. Anaes. Soc. J. 5:154, 1958.
23. Elam, J.O.: Channeling and overpacking in carbon dioxide absorbers. Anesthesiology 19:403, 1958.
24. Neff, W.B.: Annotations on the handling of carbon dioxide absorbing substances. Anesthesiology 3:688, 1942.
25. Brown, E.S., Seniff, A.M., and Elam, J.O.: Carbon dioxide elimination in semiclosed systems. Anesthesiology 25:31, 1964.
26. Sharp, J.H., Trudell, J.R., and E.N.: Volatile metabolites and decomposition products of halothane in man. Anesthesiology 50:2, 1978.
27. Breck, D.: Zeolite Molecular Sieves: Structure, Chemistry and Use. New York, Wiley Interscience, 1974, pp. 634–637.
28. Reventos, J., and Lemon, P.G.: The impurities of flurothane. Brit. J. Anaesth. 37:716, 1965.
29. Grodin, W.K., and Epstein, R.A.: Halothane adsorption complicating the use of soda-lime to humidify anaesthetic gases. Brit. J. Anaesth. 54:555, 1982.
30. Grodin, W.K., Epstein, M.A.F., and Epstein, R.A.: Soda lime adsorption of isoflurane and enflurane. Anesthesiology 62:60, 1985.
31. Eger, E.I., II, and Strum, D.P.: The adsorption and degradation of isoflurane and I-653 by dry soda lime at various temperatures. Anesth. Analg. 66:1312, 1987.
32. Grodin, W.K., Epstein, M.A.F., and Epstein, R.A.: The mechanism of halothane adsorption by dry soda lime. Brit. J. Anaesth. 54:561, 1982.
33. McCauley, J.: Trichloroethylene and trigeminal neuralgia. Brit. Med. J. 2:713, 1943.
34. Atkinson, R.S.: Trichloroethylene anaesthesia. Anesthesiology 21:67, 1960.
35. Cohen, E.N., and Van Dyke, P.A.: Metabolism of volatile anesthetics: Implications for toxicity. Reading, MA, Addison-Wesley, 1977.

19

ENDOTRACHEAL ANESTHESIA: I. BASIC CONSIDERATIONS

EARLY CONTRIBUTORS TO ENDOTRACHEAL ANESTHESIA[1]

1000— Avicenna. First reported human tracheal intubation (Arabian)[1a]
1543—A. Vesalius performed intubation of animal trachea[1b]
1667—Robert Hooke demonstrated the technique of intubation to the Royal Society of London[1c]
1792—Curry performed the first human endotracheal intubation (tactile method)[1d]

MODERN FOUNDATIONS OF THE ENDOTRACHEAL TECHNIQUE[1,2]

1858—John Snow used the tracheotomy technique in the rabbit with a wide-bore tube and to-and-fro breathing from reservoir bag[2a]
1871—Friedrich Trendelenburg[2b] used Snow's technique in humans but added an inflatable cuff to prevent aspiration of blood during operations on upper air passages.
1880—William MacEwen of Glasgow performed endotracheal anesthesia as is known today.[2c] He inserted a curved metal tube through the mouth into the trachea by the sense of touch. Anesthesia was administered through the tube with chloroform, and pharyngeal packing was used to prevent aspiration
1887—J. O'Dwyer[2d] and G. E. Fell performed their classic work on oral intubation of the trachea for diphtheria membrane obstruction and treatment of apnea from opium poisoning
1893—V. Eisenmenger[2e] modified a metal orotracheal tube to have an inflatable cuff with a pilot balloon to indicate degree of inflation
1895—R. Kirsten[2f] originated the laryngoscope and the art of direct laryngoscopy, but the tactile method and insufflation prevailed until 1910
1900–1910—Franz Kuhn of Cassel, Germany,[2g] a surgeon, used a flexible coil of metal to provide an orotracheal airway for surgery of upper air passages. He employed and taught most principles of inhalation endotracheal

anesthesia, but the insufflation technique remained the vogue

1910—C. A. Elsberg[2h] of Mount Sinai Hospital, New York City, taught and practiced direct laryngoscopy and intubated the trachea with a metal endotracheal tube but continued the insufflation technique of anesthesia

1910—G. M. Dorrence[2i] reintroduced the cuff. He constructed a metal tube with a cuff for treatment of injuries of the chest and lungs and used the inhalation anesthesia technique

1911—Paluel Flagg[2j] developed a flexible, coiled metal spiral endotracheal tube covered with a sheath of penrose drain. He developed a laryngoscope for anesthesiologists for direct laryngoscopy. The inhalation technique as we know it today, in contrast to the insufflation technique prevailing, was described in his text, *The Art of Anesthesia*. Subsequently, the insufflation technique was displaced by the inhalation technique

1914–1918—I. W. Magill[2k] and E. S. Rowbotham[2l] developed a single wide-bore endotracheal tube and the technique of blind nasotracheal intubation for the British Army Plastic Unit during World War I. Magill originated an intubating forceps to guide tubes into the trachea

1928—A. Guedel and R. Waters[2m] designed an endotracheal tube and balloon cuff with a piolet tube to seal off the trachea from the upper airway

DEFINITION.[3,4] *Endotracheal anesthesia* may be defined as the administration of an anesthetic agent through a tube into the trachea via the nose or mouth. It implies that inhalation of agents as well as exhalation occurs through the tube, *ie*, to and fro.[5] The tube is merely an extension of the trachea. The term *endotrachea* is derived from the Greek, meaning "inside" and "rough" and refers to the designation of the trachea by the ancients as the rough vessel.

Tracheal insufflation anesthesia may be defined as the administration of anesthetic agents and gases into the trachea with the exhalation of the agents and respiratory gases around the tube.[6] It implies that the gases are provided directly into the respiratory tract at a continuous flow rate; also, the tube is smaller than the natural respiratory passage.

HISTORICAL DEVELOPMENT.[1] The first counterpart of the present-day technique was performed in 1880 by William MacEwen, who removed a tumor from the base of a patient's tongue; the patient was under chloroform anesthesia administered through a metal tube inserted into the trachea by the sense of touch.[2c] Simultaneously, Joseph O'Dwyer[2d] relieved laryngeal obstruction of diphtheritic origin by means of a tube inserted by touch into the trachea.

Development of the endotracheal technique was stimulated by the need for (1) safe anesthesia during operations on the head, neck, and oral cavity, particularly manifested by European surgeons; and (2) controls of respiration during thoracic surgery coming from surgeons in the United States.

The first period of development (1900–1910) was largely influenced by the work of Franz Kuhn, who used a tube of coiled flat metal 12 to 15 cm in length that he inserted into the trachea with a curved introducer by touch. After insertion of the tube, Kuhn used gauze soaked in oil to pack off the pharynx.

The second period of development revolved around the so-called insufflation method of anesthesia administration, which originated from the need to maintain an expanded lung during surgical pneumothorax. In New York, in 1909, Meltzer and Auer advanced this technique and showed that when a catheter is inserted through the larynx as far as the bifurcation of the trachea and air is blown into the catheter, full oxygenation of blood occurred and the lung would remain expanded when the chest was opened. This was called a high-pressure technique; gas exchange actually depended on a flushing principle.

A third period of development ensued with the advent of World War I not only in technique but also in physiology. The insufflation technique obviously lacked a great deal in maintaining normal respiratory physiology, and there was a return to true endotracheal respiration stimulated by the efforts of Magill and Rowbotham, anesthetists for the British Army Plastic Unit. They inserted a wide-bore rubber tube into the trachea, through which the patient not only inhaled but exhaled—the anesthetic system was semiclosed.

Unit 1912, the development of endotracheal anesthesia proceeded independently of progress in the field of laryngoscopy, especially the invention of the laryngoscope. The work of Chevalier Jackson[7] revolutionized laryngologic and endoscopic procedures, but the anesthesiologists had neglected the aid of the laryngoscope. In this year, Elsberg reported his use of Jackson's instrument in endotracheal anesthesia and laryngeal intubation and ushered in modern endotracheal anesthesia.[8] The laryngoscope now served to reduce the uncertainty, inaccuracy, and trauma of blind intubation.

FUNCTIONAL ANATOMY OF THE LARYNX

TOPOGRAPHIC LOCATION. Situated anterior to the bodies of C4, C5, and C6, the larynx commands the entrance to the pulmonary system[9] (Fig. 19–1). It is a strong muscular organ that is primarily a valve of the respiratory tract.[10] On this basis the ability to produce sound has evolved, and the larynx is pop-

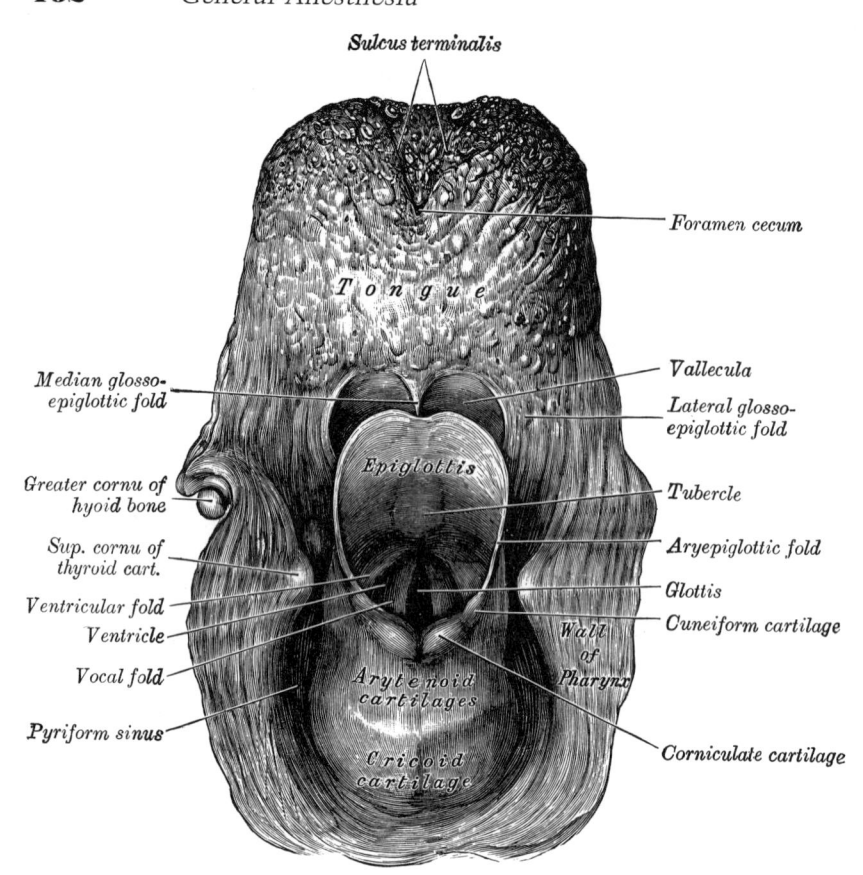

FIG. 19–1. The entrance to the larynx, viewed from behind. From Gray, H.: Anatomy of the Human Body, 30th ed. Edited by C.D. Clemente. Philadelphia, Lea & Febiger, 1985.

ularly known as the voice box. Analysis of the action of the larynx reveals its role in respiration, circulation, and maintenance of intrathoracic pressure.

FRAMEWORK (Fig. 19–2).[11] Structurally, the larynx is in the form of a box composed of nine cartilages, connected by ligaments and moved by nine muscles. There are three single cartilages and three paired cartilages.

The cricoid cartilage is a complete ring atop the trachea. It is signet shaped with the broad aspect posteriorly. Connected with the external portion of the anterior ring is the thyroid cartilage, which consists of two quadrilateral plates or laminae that fuse anteriorly in the midline; the upper border of this fusion projects forward and is popularly called the Adam's apple. A thyroid–cricoid joint exists between the two. The epiglottic cartilage is a curved, leaf-shaped structure whose upper rounded free border projects into the pharynx. The lower stalk is attached to the thyroid laminae at the inner angle by the thyroepiglottic ligament. The anterior surface of the epiglottis is attached to the hyoid cartilage by the hyoepiglottic ligament and thereby to the base of the tongue.

The portion of the epiglottis lying between these two points forms part of the anterior wall of the larynx. This intralaryngeal portion is termed the *paraglottis*. Laterally, it receives the attachment of the aryepiglottic folds and the quadrangular membrane. Anterior to this part and occupying the space above the thyroid cartilage and behind the thyrohyoid membrane is a wedge of fatty tissue called the *preepiglottic body*. This structure is important in the closure of the glottis.

Of the paired cartilages, the arytenoids are most important. They are modified pyramids with three pronounced angles: (1) sharp anterior vocal process, (2) a blunt lateral muscular process, and (3) a recurved superior or apical process. The undersurface sits on the upper border of the lamina or signet of the cricoid cartilage. A joint exists between the two so that the arytenoid can glide laterally, medially, forward and backward and can rotate. Attached to the apex of each arytenoid are the cone-shaped corniculate cartilages; situated slightly posterior to the apex are the elongated, clublike cuneiform cartilages.

THE HYOID BONE. Essential to the anatomy of the larynx is its connections to extrinsic structures. The larynx is suspended from the skull via an intermediate scaffold, the hyoid bone. This hyoid bone is attached to the skull by two stylohyoid ligaments at the lesser cornua. This horseshoe-shaped structure is at the base of the tongue, and it can be moved in all directions by action of the tongue, the strap

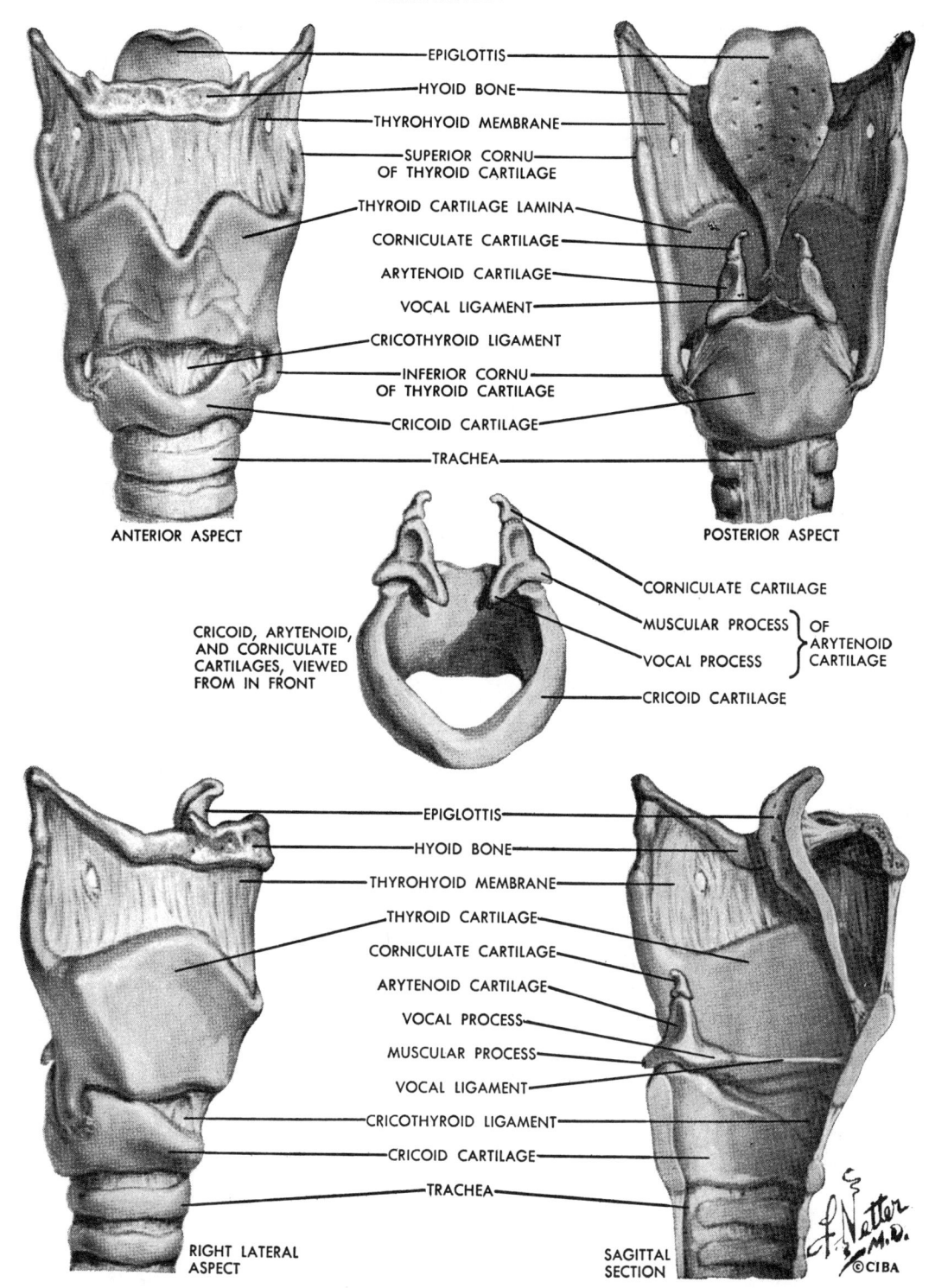

FIG. 19–2. Framework of the larynx cartilages and membranes. From Netter, F., and Saunders, W.H.: The Larynx. Ciba Clinical Symposia, 1965.

muscles of the neck, and the pharyngeal muscles. The hyoid is fixed dorsally to the conjoined tendon of the pharyngeal constrictor muscles, which are, in turn, fixed to the prevertebral fascia.

The thyroid cartilage is suspended from the anterior portion of the hyoid bone by three hyothyroid ligaments: the median hyothyroid ligament and two lateral ligaments, which arise from the greater cornua of the hyoid.

The epiglottis, in turn, is suspended from the posterior aspect of the hyoid bone. Thus, the epiglottis hangs "like the lid of a bin" from the hyoid by the hyoepiglottic ligament. The thyroepiglottic ligaments—the median and two lateral—act as hinges, and the hyoepiglottic ligament acts as a lever for the lid.

MEMBRANES AND LIGAMENTS (SEE FIG. 19–2).[11] There are *nine* membranes and ligaments (Table 19–1). These are divided into those connecting the larynx to surrounding structures and those that are intrinsic.

Two membranes are important in the fixation of the cartilages to surrounding structures. The first is the cricotracheal membrane, which attaches the lower border of the cricoid to the first tracheal ring. It is the structure to be identified in performing transtracheal anesthesia. Second is the thyrohyoid membrane, which attaches the upper border of the thyroid to the hyoid bone. The hyoepiglottic ligament, of lesser importance, is located at the base of the tongue and runs from the hyoid cartilage to the epiglottis.

Interconnecting the intrinsic cartilages of the larynx to each other are two chief membranes and two ligaments. *Of prime importance is the cricothyroid (cricovocal) membrane;* the lower border is attached to the entire length of the upper border of the cricoid arch from the arytenoid attachment posteriorly to the thyroid cartilage anteriorly. This membrane slopes upward and inward like an inverted funnel. The upper free border is the vocal fold or vocal cord and contains yellow elastic tissue called the *vocal ligament*. This ligament runs horizontally from the vocal process of the arytenoid forward to the angle of the thyroid laminae at its midpoint. It is pale and pearly white. *The second membrane is the quadrangular membrane* running from the lateral border of the epiglottis back to the lateral border of the arytenoids. The upper edge of this membrane is thick and free and is termed the *aryepiglottic fold* or *ligament;* the lower edge is relatively free and thickened by fibrous tissue into the vestibular fold or ligament (ventricular fold) or false vocal cord. This vestibular fold is capable of strong approximation with its opposite mate and effectively prevents entrance to the glottis.

TABLE 19–1. MEMBRANES AND LIGAMENTS

1. Hyothyroid ligaments (3) 2. Hyoepiglottic ligament 3. Hyothyroid membrane	Upper extrinsic attachments to surrounding structures—the hyoid scaffold

4. Thyroepiglottic ligament
5. Thyrocricoid membrane and ligament
6. Quadrangular membrane; aryepiglottic folds
7. Vestibular (ventricular) folds—edge thickens to a ligament, or false cords
8. Vocal (cricothyroarytenoid) folds—membrane edge thickens to a ligament—the true cords
9. Cricotracheal membrane to surrounding structures

In accordance with the original purpose of the larynx as a valve of the respiratory tract, inlet and outlet portions may be defined. Thus, the vocal cords act as inlet valves, while the ventricular folds, or false cords perform the function of outlet valves.[10] A lateral ballooning of the larynx between the vestibular and vocal folds forms the laryngeal sinus or ventricle of Morgagni.

COMPARTMENTS OF THE LARYNX (FIG. 19–3).[9] The fissure between the vocal folds or true cords is termed the *rima glottis*. It divides the laryngeal cavity into two main compartments: (1) The upper portion is the vestibule, which extends from the laryngeal outlet to the vocal cords. It includes the laryngeal sinus, sometimes referred to as the *middle compartment*. (2) The lower compartment extends from the vocal folds to lower border of the cricoid cartilage and thence is continuous with the trachea.

It is apparent from the structural framework that the vocal cords are partly cartilaginous and partly membranous. Specifically, the anterior two thirds is membranous and posterior one third is cartilaginous.

INTRINSIC MUSCLES.[9,11] There are nine muscles controlling the movements of the laryngeal framework (Fig. 19–4). Their names offer sufficient information to describe their origin and insertion. From the practical standpoint they may be classified according to the primary function they perform (Fig. 19–5):

1. Abductors: posterior cricoarytenoid muscles (paired)
2. Adductors: lateral cricoarytenoids (paired); interarytenoid muscle
3. Relaxor: thyroarytenoid (paired)—the medial portion is called the *vocalis muscle*. This muscle is applied to the vocal and vestibular ligaments. On

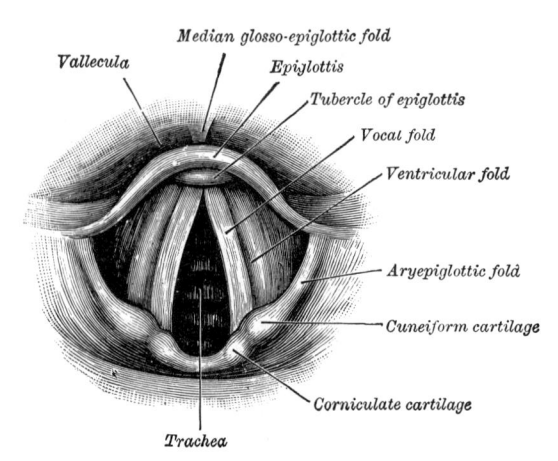

FIG. 19–3. Compartments of the larynx. From Gray, H.: Anatomy of the Human Body, 30th ed. Edited by C.D. Clemente. Philadelphia, Lea & Febiger, 1985.

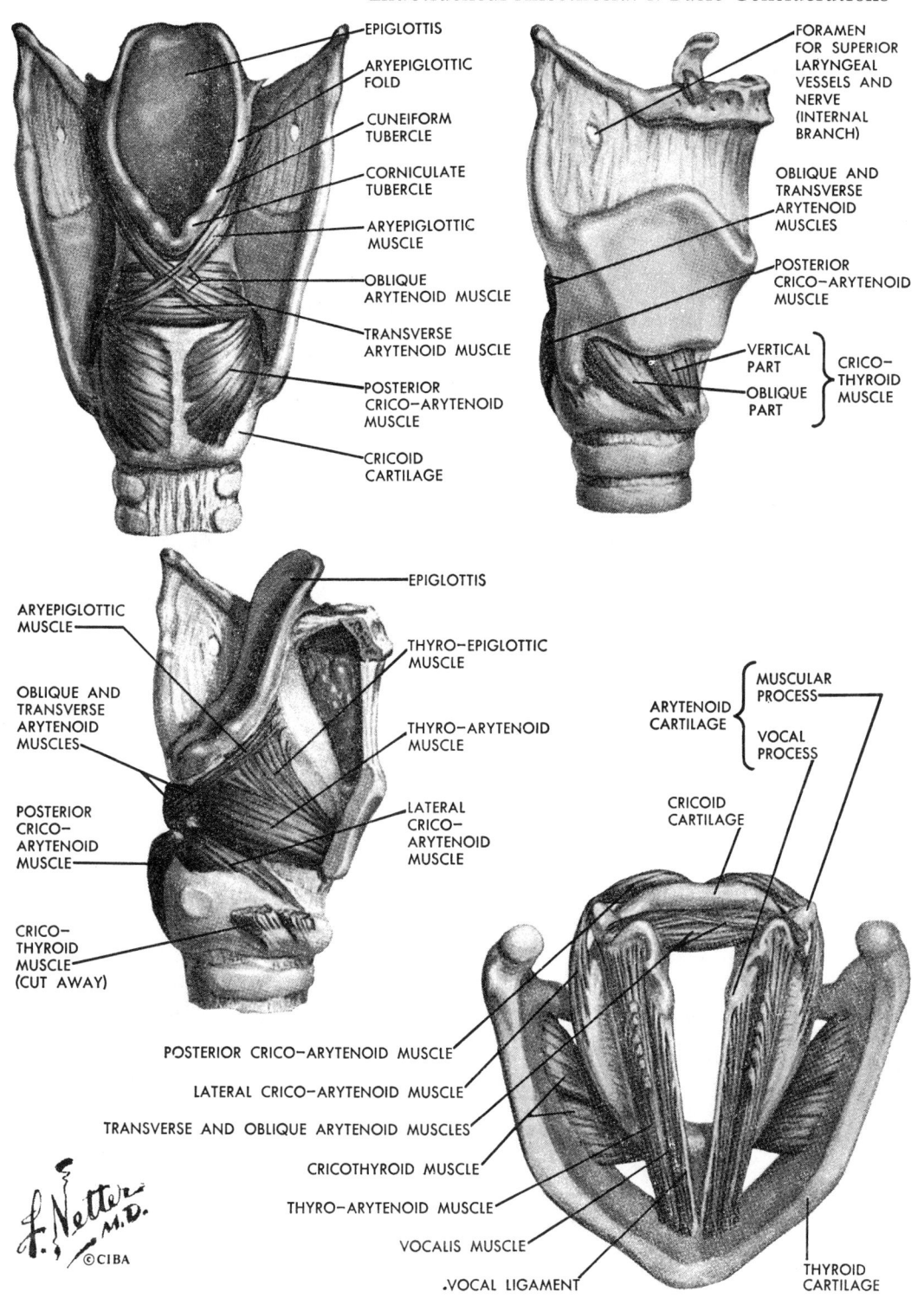

FIG. 19–4. Intrinsic muscles of larynx. From Netter, F.H., and Saunders, W.H.: The Larynx. Ciba Clinical Symposia, 1965.

strong contraction it is capable of closing the vestibule
4. Tensor: cricothyroid (paired)

The laryngeal muscles are all innervated by the recurrent laryngeal nerve of the vagus, with one exception.[12] The cricothyroid muscle is supplied by motor fibers in the superior laryngeal nerve (Fig. 19–6).

FUNCTIONS OF THE LARYNX.[10,13] Provides a valvular air passage to pulmonary system; (2) acts as a "watchdog" to the respiratory tract; (3) participates

ACTION OF CRICOTHYROID MUSCLE

ACTION OF POSTERIOR CRICO-ARYTENOID MUSCLES

ACTION OF LATERAL CRICO-ARYTENOID MUSCLES

ACTION OF ARYTENOIDEUS MUSCLE

ACTION OF VOCALIS AND THYRO-ARYTENOID MUSCLES

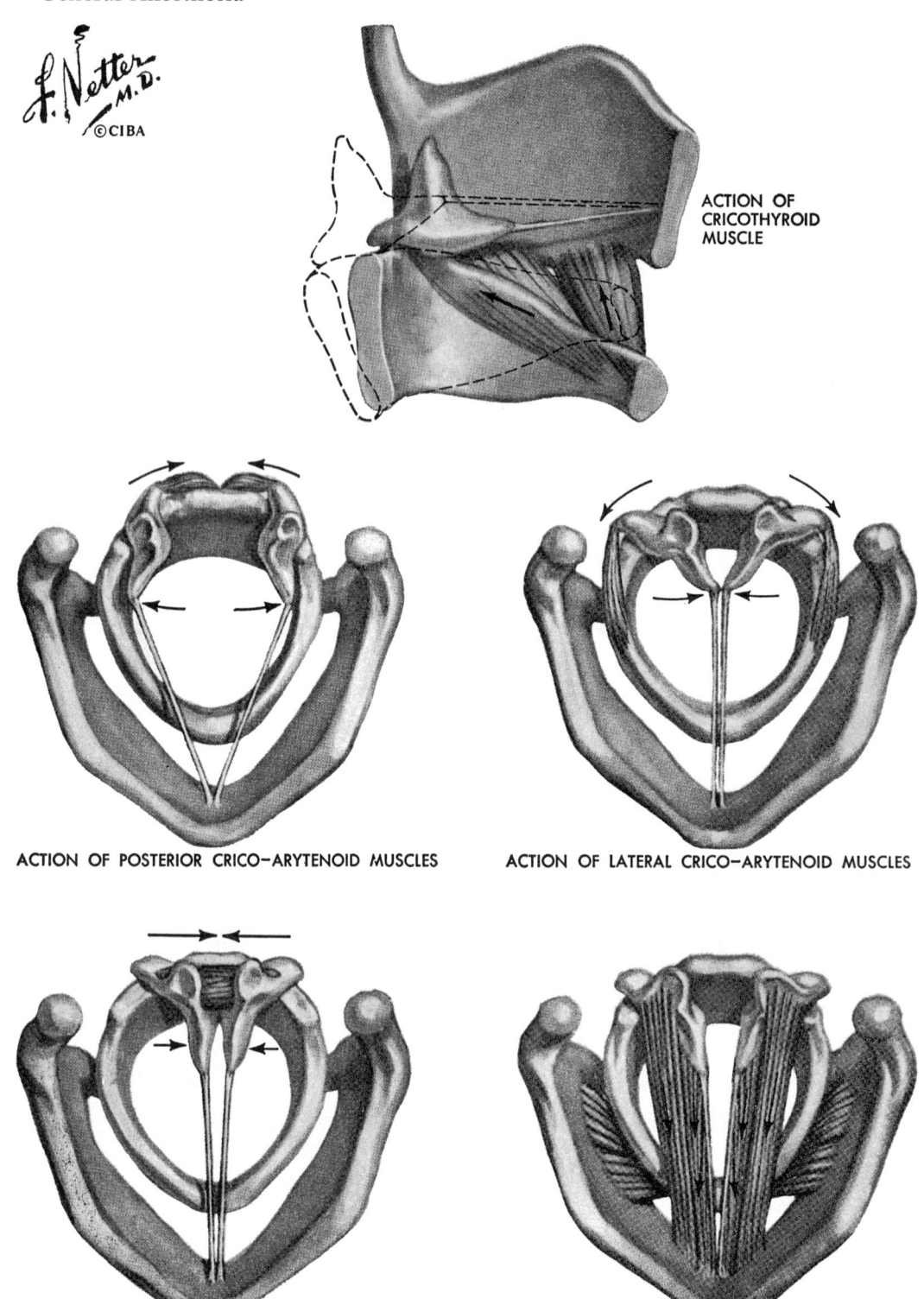

FIG. 19–5. Action of the Intrinsic Muscles. (From *The Larynx* by Frank O. Netter, M.D. and W. H. Saunders, M.D., Ciba Clinical Symposia, 1964.)

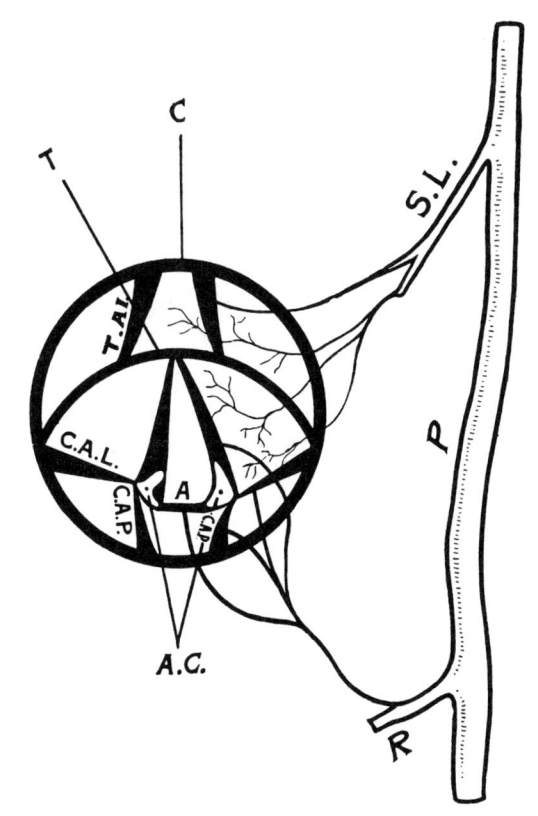

FIG. 19–6. Intrinsic muscles of the larynx and nerve supply. *P*, the vagus nerve; *R*, recurrent laryngeal nerve; *S L*, superior laryngeal nerve; *A C*, arytenoid cartilages; *T*, thyroid cartilage; *C*, cricoid cartilage; *A*, interarytenoid muscle; *C A P*, posterior cricoarytenoid muscle; *C A L*, lateral cricoarytenoid muscle; *T A I*, internal cricothyroid muscles.[9]

in the cough act to build up intrapulmonary tension; and (4) regulates intrapulmonary tension and thereby influences intrathoracic tension.

MOVEMENT OF THE LARYNX.[12,13] The entire larynx moves during respiration. It falls during inspiration and rises on expiration.

The positions of the vocal cords during various phases of action are important. At rest the cords are slightly abducted. The anterior intermembranous portion is triangular with the apex forward, whereas the intercartilaginous portion is rectangular. During resting respiration or inspiration, the cords are slightly adducted initially, then become slightly abducted. During a forced inspiration or hyperventilation, the cords are markedly abducted in both portions so that the glottis is lozenge shaped because of the pronounced action of the posterior cricoarytenoid muscle. When a high-pitched voice is desired or the tracheobronchial tree is stimulated by irritants, the lateral cricoarytenoids rotate the arytenoid cartilage medially; simultaneously, the interarytenoids approximate the arytenoid cartilages posteriorly. The total effect is an approximation of both portions of the rima glottis. The cadaveric position is that halfway between abduction and adduction.

An important law regarding the innervation of the intrinsic muscles of the larynx has a practical application in thyroid surgery. If the recurrent laryngeal nerve is accidentally injured or severed, respiratory difficulties may ensue in the postoperative period. Semon's law states that the abductor nerve fibers will degenerate before the adductor nerves.[12] Therefore, observation of the vocal cords will reveal an enhanced cord adduction that may progress to marked closure in the first 12 to 24 hours. Only later will adductor paralysis develop and the cords attain the cadaveric position.

EXTRINSIC UPPER AIRWAY MUSCULATURE.[12] Musculature extrinsic to the larynx contributes to the movement and function of the laryngeal muscles. There are 24 pairs of striated muscles surrounding the upper airway, and many appear to have an automatic cyclic motor activity in phase with respiratory muscles.[14] Respiratory activation stabilizes the system and provides patency. If contraction of these muscles is out of phase with respiratory muscle activity, air-flow resistance is increased.[15]

Patency of the upper airway with an obstructive ventilatory defect may be seen in patients with extrapyramidal disorders.[16] This has been observed in over one third of patients with parkinsonism but is also seen in other disorders such as athetosis and chorea. It is also seen in such syndromes as familial dysautonomia (Riley-Day) and the Shy-Drager conditions. In these and other abnormalities and diseases, abnormal contractions and involuntary movements of the striated muscles of the upper airway and supraglottic area as well as involuntary movements of the glottis can be observed under fiberoptic visualization. Usually a reduction of the glottic chink is present. In these patients, the forced expiratory volume in 1 second (FEV_1) is frequently reduced.

REGULATION OF SKELETAL MUSCLES OF THE UPPER AIRWAY. Regulation of respiration involves the coordination of the innervated skeletal muscles of both the upper airway and of the thorax–diaphragm system.[15,16] Chemoreceptors of the carotoid body and of the medullary centers work with locally mediated pulmonary-volume feedback mechanisms superimposed on pontomedullary pacemakers. During the latter part of expiration and prior to inspiration, activation of the cricothyroid, lateral cricoarytenoid, and thyroarytenoid muscles narrows the glottic opening and stabilizes the lung volume and maintains proper functional residual capacity (FRC).

A fraction of a second before inspiration, there is a fall in airway resistance with activation of the posterior cricoarytenoid muscle preparing the airway for easy entrance of air, whereupon there is activation of the diaphragm and intercostal muscles.[15,17]

During mild hypoxia, laryngeal constrictor muscle activity is enhanced to further increase airway resistance on expiration.[18] During hypercapnia, muscles opening the glottis dominate during both inspiration and expiration to minimize airway resistance throughout the respiratory cycle.[18]

In sleep, glottic closure during latter part of exhalation is diminished; hence, FRC is decreased. Upper airway pharyngeal muscles lose tone and narrow the nasopharynx and hypopharynx.[17,19]

CLOSURE OF THE LARYNX.[19,20] Rhythmic widening and narrowing of the glottis occurs during normal respiration. On opening of the glottis, the entire vocal process of the arytenoid moves laterally, remaining parallel to its opposite number. There is no rotation except at the extreme lateral end of its excursion when some divergence of the vocal process appears. Simultaneously, there is a downward–upward excursion of the larynx with respiration, and this accompanies contraction of the "strap muscles" of the neck, *ie,* sternothyroid and sternohyoid. During swallowing, coughing, and straining, there is also upward movement of the larynx. This brings the larynx under the shelter of the epiglottis and the tongue.

LARYNGEAL CLOSURE PROGRESSION.[20] In coughing, swallowing, severe laryngospasm, and the Valsalva maneuver, a series of complex movements is involved in closure of the larynx. These movements occur in a definite sequence and may be analyzed into three components.

First, is the shutter mechanism or simple glottic closure. This is accomplished by the intrinsic muscles of the larynx causing adduction of the vocal cords. This group of muscles is primarily concerned with phonation and is arranged to permit delicately controlled tension, thickness, and length of vocal cords. During normal respiration, approximation of the vocal cords may occur independently of the other movements to be described. A tendency to closure at the very beginning on normal inspiration is to be noted.

During general anesthesia with loss of skeletal muscle tone, the laryngeal muscles are weakened and vocal cord abduction is reduced while gas flow through the glottis remains essentially unchanged; as a consequence, of the Bernoulli effect the vocal cords may become adducted simply by virtue of the gas flow. In fact, the vocal cords assume a concave upper surface and appear as cusplike valves. Thus, inspiratory stridor may develop.

Expiratory stridor may occur as a response to unpleasant somatic sensory stimulation during surgery. It is a "vocal protest against too little anesthesia." It is accompanied by vigorous respiration.

Second is the adduction of the false cords. *Homo sapiens* is the only species possessing an aryepiglotticus muscle. Essentially, it is a muscle of phonation similar to the intrinsic muscles. By appropriate stimulation of the free edge of the aryepiglottic folds, the false cords or vestibular folds become adducted. With prolonged stimulation the aryepiglottic folds become invaginated by action of the thyroepiglotticus muscles (attached below to isthmus of thyroid cartilage and laterally inserted into the quadrangular membrane).

The combined action of adduction of the vocal cords and of the false cords obliterates the lateral ventricles or vestibule of glottis. In speaking, the aryepiglottic folds become taut, smooth, and high. This produces a deep supraglottic cavity for regulating resonance.

Third is the ball-valve mechanism (Fig. 19–7). The paraglottis (intralaryngeal portion of the epiglottis with the preglottic body of fatty tissue) is squeezed by the ascent of the larynx and the reduction of the distance between the thyroid cartilage and hyoid bone. The paraglottis bulges backward. The false cords, which also rise with the larynx, are brought into contact with the paraglottic bulge. The false cords, which may or may not actively approximate, form a valve seat for the bulging paraglottis. Thus, laryngeal closure is completed.

ENDOTRACHEAL TUBES

TERMINOLOGY.[21–25] An endotracheal tube is one through which anesthetic gases or vapors as well as the respiratory gases are conveyed into and out of the trachea. The end of the tube, which is situated in the trachea of the patient, has been designated as the *tracheal end* or *distal end.* The other end, which projects from the patient and is intended to be connected to the breathing system, is called the *machine end* or *proximal end.* The bevel of the tube is the angle at which the tracheal end of the tube is cut.

The tip of the tracheal end of the tube is bevelled. Bevels face either right or left when the concavity of the tube is viewed in its longitudinal axis and are designed to act like a simple wedge to pass through the vocal cords. A simple bevelled tip is the *Magill tip.* When an opening (eye) in the tube is present on the opposite side to the bevel, it is designated as a *Murphy tip endotracheal tube.*

CONSTRUCTION MATERIALS. Four materials have been used in the manufacture of endotracheal tubes: metal, natural rubber, synthetic rubber, and plastics.

The earliest tubes introduced by Kuhn[15] were metal modifications of the rigid bronchoscope. These were considered too traumatic and too difficult to manipulate, requiring that the head be moved in the classic bronchoscopic position, and

FIG. 19–7. Sagittal section to illustrate the action of the laryngeal ball valve. *A*, open. *B*, closed. During laryngeal closure the preepiglottic body (*PB*) is squeezed between the hyoid bone (*H*) and thyroid cartilage (*T*). The paraglottis buckles and is forced against the upper surface of the false cords (*FC*). From Fink, B.R.: The mechanism of closure of the human larynx. Trans. Am. Acad. Ophthalmol. Otol., *60*:117, 1956.

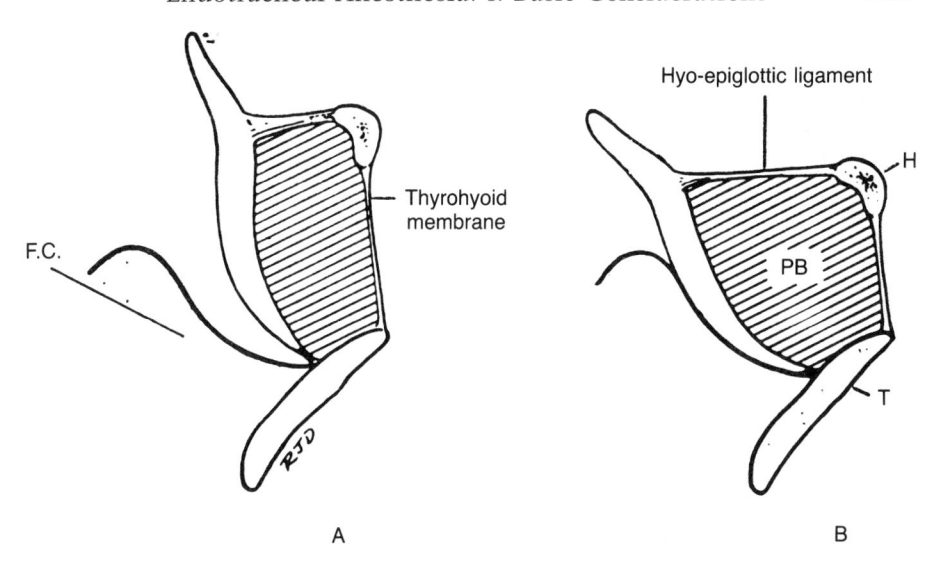

were abandoned. Flagg,[26] however, who practiced modern inhalation anesthesia, with the advice of Chevalier Jackson, constructed a flexible tube of metal coils covered by penrose rubber tubing, with a tracheal tip part of solid metal.[26,27] Woodbridge shortened the tip so that the entire tube was flexible.[28] These tubes are not used today.

Meanwhile, the experiences of Magill and Rowbotham as anesthetists in the British Army Plastic Unit (Sir Harold Gillies, Commander) in World War I (1914–1918) resulted in the development of soft, wide-bore natural rubber tubes for endotracheal intubation.[29,30] The rubber Magill tube quickly revolutionized endotracheal anesthesia.

In the years between 1944 and 1950, plastic tubes of vinyl material were introduced.[31] These tubes were initially white opalescent, but further processing produced a translucent material.

Currently, tubes are manufactured of various plastic materials or of synthetic rubber.[32]

STANDARDIZATION. Confusion arose after World War II as to size and construction of the endotracheal tube for anesthesia, because bronchoscopes were designated in terms of outside diameter (OD) in millimeters and semirigid tubes in the French catheter gauge, whereas the Magill tubes were arbitrarily numbered from 00 to 10. To eliminate the chaos and provide some standardization, a committee was appointed in 1954 by Steven Martin, president of the American Society of Anesthesiologists, entitled Committee on Standardization of Anesthesia Equipment and chaired by the author.[33] The committee recommended that the American Standards Association (later named the American National Standards Institute [ANSI]) be requested to coordinate the efforts of various interested parties—anesthesiologists, manufacturers, investigators—with the purpose of standardizing equipment.

A general conference was held in Boston on November 3, 1955, and a sectional committee, Z-79, was formed. Organization of the Z-79 committee was completed on December 8, 1956, in New York, with the American Society of Anesthesiologists as sponsor. The committee's first project was to standardize endotracheal tubes. This resulted in the first American Standards Specifications for Anesthesia Equipment: Endotracheal Tubes, approved April 22, 1960. Subsequently, this became the basis for development of an international standard.[19a]

PERFORMANCE CRITERIA FOR TUBES.[34,35] Performance specifications have been recommended by a joint group of investigators, inventors, and manufacturers. The goal is to provide endotracheal products designed to minimize misuse and to provide safe function. To this end, criteria have been prepared for tubes, cuffs, and the tube-cuff unit. These performance criteria for an ideal tube encompass the following specifications:

1. Inertness—A nontoxic, nonallergic substance capable of resisting deterioration from chemical sterilization or autoclaving
2. Surface characteristics of smoothness to avoid damage to the mucosa
3. Inner surface smooth and nonwettable to prevent secretion build-up; should allow suction catheters to pass freely
4. Nonflammable and conductive
5. Transparent
6. Easily sterilized*
7. Low durometer or kinkability; should maintain shape and not be easily compressed by position

---

* Disposable plastic endotracheal tubes are available. If properly cleaned and sterilized, however, they can be reused several times to reduce expenses.

in anatomic path; should not be compressed by inflated cuff; no critical reduction in cross-sectional area from anatomic bending; nonocclusion by torsion or kinking

8. Sufficient strength to allow thin wall construction with comparatively large internal diameter (ID) and ability to retain a curved shape
9. Thermoplasticity to conform to anatomic passageway and to be self-centering within the trachea
10. Exertion of low pressures on areas of contact with pharynx, larynx, and vocal cords
11. Nonreactive with lubricants or anesthetic agents
12. Tubes should be clearly marked according to ID of the lumen and progress in size by 0.5-mm increments
13. Radiographic and light-visible markings indicating proper length of tube insertion
14. A range of sizes should be available to satisfy most needs
15. Noninjurious catheter tip regardless of contact and nonocclusive by contact
16. 15-mm male fitting designed to avoid accidental disconnection from tube or respirator
17. Radiopaque to demonstrate in vivo tube position

RESISTANCE FACTORS.[36,37] These are determined by Poiseuille's law of flow of fluids in tubular systems (see Chapter 4).

Internal Diameter. ID is the most important factor in determining resistance. As the internal radius (r) diminishes, the resistance increases by an exponential power of 4 (i.e., r^4).

Length of Tube. Resistance is proportional to length of tube and decreases as length decreases. Because the length of endotracheal tubes used is within a range proscribed by the anatomy, this factor is of minor consequence. Most tubes, however, are supplied in lengths greater than 26 cm and should be trimmed to a functional and working length. This will decrease dead space and limit external kinking.

Contour and Connections. If the curvature of the tube is increased, resistance increases with high air flows. Curved slip joints[38] and curved breathing system connectors offer greater resistance. Right-angled units offer the greatest resistance because of turbulent air flow. Gradual curves of connectors are desired.[38]

RESISTANCE TO AIR FLOW IN ENDOTRACHEAL TUBES. The tube with the largest lumen and whose OD permits tracheal insertion without undue trauma will have the least resistance. Such resistance is based on the principles of fluid (air) flow in tubes of varying diameter. Poiseuille's law and the character of the air flow, whether laminar or turbulent, are fundamental. High flow rates and curves in the passageway by improper connectors result in turbulent flow. Excessive dead-space introduces an inefficient system (see Chapter 4).

Effect of Tube Size on Alveolar–Arterial Oxygen Difference. Whether the largest and presumably freest airway with the least resistance is the best airway has been questioned. On the basis of some work by Frumin, raising the airway resistance during expiration from -5 to $+5$ mm Hg increased the arterial oxygen tension by 10 mm Hg. The insertion of a 3-mm orifice tube, expiratory resistance increased the oxygen tension on an average of 7 mm Hg.

Logically, it can be assumed that the raised airway pressure is transmitted to the alveolar spaces with some compression of the pulmonary capillary bed but exposure of a larger alveolar surface to the capillaries. In essence, the mechanism may be one of increasing the ventilation–perfusion ratio from 0.8 to a ratio close to 1.0. Thus, venous admixture would be decreased.

Conversely, if the airway expiratory resistance is decreased, as when the larynx (the pulmonary valve) is removed by an endotracheal tube or by tracheostomy, there may be pulmonary capillary congestion a consequently lowered alveolar ventilation–capillary perfusion ratio. Thus, more nonoxygenated blood could pass by the alveolar bed and produce venous admixture. At any rate, it appears some venous admixture does occur if the airway pressure is lowered and a degree of hypoxemia is possible. This set of circumstances would be possible in open endotracheal systems. It is unlikely, however, in a closed or semiclosed system when the mechanical features of the system would balance the effect of the large endotracheal tube.

DESIGNATION OF SIZES (TABLE 19–2). Three systems are customarily used to designate the size of catheters: (1) the French catheter gauge; (2) external diameter (ED) in millimeters; and (3) ID in millimeters (American, British and ISA standard)

For endotracheal tubes, the ID is specified. The size of bronchoscopes and metal tubes has been customarily designated by the ED expressed in millimeters, whereas semirigid and rubber catheters in urologic use have been designated in French catheter gauge, which is a number that is three times the ED.

The French Catheter System.[40] The French gauge system for designating size of catheter was developed by Joseph Frederick Charrière (1803–1876), a French instrument maker. He graded the size of urethral sounds, cervical dilators, and catheters according to the ED. This French system has also been

TABLE 19–2. COMPARISON OF VARIOUS SCALES USED TO DESIGNATE THE SIZE OF ENDOTRACHEAL TUBES

Standard ID Scale (mm)	ED Scale (mm)	French Gauge*
2.5	4.3	13
3.0	4.7	14
3.5	5	15
4.0	5.3	16
4.5	5.7	17
5.0	6	18
5.5	6.3	19
5.5	6.7	20
6.0	7	21
6.5	7.3	22
7.0	7.7	23
7.5	8	24
8.0	8.3	25
8.0	8.7	26
8.5	9	27
9.0	9.3	28
9.0	9.7	29
9.5	10	30
10.0	10.7	32
10.0	11	33
10.5	11.3	34
11.0	12	36
12.0	13	39

* Equals ED × 3, not external circumference.
Abbreviations: ID = internal diameter; ED = external diameter.

adopted for tubular instruments, such as bronchoscopes and endotracheal tubes.

Each French unit differs by approximately 0.33 mm in ED from adjacent units (18 French = 6 mm). The system thus designates the ED of a tube. To convert the French size to ED, divide by 3; to convert the ED in mm to French size, multiply by 3. (Note that this French size is not the circumference.)

Size is Determined by Charrière's Filière:

1. A metal plate with 30 perforations originally; later, 40 perforations
2. Each perforation varies from the adjacent one by 0.33 mm in diameter (3 French = 1 mm)
3. The size of the holes ranges from 0.3 mm to 1.6 cm. Thus, each perforation represented a French gauge catheter size.

It should be pointed out that the size of bronchoscopes and metal tubes has been customarily designated by the external diameter expressed in millimeters, while on the other hand, semirigid and rubber tubes have been designated in terms of French Catheter Gauge, which is a number that is 3.0 times the external diameter.

CLASSIFICATION OF ENDOTRACHEAL TUBES. Tubes are classified on the basis of construction and purpose. The commonly and currently used tubes are listed in the next column.

- *Standard single-lumen (semisoft tubes made of rubber or plastic):* Magill, Murphy, Cole
- *Semirigid tubes:* armored or anode (LA); partial spiral sway tube (Hatano)
- *Preshaped tubes:* RAE (Ring-Adair-Elwyn); Saklad-Dwyer-Lindholm
- *Special tubes:* Laser-shield; Endotrol (NCC-Mallincrodt, Inc.)

MARKINGS.[22,23] Endotracheal tubes are marked in accordance with recommendations of ANSI Committee Z-79.[24]

The markings are situated on the beveled side above the cuff as follows:

- Type of tube: oral or nasal or oral/nasal
- Size: ID in millimeters
- Length of tube in centimeters, measured from the tracheal end, noted by small lines or arrows indicating varying lengths in centimeters (usually 16, 20, 22, 24, 26)
- ED or OD may also be indicated.
- Manufacturer's name or trademark
- Z-79—designates tubes complying with ANSI standards.
- Implantation tested (IT) or Z-79—indicates tube has been tested for tissue toxicity
- Opaque lines may also be included at the tracheal or distal portion of tubes.
- Precautions are usually noted: "Disposable; Do Not Reuse"

THE STANDARD TUBE (MAGILL TYPE) (ANSI Z-79) (FIG. 19–8).[21–23] Adoption of the ANSI specifications, developed by the Z-79 Committee of the American Society of Anesthesiologists, has resulted in standards for size, length, and curvature. All dimensions follow the metric system as the standard of measurement. The International Organization for Standardization (ISO) has drafted specifications almost identical to ANSI (ISO/TC 121/SC, 1984).

Size of Tubes—Bore. Sizing is according to the ID of the tubes in millimeters marked on the bevel side. The number of sizes is determined by increments of 0.5 mm in the ID and is limited only by practice requirements. Thus consecutive sizes may vary by 0.5 mm in ID and range from 2.0 mm to 20.0 mm ID.

Curvature of Tubes. Based on the anatomic requirements, certain distinctions are noted between tubes designated for oral use (Fig. 19–8) versus nasal insertion (Fig. 19–9). The distinction concerns (1) the sharper curve of the oral tube versus the nasal and (2) the difference in the angle of the bevels.

Oral tubes should have a radius of curvature of 14 cm ± 10%; the nasal tubes a radius of curvature of 20 cm ± 10%.

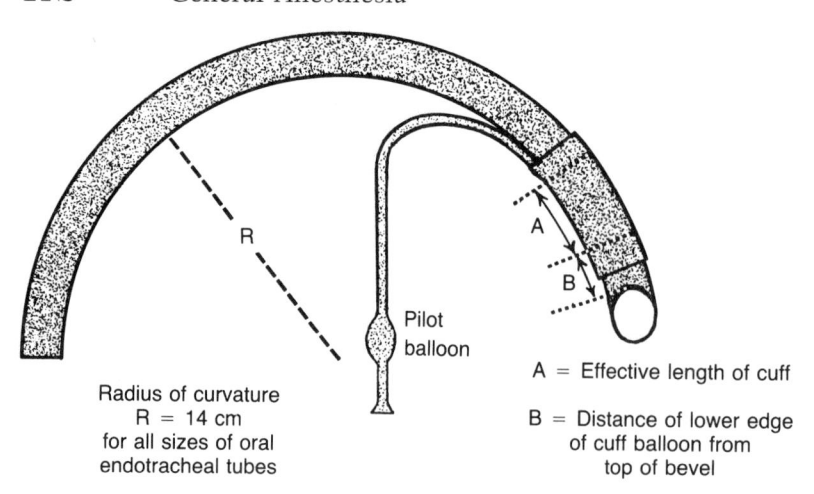

FIG. 19-8. Specifications of the oral-cuffed endotracheal tube (ANSI Z-79).

Bevel. The bevel is defined as the slanted part of the tube at the tracheal end. It is designated in degrees as the acute angle between the plane of the bevel and the longitudinal axis. The bevels of the tube should be such that the oral tube bevel is more blunt or obtuse and the nasal tube bevel more acute.

An oral tube should have a minimum bevel angle of not less than 45 degrees in relation to its long axis. A nasal tube should have a minimum bevel angle of not less than 30 degrees in relation to its long axis.

The standard actually specifies a bevel of 38 ± 8 degrees for oral tubes. The oral tubes available have angles from 38 to 56 degrees.[41]

ANATOMIC MEASUREMENTS OF THE LARYNX—GUIDE TO TUBE BORE SIZE (TABLE 19-3). The size of the laryngeal passage is measured by the anterior-posterior (AP) diameter at the vocal cords or the rima glottis opening. This varies with age and size of the patient.[34,35] Throughout the neonatal period and infancy, the cricoid ring represents a narrower AP diameter by about 1.0 mm. By 10 years of age, the AP diameter of the rima glottis is smaller than the cricoid diameter or the tracheal diameter. In the infant, the glottic opening is largely intercartilagenous, whereas the membranous portion may be only 50% or less. The stiff interarytenoid portion is thus quite vulnerable to trauma and edema.

LENGTH OF TUBES. An endotracheal tube is a substitute passageway for the normal upper airway of a patient. Most tubes are supplied from the manufacturer longer than necessary, and they are marked in centimeters from the tip of the tracheal end. It is advisable to cut off any excess length so that a tube is not advanced too far (into a stem bronchus) and to prevent kinking at the nose or mouth.

For a given patient, the appropriate length of a tube should be determined before intubation. First, the actual length is dependent on the anatomic measurements of the upper airway passage—the larynx and the trachea (Table 19-4).[42-44] A tube should be inserted into the midtrachea, usually a distance of 4 to 5 cm, so that the cuff is in the trachea. Second, the mechanical needs for use of the tube are considered. The tube should also extend 2 to 4 cm outside the lips to accommodate the slip-joint or straight connector and to permit attachment to other connectors and the breathing circuit.

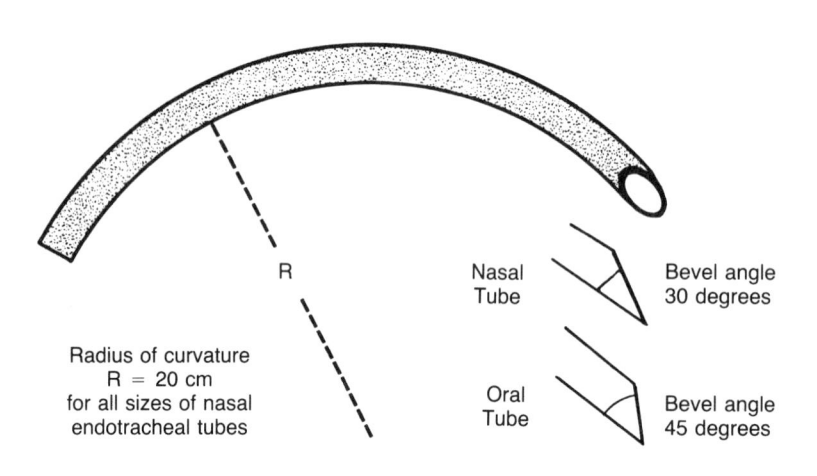

FIG. 19-9. Specifications of the nasal endotracheal tube.

TABLE 19-3. ANATOMY OF LARYNX—GUIDE TO BORE OF ENDOTRACHEAL TUBES

Age	Internal AP Diameter of Rima Glottis (mm)	Length of Ligamentous Portion of Vocal Cord (mm)
Newborn (FT)	5.0–7.0	3.0–4.0
1 month	7.5	4.0
6 months	8.0	5.0
1 year	8.5	5.0
5 years	10.0	7.5
10 years	12.0	9.5
15 years	14.0	10.0
20 years	23.0	17.0

Abbreviations: FT = full-term; AP = anterior–posterior.

Length can be estimated clinically by laying the tube alongside the patient's neck and noting that it extends from the lips to some point at or below the cricoid cartilage and not beyond the bifurcation of the trachea; the bifurcation can be topographically located at the angle of Louis (Ludwig) or the second costal cartilage.

ANATOMIC MEASUREMENTS—GUIDE TO LENGTH OF TUBE.[44] Certain measurements of airway and laryngotracheobronchial anatomy are of practical importance to the anesthesiologist engaged in endotracheal intubation. In the adult weighing 70 kg, the following are working values:

- Mean distance from lips to carina: males, 28.5 cm; females, 25.2 cm
- Mean distance from base of nose to carina: males, 31.0 cm; females, 28.4 cm
- Distance from lips to vocal cords: males, 12–16 cm; females, 10–14 cm
- Upper edge of larynx to lower edge of cricoid: mean 4–6 cm
- Mean length of trachea (vocal cords to carina): males, 12–14 cm; females, 10–14 cm

In adults, any tube over 24 cm in length will likely be suitable, because it can extend from 2 to 3 cm outside the lips to the vocal cords and can be inserted through the vocal cords a distance of 4 to 5 cm, which is desirable in the adult.

Tracheobronchial Angles. The angles at which the stem bronchi diverge from the trachea at the carina have been studied at autopsy and radiographically.

TABLE 19-4. ANATOMIC MEASUREMENTS OF AIRWAY FOR DETERMINING LENGTH OF ENDOTRACHEAL TUBE

Age	AP Diameter of Trachea* (mm)	Teeth to Cords† (cm)	Teeth to Carina‡ (cm)	Length of Trachea (cm)
Neonates				
Premature		7	10	2.5
Term	4	8	12	4
1–6 months	5	8.5	13	4.5
6–12 months	6	8.5	13	4.5
1–2 years	7	9	14	5
2–3 years	8	9	14	5
3–6 years	9	9.5	15	5.5
6–9 years	9	10	16	6
2–12 years	9	11.5	17	6
14 years	10	12	18	6
16 years	11–15	14	22	8
Adults				
Female	14–20	14–16	23–30	10
Male	18–25	15–18	25–32	12

* Data from Butz, R.O., Jr.: Length and cross section growth patterns in human trachea. Pediatrics, *42*:336, 1968.
† Data from McIntyre, J.W.R.: Endotracheal tube for children. Anaesthesia, *12*:94, 1957.
‡ Data from Schellinger, R.R.: The length of the airway to the bifurcation of the trachea. Anesthesiology, *25*:169, 1964.

Abbreviation: AP = anterior–posterior.

In his classic *Anatomy of the Lung*, W. S. Miller cites the studies of Kobler and Von Hovarka in stating that the angle of divergence averages 70 degrees in adults.[45] The adult right bronchus makes an average angle of 25 degrees with the long axis of the trachea, and the left bronchus an average angle of 35 degrees.[46] Also, the carina is not in the midline but to the left.[47,48]

In neonates (1) radiographic studies[46] show a range of right bronchial angles of 10 to 35 degrees and left bronchial angles of 38 to 45 degrees; (2) measurements by Brown[49] are reported as follows: right bronchial angle of 30 degrees with the tracheal axis and 47 degrees for the left bronchus with the tracheal axis; (3) measurement of the angles from bronchial intubation of anesthetized neonates by Kubota[47] reveals an overall tracheal angle of bifurcation of approximately 80 degrees (angle between stem bronchi). The right bronchial angle of divergence measures approximately 32 degrees and the left bronchus an angle of 46 degrees with the tracheal axis;[47] (4) Cleveland[48] gives the mean of the right bronchial angle as 26 degrees and of the left bronchial angle as 33 degrees in children and up to 18 years of age.

SELECTION OF TUBE. In the selection of an endotracheal tube, with regard to the bore, the actual bore size is determined by anatomic measurements (Table 19–5). One should also be guided by the axiom that the largest tube with the least internal resistance to flow, which will fit the patient's glottis without force, will provide the best airway.

In general, infants will take tubes varying in bore from 2.5 to 5.0 mm ID (12 to 19 French); children's sizes range from 3.5 to 7.0 mm ID (16 to 24 French) and adults in sizes from 6.0 to 10.0 mm ID (28 to 40 French).

A simple guide giving the ranges in sizes for both the bore and length is presented in Table 19–6. The length of tube chosen depends on the age and size of the patient.

TUBES FOR NASAL INTUBATION (SEE FIG. 19–9). These tubes are about 2.0 cm longer than the oral tubes. The bore should be about ID 0.5 to 1.0 cm smaller.

In selecting a tube for nasal intubation, the side to which the bevel faces is important. A tube with bevel facing the left should be used for insertion into the right nares, whereas the tube with bevel facing the right should be introduced into the left nostril. This allows the bevel to slide along the flat nasal septum. A bevel facing otherwise may easily engage the turbinates and cause excessive trauma. Determination of the side to which the bevel faces is made by holding the tube with the concave aspect upward.

THE MURPHY TYPE TUBE (FIG. 19–10). This tube defines a standard-type tube (Magill or other) with an oval hole in the side of the wall opposite the bevel side and above the upper level of the bevel.[50] The hole is called the *Murphy eye*. The area of such an opening should not be less than 80% of the cross-sectional area of the tube lumen, so that it is effective as a ventilation port if the bevel is occluded (ANSI and ISO standards).

ANODE OR ARMORED TUBES (FIG. 19–11). Anode tubes are specially constructed tubes reinforced by means of a spiral of metal wire or nylon filament.[51] The spiral is embedded between layers of rubber, latex, or plastic in such a manner that the spiral is covered internally and externally. The spiral does not extend to either end, leaving the tip and bevel free of the spiral and composed only of the tube material. Only the proximal machine end of the tube material is of sufficient length to accommodate a straight slip-joint (straight tube connector). Care must be taken to be sure that the slip-joint completely fills the machine end of the tube. The entire connector should abut on the point where the spiral begins; otherwise, pinching and kinking can occur at the juncture.[52]

Indications for this type of endotracheal tube include the following:

1. Most head and neck surgery
2. Maxillofacial surgery—"commando" procedures
3. Intracranial neurosurgery
4. Abnormal positions, including hyperflexion of head on chest, prone position, and procedures entailing severe hyperextension

TABLE 19–5. ANATOMY OF THE LARYNX AND TRACHEA (AVERAGE DIMENSIONS) AS A BASIS FOR SELECTION OF ENDOTRACHEAL TUBES[42–44,46]

	Adult Male	Adult Female	Child (6 years of age)	Infant
Diameter of the trachea (mm)	20	15	8	5
Diameter of larynx-glottis (AP) (mm)	24	18	10	6
Length of the trachea (cm)	14	12	8	6
Distance from upper teeth to carina (cm)	28	24	17	13

Abbreviation: AP = anterior–posterior.

TABLE 19-6. GUIDE TO SELECTION OF ENDOTRACHEAL TUBE SIZES* AND LENGTH[†]

	Bore (ID) (mm)	Orotracheal Length[‡] (cm)
Infants		
0–1 years	2.5–4.0	10–14
Children		12–20
1–5 years	3.5–5.0	16–24
5–15 years	5.0–7.0	
Adults		
20–60 years		
Female	8.0	22
Male	8.5	24
60+ years		
Female	8.5	24
Male	9.0	24

* Each size tube should be available in three lengths: short, medium, long.

[†] Lengths are measured from midpoint of the bevel of tube to machine end. Length will permit placement of tube in midtrachea.

[‡] For nasotracheal tubes, add 2–3 cm in length.

5. Surgery entailing compression of the neck or airway

The advantage of this tube is the lack of kinkability. These tubes can be tied in a single loop without kinking or compression. Only extraordinary force will distort the tube.

In application, a stylet is placed in the lumen to the bevel, but not beyond the tip, to provide stiffness and control of movement. The stylet should be fashioned in a small curvature with a "J" end and be well lubricated for ease of insertion and removal.

Forceps should be avoided when directing the introduction of the tube; their strong use may damage the spiral coils.

COLE TUBE (FIG. 19–12). This tube was designed by Cole for pediatric patients, especially infants and young children.[53,54] The patient end has a small bore

FIG. 19–10. Tracheal tube tips. *Left*, Magill tube. *Right*, Murphy tube. From Dorsch, J., and Dorsch, B.: Understanding Anesthesia Equipment, 2nd ed. Baltimore, Williams & Wilkins, 1984, p 357.

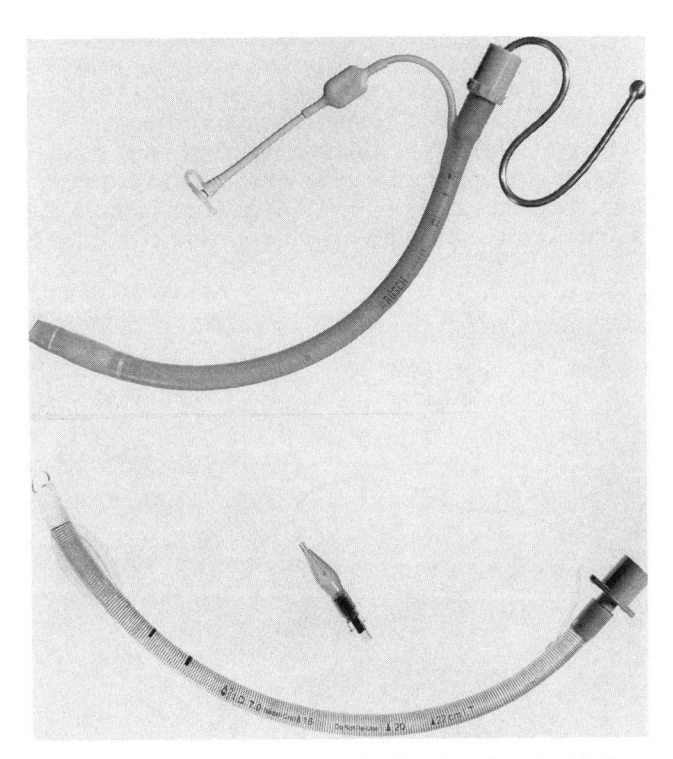

FIG. 19–11. Anode or armored tube. Spiral embedded endotracheal tube, nonkinkable or noncollapsible with ordinary use. *Upper*, low-volume–high-pressure cuff. *Lower*, high-volume–low-pressure cuff. Note that a stylet is necessary. (Courtesy P. Johnson, University of Illinois at Chicago).

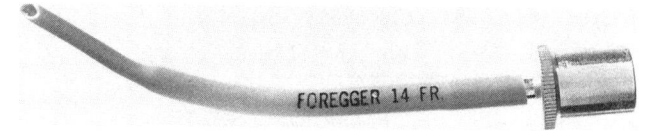

FIG. 19–12. The Cole tube. Useful in pediatric practice. Note the small size (bore) of tracheal segment and the larger size of supraglottic segment. The shoulder is between the segments. (Photo Courtesy P. Johnson, University of Illinois at Chicago).

to be accommodated through the larynx and into the trachea. The upper or proximal portion is of a wider bore. Between these two segments is a tapered part forming a shoulder, which should fit snugly into the supraglottic area but not press on the glottis. The shoulder serves to prevent advancement into the lower part of the trachea or into a stem bronchus.

Sizes are designated for the tracheal or patient end by the ID scale. They range from ID 2.0 mm (12 French) to ID 5.0 mm (18 French).

The bevel of this tube is set at 45 ± 8 degrees in relation to the axis of the tube and the opening faces to the left when viewed toward the concave aspect from the machine end.

Generally, the resistance to air flow of these tubes is less than that of tubes with a constant lumen.[38] Although the wide bore segment offers a slight increase in dead space, it is insignificant.[55]

CONTOURED, PRESHAPED TUBE (LINDHOLM) (FIG. 19–13). In 1949, Dwyer[56] proposed a modification of the standard Magill-type tube to conform to the anatomy of the upper airway. It was designed to minimize the traumatic effects of the curvature of the standard tube, which tends to exert backward pressure on the cartilages of the posterior commissure (the arytenoids) and to be angled anteriorly after passage through the vocal cords to exert a pressure and mucosal erosion on the anterior tracheal wall. By providing a second posterior curve in the lower part of the tube and thereby producing an S-shaped tube, the pressure effects are minimized.

Lindholm[57] has popularized these concepts in an improved anatomically shaped tube (Lindholm tube), which modifies the original design further and incorporates a high-volume–low-pressure cuff.

ENDOTROL TRACHEAL TUBE (NCC DIVISION, MALLINCKRODT, INC.) (FIG. 19–14). A tip-control system is incorporated in this plastic tracheal tube to change the direction of the tip. A cable extends from a ring-loop at the proximal machine end of the tube just below the slip-joint connector. While holding the tube between the thumb and second finger of the hand, the index finger is placed through the ring. Pulling the ring causes a change in the radius of curvature of the tube, principally at the tip of the tube, which then moves anteriorly. This is useful when laryngoscopy is difficult and only the epiglottis is easily seen.

THE PREFORMED RAE* TUBES (FIG. 19–15).[58] These tubes are molded so that a smooth bend is produced at the divergence of the tube from the mouth or nose. Two versions are available: one for orotracheal use and the other for nasotracheal. The pediatric tubes are uncuffed but have two lateral ports near the lip: one above the bevel and the other opposite the bevel. The adult preformed tubes are cuffed (NCC, low-pressure cuff) and have a Murphy eye-port opposite the bevel to provide for ventilation if the bevel is occluded.

The nasotracheal tube is slightly longer than the oral tube.

* Named after the designers Ring-Adair-Elwyn.

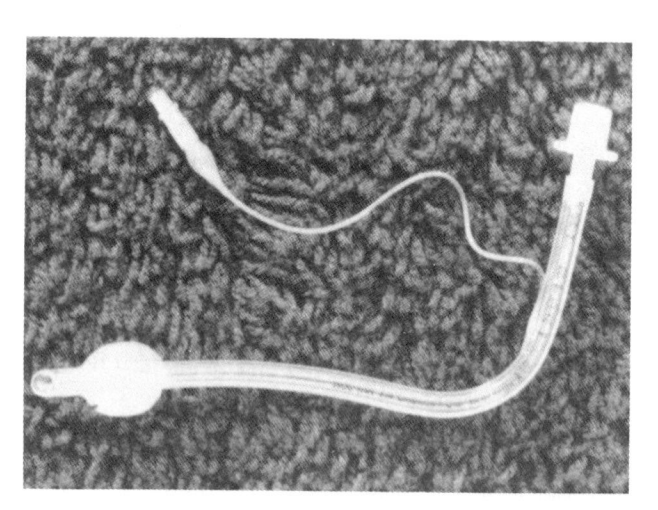

FIG. 19–13. Preshaped endotracheal tube (Dwyer-Saklad-Lindholm) Improved Lindholm tube with a high-volume, low-pressure cuff. From Dorsch, J., and Dorsch, B.: Understanding Anesthesia Equipment, 2nd ed. Baltimore, Williams & Wilkins, 1984.

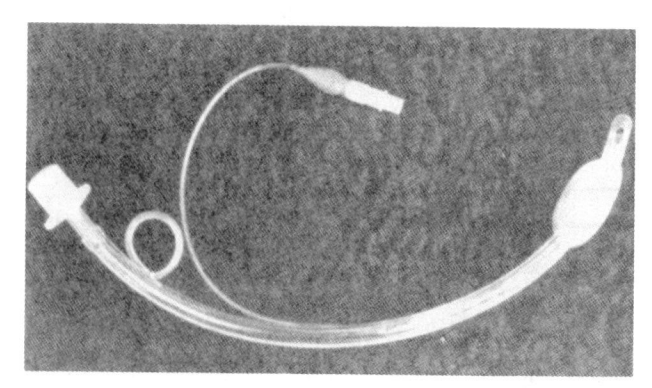

FIG. 19–14. Endotrol tracheal tube. See text. From Dorsch, J., and Dorsch, B.: Understanding Anesthesia Equipment, 2nd ed. Baltimore, Williams & Wilkins, 1984.

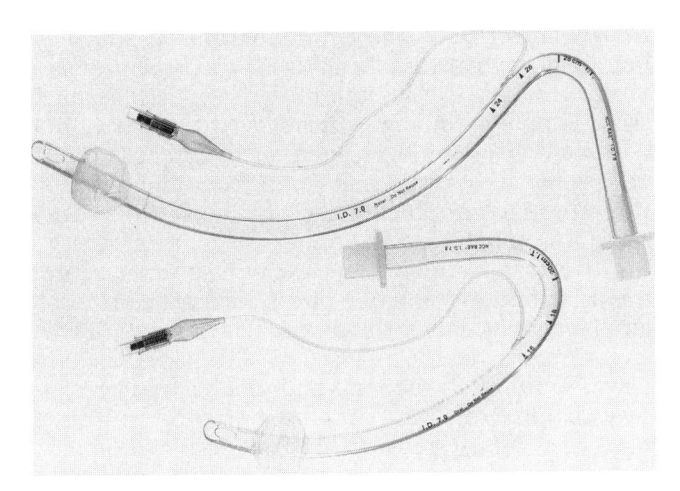

FIG. 19–15. Preformed RAE tube. *Upper,* tube for nasotracheal use. *Lower,* tube for orotracheal intubation. (Courtesy P. Johnson, University of Illinois at Chicago).

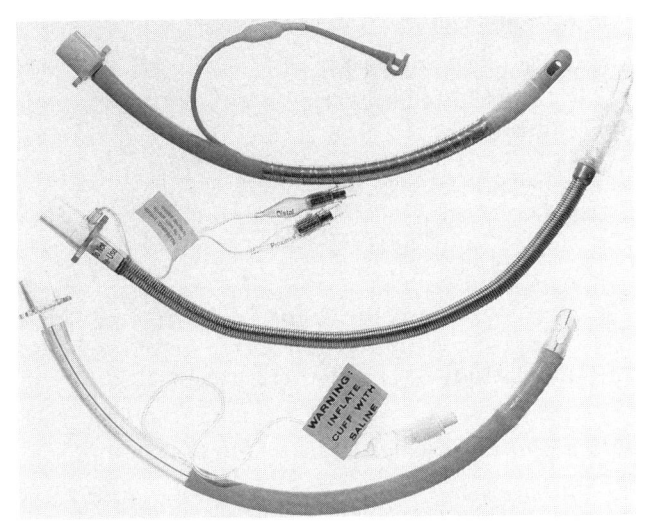

FIG. 19–16. Endotracheal tubes for laser surgery. *Upper:* standard red rubber Murphy tube wrapped with metallic tape. *Middle:* Xomed silicon rubber tube coated with a metallic veneer. *Lower:* Double-cuff metal spiral endotracheal tube, a modification of the Norton tube.

The size of these tubes covers ranges for pediatric patients and for adult use, according to ID of the lumen.

These tubes are designed for use during surgery of the head, face, or neck. The oral tube has an acute angle-bend placed at a point of emergence from the mouth and extending downward. Surgery of the head, face, and nose is permitted without encroachment by the anesthesia airway.

The nasal tube has an acute upward bend at the place of emergence from the nose. Maxillomandibular, oral, dental, and neck surgery are facilitated. Careful studies by Ring[50] have established practical and generally safe lengths for each size tube. Nevertheless, individualization of the airway of each patient is necessary to avoid bronchial intubation.

LASER-SHIELDED ENDOTRACHEAL TUBE (FIG. 19–16). Plastic and rubber can be ignited by the heat of laser beams.[59] Rubber tubes are readily damaged, but plastic tubes, such as the polyvinylchloride (PVC) type of composition, may actually catch fire.[60,61] These tubes have not been used. For the rubber tube, the usual early method of protection was a wrapping of aluminum foil completely over the rubber tube. This was applied to the main shaft and cuff.[62,63]

To withstand the heat of the laser beam and avoid ignition, tubes are currently formed of a material of silicone impregnated with metal particles (aluminum oxide). All cuffs should be inflated with saline, because an air interface may result in some fire or, principally, bursting of the cuff.

SPECIALLY DESIGNED ENDOTRACHEAL TUBES FOR LASER SURGERY (SEE FIG. 19–16). Specially designed endotracheal tubes have virtually eliminated the need to adapt the standard endotracheal tubes by wrappings for laser microlaryngeal surgery.[64]

First Endotracheal Tube. The first endotracheal tube for laser airway surgery was the standard red rubber tube with latex rubber cuff, wrapped with a spiral overlay of metallic tape from the upper portion of the cuff joined up to 5 cm superiorly along the tube (Fig. 19–16, *upper*).

Advantages:
- Reusable after proper cleansing techniques
- Nonflammable, although it may be punctured by the laser beam

Disadvantages:
- Difficult to wrap the tube smoothly and have tape adhere
- Tape may crumble or fragment

The Norton Spiral Metal Tube.[65] This tube, resembling a "gooseneck" lamp stand, without a cuff, was then developed. Although totally noncombustible and reusable after proper cleansing techniques, there were too many disadvantages:

- Total airway seal not possible—no cuff
- Tube leakage through spiral joints
- Rough exterior surfaces
- Very rigid
- Expensive

Modified Spiral Metal Tube.[66] This is a modified spiral metal tube with spirals encasing another tube and a double cuff (Fig. 19–16, *lower*). The purpose of the double cuff is to provide a continuous leakproof system if one of the cuffs is perforated by the laser beam.

Advantages:

- Totally noncombustible
- Two cuffs for added safety
- Disadvantages
- Expensive single use
- Rough surface
- Rigid

Silicone Rubber Tube—Metallic Coating.[67] A recent development is the Xomed laser tube, which is a silicone rubber tube coated with a metallic veneer that is resistant to burning (Fig. 19–16, *middle*).

Other Considerations in Laser Surgery

1. All operating room personnel wear protective glasses to deflect stray laser beams.
2. Patient's eyes are protected with damp eye pads.
3. All drapes should be cloth or nonflammable paper.
4. Endotracheal tube cuff filled with methylene blue–dyed sterile water in case of cuff puncture with laser beam to reveal a leaking system and potential aspiration.

TISSUE REACTION TO TUBE MATERIAL.[68,69] Irritation of the laryngotracheal mucosa may occur after the use of some plastic tubes. Three causes are recognized: (1) the stabilizer compounds in the plastics; (2) toxic substances formed in gas sterilization; and (3) detergent residues.

Plastic tubes are usually constructed of polymers (polyvinyl; polyethylene) compounded by a primary plasticizer (tributyl acetyl citrate; dialkyl phthalate sebacate), and a stabilizer (organotin). The organotins are leachable and cause toxic tissue inflammatory reactions.[69,70]

Because tissue reactions can occur, the specifications for endotracheal tubes and other catheters for patient contact should be tested for tissue toxicity.[70,71] The specification of the US military is suitable and requires that the tube material be implanted into rabbit muscle according to the US Pharmacopeia (USP) implantation test.[72,73]

CARE OF TUBES. Endotracheal tubes of plastic or rubber should be left in a cool place and out of sunlight. To maintain their curve and shape, they should be stored in a circular receptacle or a curved plastic container.[74] A small, wooden convex rack may be constructed corresponding to the curve of the endotracheal tubes and the concave surface of the tubes may then be laid on the rack.[75]

It is important that when handling disinfected equipment, anesthetists should maintain personal cleanliness or concurrent disinfection, especially of their hands.

Reusable Tubes. Although many tubes supplied by manufacturers are marked with such precautions as "one time use," "do not reuse," or "disposable," there is no convincing evidence that tubes may not be reused if properly cleaned and sterilized. Other disposable items, such as connectors and adapters that are made of plastic, can also be sterilized and reused.

In western countries, the use of disposable equipment is common practice but has expanded to such an extent that one of the original advantages of cost containment has been lost. In Third World countries, equipment such as endotracheal tubes, airways, connectors, and breathing circuits, if available, are regularly reused. It is necessary to employ techniques of asepsis under unfavorable conditions of a poor economy and inadequate supplies, including the military field.

Antisepsis.[76,78] Proper cleaning and care of tubes and other equipment, especially connectors and adapters, is a threefold process that includes the following:

1. Mechanical cleansing
2. Sterilization
    a. Autoclaving (steam sterilization)
    b. Gas sterilization
    c. Chemical
3. Storage in sterile packages

It is critical that the anesthetist and technical personnel maintain concurrent disinfection of their hands. The cleansing method must consistently remove the bacteria commonly involved in cross-contamination, namely *Pseudomonas, Serratia, Klebsiella,* and *Staphylococcus aureus.*[77] All should be conscientious and knowledgeable about contamination and the disinfection process. This is necessary to avoid being a carrier. Such skin and hand disinfections can be achieved by scrubbing prior to handling clean and sterile equipment.

Thorough cleansing in soapy water and mechanical scrubbing represent the most important steps in physically removing gross contamination of equipment.[78] *This should be done directly after use.* Endotracheal tubes should be meticulously cleaned, disinfected, and rendered sterile. After scrubbing the outside of the tube, the inside should be similarly scrubbed with a test tube brush. Dirty and contaminated tubes are one of the major causes of laryngeal edema and inflammation, as well as tracheitis.

The tube and other accessories, once mechanically cleaned, should be thoroughly dried. Packaging is carried out aseptically, which is then submitted to sterilization or pasteurization (automatic washing machine with water at 77°C). Steam sterilization is the most effective measure, but ethylene oxide sterilization is a common procedure. It is effective and does not cause deterioration of equipment. If neither of these two methods is available, chemical sterilization must be used.

Chemical Disinfection.[79,80] For chemical disinfection, the agent should have a wide spectrum of activity. It should be bactericidal, tuberculocidal, viricidal and fungicidal. At the same time, deterioration of equipment should not occur, and any residue should not be obnoxious or harmful. Four types of broad spectrum chemical disinfectants are available: (1) quaternaries, (2) synthetic phenolics, (3) iodophors and (4) alcohols.

Quaternaries are surface-acting agents. They will combine with organic material and lose activity. They are bactericidal for gram-positive and gram-negative organisms but are not tuberculocidal. However, when combined with alcohol the breadth of activity is increased. Solutions of these agents must be used generously. They are not irritating and non-toxic. But rubber materials become sticky.

Substituted phenols are effective against gram-negative and gram-positive bacteria and against the tubercle bacilli. They impregnate rubber and make the surface irritating.

Iodophors are iodine complexes. They are effective against gram-negative and gram-positive bacteria and tubercle bacilli. In addition, they are viricidal. Surfaces are not stained.

Alcohols, both ethyl and propyl, are bactericidal and tuberculocidal. These are useful for disinfection of small items of equipment such as connectors, laryngoscope blades, etc. They are not economically useful for cleaning surfaces of equipment, floors and walls.

For routine antisepsis, tubes may be immersed in a weak germicidal solution such as 70% ethyl alcohol, or an orthophenylphenol solution for 1 hour. Then the tubes must be thoroughly rinsed in sterile water.

Bacteriologic studies of tubes contaminated by patients have been carried out after the tubes were cleansed by scrubbing with pHisoHex. Culture studies of the tubes failed to reveal the presence of the usual respiratory bacteriologic flora. These studies also revealed that after diligent scrubbing with pHisoHex the tubes were found to be consistently sterile within 30 minutes.[75]

Similar studies[76] comparing pHisoHex with other agents revealed that scrubbing of masks and tubes with pHisoHex resulted in sterile equipment; all other agents resulted in varying failures. The pHisoHex must be assiduously rinsed from the tube since the lanolin may cause deterioration of the tube.

Tubes contaminated by tubercle bacilli should be cleansed in two steps: first, they should be mechanically scrubbed, and secondly they should be disinfected by soaking in a tuberculocidal solution for 1 hour. It has been found that after mechanical cleansing of tubes exposed to tubercle bacilli that about 15% are still contaminated. If these tubes are then placed in a tuberculocidal solution, no positive cultures can be obtained from the surface. Two such solutions are available:

1. An alcohol formaldehyde solution (Livingstone Solution),
2. Orthophenylphenol solutions.[81]

The formaldehyde solution has the following composition:

Formaldehyde (38% solution)	210 ml.
Water	606 ml.
Alcohol (95% q s ad)	4000 ml.

Following such bactericidal treatment, the tubes must be thoroughly rinsed in sterile water and then air dried. Formaldehyde is an excellent germicide and is effective as used above. But it tends to polymerize on surfaces. This can irritate the tracheobronchial mucosa. Thus, thorough rinsing is mandatory. Disinfection is best accomplished by autoclaving. However, most tubes deteriorate under steam sterilization, and therefore, gas sterilization has become a preferred method. If neither is possible, chemical sterilization may be used.

Glutaraldehyde.[82,83] This is one of the most widely used and effective chemical disinfectants for anesthesia equipment. It is available in alkaline, acid, and neutral formulations.

These solutions have extensive bactericidal, virucidal, and fungicidal action. Neutral formulation is also tuberculocidal and effective against some viruses at room temperature in 10 minutes. This formulation has corrosion inhibitions and so can be used for steel and delicate lensed instruments. It can be used for disinfecting rigid and flexible endoscopes. Gloves should be worn when using this form.

The *acid formulation* 2% is effective at room temperature against most bacteria, viruses, and fungi in 10 minutes. Tubercle bacilli are killed at 60°C in 20 minutes and spores in 60 minutes. Rubber, plastic, steel, and lensed instruments can be disinfected, but this solution should not be used on plated metal instruments. It does not irritate the hands, eyes, or nostrils nor stain the skin. Gloves need not be worn.[84]

The *alkaline formulations* are buffered at the time of use to a pH of 7.5–8.5. These are widely used in surgical suites in a special automatic unit called the Cidematic. These formulations have an irritating odor and may irritate the skin. Rubber gloves must be worn. Disinfection of endotracheal tubes by the alkaline formulations may cause laryngitis (pseudomembranous).[85] Sticking of relief valves has been reported.[86]

Gas Sterilization.[80,87] A number of anesthetic and surgical items of equipment, such as endoscopic instruments, do not tolerate steam sterilization. Ethylene oxide sterilization has been found to be effective and satisfactory for these items as well as for endotracheal tubes, either rubber or plastic. Varying concentrations of ethylene oxide from 10% to 20%, mixed with carbon dioxide, have been found efficient. Usually the following conditions prevail in the sterilization chamber:[88]

1. A concentration of ethylene oxide of about 450 mg/L
2. Adequate moisture through a humidity maintained at 45% to 50%
3. A temperature of 130°F
4. Exposure periods of 2 to 6 hours

For maximum efficiency, the equipment must be packaged in a film that is permeable to gas and moisture. Polyethylene bags or muslin are preferred. Overloading of the sterilizer must be avoided.

After sterilization, an air wash of the chamber is desirable. Many items of a rubber or plastic nature are penetrated by the ethylene oxide and thus must be removed.

Hazards of Gas Sterilization.[88,89] The possible toxic hazard from plastics such as polyvinyl chloride (PVC) sterilized by ethylene oxide is emphasized. When PVC catheters are washed with saline solution and then gas sterilized, a toxic and persistent reaction product, ethylene chlorhydrin, is formed; the amount of this substance is increased when tubes are preirradiated by the manufacturers. It has been suggested that irradiation-sterilized tubes be discarded after use and not gas sterilized for reuse.

Tubes must be thoroughly dry before packaging and sterilization. Ethylene oxide may combine with moisture to form ethylene glycol.

"Degassing" of standard tubes (not irradiated) may be accomplished by storing for 1 week after gas sterilization or by exposing the tubes after sterilization to a high vacuum of 30 in of mercury for 2 hours to remove the ethylene oxide.

Ethylene oxide, chlorhydrin, and the ethylene glycol are all tissue irritants. If not removed, ethylene oxide may be released later under use and cause erythema and edema of tissues.

Recommendations[80,88]

1. Correct initial cleaning: Thorough washing with running water, then distilled water, is essential to remove soaps and detergents
2. Thorough drying before sterilization
3. Do not soak tubes in antiseptic solutions
4. Do not resterilize with ethylene oxide gamma ray sterilized items
5. Adequate degassing time: 7 days at room air temperature; 24 hours with heat plus vacuum

THE LARYNGOSCOPE*

Safe and practical methods of endotracheal and endobronchial intubation rest firmly on the foundation of visualization of the larynx—the doorway to the tracheobronchial tree. Prior to 1885, the larynx was traditionally viewed by indirect methods using mirrors, and it was considered impossible to directly view the larynx because of the geometric relationship between the mouth and vocal cords. Little attention was paid to the mechanical interrelationship between the base of the tongue, the hyoid and the epiglottis, and the mobility of the neck.

During 1895, Alfred Kirstein in Berlin became interested in obtaining a direct view of the larynx.[90] He first used an oesophagoscope, and by slowly withdrawing the instrument from the esophagus, then firmly displacing the root of the tongue and elevating the epiglottis in an anterior direction, he was able to obtain a full view of the larynx. Kirstein fully appreciated the importance of the position of the head and the articulation at the atlanto–occipital junction to achieve the "sniffing of the air" position for airway laryngoscopy and intubation.

Kirstein later shortened the oesophagoscope, applied a hand lamp with a prism to redirect light by 90 degrees, and used the attached hand lamp as a handle. This he called his *autoscope* and was able to visualize the larynx readily and reproducibly and so demonstrated his technique. Thus was created the direct vision laryngoscope, as well as the principles of laryngoscopy.[91]

As a laryngologist, Kirstein intended his instrument to serve the requirements of his specialty. Anesthesiologists neglected this aid and continued to depend on blind nasal or oral tactile methods until about 1910.

In 1907, Chevalier Jackson introduced the separable laryngoscope with a "U" handle.[92] This was adopted in 1912 by Elsberg in New York for his anesthesia practice. The laryngoscope soon came to be recognized by many anesthetists as an important adjunct to intubation.[93,94] Flagg was a particular advocate of endotracheal intubation in anesthesia practice and in resuscitation to provide an airway.[95] He popularized direct vision laryngoscopy and developed a straight-blade–detachable laryngoscope. The application of the laryngoscope for the purpose of anesthesia and the many subsequent modifications of the instrument have served to reduce the uncertainty, inaccuracy, inconvenience, and trauma of laryngeal visualization and tracheal intubation.

---

* Credit for the material in this section is given to Dr. Barnett A. Greene and Dr. Bernard S. Goffen. "The Evolution of the Anesthesiologist's Laryngoscope," presented at the Postgraduate Assembly of the New York State Society of Anesthesiologists in 1955, is a classic compilation of source material, chiefly from the ASA Wood Library Museum of Anesthesiology, Park Ridge, IL.

Endotracheal Anesthesia: I. Basic Considerations **481**

Subsequent developments have been related to improvements in the three principal components of the instrument, which became known as the laryngoscope.

COMPONENT PARTS[96]

A laryngoscope is composed of three basic parts: the blade, the handle, and the light.

The blade is divisible into three components: a spatula, a flange, and a tip. The seemingly endless variations in laryngoscopes fall into a reasonable pattern of permutations and combinations of these various parts (Fig. 19–17) (See appendix).

THE SPATULA.[96] The spatula serves to compress and manipulate the soft tissues and lower jaw so that a direct line of vision may be achieved to the epiglottis and larynx. The long axis of the spatula may be entirely straight or curved in part or all of its length. The straight blade has always remained a favorite.[97] The curved spatula was first devised by Kirstein, then was reintroduced by Janeway in 1913 and popularized by Macintosh in 1943;[98] the curve was more pronounced than in Kirstein's model and was intended to prevent tilting of the spatula on the patient's upper teeth (Fig. 19–17). The curvature of the blade would presumably result in loss of view of the glottis if traction were improperly made along a line other than that of the handle. In Cassels's[99] opinion, however, the deep curve serves this purpose more satisfactorily by providing extra space between the spatula and teeth when the tip of the blade touches the soft tissues of the mouth. Indeed, the deep curve permits so much elevation of the spatula before it contacts the upper teeth that Macintosh insisted that the tip of the blade need not engage the epiglottis but should be inserted only as far as

MACINTOSH LARYNGOSCOPE
Original design. By lifting the base of the tongue, indirectly raises the epiglottis.

MILLER LARYNGOSCOPE
Developed in conjunction with Robert A. Miller, M.D., of San Antonio, Texas; this blade is universally popular.

LARYNGOSCOPE HANDLE

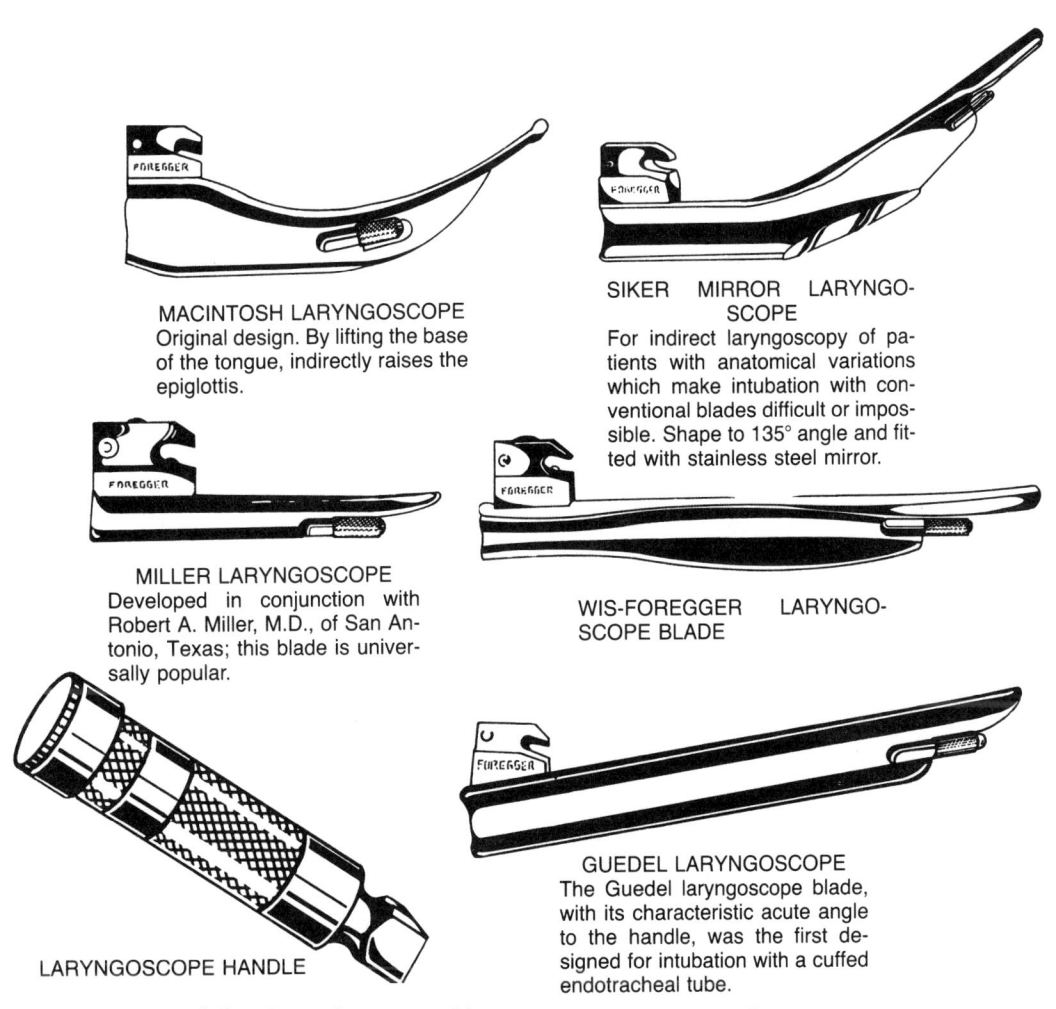

SIKER MIRROR LARYNGOSCOPE
For indirect laryngoscopy of patients with anatomical variations which make intubation with conventional blades difficult or impossible. Shape to 135° angle and fitted with stainless steel mirror.

WIS-FOREGGER LARYNGOSCOPE BLADE

GUEDEL LARYNGOSCOPE
The Guedel laryngoscope blade, with its characteristic acute angle to the handle, was the first designed for intubation with a cuffed endotracheal tube.

FIG. 19–17. Useful and popular types of laryngoscopes. Courtesy of Foregger Co., Inc.

the angle between the base of the tongue and the epiglottis.[100]

The deep curve of the Macintosh blade sometimes interferes with visualization of the anterior and middle portions of the rima glottis. As a compromise, other clinicians both before and after Macintosh, have tried to obtain the advantages of a curved spatula by reducing the entire curve (Cassels, 1942; Parrott, 1951); restricting the curve to the distal part of the blade (Janeway, 1913; Goffen, 1955); or up-tilting the distal extremity of a straight blade (Elam, 1935; Melbourne, 1952; Searles, 1950; Fink, 1954).

THE FLANGE.[96] The flange is the portion of the blade that projects from the edge of the spatula and serves to guide instrumentation and to deflect interfering tissues. The flange is part of the *cross-sectional shape* of the blade. This may vary from a simple flat or slightly curved form, like a tongue depressor without a flange, to a completely closed tube or "O"-shaped blade. Intermediate types of cross-sectional curves may resemble a "C," a flattened "C," a "U" turned on its side, or a "Z" in reverse.

Completely closed tube-blades or O-shaped blades were used by the early laryngologists because they were already accustomed to working with the esophagoscopes devised in the late 19th century. The completely closed tube of the laryngoscope was then slotted or segmented to facilitate its removal after the introduction of a bronchoscope. Later, as the laryngoscope became more commonly used for orotracheal intubation than for assistance in nasotracheal intubation, the permanently open slot became a fixed part of all laryngoscopes for the anesthesiologist.

The O-shaped tube-blade became C-shaped with the removal of the lateral segment. The Flagg and Magill laryngoscopes are the best-known examples of this type. The C shape has been flattened in its upper or spatula portion by Elam (1935), Murphy (ca. 1940), Miller (1941), and Sanders (1947) to decrease the volume of space occupied by the blade in the mouth. By flattening both the upper and lower curves of the C, a so-called lateral U shape is produced. This was introduced by Bruening in 1909, and it remains popular in the form of the Guedel blade and its numerous modifications. The flat upper and lower surfaces are less traumatic, less wasteful of space, and provide a greater working area between and lateral to the flanges of the blade.

The trend toward the use of larger endotracheal tubes, which require more space for manipulation, and the availability of muscle relaxants, which more readily provide optimum conditions for the laryngoscopy and intubation, have favored progressive simplification of design by the removal of portions of the flange and spatula. This has, therefore, tended to decrease the weight and traumatic potentialities. These changes began with the Bruening instrument (1909) in which the distal portion of the blade was reduced to a flat spatula. Guedel (1928) narrowed and tapered the inferior flange or wall of his instrument. The Waters-Hipple blade (ca. 1940) eliminated a large segment of the inferior flange and widened the diameter of the middle third of the blade to increase the available working area.

Seldon (1938) eliminated the inferior wall by rotating it 180 degrees to serve as a projecting flange; the shape was now a reverse Z. The inferior flange was no longer in the line of view nor did it circumscribe the working space; yet, as a lateral flange, it still deflected the soft tissues. Bennett (1943) eliminated the inferior flange completely and reduced the lateral flange markedly to form a shallow reversed L (⌐). Although Bennett, like Seldon, devised his laryngoscope for mouths narrowed by trismus and edema, the instrument has been found useful in normal patients. With its complete elimination of the lateral wall, the Galasso blade has completed the full cycle to the original spatula pattern of Kirstein.

BLADE TIP.[96] The tip of the blade either directly or indirectly elevates the epiglottis out of the line of vision into the larynx. To retain the epiglottis more securely, the tip has been ridged, curved, slotted, and even hooked (Fink, 1955, Fig. 19–18). To avoid trauma, the tip has been blunted and thickened. Other solutions of these problems include the devising of bifid tips to enter the valleculae by straddling the epiglottis (Kirstein, Bowen-Jackson) and the fashioning of curved or angled blades to elevate the epiglottis indirectly by pressure at the junction of tongue and epiglottis (Kirstein, Macintosh, Evans, Parrott).

HANDLE.[101] Two main categories of handles are in use among anesthetists, namely the L-type and the U-type instruments.

In the L-type of instrument, as in the early esophagoscopes, the handle started as a right-angled structure. This has been most popular among anesthetists, and several models contain a modification of the angle of the handle to the blade. Thus, some are at an acute angle (72 degrees in Guedel), and others at an obtuse angle (100 degrees in Bowen-Jackson; 135 degrees in Macbeth-Bannister).

Jackson introduced the U-type of instrument by adding to the original Kirstein model handle a bar parallel to the blade.[92]

The laryngoscope may be further classified according to the method of attachment of the blade to the handle; thus, a permanently attached blade, folding blades including "hook-on;" types, and interchangeable blades are available.

Each modification of the handle has been proposed with the claim of diminishing the tendency to use the upper incisors as a fulcrum. One undeniable advantage of the L type, especially in the fold-

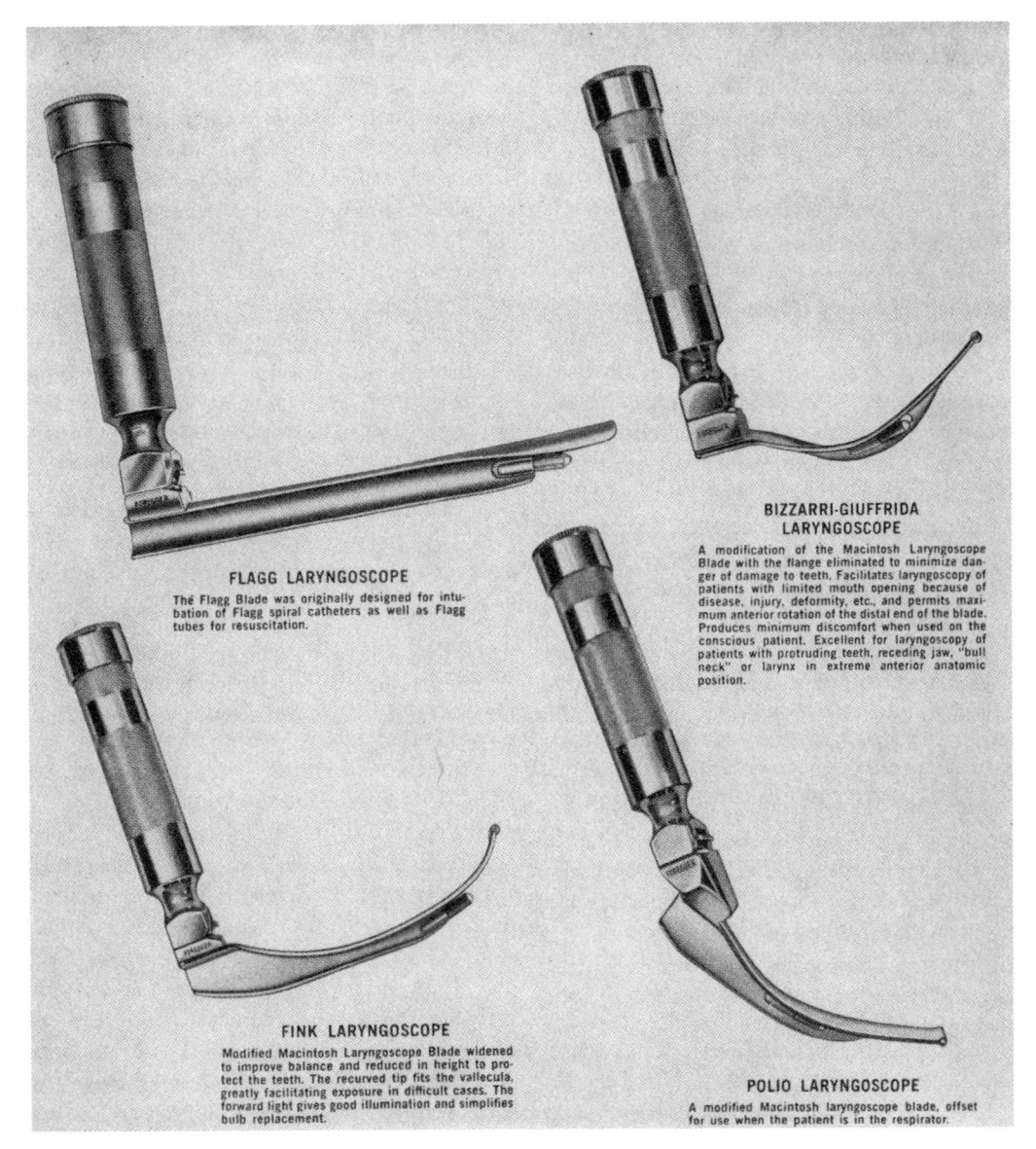

FIG. 19-18. Laryngoscopes for special purposes. Courtesy of Foregger Co., Inc.

ing models, is the decreased bulk and weight. The obtuse-angled handle facilitates the entrance of the blade in the presence of a body cast or operating table screen.

The handle in the early Kirstein and Bruening proximally lighted instruments contained the light source but not the battery. The Mörch instrument has both in the handle. The Janeway scope (1913), the first fashioned specifically for anesthetists, was also the first to incorporate the battery in the handle. Since then, the handle as a battery container has become standard for anesthetist laryngoscopes.

LIGHTING. The earliest instruments used proximal lighting, ie, the source of light emanated from a point between the scope and the observer. Headmirror, head-lamp, and electric light directed by prism or mirror were among the sources employed. Because the distance traversed is short, this method is effective, particularly with nonreflecting blade surfaces. (Unpolished, tarnished brass was used by the early German endoscopists for their instruments; Chevalier Jackson did likewise on his return to this country from Germany.)

Einhorn's invention of the electric light bulb carrier (1902) enabled Jackson to introduce distal lighting for laryngoscopy in 1907. Distal lighting has continued to be the most popular method. In recent years, however, a return to some form of proximal lighting has appeared.

In the Mörch's scope (1951), the light bulb is in the battery handle, as mentioned, to permit the detachable blade to be sterilized without fear of damage to the electrical system. Semiproximal lighting appears in the Negus (1932), Macbeth-Bannister (1944), and Magill (ca. 1950) laryngoscopes to obtain more diffuse light and to avoid the possibility of disturbance or damage to the light bulb.

The explosion hazard remained a problem that two instrument makers, Longworth and Cameron, have diminished by modifications of the electrical systems.

LEAK-PROOF INHALATION ANESTHESIA SYSTEMS

PURPOSE. The purpose of providing a leak-proof anesthetic system is twofold: (1) to provide control of ventilation without leaks, and (2) to protect the tracheobronchial tree from aspiration of foreign material.

Two methods have been employed to effect an airtight endotracheal seal. One is the pharyngeal pack and the other is the inflatable cuff.

Pharyngeal Packing. In the early use of endotracheal tubes, as for diphtheria, O'Dwyer[102] pointed out the dangers of aspiration. In 1893, Madyl[103] devised and used a laryngeal tube for otorhinolaryngeal surgery but overcame the dangers of aspiration of blood and debris by tightly packing the pharynx with gauze. Pharyngeal packing then became a common method of protecting the airway until Guedel[104] popularized the endotracheal tube cuff.

The pharyngeal pack has been used under special circumstances. Preference for this method is based chiefly on alleged disadvantages and certain rare and highly questionable complications of the inflated cuff. The concept of pharyngeal packing to secure a leak-proof airway is simple and obvious. The material used as a seal consists of a role or strip of soft gauze. This is impregnated with a lubricant such as petroleum jelly. Dry gauze or gauze saturated with saline solution is inadequate and abrades the mucosa, thereby leading to postintubation pharyngitis.

The technique of placing the gauze consists of inserting the strip either under vision with forceps or blindly by means of the index finger. Most effective packing is achieved by introducing the gauze into one side of the pyriform sinus. The strip is then carried across the pharynx to the opposite sinus. Three-inch segments are then alternately and firmly swung back and forth in the pharynx behind the endotracheal tube. Tightness of the system will depend upon the care and firmness with which the packing is introduced.

Although the chief advantage in the use of packing is as a substitute for cuffs, at the same time there are some definite disadvantages and complications that do occur when the pack is used. The gauze pack does not reduce the incidence or extent of regurgitation into the pharynx, nor does it protect against pulmonary aspiration after regurgitation occurs. In Adriani's series,[105] the incidence of aspiration was the same in patients with an endotracheal tube and pharyngeal pack as in a comparable group of nonintubated patients. Furthermore, packing does not consistently afford satisfactory closure, and air leakage frequently occurs on compressing the breathing bag with pressures ordinarily used in clinical anesthesia. Other major disadvantages of pharyngeal packing include abrasion of the oral mucosa; laceration of the uvula and frenulum of the tongue; accumulation of secretions in the pharynx (absorbent capacity of a pack is not great); compression of soft endotracheal catheters by tight packs; and failure to recover a pack at the conclusion of an anesthetic resulting in postanesthesia obstruction.

INFLATABLE ENDOTRACHEAL CUFFS

HISTORY. Inflatable endotracheal cuffs and tracheal tubes were developed concomitantly. Trendelenberg[106] described a tracheostomy tube with inflatable cuff in 1871, and Eisenmenger[107] introduced the first metal endotracheal tube with cuff in 1893. Both had inflatable rubber cuffs at their distal ends. In 1910, Dorrance[108] constructed a tracheal tube—inflatable cuff unit similar to those used today. In 1914 to 1918, Rowbotham and Magill[109] developed the uncuffed wide-bore rubber endotracheal tube, and in 1928 to 1930, Guedel and Waters[104] added a rubber inflatable cuff, similar to Dorrance's cuff, to the Magill tube. In 1943, Grimme and Knight[110] described an extratracheal retroepiglottic cuff. In the same year, Macintosh[100] developed a self-inflating endotracheal cuff.

From 1940 to 1950, home-made cuffs of surgical drain tubing, rubber dam, or condoms enclosing small urethral catheters for inflation were cemented to endotracheal tubes. Cuffs and pilot tubes were also manufactured separately and slipped on the tube by the anesthesiologist.[111] Until the early 1950s, these developments remained largely ignored; uncuffed endotracheal tubes were used with packing. During the 1952 polio epidemic in Copenhagen, cuffed endotracheal tubes and intermittent positive-pressure–controlled ventilation were generally used.[112,113] By 1956, some standards for both tube and cuff construction were established, and in the 1960s they became standard practice. Thinner, pliable plastic cuffs of various materials and designs replaced the thick rubber or latex cuffs by 1960.[114]

PURPOSE. Endotracheal cuffs are used to provide a no-leak inhalation system, to allow positive-pressure ventilation, to prevent aspiration of foreign material into the lungs, and to center the tube in the trachea.

THE CUFF SYSTEM. The endotracheal cuff system consists of an inflatable sleeve of pliable material

FIG. 19–19. Types of high-pressure, low-volume endotracheal cuffs, both single- and double-wall type. From Guedel, A.E., and Waters, E.M.: A new intratracheal catheter. Anesth. Analg., 7:238, 1928. (Courtesy Foregger Co. Inc.)

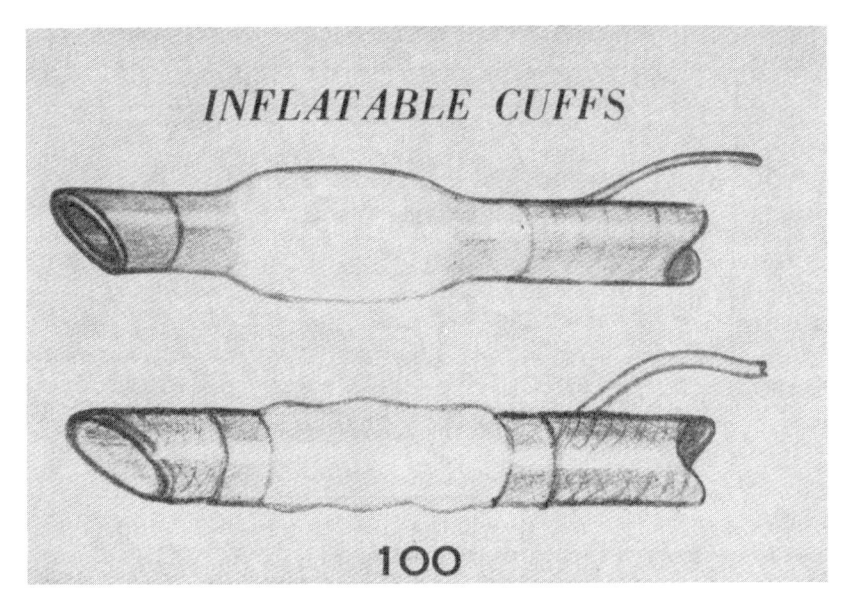

attached to the distal portion of the endotracheal tube, an inflating tube, and a pilot balloon (Fig. 19–19) (see section on standard endotracheal tube). When inflated, the cuff distends and seals the air passage around the endotracheal tube. The pilot balloon indicates the degree of inflation or deflation of the cuff. Modern endotracheal tubes have a one-way inflating valve attached to the free end of the inflating tube to prevent loss of air when the cuff is inflated.

CHARACTERISTICS OF CUFFS.[115,116] Cuffs and endotracheal tubes are made of the same material; the cuffs are built into the distal part of the patient end of the tube. Since 1970, plastic cuffs have replaced rubber and latex cuffs.

The length of the cuff varies with the size of the tube. Generally, tubes of smaller bore are of shorter length and have an appropriately sized cuff. A cuff should distend symmetrically until a no-leak seal is achieved at cuff pressures of 20 to 30 mm Hg—this is called the *seal point*. When a properly sized endotracheal tube is used, the seal point is achieved when the cuff has expanded to 1.5 times the ED of the tube.[115a]

TYPES OF CUFFS.[115,117] There are two types of endotracheal cuffs: high pressure (HP) and low pressure (LP). The HP cuffs are low volume (LV), i.e., they become totally inflated when LVs of air are injected into them (see Fig. 19–19). The LP cuffs require a much greater volume of air to become fully expanded. Two sub-types of LP cuffs are available: those that require a high volume (LPHV) of 20 ml or more of air and those that require a lower volume (LPLV) of 10 ml or less of air. Table 19–7 compares the characteristics of the various types of cuffs.

The LP cuffs have thinner, more compliant walls and a larger area of contact with the tracheal wall than the HP cuffs. When inflated to seal point, the more compliant LP cuffs do not deform the shape of the trachea, whereas the HP cuffs exert such pressure on the tracheal wall that the normal tracheal contour is deformed (Fig. 19–20). Cuff compliance plays an important role in the prevention of serious tracheal complications after intubation, particularly in long-term intubation, when the trachea may constrict or become more rigid as a result of autonomic reflexes.[118]

One of the advantages of LP cuffs is that the intracuff pressure at seal point is almost equal to the lateral pressure exerted by the inflated cuff on the wall of the trachea.[119] One disadvantage is that LP cuffs, particularly the LPHV cuffs, are bulkier than HPLV cuffs and may hinder the visualization of the vocal cords at laryngoscopy.

TRACHEAL WALL PRESSURES.[120,121] Ordinarily, under resting conditions, the capillary perfusion of the tracheal mucosa is 0.3 ml · g^{-1} · min^{-1} (60% of the cerebral perfusion of 0.5 ml · g^{-1} · min^{-1}) and the perfusion head pressure is 22 mm Hg. When a cuff is inflated in the trachea, there is a linear decrease in the perfusion. It becomes reduced when the lateral pressure on the tracheal wall attains 30 cm H$_2$O (22 mm Hg) and ceases completely at 50 cm H$_2$O (42 mm Hg) in humans. Excessive lateral tracheal-wall pressure causes ischemia of the mucosa anteriorly over the cartilages but may include deeper mucosal layers and posteriorly at the membranous portion of the trachea.[122,123] The intercartilaginous mucosa is spared, but the cilia of the overlying mucosa are destroyed.

One must distinguish between the intracuff pressure and the cuff to tracheal wall contact pressure—the CT pressure. The *intracuff pressure* produced by

TABLE 19-7. CHARACTERISTICS OF ENDOTRACHEAL CUFFS

	HPLV	LPHV	LPLV
Cuff wall	Rigid	Pliable	Pliable
Diameter	Small	Large	Small
Residual volume	Small	Large	Small
Contact area with trachea	Small	Large	Small
Intracuff pressure at seal	High	Low	Low
Tracheal wall pressure	High	Low	Low
Ratio intracuff pressure Tracheal wall pressure	>1	<1	1
Rise in intracuff pressure Per ml injected	Steep	Slow	Slow

Abbreviations: HP = high pressure; LP = low pressure; HV = high volume; LV = low volume. Adapted from Dorsch, J.A., Dorsch, S.E.: Understanding Anesthesia Equipment, 2nd ed. Baltimore, Williams & Wilkins, 1984.

inflating the conventional endotracheal cuff to effect a seal against intraairway pressures of 15 to 20 mm Hg can range between 90 and 220 mm Hg. Most of this pressure is expended in overcoming the elasticity of the cuff material, and the wide range in pressures is the result of characteristics of the cuff. Thus, the pressures in new cuffs are generally higher; in latex cuffs, smaller pressures are required.

Although most of the intracuff pressure is expended in inflating the cuff and overcoming elastic resistance, a small portion of the pressure is exerted by the cuff laterally on the wall of the trachea. This is the cuff-to-wall tracheal pressure (CT pressure). This pressure varies between 10 to 25 mm Hg and approximates the mean capillary blood pressure. Thus, there is a risk of pressure ischemia in routine cases. A high cuff pressure of 320 mm Hg may also cause rupture of the trachea, as demonstrated in cadavers.

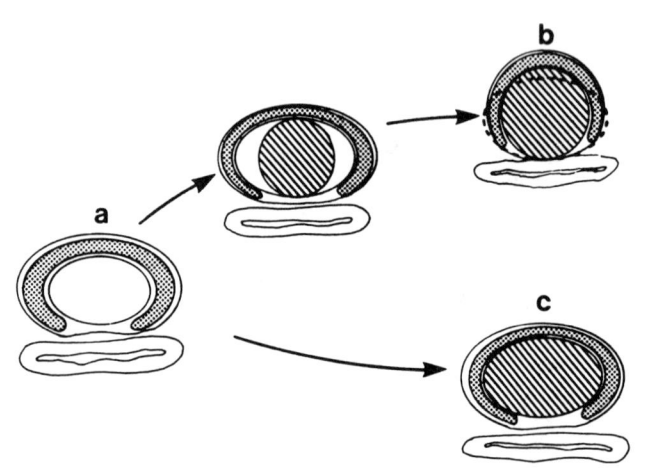

FIG. 19-20. The trachea and the cuff. a, Normal trachea and oesophagus. b, High-pressure cuff distorts the trachea and makes the tracheal contour the same as the shape of the cuff. c, Soft low-pressure cuff conforms to the normal tracheal lumen. From Cooper, J.D., and Grillo, H.C.: Analysis of problems related to cuffs on intratracheal tubes. Chest, 62:215, 1972.

In HPLV cuffs, there is a direct relationship between intracuff pressures and the volume of air injected into the cuff. The seal point is reached with small volumes (4 to 6 ml) and intracuff pressures reach more than 100 mm Hg. Most of the pressure is expended in overcoming the elastic resistance of the low-compliant cuff, whereas the mucosal wall contact pressure at seal will amount to 25 to 30 mm Hg (Fig. 19-21).[105]

In LP cuffs, the relationship between intracuff pressure and volume of air is not linear.[124] The seal point is reached with injected volumes varying from 10 ml (LPLV cuffs) to as high as 30 ml (LPHV cuffs), depending on the size, design, and the plastic material used in the cuff.[124a] LPHV cuffs inflated to pressures less than 30 cm H_2O (22 to 25 mm Hg) function as an air cushion and allow a substantial part of the arterial pressure to provide perfusion to surface mucosal capillaries and even those entering cartilages.[125] The intracuff pressure at seal point rarely exceeds 20 mm Hg. When minimal volumes are added, however, the lateral tracheal wall pressure may rise rapidly to higher levels.[126] Furthermore, when N_2O is administered, the intracuff pressure increases,[127] and the rate of increase is faster than in HP cuffs.[128]

Several investigators found no difference in lateral tracheal wall pressures to support the claimed superiority of LPHV cuffs over LPLV cuffs.[126]

There seems to be a relationship between cuff residual volume and tracheal wall pressures. Residual volume is the amount of air remaining in the cuff when the inflating tube is open to the atmosphere. Studies in model tracheas have shown that when the ratio of tracheal seal volume–cuff residual volume is 1 or less, the tracheal wall pressure is less than 35 mm Hg.[116,129]

FACTORS THAT AUGMENT TRACHEAL WALL PRESSURE. Many factors may interfere with intracuff and tracheal wall pressures in addition to the intrinsic cuff characteristics.[130]

FIG. 19-21. Curves showing relationship between intracuff pressure and lateral pressure exerted by cuff on tracheal wall as volume of air distending cuff is increased. From Adriani, J., and Phillips, M.: Use of endotracheal cuff: Some data pro and con. Anesthesiology, 18:1, 1957.

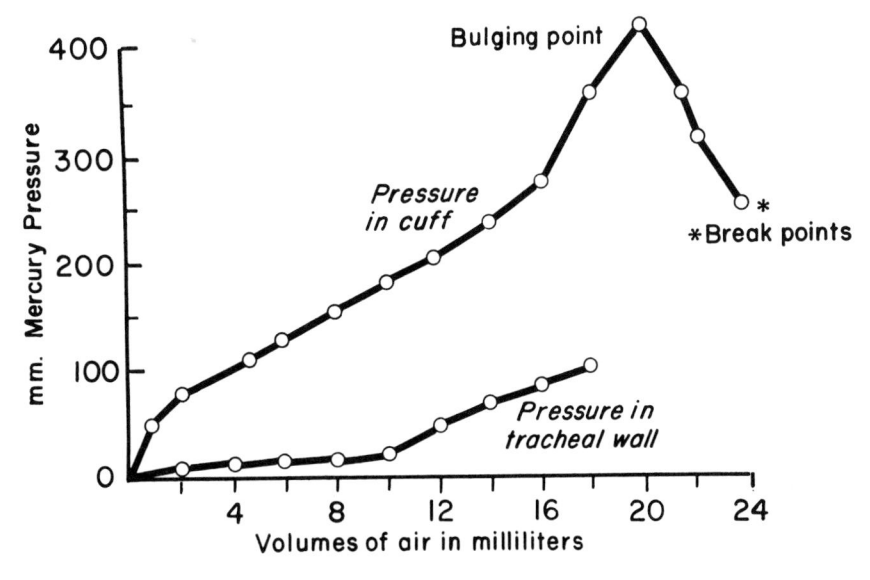

1. *Position of the head:* In the normal position of the head, the tracheal wall pressure is greater on the cartilaginous anterior wall and minimal in the posterior membranous wall; when the head is slightly flexed, the pressure difference is reduced and may be even reversed on hyperflexion of the neck. This explains why cuff damage to the tracheal mucosa is usually more severe anteriorly. A neutral position (straight cervical vertebrae) is advised.
2. *Cough:* Coughing changes the shape of the trachea (flattens the AP dimension of the trachea), compresses the inflated cuff, and raises intracuff and tracheal wall pressures (Fig. 19-22).[131]
3. *Controlled ventilation:* The intratracheal positive pressure during inspiration is transmitted to the inflated cuff and raises the tracheal wall pressure (Fig. 19-23).[130] Intracuff pressure is also raised when the patient "fights" the ventilator (Fig. 19-24).
4. *Gas mixtures:*[127,128,132] When the cuff is inflated with air and the patient inhales gas mixtures containing N_2O of 50% or more, intracuff pressure may rise 1.35 to 5 times and the volume within the cuff may increase 42% to 89% (Fig. 19-25).[128,133,134] Intracuff pressure during 2 hours in a patient receiving 67% N_2O and 33% O_2 at 20° C may increase 14 to 20 mm Hg.[135] The rate of diffusion into the cuff varies with the thickness of the cuff and the N_2O partial pressure.[136] Oxygen and other gases also diffuse through thin-walled plastic cuffs.[127]

Several techniques have been proposed to reduce the effect or to limit the diffusion of N_2O into the cuff:[132] (1) inflate the cuff with the same mixture as that inspired;[137] (2) inflate the cuff with saline; (3) inflate the cuff with air and monitor the intracuff pressure, adjusting it as needed; (4) inflate the cuff with air and use devices that limit the intracuff pressure; and (5) intermittently deflate the cuff (every 1 to 2 hours) for 10 to 15 seconds and reinflate to seal point.[138]

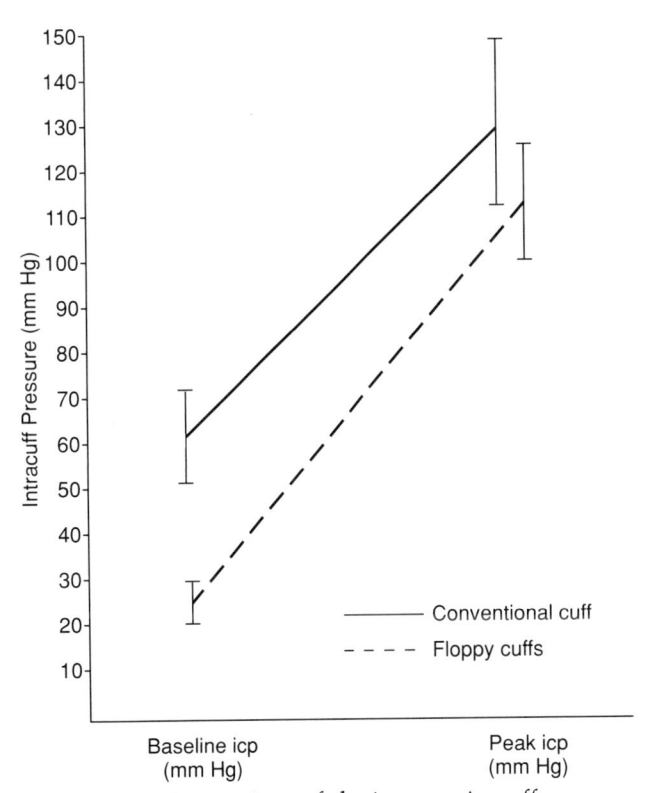

FIG. 19-22. Comparison of the increase in cuff pressure with coughing. (Bars represent s.e. mean.) From Jacobsen, L., and Greenbaum, R.: A study of intracuff pressure measurements, trends, and behavior in patients during prolonged tracheal intubation. Br. J. Anaesth., 53:97, 1981.

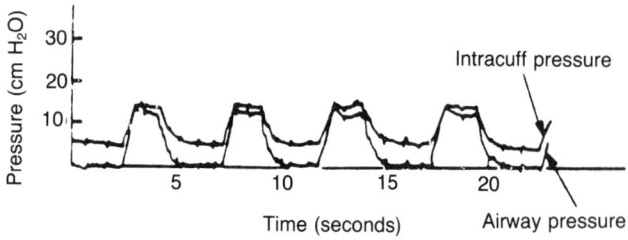

FIG. 19–23. Variation of intracuff and airway pressure for a high-volume cuff in a patient. The small superimposed changes in pressure are due to cardiac displacement. From Crawley, B.E., and Cross, D.E.: Tracheal cuffs: A review and dynamic pressure study. Anaesthesia, *30:*4, 1975.

SUMMARY. Increases in intracuff pressures caused by various factors are well documented. Recommendations have been made to monitor intracuff pressures, and devices are available to prevent undue high pressure. Nevertheless, these facts seem to be ignored by most clinicians, and little effort is made to control intracuff pressures during endotracheal anesthesia. The lack of monitoring intracuff pressure during long-term endotracheal intubation is more dangerous.[105]

RULES FOR INFLATING CUFFS.

1. Inflate slowly.
2. Use the minimal volume of air necessary to obtain a no-leak tracheal seal. This volume is usually 4 to 6 ml for HPLV cuffs, but varies greatly, from 10 to 30 ml in LP cuffs.
3. Check the seal point of inflation of the cuff by auscultation at the suprasternal notch and do not rely on the absence of leaking sounds or the "feeling of the bag."
4. Monitor intracuff pressure after inflation. Do not exceed a pressure of 30 cm H_2O. At this cuff pressure, the lateral tracheal wall pressure is 22 mm Hg. Seal point is usually reached at intracuff pressures lower than 25 cm H_2O in LP cuffs.
5. Monitor intracuff pressure frequently during anesthesia or long-term intubation.

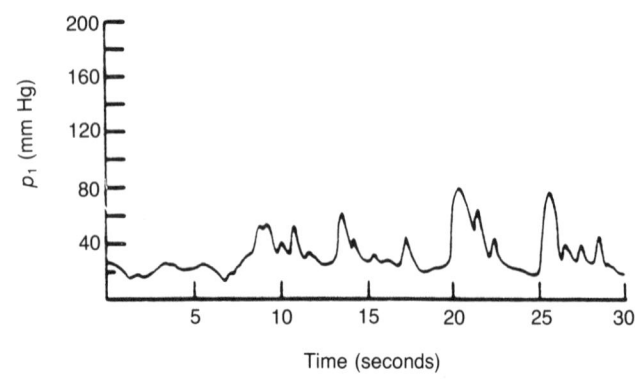

FIG. 19–24. The effect of fighting the ventilator on tracheal wall pressure. From Crawley, B.E., and Cross, D.E.: Tracheal cuffs: A review and dynamic pressure study. Anaesthesia, *30:*4, 1975.

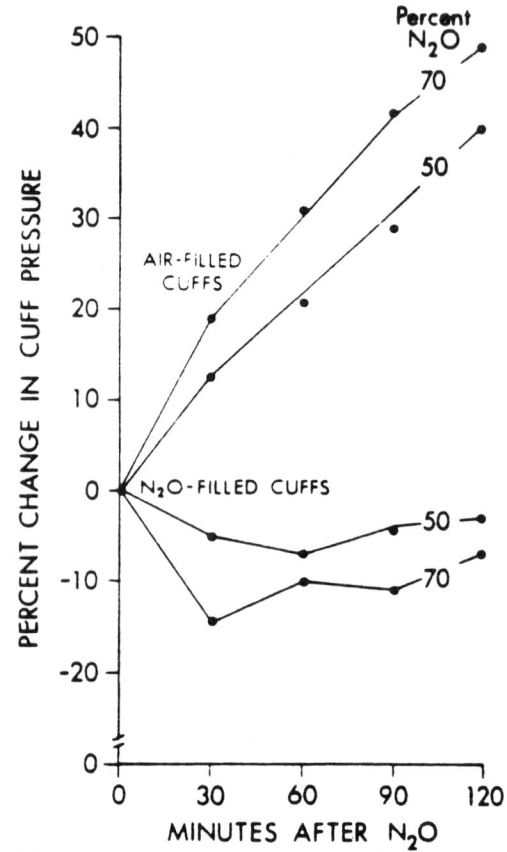

FIG. 19–25. Percent change in endotracheal cuff pressure before and after exposure to 50 and 70 percent nitrous oxide. Note that pressure change is proportional to nitrous oxide concentration and that cuffs filled with nitrous oxide show no increase in pressure. From Munson, E.S.: Nitrous oxide and body air space. Middle East J. Anesthesiol., *7:*193, 1983.

MANAGEMENT OF INFLATED CUFF. Several problems are associated with the inflated cuff. These include the overinflation and occlusive bulging; excessive intracuff pressure and pressure on the tracheal wall; occurrence of sore throat postoperatively; and risk of aspiration. Several techniques have been proposed to limit these problems and complications (Table 19–8).[139]

MONITORING CUFF PRESSURE. Monitoring intracuff pressures is a valuable procedure to prevent complications caused by overinflated cuffs.

A simple method consists of a water[110] or aneroid[119] manometer and a syringe connected to the endotracheal inflating tube via a three-way stopcock (Fig. 19–25). To inflate the cuff, turn the stopcock so that the channel is open between the syringe and the

TABLE 19–8. TECHNIQUES TO MANAGE INFLATED CUFFS

TECHNIQUE	COMMENTS
Intermittent cuff deflation	Not necessary with the use of modern high-volume cuffs
Small leaks around the cuff	Not necessary with the use of modern high-volume cuffs; risk of aspiration of pharyngeal contents
Intermittent measurement and adjustment of cuff pressure	Requires measuring system; should be routine in clinical practice
Inflate cuff with the inspired gas mixture	Prevents inspired gas diffusion into the cuff (N_2O anesthesia)
Cuff with pressure-control balloon (Lanz tube)	Prevents rises or falls in intracuff pressure (N_2O anesthesia)
Pressure-limiting devices	Avoid excessive rise of cuff pressure during N_2O anesthesia
Self-inflating cuffs	Tracheal wall pressure equals airway pressure in inspiration; risk of aspiration on expiration
Foam cuffs	Exert very low pressure on the tracheal wall; risk of aspiration

Adapted from Latto, I.P., and Rosen M. (eds): Difficulties in Tracheal Intubation. England, Bailliere Tindall, 1985.

cuff. After injecting the intended volume of air into the cuff, turn the stopcock so that the syringe channel is closed and the channel between the manometer and cuff is open. The intracuff pressure is then measured either in cm H_2O or mm Hg. It should be adjusted to 30 cm H_2O or 20 mm Hg.

If there is a leak, the endotracheal cuff (and tube) is too small for the trachea and should be changed. If an LP cuff is inflated to a pressure exceeding 30 cm H_2O to obtain a seal point, leakage may be occurring along longitudinal folds of the cuff. Usually with LPHV cuffs, the smaller volume cuff (10 ml) will solve the problem.

Intracuff pressures should be monitored frequently during the time that the patient remains intubated; several readjustments may be required to avoid excessive lateral tracheal wall pressure.

DEVICES TO LIMIT INTRACUFF PRESSURE. Many devices have been used to limit the intracuff pressure automatically.

Stanley[140] described a pressure relief valve in the shape of a T. One end of the cross of the T attaches to the inflating tube of the cuff and contains a spring-loaded check valve that prevents cuff inflation or deflation unless a syringe is connected to the other end. The upright portion of the T contains the pressure-relief valve. An index mark on the cap of this valve can be aligned with one of eight pressure-relief set points—markings around the periphery of the body of the valve. The setpoints are calibrated so that the valve opens at various pressures, from 22 mm Hg to over 200 mm Hg. Several similar pressure-limiting valves are commercially available.

McGinnis[141] and Macgovern[142] developed a pressure-regulating system consisting of a pressure-limiting balloon connected to a volume-regulating check valve and the inflating tube of the endotracheal cuff (Fig. 19–26). The balloon is made of compliant natural rubber with a wall thickness of 0.08 cm and a diameter of 2.5 cm. When inflated, the intraballoon pressure reaches a peak of 26 cm H_2O (20 mm Hg) and maintains this maximum pressure even after the injection of additional volumes of air. When the tip of a 20-ml syringe containing air is coupled to the end of the check valve, the connection between syringe balloon and cuff opens. Air is injected into the system and inflates both cuff and balloon. As inflation proceeds, the intracuff and intraballoon pressures are equal. When the balloon is fully expanded, the intracuff pressure does not exceed 26 cm H_2O. The uncoupling of the syringe automatically closes the cuff-balloon connection.

To check the intracuff pressure, one simply has to press the check valve with a syringe or other device. If the intracuff pressure exceeds 26 cm H_2O, air will flow from cuff to balloon and back. The thin-walled, pressure-limiting rubber balloon is enclosed in a much larger plastic balloon as a safety precaution. This pressure-limiting system has been incorporated in the Lanz tubes (Lanz Medical Products Co., Monroeville, PA).

Kim[136] described a tracheal tube cuff pressure stabilizer (TTCPS). TTCPS comprises a piece of transparent Plexiglas or plastic tubing measuring 1.5 cm ID and 50 cm height, a disposable central venous pressure (CVP) manometer, a vent needle, a three-way stopcock, a continuous flow system (CFS Intraflo), and extension tubing. The transparent Plexiglas serves as a water container and the other parts are assembled to function as a water manometer. The height of the fluid level, shown on the graduated marks on the CVP manometer immersed in the water reservoir will be the intended maximum in-

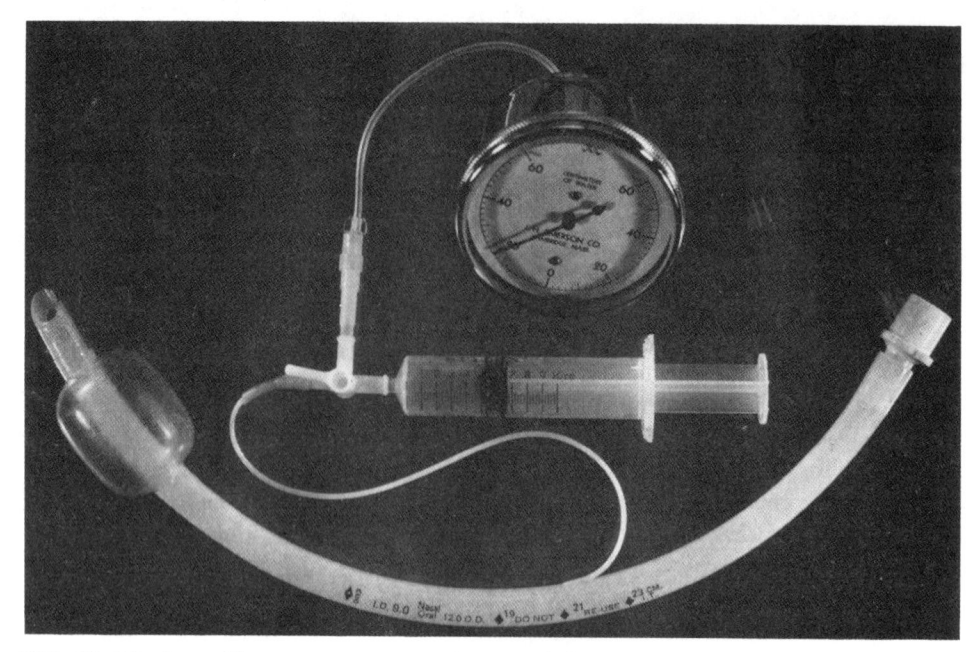

FIG. 19–26. Aneroid pressure gauge, syringe, and three-way stopcock for measurement of intracuff pressure. From Carroll, R.G., and Grenvick, A.: Proper use of large diameter, large residual volume cuffs. Crit. Care Med., 1:153, 1973.

tracuff pressure in cm H$_2$O. After the cuff is inflated, the port of the inflating tube is connected to the TTCPS. By pulling the rubber band of the CFS Intraflo, the excess amount of air, if any, bubbles out until the intracuff pressure is adjusted to the predetermined maximum pressure.

COMPLICATIONS. The complications of the use of endotracheal cuffs are discussed in this section.

Aspiration of Pharyngeal Contents. Aspiration of pharyngeal contents during anesthesia and long-term intubation with cuffed endotracheal tubes has been studied by placing dye in the lower pharynx and tracking its passage to the trachea beyond the inflated cuff. The reported incidence of aspiration of dye when HPLV cuffs are used is zero.[143–146] In these HPLV cuffs, however, the inflation to seal point may generate intracuff pressures in excess of 60 mm Hg. When LPHV cuffs were studied, the incidence of aspiration varied from 16%[147] to 100%.[143,146]

High-volume cuffs have diameters ranging from 1.5 to 2 times the average diameter of an adult male trachea. When inflated to seal point within the trachea, the pliable cuff walls develop folds or wrinkles (Fig. 19–27). Pharyngeal or tracheal secretions accumulated above the cuff may find their way down the trachea. The ease and amount of aspiration depend on the viscosity of the liquid, the hydrostatic pressure of the liquid above the cuff, and the size of the folds or wrinkles. To avoid cuff wall folding, the diameter of the cuff at residual volume should approximate the diameter of the trachea.[146] Wrinkles also may be prevented by overinflation. This is often done during short-term intubation for surgery, without evident serious complications. For long-term intubations, cuff pressures must be controlled accurately.

Sore Throat. The reported incidence of sore throat after endotracheal intubation varies from 6.6% to 90%, with an average value of 40% to 60%.[148] Many factors are individually contributing causes, such as dry inspired gases, use of succinylcholine or cholinergic drugs, oropharyngeal airways, trauma at laryngoscopy or intubation, characteristics of the tube, lubricants on the tube, coughing, and bucking.[149,150]

It seems that endotracheal cuffs, when used correctly, may influence only minimally the occurrence of sore throat. It has been shown, however,

FIG. 19-27. Lanz tube (*a*) with cuff and balloon inflated. *b.* The Lanz tube valve. *A:* A syringe is inserted into the Lanz valve and approximately 30 ml air is injected. The syringe is then removed. A cuff pressure not exceeding 25 mmHg is automatically provided. *B:* The valve system automatically keeps the cuff pressure below 25 mmHg for the duration of intubation. *C.* A special valve mechanism (*a*) regulates the speed of pressure release from the cuff to the latex balloon. The thin latex balloon expands and contracts within the operating range with no change in internal pressure. If the tracheal cuff pressure exceeds the balloon pressure the balloon expands and controls the cuff pressure. If the cuff pressure falls the balloon contracts forcing volume into the cuff maintaining a low-pressure seal. From Macgovern, G.J., et al: An engineering analysis of intratracheal cuffs. Anesth. Analg., *50*:557, 1971.

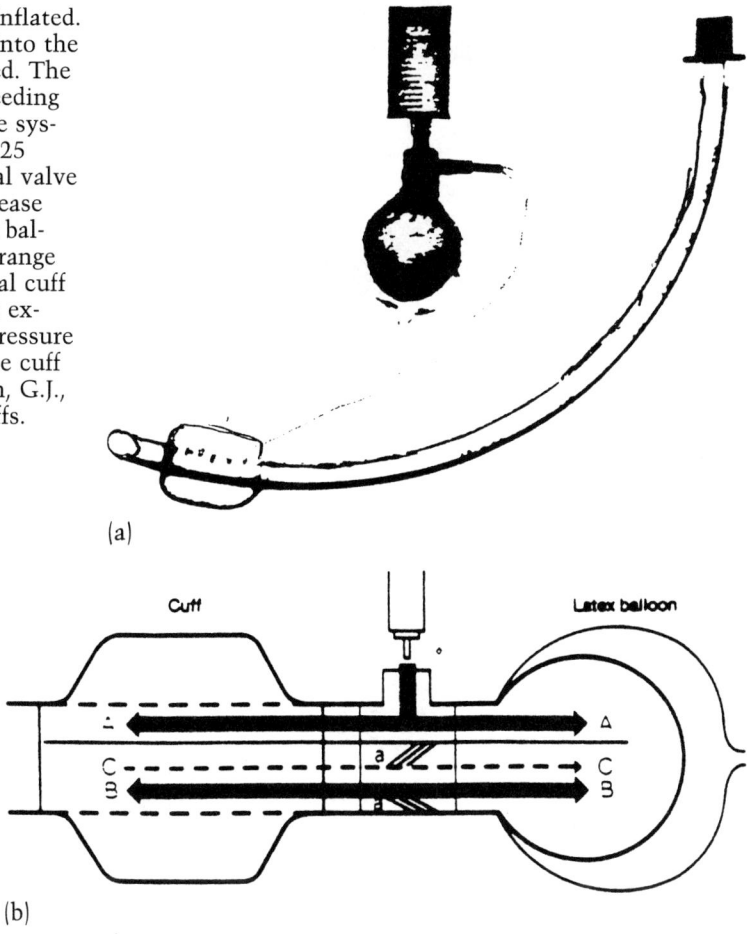

that lessening the area of contact between the cuff and the tracheal wall (cuffs with smaller residual volumes) reduces somewhat the incidence of sore throat.[148] It also seems logical that intracuff pressure should not exceed the minimum necessary to obtain a no-leak seal, and it should be monitored frequently to avoid rises because of diffusion of N_2O into the cuff.

Other Complications. Many other complications related to endotracheal cuffs have been reported; they are largely the result of improper use and cause either obstruction of the airway or pressure-ischemic lesions on the tracheal wall.

Irregular expansion of the cuff may push the bevel of the endotracheal tube against the tracheal wall, causing obstruction of the airway (Fig. 19-28A).[151]

An overinflated cuff may bulge over the tip of the tube[152] (Fig. 19-28B) or compress the lumen of the tube (Fig. 19-29),[153] resulting in partial or total tube obstruction. The former is more likely to occur when the distance from the distal end of the cuff and the tip of the tube is too short. The latter is more common when small-diameter endotracheal tubes are used or when the plastic wall of the tube is defective and weak.

Overexpansion of the cuff after long surgical procedures under N_2O–O_2 anesthesia will cause pressure ischemia and ulcerations on the tracheal wall.[154] A tracheal wall pressure of 20 mm Hg (26 cm H_2O) during 15 minutes results in superficial nonprogressive mucosal damage.[155] At 50 mm Hg (65 cm H_2O), there is partial denuding of the basement membrane, and at 100 mm Hg (130 cm H_2O) after 4 hours, the lesion is almost down to the cartilage, with possible bacterial invasion.[125] The use of low-pressure cuffs reduces drastically but does not prevent the incidence or severity of the ulceration. Intracuff pressure must be measured and monitored.

The cuff may be placed too close to the subglottic region or actually within the glottic chink. When inflated, it will cause direct vocal cord damage or compression of the recurrent laryngeal nerve.[156] These nerve endings run in the submucosa on the medial aspect of the thyroid cartilage.[157] Rupture of an overinflated cuff has been reported to cause a fatality.[158]

A common cause of difficulty in extubation is failure of cuff deflation. In most cases, it is the result of obstruction of the inflating tube distal to the pilot balloon. Clamping, biting by the patient, and mal-

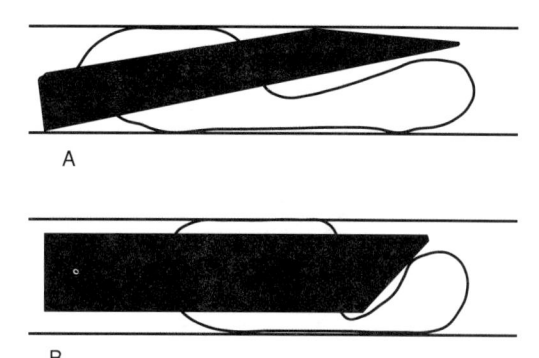

FIG. 19–28. Causes of tracheal tube obstruction: A. The bevel of the tube is pointed against the wall of the trachea by an eccentrically inflated cuff (Seuffert). B. The cuff has ballooned over the end of the tube (Hartnett).
References:
1. Seuffert and Urbach: Can. Anaesth. Soc. J., 15:300, 1968.
2. Hartnett, J.S.: J. Am. Assoc. Nurse. Anesth., 38:31, 1980.
Courtesy Dorsch, J.A., and Dorsch, S.E.: *Understanding Anesthesia Equipment*, 2nd ed. Baltimore, Williams & Wilkins, 1984. With permission.

positioned connectors (in spiral tubes) may cause the inflating tube to adhere to itself. If the inflating tube cannot be cut below the obstruction, one viable solution is to pull the endotracheal cuff close to the vocal cords and puncture it with a needle introduced through the cricothyroid membrane.[159,160] Another solution is to relax the vocal cords (succinylcholine) enough to accept the passage of the inflated cuff without trauma.

Cases have been reported when the inflating tube of nasotracheal cuffed tubes have become entangled around a nasogastric tube or a turbinate, rendering the extubation extremely difficult.

SPECIAL CUFFS

1. *Self-inflating cuffs:* Self-inflating cuffs,[161] also called parachute cuffs,[162] do not have an inflating tube. The tube distends automatically during the inspiratory phase of positive-pressure ventilation through holes cut in the endotracheal tube beneath the cuff, thus preventing undue pressure on the tracheal wall. This cuff does not protect the airway from aspiration of foreign material during expiration or spontaneous ventilation. Furthermore, the holes in the endotracheal tube may become blocked by mucus, secretions, blood, or plugs.

2. *Foam cuffs:* Kamen[163] described a low-pressure polyurethane foam cuff enclosed in a tight latex sheath covering. When a negative pressure (suction) is applied to the inflating tube, the cuff collapses so that it passes through the glottis. Releasing the negative pressure and opening the inflating tube to the atmosphere allows the cuff to inflate and make contact with the tracheal wall. Intracuff pressure is zero and lateral tracheal wall pressure is 15 mm Hg. There are no leaks during positive-pressure ventilation until the peak pressure exceeds 30 cm H$_2$O.

3. *Retroepiglottic cuff:* Grimm[110] described a large extratracheal cuff to be placed in the retroepiglottic space above the larynx, which provided adequate protection from aspiration. The retroepiglottic space in the hypopharynx is bounded by the anterior surface of the epiglottic base of the tongue and the lateral segments of the pharyngeal wall. It is approximately the size of a golf ball and, presumably, it serves as a reservoir for the food bolus just prior to swallowing. It accommodates a cuff of large dimensions, providing a contact area with the mucosa of about 15 cm^2. This large cuff, when inflated, provided a no-leak seal at intracuff pressures much lower than the endotracheal cuffs, probably aided by the surfactant in the pharyngeal wall.[164] It seems that the role of surface tension in relation to endotracheal cuff seals or pressures has not been appreciated in recent evaluations. Tracheal complications could be eliminated by transferring the cuff to the preglottic area.

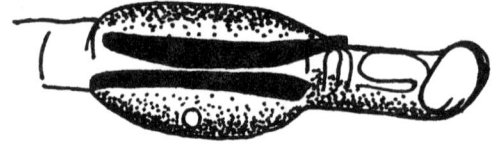

FIG. 19–29. Reduction of tube lumen by cuff. Inflation of the cuff caused narrowing of the tube lumen which persisted after the cuff was deflated (Ketover).
References:
Ketover and Feingold: Anesthesiology 48:108, 1975.
Courtesy Dorsch, J.A., and Dorsch, S.E.: *Understanding Anesthesia Equipment*, 2nd ed. Baltimore, Williams & Wilkins, 1984. With permission.

PERFORMANCE SPECIFICATIONS FOR ENDOTRACHEAL CUFFS. Performance specifications for endotracheal cuffs have been recommended by a group of investigators, inventors, and manufacturers to provide safe function and to minimize misuse of cuffs and tube-cuff units.[121] These criteria are as follows:

- **Performance Criteria for Cuffs**
    Complete protection from aspiration
    No-leak ventilation
    Noninjurious pressure to the ciliated tracheal mucosa
    Chemically nonirritating
    Signalling features to indicate underinflation or overinflation of cuff
    Automatic features to limit pressure on mucosa
    Ruggedness and reliability in function despite untrained users

Ease and reliability in measuring tracheal mucosal pressure

Ease of adjustment of tracheal mucosal pressure to the minimum that will prevent aspiration in the individual patient (test with Evans blue instilled above cuff—suction below)

Cuff must gently conform to but not distort tracheal anatomy

Progressive tracheal dilatation should be avoided or minimized

Cuff should not lose or gain resting internal pressure and volume in clinical use

- **Performance Criteria for Cuff-Tube Unit**

    Structurally joined to eliminate any unplanned separation of components; cuff, tube, pilot tube, and 15-mm taper

    Pilot balloon must not act as flap valve restricting removal of air from cuff

    Cuff must not act as flap valve restricting exit of air

    Simple, reliable, low resistance, nonleaking two-way air valve or stopcock

    Pilot balloon, valve and associated devices must not produce injury if dragged across patient's eyes and face

    Positive securement of tube in nose or mouth even in edentulous patients

    Optional provision of capability for speaking while on tracheostomy unit

    Tube not occlusive by teeth clenching; teeth should be cushioned by the tube or a securing unit

    Immediate simple signal of air flow blockage, as by cessation of breath-fogging of transparent tube or connector

    Tube not occlusive by devices that secure tube to mouth or nose

    Ease of insertion under emergency conditions

    Protection of tracheal structures from torsion

    Minimal length of effective external lever arms

    Provision for dual swivel

    Simple effective locks for 15-mm taper fittings

    Position of cuff in trachea should be adjustable to avoid exacerbating tracheal dilatation or mucosal damage caused by previous devices

    The unit should be packed sterile and should be resterilizable without alteration of original performance characteristics or tissue toxicity

    The placement and characteristics of the cuff must preclude the possibility of herniating the cuff over the distal end of the tube

    Simplicity of design for complexity of function

ADJUNCTIVE EQUIPMENT

CONNECTORS AND ADAPTERS

TERMINOLOGY. Any fitting that connects directly to an endotracheal tube is called an *endotracheal tube connector*.[165] According to ANSI standards, the size of the connector is identified by the nominal size (OD in millimeters) of the machine end of the fitting, which connects with components of the breathing circuits. All other fittings are called *adapters* with appropriate descriptive terms. In addition, the end of any component part nearest the patient is called the *patient end*, and the end nearest the machine is called the *machine end*. This terminology eliminates the confusing terms distal and proximal.

METHODS OF CONNECTION. After endotracheal intubation, the patient may be connected to the anesthesia apparatus in one of two ways:

1. By connecting the anesthesia apparatus directly to the endotracheal tube or breathing system
2. By placing the mask over the tube and face. This is not usually done, but may be used as a temporary stop gap until appropriate conditions and equipment are present.

Connectors

A wide variety of connectors is available. The simplest arrangement with the fewest pieces is the best assembly.

A connector to be fitted into the machine end of the endotracheal tube is a slip joint. This is the nontapered male end or patient end and is available in a range of sizes for all bore sizes of endotracheal tubes. The machine end is also a male connector and is designated as the normal 15-mm connector and is the common size for all tubes. The outer surface is tapered. This slip joint is available both straight and curved; the straight is the customarily used type. The appropriately sized connectors should be fitted snugly into the tracheal tube up to the knurl. Ideally, the slip joint should rest between the teeth. A tube that protrudes any distance greater than 3 to 4 cm out of the mouth of an adult is subject to kinking and displacement.

Straight connectors should be used for infants and children, at least to age 6 years.

SPECIFICATIONS FOR CONNECTORS. Many forms have been devised and are usually of plastic or metal. These are designed to connect the endotracheal tube to the inhalation system or other anesthesia machine component. In the ANSI Standards program, the machine end of the connector has been specified to be a nominal 15-mm size connection (Internal Diameter). Thus, the 11-mm connector, or Adams connector, is nonstandard.

Among the connectors classified and designated are the following:

1. *Straight endotracheal tube connector* (nominal 15 mm/0.609 in): The length of the patient end is approximately 17.5 mm, plus the internal *radius* in mm (Fig. 19–30).

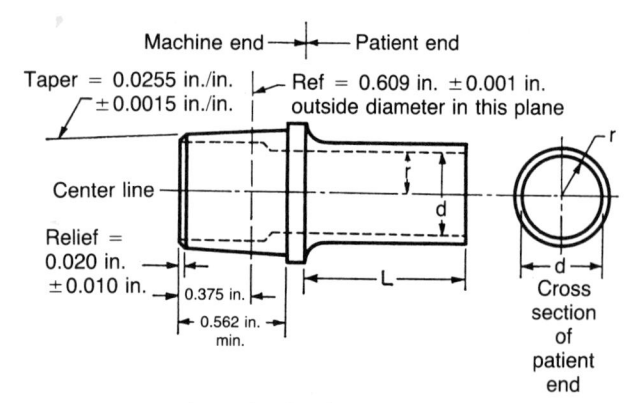

FIG. 19–30. Endotracheal-tube straight connector (nominal 15 mm/0.609 in). REF = gaging reference point; L = length of patient end = (17.5 mm + r) ± 1.5 mm; r = internal radius, patient end; d = internal diameter, patient end. American Standard Specification Z–79.2-1961. Courtesy of the American Standards Association.

Synonyms: slip joint; Adams Connector (11 mm).

2. *Right-angle curved endotracheal tube connector* (nominal 15 mm/0.609 in): An included angle of 90 degrees and straight portion having a length of 8 mm, plus the ID (Fig. 19–31).
Synonyms: Rovenstine elbow, Magill elbow (both ends the same).

3. *Acute-angle curved endotracheal tube connector* (nominal 15 mm/0.609 in): An included angle of 60 degrees. The straight portion shall have a length of 8 mm plus the ID (Fig. 19–32).
Synonyms: obtuse elbow; elbow with suction nipple.

Most items are available in all sizes as far as the male end or patient end that goes into the tube is concerned. Indeed, the ID in millimeters has been accepted as the method for designating and identifying a connector.

The sizes graduate in a series by 0.5-mm increments up to and including the 3.0 mm unit *and in 1.0-mm increments* above 3.0 mm. Such sizes are intended to permit ready insertion of the connection into its like-numbered endotracheal tube to provide secure engagement.

Although a mask may be adapted to the patient's face after intubation and special masks are available for such (Arrowood Mask), and anesthesia continued, it is preferable to provide a direct connection.

Adapters

A wide variety of adapters are available for many purposes (Fig. 19–33). An adapter may be defined as any fitting that joins an endotracheal tube connector to a valve, a circuit water condensor, or a breathing circuit system; a mask to a Y piece; or one component to another component. The unit is designated as *adapter* with the appropriate descriptive term.

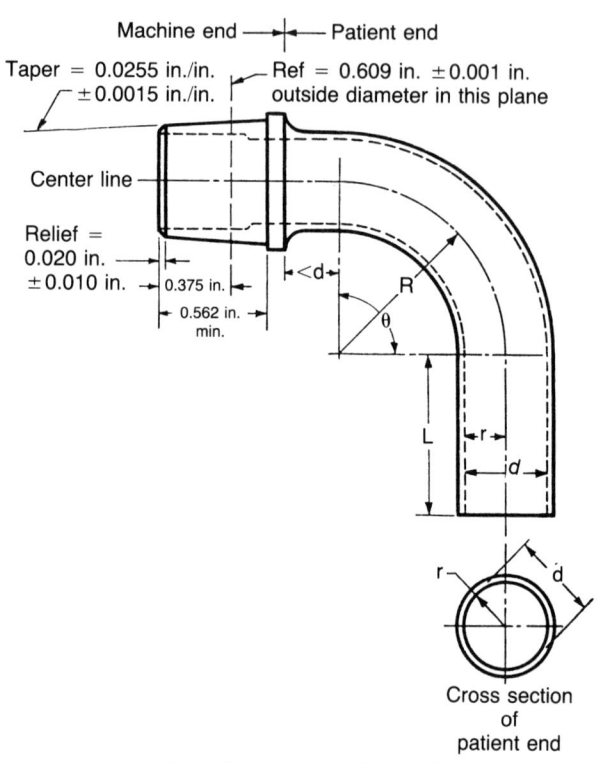

FIG. 19–31. Endotracheal tube right-angle curved connector (nominal 15 mm/0.609 in). REF = gaging reference point; R = radius of center line of curve; θ = included angle = 90.0 ± 5.0 degrees; L = length of patient end, straight portion = (8.0 mm + d) ± 1.5 mm; r = internal radius, patient end; d = internal diameter, patient end. American Standard Specification Z–79.2-1961. Courtesy of the American Standard Association.

Although a necessity in an endotracheal anesthesia system, the connectors nevertheless represent added resistance and increased dead space. The extent of resistance and dead space should be minimized as follows:

1. A straight-type connector should be used if possible because resistance is minimal.
2. The largest connector possible should be inserted into the exposed end of the endotracheal tube. If the tube is made to bulge slightly it is probable that the connector's internal surface will be closely in line with that of the tube.
3. There is a marked difference in many connectors between the ID and ED. The important feature is the ID. The difference is due to construction material and the thickness of the wall. Strong material will allow thin-walled items.
4. The ideal angled connector should have smoothly rounded inner and outer bends to form a 90-degree arc. The bend should have a radius 6 to 7 times that of the straight section of connector to diminish resistance and reduce turbulence.

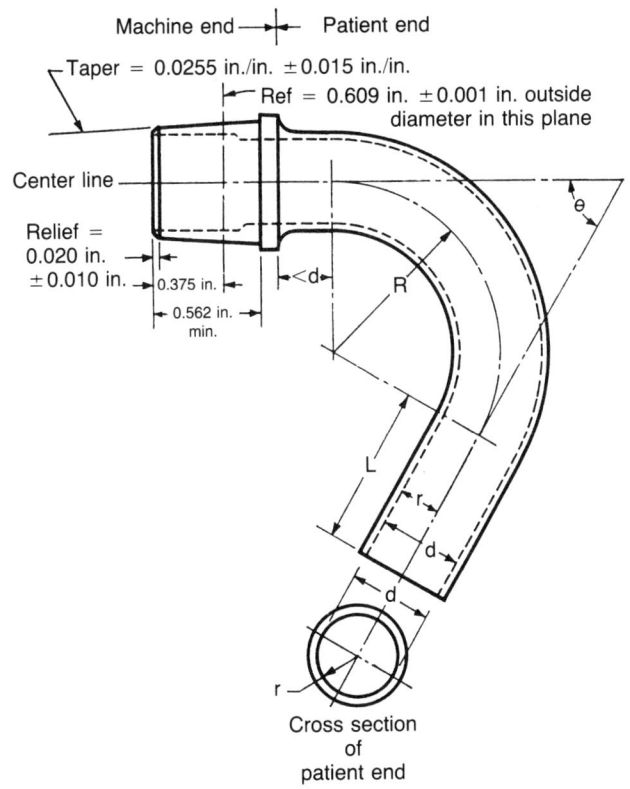

FIG. 19-32. Endotracheal-tube connector acute-angle curved (nominal 15 mm/0.609 in). REF = gaging reference point; R = radius of center line of curve; θ = included angle = 60.0 ± 5.0 degrees; L = length of patient end, straight portion = (8.0 mm + d) ± 1.5 mm; r = internal radius, patient end; d = internal diameter, patient end. American Standard Specification, Z-792-1961. Courtesy of the American Standard Association.

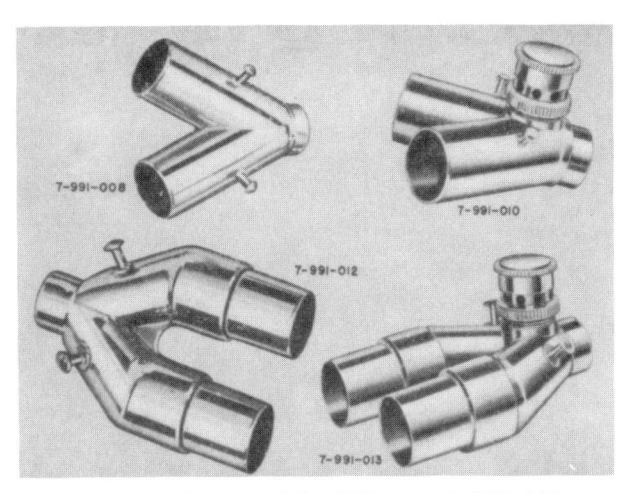

FIG. 19-33. Adapters of the "Y" type. 7-991-008. Adapter Y piece for use with standard 15-mm male catheter connectors and elbow adapters. 7-991-012. Universal Adapter Y piece permits connection of 15-mm male adapters and connectors to breathing tubes. These type adapters are available in plastic and as disposable units.

Other Adjunctive Equipment

STYLETS (FIG. 19-34). Made of malleable metal or plastic, stylets are designed to improve the curvature and to stiffen a tracheal tube. They are placed within the lumen of the tube after lubrication, which facilitates introduction and withdrawal. The end of the stylet should not extend beyond the bevel of the tube.

1. Bishop-Grillo stylet—adjustable in length; precludes an airway; designed to fit endotracheal tubes securely until intubation is complete
2. Metal stylet—with or without suction tip
3. Knitting needles
4. Copper stylet—soft, malleable wire
5. Flexiguide[166]

Introduction of soft oral tubes and of sloppy anode tubes is facilitated by a stylet. More rigid plastic tubes may be curved at the patient end by a J shaping of the stylet so as to provide an anterior direction under the epiglottis when visualization of the larynx is difficult or when anatomy is distorted.[166]

The Flexiguide[167] is a useful adjunct for both stiffening an endotracheal tube and as an introducer or guide through the vocal cords into the trachea, over which the tracheal tube is passed. The assembly is composed of a handle, thumb ring, notched inner rod, and outer tube. The ring can be manipulated and enables the operator to maneuver the flexible 5 in of the distal tip as needed in an AP plane. If the tip is inserted the length of the selected endotracheal tube and 2 in beyond, it can be introduced during laryngoscopy through the vocal cords and into the trachea to form a guide to the advancement of the endotracheal tube. This type stylet must also be lubricated.

MOUTH PROPS (FIG. 19-35). The purpose of these devices is to separate and maintain the teeth apart; to protect the teeth and to prevent closure of mouth and biting the tube. Several types are available, including metal gags or composition blocks. The following are examples:

1. Bite blocks
   a. Rolled gauze
   b. Rubber spool
   c. DeFord rubber mouth prop
   d. Bakelite wedge
   e. The oral dental screw
2. Mouth gags—Denhardt; Davis
3. Plastic dental protectors

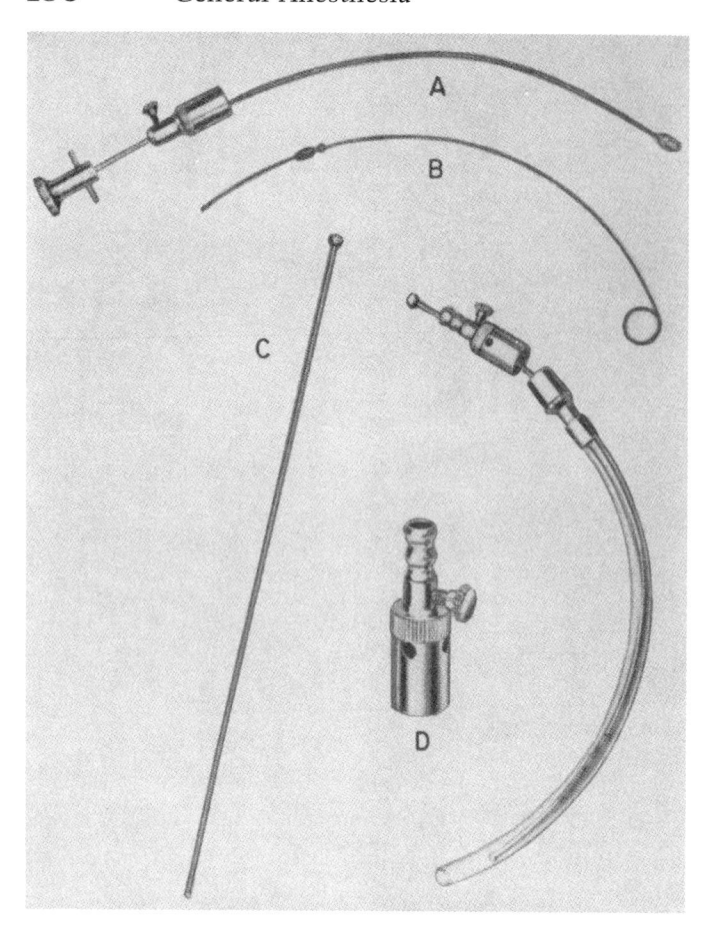

FIG. 19–34. Types of stylets. *A*, Bishop-Grillo stylet: flexible stainless steel with adjustable catheter stop. *B*, Foregger infant stylet with adjustable stop. *C*, Copper wire stylet. *D*, Guiffrede catheter stop, free and in position.

An oropharyngeal airway is frequently placed beside the endotracheal tube; however, this presents the hazard of the tip impinging on the endotracheal tube in the pharynx and compressing the tube.

TOOTH PROTECTORS. Dental trauma is a frequent complication associated with laryngoscopy and endotracheal intubation and is also the most frequent anesthesia-related cause of litigation. Damage to teeth is caused by direct pressure of the laryngoscope against the teeth when laryngoscopy is performed with levering or prying instead of a lifting maneuver. Because the flange of the widely used laryngoscopic blades is located on the left side, it is evident that the left central incisor of the maxilla is most frequently involved. Dental trauma also occurs during the recovery period when patients may bite on an oropharyngeal airway or an endotracheal tube; patients may grind their teeth while in a semiconscious state and inadvertently cause damage.

Certain clinical factors predispose to dental trauma: mandibulofacial abnormalities; conditions recognized as a cause of difficult intubation (obesity; robust, muscular and short-necked patients; cervical vertebral abnormalities; burns); and intubation for emergencies. These present technical difficulties the risk of which is greatly increased with the presence of the following:[168] carious or loose teeth; injury; malnutrition; periodontal disease; fixed dentures; presence of crowns and restorations; vulnerability in the very young and the elderly; vulnerability of gums to trauma in the edentulous patient; and oral disease that weakens support of teeth.

For elective surgery in the presence of extensive dental disease, dental consultation and dental hygienic repair should be instituted. To prevent or minimize dental trauma or to protect the gums, various devices to protect the teeth and gums have been proposed. These include the following:[169]

1. Simple pads of adhesive tape molded over the upper central incisors
2. An adhesive bandage composed of gelatin, pectin, methylcellulose, and polyisobutylene. This is supplied in a thin wafer molded over the teeth[169]
3. Mouth guards—rubber or plastic; plastic moulding compound molded to fit

Procedure After Injury

- Write a note in the patient's medical record
- Attempt to retrieve a dislodged loose tooth
- Radiologic examination is needed if a tooth is lost
- Inform the patient or family
- Preserve a loose tooth in saline
- Preanesthesia, inform the patient of increased risk of injury when vulnerable conditions exist

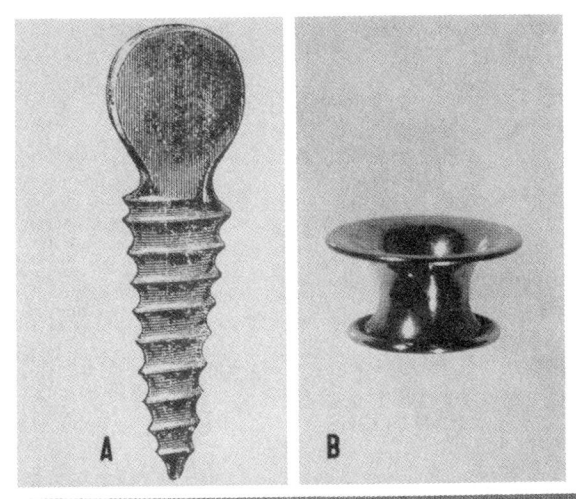

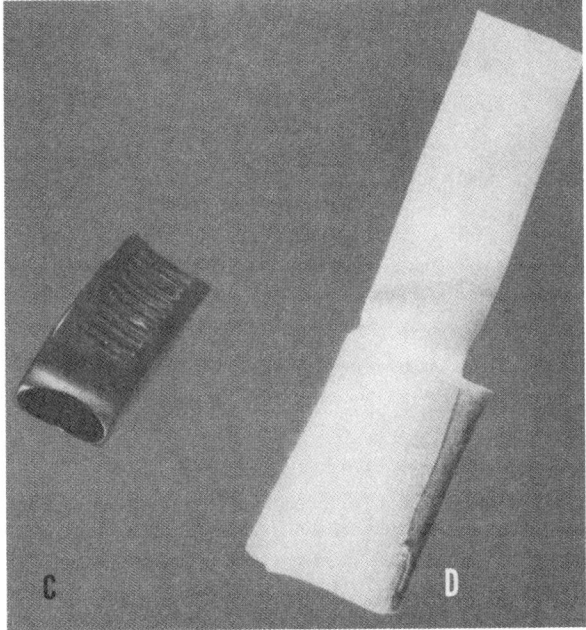

FIG. 19–35. Types of bite blocks. *A*, Plain oral screw. *B*, Bakelite spool. *C*, Jackson wedge. *D*, gauze roll–adhesive covering.

Disadvantages. The hampering effect of protectors on the performance of intubation has been studied. Aromaa[170] found that prototypes of commonly used protectors do not guarantee against dental damage. Furthermore, visualization of the oropharyngeal and laryngeal structures is limited and is a problem in 15% of the procedures. There is decreased space in the oral cavity for manipulations, and in emergencies (rapid-sequence maneuver), time is lost in providing a protector.

Conclusion. When dental problems are identified at the time of preanesthetic assessment, it is prudent to have a dental consultation or to inform the patient of a clear risk of dislodgement of a tooth. Of great importance is the fact that with correct training followed by practice and experience, the frequency of dental trauma is minimal and is much less than 1%.

INTUBATING FORCEPS (FIG. 19–36).[171] The purpose of such forceps is as follows:

1. To guide the endotracheal tube into the glottis (particularly nasal tubes that have been advanced into the pharynx)
2. To guide Levine tubes into the esophagus
3. To insert pharyngeal packing

Two types of forceps have been designed and are in common use, namely the Magill (military) forceps and the Rovenstine modification. Lundy and Trovell have attached a laryngoscope light to the blade of the forceps to aid in lighting the pharynx.

SUCTION CATHETERS. Small catheters of various types may be used for the special purpose of "tracheal toilet" (Table 19–9). Such cleaning may be required during surgery or following anesthesia. It is especially necessary when secretions are excessive or when infections produce the "wet lung" picture.

Among the catheters available are the following:

1. Standard urethral rubber catheters: Sizes 14 to 16 for adults and sizes 10 to 12 to 14 for children
2. Whistle-tip catheters; large lumen desirable
3. Silk woven catheters
4. Urethral catheters for children
5. Plastic catheters

These catheters may be joined to the main suction tubing by a glass adapter or a plastic-tapered Vitax connector.

LUBRICANTS.[172] An ointment containing a topical anesthetic is preferred and should be applied in a thin coat. It remains on the tube for many hours, and most of the lubricant can be recovered. Approximately 0.5 ml of ointment will adequately lubricate endotracheal tubes in sizes 30 to 38 French. After 2 hours in situ, the amount of ointment recovered, when the tubes are removed, is approximately 0.33 ml. Thus, less than 0.25 ml is lost. It is estimated that 60 to 100 ml of oil is needed to produce a pneumonia. The possibility of developing oil pneumonia is so remote that it should not be considered.

The topical anesthetic is desirable and diminishes cord activity and, hence, glottic trauma; there are no reports of reactions to the topical agent used in this manner. Water-soluble jellies are useful for nasal intubation in addition to the coat of ointment. The water-soluble lubricants tend to dry out and become gritty; they may cause adherence of mucosa to the endotracheal tube.[173]

Loeser's studies[172,174] of the incidence of sore throat as related to lubricants and cuff design have revealed high incidence and severity of sore throat

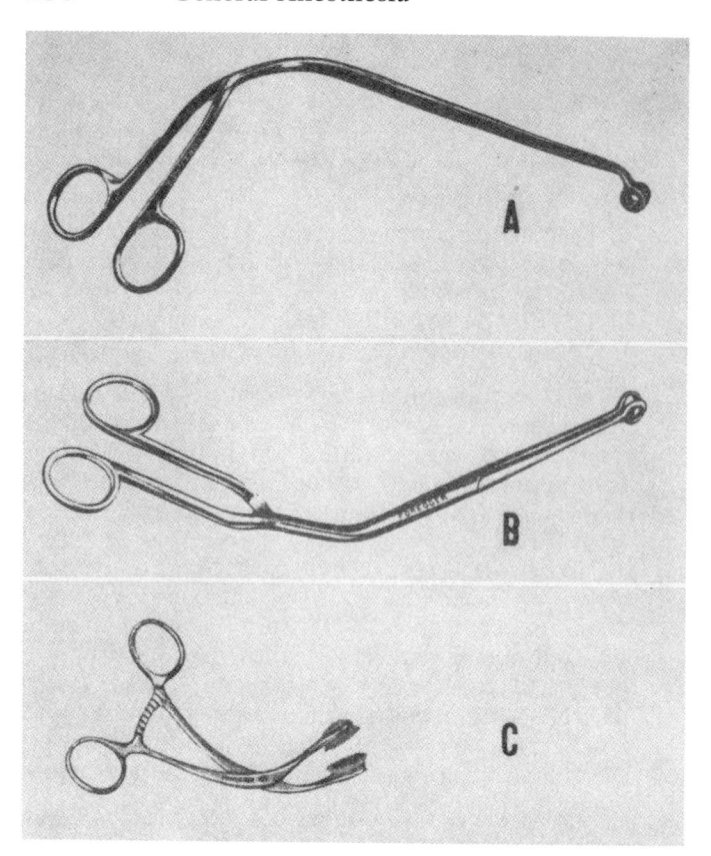

FIG. 19–36. Forceps for use in endotracheal intubation. *A*, A modification by Rovenstine of the Magill forceps to be used with all types of catheters as well as Magill tubes. *B*, Magill, military. *C*, Tongue forceps with rubber cushion.

when 4% lidocaine jelly is used. A lower incidence—about 40%—was found with the lidocaine–saline solution or saline wetting of the tube alone. Large-volume cuffs without lubricant were associated with an incidence of 46% sore throat, whereas the use of low-volume cuffs without lubricant (sterile water wash) resulted in an incidence of 15% sore throat.

In a follow-up study (Table 19–10), Surgilube (water-soluble jelly) was associated with an incidence of sore throat of 16% to 30%, depending on the type of cuff design. In the same study, 5% lidocaine jelly was associated with sore throat in 24% to 58% of patients.

SECURING ENDOTRACHEAL TUBES WITH TAPES. Securing endotracheal tubes in proper position is of extreme importance in the endotracheal technique. It is usually accomplished by looping an adhesive tape about the endotracheal tube and then fixing the tape to the patient's face. Five different types of fixation tapes are commonly used:

1. Silk surgical adhesive tape (nonallergenic)
2. Plastic waterproof adhesive tape
3. Dermiclear (transparent tape—Johnson & Johnson)
4. Curity (cloth adhesive tape—Kendall)
5. Micropore surgical tape

TABLE 19–9. BASIC DIMENSIONS OF SUCTION CATHETERS

Outside diameter			Minimum effective length (L)		
mm	Tolerance	Nearest Charrière size* equivalent	Short (mm)	Medium (mm)	Long (mm)
1.5	±0.15	5	250	350	500
2.0	±0.15	6	250	350	500
2.5	±0.25	8	250	350	500
3.0	±0.25	9	250	350	500
4.0	±0.25	12	250	350	500
5.0	±0.25	15	250	350	500
6.0	±0.25	18	250	350	500

* Refers to nearest Charrière gauge equivalent.
From Rosen, M., and Hilliard, E.K.: The use of suction in clinical medicine. Br. J. Anaesth., 32:486, 1960.

TABLE 19-10. INCIDENCE (%) AND SEVERITY (MEAN ± SD) OF POSTOPERATIVE SORE THROAT IN 600 PATIENTS (50 PATIENTS IN EACH GROUP) FOLLOWING ENDOTRACHEAL INTUBATION

Cuff* Tracheal Contact Length (mm)	Cuff	Incidence (%) and Severity (0–3)		
		None	Surgilube	5% Lidocaine
20 ± 1.0	Double Contour	12%	16%	24%
		0.12 ± 0.33	0.20 ± 0.50	0.32 ± 0.65
29 ± 1.4	Lo Pro	30%	20%	30%
		0.32 ± 0.51	0.30 ± 0.68	0.30 ± 0.46
29 ± 1.4	Taper	26%	30%	38%
		0.30 ± 0.58	0.34 ± 0.56	0.36 ± 0.60
37 ± 2.5	Hilo	26%	30%	58%
		0.30 ± 0.54	0.36 ± 0.60	0.74 ± 0.80†

* Measurements obtained from five cuffs of each of the endotracheal tubes studied.
† $P < 0.05$, Bonferroni test when compared with all other groups.
From Loeser, E.A., et al.: The influence of endotracheal tube cuff design and cuff lubrication on postoperative sore throat. Anesthesiology, 58:376, 1983.

The adhesive bond of these tapes to different types of endotracheal tubes has been studied by Fenje[175] and Steward.[176] Silk tape provides best adherence to most type tubes and shows the greatest strength in resisting separation. Plastic waterproof adhesive tape was found to be the next most adherent, especially to the Portex Blue endotracheal tube. Other tapes, such as the Dermiclear, cloth, and micropore have poor adhesive quality.

Tube material influences the strength of bonding. Silk tape adheres strongly to clear tubes, Portex or NCC* but has limited strength to resist separation when applied to Portex Blue tubes.

Silicone material or silicone rubber reinforced tubes limits the ability of most tapes to adhere to the tube. Silk appears to have some utility. An alternative technique to provide a bonding surface to the reinforced spiral tubes, however, is to wrap the endotracheal tube with "operative site" surgical covers over the area to which tape is applied.

Treatment of the silicone tubes first with tincture of benzoin or skin-bond cement fails to provide a bonding surface. Tightly wrapping several loops of surgical silk around the reinforced tube to provide an adhesive surface[176] has not been satisfactory, and the silk tends to slip.

It is recommended that the silk-type surgical adhesive tape be used. Once the tape material is secured to the endotracheal tube, it is then applied to the patient's face (or forehead). The tape should be nonallergenic. Pretreatment of the facial skin to provide an adhering surface should be done with extreme care. A diluted tincture of benzoin may be used.

PRINCIPLE OF PROPER TRACHEAL PLACEMENT. The safe (anatomically neutral) position for the tip of an endotracheal tube when inserted should be in the midtrachea. This will avoid either bronchial intubation or inadvertent tracheal extubation. The tip of the tube should be a safe distance above the carina and a sufficient distance below the vocal cords.

Clinical confirmation of a tracheal position is determined by auscultation of both lung fields anteriorly over the superior lobe or the upper lobe in the subclavicular area and in the midaxillary region of infants. While ventilating the patient, breath sounds should be heard and thoracic cage movements observed bilaterally. Pulmonary compliance should be easy. Auscultation over the epigastrium should not reveal gurgling sounds. Capnography is desirable.

After securing the endotracheal tube, it is important to maintain the head in an anatomically neutral position. Neck flexion causes the tip of an endotracheal tube to move caudad further into the trachea, whereas neck extension results in an upward movement.[177]

Bloch[178] has proposed that, in children, after a tracheal position has been determined that the tube should be advanced until it passes the carina and enters the mainstream bronchus. When normal clinical observations will return, auscultation of the chest will reveal breath sounds only on one side and absence on the opposite side, usually the left. Unilateral decrease in thoracic cage movements and decreased compliance will be appreciated. The tube should then be withdrawn about 2 cm.

SUCTION CATHETERS—RATIONAL USE.[179] Standards for suction catheters used for clearing the tracheobronchial tree through endotracheal tracheostomy tubes have been developed by the International Standards Committee (Org. TC 121 Subcommittee).[180] First, the sizes of the suction catheters are designated by the outside diameter (OD) expressed in millimeters. In addition, the lengths of the catheters are classed as short, medium, or long. The size of a catheter is thus expressed as the OD in mm (or Charrière size; French gauge), and the usual length as 500 mm.

* National Catheter Company. Division of Mallinckrodt, Inc.

TABLE 19–11. BASIC DIMENSIONS OF SUCTION CATHETERS

Outside diameter			Minimum effective length		
mm	Tolerance	Nearest Charrière size* equivalent	Short (mm)	Medium (mm)	Long (mm)
1.5	±0.15	5	250	350	500
2.0	±0.15	6	250	350	500
2.5	±0.25	8	250	350	500
3.0	±0.25	9	250	350	500
4.0	±0.25	12	250	350	500
5.0	±0.25	15	250	350	500
6.0	±0.25	18	250	350	500

* Nearest Charrière gauge equivalent.
From Rosen, M., and Hilliard, E.K.: The use of suction of clinical medicine. Br. J. Anaesth., 32:486, 1960.

The basic dimensions of suction catheters have been tabulated in terms of both the OD and the minimum effective length (Table 19–11). The more common expression for the size of a catheter is that of the French gauge or Charrière size.

The French catheter gauge, or the Charrière system, is related to the OD; and not related to the outside circumference of a catheter. Thus, the French gauge system is a simple multiple of the OD, i.e., it is three times the OD (or the nearest whole number equivalent). For example, if the OD is 3 mm, the French gauge is #9 French or #9 Charrière. Likewise, a 6-mm OD catheter is an 18-French gauge type catheter. Conversely, 1 Charrière (or French gauge) unit equals 0.33 mm.

The size of the catheter used should not occupy more than half of the ID of the endotracheal or tracheostomy tube (Table 19–12). When a larger catheter whose OD size is greater than one-half the ID of an endotracheal tube (sizes designated by ID measurement) is inserted into a given endotracheal tube, physiologic disturbances are caused by the application of suction force to the tracheobronchial tree, and this may be dangerously accentuated.[179a] Hypoxia is a frequent complication during endotracheal suctioning. Graff recommends the use of a catheter that provides alternately suctioning and oxygen[179b] (Neo-cath, Pulmonary Medical Devices, Atlanta, Ga.).

PEDIATRIC CONSIDERATIONS FOR ENDOTRACHEAL ANESTHESIA

Infants and young children differ anatomically, physiologically, and pharmacologically from adults.[181] A better understanding of pediatric anesthesia-related problems has resulted in reduced morbidity and mortality.

Anesthesia-related mortality in children 1 to 10 years of age at Boston Children's Hospital between 1959 and 1966 was about 1/5,000 and between 1968 and 1978 about 1/14,000.[182,183]

Most deaths occur in the neonatal period and are related to airway complications. Most anesthetic deaths are preventable.

To provide safe anesthetic care, it is necessary that certain anatomic and physiologic differences between children and adults be recognized. These should be reviewed in depth in pediatric texts and in texts on pediatric anesthesia.[184,185]

COMMENTS. Some general features are noted. The weight of the average full-term normal newborn is 3 kg. The birth weight doubles at 3 months and triples at 1 year (10 kg). Beyond that, weight increases 2 kg/year until age 6.

Infants have a larger body surface area (BSA). The neonate is 1/25th the weight of an adult, but BSA is 1/9th that of an adult. The head is large, the neck is short, and the chin recedes.

Neonates are obligate nasal breathers. The epiglottis is positioned higher in the pharynx and contacts the soft palate, making oral breathing difficult. The high position of the epiglottis helps create two separate channels, one for breathing and one for swallowing.

The lungs are underdeveloped; they continue to develop after birth. The number of alveoli continues to increase to 6 years of age, at which time the number is approximately that of the adult. Expansion of individual alveoli continues, however, functional development continues until the age of 18 years.

ANATOMY OF THE LARYNX.[186] Anatomically, the infant larynx differs from the adult in several important respects. It is situated more cephalad than in the adult and during development comes to occupy a position lower in the neck (Fig. 19–36). At birth, the lower border of the cricoid cartilage is opposite the upper border of C4, while at 6 years it is at C5; at about 13 years of age the cricoid cartilage comes to occupy the adult position or the level of C7. The rima glottis, is one or two vertebrae higher. Thus, in the newborn child it is opposite C3 and C4 and

TABLE 19-12. SELECTION OF SUCTION CATHETER ACCORDING TO SIZE OF ENDOTRACHEAL TUBE

Age or weight	Endotracheal tube size			Suction catheter (French)
	Internal diameter (mm)	External diameter (French)	Length (cm)	
Under 1500 g	2.5 uncuffed	12	8	4
Newborn-6 mo	3.0 uncuffed	14	10	4
6-18 mo	3.5 uncuffed	16	12	6
18 mo-3 yr	4.0 uncuffed	18	14	6
3-5 yr	4.5 uncuffed	20	16	8
5-6 yr	5.0 uncuffed	22	16	8
6-8 yr	5.5 cuffed	24	18	10
8-10 yr	6.0 cuffed	26	18	10
10-12 yr	6.5 cuffed	28	20	12
12-14 yr	6.5 cuffed	28	20	12
14-16 yr	♂ 7.0 cuffed	30	22	12
	♀ 6.5 cuffed	28		
16-21 yr	♂ 7.5 cuffed	32	22	12
	♀ 7.0 cuffed	30		

NOTE: Endotracheal tube should fit so as to allow full expansion of both lungs on manual inflation but allow a definite leak with pressure of 20 to 25 cm H_2O.

The appropriate suction catheter in the OD or French scale is smaller than the ID of the endotracheal tube by approximately one third.

From Rosen, M., Hilliard, E.K.: Use of suction in clinical medicine. Br. J. Anaesth., 32:486, 1960.

occupies the adult level opposite C5 after the age of 13 years.

Comparison of the anatomic structures of the larynx in the adult and infant show the differences listed (Fig. 19-37). The epiglottis is relatively longer, stiffer and "U"- (omega) or "V"-shaped, in contrast to the flexible flat structure in the adult. Because the hyoid bone in the infant is intimately attached to the thyroid cartilage, the adjacent base of the tongue tends to depress the epiglottis, causing it to protrude further into the pharyngeal cavity. The epiglottis thus makes a 45-degree angle from the anterior wall, while in the adult it is more erect because of separation of the thyroid and hyoid cartilages.

The cricoid cartilage is a complete ring, and in the infant is the narrowest point in the upper respiratory tract. It is the only nonexpansile structure in the upper airway. Because the posterior plate-like portion (lamina or signet) is inclined posteriorly at its superior aspect, the larynx becomes funnel shaped. Thus, the lower border or ring portion of the cricoid may be smaller than the rima glottis or the internal diameter of the trachea.

The arytenoid cartilage presents some interesting details in the infant of importance in endoscopy. The vocal process of this cartilage represents about half of the vocal cord length, while in the adult it may be only one fourth. The remaining portion is ligamentous. Further, the vocal process inclines downward into the trachea so that the vocal cord is concave. Because the cartilaginous part is relatively rigid the rima glottis may be limited in size.

The mucous membrane is composed of both squamous and ciliated columnar epithelium; the squamous epithelium lines the supraglottic portion of the larynx down to and including the vocal cords and is tightly bound down by fibrous tissue. Columnar epithelium lines the entire cavity of the larynx below the rima glottis. (It is also found in the laryngeal ventricle and inferior parts of the vestibule.) Because it is loosely attached to submucous tissue, it is prone to become edematous and abraded.

POSITION OF LARYNX TOPOGRAPHICALLY IN INFANTS AND CHILDREN.[187] At birth, all upper airway structures are high in the neck. The tip of the epiglottis is at the level of the middle of C1; the hyoid at the level of C2-C3, and the glottis at C3 (Table 19-13). In the neonate, the tip of the epiglottis is able to contact the uvula and soft palate and makes the infant an obligate nasal breather; the infant is thus able to swallow and breath at the same time. After 6 months, this situation is no longer present in the human but is a persistent feature of all other primates.

An elegant study by Westhorpe shows that between birth and 3 years there is a marked descent of all airway structures in the neck (Fig. 19-38). By three years, the epiglottis is at the level of C3 and the hyoid cartilage at the disc between C3 and C4, while the glottis has descended to a level between C4-C5 (Fig. 19-39). A view of the glottis up to the age of 2 years also reveals that it is angled anteriorly, coupled with a downward slope of the arytenoids. The cords, therefore, have a concave appearance.

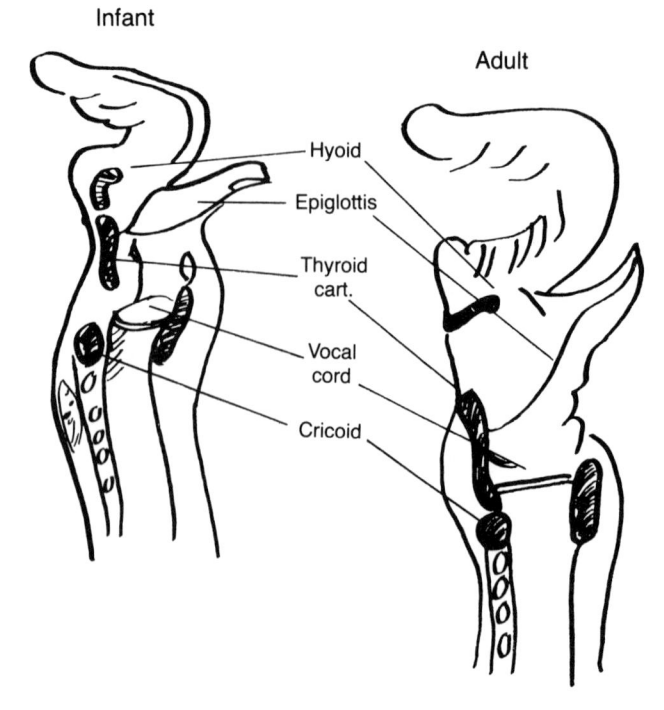

INFANT

Tongue—relatively larger
Larynx—more cephalad
Epiglottis—"U" shaped short, stiff, close to base of tongue and more horizontal
Hyoid and Thyroid—cartilages intimately close
Glottis—one-half is cartilaginous
Arytenoid—inclined inferiorly. Vocal cords concave
Cricoid—plate inclined posteriorly to form a funnel

ADULT

Tongue—relatively smaller
Larynx—more caudad
Epiglottis—flat, flexible and more erect

Hyoid and Thyroid—cartilages separated
Glottis—one-fourth is cartilaginous
Arytenoid—horizontal and cords horizontal
Cricoid—plate vertical

FIG. 19–37. Comparison of the infant and adult larynx. Adapted for Eckenhoff, J.E.: Some anatomic considerations of the infant larynx influencing endotracheal anesthesia. Anesthesiology, 12:407, 1951.

Laryngoscopic view of the larynx reveals that it is funnel shaped because of the narrow subglottic (cricoid) area. The adult larynx is cylindrical shaped (Fig. 19–40).

Lateral radiographs of the skulls and cervical spines of infants and children provide much information about the airway anatomy, which facilitates intubation. The topographic relation of the larynx to the cervical vertebrae will determine the intubation angle achieved by head positioning and by the technique of laryngoscopy (see Fig. 19–39).

In the neonate and the infant under 2 years of age, there are essentially no intervertebral joints above the level of the larynx that can be flexed. Hence, there is no advantage of visualization of the glottis by flexing the head on a pillow, as in the adult. In positioning the head, a "doughnut roll" can be placed under the occiput to keep the head from rolling.

In children 2 to 6 years of age, some increased angulation of the airway axes of 1 to 2 degrees can be achieved, with improved visualization of the glottis by placing the head on a low pillow (or folded sheet).

In children after 6 years of age and up to puberty, improved visualization can be achieved by flexing the head progressively. This is accomplished by increasing the height of the pillow up to the adult height of 2 to 3 inches.

AIRWAY DIFFERENCES IN THE NEWBORN. Differences between the newborn and older children or the adult are summarized as follows:

1. High position of larynx located in premature at mid-C3; in the infant at C3–C4; adult at C5–C6. Larynx when viewed is funnel shaped.
2. Tongue: Large in proportion to oral cavity and easily obstructs oral airway.
3. Shape of epiglottis: Stubby and V-shaped or omega-shaped. In adult, it is thin, flat, and floppy.
4. Angulation of vocal cords: Adult axis perpendic-

TABLE 19-13. LEVEL OF LARYNGEAL STRUCTURES IN RELATION TO CERVICAL VERTEBRAE (C) OR INTERVERTEBRAL DISCS

Age (yr)	Tip of epiglottis	Hyoid	Glottis	Cricoid (inferior margin)
0	mid C1	disc 2-3	mid C3	sup C4
6/12	mid C2	mid C3	disc 3-4	mid C4
1	disc 2-3	inf C3	mid C4	disc 4-5
2	mid C3	disc 3-4	mid C4	mid C5
3	mid C3	disc 3-4	disc 4-5	mid C5
4	mid C3	disc 3-4	disc 4-5	mid C5
6	mid C3	disc 3-4	disc 4-5	mid C5
8	mid C3	disc 3-4	disc 4-5	mid C5
10	inf C3	sup C4	disc 4-5	mid C5
Adult	inf C3	sup C4	mid C5	disc 6-7

From Westhorpe, R.N.: The position of the larynx in children and its relationship to the ease of intubation. Anaesth. Intensive Care, 15:384, 1987.

ular to axis of trachea; in infant and young child, posterior attachment of cords and higher trachea causes glottis to be angled downward, toward the trachea; after 8 to 10 years of age, angulation is that of adult, being perpendicular to trachea.

5. Epiglottis is more horizontal and angled backward in the infant; in contrast, the epiglottis in older children and adults is more erect and parallel to the axis of the trachea.

6. Cricoid cartilage and subglottic area is the narrowest point in the airway and is nonexpansive.

AIRWAY ASSESSMENT—INFANT. Several anatomic features of the newborn and infant differing from the adult must be considered in the management of the airway.[183,189]

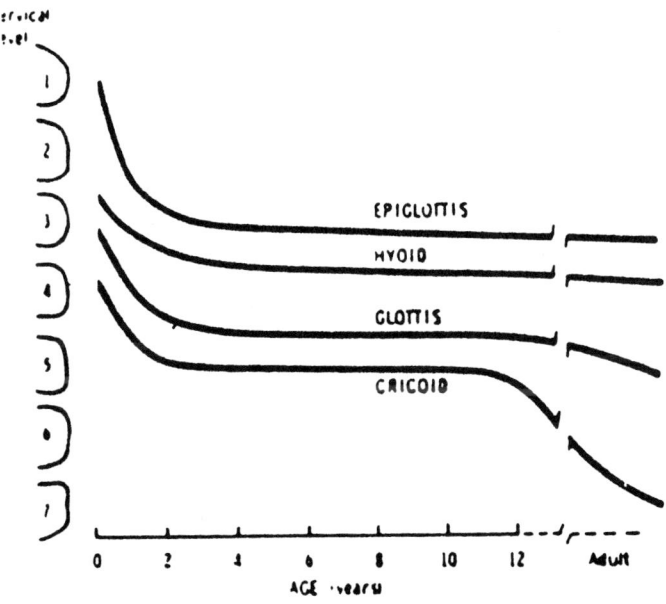

FIG. 19-38. The level of laryngeal structures at different ages, in relation to the cervical spine. From Westhorpe, R.N.: The position of the larynx in children and its relationship to the ease of intubation. Anaesth. Intensive Care, 15:384, 1987.

Skull. At birth, it is relatively enormous. There is no need for a pillow to place head in sniffing position. A small "doughnut," however, is necessary to stabilize the head.

Mouth. Small with weak muscles. The maxilla is short. The level of the upper gum is opposite C1.

Lips. These are large with the frenulum of the upper lip tight to the gums.

Teeth (Table 19–14). These are primary or deciduous, with different times of eruption and shedding.[188] Care is necessary to avoid trauma to the gums or to dislodge teeth. If a tooth is loose or inadvertently loosened, it should be removed to avoid swallowing or aspiration.

Tongue. The tongue is large. At rest, it fills the entire oral cavity and touches the soft palate. The airway may be occluded by the tongue pushing the palate to the posterior pharyngeal wall.

Palate. The hard palate is short, while the soft palate is long, thin, and delicate. The uvula tip (posterior edge) extends behind the tongue into the pharynx almost to the epiglottis, and may make contact with the epiglottis.

Mandible. A receding jaw is to be seen. It is horizontal without an ascending ramus. The glenoid fossa is shallow and lies in an AP plane to accommodate the mandible. With growth and the development of an ascending ramus, the glenoid fossa develops into a socket and shifts to a horizontal plane.

The mandible is easily displaced, being limited only by ligamentous suspension. It may shift behind the maxilla.

Maxilla and Facial Structure. Facial bones are in the process of rapid development. Suture lines have not become cemented, and displacement is easy.

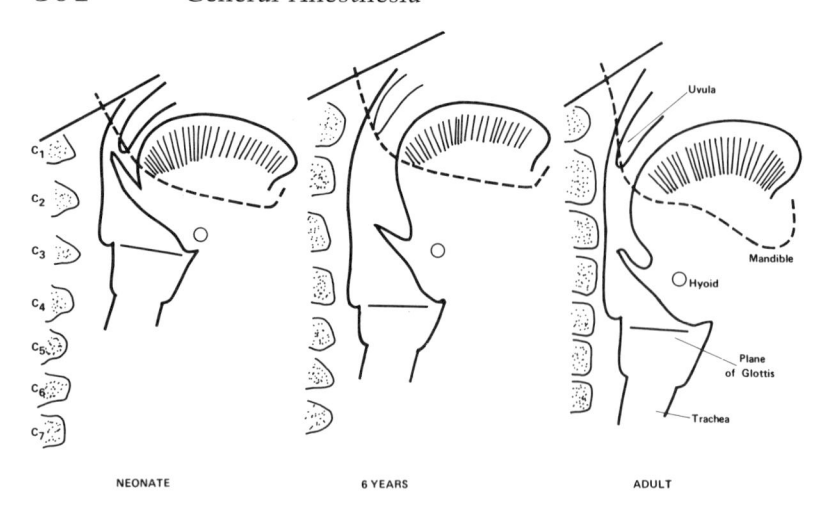

FIG. 19-39. Diagrammatic representation of relative positions of upper airway structures in the newborn, the 6-year-old child, and the adult. From Westhorpe, R.N.: The position of the larynx in children and its relationship to the ease of intubation. Anaesth. Intensive Care, *15*:384, 1987.

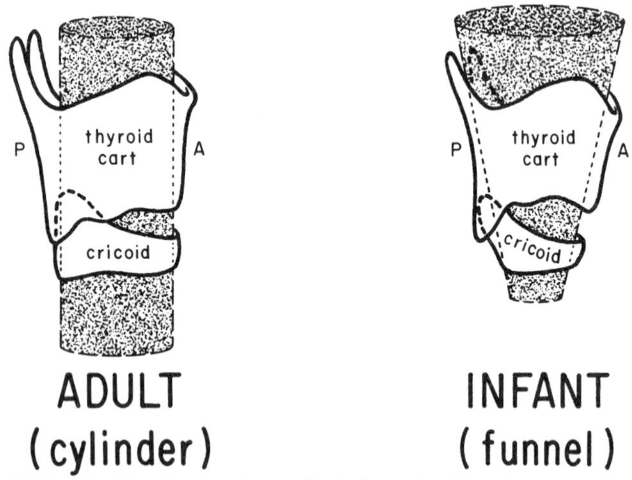

FIG. 19-40. Comparison of adult and infant larynx. The infant larynx is funnel-shaped, due to the narrow subglottic area (cricoid ring). By contrast, the adult larynx resembles a cylinder. From Coté, C., and Todres, I.D.: The Pediatric Airway. In *A Practice of Anesthesia for Infants and Children.* J.F. Ryan, I.D. Todres, C. Coté, N.G. Goudsouzian, eds. Grune and Stratton, 1988. Courtesy of Charles Coté. With permission.

INDICATIONS FOR ENDOTRACHEAL TECHNIQUE.[188,189] An endotracheal airway should be employed whenever it is expected that difficulty will be experienced in keeping the respiratory passages patent. The tube may be inserted either orally or nasally, depending on the circumstances of the operation. Nasotracheal intubation, however, is more difficult to perform in the infant than in children or adults, and this route should be avoided, if possible.

The indications for the use of an endotracheal tube in pediatric anesthesia may be considered under three headings: mandatory, preferable, or optional. The decision is based on the problems involved, the potential of the surgery interfering with anesthesia, and the control of airway and proper inspiration.

Generally, an endotracheal airway is mandatory for most surgical procedures: head and neck surgery, intracranial neurosurgery, oral-pharyngeal procedures, including tonsillectomy, oral-dental procedures, thoracic surgery, and abdominal surgery.

It is also mandatory for general anesthesia in most orthopedic procedures.

It is required in long surgical procedures and whenever the surgical position is other than supine. Premature infants requiring ventilatory support and who are to have a surgical procedure should have an endotracheal airway. A few short procedures under 3 to 5 minutes may be performed safely by a competent and experienced anesthesiologist. Examples include circumcision, incision and drainage of peripheral abscesses, and some diagnostic procedures—in the absence of a full stomach.

PEDIATRIC ENDOTRACHEAL TUBES.[189,190] Endotracheal tubes for infants and children are of necessity small.[191-194] The selection of the proper tube should provide a snug fit to ensure delivery of a set tidal volume and to minimize soilage of the lower respiratory tract.[195] Tubes that are too tight (no air leak) and larger than the diameter of the cricoid ring are associated with serious postintubation croup.[196] These tubes are generally without cuffs, because the latter will tend to increase the size of the tube and the consequences of mucosal trauma and edema.[192-194]

Several objectives should be kept in mind to provide an efficient, effective airway, the following are desirable: (1) minimal resistance, (2) a minimal leak to reflect that the tube is not tight and possibly glottic edema forming, (3) ensure delivery of a set tidal volume; and (4) that the positive inspiratory pressure is sufficient to deliver the necessary tidal volume, yet providing a minimal leak.[197]

TABLE 19-14. PRIMARY OR DECIDUOUS TEETH

	Calcification		Eruption		Shedding	
	Begins at (fetal mo.)	Complete at (mo)	Maxillary (mo)	Mandibular (mo)	Maxillary (yr)	Mandibular (yr)
Central incisors	5th	18–24	6–8	5–7	7–8	6–7
Lateral incisors	5th	18–24	8–11	7–10	8–9	7–8
Cuspids	6th	30–36	16–20	16–20	11–12	9–11
First molars	5th	24–30	10–16	10–16	10–11	10–12
Second molars	6th	36	20–30	20–30	10–12	11–13

Sexes are combined although girls tend to be slightly advanced over boys.
Averages are approximate values derived from various studies.
From Nelson, W.: Textbook of pediatrics, 1964. *In* Headings, D.L.: The Harriet Lane Handbook, 7th ed. Chicago, Year Book Medical Publishers, 1975.

Leak pressure is defined as the inspiratory pressure needed to cause an audible escape of gas around the endotracheal tube.

Guidelines and Variables

1. A tube should be selected that passes through the cricoid ring, which is the narrowest part of the pediatric laryngotracheal diameter. Chodoff[195] suggests that a tube one size smaller than one which passes the vocal cords but is tight on advancement through the cricoid into the trachea should be employed.
2. The leak should occur at pressures between 20 and 25 cm H$_2$O. A leak at greater pressure is associated with increased postintubation croup.[196,198]
3. During complete paralysis, leak pressure has been determined to be about 17 cm H$_2$O in a paralyzed patient. As paralysis decreases, the leak pressure increases to 30 cm H$_2$O on recovery of the neuromuscular junction.[197]
4. The head should be in a neutral position. Turning the head from a neutral position increases the pressure needed for a leak and increases resistance to air flow in the tube. The supraglottic soft tissues passively envelope the tube and restrict air flow to some extent.
5. In the unparalyzed patient, the glottic and supraglottic muscle tone is increased against the outer wall of the endotracheal tube. Another feature is the action of the cricopharyngeus muscle, which is attached to the cricoid ring and blends with the esophageal musculature. Increased tone of the cricopharyngeus muscle results in drawing the esophagus anteriorly against the posterior surface of the trachea and may angle or compress an endotracheal tube.

Airway Resistance In Pediatric Tubes.[199] Endotracheal tubes for infants and children have a ratio of wall thickness to tube diameter much greater than in larger tubes. This leads to a high increase in airway resistance. The resistance, however, is not fixed but is a function of the air flow through the tube and is determined by a difference in the pressure gradient across the tube.[200a] This can be carried out with different flows through the tube. The pressure–flow ratio or quotient reflects resistance. In addition, with smaller tubes and with increased flow, there is to be expected nonlaminar flow, which imposes an additional element of work. During quiet respiration in the newborn, maximal flow has been determined to be approximately 4 L/min.[200b] Upper airway resistance in the newborn has been estimated to be between 1.0 and 3.0 kPa/L/s; i.e., 22.5 mm Hg/L/s in the spontaneously breathing newborn.[201] It is thus considered that spontaneous ventilation through tracheal tubes with resistance exceeding 3.0 kPa/L/s increases respiratory work.

In a careful study of airway resistance, Blom[202] has determined the pressure–flow quotient at flows of 4.0 L/min of different endotracheal tubes (Table 19–15). It is evident that, in the two commonly used ID size endotracheal tubes, the 3.0 mm ID always represents a higher resistance profile. The RAE nasal and oral endotracheal tubes,[194] with their incorporated angle of less than 90 degrees and with lengths of 3.0 to 6.0 cm, have a resistance to gas flow that may have serious consequences if ventilation is spontaneous during anesthesia. It may also present problems in weaning from artificial ventilation. Not only the RAE and Rüsch nasotracheal tubes of 3.0 mm ID but also the oral tracheal tubes presented a flow resistance exceeding 3.0 kPa/L/s, with air flows of 4.0 L/min. From this study, these particular tubes should be used only with assisted or controlled ventilation. On the other hand, the Mallinckrodt pediatric and the Portex Plain endotracheal tubes of ID of 3.0 and 3.5 mm at flows of 4.0 L/min, had R values of less than 3.0.

PEDIATRIC ENDOTRACHEAL TUBE CUFFS. In pediatric anesthesia practice, the uncuffed endotracheal tube

TABLE 19–15. THE VARIATION OF THE PRESSURE–FLOW QUOTIENT R kPa/L/s AT FLOW OF 4 L/MIN OF 10 TRACHEAL TUBES OF EACH CATEGORY: RAE IN PRE-MOULDED LENGTHS, RÜSCH, PORTEX, MALLINCKRODT IN 11-CM LENGTH.

Tracheal tube	Mean	Standard deviation	Range
ID 3.0 mm (n = 10)			
RAE nasal	5.288	.081	(5.18–5.48)
RAE oral	4.725	.087	(4.58–4.80)
Rüsch	3.600	.079	(3.45–3.68)
Mallinckrodt	2.783	.130	(2.63–2.93)
Portex	2.805	.088	(2.70–2.93)
ID 3.5 mm (n = 10)			
RAE nasal	2.475	.050	(2.40–2.55)
RAE oral	2.423	.106	(2.25–2.55)
Rüsch	2.048	.087	(1.95–2.18)
Mallinckrodt	1.238	.081	(1.13–1.35)
Portex	1.643	.090	(1.58–1.80)

From Blom, H., Rytlander, H., and Wisborg, T.: Resistance of trachael tubes 3.0 nd 3.5 mm internal diameter: A comparison of four commonly used types. Anaesthesia 40:885, 1985.

is commonly used. Generally, the risk of pulmonary aspiration of gastric contents is infrequent; in the infant and young child under 5 years of age, the proper sized endotracheal tube will be sufficient and snug to prevent aspiration. It is also recognized that an uncuffed tube minimizes postintubation stridor. Furthermore, the funnel-shaped laryngeal and tracheal structure in infants by its design limits aspiration. An audible leak is also a factor in limiting build-up of pulmonary pressure and the exsufflation around the tube aids in blowing away the secretions or extraneous fluids in the supraglottic region.

Experience generally indicates that when endotracheal tubes of 5.5 mm ID or larger are employed a cuff is undesirable.[203] This size is likely to be used in children over 5 years of age. At this age and with this size of tube, the risk of pulmonary aspiration is greater, and the cuff should be inflated only to the point when a leak is audible at the end of a positive-pressure inflation.

SELECTION OF TUBE. The endotracheal tube employed in a given case should be of suitable diameter and length.[204,205] Both specifications are determined by anatomic conditions (See Table 19–4). Anatomic variations are significant, and these measurements should be used as guidelines.[206,207,208]

Proper Size or Diameter of the Tube. Tube size is governed by consideration of the AP diameter of the glottis.[207] In the newborn, this is about 5 mm, and at 1 year of age about 6 mm. Thereafter, the AP diameter increases about 0.5 mm for each year of life until the age of 10 to 12 years. During adolescence, there is more rapid change to attain average adult measurements of 1.5 to 2.2 cm in men and 1.2 to 1.8 cm in women. The average expected diameter of tubes at various age levels is presented for neonates (Table 19–16) and for children (Table 19–17), and, based on these values, tubes of proper diameter are chosen.

Formula for Size. One rule of thumb useful in selecting the size of tubes for children over 1 year of age is that of Cole's.[209] Originally, the formula provided the size (OD) in the French catheter gauge system. This has been modified by Butz;[207] the current formula for tube size is based on the ID system and is as follows:

$$\text{ID Bore (mm)} = 4.0 + \frac{\text{Age}}{4}$$

Proper Length of Endotracheal Tube.[207] This is governed by consideration of the distance from the incisor teeth to the vocal cords; the length of the trachea; and the proximal mechanical needs to adapt to the breathing system. The trachea in the normal, well-developed newborn measures about 2.5 to 4.0 cm in length. This increases with age; the average lengths of tracheas have been measured (Table 19–18).[207,208] Similarly, the distance from the central incisor teeth to the vocal cords has been measured in children of different age groups (Table 19–19).[210] These anatomic values are noted above.

Formula of Length. A rule of thumb useful in selecting a tube of appropriate length for orotracheal placement is that of Levine[211] as follows:

$$\text{Length of the tube (cm)} = \frac{\text{Age in years}}{2}$$

CLINICAL METHODS FOR DETERMINING LENGTH OF TUBE. Three clinical methods have been employed to determine the length of tube required that will not reach the carina and yet not slip out of the glottis. These depend on the average distance from

TABLE 19-16. EXPERIENCE STANDARDS: I. APPROXIMATE ENDOTRACHEAL TUBE BORE SIZE* AND LENGTH† FOR INFANTS AND CHILDREN UNDER 3 YEARS OF AGE

Age	Weight (kg)	Internal Diameter (mm)	French Gauge	Length of Orotracheal Tube† (cm)	Suction Catheter (French)
Premature	< 1.5	2.5	12	8–9	5
Preterm	1.5–2.5	3.0	13	10	6
Term	> 2.5	3.5	14	11	6
3–6 months	4.0–6.0	3.5	14–15	11	8
6–12 months	6.0–8.0	4.0	16	12	8
1–2 years	8.0–12.0	4.5	18	13	8
2–3 years	12.0–16.0	5.0	18	14	10

* Each size tube should be available in three lengths: short, medium, and long.
† Lengths are measured from midpoint of the bevel of tube to machine end. Length will permit placement of tube in midtrachea, and should allow full expansion of both lungs and a leak at a pressure of 20 to 25 cm H₂O.
‡ For nasotracheal tubes, add 2 cm in length.
Data from Leigh, M.D., and Belton, M.K.: Pediatric Anesthesiology, 2nd ed. New York, Macmillan, 1960; and Smith, R.M.: Anesthesia for Infants and Children, 4th ed. St. Louis, C.V. Mosby, 1980.[204,205]

incisor teeth to vocal cords as a variation with age (see Table 19–18).[210]

External (Topographic) Measurement.[204] Several catheters of different sizes within the estimated range of diameter are selected. Three variations in length of each size are made available. The actual length of tube required is estimated by measuring the distance from the nares to the ear lobe and adding 3 cm. Another method is to lay the tube alongside the patient's neck from incisor teeth to middle of thyroid cartilage and add 3 cm to the measurement. In either case, the measured distance is usually 1 cm greater than the actual distance from incisor teeth to vocal cords but may show wide variations. The added 3 cm allows for the distance the tube extends through the glottis and into the trachea as well as the length extending outside the teeth. Thus, a proper choice depends on astute estimation and experience, and a further selection may be necessary at the time of laryngoscopy.

To perform topographic measurements in infants and children, the following methods may be used:

1. For orotracheal tubes
   a. Measure along neck from midthyroid to lips, then add 2 cm for infants or 3 cm for children.
   b. Measure the distance from the ear lobe to nose tip, then add 2 cm for infants or 3 to 5 cm for children.
2. For nasotracheal tubes
   a. In children aged 1 to 4 years, measure the distance from the ear lobe to nose tip, then multiply by 1.25.
   b. In children aged 4 to 12 years, measure the distance from the ear lobe to nose tip, then multiply by 1.5.

TABLE 19-17. EXPERIENCE STANDARDS: II. GUIDE TO CHOICE OF ENDOTRACHEAL TUBE* IN CHILDREN AGED 3 TO 12 YEARS

Age (yr)	Standard Internal Diameter (mm)	External Diameter (mm)	French Gauge	Length† (cm)	Connectors (slip joints) (mm)
3–6	4.5	6.7	20	14 15 16	6.0
	5.0	7.3	22		7.0
	5.5	8.0	24		7.0
6–9	5.5	7.3	22	16 17 18	8.0
	6.0	8.0	24		8.0
	6.5	8.7	26		8.0
9–12	6.0	8.0	24	18 19 20	9.0
	6.5	9.3	26		9.0
	7.0	9.0	28		10.0

* Each size tube should be available in three lengths: short, medium, and long.
† Lengths are measured from midpoint of the bevel of tube to machine end. For nasotracheal tubes, add 2–3 cm in length. Length will permit placement of tube in midtrachea.
Data from Leigh, M.D., and Belton, M.K.: Pediatric Anesthesiology, 2nd ed. New York, Macmillan, 1960.

TABLE 19-18. TRACHEAL LENGTH IN INFANTS AND CHILDREN

Age (yr)	Length (cm)
Premature	2.5
Full term	3.0
1 month	3.7
2 months	4.5
1 year	4.8
2 years	5.4
3 years	5.8
5 years	6.0
10 years	7.0
15 years	7.5

Modified from Butz, R.O., Jr.: Length and cross section growth patterns in human trachea. Pediatrics, *42*:336, 1968; and Shellinger, R.R.: The length of the airway to the bifurcation of the trachea. Anesthesiology, *25*:169, 1964.

TABLE 19-19. DISTANCE FROM INCISOR TEETH TO VOCAL CORDS RELATED TO AGE

Age (yr)	Distance (cm)
1	8
2	9
3	9
4	9.5
5	10
6	10
7	10.5
8	11
9	11
10	11.5
11	12
12	12

Data from McIntyre, J.W.R.: Endotracheal tube for children. Anaesthesia, *12*:94, 1957.[210]

Calculated Lengths.[210] An average length of tube for orotracheal intubation can be calculated for various ages from anatomic measurements, i.e., the average distances from incisor teeth to vocal cords and vocal cords to carina (see Table 19-18).

The length of tube required for children over 1 year of age is determined by adding the following:

1. The average distance from incisor teeth to vocal cords plus the distance into midtrachea
2. The length of larynx below the vocal cords, i.e., 1 to 2 cm
3. The distance the tube should extend into midtrachea, i.e., 1 cm
4. The length of the bevel of the tube, i.e., 0.5 cm
5. The minimum distance the tube should extend outside teeth, i.e., 1 cm.

Therefore, the length of tube is the average teeth to cord distance plus 4 cm. These lengths are somewhat shorter by 1 to 2 cm than the length determined by topographic measurement.

Sternal Measurement Technique. Schellinger[208] has studied the length of the airway from the incisor teeth (or base of nose) to the carina. This bears a close correlation with the external or topographic measurement from the cricothyroid (CT) notch to the tip of the xiphoid. The CT notch to xiphoid distance in centimeters provides a safe estimate of the maximal length of a nasotracheal tube, whereas this same distance *less* 2 cm provides a safe estimate of the maximal length of an orotracheal tube.

LARYNGOSCOPY.[205] Laryngoscopy in children requires more delicacy and precision than in the adult because (1) the larynx is situated higher than in the adult; (2) the tongue is relatively larger; (3) the epiglottis is depressed so it occupies more of the pharyngeal cavity and it is short, stiff, and U shaped; and (4) the vocal cords are more concave.

Visualization of the cords is usually accomplished in the following manner: with the head in the neutral position, the "L" laryngoscope is introduced into the mouth near the right side with the handle pointing toward the right shoulder. As the blade is passed into the oral cavity and brought to a perpendicular plane, the handle is swung into the midline. When the epiglottis is seen, it is elevated by the tip of the blade. This may be difficult to accomplish with newborn; therefore, the blade may be passed into the postcricoidal space, i.e., into the esophageal entrance, and slowly withdrawn until the arytenoids come into view. Elevation of the blade tip usually exposes the cords.

Practical Guides for Laryngoscopy and Intubation

1. No pillow is necessary for the sniffing position (large head makes up for it).
2. A straight blade with a wide tip is ideal for intubation because it holds the tongue better and elevates the epiglottis firmly (the Miller blade provides a better view).
3. Avoid traumatizing the anterior commissure; the cords are slanted anteriorly, and the posterior commissure is more caudad than the anterior commissure; stylets are more likely to injure the larynx and are unnecessary.
4. Use an endotracheal tube that allows full expansion of both lungs on manual inflation but allows a definite leak at 20 to 25 cm H_2O of inflation pressure. Use of a large tube can cause croup (common in children 1 to 4 years of age). Use of a small tube increases airway resistance.
5. Do not use cuffed tubes for children less than 6 years of age.
6. Use a humidifier to prevent inspiration of secretions that result in occlusion of the lumen.
7. The nasopharynx should be gently suctioned prior to extubation; avoid temperature probes and unnecessary tubes through the nose.

8. Empty the stomach after intubation and prior to extubation. Extubate while the child is fully awake.

Introduction of the Tube. Under vision, the tube is directed toward the glottis. The bevel should parallel the cords. Introduction through the cords is facilitated by gentle rotation. This is preferable to a straight thrust. Advancement beyond the cords may be impeded by the cricoid ring; if this, a smaller tube should be used, otherwise pressure ischemia of mucous membrane may occur with reactive edema or, after prolonged use, necrosis and ulceration. The trachea in the normal, well-developed newborn measures about 2.5 to 4 cm in length. The length of tube below the vocal cords for patients under 6 months should not be more than 1 cm; for patients up to 1 year, not more than 2 cm.

The tip of the endotracheal tube should not reach the carina nor should it be in danger of slipping above the vocal cords.[186,205] Cuffs should not be used in infants—pharyngeal packs are satisfactory and, when properly placed, will prevent aspiration.

SECURING ENDOTRACHEAL TUBES. A tube should be taped at the machine end of the tube at a distance of approximately three times the ID, from the lip of the patient.[212] For example, a 4.0 mm endotracheal tube should be secured at the proximal end of the tube about 1 cm from the lip of the patient. The silk-type adhesive tape is recommended.[175] It is looped about the endotracheal tube and the ends then applied firmly to the upper lip or the chin.

After securing the endotracheal tube, it is important to maintain the head in an anatomically neutral position. Neck flexion causes the tip of an endotracheal tube to move caudad further into the trachea, whereas neck extension results in an upward movement.[213] Rotation of the head in an infant may cause a cephalad movement up to 1.2 cm.[214] Radiologic studies of the tip of the tube show that flexion of the neck will cause the endotracheal tube to advance up to 0.5 cm into the trachea, whereas extension results in upward movement of up to 2 cm.[215] The mean range of full movement of an orotracheal tube was found to be 1.43 cm ± 0.480 SD, and the range of a nasotracheal tube was found to be 1.68 cm ± 0.59 SD.

Bloch[178] recommended the following technique: (1) that the tracheal position of the tube after insertion be determined by clinical criteria; (2) that the tube be advanced into a stem bronchus and clinical evidence of this then adduced; and (3) the tube is then withdrawn 2 cm and will be about this distance above the carina. Radiologic evidence has supported the safety and correctness of this maneuver.

SUCTIONING OF ENDOTRACHEAL TUBES.[216] In suctioning endotracheal tubes in infants and young children, it is important not to occlude the lumen of the endotracheal tube with the suction catheter, because this will exhaust lung air and lead to atelectasis.

Two principles in suctioning should be followed:

1. Use a suction catheter size with an OD less than one-half the endotracheal tube ID (catheter OD is less than 50% of the tube ID). For example:
    a. For a 3 mm endotracheal tube, use an uncuffed No. 5 French suction catheter. The OD of the 5 French catheter is about 1.6 mm.
    b. For a 4 mm endotracheal tube, use an uncuffed No. 6 French suction catheter. The OD of the 6 French catheter is about 2 mm.
2. Use low-pressure, high-flow suction briefly and intermittently until clear (less than 10 cm H_2O).

EFFECT OF AIRWAY EDEMA.[217] When airway edema occurs, resistance to air flow is different in children and adults. In an adult, if 1 mm of edema occurs within the larynx, trachea, or airway, it reduces the cross-sectional area by 44% and increases the resistance to air flow threefold. The same degree of edema occurring in an infant's airway reduces the cross-sectional area by 75% and increases the resistance to air flow sixteenfold (Fig. 19–41). These data represent laminar flow. If they represented turbulent flow, as would occur with airway obstruction, resistance to breathing may be increased by as much as thirtyfold.

Thus, proportional degrees of edema cause much more airway obstruction in a pediatric patient than in an adult. In turn, this edema and obstruction markedly increase the work of breathing, eventually causing respiratory failure.

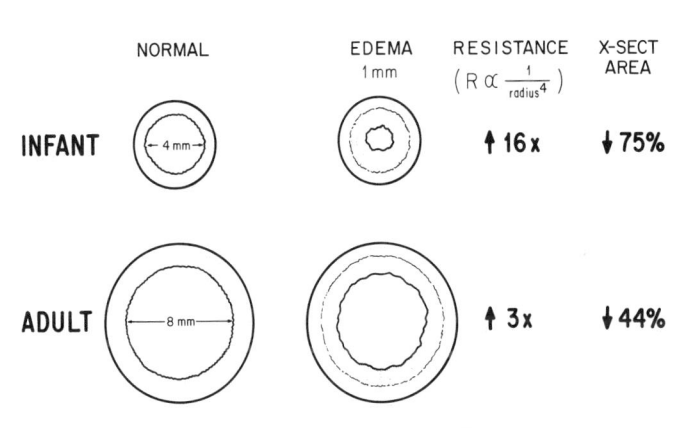

FIG. 19–41. Effects of airway edema on flow resistance and cross-sectional area. There are greater proportional changes in cross-sectional area and airway resistance with equivalent circumferential edema in the infant than in the adult. From Coté and Todres: The Pediatric Airway. In *A Practice of Anesthesia for Infants and Children*. J.F. Ryan, I.D. Todres, C.J. Coté, N.G. Goudsouzian, eds. Grune and Stratton, 1985. Prints, courtesy of Charles Coté. With permission.

STRIDOR.[218] Noisy respiration, termed *stridor*, is obstructed respiration. It may occur on inspiration or expiration. Causes of stridor can be congenital, as often seen in pediatric patients, or acquired (Table 19–20).[219] Inspiratory stridor is the result of either mechanical block or noxious inhaled substances.[220] The most frequent block is caused by backward displacement of the tongue into the pharynx, with or without compression of the soft palate against the pharynx. Forward movement of the mandible alleviates the condition. Noxious stimuli include saliva, blood, and foreign bodies in the process of being aspirated. Dusty air or irritating breathing mixtures also provoke protective laryngeal closure, as does either extremely hot or cold air. The closure resulting from noxious influences is called *laryngospasm* and may be progressive from simple vocal cord adduction on inspiration through vestibular fold closure to complete ball valve block, depending on the intensity of the stimulus.

TABLE 19–20. CAUSES OF STRIDOR IN THE PEDIATRIC PATIENT

Congenital stridor
  Craniofacial dysmorphology (with micrognathia and glossoptosis)
    Pierre Robin syndrome
    Treacher–Collins syndrome (mandibulofacial dysostosis)
    Hallerman–Streiff (oculomandibular)
    Möbius syndrome
    Delange syndrome
    Freeman–Shelton (whistling face)
  Macroglossia
    Beckwith's syndrome
    Congenital hypothyroidism
    Glycogen storage diseases
    Down syndrome
    Diffuse muscular hypertrophy of the tongue
    Localized lingual tumors
  Laryngomalacia
  Congenital subglottic stenosis
  Congenital laryngeal webs
  Laryngotracheoesophageal cleft
  Congenitial vocal-cord paralysis
  Vascular rings and slings
  Congenital tracheal anomalies
  Congenital calcification of tracheal cartilage
  Congenital tumors and cysts
    Congenital subglottic hemangioma
    Laryngeal lymphangioma and cystic hygroma
    Cysts and laryngoceles
    Miscellaneous congenital tumors
  Birth trauma—edema
  Metabolic stridor: Laryngysmus stridulosa
  Immunologic stridor—hereditary angioneurotic edema
  Neurogenic stridor—reflex laryngospasm
Acquired stridor
  Infectious stridor
    Epiglottitis
    Croup
    Acute spasmodic laryngitis
    Diphtheria
    Retropharyngeal abscess
  Immunologic stridor—juvenile rheumatoid arthritis
  Trauma
    Foreign bodies
    Iatrogenic stridor
      Postintubation
      Postinstrumentation
      Postoperative
    External trauma
    Thermal and chemical trauma
  Neoplasia
    Laryngeal papillomatosis
    Miscellaneous tumors and nodes

From Maze, A., and Bloch, E.: Stridor in pediatric patients. Anesthesiology, 50:132, 1980.

REFERENCES

1. Gillespie, NA: The evolution of endotracheal anesthesia. J. Hist. Med. and Appl. Sci., I(#4):583–595. Edited by Henry Schuman. New York, G. Banta Pub. Co., Wisconsin, 1946.
1a. Avicenna. Liber Canonis, Lib 3, Fen 9; 1507:137–8, Venice.
1aa. Brandt, L.: Anesth. Analg., 66:1198, 1987.
1b. Vesalius, A.: *De Humani Corporis Fabrica*, 1st ed. Basel, Switzerland, 1543, pg. "658." The passage in question begins on line 47 of the penultimate page of the book. Owing to a typographical error, the page is numbered 658, whereas it should be numbered 662.
1c. Hooke, R.: Preserving animals alive by blowing through their lungs with bellows. Phil. Trans. Roy. Soc., 2:539, 1667.
1d. White, G.M.J.: The first endotracheal intubation. Br. J. Anaesth., 32:235, 1960.
2. Waters, R.M., Rovenstine, E.A., Guedel, A.E.: Endotracheal anesthesia and its history. Anesth. Analg., 12:196, 1933.
2a. Snow, J.: *On Chloroform and Other Anaesthetics*. London, J. Churchill, pg. 117, 1858.
2b. Trendelenberg, F.: Tamponade de trachea. Arch. Klin. Chir., 12:121, 1871.
2c. Macewen, W.: Clinical observations on the introduction of tracheal tubes by the mouth instead of performing tracheotomy. Br. Med. J., 2:122, 163; 1880.
2d. O'Dwyer, J., Fell, G.E.: Fifty cases of croup in private practice treated by intubation of the larynx with a description of the method and of the dangers incident thereto. Med. Rec., 32:577, 1887.
2e. Eisenmenger, V.: Zur Tamponade des Larynx nach Prof. Maydl. Wien. Med. Wschr., 43:199, 1893.
2f. Kirstein, A.: Die autoskopie des Kehlkopfs und der Luft rohre. Berl. Klin. Wchnscher., 32:476, 1895.
2g. Kuhn, F.: Die perorale Intubation. Zbl. Chir., 28:1281, 1901.
2h. Elsberg, C.A.: The value of continuous intratracheal insufflation of air (Metzer) in thoracic surgery. Med. Rec., 77:493, 1910.
2i. Dorrence, G.M.: On the treatment of traumatic injuries of the lungs and pleura with the presentation of a new intratracheal tube for use in artificial respiration. Surg. Gynecol. Obstet., 11:160, 1910.
2j. Flagg, P.: *The Art of Anesthesia*. Philadelphia, J. B. Lippincott Co., 1916.
2k. Rowbotham, E.: Intratracheal anesthesia by the nasal route for operations on the mouth and lips. Br. Med. J., 2:590, 1920.
21. Magill, I.W.: Appliances and preparation: Forceps for intratracheal anaesthesia. Br. Med. J., 2:670, 1920.
2m. Waters, R.M., Guedel, A.F.: A new intratracheal catheter. Curr. Res. Anesth. Analg., 7:238, 1928.

3. Gillespie, N.A.: *Endotracheal Anesthesia*, 3rd ed. Chapter 1: History of endotracheal anesthesia, pp. 1–24. Edited by Bamforth and Siebecker. Madison, University of Wisconsin Press, 1963.
4. Magill, I.W.: Endotracheal anesthesia. Am. J. Surg., 34:450, 1936.
5. Kuhn, F.: Die perorale Intubation. Berlin, S. Karger, 1911.
6. Meltzer, S.J., Auer, J.: Continuous respiration without respiratory movements (insufflation method). J. Exp. Med., 11:622, 1909.
7. Jackson, C.: The technique of insertion of intratracheal insufflation tubes. Surg. Gynecol. Obstet., 17:507, 1913.
8. Elsberg, C.A.: Intratracheal insufflation anesthesia: Its value in thoracic and in general surgery. N.Y. J. Med., 12:524, 1912.
9. Gray, H.: *Anatomy of the Human Body*, 30th ed. Edited by C.D. Clemente. Philadelphia, Lea & Febiger, 1985.
10. Negus, V.E.: *The Comparative Anatomy and Physiology of the Larynx*. New York, Hafner Publishing Co., 1949.
11. Netter, F., Saunders, W.H.: The larynx. Ciba Clinical Symposia, 1965.
12. Ballenger, H.C.: *A Manual of Otology, Rhinology and Laryngology*, 4th ed. Philadelphia, Lea & Febiger, 1954.
13. Vandam, L.D.: The functional anatomy of the lung. Anesthesiology, 13:130, 1952.
14. Proctor, D.F.: All that wheezes . . . Am. Rev. Respir. Dis., 127:261, 1983.
15. Scharf, S.M., Feldman, N.T., Goldman, M.D., et al.: Vocal cord closure: A cause of upper airway obstruction during controlled ventilation. Am. Rev. Respir. Dis., 117:391, 1978.
16. Vincken, W.G., Gauther, S.G., Dollfuss, R.E., et al.: Involvement of upper-airway in extrapyramidal disorders: A cause of air flow limitation. New. Engl. J. Med., 311:438, 1984.
17. Megerian, D., Ryan, A.T., Sherrey, J.H.: An electrophysiological analysis of sleep and respiration of rats breathing different gas mixtures: Diaphragmatic muscle function. Electroencephalog. Clin. Neurophysiol., 50:303, 1980.
18. Onal, F., Lopata, M., O'Connor, T.D.: Diaphragmatic and genioglossal electromyogram responses to CO_2 rebreathing in humans. J. Appl. Physiol., 50:1052, 1981.
19. Phillipson, E.A.: Control of breathing during sleep. Am. Rev. Respir. Dis., 118:909, 1978.
20a. Fink, B.R.: The mechanism of closure of the human larynx. Trans. Am. Acad. Ophthalmol. and Otol., 60:117, 1956.
20b. Fink, B.R.: *The Human Larynx: A Functional Study*. New York, Raven Press, 1975.
21. American Standards Specification of Anesthesia Equipment—Endotracheal Tubes: American Standard Z79.1. Sponsored by the American Society of Anesthesiologists, 1960.
22. American Standards Association: Specifications for anesthetic equipment. Endotracheal tube connectors and adaptors. Z79.2, 1961.
23. *American National Standard for Anesthetic Equipment—Endotracheal Tubes:* ANSI Z79.14–1980. New York, American National Standards Institute, 1980.
24. American National Standard for Anesthetic Equipment—Tracheal Tubes: ANSI Z79.14–1983. New York, American National Standards Institute, 1983.
25. ISO Technical Committee TC 212, 1983.
26. Flagg, P.J.: *The Art of Anesthesia*. Philadelphia, J. B. Lippincott Co., 1912.
27. Flagg, P.J.: A simplified method of intratracheal ether anesthesia. Anesth. Analg., 8:327, 1929.
28. Woodbridge, P.D.: A flexible metal tube for intratracheal anesthesia. Anesth. Analg. (Suppl), 13:68, 1934.
29. Rowbotham, E.: Intratracheal anaesthesia by the nasal route for operations on the mouth and lips. Br. Med. J., 2:590, 1920.
30. Rowbotham, E., Magill, I.W.: Anaesthetics in the plastic surgery of the face and jaws. Proc. Roy. Soc. Med. (Anaesth), 14:17, 1921.
31. Gordon, R.A., Ainslie, E.H.: Experience with vinyl-plastic endotracheal tubes. Anesthesiology, 6:359, 1945.
32. Hunter, A.R.: Vinyl Portex endotracheal tubes. Br. J. Anaesth., 19:128, 1945.
33. Collins, V.J.: Committee on Standards, American Society of Anesthesiologists, 1955 (See Gillespie NA, (#3), 3rd ed. 1963, p. 39).
34. Carroll, R.G., Kamen, J.M., Grenvick, A., et al.: Recommended performance specifications for cuffed endotracheal and tracheostomy tubes: A joint statement of investigators, inventors and manufacturers. Crit. Care. Med., 11:155, 1973.
35. Shupak, R.C., Deas, T.C.: The ideal tracheal tube. Proceedings of a Workshop on Tracheal Tubes, Valley Forge, PA, April 30–May 1, 1981, pp. 103–106.
36. Orkin, L.R., Siegel, M., Rovenstine, E.A.: Resistance to breathing by apparatus used in anesthesia. Endotracheal equipment. Anesth. Analg., 33:217, 1954.
37. Gallon, S.: The resistance of endotracheal connectors. Br. J. Anaesth., 29:160, 1957.
38. Brown, E.S.: Resistance factors in pediatric endotracheal tubes and connectors. Anesth. Analg., 50:355, 1971.
39. Frumin, M.J., Lee, A.S.J., Papper, E.M.: New valve for nonrebreathing systems. Anesthesiology, 20:383, 1959.
40. *Dorland's Medical Dictionary*, 26th ed. Philadelphia, Saunders Publishing Co., 1981.
41. Bernhard, W.N., Yost, L., Turndorf, H., et al.: Cuffed tracheal tubes—physical and behavioral characteristics. Anesth. Analg., 61:36, 1982.
42. Butz, R.O., Jr.: Length and cross section growth patterns in human trachea. Pediatrics, 42:336, 1968.
43. McIntyre, J.W.R.: Endotracheal tube for children. Anaesthesia, 12:94, 1957.
44. Schellinger, R.R.: The length of the airway to the bifurcation of the trachea. Anesthesiology, 25:169, 1964.
45. Miller, W.S.: *The Lung*. Springfield, IL, Charles C. Thomas Publishers, 1937; p. 21.
46. Meschan, I.: *An Atlas of Normal Radiographic Anatomy*. Philadelphia, W. B. Saunders, 1968; p. 450.
47. Kubota, Y., Toyoda, Y., Nagata, N., et al.: Tracheo-bronchial angles in infants and children. Anesthesiology, 64:374, 1986.
48. Cleveland, R.H.: Symmetry of bronchial angles in children. Radiology, 133:89, 1979.
49. Brown, T.C.K., Fish, G.C.: *Anaesthesia for Children*, 1st ed. Melbourne, Blackwell Scientific Publications, 1979; p. 3.
50. Murphy, F.J.: Two improved intratracheal catheters. Anesth. Analg., 20:102, 1941.
51. Hargrave, R.: An improved catheter for endotracheal nitrous oxide oxygen anaesthesia. Can. Med. Assoc. J., 26:218, 1932.
52. Hargrave, R.: Intratracheal nitrous oxide-oxygen anesthesia. Anesth. Analg., 8:103, 1929.
53. Cole, F.: An endotracheal tube for babies. Anesthesiology, 6:627, 1945.

54. Cole, F.: A new endotracheal tube for infants. Anesthesiology, 6:87, 1945.
55. Glauser, E.M., Cook, C.K., and Bougas, T.P.: Pressure-flow characteristics and dead spaces of endotracheal tubes used in infants. Anesthesiology, 22:339, 1961.
56. Dwyer, C.S., Kronenberg, S., and Saklad, M.: The endotracheal tube: A consideration of the traumatic effects with a suggestion for the modification thereof. Anesthesiology, 10:714, 1949.
57. Lindholm, C.E.: Experience with a new orotracheal tube. Acta Otolaryngol., 75:389, 1973.
58. Ring, W.H., Adair, J.C., and Elwyn, R.A.: A new pediatric endotracheal tube. Anesth. Analg., 54:273, 1975.
59. Konchigeri, H.N., and Shaker, M.H.: Anesthesia for intralaryngeal laser surgery. Can. Anaesth. Soc. J., 21:343, 1974.
60. Snow, J.C., et al.: Fire hazard during CO_2 laser microsurgery on the larynx and trachea. Anesth. Analg., 55:146, 1976.
61. Hirschmann, C.A., and Smith, J.: Indirect ignition of the endotracheal tube during carbon dioxide laser surgery. Arch. Otolaryngol., 106:639, 1980.
62. Ossof, R.H., et al.: Comparison of tracheal damage from laser-ignited endotracheal tube fires. Ann. Otol. Rhinol. Laryngol., 92:333, 1983.
63. Lejeune, F.E., et al.: Heat sink protection against lasering endotracheal cuffs. Ann. Otol. Rhinol. Laryngol., 91:606, 1982.
64. Kalhan, S.B., and Cascorbi, H.F.: Anesthetic management of laser microlaryngeal surgery. Anesthesiol. Rev., 8:23, 1981.
65. Norton, M.L., and deVos, P.: A new endotracheal tube for laser surgery of the larynx. Ann. Otol. Rhinol. Laryngol., 87:554, 1978.
66. Patil, V., Stehling, L.C., and Zauder, H.L.: A modified endotracheal tube for laser microsurgery. Anesthesiology, 51:571, 1979.
67. Hayes, C.M., Gaba, D.M., and Goode, R.L.: Incendiary characteristics of a new laser-resistant endotracheal tube. Otol. Head Neck Surg., 95:37, 1986.
68. Little, K., and Parkhouse, J.: Tissue reactions to polymers. Lancet, 2:857, 1965.
69. Guess, W.L., and Stetson, J.B.: Tissue reactions to organotin-stabilized polyvinyl chloride (PVC) catheters. J.A.M.A., 204:580, 1968.
70. Guess, W.L.: Tissue testing of polymers. Int. Anesthesiol. Clin., 8:70, 1969.
71. Rendell-Baker, L.: Irritation from plastic endotracheal tubes. ASA Newsl., March, 1968.
72. Rendell-Baker, L.: Hazards of prolonged intubation and tracheotomy equipment (editorial). J.A.M.A., 204:624, 1968.
73. U. S. Pharmacopeia, XVII, p. 905. U. S. Pharmacopeial Convention, Rockville, MD, 1955.
74. Adams R., et al.: Control of infection within hospitals. J.A.M.A., 169:1557, 1959.
74a. Gillespie, N.A.: *Endotracheal Anesthesia*, 3rd ed. Bamforth, B.J., Siebecker, K.L. (Ed.) Madison, University of Wisconsin Press, pp. 66–68, 1963.
75. Keet, J., Collins, V.J.: Cleaning and disinfection of endotracheal tubes. Resident's Thesis, 1963. St. Vincent's Hospital Medical Center, New York.
76. Gross, G.L.: Decontamination of anesthetic apparatus. Anesthesiology, 16:903, 1955.
77. Kundsin, R.B., Walter, C.W.: Asepsis for inhalational therapy. Anesthesiology, 23:507, 1962.
78. Barry, A.E., Noble, M.A., Marrie, T.J., et al.: Cleaning of anaesthesia breathing circuits and tubings: A Canadian survey. Can. Anaesth. Soc. J., 31:572, 1984.
79. Spaulding, E.H.: Chemical disinfection and antisepsis in the hospital. J. Hosp. Res., 9:7, 1972.
80. Dorsch, J.A., Dorsch, S.E.: *Understanding Anesthesia Equipment: Construction, Care and Complications*, 2nd ed. Chapter 15: Cleaning and sterilization. Complications and hazards, pp. 426–429. Baltimore, Williams and Wilkins, 1984.
81. Livingstone, H., Hendrick, F., Holicky, I., et al.: Cross infections from anesthetic face masks. Surgery, 9:433, 1941.
82. *Ethylene Oxide Use in Hospitals. A Manual for Health Care Personnel.* American Society for Hospital Central Service Personnel of the American Hospital Association, 840 N. Lake Shore Drive, Chicago, Illinois, 60611, 1982.
83. Borick, P.M.: Chemical sterilizers (chemosterilizers). Adv. Appl. Microbiol., 10:291, 1968.
84. Roberts, R.B.: The anaesthetist, cross-infection and sterilization techniques—a review. Anaesth. Intens. Care, 1:400, 1973.
85. Belani, K.G., Priedkalns, J.: An epidemic of pseudomembraneous laryngotracheitis. Anesthesiology, 47:530, 1977.
86. Mostafa, S.M.: Adverse effects of buffered glutaraldehyde on the Heidbrink expiratory valve. Br. J. Anaesth., 52:223, 1980.
87. Ethylene oxide sterilization. Hospitals, 45:99, 1971.
88. American National Standards Institute Sectional Committee Z-79 and ASA Subcommittee on Standardization: Ethylene oxide sterilization of anesthesia apparatus. Anesthesiology, 33:120, 1970.
89. Hazards associated with ethylene oxide sterilization. N.Y. State J. Med., 69:1319, 1969.
90. Kirstein, A.: Die Autoskopie des Kehlkopfs und der Luftrohre. Berl. Klin. Wchnschr., 32:476, 1895.
91. Hirsch, N.P., Smith, G.P., and Hirsch, P.O.: Alfred Kirstein: Pioneer of direct laryngoscopy. Anaesthesia, 40:38, 1986.
92. Jackson, C.: Instrumental aids to bronchoscopy and oesophagoscopy. Laryngoscope, 17:492, 1907.
93. Janeway, H.H.: Intratracheal anesthesia from the standpoint of the nose, throat and oral surgery with a description of a new instrument for catheterizing the trachea. Laryngoscope, 23:1082, 1913.
94. Magill, I.V.: An improved laryngoscope for anesthetists. Lancet, 1:500, 1926.
95. Flagg, P.J.: The exposure and illumination of the pharynx and larynx by the general practitioner: A new laryngoscope designed to simplify the technique. Arch. Otolaryngol, 8:716, 1928.
96. Greene, B.A., and Goffen, B.S.: The evolution of the anesthesiologist's laryngoscope: A compilation of source material from Wood Library Museum of Anesthesiology. Postgraduate Assembly of New York State Society of Anesthesiology. New York, 1955.
97. Miller, R.A.: A new laryngoscope. Anesthesiology, 2:317, 1941.
98. Macintosh, R.R.: An improved laryngoscope. Br. Med. J., 2:914, 1941.
99. Cassels, W.H.: Advantages of a curved laryngoscope. Anesthesiology, 3:580, 1942.
100. Macintosh, R.R.: A new laryngoscope. Lancet, 1:205, 1943.
101. Wiggin, S.: A new modification of the conventional laryngoscope. Anesthesiology, 5:61, 1944.
102. O'Dwyer, J.: Fifty cases of croup in private practice treated

by intubation of the larynx, with a description of the method and of the dangers incident thereto. Med. Record, 32:557, 1887.
103. Maydl, K.: Über die Intubation des Larynx als Mittel gegen das Einfliessen von Blut in die Respirationsorgane bei Operationen. Wien Med. Wschr., 43:57, 102, 1893.
104. Guedel, A.E.: and Waters, R.M.: A new intratracheal catheter. Anesth. Analg., 7:238, 1928.
105. Adriani, J., and Phillips, M.: Use of endotracheal cuff: Some data pro and con. Anesthesiology, 18:1, 1957.
106. Trendelenburg, F.: Beitrage zur den operationen an den Luftwegen tamponade der trachea. Arch. J. Klin. Chir., 12:221, 1871.
107. Eisenmenger, V.: Zur Tamponnade des Larynx nach Prof Maydl. Wien Med. Wschr., 43:199, 1893.
108. Dorrance, G.M.: On the treatment of traumatic injuries of the lungs and pleura, with the presentation of a new intratracheal tube for use in artificial respiration. Surg. Gynecol. Obstet., 11:160, 1910.
109. Rowbotham, E.S., and Magill, I.W.: Anaesthetics in the plastic surgery of the face and jaws. Proc. Roy. Soc. Med. (Anaesth.), 14:17, 1921.
110. Grimm, J.E., and Knight, R.T.: An improved endotracheal technic. Anesthesiology, 4:6, 1943.
111. Cassels, W.: An easy method of putting inflatable cuffs on endotracheal tubes. Anesthesiology, 5:526, 1944.
112. Mörch, E.T., Saxton, G.A., and Gish, G.: Artificial respiration by the uncuffed tracheostomy tube. J.A.M.A., 160:864, 1956.
113. Ibesen, B.: The anaesthetist viewpoint on the treatment of respiratory complications in poliomyelitis during the epidemic in Copenhagen. Proc. Roy. Soc. Med., 47:72, 1952.
114. Jackson, R.R., and Rokowski, W.J.: An endotracheal tube with cellophane cuff. J.A.M.A., 199:756, 1967.
115. Carroll, R.G., Hedden, M., and Safar, P.: Intratracheal cuffs: Performance characteristics. Anesthesiology, 31:275, 1969.
115a. Carroll, R.G., Hedden, M., and Safar, P.: Evaluation of tracheal tube cuff designs. Crit. Care Med. 1:45, 1973.
116. Chandler, M., and Crawley, B.E.: Rationalization of the selection of tracheal tubes. Br. J. Anaesth., 58:111, 1986.
117. Dorsch, J., and Dorsch, S.: Understanding Anesthesia Equipment, 2nd ed. Baltimore, Williams & Wilkins, 1984.
118. Cooper, J.D., and Grillo, H.C.: Analysis of problems related to cuffs on intratracheal tubes. Chest, 62:21S, 1972.
119. Carroll, R.G., and Grenvick, A.: Proper use of large diameter, large residual volume cuffs. Crit. Care Med., 1:153, 1973.
120. Carroll, R.G., McGinnis, G.E., and Grenvick, A.: Performance characteristics of tracheal cuffs. Int. Anesthesiol. Clin. 12:111, 1974.
121. Carroll, R.G.: et al: Recommended performance specifications for cuffed endotracheal and tracheostomy tubes: A joint statement of investigators, inventors and manufacturers. Crit. Care Med., 11:155, 1973.
122. Dobrin, P., and Canfield, T.: Cuffed endotracheal tubes: mucosal pressures and tracheal wall blood flow. Am. J. Surg., 133:562, 1977.
123. Seegobin, R.D., and Van Hasselt, G.L.: Endotracheal cuff pressure and mucosal blood flow: endoscopic study of effects of four large volume cuffs. Br. Med. J., 288:985, 1984.
124. Mehta, S.: Safe lateral wall cuff pressure to prevent aspiration. Ann. R. Coll. Surg. (Eng.) 66:426, 1984.
124a. Bernhard, W.N., et al.: Adjustment of intracuff pressure to prevent aspiration. Anesthesiology 50:363, 1979.
125. Nordin, U., Lindholm, C.E., and Wolgast, M.: Blood flow in the rabbit tracheal mucosa under normal conditions and under the influence of endotracheal intubation. Acta. Anaesthesiol. Scand., 21:81, 1977.
126. Kim, J.M., Mangold, J.V., and Hacker, D.C.: Laboratory evaluation of low pressure tracheal cuffs: Large volume vs. low volume. Br. J. Anaesth., 57:913, 1985.
127. Mehta, S.: Effects of nitrous oxide and oxygen on tracheal cuff gas volume. Br. J. Anaesth., 53:1277, 1981.
128. Stanley, T.H.: Nitrous oxide and pressures and volumes of high and low pressure endotracheal tube cuffs in intubated patients. Anesthesiology, 42:637, 1975.
129. Tonnesen, A.S., Vereen, L., and Arens, J.F.: Endotracheal cuff tube residual volume and lateral pressure in a model trachea. Anesthesiology, 55:680, 1981.
130. Crawley, B.E., and Cross, D.E.: Tracheal cuffs. A review and dynamic pressure study. Anaesthesia, 30:4, 1975.
131. Jacobsen, L., and Greenbaum, R.: A study of intracuff pressure measurements, trends and behavior in patients during prolonged tracheal intubation. Br. J. Anaesth., 53:97, 1981.
132. Stanley, T.H., Kawamura, R., and Graves, C.: Effects of nitrous oxide on volume and pressure of endotracheal tube cuffs. Anesthesiology, 41:256, 1974.
133. Munson, E.S.: Transfer of nitrous oxide into body air cavities. Br. J. Anaesth., 46:202, 1979.
134. Munson, E.S.: Nitrous oxide and body air space. Middle East J. Anaesthesiol., 7:193, 1983.
135. Raeder, J.C., Borchgrevink, P.C., and Selfevold, O.M.: Tracheal tube pressures: The effects of different gas mixtures. Anaesthesia, 40:444, 1985.
136. Kim, J.M.: The tracheal tube cuff pressure stabilizer and its clinical evaluation. Anesth. Analg., 59:291, 1980.
137. Konchigeri, H.N., and Lee Y.E.: Preventive measure against nitrous oxide induced volume and pressure changes of endotracheal tube cuffs. Middle East J Anesthesiol., 5:369, 1979.
138. Collins, V.J.: Principles of Anesthesiology, 2nd ed. Philadelphia, Lea & Febiger, 1977.
139. Latto, I.P., Rosen M. (Eds.): Difficulties in Tracheal Intubation. England: Bailliere Tindall, p. 71; 1985.
140. Stanley, T.H., Foote, J.L., and Liu, W.S.: A simple pressure relief valve to prevent increases in endotracheal cuff pressure and volume in intubated patients. Anesthesiology, 43:478, 1975.
141. McGinnis, G.E., et al.: An engineering analysis of intratracheal cuffs. Anesth. Analg., 50:557, 1971.
142. Macgovern, G.J., et al.: The clinical and experimental evaluation of a controlled-pressure intratracheal cuff. J. Thorac. Cardiovasc. Surg., 64:747, 1972.
143. Bernhard, W.N., et al.: Adjustment to intracuff pressure to prevent aspiration. Anesthesiology, 50:363, 1979.
144. Bernhard, W.N., et al.: Cuffed tracheal tubes: Physical and behavioral characteristics. Anesth. Analg., 61:36, 1982.
145. Bernhard, W.H., et al.: Just seal intracuff pressures during mechanical ventilation. Anesthesiology, 57:A145, 1982.
146. Seegobin, R.D., and Van Hasselt, G.L.: Aspiration beyond endotracheal tubes. Can. Anaesth. Soc. J., 33:273, 1986.
147. Bone, D.K., et al.: Aspiration pneumonia: Prevention of aspiration in patients with tracheostomies. Ann. Thorac. Surg., 18:30, 1974.
148. Loeser, E.H., et al.: Reduction in postoperative sore throat with new endotracheal tube cuffs. Anesthesiology, 52:227, 1980.
149. Jensen, R.J.: Sore throat after operation: Influence of tra-

cheal intubation, intracuff pressure and type of cuff. Br. J. Anaesth. 54:453, 1982.
150. Stenqvist O., Nilsson K.: Postoperative sore throat related to tracheal tube cuff design. Can. Anaesth. Soc. J. 29:384, 1982.
151. Seuffert, G.W., and Urbach, K.F.: An additional hazard to endotracheal intubation. Can. Anaesth. Soc. J., 15:300, 1968.
151a. Perel, A., et al.: Collapse of endotracheal tubes due to overinflation of high pressure cuffs. Anesth. Analg., 56:731, 1977.
152a. Chan, M.C.J.: Collapse of endotracheal tubes. Anaesth. Intensive Care, 9:289, 1981.
152b. Hartnett, J.S.: Aberrant inflation of disposable endotracheal tubes with complete airway obstruction. J. Am. Assoc. Nurse Anesth., 38:37, 1980.
153. Ketover, A.K., and Feingold, A.: Collapse of a disposable tube by its high-pressure cuff. Anesthesiology, 48:108, 1975.
154. Paegle, R.D., Agnes, S.M., and Davis, S.: Rapid tracheal injury by cuffed airways and healing with loss of ciliated epithelium. Arch. Surg., 106:31, 1973.
155. Hackl H., Koenig G.: Experimental investigations concerning resistance of the trachea against inflatable cuffs. Der Anesthetist 8:134, 1961.
156. Ellis, P.D.M., and Pallister, W.K.: Recurrent laryngeal nerve palsy and endotracheal intubation. J. Laryngol. Otol., 89:823, 1975.
157. Hahn, F.W., Jr., Martin, J.T., and Lillie, J.C.: Vocal-cord paralysis with endotracheal intubation. Arch. Otolaryngol., 92:226, 1970.
158. Lennon, B.B., and Rovenstine, E.A.: Fatality following rupture of inflatable cuff in endotracheal airway. Anesth. Analg., 18:217, 1939.
159. Gould, A.B., and Seldon, T.H.: An unusual complication with a cuffed endotracheal tube. Anesth. Analg., 47:239, 1968.
160. Tashayod, M., and Oskoni, B.: A case of difficult intubation. Anesthesiology, 39:337, 1978.
161. Macintosh R.R.: Self-inflating cuff for endotracheal tubes. Br. Med. J. 2:234, 1978.
162. Merav, A.D.: Low-pressure "parachute" endotracheal cuff. N.Y. St. J. Med., 71:1926, 1971.
163. Kamen, J.D., and Wilkinson, C.J.: A new low pressure cuff for endotracheal tubes. Anesthesiology, 34:482, 1971.
164. Elam, J.O., and Johnson, E.R.: Another look at endotracheal cuff behavior. Lecture Course, Department of Anesthesiology, University of Texas, Southwestern Medical School, Dallas, Texas, 1978.
165a. Tracheal Tube Connectors and Adapters ANSI Z79.2, 1976, American National Standards Institute, 1430 Broadway, New York, N.Y. 10060.
165b. Standards for 22 mm Anesthesia Breathing Circuit Connectors Pamphlet M-1, Compressed Gas Association, Inc. 500 Fifth Ave. New York, N.Y. 10036, 1972.
166. Salem, M.R., Mathubithian, M., and Bennett, E.J.: Difficult intubation. N. Engl. J. Med., 295:879, 1976.
167. Rao, T.L.K., et al.: Experience with a new intubation guide for difficult tracheal intubation. Crit. Care Med., 10:882, 1982.
168. Wright, R.B., and Manfield, F.F.V.: Damage to teeth during the administration of general anesthesia. Anesth. Analg., 53:405, 1974.
169. Rosenberg, M., and Bolgla, J.: Protection of teeth and gums during endotracheal intubation. Anesth. Analg., 47:34, 1968.
170. Aromaa, U., et al.: Difficulties with tooth protectors in endotracheal intubation. Acta Anaesthesiol. Scand., 32:304, 1988.
171. Magill, I.W.: Forceps for endotracheal anesthesia. Br. Med. J., 2:670, 1920.
172. Loeser, E.A., et al.: The influence of endotracheal tube cuff design and cuff lubrication on postoperative sore throat. Anesthesiology, 58:376, 1983.
173. Granatelli, A.: Studies at Bellevue Hospital, N.Y., N.Y. 1959 Personal Communication.
174. Loeser, E.A., et al.: Postoperative sore throat: Influence of tracheal tube lubrication versus cuff design. Can. Anaesth. Soc. J., 27:156, 1980.
175. Fenje, N., and Steward, D.J.: A study of tape adhesive strength on endotracheal tubes. Can. J. Anaesth., 35:198, 1988.
176. Steward, D.J.: Fixation of reinforced silicone tracheal tubes. Anesthesiology, 63:334, 1985.
177. Conrady, P.A., Goodman, L.R.: Alteration of endotracheal tube position. Crit. Care Med., 4:8, 1976.
178. Bloch, E.C., Ossey, K., and Ginsberg, B.: Tracheal intubation in children: A new method for assuring correct depth of tube placement. Anesth. Analg., 67:590, 1988.
179a. Rosen, M., and Hilliard, E.K.: The use of suction in clinical medicine. Br. J. Anaesth., 32:486, 1960.
179b. Graff, M., et al.: Prevention of hypoxia and hyperoxia during endotracheal Suctioning. Crit. Care Med., 15:1133, 1987.
180. ISO Technical Committee TC 212, 1983.
181. Marchildon, M.B.: Physiologic considerations in the newborn surgical patient. Surg. Clin. North Am., 56:245, 1976.
182. Downes, J.J., and Raphaely, R.: Pediatric intensive care. Anesthesiology, 43:242, 1975.
183. Nelson, W.: Textbook of Pediatrics. In The Harriet Lane Handbook, 7th ed. Edited by D.L. Headings. Chicago, Year Book Medical Publishers, 1975.
184. Smith, R.M.: Anesthesia for Infants and Children, 4th ed. St. Louis, C.V. Mosby, 1980.
185. Gregory, G.A.: Pediatric Anesthesia. New York, Churchill Livingstone, 1983.
186. Eckenhoff, J.E.: Some anatomic considerations of the infant larynx influencing endotracheal anesthesia. Anesthesiology, 12:407, 1951.
187. Westhorpe, R.N.: The position of the larynx in children and its relationship to the ease of intubation. Anaesth. Intensive Care 15:384, 1987.
188. Stephen, C.R.: Technics in pediatric anesthesia: The nonrebreathing method. Anesthesiology, 13:77, 1952.
189. Ryan, J.F., et al.: A practice of Anesthesia for Infants and Children. Orlando, Grune and Stratton, p. 39; 1986.
190. American National Standard for Anesthetic Equipment—Tracheal Tubes. ANSI Z79.14–1983, American National Standards Institute, 1430 Broadway, New York, NY 10018.
191. Shupak R.C., Deas T.C.: The ideal tracheal tube. Proceedings of a Workshop on Tracheal Tubes, Valley Forge, Pa., April 30–May 1, 1981. pp. 103.
192. Cole F.: An endotracheal tube for babies. Anesthesiology, 6:627, 1945.
193. Cole, F.: A new endotracheal tube for infants. Anesthesiology, 6:87, 1945.
194. Ring, W.H., Adair, J.C., Elwyn R.A.: A new pediatric endotracheal tube. Anesth. Analg., 54:273, 1975.
195. Chodoff, P., and Helrich, M.: Factors affecting endotracheal tube size: A statistical analysis. Anesthesiology, 28:779, 1967.
196. Lee, K.W., Templeton, J., and Dougal, R.M.: Tracheal tube

size and postintubation croup in children. Anesthesiology, 53:S325, 1980.
197. Finholt, D.A., Henry, D.B., and Raphaely, R.C.: Factors affecting leak around endotracheal tubes in children. Can. Anaesth. Soc. J., 32:326, 1985.
198. Koka, B.V., et al.: Postintubation croup in children. Anesth. Analg., 56:501, 1977.
199. Brown, E.S.: Resistance factors in pediatric endotracheal tubes and connectors. Anesth. Analg., 50:355, 1971.
200a. Glauser, E.M., Cook, C.K., Bougas, T.P.: Pressure-flow characteristics and dead spaces of endotracheal tubes used in infants. Anesthesiology, 22:339, 1961.
200b. Swyer, P.R., Reiman, R.C., and Wright, J.J.: Ventilation and ventilatory mechanics in the newborn. J. Pediatr., 56:612, 1960.
201. Polgar, G.: Airway resistance in the newborn infant. J. Pediatr., 59:915, 1961.
202. Blom, H., Rytlander, M., and Wisborg, T.: Resistance of tracheal tubes 3.0 and 3.5 mm internal diameter: A comparison of four commonly used types. Anaesthesia, 40:885, 1985.
203. Roy, W.L.: Intraoperative aspiration in a paediatric patient. Can. Anaesth. Soc. J., 32:639, 1985.
204. Leigh, M.D., and Belton, M.K.: Pediatric Anesthesiology, 2nd ed. New York, Macmillan, 1960.
205. Smith, R.M.: Anesthesia for Infants and Children, 4th ed. St. Louis, C.V. Mosby, 1980.
206. Ballantine, R.I.W., and Jackson, I.: Pediatrics, Vol. I, Abt IA. Philadelphia, W.B. Saunders, 1923, p. 345.
207. Butz, R.O. Jr.: Length and cross section growth patterns in human trachea. Pediatrics, 42:336, 1968; Am. Acad. Peds., 1968.
208. Shellinger R.R.: The length of the airway to the bifurcation of the trachea. Anesthesiology, 25:169, 1964.
209. Cole, F.: Correspondence. Anesthesiology, 14:506, 1953.
210. McIntyre, J.W.R.: Endotracheal tube for children. Anaesthesia, 12:94, 1957.
211. Levine, J.: Endotracheal tube in children. Anaesthesia, 13:40, 1958.
212a. Richards, S.D.: A method for securing pediatric endotracheal tubes. Anesth. Analg., 60:224, 1981.
212b. Steward, D.J.: Fixation of reinforced silicone tracheal tubes. Anesthesiology, 63:334, 1985.
213. Toung, J.K., et al.: Movement of the distal end of the endotracheal tube during flexion and extension of the neck. Anesth. Analg., 64:1030, 1985.
214. Kuhns, L., and Poznanski, A.: Endotracheal tube position in the infant. J. Pediatr., 78:991, 1971.
215. Todres, I.D., et al: Endotracheal tube displacement in the newborn infant. J. Pediatr., 89:126, 1976.
216. Rosen, M., Hilliard, E.K.: The use of suction in clinical medicine. Br. J. Anaesth., 32:486, 1960.
217. Coté, C., Todres, I.D.: The pediatric airway in A Practice of Anesthesia for Infants and Children, J.F. Ryan, I.D. Todres, C.J. Coté, N.G. Goudsouzian, Eds. Orlando, Grune & Stratton, 1985.
218. Abbott, T.R.: Complications of prolonged nasotracheal intubation in children. Br. J. Anaesth. 40:347, 1968.
219. Maze, A., Bloch, E.: Stridor in pediatric patients. Anesthesiology, 50:132, 1980.
220. Holinger, P.H., Johnston, K.C.: Factors responsible for laryngeal obstruction in infants. J.A.M.A., 143:1229, 1950.

APPENDIX

Originator	Date	SPATULA Straight	SPATULA Curved	FLANGE CROSS-SECTION Semi-flat —	FLANGE CROSS-SECTION Flat —	FLANGE CROSS-SECTION "O" type O	FLANGE CROSS-SECTION "C" type C	FLANGE CROSS-SECTION Flat "C" U	FLANGE CROSS-SECTION "U" type ∪	FLANGE CROSS-SECTION "Z" type N	BLADE-TIP Flat	BLADE-TIP Curved	BLADE-TIP Uplift
Kirstein	1895	x		x								x	x
Kirstein	1896		x		x						x		
Killian	1904	x				x						x	
Jackson	1907	x				x					x		
Jackson (Diagnostic)	1907	x				x						x	
Jackson	1907	x				x						x	
Bruening	1909	x							x		x		
Hill	1909	x					x					x	
Jackson (Oval)	1913	x					x					x	
Janeway	1913		x			x						x	
Janeway	1913		x			x						x	
Magill	1920	x					x				x		x
Guedel	1927	x							x			x	
Flagg	1928	x					x					x	
Elam	1935	x						x			x		x
Seldon	1938	x								x	x		
Miller	1941		x					x				x	
Murphy	1941	x						Flat x				x	x
MacIntosh	1943		x						x		x		
Bennett	1943	x									x	x	
Searles	1950	x		x								x	x
Fink	1955		x						x		x		

			HANDLE			LIGHT			
Ridge	Slot	Hook	U type	L type	Angle if other than 90°	Proximal	Distal	Internal	COMMENT
			x			x			Fashioned from a tube by removal of a segment from its length
			x			No intrinsic light			Used to elevate epiglottis indirectly
			x			No intrinsic light			Separable to facilitate introduction of bronchoscope
			x			No intrinsic light			Separable to facilitate introduction of bronchoscope
			x				x		Primarily for laryngoscopy; uses the Einhorn light carrier; not separable
			x				x		Used prior to and as aid to bronchoscopy
			x			x			Side opening is an aid to instrumentation
			x					x	Side opening is an aid to instrumentation
			x				x		Popular as aid to tracheal intubation after 1913
				x			x		For anesthetists—tube was passed through lumen; telescope and prism used
				x			x		Telescope and prism eliminated in this model; battery contained in handle
			x					x	Originally used mainly to aid nasotracheal intubation
				x	72°		x		Accommodates large-diameter tubes for orotracheal intubation
				x			x		Intended originally for passing Flagg tubes through bore of laryngoscope
			x					x	Tip uplift improves visibility and ease of intubation
				x			x		Aid to nasotracheal intubation when mouth cannot be opened widely
x				x			x		For patients with long narrow "rabbity" oral cavity
				x			x		For partial ankylosis of jaw
				x				x	Indirect technique used to elevate epiglottis
				x	72°		x		For severe ankylosis of jaw
				x			x		Dually lighted; for right- or left-handed operator
				x			x		Used like curved Macintosh

20

ENDOTRACHEAL ANESTHESIA: II. TECHNICAL CONSIDERATIONS

EVALUATION OF THE AIRWAY

PREINTUBATION EVALUATION. The anesthesiologist should anticipate difficulties in intubating patients and should recognize obstacles before beginning the procedure. The following considerations are crucial:

1. Patient history of vocal or nasal difficulties and of operations of the eye, nose, mouth, or throat.
2. Anatomic developmental syndromes (see Appendix)
   a. Recognize facial abnormalities.
   b. Note existence of congenital syndromes; most are symmetric. The following are illustrative:
      (1) *Hypertelorism* is caused by an enlarged sphenoid bone with wide nasal bridge. Exophthalmos is present; eyes are wide apart as a result of embryologic arrest in migration of orbits; and it is associated with mental retardation.
      (2) *Crouzon's disease,* caused by the premature closure of cranial sutures, consists of hypertelorism with well-developed mandible, hypoplastic maxilla, prominent nose, and mild facial hypoplasia.
      (3) *Apert's syndrome* combines abnormalities of Crouzon's disease with webbed fingers and toes. This syndrome and Crouzon's malformation are inherited as a dominant Mendelian disorder.
      (4) *Treacher-Collins syndrome* consists of mandibulofacial synostosis as a result of maldevelopment of first branchial arch (receding jaw). There is a hypoplastic mandible with macrostomia, choanalatresia, and generalized underdevelopment.
      (5) *Pierre-Robin syndrome* includes underdeveloped mandible (micrognathia) with microstomia, glossoptosis, posterior displacement of the tongue, relative macroglossia, and cleft palate (50%).
      (6) *Klippel-Feil syndrome* is associated with synostosis of the cervical vertebrae.
      (7) *Ellis van Creveld Dwarfism* is a syndrome of chondroectodermal dysplasia, which is

a form of dwarfism that appears in Amish people. Characteristics include a hypoplastic maxilla, hepatosplenomegaly, and polydactylism. A congenital cardiac defect is present—usually a single atrium or a septal defect.

(8) *Arnold-Chiari deformity* is a premature closure of the cranial sutures producing craniosynarthrosis, which results in an elongated but flattened medulla oblongata and cerebellum, with protrusion through the foramen magnum into the spinal canal. The condition is associated with spina bifida occulta and meningomyelocele. Extreme care in moving the head during intubation is mandatory.

3. Clinical review of airway
   a. Patency of nares: determine by inspection and by sniffing; note obstructions or deviated septa (Fig. 20-1).
   b. Examination of jaws: note any restrictions, ankylosis, or trismus under or overgrowth (Fig. 20-2).
   c. Examine oral cavity for size of tongue, condition of teeth, and the ability to protrude the tongue (Fig. 20-3).
   d. Flexion–extension ability of neck (Fig. 20-4 and Fig. 20-5).
   e. Deviation or compression of trachea—detected by inspection of the neck and review of roentgenograms
   f. Action of vocal cords—evaluation of quality of voice
   g. Indirect laryngoscopy

STANDARD PROCEDURE FOR AIRWAY ASSESSMENT. In the presence of facial and neck deformities, the anesthesiologist readily anticipates difficulties in airway management and endoscopic manipulation. When subtle anatomic abnormalities exist, they can cause difficulty in management.

A complete evaluation of the mouth, nose, pharynx, neck, and head therefore, is necessary to reveal potential problems, and it is recommended that a standard procedure (Table 20-1) be followed.

Application of Standards. The predictive value of a difficult intubation is based on abnormal anatomic conditions. A single factor may make laryngoscopy and intubation difficult. A combination of factors, however, is usually present.

The following conditions present an ideal situation for intubation (see Fig. 20-8):

1. A mobile mandible without temporomandibular joint limitation (Fig. 20-6)
2. A mouth that opens widely—at least 3 fingerbreadths in an adult (Fig. 20-7)
3. Clear visualization of the mouth, pharynx, and faucial pillars
4. Normal size of intraoral cavity and tongue
5. Full range of motion of head and neck
6. No pathology

Table 20-2 presents a clinical checklist for evaluation of intubation conditions, the so-called "table of T's."

INDICATORS OF DIFFICULT INTUBATION. The classic signs alerting the operator to difficulty of intubation are as follows:

1. Poor flexion–extension mobility of the head on the neck[1,2] (see Fig. 20-9)
2. A receding mandible[3] and presence of prominent teeth (Fig. 20-10)
3. A reduced atlanto–occipital distance; a reduced space between C1 and the occiput[4]
4. Large tongue size[5,6]—related more to the ratio of

FIG. 20-1. Anterior viewing and palpation of neck. Pathology of the neck should be first identified. If absent, three measurements of size and distance should be noted or made: the pointed chin (narrow submental angle), the hypomental distance (HM), and the thyromental distance (TM). Difficult intubation is likely if HM is less than 5 cm and/or TM is less than 6 cm. From McIntyre, J.W.R.: Continuing medical education: The difficult tracheal intubation. Can. J. Anaesth., 34:204, 1987.

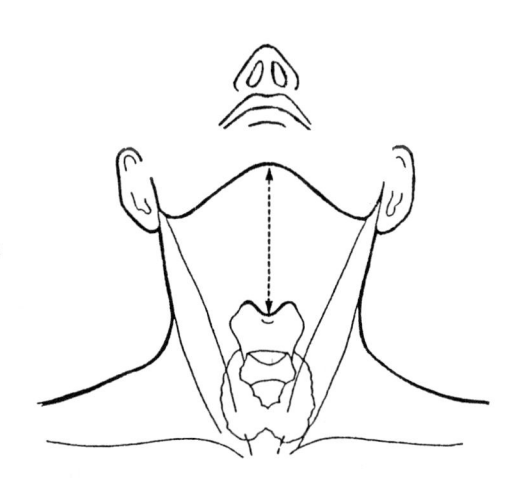

	Yes	No
Nasal Passages Clear		
Submental Angle Narrow		
Submental Swelling		
Submandibular Swelling		
Suprathyroid Notch to Chin Distance <6 cm		
Trachea Deviated		
Neck Swelling		
Neck Scarring		
Antesternal Mass		

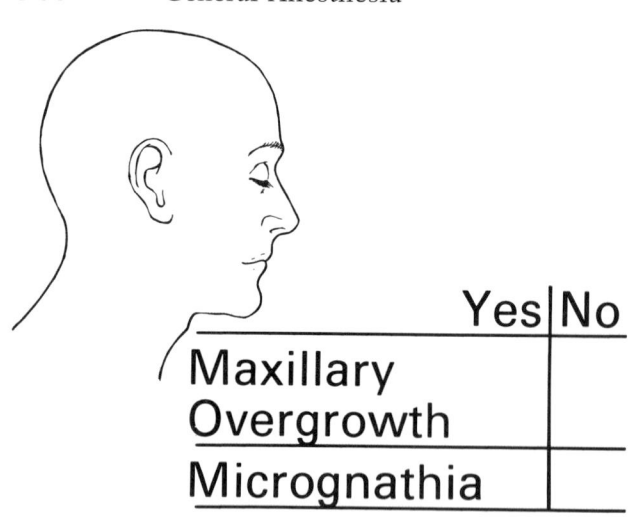

FIG. 20–2. Lateral/anterolateral viewing. From McIntyre, J.W.R.: Continuing medical education: The difficult tracheal intubation. Can. J. Anaesth., *34:*204, 1987.

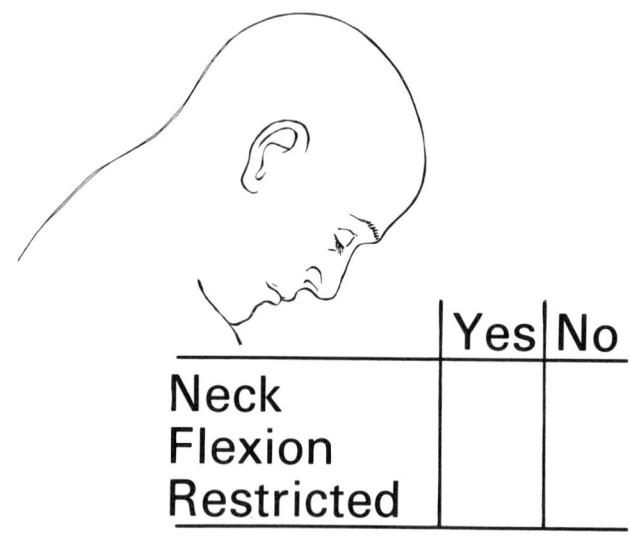

FIG. 20–4. Neck flexion. From McIntyre, J.W.R.: Continuing medical education: The difficult tracheal intubation. Can. J. Anaesth., *34:*204, 1987.

the anterior length of the tongue to the length of the chin or mandible

In 1983, Nichol[7] reported that when the head is extended there is an anterior bowing of the cervical spine, as demonstrated by x-ray. This has been widely interpreted as "the anterior larynx;" however, the cervical spine bowing is related to the failure to place the head in a "sniffing position," and "lifting" with the laryngoscope blade—not prying. In the absence of unusual spinal abnormalities, the sniffing–lifting sequence will straighten the cervical spine and reduce any forward thrust on the larynx. (And the larynx will always remain anatomically anterior to the spine!)

Other abnormalities can occasionally cause difficulty, but these are readily recognized and the intubation technique then appropriately planned. Such conditions are poor mouth opening, prominent maxilla, narrow palate, oropharyngeal tumors, and neck scarring from burrs, trauma, or postsurgical distortion.

Analysis of Anatomic Factors. In an analysis by Bellhouse[8] of some 22 of the varying anatomic factors and measurements of the airway in patients who are hard to intubate, difficulty was clearly related to reduced head extension, reduced chin protrusion, and increased tongue size. According to this

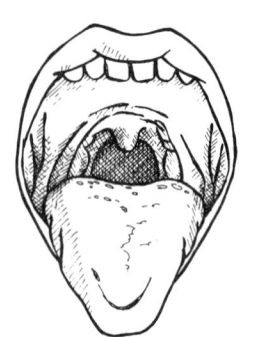

FIG. 20–3. Viewing of mouth, teeth, and oral cavity. Opening of mouth by a minimum of two fingers in average adult should be noted and the visualization of structure assessed on Mallampati score. From McIntyre, J.W.R.: Continuing medical education: The difficult tracheal intubation. Can. J. Anaesth., *34:*204, 1987.

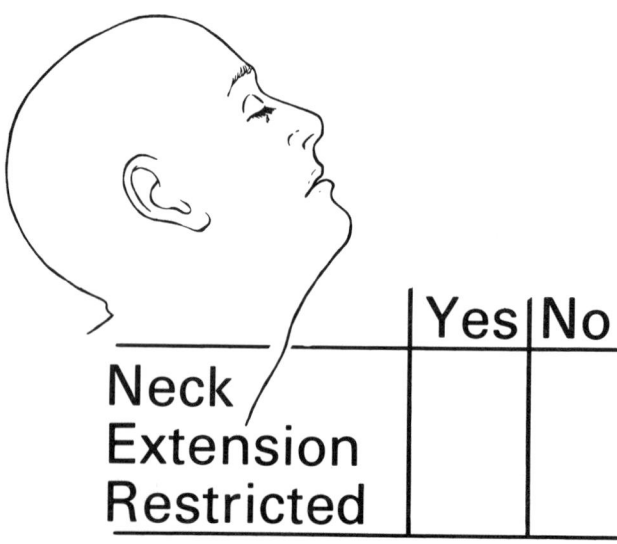

FIG. 20–5. Neck extension. From McIntyre, J.W.R.: Continuing medical education: The difficult tracheal intubation. Can. J. Anaesth., *34:*204, 1987.

TABLE 20–1. SIX STANDARDS IN THE EVALUATION OF AIRWAY

- Temporomandibular mobility *(one finger)* (Fig. 20–6)
- Inspection of mouth and oropharynx and classifying these features on the Mallampati* score *(two fingers)* (see Fig. 20–2)
- Measurement of mandibular length from chin (mental) to hyoid—4 cm in adult *(three fingers)* (Fig. 20–7)
- Measurement of distance from chin to thyroid notch—5 to 6 cm *(four fingers)* or greater in adult (Fig. 20–8)
- Ability to flex head toward chest, extend head at atlanto-occipital junction, and rotate head right and left *(five movements)* (Fig. 20–9)
- Symmetry of nose and patency of nasal passage

* See discussion in text.

study, the following can be assessed at the bedside without the aid of indirect laryngoscopy:

1. Failure to see the soft palate in the seated position when the mouth is fully opened and the tongue protruded, or failure to see the uvula under the above conditions[5]
2. Atlanto–occipital extension reduced by more than one third because of an abnormal atlanto–occipital joint (in a normal atlanto–occipital joint, 35 degrees of extension are possible).[1,2] Radiologically, there is reduced space between C1 and the occiput (see Fig. 20–9).
3. A recessed chin (reduced mandibular protrusion or size) so that less than 2.5 cm lies in front of the line of vision[3] (see Fig. 20–10)
4. Large tongue size, more related to the ratio of the anterior length of the tongue to the length of the chin [6,8]

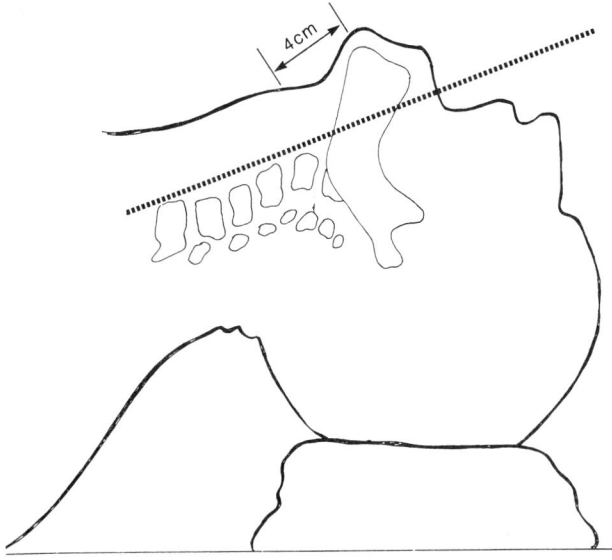

FIG. 20–7. The hyoid–chin measurement: The distance in the adult should be at least 6 cm, or three fingerbreadths. From McIntyre, J.W.R.: Continuing medical education: The difficult tracheal intubation. Can. J. Anaesth., *34*:204, 1987.

PREDICTION OF DIFFICULT INTUBATION ON LARYNGOSCOPY.[9] On laryngoscopy, difficulty in intubation can be assessed according to degrees of difficulty that are classified into four grades. This assumes that laryngoscopy is properly performed and that adequate relaxation exists. The classification is as follows: (1) glottis visible (almost entirely); (2) only the posterior commissure of the glottis is visible; (3) no part of the glottis but the epiglottis is visible; or (4) the epiglottis is not visible. These observations are

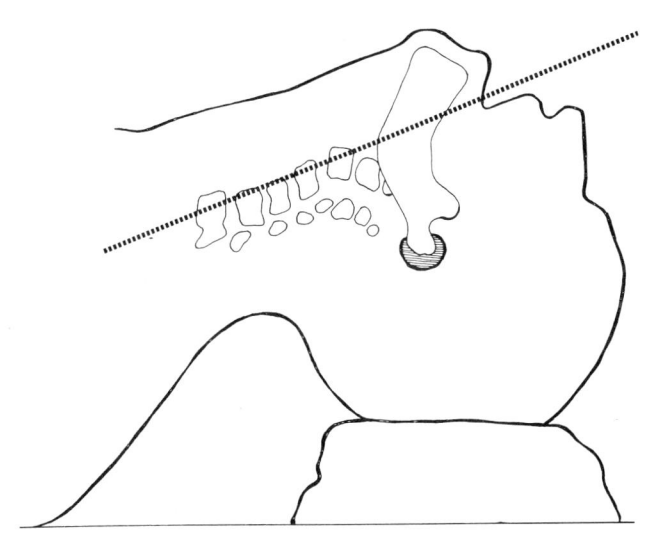

FIG. 20–6. Temporomandibular mobility. From McIntyre, J.W.R.: Continuing medical education: The difficult tracheal intubation. Can. J. Anaesth., *34*:204, 1987.

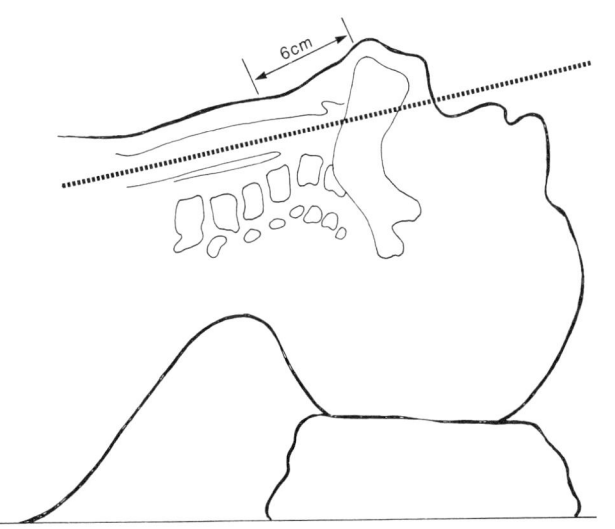

FIG. 20–8. Ideal situation. From McIntyre, J.W.R.: Continuing medical education: The difficult tracheal intubation. Can. J. Anaesth., *34*:204, 1987.

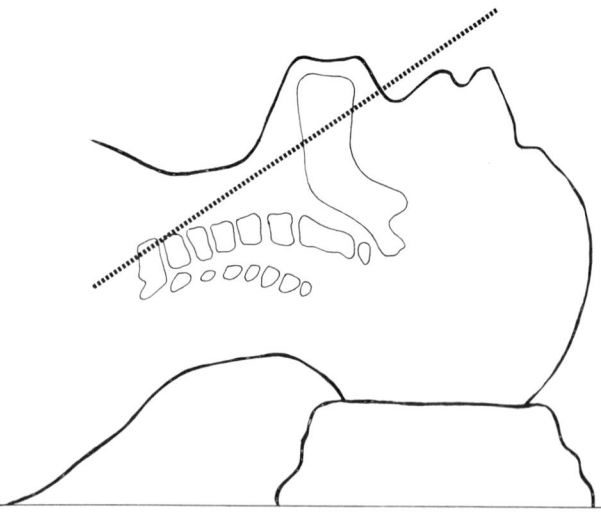

FIG. 20–9. Rigid cervical spine. The curved Macintosh blade is the choice. Lifting of the mandible away from the face at a 45-degree angle is necessary. The nasotracheal route or placement of a retrograde catheter inserted below the cricoid and advanced into the pharynx and mouth can serve as a thread. Fiberoptic bronchoscopy should be available as back-up. From McIntyre, J.W.R.: Continuing medical education: The difficult tracheal intubation. Can. J. Anaesth., 34:204, 1987.

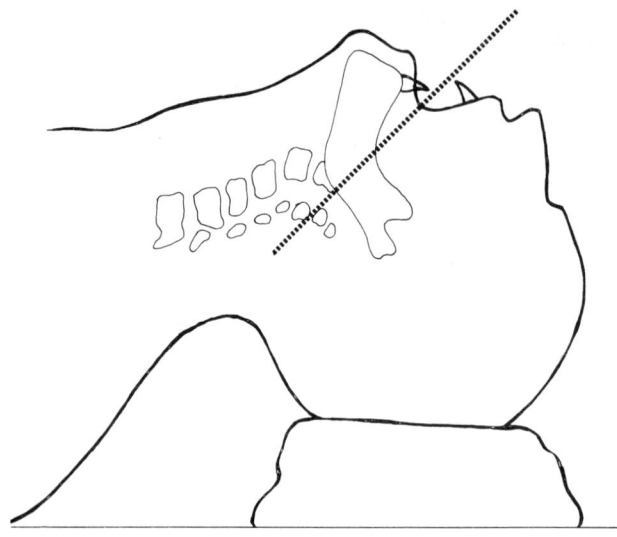

FIG. 20–10. Prominent teeth. The Macintosh blade is the choice. Lifting the mandible at an angle of 45 degrees away from face is necessary. From McIntyre, J.W.R.: Continuing medical education: The difficult tracheal intubation. Can. J. Anaesth., 34:204, 1987.

confirmatory of the bedside preoperative evaluation and score of Mallampati.

It is evident that classes 3 and 4 often represent conditions in which there is ankylosis of the mandible or neck, oral pathology with tumors or infection, and the condition of the epiglottis and edematous tongue.

The Macintosh laryngoscope has a total curve of almost 30 degrees and can negotiate most tight oropharyngeal corners.[8] Sometimes it cannot elevate the hyoid bone and, hence, the epiglottis, especially when the latter is floppy.[10] Under these circumstances, a straight-blade technique will solve the problem by directly lifting the epiglottis.

TABLE 20–2. TABLE OF T's: A CLINICAL CHECKLIST FOR EVALUATION OF INTUBATION CONDITIONS

1. Teeth
2. Tongue (swallowing)
3. Tonsils (sore throats)
4. Temporomandibular joint
5. Torticollis (flexion-extension-rotation of neck)
6. Thyroid notch
7. Trachea
8. Tumors
9. Turbinates (snuffing)
10. Tuberculum pharygneum
11. Talk (voice)
12. Tales (history)

From Zymslowski, W.P., and Janfaza, P.: The T's of endotracheal intubation. Anesthesiology, 58:107, 1983.

SUMMARY OF ANATOMIC FACTORS THAT CAUSE DIFFICULT INTUBATION. Superficial anatomical features:

- Short, muscular neck
- Restricted flexion and extension of neck
- Poor mobility of mandible with temporomandibular joint stiffness or limitation
- Receding mandible ("Andy Gump" jaw) (micrognathia) and obtuse mandibular angles
- Maxillary overgrowth

Anatomical measurements:

- Suprahyoid notch to chin distance short (less than 6 cm or three fingers in adult men)
- Thyroid notch to chin less than 7 cm or four fingers in adult male weighing 70 kg
- Full set of teeth; large or loose teeth
- Protruding maxillary incisor teeth ("buck teeth")

Oropharyngeal anatomy:

- Mouth opening restricted or narrow
- Oral cavity narrow and space restricted for maneuvering laryngoscopic blade
- Palate long or highly arched
- Faucial pillars not readily seen
- Large tongue
- Uvula not visualized
- Enlarged tonsils
- Patency of nares poor

PREDICTION OF DIFFICULT INTUBATION BY MALLAMPATI SCORE. Anatomic abnormalities, as well as pathologic conditions of the head, oral cavity, and neck are obvious situations that indicate that laryngoscopy and intubation would be difficult. One

FIG. 20–11. Correlation Between Visibility of Pharyngeal Structures and Exposure of Glottis by Direct Laryngoscopy According to Number of Patients (%). From Mallampati, S.R., et al.: A clinical sign to predict difficult tracheal intubation: A prospective study. Can. Anaesth. Soc. J., 32:429, 1985.

Visibility of Structures	Laryngoscopy Grade			
	Grade 1	Grade 2	Grade 3	Grade 4
Class 1 155(73.8%)	125(59.5%)	30(14.3%)	—	—
Class 2 40(19%)	12(5.7%)	14(6.7%)	10(4.7%)	4(1.9%)
Class 3 15(7.14%)	—	1(0.5%)	9(4.3%)	5(2.4%)

Class 1: Faucial pillars, soft palate, and uvula could be visualized. *Class 2:* Faucial pillars and soft palate could be visualized, but uvula was masked by the base of the tongue. *Class 3:* Only soft palate could be visualized. *Grade 1:* Glottis (including anterior and posterior commissures) could be fully exposed. *Grade 2:* Glottis could be partly exposed (anterior commissure not visualized). *Grade 3:* Glottis could not be exposed (corniculate cartilages only could be visualized). *Grade 4:* Glottis including corniculate cartilages could not be exposed.

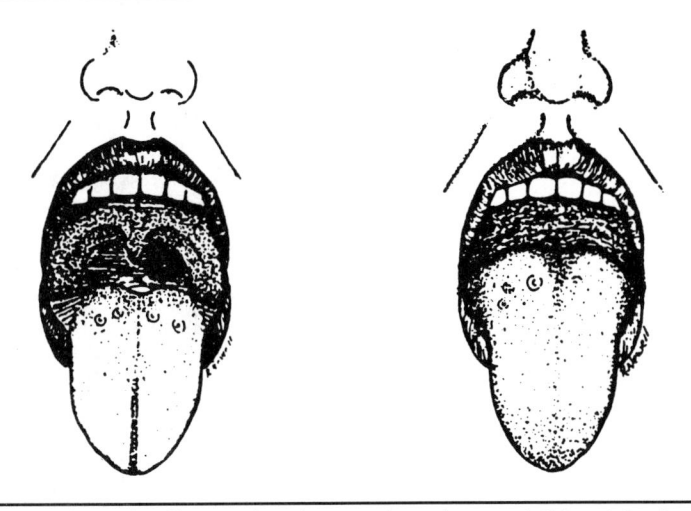

Left: Note that faucial pillars, soft palate, and uvula are visible; *right*, in this patient, these pharyngeal structures are not visible.

clinical sign that can be used to predict a difficult laryngoscopy is concealment of the faucial pillars as well as the uvula by the base of the tongue (see Fig. 20–3 and Fig. 20–11). This is particularly evident when the tongue is disproportionately large for the oral cavity and offers some obstruction to visualization of the larynx. It is a key sign in the standards of evaluation.

Examination is carried out as follows. In the preoperative examination, patients, while seated, are asked to open their mouth and protrude their tongue as far as possible. Assessment of the visualization of the oropharyngeal cavity will allow the anesthesiologist to place the patients' airway in one of three classes, according to Mallampati: class I—faucial pillars, soft palate, and uvula readily visualized; class II—faucial pillars and soft palate visualized, but the uvula masked by the base of the tongue; and class III—only soft palate easily visualized.

Extent of Exposure of Glottis on Direct Laryngoscopy. This factor has been rated on a scale of 1 to 4: grade 1—glottis, including the anterior and posterior commissures, fully exposed and visualized; grade 2—glottis partially exposed and visualized; anterior commissure not visualized; grade 3—glottis not exposed and commissures not visualized; only the corniculate cartilages visualized; and grade 4—neither glottis nor corniculate cartilages are visualized. The epiglottis tip may be observed.

SPECIAL CONDITIONS CONTRIBUTING TO DIFFICULT INTUBATION.[11]

EPIGLOTTIC ABNORMALITIES. Many abnormalities of the epiglottis render visualization of the glottis incomplete or impossible.[12] These may be considered under the headings of: congenital defects (bifid; hypoplastic; absent); tumors (sarcoid; cysts[12]; lingual–epiglottic cysts); infective (epiglottitis; tuberculosis; edema with upper respiratory infection); and structural (abnormal size and angulation).[13]

DYSFUNCTION OF TEMPOROMANDIBULAR JOINT.[14] A number of clinical conditions result in a stiff temporomandibular joint or immobility as a result of disorders in surrounding structures. These conditions should be determined by both history and examination. Examination of the temporomandibular joint should be performed correctly by placing the thumb of one hand behind the ear lobe and the index finger of the same hand anterior to the tragus into the coronoid process and pressing deep into the joint. The patient should be asked to open and close the mouth and "wiggle" the jaw.

The following is a summary of temporomandibular joint dysfunctions:

1. Indirect (false) ankylosis due to:
    a. Burns
    b. Trauma
    c. Radiotherapy
    d. Malformation or fracture of coronoid process
    e. Myopathy of temporalis muscle
    f. Trismus-infections (local organisms) (viral "flu")
    g. Following surgery of head and neck or craniotomy (temporal fossa) (see below)[15]
2. Direct (true) ankylosis due to:
    a. Polyostotic fibrous dysplasia
    b. Diabetic "stiff joint" syndrome
    c. Miscellaneous

Ankylosis of the Temporomandibular Joint (Postcraniotomy).[15]

One overlooked cause of difficult intubation is the ankylosis of the temporomandibular joint, which frequently develops after temporal craniotomy. Surgery in the region of the temporal fossa often results in contracture of the temporalis muscle with "pseudoankylosis" of the jaw. Causes of the contracture include postincisional scar formation in skin and muscle; Volkmann's contracture due to ischemia of the muscle; or hematoma or fluid accumulation. It is recommended that passive and active jaw exercises be started after surgery and that these postcraniotomy patients be carefully evaluated for subsequent anesthetics.[15]

LARYNGEAL CYSTS. Cysts of the larynx are infrequently encountered, and the true incidence is unknown. They are usually asymptomatic and benign. They are readily classified according to their position and according to the pathologic process that results in cyst formation. De Santo[16] reviewed a 10-year experience at the Mayo Clinic and classified these cysts into three categories, based on anatomic location and probable pathogenesis. These are as follows.

Ductal Cysts.
These cysts represent the most common type; they are located at the lingual surface of the epiglottis or at the free margin of the vocal cords.

Saccular Cysts.
These cysts comprise about 24% of those encountered. They are usually congenital and are found in the ventricle and the lateral portion of the larynx, including the free margin of the vocal cords, the arytenoid area, and the aryepiglottic folds, as well as the pyriform sinus. These cysts originate from the epithelial surface and usually contain mucus or air.

Thyroid Cartilage Foramenal Cysts.
These cysts are usually related to the thyroid cartilage and connected with the aryepiglottic folds and the arytenoid.

Although most of the laryngeal cysts are benign, they may be associated with carcinoma. Trauma, inflammation, or fibrosis may create a cyst.

If there is reason to suspect some form of obstruction, and if there is a voice change, careful examination in the awake patient is indicated. A lateral radiograph may be necessary to determine the extent of cysts and whether they are large and create any laryngeal deformity.

DIABETIC "STIFF JOINT SYNDROME".[17] This syndrome consists of the following: juvenile onset diabetes mellitus, short stature (nonfamilial), waxy skin, and joint contractures. The fourth and fifth phalangeal joints are the small joints frequently involved. Large joints, as of the cervical spine, are rarely involved, but limited motion at the atlanto–occipital joint may be seen with limited motion of extension and flexion of the head. This represents a cause of difficult laryngoscopy and intubation. Nasotracheal blind technique has been used successfully, but fiberoptic placement technique is recommended.

CALCIFIED STYLOHYOID LIGAMENTS.[18] An unusual condition of uncertain cause is the occurrence of calcified stylohyoid ligaments. This may be manifested by a crease over the hyoid bones; the condition can be observed in a radiologic examination. Laryngoscopy is difficult because of the inability to lift the epiglottis from the posterior pharyngeal wall because of its firm attachment to the hyoid by the hyoepiglottic ligament. Simultaneously, there is the splinting effect that the calcified ligaments have on the surrounding neck tissues.

When difficulty in lifting the epiglottis with a Macintosh blade is encountered, the following steps are recommended:

- Use a straight blade.
- Use a stylet with a small "hockey-stick" molding at the tip.
- Do an awake intubation if the condition is recognized in advance.

- Use blind intubation by following air sounds with patient spontaneously breathing.
- Use fiberoptic laryngoscopic technique.

KLIPPEL-FEIL SYNDROME[19] Patients with this syndrome are vulnerable to cervical spinal cord injury and the risk of neurologic damage during laryngoscopy and intubation. Significant features for anesthesia include Klippel-Feil syndrome, fusion of the cervical spine, a short neck, and elevated small scapula. Rapid rotation of the head and neck may precipitate a syncopal attack. Other associated abnormalities include spina bifida, cardiovascular anomalies, cleft palate, diminished neuromuscular capacity, and sleep ventilatory disorders.

FIBROUS DYSPLASIA (POLYOSTOTIC).[20] This is a disorder characterized by expanding fibro-osseous lesions in bone. Structural changes involve fractures from minor trauma of any bone, including the mandible. Rough laryngoscopy can be the cause of mandibular fracture. Spinal distortion with collapse of vertebrae and severe kyphoscoliosis occurs; this precludes spinal anesthesia.

In addition to the bony changes, there are endocrine abnormalities. Acromegaly, hyperparathyroidism, hyperthyroidism, and Cushing's syndrome are common. There may be significant salivation and mucus secretion.

Routine laryngoscopy and intubation are difficult, especially because of the macrognathia, but an endotracheal airway can be provided. When there is careful assessment of the existing anatomic problem, recognition of the risk and judicious planning can follow. Alternative techniques and preparations should be planned and include (these recommendations are also pertinent to acromegaly):

- Awake intubation under topical anesthesia.
- Explanation of the need to the patient and informing the patient of the steps in the procedure to secure cooperation.
- Standard monitoring: electrocardiogram, automatic blood pressure measurement, pulse oximeter.
- Premedication: tranquilization only IV, with small doses of midazolam and an opioid
  - Small doses of fentanyl (50 µg) or sufentanil (5.0 µg)
  - A generous dose of anticholinergic: atropine, 0.6 to 0.75 mg, in younger patients or glycopyrrolate 0.4 to 0.5 mg in patients over 50 years of age.
- Use a fiberoptic laryngoscope or bronchoscope as an introducer for the appropriate size endotracheal tube—longer than usual 30 cm.
- After securing the endotracheal airway, anesthesia can be induced and relaxation provided.

PARADOXIC VOCAL CORD MOTION. Acute airway obstruction manifested by stridor in the adult is uncommon. Causes include foreign body aspiration, infectious processes, anaphylactic reactions, trauma, vocal cord paralysis, and masses involving the larynx or adjacent structures. Airway obstruction in the adult or adolescent without diagnostic findings is rare.[21] Such functional stridor with acute dyspnea has been reported. On laryngoscopy, many of these patients show paradoxic vocal cord motion and this has been described as a syndrome.[22]

The clinical features are as follows: a history of chronic respiratory complaints, most commonly in women, including an asthma-like condition, hay fever, and allergic rhinitis. A triad of wheezing, nasal polyps, and aspirin sensitivity is reported, which is also seen in about 10% of asthmatic patients. Often a stress-related psychiatric history is present. Direct laryngoscopy reveals the following paradoxic vocal cord motion: adduction of the true vocal cords on inspiration and abduction on exhalation.

Anesthetic Considerations.[23] Patients should have a complete otolaryngologic evaluation as well as a psychiatric consultation prior to any anesthesia. Preanesthetic medication should be generous, and tranquilizers of the shorter acting phenothiazines (promethazine) or a benzodiazepine are recommended. If wheezing is a common feature, preoperative oral thiophylline, a beta$_2$-adrenergic agonist (terbutaline or metaproterenal) and aerosols of beclomethasone and metaproterenol are recommended.

- Regional anesthesia is recommended to avoid intubation.
- When general anesthesia is required, mask anesthesia is usually sufficient for minor procedures.
- When muscle relaxants and endotracheal anesthesia are indicated, the patient should be intubated in surgical planes of stage III, accompanied by IV lidocaine.
- Extubation should be accomplished while the patient is in light surgical planes but breathing spontaneously.
- Paradoxic airway obstruction is likely to occur in the postoperative period and seems related to both pain and general stress. Laryngoscopy should be performed to confirm paradoxic vocal cord motion.
- Postoperative respiratory therapy should include a helium–oxygen mixture to reduce turbulent gas flow at the vocal cords.
- If stridor is persistent despite conservative management, tracheostomy should be considered.

SPINE ABNORMALITIES.[24] Commonly encountered spinal abnormalities include cervical spine disease, injuries to the cervical spine (Fig. 20-9), and decreased distance between occipital and spinous process of C2 (axis) vertebra (often called the atlanto–occipital distance[25]) or the atlanto–occipital gap.[26]

TECHNIQUES OF INTUBATION

PREINTUBATION PREPARATION

1. Preliminary clearing of air passages
   a. Voluntary cough
   b. Nose blowing
2. Use of a mouthwash and gargle for reducing bacterial flora of mouth and throat
3. Use of topical vasoconstrictor when indicated
4. Preparation of equipment and selection of tubes; ointment with topical anesthetic is preferred for lubrication
5. Preoxygenation (see Chapter 16)
6. Ability to assist ventilation should be assessed before paralysis is induced

EQUIPMENT SET-UP. A tray for endotracheal anesthesia should be set up for each case. The preparation of this equipment should be meticulous and orderly. Ten items are noted as follows:

1. Laryngoscopes—one for backup and two-size blades
2. Tubes—selected sizes; one smaller than that estimated for appropriate size
3. Lubricant for tube—an anesthetic ointment
4. Forceps (introducing)—Magill
5. Bite block (pharyngeal airway)
6. Adhesive tape—two strips 0.5 inch wide, 10 inches long; ends tucked in
7. Suction—Yankauer sucker (plastic); catheter—proper size
8. Connectors
9. Pharyngeal pack may be needed in infants or children
10. Syringe—10 ml with blunt needle for inflating cuffs on tubes

Accessory items include:

1. Spray for topical anesthetics
2. Stylette for flexible tubes as anode (flexometallic; metal-spiral) tube

STANDARD METHODS OF INTUBATION AND ALTERNATIVES

1. Direct-vision orotracheal intubation
2. Nasotracheal intubation—blind (Magill) or visually assisted
3. Tactile intubation technique (insertion of tube by touch)
4. Awake intubation with topical anesthesia
5. Retrograde intubation
6. Fiberoptic intubation
7. Use of small suction catheter as a guide for the proper tube

Alternatives. Do *not* persist when extraordinary difficulties exist, but ventilate and awaken patient. If critical, insert a large-bore needle or cricotrachealtome through the cricotracheal or the first tracheotracheal membrane, not through the cricothyroid membrane.*[27]

Choice of Method. At the time of the preoperative visit, decisions must be made concerning the route of intubation—oral or nasal; whether intubation will be performed in an awake or unconscious state; and the type of anesthesia—general with relaxants.

DIRECT-VISION OROTRACHEAL INTUBATION

ANESTHESIA. Orotracheal intubation may be performed under either good general anesthesia or topical anesthesia. The general anesthesia must be deep enough to relax the mandibular muscles and to obtund the pharyngeal and laryngeal reflexes (stage III, plane 3 anesthesia). When these conditions prevail, laryngoscopy is facilitated and the glottis easily viewed.

The apneic relaxant technique is a popular method for intubation under general anesthesia. The production of light anesthesia is accompanied by a muscle relaxant. Succinylcholine has been a popular relaxant.[28] The newer muscle relaxants (vecuronium, atracurium) however, are preferred and can rapidly provide conditions for intubation if the "priming" technique is used. These agents avoid the adverse effects of succinylcholine and provide continuing relaxation for surgical needs. Generally, apnea or hypoventilation ensues.

In either the deep anesthesia technique or the relaxant apneic technique, unforeseen circumstances may be faced:

1. Distorted anatomy
2. Light failure of the laryngoscope
3. Lack of skill for the situation
4. Others (Table 20-3)

These conditions lead to hypoxia, which can be minimized by oxygenation just prior to laryngoscopy.

Lachman[29] showed that if patients inhaled 100% oxygen for 3 minutes, the blood arterial oxygen saturation remained at almost 100% for 10 minutes. This contrasts with the saturation in patients who were not ventilated with oxygen in whom saturation fell rapidly to dangerous levels during apnea or when patients were breathing only room air (average drop, 15%). During short periods of apnea (without prior oxygenation), disorders of heart rate and rhythm are pronounced.[30a] Oxygenation prior to production of apnea will delay electroencephalographic depression for 12 minutes.[30b]

Thus, prior oxygenation provides a pulmonary

---

* Introduction of large-bore needles through the cricothyroid membrane is associated with subglottic and glottic injury and is not likely to be effective if the obstruction is laryngeal.

TABLE 20-3. COMMON ERRORS IN OROTRACHEAL INTUBATION

Step	Error
Position	Axes not aligned
Opening of mouth	Mouth not wide open
Insertion of blade	Choosing wrong size or wrong blade; blade not inserted on right side of tongue.
Exposure of vocal cords	Leverage rather than lifting
Introduction of tube	Obscuring line of vision of tube; failure to maintain natural curve of tube; angulation of trachea due to excessive traction.

From Salem, M.R., Mathrubhutham, M., and Bennett, M.J.: Difficult intubation. N. Engl. J. Med., 295:879, 1976.

reservoir of oxygen. The procedure enhances safety, increases the time for manipulations, and delays hypoxemia and cerebral depression.

RELAXANTS FOR INTUBATION. The dose of succinylcholine for the purpose of intubation is 1 mg/kg. Smaller doses are not too effective, and larger doses are unnecessary. Pretreatment by an average dose of 3 mg of d-tubocurarine or 1 mg of either vecuronium or pancuronium 3 minutes prior to administration of succinylcholine is necessary to minimize fasciculations. Optimal conditions ensue in 40 to 50 seconds. Assessment of proper conditions is guided by lack of fasciculations; cessation of spontaneous respiration; relaxation of neck and jaw muscles; and, most important, observation of motionless vocal cords.[31] In children, preliminary curarization is usually not necessary, because they tolerate depolarizing drugs well and fasciculations are minimal.

Facilitating intubation by d-tubocurarine alone is slow under urgent circumstances. In second plane stage III anesthesia depth (halothane, enflurane, isoflurane), however, a dose of 0.1 to 0.15 mg/kg will produce apnea and excellent relaxation in 2 to 3 minutes. The curonium derivatives—pancuronium and alcuronium—are satisfactory. A dose of pancuronium of 0.13 mg/kg or alcuronium 0.24 mg/kg will produce excellent conditions in 50 to 60 seconds, respectively.

The intermediate-acting nondepolarizing agents (vecuronium or atracurium) are preferred. When the priming technique using a dose one tenth to one fifth the full dose occurs 3 minutes prior to the administration of the remainder of the calculated dose, a more rapid production of relaxation is achieved.

POSITION OF HEAD. To perform laryngoscopy, it is necessary to bring the passageway *from* the incisor teeth *to* the larynx and trachea into a straight line. Examination of this passageway reveals three directional axes (Fig. 20–12):[32]

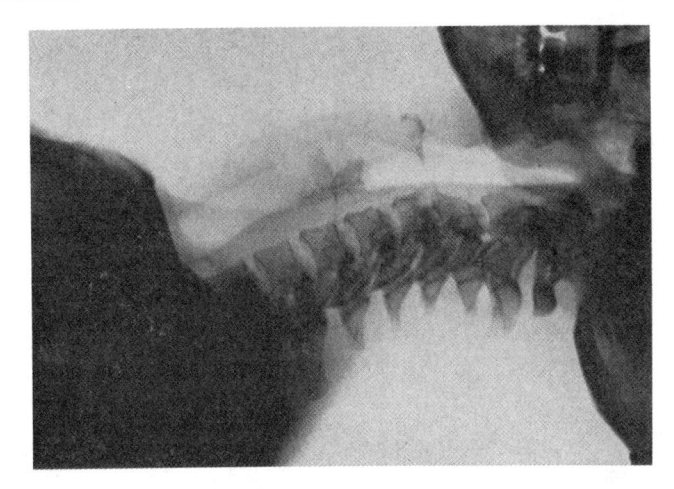

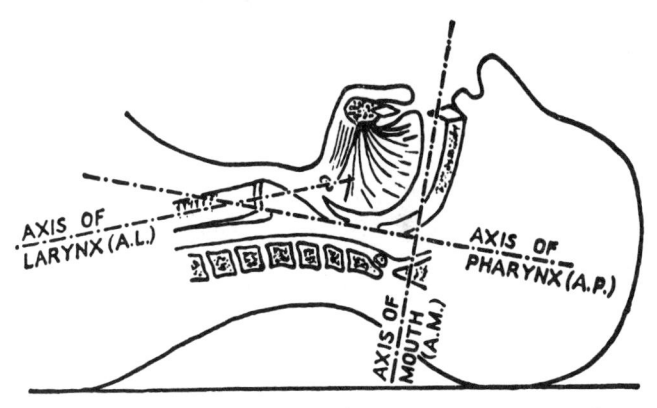

FIG. 20–12. The three axes of air passageway to trachea showing the relative position of the mouth, pharynx, and larynx with patient lying flat. From Bannister, F.B., and Macbeth, R.: Direct laryngoscopy and tracheal intubation. Lancet, 1:651, 1944.

1. The axis of the cavity of the mouth
2. The axis of the cavity of the pharynx
3. The axis of the larynx and trachea

The oral axis forms a right angle with that of the pharynx. The pharyngeal axis, in turn, crosses that of the larynx obtusely, as illustrated. The problem of bringing all axes into a straight line is simply one of mechanics and can be accomplished by placing the patient's head in the proper position. Two approaches have been used.

The Classic Position of Jackson. This position provides the conditions for what is termed *suspension laryngoscopy*. The patient is placed supine with shoulders near the edge of the table and with a sandbag pillow under the shoulders. Both head and neck are in full extension. As originally described by Jackson in 1913, "the patient's head must be in full extension with vertex firmly pushed down toward the feet of the patient, so as to throw the neck upward and bring the occiput down as close as possible beneath the cervical vertebrae."[33]

528   General Anesthesia

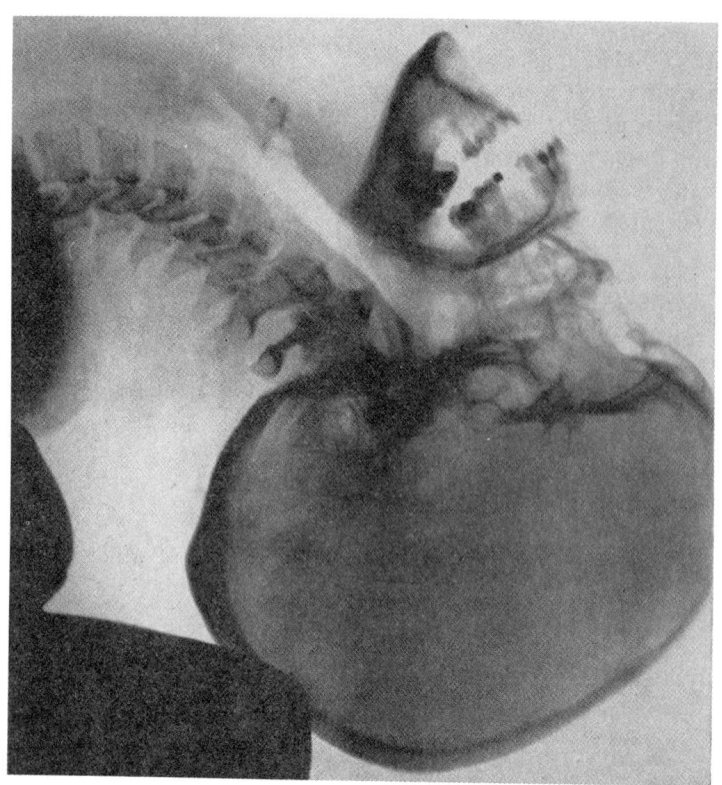

FIG. 20–13. Classic position for laryngoscopy showing the effect of extension of the neck on the three axes of the air passageway. From Bannister, F.B., and Macbeth, R.: Direct laryngoscopy and tracheal intubation. Lancet, *1*:651, 1944.

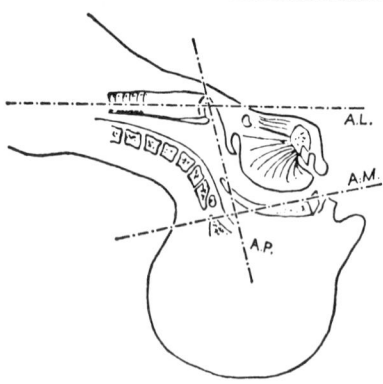

The effect of this maneuver on the axes of the passageway is illustrated in Figure 20–13. With this position, when the tongue and epiglottis are lifted forward to align the pharyngeal and laryngeal axes, the extension is undone. It is evident that this is a complex and illogical approach. Furthermore, when the laryngoscope blade is introduced into the pharynx, the view is that of the esophagus and posterior part of the larynx. The epiglottis usually obstructs vision. To observe the anterior portion of the larynx and glottis, the tongue and epiglottis must be elevated and the scope must be pivoted on the teeth. Such leverage is frequently strong and, therefore, hazardous. It is condemned.

The Amended Position. An entirely different approach to aligning the axes of the passageway involves raising the head off the table and leaving the shoulders on the table. If the head is raised about 5 cm by placing a pillow beneath the occiput, the pharyngeal and laryngeal axes immediately coincide (Fig. 20–14).

The cervical spine is now straight. Furthermore, this position lessens the tension on neck muscles and decreases the actual distance from teeth to glottis. The alignment may be called the "sniffing position." This position of the head has the same relation to the body as that of soldiers standing at attention with their jaw jutting forward on their shoulders. Again, it is evident that this is the anatomically correct position for alignment of the passageway and, therefore, proper for laryngoscopy and intubation.

Next, the head is extended at the atlanto–occipital joint (Fig. 20–15). All axes will be in alignment now, but the tongue and epiglottis will encroach on the

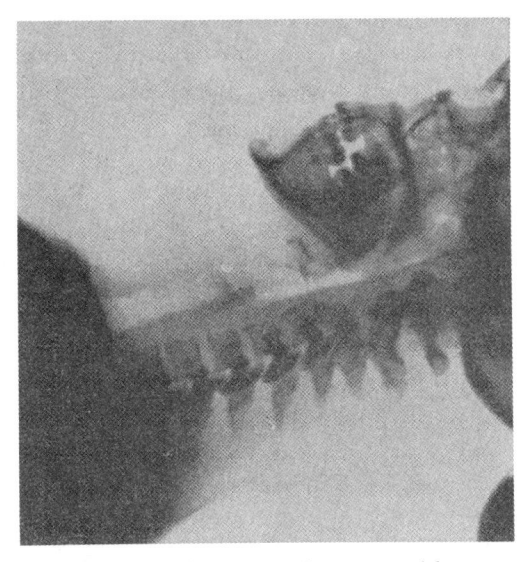

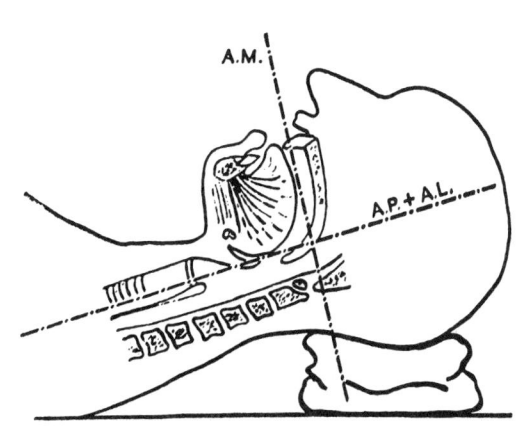

FIG. 20–14. Axes of the pharynx and larynx may be made to coincide when the head is raised. The cervical spine is also straightened. From Bannister, F.B., and Macbeth, R.: Direct laryngoscopy and tracheal intubation. Lancet, *1*:651, 1944.

passage. The laryngoscope blade lifts these structures and an unobstructed view is obtained. The vector of the lifting force by the arm should be at about a 45° angle away from the operator. Actually, the patient's head is suspended by the laryngoscope blade contacting the base of the tongue and with the tip behind the epiglottis. *Do not pry or use a leverage motion against the teeth as a fulcrum.*

At this time, the novice will often complain that the "larynx is anterior." This is anatomically a fallacious statement and the problem is related to improper leverage—prying. The *lifting* motion must be improved; the tendency to have an associate press the larynx posteriorly merely distorts visualization further. To facilitate visualization of the larynx and permit easy introduction of an endotracheal tube, the "Salem maneuver" is recommended.[36] This consists only of *cephalad* displacement of the larynx (not posterior pressure). This maneuver can be combined with the Sellick maneuver.

LARYNGOSCOPY

POSITION OF OPERATOR. The laryngoscopist should stand at the head of the table and above the patient's head, while the patient is lying supine. The laryn-

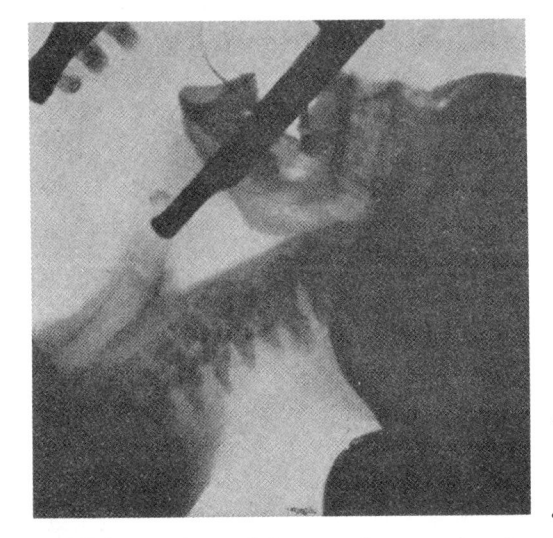

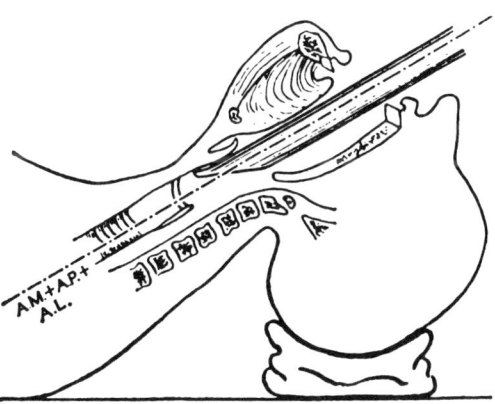

FIG. 20–15. Axis of the mouth is now made to coincide with the other axes by extension of the head at the atlanto–occipital junction. From Bannister, F.B., and Macbeth, R.: Direct laryngoscopy and tracheal intubation. Lancet, *1*:651, 1944.

goscopist should stand at the patient's head. The optimal height of the patient's head for laryngoscopy and intubation is at the xiphoid of the operator. This may or should vary with the sightedness of the operator (near or far). It is mechanically more efficient if the operator is not required to bend down and if the laryngoscope arm is flexed and at right angles to the body—better leverage is thereby obtained. The operating table should be adjusted accordingly.

POSITION OF PATIENT ON TABLE. The patient should be supine, and the height of the table should be adjusted so that it is at the level of a laryngoscopist's xiphoid. Modification may be necessary for those requiring eye glasses. This position of the table permits laryngoscopists to stand comfortably and to allow them to suspend the mandible and larynx with the straight blade laryngoscope held in the left hand with the arm flexed and their left elbow relatively close to their body.

The circulating nurse should be requested to dim the room lights at this time; this provides a better focus of the laryngoscope light and better vision for the laryngoscopist.

HOLDING THE LARYNGOSCOPE. The handle of the laryngoscope should be held in the left hand. After cocking the blade on the handle, the convex surface of the blade should be viewed and the flange noted to the left; the light mechanism should be checked. With the handle in the left hand, the dominant right hand (in right-handed operators) is free to carry out a variety of manipulations, including parting the lips and opening the mouth.

LARYNGOSCOPY PROCEDURE (Fig. 20–16). Laryngoscopy is accomplished in three steps.

Insertion of Laryngoscope Blade Into Mouth. As a principle, the thinnest part of the laryngoscope blade (spatula) should be inserted into the mouth. When the commonly used blades are viewed at the convex or posterior surface while holding the handle in the "ready" position, the flange is noted on the left side of the blade, and this side presents a thicker dimension than the thin right edge. The insertion in the midline, and especially on the left side of the mouth, means that the thicker part of the blade is introduced and is not a sensible approach. It is evident that the blade should be slightly rotated clockwise and that the handle be allowed to dip to the right shoulder.

The thumb and index finger of the right hand open the mouth. As the thumb pushes the mandible downward, the index finger "rolls away" the lower lip. The mandible may then be picked up by the thumb and index finger. The blade should then be inserted into the open mouth between the teeth *into the right side* of the mouth, along the *right* lingual edge toward the right molar teeth and the base of the tongue. The handle is then rotated from the right shoulder to the midline, and the blade advanced over the tongue into the pharynx, while the tongue is displaced to the left and is maintained out of the line of vision by the flange of the laryngoscope.

Visualization of Epiglottis. As the tip of the laryngoscope reaches the base of the tongue, the operator now advances the laryngoscope slowly and atraumatically with the left hand, while the right hand with the thumb inside the mandible pulls the lower jaw up over the blade. This is continued until the epiglottis is viewed. This structure is considered to be a most important landmark, and a slight lift of the handle upward and forward at 45 degrees will reveal the tip of the epiglottis.

Elevation of Epiglottis—Straight-Blade Technique. When brought into view, the laryngoscope is advanced so that the tip of the blade comes to lie behind the epiglottis, whereupon the epiglottis is picked up and the entire jaw lifted upward without prying. The glottis will now come into view (Fig. 20–17).

This right-sided insertion into the mouth is especially useful and necessary in robust, muscular patients, in the obese or heavy bosomed patients, and those patients with kyphosis or scoliosis. The incisor teeth are less likely to be scratched or chipped. At the time when "iron lungs" were used to ventilate polio patients, this maneuver was widely used. A special "polio laryngoscope" was designed by Rovenstine, so that the handle itself extended at a right angle to the blade.

In patients unable to open their mouth widely due to severe pharyngitis, swollen tongue or Ludwig's angina, or submandibular fascitis, a flat, thin blade without a flange, such as the Galasso blade, is recommended.[34]

Laryngoscopy—Curved Blade, Macintosh Technique (Fig. 20–18). Normally, the straight blade is passed beyond and posterior to the epiglottis to elevate the epiglottis. Two hazards are present: injury to upper teeth, and laceration of posterior pharyngeal wall.

The curved blade of Macintosh is designed to fit into the angle made by the base of the tongue and epiglottis (Fig. 20–18 *A* and *B*). When the scope is lifted, the base of the tongue is pushed upward. The epiglottis, being attached to the base of the tongue, is also drawn upward, and the larynx comes into view (Fig. 20–18 *C* and *D*). The epiglottis is not directly manipulated.

INTUBATION. After the larynx has been exposed, the selected and well-lubricated endotracheal tube is inserted. This should be done in one continuous sweeping motion, with the tube held like a pen. The tube should be passed during the inspiratory phase

FIG. 20–16. Four-step technique of intubation with straight laryngoscope blade:
1. Insertion of laryngoscope.
2. Visualization of epiglottis.
3. Lifting motion, *not prying*, after epiglottis has been "picked up."
4. Insertion of endotracheal tube.

From Thomas, G.: Technique in intubation anesthesia. Anesth. Analg., *17*:301, 1938.

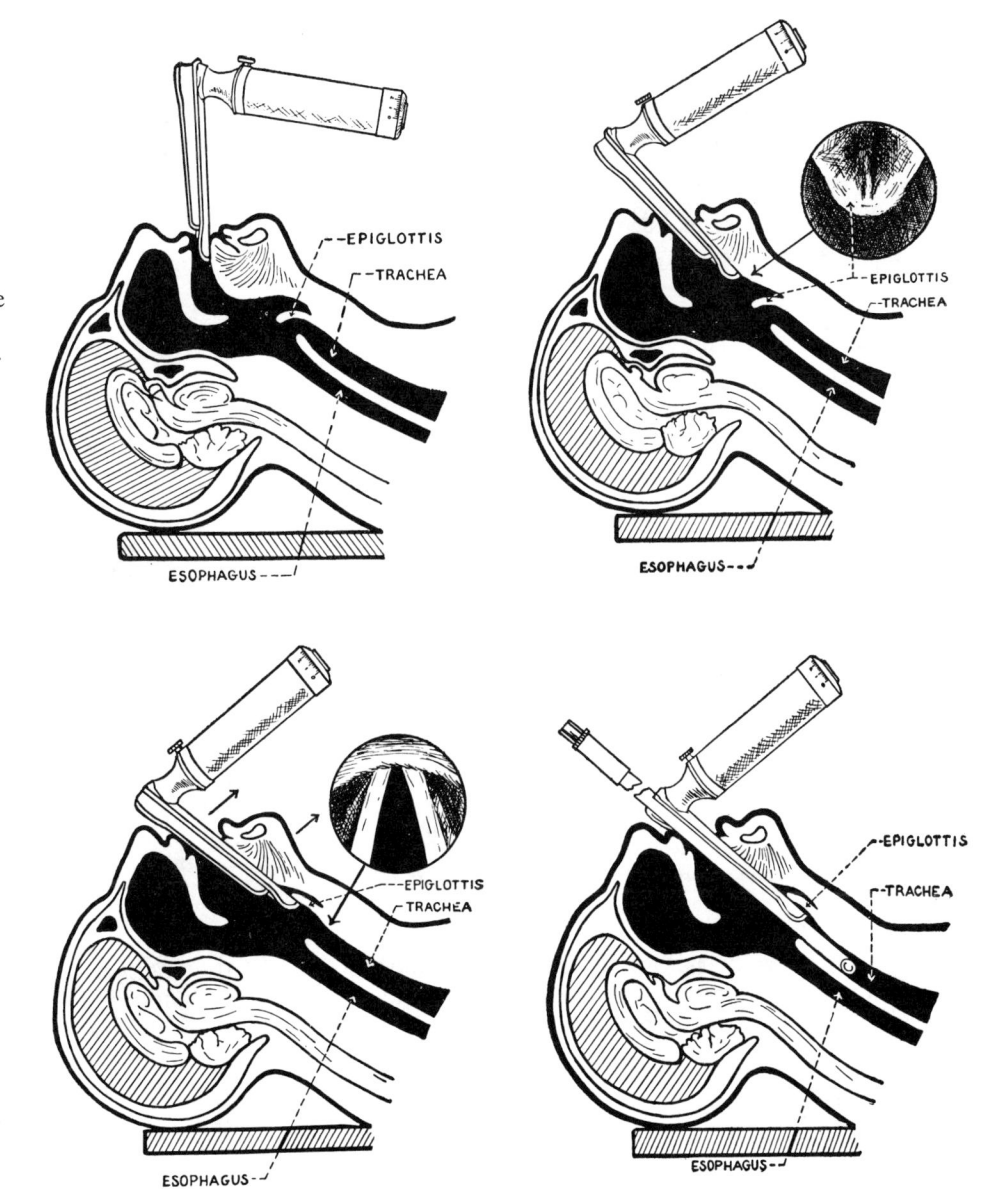

of respiration when phonation is absent. Obviously, a tube will pass into the trachea most easily when abduction of the vocal cords is greatest. This occurs during deep inspiration or hyperventilation and can be produced by slight carbon dioxide excess, but this is not recommended.

Magill[35a,35b] stressed the importance of introducing the endotracheal tube during inspiration, and it is certainly easy to introduce a tube as a patient gasps following laryngospasm. Many tubes can be inserted during an explosive cough, however, when the vocal cords are markedly abducted.

As soon as the tube is inserted, a mouth prop should be placed between the teeth, the laryngoscope removed, and the pharynx packed or the cuff inflated.

Throughout all these maneuvers, the endotracheal tube should be held securely in the fingers of one hand; on completion of the above steps the tube can be anchored by adhesive strips around the bite block and crossed over the face to prevent the tube from either slipping out of the trachea or entering it further (Fig. 20–19). Next, connections should be made with the inhalation breathing circuit and anesthetic apparatus. Respiratory excursions and movement of the chest should be noted from either spontaneous breathing or mechanical ventilation.

Assessment of Conditions at Intubation. Intubating conditions depend on several factors: depth of anesthesia or adequacy of topical anesthesia, degree of muscle relaxation, patient comfort–cooperation index, anatomic class of upper airway,[5a] and, above all, the skill of the endoscopist. These con-

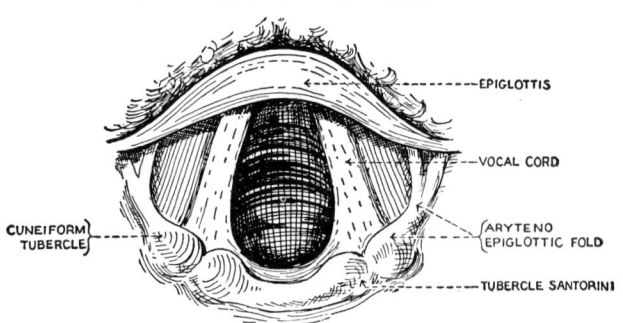

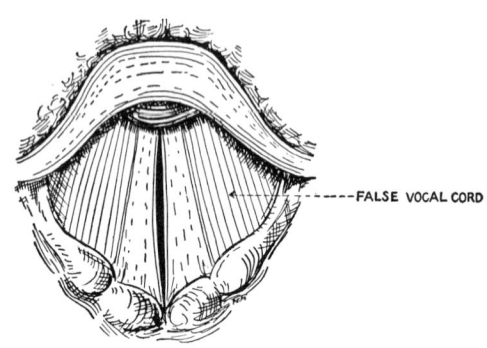

FIG. 20-17. Technique of intubation. Laryngoscopic view of larynx with glottis widely open (*upper*) and widely closed (*lower*). From Thomas, G.: Technique in intubation anesthesia. Anesth. Analg., *17*:301, 1938.

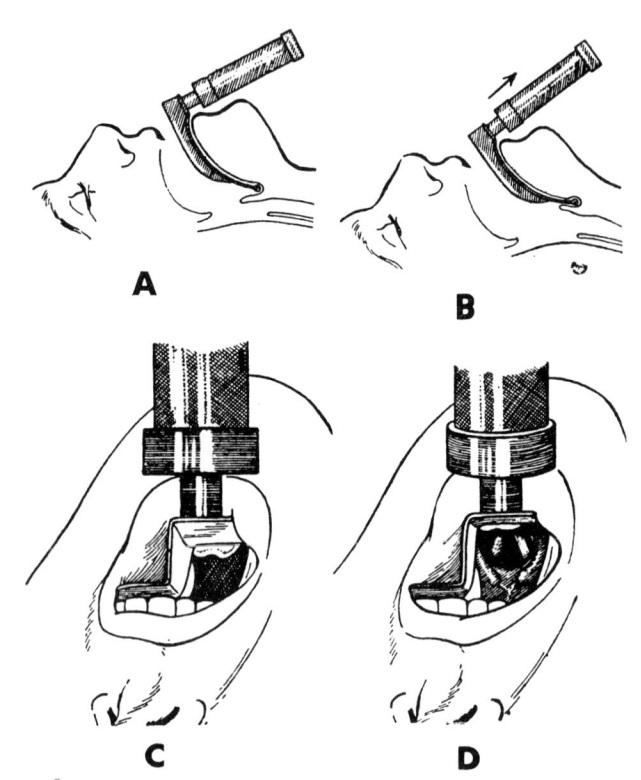

FIG. 20-18. Curved blade laryngoscopy (Macintosh). *A* and *C*, Position of blade tip and view obtained before lifting laryngoscope. *B* and *D*, Position of blade and view when laryngoscope is lifted in direction of arrow.

ditions have been classified according to a grading system that characterizes the conditions as excellent, satisfactory, fair, or poor, as shown in Table 20-4.[31b]

INDICATIONS OF SUCCESSFUL INTUBATION. After intubation, examination of the chest by inspection and by auscultation must be performed. Both lung fields should aerate well.

Particular attention should be paid to auscultation of the apical areas of the superior lobes. In the adult, it is not necessary to auscultate other areas of the chest.

Some Immediate Signs of Tracheal Intubation.

1. Often there is an immediate cough or reflex breath-holding followed by a panting type of respiration.
2. Warm breath may be felt at the machine end of the endotracheal tube when the patient is breathing spontaneously or the chest is compressed.
3. Auscultation of chest—blowing type of breath sounds may be heard.
4. The lungs may be inflated by immediately connecting the tube to the breathing system and manual inflation accomplished. (Direct mouth-to-tube inflation is condemned.) If the tube is not in the trachea, the upper part of the chest will not expand and the abdomen may bulge. There is more resistance to blowing when the tube is in the esophagus than when in the trachea.
5. Free excursions of the rebreathing bag indicate a clear airway, if the patient is breathing spontaneously.
6. If the patient is paralyzed and being mechanically ventilated, the ventilator will operate smoothly and without clatter, provided the system has no leaks.

Additional Indications of Intubation. Other indications that the trachea has been successfully intubated are listed in Table 20-5.

Tactile Verification of Position of Endotracheal Tube.[37] A simple tactile technique for verification of placement of the endotracheal tube follows a modification of the essential steps of tactile intubation.

In this verification maneuver, however, it is easier for right-handed operators to introduce the index finger only of their right hand into the left side of the patient's mouth and over the left lateral margin of the tongue, down into the left pharyngeal space. The left hand remains outside of the mouth and is

TABLE 20-4. CLASSIFICATION OF CONDITIONS AT INTUBATION

Grade	Characteristics
A	*Excellent:* flaccid relaxation of jaw muscles; mouth wide open; good cord visualization; cords well separated—abducted; no bucking at intubation
B	*Satisfactory:* mouth easily opened; jaw muscles well relaxed; good cord visualization; slight cord movement when touched but abducted; minimal bucking at intubation
C	*Fair:* conditions less favorable; jaw muscles not well relaxed; cord visualization fair but allowing intubation; bucking on intubation
D	*Impossible:* poor relaxation of jaw and resistance to opening mouth; poor cord visualization or none; cords adducted if viewed; superior pharyngeal constrictor muscle activity; patient unable to be intubated or, if intubated, marked bucking and body movement

Modified from Lund, I., and Stovner, J.: Experimental and clinical experiments with a new muscle relaxant. Acta Anesthesiol. Scand., 6:85, 1962.[31b]

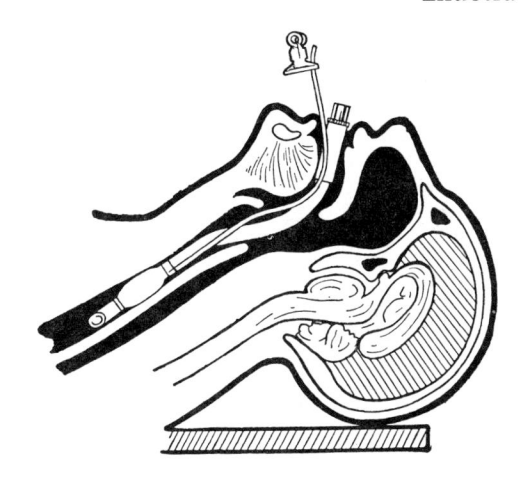

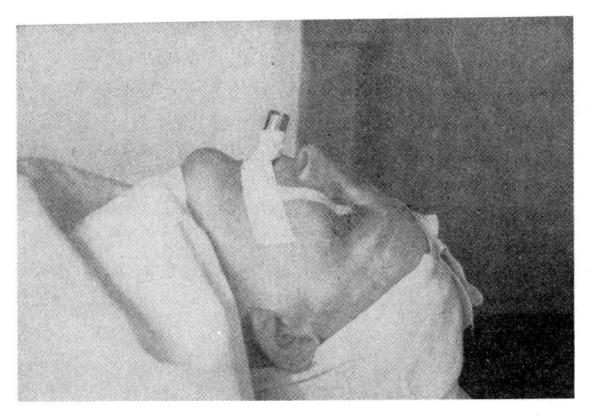

FIG. 20-19. Technique of intubation. *Upper,* section of head showing endotracheal tube in place with cuff inflated. *Lower,* patient's face showing endotracheal tube anchored at mouth with adhesive.

used to manipulate the neck: first, the hyoid is manipulated in the upper part of the neck by moving it first to the right and then to the left; second, the larynx is similarly moved in a rotary fashion. These actions serve to make these structures palpable to the right index finger placed in the pharynx. The index finger is curled medially toward the interarytenoid groove, while the neck is moved with the left hand. The endotracheal tube will be palpable anterior to the arytenoid groove.

POSITION OF ENDOTRACHEAL TUBE IN TRACHEA. The ideal positon of the tip of an endotracheal tube in the adult man weighing 70 kg is 5 to 7 cm above the carina, ie, the tip of the tube should be in the midtrachea. The carina is usually demonstrable at the level of T5 or T6 but may be 1 vertebral body above or below this level. The glottis is likewise demonstrable in radiologic examinations at the level of C5 or C6. The cricoid cartilage is usually at C6.

Goodman[38,39] has studied radiologically the effect of head movements on the position of an endotracheal tube. Flexion of the head or neck causes a descent of the tip of the tube approximately 2 cm in the adult man; extension of the neck from a neutral position causes an ascent of the tube by 3 cm.

Further study of the effects of neck flexion and extension on position of the cords and carina demonstrate the following:

- Position of the carina only slightly changes with respect to the thoracic vertebrae (Fig. 20-20).
- Flexion causes the tip of an endotracheal tube to move preferentially downward to the right main bronchus.
- Flexion causes the vocal cords to be slightly displaced downward.
- Neck extension causes dramatic position changes—the vocal cords move superiorly from a level of C5 to C4; this increases the distance from the cords to carina (Fig. 20-21). More importantly, the distance from the lips to the vocal cords increases from 13.3 cm to 15.5 cm.

Thus, neck flexion risks accidental endobronchial intubation, whereas neck extension risks accidental extubation. Therefore, any change in patient position, especially in turning the body, movement of the head, or placing the patient prone, requires that the position of the endotracheal tube be checked. Auscultation should be completed promptly.

MECHANICAL COMPLICATIONS. Obstruction can be produced by simple mechanical factors. Deformation of the relatively smooth curve of the endotracheal tube over the curves and axes of the anatomic airway—oral to pharyngeal, pharyngeal to laryngeal—can occur.[40] Kinking of the tube can occur as a result of unusual head position. Displacement of the tube may occur from hyperextension or flexion of the head, moving the head, or inadequate fixa-

534 General Anesthesia

TABLE 20-5. SIGNS OF ENDOTRACHEAL INTUBATION

1. Visualization of passage of tube (and cuff) through glottis during laryngoscopy.
2. Movement of chest and reservoir bag when patient is breathing spontaneously.
3. Movement of chest on manual inflation in apneic or paralyzed patient, followed by expansion of reservoir bag on passive exhalation. *Fogging* of clear plastic tubes should be noted on exhalation.
4. Burping sign: Before inflation of the cuff, manual inflation should be accompanied by easy expansion of chest if the tube is in the trachea. If it is in the esophagus, a typical "burp" will ensue.
5. Auscultation of anterior chest wall in the 2nd–3rd interspace 1 inch from the manubrium for apical segments of superior lobes, during manual inflation of lungs should be considered as follows:
   a. Breath sounds should be equal bilaterally.
   b. Wheezes and bronchi are often adventitious.
   c. Normal vesicular sounds heard during spontaneous breathing or during careful manual inflation of the lungs is usually proof of proper placement of the tube.
   d. Auscultation of midaxillary space should also be performed for infants and children.
6. If anesthesia is light, patient may "buck" when tube enters the trachea, an obvious sign of placement, but undesirable. There are "irritant receptors" in the airway and trachea. Stimulation, therefore, causes the bucking and bronchoconstriction. The bucking, to some extent, but the bronchoconstriction especially, can be attenuated by atropine.[38]
7. Do not inflate lung by mouth-blowing into endotracheal tube. This may be hazardous to the anesthetist, who may aspirate bacterial contaminants or foreign particulate matter from the patient's respiratory system.
8. Negative findings include the following:
   a. No distention of stomach.
   b. No significant tachycardia.
   c. No cyanosis.
   d. No burping on bag pressure with tube assembly connected.
9. Monitoring gases include the following:
   a. End-tidal CO_2 monitoring—normal range of Pa_{CO_2}.
   b. Monitoring of oxygenation by oximetry—may detect endobronchial intubation.
10. Roentgenography: Not a routine; useful with endobronchial tubes and long-term recovery and intensive care.

tion.[41] The process of "tongueing" by patients lightly anesthetized has been considered. Tracheal motion has also been demonstrated during apnea and mechanical ventilation.[42] In prolonged intubation, especially with soft plastic endotracheal tubes and low-pressure–large-volume cuffs, dislocation of the orotracheal tube may occur during intermittent positive-pressure ventilation: during inflation, a force is applied to the tracheal side of the cuff, which is greater than the atmospheric pressure above the cuff, and this may cause displacement upward of the tube into the larynx or even into the pharynx. Frequently, the cuff may be forced upward through the larynx.[43]

ESOPHAGEAL INTUBATION. Misplacement of the endotracheal tube into the esophagus has been recognized as a complication of endotracheal intubation since 1915, when noted by Paluel Flagg in *The Art*

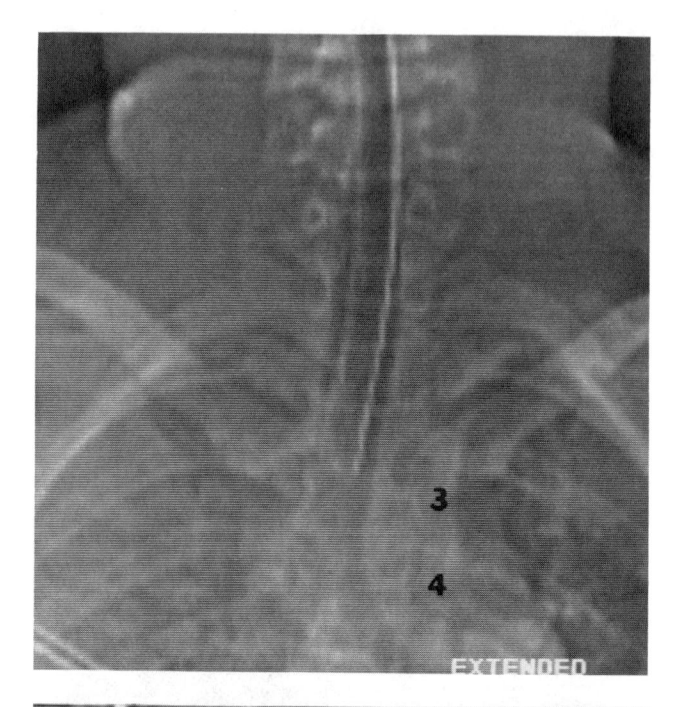

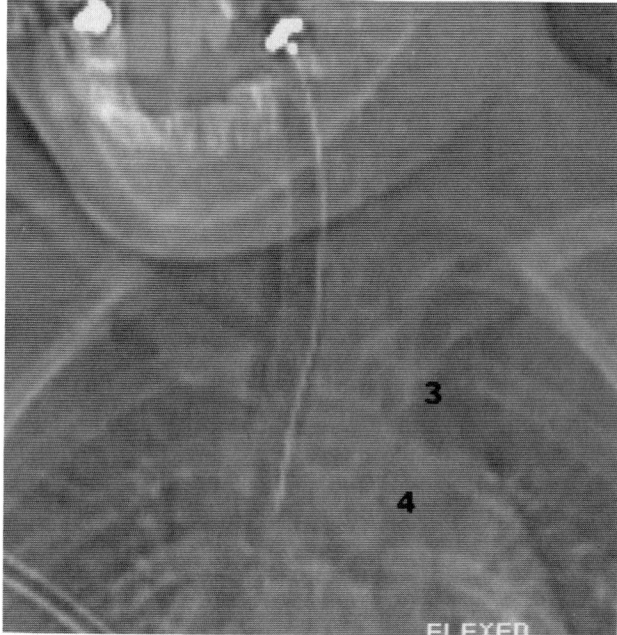

FIG. 20-20. With the neck in the extended position, the endotracheal tube tip lies above the carina (*upper*), but during flexion (*lower*), the tip moves downward toward the right main bronchus. Note the minimal movement of the carina relative to T3 and T4. From Goodman, L.R.: Radiological evaluation of patients receiving assisted ventilation. J.A.M.A., 245:858, 1981.

of Anesthesia.[44] One of the first detailed reports of esophageal intubation was that of Edward[45] in 1938. A tube inadvertently placed in the esophagus at the time of anesthetic intubation was attached to a high-pressure oxygen source and the stomach ruptured. The patient died of sepsis postoperatively.

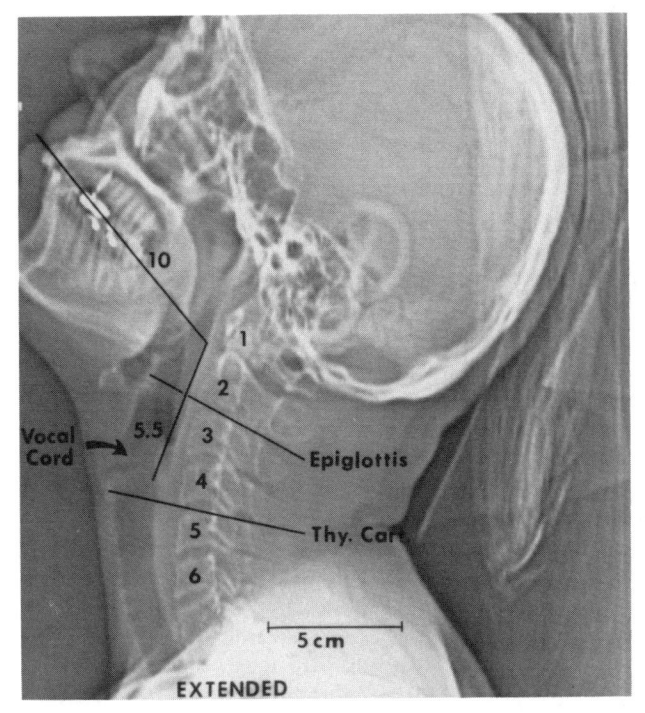

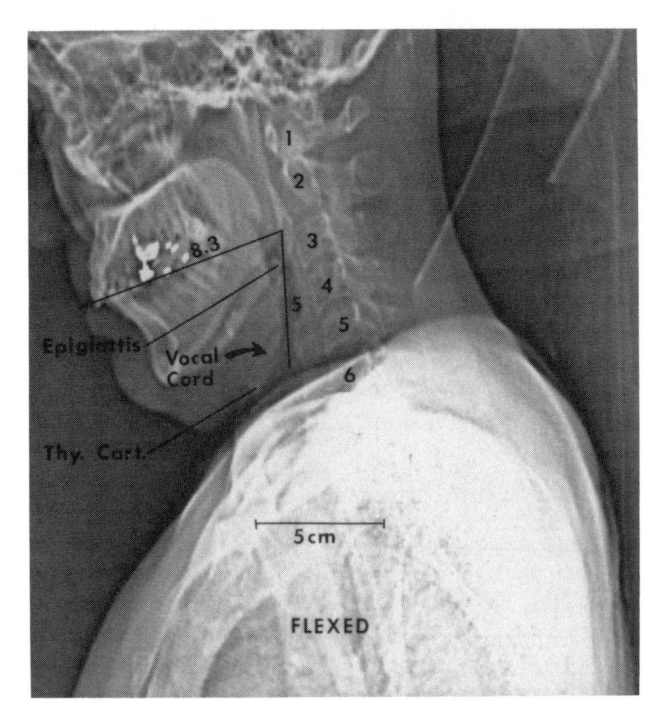

FIG. 20–21. Computed tomography scans of C1–C6 and upper and middle airways in an adult with the neck extended (*left*) and flexed (*right*). Note some upward displacement (distance in cm) of the cords as a result of head and neck extension (C5 to C4). Also note the larger increase in distance from incisors → oropharynx → cords during extension. From Goodman, L.R.: Radiological evaluation of patients receiving assisted ventilation. J.A.M.A., 245:858, 1981.

Accurate placement of a tube in the trachea and verification of its position are critical. A misplacement should be diagnosed by the several methods previously outlined. The tragedy is that esophageal intubation may go unrecognized until disaster occurs with cardiac arrest.

The frequency of esophageal intubation is not known, but unrecognized esophageal intubation is either a contributing or main cause of anesthetic morbidity and mortality. In Keenan's[46] study of cardiac arrest attributed to anesthesia, about 15% were the result of unrecognized esophageal intubations.

Utting's[47] report of anesthetic accidents in the United Kingdom revealed that faulty technique was the principal cause of death in about half the cases and that inadvertent esophageal intubation was the usual mode. An Australian investigation[48] of anesthetic mortality revealed that about 70% of deaths were related to airway management, and esophageal intubation was identified as the principal or contributing factor.

Fatalities may not be the only outcome. The occurrence of cardiac arrest imposes a serious burden on all involved. The frequency of neurologic damage is also a devastating result.

Detection techniques for esophageal intubation have been reviewed by Birmingham,[49] who found that although direct visualization of the entrance of the endotracheal tube through the glottis into the trachea is the cornerstone of skillful technique, it is not an absolute guarantee of proper placement. Many "slips" can occur postintubation. Inadvertent displacement may occur while securing the tube, connecting the tube to the breathing circuit, moving the patient's head, and positioning the patient.

A second reliable detection technique is that of capnography;[50] however, it too has many drawbacks.

Most other techniques of detection of a malpositioned tube outside the trachea have been reported to fail on occasion (see Table 20–5).

Some strategies for detection of esophageal misplacement are uncommon, unreliable, impractical, and wasteful of precious time when there is a sense of uncertainty. These include pressing on the sternum and noting the sound of expelled air (it can be air escaping from the esophagus); detecting condensation of water vapor in the wall of the tube lumen; noting the appearance or gurgling sound of gastric contents in the tube (it may be bloody secretions from the upper air passages in a correctly placed tube); or using pulse oximetry (too late).

Some cumbersome or sophisticated techniques include chest radiography, fiberoptic bronchoscopy, and Eschmann endotracheal tube introducers.

Comment. When uncertain about the placement of a tube in the trachea and the simple, readily applied detection techniques—auscultation of the chest, movement of the chest on positive-pressure inflation without a burp—it is recommended that laryngoscopy be again performed (perhaps by an experienced anesthesiologist). If the tube is not visualized through the vocal cords, it should be removed and the patient reintubated again by a more experienced anesthesiologist.

NASOTRACHEAL INTUBATION

The nasal route is needed in many oral–dental, maxillary–mandibular, head and neck, or facial surgical procedures. Intubation of the trachea can be accomplished by direct vision or by the blind technique.

Direct-Vision Nasotracheal Intubation

Nasotracheal intubation can be a planned procedure but is also employed when advancement by the blind technique through the vocal cords into the trachea is not easily accomplished. The following are considerations for this technique:

- The preparation of equipment and choice of tubes, the anesthetic requirements, the position of the head, and the preparation of the patient with attention to the nasal passageway are identical to the blind nasal technique (see later discussion). Shrinkage of the nasal mucosa by decongestants—cocaine—is recommended to provide topical anesthesia also.
- A well-lubricated tube (the Rae tubes are the choice) is inserted along the floor of the nasal cavity over the hard and soft palate into the pharynx. This is usually noted as a distinct "give."
- At this point, laryngoscopy is performed identical in technique to that described by orotracheal intubation.
- The endotracheal tube will be visualized in the hypopharynx and can now be manipulated by means of a Magill forceps. The tube is grasped by the forceps and directed toward the larynx while the proximal end of the tube is advanced through the nose and pharynx into the glottis and passed through. The tube can be regrasped at a higher point and passed the desired distance into the trachea.

Blind Nasotracheal Intubation

PREPARATION. A patient to be intubated nasally should be questioned beforehand to determine through which nostril breathing is easier. At the same time both nostrils should be examined and patency assessed by the sniffing test. Premedication is not varied from the usual.

ANESTHESIA. Blind intubation can be accomplished in any plane of general anesthesia. It is generally required, however, that the patient be breathing spontaneously. Deep planes of anesthesia are not necessary and actually one of the advantages of the technique is that a light plane of anesthesia is more satisfactory. Other requirements for successful blind intubation are hyperpnea and intubation during expiration.

POSITION OF HEAD. The relaxed or amended endoscopy position of the head is required; sharp extension of the head is to be avoided. In practice it is recommended that one err on the side of slight flexion of the head forward toward the chest.

PROCEDURE. *First,* choose a moderately stiff endotracheal tube with a wide (not a sharp curve). For example, a 25-cm tube should have a curve that subtends at least a 60-degree angle. The average adult male nares will admit a 12-mm outside diameter (OD) catheter; the female nares will admit a 10-mm OD catheter. Lubricate the tube with a thin coat of ointment and then a generous amount of water-soluble jelly.

Second, apply a topical anesthetic (cocaine preferable) to the more patent nares to shrink the mucosa.

Third, introduce the well-lubricated tube along the floor of the nose with the bevel facing the nasal septum into the hypopharynx (Figs. 20–22, 20–23, and 20–24). A tube introduced through the right nostril will cross the hypopharynx and contact the left pharyngeal wall. It is, therefore, recommended that the head be slightly abducted to the left of the midline. This will line up the passageway from nares through pharynx to glottis and trachea. On the other hand, tubes introduced into the left nares will cross the hypopharynx to contact the right pharyngeal wall. Again, abducting the head toward the right will line up the passageway (Fig. 20–25).

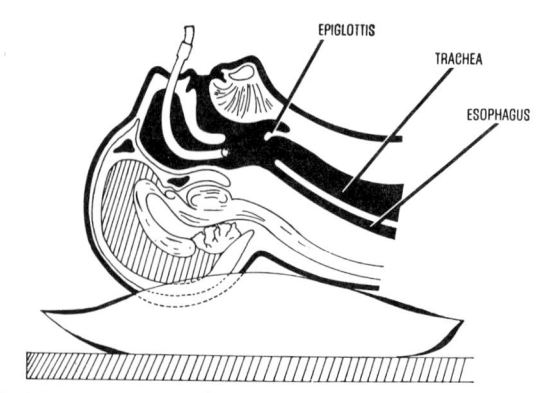

FIG. 20–22. Nasotracheal intubation. Step 1. A well-lubricated endotracheal tube is introduced along the floor of the nose with the bevel facing the nasal septum.

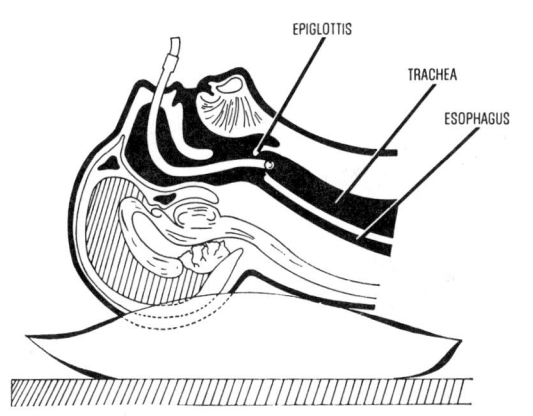

FIG. 20–23. Nasotracheal intubation. Step 2. The endotracheal tube is advanced through the nostril into the hypopharynx to a point just above the glottic opening.

Fourth, hold the ear close to the end of the tube and note the type of breathing. The operator is guided from this point exclusively by hearing the breath sounds. *Advance the tube as long as breathing is tubular in quality.*

Fifth, introduce tube through glottis by slight rotation. It is favored during expiration; at this time cords are slightly abducted and the laryngeal reflex is less active.

INCORRECT PLACEMENT. The natural curve of the endotracheal tube should be continuously kept in mind. The most common difficulty is to have the tube impinge in the sulcus between the base of the tongue and the epiglottis (Fig. 20–26) or on the anterior commissure and be stopped. This is usually the result of too sharp extension of the head. Similarly, the tube will be stopped if it comes to rest on the closed glottis during laryngospasm.

Other nontracheal positions that a tube may take are in the esophagus (Fig. 20–26) and in the pyriform sinus. Lateral deflection of the tube may be overcome by abduction of the head.

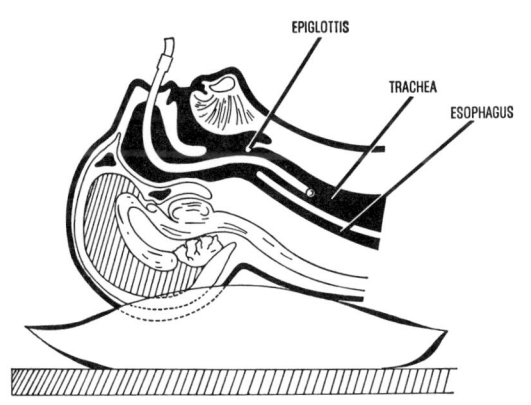

FIG. 20–24. Nasotracheal intubation. Step 3. The endotracheal tube is advanced while the operator is listening to breath sounds. It is advanced as long as breathing is tubular in quality until it is in the trachea.

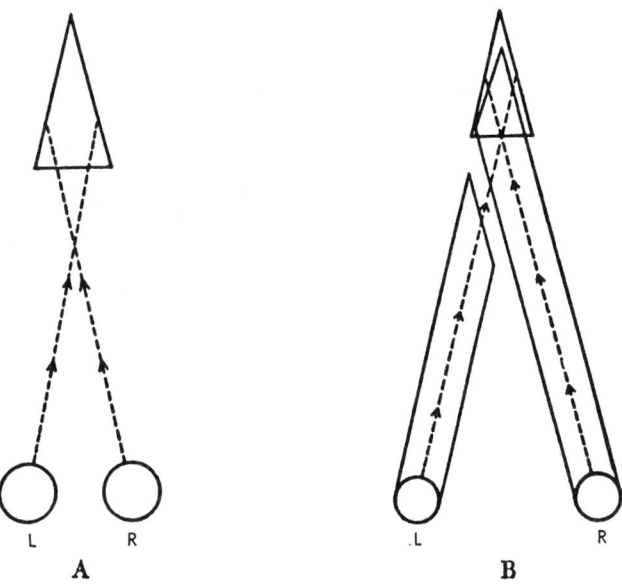

FIG. 20–25. Nasotracheal intubation, showing the direction taken by tubes inserted into the left and right nostril as they advance through the pharynx. Note the tubes cross the hypopharynx to contact the opposite pharyngeal wall. From Gillespie, N.A.: Endotracheal Anesthesia, 3rd ed. Edited by Bamforth and Siebecker. Madison, University of Wisconsin Press, 1963.

MANEUVERS TO CORRECT DEVIATIONS. If blind intubation is unsuccessful after a few "passes," then expose the glottis with laryngoscope and direct the tube between the cord under vision (Fig. 20–27). The tube is in good position if the quality of sounds is tubular and the sounds continue to increase in intensity until a maximum is attained when tube is in the trachea. If sounds diminish or disappear, the tube is no longer aimed at the rima glottidis and should be withdrawn and readvanced.

ADVANTAGES. The advantages of nasotracheal intubation include the following:

- Useful for long-term intubation and ventilatory care
- Easily secured
- Minimal chance of kinking
- Greater comfort in awake patient
- Less chance of semiconscious or awake patient biting the tube and causing occlusion
- Minimal oropharyngeal secretions, especially in awake patients
- Oral feeding possible during long-term intubation in intensive care units

DISADVANTAGES. Disadvantages of nasotracheal intubation include the following:

- Damage to nasal tissues
  - Perforation of nasal septum
  - Dislodgement of adenoses

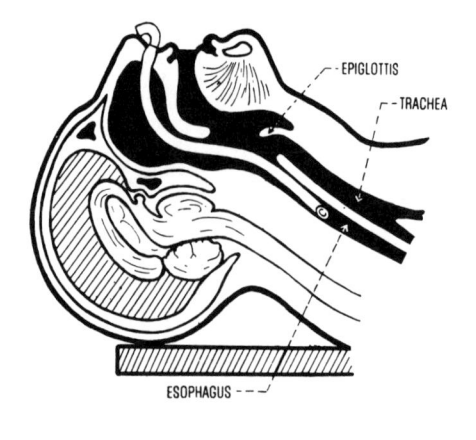

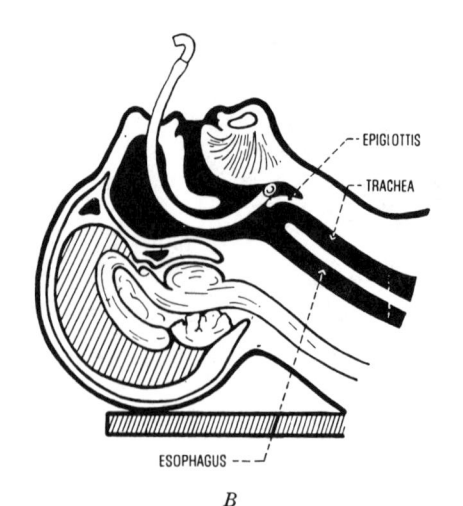

FIG. 20–26. Technical complications of nasotracheal intubations. A, One complication, the tube in the esophagus. B, The tube entering the sulcus between the base of the tongue and the epiglottis.

- Epistaxis frequent
- Eustachian tube obstruction
- Occurrence of localized infections and sinusitis
- Higher incidence of bacteremia
- Higher pulmonary infections (questionable)
- Smaller-sized endotracheal tube than for oral intubation
- Suctioning of tracheal secretions more difficult

TACTILE TRACHEAL INTUBATION

The tactile method of intubation was developed and practiced by Macewan[51] in 1880 and is the first technique developed for endotracheal intubation without tracheostomy (as by Trendelenberg) or the use of the laryngoscope. The technique was also advocated by Sykes[52] in 1937 as a method of simplicty without the need for instruments. But, by 1950 simple practical laryngoscopes were available, especially the Macintosh curved blade. This made the visual technique easy, more certain, rapid, accurate, and clean.

DESCRIPTION OF THE TACTILE METHOD. In the tactile method, preparation by the operator consists of wearing standard surgical gloves. Topical anesthesia in a tranquil patient is needed. The method can be used in a deeply comatose patient in an emergency or when deep anesthesia and relaxation are present. Long, sensitive fingers are important.

The operator stands to the left of the patient's head and faces the patient—face-to-face. The patient's mouth is opened and the index and middle

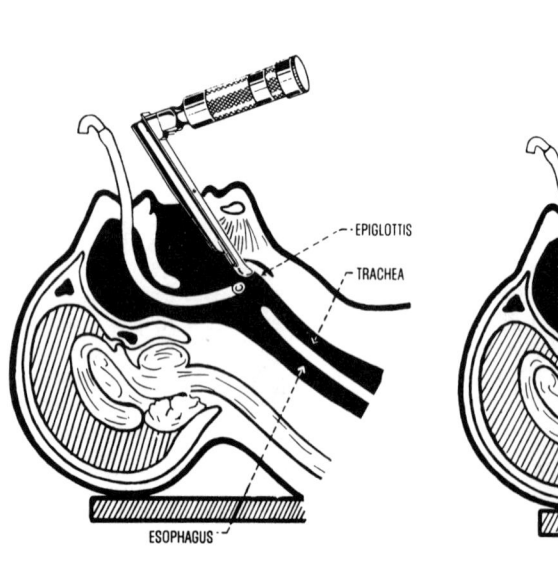

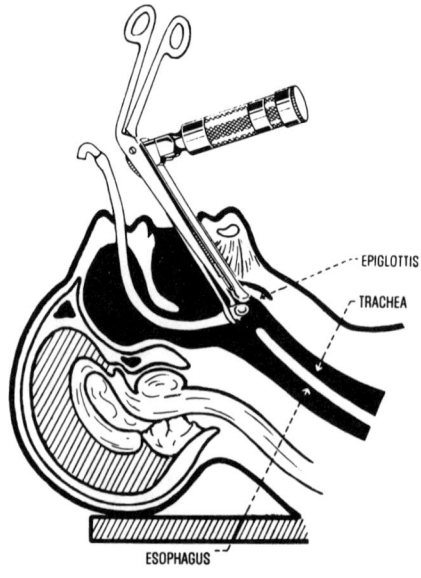

FIG. 20–27. Maneuver to place tube correctly. A, The epiglottis is retracted, exposing the glottis. An attempt is then made to introduce the tube into the larynx. B, Should failure arise (A), the end of the tube is grasped with Magill's forceps and threaded into the larynx as shown.

fingers of the left hand, palm side down are inserted into the patient's mouth in the midline. The fingers are spread and passed over the tongue into the pharynx—the index finger to the left side of the tongue into the pharynx—the index finger to the left side of the tongue and the middle finger over the right side of the tongue. As the fingers are advanced to the base of the tongue (radix linguae), each finger tends to lie in the vallecula of the tongue and the hyoid may be palpable. In the midline, a fold from the base of the tongue to the epiglottis is easily identified (plica glosso-epiglottica mediana). The left hand now retracts the tongue forward. At this point, the right hand introduces the curved endotracheal tube into the mouth and pharynx. The index finger of the right hand can now direct the tube under the epiglottis and away from the posterior pharynx and into the supraglottic funnel. By advancing the index finger further into the pharynx and curving it medially and anteriorly, it will lie behind the interarytenoid groove; and the endotracheal tube will be palpable anterior to both.

The procedure is detailed, but all these motions could be deftly accomplished in 5 to 10 seconds, with practice.

USE IN COMATOSE TRAUMA PATIENTS. In deeply comatose trauma patients with possible cervical spine injury and in situations where laryngoscopic visualization may be thoroughly obscured by blood or vomitus, the tactile technique may be employed. In these patients, airway management is of importance. One advantage is that the technique can be accomplished with minimal movement of the head and neck. It may also be accomplished in paralyzed patients in need of airway and who are obese and short necked.[53]

The technique consists of the following:

1. Palpating the epiglottis with the middle and index fingers of the left hand.
2. Guiding an endotracheal tube with a slightly curved distal portion, the so-called "J curve," to the epiglottis.
3. The tube tip is displaced behind the epiglottis as the tongue and jaw are lifted.
4. At this point, the tube can slip through the vocal cords. *Note:* The epiglottis is relatively easily palpated, and pushing the corner of the mouth sideways and anteriorly will facilitate the digital contact. A stylette may be used to provide the J curvature to the endotracheal tube.

OTHER USES. In patients with submandibular abscesses or large intraoral or pharyngeal tumors, the tactile technique is also a useful and successful approach. Topical anesthetization is necessary, and the procedure is performed before the patient is critically obstructed or comatose.

INTUBATION IN THE CONSCIOUS STATE

Many situations arise where in the interests of safety, general anesthesia followed by intubation is precluded. These patients are provided with topical anesthesia of the hypopharynx, larynx, and trachea followed by insertion of the endotracheal tube transorally or nasally. In the latter case additional anesthesia of nares must be provided.

INDICATIONS. Intubation in the conscious state is indicated in the following circumstances:

1. Head and neck surgery in patients with distorted anatomy, markedly compromised airway, or ankylosis of the jaw—in these cases, as soon as patients are lightly anesthetized, they are prone to obstruction and the statistical chances of severe hypoxia are great (despite the skill of the best anesthesiologist).
2. Semicomatose patients from head trauma or poisoning—these patients often need an airway but are reflexly active enough not to tolerate one.
3. Neurosurgical cases with neck fractures or skull fractures wherein movements or raising intracranial pressure are undesirable.
4. Prolonged intestinal obstruction with marked distention and little or no effective decompression—these patients often regurgitate and aspirate when anesthetized. Preliminary intubation and establishment of a leak-proof airway with cuff—not pack—will avoid the lethal effect of aspiration.

NERVES INVOLVED IN TOPICAL ANESTHESIA. The innervation of the oropharynx and larynx is as follows:

1. Nerves of tongue
   a. Sensation of anterior two thirds (lingual branch of mandibular nerve)
   b. Taste sensation of anterior two thirds (chorda tympani of facial nerve)
   c. Base and sides, general sense and taste (lingual branch of glossopharyngeal nerve)
   d. Root of tongue (superior laryngeal nerve)
2. Nerves of pharynx
   a. Oral part
   b. Laryngeal part
   c. Filaments of glossopharyngeal unite with branches from vagus and sympathetic opposite the constrictor pharyngius media muscle to form the pharyngeal plexus.
3. Nerves of larynx
   a. *Superior laryngeal*—Internal branch pierces the posterior portion of hyothyroid membrane above the superior laryngeal vessels at the greater cornu of the hyoid cartilage. It divides into three branches distributed to both surfaces of the epiglottis, the aryepiglottic fold, and the mucosa over back of larynx

b. *Recurrent laryngeal*—Passed upward beneath lower border of inferior pharyngeal constrictor muscle immediately behind the cricothyroid joint. A few filaments with sensory components communicate with the superior laryngeal over the back of the larynx.
4. Nerves of trachea—derived from vagus and the recurrent laryngeal as well as sympathetics.

BLOCK AT BASE OF PALATOGLOSSAL ARCH. The gag reflex consists of an afferent input over the glossopharyngeal nerve, which is elicited by firm pressure on the root of the tongue (radix lingual) where submucosal pressure receptors are located.[54a]

For purposes of laryngoscopy and the abolition of the gag reflex, a local anesthetic agent may be injected at the base of the palatoglossal arch.[54b] This is the ridge extending from the lateral pharyngeal wall to the lateral margin of the tongue known as the *anterior tonsillar pillar*. Insertion of a short needle is slightly lateral to the margin of the root of the tongue, at the point where it joins the floor of the mouth. A dose of 2 ml of 2% lidocaine is slowly injected and the procedure repeated on the opposite side. The result of this block will be manifest in a few minutes, with complete anesthetization of the posterior third of the tongue. This will allow manipulation of the tongue and direct laryngoscopy with minimal discomfort.

TECHNIQUES OF TOPICAL ANESTHESIA. The nerves of the pharynx and glottic region can be anesthetized by two routes: the transoral and the extraoral.

Transoral Anesthetic Technique. This technique consists of application by *spraying* a topical anesthetic solution to the mucosa to block the nerve terminals; this is followed by application of cotton pledgets soaked in a solution of a topical anesthetic to the pyriform sinus for 3 minutes (pledgets should be firmly grasped by a laryngeal Jackson forcep).

Extraoral Anesthetic Technique. This technique is a block of the superior laryngeal nerve. A 2-inch needle is inserted at the *greater cornua*, and 2 ml of a local anesthetic are injected.

The glottic and tracheal region can be anesthetized by the following two routes:

1. Placing of pledgets directly on cords, followed by direct introduction of an anesthetic solution inserted into the trachea through the mouth via a cannula.
2. Transtracheal injection.

TRANSTRACHEAL TECHNIQUE.[55]

Instruction. Patient is instructed not to cough, talk, or swallow while needle is in place.

Position. Patient position is supine with head hyperextended.

Landmarks. The cricoid cartilage is identified as is the first tracheal ring below. The **cricotracheal** interspace is the site for injection.

(The triangular area between the thyroid and cricoid cartilage is called the *cricothyroid membrane* or *conus elasticus*, and is composed of yellow elastic tissue. It is close to the glottis in the subglottic space, and a needle inserted at this point may injure the vocal cords.)

Procedure (Fig. 20–28). After cleaning the skin and preparing the site with an antiseptic, infiltrate the skin overlying the cricotracheal membrane with 1% lidocaine. Prepare a 23-gauge 1.5-in needle with an attached 2-ml syringe filled with a topically effective anesthetic. Recommended agents are cyclaine 5% or tetracaine 2%. Cocaine is not desirable because of occasional subcutaneous deposits with severe irritation.

The needle is inserted in the midline and advanced perpendicularly to the skin through the cricotracheal membrane until lack of resistance is appreciated, indicating an intratracheal position. Confirm this by aspirating air before making injection. Quickly empty the syringe and withdraw. Instruct patient to cough vigorously to spread the solution. Further anesthesia of the mouth, pharynx, and supraglottic area is obtained with a spray.

AWAKE NEONATE AND LARYNGOSCOPY. Awake laryngoscopy in the neonate is a common procedure for intubation when resuscitation and intense respiratory care are needed. The technique of preoxygenation for a period of 2 minutes is usually accompanied by breath-holding, bradycardia, and cyanosis. There are significant decreases in heart rate, systolic blood pressure, and transcutaneous oxygen tension. This decrease in heart rate occurs despite prior administration of atropine. Transcutaneous oxygen tension may fall dramatically by 80%.[56,57]

Intracranial pressure also greatly increases in the awake neonate and infant during laryngoscopy and intubation. Such an increase may cause intraventricular and intracranial hemorrhage. The increase in intracranial pressure correlates with the increases in arterial and central venous pressures.

In quiet, undisturbed infants, the intracranial pressure has been measured and shows some variability with age from 7 mm Hg to 8.2 mm Hg in ages 28 to 40 weeks. During orotracheal intubation, there is a significant increase in intracranial, both in the awake and anesthetized infant.[58]

Anterior fontanelle pressure (AFP) can be measured by a noninvasive technique using the Ladd transducer,* and these measurements correlate

---

* Ladd Research Institute, Burlington, Vt.

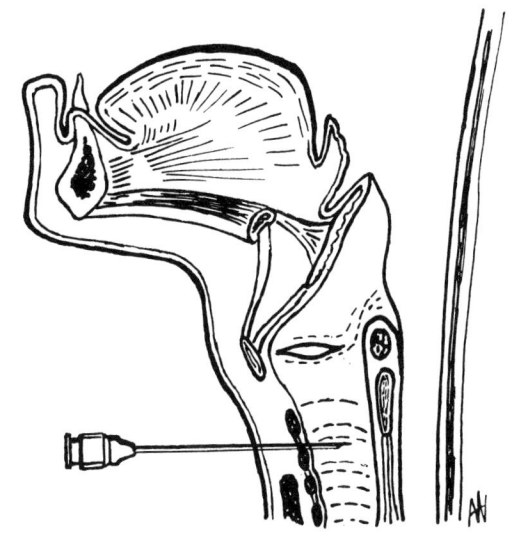

FIG. 20–28. Transtracheal technique of topical anesthesia, showing the insertion of the anesthetic needle through the cricotracheal membrane. This route is preferred. Other techniques specify the introduction of the needle through the cricothyroid membrane, but this can produce injury to the vocal cords.

closely with intracranial pressure.[59] In undisturbed infants, the AFP values are within a range of 8 to 9 mm Hg. With crying, AFP greatly increases to 15 to 20 mm Hg. In infants less than 8 weeks' postnatal age, laryngoscopy and intubation significantly increase systolic blood pressure and AFP. AFP increases to 30 to 35 mm Hg in the awake infant and to 15 ± 18 mm Hg in the lightly anesthetized infant.

Although anesthesia attenuates the intracranial and AFP response to intubation, many neonates have pressures above 25 mm Hg. It has been demonstrated that the increase in pressure is significantly minimized by muscle paralysis with small doses of pancuronium, which prevent coughing or increased intrathoracic pressure.[60] During tracheal suctioning, White[61] has shown a greater attenuation of the rise in intracranial pressure than other strategies, such as pretreatment with fentanyl or thiopental.

Recommendations. To avoid these adverse respiratory and hemodynamic changes, it is recommended that there be continuous oxygenation throughout laryngoscopy. This can be accomplished by a modified laryngoscope blade (oxyscope), which permits insufflation of 100% oxygen continuously into the supraglottic space. With this technique, no significant hemodynamic changes are observed. Both the Miller and Macintosh No. 0 and No. 1 blades have been modified for this purpose.

Light inhalation anesthesia should be provided to prevent crying and struggling, as well as to attenuate the rise in intracranial and AFP during intubation.

Consideration should also be given to the use of intramuscular succinylcholine prior to intubation or to suctioning the trachea of the infant. Although succinylcholine may itself increase intracranial pressure, the extent is limited when compared to the risks otherwise occurring during airway management.

CERVICAL FRACTURES AND INTUBATION. Intubation of the trauma victim with fracture of the cervical spine, with or without an unstable cervical spine or dislocation, poses serious technical problems. Existing neurologic function should be preserved and the patient should be protected from injury related to manipulation of the head for intubation. It is estimated that 10% of severe head injuries have associated cervical spine injuries. Of patients with cervical spine fracture or dislocation, including atlanto–occipital subluxation, about 14% have neurologic deficits. It is also estimated that 30% to 65% of patients with isolated head trauma will be hypoxic. In many of these patients, respiratory insufficiency is present and airway and ventilatory management is necessary.

Axial traction of the cervical spine is usually used to stabilize the spine. For orotracheal intubation, this introduces a difficult positional problem for laryngoscopy. The usual maneuvers for laryngoscopy are a risk to cause neurologic damage. The effect of axial traction during intubation has been studied radiologically by Bivins.[62] The effect of axial traction alone was shown to produce posterior subluxation at the fracture site at C6–C7 of 4 mm in patients without instability and a mean of 9 mm of distraction in those with instability.

When orotracheal intubation without axial traction is performed, anterior subluxation at the fracture site (C6–C7 type) of a mean of 31 mm occurs.

When orotracheal intubation with axial traction is performed, there is increased distraction by 14 mm and anterior subluxation by 18 mm in the C6–C7 injury.

From this revealing study, it is evident that in-line axial traction may itself be hazardous, especially when intubation is unavoidable and the orotracheal technique is elicited. It is recommended by Bivins[62] that nasotracheal route be used for intubation in patients with cervical spine fractures. This can be accomplished with topical anesthesia; such anesthesia should also be used in the comatose patient. The patient's head should be maintained in the neutral position. An experimental study by Aprahamian[63] demonstrated that nasotracheal intubation without cricoid pressure resulted in less movement of the patient than orotracheal intubation. The intubation procedures must be determined by the presence of other injuries of the face and jaw and of blood or vomitus in the nasopharyngeal or oropharyngeal passageway.

TECHNICAL DIFFICULTIES OF INTUBATION. These difficulties are associated chiefly with physical differences in patients: those with short, thick necks present a technical challenge because the passage from the mouth to the trachea cannot be easily straightened. Thus, the use of a straight-blade laryngoscope is not recommended. In such situations, the curved blade of the Macintosh variety or the Fink blade is useful.

Care must be exercised to avoid dental injury. The upper central incisors are prone to contact with the laryngoscope. The proper technique requires that there be a lifting force exerted through the laryngoscope handle—the *tendency to pry must be avoided*. A strip of adhesive placed about the upper teeth is a precautionary guide only and may minimize chipping.

Ankylosis of jaws or masseter spasm present obvious problems. It is difficult to open the patient's mouth and separate the jaws sufficiently to admit the straight laryngoscope blade. A curved blade can often be admitted; the nasotracheal route is sometimes the best solution, and intubation would be accomplished blindly. If it is anticipated that intubation will be inordinately difficult, conscious blind intubation or tracheostomy should be used.

Cass[1] summarizes six common anatomic causes of difficult intubation, as follows:

1. Short muscular neck with full set of teeth
2. Receding jaw with obtuse mandibular angles
3. Protruding upper incisor teeth associated with relative overgrowth of the premaxilla
4. Poor mobility of mandibles
5. Long, high-arched palate associated with a long narrow mouth
6. Increased alveolar mental ridge distance requiring wide opening of mandible for insertion of laryngoscope

ANATOMY OF CRICOTHYROID/CRICOTRACHEAL MEMBRANE (GRAY'S ANATOMY). The cavity of the larynx extends from the laryngeal inlet (glottic chink) to the level of the *lower* border of the cricoid cartilage. The anterior part of this cavity is the cricovocal membrane, represented in its more central area by the cricothyroid ligament, which is thick and subcutaneous and connects the contiguous margins of the thyroid and cricoid cartilages. The following is evident: (1) that the vocal cords extend anteriorly to the cricoid cartilage arch, and the anterior part is actually the cricothyroid ligament; any entrance through the thick cricothyroid ligament either may pass into the laryngeal cavity or may be above the vocal cords proper; if the entrance is not in the midline, a needle will sequester in the lateral recesses below the vocal cords and laryngeal inlet and impinge laterally on the cricovocal membrane with damage to the vocal ligament. (2) Furthermore, the upper part of the cricovocal-cricothyroid ligament is crossed by a small arterial arch formed by the junction of two cricothyroid arteries. An advancing needle can and has ruptured this artery, causing bleeding or an obstructive hematoma.

Another consideration is the position of the isthmus of the thyroid gland. It normally covers the second and third tracheal rings. Thus, entrance into the trachea above the first tracheal ring avoids damage to the thyroid gland.

SITE OF SUBGLOTTIC PUNCTURE.[64c] From the anatomical considerations, the safest and most effective site for puncture into the trachea should be below the structure of the larynx and is the *cricotracheal membrane*. After retrograde placement of a guide catheter, the passage of an endotracheal tube over the guide catheter or by "guided pulling" of the endotracheal tube *ensures* the tube's placement in the trachea, i.e, it allows advancement *past* the vocal cords, into the trachea. It does not become caught on the upper surface of the vocal cords, does not kink, and does not damage the cricoid-thyroid arterial arch.

RETROGRADE INTUBATION.[64] Retrograde intubation is a technique in which a guide is passed into the trachea and then advanced upward through the vocal cords to emerge into the mouth or nose. An endotracheal tube is then passed over the guide until it enters the trachea. The first report of this technique was presented in 1960 by Butler.[64] Nevertheless, the technique had been used by the head and neck service at Doctors' Hospital in New York City (Dr. D. Burdick) and at St. Vincent's Hospital in New York City (Drs. J. Conley and A. Smessaert) to provide an airway for "commando" procedures). It was selected for upper airway cancer when the obstructive condition and pathology precluded ordinary intubation technics and tracheostomy was not desired.

Types of Guides. The guides used should possess four important characteristics: (1) small enough to pass through an 18-gauge needle; (2) long enough to enter at the upper trachea and emerge at the mouth or nose (a 20- to 30-cm length is sufficient for adults; (3) flexible enough to bend along a given pathway and be manipulated to follow the path of least resistance and (4) stiff enough to follow the internal anatomy of the upper airway and to pass through the nose, enter the upper airway and emerge at the nose or into the mouth.

Three types of guides commonly used and recommended are as follows:

1. *Ureteral catheters*—these are small and flexible, but stiff enough to advance upward along the internal anatomy. They are particularly useful when nasal intubation is planned.
2. The *flexible-tipped Seldinger wire*—this is stiff

enough to follow the internal anatomy and is advantageous when nasal intubation is planned. The Swan-Ganz introducer wire is also recommended.[64b]

3. Small *epidural catheters* of the polyvinylchloride type, 25-gauge, 30 cm, with an introducing wire in place—this catheter is readily available and flexible enough, with some degree of floppiness, so that it enters the mouth and can be retrieved from the mouth and so withdrawn.

Procedure. The above equipment should be displayed with all the instruments for intubation, including proper laryngoscopes, curved and straight blades, and Magill forceps. An 18-gauge needle is introduced into the trachea below the cricoid cartilage and angled 45 degrees cephalad.

The selected guide wire or catheter is introduced through the needle and advanced upward through the vocal cords into the pharynx. Further advancement permits the catheter to follow into the nasopharynx with the stiffer type of guide when the head is slightly flexed. The more floppy type epidural catheter, when used with the wire withdrawn 1 to 2 cm, permits easier advancement into the mouth.

If the head is extended, advancement will usually be into the oropharyngeal cavity and into the mouth.

When the guide wire or catheter is brought out of the nose or mouth, the appropriate size of endotrcheal tube is then passed over the guide wire. During the introduction of the endotracheal tube, the guide wire is held relatively taut. The endotracheal tube is then advanced over the guide wire to the glottic opening. The chief resistance that is encountered is usually the result of difficulty or failure to enter the larynx.

When the endotracheal tube is approximately at the level of the vocal cords, the 18-gauge needle should be removed. It is emphasized that the catheter, once passed through the needle in an upward direction, should never be withdrawn through the standard 18-gauge introducing needle to avoid the shearing or breaking of the catheter by the bevel of the needle.

Indications. Retrograde intubation is indicated whenever extremely difficult or impossible intubation conditions are anticipated, such as (1) major congenital deformities of the face and neck structures; (2) the large oropharyngeal tumors, including abscesses (Ludwig's abscess); or (3) extensive scarring of upper airway from flame burns or sclerosing chemicals (lye).

Preoperative Assessment. The assessment should include the usual standard airway evaluation, indirect or direct laryngoscopy, and preoperative mouth and throat cultures. Contamination of the lower respiratory tract is more frequent with this technique.

GUIDED PULLING—MODIFIED RETROGRADE TECHNIQUE.[64c] This technic is performed as follows:

- Local anesthetic infiltration over the *cricotracheal* membrane.
- Midline puncture of the membrane with 16G Touhy needle.
- Introduction of a 19G epidural catheter through the needle, then upward direction of the catheter.
- Advancement of catheter cephalad and retrieval from the mouth.
- For nasotracheal intubation, a second catheter is introduced through the nose into the mouth and also retrieved from the mouth; the two catheters are tied together and the retrograde laryngeal catheter is drawn upward, out through the nose, and untied from the second (nasal) catheter.
- The laryngeal catheter guide is now affixed to the endotracheal tube by a gliding knot through the side hole (the Murphy eye). This is a gliding knot (see Fig. 20–29).
- The endotracheal tube is now pulled downward by the catheter outside this trachea while simultaneously being gently thrust downward.
- The catheter is removed by cutting it at the puncture site and then pulling it out of the nasal end of the tracheal tube. This is easily accomplished because of the gliding nature of the knot.

BOUGIE GUIDE FOR TRANSORAL INTUBATION. The use of a gum elastic bougie as a guide for the introduction of an appropriate-size tube into the trachea was described in 1949 by Macintosh.[65] It is used when visualization of the vocal cords is difficult or impossible. The technique involves two phases: (1) the placement of the bougie transorally into the trachea; and (2) the threading of the selected tracheal tube over the bougie into the trachea. A 13- or 14-French gauge, 60-cm (24-in) gum elastic bougie marked at 5-cm intervals is used. The bougie should be molded to provide concave anterior curvature so that the tip will snap or click along the inner surface of the anterior tracheal wall.

Clues to the placement of the bougie are the following:[66]

1. As the bougie passes through the glottic chink and slides along the tracheal rings, a "washboard" effect may be felt or appreciated as gentle snaps (called *clicks*).
2. If the bougie is in the trachea, its advancement may encounter resistance and be foreshortened as it passes deeply into the stem bronchi. If in the esophagus, the bougie may be advanced its full length without any resistance.
3. A cough reflex may be elicited as the bougie advances into the trachea.

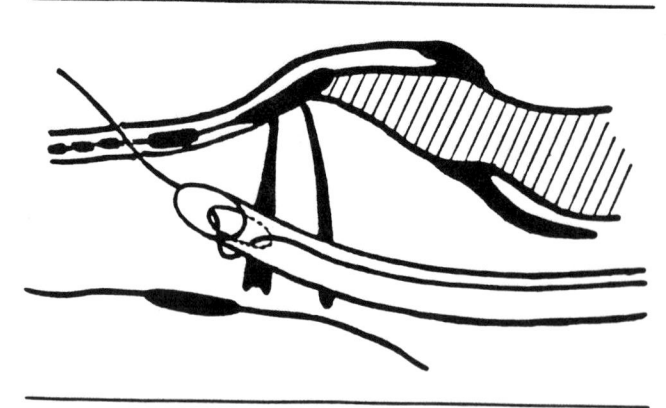

FIG. 20–29. Cross-section of larynx and trachea, with the tracheal tube pulled down by the catheter guide into correct position. The catheter exit is at the level of the *cricotracheal membrane.* From Abou-Madi, M.N., Trop, D.: Pulling versus guiding: A modification of retrograde guided intubation. Can. J. Anaesth., 36:336, 1989.

Technique. Laryngoscopy is always performed and at least the base of the tongue or upper lip of the epiglottis is seen or estimated. The bougie is then introduced posterior to the epiglottis as seen or imagined.

As it advances through the aperture of the vocal cords, a cough may be elicited, and as it passes along the anterior trachea, the mild snapping or clicking noted as a clue can be felt as the tip passes each tracheal ring.

In a study of the signs of bougie placement, Kidd[67] found the signs suggested by Sellers[66] to be reliable. Clicks were felt in 90% of tracheal placement. The bougie was held up when a distance from the lips of 24 to 40 cm had been reached. When in the esophagus, no clicks were observed and no resistance encountered even when the full length of the bougie had been introduced.

The placement of the bougie is the key to intubation. Once it is in the trachea, the endotracheal tube is simply threaded over the bougie guide, and its entrance through the vocal cords and into the trachea is readily appreciated.

FIBEROPTIC INTUBATION

The concept of fiberoptics, defined as the transmission of pictures via bundles of glass fibers, was first introduced in 1927 by John L. Baird.[68] About 30 years elapsed before the first application in medicine, when Hirschowitz[69] used a flexible gastroscope to inspect duodenal ulcers. In 1967, Murphy[70] used a fine-caliber, flexible-glass–fiber choledochoscope as an optical stylet to intubate several patients. Meanwhile, industry offered the medical profession an optic instrument tailored to the specialty.

PRINCIPLES OF FIBEROPTIC LIGHT TRANSMISSION. When a glass rod is exposed to high heat and stretched, the glass changes to a long fine thread, a flexible fiber measuring between 5 and 25 μ in diameter. The fibers retain the property of glass to transmit light and images along its length and are designated as *core fibers.* To insulate a core fiber optically, it is coated with a layer of melted glass, which has a lower refractive index, a process called *cladding.*

This process ensures that light entering at the end of the glass rod or fiber travels through the fiber and is repeatedly reflected internally as it strikes the cladded glass (Fig. 20–30). When a large number of these fibers of the smallest diameter are fastened together tightly at both ends, a flexible bundle is formed with a compact, regular arrangement of glass fibers at one end of the bundle, which is precisely the same at the other end (coherent bundle). This is the image-transmitting bundle. The resolution of the image depends on the regularity, density, and compactness of the fibers, as well as fiber size. The light-transmitting bundle consists of fibers about 25 μ in diameter and are not arranged in any precise order (the incoherent bundle).

STRUCTURE OF THE FIBEROPTIC SCOPE (FIG. 20–31).[71] A fiberoptic unit has two types of fiberoptic bundles. One type is the incoherent glass fiber bundle, which transmits light from an external source along the guide cable through the control handle and then through the insertion cord to the tip of the instrument. A second shorter, coherent fiberoptic bundle transmits the reflected light from an image back through the insertion cord to the control handle, where a series of lenses and an eyepiece allow viewing of the image (Fig. 20–32). The scope is also designed with coordinated rotation, so that rotation of the handle causes rotation of the tip of the scope, allowing full 360-degrees viewing. A working channel is provided through which the operator can inject drugs, air, or oxygen, aspirate fluids, or pass a biopsy instrument.

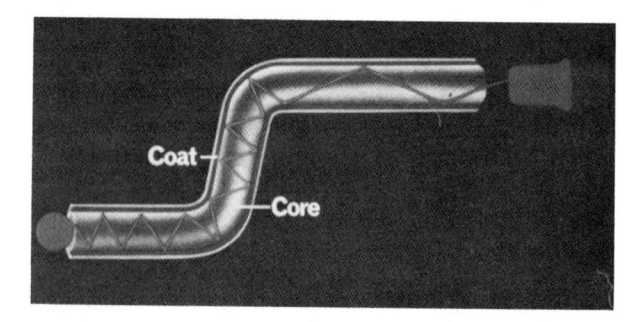

FIG. 20–30. Representation of the path taken by a beam of light entering and exiting a glass fiber. From Patil, V.U., Stehling, L., and Zauder, H.L.: Fiberoptic Endoscopy in Anesthesia. Chicago, Year Book Medical Publishers, 1983.

FIG. 20–31. Flexible fiberoptic laryngoscope. *A*, tip deflection control knob. *B*, eyepiece. *C*, diopter adjustment ring. *D*, working channel sleeve and plug. From Dripps, R.D., Eckenhoff, J.E., and Vandam, L.D.: Introduction to Anesthesia: The Principles of Safe Practice, 6th ed. Philadelphia, W.B. Saunders, 1982.

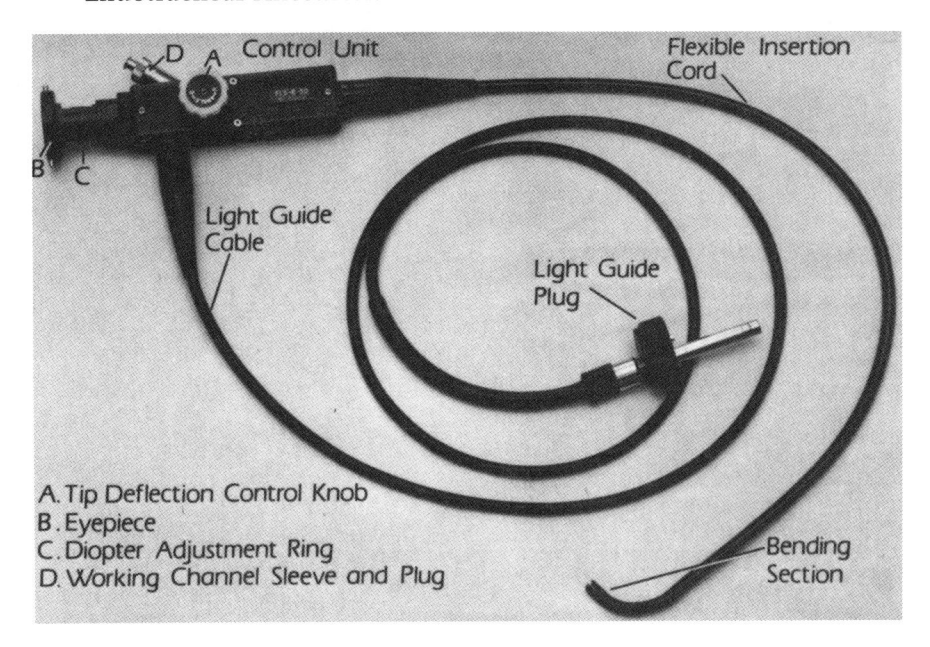

INDICATIONS FOR FIBEROPTIC BRONCHOSCOPY. Therapeutic indications include foreign body aspiration, difficult endotracheal intubation, hemoptysis, and acute lobar collapse.

Diagnostic indications include localized wheeze; atelectasis; unresolved pneumonia; chest radiograph suggestive of neoplasia; abnormal sputum cytology; recurrent laryngeal nerve palsy; phrenic nerve paralysis; chronic cough; hemoptysis; diffuse lung disease; bronchography; and the checking of the position of a double-lumen tube.

PREPARATION OF THE PATIENT. Appropriate sedation and tranquilization are recommended according to the patient's needs. The technique can be applied in the awake patient using appropriate topical and regional anesthesia or in the anesthetized patient.

PREPARATION OF EQUIPMENT. Some guidelines must be followed before using the fiberoptic endoscope:

- Check light source and endoscope
- Apply antifog agent to lens
- Focus lens prior to use
- Lubricate insertion tube
- Cut endotracheal tube to correct length
- Insert endoscope into endotracheal tube*

MANIPULATION OF THE INSTRUMENT.[72] All flexible fiberoptic instruments tie incoming and outgoing fiberoptic bundle strands, the suction channel, and flexion cables into a slender tube of varying length (30 to greater than 100 cm).

A fiberoptic conduit brings light from a remote

*The Carden bronchoscopy tube may be used. It is specially designed for fiberoptic bronchoscopy. The machine end is larger than the patient end and is somewhat funnel shaped similar to the Cole tube. This feature enables one to more easily insert the fiberoptic bronchoscope and lessens the resistance to passage of the bronchoscope. Carden, E., Ray, P.: Special new low resistance to flow tube and endotracheal tube adapter for use during fiberoptic bronchoscopy. Ann. Oto. Rhinol. Laryngol. 24:631, 1975.

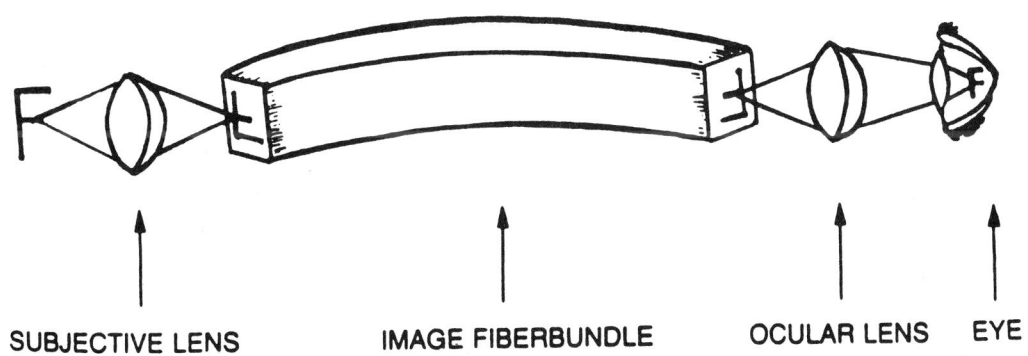

FIG. 20–32. The image, inverted by the distal lens, is restored to its proper orientation by the ocular lens. From Patil, V.U., Stehling, L., and Zauder, H.L.: Fiberoptic Endoscopy in Anesthesia. Chicago, Year Book Medical Publishers, 1983.

source, and other bundles of fiberoptic strands conduct a reflected image back from the working tip.

Fiberoptic strands are flexible but cannot be kinked or twisted. They are tied into a small "umbilical cord" from the optic head to the working tip. The operator must hold an objective lens, the "optic head," at one end of the instrument while manipulating a flexible tip with the other.

Because of the limited OD needed for airway endoscopes, control cables are only placed along two sides of the instrument and flexion can only be achieved in one plane (Fig. 20-33). Thus, the instrument must be rotated as a unit if the tip is to be redirected in another plane and, because it is flexible, it must be advanced and withdrawn from a point that is closest to the working tip.

The control head must be held close to the eye with one hand (the dominant hand) while the instrument is positioned with the other (Fig. 20-34). The dominant hand rotates the entire instrument around its central axis while the thumb controls the tip deflection lever and the forefinger intermittently occludes the external suction bypass, allowing suction via the instrument. The other hand allows the tip to rotate passively while controlling the depth to which it has been advanced in the airway.

Experience with fiberoptic instruments increases the success rate and decreases procedure time; however, a number of circumstances may complicate the procedure and are considered in the following section.

PROCEDURE—RECOMMENDATIONS. Successful fiberoptic intubation requires controlled conditions and a stable patient:

- An awake patient is desired and sedatives or small doses of narcotic drugs are useful. Topical anesthesia and vasoconstrictors are necessary. Gentle technique must be followed.
- First attempts with a fiberoptic instrument in supine patients under general anesthesia compounds the difficulty for a beginner, because the natural airway is narrowed in a supine patient. With the patient under general anesthesia, it often requires two operators to perform successful endoscopy, despite mechanical retraction of the tongue, a Patil endoscopy mask, or endoscopy oral airway.
- In contrast, the awake patient who is in a sitting position will swallow secretions, maintain the airway, and follow commands if managed appropriately. The sitting position allows good opening of the pharynx to give the endoscope tip a field of vision.
- Because the ability to visualize the airway indirectly by use of a mirror or directly by a flexible instrument that can pass around corners does not reliably predict the oropharyngeal site of the scope, direct laryngoscopy with a standard laryngoscope may be used for initial placement of the fiberoptic endoscope into the hypopharynx or supraglottic region.
- Secretions may obscure the imaging and must be controlled by prior anticholinesterases and suctioning. Swallowing may direct the tip into pockets of tissues and lose the view from the midline passageway.
- Disorientation in visualizing the airway through the fiberoptic scope is best resolved by withdrawing the tip slightly and examining the anatomic area with gentle up-and-down tip deflection.
- Too rapid advancement of the fiberoptic scope will cause a rapid change in sequence of airway anatomy and cause a loss of orientation.
- Successful fiberoptic procedure requires preoperative preparation, a plan of management, and constant contact with the patient and postoperative follow-up. Control of the situation with good patient rapport is essential.

Technique of Tracheal Intubation. Introduce endoscope into pharynx; maintain in midline and advance 8 to 10 cm. Look into the endoscope and

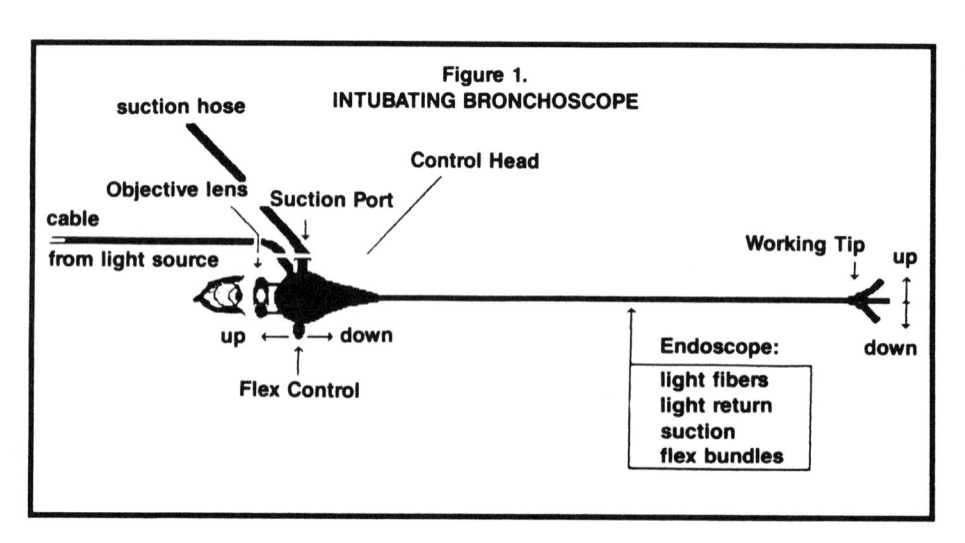

FIG. 20-33. Intubating bronchoscope. In any one plane, viewing is achieved by up-and-down flexion of tip. Illustration courtesy of Patil, V.U., Stehling, L., and Zauder, H.L.: Anesthesiology News, 13:#17, 51, 1987.

FIG. 20–34. The intubating bronchoscope rotates as a unit to allow flexion in all planes. Illustration courtesy of Patil, V.U., Stehling, L., and Zauder, H.L.: Anesthesiology News, 13:#17, 51, 1987.

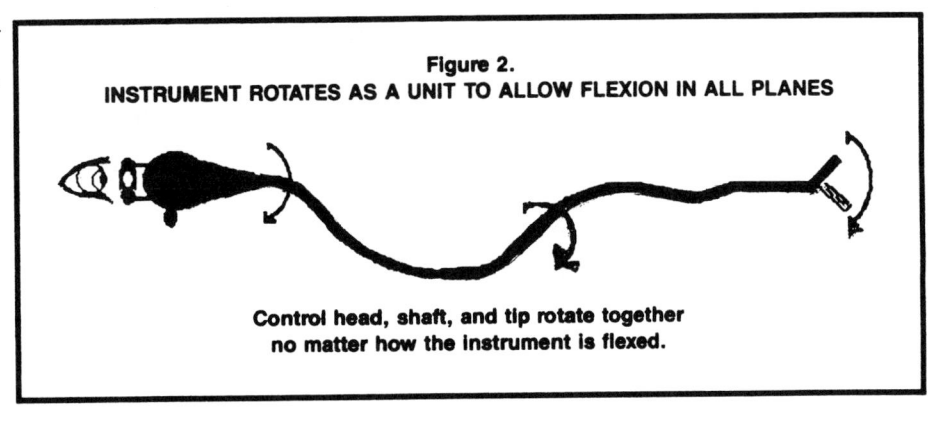

identify structures, namely, the epiglottis. Flex tip downward to visualize the posterior commissure and advance under the epiglottis. Flex the tip of the endoscope upward to visualize the larynx. Rotate the distal end of the insertion tube toward midline, if necessary. Pass the fiberoptic tube through the vocal cords; return the tip of the endoscope to a neutral position and advance. Position the endoscope tip in the trachea midway between the vocal cords and the carina and thread the endotracheal tube. Thread the endotracheal tube into the trachea over the fiberoptic scope.

NASAL APPROACH.[73] Nasal mucosal vasoconstriction by cocaine or phenylephrine is used to decrease bleeding. The endoscope is passed through the nostril directly or through a rubber nasal airway, which is split longitudinally (Fig. 20–35). Once the endoscope is advanced into the trachea, the airway is removed and the endotracheal tube threaded over the inserted endoscope. Deviation of the nasal septum, causing displacement of the endotracheal tube, is overcome by slight internal rotation of the tube.

ORAL APPROACH.[72] A standard-size ID endotracheal tube is used. The potential for tissue trauma and bleeding is lower during orotracheal intubation, but it is difficult to thread the endotracheal tube once the endoscope is within the trachea, because of the acute angle formed by the oropharynx and trachea. This problem can be overcome by retraction of the tongue and protrusion of the mandible. If the bevel of the tube is caught at the level of the epiglottis or aryepiglottic folds, slight rotation of the endotracheal tube, combined with forward displacement of the tongue, will usually disengage the tube and allow it to slide through the vocal cords.

The largest endoscope that will fit easily into the endotracheal tube should be used; it is more difficult to thread a larger endotracheal tube over a small, flexible endoscope.

CARE OF THE INSTRUMENT.[73] The fiberoptic scope is a delicate instrument that must be handled with care. The endoscope must be protected from a patient's bite with teeth or gums by the use of some type of bite block. The angle mechanism for tip deflection is frequently broken by an inexperienced operator. Never force the deflection of the tip if resistance is felt. Do not use the angle mechanism within the confines of an endotracheal tube.

Cleaning Instruments. For cleaning, follow the manufacturer's directions. The working channel should be thoroughly flushed with water as soon as the procedure is completed so that secretions and blood are not allowed to dry. The external surface

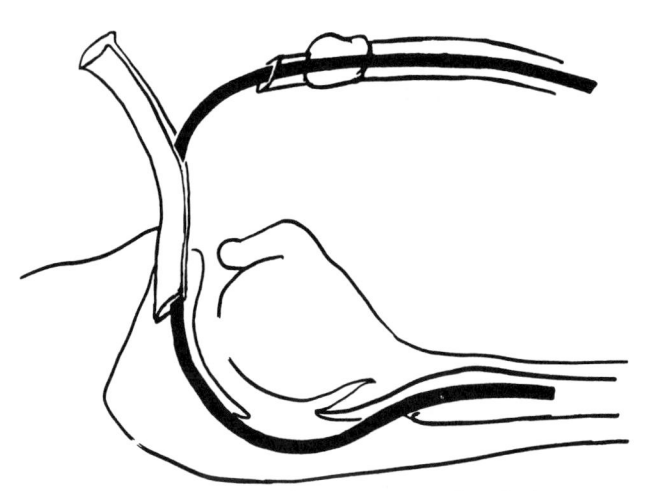

FIG. 20–35. Tissue trauma is minimized and placement of the insertion tube is facilitated if the latter is threaded into a nasal airway prior to passage. The airway should be slit longitudinally before insertion of the instrument to permit removal of the airway without altering the position of the insertion tube. The tip of the insertion tube must not protrude through the end of the airway when passed through the nose. This technique is especially useful when using a pediatric bronchoscope because of the delicacy of the instrument. From Patil, V.U., Stehling, L., and Zauder, H.L.: Fiberoptic Endoscopy in Anesthesia. Chicago, Year Book Medical Publishers, 1983.

of the control unit and light guide cable should be wiped with a sponge dampened with 70% alcohol. The external surface of the insertion cord should be washed with soap and water and then immersed in glutaraldehyde solution for 10 to 30 minutes for disinfection. The glutaraldehyde solution should be aspirated with a syringe into the working channel to disinfect it for 10 to 30 minutes. This soaking can be done in special basins or containers manufactured for this purpose. Thoroughly flush the working channel and insertion cord with water, then 70% alcohol. Aspirate air to dry the channel. The endoscope should be thoroughly dry inside and out prior to storage.

Alternatively, the endoscope can be sterilized with ethylene oxide gas.

COMPLICATIONS. Table 20–6 lists the complications associated with fiberoptic intubation.

PROTECTION OF AIRWAY—SELLICK MANEUVER

The problems of regurgitation, vomiting, and aspiration are frequently encountered in emergency circumstances and often in elective anesthesia care.

A patient with a full stomach is at great risk for regurgitation and aspiration. To secure the airway against pulmonary aspiration becomes a primary objective for safe general anesthesia. It is usually accomplished by a rapid-sequence technique, and this is commonly chosen. Intravenous agents are used for rapid induction at fairly large doses, with the simultaneous production of full paralysis by the use of muscle relaxants. A priming technique with nondepolarizing drugs is recommended; succinylcholine is also commonly used but is attended with a number of hazards, such as an increase in intragastric pressure and cardiac arrhythmias. Full paralysis will, of course, prevent vomiting but will not prevent regurgitation.

To contribute to the safety of the rapid-sequence induction and to minimize regurgitation of gastric material reaching the pharynx and upper airway, Sellick[74a] in 1961 demonstrated the effectiveness of cricoid compression. The maneuver consists of temporary occlusion of the upper esophagus by firm backward pressure on the cricoid ring against the bodies of the cervical vertebrae, usually C5 to C7. The compression force should be slightly off center to the left but uniform.

EFFICIENCY OF THE SELLICK TECHNIQUE. The efficacy of the maneuver has been demonstrated in adults by Fanning[75] and in children by Salem.[76] Significant complications of the technique itself have not been observed.[74b] The technique, however, may be poorly performed and occlusion incomplete. Two factors are important in the correct application: (1) The direction of the force—this must be uniformly and completely against the vertebral bodies of C6 and C7. In children, the cricoid is slightly higher in topographic location to the vertebral bodies; and (2) The amount of pressure—the force needed to occlude the esophagus is represented by approximately the equivalent of 4.5 kg[77] and considered to be sufficient weight to produce the desired effect in most patients.

To facilitate a uniform pressure, a cricoid yoke device has been introduced by Lawes.[78,79] This is designed to produce consistent and reproducible cricoid pressure. It introduces another device requiring manipulation, however, and minimizes the simplicity of the original Sellick maneuver.

Frequently, a nasogastric tube is present in these patients, and the competence of the esophagogastric valvular mechanism (esophageal sphincter) may be compromised, allowing a greater volume of regurgitant material. Under these circumstances, there is concern about the ability of the Sellick maneuver to prevent gastric contents reaching the pharynx. In an elegant study, Salem[80] has demonstrated that cricoid compression will seal off the esophagus from the pharynx and upper airway. Further, insertion of a nasogastric tube prior to the beginning of anesthesia in patients with an overdistended stomach clearly fails to reduce intragastric pressure. Emptying a full stomach, as in those patients who have recently eaten and prior to emergency surgery, by an oropharyngeal large-bore tube, may be advisable. This is particularly applicable with the onset of labor in those patients who have just eaten.[81]

The nasogastric tube of the plastic type is not occluded by cricoid pressure. These tubes are quite firm. This is in contrast to the ability to readily occlude, by slight pressure, the soft latex nasogastric tubes. It is, therefore, recommended that because there is no leakage from the esophagus along the

TABLE 20–6. COMPLICATIONS ASSOCIATED WITH FIBEROPTIC INTUBATION

Category	Signs and Symptoms
Premedication	Respiratory depression
	Hypertension or syncope
	Hyperexcitement
Local anesthesia	Laryngospasm
	Bronchospasm
	Seizures
	Cardiorespiratory arrest
Bronchoscopy	Bronchospasm
	Laryngospasm
	Hypoxemia
	Cardiac arrhythmias
	Fever
	Pneumonia
Biopsy-brush procedures	Pneumothorax
	Hemorrhage
	Pneumonia

course of the nasogastric tubes into the pharynx, the nasogastric tubes should be left unclamped.[80a]

FACILITATION OF INTUBATION (SALEM TECHNIC).[80b] Cephalad (upward) displacement of the larynx has been demonstrated to facilitate visualization of the vocal cords and intubation of the trachea. This can be combined with the Sellick maneuver.

SHARED AIRWAY: TUBES AND AIRWAY FOR ENDOSCOPIC AND OROLARYNGOTRACHEAL PROCEDURES. The shared airway presents a challenge in control of ventilation by the anesthesiologist because the endoscopist and laryngologist must visualize the anesthesiologist's operative field. Strategies to accomplish both purposes with safety include the following:

1. Small-diameter endotracheal tubes (4.5 to 6 mm for the adult)—These are placed in the posterior commissure in the interarytenoid space[82a]
2. A tracheal insufflation anesthetic technique with exhalation occurring around the fresh gas-flow delivery tube—Obstructive pathology must not be present
3. Jet injector technique[82b]

Special Problems of Laser Surgery (Table 20–7). Laser surgery involves the use of energy from a coherent light beam. The term laser is an acronym for *light amplification by stimulated emission radiation.* Ordinary light contains many different wave lengths in varying phases and is incoherent. The laser beam is coherent, all waves being of a single frequency and in phase and can be precisely aimed and used as a surgical cutting tool. The materials used as substances for production of a laser beam when energized are gases such as argon, helium-neon, and carbon dioxide; solids, such as the ruby, are also used. The low-energy state of these substances is excited by electricity or by ordinary light, and when the molecules of the substrate are energized, they emit a powerful coherent concentrated light beam.

Two types of lasers are in current use: (1) the CO_2 laser, which is used to remove laryngeal papillomas, polyps, nodules, and cysts; this has a wave length of 10.6 μ in the infrared region; the beam is absorbed by all tissues and destroys membranes and cells; and (2) the argon laser beam, which is selectively absorbed by pigmented tissues and is used to repair retinal detachment and to remove nevi.

The thermal effects of lasers on endotracheal tubes has posed problems. Either the plastic or rubber tubes may be perforated, burned, or charred. Red rubber tubes are more easily ignited or charred than vinyl tubes,[83] while the vinyl tube is easily perforated.[84]

Protection of the Tube. Several proposals that have been made to protect endotracheal tubes from damage or fire include aluminum foil wrapping,[85a] moist muslin wrapping,[85b] application of moist cottonoids, and use of flexible stainless steel (matte finished) endotracheal tubes.[86]

In general, uncuffed red rubber tubes wrapped in aluminum foil appear to be satisfactory for children. For adults, the moist muslin wrapped tube is the more satisfactory.[87] Some of the problems are that aluminum foil deflects laser beams and increases kinkability. Its sharp edges may injure mucosa. Also, wrapping increases bulk, and cuffs are still vulnerable.

EVALUATION OF TRAUMA TO LARYNX FROM ACCIDENTS.[88a,88b] Following accidents and associated trauma to the head and neck, the larynx of a patient scheduled for surgery should be carefully evaluated. The ordinary techniques of assessment should be completed, including indirect laryngoscopy. Mobility of the neck should be estimated and the integrity of the laryngeal lumen should be determined. Soft-tissue x-rays of the neck and cervical spine are important. When indicated, xero-radiography may provide evidence of soft-tissue injury. Computed tomography scanning has been used to diagnose fractures of the thyroid cartilage or cricoid ring, as well as to assess the patency of the airway.[88c]

Four varieties of laryngeal trauma are frequently encountered: (1) supraglottic laryngeal fracture—the epiglottis is displaced posteriorly but the vocal cords may be spared; (2) cricotracheal separation—the larynx and trachea are distracted and usually subluxated. If there is complete separation of the larynx from the trachea, a fatality is usual; (3) midline

TABLE 20–7. ANESTHETIC PROBLEMS AND SOLUTIONS IN LARYNGEAL LASER SURGERY

Anesthetic Problems	Solutions
Shared airway	Small-diameter endotracheal tubes or use of jet injector cannulae to keep out of surgical field
Perforation or burning of endotracheal tubes or jet injector cannulae	Red rubber tubes wrapped with aluminum tape or muslin. Nonflammable jet injector cannulae
Perforation of endotracheal tube cuff	Packing moist cottonoids between cuff and glottis
Drying of muslin, wrapping, and cottonoids	Multiperforated epidural catheter placed alongside tube prior to wrapping, and constantly irrigated
Harmful effects of laser beam on eyes	Protection of patients' eyes with eye shields. Protection of personnel eyes with glasses
Need for immobile surgical field	Paralysis or deep anesthesia with controlled ventilation

From Konchigeri, H.N., and Shaker, M.H.: Anesthesia for intralaryngeal surgery. Can. Anaesth. Soc. J., 21:343, 1974.

vertical fractures—these will damage the anterior commissure and usually separate the thyroid plates from the midline; and (4) the laryngeal skeleton itself may be shattered with multiple fractures of the cricoid, thyroid, or even the arytenoid cartilages in older patients when there may be extensive calcification of the laryngeal skeleton.

Problems Encountered. Some problems associated with laryngeal trauma include obstruction of the airway from displacement of teeth, soft tissues, structures of the larynx, and bone-fracture fragments of maxilla and mandible; separation of the trachea from the larynx at the cricoid; displacement of the epiglottis due to supraglottic laryngeal fracture; injury or fracture of the cervical spine with limitation to flexion–extension of the head; surgical emphysema—soft tissues and compartments of neck, mediastinal emphysema; and coma from concomitant head injury.

Management of Airway. [88] A general recommendation for patients with head and neck trauma is to establish an airway while the patient is awake, using a local or topical anesthesia. In the unconscious patient, a local or topical anesthesia is preferred and needed.

- Oral tracheal intubation may be readily accomplished in most circumstances with good topical anesthesia and a cooperative patient. Minimal tranquilization but *not* sleep can be achieved with low doses of diazepam or ketamine.
- In the absence of stridor and noisy respirations in severe, major head and neck injury and in presence of easy respiration and careful assessment of the upper passageways, intubation may be accomplished after induction of general anesthesia.
- Nasal intubation may be desired in mandibular fractures, but after careful assessment of the overall anatomic condition.
- When the airway is severely compromised* from trauma (or infection or tumor), a preliminary tracheostomy with local anesthesia is recommended.

TRANSTRACHEAL VENTILATION. An airway and pulmonary ventilation can be accomplished in an emergency and when the upper airway is blocked by the insertion of a large-bore needle (10 to 12 gauge) or trocar directly into the trachea. One need not look for sophisticated devices such as a cricothyretome or do a tracheostomy. The effective use of large-bore needles and percutaneous transtracheal ventilation was first described by Jacoby and Hamelberg in 1951.[88d]

The needle should be placed below the cricoid ring and puncture accomplished through the cricotracheal membrane or the next tracheotracheal membrane. Intermittent positive pressure through the delivery tube from an anesthesia machine or from a simple assembly of an oxygen cylinder-pressure gauge-flowmeter. A jet type of application can be simulated.[88e]

INDICATIONS AND ADVANTAGES OF ENDOTRACHEAL INTUBATION

An endotracheal tube should be looked on as another airway, albeit the most effective and desirable one. The application of the technique and the introduction of a tube into the trachea should be looked on only as another device for safe anesthetic management of the patient. Whenever an indication exists, the endotracheal airway should be used. Disadvantages are insignificant in view of the overwhelming advantages.

INDICATIONS. Use of the endotracheal technique is indicated when general anesthesia is administered where the anesthetist must either *assure* a good patent airway or *be able to* control or assist respirations as desired. Table 20–8 summarizes the varying degrees of necessity for endotracheal intubation.

ADVANTAGES. The following objectives are achieved by an endotracheal airway:

1. Provides a free unobstructed airway—eliminates obstruction due to relaxed tongue, pharyngeal tissue, and laryngospasm.
2. Decreases respiratory effort because of the freedom of air flow.
3. Provides control of airway—to maintain an airway when the head is inaccessible to the anesthetist, an endotracheal tube is the only reliable means.
4. Increases relaxation—the better relaxation for abdominal surgery during endotracheal anesthesia results from the smooth and minimal diaphragmatic effort occurring with the free airway.
5. Prevents aspiration—an endotracheal tube with cuff during surgery of the head, neck, or oral cavity is the main safeguard against aspiration of blood, teeth, and tissues. Similarly, aspiration of intestinal contents during abdominal procedures for intestinal obstruction is minimized.
6. Controls ventilation—in open-chest surgery, collapse of the lung and mediastinal flutter are most easily overcome by means of an endotracheal tube. Similarly, any of the respiratory derangements possible in intrathoracic work may be controlled without hypoxia developing.
7. Assists respiration—best accomplished with the aid of an endotracheal tube; it is particularly desirable during surgery in lithotomy, Trendelenburg and prone positions.
8. Facilitates resuscitation—when an endotracheal tube is in place, sudden respiratory and car-

---

*Respiration is noisy (stridor) and accessory muscles are used.

TABLE 20-8. INDICATIONS FOR ENDOTRACHEAL INTUBATION

Group	Indication

I	Intubation mandatory
	Patient's life depends on use of endotracheal tube. No patient in this group should be operated upon under general anesthesia without intubation
	  1. Intracranial operations
	  2. Intrathoracic operations
	  3. Prone position—major operation
	  4. Operation in presence of intestinal distention or recent feeding
	  5. Major head and neck surgery
	  6. Intraoral surgery, including tonsillectomy
	  7. Major intraabdominal surgery

II	Intubation preferable
	Intubation affords a greater safety or superior operating conditions. With a capable anesthesiologist, the advantages far outweigh the minor complications.
	  1. Minor head and neck surgery
	  2. Minor surgery of abdominal wall and thoracic wall.
	  3. Positions compromising physiology (eg, kidney position)

III	Intubation optional
	Advantages and disadvantages balanced (usually short procedures)
	Done at option of anesthetist and related to skill and experience
	  1. Minor surgery of extremities and superficial torso
	  2. Minor superficial surgery of head and neck
	In nearly all other procedures, intubation is not justified.

IV	No intubation

Modified from Smith, R.: Indications for endotracheal intubation. Curr. Res. Anesth. Analg., 33:107, 1954.

diovascular complications are more quickly treated and oxygenation is better effected.

9. Removes the anesthetist and apparatus from surgical field.

10. Diminishes dead space—content of the mouth–nose–pharynx is between 60 and 75 ml, whereas that of a No. 10 Magill tube, from where it enters the glottis to the lips, is 14 ml. If there is a direct connection with the source of anesthetic mixture and the machine without a *mask*, there is further reduction in dead space otherwise imposed by the face mask of some 100 to 150 ml. It is thus evident that the use of a face mask after intubation is illogical.

DISADVANTAGES. It is emphasized that the difficulties associated with endotracheal intubation are insignificant in view of the overwhelming advantages. Disadvantages are all mechanical and are either of technique or maintenance. These are summarized as follows, although many of these alleged disadvantages are questionable:

1. Requires technical skill on the part of the operator
2. Requires thorough knowledge of anatomy and physiology of respiration
3. Deeper anesthesia is needed more than may be required for the surgery
4. Induction is longer
5. Tube may kink
6. Leaks may occur if packing is poor
7. Arrhythmias sometimes occur
8. Traumatic complications occur
9. Intubation under light anesthesia may provoke cough, breath-holding, or bronchospasm

EXTUBATION

As important for overall patient welfare as intubation is the proper removal of the endotracheal tube, referred to as *extubation*. A dilemma and controversy exist between extubation in deep levels of general anesthesia or extubation when the patient is awake. Each carries definite hazards.

A middle course is recommended. It is generally agreed that extubation should be performed in light stages of anesthesia—the stage of unconsciousness or stage of analgesia—and that there should be spontaneous central respiratory control. Thus, two goals are to be achieved: (1) the time of postextubation and postanesthesia respiratory depression will be short, and (2) the time interval of depressed protective laryngeal and pharyngeal reflexes will be reduced. The anesthetist avoids two serious and historically fatal complications of general anesthesia, the respiratory depression or ventilatory hypoxia and the hazard of pulmonary aspiration, both related to deep levels of anesthesia. It is important to also be aware of medications not yet eliminated, which can delay the return to consciousness (Table 20–9).

Some practical suggestions, when extubation is to be accomplished while the patient is still under the waning influence of general anesthesia, are as follows:

TABLE 20-9. DELAYED RETURN TO CONSCIOUSNESS

Premedications
  Benzodiazepines
  Neuroleptics
  Barbiturates
  Narcotics
Other Medications
  Lidocaine
  Monoamine oxidase inhibitors
  Cimetidine
  Some antihypertensives
Patient-administered medication

From Civetta, J.M.: Perioperative effects of anesthesia. Curr. Rev. Clin. Anesth., 8:Lesson 16, March 1988.

1. Use an anesthetic lubricant on endotracheal tube before the procedure to diminish laryngospasm (Americaine; Nupercainal ointment).
2. Wash out volatile agents.
3. Timing of procedure: Extubate at level of anesthesia—either 1st plane, stage III, Guedel or a level of unconsciousness, stage II.
4. Use a strategy to protect against bucking (IV lidocaine).
5. Begin reversal of relaxants so the antagonist effect is complete first, before extubation and awakening.

Associated difficulties must be recognized when extubation is performed in extremely light planes when the patient begins to swallow or during actual awakening. A paroxysm of coughing or laryngospasm may negate all efforts at maintaining good physiology. It is necessary to prevent the effects of both bucking and laryngospasm. Clinical experience will enable the anesthetist to individualize each patient's care and estimate the proper course to pursue (Fig. 20-36).

Other difficulties associated with extubation while the patient is still unconscious are related to poor muscle relaxation and include rigidity of the jaw and raised intraabdominal pressure. The first makes tracheobronchial toilet inadequate and the second may foster regurgitation, aspiration, and pulmonary morbidity. Furthermore, the raised intraabdominal pressure is the result of the bucking phenomenon and, if violent, may cause tearing of sutures and wound disruption.

An alternative to attaining an appropriate anesthetic depth is to allow the patient to recover to a level of unconsciousness, stage II or stage I of analgesia, and employ a short-acting muscular relaxant. When the time is propitious to proceed with extubation, a dose of succinylcholine calculated to just produce apnea is injected.[28] The remainder of the steps of extubation are then complete.

COMPLICATIONS OF EXTUBATION. Extubation should proceed at the conclusion of anesthesia so that an unobstructed, normal airway and spontaneous, normal respiration can be quickly reestablished. At the same time, care must be exercised to avoid complications. Three complications should be anticipated and efforts made by properly planned procedure to prevent their occurrence, as follows:

1. Apnea and breath-holding
2. Laryngospasm
3. Bucking, if tube is still in place, or coughing when the tube is removed

These complications are accompanied by ventilatory inadequacy with cardiovascular effects, hypoxemia, and hypercarbia. They are related to light levels of anesthesia. If a patient is brought to a level of anesthesia (stage III, plane 1) with reversal of relaxants and spontaneous breathing while the tube is in place, these complications are avoided or short lived.

Clearing of pharyngeal and tracheal secretions is necessary before the removal of a tube. A careful tracheobronchial toilet is recommended. A tube should be removed gently and gradually to reduce the incidence and severity of complications.

Allowing a patient to awaken with a tube in place carries with it significant disadvantages. The discomfort is well recognized, while some anxiety or panic may be manifested when a patient cannot talk.

The use of succinylcholine to prevent or overcome spasm and coughing at this time is a critical technique or a substitute for good technique and carries with it the dangers of succinylcholine side effects.

BUCKING PHENOMENON. Bucking is defined as a modified cough, because the presence of the endotracheal tube between the vocal cords prevents the development of a full head of intrapulmonary pressure (the tussic squeeze action of Coryllos).[89a] The diaphragmatic, thoracic, and abdominal muscles are usually all contracted.

Bucking may occur during the maintenance of anesthesia or during recovery and extubation. During surgery, it is related to the following conditions:

- Too light an anesthetic or the waning of topical anesthesia
- Sudden changes in surgical technique, such as traction on the viscera or further exploration

Bucking → Hypoxia / Increased cerebrospinal fluid pressure—cerebral congestion / Increased intraabdominal tension

Laryngospasm → Hypoxia / Increased intracranial pressure / CO_2 retention

FIG. 20-36. Complications to be prevented in the extubation procedure.

- Inadequate levels of muscle relaxants
- Shifting of the endotracheal tube and tube touching the carina

Studies have been carried out in volunteers with endotracheal tubes in place and measurements made of the various parameters related to coughing. Gal[89b] has determined that although endotracheal intubation does not impair the ability to generate normal pressures during bucking (coughing), there is, nevertheless, an alteration in the timing of pressure and air flow through the bronchiotracheal passageways such that the modified cough simply resembles a normal forced expiration. Thus, the resistance of the tube and its noncollapsibility did not allow maximum flows to be reached despite increased effort and high lung volumes. At low lung volumes, the increased effort that is possible did produce some compressive narrowing of the large airways distal to the tubes, and such tussive squeeze did transport secretions into the area of the trachea. With the failure of a high flow rate needed to achieve good linear velocities, however, clearing of secretions was not accomplished. In fact, the secretions are likely to accumulate at the area around the end of the endotracheal tube.

Alterations in cardiac and vascular parameters on endotracheal extubation have been studied. It is well known that on intubation, arrhythmias are a frequent complication, and many techniques are employed to minimize or prevent such cardiac as well as blood pressure changes. In the study by Dhamee,[90] it appeared that on extubation, without any particular effort to control cardiac activity, arrhythmias are likely to be seen in about 20% of patients. It is of importance, however, to realize that although at the first minute immediately following extubation there are few recognized cardiovascular changes, nevertheless, by 5 minutes there is a decrease in cardiac rate and a lowering of the rate pressure product (RPP). This result may be related to the fact that the irritation effect of the endotracheal tube is removed and that electrocardiographic changes are thus less likely to be observed. It is recommended that despite the absence of arrhythmias, careful observation of cardiac rhythm and blood pressure be carried out during and after extubation.

TIMING OF EXTUBATION. As during intubation, the awake or lightly anesthetized patient will exhibit physiologic and mechanical disturbances when the tube remains in situ or is removed. It is, therefore, desirable to remove the tube at an optimal time. Early extubation refers to the removal of the endotracheal tube while the patient is still partially anesthetized and breathing spontaneously. This is preferable to allowing the patient to awaken and readily respond to verbal commands ("open your eyes," "take a deep breath," etc.). It avoids most of the undesirable effects, such as bucking, laryngospasm, coughing and increased intracranial pressure, yet does not cause any increase in postoperative pulmonary complications. As soon as the tube is removed, the patient may have assisted ventilation by bag and mask. This applies even to high-risk patients. A comparison of early extubation and mask ventilation versus maintenance of intubation as a prophylactic measure showed no significant differences in postanesthetic morbidity or mortality: continued endotracheal intubation into the recovery period did not diminish respiratory complications, improve gas exchange, or decrease intrapulmonary shunt.[91]

With early extubation, functional residual capacity returns to normal more quickly and patients are more comfortable. Extubation is accomplished when the patient has a respiratory rate of less than 30 breaths per minute and maintains a blood pH of 7.3 or more. An additional criterion is the measurement of inspiratory force. An ability to exert an inspiratory force of -20 to -30 cm H_2O also indicates a capacity to cough.[92] Measurement can be made by attaching a simple manometer to an endotracheal tube (cuff inflated) or to a fitted mask. The Boehringer manometer is available for this purpose. This criteria can be applied in the operating room as well as in recovery or intensive care areas. Relaxants should be reversed and train-of-four present with twitch height approximately equal.

SUPPRESSION OF BUCKING. Suppression of the bucking phenomenon (modified cough) after endotracheal intubation is a desirable objective with amelioration of the undesirable autonomic responses. It is also an objective at the time of tracheal suctioning and extubation.[93]

In 1950 Burstein[93] showed that the IV administration of 100 mg procaine 1 to 5 minutes before endotracheal intubation decreased the incidence of cardiac arrhythmias of sympathetic response (hypertension) and the occurrence of coughing (bucking). Taylor[94] demonstrated that a continuous IV procaine drip of 10 to 60 mg/hr could supplement general anesthesia and reduce the bucking phenomenon and the sympathetic responses.

In 1963 Steinhaus[95] demonstrated that IV lidocaine was an effective cough suppressant to movement in the trachea of the endotracheal tube. Hamill[96] has clearly demonstrated that the IV administration of lidocaine in contrast to laryngotracheal instillation is the more effective route.

The optimal effective dose of lidocaine and the time interval between administration and application of the tracheal stimulus for effective action needed to suppress the response to laryngoscopy, intubation, and extubation have been carefully defined.[97]

The Dose. Suppression by lidocaine is dose dependent. The incidence of coughing decreases with increasing doses. With 1 mg/kg of body weight, the incidence of coughing is 30%; at 1.5 mg/kg, the incidence is 20%. The optimal dose is 2 mg/kg, IV, to suppress coughing completely.

The Time. Complete suppression occurs at 1 to 2 minutes with the optimal dose and continues for 3 minutes. Thereafter, there is some depression of the laryngeal and tracheal cough response, whereas at 7 minutes this depression is insignificant.

The Effective Plasma Level. Plasma levels of 3 μg/ml or more are associated with complete suppression (4 μg/ml). With the doses described, no serious side effects are noted in healthy persons.

Use in Other Endoscopic Procedures. IV doses of 100 to 200 mg of lidocaine (2 ml of 1% solution) successfully suppress bucking and coughing during bronchoscopy under general anesthesia, without resorting to deep planes of surgical anesthesia.[98]

In bronchoscopic examinations under general anesthesia, IV lidocaine has also been useful in providing good contrast distribution and smooth nonbucking conditions.[99]

Supression of Adverse Effects of Extubation. Extubation can be smooth, with minimal or no bucking or subsequent laryngospasm, if an IV dose is administered 1 to 2 minutes before tracheobronchial toilet, suctioning, and subsequent removal of the endotracheal tube.

Laryngospasm postextubation is controlled by doses of IV lidocaine. This is also recommended for children.[100] It has been demonstrated by Leicht[101] that when children begin to swallow on emergence, the administration of lidocaine at doses of 1.5 mg/kg is not effective. Two considerations derive from this observation: (1) the dose should be 2 mg/kg; and (2) the time of administration should be while the patient is lightly anesthetized and breathing but before swallowing or the gag reflex appears.[101]

Intraocular Pressure.[102] Tracheal intubation during general anesthesia (stage III, plane 1) and with nondepolarizing muscle relaxants is accompanied by elevation in intraocular pressure, which may average 35% above baseline and only partially related to coughing. In patients who do not cough, the same percent elevation also occurs. Thus, part of the rise in intraocular pressure can be attributed to autonomic reflex stimulation. DeJong[103] has demonstrated that both cough and autonomic reflexes can be suppressed by IV lidocaine with doses of 2 mg/kg. The mechanism of the suppression is the inhibiting action of lidocaine on the polysynaptic spinal reflexes when no cardiovascular depression exists.[103]

Drenger[102] has demonstrated that the administration of lidocaine in doses of 2 mg/kg 2 minutes prior to laryngoscopy and intubation attenuates the elevation of intraocular pressure as it also attenuates coughing and autonomic responses. With this dose at the proper time the intraocular pressure elevation may only be 5% to 10%, which contrasts with the 35% elevation in the absence of lidocaine treatment.

Other Local Agents. *Cocaine.* Topical cocaine has been used as an agent to suppress coughing and bucking. It is the drug of choice among many otorhinolaryngologists for laryngeal and bronchoscopic examinations. It is also used in anesthesia practice for nasal intubation in the awake state and for laryngoscopy. Advantage is taken of the ability to produce local vasoconstriction of the air passages. It is available as a 4% solution and can be applied with cotton swabs to the pyriform sinuses or as a spray to the pharyngeal and laryngeal mucous membranes. The topicalization should be done at least 5 minutes prior to induction of anesthesia to allow adequate time for the anesthetic effect. With a concentrated solution of 10%, (2.0 ml) surface anesthesia is evident in 2 to 5 minutes. With a 4% (4.0 ml) solution, at least 10 minutes should be allowed for the onset of the anesthesia. The dose should be limited to approximately 200 mg at a single setting.

The drug should not be administered to patients with a history of hypertension of coronary artery disease. The effect of cocaine in blocking the reuptake of endogenous catecholamines at the nerve terminals and thereby potentiating the effect of catecholamines on adrenergic receptors should be recognized. This is the mechanism that is the basis for severe systemic toxicity, not only hypertension and tachycardia, but convulsions and death.

It is also important that cocaine should not be administered to patients who will subsequently receive halothane anesthesia.

Burstein[93] reported on the use of cocaine topicalization of the upper air passages with 10% cocaine spray. In this study, patients still developed arrhythmias and patients also coughed or bucked after being intubated.

Tetracaine. Tetracaine in concentrations of 0.5% to 2% solution is widely used in providing topical anesthesia of the upper airway by spray, by cotton swabs to the pyriform sinuses, or by a microatomizer for the larynx and trachea. This drug is widely used and is the usual choice for bronchoscopy and bronchography. A solution of 1% to 2% concentration is used. It produces adequate topical anesthesia of the upper airway in 5 to 10 minutes, with a duration of action of 1 hour. Carabelli[104] has suggested the use of 0.25% tetracaine solution for topical use, but the onset is delayed and anesthesia is spotty.

In anesthesia practice, a spray of 1% to 2% tetracaine delivered by an atomizer and application by pledgets to the pyriform sinuses permits laryngoscopy in 5 to 10 minutes and produces excellent topical anesthesia. If, in addition, there is administration of 1 or 2 ml of the tetracaine solution translaryngeally or transtracheally, there is minimal response to intubation.

Procaine. IV procaine drip has been used to supplement general anesthesia and to minimize the consequences of intubation. Taylor[94] observed a decrease in cardiac arrhythmias and hypertensive responses, as well as a minimization of coughing; however, he also noted frequent hypotension and circulatory depression. The IV administration of procaine does result in falls in blood pressure in over 50% of patients. Although these changes were small, it is evident that procaine has a myocardial depressant action. A certain degree of unpredictability and the side effects have resulted in discontinuing the use of IV procaine for the control of bucking and coughing.

PROCEDURE OF EXTUBATION. To accomplish the various goals mentioned (see Fig. 20–35), the following steps are recommended. They are all employed with variations by different clinicians but the objectives remain the same:

1. *Maintain an appropriate light anesthetic depth* (stage III, Plane 1) with the patient showing spontaneous respiration and minimal residual muscular relaxation. To avoid bucking: administer 1 to 1.5 mg/kg lidocaine (1 ml of 1% for 70 kg man) 2 minutes before the start of the procedure to suppress bucking, postintubation coughing, and laryngospasm in both adults and children.[101]
2. *Perform pharyngeal and supralaryngeal cleansing* under vision with Yaukauer suction tip (Pharyngeal–laryngeal toilet [PLT]).
3. *Ventilate patient* about one half minute with oxygen.
4. *Suction the trachea (and bronchi if indicated) gently* with an appropriate size suction catheter and an open suction system (no more than 5 seconds). Keep suction off until tip is in position. If secretions are plentiful, repeat the procedure. Remember that small amounts of secretions accumulate in the subglottic region and in the area above the inflated cuff.
5. *Reconnect with breathing circuit and ventilate the patient* with 50% air and 50% oxygen. Deflate cuff and continue to assist ventilation with mild positive pressure. Do not inhibit Hering-Breuer reflex with high positive pressure. Encourage spontaneous breathing. Do not overventilate.
6. *Monitor neuromuscular junction block with train-of-four* for residual paralysis. Reverse as indicated.
7. *Disconnect the anesthesia system from the endotracheal tube.* Insert the suction catheter just beyond the tip of the endotracheal tube, leaving the Y system open and maintain in this position.
8. *The endotracheal tube with suction catheter is then slowly (3 to 5 seconds) withdrawn* with the Y system intermittently closed and suction on. (Most experience indicates that rapid removal provokes more intense response and does not remove secretions.) *Note:* Most suction units provide a high flow–low pressure system.
9. *Ventilate or assist spontaneous efforts of the patient immediately* with bag and mask and 50% air and 50% oxygen.
10. *Inspect vocal cords and complete pharyngeal toilet,* if necessary. Insert oropharyngeal (or nasopharyngeal) airway, if indicated.

The application of positive pressure during extubation and the concept of the "pseudo-cough" is without foundation of efficacy in children or adults with a normally developed chest–diaphragm system. This procedure is hazardous, because secretions will be left in the subglottic and immediate supraglottic region. To have effective expulsion of tracheobronchial secretions, an intrapulmonary pressure of over 80 mm Hg must be developed and followed by an active "tussic" squeeze—not likely in the patient emerging from anesthesia.

SUCTION CATHETERS. Standards for suction catheters used for clearing the tracheobronchial tree through endotracheal and tracheostomy tubes have been developed by the International Standards Committee (Org TC 121 Subcommittee).[105]

In the use of these suction catheters, it is recommended that the size of the catheter should not be more than half of the *inside* diameter (ID) of the endotracheal or tracheostomy tube (Table 20–10). When a larger catheter whose ID size is greater than one-half the ID of an endotracheal tube (sizes designated by ID measurement) is inserted into a given endotracheal tube, physiologic disturbances are caused by the application of suction force to the tracheobronchial tree, and this may be dangerously accentuated.[106]

EXTUBATION IN SPECIAL CIRCUMSTANCES. Many conditions requiring prolonged ventilatory support are encountered in nonanesthesiologic circumstances. Included are coma from poisoning; paralysis (tetraplegia) from trauma; adult respiratory distress syndrome; tumors of the upper airway; and infections of the upper air passages. The latter is represented by abscesses of dental origin, inflammatory conditions of the fascial planes of the neck (Ludwig's angina), pharyngeal and palatine infections, and

TABLE 20–10. SELECTION OF SUCTION CATHETERS CORRESPONDING TO ENDOTRACHEAL TUBE SIZES

Inside Diameter, mm Size of Endotracheal Tube	Outside Diameter of Catheter mm Tolerance	Nearest French Size* Suction Catheter
4.0 (Fr 12)	1.0 ± 0.15	4
4.0 (Fr 14)	1.5 ± 0.15	4
4.0 (Fr 14)	2.0 ± 0.15	6
5.0 (Fr 16–18)	2.5 ± 0.25	8
6 (Fr 20–24)	3.0 ± 0.25	9
8 (Fr 24–28)	4.0 ± 0.25	12
10 (Fr 32)	5.0 ± 0.25	15
23 (Fr 36)	6.0 ± 0.25	18

*Refers to nearest Charrière gauge equivalent.
Modified from: Rosen, M., Hilliard, K.K.: The use of suction in clinical medicine. Brit. J. Anaesth. 32:486, 1960.
Substitutes for the smaller suction catheters are short lengths of plastic epidural catheters. The ED of these is less than 1.5 mm.

epiglottitis. Infections are usually accompanied by fever.

Extubation should basically rely on the establishment of reasonable neuromuscular control and mechanical capacity to sustain without fatique spontaneous respiration. In the case of infection, not only should these parameters be present, but any swelling shoud have subsided and the temperature should have returned to normal for 24 hours. Even then, extubation should only be performed following visual inspection of the laryngeal and pharyngeal passageway.[107]

REFERENCES

1. Cass, N.M., James N.R., and Lines, V.: Difficult direct laryngoscopy complicating intubation for anaesthesia. Br. Med. J., 1:488, 1956.
2. Brechner, V.L.: Unusual problems in the management of airways. I. Flexion–extension mobility of the cervical spine. Anesth Analg, 47:362, 1968.
3. Block, C., and Brechner, V.L.: Unusual problems in airways management. II. The influence of the temporomandibular joint, the mandible and associated structures on endotracheal intubation. Curr. Res. Anesth., 50:114, 1971.
4. White, A., and Kander, P.L.: Anatomical factors in difficult direct laryngoscopy. Br. J. Anaesth., 47:468, 1975.
5a. Mallampati, S.R., et al: A clinical sign to predict difficult tracheal intubation: A prospective study. Can. Anaesth. Soc. J., 32:429, 1985.
5b. McIntyre J.W.R.: Continuing medical education: The difficult tracheal intubation. Can. J. Anaesth., 34:204, 1987.
6. Samsoon, G.L.T., and Young, J.R.B.: Difficult tracheal intubation: A retrospective study. Anaesthesia, 42:487, 1987.
7. Nichol, H.C., and Zuck, D.: Difficult laryngoscopy: the "anterior" larynx and the atlanto–occipital gap. Br. J. Anaesth., 55:141, 1983.
8. Bellhouse, C.P., and Dore, C.: Criteria for estimating likelihood of difficulty of endotracheal intubation with the Macintosh laryngoscope. Anaesth. Intens. Care, 16:329, 1988.
9. Cormack, R.S., and Lehan, J.: Difficult tracheal intubation in obstetrics. Anaesthesia, 39:1105, 1984.
10. Boidin, M.P.: Airway patency in the unconscious patient. Br. J. Anaesth., 57:306, 1985.
11. Salem, M.R., Mathrubhutham, M., and Bennet, E.J.: Difficult intubation. N. Engl. J. Med., 295:879, 1976.
12. Bachman, A.L.: Benign, non-neoplastic conditions of the larynx and pharynx. Radiol. Clin. North Am., 16:273, 1978.
13. Hotchkiss, R.S., et al.: An abnormal epiglottis as a cause of difficult intubation: Airway assessment using magnetic resonance imaging. Anesthesiology, 68:140, 1988.
14. Block, C., and Brechner, V.L.: Unusual problems in airway management. II. The influence of the temporomandibular joint, the mandible, and associated structures on endotracheal intubation. Anesth. Analg., 50:114, 1971.
15. Coonan, T.J., et al.: Ankylosis of the temporomandibular joint after temporal craniotomy: A cause of difficult intubation. Can. Anaesth. Soc. J., 32:2, 1985.
16. De Santo, L.W., Define, K.D., and Weiland, L.H.: Cysts of the larynx: Classification. Laryngoscope, 80:145, 1970.
17. Salzarulo, H.H., and Taylor, L.A.: Diabetic "stiff joint syndrome" as a cause of difficult endotracheal intubation. Anesthesiology, 64:366, 1986.
18. Akinyemi, O.O., and Elegbe, E.O.: Difficult laryngoscopy and tracheal intubation due to calcified stylohyoid ligaments. Can. Anaesth. Soc. J., 28:80, 1981.
19. Naguib, M., Farag, H., and Ibrahim, A.E.W.: Anaesthetic considerations in Klippel-Feil syndrome. Can. Anaesth. Soc. J, 33:1, 1986.
20. Strauss, E.J., Poplak, T.M., and Braude, B.M.: Anaesthetic management of a difficult intubation. S. Afr. Med. J., 68:414, 1985.
21. Cormier, Y.R., Camus, P., and Desmeules, M.J.: Non-organic acute upper airway obstruction: Description and a diagnostic approach. Am. Rev. Respir. Dis., 121:147, 1980.
22. Appelblatt, N.H., and Baker, S.R.: Functional upper airway obstruction: A new syndrome. Arch. Otolaryngol., 107:305, 1981.
23. Hammer, G., Schwinn, D., and Wollman, H.: Postoperative complications due to paradoxical vocal cord motion. Anesthesiology, 66:686, 1987.

24. Brechner V.L.: Unusual problems in the management of airways: I. Flexion-extension mobility of the cervical vertebrae. Anesth. Analg. 47:362, 1968.
25. Patil, V.O., Stehling, L.C., and Zauder, H.L.: Predicting the difficulty of intubation utilizing an intubation gauge. Anesth. Rev., 10:32, 1983.
26. Nichol, H.C., and Zuck, D.: Difficult laryngoscopy: The "anterior" larynx and the atlanto–occipital gap. Br. J. Anaesth, 55:141, 1983.
27. Spoerel, W.E., Narayanan, P.S., and Singh, N.P.: Transtracheal ventilation. Br. J. Anaesth., 49:932. 1971.
28. Lambie, R.S., Pfaff, F.: The use of succinylcholine during endotracheal intubation. Anesthesiology, 7:47, 1956.
29. Lachman, R.J.: Long, J.H., and Krumperman, L.W.: Changes in blood gases associated with various methods of induction for endotracheal anesthesia. Anesthesiology, 16:29, 1955.
30a. Nahas, G.G.: Heart rate during short periods of apnea in curarized dogs. Am. J. Physiol., 187:302, 1956.
30b. Fujimori, M., and Virtue, R.W.: The value of oxygenation prior to induced apnea. Anesthesiology, 21:46, 1960.
31a. Hey, V.M.F.: Relaxants for endotracheal intubation. Anaesthesia, 28:32, 1973.
31b. Lund, I., Stovner, J.: Experimental and clinical experiments with a new muscle relaxant. Acta Anaesthesiol. Scand., 6:85, 1962.
32. Bannister, F.B., and Macbeth, R.: Direct laryngoscopy and tracheal intubation. Lancet, 1:651, 1944.
33a. Jackson, C., and Jackson, D.L.: The Larynx and Its Diseases. Philadelphia, W.B. Saunders, 1937.
33b. Jackson, C.: The technique of insertion of intratracheal insufflation tubes. Surg. Gynec. Obstet., 17:507, 1913.
34. Bennett, J.H.: Anesthetic management for drainage of abscess of submandibular space (Ludwig's angina). Anesthesiology, 4:25, 1943.
35a. Magill, I.W.: Endotracheal anesthesia. Am. J. Surg., 34:450, 1936.
35b. Magill, I.W.: Anesthesia in endoscopy. J. Laryngol. Otol., 54:425, 1939.
36. Salem, M.R., et al.: Cephalad displacement of the larynx facilitates intubation. Anesthesiology, 67:3, 1987.
37. Charters, P., and Wilkinson, K.: Tactile orotracheal tube placement test: A bimanual tactile examination of the positioned orotracheal tube to confirm laryngeal placement. Anesthesia, 42:801, 1987.
38. Mirakur, R.K., et al.: IM or IV atropine for the prevention of oculocardiac and other reflexes. Br. J. Anaesth., 54:1059, 1982.
39a. Goodman, L.R.: Radiological evaluation of patients receiving assisted ventilation. J.A.M.A., 245:858, 1981.
39b. Goodman, L.R., and Putman, C.E.: Intensive Care Radiology. St. Louis, C.V. Mosby, 1978.
40. Lindholm, E.E., and Carroll, R.G.: Evaluation of tube deformation pressure in-vitro. Crit. Care Med., 3:196, 1975.
41a. Conrardy, P.A., Goodman, L.R., and Singer, L.F.: Alteration of endotracheal tube position. Crit. Care Med., 4:8, 1976.
41b. Toung, T.J.K., Grayson R., Saklad, J., et al: Movement of the distal end of the endotracheal tube during flexion and extension of the neck. Anesth. Analg., 64:1029, 1985.
42. Scarpelli, E.M., Real, F.J.P., and Rudolph, A.M.: Tracheal motion during eupnea. J. Appl. Physiol., 20:473, 1965.
43. Ripoll, I., et al.: Spontaneous dislocation of endotracheal tubes. Anesthesiology, 49:50, 1978.
44. Flagg, P.: The Art of Anesthesia. Philadelphia, J.B. Lippincott, 1916.
45. Edward, E.: Death on the table. Br. J. Anaesth., 15:87, 1938.

46. Keenan, R.L., and Boyan, C.P.: Cardiac arrest due to anesthesia: A study of incidence and causes. J.A.M.A., 253:2373, 1985.
47. Utting, J.E., Gray, T.C., and Shelley, F.C.: Human misadventure in anaesthesia. Can. Anaesth. Soc. J., 26:472, 1979.
48. Holland, R.: Anesthesia-related mortality in Australia. In International Anesthesiology Clinics. Edited by E.C. Pierce and J.B. Cooper. Boston, Little, Brown, 1984, p. 61.
49. Birmingham, P.K., Cheney, F.W., and Ward, R.J.: Esophageal intubation: A review of detection techniques. Anesth. Analg., 65:886, 1986.
50a. Linko, K., Paloheimo, M., and Tammisto, T.: Capnography for detection of accidental oesophageal intubation. Acta Anaesthesiol. Scand., 27:199, 1983.
50b. Murray, I.P., Modell, J.H.: Early detection of endotracheal tube accidents by monitoring carbon dioxide concentration in respiratory gas. Anesthesiology, 59:344, 1983.
51a. Macewen, W.: Clinical observations on the introduction of tracheal tubes by the mouth instead of performing tracheotomy or laryngotomy. Br. Med. J., 2:122, 1880.
51b. Trendelenberg, F.: Tamponade & trachea. Arch. Klin. Chir., 12:121, 1971.
51c. Kuhn, F.: Die perorale intubation. Zbl. Chir., 28:1281, 1901.
52a. Sykes, W.S.: Oral endotracheal intubation without laryngoscopy: A plea for simplicity. Anesth. Analg., 16:133, 1937.
52b. Siddal, W.J.W.: Tactile orotracheal intubation. Anaesthesia, 21:221, 1966.
53. Stewart, R.: Tactile method of oral intubation in comatose trauma patients. Ann. Emerg. Med., 13:175, 1984.
54a. Woods, A.M., and Lander, C.J.: Abolition of gagging and the hemodynamic response to awake laryngoscopy (abstract). Anesthesiology, 67:2204, 1987.
54b. Barton, S., and Williams, J.D.: Glossopharyngeal nerve block. Archs. Otolaryngol., 93:186, 1971.
55. Bonica, J.: Transtracheal anesthesia for endotracheal intubation. Anesthesiology, 10:736, 1949.
56. Hinkle, A.J.: Laryngoscopy in the awake neonate. Anesthesiol. Rev., 13:43, 1986.
57. Todres, I.D., and Crone, R.K.: Experience with a modified laryngoscope in sick infants. Crit. Care Med., 9:128, 1981.
58a. Vidyasagar, D., and Raju, T.N.K.: A simple non-invasive technique of measuring intracranial pressure in newborn (LADD transducer). Pediatrics, 59:957, 1977.
58b. Raju, T.N.K., et al.: Intracranial pressure during intubation and anesthesia in infants. J. Pediatr., 96:860, 1980.
59. Stow, P.J., et al.: Anterior fontanelle pressure responses to tracheal intubation in the awake and anesthetized infant. Br. J. Anaesth., 60:167, 1988.
60. Kelly, M.A., and Finer, N.N.: Nasotracheal intubation in the neonate: Physiologic responses and effects of atropine and pancuronium. J. Pediatr., 105:303, 1984.
61. White, P.F., et al.: A randomized study of drugs for preventing increases in intracranial pressure during endotracheal suctioning. Anesthesiology, 57:242, 1982.
62. Bivins, H.G., et al.: The effect of axial traction during orotracheal intubation of the trauma victim with an unstable cervical spine. Ann. Emerg. Med., 17:25, 1988.
63. Aprahamian, C., et al.: Experimental cervical spine injury model: Evaluation of airway management and splinting techniques. Ann. Emerg. Med., 13:21, 1984.
64a. Butler, F.S., and Cirillo, A.A.: Retrograde tracheal intubation. Anesth. Analg., 39:333, 1960.
64b. Roberts, K.W.: New use for Swan-Ganz introducer wire. Anesth. Analg., 60:67, 1981.
64c. Abou-Madi, M.N., Trop, D.: Pulling versus guiding: A mod-

ification of retrograde guided intubation. Can. J. Anaesth., 36:336, 1989.
65. Macintosh, R.R.: An aid to oral intubation. Br. Med. J., 1:28, 1949.
66. Sellers, W.F.S., and Jones, G.W.: Difficult tracheal intubation. Anaesthesia, 41:93, 1986.
67. Kidd, J.F., Dyson, A., and Latto, I.P.: Successful difficult intubation. Anaesthesia, 43:437, 1988.
68. Baird, J.L.: British Patent Specification #N020969/27, 1927.
69. Hirschowitz, B.I., et al.: The fiberscope. Gastroenterology, 35:50, 1958.
70. Murphy, P.: A fiber-optic endoscope used for nasal intubation. Anaesthesia, 22:489, 1967.
71. Patil, V.U., Stehling, L., and Zauder, H.L.: Fiberoptic Endoscopy in Anesthesia. Chicago, Year Book Medical Publishers, 1983.
72a. Raj, P.P., et al.: Technics of fiberoptic laryngoscopy in anesthesia. Anesth. Analg., 53:708, 1974.
72b. Ovassapian, A., Dykes, M.H.M., and Golman, M.E.: Fiberoptic nasotracheal intubation: A training program. Anesthesiology, 53:S354, 1980.
72c. Ovassapian, A., et al.: Fiberoptic nasotracheal intubation. Anesth. Analg., 62:692, 1983.
73. Murphy, P.: The fiberoptic laryngoscope. Anesthesiol. Rev., 8:23, 1981.
74a. Sellick, B.A.: Cricoid pressure to control regurgitation of stomach contents during induction of anaesthesia. Lancet, 2:404, 1961.
74b. Sellick, B.A.: Rupture of the esophagus following cricoid pressure? Correspondence. Anaesthesia, 37:213, 1982.
75. Fanning, G.L.: The efficacy of cricoid pressure in preventing regurgitation of gastric contents. Anesthesiology, 32:553, 1970.
76. Salem, M.R., Wong, A.Y., and Fizzoti, G.F.: Efficacy of cricoid pressure in preventing aspiration of gastric contents in paediatric patients. Br. J. Anaesth., 44:401, 1972.
77. Wraight, W.J., Chamney, A.R., and Howells, T.H.: The determination of an effective cricoid pressure. Anaesthesia, 38:461, 1983.
78. Lawes, E.G., et al.: The cricoid yoke: A device for producing consistent and reproducible cricoid pressure. Br. J. Anaesth., 58:925, 1986.
79. Lawes, E.G.: Cricoid pressure with or without the "cricoid yoke." Br. J. Anaesth., 58:1376, 1986.
80a. Salem, M.R., et al.: Cricoid compression is effective in obliterating the esophageal lumen in the presence of a nasogastric tube. Anesthesiology, 63:443, 1985.
80b. Salem, M.R., et al.: Cephalad displacement of the larynx facilitates intubation. Anesthesiology, 67:3, 1987.
81. Cohen, S.E.: Aspiration syndromes in pregnancy. Anesthesiology, 51:375, 1979.
82a. Reiman, J.: Use of small interarytenoid endotracheal tubes for anesthesia in pharyngeal and laryngeal surgery. Section on Anesthesia. New York, A.M.A. Convention, 1952.
82b. El-Baz, N., et al.: High frequency ventilation with an uncuffed endotracheal tube. J. Thorac. Cardiovasc. Surg., 84:823, 1982.
83. Hirschman, C.A., and Smith, J.: Indirect ignition of the endotracheal tube during carbon dioxide laser surgery. Arch. Otolaryngol., 106:639, 1980.
84. Konchigeri, H.N., and Shaker, M.H.: Anesthesia for intralaryngeal laser surgery. Can. Anaesth. Soc. J., 21:343, 1974.
85a. Snow, J.C., et al.: Fire hazard during CO_2 laser microsurgery on the larynx and trachea. Anesth. Analg., 55:146, 1976.
85b. Patil, V., Stehling, L.C., and Zauder, H.L.: A modified endotracheal tube for laser microsurgery. Anesthesiology, 51:571, 1979.
86. Norton, M.L., and deVos, P.: A new endotracheal tube for laser surgery of the larynx. Ann. Otol. Rhinol. Laryngol., 87:554, 1978.
87. Kalhan, S.B., and Cascorbi, H.F.: Anesthetic management of laser microlaryngeal surgery. Anesthesiol. Rev., 8:23, 1981.
88a. Bogatz, M.S., and Katz, J.A.: Airway management of the trauma patient. Semin. Anesth., 4:114, 1985.
88b. Flood, L.M., and Astley, B.: Anaesthetic management of acute laryngeal trauma. Br. J. Anaesth., 54:1339, 1982.
88c. Mancuso, A.A., and Hanafee, N.N.: Computed tomography of the injured larynx. Radiology, 133:139, 1979.
88d. Jacoby, J.J., Hamelberg, W., et al.: A simple method of artificial respiration. Am. J. Physiol., 167:798, 1951.
88e. Benumof, J.L., and Scheller, M.S.: The importance of transtracheal jet ventilation in the management of difficult airway. Anesthesiology, 71:769, 1989.
89a. Gal, T.J.: Effects of endotracheal intubation on normal cough performance. Anesthesiology, 52:3241, 1980.
89b. Coryllos, P.N.: Action of the diaphragm in cough: Experimental and clinical study in humans. Am. J. Med. Sci., 194:523, 1937.
90. Dhamee, M.S., and Ghandi, S.K.: Alterations in cardiac parameters on endotracheal extubation. Anesthesiol. Rev., 11:35, 1984.
91. Shackford, S.R., Virgilio, R.W., and Peters, R.M.: Early extubation versus prophylactic ventilation in the high risk patient: A comparison of postoperative management in the prevention of respiratory complications. Anesth. Analg., 60:76, 1981.
92. Ayoub, A.H., and Aldridge, J.: Inspiratory force as a criterion for extubation and discharge from recovery room. Resp. Care, 22:594, 1977.
93a. White, P.F., et al.: A randomized study of drugs for preventing increases in intracranial pressure during endotracheal suctioning. Anesthesiology, 57:242, 1982.
93b. Burstein, C.L., Woloshin, G., and Newman, W.: Electrocardiographic studies during endotracheal intubation. II. Effects during general anesthesia and intravenous procaine. Anesthesiology, 11:299, 1950.
94. Taylor, I.B., et al.: Intravenous procaine: An adjuvant to general anesthesia: A preliminary report. Anesthesiology, 11:185, 1950.
95. Steinhaus, J.E., and Gaskin, L.: A study of lidocaine as a suppressant of cough reflex. Anesthesiology, 24:285, 1963.
96. Hamill, J.F., et al.: Lidocaine before endotracheal intubation: Intravenous or laryngotracheal? Anesthesiology, 55:578, 1981.
97. Yukioka, H., et al.: Intravenous lidocaine as a suppressant of coughing during tracheal intubation. Anesth. Analg., 64:1189, 1985.
98. Blancato, L.S., Peng, A.T.C., and Alonsabe, D.: Intravenous lidocaine as an adjunct to general anesthesia for endoscopy. Anesth. Analg., 48:224, 1969.
99. Smith, F.R., and Kundahl, P.C.: Intravenously administered lidocaine as cough depressant during general anesthesia for bronchography. Chest, 63:427, 1973.
100. Baraka, N.: Intravenous lidocaine controls extubation laryngospasm in children. Anesth. Analg., 57:506, 1978.
101. Leicht, P., Wisborg, T., and Chraemmer-Jørgensen, B.: Does intravenous lidocaine prevent laryngospasm after extubation in children? Anesth. Analg., 64:1193, 1985.

102. Drenger, B., et al.: The effect of intravenous lidocaine on the increase in intraocular pressure induced by tracheal intubation. Anesth. Analg., *64*:1211, 1985.
103. DeJong, R.H.: Physiology and Pharmacology of Local Anesthesia. Springfield, IL, Charles C. Thomas, 1970, p. 144.
104. Carabelli, A.A.: The use of tetracaine in subposologic quantities for bronchoscopy and bronchography. Anesthesiology, *13*:169, 1952.
105. ISO Technical Committee, Subcommittee 121, 1984.
106. Rosen, M., and Hilliard, E.K.: The use of suction in clinical medicine. Br. J. Anaesth., 32:486, 1960.
107. Rothstein, P., and Lister, G.: Epiglottitis—duration of intubation and fever. Anesth. Analg., *62*:785, 1983.

APPENDIX: SYNDROMES ASSOCIATED WITH UPPER AIRWAY ABNORMALITIES

Disorder or Syndrome	Cause of Difficult Intubation	Salient Features
Syndromes with Features of Micrognathia (Hypoplastic Mandible)		
Aglossia-adactylia	Micrognathia Intraoral bands	Agenesis of distal limb segment (digits in particular) Dental anomalies
Aminopterin-induced	Micrognathia	Low birth weight Cranial dysplasia Abnormal facies Limb anomalies
Arthochalasis multiplex congenita	Micrognathia	Congenital joint flaccidity with recurrent dislocation Associated anomalies include hydrocephalus and deformed feet
Arthrogryposis	Hypoplastic mandible Temporomandibular fusion	Multiple joint contracture at birth
Bird-headed dwarf	Micrognathia	Bird-headed appearance Low-set ears Highly arched or cleft palate Genitourinary anomalies
C syndrome of multiple congenital anomalies	Micrognathia	Short stature Hypoplastic metacarpals and phalanges Soft-tissue syndactyly
Cerebro-costo-mandibular	Micrognathia Inadequate tracheal airway due to insufficient support from partially collapsed tracheal cartilages	Dorsal rib gaps consisting of fibrous or cartilaginous tissues, causing respiratory distress due to flail chest
Cornelia de Lange	Micrognathia Occasionally, choanal atresia	Microbrachycephaly Characteristic facies (low hairline, heavy confluent eyebrows) Marked mental, motor, and social retardation Limb anomalies
Cri du chat	Micrognathia	Severe growth and mental retardation Cat-like cry Muscular hypotonia Various central nervous system, cardiac, genitourinary, and vertebral anomalies
De Morsiers	Hypotonia, spasticity seizures	Congenital optic nerve hypoplasia Pituitary dysfunction hyponystagmus Small stature Some-mental retardation
Diastrophic dwarfism	Micrognathia Cervical kyphosis	Micromelic dwarfism Hichhiker's thumb Flexion contractures in peripheral joints Scoliosis Deformed ear lobes
DiGeorge's	Hypoplastic mandible	Unusual facies Hypocalcemic tetany in newborns Frequent respiratory infections Absent thymus Aortic arch anomalies, esophageal atresia, tracheal and esophageal fistulas, congenital heart disease

Disorder or Syndrome	Cause of Difficult Intubation	Salient Features
Ellis-Van Creveld	*See assessment in text*	
Goldenhar's	Hypoplastic mandible	Epibulbar (lipo) dermoids Hypoplastic maxilla and temporal bones Vertebral anomalies
Hemifacial microsomia	Unilateral micrognathia Unilateral neck shortness	Unilateral hypoplasia with aplasia of ear, preauricular skin tag Unilateral hypoplastic maxilla Rarely, pulmonary agenesis, on affected side
Hypertelorism	Hypoplastic mandible Enlarged maxilla Macroglossia	Widely separated eyes Enlarged splenoid bone Mental retardation
Idiopathic hypercalcemia	Micrognathia	In infancy: anorexia, vomiting, constipation, hypotonia, physical retardation Supravalvular aortic stenosis Mental retardation
Klippel-Feil	Short or "absent" neck Decreased mobility of head in patients with atlanto-occipital fusion Micrognathia	Fused cervical or cervicothoracic vertebrae Hemivertebrae Deafness (30%) Webbed neck Torticollis
Larsen's	Micrognathia Floppy epiglottis, arytenoid and tracheal cartilage secondary to diminished cartilage rigidity	Dislocated elbows, hips and knees
Mickel's	Micrognathia Short neck	Occipital encephalocele Cleft lip and palate Polydactyly Polycycstic kidneys Limb, cardiovascular, and gastrointestinal anomalies
Melnick-Needles	Micrognathia	Failure to thrive Sclerosis at base of skull and mastoids Tall upper cervical vertebrae Metaphyseal flaring
Noonan's (Male-Turner)	Micrognathia Short neck	Short stature with delayed puberty
Opitz-Frias	Hypergnathia High arched palates Hypertelorism Suoqeatten steious	Many patients with mild mental retardation Epicanthal folds, ptosis of eyelids (60%) Congenital heart disease
Pierre Robin	Micrognathia Glossoptosis	Cleft palate Limb anomalies Congenital heart disease Absent gag reflex
Polyostotic fibrous dysplasia Craniofacial	Macrognathia	Craniofacial distortius Macrognathia

Disorder or Syndrome	Cause of Difficult Intubation	Salient Features
Syndromes With Features of Micrognathia (Hypoplastic Mandible) *(Continued)*		
Smith-Lemeli-Opitz	Micrognathia Short neck	Microcephaly with moderate to severe mental retardation Hypotonia at birth with progressive spasticity Genitourinary anomalies in males Other anomalies include cleft palate, cataract, syndactyl second and third toes
Treacher Collins	Hypogenesis or agenesis of mandible Occasional choanal atresia	Hypoplastic malar bones Malformed ears with conductive deafness Antimongoloid slant Congenital heart disease Underdeveloped paranasal sinuses and mastoids
Trisomy 13	Micrognathia	Typical facies: microcephaly, large broad nose, clift lip and palate, hyper- or hypo-telorism, malformed and low-set ears, anophthalmia or microphthalmia Digital anomalies "Rocker-bottom" feet Severe mental retardation
Trisomy 18	Micrognathia Small triangular mouth with short upper lip	Physical and mental retardation Muscular hypertonicity Shield deformity of chest Second finger overlapping third Foot deformities ("rocker-bottom") Anomalies of cardiovascular, gastrointestinal, and genitourinary systems
Trisomy 21	Atlanto-axial instability	
Trisomy 22	Micrognathia	Microcephaly Preauricular skin tags Cleft palate Mental and growth retardation Congenital heart disease
Turner's	Relatively small mandible Short neck	Short stature Transient lymphedema of hands and feet in infancy Shield chest, widely spaced hypoplastic nipples Cubitus nalgus Congenital heart disease (coarctation of aorta, 15%) Ovarian dysgenesis Hearing defect
Ulrich-Feichtiger	Micrognathia	Mask-like facies with depressed nose Eye anomalies External ear deformations, deafness Limb anomalies Genitourinary anomalies
Wolf's	Micrognathia	Mental and growth retardation Craniofacial anomalies Cleft lip and/or cleft palate
Syndromes Characterized by Macroglossia and a Small Mouth		
Beckwith-Wiedemann	Macroglossia	Omphalocele or umbilical hernia Gigantism with visceromegaly Hypoglycemia Malignant neoplasms

Disorder or Syndrome	Cause of Difficult Intubation	Salient Features
Cowden's (multiple hamartomas)	Hypoplastic mandible Microstomia	Bird-like face Gastrointestinal polyps (in 50%) Breast, mucosal, and cutaneous lesions
Down's (mongolism)	Microstomia Protruding tongue	Hypotonia Epicanthal folds Mental and motor retardation Congenital heart disease
Hurler's	Macroglossia	Grotesque facial features Severe mental retardation Coarse hair, corneal opacities Thoracolumbar gibbus, flexion contractures Hepatosplenomegaly Deficiency of α-L-iduromidase
Kocher-Debré-Sémélaigne (cretinism with muscular hypertrophy)	Large tongue	Myxedema Retarded intellectual, physical, osseous and dental development Generalized increase in muscle mass
Pompe's (glycogen storage disease Type III)	Macroglossia	Hypotonicity Mental retardation Cardiomegaly Deficiency of α-1,4-glucosidase

Syndromes Characterized by Small Mouth and Other Abnormalities

Freeman-Sheldon (whistling face)	Microstomia Short, broad neck Mild pterygium colli	Ulnar deviation bands, finger contractures, non-opposable thumbs
Glossopalatine ankylosis, microglossia, hypodontia, and anomalies of the extremities	Attachment of tongue to hard palate or upper alveolar ridge Anklyosis of temporomandibular joint	Anomalies of the extremities
Grieg's	Macroglossia Extreme width between eyes	Enlarged sphenoid Ocular hypertelorism Mental retardation Webbed neck Congenital heart disease
Hallerman-Streiff	Microstomia Micrognathia	Dyscephaly (scapho- or brachycephaly) Small face, small pinched nose Microophthalmia, blue sclerae Hypotrichosis Proportionate dwarfism
Otopalatodigital	Microstomia	Frontal bossing, prominent occiput Cleft palate Deafness Carpal, tarsal, and digital anomalies

Syndromes Characterized by Temporomandibular Joint Dysfunction

Dutch-Kentucky	Decreased ability to open mouth Trismus of masticatory muscles	Genetic autosomal dominant Flexion deformity of fingers occurring with wrist extension (Pseudocamptodactyly)
Ophthalmo-mandibulo-melic	Jaw anomalies Temporomandibular fusion, a lack of the carotid proces, obtuse mandibular angle	Limb anomalies Blindness from corneal opacities
Still's	Fusion of cervical spine	Arthritis Fever, weakness, weight loss Pneumonitis, pericarditis

Disorder or Syndrome	Cause of Difficult Intubation	Salient Features
Syndromes Characterized by Temporomandibular Joint Dysfunction *(Continued)*		
Temporomandibular joint	Limitation of motion of temporomandibular joints	Pain and limitation of motion of temporomandibular joints Muscle spasm Degenerative changes in temporomandibular joints
Syndromes That May Prohibit Nasotracheal Intubation		
Choanal atresia	Nasal passage obstruction	If bilateral, severe respiratory distress occurs, especially during feeding
Crouzon's craniofacial dysostosis	Narrow nasopharynx and oropharynx	Acrocephaly with parrot-beaked nose Hypertelorism with bilateral exophthalmos Airway obstruction with cor pulmonale
Syndromes in Which Stomatitis Is a Feature		
Behçet's	Aphthous stomatitis	Genital ulcers Uveitis with hypopyon Enterocolitis with ulcerations (40%) Deep vein thrombosis, pulmonary embolism, intracranial thrombophlebitis
Letterer-Siwe	Stomatitis	Hepatosplenomegaly Skin rash Fever Lymphadenopathy Bleeding, anemia

From Orkin, F.K., and Cooperman, L.H.: Complications in Anesthesia, Philadelphia, J.B. Lippincott, 1983.

ENDOTRACHEAL ANESTHESIA: III. COMPLICATIONS

COMPLICATIONS OF INTUBATION

With clinician skill and experience, the incidence of intubation complications becomes minimal. Most local sequelae result from trauma, are mild in degree, and are of little consequence. Subjective complaints must be treated and comfort provided.

Mishaps are related to (1) equipment, (2) the intubation process, and (3) late sequelae (Table 21–1). The types of complications are both physiologic and anatomic and may occur immediately or be delayed.[1] Early complications are listed in Table 21–2.

CLINICAL DESCRIPTION.[2] Most complications of intubation are related to a physiologic stress reaction or anatomic mechanical damage. Consideration must be given to the mechanism, the time of occurrence during the anesthesia, the acuteness or chronicity, and the severity of the damage.

Etiology. Some common causes of endotracheal anesthesia complications include mechanical–traumatic; pathophysiologic–reflex or neurogenic; allergic; and pharmacochemical (topical anesthetics; tube lubricants).

Timing of Occurrence. It is necessary to identify the time when a complication occurs or is induced in relation to the sequence of the intubation procedure. Pathophysiologic complications are usually immediate and are related to the pharmacologic agents used to provide conditions for laryngoscopy at the time of placement of the endotracheal tube and, later, at the time of extubation, or to mechanical stimulation of reflexogenic zones by the laryngoscope or the tube. Trauma also occurs at the time of laryngoscopy and intubation and has a mechanical basis; the consequences are observed and diagnosed after extubation. Some traumatic insults may not be readily apparent, and complaints may not be expressed for hours or days after the patient awakens.

566 *General Anesthesia*

TABLE 21–1. COMPLICATIONS OF ENDOTRACHEAL ANESTHESIA

Mishaps of equipment
  Tube:
    Kink, collapse—respiratory obstruction
    Bore too small—respiratory obstruction
    Too long—increased dead space
    Layers of latex tube may peel off, forming flap
  Stylet:
    Plastic—may break and free in trachea or bronchus
    Too long—may lacerate larynx or trachea
  Laryngoscope:
    Bulb may go out or be too dim
    Bulb may drop off free in airway
  Cuff:
    Pressure kills ciliated tracheal lining (cilia not active in raising mucus)
    May overlap end of tube with obstruction
    May collapse soft tube
  Lubricant:
    Oil or petrolatum can cause lipoid pneumonia
    Water may cause edema
    Water-soluble jellies may dry and abrade cords
    Anesthetic jellies—usable
  Pack:
    Shreds of gauze in airway
    Pack may be left in inadvertently
    Pressure on larynx may cause edema
Mishaps of intubation
  Trauma:
    Trauma to teeth, lips, gums, dentures, etc.
    Stretched pharyngeal muscles—subluxation of jaw
    Trauma to larynx, epiglottis; laceration of pharynx (divots)
    Trauma to any part of throat or airway
    Nosebleeding
    Tracheal trauma leading to mediastinal emphysema and mediastinitis
  Reflex disturbances:
    Cardiac arrhythmias due to vagovagal reflexes.
      Apnea (breathholding)
      Laryngospasm
      Coughing, bucking
  Position:
    Too far in—right bronchus, atelectasis left (Fig. 21–1).
    Bevel against tracheal wall (Figs. 21–2, and 21–3)
    Not far enough—cuff between cords
  Foreign body:
    Between cords (tube, etc.)—edema, erythema
    Pressures of tube anteriorly or posteriorly—tracheal wall necrosis
Postanesthetic complications
  Laryngitis:
    Hoarseness—not common; watch carefully
  Tracheitis:
    Sensation of constriction in neck; persistent cough—treat with codeine
  Edema of larynx:
    Rare; serious—reintubate
  Infections:
    Due to contaminated tubes
  Ulcers of larynx
  Granulomas
  Respiratory morbidity:
    Pneumonia
  Surgical emphysema

Anatomic Complications. The anatomic problems may occur during the procedure of positioning the head for laryngoscopy, during the act of laryngoscopy, and during introduction of the endotracheal tube. These complications must be related topographically to the site of the lesions. Trauma at this time may be readily recognized, as when teeth are damaged or nasal bleeding or misplacement of the tube occur. Delayed anatomic complications may be recognized after extubation and may range from mild sore throat to severe glottic edema. Chronic conditions may only be recognized after several days, including ulcers, granulomas, and infections of the vocal cords.

Pathophysiologic Complications (Neurogenic Reflexes). These complications are of three types: (1) laryngovagal (bradycardia); (2) laryngosympathetic (hypertension); and (3) laryngospinal (hypotension; splanchnic reflex). The clinical picture is that of adverse cardiovascular or respiratory system responses.

Clinical Character. Incidence should be classified as common or rare; the severity of the complication and the chronicity; and the immediate treatment or subsequent need for otolaryngologic or surgical care. Two or more complications may be induced simultaneously and coexist for varying periods of time. The duration should be anticipated and a prognosis established.

PATHOPHYSIOLOGIC AND REFLEX COMPLICATIONS

Respiratory Effects

Premature performance of laryngoscopy and intubation is frequently accompanied by three immediate respiratory complications that occur not only when the patient is asleep and not anesthetized but also when the depth of anesthesia is light. The following complications are immediate and often are associated with acute trauma to the upper airway (Table 21–3):

1. *Apnea*—may be from respiratory inhibition or reflex breathholding; occurs in light planes.
2. *Laryngospasm and bronchospasm*—spasm of the laryngeal muscles may occur while a tube is in the trachea. Because of the interposing tube, the situation may not be apparent but the vocal cords may be contracting against the tube and producing mechanical trauma of the cords (occurs in light planes of anesthesia).
3. *Obstruction*—kinking, displacement, or biting of the tube; bevel against tracheal wall; bleeding and secretions; inadvertent introduction of foreign bodies.

TABLE 21–2. EARLY COMPLICATIONS OF TRACHEAL INTUBATION

	During Intubation	With Tube in Place	During Extubation
Traumatic—mechanical	*Direct* Fracture–luxation of cervical spinal column (spinal cord injury) Eye trauma Epistaxis Tooth trauma Laceration of pharynx or larynx Perforation of esophagus or pharynx Retropharyngeal dissection Subcutaneous or mediastinal emphysema Arytenoid dislocation Aspiration (blood, tooth, laryngoscope bulb, gastric contents, tumor tissue, adenoid) *Indirect* Pneumothorax Esophageal intubation (gastric distention; swallowed tube) Bronchial intubation (hypoxemia)	Fracture–luxation of cervical spinal cord Ventilatory obstruction Rupture of trachea Emphysema, pneumothorax Ruptured cuff Tracheal bleeding Aspiration Trauma to subglottis by inflated cuff Recurrent nerve paralysis, malposition of cuff (subglottic and intraglottic) Denudation of tracheal mucosa (cilia) Bacteremia (nasotracheal)	Trauma to glottis by inflated cuff Difficult or impossible extubation Ventilatory obstruction

Pathophysiologic (reflex)	Pharyngeal spasm
	Laryngeal spasm
	Bronchospasm
	Bucking–coughing
	  Increased intraocular pressure
	  Increased intracranial pressure
	Cardiac arrhythmias
	Arterial hypotension
	Arterial hypertension
			Bucking–coughing
			Laryngeal spasm

Modified from Blanc, V. F., and Tremblay, N. A. G.: The complications of tracheal intubation. Anesth. Analg. 53:203, 1974.

LARYNGOSPASM

DEFINITION.[3] Laryngospasm is spasm of the adductor muscles (arytenoids, lateral cricoarytenoids, and cricothyroid) of the vocal cords that causes obstruction to respiration. It may be partial or complete. If partial, there will be crowing, grunting, or wheezing, especially on inspiration. If complete, apnea occurs and there is an inability to inflate the lungs.

The overall incidence of laryngospasm is about 8 in 1000 patients.[4] In children ages 1 to 9 years, it is approximately 17 in 1000, whereas infants have the highest incidence, more than three times that of any other age group.[5]

INCIDENCE. Certain conditions are associated with a greatly increased incidence, especially in the absence of adequate anesthesia. These include the following:

- Oral endoscopy or esophagoscopy
- Introduction and presence of a nasogastric tube
- Presence of respiratory tract infection

On extubation, especially if performed while the patient is awakening, it is almost always observed.

CLASSIFICATION.[3]

First Degree. This is a simple protective reaction with adduction of true cords in apposition because of irritants. It is most common and least harmful.

TABLE 21–3. IMMEDIATE COMPLICATIONS OF INTUBATION

Apnea
Laryngospasm and bronchospasm
Kinking of endotracheal tube
Biting of tube by patient
Displacement of tube
Aspiration of mucus, blood, or vomitus about sides of tube due to poor packings or cuffs

Treatment is not necessary, and the problem will correct itself.

Second Degree. This is a more extensive protective reaction with apposition of false cords. The aryepiglottic folds are in spasm and block the view of the true cords. This is not a serious problem in healthy persons and will resolve. Pulling the jaw forward favors release of the spasm. Oxygen should be administered when the spasm breaks.

Third Degree. All muscles of the larynx as well as the pharynx are in spasm; the larynx is tipped forward to the epiglottis. Change in head position and a painful stimulus often cause release; however, it is usually necessary to intubate and occasionally perform a tracheostomy.

Fourth Degree. The epiglottis is incarcerated in the upper part of the larynx.

MECHANISM. The classification by Rovenstine[6] has been supported by the studies and description of laryngospasm by Fink[7] (see Fig. 21–1). With the aid of lateral x-rays of the neck, computed tomography, scans and electromyography, he described laryngeal closure as occurring at three anatomic levels:[8] (1) the true vocal cords may simply act like a shutter mechanism and may be the only action—this causes stridor; (2) the false vocal cords (or vestibular folds) and the true cords may become apposed in midline and produce a more persistent closure[9]; and (3) the supraglottic folds—the aryepiglottic membranes—become rounded and fold inward with posterior displacement of the epiglottis. As these tissues are drawn into the laryngeal inlet, a ball-valve effect is created. Shortening of the thyrohyoid muscle is engaged in this action, tilting the larynx toward the epiglottis and the whole backward into the glottic chink.

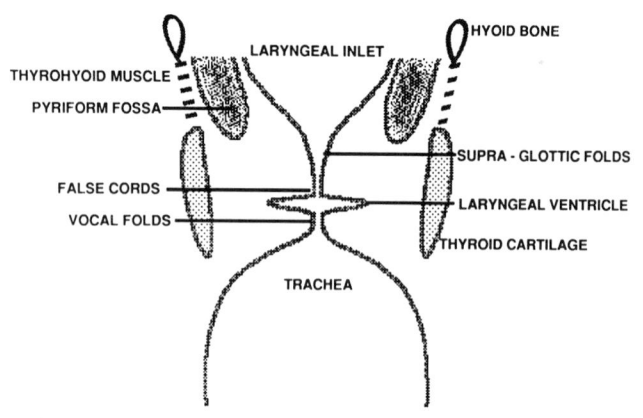

FIG. 21–1. Sectional view of larynx. Adapted from Fink BR. The etiology and treatment of laryngeal spasm. Anesthesiology 17:569, 1976. Modified by Roy and Lerman: Can. J. Anaesth., *35*:93, 1988.

The laryngeal closure may be sequential and in large measure related to the intensity or duration of stimulation or a varying background of anesthetic drug interaction and depth. Once laryngospasm is excited, the degree of laryngeal closure continues long after cessation of the stimulation.[10]

In consideration of the laryngeal reflex of Kratschmer, noxious stimulation of the glottic region sends afferent impulses over the superior laryngeal nerves.[11] Strong noxious stimulation of the pharynx and base of the tongue sends these afferent impulses over sensory branches of the glossopharyngeal nerve.[12]

The efferent arc of the reflex is rapidly activated via the recurrent laryngeal nerve and motor nerves to the pharynx. The extrinsic strap muscles of the neck are activated by the hypoglossal nerve.

CAUSES.[4]

1. Laryngospasm seen during induction of anesthesia is invariably related to untimely introduction of an inhalation agent, inappropriate preanesthetic medication, and premature insertion of airways. All are basically related to inadequate anesthesia technique or anesthetic depth.
2. Drugs with parasympathetic action may induce laryngospasm, which may occur with large doses even in the absence of premedication.[13] Light thiopental is a good example.[14,15] Induction doses produce a stage II sleep, but this depth does not depress the laryngeal reflex and even sensitizes the reflex. Hence, insertion of an airway is not accommodated. In deep barbiturate hypnosis, however, synaptic transmission in the supralaryngeal nerve is reduced and spasm may be released but delayed. This approach requires an overdose. Succinylcholine initially may cause adduction of cords, but this is short lived and terminated by 1 minute after onset of action. Methohexital is also associated with occasional bouts of laryngospasm, as well as sneezing episodes during induction.
3. Of the inhalation agents, diethyl ether classically is prone to produce laryngospasm if the patient is allowed to inhale concentrations greater than 3% too early before some sedation or sleep is produced. Nitrous oxide does not induce laryngospasm. Volatile agents are capable of exciting laryngospasm, especially in children when they are not tranquilized and the inhalation agent is used for induction.[16] Isoflurane is more likely to induce laryngospasm, whereas enflurane and halothane infrequently do so.
4. Mechanical stimulation factors include (a) endogenous substances, such as saliva, loose teeth, regurgitated gastric contents, blood, and mucus secretions, are capable of eliciting a laryngospasm; and (b) exogenous foreign substances, such as dust in the breathing circuit, soda lime

dust, pharyngeal airways, laryngoscopic stimulation, suction catheters or Yankauer tips, will induce spasm of the larynx (or bronchospasm) when making contact with laryngeal or paralaryngeal structures.
5. Reflexes, including stretching of the anal or vaginal sphincters or dilatation of the cervical canal, will elicit a laryngospasm; strong traction on visceral organs during intraabdominal surgery will elicit a response under light anesthesia but will not result in obstruction if an endotracheal tube is in place.

DIAGNOSIS. Incomplete closure (first- and second-degree laryngospasm) is associated with stridorous respiratory noises intermittently. These are audible, but air movement can be better detected through a precordial stethoscope.

Complete closure is rare. The usual signs of respiratory obstruction are seen, including vigorous respiratory efforts, tracheal tug, paradoxic chest wall motion, and spasmodic abdominal (diaphragmatic) movements. But with all this, respiratory sounds are absent, (so a precordial stethoscope must be used routinely).

PREVENTION. Prepare patients with appropriate premedication and eliminate anxiety. Provide a steady state of anesthesia—not just sleep—either with a volatile agent or a complete balanced neurolept-narcotic technique.

Remove foreign substances before starting anesthesia. (Management of patients with head trauma and intraoral bleeding or a full stomach are discussed elsewhere.)

MANAGEMENT

Incomplete Closure

1. Remove irritant stimuli; stop endoscopic and surgical manipulation
2. Deepen the level of anesthesia
3. Facilitate ventilation by gentle positive airway pressure with a well-fitted face mask

Most first- and second-degree laryngospasms are self limiting. Overzealous, vigorous attempts to ventilate will aggravate the block. Hypoxia or asphyxia depresses reflex neural activity and may terminate laryngospasm.[12]

Complete Airway Obstruction (third-degree spasm)

1. Lift the chin while the head is on a pillow or displace jaw forward by applying pressure to the ascending rim of the mandible just behind the angle.
2. Alternately lifting and relaxing the chin will stretch and relax the strap muscles of the neck, especially the hypothyroid muscle (the brace reflex).[17]
3. Spray 4% cocaine into the pharynx and onto the cords.
4. Attempt to facilitate ventilation by gentle airway pressure via mask.
5. When conservative measures are not effective in breaking spasm within 1 minute, then a muscle relaxant should be given intravenously. Succinylcholine, 1.5 mg/kg, is injected. If venous access is not immediately available, intramuscular injection of succinylcholine, 4 mg/kg, is effective in 60 to 75 seconds. The laryngeal apparatus relaxes; ventilation should be given with bag and mask. Intubation may be necessary.
6. Insertion of a large-bore or cricothyroid needle through the cricotracheal space will provide an avenue for oxygen insufflation. The use of the cricothyrotome through the cricothyroid membrane is hazardous due to the proximity of subglottic stimulation and cords.
7. Tracheostomy is a last resort, but with cool, calm management and a plan of action, this procedure is rarely needed.

In the presence of complete obstruction (third-degree), forceful application of positive airway pressure via a filled face mask will not break the spasm or the obstruction but will enhance the obstruction by distending the pyriform fossae on each side of the larynx and press the aryepiglottic folds more firmly toward the midline, causing marked obstruction with bradycardia. The distribution of forces by this common maneuver and its ineffectiveness have been emphasized by Fink.[7] Furthermore, the oxygen under high positive pressure usually passes into the stomach and the distention elevates the diaphragm.

BRONCHOSPASM.

DEFINITION.[3] Bronchospasm is a lower airway obstruction that results from constriction of the bronchiolar muscles of the secondary and tertiary bronchial branches. The diagnosis should be made in the absence of a mechanical obstruction of the airway, such as foreign bodies, secretions, or blood, or complications associated with the use of pharyngeal devices or endotracheal tubes. Various clinical criteria have been used to make the diagnosis.

The occurrence of expiratory wheezing, a reduced tidal volume, the use of accessory muscles, forceful expiratory contractions, and an increase in peak airway pressures during ventilation are classic signs.[18] For true bronchospasm, the bronchoconstriction should require treatment with a bronchodilator.[19] In the study by Olsson,[20] only an anesthetic notation on the record was used for computing incidence (see following discussion), but the checking was based on clinical criteria.

MECHANISM. Bronchospasm is triggered by mechanical stimulation, especially of the laryngotracheal areas. Tracheal and carinal areas are perhaps the most sensitive and evoke intense protective coughing, bucking, and spasm. Laryngeal and glottic stimulation may not only evoke varying degrees of laryngospasm, but if the stimulus is of sufficient intensity, bronchospasm may be induced.

INCIDENCE.[20] The overall incidence of bronchospasm in the course of administering anesthesia is approximately 1.6 in 1000 anesthetics.

The higher overall incidence that occurred in the age group 0 to 9 years was 4 in 1000. When the following conditions existed, the rate was greatly increased, presumably because of a greater reactive airway:

- Respiratory infection (41 in 1000)
- Pathologic electrocardiogram (24 in 1000)
- Obstructive lung disease (22 in 1000)
- ASA physical status III (24 in 1000)
- Oral endoscopy/tracheal intubation (9 in 1000)
- Rectal instillation of anesthetic drugs (35 in 1000)

There is also a higher incidence in certain spinal operations as well as oral endoscopic surgery, tonsillectomy, and diagnostic encephalography or myelography.

In the age group of 50 to 69 years, the incidence is higher than the average, at 1.8 in 1000 or 1 in 550 anesthetics. This incidence has been reported to be greatly increased when clinical conditions such as the following exist preanesthestically:

- Presence of airway obstruction (tumors, foreign body) (9 in 1000)
- Obstructive lung disease (7.7 in 1000)
- Previous myocardial infarction (5.5 in 1000)
- During and after bronchoscopy (7.6 in 1000)
- During and after mediastinoscopy (7.8 in 1000)

COMMENT. The incidence of bronchospasm is lower for anesthetics administered during the early morning but higher for anesthetics in the afternoon and evening. Allergies in children are related to a lower incidence, whereas an increased incidence is noted in the older age group. Insufficient preanesthetic medication resulted in a higher incidence in children, especially boys.

Obstructive Mechanical Hypoxemia

Hypoxemia and signs of respiratory obstruction related to endotracheal intubation are mechanical in nature. The following common conditions are representative.

- Displacement of tube downward or out of the larynx[21]
- Esophageal intubation[22]
- Inadvertent unrecognized bronchial intubation (see Fig. 21–2)[23]
- Kinking of the endotracheal tube from malpositioning in the prone position and bevel impinging on the tracheal wall (see Fig. 21–3). Figure 21–4 illustrates the use of a nonkinkable tube.[24]
- Biting of the tube in patients not adequately anesthetized or paralyzed[25,28]

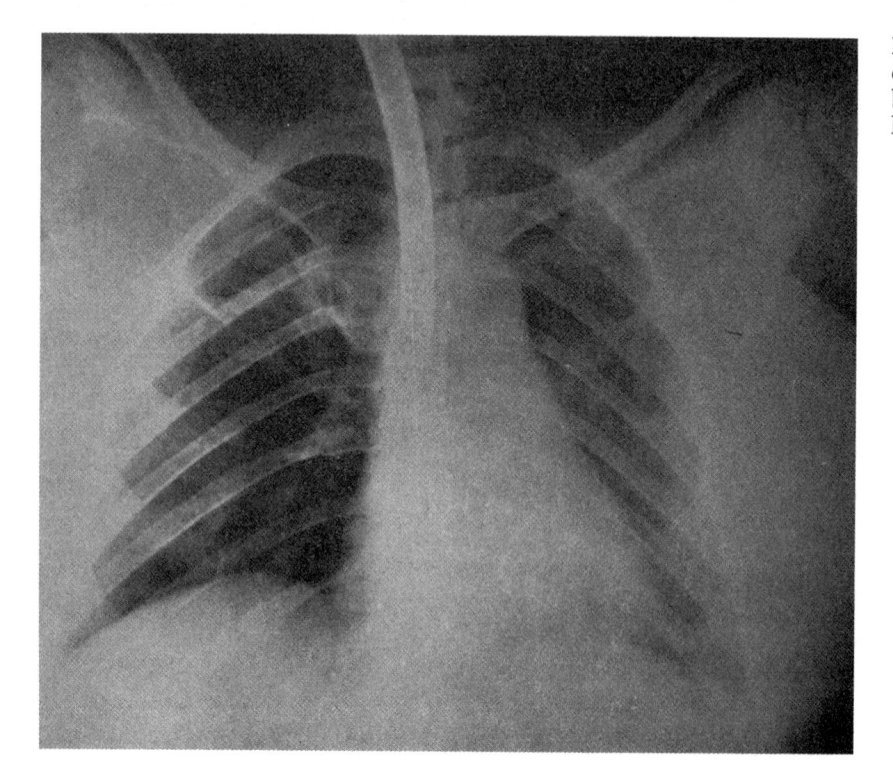

FIG. 21–2. Radiograph of patient with endotracheal tube misplaced in right bronchus. Note the haziness of the left lung and the developing atelectasis.

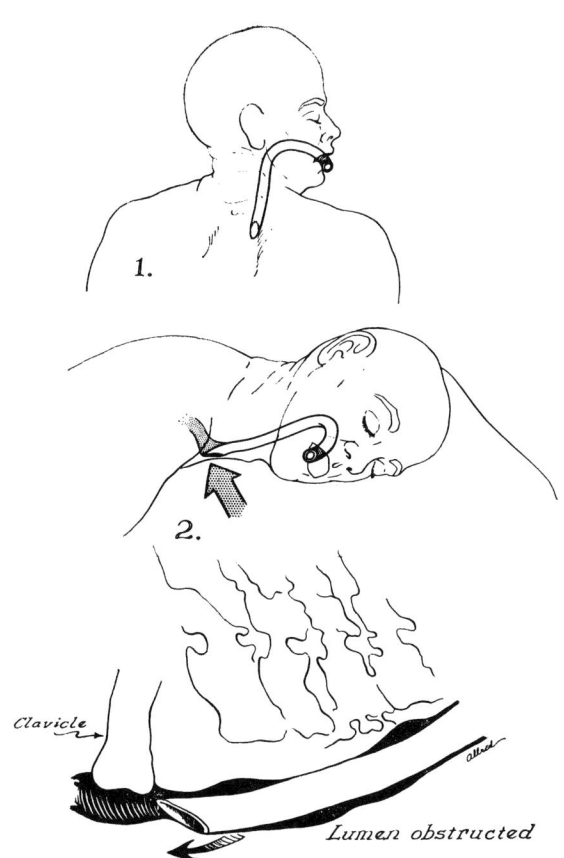

FIG. 21-3. Complication of intubation showing impingement of bevel against tracheal wall due to prone position with head rotated. Courtesy of Dr. R. C. Thompson.[27] In 1. the head is hyperflexed and rotated; 2. the head and neck are hyperextended and rotated.

- Foreign body obstruction of the lumen of the tube[26]
- Impingement of bevel against tracheal wall in the supine position usually due to excess extension of head (Fig. 21-5) or rotation of head in prone position (see Fig. 21-3).[27]
- Overinflated cuffs (Fig. 21-6 and Fig. 21-7).[29]

Cardiovascular Effects

A marked cardiovascular response with a rise in blood pressure and increase in pulse is often encountered during endotracheal intubation. This was first described in 1950 by Burstein.[30] The response is usually most evident during laryngoscopy and manipulation of the epiglottis.[31] The systolic pressure may increase a mean of 45 mm Hg. It is usually accompanied by pulse rate changes, especially sinus and even ventricular tachycardia.[32] Although the response may be transient, it is invariable, significant, often persistent, and of great concern. Sensitive receptor areas of the epiglottis, when mechanically stimulated, particularly evoke the reflex response.[33] Baumgartner[34] and Wycoff[35] have demonstrated that succinylcholine will produce a transient rise in blood pressure, usually accompanied by slowing of the pulse. Rapid rates, however, do occur, and serious arrhythmias from single doses of succinylcholine have been observed.[34]

EARLY TREATMENT. The blood pressure rise can be minimized by increasing the depth of anesthesia or by hyperventilation. Burstein[32] also demonstrated that topical anesthesia will minimize the rate changes and arrhythmias.

Topical anesthesia greatly minimizes the reaction but does not completely abolish the responses. It is probable that deep pressure on the base of the tongue and neck muscles is also responsible.

Premedication with belladonna drugs does not significantly alter the incidence or degree of bradycardia during laryngoscopy except in infants and children.

Table 21-4 summarizes the techniques used to control blood pressure and arrhythmia response to laryngoscopy and intubation.[36-60]

EFFECT ON PULMONARY CIRCULATION.[61a] Pulmonary circulation is adversely affected when patients are lightly anesthetized and paralyzed and endotracheal intubation is carried out. There is a marked bronchiolar constriction as well as constriction of the pulmonary arterial bed.[61b] This reduces alveolar perfusion and produces a significant pulmonary shunt.[39a,39b,61]

RESPONSE IN PATIENTS WITH CORONARY ARTERY DISEASE. More frequent and more pronounced tachycardia and hypertension are observed during intubation of patients with valvular heart disease and especially coronary artery disease. Systolic, diastolic, mean arterial pressure (MAP), and the rate-pressure product (RPP) are all elevated. Such elevations are highly significant in patients with coronary artery disease. In these patients there is also a twofold elevation in plasma norepinephrine but no change in epinephrine levels.[39a]

EFFECT OF INTRAVENOUS INDUCTION DRUGS. Various intravenous induction drugs for production of unconsciousness (UD$_{95}$) do not attenuate the cardiovascular response to laryngoscopy, and elevations of blood pressure, both systolic and diastolic, and some increase in heart rate occur. The elevation of blood pressure is associated with norepinephrine release, whereas the changes in heart rate are epinephrine related.[62]

Catecholamine levels change significantly. Norepinephrine levels may double on laryngoscopy and intubation (from 160 to 300 pg/ml) and continue for 4 to 8 minutes; epinephrine levels may quadruple from 70 to 280 pg/ml. Simultaneously, an endocrine stress is evident by an increase in beta endorphins of 15 pg/ml.[63]

572 *General Anesthesia*

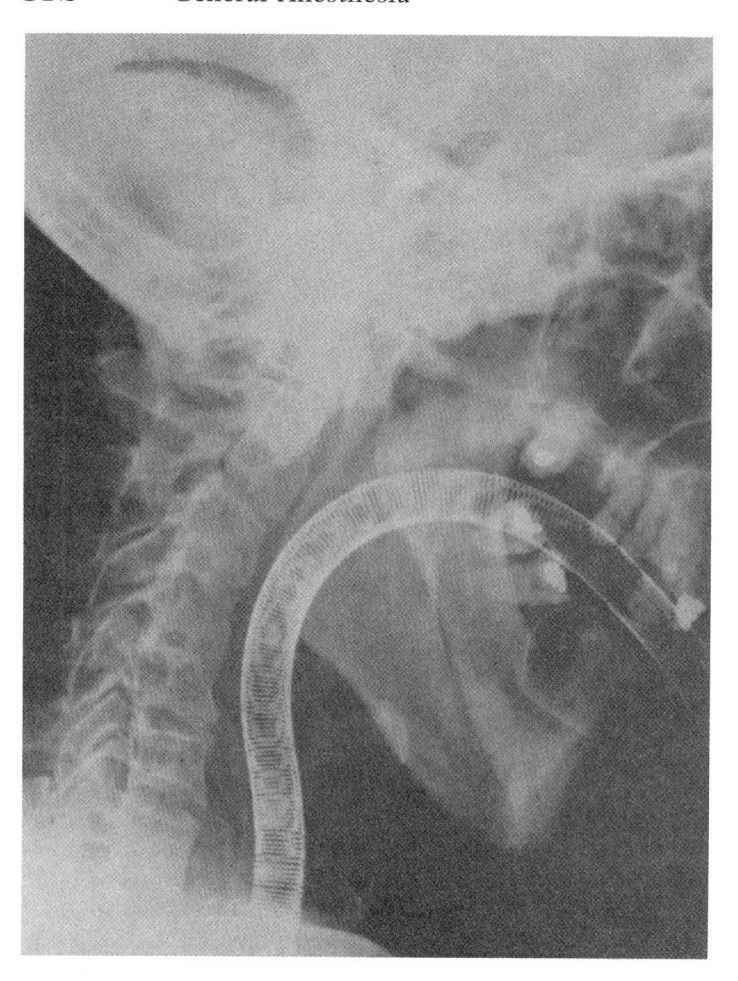

FIG. 21–4. A nonkinkable tube (anode or LA metal spiral) in place. Exaggerated flexion of head on the chest does not kink tube. Obstruction noted in Figures 21–2 and 21–3 is also avoided by this tube.

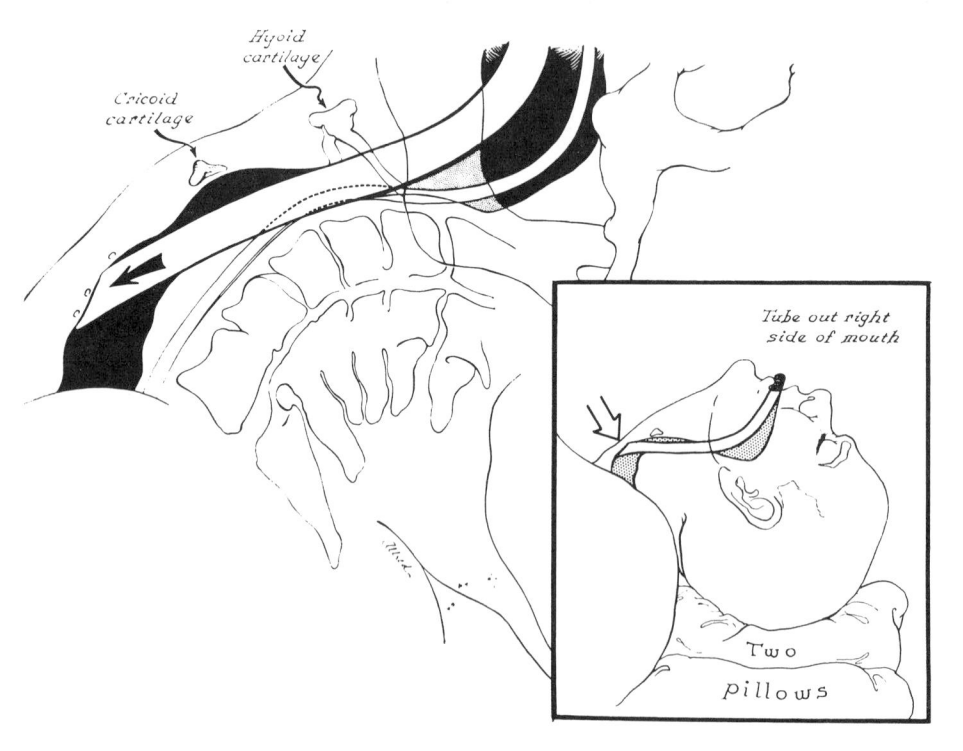

FIG. 21–5. Complication of intubation showing impingement of the bevel of the endotracheal tube against the tracheal wall due to extended position of head. In supine position; also shows kinking due to forward force of cervical vertebrae. After intubation with soft tubes, the head should be maintained in a natural position. Courtesy of Dr. R. C. Thompson.

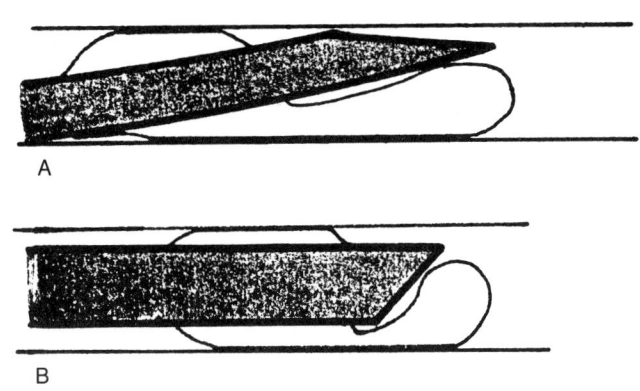

FIG. 21–6. Two causes of tracheal tube obstruction. *A,* the bevel of the tube is pushed against the wall of the trachea by an eccentrically inflated cuff. *B,* the cuff has ballooned over the end of the tube. From Dorsch, J.A. and Dorsch S.E.: Understanding Anesthesia Equipment, 2nd ed. Baltimore, Williams & Wilkins, 1984.

One exception to the above rule is that two benzodiazepines are partially effective: diazepam (oral and intravenous), as well as midazolam, does block the autonomic sympathetic outflow.[64]

EFFECT OF ANESTHETIC AGENTS ON CARDIOVASCULAR RESPONSES.[65] A study of four anesthetic techniques with inhaled agents on hemodynamic responses to endotracheal intubation has shown the following:

- Neither halothane–nitrous oxide–oxygen nor nitrous oxide–oxygen–intravenous morphine altered the hypertensive or cardiac response.
- On the other hand, the enflurane–nitrous oxide–oxygen technique and the neurolept–narcotic (fentanyl)–nitrous oxide–oxygen technique were effective in attenuating the hemodynamic response.

MECHANISM. The cardiovascular response to the act of tracheal intubation is a reflex phenomenon with the afferent stimuli carried over both glossopharyngeal and vagal pathways. Such stimuli activate suprasegmental and hypothalamic sympathetic centers to cause a peripheral sympathoadrenal response with release of adrenaline and noradrenaline. Within 1 minute of laryngoscopy alone, there is a hypertensive response with only slight increases in cardiac rate.[66]

The cardiovascular changes and catecholamine release should be divided into two phases, differentiating the act of laryngoscopy and its effects from the act of tracheal insertion of an endotracheal tube (or of a catheter or bronchoscope), as shown by Shribman.[67] Laryngoscopy alone without intubation provides a supraglottic pressor stimulus with significant increases in both systolic and diastolic pressures from a cental level of a stable anesthetic state, as well as increases above the preinduction control levels (Fig. 21–8). Increases in heart rate are slight and not significant from laryngoscopy alone.

Accompanying the pressure response within the same minute of appearance of the cardiovascular response is a significant increase in plasma noradrenaline and adrenaline (Figs. 21–9 and 21–10).

The second phase, or the act of intubation and placement of an endotracheal tube in the trachea or of a catheter, stimulates infraglottic receptors and evokes an additional cardiovascular response with a further increase in catecholamines. The pressor response is much greater, increasing by 36% from postinduction control levels. The heart rate also now significantly increases by about 20% with the act of tracheal intubation, whereas, as noted earlier, there is little rate response to laryngoscopy alone.

Accompanying these cardiovascular changes are rapid and significantly greater increases in both adrenaline and noradrenaline with the introduction of the tube into the trachea (Figs. 21–9 and 21–10).[68]

Derbyshire[69] has shown that 1 minute after laryngoscopy and intubation, the MAP increases by about 35% and the heart rate increases about 18% over the control levels. These cardiovascular changes are accompanied by elevations in plasma catecholamines: noradrenaline increases 45% and adrenaline 40%.

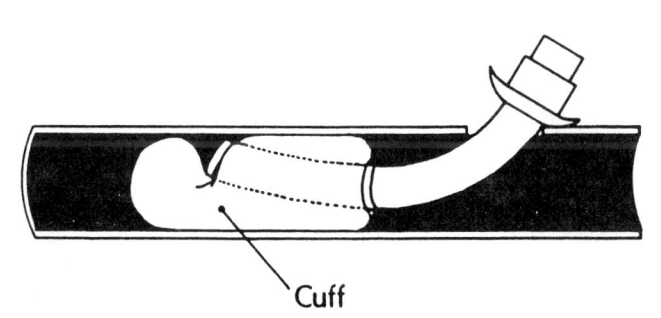

FIG. 21–7. Schematic representation of cuff herniating over end of tracheostomy tube and causing obstruction (see text). From Shapiro, B. Clinical applications of respiratory care. Chicago, Year Book Medical Publishers, 1975.

TECHNIQUES OF HEMODYNAMIC CONTROL

There are many approaches to minimize the hemodynamic adverse responses to laryngoscopy and intubation. Essentially, they can be reduced to the three following groups based on the reflex arc:

1. *Block of the sensory peripheral receptors and the afferent input:* Block of sensory receptors and of afferent nerves is accomplished by topical application and infiltration of nerves. Of the topical surface anesthetics, tetracaine (1% to 2%)[30] and cocaine (4%) are preeminent.[35,36] Dyclonine (1%) has been found to be an excellent and safe

TABLE 21–4. TECHNIQUES USED FOR CONTROL OF PRESSOR AND ARRHYTHMIA RESPONSE TO LARYNGOSCOPY AND INTUBATION

Technique	Reference
Topical Anesthesia (tetracaine 1%, cocaine 4%)	Burstein[30] (1950); Wycoff[35] (1960); Denlinger[36] (1974)
Anesthesia surgical depth	King[31] (1951) Forbes[37] (1970)
Regional block of the larynx and tetracaine, topical	Wycoff[35] (1960)
Lidocaine	
Topical	Denlinger[36] (1974); Abou-Madi[38] (1975); Stoelting[39a,39b] (1977,1978); Kautt[40,41] (1982)
Intravenous (1.5 mg/kg)	Steinhaus[42,43] (1970); Denlinger[44] (1976); Abou-Madi[45] (1977)
Fentanyl pretreatment (5 μg/kg)	Dahlgren[46] (1984)
Beta-adrenergic block	
Propranolol (nonselective)	Prys-Roberts[47a,47b] (1971, 1973)
Practolol (cardioselective)	Wycoff[35] (1980); Siedlecki[48] (1975)
Metoprolol (4 mg) (cardioselective)	Coleman[49] (1980)
Antihypertensive drugs (ganglionic)	
Trimethaphan	De Vault[50] (1960)
Phentolamine	Siedlecki[48] (1975)
Antihypertensive drugs (peripheral)	
Sodium nitroprusside	Stoelting[51] (1979)
Hydralazine (0.4 mg/kg)	Davies[52] (1981)
Nitroglycerin	
Topical	Kamra[53] (1986)
Intranasal	Dich-Nielsen[54] (1986)
Nifedipine sublingual (10 mg)	Kale[60] (1988)
Antihypertensive drugs (central)	
Droperidol (0.5 μg/kg)	Curran[55] (1980)
Clonidine, oral (4 μg/kg)	Flacke[56] (1987); Ghigone[57] (1987)
Low-dose thiopental (1.5 mg/kg)–lidocaine (4 mg/kg)–diazepam	Ackerman[58] (1984)
Topical lidocaine 10% nasally for nasal intubation	Hartigan[59] (1984)
Minimize the time of laryngoscopy (<15 s)	Burstein[30] (1952); Stoelting[39] (1978)

agent.[70,71] Topical 4% lidocaine, while widely used including the 10% solution,[59] is a relatively poor topical agent and is little more effective than procaine 4%.[36,38–41] Nerve block of the superior laryngeal nerves is easily accomplished. After a latent period of 2 to 4 minutes, excellent sensory anesthesia of the larynx is obtained. This has the advantage of prevention of the bombardment of the central nervous system with noxious stimuli, a part of anociception.

2. *Block of the central mechanisms of integration of sensory input:* Central nervous system block is achieved by narcotic drugs such as fentanyl[46] and morphine pretreatment and neurolept agents such as droperidol for hypothalamic block,[55,58] but the most effective approach is adequate general anesthesia at the surgical levels of stage III.[31,32]

3. *Block of the efferent pathways and the effector receptors:* Methods of attenuating the hemodynamic stress responses are voluminous. Intravenous lidocaine sedates the cardiac mechanisms to diminish tachycardia, and large doses may obtund the blood pressure responses.[42–45] Propranolol and other beta-adrenergic blocking agents block the cardiac responses but do not adequately reduce hypertensive responses.[47–49] Ganglionic sympathetic block has been tried with trimethaphan[50] and phentolamine.[48] Direct arteriolar block of smooth musculature of the arterioles with hydralazine[52] or nitroprusside[51] minimizes blood pressure elevations. Calcium channel blockers of the nifedipine type are especially effective.[60]

CONCLUSION. It is evident that no single drug or technique is satisfactory in preventing the undesirable hemodynamic effects of laryngoscopy and endotracheal intubation. Most approaches are directed at controlling the reactions to stress rather than the stress stimuli or their central nervous system recognition.

At the present time, the most satisfactory and effective technique is to provide a surgical stage of

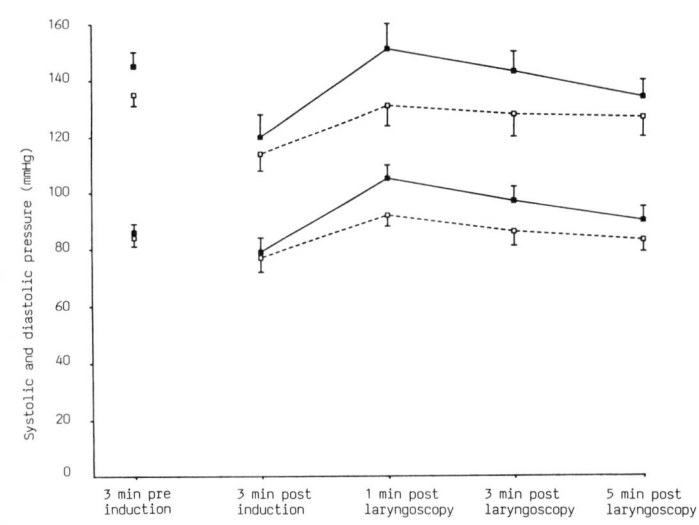

FIG. 21–8. Systolic and diastolic arterial pressures (mean ± SEM) in both groups before induction, and for the 5-min period after laryngoscopy. □- - -□ = Laryngoscopy only (n = 12); ■——■ = laryngoscopy and intubation (n = 12). From Shribman, A.J., Smith, G., and Achola, K.J.: Cardiovascular and catecholamine responses to laryngoscopy with and without tracheal intubation. Br. J. Anaesth., 59:295, 1987.

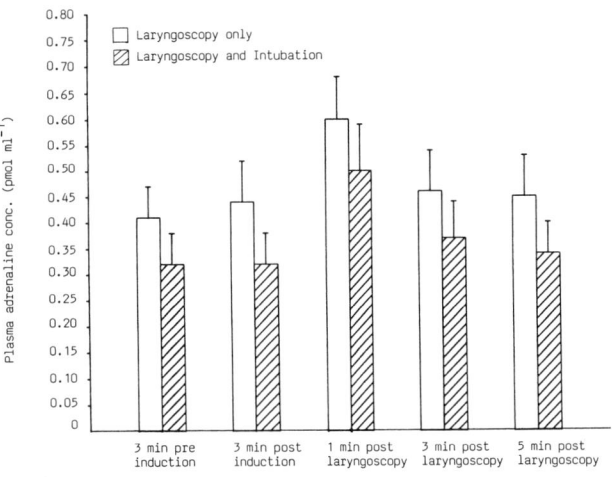

FIG. 21–10. Plasma adrenaline concentrations (mean ± SEM) in both groups at each stage of the study. n = 12 (both groups). From Shribman, A.J., Smith, G., and Achola, K.J.: Cardiovascular and catecholamine responses to laryngoscopy with and without tracheal intubation. Br. J. Anaesth., 59:295, 1987.

anesthesia as with a general inhalation volatile agent accompanied by muscle paralysis or, alternatively, with a sedative–neurolept–narcotic combination with nitrous oxide–oxygen and a muscle relaxant.

Recommendations, therefore, are three:

1. Stage III levels of anesthesia[30,31,37]
2. Laryngotracheal topical anesthesia with an effective topical agent, such as 2% tetracaine,[35] or nerve block anesthesia with lidocaine 1%
3. Minimal duration and intensity of airway manipulation, i.e., skilled laryngoscopy and manipulation for less than 20 seconds[39]

Evaluation of Techniques of Hemodynamic Control

INTRAVENOUS LIDOCAINE. Intravenous lidocaine is effective in the prevention of arrhythmias and hypertension as well as other aspects of anesthetic care (Table 21–5). In the intravenous infusion drip technique of lidocaine anesthesia, the antiarrhythmic and antihypertensive effects are notable. A bolus injection of 1.5 mg/kg lidocaine 2% solution, however, can be given about 90 seconds (and at 3 minutes) prior to laryngoscopy and is effective in minimizing undesirable cardiovascular responses.[44] Attenuation is optimal when administered at 2.5 to 3 minutes preintubation.[71] This dose provides an arterial lidocaine level of 2.5 to 5 μg/ml, which significantly attenuates the cardiovascular response.

In women with pregnancy-induced hypertension and toxemia, intravenous lidocaine does not completely attenuate cardiovascular responses to laryngoscopy and intubation. Transfer to the fetus of the lidocaine can result in induced venous levels of about one-half of the maternal blood level, but the fetal hepatic concentration is at least three times that of the maternal hepatic concentration.[72]

The rise in intraocular pressure, which occurs during laryngoscopy and intubation when a state of

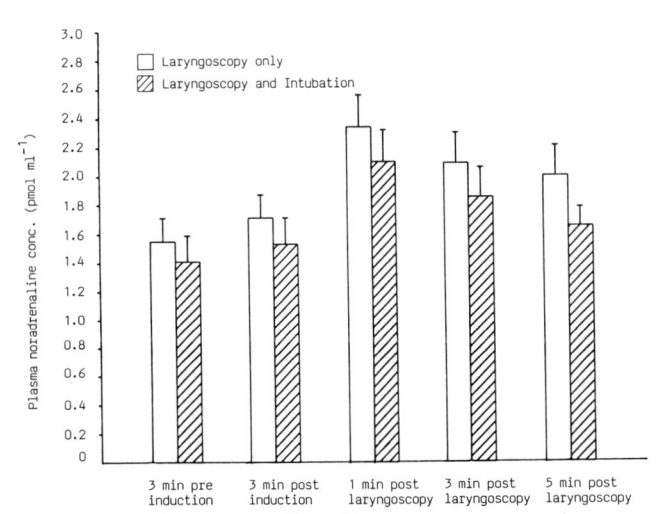

FIG. 21–9. Plasma noradrenaline concentrations (mean ± SEM) in both groups at each stage of the study. n = 12 (both groups). From Shribman, A.J., Smith, G., and Achola, K.J.: Cardiovascular and catecholamine responses to laryngoscopy with and without tracheal intubation. Br. J. Anaesth., 59:295, 1987.

TABLE 21-5. USES AND ADVANTAGES OF INTRAVENOUS LIDOCAINE

Decreases anesthetic requirements—reduces MAC values; potentiates nitrous oxide, halothane at blood levels of 3–6 μg/ml[74]
Suppresses cough reflex on intubation[43,75]
Suppresses cough during bronchoscopy[76,77]
Attenuates circulatory response to intubation[45,78,79]
Prevents increases in intracranial pressure on intubation[80,81]
Suppresses increases in intraocular pressure after intubation[82]
Controls extubation cough and laryngospasm in children[83] and adults[84]
Antiarrhythmia action[85]

adequate anesthesia with relaxation is not present, can be attenuated with intravenous lidocaine 1.5 mg/kg. This has been successful in children.[73]

A combination of drugs consisting of lidocaine with low-dose thiopental, 1.5 mg/kg, and diazepam, all administered intravenously 2 to 4 minutes prior to laryngoscopy, has been reported to obtund hypertensive patients; however, hypotension may occur.[58]

TOPICAL ANESTHESIA. Topical anesthesia of the pharynx and larynx with a potent topical agent, such as tetracaine 1% to 2% or dyclonine, appears to be the most effective technique of obtunding adverse cardiovascular responses.[35] The topical agent is preferably sprayed on the larynx 1 to 2 minutes prior to intubation and additionally sprayed during initial laryngoscopy.[36]

INTRAVENOUS FENTANYL. Fentanyl in doses of 6 μg/kg 2 minutes prior to intubation will attenuate hemodynamic responses; smaller doses have essentially no effect; and larger doses of 15 μg/kg are required to abolish the responses significantly.[40,41,46]

Fentanyl preloading by 2 to 3 minutes at a dose of 6 μg/kg does obtund but not abolish the sympathetic and endocrine response (stress) to intubation. Cork[63] determined that in rapid-sequence induction, the UD_{95} dose of thiopental can be reduced with fentanyl preloading. At the same time, plasma beta endorphins do not increase, whereas in control subjects (no fentanyl) there is an increase in immunoreactive plasma levels by 15 pg/ml. Total catecholamines do not increase on intubation; epinephrine may increase, but norepinephrine may decrease from control levels.

Different doses of fentanyl of approximately 6, 11, and 15 μg/kg have been compared for their effect on MAP and common carotid blood flow. Only the 15-μg/kg dose effectively prevented elevations of arterial pressure and maintained a normal blood flow.[86] Higher doses, such as 25 to 100 μg/kg, are not more effective and may produce hypotension as well as postoperative respiratory depression and neurologic depression.[87]

TOPICAL LIDOCAINE. Application of lidocaine 4% by aerosol spray to oropharyngeal and laryngeal mucous membranes or gargling with viscous lidocaine attenuates partially the hypertensive effect of laryngoscopy but not the cardiac rate nor the further hypertensive response to tracheal intubation.

Effect on Catecholamines. In Derbyshire's studies,[66] 4% lidocaine failed to attenuate significantly the cardiovascular responses induced by laryngoscopy and intubation. In addition, no significant effect on the sympathoadrenal axis and release of catecholamines was observed: (1) noradrenaline continued to increase to 40% to 50% above resting levels (this is similar to the increases seen without topical lidocaine) and (2) plasma adrenaline levels in patients treated with topical lidocaine showed a greater increase over that in patients not treated.

For nasal intubation, Hartigan[59] has suggested the use of 10% lidocaine topically applied to both nostrils. This appeared to be more effective than 1.5 mg lidocaine intravenously, but elevations of blood pressure did occur and lasted up to 4 minutes. Blood levels of lidocaine were not determined, and it is likely that rather toxic levels might be reached with the concentrated topical lidocaine.

It is concluded that topical lidocaine is relatively ineffective in preventing the hemodynamic effects of laryngoscopy and intubation.[41] The mucosal anesthesia produced by 4% lidocaine is inadequate at best.

TRANSLARYNGEAL LIDOCAINE. Use of this technique before endotracheal intubation has been shown not to alter significantly the cardiovascular responses to endotracheal intubation.[78,88] A less-persistent pressor response was the sole effect of translaryngeal lidocaine when compared with intravenous administration.[89] It is suggested that the translaryngeal administration attenuates cardiovascular responses due to absorption into the circulation.[39a] One study shows that placement of 5% lidocaine ointment on the endotracheal tube may result in plasma lidocaine levels of up to 2 μg/ml.[90]

BETA-ADRENORECEPTOR BLOCK. $Beta_2$ adrenergic block has been proposed and used by Prys-Roberts[47b] to allay the pressor and rate response to laryngoscopy. Initially, propranolol was used, but cardioselective $beta_2$ blockers, such as metoprolol, have been recommended and used.[49] Some amelioration of the undesirable response was noted. The technique consists of either long-term propranolol therapy or administration intravenously of 0.1 to 0.2 mg/kg 3 minutes prior to laryngoscopy. Chronic propranolol therapy is nonspecific and although heart rate may be minimized and the myocardial contractility reduced, there is an additional attenuation of the effects of the anesthetic procedure with administration of small doses prior to laryngoscopy and intubation. Most experience, however, demonstrates that the hemodynamic responses are relatively unaltered by this technique and that the use of beta blockers does not ensure protection against increases in MAP or heart rate.[91]

Esmolol. This newer beta-adrenoreceptor antagonist has been found effective in attentuating hemodynamic responses to laryngoscopy and intubation. This is a cardioselective type of beta-receptor block that antagonizes the effects of a generalized increase in sympathetic activity.[92] It is a water-soluble isopropylaminopropoxyphenyl derivative. Because of its ester linkage, it is rapidly hydrolyzed in blood by esterases. In vitro inhibition of plasma cholinesterase occurs, but this esterase's activity is not altered in vivo.[93]

Esmolol has a rapid onset of action within 3 minutes and a short duration of action, with the peak plasma concentration reduced by one-half at 10 minutes; by 25 minutes the plasma esmolol is hardly detectable. The elimination half-life is 9 minutes.[94]

Administration and dosage have been studied in patients by Menkhaus.[95] A loading dose of 500 µg/kg/min is administered over a period of 1 minute. A maintenance dose of 100 µg/kg/min by continuous infusion follows for an additional 5 minutes. The esmolol is first given at time of induction and continued by infusion, so that laryngoscopy is accomplished approximately 3 minutes after the start of the infusion. Larger doses do not improve the hemodynamic condition at the time of laryngoscopy and intubation; however, there is an increase in plasma norepinephrine at the time of laryngoscopy, intubation, and onset of surgery. Attenuation of deleterious hemodynamic response to endotracheal intubation and surgical stimulation occurs. It has been effective during light balanced anesthesia with intravenous drugs, including (1) diazepam–50% N_2O–O_2–pancuronium;[95] (2) ketamine;[96] (3) fentanyl–pancuronium;[97a,97b] (4) thiopental–enflurane (light).[98]

Although serum concentrations of catecholamine, specifically norepinephrine, were elevated, no significant changes in cardiac rate occurred. In the fentanyl–pancuronium technique, a statistically significant but transient increase in pulmonary capillary wedge pressure occurred after intubation.[97a]

In patients not on beta-blocker therapy, there may be a slight decrease in cardiac rate during esmolol infusion.[99]

MISCELLANEOUS TECHNIQUES.

Topical Nitroglycerin. Application of a 2% nitroglycerin ointment to the forehead of patients about 12 minutes prior to intubation has been reported to attenuate the pressor response to intubation.[53] The ointment is rubbed over an area of 10 × 5 cm; each 2.5-cm length contains 15 mg glyceryl trinitrate. A rise in systolic pressure of about 25 mm Hg occurred in the control group and existed for 4 minutes, but a rise of only 7.5 mm Hg occurred in the treatment group. Some side effects reported by other investigators included nasal congestion, headache, dizziness, and some hypotension. With Kamra's technique,[53] not one of these effects were detected.

Intranasally administered nitroglycerin produces some attenuation of the pressor response and a slight increase in heart rate.[54] A study of the data, however, shows that the systolic pressure is significantly increased from about 100 mm Hg at the time of established anesthesia to about 130 mm Hg after intubation. Further, composite plots of MAP and RPP show significant elevations from the values when anesthesia is established to the values after intubation of 75 mm Hg to about 100 mm Hg and RPP of about 1000 to 1800 kPa. A combination of intravenous lidocaine and nasal nitroglycerin provided better effect. The technique affords some attenuation of cardiovascular response but is not significantly better than many other strategies.[54]

Clonidine. Clonidine is a centrally acting antihypertensive agent that has become an important therapeutic agent in the management of hypertension. Several of its pharmacologic attributes suggest a broad usefulness in anesthesia practice, because of the following effects:[100]

- Reduction of central sympathetic outflow, thereby modulating presynaptic transmitter release[101]
- Suppression of central noradrenergic hyperactivity due to stress[102]
- Decrease in minimum alveolar concentration (MAC) values for anesthetic agents such as halothane, enflurane, isoflurane (40% reduction)[103,104]
- Decrease in UD_{50} values for intravenous thiopental and narcotics[105]
- Reduction in dose of narcotic needed to attenuate reflex cadiovascular responses to intubation
- No adverse effect on bronchomotor tone[106]
- Analgesic action when administered epidurally[107]

Clinical Use in Anesthesia. Clonidine has been found to be an excellent agent to provide hemodynamic stability,[104] especially in patients with hypertension, and to reduce reflex cardiovascular responses on intubation and during surgical manipulations.

Clonidine is administered as an oral drug in doses of 4 µg/kg as part of preanesthetic medication 1.5 hours before induction. During various elective surgical procedures, the heart rate stabilizes in a range of 70 to 80 beats per minute, and blood pressure responses to intubation, surgical manipulation, and during recovery shows minimal elevations compared with controls.[105] A further advantage is the reduction of isoflurane requirements by 40%, as determined by end-expiratory concentration.

In the study by Flacke,[108] using narcotic-type anesthesia for management of coronary artery bypass graft surgery, the dose requirement of sufentanil was reduced by 40%. The need for control of intraoperative and postoperative blood pressure was halved. Plasma catecholamine levels were consistently reduced.

In Orko's study[109] of normotensive patients, clonidine was associated with an increase of systolic arterial pressure of 42 mm Hg and a heart rate increase of about 18 beats per minute. More important was the reported high incidence of hypotension and significant bradycardia, which persisted during anesthesia and into the recovery period. Orko concluded that clonidine has some advantage in a hyperdynamic response to intubation and definite disadvantages in bradycardia and persistent hypotension postoperatively.

Conclusion. Clonidine provides several clinical advantages and is evidently quite effective in hypertensive patients submitted either to general-type or bypass surgery. Longnecker[100] has described the lability of blood pressure with both anesthetic and surgical manipulations that produces anesthesia records with peaks and valleys as "alpine anesthesia." Clonidine appears to flatten the peaks.

In normotensive patients, the occurrence of bradycardia and episodes of hypotension requires that the drug be used with caution and perhaps in smaller doses.

Recommendations. As mentioned earlier, a summary of techniques used to prevent hypertensive episodes and arrhythmias is presented in Table 21–4. Of the miscellaneous techniques proposed, the following three are most effective:

1. Complete regional nerve block and topical anesthesia with a potent agent (tetracaine; cocaine), combined with sedation employing diazepam or midazolam
2. General anesthesia with potent inhalation agents—enflurane and isoflurane are effective when supplemented
3. The use of intravenous lidocaine as a supplement and pretreatment with fentanyl clonidine, or nifedipine.

A review of the literature reveals little evidence that intravenous lidocaine does little more than produce a modest attenuation of the hemodynamic responses to laryngoscopy and intubation.[110]

TABLE 21–6. CAUSATIVE FACTORS

1. Anatomical conditions and tube configuration
   a. shape
   b. bore
2. Motor activity of vocal cords (hammer-anvil-Jackson)
3. Inflated cuff
4. Movement between tube and cords[113,114]
5. Nature of tube surface
6. Biological properties of material
7. Products of sterilization
8. Clinical—poor physical status
9. Length of intubation
10. Damage = Time X (mechanical + physical + chemical)

TRAUMATIC ANATOMIC–ANESTHETIC COMPLICATIONS

PREDISPOSING CONSTITUTIONAL FACTORS[111,112]
(Table 21–6)

Age. The infant is the most vulnerable patient to injuries. Re-emphasis on the size of the laryngeal structure and of the tube is essential. The cricoid is the narrowest part of the laryngeal passageway. A 1-mm edema of the mucosa will diminish the lumenal diameter (more than 50%) and area so that air flow will be restricted, turbulent, and require greater increased respiratory effort. Small tubes that can be accommodated through the cricoid ring are the objective. Tubes that pass through the vestibule and vocal cords may not pass through the ring.

The elderly patient is also at greater risk. There is frequent dehydration, anemia, avitaminosis, fragile bony structures, osteoporosis, and atrophic mucosa. The tolerance of tissues to trauma is limited.

Sex. The incidence of complications is higher in women because the size of the airway passages is smaller and the mucous membranes are thinner than in men. In adult women, a tube 0.5- to 1-mm smaller than for a man of similar build should be used.

Physical Habitus (Body Build). The robust pycnic patient with a short, thick, muscular neck is more difficult to laryngoscope and to intubate, when compared with the asthenic or lean patient.

Any factor that increases the difficulty of laryngoscopy and of intubation increases the risk of mechanical trauma and complications.

Structural Abnormalities. A wide variety of congenital or acquired anatomic abnormalities of the head, face, mouth, larynx, neck, and skeletal muscles increase the difficulty of laryngoscopy. These have been enumerated in Chapter 20.

Such conditions as upper airway infections, abscesses, tumors, or deformities or previous injuries to the face or jaw will limit opening of the mouth or displace or compress the air passage. Even an indwelling gastric tube running through the pharynx may distort the normal conditions. A gastric tube in situ for several days may cause erosion of the soft tissues, as well as the cricoid cartilage.

Physical Condition of Patient. Chronic debility and acute illness, dehydration, enemia, and malnutrition at any age all render a patient more vulnerable to trauma and less able to heal damaged structures.

CLINICAL FACTORS.[111]

Infections. Infection of the oropharyngeal passageway, or the "dirty mouth" syndrome, leads to more chronic and progressive infections, ulceration, and tissue destruction.

Duration of Intubation. The incidence of more serious laryngotracheal injury and complications is increased with longer periods of intubation.

Size of the Endotracheal Tube. Tubes with an outer diameter larger than the laryngeal lumen or that must be forced through the glotti chink will cause inordinate immediate and progressive damage.

Shape of the Endotracheal Tube. The shape of the tube is significant. Because the usual Magill tube or other commonly used endotracheal tube is curved in one direction, it follows that when inserted into a relatively straight passage, namely the trachea and pharyngeal axis, there will be three points of pressure. This is particularly so after nasotracheal intubation. These pressure points are the posterior pharyngeal wall, the posterior commissure of the larynx, and the inner surface of the anterior tracheal wall.

Traumatic Technique. Rough or clumsy handling of the laryngoscope is an obvious cause of damage to anatomic structures. Repeated attempts at insertion of either the laryngoscope into the mouth or the tube toward the larynx increase the damage and the incidence of complications. The presence of blood on the tip or the laryngoscope blade attests to trauma.

Cuff Pressure. Inflation of a cuff should achieve an even ballooning without bulges in the cuff. This is accomplished by a steady, timed injection of a volume of air to fill the cuff, determined and tested in advance. (Sudden inflation pressures lead to bulges.) The pressure should be sufficient to provide an airtight system but not to exceed mucosal circulation.

Vocal Cord Motion.[113] Inadequate depth of anesthesia and insufficient sensory block of the vocal cord muscle result in continuous sensory stimulation of the supralaryngeal nerves and a reaction of cord adduction against the tube. Respiratory and phonatory activity with the tube in situ may occur. This also is related to inadequate depth of anesthesia. Glottic movement also occurs during swallowing or coughing and also during muscular paralepis.[189]

Movement of the Endotracheal Tube. Positioning of the patient's head will move the tube downward or upward against the vocal cord mucosa. Motion of a tube may occur as a result of ventilator cycling motion, thereby causing tube movement up and down, and compliance changes.[114]

SPECIFIC TRAUMATIC ANATOMIC COMPLICATIONS

Many traumatic complications are evident at the time of laryngoscopy and intubation. They are more manifest and accompanied by patient complaints in the postanesthetic period, however. Some are delayed in their severity and may become chronic.

LACERATION AND ULCERATION[115] Laceration and ulceration of lips, mouth, and pharynx are relatively frequent occurrences as a result of inept technique and rough handling of the laryngoscope. Abrasions are frequent and may lead to an infection and ulceration. This most often results from inexperience or lack of practice.

INJURY TO TEETH AND GUMS.[115a,115b,116] Chips of the incisor teeth are the more frequent injury. A good, relaxed tone of the masticatory and facial muscles and careful introduction of the laryngoscope into the mouth are essential. Masseter muscle relaxation following succinylcholine should be carefully estimated. Various types of rubber or plastic tooth guards or stints are available; taping of the teeth has been used. These may only provide a false sense of security. Bite blocks should be placed at the side of the mouth between the premolars and molars. Pharyngeal airways must not be used as bite blocks!

Loose or capped teeth are prone to dislodgement or injury. These should be reported and recorded on the preanesthetic visit. The patient should be made aware of the risk. A broken tooth part should be recovered and saved as a specimen. If a loose tooth is present, the patient should be informed that it may be necessary to extract it at the time of anesthesia.

DISLOCATION OF THE MANDIBLE.[117] Normally, on wide opening of the mouth, the condyle of the mandible projects forward and downward. In the presence of lax temporomandibular ligaments, the coronoid process may "pop out" of the glenoid fossa of the temporal bone. The dislocation is a frequent occurrence in an exaggerated yawn.

When the condyle pops out during laryngoscopy, it is necessary to reduce the dislocation.

Reduction of a dislocation of the mandible can be accomplished by the following maneuvers: (1) downward pressure of the posterior teeth of the mandible through the open mouth; (2) lifting the chin; and (3) displacing the entire mandible posteriorly. These are done in sequence.

ATLANTOAXIAL SUBLUXATION[118] (see "Complications in the Pediatric Patient").

SORE THROAT: PHARYNGITIS AND LARYNGITIS.[119] Sore throat is a most common complication and a complaint in most patients who are laryngoscoped. The actual soreness may emanate from the pharynx, supraglottic, laryngeal, or tracheal sites. It may be severe in almost 10% of patients and is accompanied by difficulty in swallowing. Sore throat is related to the extent of the contact of the pharynx with the laryngoscope and the number of attempts at insertion of the endotracheal tube, as well as other factors (Table 21–7) (Usually, the condition subsides in 2 to 4 days. Treatment is symptomatic with throat lozenges and humidification of air.)

The overall incidence of injury to the larynx with pharyngitis, laryngitis and sore throat is about 6% following short-term intubation. A common early complication is hematoma of the vocal cords, which represents 4.5% of the injuries. Laceration of the vocal cords also occurs in approximately 1 in 1000 instances of intubation.

The occurrence of sore throat has been found also to be associated with the size of the endotracheal tube (oversized)[120a] and with the length of cuff in contact with the trachea. As tracheal cuff length increases, the incidence and severity of pharyngitis, laryngitis, and tracheitis increases. Lubrication of the tubes and cuffs is also a factor.[120b] Lidocaine jelly is especially associated with a high incidence of sore throat (24% or more) (Table 21–8) in contrast to the Surgilube incidence of 16%.[121]

Sore throat, hoarseness, and myalgia occur after bolus injections of succinylcholine (1 mg/kg). In the study by Capan, only mask inhalation anesthesia with N_2O–O_2 following thiopental and fentanyl induction was employed without laryngoscopy or intubation. In the 6 to 12-hour postoperative period, 10% of patients had sore throat and 18% developed myalgia. If d-tubocurarine was employed and followed by a dose of succinylcholine, 1.5 mg/kg, the incidence of sore throat was reduced to 5% and myalgia to 10%. Hoarseness developed in 15% of most groups and was apparently related to dry anesthetic gases. Humidification reduced hoarseness.

EPIGLOTTITIS.[123] Occasionally, an acute epiglottitis may occur postanesthetically in children and adults. The common bacterium encountered is *Hemophilus influenzae* type B, which may be cultured from the epiglottis or blood. The presenting symptom is rapidly developing respiratory distress from obstruction that is in part relieved by sitting. When patients are suspected of having epiglottitis, they should be admitted to an intensive care respiratory care unit and equipment (especially a rigid bronchoscope) readied for emergency intubation or tracheostomy.[124] An otolaryngologist should be consulted to inspect the upper airway. If distress is progressing, patients can be taken to the operating room and anesthetized in the sitting position with an inhalation technique using halothane. Nasal intubation can be accomplished without muscle relaxants. The tube should be smaller than the usual size for a given patient. Heated and humidified oxygen–air mixtures should be administered, and antibiotic treatment with ampicillin, 200 mg/kg/d, or chloramphenicol, 100 mg/kg/d, should be initiated. Surveillance should be continued until the inflammatory epiglottic process subsides as determined by inspection and lack of complaint.

OTHER EPIGLOTTIC COMPLICATIONS. The groove between the base of the tongue and the epiglottis may be extensively traumatized by forceful application of Macintosh laryngoscope blades. The underlying hyoepiglottic ligament may be damaged, and eventual scar formation at this site can immobilize and flatten the epiglottis. In the use of the straight laryngoscope blades, injury to the posterior mucosa of the epiglottis is not unusual.

LARYNGITIS. This complication may occur as a localized phenomenon of the cords or may be extensive and include the entire vestibule of the larynx and the false cords. It may be manifested as reddening, congestion, edema, and submucosal hemorrhage. The patient complains of hoarseness and tightness in the throat. A cardinal sign is inspiratory stridor of mild degree. It is generally self limiting and recovery is spontaneous in 3 to 5 days. The reported incidence is about 45%, but only 5% is severe.[119]

Causes include (1) a mechanical trauma to vocal cords, as by rough maneuvering of the endotracheal tube, too large a tube, or failure to advance the tube

TABLE 21–7. FACTORS IN DEVELOPMENT OF UPPER AIRWAY IRRITABILITY AND "SORE THROAT"

Traumatic laryngoscopy
Long endotracheal tube cuffs
Inappropriate tube curvature
Stiff construction of tubes
Large-volume cuffs
Lubrication with lidocaine jelly
Succinylcholine
Light level of anesthesia (stage II)

TABLE 21-8. MEAN INCIDENCE AND SEVERITY (0–3 ± SD) POSTOPERATIVE SORE THROAT

Group	Tube	Lubricant	Incidence (%)	Severity (0–3)
I	Uncuffed	4% lidocaine jelly	90*	2.10 ± 0.8*
II	Uncuffed	4% lidocaine solution	40	0.45 ± 0.6
III	Uncuffed	Saline solution	40	0.40 ± 0.4
IV	Large volume cuff	None	46	0.49 ± 0.6
V	Low volume cuff	None	25‡	0.31 ± 0.4
VI	None (mask)	None	15†	0.20 ± 0.3

*P < 0.001 as compared with all other groups utilizing the Chi square test.
†P < 0.01 as compared with all other groups utilizing the Chi square test.
‡P < 0.05 as compared with all other groups utilizing the Chi square test.
From Loeser, E.A., et al.: Postoperative sore throat: Influence of tracheal tube lubrication versus cuff design. Can. Anaesth. Soc. J., 27:156–158, 1980.

with the bevel parallel to the cords[113]; (2) movement of the cords during anesthesia against the tube due to inadequate anesthesia—the junction between the membranous and cartilaginous parts of the vocal cords at the site of the vocal process of the arytenoids is particularly susceptible to abrasion and ulceration[114]; (3) irritation by particulate matter or inadvertent chemical contaminants in the breathing atmosphere; (4) irritation by lubricants applied to tube; (5) chemical response to leachable agents in plasma material of tubes (stabilizes organization of polyvinylchloride); and (6) reaction to products formed during ethylene oxide sterilization.[125,126]

Treatment. Treatment consists of painting the traumatized area with an anesthetic-antiseptic solution. Troches of sulfa drugs and antibiotics are available, and ordinary lozenges afford great relief. The accompanying edema may be ameliorated by spraying with epinephrine 1:10,000 dilution. In severe edema, multiple punctures of the area occasionally will release the fluid. The patient must be watched carefully, and tracheostomy must be performed if conservative measures fail.

LARYNGEAL EDEMA.[127] (Fig. 21–11). This may occur at any time throughout the endotracheal and extubation anesthesia period. Initial roughing of the laryngeal mucosa and intubation trauma may cause congestion followed by edema. The edema may be located at any point of the laryngeal structure and should be identified as principally supraglottic, at the vocal cords, or subglottic.[128] Causes are the same as those producing laryngitis. Edema may occur as a predominant finding, with little or no inflammation. When congestion and edema exist, there may be a progression to advanced inflammation with exudation into the loose connective tissue structure of the submucosa of the larynx. This is an advanced form of laryngitis and is serious. The cardinal sign is loud, high-pitched inspiratory stridor.

Supraglottic Edema.[129] This is usually located in the area between the epiglottis and the base of the tongue and the aryepiglottic folds. Swelling can be rapid, and the tissues can bulge into the laryngeal inlet or vestibule, causing serious respiratory obstruction.

Edema of the vestibular folds or false cords may occur rapidly during laryngoscopy and obscure vision of the true cords.

Glottic Edema. Glottic edema occurs in the loose areolar-type tissue underlying the mucous membrane covering the vocal cords; the area readily swells and is referred to as *Reinke's space*. Edema of the loose tissue between the cords and the vestibular folds, i.e., in the vestibule of Morgagni, will limit the air passage and obscure the vision of the vocal cords.

Subglottic Edema. This is generally more serious; it is not readily recognized on examination, as is supraglottic and glottic edema. Extravasation of fluid is relatively easy because of the loose submucosal connective tissue. Because this area is enclosed within the cricoid cartilaginous ring, the degree of obstruction of the air passage can be great. In infants and children, it is an especially dangerous complication.

Prevention. Sterilized endotracheal tubes, clean laryngoscope blades, and aseptic technique in handling tubes and instruments are essential. Application of lubricants to tubes should be aseptic. The anesthesiologist should scrub hands before proceeding.

Treatment. Mild edema may not require extraordinary therapy and will be self limiting. Resolution is slow, however, because there is sparse lymphatic drainage of the region. Pulse oximetry is desired in infants and children to detect obstructive phenomena. Humidification of breathing mixture by means of nebulized mist is beneficial. A spray of racemic epinephrine solution is useful in reducing the edema, and steroid therapy is usually indicated.

If significant edema occurs in the infant or child,

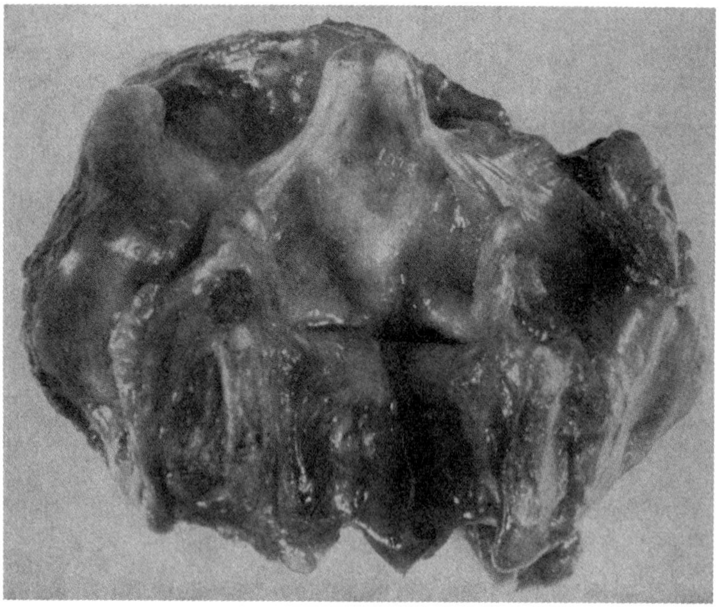

FIG. 21-11. Edema of the larynx, especially of the subglottic region on the left, as a complication of intubation. The larynx is split and is seen from the posterior.

reintubation should be performed and antibiotics should be administered. Dexamethasone is a valuable adjunct.

SUPRAGLOTTIC OBSTRUCTIVE EDEMA.[129a,129b] Upper airway obstruction can occur from improper or traumatic manipulation of the upper airway. Both pharyngeal and supraglottic edema or hematoma have been reported. One mechanism results from a forceful flexed neck position, in which a compression force vector on the soft tissues of the neck transects the airway through the epiglottis and arytenoids (Fig. 21–12). This has resulted in marked epiglottic and aryepiglottic edema. The mechanism is possibly due to venous obstruction, ischemia, and transudation of fluid.

ULCERS OF THE LARYNX.[111,113] Ulceration of the vocal cords occurs and is caused by contact of the endotracheal tube denuding the surface of the cords (Table 21–9). The occurrence is not necessarily related to overt trauma or difficult intubation. A raw, reddened surface of the cords is not unusual, but a persistence and failure in healing are infrequent. The ulcerations are seen at the posterior region of the glottis, at the junction of the cartilaginous and membranous portions of the vocal cords, which is a particularly vulnerable site. The vocal process of the arytenoid cartilage at this junction is vulnerable because it is subject to active adduction during light anesthesia, to contact with each other on coughing or phonation, or to constant action against the indwelling endotracheal tube.[113] The vocal cord process is also the site for voice abuse. The posterior location of the lesion is also due to the forces acting by the tube at this point. The curved endotracheal tube is forced posteriorly by the triangular shape of the glottis and the curvature of the cervical spine, which forces the cricoid forward and the tube backward. The tube is thus deformed into an S shape from the posterior pharynx and impinges on the posterior laryngeal commissure, which acts as a fulcrum.

Prevention. After laryngoscopy and intubation, it is important that the patient's head be left on a pillow in the sniffing position so that the cervical spine is straight. This position will modify the pressure on the posterior laryngeal wall.

ASSESSMENT OF DAMAGE

Because the laryngotracheal damage occurring after use of endotracheal tubes needs to be properly evaluated, a scoring system has been proposed (Table 21–10).[136] The larynx is divided into two halves, right and left, and into six anatomic regions. Each region is scored on a three-point system for: (1) the area of edema or submucosal hemorrhage (or both); (2) the area of inflammation; (3) the area of ulceration; and (4) the depth of ulceration (Table 21–11).

Regions 1 to 4 (see Table 21–10) are given a score of 3 each with involvement of more than half of the total area, a score of 2 with involvement of one fourth to one half, and a score of 1 with less than one fourth. *Region 5* is given a score of 3 with involvement of more than 2 cm^2, a score of 2 with 1 to 2 cm, and a score of 1 with less than 1 cm^2. In *region 6*, a score of 3 is given when four or more tracheal rings are involved; a score of 2 when 2 to 4 rings are involved; and a score of 1 when less than 2 rings are involved. The *depth* of ulceration is scored 3 when cartilage is ex-

TABLE 21-9. TYPES OF LESIONS

1. Ulceration of larynx
   Posterior parts
   Less often large doses of curare
2. Medial side of arytenoid
   Ulceration
   "Hammer and anvil" type
   Perichondritis (2/3 at autopsy)
   To cartilage (1/3)
3. Subglottic reaction
   Children under 10 years
   Cricoid ring
   Loose subglottic tissue
   Posterior location
   Oversized tube
   Chondritis
4. Ulceration of trachea
   Anterior wall
   Type of tube
   Ulceration
5. Middle part of trachea
   Cuff damage
   Tip of tube-Anterolateral
   Rupture

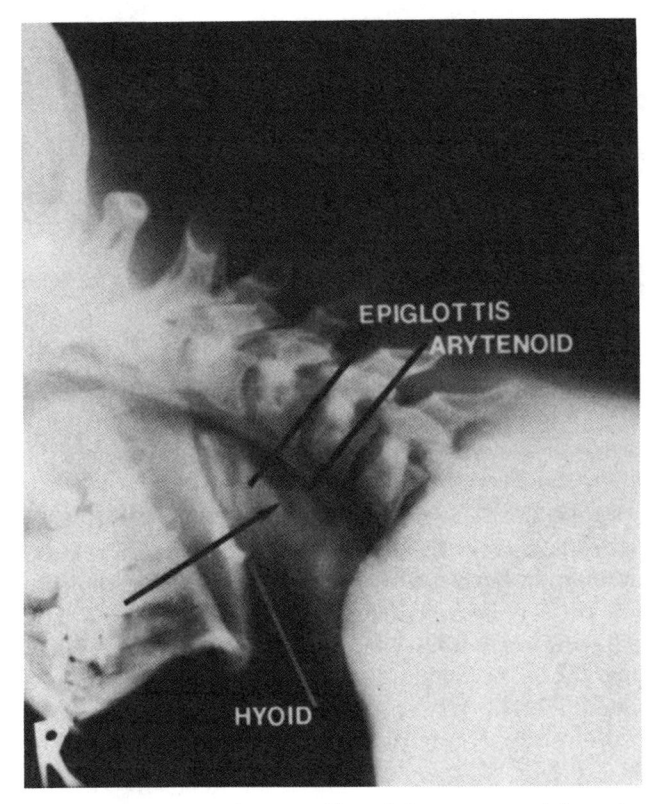

FIG. 21-12. Convalescent film of the airway with neck acutely flexed. The arrow indicates the compression force vector that transects the airway through the epiglottis and arytenoids. From Bennett, R.L., Lee, T.S., and Wright, B.D.: Airway-obstructing supraglottic edema following anesthesia with the head positioned in forced-flexion. Anesthesiology, 54:78, 1981.

posed, 2 when ulceration is intermediate, and 1 when ulceration is superficial. A maximum total score for any region is thus 12, and for the entire laryngotracheal area is 144.

GRANULOMAS OF THE LARYNX.[130-132] Ulcer granulomas of the vocal cords generally are rare.[130] Following endotracheal intubation, they are more rare. In one large series of granulomas, only 18% had a history of anesthetic intubation.[130] In the other patients, causative factors could not be readily identified, but anesthesia had not been part of the history; only upper respiratory infections and voice abuse were frequent pre-existing factors.

Symptoms are those of partial airway block, presenting as hoarseness, stridor, cough, and sore throat. These are the symptoms of laryngitis and ulceration, which are preceding conditions.

The incidence of granulomas has been reported to be between 1 in 1000[133] and 1 in 10,000.[134] Women are predominantly vulnerable, with a frequency 10 times that of men.

Granulomas develop on one or both vocal processes, as a result of contact ulceration that fails to heal.[135] (Fig. 21-13) The granulation tissue persists (Table 21-12) and may form polypoid masses.[137] Because both ulceration and granuloma formation can occur after a short period of intubation or after a prolonged intubation, it appears that duration of intubation is not a determinant.

Prevention. Prevention includes sterile endotracheal tubes, aseptic and gentle technique of intubation, appropriately sized lubricated tubes, adequate general anesthesia, topical anesthetic tube ointment, and minimal movement of the tube (avoiding movement of the head; maintaining the sniff position by a shallow pillow under the head).

PERICHONDRITIS OF LARYNGEAL CARTILAGES.[138] Perichondritis of the laryngeal cartilages may also occur after even mild degrees of vocal cord trauma and ulceration. It is more common when the larynx has been markedly traumatized to the extent that the cartilages are exposed or the endotracheal tube

TABLE 21-10. SCORING FOR LARYNGOTRACHEAL DAMAGE

Regions Scored	Types of Damage in Each Region Scored with 1, 2 or 3 Each
1. Epiglottis	(1) Submucosal hemorrhage or edema or both, area involved
2. Arytenoid	(2) Inflammation, area involved
3. Vocal cords, superior	(3) Ulceration, area involved
4. Vocal cords, inferior	(4) Ulceration, depth
5. Subglottic area	
6. Trachea	

From Hedden, M., et al: Laryngotracheal damage after prolonged use of orotracheal tubes in adults. J.A.M.A., 207:703, 1969.

TABLE 21-11. CLASSIFICATION OF DAMAGE
Basis of Circumference and Depth

I	Hyperemia-edema (no ulcer)
II	Superficial ulceration of mucosa less than ⅓ circumference
III	Superficial > ⅓ of circumference
	Deep ulceration < ⅓ of circumference
IV	Deep ulceration > ⅓ of circumference
	Deep ulceration with exposed cartilage

TABLE 21-12. HEALING LESIONS

1. Primary Epithelialization (⅔)
2. Granuloma Formation (⅓) (Secondary)
   - None in infants
   - Mostly right side
   - Localization on cords
   - Surgical—often pedunculated
   - Regress spontaneously (95%)
   - Conservative therapy
   - Time of healing 60 days (1–10 mo.)
3. Fibrous Scar
   - Stenosis X-Sect 30%
   - Frequency 0.5%
   - Infants 6.7% (4.4% subglottic)
   - Glottic webs
4. Vocal Disturbances

From Way, W. L., Sooy, F. A.: Histologic changes produced by endotracheal intubation Ann. Otolaryngol, 74:799, 1965.

has been in situ for more than 4 days. The ulceration and inflammatory process penetrate into the deeper tissue, including the underlying cartilages. Bacterial infection may occur.

TRACHEITIS.[139,140] Tracheitis is an infrequent, serious complication of endotracheal intubation. It occurs more often with stiff tubes. The injury usually is to the anterior luminal surface of the trachea. Impingement of the tip of the tube on this surface results in abrasion of the mucosa and a nonspecific inflammatory response. A major cause is poor positioning of the head in the extended position (no occipital pillow), so that the tube is angulated anteriorly into the trachea. This malposition also causes the tube to press against the posterior commissure, which acts as a fulcrum.

The patient has a constricting sensation in the neck and is plagued by coughing. Codeine is most helpful. Soothing measures such as steam inhalations and expectorants are indicated.

Prevention. Proper head positioning of a patient is fundamental. A contributing preventive measure is to use nonkinkable tubes when patients are placed in positions other than the supine. Indications for such a tube include the prone, lateral, and various neurosurgical positions where the head may be hyperextended or hyperflexed (see Fig. 21–5).

SUBGLOTTIC AND TRACHEAL STENOSIS.[138,141] Narrowing of the trachea in the subglottic region or lower is related to prior trauma by the endotracheal tube or to the inflated cuff. This is usually progressive, with ulceration followed by edema, exudation, and fibroblastic proliferation. Damage to the underlying cartilage may also develop. The stenosis is due to the fibroplastic reaction and scar formation during the final stage of the healing process.[142]

Most subglottic pathologic changes are associated with improperly placed tubes and inflated cuffs. A tube that is not advanced into the trachea so that the cuff is located in the trachea will permit the cuff, when inflated, to impinge on the subglottic area or even partially balloon into the glottic chink.

The same type of pathologic change can occur in the trachea. When the adult tracheal lumen is reduced to about 25% of its diameter, symptoms develop.

Duration of intubation is a significant contributing factor, and after 3 to 4 days the incidence ranges from 1 to 4%.

Treatment. When symptoms occur, treatment is initially by surgical dilitation. Laser surgery has become a corrective tool. Photoresection of the stenotic region under direct vision offers a less invasive technique.[143] When this is ineffective, a permanent tracheostomy is indicated, or resection and anastomosis may be considered. Extensive lesions may require stage repair or even tracheal resection.

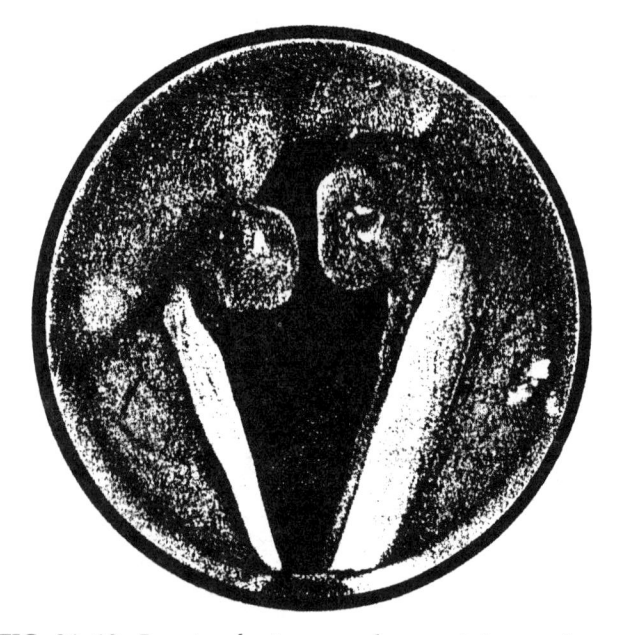

FIG. 21–13. Post-intubation granulomas of the vocal folds. Their position at the junction of the ligamentous (white) and cartilaginous portions of the folds is typical. (Becker, W., Buckingham, R.A., Holinger, P.H., et al.: Atlas of otorhinolaryngology and bronchoesophagoscopy. Stuttgart, Georg Thieme Verlag, 1969) Reproduction from Orkin, F.K., and Cooperman, L.H.: Complications in Anesthesiology. J.B. Lippincott Co., Philadelphia, 1983.

In the situation requiring prolonged intubation, incipient tracheal damage should be suspected. When there is positional leak in the system, there is a need for increased volume of air in the cuff to achieve a seal to prevent an episode of "silent" aspiration of gastric contents into the trachea. The increased pressure increases the subglottic damage.

RUPTURE OF THE TRACHEA.[140] *Tracheomalacia,* or softening and degeneration of the cartilage of the tracheal rings, may result from prolonged intubation, especially in debilitated patients. Subsequent rupture may occur but is a rare event.

More frequently, the posterior membranous portion of the trachea may be stretched. If extensive, it may make up over one half of the circumference of the trachea. Bulging or herniation may occur and even extend laterally to near the superior vena cava. In emphysema the membranous portion may already be thin and inelastic and the cross section changed from a circle to an oval.[144] Tears with leaks may occur during anesthesia, and edema of pneumothorax or mediastinal emphysema may exist.

PERFORATION OF THE HYPOPHARYNX (OR PYRIFORM SINUS). Perforations of the hypopharynx, pyriform sinus, and esophagus have been described.[145–148] Most of the cases appear to occur during anesthesia for planned surgery, especially if there is evidence of a difficult airway.[146] Some cases are related to efforts at resuscitation under suboptimal conditions. Perforation of the esophagus has also been described and can occur with traumatic nasogastric intubation.[149]

The consequences of such perforation vary from cervical emphysema to severe respiratory distress, mediastinitis, pneumothorax, and mediastinal empyema. The mortality rate due to mediastinitis is about 50%. Hence, it is important that early diagnosis and management be carried out (see section entitled "Surgical Emphysema").

The diagnosis of perforation should be suspected when a patient complains of dysphagia postoperatively and when there is neck pain following a difficult intubation. Three technical features are usually associated with this complication, namely, difficult laryngoscopy, attempts at blind nasal intubation, and the use of a stylet. There is usually increased salivation seemingly related to the discomfort of swallowing.

Subcutaneous emphysema in the neck region is an early sign, and it becomes very prominent when the patient coughs. Spontaneous closure of a perforation is unusual, and conservative therapy increases the risk of mortality. The diagnosis may be confirmed when a radiograph is taken following the swallowing of a contrast media. A chest radiograph will frequently show widening of the mediastinum. Following the swallowing of a contrast media, a tracheoesophageal fistula may be easily demonstrated. Delay in closure of the perforation will often lead to a mediastinal abscess and the development of sepsis, with an elevated temperature. Treatment consists of early operation and closure of the perforation, which, if delayed for more than 12 hours, has been associated with a mortality rate of 56%.

UNUSUAL AND CHRONIC COMPLICATIONS (Table 21–13)

LINGUAL NERVE INJURY.[150,151] Paresis of the lingual branch of the glossopharyngeal nerve has been reported. Numbness and weakness of the tongue with some difficulty in swallowing are the chief complaints. The condition may last for 1 to 2 weeks.

Injury to the hypoglossal nerve may also occur, resulting in transient paralysis of the hyoglossal muscle of the tongue.

The mechanism for these injuries is forceful compression by the laryngoscope blade against the base of the tongue, especially with improper application of the curved Macintosh blade.

RECURRENT LARYNGEAL NERVE PARALYSIS.[152,153] Recurrent laryngeal nerve paralysis may occur following endotracheal intubation. Characteristically, it occurs in the elderly and consequent to intubation and lasts 24 to 48 hours. After extubation, patients have severe hoarseness, and immediate examination reveals right vocal cord paralysis with the right cord in a paramedian position.[154] In the instances reported, the endotracheal tubes were an appropriate size and no difficulties were encountered on intubation. Evidence of abrasion or damaged vocal cord tissue was not observed. The paralysis may continue for 6 to 8 weeks and usually clears in 2 to 3 months.

The cause of this complication is evidently due to a pressure neuropraxia from overinflated endotracheal tube cuffs. Ellis[155] studied the anatomic relationship of inflated cuffs to the laryngeal structures and the motor innervation of the cords. At the level of the cricoid cartilage, the right recurrent nerve divides into anterior and posterior branches, and it is at this point that the anterior branch is vulnerable to pressure. He demonstrated that this branch can be compressed between the cuff of the endotracheal tube and the lamina of the thyroid cartilage. This is particularly so if the cuff is asymmetrically inflated,

TABLE 21–13. LATE DAMAGE—LARYNX
Adults 5% Infants 7% None after 2 years

1. Paresis (internus-transversus)
2. Subglottic Granuloma—Membranes
3. Atrophic scars on vocal process
4. Cysts
5. Stenosis
6. Vocal Disturbances

so that a portion impinges on the subglottic region or is inflated within the glottic chink.

ARYTENOID CARTILAGE DISLOCATION.[156] Hoarseness and pain on swallowing after endotracheal intubation may be related to a rare cause of arytenoid cartilage dislocation or subluxation of the cartilages.[157] This is caused by direct trauma of the endotracheal tube impacting on the posterior commissure and traumatizing the intercartilaginous portion of the vocal cords, invariably on the left side.[158]

FUSION (SYNECHIA) OF VOCAL CORDS. This rare complication has been reported by Kirchner[141] following endotracheal intubation. When trauma to both vocal cords with denudation and loss of mucous membrane occurs, the healing process may be accompanied by union of the cords at the raw surface edges. It is likely to follow extensive ulceration of the cords and is often related to endotracheal intubation followed by tracheostomy.

Glottic dilitation can relieve the airway obstruction, but surgical separation has been needed; in some instances, membranes or webs may also develop where laryngeal or tracheal ulceration has occurred.

SUBGLOTTIC MEMBRANE.[159] Thin subglottic membranes may develop in the postoperative period. Usually, these are seen about 24 to 48 hours after extubation in obese or short-necked patients and those with a narrow tracheal lumen. Use of a cuffed tube or a tube larger than necessary is a factor. The pseudo-membrane is usually due to slough of the tracheal mucosa from the endotracheal tube denuding the tracheal surface or to accumulation of inspissated secretions in the subglottic region.[160]

Signs of respiratory obstruction with crowing noises and dyspnea develop. On examination, the vocal cords are normal, but adherent webs and membranes in the subglottic region are noted crossing the tracheal lumen and partially occluding the lumen. In debilitated patients, the webs may become thickened and produce more serious obstruction. Removal can be accomplished through a bronchoscope.

DENUDATION OF TRACHEAL MUCOSA (CILIARY DAMAGE).[160,161] Tracheal tubes even for short-term use cause damage to the epithelium and cilia of the trachea. The surface of the trachea normally has the appearance of a waving field of wheat (by scanning electron microscopy), but after 2 hours with either uninflated or air-filled cuffs, the cilia are flattened and crushed. After 6 hours, there is necrosis and slough, and 2 days are required before regeneration is apparent.[162,163]

After long-term use (24 to 48 hours or more), the mucosa is not only damaged and denuded but squamous cell metaplasia occurs during the repair process (Fig. 21–14).

TRAUMA OF INFLATED CUFFS.[164] The complications associated with overinflation of the inflatable cuff are related to ischemia and pressure necrosis. The fact that the pressure exerted against the tracheal mucosa even by a properly inflated cuff equals and often exceeds capillary blood pressure explains the mechanism of mucosal damage. In addition, this is usually superimposed on other factors. Thus, rupture of the trachea is correlated with the presence of debility, generalized arteriosclerosis, or pre-existing tracheitis.[165] The causes of trauma includes contusion, hemorrhage of the tracheal wall, mucosal sloughs, and rupture.

RESPIRATORY TRACT INFECTION.[166,167] Contamination of the tracheobronchial tree can occur in the process of introducing the endotracheal tube (or fiberoptic tube) by carrying oropharyngeal bacteria along with the tube as it advances into the trachea.[168] The following tracheal protective mechanisms are impaired by the process of intubation:

1. Anesthetic agents—reduce ciliary action
2. Mechanical denudation of mucosa of the trachea by the endotracheal tube
3. Reduced immune and inflammatory responses. As a consequence, nonresident bacteria are more capable of gaining "hold." Predisposing to this are prolonged anesthesia and debilitated patients

Prevention can be accomplished in part by preanesthetic oropharyngeal hygiene carried out on awakening or 1 to 2 hours preanesthesia. Dental care and gargling with a bland solution are all that are required. Tracheal aspirates in patients after such a regimen show a marked reduction in the number of bacterial colonies compared with patients not practicing oropharyngeal hygiene.

Respiratory Morbidity.[165] The relationship of endotracheal anesthesia to respiratory morbidity and pneumonia has been studied. No valid difference can be demonstrated in the incidence of respiratory complications between intubated and nonintubated patients, when a paired analysis as to similar age, physical status, and procedure is performed.

Generally, the nature of the operative procedure and the preoperative condition of the patient are more important than the anesthetic methods. Patients with any pre-existing respiratory disease show a higher incidence of both major and minor complications after intubation, and this incidence is greater after nasal intubation than oral intubation. In the normal subject, little difference in the morbidity between the two routes of intubation has been determined. Technical difficulties in intubation and trauma in intubation increase the complication rate.

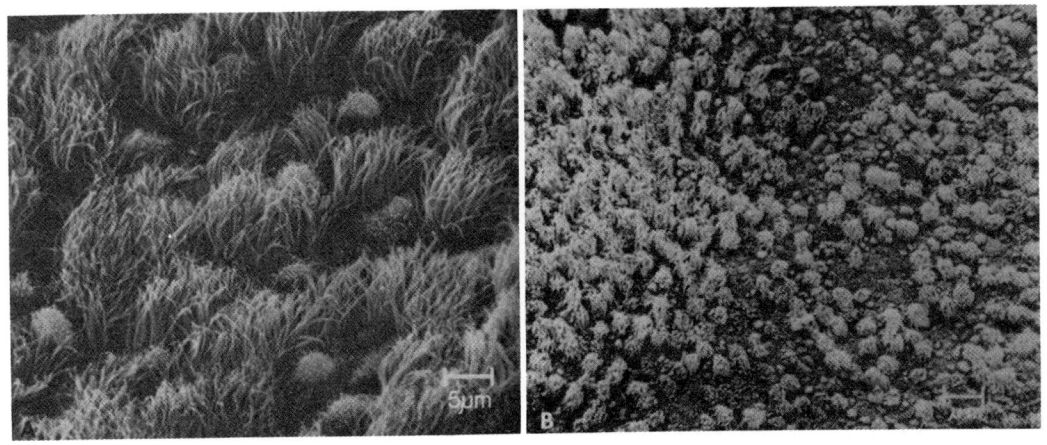

FIG. 21-14. A, normal human trachea. B, trachea from patient 8 days after endotracheal intubation; note almost complete loss of cilia and tendency toward squamous metaplasia (original magnification × 2500). From Klaine, A.S., et al: Surface alterations due to endotracheal intubation. Am. J. Med., 58:674, 1975.

Oropharyngeal bacteria not ordinarily present in the trachea can be introduced into the trachea. In addition, there is usually an overall increase in the number of bacteria in the larynx and trachea. To some extent, this can be limited by the use of a lubricant containing a sulfonamide to decrease the extent of contamination.[168] More desirable are good oral hygiene and dental care. Use of a mouthwash several times on the preoperative day and on the morning of surgery is effective in reducing tracheal contamination. This is especially important in patients with carious teeth and vitamin deficiency; when endotracheal anesthesia is planned, the anesthetist can include an order for oral hygiene care and use of mouthwash on the evening before and the morning of surgery. The recovery of tracheal bacteria after intubation is sharply reduced by prior gargling compared to recovery rate in controls.[168b]

PROLONGED INTUBATION AND PULMONARY INFECTION. When endotracheal tubes are allowed to remain in situ in critical care patients for more than 2.5 days and continued for several days (average 9 days), the inner surface becomes coated with a confluent amorphous mass.[169] This provides a nidus for bacterial growth. The normal throat flora can be cultured early. Subsequently, a variety of Gram-positive and Gram-negative bacteria (Proteus type) can be cultured. The biofilm that develops on the surface of the plastic tubes is a polysaccharide with embedded organisms, such as *Staphylococcus epidermides*, *S. aureus*, and *Pseudomonas*. These are producers of a polysaccharide substance termed *glycocalyx*, which effects adhesion to synthetic plastic surfaces. In this matrix, polymicrobial flora colonize.

When catheter suction of the tracheobronchial trees is employed, portions of the biofilm can be dislodged in the trachea and seed the pulmonary tree, producing a nosocomial infection.

INTRAOPERATIVE BACTEREMIA. Tracheal intubation has been associated with bacteremia (Table 21-14). Positive blood cultures have been reported after both orotracheal[170,171] and nasotracheal placement of tubes.[170,172] Orotracheal intubation is associated with an incidence of less than 3% if atraumatic, but the incidence is more than doubled if laryngoscopy and insertion of the tube are rough or traumatic.

Nasotracheal intubation is associated with a much higher incidence, about 17%, of bacteremia,[172] and it is recommended that prophylactic antibiotics be used. It appears that the cuffed endotracheal tube passed through the nose is also more likely to produce bacteremia. Transient bacteremia may occur, even when topical vasoconstrictors are used to shrink the mucosa and even in the absence of trauma.[173]

Instrumentation of the upper airway by a number of procedures can cause bacteremia:[174,175] catheter or Yankhauer oropharyngeal suctioning, if vigorous; tracheobronchial suctioning through the endotracheal tube; oropharyngeal manipulation for laryngoscopy or bronchoscopy; during esophageal gastroscopy[176]; and difficult passage of nasogastric or orogastric tubes.[149]

In susceptible patients—those with nasal infections, "runny noses," chronic sinusitis, and debilitated conditions—prophylactic antibiotic therapy is warranted in the circumstances when nasotracheal intubation is to be performed.

Portal of Entry. The normal flora of the oropharyngeal cavity or nose can enter the circulation through abrasions or lacerations of the pharyngeal or nasal mucosa. Entry can also occur through in-

TABLE 21-14. BACTEREMIA* FOLLOWING VARIOUS INSTRUMENTATION AND MANIPULATIONS OF UPPER AIRWAY

	Incidence of (%) Bacteremia
Orotracheal intubation[170,171]	<3
If traumatic	7
Nasotracheal intubation[170,172]	17
Tracheal cuffed tubes[172]	22
Suctioning through endotracheal tube in newborn frequent	50
Nasotracheal intubation for dental surgery	
In presence of periodontitis[174]	33
For elective dental restorative procedures in pediatric patient[175]	12
For dental and maxillofacial surgery[173]	5.5
Gastrointestinal endoscopy[174]	8
Bronchoscopy, rigid (febrile patients)[177]	33
Bronchoscopy, fiberoptic (afebrile patients)[178]	0

* Positive blood culture.

jured tracheal mucosa when abraded, scratched, or injured by stylets or following over-inflation of cuffs with ensuing mucosa sloughs.

Transfer of nasopharyngeal commensals into the trachea by passage of the endotracheal tube is also an implicated portal. Injured gums, diseased gums and/or dislodged teeth are important sites of bacterial entrance.

Microorganisms Cultured. The organisms usually cultured belong to the *Streptococcus viridans* group. *Hemophilus influenzae* is also a frequently cultured bacterium. It is surprising that no skin contaminants, such as the staphylococcus group, are likely to be cultured.

Prophylaxis. Antibiotics are recommended in susceptible patients prior to anesthesia. Technical precautions include the avoidance of rough instrumentation in endoscopy and careful and delicate manipulation of the oral airway, including insertion of the pharyngeal or Guedel airway. Oral hygiene, dental care, and gargling preoperatively[168a,168b] will diminish the numbers of orotracheal commensals. The use of nasal vasoconstrictors to shrink the mucosa may ease the passage of nasopharyngeal or nasotracheal tubes and diminish trauma. Evidence in reducing bacteremia by this means, however, is scanty. In Dinner's study,[173] it has not been found effective in reducing bacteremia; however, it is reasonable that the vasoconstrictor will diminish trauma.

SURGICAL EMPHYSEMA.[180-181] Abrasions of the pharyngeal mucosa or of the glottic tissues followed by relatively high intrabronchial pressure of 40 mm Hg can produce surgical emphysema.[182] Characteristically, the patient develops air under the subcutaneous tissues of the neck, which may progress into the superficial tissues of the chest and axilla. This produces a gruesome appearance with cyanosis. Further extension along the fascial planes into the mediastinum may readily occur with impaired respiration and subsequent pneumothorax (Fig. 21-15).

A second mechanism involves the establishment of a portal of entry of air from alveoli into the perivascular sheaths. A gradient of air pressure must then be established between the two. This is related to rupture of the surface of the alveoli into the pulmonary interstitium and progression centrally along blood vessels.

Initially, high pressure of 400 mm Hg is required, but once a break occurs, much smaller intraalveolar pressures of 5 mm Hg or less will suffice to perpetuate the condition.[183] The air makes tracts along smaller blood vessels into the hilum of the lung, thence into the mediastinum to produce mediastinal emphysema. Further extension into the neck and chest as well as into the retroperitoneal tissue spaces occurs. This is the classic pathogenesis of interstitial mediastinal emphysema described by Macklin.[183]

TENSION PNEUMOTHORAX.[184] Following traumatic laceration or perforation of the pharynx or pyriform sinus, a pneumothorax may occur and progress to a tension pneumothorax. This is noted by instability of the chest and both respiratory and circulatory impairment. Distended neck veins are seen, along with chest hyperresonance and distant breath sounds. It is more likely when high positive end-expiratory pressures are used to ventilate the patient.

Complications Specifically Related to Nasotracheal Intubation

LACERATION OF NASAL MUCOSA. In traumatic nasotracheal intubation, three complications may ensue: nasal hemorrhage, fracture of the turbinates, and dissection of the tube beneath the mucosa and into the retropharyngeal space. Symptoms consist of cough, hemoptysis, and cyanosis. Abscess formation

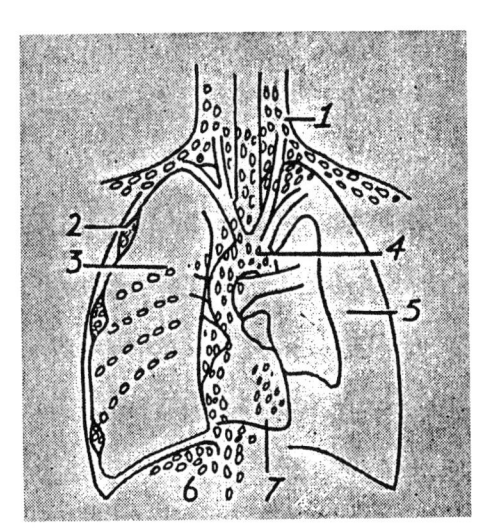

FIG. 21–15. Surgical emphysema. Shows escape of air following rupture of lungs. 1. Subcutaneous emphysema; 2. subpleural bleb; 3. pulmonary interstitial emphysema; 4. mediastinal emphysema; 5. pneumothorax; 6. pneumoperitoneum; 7. air embolism to heart. Similar distribution may occur following pharyngeal or laryngotracheal injury with air dissection into mediastinum and pulmonary interstitial space. Positive airway pressure is a usual factor. From Dripps, R.D., Eckenhoff, J., Vandam, L: Introduction to Anesthesia, 7th ed. Philadelphia, W.B. Saunders Co., 1988.

is likely to follow; nonpulmonary emphysema can ensue.

RETROPHARYNGEAL DISSECTION. After laceration of the nasal or pharyngeal mucosa by the laryngoscopy or the tube itself, persistence in advancing the endotracheal tube against resistance may result in retropharyngeal dissection.[182]

NASAL BLEEDING (EPISTAXIS). This is due to large tubes used in nasotracheal intubation and can be prevented by prior use of decongestants. Appropriate size of the tube should be determined by observation and a trial of insertion. If a significant force is apparently needed, switch to a smaller tube. Good lubrication and proper technique are essential. Epistaxis occurs occasionally in adults but is frequent in children and common in infants.

STRICTURE OF NOSTRIL. A large, tight-fitting nasotracheal tube can abrade the nasal mucosa and compress the lining of the nose, thereby producing inflammation. In the healing process, fibrous tissue may advance to scar formation and stricture, more commonly in infants and children than adults.

SINUSITIS. The problem of sinusitis is associated with nasotracheal intubation and is caused by blocking of the maxillary and frontal sinus openings into the nose under cover of the middle turbinate (ethmoid infundibulum). Compression of the middle turbinate against the lateral wall and the sinus openings, coupled with congestion and edema, will block the openings.

Acute maxillary sinusitis may develop with facial pain and unexplained postoperative fever.[185] Contributing factors include prolonged nasal intubation, the simultaneous use of nasogastric tubes and nasotracheal tubes, and the inability of the patient to complain and localize the site of discomfort.[186a] An acute sinusitis may occur from a nasogastric tube in the absence of nasotracheal intubation. An incidence of 6.5% is usual after short-term anesthesia. However, if intubation is prolonged, the incidence rises from 26% at 1 to 2 days, and within 3 days *all* patients have radiological and bacteriological evidence.[186b]

Treatment is symptomatic. Nasogastric tubes should be removed as early as possible. Nasal decongestant sprays with a vasoconstrictive action (phenylephrine 1%) are helpful, along with humidification.

COMPLICATIONS IN THE PEDIATRIC PATIENT

Three complications that are relatively common and are related to tracheal intubation in infants are croup (stridor), subglottic stenosis, and perforation or laceration of the pharynx, esophagus, and trachea.[187]

The factors related to these complications (Table 21–15) are traumatic technique; the use of tubes that are too large; rigidity of tracheal tubes, which may be ameliorated by warming the tubes to 30°C; the use of stylets; the skill of the intubator; excessive external laryngopressure on the cricoid; anatomic abnormalities; extensive hyperextension of the head; overinflation of cuffs; and the use of cuffs in infants.

CROUP (STRIDOR). This condition was first described as a clinical entity by Francis Home, a Scottish physician, in 1765.[188a] The word *croup* is Scottish for an acutely sore throat. This throat inflammation was probably diphtheria related. It was suggested that the trachea be entered to prevent suffocation.

This condition, defined as an infection of the larynx in infants and children, can be distinguished from epiglottitis by physical findings (see Table 21–15).[188b] Croup is characterized by the complaint of a sore throat and signs of difficult and noisy respiration, i.e., stridorous-type breathing, a hoarse voice, and a harsh, high-pitched cough. Classically, it is a laryngotracheobronchitis occurring in infants and children and, in recent years, known to be caused by parainfluenza virus types I and II. It is, however, more related to any type of upper respiratory infection or acquired from trauma and irritation essen-

590 General Anesthesia

TABLE 21-15. PHYSICAL FINDINGS IN CROUP AND EPIGLOTTITIS

Physical Findings	Croup	Epiglottitis
Protective posture	Absent	Present
Fever	Low	High
Cyanosis	Usually absent	Usually present
Stridor	Present	Mild to none
Nasal flaring	May develop	Usually present
Retractions	Initially mild when occur	Initially marked
Diaphragmatic and abdominal excursions	Not usually apparent	Marked
Heart rate	Sinus tachycardia	Sinus tachycardia, bradycardia with severe hypoxia and preceding cardiac arrest
Respiratory rate	Tachypnea	Tachypnea

From Diaz, J.H.: Croup and epiglottitis in children: The anesthesiologist as diagnostician. Anesth. Analg., 64:621, 1985.

tially of the vocal cords, producing a basic laryngitis, and may indeed be due to voice abuse. It is particularly related in anesthesia practice to traumatic laryngoscopy and intubation, as well as the use of endotracheal tubes larger than can be accommodated properly through the vocal cords. It is seen in adults as well as children.

Factors in anesthesia practice leading to this condition include traumatic endotracheal intubation, the use of oversized tubes, more particularly in infants and children, and the use of cuffed tubes. The incidence is increased when cuffed tubes are used. Overinflation of cuffs is a contributing factor.

Prevention. In infants and young children, uncuffed tubes should probably be used. In all instances, even in older children when a cuff is necessary, a slight leak should be provided. First, determine the inspiratory pressure producing control of ventilation, but not more than 30 cm H_2O. This ventilatory pressure should then be reduced so that an audible escape of air is permitted. Inspiratory pressures of 14 to 20 cm H_2O are usually sufficient. The patient's head should be kept in a neutral position; turning the head to the side increases the pressure needed for a leak from 14 to 24 cm H_2O. These patients should be kept paralyzed and not breathing spontaneously. Despite this, there is some motion of the vocal cords, and Scarpelli has demonstrated that there is tracheal motion during eupnea.[189]

Diagnosis. The degree of upper airway obstruction caused by croup or epiglottitis should be assessed and scored (Table 21-16).[190]

Treatment. This should be adjusted according to the degree of obstruction or the anticipated progression. An advanced degree of obstruction not responding to inhalation therapy with humidified oxygen and antibiotics may require the insertion of an artificial tracheal airway. An orotracheal airway may be used preferentially but a tracheostomy airway may be necessary.[132]

ATLANTOAXIAL SUBLUXATION. Atlantoaxial instability is a rare disorder that occurs in children. It is usually secondary to infections, collagen vascular disorders, or steroid therapy. In children with trisomy 21, the incidence of instability ranges from 14% to 22%.[191] When instability is determined, there is an increased incidence of subluxation, as first noted in 1965 by Tishler.[192a] A small percentage of these children, approximately 15% of those with instability, may become symptomatic.[192b]

In several situations, particularly when these children participate in vigorous physical activities, subluxation occurs and is symptomatic.[193] Subluxation is also likely to occur when these children are submitted to surgical intervention, particularly for developmental abnormalities. Should subluxation occur, there is significant danger of neurologic complications. For 31% of patients who develop subluxation, surgical correction produces little or no symptomatic improvement.

It is important, therefore, to screen the patients with Down syndrome for instability of the neck.[194] Lateral roentgenograms of the neck in flexed, extended, and neutral positions should be included. If the distance between the anterior arch of the atlas and the adjacent odontoid process exceeds 5 mm, the diagnosis of atlantoaxial instability can be made.[197a]

Management includes radiologic assessment and avoidance of neck flexion.[194] It has been further suggested that when cervical instability is determined to be present, posterior cervical spinal fusion should be performed prior to any other surgical procedure. The use of cervical braces may be employed for the short term.[191]

PALATAL GROOVE FORMATION IN NEONATES.[195] The presence of orotracheal tubes in neonates and infants is often accompanied by damage or pressure. Long-term use is associated with palatal groove formation, acquired cleft palate, and defective primary dentition. The incidence in the neonate is greatest when a tube is required for more than 15 days. A

TABLE 21-16. DOWNES SCORING SYSTEM FOR UPPER AIRWAY OBSTRUCTION

Physical Finding	Score*		
	0	1	2
Stridor	None	Inspiratory	Inspiratory and expiratory
Cough	None	Hoarse cry	Bark
Retractions and nasal flaring	None	Flaring and suprasternal retractions	Flaring and suprasternal, subcostal, intercostal retractions
Cyanosis	None	In air	In 40% O$_2$
Inspiratory breath sounds	Normal	Harsh, with wheezing or rhonchi	Delayed

* Maximum score is 10. Normal score is 0. Score of 4 or more requires therapy. Patient with score of 7 or more not responding to medical management may require immediate insertion of an artificial tracheal airway. From Downes, J.J., Godinez, R.I.: Acute upper airway obstruction in the child. American Society of Anesthesiologists refresher courses in anesthesiology, vol 8. Philadelphia, J.B. Lippincott, 1980;29.

significant impression and complication, however, can occur within 1 day. It is noted that the use of orogastric feeding tubes for up to 50 days has not been associated with palatal groove formation. Thus, the position of the endotracheal tube in the oral cavity becomes of importance. The tube usually rests against the center of the hard palate. The median palatal suture is a fibrous articulation without fusion. The continuous pressure of the endotracheal tube against this median palatine suture is most likely to result in a palatal groove due to the continuous pressure. Duration of orotracheal intubation and the associated palatal groove formation have been reviewed in a careful study that reports an overall incidence of approximately 48%. In neonates requiring a tube for more than 2 weeks, the incidence was determined to be 87%.[194]

PERFORATION OF AIRWAY. Tracheal perforation is a serious complication and should be considered when there is difficulty in ventilation of the neonate following intubation. Surgical emphysema or pneumothorax may be manifest. Immediate replacement of the tube in the tracheal lumen often will resolve the situation. Surgical correction, however, is frequently necessary.[195]

PROLONGED NASOTRACHEAL INTUBATION IN PEDIATRIC PATIENTS.[196] Prolonged nasotracheal intubation is an alternative to tracheostomy for establishing and maintaining an artificial airway. It has been found to be safe and extremely valuable in treating infants and children with respiratory failure requiring mechanical ventilation. A review of tracheostomy in children reveals that the intraoperative complication rate varies between 10% and 20%.[197] In the report by Oliver, the average incidence was determined to be 16% and included pneumothorax and pneumomediastinum and other traumatic injuries, as well as hemorrhage. If the tracheostomy is performed over a nasotracheal tube, however, these serious complications occur in less than 4% of patients.[197]

The major complication following prolonged nasotracheal intubation in patients with pulmonary disease requiring ventilatory care is subglottic stenosis. This has been reported in about 3% of the patients who had prolonged nasotracheal intubation.

Other significant complications observed following extubation included edema, ulceration of the vocal cords, perichondritis, granulation reaction, and granuloma formation.

In patients with upper airway obstruction, such as laryngotracheobronchitis, the incidence of complications from prolonged nasotracheal intubation is significantly higher than tracheostomy. Both subglottic granulomas and subglottic stenosis, as well as papillomas, are more frequent occurrences. Because of the significant number of complications in patients with upper airway disease, prolonged nasotracheal intubation is not recommended in children with croup.[198]

REFERENCES

1. Blanc, V.F., Tremblay, N.A.G.: The complications of tracheal intubation. A new classification and review of literature. Anesth. Analg., 53:203, 1974.
2. Applebaum, E.L., Bruce, D.L.: *Tracheal Intubation.* Philadelphia, W.B. Saunders Co., 1976.
3. Burstein, C.L.: *Fundamental Considerations in Anesthesia.* New York, The Macmillan Company, 1952.
4. Olsson, G.L., Hallen, B.: Laryngospasm during anaesthesia: A computer-aided incidence study in 136,929 patients. Acta. Anaesth. Scand., 28:567, 1984.
5. Roy, W.L., Lerman, J.: Laryngospasm in paediatric anaesthesia. Can. J. Anaesth., 35:93, 1988.
6. Rovenstine, E.A.: New York Postgraduate Medical School and Bellevue Hospital, Manual of Instruction. Department of Anesthesiology, 1946.
7. Fink, B.R.: The etiology and treatment of laryngeal spasm. Anesthesiology, 17:569, 1956.
8. Fink, R.B.: The mechanism of closure of the human larynx. Trans. Am. Acad. Ophthalmol. Otolaryngol., 60:117, 1956.
9. Keating, V.J.: Anaesthetic emergencies. In: *General Anaesthesia,* 2nd ed. Evans, F.T., Gray, T.C., eds. Volume 2, Chapter 25, pp. 522–3. London, Butterworths, 1965.

10. Rex, M.A.E.: A review of the structural and functional basis of laryngospasm and a discussion of the nerve pathways involved in the reflex and its clinical significance in man and animals. Br. J. Anaesth., 42:891, 1970.
11. Hinkle, J.E., Tantum, K.R.: A technic for measuring reactivity of the glottis (Kratschmer Reflex). Anaesthiology, 35:634, 1971.
12. Suzuki, M., Sasaki, C.T.: Laryngeal spasm: A neurophysiologic redefinition. Ann. Otol., 86:150, 1977.
13. Burstein, C.L., Rovenstine, E.A.: Respiratory parasympathetic action of some shorter-acting barbiturates and derivatives. J. Pharmacol. Exp. Therap., 63:43, 1938.
14. Horita, A., Dille, J.M.: Observations on the action of thiopental (Pentothal®) on the laryngeal reflex. Anesthesiology, 16:848, 1955.
15. Barron, D.W., Dundee, J.W.: Clinical studies of induction agents. XVII: Relationship between dosage and side effects of intravenous barbiturates. Br. J. Anaesth., 39:24, 1967.
16. Fisher, D.M., Robinson, S., Brett, C.M., et al.: Comparison of enflurane, halothane, and isoflurane for diagnostic and therapeutic procedures in children with malignancies. Anesthesiology, 63:647, 1985.
17a. Reid, L.C., Brace, D.E.: Reflexes from the mouth, trachea and esophagus which stimulate respiration. Anesthesiology, 4:345, 1943.
17b. Widdicombe, J.G., Kent, D.C., Nadel, J.A.: Mechanisms of bronchoconstriction during inhalation of dust. J. Appl. Physiol., 17:613, 1962.
18. Barbee, W.H.: Bronchospasm in the operating room. Anesthesiology, 47:478, 1978.
19. Sprague, D.H.: Treatment of intraoperative bronchospasm with nebulized isoetharine. Anesthesiology, 46:222, 1977.
20. Olsson, G.L.: Bronchospasm during anaesthesia: A computer-incidence study of 136,929 patients. Acta. Anaesth. Scand., 31:244, 1987.
21. Goodman, L.R.: Radiologic evaluation of patients receiving assisted ventilation. JAMA, 245:858, 1981.
22. Birmingham, P.K., Cheney, F.W., Ward, R.J.: Esophageal intubation. Anesth. Analg., 65:886, 1986.
23. Stirt, J.A.: Endotracheal tube misplacement. Anaesth. Intens. Care, 10:274, 1982.
24. Conrardy, P.A. et al.: Alteration of endotracheal tube position: Flexion and extension of the neck. Crit. Care. Med., 4:7, 1976.
25. Powell, D.R.: Obstruction to endotracheal tubes. Br. J. Anaesth., 46:252, 1974.
26. Peers, B.: Foreign bodies in endotracheal tubes. Anaesth. Intens. Care, 3:267, 1975.
27. Thompson, R.C.: Obstructed endotracheal tube demonstrated by roentgenogram. JAMA, 162:194, 1956.
28. McTaggert, R.A. et al.: Another cause of obstruction in an armoured endotracheal tube. Anesthesiology, 59:164, 1983.
29. Dorsch, J.A., Dorsch, S.E.: *Understanding Anesthesia Equipment*, 2nd ed., pp. 379–400. Baltimore, Williams & Wilkins, 1984.
30. Burstein, C.L., Lopinto, F.J., Newman, W.: Electrocardiographic studies during endotracheal intubation. I. Effects during usual routine technics. Anesthesiology, 11:224, 1950.
31. King, B.D., Harris, L.C., Greifenstein, F.E. et al.: Reflex circulatory responses to direct laryngoscopy and tracheal intubation performed during general anesthesia. Anesthesiology, 12:556, 1951.
32. Burstein, C.L., Woloshin, G., Newman, W.: Electrographic studies during endotracheal intubation. II. Effects during general anesthesia and intravenous procaine. Anesthesiology, 11:299, 1950.
33. Reid, L.C., Brace, D.E.: Irritation of the respiratory tract and its reflex effect upon the heart. Surg. Gynecol. Obstet., 70:157, 1940.
34. Baumgartner, L., Collins, V.J.: Succinylcholine effect on blood pressure and pulse during intubation. CAC: St. Vincent's Hospital, New York, June, 1952.
35. Wycoff, C.O.: Endotracheal intubation: Effects on blood pressure and pulse rate. Anesthesiology, 21:153, 1960.
36. Denlinger, J.K., Ellison, N., Ominsky, A.J.: Effects of intratracheal lidocaine on circulatory responses to tracheal intubation. Anesthesiology, 41:409, 1974.
37. Forbes, A.M., Dally, F.G.: Acute hypertension during induction of anaesthesia and endotracheal intubation in normotensive man. Br. J. Anaesth., 43:618, 1970.
38. Abou-Madi, M.N., Keszler, H., Yacoub, O.: A method for prevention of cardiovascular reactions to laryngoscopy and intubation. Can. Anaesth. Soc. J., 22:316, 1975.
39a. Stoelting, R.K.: Circulatory response to laryngoscopy and tracheal intubation with or without prior oropharyngeal viscous lidocaine. Anesth. Analg., 56:618, 1977.
39b. Stoelting, R.K.: Blood pressure and heart rate changes during short duration laryngoscopy for tracheal intubation: influence of viscous or intravenous lidocaine. Anesth. Analg., 57:197, 1978.
40. Kautto, U.-M.: Attenuation of the circulatory response to laryngoscopy and intubation by fentanyl. Acta. Anaesth. Scand., 26:217, 1982.
41. Kautto, U.-M., Heinonen, J.: Attenuation of circulatory response to laryngoscopy and tracheal intubation: a comparison of two methods of topical anaesthesia. Acta. Anaesth. Scand., 26:599, 1982.
42. Steinhaus, J.E.: Pharmacology of intravenous local anesthetics. Acta. Anaesth. Scand., 36:71, 1969.
43. Steinhaus, J.E., Gaskin, L.: A study of intravenous lidocaine as a suppressant of cough reflex. Anesthesiology, 2:285, 1963.
44. Denlinger, J.K., Messner, J.T., D'Orazio, D.J., et al.: Effect of intravenous lidocaine on the circulatory response to tracheal intubation. Anesth. Rev., 3:13, 1976.
45. Abou-Madi, M.N., Keszler, H., Yacoub, J.M.: Cardiovascular reactions to laryngoscopy and tracheal intubation following small and large intravenous doses of lidocaine. Can. Anaesth. Soc. J., 24:12–19, 1977.
46. Dahlgren, N., Messeter, K.: Treatment of stress response to laryngoscopy and intubation with fentanyl. Anaesthesia, 36:1022, 1981.
47a. Prys-Roberts, C., Greene, L.T., Melcohe, R., et al.: Studies of anaesthesia in relation to hypertension. II. Haemodynamic consequences of induction and endotracheal intubation. Br. J. Anaesth., 40:531, 1971.
47b. Prys-Roberts, C., Foex, P., Biro, C.P., et al.: Studies of anaesthesia in relation to hypertension. V. Adrenergic beta-receptor blockade. Br. J. Anaesth., 45:671, 1973.
48. Siedlecki, J.: Disturbances in the function of cardiovascular system in patients following endotracheal intubation and attempts of their prevention by pharmacological blockade of sympathetic system. Anaesth. Resus. Inten. Ther., 3:107, 1975.
49. Coleman, K.S., Jordan, C.: Cardiovascular response to anaesthesia: Influence of beta-adreno-receptor blockade with metoprolol. Anaesthesia, 35:972, 1980.
50. De Vault, M., Griefenstein, F.E., Harris, L. C., Jr.: Circu-

latory responses to endotracheal intubation in light general anesthesia—the effect of atropine and phentolamine. Anesthesiology, 21:360–362, 1960.
51. Stoelting, R.K.: Attenuation of blood pressure response to laryngoscopy and tracheal intubation with sodium nitroprusside. Anesth. Analg., 58:116, 1979.
52. Davies, M.J., Cronin, K.D., Cowie R.W.: The prevention of hypertension at intubation (hydralazine). Anaesthesia, 36:147, 1981.
53. Kamra, S., Wig, J., Sapra, R.P.: Topical nitroglycerine: A safeguard against pressor responses to tracheal intubation. Anaesthesia, 41:1087, 1986.
54. Dich-Nielsen, J., Hole, P., Lang-Jensen, T., et al.: The effect of intranasally administered nitroglycerin on the blood pressure response to laryngoscopy and intubation in patients undergoing coronary artery by-pass surgery. Acta. Anaesth. Scand., 30:23, 1986.
55. Curran, J., Crowley, M., O'Sullivan, G.: Droperidol and endotracheal intubation attenuation of pressor response to laryngoscopy and intubation. Anaesthesia, 35:290, 1980.
56. Flacke, J.W., Bloor, B.C., Flacke, W.E., et al.: Reduced narcotic requirements by clonidine with improved hemodynamic and adrenergic stability in patients undergoing coronary bypass surgery. Anesthesiology, 67:909, 1987.
57. Ghignone, M., Calvillo, O., Quintin, L.: Anesthesia and hypertension: The effect of clonidine on perioperative hemodynamics and isoflurane requirements. Anesthesiology, 67:3–10, 1987.
58. Ackerman, W.E., Kochansky, S.E., et al.: Lidocaine-low dose thiopental to control blood pressure lability during induction, laryngoscopy and intubation in hypertensive patients. Anesth. Rev., 11:18, 1984.
59. Hartigan, M.L., Cleary, J.L., Gross, J.B., et al.: A comparison of pretreatment regimens for minimizing the haemodynamic response to blind nasotracheal intubation. Can. Anaesth. Soc. J., 31:497, 1984.
60. Kale, S.C., et al.: Nifedipine prevents the pressor response to laryngoscopy and tracheal intubation in patients with coronary artery disease. Anaesthesia, 43:495, 1988.
61a. Fox, D.J., Sklar, G.S., Hill, C.H., et al.: Complications related to the pressor response to endotracheal intubation. Anesthesiology, 47:124, 1977.
61b. Nadel, J.A., Widdicombe, J.G.: Reflex effects of upper airway irritation on total lung resistance and blood pressure. J. Appl. Physiol., 17:861, 1962.
62. Takki, S., Tammisto, T., Nikki, P., et al.: Effect of laryngoscopy and intubation on plasma catecholamine levels during intravenous induction of anaesthesia. Br. J. Anaesth., 44:1323, 1972.
63. Cork, R.C., Weiss, J.L., Hameroff, S.R., et al.: Fentanyl preloading for rapid-sequence induction of anesthesia. Anesth. Analg., 63:60, 1984.
64. Zsigmond, E.K., Winnie, A.P., Raza, S.M., et al.: Nalbuphine as an analgesic component in balanced anesthesia for cardiac surgery. Anesth. Analg., 66:1155, 1987.
65. Bedford, R.F., Marshall, W.K.: Hemodynamic response to endotracheal intubation. Anesthesiology (Suppl), 61:A270, 1981.
66. Derbyshire, D.R., Smith, G., Achola, K.J.: Effect of topical lignocaine on the sympatho-adrenal responses to tracheal intubation. Br. J. Anaesth., 59:300, 1987.
67. Shribman, A.J., Smith, G., Achola, K.J.: Cardiovascular and catecholamine responses to laryngoscopy with and without tracheal intubation. Br. J. Anaesth., 59:295, 1987.
68. Kumar, S.M., Kothary, S.P., Zsigmond, E.K.: The effect of pancuronium on plasma-free norepinephrine and epinephrine in adult cardiac surgical patients. Acta. Anaesth. Scand., 22:423, 1978.
69. Derbyshire, D.R., Smith, G.: Sympathoadrenal responses to anaesthesia and surgery. Br. J. Anaesth., 56:725, 1984.
70. Adriani, J., Zepernick, R.: The comparative potency and effectiveness of topical anesthetics in man. Clin. Pharmacol. Therap., 5:49, 1964.
71. Ritchie, J.M., Greene, N.M.: Local anesthetics. Chapter 15 in: The Pharmacological Basis of Therapeutics, 8th Edition (Goodman, Gilman, Eds). New York, Pergamon Press, 1990.
71a. Tam, S., Chang, F., Campbell, J.M.: Attenuation of circulatory responses to endotracheal intubation using intravenous lidocaine: Optimal time of injection. Can. Anaesth. Soc. J., 32:565, 1985.
71b. Tam, S., Chang, F., Campbell, J.M.: Optimal time of injection before tracheal intubation. Anesth. Analg., 66:1036, 1987.
72. Finster, M., et al.: The placental transfer of lidocaine and its uptake by fetal tissue. Anesthesiology, 36:159, 1972.
73. Roy, W.L., Lerman, J.: Laryngospasm in paediatric anaesthesia. Can. J. Anaesth., 35:93, 1988.
74. Himes, R.S., DiFazio, C.H., Burney, R.G.: Effects of lidocaine on the anesthetic requirements for nitrous oxide and halothane. Anesthesiology, 47:437, 1977.
75. Poulton, T.J., James, F.M., III: Cough suppressions by lidocaine. Anesthesiology, 50:470, 1979.
76. Yukioka, H., Yoshimoto, N., Nishimura, K., et al.: Intravenous lidocaine as a suppressant of coughing during tracheal intubation. Anesth. Analg., 64:1189, 1985.
77. Christensen, V., Ladegaard-Pedersen, H.J., Skovsted, P.: Intravenous lidocaine as a suppressant of persistent cough caused by bronchoscopy. Acta. Anaesth. Scand., 67 (Suppl):84, 1978.
78. Hamill, J.F., Bedford, R.F., Weaver, D.C., et al.: Lidocaine before endotracheal intubation: intravenous or laryngotracheal? Anesthesiology, 55:578, 1981.
79. Tam, S., Chung, F., Campbell, M.: Intravenous lidocaine: Optimal time of injection before tracheal intubation. Anesth. Analg., 66:1036, 1987.
80. Donegan, M.F., Bedford, R.F.: Intravenously administered lidocaine prevents intracranial hypertension during endotracheal suctioning. Anesthesiology, 52:516, 1980.
81. Bedford, R.F., Winn, H.R., Tyson, G., et al.: Lidocaine prevents increased ICP after endotracheal intubation. In: Schulman, K., Mamarou, A., Miller, J.D., et al, eds. Intracranial Pressure IV. Berlin, Springer, pp. 595–8, 1980.
82. Drenger, B., Peer, J., Venezra, D., et al.: The effect of intravenous lidocaine on the increase in intraocular pressure induced by tracheal intubation. Anesth. Analg., 64:1121, 1985.
83. Baraka, A.: Intravenous lidocaine controls extubation laryngospasm in children. Anesth. Analg., 57:506, 1978.
84. Wallin, G., Cassuto, J., Högström, S., et al.: Effects of lidocaine infusion on the sympathetic response to abdominal surgery. Anesth. Analg., 66:1008, 1987.
85. Collinsworth, K.A., Kalman, S.M., Harrison, D.C.: The clinical pharmacology of lidocaine as an anti-arrhythmic drug. Circulation, 50:1217, 1974.
86. Chen, C.T., Toung, T.J.K., Donham, R.T., et al.: Fentanyl dosage for suppression of circulatory response to laryngoscopy and endotracheal intubation. Anesthesiol. Rev., 13:37, 1986.
87. Shupak, R.C., Harp, J.R., Stevenson-Smith, W., et al.: High

dose fentanyl for neuroanesthesia. Anesthesiology, 58:579, 1983.
88. Kraut, R.A.: A comparison of intravenous and laryngotracheal lidocaine before endotracheal intubation. Anesth. Prog., Mar/April:34, 1983.
89. Viegas, O., Stoelting, R.K.: Lidocaine in arterial blood after laryngotracheal administration. Anesthesiology, 43(4):491, 1975.
90. Sellers, W.F.S., Dye, A., Harvey, J.: Systemic absorption of lignocaine ointment from tracheal tubes. Anaesthesia, 40:483, 1985.
91. McCammon, R.L., Hilgenberg, J.C., Stoelting, R.K.: Effect of propranolol on circulatory responses to induction of diazepam-nitrous oxide anesthesia and to endotracheal intubation. Anesth. Analg., 60:579, 1981.
92. Zaroslinski, J., Borgman, R.J., O'Donnell, J.P., et al.: Ultra short acting beta blockers: A proposal for treatment of the critically ill patient. Life Sci., 31:899, 1982.
93. Barabas, E., Zsigmond, E.K., Kirkpatrick, A.F.: The inhibitory effect of esmolol on human plasma cholinesterase. Can. Anaesth. Soc. J., 33:332, 1986.
94. Sum, C.Y., Yacobi, A., Kartzinel, R., et al.: Kinetics of esmolol, an ultra short acting beta blocker, and of its major metabolite. Clin. Pharmacol. Ther., 34:27, 1983.
95. Menkhaus, P.G., Reves, J.G., et al.: Cardiovascular effects of esmolol in anesthetized humans. Anesth. Analg., 64:327, 1985.
96. Gold, M.I., Brown, M.S., Selem, J.S.: The effect of esmolol on hemodynamics after ketamine induction and intubation. Anesthesiology, 61:A19, 1984.
97a. Newsome, L.R., Roth, J.V., Hug, C.C., Jr., et al.: Esmolol attenuates hemodynamic responses during fentanyl-pancuronium anesthesia for aortocoronary bypass surgery. Anesth. Analg., 65:451, 1986.
97b. Girard, D., Thys, T.M., Kaplan, J.A., et al.: Hemodynamic effects of esmolol during fentanyl anesthesia for CABG. Anesth. Analg., 64:217, 1985.
98. Zsigmond, E.K., Kirkpatrick, A.F., Barabas, E., et al.: Pharmacodynamics and pharmacokinetics of esmolol infusions during thiopental induction and intubation. Anesthesiology, 63:A61, 1985.
99. Korenaga, G.M., Kirkpatrick, A.F., Lord, J.G., et al.: Effect of esmolol on tachycardia induced by endotracheal intubation. Anesth. Analg., 64:238, 1985.
100. Longnecker, D.E.: Alpine anesthesia: Can pretreatment with clonidine decrease the peaks and valleys? Anesthesiology, 67:1, 1987.
101. Langer, S.Z., Cavero, I., Masinghaun, R.: Recent development in noradrenergic transmission and its relevance to the mechanism of action of certain antihypertensive agents. Hypertension, 2:372, 1980.
102. Quintin, L., Gonon, E., Buda, M., et al.: Clonidine modulates locus coeruleus metabolic hyperactivity induced by immobilization in behaving rats. Brain Res., 362:366, 1986.
103. Bloor, B.C., Flacke, W.E.: Reduction in halothane anesthetic requirement by clonidine, an alpha-adrenergic agonist. Anesth. Analg., 61:741, 1982.
104. Ghignone, M., Calvillo, O., Quintin, L.: Anesthesia and hypertension: The effect of clonidine on perioperative hemodynamics and isoflurane requirements. Anesthesiology, 67:3–10, 1987.
105. Ghignone, M., Quintin, L., Duke, P.C., et al.: Effects of clonidine on narcotic requirements and hemodynamic response during induction of anesthesia and endotracheal intubation. Anesthesiology, 64:36, 1986.
106. Anderson, R.G.G., Ekstrom, T., Gundstrom, N., et al.: Inhibitory effects of an alpha-$_2$ adrenoreceptor agonist, clonidine, on bronchospastic response in guinea-pig and man. Acta. Physiol. Scand. (Suppl) 124, 1985.
107. Tamsen, A., Gordh, T.E.: Epidural clonidine produces analgesia. Lancet, 2:231, 1984.
108. Flacke, J.W., Bloor, B.C., Flacke, W.E., et al.: Reduced narcotic requirements by clonidine with improved hemodynamic and adrenergic stability in patients undergoing coronary bypass surgery. Anesthesiology, 67:909, 1987.
109. Orko, R., Pouttu, J., Ghignone, M., et al.: Effect of clonidine on haemodynamic responses to endotracheal intubation and on gastric acidity. Acta. Anaesth. Scand., 31:325, 1987.
110. Chraemmer-Jørgensen, B., et al.: Lack of effect of intravenous lidocaine on hemodynamic responses to rapid sequence induction of general anesthesia: A double-blind controlled clinical trial. Anesth. Analg., 65:1037, 1986.
111. Lindholm, C.-E.: Prolonged endotracheal intubation. Acta. Anaesth. Scand. Supplement, 33:1–131, Chapter 8, Relevant statistical data, p. 92–102, 1969.
112. Applebaum, E.L., Bruce, D.L.: Chapter 8: Complications, pp. 77–80. In: *Tracheal Intubation.* Philadelphia, W.B. Saunders, 1976.
113a. Bergstrom, J., Moberg, A., Orell, S.R.: On the pathogenesis of laryngeal injuries following prolonged intubation. Acta. Otolaryngol., 55:342, 1962.
113b. Dedo, H.H.: The paralyzed larynx. An electromyographic study in dogs and humans. Laryngoscope, 80:1455, 1970.
114. Cooper, J.D., Grillo, H.C.: The evolution of tracheal injury to ventilatory assistance through cuffed tubes. Ann. Surg., 169:334, 1969.
115a. Boice, J.B., Krous, H.F., Foley, J.M.: Gingival and dental complications of orotracheal intubation. JAMA, 236:957, 1976.
115b. Wright, R.B., Manfield, F.F.V.: Damage to teeth during the administration of general anesthesia. Anesth. Analg., 53:405–8, 1974.
116. Dornette, W.H.L.: Care of the teeth during endoscopy and anesthesia. Clin. Anesth., 8:217, 1972.
117. Sosis, M., Lazar, S.: Jaw dislocation during general anesthesia. Can. J. Anaesth., 34:407, 1987.
118. Williams, J.P., Somerville, G.M., Miner, M.E., et al.: Atlanto-axial subluxation and trisomy-21: Another perioperative complication. Anesthesiology, 67:253, 1987.
119a. Baron, S.H., Kohlmoos, H.W.: Laryngeal sequelae of endotracheal anesthesia. Ann. Otol., 60:767, 1961.
119b. Peppard, S.B., Dickens, J.H.: Laryngeal injury following short-term intubation. Ann. Otol. Rhinol. Laryngol., 92:327, 1983.
120a. Stout D.M., Bishop, M.J., Swersteg, J.F., et al.: Correlation of endotracheal tube size with sore throat and hoarseness following general anesthesia. Anesthesiology, 67:419, 1987.
120b. Loeser, E.A., Kaminsky, A., Diaz, A., et al.: The influence of endotracheal tube cuff design and cuff lubrication on postoperative sore throat. Anesthesiology, 58:376, 1983.
121. Loeser, E.A., Stanley, T.H., Jordan, W., et al.: Postoperative sore throat: Influence on tracheal tube lubrication versus cuff design. Can. Anaesth. Soc. J., 27:156, 1980.
122. Capan, L.M., Bruce, D.L., Patel, K.P., et al.: Succinylcholine induced postoperative sore throat. Anesthesiology, 59:202, 1983.
123. Andreassen, U.K., Husum, M.T., Leth, N.: Acute epiglottitis in adults. Acta. Anaesth. Scand., 28:155, 1984.

124. Shapiro, J., Eavey, R.D., Baker, A.S.: Adult supraglottitis: A prospective analysis. JAMA, 259:563, 1988.
125. Rendell-Baker, L.: Hazards of prolonged intubation and tracheotomy equipment. Editorial. JAMA, 204:624, 1968.
126a. Stetson, J.B., Whitbourne, J.E., Eastman, C.: Ethylene oxide degassing of rubber and plastic materials. Anesthesiology, 44:174, 1976.
126b. Stetson, J.B., Guess, W.L.: Causes of damage to tissues by polymers and elastomers used in fabrication of tracheal devices. Anesthesiology, 33:635, 1970.
127. Donnelly, W.H.: Histopathology of endotracheal intubation. Arch. Pathol., 88:511, 1969.
128. Biller, H.F., Harvey, J.E., Bone, R.C., et al.: Laryngeal edema—an experimental study. Ann. Otol., 79:1084, 1970.
129a. Bennett, R.L., Lee, T.S., Wright, B.D.: Airway-obstructing supraglottic edema following anesthesia with the head positioned in forced-flexion. Anesthesiology, 54:78, 1981.
129b. Grundy, E.M., Bennett, E.J., Schmidt, G.B.: Causes of acute airway obstruction. Anesth. Rev., 4:47, 1977.
130. New, G.B., Devine, K.D.: Contact ulcer granuloma. Arch. Otorhinolaryngol, 58:548, 1949.
131. Jackson, C.: Contact ulcer granuloma and other laryngeal complications of endotracheal anesthesia. Anesthesiology, 14:425, 1953.
132. Holinger, P.H., Johnson, K.C.: Contact ulcer of the larynx. JAMA, 172:511, 1960.
133. Howland, W.S., Lewis, J.J.: Mechanisms in the development of post-intubation granuloma of the larynx. Ann. Otol., 65:1006, 1956.
134. Snow, J.C., Harano, M., Balough, K.: Postintubation granuloma of the larynx. Anesth. Analg., 45:425, 1966.
135. Pullen, F.W., II: Postintubation tracheal granuloma. Arch. Otolaryngol., 92:340, 1970.
136. Hedden, M., Ersoz, C.J., Donnelly, W.H., et al.: Laryngotracheal damage after prolonged use of orotracheal tubes in adults. JAMA, 207:703, 1969.
137. Way, W.L., Sooy, F.A.: Histologic changes produced by endotracheal intubation. Ann. Otol., 74:799, 1965.
138. Gross, C.W., Gros, J.C.: Rare complications after prolonged translaryngotracheal intubation. Ann. Otol., 80:583, 1971.
139. Hilding, A.C.: Laryngotracheal damage during intratracheal anesthesia. Ann. Otol., 80:567, 1971.
140. Thompson, D.S., Read, R.C.: Rupture of the trachea following endotracheal intubation. JAMA, 204:137, 1968.
141. Kirchner, J.A., Sasakic, T.: Fusion of the vocal cords following intubation and tracheostomy. Trans. Am. Acad. Ophthalmol. Otolaryngol., 77:88, 1973.
142. Jackson, C.: High tracheostomy and other errors. The chief causes of chronic laryngeal stenosis. Surg. Gynecol. Obstet., 32:392, 1921.
143. Finch, J.S.: Intubation tracheal injury. Curr. Rev. Clin. Anes., 5(16):1985.
144. Ranier, W.G.: Major airway collapsibility in the pathogenesis of obstructive emphysema. J. Thorac. Cardiovasc. Surg., 46:559, 1963.
145. Dubost, C., Kaswin, D., Duranteau, A., et al.: Esophageal perforation during attempted endotracheal intubation. J. Thorac. Cardiovasc. Surg., 78:44, 1979.
146. O'Neill, J.E., Griffin, J.P., Cottrell, J.E.: Pharyngeal and esophageal perforation following endotracheal intubation. Anesthesiology, 60:487, 1984.
147. Hirsch, M., Abramowitz, H.B., Shapiro, S., et al.: Hypopharyngeal injury as a result of attempted endotracheal intubation. Radiology, 128:37, 1978.
148. Wengen, D.F.A.: Piriform fossa perforation during attempted tracheal intubation. Anaesthesia, 42:519, 1987.
149. Norman, E.A., Sosis, M.: Iatrogenic oesophageal perforation due to tracheal or nasogastric intubation. Can. Anaesth. Soc. J., 33:222, 1986.
150. Teichner, R.L.: Lingual nerve injury: A complication of orotracheal anesthesia. Br. J. Anaesth., 43:413, 1971.
151. Jones, B.C.: Lingual nerve injury: A complication of intubation. Br. J. Anaesth., 43:730, 1971.
152. Hahn, F.W., Jr., Martin, J.T., Lillie, J.C.: Vocal-cord paralysis with endotracheal intubation. Arch. Otol., 92:226, 1970.
153. Lim, E.K., Chia, K.S., Ng, B.K.: Recurrent laryngeal nerve palsy following endotracheal intubation. Anaesth. Intensive Care, 15:342, 1987.
154. Holley, H.S., Gildea, J.E.: Vocal cord paralysis after tracheal intubation. JAMA, 215:281, 1971.
155. Ellis, P.D.M., Pallister, W.K.: Recurrent laryngeal nerve palsy and endotracheal intubation. J. Laryngol. Otol., 89:823, 1975.
156. Nicholls, B.J., Packham, R.N.: Arytenoid cartilage dislocation. Anaesth. Intensive Care, 14:196, 1986.
157. Kambic, V., Radsel, Z.: Intubation lesions of the larynx. Br. J. Anaesth., 50:587, 1978.
158. Quick, C.A., Merwin, G.E.: Arytenoid dislocation. Arch. Otolaryngol., 104:267, 1978.
159. Etsten, B., Mahler, D.: Subglottic membrane: A complication of endotracheal intubation. NEJM, 245:957, 1951.
160. Muir, A.P., Straton, J.: Membraneous laryngo-tracheitis following endotracheal intubation. Anaesthesia, 9:105, 1954.
161. Klainel, A.S., Turndorf, H., Wu, W.-H., et al.: Surface alterations due to endotracheal intubation. Am. J. Med., 58:674, 1975.
162. Keane, W.M., et al.: Complications of intubation. Ann. Otol. Rhinol. Laryngol., 91:584, 1982.
163. Kumar, S.M., Pandit, S.K., Cohen, P.J.: Tracheal laceration associated with endotracheal anesthesia. Anesthesiology, 47:298, 1977.
164. Paegle, R.D., Agnes, S.M., Davis, S.: Rapid tracheal injury by cuffed airways and healing with loss of ciliated epithelium. Arch. Surg., 106:31, 1973.
165. Hackl, V., Konig, G.: Experimental investigations concerning resistance of the trachea against inflatable cuffs. Der Anesthetist, 8:134, 1961.
166. Gillespie, N.A., Conroy, W.A.: Endotracheal anesthesia—the relation of nasotracheal and orotracheal intubation to respiration morbidity. Anesthesiology, 2:28, 1941.
167. Gillespie, N.A.: The relation of intubation to postoperative respiratory complaints. Anaesthesia, 6:206, 1951.
168a. Beck, H., Preisler, O.: Laryngeal and tracheal flora before and after intubation. Der Anaesthesist 8:110, 1959.
168b. Collins, V.J., Klatskin, D.: The advantage of preanesthetic gargling in reducing tracheal bacterial contamination. Cook County Hospital Dental Anesthesia Practice. Procedure Manual, 1968.
169. Sottile, F.D., Marrie, T.J., Prough, D.S., et al.: Nosocomial pulmonary infection: Possible etiologic significance of bacterial adhesion to endotracheal tubes. Crit. Care Med., 14:265, 1986.
170. Berry, F.A., Jr., Blankenbaker, W.L., Ball, C.G.: Comparison of bacteremia occurring with nasotracheal and orotracheal intubation. Anesth. Analg., 52:873, 1973.
171. Gerber, M.A., Gastanaduy, A.S., Buckley, J.J., et al.: Risk of bacteremia after endotracheal intubation for general anesthesia. South Med. J., 73:1478, 1980.
172. McShane, A.J., Hone, R.: Prevention of bacterial endocarditis: Does nasal intubation warrant prophylaxis? Br. Med. J., 292:26, 1986.

173. Dinner, M., Tjeuw, M., Artusio, J.F., Jr.: Bacteremia as a complication of nasotracheal intubation. Anesth. Analg., 66:460, 1987.
174. Baltch, A.L., Pressman, H.L., Hammer, M.C., et al.: Bacteremia following dental extractions in patients with and without penicillin prophylaxis. Am. J. Med. Sci., 283:129, 1982.
175. Berry, F.A., Jr., Yarbrough, S., Yarbrough, N., et al.: Transient bacteremia during dental manipulation in children. Pediatrics, 51:476, 1973.
176. Baltch, A.L., Buhac, I., Agrawal, A., et al.: Bacteremia after gastrointestinal endoscopy. Arch. Intern. Med., 137:594, 1977.
177. Burman, S.O.: Bronchoscopy and bacteremia. J. Thorac. Cardiovasc. Surg., 40:635, 1960.
178. Smith, R.P., Sahetya, G.K., Baltch, A.L., et al.: Bacteremia associated with fiberoptic bronchoscopy. N.Y. State J. Med., 83:1045, 1983.
179. Brandstater, B., Muallem, M.: Atelectasis following tracheal suction in infants. Anesthesiology, 31:468, 1969.
180. Marcotte, R.J., Phillips, F.J., Livingstone, H.J.: Differential intrabronchial pressures and mediastinal emphysema. J. Thorac. Surg., 9:346, 1940.
181. Spence, M.: Surgical emphysema during anesthesia. Anesthesia, 10:50, 1955.
182. Smith, R.H., Pool, L.L., Volpitto, P.P.: Subcutaneous emphysema as a complication of endotracheal intubation. Anesthesiology, 20:714, 1959.
183. Macklin, M.T., Macklin, C.C.: Malignant interstitial emphysema of the lungs. Medicine, 23:281, 1944.
184. Padovan, I.F., Davison, C.A., Henschel, E.O., et al.: Pathogenesis of mediastinal emphysema and pneumothorax following tracheostomy. Exper. Chest, 66:553, 1974.
185. Knodel, A.R., Beekman, J.F.: Unexplained fever in patients with nasotracheal intubation. JAMA, 248:865, 1982.
186a. Willatts, S.M., Cochrane, D.F.: Paranasal sinusitis: a complication of nasotracheal intubation. Br. J. Anaesth., 57:1026, 1985.
186b. Hansen, M., et al.: Incidence of sinusitis in patients with nasotracheal intubation. Br. J. Anaesth., 61:231, 1988.

187. Maze, A., Bloch, E.: Stridor in pediatric patients. Anesthesiology, 50:132, 1980.
188a. Home, F.: An enquiry into the nature, cause and cure of croup. Edinberg, Kincaid and Bell, 1965.
188b. Diaz, J.H.: Croup and epiglottitis in children: The anesthesiologist as diagnostician. Anesth. Analg., 64:621, 1985.
189. Scarpelli, E.M., Real, F.J.P., Rudolph, A.M.: Tracheal motion during eupnea. J. Appl. Physiol., 20:473, 1965.
190. Downes, J.J., Godinez, R.I.: *Acute Upper Airway Obstruction in the Child.* American Society of Anesthesiologists Refresher Courses in Anesthesiology, Vol. 8. Philadelphia, J.B. Lippincott, p. 29, 1980.
191. Williams, J.P., Somerville, G.M., Miner, M.E., et al.: Atlanto-axial subluxation and trisomy-21: Another perioperative complication. Anesthesiology, 67:253, 1987.
192a. Tishler, J., Martel, W.: Dislocation of the atlas in mongolism. Radiology, 84:904, 1965.
192b. Pueschel, S.M., Herndon, J.H., Gelch, M.M., et al.: Symptomatic atlanto-axial subluxation in persons with Down syndrome. J. Pediatr. Orthop., 4:682, 1984.
193. Committee on Sports Medicine: Atlantoaxial instability in Down syndrome. Pediatrics, 74:152, 1984.
194. Kobel, M., Creighton, R.E., Steward, D.J.: Anaesthetic considerations in Down's syndrome: Experience with 100 patients and a review of the literature. Can. Anaesth. Soc. J., 29:593, 1982.
195. McLeod, B.J., Sumner, E.: Neonatal tracheal perforation: A complication of tracheal intubation. Anaesthesia, 41:67, 1986.
196. Allen, T.H., Steven, I.M.: Prolonged nasotracheal intubation in infants and children. Br. J. Anaesth., 44:835, 1972.
197. Othersen, H.B.: Intubation injuries of the trachea in children. Ann. Surgery, 189:601, 1979.
198. Striker, T.W., Stool, S., Downes, J.J.: Prolonged nasotracheal intubation in infants and children. Arch. Otolaryngol., 85:210, 1967.

22

ENDOBRONCHIAL TECHNIQUE

HISTORY

1932—Gale and Waters described endobronchial anesthesia[1]

1936—Magill performed endobronchial anesthesia under vision with a small bronchoscope inside a long endotracheal tube[2]

1936—Rovenstine devised a long rubber endotracheal tube with two inflatable cuffs for intubatins one bronchus and sealing off the other bronchus[3]

1938—Crafoord sealed off diseased lungs with tampons[4]

1948—Ruth used long spiral metal tubes (Woodbridge type) with an inner bronchoscope for visual endobronchial intubation[5]

1952—Bonica described the use of long rubber Magill tubes in endobronchial intubation[6]

1953—Carlens introduced the double-lumen endobronchial tube for use in anesthesia[7,8]

Historically, occlusion of the bronchus on the diseased side by use of tampons or bronchial blockers was the first technique that provided satisfactory conditions permitting successful open thoracic surgery. The procedure was time consuming and cumbersome. Single-lumen catheters were then used with double cuffs often placed under vision. More controllable surgical conditions, as well as controlled ventilatory physiology, have been achieved by the double-lumen catheter techniques, which are dependable and have become the standard of practice.

To prevent transbronchial spread of disease or secretions during pulmonary surgery, three principal approaches have been used:*

1. Occluding the main bronchus of the diseased lung by tampon[4] or by an inflatable balloon blocker[2,9a] (Fig. 22–1A and 22–1B).

---

* The prone position for surgery under endotracheal anesthesia was first employed by Overholt in performing various intrathoracic pulmonary procedures. (Overholt, R.H. et al: Pulmonary resection in the treatment of tuberculosis. J. Thorac. Surg., 15:384, 1946.)

FIG. 22–1. Development of techniques of endobronchial anesthesia. *A*, Magill's technique of plugging diseased bronchus with fine suction catheter equipped with small inflatable cuff. *B*, Crafoord's technique of one-lung anesthesia by plugging bronchus with gauze tampon. *C*, Rovenstine's technique employing a long double-cuffed tube for endobronchial intubation. *D*, Carlens technique using a double-lumen and cuffed endobronchial tube.

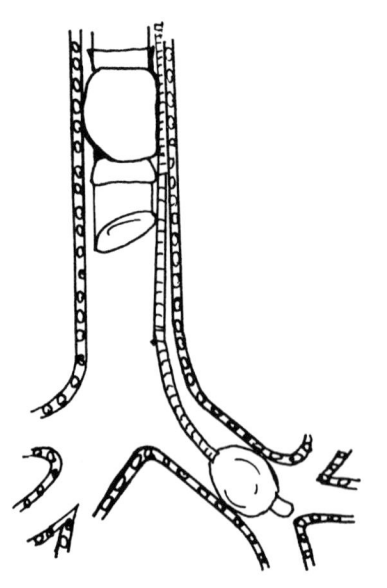

A, Magill Bronchial Blocker

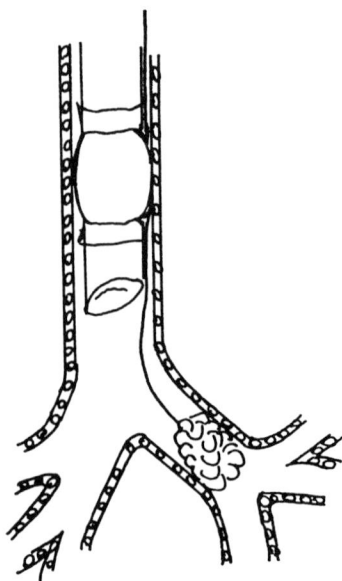

B, Crafoord Tampon

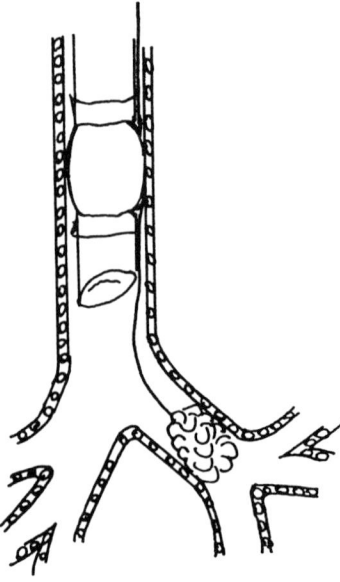

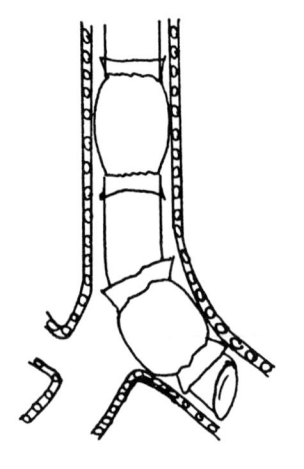

C, Rovenstine's Two Cuff Technic

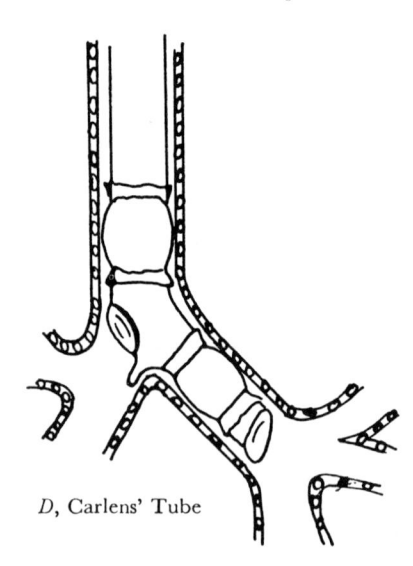

D, Carlens' Tube

2. Occluding the main bronchus of the diseased lung by a double-cuffed, long, single-lumen endotracheal tube inserted into the bronchus of the healthy lung (Rovenstine "two-cuff") (Fig. 22–1*C*).[3]
3. Separating the healthy lung from the diseased lung by a double-lumen endobronchial tube (Carlens' classic technique[8]) (Fig. 22–1*D*). Other special double-lumen endobronchial tubes are available.

Closed endobronchial anesthesia was suggested in 1932 by Gale and Waters as a technique for "sealing off" a diseased lung from the contralateral sound lung.[1] In 1936, Magill described the performance of endobronchial anesthesia using a bronchoscope of suitable size inside a long Magill tube carrying an inflated cuff. Magill[2] also described a second method where a fine suction catheter equipped with an inflatable cuff was introduced into the bronchus of the diseased lung to act as a plug or bronchial blocker when inflated. A long endotracheal tube was then inserted deep into the trachea but not into the other bronchus and its cuff inflated. At best, the technique requires a short procedure, is cumbersome, and does not assure control. The blocker frequently may slip during positioning of the patient or if the patient coughs. It is no longer used.

In 1936, Rovenstine[3] described an endobronchial technique using a semirigid catheter fitted with two inflatable cuffs. One cuff was placed within an inch of the open end of the tube; the second was separated from the first by about 2 inches. The catheter was introduced blindly into the selected bronchus and the distal cuff inflated, thereby sealing this lung from the opposite side. When bilateral ventilation was desired, the distal cuff was deflated and the proximal inflated to provide a simple endotracheal set-up.

In 1938, Crafoord accomplished one-lung anesthesia by introducing a gauze tampon into the bronchus of the diseased lung.[4]

In 1948, Ruth[5] designed an endobronchial airway that combined a noncollapsible tube of coiled wire whose obturator was a special bronchoscope. The tube was essentially an elongated Woodbridge endotracheal tube.

Bonica[6] has modified the Magill endobronchial airway for right or left bronchial intubation. He used a single seam cuff and a lip along the convexity to facilitate insertion into the bronchus and not to occlude the eparterial bronchus.

Many other modifications of a single-lumen tube using cuffs to seal one lung from the other have been suggested. However, attention will be directed at current practices.

ENDOBRONCHIAL INTUBATION TECHNIQUE

INDICATIONS.[6,10b,11b] The purpose of endobronchial anesthesia is to prevent transbronchial spread of disease or secretions or to seal off pulmonary leaks. The indications for endobronchial anesthesia include lung abscess, bronchiectasis, and bronchopleural fistula. Table 22–1 lists additional indications.[10b]

ADVANTAGES. In addition to the advantages offered by use of the endotracheal tube, the endobronchial tube seals off the sound lung from the diseased lung with the following results:

1. Secretions, abscess, fluids, and blood are prevented from flowing into the healthy lung and drowning the patient.[13]
2. Contamination is prevented.
3. Loss of anesthetic gases through a bronchopleural fistula is prevented.

Definite advantages are to be found in lung resections. These are summarized as follows:[8,10b,11a]

1. The diseased lung may be deflated to provide better operating field conditions without interfering with ventilation of the sound lung.
2. The surgical lung can be inflated when intersegmental planes are developed.
3. The bronchus can be divided without interfering with the anesthesia.
4. It is unnecessary to apply a clamp to the proximal part of the bronchus and, hence, tissue injury is avoided.
5. The surgeon may easily inspect the open bronchus.
6. Carinal resections and bronchotomies can be performed more safely.

TABLE 22–1. INDICATIONS FOR ONE-LUNG ANESTHESIA

Absolute
  Prevention of spillage or contamination from diseased to nondiseased lung
    Infection—abscess; bronchiectasis; hyatid cyst
    Massive hemorrhage
  Control ventilation distribution
    Bronchopleural fistula
    Bronchopleural cutaneous fistula
    Giant unilateral lung cyst; bullous emphysema
    Tracheobronchial trauma; rupture; tears
  Unilateral bronchopulmonary lavage
    Pulmonary alveolar proteinosis
Relative
  Surgical exposure—high priority
    Thoracic aortic aneurysm
    Pneumonectomy
  Surgical exposure—low priority
    Esophageal resection
    Lobectomy—upper
    Segmental resection
  Occluding pulmonary emboli
Miscellaneous
  Treatment of refractory atelectasis

Modified from Kaplan, J.A.: Thoracic Anesthesia. New York, Churchill Livingstone, 1983.

7. Level of anesthesia can be maintained even while the diseased lung is being suctioned.
8. Some hypoxia occurs on the basis of venous admixture. Because the occluded lung will have no ventilation but will still have some perfusion, this unoxygenated blood will mix with that from the opposite side and the result will be blood with lowered O_2 content.

ANATOMIC PRINCIPLES. For successful performance of endobronchial intubation, the operator must have knowledge of normal bronchial anatomy and an awareness of anatomic deformities due to pathology. Chest roentgenograms should be studied for tracheal deviation and mediastinal shift, especially in presence of atelectasis or pneumothorax.

Generally, the distance along the right bronchus from the carina to the first branch is quite small, and introduction of a tube into the right stem bronchus will occlude the right eparterial bronchus. Intubation of the left bronchus does not present a similar difficulty (Fig. 22–2).

Some anatomic measurements of importance in this procedure are as follows:

1. Distance along the right main stem bronchus from carina to the first bronchial branch
  Mean 1.5 cm
  Range 0.5–2.5 cm
2. Distance along the left main stem bronchus from carina to the first bronchial branch
  Mean 5 cm
  Range 4–6 cm

Preparation of a patient for endobronchial intubation requires heavy atropinization. Intubation is

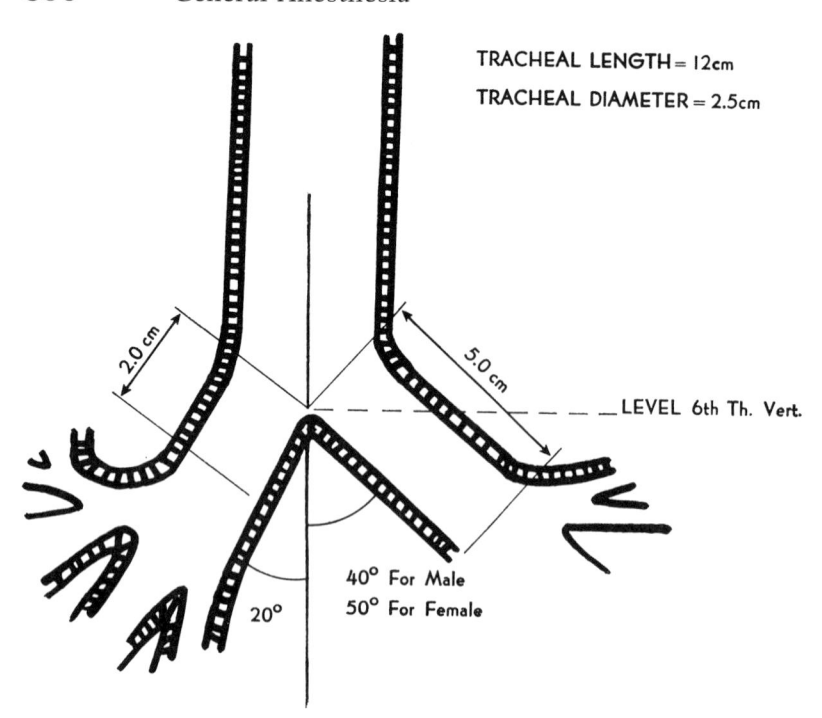

FIG. 22–2. Anatomy of main stem bronchi. The left main stem is long enough to permit insertion of a tube with inflatable cuff without obstructing upper lobe bronchus. Tracheal length is 12 cm; tracheal diameter is 2.5 cm.

performed during deep anesthesia or following thorough topical anesthesia. The technique of transtracheal cocainization of the tracheobronchial tree is suitable to the latter.

After intubation of the bronchus, auscultation of the chest will reveal the correctness of intubation. Care must be exercised in positioning the patient to avoid displacement of the tube.

CLASSIFICATION OF TECHNIQUES. The techniques of endobronchial intubation are related to the design of tubes used to achieve the primary objectives of endobronchial intubation: to seal off a diseased lung from the healthy lung and to provide one-lung ventilation for surgical purposes (Table 22–2).

1. Single-lumen endobronchial techniques
   a. Blind
      (1) With Magill balloon-tipped blocker
      (2) Rovenstine double-cuffed long endotracheal tube
      (3) Bonica standard Magill long tube with one cuff
   b. Direct visual placement into bronchus using a rigid small bronchoscope or a fiberoptic bronchoscope inside a long (36-cm) endotracheal tube
2. Double-lumen catheter method
   a. Carlens catheter intubation
   b. Robertshaw-type catheter (Robertshaw; National; Rusch)
3. Awake bronchial intubation with long (30-cm) standard endotracheal tube; may have value in an emergency[6]

Of the single-lumen endobronchial techniques, the Magill tube with a balloon-tipped blocker and the Rovenstine double-cuffed tube, developed out of designs by Gale and Waters, are of historical interest.

Of the techniques developed since 1936, only the double-lumen endobronchial method has become the standard of practice. Discussion is thus limited to the classical bronchial intubation with the Carlens catheter (with hook) and with the Robertshaw-type endobronchial tube (Robertshaw tube and Broncho-Cath [National Catheter Corporation]).

PRELIMINARY PREPARATION. All equipment needed for endobronchial intubation is prepared and checked.

- Cuffs should be tested by inflation while under water and observed for leaks and then deflated.
- Connections should be available and checked (Carlens or Cobb connectors).
- Two sizes of endobronchial tubes should be available.
- A Macintosh-type laryngoscope with two sizes of curved blades is recommended, because it provides maximum exposure of the orolaryngeal airway and the widest space for introduction of the endobronchial tube.
- A malleable stylet may be inserted properly to the tip of the tube.
- Tubes should be well lubricated. A lubricant with a potent topical anesthetic, such as tetracaine or Nupercainal ointment, is first applied in a thin coat. A water-soluble jelly is then applied.

TABLE 22–2. ENDOBRONCHIAL TUBES

Magill endotracheal tube and the Magill bronchial balloon blocker (1936)
Single-lumen endobronchial tubes
- Gale and Waters (1932)[1]
- Magill endobronchial tube with bronchial cuff and no tracheal cuff (1936)[2]
- Rovenstine's double-cuffed endotracheal tube (1936): one tracheal cuff; one endobronchial cuff[3]
- Macintosh-Leatherdale left-sided tube for right thoracotomy (1955)[9a]
- Macintosh-Leatherdale with right side port and left bronchial blocker for left thoracotomy (1956)[9a]
- Gordon-Green right-sided tube (1957) with modified cuff[9b]
- Use of long endotracheal tube technique (1952)[6]

Double-lumen endobronchial tubes (four types):
- Carlens catheter—left-sided intubation (1949),[7] used principally for right thoracotomy but can be used for left thoracotomy by occluding the inlet to the left lumen
- White catheter, right sided (1960)[9c]
- Bryce-Smith catheter, right and left sided (1959)[9c,9d]
- Robertshaw type, right and left sided (1962),[14] and Broncho-Cath (1983)[10b]

SELECTION OF TUBE. The selection of a proper-sided tube is dictated by the surgical requirements and the disease condition.

For operations on the right lung, ventilation of this lung is not required (the lung is isolated), while the left lung must be ventilated; therefore, a left-sided double-lumen tube is used to intubate the left stem bronchus and is the most commonly used tube for right thoracic surgery.

For operations on the left lung, which will not require ventilation while the right lung is ventilated, a right-sided double-lumen endobronchial tube is used. Intubation of the right stem bronchus with a right-sided tube, however, carries the risk of obstruction of the right epiarterial bronchus and incomplete ventilation in the right upper lobe, particularly the apical segments. To avoid this risk, the left-sided tube can be used and provides equally satisfactory conditions for maintaining ventilation.

Use of Left-Sided Endobronchial Tube For Left-Sided Surgery. The left-sided double-lumen endobronchial tube of the Robertshaw type can be used for left lung surgery and left thoracic surgery. An important caution is to withdraw the endobronchial tube into a tracheal position if clamping or ligation of the left main stem bronchus is surgically necessary, as in pneumonectomy.[10a,10b]

Contraindication. In the presence of pathologic conditions at or around the left-sided proximal portion of the left main stem bronchus or carinal lesions encroaching on the stem bronchus, a left-sided tube for left-sided surgery is contraindicated.

SIZE OF TUBE (Table 22–3). For female adult patients, the Carlens tube of French catheter gauges No. 35 or 37 (external diameter [ED] 11 and 13 mm), the medium-sized Robertshaw and/or the Broncho-Cath French sizes 35 or 37 are selected.

For adult male patients, the Carlens tube in sizes 39 and 41 French, the Robertshaw large-sized tube and the Broncho-Cath french sizes 39 or 41 (ED 14 and 16 mm) are usually used. However, the medium-sized Robertshaw will be satisfactory in a majority of males and is technically easier to use.

For adolescents, the No. 35 French Carlens tube or the small Robertshaw tube is chosen. For smaller children, a small French-28 catheter is available.

ANESTHESIA CONSIDERATIONS. Topical anesthesia of the upper airway and laryngobronchial passages, as for bronchoscopy, is complete. The customary anesthesia is induced intravenously and established with a narcotic or volatile agent. The patient is then completely paralyzed (it is recommended that there be few or no twitches following tetanic stimulation (vecuronium is preferred)).

ENDOBRONCHIAL INTUBATION PROCEDURE. It is helpful to consider that with all the endobronchial tubes, the technical procedure of intubation is accomplished in three steps: (1) insertion through the vocal cords, (2) advancement in the trachea toward the carina, and (3) insertion into a stem bronchus.

BLIND ENDOBRONCHIAL TECHNIQUE WITH THE SINGLE-LUMEN LONG ENDOTRACHEAL TUBE. Either bronchus can be successfully intubated blindly, but there are slight variations of technique that must be observed. The tube employed is a standard rubber Magill tube in its original length as supplied by the manufacturer. This may be 36 to 42 cm. For the left bronchus the bevel should face the left when the tube is held in position. For the right bronchus the bevel should face toward the right and in addition should be further cut so that a longer lip is produced and the bevel opening is about 3 cm long.

Right Bronchial Intubation. Performing right bronchial intubation is relatively easy. Obstruction of the right eparterial bronchus must be avoided. The long bevel tube described above accomplishes this goal. The tube is well lubricated with an anesthetic ointment. Introduction into the trachea is accomplished under vision with a laryngoscope. Advancement is performed with the tube in the midline or slightly rotated so that the convexity is just to the left of the midline. When the tip enters the right bronchus, some resistance is encountered. After checking the position of the tube, the cuff is inflated and should effectively seal the right lung from the opposite side.

Left Bronchial Intubation. The tube with left-sided bevel is introduced by aid of the laryngoscope into the trachea. The catheter is rotated counterclockwise so that the convexity is to the right and the

TABLE 22-3. DOUBLE-LUMEN ENDOBRONCHIAL CATHETERS

Tube	Date	Construction	Size (French Gauge)	Problems
Carlens	1949	Red rubber	35, 37, 39, 41	Left only; low-compliant cuff
White	1960	Red rubber, molded bonded cuff; right side; cuff slotted for ventilation of right upper lobe	37, 39, 41	Equivalent to Carlens; difficult to place; the "carinal hook" or lip slips
Robertshaw	1962	Red rubber, extruded, bonded cuff; right cuff slotted	Small, medium, large	For both right and left intubation; low-compliant cuff; ED/ID ratio high (thick-walled)
Broncho-Cath	1978	Polyvinylchloride	35, 37, 39, 41	No right-sided catheter; kinks (rotates) easily; high-pressure cuff when overinflated.

Modified from Kaplan, J.A.: Thoracic Anesthesia. New York, Churchill Livingstone, 1983.

concavity is to the left. The tip of the catheter and the bevel will now slide down the left wall of the trachea and enters the bronchus. Further advancement causes the tube to jam into the left lower lobe bronchus. It should be slightly withdrawn and the catheter rotated back into a midline position with the bevel facing the left lateral (Fig. 22-3).

CARLENS CATHETER TECHNIQUE

Description of Carlens Catheter. The double-lumen catheter originally constructed by Carlens for bronchospirometry (Fig. 22-4) has been adapted to anesthesia practice.[7] The catheter is designed for left-sided endobronchial intubation. This catheter is made of rubber and is obtainable in four sizes. The lumen of each side of the catheter has a diameter of 7 or 8 mm for men and 6 or 7 mm for women. The total EDs are 13 or 16 and 11 or 12 mm, respectively (Fig. 22-5). The cross-section of each lumen is D-shaped. The lumina are side by side, forming a double-D mirror image in cross-section. The long portion of the tube, the bronchial luminal side, enters the left bronchus. An opening on the right side of the tube above the bronchial tip, the terminal part of the right lumen or tracheal limb, provides mainstream ventilatory access to the right stem bronchus and right lung.

Procedure for Carlens Catheter Intubation.[8] Anesthesia in the operating room is usually general, and the tube is introduced under vision. The Macintosh laryngoscope is the most satisfactory. A straight metal stylet in the tube is desirable. The rubber carinal hook is tied close to the catheter with a moistened silk thread in a slipknot. This facilitates introduction through the glottis, which is accomplished by a slight rotating movement to the right, so that the hook is toward the posterior commissure.

A right opening in the tube is essentially in the trachea, faces the right stem, and provides access to the right stem. Two cuffs are present: one on the long bronchial tube extension and a tracheal cuff above the right side opening of the tracheal part.

The catheter then moves through the glottis and

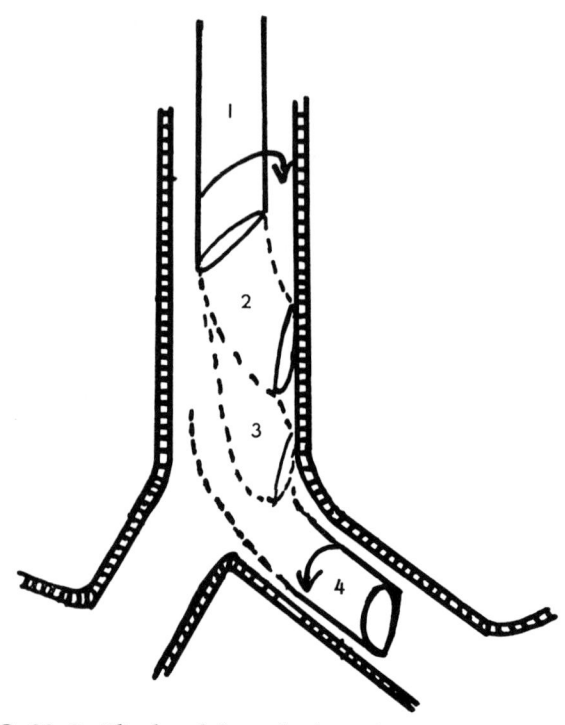

FIG. 22-3. Blind endobronchial intubation. Steps 1-4 show the advancement of the tube into the left bronchus. Note rotation in steps 1 and 4.

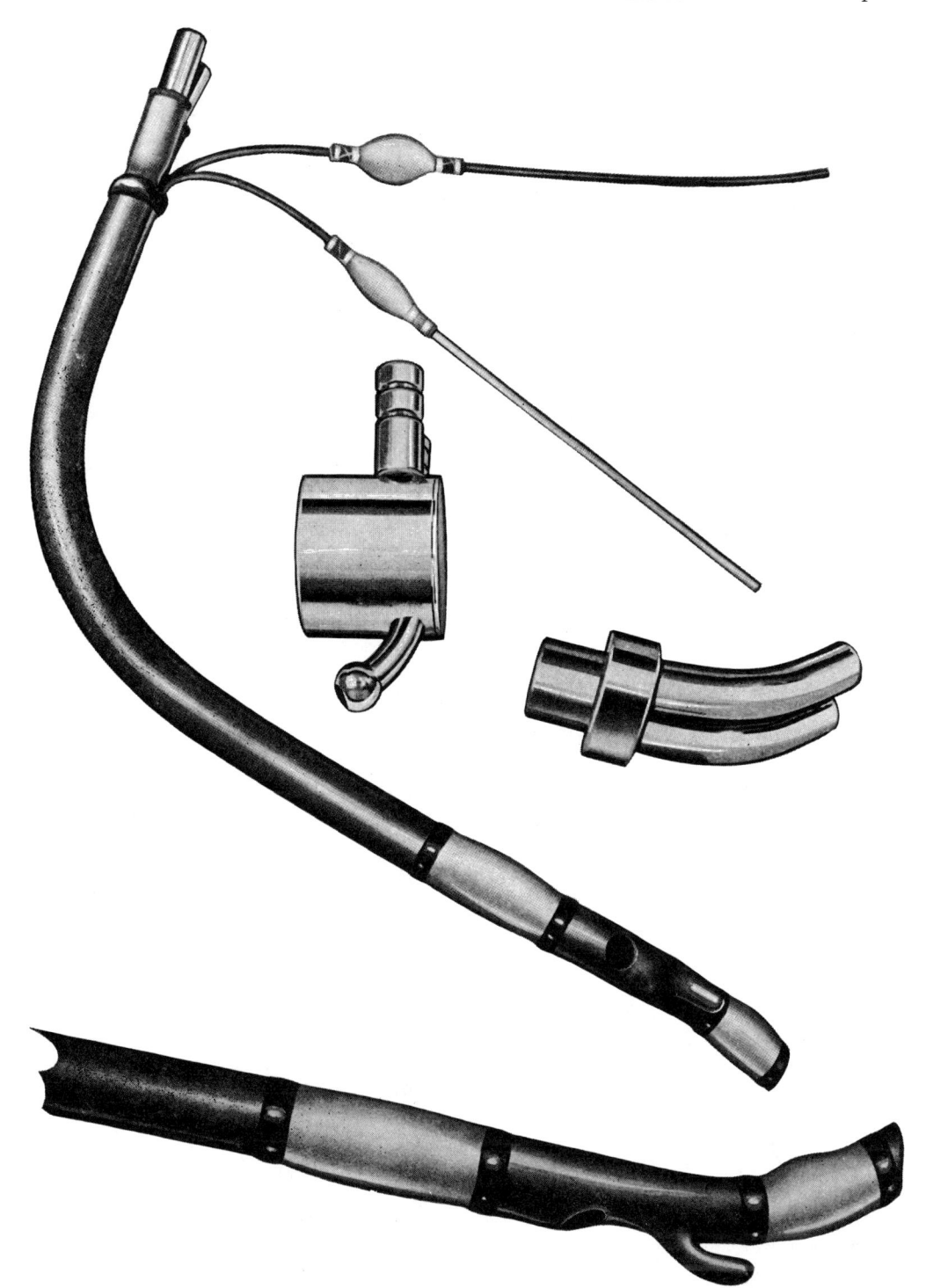

FIG. 22–4. Carlens double-lumen intrabronchial catheter, showing complete tube with adapter in position, standard adapter with slip joint connection, and 15-mm connector. *Lower*, close-up of catheter tip with carinal hook. (Courtesy of the Foregger Company.)

down the trachea. It tends to turn toward the left and the stylet should be removed at this time. During the period of advancement, the tip of the catheter can be felt to exert slight pressure on the tracheal wall. As the tip approaches the left bronchus, the sensation of resistance disappears. Further advancement of a few millimeters enables the operator to feel the hook engage the carina. By gentle pressure, this engagement can be made firm and the cuffs are then inflated. The pressure should be just

604 General Anesthesia

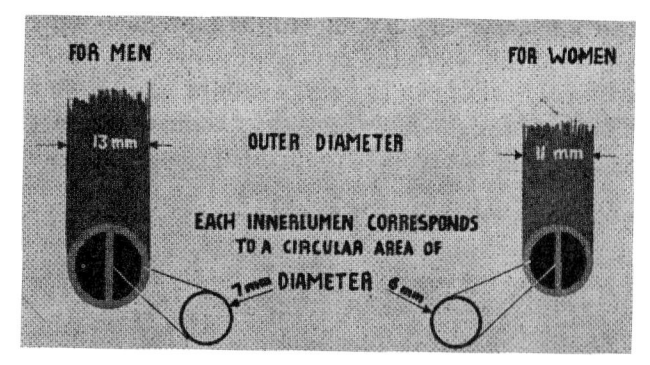

FIG. 22–5. Diagram of cross-sections of the double-lumen catheters. The catheter is made of rubber in four sizes. From Björk, V.O., Carlens, E., and Friberg, O.: Endobronchial anesthesia. Anesthesiology, *14*:60, 1953.

sufficient to prevent leakage. The catheter is maintained in the correct position by the hook and by the inflated cuffs (Fig. 22–6).

WHITE DOUBLE-LUMEN ENDOBRONCHIAL CATHETER[9c] **(Fig. 2–7).** This endobronchial catheter with a carinal hook was designed to be used for intubation of the right bronchus and so supplements the left sided Carlens tube. The bronchial cuff is identical to that of the right-sided Robertshaw bronchial tube.[10b]

The technique of intubation follows the procedure for Carlens tube intubation[8] or the El-Etr alternative

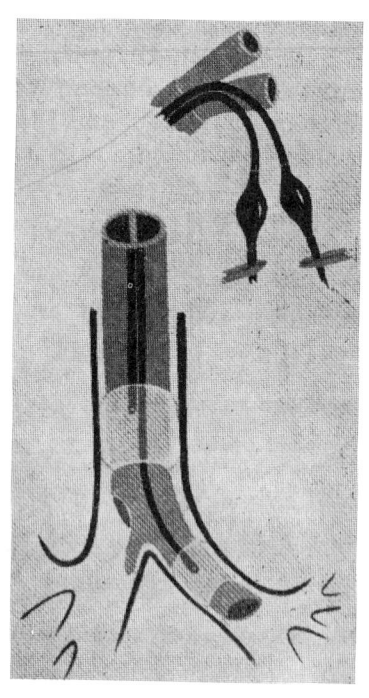

FIG. 22–6. The double-lumen catheter in place. Note the rubber hook engaging the carina. From Björk, V.O., Carlens, E., and Friberg, O.: Endobronchial anesthesia. Anesthesiology, *14*:60, 1953.

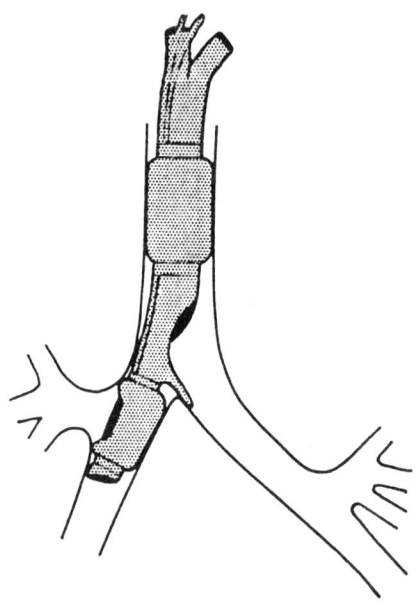

FIG. 22–7. White double-lumen endobronchial tube. From Kaplan, J.A.: Thoracic Anesthesia. New York: Churchill Livingstone, 1983.

technique[12] for insertion through the vocal cords (see following discussion).

ALTERNATIVE INSERTION. Double-lumen endobronchial tubes with carinal hooks (Carlens; White) can be inserted into the trachea without first tying the hook to the tube by a slip knot. This is accomplished as follows (Fig. 22–8):[12]

- The tube tip only is first inserted through the vocal cords with the hook facing posteriorly under laryngoscopic vision.
- After the tip passes through the vocal cords, the tube is rotated (clockwise) 180 degrees and advanced through the vocal cords with a rotary motion, so that the hook faces anteriorly and the tube and hook area becomes positioned below the cords.
- Once through the vocal cords, the tube is rotated an additional 90 degrees so that the hook faces laterally.
- Advancement of the tube will place the tube in the appropriate left bronchus and then allow the hook to engage the carina.

DESCRIPTION OF THE ROBERTSHAW ENDOBRONCHIAL TUBE (Fig. 22–9).[14] The Robertshaw tube is the most commonly used double-lumen tube. The lumina are D-shaped, placed side by side, and designed for the largest possible lumen to facilitate suctioning and reduce resistance to air flow. Both left-sided and right-sided tubes are available; they are constructed with two curves 90 degrees apart and no carinal hook. These tubes are relatively inexpensive and may be reused.

FIG. 22–8. The alternate technique of insertion of the Carlens double-lumen tube. The tip is passed through the vocal cords and then rotated 180 degrees to the right. When the hook passes through the larynx, the tube is rotated a further 90 degrees to the right for placement on the carina. From El-Etr, A.A.: Improved technique for insertion of the Carlens catheter. Anesth. Analg. (Cleve), *48*:738, 1969.

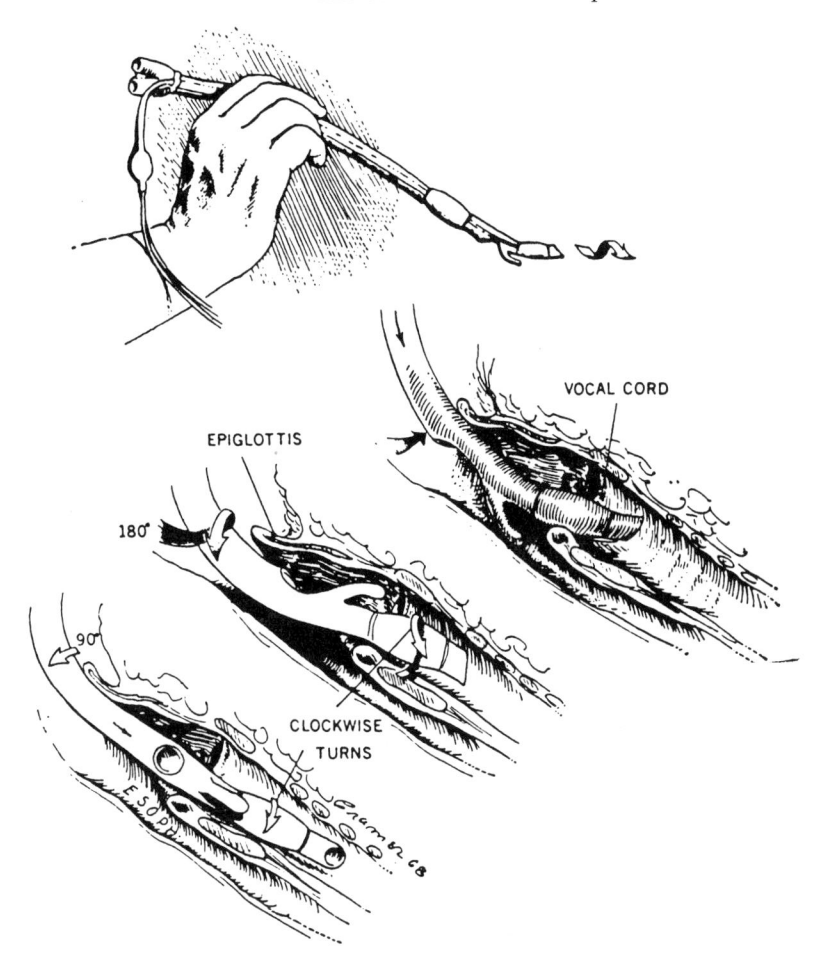

Left Endobronchial Tube. In viewing the concavity of the left-sided tube from above, it is noted that the tip curves to the left. This is the long part of the tube and contains the bronchial lumen. It is fitted with a small cuff known as the *bronchial cuff.* A second cuff, the *tracheal cuff,* surrounds the entire tube and is situated more proximally. The tip of the tube, which enters the left bronchus, is angled to the left from the main tracheal shaft by 45 degrees. Between the two cuffs is an opening in the right side of the tube where the right lumen terminates.

Right Endobronchial Tube. In viewing the concavity of the right-sided Robertshaw endobronchial tube from above, the tip of the tube is seen to curve to the right by about 30 degrees. To this tip is attached the right endobronchial cuff, with a slot facing laterally to allow inflation of the right upper lobe with minimal upper lobe occlusion and with a wide zone of inflation above and around the slot for a more reliable seal. Thus, the right lumen terminates both at the side port (slot) to the upper lobe and at the tip for ventilation of the middle and lower lobes. A second cuff—the tracheal cuff—is located more proximally on the tube and surrounds the entire tube.

Accurate placement of this tube is necessary. The risk of inadequate ventilation of the right upper lobes is still present and, in practice, the left-sided Robertshaw tube is often used in left thoracic surgery, as well as for right thoracic surgery.[10a]

DESCRIPTION OF BRONCHO-CATH DOUBLE-LUMEN TUBE (Fig. 22–10). The Broncho-Cath tube is essentially the same as the classic Robertshaw tube, with some refinements. Intubation of the stem bronchi with this tube is the same. The following are features of the Broncho-Cath:

- Recommended for single use
- No carinal hook
- For left or right main stem bronchial intubation
- Material is clear polyvinylchloride
- The lumina are D-shaped and side by side
- Cuffs are thin-walled, with low pressure characteristics
- Color coded (blue) for bronchial lumen (main stem) tubes
- Sizes French 35 and 37 (for females); 39 and 41 (for males)
- A smaller size (French 28) is available for children
- Radiopaque markers are located:
  On *left-sided tube,* one marker encircling tube above bronchial cuff (4 cm from distal tip)

606 General Anesthesia

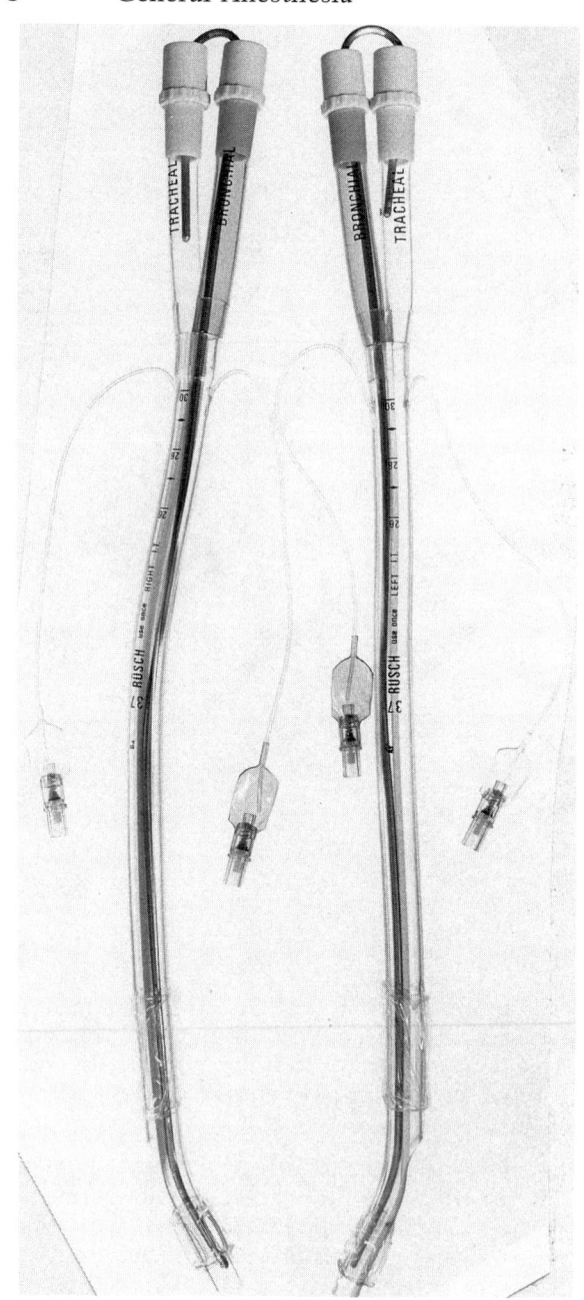

FIG. 22–9. Robertshaw double-lumen endobronchial tubes. Clear plastic construction of polyvinylchloride by Rusch. Left-sided tube (*left*) and right-sided (*right*).

On right-sided tube, two markers encircling the tube at the upper end of the cuff 2 cm from the eye and encircling the eye or slot of the bronchial segment.

PROCEDURE—ROBERTSHAW-TYPE TUBE. The Robertshaw tube is the most commonly used endobronchial tube.[10,10b,11b] Bronchial intubation with the left-lung endobronchial tube is accomplished easily. The tube can be introduced without a stylet as follows:

1. Insertion through vocal cords
   a. Pass the tube with the distal curve or tip facing anteriorly (concave anteriorly). The proximal curve or concavity of the shaft faces to the right (Fig. 22–11).
   b. When the tip passes the larynx, it is rotated 90 degrees to the left, i.e., counterclockwise, so that the tip faces the left wall of the trachea; the proximal curve or shaft of the tube is now concave anteriorly.
2. Advancement in the trachea
   a. The tip slips along the tracheal wall with minimal resistance until most of the tube has been introduced.
3. Insertion into stem bronchus
   a. When moderate resistance to further advancement is encountered, the tip is in the stem bronchus. Occasionally, a flip or loss of resistance may be experienced as the tube enters the stem bronchus, when further advancement meets with significant resistance and the tube is now firmly seated.

Principle. Throughout the procedure of endobronchial intubation, laryngoscopy with the Macintosh blade should be continued until the tube is considered in the proper bronchus. This is necessary so that the proximal part of the tube can be advanced through the upper airway passages with some degree of ease.

Insertion of Right-Sided Tube. For insertion of a right-sided tube into the right stem bronchus, the only difference in technique is related to the passage through the vocal cords when a stylet is not used. Again, the principle is that the tip of the tube should face anteriorly and the distal curve be concave anteriorly. This means that the proximal end of the tube should be to the operator's left and the curve of the shaft be concave to the left. When the tip passes through the glottis, it is now rotated about 90 degrees to the right, or clockwise, so that the tip faces the right tracheal wall.

Alternative Procedure With Use of Stylet. A malleable stylet may be used and is inserted into the bronchial lumen of the double-lumen catheter. It should be well lubricated and molded so that the tip of either the left or right endobronchial tube is shaped to face anteriorly, but in the same curvature of the concavity of the shaft.

Once the tip of the tube has passed through the vocal cords, the stylet is immediately removed. Unless the stylet is lubricated with a thin coat of an ointment or gel, it will be difficult to remove.

Awake Intubation. The Carlens catheter may also be introduced under good topical anesthesia while the patient is conscious (see awake endotracheal intubation for topical anesthesia procedure, Chapter 20). Position and technique are the same as de-

FIG. 22–10. Right- and left-sided Robertshaw double-lumen endobronchial tubes are shown. *A* and *C* show a picture and a schematic of a right-sided tube and *B* and *D* a picture and schematic of a left-sided tube. From Kaplan, J.A.: Thoracic Anesthesia. New York, Churchill Livingstone, 1983.

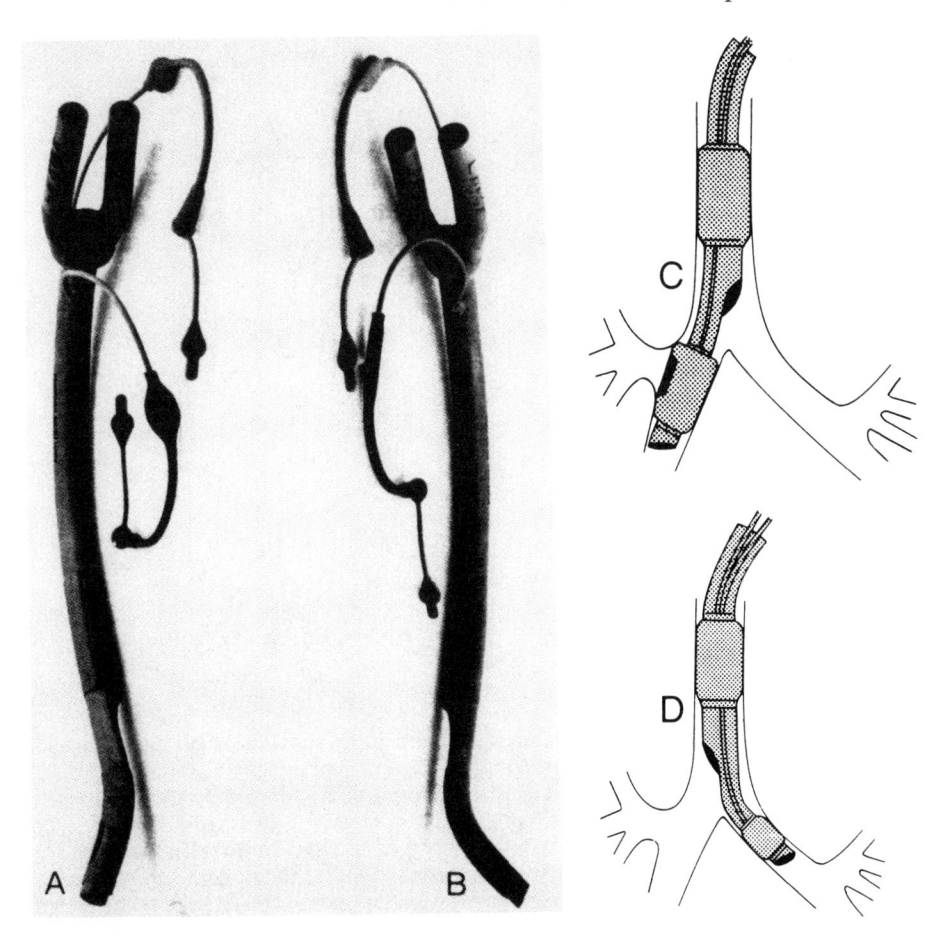

scribed above for introduction during general anesthesia. In the clinic, the catheter may be introduced while patients are sitting with their head forward in the "sniffing attitude." Visualization is accomplished by indirect mirror laryngoscopy while a curved stylet is employed.

Once the catheter is in situ, it is possible to apply suction and administer anesthesia to each lung separately.

Connector. A special connector must be fitted to the proximal end of double-lumen endotracheal tubes and then attached to the anesthesia breathing circuit. The Cobb-type connector (Fig. 22–12) is commonly used. This allows the following procedures:

- Diversion of anesthetic gases from bilateral to unilateral lung ventilation
- Each lumen to be opened alternately to the atmosphere.
- Each lung to be opened to continuous positive airway pressure or to be ventilated separately
- Introduction of suction catheters selectively to each lung

Selection of Side to Intubate. Intubation of the nonoperative stem bronchus or the dependent lung in the lateral position is usual and advised. When using the double-lumen endobronchial tubes, intubation of the stem bronchus of the lung to be operated on, which is usually uppermost in the lateral position, may result in poor function of the tubes. Kaplan[10b] has identified the following difficulties if the operative lung stem bronchus is intubated:

- Displacement of the bronchial limb of the tube by mediastinal compression or surgical manipulation
- Intermittent occlusion of the tracheal lumen against the most dependent lateral tracheal wall to cause a ball-valve obstruction to gas flow. This may cause wheezing, prolonged expiratory flow, and hypercarbia.

POSTINTUBATION MANAGEMENT

CHECKING THE TUBE POSITION.[13] To assure proper positioning of the endobronchial tube and functional separation of the two lungs, a set procedure should be followed as the cuffs are sequentially inflated and deflated and lung ventilation tested by positive pressure. The proximal bronchial and tracheal limbs of the tube should be alternately clamped and one-lung ventilation confirmed.

The clinical methods used to assess the tube position consist of:

608 *General Anesthesia*

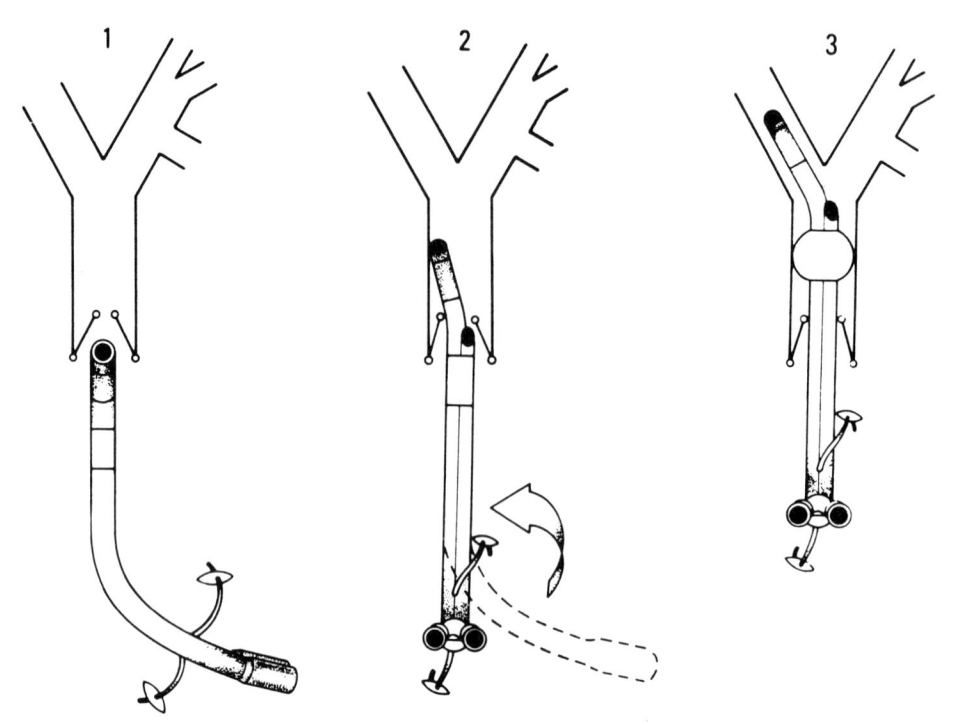

FIG. 22–11. Schematic diagram of the passage of the left lung Robertshaw tube. The distal curvature should be concave anteriorly initially (as tube tip advances through glottis), and the proximal curve should be off to the right and parallel to the floor (in the supine patient). After the tube tip passes the vocal cords, the entire tube should be rotated 90 degrees so that the proximal curvature is now concave anteriorly and the distal curvature is off to the left and parallel to the floor. The tube should be pushed in until a moderate resistance to further passage is encountered and most of the tube is inside the mouth (close to the parting of the individual lumens from the common molding). From Kaplan, J.A.: Thoracic Anesthesia. New York, Churchill Livingstone, 1983.

- Visual inspection of chest wall motion,
- Auscultation of the chest at the different times when the two cuffs are alternately inflated and deflated,
- Auscultation of the chest at times that the tracheal and bronchial lumina are alternately clamped.

Confirmation of tracheal and endobronchial position can be obtained by fiberoptic endoscopy. This has become a routine procedure as a check. Radiographic evidence may also be obtained.

Primary objectives in checking the position of the tube are the following:

1. To check proper tracheal placement and function of the tracheal cuff
2. The check endobronchial position and function of the bronchial cuff
3. To be able to ventilate each lung independently and to isolate one lung from the other

Cuffs should be inflated slowly. The bronchial cuffs are relatively small-volume cuffs, especially the left main stem bronchial cuff; no more than 3 to 5 ml of air should be used for inflation.

After placement of the double-lumen tube is the usual blind fashion, the tracheal and bronchial cuffs are inflated sequentially and the limbs of the endobronchial tube are occluded according to one of two techniques:

1. *Classic Technique (minimal leak; sequential inflation of cuffs)*[13–15]
   a. Tracheal cuff inflation (first). Ventilation through the double-lumen limbs should now permit bilateral lung expansion; confirm by inspection of the chest wall and by auscultation. If not, withdraw 2 to 3 cm and repeat (Fig. 22–13A).
   b. The tracheal limb of the catheter is then clamped and the tracheal cuff deflated. Ventilation through the endobronchial limb of the catheter is continued and leaks observed.
   c. The endobronchial cuff is then inflated (second) with sufficient air, usually 1 to 3 ml, to prevent leaks. With left-sided endobronchial tubes, only the left lung fields should now expand and reveal unilateral breath sounds (Fig. 22–13B).
   d. The tracheal limb is now unclamped and the

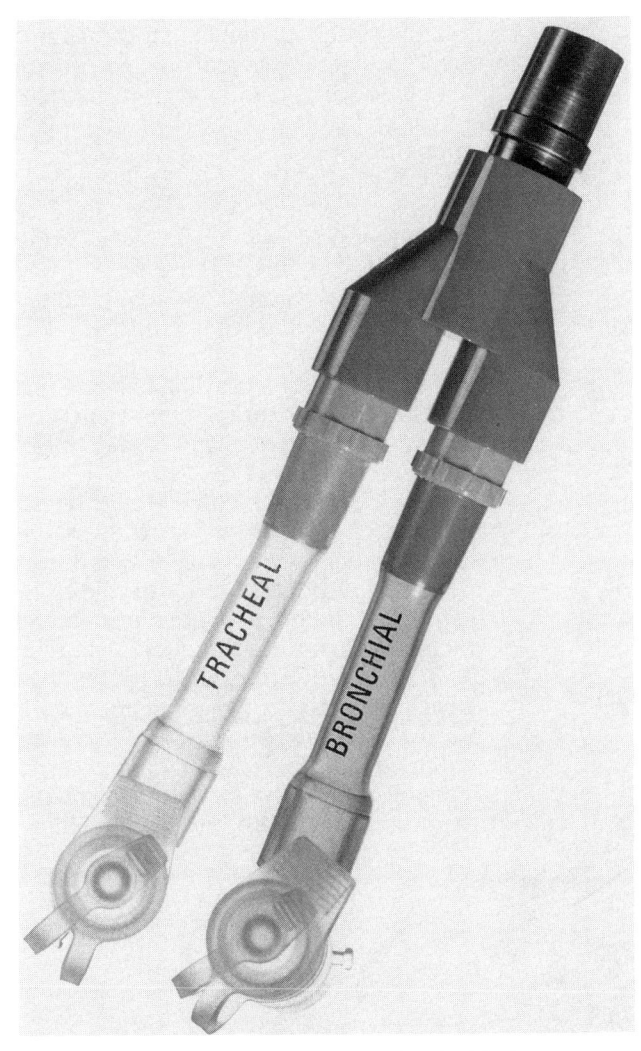

FIG. 22–12. Cobb-type connector for double-lumen endobronchial tubes.

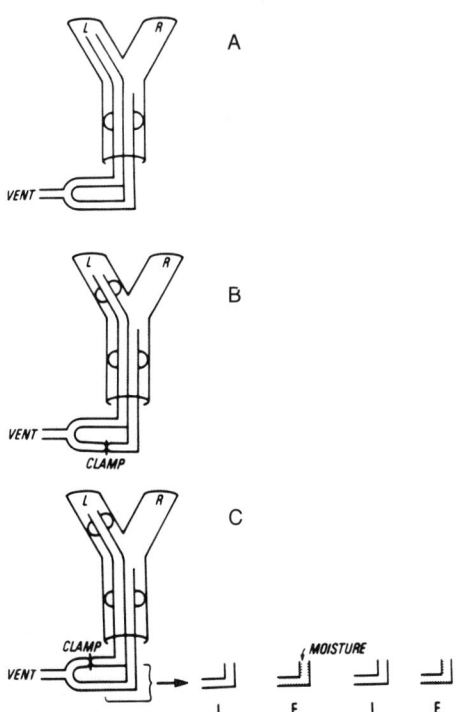

FIG. 22–13. Schematic representation of one technique to ensure proper functioning of a left-sided double-lumen endotracheal tube. (A) Proper tracheal placement; 1. Inflate tracheal cuff. 2. Ventilate. 3. Both lungs should be ventilated. 4. If not, withdraw and repeat. (B) Proper functioning of left side; 1. Clamp tracheal limb and tracheal cuff. 2. Ventilate through bronchial limb and observe leaks. 3. Clamp bronchial cuff. 4. Only lung on intubated bronchial side should expand and reveal breath sounds. (C) Proper functioning of right side; 1. Clamp endobronchial limb. 2. Ventilate through the tracheal limb; only the lung on nonintubated bronchial stem should expand or reveal breath sounds. The bottom panel indicates that during inspiration, respiratory gas moisture disappears and during exhalation the clear plastic tubing of the double-lumen tube fills with respiratory gas moisture. Modified from Benumof, J.: Physiology of the open chest and one-lung anesthesia. In Thoracic Anesthesia. Edited by J. Kaplan. New York, Churchill Livingstone, 1983.

ability to inflate lungs reconfirmed. Further assurance of the position of the tube can be ascertained by clamping the endobronchial limb. Ventilation through the tracheal limb should permit expansion of right lung fields only with left side endobronchial tubes (Fig. 22–13C).

2. *Brodsky Technique (using sequential clamping of proximal luminal limbs).*[16]
   a. After endobronchial placement of left-sided endobronchial tube, *both* the tracheal and endobronchial cuffs are inflated—the tracheal cuff is inflated with 3 to 4 ml of air, while the endobronchial cuff is inflated with 1 to 3 ml of air. The patient is then ventilated and the following are noted:
      (1) Bilateral chest wall movement
      (2) Fogging of both lumens of the double-lumen catheter
      (3) Air sounds on auscultation over both lung fields
   b. To assure proper placement of the left-sided double-lumen catheter, the limbs of the tube are alternately clamped, while both cuffs remain inflated:
      (1) The tracheal (right) limb is occluded; with left side endobronchial intubation, breath sounds should be heard only on the left.
         - *Malpositions*
           - If sounds are heard over the right lung (lower lobes) only, while ventilating through the endobronchial (left) limb, the endobronchial lumen of the catheter is in the right bronchus. This is a frequent displacement (Fig. 22–14).
           - If breath sounds are heard on both sides,

clamped and the patient then ventilated through the right tracheal lumen. Breath sounds should be heard only over the right lung fields (Fig. 22-15).
  • *Malpositions*
    • If there is difficulty in ventilating and marked resistance to air flow, and if no breath sounds are heard over either lung fields, the tip of the tube is either in the trachea or has been advanced too deep into the left stem bronchus (Fig. 22–16).
    • In the latter deep situation, the tracheal cuff is over the right stem bronchus and partially (or entirely) in the left bronchus (see Fig. 22–16A).
    • The endobronchial cuff should be deflated: a) if the tip of the tube is too deep—breath sounds will be heard over the left lung fields and not on the right (Fig. 22–16B) and b) if the tip is in the trachea and the endobronchial cuff is deflated—ventilation through the tracheal limb will allow gas to enter both lungs and breath sounds will be heard on both sides (Fig. 22-17).
  • *Correction of Position.* To position the tube properly, deflate both cuffs. Under

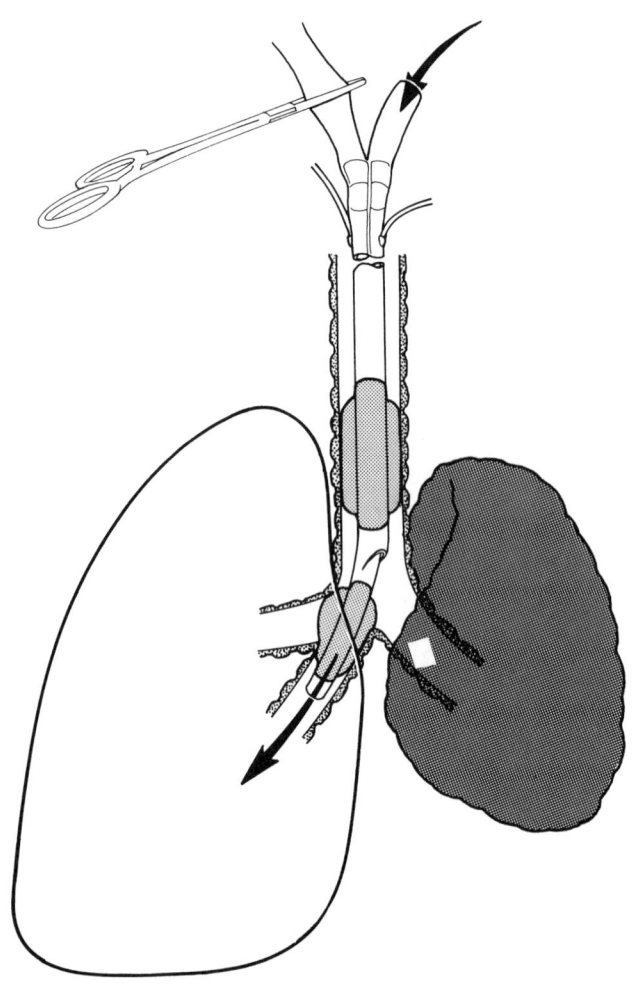

FIG. 22–14. Both the tracheal and endobronchial cuffs are inflated and the right (tracheal) lumen is occluded. If breath sounds are heard only over the right lung while ventilating through the left (endobronchial) lumen, a right endobronchial intubation has occurred. From Brodsky, J., and Marks, J.B.D.: A simple technique for accurate placement of double-lumen endobronchial tube. Anesthesiol. Rev., *10*:26, 1983.

while ventilating through the endobronchial tube, then the tip of the tube is above the carina.
  • *Correction of Position*
(1) When the diagnosis of intubation of the right bronchus with a left-sided endobronchial tube is made, both cuffs should be deflated and the tube withdrawn. Intubation of the left bronchus should now be again attempted.
(2) When the diagnosis of tube placement is that the bronchial limb is above the carina, both cuffs should be deflated and the tube advanced into the left bronchus.
(3) The endobronchial limb (left limb of left side endobronchial catheter) on the catheter mount of the double-lumen tube is

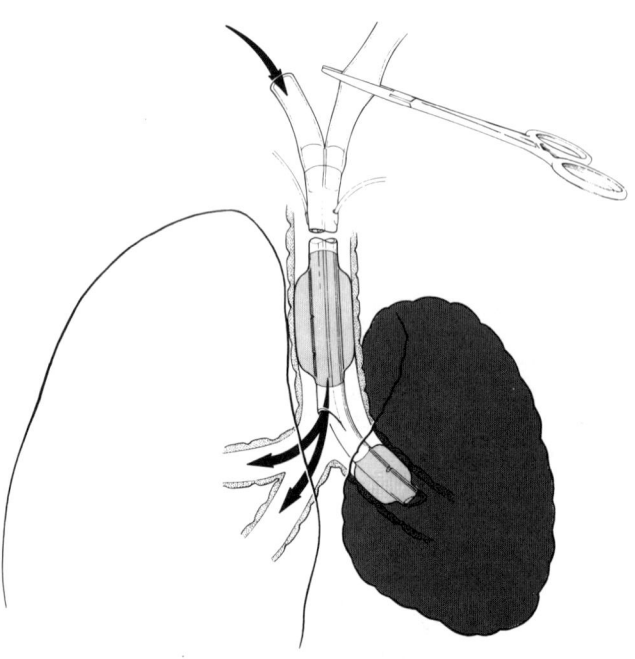

FIG. 22–15. Both the tracheal and endobronchial cuffs are inflated and the left (endobronchial) lumen is occluded. If breath sounds can only be heard over the right lung while ventilating through the right (tracheal) lumen, then the tube is in the correct position. From Brodsky, J., and Marks, J.B.D.: A simple technique for accurate placement of double-lumen endobronchial tube. Anesthesiol. Rev., *10*:26, 1983.

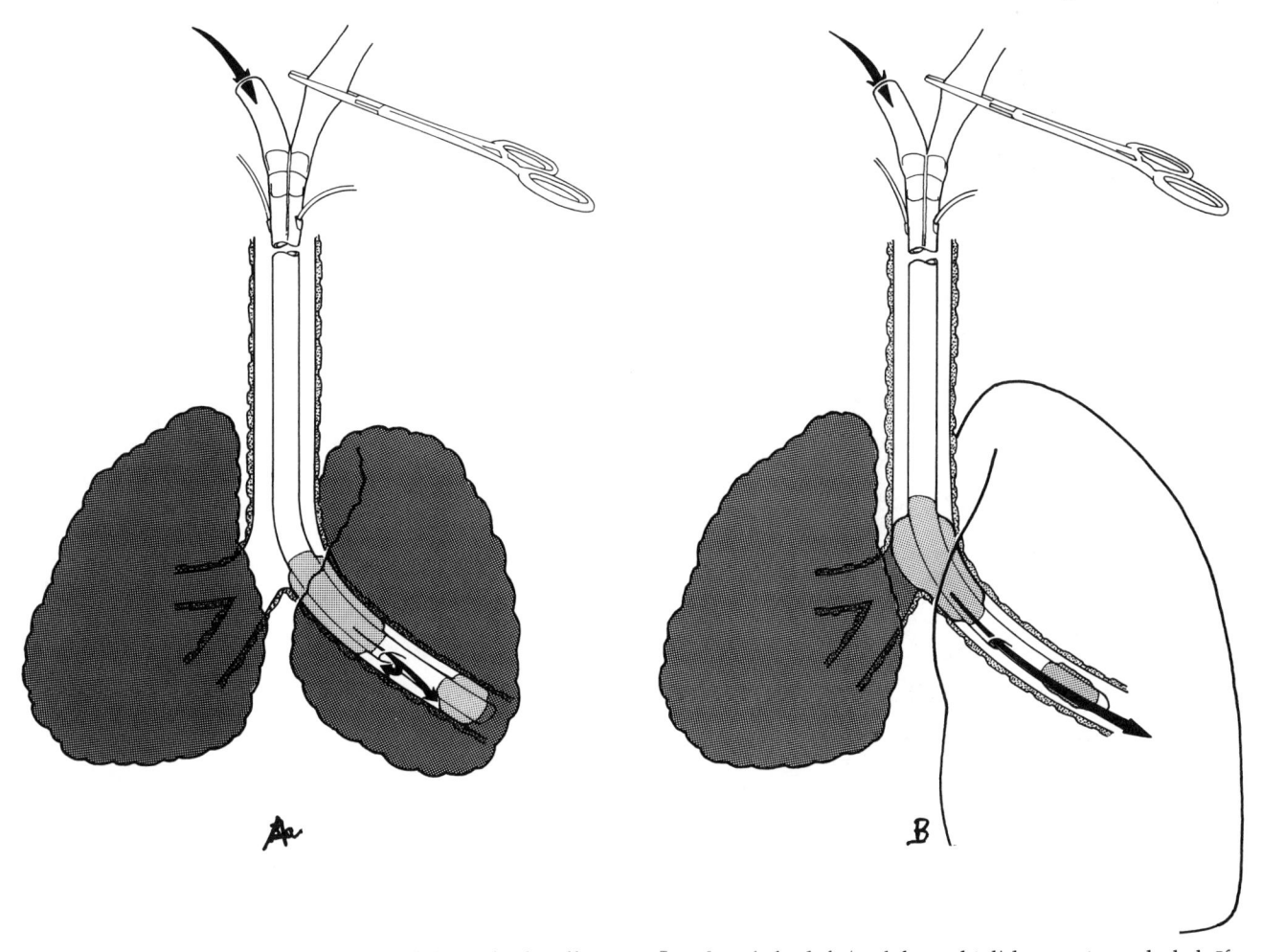

FIG. 22–16. Both the tracheal and endobronchial cuffs are inflated and the left (endobronchial) lumen is occluded. If you cannot ventilate through the right (tracheal) lumen (A) the endobronchial cuff is then deflated. If the tube is too deep, breath sounds will now be heard only over the left lung while ventilating through the right lumen (B). From Brodsky J., and Mark, J.B.D.: A simple technique for accurate placement of double-lumen endobronchial tube. Anesthesiol. Rev. 10:26, 1983.

the first condition, the tube should be advanced, while under the second condition, the tube should be withdrawn. After these maneuvers, both cuffs are reinflated and tests repeated according to the original procedure.

ERRORS IN PLACEMENT.[16,17] Clinical assessment of the position of double-lumen endobronchial tubes does not assure that the placement is correct. In the study by Smith[17], when flexible fiberoptic bronchoscopy (FFB) observations were made to determine tube position and patency, almost 50% were not in an optimal position. Among the complications, the following were noted:

1. The inabilty to visualize endobronchial cuff when making observations through the tracheal lumen by FFB. The tube had been advanced too far beyond the carina into the left stem bronchus (26%).
2. Failure to ventilate the left upper lobe. The tube had been advanced too far. FFB enabled the operator to withdraw the tube approximately 1 cm and permit left upper lobe ventilation.
3. Herniation of the bronchial cuff over the carina was noted in 17% of patients. This may cause the endobronchial lumen to slip out of the left stem to obstruct the unintubated bronchus, preventing ventilation or collapse of the right lung in right thoracotomy.
4. Narrowing of the bronchial lumen by pressure of the inflated cuff on the bronchial lumen.

Fiberoptic bronchoscopy allows accurate confirmation of the position of endotracheal tubes and facilitates repositioning.[18] It is recommended when double-lumen endobronchial tubes are used.

612   *General Anesthesia*

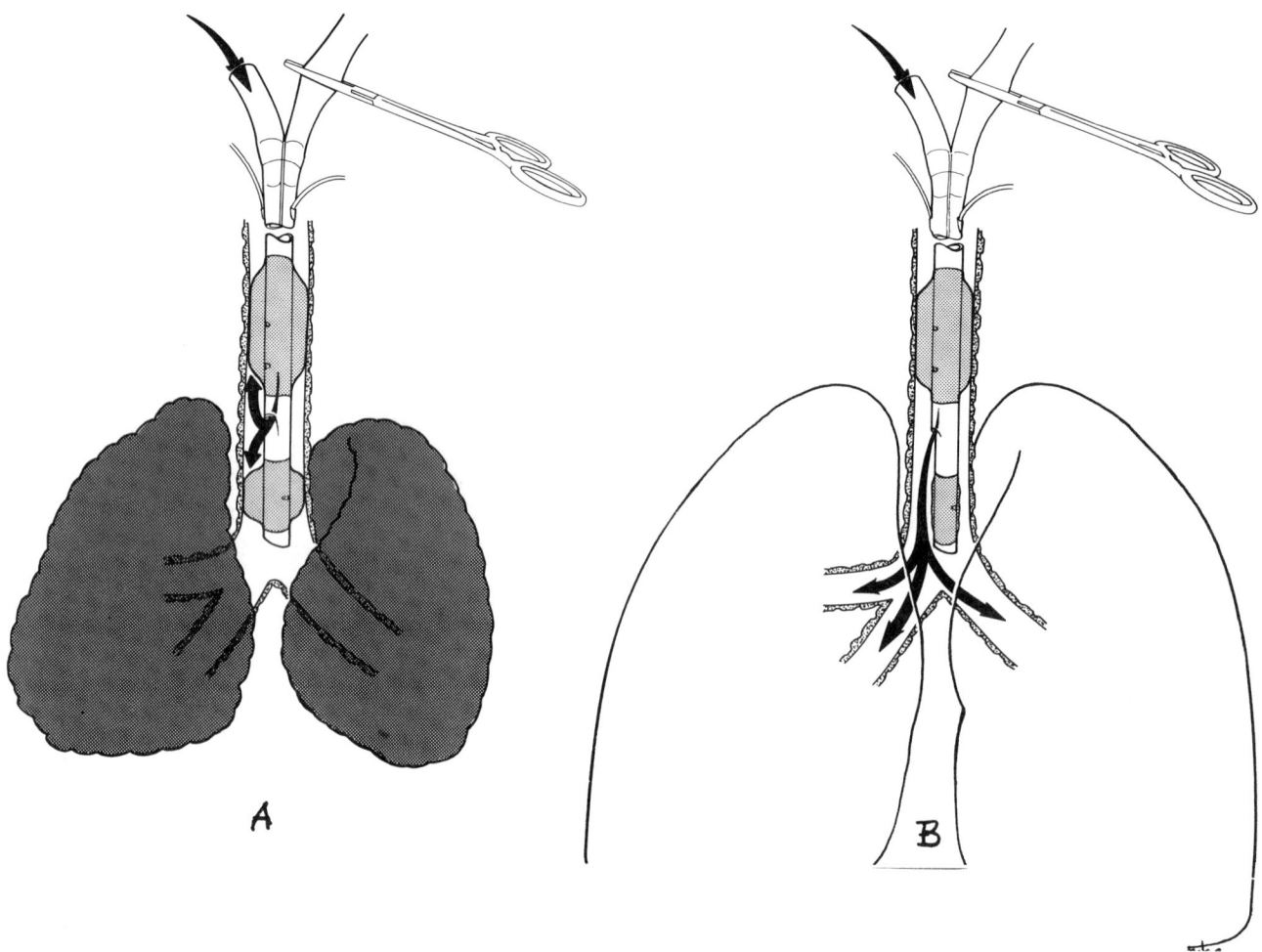

FIG. 22–17. Both the tracheal and endobronchial cuffs are inflated and the left (endobronchial) lumen is occluded. If you cannot ventilate through the right (tracheal) lumen (*A*), the endobronchial cuff is then deflated. If the tube is not far enough into the left bronchus, breath sounds will now be heard over both the right and left lungs while ventilating through the right lumen (*B*). Brodsky, J., and Marks, J.B.D.: A simple technique for accurate placement of double-lumen endobronchial tube. Anesthesiol. Rev., *10:*26, 1983.

USE OF FIBEROPTIC BRONCHOSCOPE. The FFB is useful to confirm the placement of an endobronchial tube after "blind" endobronchial intubation and to assist in the placement of endobronchial tubes.

Placement of Endobronchial Tube by FFB.[18] After endotracheal placement of the endobronchial tube, the FFB is introduced into the bronchial lumen of the double-lumen endobronchial catheter. The FFB is advanced into the left stem bronchus. The catheter is then guided over the FFB into the left stem bronchus. The FFB is removed and then inserted into the tracheal right lumen. The proximal edge of the bronchial cuff is visualized and is placed about 1 cm distal to the carina into the left bronchus. The FFB is removed and the cuffs inflated—first, the bronchial and second the tracheal—using the minimal leak technique. Isolation of the lungs is then checked by the technique of alternate clamping of the right and left lumens at the catheter mount.

MANAGEMENT OF VENTILATION DURING SURGERY[11a,11b]

The following is an outline of ventilatory management during thoracic surgery when the endobronchial tube is properly placed and the patient properly positioned on the operating table. Care must be taken in moving a patient from the supine to the lateral position. Flexion or extension of the head must be avoided, otherwise the endobronchial tube may be easily displaced. The placement of the tube must be checked again once the surgical positioning is completed.

1. Both lungs should be ventilated until the pleural cavity on the surgical side of the chest is about to be entered.
2. At this point, the proximal limb of the tube's lumen to the operated side is occluded and ventilation of the unoperated side alone is continued.
3. Begin one-lung ventilation with a tidal volume of 10 ml/kg of body weight and adjust later after obtaining blood gases.
4. Adjust the tidal volume first and rate second, so that the Pa_{CO_2} is maintained at about 40 mm Hg[19,20]
5. Ventilate with 50% oxygen ($F_{I_{O_2}}$ = 0.5).[21,22a] Ventilation with 100% oxygen may increase dependent atelectasis due to denitrogenation.
6. Monitor arterial P_{O_2} and P_{CO_2} blood gases frequently and continuously.
7. Consult with the surgeon on early arterial clamping to the diseased segment or lobe. The pulmonary artery is clamped for pneumonectomy.
8. In the presence of hypoxemia:
   a. Increase tidal volume at least 15 ml/kg of body weight to ventilated (dependent) lung[22,23]
   b. Increase $F_{I_{O_2}}$ to 1.0 for brief periods.
   c. Application of 5 to 10 cm positive end-expiratory pressure (PEEP) to ventilated (dependent) lung may be associated with decreased oxygenation.[22b]
   d. If necessary, unclamp proximal limb of the tube lumen to operated side and increase tidal volume to about 15 ml/kg.

THE QUIET SURGICAL FIELD—APNEIC OXYGENATION TECHNIQUE. If a completely quiet surgical field is required, a period of up to 20 minutes to apnea can probably be provided under the following conditions:

1. Patient is hyperventilated with 100% oxygen for 5 minutes for full lung expansion. This will provide an increased pulmonary volume of oxygen by reducing carbon dioxide to Pa_{CO_2} and PA_{CO_2} values to 15 to 20 mm Hg. Pulmonary CO_2 volume may be reduced from 5.5% to 2%; water content reduced to 3%; and pulmonary oxygen volume increased by filling the inspiratory reserve volume.
2. Oxygenation of pulmonary blood will continue by diffusion—the principle of mass movement from site of high gradient partial pressure (lung) to a site of lower partial pressure.
3. Carbon dioxide will increase during the apneic period. From a Pa_{CO_2} level of 10 to 15 mm Hg, CO_2 will increase about 6 mm the first minute, 4 mm the second minute, and 2 and 3 mm/min thereafter.

The above conditions pertain to patients in generally good health. Typical patients for thoracic surgery are not in good health and apneic periods should be limited to 10 minutes.

PHYSIOLOGY OF ONE-LUNG VENTILATION*

Surgical pneumothorax significantly alters pulmonary physiology, and this is further complicated by the lateral position used for thoracic operations.[†] The change in ventilation and perfusion of both lungs is of importance in determining the net gas-exchange efficiency during thoracotomies.[11b,24]

In the lateral position, the dependent lung is compressed due to restriction of the size of the lungs by the mediastinum shifting downward, limited motion of the chest wall, and upward displacement of the diaphragm by the abdominal contents. The opposite is true in the up-lung, on the operated side, which will have an increased compliance and will move more freely than the dependent lung and be preferentially ventilated in the absence of chest wall containment.

In the lateral position, the pulmonary circulation is simultaneously altered. Due to gravitational influence, the dependent lung will be preferentially perfused and receive a larger percentage of the cardiac output than the up-lung.

The net effect is that the up-lung will be overventilated and underperfused, and the down-lung will be underventilated and overperfused. This leads to disturbances in ventilation–perfusion relationships that are sometimes difficult to correct during thoracotomies.

It is evident that arterial oxygenation is affected by two main factors: (1) pulmonary blood flow through the unventilated lung (compulsory shunt), and (2) oxygenation efficiency of the ventilated lung.

EFFECT OF ONE-LUNG VENTILATION ON SHUNT. During one-lung anesthesia, blood flow continues in the unventilated up-lung and a compulsory shunt remains, resulting in a reduction of mainstream arterial oxygen tension. Several compensatory mechanisms, however, reduce the amount of blood flow in the unventilated up-lung:[25]

1. Gravitational redistribution of blood flow away from unventilated lung to dependent lung[25]
2. Actual compression of pulmonary vasculature in the open chest by atmospheric collapse of the lung and by elastic recoil and resistance to flow by the contracted parenchymal tissue itself[25,26]
3. By reflex hypoxic pulmonary vasoconstriction (HPV), an autoregulatory phenomenon[25]

---

* This section was written with collaboration of Dr. Adel El-Etr.
† These physiologic changes also occur in the lateral decubitus position in the closed-chest patient but are exaggerated when the upper thorax is open.

4. By surgical ligation of pulmonary vessels, which further restricts blood flow to the operative region and diverts the blood to dependent ventilated regions[27]
5. In one-lung ventilation, collapse of the lung being operated on is more complete. This minimizes routine lung manipulation and avoids the occasional need for severe retraction of the lung and torsion of large blood vessels.

***Reflex Hypoxic Pulmonary Vasoconstriction.*[28]**
There is ample evidence that this phenomenon of HPV occurs in humans. Ventilation with a hypoxic gas mixture, or atelectasis of one lung or one lobe, generally causes a 30% to 40% diversion in the first instance, and in the condition of atelectasis, a 50% to 60% diversion of blood flow away from hypoxic to nonhypoxic areas of the lungs. This minimizes transpulmonary shunt. During one-lung anesthesia for thoracotomies, active vasoconstriction in the collapsed lung due to regional alveolar hypoxia diverts blood flow away from hypoxic regions of the upper lung and, thereby, serves as an autoregulatory mechanism that protects the arterial oxygen tension and adjusts regional ventilation–perfusion relationships. Ligation of pulmonary vessels during resections also diverts blood away from the operated side and increases blood flow to the dependent, unoperated lower lung.[27]

The most significant reduction in blood flow to the nondependent lung is caused by the reflex of vasoconstriction.[29] The normal response of the pulmonary vascular bed to atelectasis is an increase in pulmonary vascular resistance in the atelectatic lung, due almost entirely to vasoconstriction. This selective increase in vascular resistance in the atelectatic lung diverts blood flow away from the atelectatic lung toward the remaining normoxic or hyperoxic ventilated lung areas. This simultaneously reduces the amount of shunt. Many clinical studies with one-lung ventilation show that the shunt through the nonventilated lung is usually reduced to a range of 20% to 25% of the cardiac output, compared with the expected 40% or 50% if a purely physical mechanism was involved. Thus, HPV is an autoregulatory mechanism that protects the arterial oxygen tension by decreasing the amount of shunt flow that can occur through the hypoxic lung.

The influence of this reflex during one-lung anesthesia has been studied extensively.[29] The reflex may be antagonized by several clinical conditions, which may directly vasodilate hypoxically constricted lung vessels. These include the infusion of vasodilator drugs, the presence of infection in the nondependent lung, and hypocarbia.

EFFECTS OF ANESTHETICS. The effects of anesthetics on HPV in intact human studies are unfolding. All intravenous anesthetics studied to date have no effect on HPV. Nitrous oxide results in a small inhibition of HPV.

It is the halogenated inhalational agents' effects on HPV in humans that are questioned. Current experience with halothane in intact human studies shows universal inhibition of HPV; however, the net effect on arterial oxygen saturation is trivial.[30] The reasons for this are the drug's other effects on determinants of HPV, such as cardiac output, pulmonary vascular pressure, bronchodilation, effect on baroreceptors, and chemical/metabolic influences.

Domino[31] has shown isoflurane anesthesia to have a direct inhibiting effect on regional HPV in dogs. Rogers[32] has shown in humans, however, that following a base anesthetic of intravenous agents, adding progressive increments of isoflurane did not alter the arterial Pa_{O_2} significantly. Coupled with this were measurements of major hemodynamic indices (cardiac output, shunt fraction [$\dot{Q}_s/\dot{Q}_t$], and pulmonary artery pressures).[33] The study concluded that the negligible changes in Pa_{O_2} indicate that isoflurane has no effect on HPV.

Because of the multiple advantages to the use of inhalational agents (bronchodilation, lowered metabolism and oxygen requirements, rapid elimination, use of high FI_{O_2}, and their being easily titratable and levels controlled for cardiovascular stability), their safety with stable one-lung ventilation has been established.[34]

One question relates to the reported increase in HPV with repeated hypoxic stimuli.[35] It was recently shown, however, that in closed-chest dogs, the initial degree of HPV was maximal and there was no potentiation of the HPV response with repeated hypoxic stimuli.[36]

EFFICIENCY OF OXYGENATION IN VENTILATED (DEPENDENT) LUNG. During thoracotomies, oxygenation efficiency of the ventilated lung is reduced by lowered functional residual capacity, lower tidal volume, and effect of gravity. The use of one-lung ventilation can actually improve the ventilation efficiency of the dependent lung. To avoid atelectasis in the dependent lung, large tidal volumes of about 12 ml/kg should be used. This will increase the functional residual capacity and hopefully avoid atelectasis without significant deterioration in the $\dot{Q}_s/\dot{Q}_t$. Smaller tidal volumes are almost invariably associated with an increase in the $\dot{Q}_s/\dot{Q}_t$.

Carbon dioxide elimination with one-lung anesthesia has been studied, and usually there is no change in CO_2 clearance if normal ventilation is maintained or slightly increased. Two-lung ventilation should be maintained as long as possible and then, when one-lung ventilation is used, large tidal volumes of 8 to 12 ml/kg are maintained for one lung, and the total minute ventilation is maintained slightly more than before to produce a Pa_{CO_2} of 40 mm Hg.[37]

SUMMARY OF PHYSIOLOGIC EFFECTS OF ONE-LUNG ANESTHESIA. One-lung anesthesia, although advantageous in many types of thoracic surgery, technically poses several physiologic disadvantages. In the open-chest patient, there is a general defective pulmonary oxygen exchange. The following physiologic gas exchange defects are identified:

1. Increased alveolar to arterial oxygen tension difference $(P[A - a]_{O_2})$ across the alveolar capillary membrane[38,39]
2. Some perfusion of collapsed non-dependent lung alveoli occurs; i.e., in the operative side and/or due to disease.[40] This continues and produces a compulsory shunt.
3. Preferential perfusion of dependent atelectatic lung segments also results in a shunt. These lung segments are compressed due to gravitational effects from mediastinal shift and compression by abdominal contents against the dependent diaphragm, thereby reducing functional residual capacity.[24]
4. Atelectasis of dependent and/or nondependent lung segments is enhanced during anesthesia due to denitrogenation (nitrogen is a space filler and has a low blood solubility); this effect is more pronounced when $F_{I_{O_2}}$ is greater than 50%; oxygen and some anesthetic gases are thereby more rapidly absorbed from alveoli.[41]
5. Antagonism of hypoxic vasoconstriction by anesthetic agents; this allows perfusion to continue or be increased with an increased $P(A - a)_{O_2}$ and an increased shunt in the presence of hypoventilated lung segments.[30] Recent studies indicate that the inhalational volatile agents minimally affect hypoxic pulmonary vasoconstriction in humans.[12,31,34]

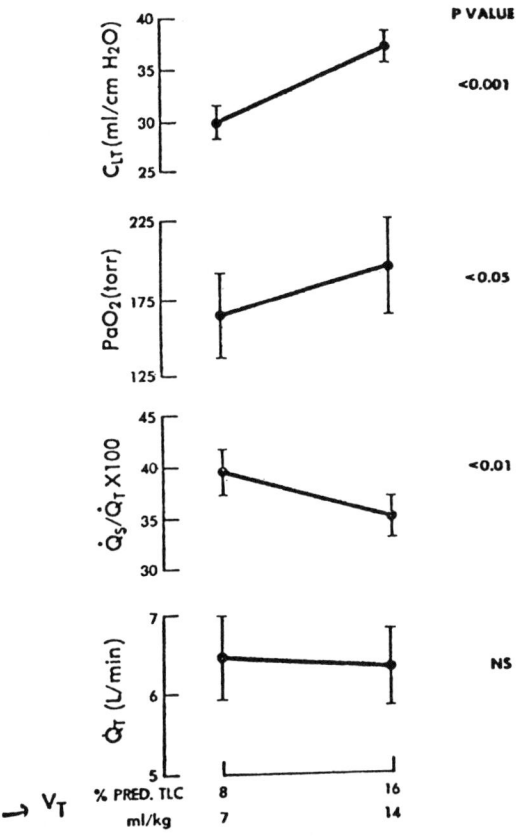

FIG. 22–18. Effect of tidal volume (V_T) during one-lung ventilation (mean ± SE, n = 13). Data were analyzed using Student's t test for paired data. C_{LT} = lung-thorax compliance; Pa_{O_2} = arterial oxygen partial pressure; $\dot{Q}_s/\dot{Q}_t$ = physiologic shunt; and $\dot{Q}_t$ = cardiac output. From Katz, J.A., et al.: Pulmonary oxygen exchange during endobronchial anesthesia: Effect of tidal volume and PEEP. Anesthesiology, 56:164, 1982.

EFFECT OF TIDAL VOLUME. The degree of impairment in Pa_{O_2} during one-lung ventilation correlates inversely with the preoperative percentage of predicted FEV_1.[37] In a study of the effect of tidal volume, it has been demonstrated that large tidal volumes of greater than 8% and approximately 16% of total lung capacity show a significant improvement in Pa_{O_2} and a decrease in $\dot{Q}_s/\dot{Q}_t$. This occurs without a significant change or effect on cardiac output, $\dot{Q}_t$. Simultaneously, there occurs an increase in lung compliance (Fig. 22–18).

The explanation of the salutary effects of increasing tidal volumes is related first to the resultant increased volume in the dependent lung. This increases intraalveolar pressure and, in turn, increases pulmonary vascular resistance. The result is twofold: (1) a recruitment of partially collapsed or atelectatic dependent alveoli, and (2) a more even redistribution of blood flow. The high tidal volume produces a physiologic balance between dependent lung recruitment of alveoli and the increased vascular resistance in the dependent lung, thereby restoring the ventilative–perfusive relationship toward normal.[37,42]

ADVERSE EFFECT OF PEEP. A study of PEEP of up to 10 cm H_2O did not provide any improvement in Pa_{O_2}, nor did it decrease the $\dot{Q}_s/\dot{Q}_t$, whether the ventilation was by mechanical or manual means.[39] Application of 10 cm H_2O PEEP applied during tidal volumes of 16% of total lung capacity also decreased Pa_{O_2} from approximately 210 mm Hg to 162 mm Hg in patients; at the same time, $\dot{Q}_t$ decreased by 10%.[23,37]

Proper placement of pulmonary artery catheters is important[23,37] in obtaining data.[43] If located in a right collapsed nondependent lung, the cardiac output may be low. If a nondependent lung is exposed the CPAP or PEEP zone 1 type, conditions may be produced in the nondependent lung with excess ventilation and minimal perfusion (Fig. 22–19).

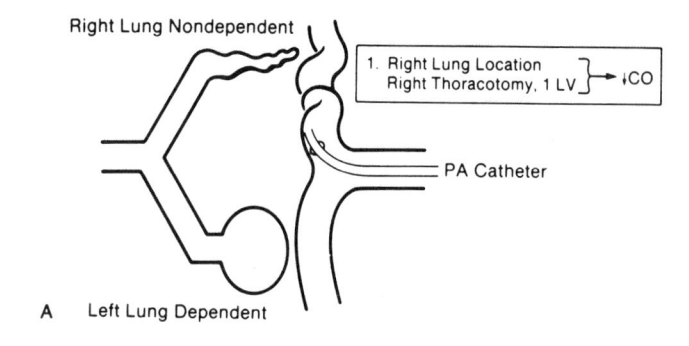

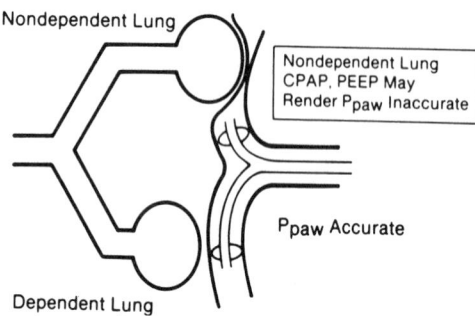

FIG. 22-19. Conditions during thoracotomy in the lateral decubitus position when pulmonary artery catheter data may be inaccurate. (A) During right thoracotomy with a pulmonary artery (PA) catheter located in the collapsed right lung (one-lung ventilation [1 LV]), the cardiac output (CO) may be lower than when the right lung is ventilated. The thermistor in the collapsed lung may be exposed to abnormal flow patterns or vascular wall interference. (B) When the pulmonary artery catheter is in the nondependent lung and the nondependent lung is exposed to CPAP or PEEP, the pulmonary artery wedge pressure (P_{paw}) may be inaccurate. Nondependent lung CPAP or PEEP may cause zone 1 conditions in the nondependent lung. The P_{paw} is probably always reasonably accurate when the pulmonary artery catheter is in the dependent lung, even if the dependent lung is exposed to PEEP. (From Benumof, J.L. *Anesthesia for Thoracic Surgery.* Philadelphia, W.B. Saunders, 1987.)

Ventilation in Lateral Position. In two-lung ventilation of patients in lateral decubitus position, closed chest, Baraka[23] has confirmed that there is better ventilation of the dependent lung than the nondependent lung, i.e., a preferential ventilation of the dependent lung to match the increased perfusion when a large tidal volume of about 15 ml/kg and an F_{IO_2} of 0.5 is used for ventilation. A normal arterial P_{O_2} and P_{CO_2} can be maintained at zero end-expiratory pressure. About 56% of tidal volume is delivered to the upper lung and 44% to the dependent lung. However, institution of PEEP (10 cm H_2O) was followed by a further increase of tidal volume up to 63% to the upper lung and a decrease in ventilation to the dependent lung down to 37% of tidal volume.

In these surgical circumstances (closed chest, lateral position), it is recommended that ventilation be accomplished with tidal volumes of 15 ml/kg of body weight, an F_{IO_2} of 0.5, and no PEEP.

It is also evident that in most situations, an F_{IO_2} of 0.5 is sufficient. Denitrogenation is less complete, and the nitrogen provides a filling effect in the alveoli to diminish atelectasis.

REFERENCES

1. Gale, J.W. and Waters, R.M.: Closed endobronchial anesthesia in thoracic surgery. J. Thorac. Surg., *1*:432, 1932.
2. Magill, I.W.: Anesthetics in thoracic surgery with special reference to lobectomy. Proc. Soc. Med., *29*:643, 1936.
3. Rovenstine, E.A.: Anesthesia for intrathoracic surgery: Endotracheal and endobronchial techniques. Surg. Gynec. Obstet., *63*:325, 1936.
4. Crafoord, C.: On technique of pneumonectomy in man. Acta. Chir. Scand., *18*:1, 1938.
5. Ruth, H.S., Grove, D.D., Keown, K.K.: Endobronchial anesthesia by means of an improved endobronchial airway. Anesthesiology, *9*:422, 1948.
6. Bonica, J.J.: Endobronchial anesthesia for intrathoracic surgery. Anesthesiology, *12*:344, 1951.
7. Carlens, E.: A new flexible double-lumen catheter for broncho-spirometry. J. Thorac. Cardiovasc. Surg., *18*:742, 1949.
8. Björk, V.O., Carlens, E., Friberg, O.: Endobronchial anesthesia. Anesthesiology, *14*:60, 1953.
9a. Macintosh, R. and Leatherdale, R.A.L.: Bronchus tube and bronchus blocker. Br. J. Anaesth., *27*:556, 1955.
9b. Green, R. and Gordon, W.: Right lung anesthesia. Anesthesia for left lung surgery using a new right endobronchial tube. Anesthesia, *12*:86, 1957.
9c. White, G.M.J.: A new double-lumen tube. Br. J. Anaesth., *32*:232, 1960.
9d. Bryce-Smith, R.: A double-lumen endobronchial tube. Br. J. Anaesth., *31*:274, 1959.
9e. Bryce-Smith, R., Salt, R.: A right-sided double-lumen tube. Br. J. Anaesth., *32*:230, 1960.
10a. Pappin, J.C.: The current practice of endobronchial intubation. Anaesthesia, *34*:57, 1978.
10b. Kaplan, J.A. (ed): *Thoracic Anesthesia.* New York, Churchill Livingstone, 1983.
11a. Benumof, J. and Alfrey, D.D.: Anesthesia for thoracic surgery. In: *Anesthesia,* 2nd ed. (Miller, R., ed). New York, Churchill Livingstone, 1986.
11b. Benumof, J.L.: Physiology of the open chest and one-lung anesthesia. Chapter 8 in: *Thoracic Anesthesia* (Kaplan, J.A., ed). New York, Churchill Livingstone, 1983.
12. El-Etr, A.A.: Improved technique for insertion of Carlens catheter. Anesth. Analg., *48*:758, 1969.
13. Björk, V.O., and Carlens, E.: The prevention of spread during pulmonary resection by the use of a double-lumen catheter. J. Thorac. Cardiovasc. Surg., *20*:151, 1951.
14. Robertshaw, R.L.: Low resistance double-lumen endobronchial tubes. Br. J. Anaesth., *34*:576, 1962.
15. Read, R.C., Friday, C.D., and Eason, C.N.: Prospective study of the Robertshaw endobronchial catheter in thoracic surgery. Ann. Thorac. Surg., *24*:156, 1977.
16. Brodsky, J.B., and Mark, J.B.D.: A simple technique for accurate placement of double-lumen endobronchial tube. Anesthesiol. Rev., *10*:26, 1983.
17. Smith, G.B., Hirsch, N.P., and Ehrenwerth, J.: Placement of double-lumen endobronchial tubes: The correlation be-

tween clinical impressions and bronchoscopic findings (unpublished data). New Haven, CT., Department of Anesthesiology, Yale University School of Medicine, 1985.
18. Ovassapian, A., Braunschweig, R., and Joshi, C.W.: Endobronchial intubation using flexible fiberoptic bronchoscope. Anesthesiology, 59:A501, 1983.
19. Flacke, J.W., Thompson, D.S., and Read, R.C.: Influence of tidal volume and pulmonary artery occlusion on arterial oxygenation during endobronchial anesthesia. South. Med. J., 69:619, 1976.
20. Khanom, T., and Branthwaite, M.A.: Arterial oxygenation during one-lung anaesthesia. 1. A study in man. Anaesthesia, 28:132, 1973.
21. Torda, T.A., et al.: Pulmonary venous admixture during one-lung anesthesia: The effect of inhaled oxygen tension and respiration rate. Anaesthesia, 29:272, 1974.
22a. Katz, J.A., et al.: Time course and mechanisms of lung-volume increase with PEEP in acute pulmonary failure. Anesthesiology, 54:9, 1981.
22b. Katz, J.A., Laverne, R.G., Fairley, H.B., Thomas, A.N.: Pulmonary oxygen exchange during endobronchial anesthesia: Effect of tidal volume and PEEP. Anesthesiology, 56:164, 1982.
23. Baraka, A., et al.: Dependent PEEP during two-lung ventilation in the lateral decubitus position. Anesth. Analg., 66:347, 1987.
24. Craig, J.O.C., Bromley, L.L., and Williams, R.: Thoracotomy and contralateral lung: A study of the changes occurring in the dependent and contralateral lung during and after thoracotomy in lateral decubitus. Thorax, 17:9, 1962.
25. Atwell, R.J., Hickam, J.B., Pryor, W.W., Page, E.P.: Reduction of blood flow through the hypoxic lung. Amer. J. Physiol., 166:37, 1951.
26. Westcoff, R.N., Fowler, N.O., Scott, R.C., et al.: Anoxia and human pulmonary vascular resistance. J. Clin. Invest., 30:957, 1951.
27. Flacke, J.W., Thompson, D.S., Read, R.C.: Influence of tidal volume and pulmonary artery occlusion on arterial oxygenation during endobronchial anesthesia. South Med. J., 69:619, 1976.
28. Aviado, D.M., Jr., Ling, J.S., and Schmidt, C.F.: Effects of anoxia on pulmonary circulation: Reflex pulmonary vasoconstriction. Am. J. Physiol., 189:253, 1947.
29. Benumof, J.L.: One-lung ventilation and hypoxic pulmonary vasoconstriction: implications for anesthetic management. Anesth. Analg., 64:821, 1985.
30. Bjertnaes, L.J.: Hypoxic induced pulmonary vasoconstriction in man: Inhibition due to diethyl ether and halothane anesthesia. Acta Anaesthiol. Scand., 22:520, 1978.
31. Domino, K.B., et al.: Influence of isoflurane on hypoxic pulmonary vasoconstriction in dogs. Anesthesiology, 64:423, 1986.
32. Rogers, S.N., and Benumof, J.L.: Halothane and isoflurane do not impair arterial oxygenation during one-lung ventilation in patients undergoing thoracotomy (abstract). Anesthesiology, 59:A532, 1983.
33. Rogers, S.N., and Benumof, J.L.: Halothane and isoflurane do not decrease Pa_{O_2} during one-lung ventilation in intravenously anesthetized patients. Anesth. Analg., 64:646, 1985.
34. Augustine, S.D., and Benumof, J.L.: Halothane and isoflurane do not impair arterial oxygenation during one-lung ventilation in patients undergoing thoracotomy. Anesthesiology, 61:A484, 1984.
35. Unger, M., et al.: Potentiation of pulmonary vasoconstrictor response with repeated intermittent hypoxia. J. Appl., Physiol., 43:662, 1977.
36. Grover, R.F.: The fascination of the hypoxic lung (editorial). Anesthesiology, 63:580, 1985.
37. Katz, J.A., et al.: Pulmonary oxygen exchange during endobronchial anesthesia: Effect of tidal volume and PEEP. Anesthesiology, 56:164, 1982.
38. Browne, R.A., Catton, D.V., and Ashworth, E.J.: A study of oxygenation during thoracotomy. Can. Anaesth. Soc. J., 15:468, 1968.
39. Tarhan, S., and Lundborg, R.O.: Carlens endobronchial catheter versus regular endotracheal tube during thoracic surgery: A comparison of blood gas tensions and pulmonary shunting. Can. Anaesth. Soc. J., 18:594, 1971.
40. Torda, T.A., et al.: Pulmonary venous admixture during one-lung anesthesia: The effect of inhaled oxygen tension and respiration rate. Anaesthesia, 29:272, 1974.
41. Nunn, J.F., et al.: Detection and reversal of pulmonary absorption collapse. Br. J. Anaesth., 50:91, 1978.
42. Finley, T.N., Hill, T.R., and Bonica, J.J.: Effect of intrapleural pressure on pulmonary shunt through atectatic dog lung. Am. J. Physiol., 205:1187, 1963.
43. Benumof, J.L.: Anesthesia For Thoracic Surgery. Philadelphia, W.B. Saunders, 1987.

CONTROL OF BREATHING BY ARTIFICIAL METHODS

This chapter has been written with the assistance of Wade Jones, Director of Respiratory Care, University of Illinois, Chicago.

The anesthesiologist may exert control over a patient's breathing by two well-defined methods: *controlled ventilation* and *assisted ventilation*. Controlled ventilation is applied when all spontaneous respiration has ceased; assisted ventilation is used to augment or assist inadequate spontaneous respiration. These methods are best performed with an endotracheal airway.

HISTORY.
1934—Classic work of Guedel on "Ether Apneas"[1]
1941—Burstein's assisted-respiration technique[2]
1945—Cournand "Studies of Effect of Positive Pressure Breathing on Cardiac Output and Circulation in Man"[3]
1946—Otis, Rahn[4,5] published compliance studies of lungs and thorax
1959—Mushin et al. published *Automatic Ventilation of the Lungs*[6]
1962—Holaday[7] published a classification of lung ventilators
1980—Mushin et al. published *Automatic Ventilation of Lungs*, 3rd Edition[6]
1991—Chatburn published "A New System for Understanding Mechanical Ventilators"[7a]

DEFINITIONS

CONTROLLED VENTILATION. Controlled ventilation is a technique that employs manual or mechanical ventilation, in which the frequency of breathing is determined by the ventilator according to preset cycling pattern without initiation by the patient. The drive of the respiratory center may be temporarily lost through (1) elevation of the response threshold of the center, by depression of the center (narcosis or deep anesthesia), or by diminution of the strength of the stimulus (lowering P_{CO_2}); or (2) peripheral muscular paralysis, which may cause the cessation of respiratory movements. Under these conditions, respiratory effort and pulmonary ventilation may be entirely supplied manually or mechanically by the anesthetist or therapist. Therefore, controlled artificial ventilation may be defined as rhythmic inflation of the lungs, 12 to 25 times per minute, with the application of 10 to 100 cm H_2O pressure to the breathing system when all spontaneous respiration has ceased.

Originally, controlled ventilation was described in 1934 by Guedel[1] as ether apneas. He emphasized the need for full morphinization to achieve apnea and the necessity of carrying on artificial ventilation.

To achieve controlled ventilation there are three requisites:[2] (1) production of apnea or its existence; (2) artificial ventilation; and (3) ability to return the patient to spontaneous respiration.

Controlled ventilation may be either passive or active. The distinction is made on the basis of the presence or absence of a spontaneous respiratory drive. Ventilation is efficiently and easily accomplished when the patient passively accepts the mechanically imposed force. This occurs when deep anesthesia or muscular paralysis is present or when a spontaneous central respiratory drive is absent. A central respiratory drive may be present and, if in synchrony with the ventilator, efficient ventilation ensues. If a respiratory drive is not synchronous with the ventilator, the patient is described as "fighting the ventilator." This may be an index of inadequate ventilator settings. Measures must be taken to attain passive acceptance by the patient of the imposed forces and permit easy ventilation. Several proper maneuvers are actively employed to achieve synchrony and/or apnea, such as reduction of carbon dioxide, hyperinflation to overstimulate pulmonary vagal receptors, correction of hypoxemia, and correction of shunting. It also may be necessary to institute measures to suppress the patient's respiratory drive by means of morphine or a relaxant to permit the ventilator to function efficiently and to stabilize ventilation.

ASSISTED VENTILATION. This is another technique of ventilation available that can be employed to achieve gas exchange.

It is the type of ventilation performed in the presence of an active respiratory center and spontaneous respiratory movement. It is performed to augment the patient's efforts and is synchronous with the patient's inspiratory efforts. Whenever assisted ventilation is carried out manually or mechanically, the patient initiates inspiration and establishes the frequency of breathing.

This method has certain advantages over controlled ventilation. There is less delay in resumption of spontaneous ventilation and there is less likelihood of alveolar or pulmonary damage. The depth of anesthesia is more easily determined. There are few adverse effects. Burstein[2] first recommended the maneuver and called it *compensated respiration.* It is described as the application of graded pressures of 3 to 40 cm H_2O to the breathing bag during anesthesia synchronous with inspiratory effort. There is complete release of any manual pressure to the breathing bag during expiration. This amount of pressure is insufficient to depress the Hering-Breuer reflex and to cause apnea.

PRODUCTION OF APNEA. There are four well-defined techniques available for the production of apnea in the anesthetic situation. All depend on a combination of diminished respiratory stimuli (removal of carbon dioxide or inhibiting respiratory drive reflexes) or raised respiratory center threshold. The relaxant drug apnea represents peripheral muscular paralysis. There are many possible modifications.

1. Diminished Stimuli (Dominant) + Raised Threshold (Accessory). Starting with a patient in light plane 2 of stage III anesthesia, the anesthetic vapor tension is increased in the rebreathing bag and, by rhythmic manual compression of the breathing bag, synchronous with inspiration, the pulmonary alveolar surface is exposed to this tension. This results in the rapid absorption of the vapor by the blood and exposes the respiratory center to high concentrations of anesthetic.

Throughout this interval of hyperventilation, carbon dioxide absorption progresses. Hence, there is a simultaneous and appreciable decrease in the blood carbon dioxide, and apnea results. Although there is both respiratory center depression and diminished carbon dioxide stimulation, there is also inhibition of the Hering-Breuer reflex from the pulmonary distension. Actually, the removal of the regulatory Hering-Breuer reflex is a predominant factor in causing the apnea, and this technique may be considered as a true vagal apnea.

Burstein[2] has demonstrated in humans that the carbon dioxide level is relatively unimportant in maintaining controlled respiration. Controlled respiration during cyclopropane anesthesia was accomplished and continued when the carbon dioxide content had risen from the preanesthetic level of 42.4 to 54.7 vol% during control.

2. Raised Threshold (Dominant) + Diminished Stimuli (Accessory). Starting with a patient in light plane 2 anesthesia, an active carbon dioxide hyperpnea is produced with a high anesthetic vapor tension in the breathing bag. The brain becomes rapidly saturated with the anesthetic, and the respiratory center is markedly depressed. At the time of estimated maximal depression (pupils widely dilated, shallow diaphragmatic respiration), the carbon dioxide absorber is placed in the breathing circuit and with the removal of the excess carbon dioxide, apnea is produced. This technique is not recommended.

3. Oxygen Apnea – Diminished Stimuli + Raised Threshold. The oxygen apnea technique requires the depression of the medullary respiratory center by full morphinization or by barbiturates plus further depression with the anesthetic agent. This leaves respiration chiefly under the control of the carotid body, stimulation of which is due to hypoxemia. If a high oxygen concentration is now added to the breathing system, the hypoxemic stimulus is removed and apnea results.

4. Relaxant Technique. The curare technique was initially developed by Hathaway. After ample medication, nitrous oxide and oxygen are administered. When plane 1 anesthesia is reached, a pharyngeal airway is inserted and the ability to inflate the lungs is tested. If clear, a dose of relaxant is administered, calculated to stop respiration. Non-depolarizing agents with a significant duration of action are chosen. A dose of 15 to 20 mg of *d*-tubocurarine is sufficient and may be repeated as necessary. Apnea of 20 to 30 minutes is produced and ventilation is then carried out by the anesthetist. Similarly, pancuronium in doses of 0.13 mg/kg is effective.

INDICATIONS FOR ASSISTED OR CONTROLLED VENTILATION. In the presence of apnea, controlled ventilation must be instituted—there is no choice. Patients with severely depressed respiration or who are tachypneic are better managed by controlled ventilation. Complete mechanical control is required for patients suffering from coma, poisoning, or in some cases, crushed chest; it is usually employed in patients following upper abdominal or open chest surgery.

Assisted ventilation is employed in less urgent circumstances. Patients should be conscious, breathing regularly at a reasonable rate, and showing good respiratory efforts. It is likely to be employed in patients suffering from chronic pulmonary disease.

PRINCIPLES OF MECHANICAL PULMONARY VENTILATION

Once apnea or a significant degree of hypoventilation is produced, the patient must be artificially ventilated. If the ventilation is completely done artificially (manually or mechanically), it is designated as *controlled ventilation* and the ventilation is set in the control mode (CMV). If the patient is breathing spontaneously and initiates inspiration at an adequate frequency of ventilation but at an insufficient tidal volume that requires artificial support, it is designated *assisted ventilation*. Ventilators are set in the assist mode (AMV). The actual ventilation will depend on the interrelationship of four variables: (1) pressure; (2) volume; (3) flow pattern; and (4) rate and time sequence. Changes in these variables will depend on patient factors of lung compliance and airway resistance as well as characteristics and settings of the ventilator. The ventilation may be either manual or mechanical. The essential objective in both are the following:

1. Ventilate normal or abnormal lungs effectively
2. Impose a minimal disturbance on cardiovascular function

In these discussions, the ventilatory *cycle* is defined as the period from the beginning of one inspiration to the beginning of the next inspiration. Three phases are recognized: in sequence, there is the inflation (inspiratory) phase, the exhalation or deflation phase, and the expiratory pause. The deflation phase and the expiratory pause together represent the expiration or expiratory period (Fig. 23–1).

PRESSURE SEQUENCES. In 1942 Barach[8-11] introduced the procedure of continuous positive pressure breathing (CPPB) for the treatment of patients with obstructive dyspnea and/or pulmonary edema. Such patients were breathing spontaneously; the pressure was applied throughout the respiratory cycle but was somewhat higher during inspiration than expiration. Subsequently, the technique of intermittent positive pressure breathing, termed *IPPB*, was introduced into aviation medicine and into respiratory care. Patients receiving IPPB are also breathing spontaneously, and the positive pressure is specifically applied to enhance or assist inspiration. Thus, the letter "B" is reserved for patients breathing spontaneously.

In 1934[10] the observation of pursed-lip breathing (PLB) in patients led to the use of expiratory resistance. The technique used spontaneously by the patient was duplicated mechanically by exhalatory resistance only during the expiratory phase. It is noted that PLB was observed by Laennec in 1830 in patients with chronic obstructive lung disease.

Appropriately, the application of positive pressure to the airway of apneic patients may be considered as ventilation (artificial) designated by the letter "V"; and the pressure may be either continuous or intermittent. Thus, one may distinguish several types of controlled ventilation.

1. Continuous positive-pressure ventilation (CPPV)[12]
2. Intermittent positive-pressure ventilation (IPPV)[13]
   a. With zero end-expiratory pressure (ZEEP)
   b. With PEEP this is equivalent to CPPV
   c. With negative end-expiratory pressure (NEEP)
3. Positive–negative pressure ventilation (PNPV)
4. End-inspiratory pause (EIP) or sustained end-inflation pressure

CPPV.[1] This is defined as continuous pressure above atmospheric at the airway opening throughout the respiratory cycle during controlled ventilation. The pressure is *not constant*. The positive compressing force on the pulmonary system is applied not only for inflation but a *smaller* definite positive force continues to be exerted during deflation. This ven-

FIG. 23–1. Phases of the respiratory cycle: During intermittent positive pressure ventilation, the operator should recognize three phases: the inspiratory, the expiratory, and the expiratory pause.

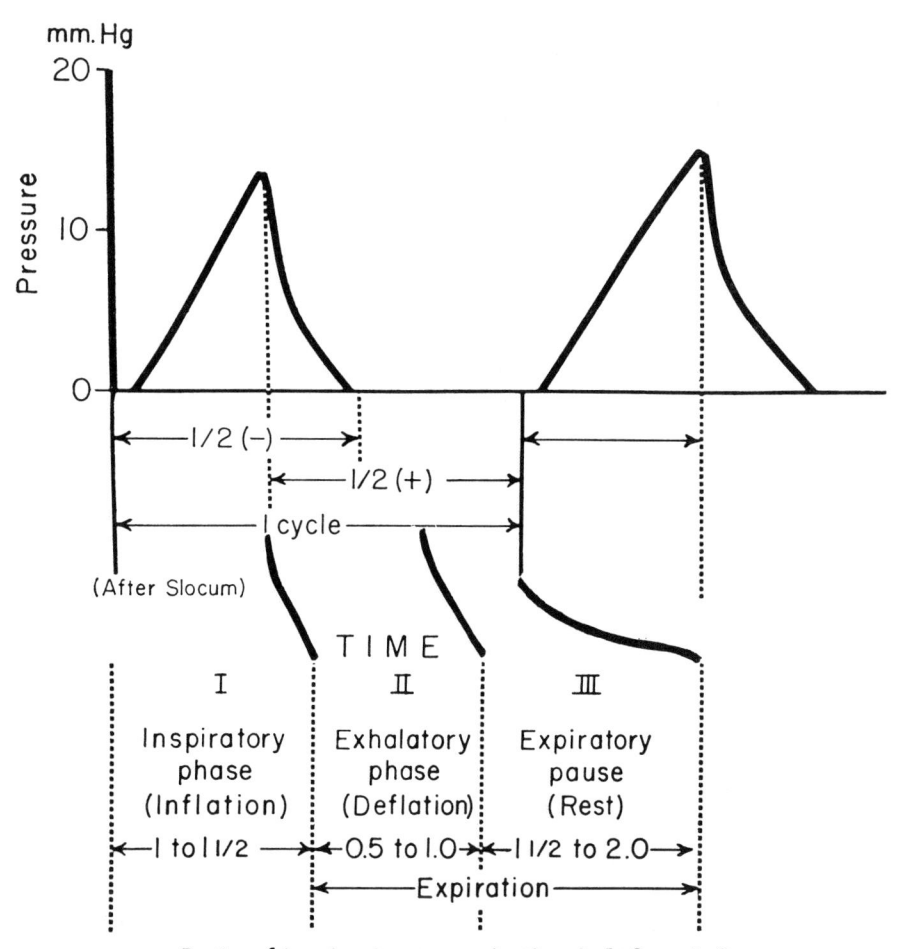

Ratio of inspiration to expiration is 1:2 or 1:3

tilation technique is indicated during anesthesia for maintaining low fractional inspired oxygen percent and normal arterial oxygenation. The procedure must be employed with caution because the circulation may be profoundly impaired, especially if hypovolemia exists.[15]

IPPV. As a form of control of ventilation this is characterized by positive pressure to the airway during the respiratory phase only. No pressure is applied during exhalation, and no end-expiratory pressure is added.

It has been proposed that during mechanical ventilation (MV) by IPPV, the type of end-expiratory pressure be designated. If no pressure is added at this time, as in classically defined IPPV, one may add the abbreviation "ZEEP," for zero end-expiratory pressure, for further clarification.[14] Exhalation is passive and no external (mechanical) pressures are applied during—the expiratory pause.

PEEP. A residual pressure above atmospheric maintained in the airways at the end of exhalation is designated as *PEEP*. This may be used during spontaneous or mechanical ventilation. During the exhalatory pause (if any), a positive pressure continues to exist; the intrapulmonary pressure is positive throughout the entire respiratory cycle.

In patients mechanically ventilated by IPPV but continuing to have severe hypoxemia, the *addition of a PEEP* of 5 to 20 cm H_2O increases arterial oxygenation. This was originally shown by Frumin.[16] The degree of increase in Pa_{O_2} is related to the resultant increase in lung volume and, specifically, functional residual capacity (FRC). A PEEP of 5 cm H_2O in patients with severe acute respiratory failure produces a mean increase in Pa_{O_2} of 68 mm Hg and FRC of 0.35 L. Rises in oxygen tension are larger in patients with initially low lung volumes and low pulmonary compliance. Consequent to PEEP pulmonary compliance is improved and FRC increases (Fig. 23-2).

The mechanisms of this effect are several: prevention of airway closure; maintenance of a normal or elevated FRC; uniform air distribution; recruitment of and inflating of atelectatic and underinflated alveoli and diminished shunting; increased pressure gradient of oxygen between alveolus and capillary; decreased interstitial and alveolar water by increasing influx into perialveolar capillaries; and

622   General Anesthesia

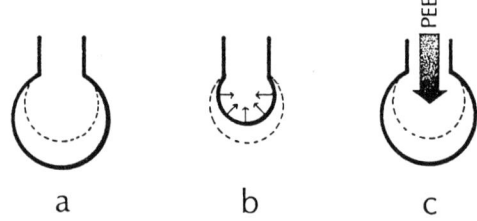

The dotted circle represents the alveolar critical volume (below which elastic forces will cause collapse). *A* represents a normal alveolus at the end of expiration. Note the FRC is above the critical volume. *B* represents an abnormal alveolus at the end of expiration; the volume is less than the critical volume and the alveolus tends to collapse. It may be stated that the FRC is below the critical volume. *C* represents alveolus *B* at the end of expiration when PEEP is applied. Note the "back pressure" prevents the alveolar volume from diminishing below the critical volume. PEEP has increased the FRC and reestablished more normal alveolar function.

FIG. 23–2. The mechanism of PEEP. From Shapiro, B. A., Harrison, R., and Trout, C.: Clinical Application of Respiratory Care. Chicago, Year Book Medical Publishers, 1975.

flattening of alveoli. One of the advantages of PEEP is the increase in Pa_{O_2} in the presence of the same or even lowered inspired oxygen tension.

As early as 1939 Barach demonstrated that mild expiratory pressures as low as 6 cm H_2O will enlarge the diameter of the bronchi; exhalation against pressures of 20 cm H_2O retards outflow of air and causes marked increase in bronchiolar size.[11] PLB will also maintain open bronchi.[10,11]

Retard exhalation is the technique of placing a resistance in the expiratory arm of a ventilator. This has the effect of PEEP.

Optimal PEEP. This is defined as that positive end-expiratory airway pressure that produces a maximal Pa_{O_2} with minimal interference with cardiovascular dynamics. It should coincide with optimal lung function. Oxygen transport should then be maximal (cardiac output × arterial oxygen content).

In conditions where the usual range of PEEP appears to be ineffective, higher PEEPs of 20 to 40 cm H_2O may be cautiously employed.[17] One must assess each increment in pressure against the response. Evidence of failing cardiac output is the end point.

Disadvantages. Excessive pressures or pressures beyond the optimum produce overdistention of alveoli. This leads to increased dead space and decreasing compliance.

Hemodynamic responses are considerable.[18] Because PEEP causes a large increase in mean airway pressure, the circulatory effects of airway pressure are exaggerated. PEEP causes a fall in cardiac index; a PEEP of 13 cm H_2O reduces cardiac index by 20%.

Use. Conditions for institution of PEEP are the following:[14]

1. Inability to maintin a Pa_{O_2} of 70 mm Hg with inspired oxygen of 50% or more during IPPV.
2. Failure to reduce pulmonary shunting by other means.
3. A normovolemic patient.
4. Low pulmonary lung volume or FRC.
5. Low compliance.

The cause of any hypoxemia should be carefully assessed. In hemorrhage, shock, or respiratory obstruction, Pa_{O_2} will not improve with PEEP and the procedure may be dangerous.

Techniques for Producing PEEP. Two techniques are used to accomplish PEEP. During CPPV in a patient on this form of positive-pressure ventilation, a positive airway pressure continues into the end-expiratory phase and so provides PEEP. During IPPV, the airway pressure reaches atmospheric pressure at exhalation and the positive pressure is intermittent. The addition of an end-expiratory pressure then produces CPPV. Thus, CPPV is IPPV with PEEP.

Continuous positive airway pressure (CPAP) is a technique for providing PEEP. The origin is as follows: if a patient is spontaneously breathing, there is a period of negative airway pressure that can trigger a positive pressure by a machine and intermittently augment inspiration. This is IPPB. A patient breathing spontaneously throughout the respiratory cycle assisted by an IPPB machine with an exhalatory pressure device at a higher than atmospheric pressure (greater than 760 mm Hg) is designated as under CPPB. CPAP describes the circuit pressure under these conditions.[19]

Many systems are available to deliver PEEP to the spontaneously breathing patient. These are grouped into demand systems and continuous flow systems using various resistors.[20] The reader is referred to the design of these systems reviewed by Kacmarek.[21]

Pressure Support Ventilation (PSV). This technique is defined as a constant positive pressure on the airways during the inspiratory phase of a patient's triggered breath. PSV has no preset tidal volume but is flow limited, not pressure limited. The degree of pressure support is regulated by the physician or respiratory care therapist.

NEGATIVE END-EXPIRATORY PRESSURE. In this technique, after a positive inflation pressure is applied a negative pressure is introduced toward the end of the exhalation phase of the cycle. As deflation is completed, the airway pressure is returned to zero during the expiratory pause.

A negative pressure applied to the airway during the latter part of expiration reduces the intrathoracic mean pressure and some theoretic cardiocirculatory advantages result.[22] Interference with cardiac output is usually less when compared to IPPV without negative pressure. In individuals with intact circulatory reflexes, the differences are insignificant.[23,24] But in patients with circulatory inadequacy, the decrease in cardiac output is less than under IPPV alone.[22] A negative expiratory pressure, however, imposes the danger of airway collapse.

INTERMITTENT POSITIVE–NEGATIVE PRESSURE VENTILATION (IPNPV). This technique consists of the sequence of intermittently applied positive pressure for lung inflation → a negative pressure throughout deflation → no pressure during the expiratory pause. It differs from NEEP in that the negative pressure is applied immediately at the conclusion of inspiration and throughout the exhalation phase, not just at the end of exhalation.

END-INSPIRATORY HOLD (EIP) PLATEAU.[18] At the end of inspiration, a maintenance of the applied inspiratory pressure for a brief time has been proposed to retain the insufflated tidal volume in the pulmonary system. Essentially, the pressure at the end of inspiration is sustained to provide a pressure plateau—a modified Valsalva maneuver. Such a technique has been recommended as a means to permit a better gas distribution in the lungs and to a better ventilation/perfusion equilibrium.

A raised mean airway pressure gives rise to measurable changes in circulation. The addition of inspiratory hold further decreases cardiac output, stroke work of both right and left ventricles, and pulmonary vascular conductance (increased vascular resistance). It is claimed that the adverse circulatory effects of inspiratory hold are not as extensive as those encountered in PEEP techniques.

WORK OF VENTILATION.[25] Work is defined as exerting a force through a distance. A force is the acceleration given to a mass. In the metric system, force may be expressed as kilopound (kp) and is the product of mass (M) × distance (L) × time squared, or MLT^2. One kp is the force that gives a mass of 1 kg an acceleration of 9.81 m/sec^2.

The work of breathing is the product of the force applied (the pressure) multiplied by the mass of air moved per unit time (the flow) multiplied by time: $W = P \times \text{flow} \times dt$. Force in breathing is the acceleration given to a mass of air by an applied pressure. It is evidenced by the movement of air or flow. Flow itself is the volume moved per unit time and is dependent on the force applied, namely pressure. Thus, the driving mechanical force in breathing is that of applied pressure or a created pressure differential.

VARIABLES OF VENTILATION

PRESSURE.[4,8] The value of the pressure applied in intermittent positive pressure depends on two factors: (1) compliance of the pulmonary system or the volume–pressure relationship, and (2) airway resistance. Each increment of pressure produces an incremental change in volume, which varies between 10 and 20 mm Hg in adults. In children, pressures of 5 to 10 mm Hg are needed, and in infants, 2 to 5 mm Hg are sufficient. These pressures not only overcome normal resistances and expand the lung, permitting good gas mixing and exchange, but also serve to maintain the apnea by inhibiting the Hering-Breuer reflex through the increase in airway pressure at the respiratory bronchioles.

Under these conditions, ventilatory control is simple and efficient. Anesthesia can be maintained in light planes without resumption of spontaneous respiratory activity. During the expiratory phase, there is complete release of pressure with return to atmospheric pressure.

VOLUME.[4,8] Each patient's minute volume should be estimated or predetermined, and a tidal volume as well as a proper rate should be calculated from this finding. The volume of gas introduced into a patient is a function of the flow rate and the time duration. Because flow is the movement of a volume of gas and determined by a force, namely, pressure, it is evident that the volume of gas delivered is proportional to pressure. That is, the respiratory work is a product of volume (or mass moved) times the pressure. In ideal circumstances, one should expect to deliver a volume of 90 to 100 ml of air for each 1 mm Hg pressure applied to the average adult pulmonary system in accordance with compliance factors. When resistance factors and other functional factors are considered, however, the volume–response relationship to a pressure increment is approximately 60 ml to each 1 mm Hg pressure, or 50 ml/1 cm of water pressure.

RATE AND TIME SEQUENCE.[13] The rate and time sequence are important to avoid adverse effects. Generally, the time of a respiratory cycle in the adult should be 3 to 5 seconds. This results in a rate of 12 to 20 inflations per minute for adults. In children, the time of a cycle is approximately 3 seconds, giving a rate of 20 per minute, and in infants, the time of a cycle may be 1 to 2 seconds, permitting a rate of 30 to 40 per minute.

Strict attention to the regulation of the inspiratory and expiratory periods according to the classic work of Cournand is required. The applied pressure should be relatively short in duration; after attaining the peak pressure, the pressure of the breathing system should be allowed to drop rapidly to atmospheric. The period of expiration must at least be as long as the inspiratory phase, but more correctly, as

624 General Anesthesia

long as the total time when a positive pressure in the pulmonary system exists. It must be of such length to allow a sufficient large number of heart beats to take place to compensate for the reduction in output that occurs during the inspiratory phase of rising pressure.

FLOW RATE AND PATTERN.[13] Flow represents the volume of gas (or mass) moving per unit time. It is determined by an applied force, which, in breathing is pressure as noted under "Work of Ventilation." The flow curve depends chiefly on the force applied to the system and the pattern by which the positive pressure is applied to the respiratory tract. It must vary with the individual patient. A flow curve is thus the net effect of the applied pressure against the compliance of the lungs, thorax, and airway resistance. If the applied pressure could continuously adjust and respond to changes in the respiratory system, an ideal artificial respiratory method would result (Fig. 23–3).

The pattern of the positive pressure application generally should be such a type and period as to provide a low mean airway pressure. Mean pressure is the mean of an infinite number of pressure recordings in the lung throughout the respiratory cycle. It is not the average of the highest and lowest pressure. It is illustrated diagrammatically in Figure 23–3.

EFFECTS OF POSITIVE AIRWAY PRESSURE

EFFECTS OF NORMAL VENTILATION ON CIRCULATION.[25] Normal ventilation influences the cardiocirculatory system. The effects are schematically represented in Figure 23–4. As inhalation occurs, a lowered intrathoracic pressure increases the inflow of blood in the pulmonary vessels. Associated with this is an increase in right ventricular stroke volume and a rise in net pulmonary artery pressure. Meanwhile, there is a limitation in the outflow of blood from the thorax. This is evidenced by a decrease in the left ventricular stroke volume and a lowering of net systemic arterial pressure.

IMMEDIATE EFFECTS OF POSITIVE AIRWAY PRESSURE ON CIRCULATION. The physiologic effects of controlled ventilation are those of positive pressure in the airway. In brief, the applied pressure on the breathing bag or by a mechanical ventilator is transmitted to the tracheobronchial tree, the alveoli, and the intrathoracic structures (including the great vessels and the esophagus). This pressure on the tracheobronchial system stimulates adverse reflexes and, on the alveoli, causes a simple mechanical impedance to circulation through the lungs. The effects of *continuous positive* pressure may be quite drastic (Fig. 23–5).

The effects of *intermittent* positive pressure respiration on circulation are likewise due to the transmission of pressure to the pulmonary system. They are hence similar to those of continuous positive pressure but are markedly reduced. There is also a compensatory interval during the deflation phase of the intermittent positive-pressure technique. This permits some compensation for any adverse effects during inspiration. The effects on the entire circulation are quite striking and reverse the normal cardiocirculatory effects of respiration (Fig. 23–6).

SUMMARY OF PHYSIOLOGIC EFFECTS OF POSITIVE-PRESSURE VENTILATION[15]

Hemodynamics. *Venous pressure increases*[25] in parallel to the rise in intrapulmonic pressure. It may be 40% of applied pressure (chest opened) or 70% of applied pressure (chest closed). Associated with the increased venous pressure is congestion and skin reddening.

Arterial pressure increases, and, like venous pressure, is due to mask pressure transmitted to pleural space.

Blood volume decreases 6% to 7% with loss of 300 ml of fluid (positive pressure of 20 cm H_2O) due to capillary filtration.

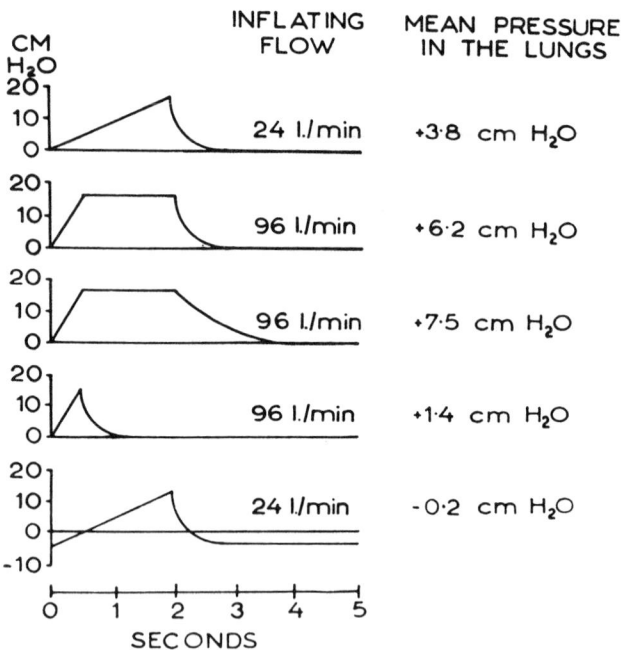

FIG. 23–3. Patterns of airway pressure, illustrating the meaning of the term *mean pressure in the lungs* during artificial ventilation. In each case, the total respiratory cycle lasts 5 sec; the tidal volume is 800 ml and the compliance is 0.05 L/cm H_2O. Hence the pressure range is 16 cm H_2O. The airway resistance is taken as 2 cm H_2O/(L/sec). From Mushin, W. W., Rendell-Baker, L., and Thompson, A. W.: Automatic Ventilation of the Lungs, 2nd ed. London, Blackwell Scientific, 1969.

FIG. 23-4. Effect of normal respiration on the cardiocirculatory system. From Cournand, A., et al: Physiologic studies of the effects of intermittent positive pressure breathing on cardiac output in man. Am. J. Physiol., *152*, 161, 1948.

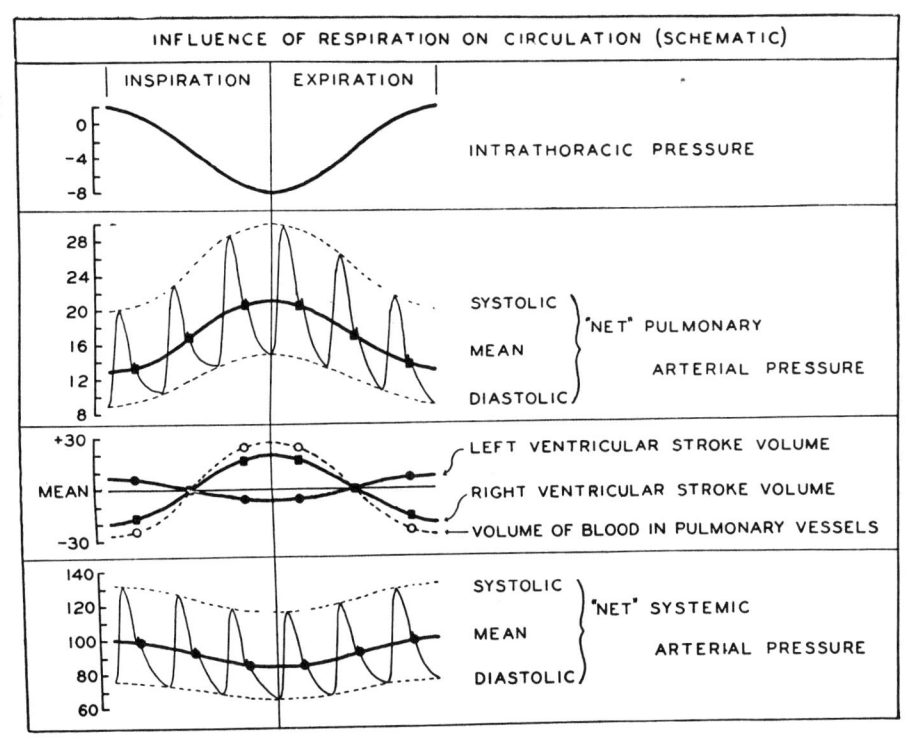

Blood flow is slowed in mesenteric veins; blood flow in finger is reduced to 73% of normal at continuous positive pressure of 22 mm Hg.[26]

Circulation time is prolonged,[5] and *cardiac output* is reduced.[27] A decrease of 1 to 1.7 L/min may occur at continuous pressure of 20 mm Hg. *Stroke volume* is reduced.[28]

Oxygen Consumption. This is increased by 15%. Impedance to filling left side of the heart and filling of right side tends to produce cardiac tamponade.[24]

Atrial Pressures. Effective atrial pressures are reduced. Normal mean pressures are 4 mm Hg for the right atrium and 8 mm Hg for the left atrium. These are reduced by one fourth to one third in mean value by intermittent positive-pressure breathing.

Systemic Blood Pressure. There is a reduction in systolic, diastolic, mean, and pulse pressures.

Pulmonary Blood Flow.[29] Lungs ordinarily have 6% of total blood volume on expiration and 9% on in-

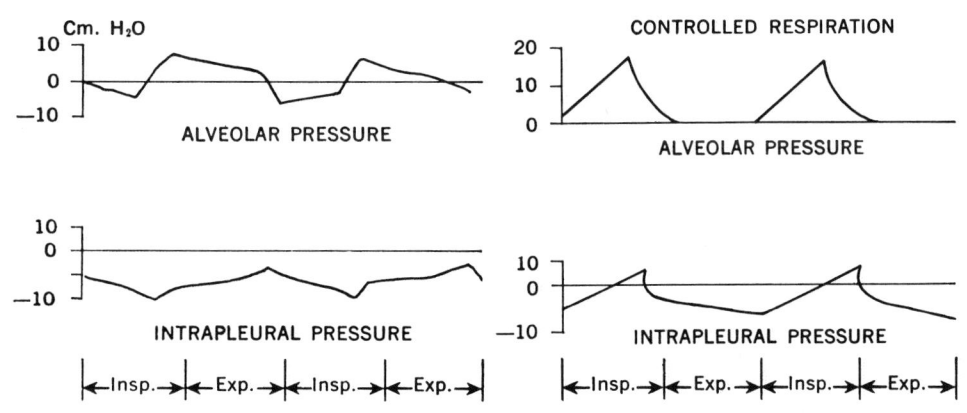

FIG. 23-5. Calculated pressure changes in alveoli and pleura during both spontaneous and controlled respiration (Insp. = inspiration; Exp. = expiration). From Mushin, W. W., Rendell-Baker, L., and Thompson, A. W.: Automatic Ventilation of the Lungs, 2nd ed. London, Blackwell Scientific, 1969.

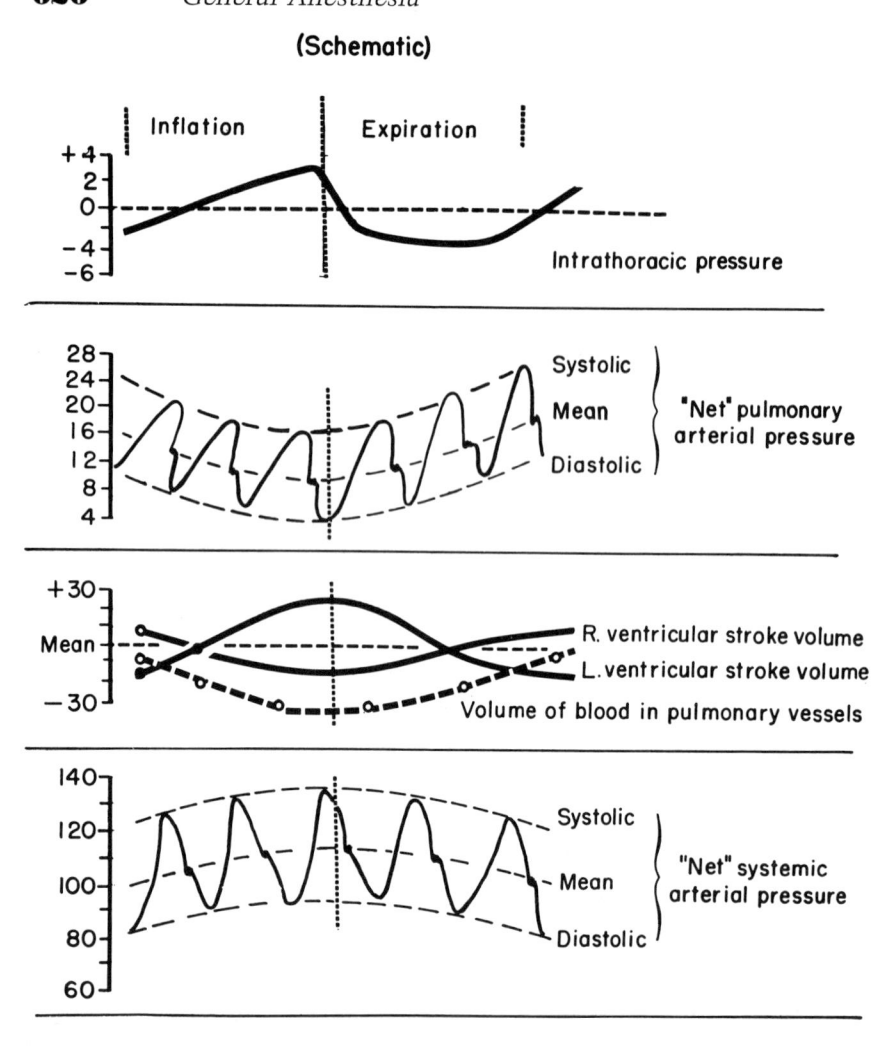

FIG. 23–6. Effect of intermittent positive-pressure ventilation on cardiocirculatory system. From Cournand, A., et al: Physiologic studies of the effects of intermittent positive pressure breathing on cardiac output in man. Am. J. Physiol., *152*, 161, 1948.

spiration. There may be as much as 20% of total volume while supine or in mitral stenosis or cardiac failure. Continuous positive pressure shifts blood from this pulmonary reservoir to extrathoracic vessels.

Pulmonary Ventilation. Continuous positive pressure increases residual air and interferes with gas mixing.[30] Reversal of normal effort relation in respiration occurs; expiration becomes active.[31]

Renal Function. Positive-pressure breathing decreases renal perfusion, glomerular filtration rate and urine formation (33% reduction). Water and sodium retention occurs. Bioassay of plasma reveals high levels of antidiuretic hormone (ADH). Osmolarity of urine increases while sodium decreases. Negative pressure breathing results in the reverse. Vagotomy diminishes the influence of pressure breathing.[32]

MECHANISM OF EFFECTS OF IPPV ON CIRCULATION. As previously noted, the effects of continuous positive airway pressure may be drastic. Those of intermittent positive pressure are qualitatively similar but quantitatively less. This is particularly true in the closed chest but surprisingly also true, to a lesser extent, in the presence of the open chest.[33]

This interference is important to the patient with an otherwise compromised circulation, *e.g.*, a patient in or near shock. The subject with a normal heart and peripheral circulation withstands increased intrapleural pressures so long as the central venous pressure can become elevated to exceed the intrapleural pressure slightly.

The circulatory interference is of three principal types:

1. *Impedance of pulmonary blood flow*[29] (Fig. 23–7): Impedance to pulmonary blood flow may occur as a result of compression of the capillary bed by raised intra-alveolar pressure. The pulmonary capillary blood pressure is approximately 12 cm H_2O. An increase in alveolar pressure to +6 cm H_2O may markedly interfere with pulmonary circulation and burden the right heart.[34,35]

2. *Impairment of "thoracic pump" factor on venous return.*[15,36]: During spontaneous respiration, a

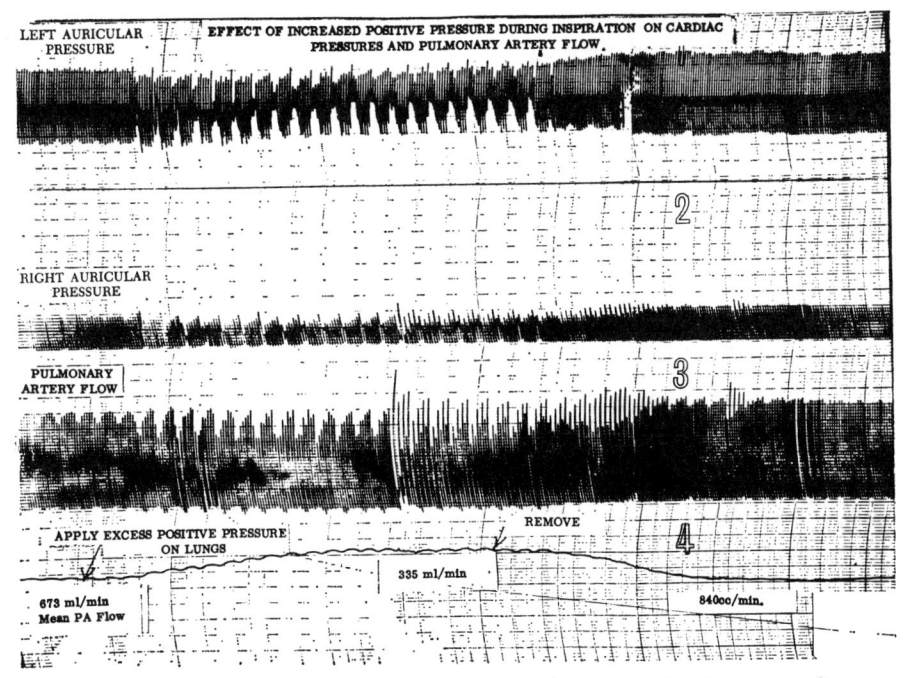

FIG. 23–7. Effect of increased positive pressure during inspiration on cardiac pressures and pulmonary artery blood flow. Note the fall in left atrial pressure due to impedance of pulmonary flow. The pulmonary artery flow falls from a mean value of 673 ml/min to 335 ml/min with an airway pressure of 16 mm Hg. Note also the fall in right atrial pressure due to the impairment of venous return.

fall in intrapleural pressure accompanied by a fall in intra-alveolar pressure occurs during inspiration. This fall in pressure is reflected in a decreased pressure in the great veins and the atria. At the height of a normal inspiration, the fall in intrapleural pressure amounts to -6 to -10 cm H_2O, whereas the fall in intraalveolar pressure amounts to -4 to 5 cm H_2O. Thus, natural ventilation provides a suction pump.

The abolition of the thoracic pump mechanism for venous return to the right heart represents a major form of interference in circulation. During controlled ventilation the intrapleural pressure may be elevated to $+3$ cm H_2O. The atria and great veins are compressed at the height of inflation and the intravascular pressure raised so as to minimize the extrathoracic–intrathoracic gradient of pressure. Venous flow into the veins and heart, cardiac output, and blood pressure decrease.[36–38]

Compensatory mechanisms may be invoked to reestablish the normal extrathoracic-intrathoracic pressure gradient. A rise in peripheral venous pressure occurs by a reflex increase in venomotor tone. This occurs if neurogenic vasomotor responses are intact (not depressed by a central nervous system drug) and blood volume is normal. Thus, either a depressed (or overanesthetized) patient or one with a reduced circulatory volume may be incapable of compensating for the adverse circulatory effects of controlled ventilation (CV-IPPV), and controlled ventilation may be hazardous.

Alpha-receptor blockade results in an increased susceptibility to changes in intrathoracic pressure.

3. *Cardiac tamponade:* When the lungs are inflated by a positive pressure and the entire intrathoracic pressure becomes positive during controlled ventilation, the increased pressure is imposed on the heart and great vessels. Subjecting these structures to such pressure tends to squeeze them and impede venous flow into the thorax.[16–20, 22–24, 39–41]

LONG-TERM EFFECTS OF IPPV. Airway pressure changes are readily transmitted to the intrathoracic structures. An increase in the intrathoracic pressure over a prolonged period (days) initiates several changes that may compensate for the circulatory changes cited, including (1) distribution of body water;[9] (2) urinary output;[40] (3) sodium excretion;[41] (4) ADH secretion (increased plasma levels).[32]

MECHANICAL INJURY TO LUNGS. Experimentally, the pressure required to rupture the exposed lung is about 40 to 80 cm H_2O.[42] When the lungs are supported in the intact thorax, pressures of 80 to 140 cm H_2O are needed. It is not unusual in everyday living to produce intrapulmonary pressures of 80 to 90 cm H_2O as during straining or coughing. These factors together with the breathing system must be evaluated in considering potential mechanical injury to the lungs. By manual means, it is most difficult to attain pressures greater than 50 to 60 cm H₂O. With mechanical ventilators, however, a high pressure can be achieved and possibly rupture alveoli. This is particularly true if there is uneven inflation in which case alveolar septa may be ruptured.[43,44]

During intrathoracic operations, there is reduced lung function and altered pulmonary air volumes.[45] Differential pressures are created often by the positive-pressure ventilation with overexpansion in some areas with rupture.[45,46]

ACUTE METABOLIC LUNG INJURY.[51] Injury to the lung can result from severe systemic disturbances with the production of toxic chemical metabolites that cause parenchymal lung damage. The endothelial cells of the pulmonary capillaries are insulted first and allow transudation of water and colloid units into the lung interstitium. The clinical picture is that of noncardiogenic pulmonary edema (NCE). Second, the alveolar epithelium shows diffuse cellular damage, particularly to type 1 alveolar cells, and is associated with an exudative process into the first interstitium of both large and small white blood cells.[48] A typical inflammatory picture is histologically observed.[49]

The damage to both endothelium and alveolar epithelium produces the clinical picture of the adult respiratory distress syndrome (ARDS).[50] Conditions commonly producing acute lung injury and ARDS include multiple trauma, shock, and sepsis. Other predisposing factors include aspiration, interstitial pneumonia, multiple transfusions, fat embolism, hypotension, prolonged extensive surgery over 8 hours in duration, and hyperoxia. Damage to type 1 cells is further associated with a loss of surfactant and consequent decreased lung compliance. Unventilated lung areas result in intrapulmonary shunting and hypoxemia, which is refractory. Type 2 cells are damaged later in the injury process and, usually, when exposed to high oxygen concentrations. Simultaneously, destruction of white blood cells from the exudative process releases mediators and aids in the formation of fibrin thrombi. The development of ARDS coincides with the malfunction of type 2 cells.[51]

Therapy.[51] The primary objective is to achieve an adequate arterial oxygen content with an FI$_{O_2}$ below 0.5 and with PEEP levels that do not significantly reduce cardiac output.[52] For NCE, improvement in gas exchange is accomplished with 5 to 15 cm H₂O PEEP, and 10 cm H₂O appears to be optimal. For ARDS, improvement is seen with higher levels of PEEP, between 10 and 30 cm H₂O, whereas the optimal response is usually seen at levels between 10 and 20 cm H₂O PEEP.[53] The application of PEEP in NCE results in dramatic improvement and the morbidity has been greatly diminished. Patients with severe ARDS continue, however, to have a high morbidity, and the mortality approaches 50% despite the present techniques of supportive care.[54] New understanding of the mechanisms involved and of newer therapies needs to be developed.[55]

PRECAUTIONS IN PRESSURE VENTILATION. To avoid both physiologic complications and structural injury, the mean airway pressure must be kept low. The mean airway pressure is defined as the mean of an infinite number of individual pressure values. It can be kept low by the following considerations:

1. The *tidal volume* required should be transferred in a brief time, i.e., inflation should last 1 to 1.5 seconds. This leaves a longer period during which there is minimal or no positive pressure and hence the mean pressure through the respiratory cycle becomes low. The ventilation force must deliver flows up to 60 L/min on demand.
2. The *time of inspiration* must be shorter than that of expiration. The time of the inspiratory phase or inspiration should be shorter than exhalation phase plus the expiratory pause. The ratio of inspiratory to expiratory time should be approximately 1:2. One may consider that the expiratory pause (when no air is flowing) should be almost as long as the inspiratory phase.
3. *Resistance to expiration* should be low. This minimizes the intra-alveolar pressure.
4. The application of *negative pressure*[22,23,25] tends to counteract the circulatory effect of positive airway pressures. The requirements for the proper application of a negative phase are several. First, an intact thorax is essential. In the open chest, a negative pressure will merely collapse the exposed lung. Second, a normal lung elasticity is necessary to respond to the suction force of the negative pressure by contracting and thereby permitting a lower extrapleural pressure to be created. Similarly, the bronchial tree should not collapse; such collapse may occur at weak points. Third, a minimal airway resistance will allow the air to be "sucked" out without trapping. Fourth, low negative pressures, −5 cm of H₂O or less, are indicated. Higher pressures evoke check-valve mechanisms at bronchioles and the lower end of the trachea. Collapse at these points may cause extensive air trapping, whereas failure of some collapse at these points may permit pulmonary edema.

VALUE OF DIFFERENT PRESSURE PATTERNS. Ventilatory patterns or pressures that are favorable to the circulation are as a rule unfavorable to the efficiency of ventilation. A rapid inspiratory flow, absence of EIP or PEEP, a long expiration, and an expiratory pause are favorable to circulation and minimally interfere with cardiac output.[56] A negative-pressure expiratory phase tends to counteract the effects of positive inspiratory pressures and to promote ve-

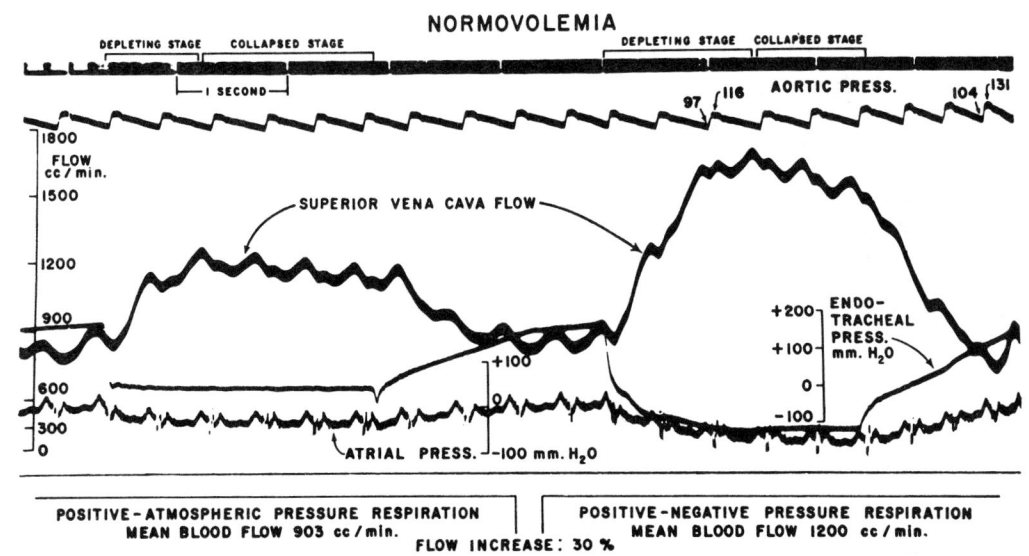

FIG. 23–8. Effect of negative airway pressure on venous return to the heart. Note the marked increase in superior vena cava flow. In hypovolemia this effect is similar and improves the cardiac output and circulation. From Brecher, G.A.: Venous Return. New York, Grune and Stratton, 1956.

nous return (Fig. 23–8).[33] The use of a negative-pressure phase may be indicated in patients with circulatory failure. In contrast, a high elevated mean mask pressure raises intrathoracic pressure, decreases venous return, impedes pulmonary blood flow, and, after several cardiac beats, may reduce cardiac output by as much as 25%.

Ventilation is *disadvantaged* by negative airway expiratory pressure. There is uneven air distribution in the lungs; airway closure tends to occur early with some air trapping. The caliber of the small- and even medium-sized bronchi is reduced, thereby increasing resistance to flow.[57,58] A low or negative airway pressure may reduce residual pulmonary volume and occasionally promote pulmonary congestion.[59]

A moderate positive expiratory pressure of 5 cm H_2O does not significantly alter pulmonary circulatory or systemic dynamics, nor does it alter cardiac output in normovolemic patients. Also, cardiac output is less likely to be altered in patients with low pulmonary compliance. Circulatory readjustments more easily occur when an expiratory pause is permitted.

INDICATIONS FOR CONTROLLED OR ASSISTED VENTILATION IN ANESTHESIA PRACTICE[60]

GENERAL[59]

1. To provide ideal working conditions of quiet and increased relaxation.
2. To correct mediastinal flutter and paradoxic ventilation.
3. To facilitate removal of anesthetic agents before the end of surgery.
4. For prolonged operations or any operation that favors atelectasis.

SPECIAL. Assisted ventilation is specifically indicated:[60]

1. During most surgical procedures under general anesthesia.
2. During decortication of lung.
3. To facilitate mixing of gases (emphysema).
4. When there is difficulty in obtaining collapse of lung on operated side.

Controlled ventilation is specifically indicated during:

1. Any need for a quiet diaphragm.
2. Dissection of lung from diaphragm or pericardium.
3. Dissection of hilar vessels.
4. Repair of diaphragmatic hernia; transpleural spleen and gastroesophageal operations.
5. Bronchiectasis.
6. In cardiac surgery—shunt operation of tetralogy type.

REQUISITES

1. Patent airway (endotracheal tube for anesthesia or respiratory care).
2. Synchronization with spontaneous breathing or muscular paralysis (with relaxant).

INDICATIONS FOR VENTILATORY SUPPORT IN CRITICAL CARE MEDICINE.[54] There are three major categories of disordered cardiopulmonary physiology managed in part by mechanical ventilatory support: (1) apnea, (2) acute ventilatory failure, and (3) impending ventilatory failure.

Apnea, when persistent, is usually due to drugs or cerebral hypoxia. It is readily diagnosed and is dominated by low arterial P_{O_2} and high Pa_{CO_2}. Absence of ventilation requires mechanical ventilatory support or manual artificial respiration initially.

Acute ventilatory failure describes the failure of the mechanical pulmonary system to adequately move air into and out of the lungs and permit exchange of gases at the capillary-alveolar level. It is a component of acute respiratory failure. Acute respiratory failure (ARF) defines this state and failure of ventilation is usually the chief cause.

Mechanical elements of breathing consists of the integrity of the structural component, the chest cage, the muscles of respiration, and the nervous system component regulating muscle performance. These are designated as *the ventilatory pump*. Failure of this system may be due to anatomic abnormalities, central nervous system depression, motor nerve disorders, and malfunctions at the myoneural junction. Ventilatory muscle fatigue is a major feature of acute respiratory failure and impending failure. These factors represent the state of *pump failure*.

Lung factors that increase the work of breathing and lead to ventilatory failure include: (1) hypoxemia causing increased respiratory drive; (2) increased airway resistance; (3) decreased lung compliance; and (4) increased physiologic dead space and/or increased functional residual capacity. These factors in various combinations denote *lung failure*.

In acute or impending ventilatory failure, the excretion of carbon dioxide is more compromised than is the oxygenation system. Hence, the condition has been historically termed *respiratory acidosis*. Blood gases are diagnostic and an arterial P_{CO_2} above 50 mm Hg, with an arterial pH below 7.3, define *ventilatory failure*.

One may summarize the clinical circumstances in the traditional term of acute respiratory failure (ARF) as resulting from two primary mechanisms, namely, failure of the intrinsic ventilatory pump or failure of gas exchange at the alveoli due to lung factors.

PROCEDURES TO DETERMINE DEPTH OF ANESTHESIA DURING CONTROLLED VENTILATION

1. Depth can be assessed by remembering the patients' behavior during induction and how quickly they are anesthetized.
2. Note ease with which apnea is produced.
3. Allow spontaneous respiration to return and note how quickly this occurs.
4. Determine whether only thoracic muscles are relaxed as shown by abdominal movement without chest movement, or if both thoracic and diaphragmatic muscles are relaxed—the latter indicates much greater depth.
5. Note compliance, the "feel of the bag." In deep planes there is little resistance.
6. Determine carbon dioxide response.
7. Note how much anesthetic has been used and determine or estimate the end-expiratory concentration of the anesthetic inhalation agents.
8. Variations in pulse rate will furnish an indication of anesthetic depth.

MANUAL ARTIFICIAL VENTILATION[12,61–63]

To bring about proper ventilation by manual means, the following basic variables must be evaluated and practical guides established.

PRESSURE VALUES. First, consideration must be given to the amount of pressure to be applied. From compliance studies under ideal circumstances, one should expect to obtain approximately 100 ml of air displacement for each 1 mm Hg pressure applied. Because some of this force must overcome resistance and friction, however, the volume resulting from 1 mm Hg of applied pressure is somewhat lower. Approximately 60 ml of air will be moved into the lung for each mm Hg pressure change (50 ml/cm H_2O). In general, the pressure varies with the individual patient's physical state and the level of anesthesia. In practice, the range of pressure is between 8 and 20 mm Hg.

RATE OF INFLATION. Next, consideration must be given to the rate with which the positive pressure is applied to the breathing bag. In general, it might be stated that the minute volume ventilation in clinical anesthesia exceeds the patient's normal spontaneous minute ventilation because of ventilatory perfusion inequalities that inevitably develop during anesthesia and artificial ventilation. Because minute volume is the product of tidal air times respiratory rate, and alveolar ventilation is more effectively accomplished by an excess of the tidal volume, a respiratory rate smaller than that in the unanesthetized state will suffice. It is recommended that the intermittent positive pressure force be applied 10 to 15 times per minute in adults and should be rhythmic. Fewer ventilations with a short inflation phase will also produce a lower mean airway pressure. For children, a rate of 20 times per minute with variations from 15 to 30 times represents an efficient value. For infants, rates of 30 to 40 times per minute are efficient.

TIME SEQUENCE OF THE CYCLE. The third consideration is that of the relationship between the inspiratory phase of the ventilatory cycle and the expiratory phase. The latter period includes an expiratory pause. From Cournand's work,[30a] it is axiomatic that the exhalation or deflation period, plus the period of rest, should be longer than the inspiratory period to compensate for any impedance to venous return and to allow restoration of circulatory dynamics. The inspiratory period or inflation phase should last from 1 to 1.5 seconds. Removing all pressure then permits exhalation to occur with minimal impedance; in the normal lung that time should be about 1 second, but in emphysema or in bronchoconstrictive disease it may last 5 seconds. After deflation, a pause should be observed denoted by inactivity before the next inflation. This expiratory phase should last as long as the inflation period. Stated another way, the period of expiration must occupy more than one half the respiratory cycle. A good rule in practice is to divide the total cycle into thirds: one third (1 to 1.5 sec) inspiratory; one third expiratory deflation, and one third for expiratory pause (rest).

PATTERN OF POSITIVE PRESSURE. The fourth consideration is that of the pattern by which the force of positive inflationary pressure is applied. This should vary with the individual patient. The anesthetist can quickly judge how readily air is entering a given pulmonary system by appreciating the changes in resistance. The pattern of pressures can then be varied accordingly. In the normal lung, one begins the application of force slowly during the first 0.5 second and then sharply and steadily attains a peak within a total of 1 to 1.5 seconds. At the height of inflation, there is complete and absolute release of any compressing force on the breathing bag. It is also important that a rebreathing bag at the end of expiration not be full because a full bag will exert significant continued, undesirable pressure on the alveoli.

Careful manual control of ventilation according to the fundamental principles outlined will furnish physiologic ventilation. The trained, informed, and experienced anesthesiologists can simulate an ideal pressure curve. Furthermore, they can individualize the patient's resistance and compliance and adapt their pressures and breathing patterns to suit the circumstances. By attention to detail and timing, cardiovascular deterioration can be avoided. It has been stated that "ventilation carefully assisted by the anesthetist squeezing the bag as the patient inspires gives an effective ventilation."[12]

Disadvantages are obvious. The manual technique requires stamina for long procedures; it may become tiresome and diminish the anesthetist's attention. At least one hand must be occupied at all times, else ventilation will suffer. Thus, the anesthetist is not too free to carry out other therapy and extensive monitoring.

MECHANICAL VENTILATION[6,63]

The devices employed for resuscitation, mechanical ventilation, and intermittent positive pressure therapy are broadly classified as ventilatory support units. In 1975 the American College of Chest Physicians (ACCP) and the American Thoracic Society (ATS) jointly proposed a series of terms and symbols on pulmonary nomenclature. The terms and symbols used in Anesthesia and Respiratory Care will be used here (see Appendix 1 at the end of the Chapter).[64]

DEFINITIONS. A ventilator is a mechanical device designed to augment or replace the patient's lung ventilatory system and spontaneous ventilation when attached to the upper airway. Ventilators are further classified into five categories, depending upon whether (1) they completely replace normal ventilatory efforts; (2) the ventilator is triggered by spontaneous breathing in between mechanical ventilation; or (3) a combination of units; as explained in the following:

1. *Controlled ventilation*: Manual or mechanical ventilation in which the frequency of breathing is determined by the ventilator according to a preset rate and the appropriate tidal volume delivered accordingly. The patient's efforts will not affect the rate. The ventilator is in the Control Mode Ventilation (CMV).
2. *Assisted ventilation*: Manual or mechanical ventilation in which the patient initiates inspiration and establishes the rate of breathing at which positive pressure is delivered, producing a tidal volume. The ventilator is in the Assist Mode Ventilation (AMV).
3. *Assist-control ventilation*: Manual or mechanical ventilation in which the minimum frequency of breathing is determined by a preset rate on the ventilator, but the patient has the option to initiate inhalation and breath at a faster rate.
4. *Intermittent mandatory ventilation (IMV)*: Periodic controlled ventilation is given, with the patient capable of breathing spontaneously between controlled breaths.
5. *Synchronized IMV (SIMV)*: Periodical controlled ventilation is given but is synchronized with the patient's inspiratory effort. The patient is able to breathe spontaneously in between the synchronized mandatory breaths.

CHARACTERISTICS OF VENTILATORS

PRINCIPLES OF OPERATION. A ventilator's function is to deliver a supply of gas to the lungs and to enhance carbon dioxide removal. The following two variables in ventilation should be considered:

632 *General Anesthesia*

1. *Volume ventilator*: The ventilator delivers a preset inspiratory volume within a specific time limit. This volume is delivered irrespective of the pressure required to deliver that volume. The volume remains constant and the pressure is variable.
2. *Pressure ventilator*: The ventilator delivers a preset inspiratory pressure. This pressure is delivered irrespective of the volume of gas going into the patient's lungs. The pressure remains constant and the volume is variable.

In practice, ventilators must be readjusted from time to time regardless of which mechanism they employ because of changes in metabolic requirements or changes in resistance and lung characteristics. Attempts have been made to devise auxiliary control mechanisms using some signal from the patient to alter respiratory frequency or inspiratory pressure. Montgomery has used the electromyogram to trigger tank and other types of respirators.[65] Frumin[66] has successfully sampled the end-expiratory air and used its P_{CO_2} to adjust peak inspiratory

BLOWER TYPE VENTILATORS
CONSTANT FORCE GENERATOR

INTRAPULMONARY GAS DISTRIBUTION: UNEVEN

HYPER-VENTILATION   HYPO-VENTILATION   PENDULUM AIR   AIRTRAPPING (EXPIRATION)

■▶ RESPIRATOR'S DRIVING FORCE ON RESPIRATORY GAS
■ GAS FLOW RATE
■ ■ ■ TOTAL RESISTANCE AGAINST INSUFFLATION (PRESSURE)

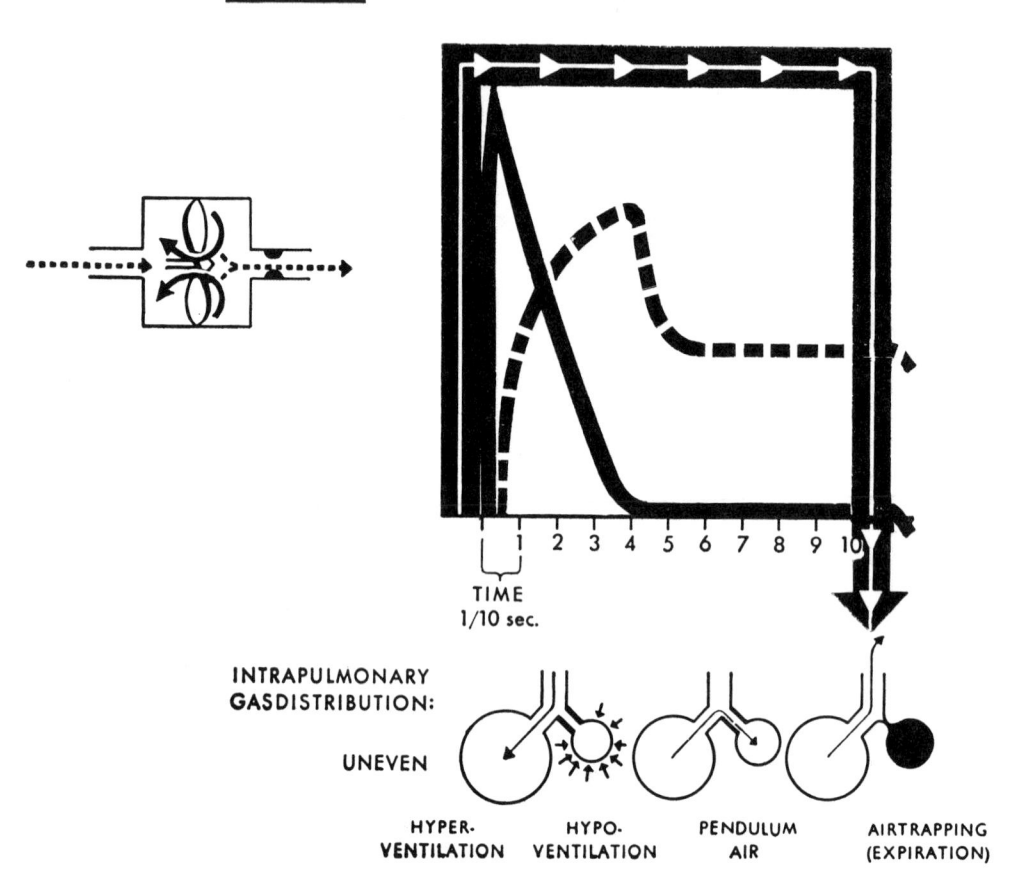

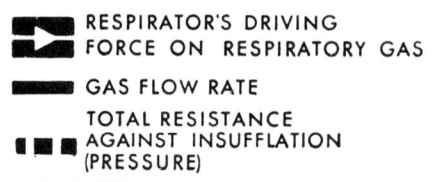

FIG. 23–9A. Illustrates principal differences in characteristics during inspiration between pressure preset type ventilators (constant force) and volume preset ventilators (increasing force). Notice the harmful effect on intrapulmonary gas distribution because the respirator's driving force on respiratory gas starts abruptly with a resulting high initial rate of gas flow which decreases when resistance increases. Compare with Figure 23–9B on facing page. Courtesy of Electro Medicinska.

Control of Breathing by Artificial Methods **633**

pressure to maintain a constant P_{CO_2} in the patient.

Changes in lung characteristics affect the performance of ventilator action. A decrease in compliance or an increase in resistance does not greatly influence a volume-cycled ventilator. But if the ventilator operates as a constant pressure generator, then the inspiratory time must be increased or the total minute ventilation will be decreased. Adjustment must be made by decreasing expiratory time or increasing the force of delivery.

Contrariwise, a pressure-cycled ventilator is generally susceptible to pulmonary changes. But if the ventilator operates as a variable-pressure generator, *i.e.*, a flow generator, then with a change in resistance or compliance there will be changes in tidal volume. In turn, there will be a compensatory increase or decrease in rate so that minute ventilation may be held constant. If the rate becomes rapid, however, a critical point is reached when only dead space will be ventilated.

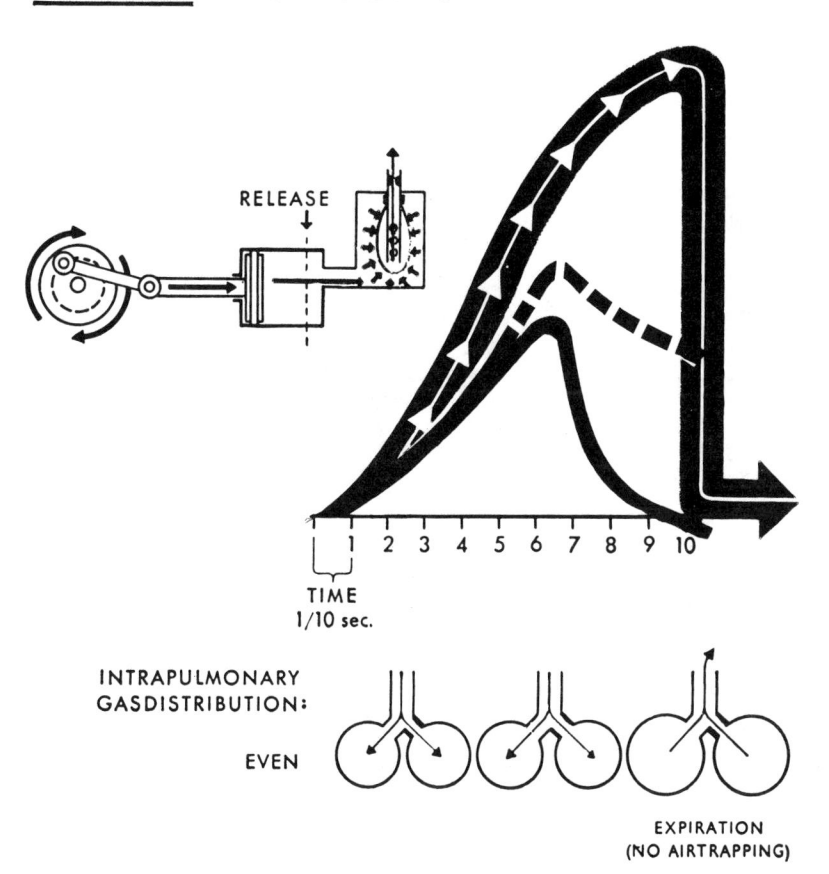

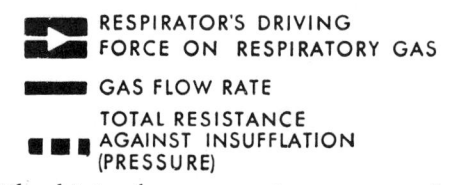

FIG. 23–9B. The driving force on respiratory gas gradually increases due to accelerating speed of the piston in the cylinder, thus causing the flow rate of the inspiratory gas to increase simultaneously with increasing resistance (increasing force generator). The effect on intrapulmonary gas distribution is even. Compare with Figure 23–9A on facing page. Courtesy of Electro Medicinska.

634 *General Anesthesia*

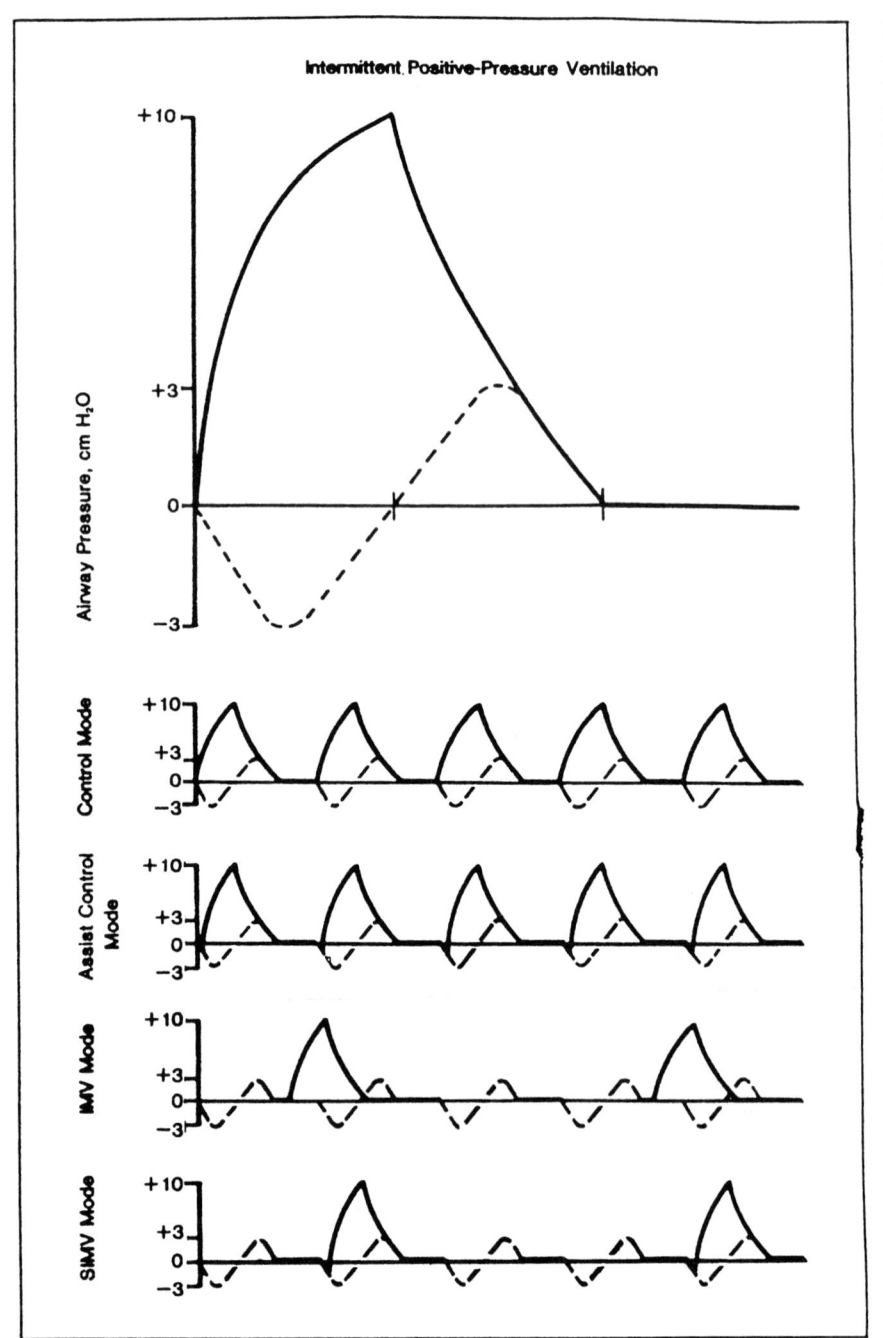

FIG. 23–10. Classic airway pressure curves for various modes of intermittent positive-pressure ventilation superimposed on the normal spontaneous airway pressure curves. IMV indicates intermittent mandatory ventilation; SIMV, synchronized IMV. From Cane, R.D., and Shapiro, B.A.: Mechanical ventilatory support. J.A.M.A., *254*:87, 1985.

CHARACTERISTICS OF INSPIRATION PHASE (Fig. 23–9). Principal differences in the characteristics of the inspiration phase of the volume preset ventilator (increasing force generator [23–9B]) compared to pressure preset ventilator (constant force generator [23–9A]) are illustrated.

PRESSURE PATTERNS. Each ventilator has a characteristic pattern to the curve showing changes in pressure during the ventilatory cycle, depending on the mode selected (Fig. 23–10).

The pressure patterns that are produced by a ventilator will be determined by the functional characteristics of the machine and by the patient's resistance to the air flow and to lung expansion. The greater the patient's resistance, the more exaggerated will be the pressure variations produced during inflation and deflation. The magnitude of pressure changes possibly generated by the machine can never exceed the fundamental capacities of the machine. For example, an instrument that is incapable of generating a vacuum can only develop intermittent positive pressures. An instrument that vents to atmosphere through a low-resistance port will not provide positive upper airway pressures during exhalation. A variety of pressure patterns, *e.g.* IPPV, PNPV, and IPPV, with a positive pressure residual can be developed by the same ventilator if it has an optimal negative-pressure phase and a variable resistance to exhalation.

CONTROL OF FLOW. Air flow into the lungs is determined by changes in airway pressure. The force generated by a ventilator is expended against (1) the elastic resistances of the lungs and thorax; (2) the nonelastic resistances of the lungs and thorax; (3) the nonelastic resistances of the tissues such as their inherent weight or inertia; and (4) the fundamental resistance offered by the air passages to the flow of air in them. If resistance is high, overall flow must be low or a greater pressure will be needed to deliver the volume of gas.

Thus, the rate and volume of air entering the lungs or the flow as well as the pattern of flow are determined by the speed of build-up of airway pressure.

CYCLING METHOD. Four methods are used to determine when the gas supply to the patient is to be interrupted. Presumably, the controls are set when an adequate volume of gas has been delivered. This cycling occurs when:

1. A predetermined volume is delivered (volume ventilator)
2. A predetermined pressure is reached (pressure ventilator)
3. After a predetermined time has elapsed
4. A predetermined safety limit is reached

In the first two, cycling to exhalation depends upon the tripping of a pressure-sensitive toggle valve. This valve may be triggered when the given volume of gas has been delivered, or triggering may occur when a maximum airway pressure is reached. If the valve is triggered by the patient's negative inspiratory effort, this valve is thrown into the inspiratory position and a volume of gas is delivered to the patient.

A ventilator that offers assisted ventilation is triggered by a subatmospheric (negative) pressure produced by a minimal inspiratory effort of the patient to open the toggle valve that allows the delivery of a volume of gas to the patient. When a *maximum inspiratory* preset pressure or preset volume is achieved in the airway, the valve is triggered into the expiratory position. Thus, by adjusting the flows, rate, pressure, or volume, the maximum inspiratory pressure or volume will determine the time of expiration and a minimum airway pressure will determine the initiation of inspiration.

In some ventilators, cycling is determined by a timing mechanism that depends on a pneumatic, electrical, or mechanical device. The maximum duration of the inspiratory phase is determined and the apparatus cycles at this time, regardless of the pressure achieved.

CONSTRUCTION ASPECTS.[25,67,68] Engineers have devised many ingenious systems for performing artificial ventilation. Compressed gas was used in early ventilators as a pneumatic control device to provide the necessary energy. The gas used to ventilate the patient is obtained from a compressed oxygen or air source. Such methods of control have been replaced by fluidically controlled devices. Electronic power control for ventilators is available.

A ventilator basically is a generator of a force applied to the pulmonary system. Because this force may be applied according to either an increasing pattern or a constant pattern, ventilators can be classified as flow generators or pressure generators that are constant or nonconstant. Table 23–1 lists other variables that are used to classify ventilators.

CLASSIFICATIONS OF VENTILATORS

FLOW GENERATORS (VOLUME PRESET TYPE).
Constant Flow Generators (Fig. 23–11). A constant flow generator has a high internal resistance to deliver a constant flow to the patient. This flow into the lung remains constant, even though the patient's resistance or compliance has changed. This type of generator produces an increasing force throughout inspiration and an increasing pressure in the lungs (Fig. 23–12).

The operating pressure of a constant flow generator can be affected if the patient's pressure comes close to or equals the operating pressure. If this

TABLE 23–1. VENTILATOR VARIABLES

INSPIRATORY PHASE
  Flow generator
    Constant
    Nonconstant
  Pressure generator
    Constant
    Nonconstant
INSPIRATORY PLATEAU
CHANGEOVER FROM INSPIRATORY PHASE TO EXPIRATORY PHASE
  Time-cycled
  Pressure-cycled
  Volume-cycled
  Secondary limit (safety limit)
EXPIRATORY PHASE
  Retard pressure
  Subambient pressure
  Threshold pressure (PEEP, ZEEP, etc.)
CHANGEOVER FROM EXPIRATORY PHASE TO INSPIRATORY PHASE
  Control
  Assist
  Assist/control
  Intermittent mandatory ventilation
  Pressure support

636 General Anesthesia

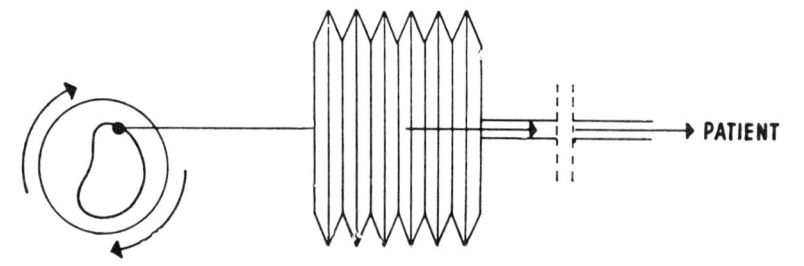

FIG. 23–11. Increasing force generator direct-acting in the patient circuit. The gas flow will be proportional to the speed of the bellows. Pressure and flow will be synchronized, and the available power will gradually increase with a maximum at peak flow. From Norlander, O.P.: Functional analysis of force and power of mechanical ventilators. Acta Anaesthesiol. Scand., 8:57, 1964.

happens, the constant flow generator becomes a constant pressure generator.

Methods in which a constant flow generator may be adapted include:

1. Blowers
2. High-pressure gas source with reducing valves
3. Compression with or without reducing valves
4. Gas injector (only if without back pressure)

The Puritan Bennett MA 1-7200, Seemens Servo Bard C, and Bourns BEAR ventilators are examples of constant flow generators.

Nonconstant Flow Generators (Fig. 23–13). A ventilator in this category has an identical flow pattern from breath to breath, regardless of changes in the patient's lung characteristics. The Emerson ventilator is a good example of a nonconstant flow generator and produces a sine wave flow into the lung developed by the use of a piston and wheel (Fig. 23–14).

CONSTANT FORCE GENERATORS (PRESSURE GENERATORS). Pressure generators, by contrast, deliver a relatively constant force throughout inspiration. Functional characteristics of flow, volume, and pressure patterns will differ depending on the *magnitude* of the force or the pressure as related to the resistance in the apparatus and, additionally, the resistance in the patient. Thus, two main modifications are recognized:

1. *Low source force (low pressure and low resistance in apparatus)*: Devices of this type generate an abrupt but constant force (Fig. 23–15). It is only slightly modified by the inertia features of the apparatus so that the driving force on the respiratory tract of the patient is relatively constant. This is seen in the pressure pattern at the mouth showing a rapid rise. As such, the device shows the functional patterns (Fig. 23–16) of a high initial flow rate followed by a steadily declining rate to zero with a coincident rapid increase in lung volume and a rapid rise in alveolar pressure.
2. *High source of pressure or force with high apparatus resistance*: Devices of this type can generate a high force that is dissipated, in part, by the apparatus so that the pressure delivered to the patient is near to the pressures developing in the alveoli. The pressure is not abrupt but is relatively constant (Fig. 23–17). This is seen in the pressure pattern at the mouth or the delivered pressure. Devices of this type show the functional pattern (Fig. 23–18) of a moderate initial flow rate followed by a slight decrease in flow rate with a coincident linear rise in lung volume and a parallel rise in alveolar pressure.

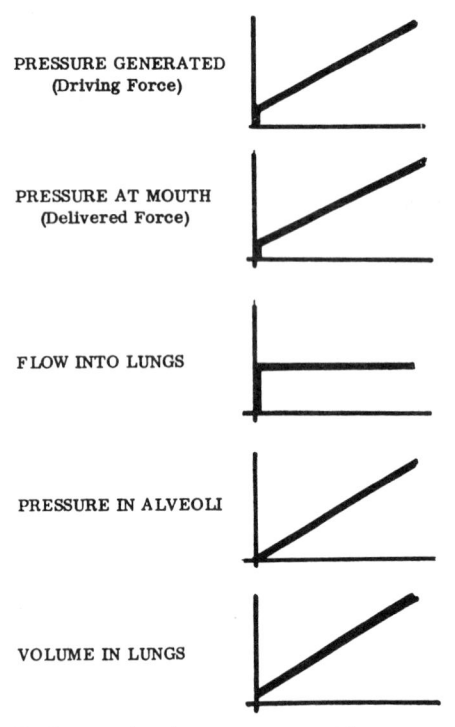

FIG. 23–12. Increasing force generator (flow generator) of constant flow type showing characteristics of the inspiratory phase: force available or pressure generated, of an increasing linear pattern, the pressure delivered, flow into pulmonary system, pressure developed in alveoli, and volume change in lungs. From Mushin, W.W., Rendell-Baker, L., and Thompson, A.W.: Automatic Ventilation of the Lungs, 2nd ed. London, Blackwell Scientific, 1969.

HUMIDIFICATION. When gases from a wall outlet or cylinder are used and delivered to the lungs, some means of humidifying the gas should be provided. The objectives are (1) to prevent the formation of crusts in the airways; (2) to minimize insensible water loss and to maintain the mucosa in a moist

Control of Breathing by Artificial Methods **637**

FIG. 23–13. Increasing Force Generator (Indirect-Acting). The force is generated by a piston in a cylinder and acts on a bag in the patient circuit. The force generated in the cylinder is utilized for complete compression of the bag. The flow generated in the patient circuit will depend on the primary force characteristics and on the compliance and resistance of the patient's lung. (After Norlander. Pub. in Acta Anes. Scand.)

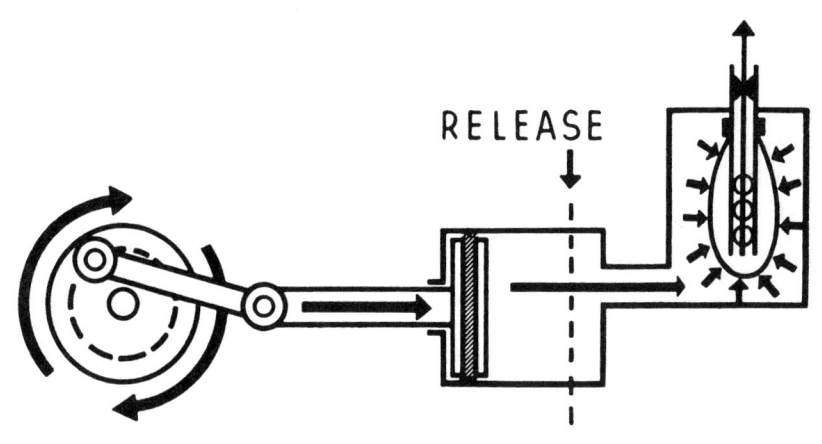

condition; and (3) to diminish inspissation of secretions.

MONITORING. It is desirable to have some means of monitoring the function of a ventilator while it is working, not only for the purpose of checking on the function of the ventilator, but to detect changes in the mechanical properties of the pulmonary tract of the patient.[67,69] Something that measures, however crudely, the volume of air forced into the patient with each stroke of a controlled pressure ventilator will provide warning of obstruction or of any changes in the airway or lungs that would increase the patient's resistances to inflation. When a controlled volume ventilator is being used, a pressure manometer leading from the upper airway will give warning of leaks or of compliance changes in the patient.

Some attention has been given to the development of monitoring systems that will warn you both visually (lights) and audibly (buzzers) in the event of a power failure, of faulty operation of the ventilator or changes in the patient's condition. This approach could lead to a false sense of security. Anesthesiologists, nurses, and respiratory care practitioners should be trained in alertness so that any change in performance or patient condition should be immediately observed.

ADVANTAGES OF MECHANICAL VENTILATORS.
For the patient:

- Safer
- Constant ventilation (rate, pressure, volume)

FIG. 23–14. Inspiratory phase: flow, volume, and pressure patterns with a sine-wave-pressure generator. From Mushin, W.W., Rendell-Baker, L., and Thompson, A.W.: Automatic Ventilation of the Lungs, 2nd ed. London, Blackwell Scientific, 1969.

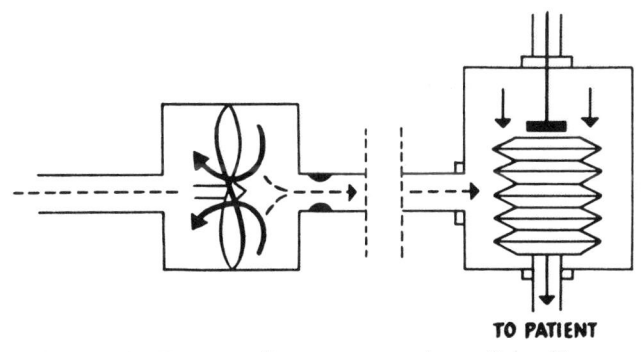

FIG. 23–15. Constant force generator (nonadjustable flow). The force is generated by a compressor of the blower type, which has a maximum output of 140 to 180 L/min without any load. From Norlander, O.P.: Functional analysis of force and power of mechanical ventilators. Acta Anaesthesiol. Scand., 8: 57, 1964.

638 *General Anesthesia*

PRESSURE GENERATED
(Driving Force)

PRESSURE AT MOUTH
(Delivered Force)

FLOW INTO LUNGS

PRESSURE IN ALVEOLI

VOLUME IN LUNGS

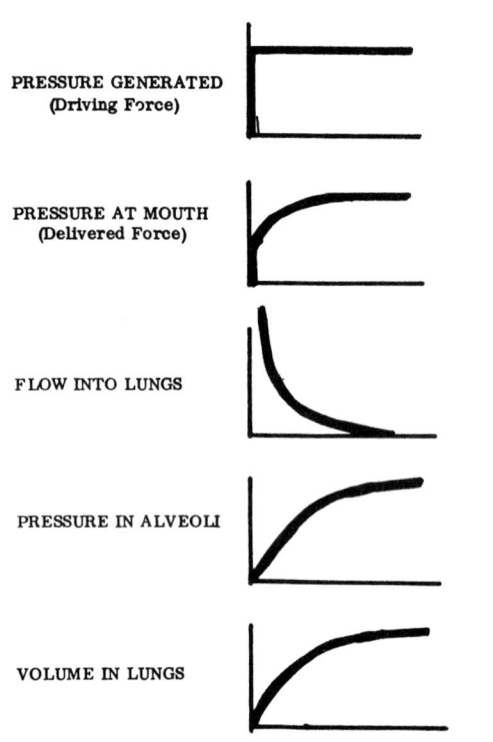

FIG. 23–16. Constant force generator (pressure generator). Generator possesses a low source of force and apparatus has low resistance. Characteristics of inspiratory phase are shown. From Mushin, W.W., Rendell-Baker, L., and Thompson, A.W.: Automatic Ventilation of the Lungs, 2nd ed. London, Blackwell Scientific, 1969.

- Less anesthetic required
- May support the circulation

For the anesthetist:

- A "third hand"
- Frees the right hand from squeezing the bag to other duties
- Blood pressure
- Pulse
- Intravenous infusions
- Charting

For the surgeon:

- Better working conditions
- Quieter operative field
- Better relaxation

DISADVANTAGES OF MECHANICAL VENTILATORS

- *Complicated*—the addition of one more piece of equipment is an added strain on the anesthetist, who must be well trained, experienced, and maintain surveillance of the ventilator variable.
- *Apnea*—apnea is produced, and the most reliable sign of anesthesia, the ventilation, is no longer available.
- *Overdosage of anesthetics*—especially of ether and relaxants; overdosage is more likely to occur if the anesthetist is not very experienced.
- *Requires a more skilled anesthetist*

REPRESENTATIVE VENTILATORS

The selection of a ventilator is determined by the purpose and circumstances of a patient's problem. A frequent question asked is "What is the best ventilator?" There is no ideal, all-purpose ventilator available today. Which ventilator is best prescribed in a given situation will depend on the nature of the patient's requirements for artificial ventilation, whether it is required for a brief period or long duration, and whether the patient's problem is associated with loss of respiratory drive, peripheral motor loss, or pulmonary disease. It will depend on who is going to operate and oversee the maintenance of the vertilator and obviously what power and compressed gas resources are available.

CHOICE OF VENTILATOR (TABLE 23–2). Pulmonary system conditions and changes in airway resistance,

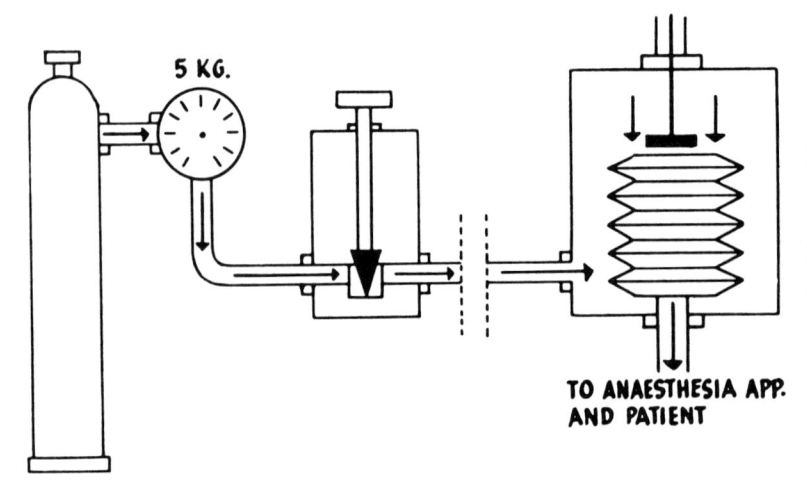

FIG. 23–17. Constant force generator (adjustable flow). The primary force is generated by the compressed gas cylinder. Through the adjustable flow resistance, a gas flow of 0–0.5 L/sec is adjusted, which compresses the bellows. The bellows–patient system contains a safety device limiting the peak pressures to about 30 cm H_2O. From Norlander, O.P.: Functional analysis of force and power of mechanical ventilators. Acta Anaesthesiol. Scand., 8: 57, 1964.

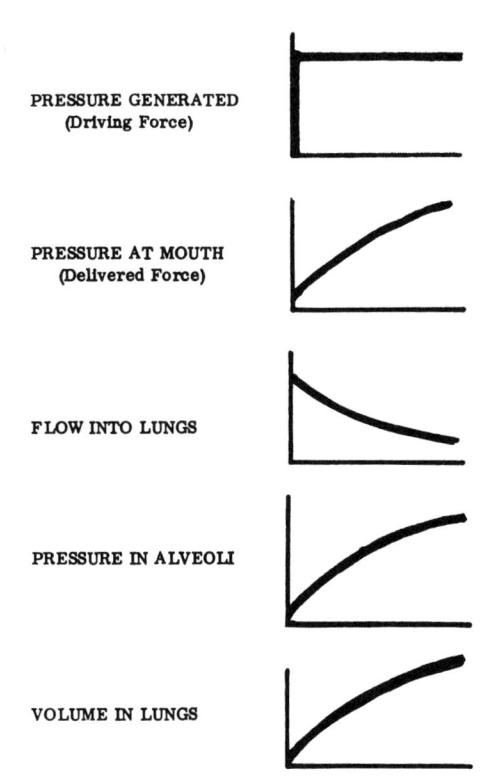

FIG. 23–18. Constant force generator (pressure generator) with high source of pressure and high apparatus resistance. Characteristics of inspiratory phase are shown. From Mushin, W.W., Rendell-Baker, L., and Thompson, A.W.: Automatic Ventilation of the Lungs, 2nd ed. London, Blackwell Scientific, 1969.

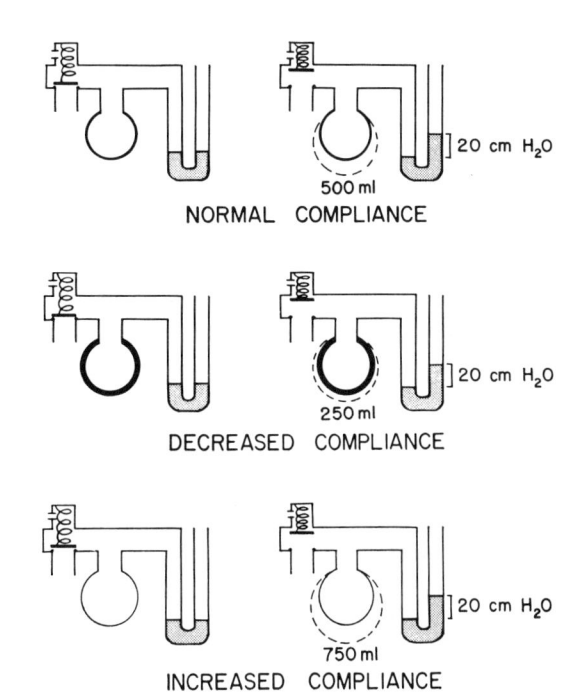

FIG. 23–19. Pressure preset ventilator. Changes in volume associated with fixed cycling pressures in the face of different compliances. From Saklad, M.: Modern Treatment, 6:1, 1969.[70]

lung compliance, pulmonary pathology, and leaks determine the choice of ventilator. Mechanical performance, monitoring, amount of force to be generated, and reliability for continuous use are other determinants.

A *pressure preset ventilator* is useful in the following circumstances: for short-term ventilation; where small airway leaks exist in the delivery system; and when compliance of lung is good while airway resistance is low. These devices compensate for small leaks, but if the leaks are large, cycling of the ventilator may not occur. If changes in resistance or compliance occur, a variable volume will be delivered. As compliance decreases, a smaller volume is delivered (Fig. 23–19).

A *volume preset ventilator* is indicated for prolonged use and for conditions of changing resistance and compliance. Generally, if resistance increases and/or compliance decreases, these devices will still deliver the set volume. In presence of airway leaks, a smaller volume will be delivered into the pulmonary system. In this circumstance the ventilator may be preset with a larger volume—enough to compensate for the leak (Fig. 23–20).

EFFECT OF CHANGE IN COMPLIANCE. Changes in volume delivered when changes in compliance occur have been studied by Saklad,[70] and his comparison of ventilators is shown in (Table 23–3). Lost gas due to compression within a ventilator system has also been studied. This is based on a milliliter of volume for each centimeter of water pressure applied to the ventilator system (Table 23–4).

The ventilator compliance can be determined by occluding the circuit outlet and have the ventilator compress a known volume into the circuit. The pressure displayed on the ventilator manometer should be noted. The compliance factor (f) is determined by dividing the known volume compressed by the pressure developed in the circuit.

$$f = \frac{volume}{pressure} = \frac{100 \text{ ml}}{40 \text{ ml}}$$
$$\cong 2.2 \text{ ml/cm H}_2\text{O}$$

EFFECT OF LEAKS. The capability to compensate for leaks represents an important difference between the two classes of ventilators. In model studies ven-

TABLE 23–2. PRESSURE VERSUS VOLUME PRESET VENTILATORS

Ventilator Type	Leaks	Compensation for Increased Resistance
Pressure limited	Yes	No
Volume limited	Yes	Yes

VOLUME PRESET – PRESSURE VARIABLE

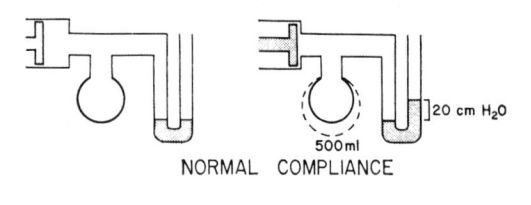

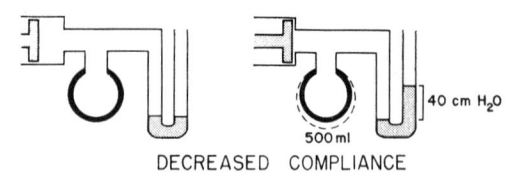

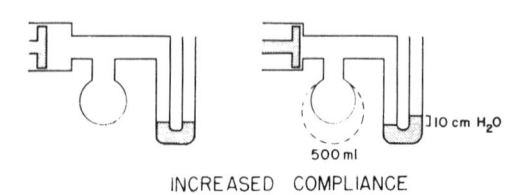

FIG. 23–20. Volume preset ventilator. Changes in pressure associated with fixed delivery in the face of different compliances. From Saklad, M.: Modern Treatment, 6:1, 1969.[70]

tilators were set to deliver 500 ml 20 times per minute to a midcompliance lung. As leaks are introduced into the system, the pressure preset ventilator (Bird Mark VII) maintains tidal volume until cycling fails. The minute volume progressively fell, however, because of decreasing ventilatory rate. Before complete failure, the minute volume was 28% of starting value (Fig. 23–21).

In volume preset ventilators (Engstrom) the tidal and minute volumes fall together. At a critical leak the ventilator continues to deliver a minute volume when the pressure ventilator is failing and is able to deliver a tidal and minute volume of 70% of starting value. Even when leaks are large, the volume ventilator delivers at least 50% of its initial volume, depending on the size of the leak.

TABLE 23–3. CHANGES IN VOLUME OUTPUT OF VENTILATORS IN FACE OF CHANGING COMPLIANCE

Ventilator	Low (ml)	Mid (ml)	High (ml)
Volume preset			
Air Shields	430	500	540
Bennett (VPS)	450	500	550
Pressure preset			
Bennett (PPS)	200	500	800
Bird (Mark VII)	225	500	820

From Saklad, M.: Modern Treatment, 6:1, 1969.[70]

TABLE 23–4. LOST GAS DUE TO COMPRESSION WITHIN VENTILATOR SYSTEM*

Ventilator	ml/cm H$_2$O
Air Shields	5.7
Bennett MA 1	7.1
Bennett PR 2	2.5
Bird Mark VII	2.2
Drager	1.0
Emerson (Post-op)	4.8
Engstrom (Adult tubing)	6.9
Engstrom (Pediatric tubing)	6.1
Ohmeda	2.4

* To determine correct tidal volume:
Multiply the factor corresponding to the ventilator by the peak pressure achieved. Subtract this from the volume delivered by the ventilator.
To determine correct minute volume:
Multiply the factor times the peak pressure and then times the ventilator rate. Subtract from minute volume delivery.
From Saklad, M.: Modern Treatment, 6:, 1969.[70]

REQUIREMENTS FOR RESUSCITATION. Automatic equipment is probably not necessary for emergency resuscitation, although an oxygen-enriched atmosphere may be desirable. Mouth to mask or mouth to airway devices can be operated comfortably and without fatigue for hours.[71] Hand-operated bellows are just as simple, efficient and reliable.

REQUIREMENTS FOR ANESTHESIA. In anesthesia, and especially for open chest work, almost any system that will compress a bellow, which is part of a closed rebreathing system or nonrebreathing system, can be used effectively because the anesthesiologist is constantly available to regulate the gas mixture and readjust the ventilator as necessary (Table 23–5). However, the total pulmonary compliance of the average anesthetized patient is subject to rather wide variations during surgery,[72,73] and controlled volume ventilators tend to insure a more even ventilation than controlled pressure ventilators. These are especially easy to use during anesthesia since each patient can be intubated and an airtight system readily can be obtained.

REQUIREMENTS FOR MEDICAL PATIENTS WITH CHRONIC PULMONARY DYSFUNCTION (TABLE 23–6). A ventilator generally should be selected on the basis of simplicity, ease of maintenance, and the underlying pulmonary difficulties of the patient. One should also consider that the ventilator might be used for long-term therapy.

The controls should be simple to operate and to understand. The less interaction there is between the functions of the ventilator, the better from the point of view of teaching respiratory care personnel to regulate a machine. For instance, in some machines, changing the maximum pressure setting will also change the cycling rate. Although this may be desirable in some situations, it is probably better to

FIG. 23-21. Changing tidal and minute volume delivery to a lung model with a compliance of 0.069 L/cm in the presence of increasing amounts of induced leakage produced by increasing number of holes of 3/32" diameter. From Saklad, M.: Modern Treatment, 6:1, 1969.[70]

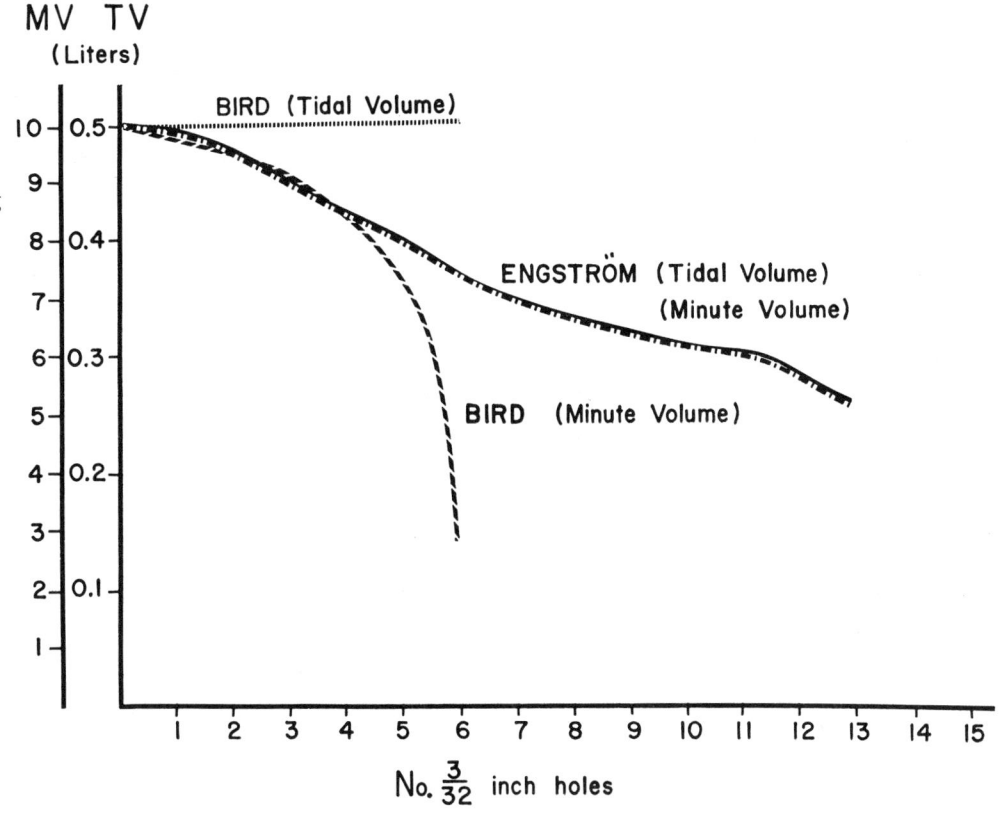

have the major parameters independently adjustable. These would include maximum pressure or volume, rate of inspiratory flow, and cycle duration.

SELECTION. For the conscious patient who breathes spontaneously but with inadequate exchange, an automatic cycling ventilator is usually most reliable. It is not necessary to provide an assistor that will follow the pattern of respiration. Most of these patients adapt quickly to the pattern of an automatic cycling machine.

The attachment to the patient should also be the simplest to maintain and the most secure possible. Although the tank-type respirator performs in a stable manner, the neck piece makes care of a low-lying tracheostomy difficult and nursing of the patient is most inconvenient. The rocking bed, for those patients who require no more than the rather minimal supportive assistance these afford, is of course the simplest.

Many patients with paralysis and others who require assistance with moderate pressures can handle pipe-stems or bite tubes comfortably for long periods while sitting up. These patients usually have to be returned to a tank respirator or rocking bed at night.

Acutely ill patients and those who require higher pressures can be treated effectively for long periods with either a snug-fitting tracheostomy tube fashioned from some soft material like a plastic or rubber or with a cuffed plastic tracheostomy tube.

All patients who can achieve reasonable arterial oxygen saturation on air should be so managed. Several nonrebreathing systems delivering room air and operating on simple and reliable principles are available.

DISCONTINUATION OF CONTROLLED VENTILATION

DEFINITION.[73a] The process of discontinuing ventilator therapy, including airway devices and inhalation therapeutic agents, on a patient dependent on a mechanical ventilator is referred to as *weaning*.

Weaning may be considered to be of three types: (1) from mechanical ventilation, (2) from artificial airways, and (3) from therapeutic gases and aerosols. Primary consideration will be given to weaning from mechanical units.

The actual process of discontinuing ventilator support falls into three stages: (1) preweaning, (2) the weaning procedure, and (3) postweaning care.

GENERAL PRINCIPLE.[74] The criteria for weaning a patient from a ventilator are the reverse of those that necessitated the use of the ventilator initially. Before initiating the actual procedure, the physician must decide that the primary determinant, that is, the pathophysiologic condition dictating the insti-

TABLE 23-5. ANESTHESIA VENTILATORS

Ventilator	Circuit	Control	Drive	Pressure Limit (cm H$_2$O)	PEEP (cm H$_2$O)	Modes of Operation
Air Shields "Ventimeter"	Double	Pneumatic	Pneumatic	40 old; 60 new	None	CMV, assist-control
Hospal 300	Double	Pneumatic	Pneumatic	40	None	CMV, assist, assist-control
Bird Ventilator Mark IVA	Double	Fluidic	Pneumatic	110	0-35	CMV, IMV, assist-control, CPAP
North American Drager AV	Double	Fluidic	Pneumatic	120	0-20	CMV
Ohio	Double	Fluidic	Pneumatic	65	0-15 adapted	CMV
Penlon Nuffield 400	Double	Fluidic	Pneumatic	60	0-20 adapted	CMV
North American Drager AV-E	Double	Electric	Pneumatic	120	2-18	CMV
Ohmeda 7000	Double	Electric	Pneumatic	65	0-20 adapted	CMV
Ohmeda Prototype	Double	Electric	Pneumatic	100	0-20 adapted	CMV
Penlon AV 500	Double	Electric	Pneumatic	70	0-20 adapted	CMV
Foregger Anesthesia	Double	Electric	Pneumatic	70	2-18	CMV
Siemens 900 D	Single	Electric	Pneumatic	120	0-50	CMV, assist-control, pressure support

From Shapiro, B.A., and Cane, R.D.: *Positive Airway Pressure Therapy: PPV and PEEP.* Anesthesiol. Clin. North Am., 5: 1, 1987.

TABLE 23-6. CRITICAL CARE VENTILATORS

Ventilator	Circuit	Control	Drive	Pressure Limit (cm H$_2$O)	PEEP (cm H$_2$O)	Modes of Operation
Monaghan 225	Double	Fluidic	Pneumatic	100	0-20	CMV, SIMV, assist-control, spontaneous, assist
Bennett MA-1	Double	Electric	Compressor	80	0-15	CMV, assist-control, IMV with adaptor, assist
Bennett MA-2, MA-2 + 2	Double	Electric	Compressor	120	0-45	CMV, assist-control, SIMV, CPAP, assist
Ohio CCV-2	Double	Electric	Rotary blower	100	0-40	CMV, SIMV, assist-control, assist, CPAP
Engstrom Erica	Double	Electric	Pneumatic	120	0-30	SIMV, CMV, CPAP, assist, assist-control, inspiratory assist, minimum mandatory ventilation
InterMed Bear I	Single	Electric	Pneumatic, compressor, backup	100	0-30	CMV, SIMV, CPAP, assist, assist-control
InterMed Bear II	Single	Electric	Pneumatic, compressor, backup	120	0-50	CMV, CPAP, SIMV, assist, assist-control
Newport E-100	Single	Electric	Pneumatic	80	0-25	CMV, IMV, assist-control, CPAP
Siemens						
900	Single	Electric	Pneumatic	100	0-50 adapted	CMV, assist, assist-control
900 B	Single	Electric	Pneumatic	100	0-50 adapted	CMV, IMV, assist, assist-control
900 C	Single	Electric	Pneumatic	120	0-50	CMV, SIMV, CPAP, assist, assist-control, pressure support

From Shapiro, B.A., and Cane, R.D.: *Positive Airway Pressure Therapy: PPV and PEEP.* Anesthesiol. Clin. North Am., 5: 1, 1987.

TABLE 23–7. GENERAL FACTORS REQUIRING CORRECTION BEFORE VENTILATOR WEANING IS INITIATED

Anemia	Arrhythmias
Reduced cardiac output	Fever
Fluid balance	Infection
(fluid overload or	Acid-base abnormalities
dehydration)	Electrolyte abnormalities
Shock	Hyperglycemia
State of consciousness	Sleep deprivation
Renal failure	Energy depletion
Secretions	Fever or shivering

tution of mechanical ventilation, is no longer present.

GENERAL CONSIDERATIONS (TABLE 23–7). In addition to the reversal or correction of the primary cause of acute respiratory insufficiency or acute respiratory failure, the clinical conditions that developed consequent to the respiratory insufficiency or were part of the primary cause, should be corrected. A chest x-ray film within normal pulmonary and structural limits, a normal oxygenation system, and a stable cardiovascular system are needed. The inspired oxygen concentration (F_{IO_2}) should be reduced so that the patient's requirements are met by an atmosphere of 50% oxygen or less ($F_{IO_2} < 0.5$).

RESPIRATORY CRITERIA (TABLE 23–8). Certain physiologic parameters must be measured that indicate that (1) the patient has the mechanical ability to sustain spontaneous ventilation and (2) there is a normal capability of the oxygenation system to supply tissue needs.

Tests of these two abilities are considered the criteria for discontinuing mechanical ventilation.

GENERAL PREPARATIONS. Weaning should be undertaken in the morning when sufficient technical and professional support are available.

1. Patient should be conscious with no residual or minimal respiratory depressants (*e.g.*, narcotics, hypnotics, muscle relaxants, etc.). Mental alertness and neurologic status should be thoroughly evaluated.
2. The patient should have been sitting up in bed or in a chair for at least 15 or 30 minutes, 3 times a day (if possible).
3. The patient should be encouraged to take oral feeding (if possible).
4. Any encumbrances (tight clothing, wrappings on the chest or abdomen) should be removed (if not needed).
5. Patient should be encouraged to wash self at bedside (if possible).

TECHNIQUE OF WEANING (Fig. 23–22)

There is no "best" way to wean any patient. Patients who require prolonged mechanical ventilation for various reasons need to be treated and weaned on an individualized basis. Most important is to have a systematic, physiologically oriented weaning procedure that does not fatigue the patient.

DISCONTINUATION OF VENTILATON (IPPV). When the usual criteria for weaning a patient from a mechanical ventilator are met and the patient manifests good spontaneous muscular efforts, discontinuation of IPPV may begin. Either a planned, gradual reduction in patient dependency on mechanical support or complete and immediate withdrawal of mechanical support may be instituted (Table 23–9).

The gradual and progressive reduction in patient dependency on a ventilator may take two courses:

1. *By Gradual Reduction of Inspiratory Pressure.* Initially an assist mode of ventilation should be instituted to replace the controlled mode. A plan of stepwise reduction of the inspiratory pressure should then be followed with or without intermediate periods of unassisted breathing.
2. *By Periods of Unassisted Spontaneous Breathing.* The IMV or SIMV mode is instituted to replace the controlled mode. As the mandatory rate

TABLE 23–8. RESPIRATORY PHYSIOLOGIC CRITERIA OF WEANING ABILITY

Variable	Value
Tests of Mechanical Capability	
Vital capacity	> 10–15 ml/kg bw
Forced expiratory volume in 1 sec	> 10 ml/kg bw
Peak inspiratory pressure	> −20 to −30 cm H_2O
Resting minute ventilation (can be doubled	
with a maximal voluntary ventilation)	< 10 L/min
Tests of Oxygenation Capability	
AaD_{O_2} on 100% O_2	< 300–350 mm Hg
Shunt fraction	< 10–20%
Dead space/tidal volume	< 0.55–0.6
Stable cardiovascular system	

644 *General Anesthesia*

```
                          CPPV
                      ↙    ↓    ↘
                 IPPV → ASSIST ← CPPB
                        MODES
                          
              IPPB ↘
                    ↘
                     HYPERINFLATION
                      IMV + PEEP
                          ↓
      AYRE-T PIECE ← ──── DISCONTINUE IMV
        MODIFIED                ↓
           ↓
      ⎛ GAS MIXTURE ⎞ ← ─────── DISCONTINUE PEEP
      ⎝ HUMIDIFIED  ⎠
           ↓
           ↓
      AMBIENT BREATHING
           ↓
      oxygen enrichment
           ↓
        air only
```

FIG. 23–22. Sequence of modalities used in weaning.

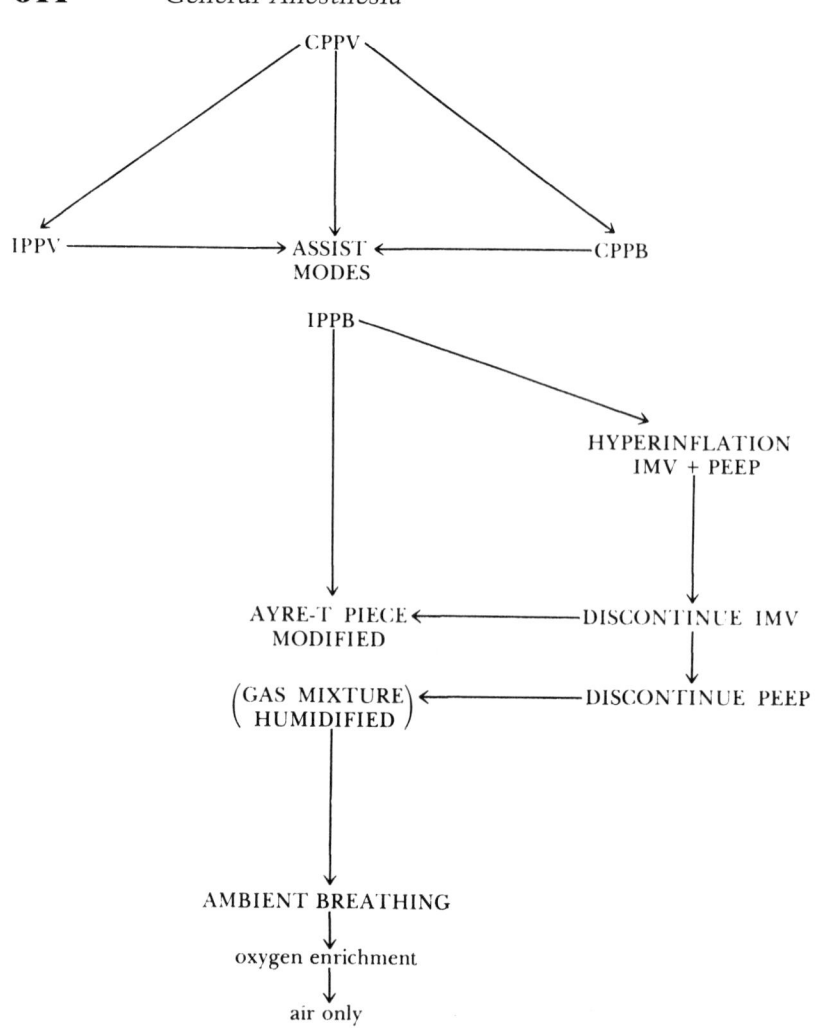

is decreased, the patients are permitted to breathe more frequently on their own, unassisted by mechanical ventilation. If the patient response is positive, the decreasing of the mechanical rate continues.

Either of these two procedures can be accomplished rapidly as at the conclusion of general anesthesia. They may require several hours in patients supported for therapeutic reasons. If any untoward or adverse effects are evident, or spontaneous breathing fails to maintain physiologic parameters, ventilator support should be immediately resumed. Careful monitoring, especially of blood gases, during this period is necessary (Table 23–10).

When a low functional residual capacity exists, there may be rapid airway closure. Under these circumstances, especially when the inspiratory pressures have been high, maintaining the patient on IPPB is recommended. Each spontaneous respiratory effort is mechanically augmented. That is, the patient is placed on an assist mode. In addition, PEEP should be provided. One can then gradually reduce the inspiratory pressure only until little or no inspiratory assistance is needed. At this point, one can gradually discontinue any CPPB.

When the dead space to tidal volume ratio $(V_{D_5}V_T)$ is high, intermittent volume ventilation should be continued. Every third or fourth breath should be augmented by the ventilator to three or four times the desired tidal volume. This augmented breath is superimposed on the patient's own respiratory rhythm, or it may synchronize with a spontaneous inhalation. It is a hyperinflation originally designated as an *artificial sigh*. The procedure of having a ventilator automatically augment pulmonary inflations, a preset number of times per minute has been termed *intermittent mandatory ventilation* (IMV).[75]

DISCONTINUATION OF CONTROLLED VENTILATION (IPPV). Most patients in critical care areas who have been on controlled ventilation by means of IPPV can be successfully and quickly weaned by the use of a T-piece technique. Besides the criteria for complete weaning, emphasis must be placed on the observation that the patient is making significant

TABLE 23–9. SEQUENCE OF MODALITIES USED IN GRADUAL WEANING*

Control Modes
    Continuous positive pressure ventilation—CPPV
    Intermittent positive pressure ventilation—IPPV
        for long term—use volume preset ventilators
    Discontinue by using assist modes
    Intermittent mandatory ventilation (IMV) or synchronized intermittent mandatory ventilation
Assist Modes
    Inspiration phrase of spontaneous breathing augmented by positive pressure—IPPB using either:
        Volume-preset ventilator *or*
        Pressure-preset ventilator
    Periods of unassisted spontaneous breathing—Discontinue assisted breathing by IPPB frequently and for lengthening periods of time
    Artificial sigh by bag or mask while breathing spontaneously
    Mechanical hyperinflation at preset intervals—intermittent mandatory ventilation—IMV
    Continuous Positive Pressure Breathing (CPPB)—spontaneous breathing augmented by positive pressure throughout respiratory cycle (CPAP)
    CPPB + IMV (designated by some as IMV + PEEP)—spontaneous breathing with positive pressure throughout respiratory cycle and with mechanical hyperinflation at preset intervals
        Discontinue hyperinflation (IMV) by gradual reduction of frequency of hyperinflation per min
        Discontinue PEEP by graded reduction of end-expiratory pressure
    Exhalatory resistance pressure by mask
T-Piece (Ayre Modified) Technique
    Patient breathing spontaneously
    Oxygen supplement humidified
Ambient Breathing
    Oxygen supplement
    Air only

* In decreasing order of mechanical support from complete control to unassisted respiratory support. This is not necessarily the order in which an individual patient may be managed.

spontaneous respiratory efforts. The mechanical support is completely withdrawn and the respiratory efforts are completely unassisted. A T-piece (modified Ayre T type) is then attached to the airway, either endotracheal tube or tracheostomy tube, and a high flow of oxygen is admitted to the system. In addition, the breathing mixture should be humidified by means of a heated nebulizer appropriately attached to the system. The $F_{I_{O_2}}$ on institution of the T-piece technique should be slightly higher than when the patient was on controlled ventilation, but preferably not above 60% oxygen. With some modern ventilators, the ventilators can be switched to a mode similar to that of an Ayre T-piece, allowing patients to breathe on their own with a known $F_{I_{O_2}}$.

DISCONTINUATION FROM CPPV (WEANING FROM PEEP).[76] In *continuous* positive pressure ventilation (CV–controlled mode of ventilation), the patient usually has an increased functional residual capacity. Because there is a positive pressure maintained during exhalation and at the end of exhalation, namely PEEP, the weaning process should begin with a reduction of the pressure exerted during the exhalatory phase and at the end of exhalation. Weaning from PEEP is indicated when AaD_{O_2} on best PEEP significantly decreases from a previous value on the same amount of end-expiratory pressure and this coincides with other signs showing improvement in compliance and slower airway closure. PEEP is then eliminated gradually by decrements of 3 to 5 cm H_2O every 2 to 4 hours until a zero-end expiratory pressure is achieved. This may require 18 to 24 hours.

The patient is then supported by a control mode of inspiratory positive pressure only; that is, IPPV. The patient is permitted to stay on IPPV for as long as 24 hours. The procedure for weaning from IPPV through assist mode to complete spontaneous breathing on a T-piece is then followed, as outlined above.

TABLE 23–10. DIAGNOSTIC SIGNS AND SYMPTOMS TO BE OBSERVED FOR SUCCESSFUL WEANING

Patient level of consciousness, patient apprehension, diaphoresis.
Blood pressure (every 5 min until patient can tolerate 15–30 min off ventilator; every 10–15 min thereafter). Reconnect patient to ventilator if there is a rise or fall in blood pressure.
Pulse and cardiac rhythm (frequency as above). A cardiac monitor is helpful during the early phase of weaning. Reconnect if ventricular rate increases by 20 beats/min or if the rate >110 in adults.
Respiratory rate (frequency as above).
Reconnect to ventilator if respiratory rate >30/min in adults.
Tidal volume ideally should be >300 ml in adults.
Arterial blood gases.

WEANING FROM ARTIFICIAL AIRWAYS.[74,76] Extubation should be performed when the indications for intubation (ventilatory assistance, protection of the airway, obstruction and tracheobronchial toilet) no longer exist.

The following checklist will help to rule out the need for an artificial airway:

1. Ventilatory reserve—adequate respiratory parameters:
    a. Tidal volume > 5 ml/kg; FVC > 15 ml/kg
    b. pH > 7.30; Pa_{CO_2} < 50; Pa_{O_2} > 60 on $F_{I_{O_2}}$ < 0.5
2. Clean tracheobronchial tree
3. Patency of the upper airway—no upper airway obstruction present. To test the presence of a patent airway in an intubated patient, deflate the cuff after meticulous pharyngeal suctioning, then ask the patient to take a deep breath and exhale it forcefully while the tube is occluded. If no obstruction is present, the patient will be able to exhale easily around the tube
4. Reflex protection of airway—the patient is able to swallow and cough effectively
5. Reserve for clearing tracheobronchial tree—this is adequate if:
    a. FVC is three times the predicted tidal volume for the patient (15 ml/kg bw).
    b. The patient is alert enough to give FVC

When all the above mentioned criteria are met, the patient can be extubated. After extubation, the patient should be placed on high humidity oxygen while blood pressure, pulse rate, respiratory rate, breath sounds, and ECG are monitored. Arterial blood gases and ventilatory parameters should be determined 30 minutes after extubation. Watch for inspiratory stridor, wheezing, diminished breath sounds, fluctuation of blood pressure and pulse rate, and acute arrhythmias.

Removal of Tracheostomy Tube. Weaning a patient from a tracheostomy airway should be done cautiously. To reinsert a tracheostomy tube under less than optimal conditions is hazardous. Tracheostomy stoma functionally close within 8 to 12 hours after decannulation, but to repeat tracheostomy carries a high surgical risk of bleeding and infection.

Three methods for testing the patient's ability to function without the tracheostomy tube while keeping the stoma patent and allowing quick and safe recannulation have been described.

1. Using a small size metal tracheostomy tube and corking the orifice.
2. Using a fenestrated tracheostomy tube, which has an opening or window cut into the outer cannulas.
3. Using a tracheal button: Keistner tube is a representative of this group. It consists of a plastic tube that maintains the patency of the tracheostomy track and has a one-way valve through which the patient inspires; expiration is through the patient's upper airway. Patency of the airway and the ability of the patient to cough and talk can be monitored while the tube maintains the stoma. If after 24 hours the patient is able to clear secretions without difficulty and without upper airway obstruction, the tracheostomy tract can be closed. Keep a regular tracheostomy tube at the bedside of the patient with a Keistner tube.

WEANING FROM OXYGEN-ENRICHED ATMOSPHERES.[76] Once a patient has been weaned from controlled ventilation and has had the trachea extubated, there is usually a persistent intrapulmonary shunt or ventilation-perfusion abnormality requiring the use of supplemental oxygen to maintain an arterial oxygen tension of 70 to 100 mm Hg.

The amount of oxygen required to produce a 70 to 100 mm Hg Pa_{O_2} can be determined by blood gas analysis while breathing known concentrations of oxygen. Because the $F_{I_{O_2}}$ on low-flow O_2 systems partially depends on the patient's tidal volume and respiratory rate, weaning should be done while the patient is on a high flow system, which gives an accurate $F_{I_{O_2}}$ independent of variations in the patient's minute volume.

The ever-present danger of CO_2 narcosis with high concentrations of inspired oxygen in patients with chronic obstructive pulmonary disease (COPD) must be kept in mind. Appropriate observations of the level of consciousness in relationship to the Pa_{CO_2} and pH must be made to guard against this possibility. Oxygen should be considered a drug and be discontinued when the patient no longer needs it. Before weaning patient from oxygen, ventilatory parameters and arterial blood gases should be measured. After 30 minutes on room air, the above mentioned measurement should be repeated. If there are no significant changes in Pa_{CO_2}, tidal volume, and respiratory rate (minute volume) noted, the patient can be weaned from oxygen completely. It is worthwhile to review the patient's past medical records, if available, to ascertain blood gas and acid-base status before the exacerbation, because the achievement of these values is the ultimate goal of therapy.

HIGH-FREQUENCY POSITIVE-PRESSURE VENTILATION

DEFINITION. High-frequency ventilation (HFV) is defined as a pattern of ventilation in which high respiratory rates and small tidal volumes approximate to or less than the patient's dead space volume are applied.[1] Although the minimum rate is not an absolute one, the HFV rate can be minimally set as a frequency greater than four times the normal respiratory rate of the subject. However, the Food and Drug Administration has proposed that the minimum rate for so-called HFV should be 150 breaths per minute minimum, whereas the maximum can be as high as 3000 changes per minute.[2]

OBJECTIVES. For respiratory insufficiency and failure, the objectives of conventional therapeutic measures are (1) to provide safe and effective support of cardiovascular function; (2) to provide adequate pulmonary gas exchange; and (3) to treat the underlying pulmonary pathologic condition.

The conventional methods consist of artificial ventilatory support, usually with increased ambient oxygen and continuous positive pressure. Frequently, IPPB and expiratory pressure techniques are employed. There are many situations, however, in which ventilation–perfusion abnormalities are not easily corrected. In addition, the use of positive pressure techniques has resulted in significant impairment of cardiovascular function. Oxygen toxicity in prolonged artificial ventilation and the problems of impairment or impedance to cardiovascular function are also concerns. One proposal to overcome especially the latter hazard is to use HFV.

HISTORY. The forerunner of HFV was that of continuous-flow apneic ventilation. In 1909, Metzer and Auer[3] used a system of apneic ventilation by high flow of fresh gas into the respiratory tract that depended on diffusion for gas exchange.[4] The subject of diffusion respiration was reviewed by Holmdahl, who introduced the term *apneic diffusion oxygenation* (ADO).[5] Frumin reported on anesthesia patients whose gas exchange depended on the principle of diffusion.[6] Oxygenation was adequate, but severe respiratory acidosis occurred.[5]

In 1957, John Emerson* patented and manufactured a machine known as the Emerson Flow Interrupter, which was capable of producing ventilatory rates of 60 to 2000 breaths per minute. In 1967, 10 years later, Sjöstrand described HFV in a range of frequencies from 60 to 100 breaths per minute, and in a report of 1969, HFV–HFPPV (high-frequency positive-pressure ventilation) was described.[7] The techniques were developed in an attempt to provide ventilatory support with adequate gas exchange that would not cause unusual hemodynamic changes or respiratory cycle–dependent shifts in blood pressure.

PHYSICS OF GAS EXCHANGE IN HFV. In ordinary breathing, gas is conveyed through a system of conduits by a gradient of pressure to the alveolar system where mixing and dispersion occurs (Brownian movement), followed by molecular diffusion.[8] The gradient of pressure is created by a lowering of the terminal airway pressure below atmospheric by a decrease in transpleural pressure accomplished by the respiratory pump. In conventional mechanical ventilation, the gradient of pressure is created by increasing the pressure in the conduit airways. In these situations, displacement of air occurs by a movement of volume approximately three times greater than the dead space or conduit system into an expansible balloon system, the alveolar system, or gas exchange system.

These traditional concepts of applied physics to the mechanics of normal or conventional mechanical ventilation are not completely applicable to HFV.[9] In HFPPV and high-frequency jet ventilation (HFJV), tidal volumes equal to or slightly less than dead space at high frequency probably use displacement to some extent.[10] But the basic exchange depends on agitated mixing and dispersion within the alveolar system (Lehr).[11] This intraregional gas mixing is coupled with "augmented" molecular diffusion.[12] Fresh gas reaches alveoli by combined convection and diffusion. In large airways, convention current is the mechanism of air movement; in the terminal airways where forward velocity of air is decreased, movement of air occurs by stream dispersion and molecular diffusion.

For ventilation at frequencies greater than 600 breaths per minute, the theory of coaxial flow can be applied.[13] In a tubular system subjugated to high velocity flow, a laminar flow occurs in the central mainstream and a turbulent flow exists at the periphery. The flow profile is parabolic. Hence, air movement can be bidirectional, with movement distally, i.e., to the alveoli in the center or mainstream, and reverse flow or exit movement occurring at the sides or periphery of the tubes. Axial movement is linearly related to velocity.[14] Beyond the named bronchi and into the wide cross-sectional area of the numbered bronchi, fluid movement is of a delta-basin river pattern with a central narrow rushing movement, presumably at a high pressure, and a peripheral backwash or reverse flow at a lower pressure per unit area.

Diffusion in alveoli is augmented by oscillatory flows. This is a well-recognized principle in the field of fluid mechanics.[15]

CLASSIFICATION OF VENTILATORS FOR HFV.[2] HFV can be accomplished by three major types of ventilators now available. Each produces gas displacement in different ways and by different mechanical systems:

1. HFPPV
    a. Uses a pneumatic valve
    b. Modified by a flow interrupter
2. HFJV
3. High-frequency oscillators (HFO)

Even though many forms of HFV have been described, the difference between each technique can be realized by the following brief descriptions:

---

* Emerson is the inventor of an apparatus for vibrating portions of a patient's airway (vibrations) with oscillations between 500 and 1500 per minute. Patent was applied for March 2, 1955. Letters of patent (patent no. 2, 918, 917) was granted December 29, 1959.

- HFPPV is the delivery of small volumes of gas at high liter flows (175 to 250 L/min) to the lungs at a rate of around 50 breaths or more per minute.[9,16,17]
- HFJV is the delivery of a pulsating gas under pressures of 5 to 50 psi to the lungs. Rates up to 150 breaths per minute can be used, with gas entrainment around the jet adding to high inspiratory flow.[18,19]
- HFO uses a reciprocating pump to deliver gas flow of a known concentration to the lungs. Rates of 5 to 40 Hz can be used, but 10 to 15 Hz are the most widely reported.[20,21]
- High-frequency flow interrupters (HFFI) are similar to jet ventilation but use rates of 100 to 200 in the adult and 300 to 400 in the infant. The gas being delivered is chopped into a pulse line pattern.[22]
- Combined high-frequency ventilation (CHFV) uses conventional mechanical ventilation and imposes HFV in the background.

FUNCTIONAL DIFFERENCES OF HFV MODALITIES (FIG. 23–23).[23,24]

HFPPV.[1,16] The mechanical system consists of a bifurcated tube with an inhalatory side arm angled to an expiratory side arm. A pneumatic valve permits unidirectional flow. At the moment of active positive pressure during inspiration, compressed gas flow is directed into the patient, while during passive inhalation, the gases are preferentially directed out the exhalation limb.[17]

The performance characteristics of this system allow the following: 50 to 150 breaths per minute; tidal volumes delivered at each breath approximating the volume of dead space; and an inspired oxygen ($F_{I_{O_2}}$) equal to that of the compressed gas.

HFJV.[18] The system for jet ventilation allows a volume of compressed gas to be delivered at high velocity to the patient's central airway via a small catheter (Fr 12 or 14) inserted into an endotracheal tube. Inspiration is active and exhalation passive. This form of HFV was introduced in 1977 by Klain and Smith.[18]

Characteristic of this system is the gas entrainment from the air in the endotracheal tube and around the tip of the catheter, caused by the high velocity or jet of air from the catheter consequent to the Bernoulli principle and Venturi effect.[19]

The tidal volume is a combination of the compressed gas flow and the entrained air. The tidal volume is slightly less than that of the dead space; the frequency ranges between 60 and 600 breaths per minute.

HFO.[20,24] HFO is characterized by a to-and-fro movement of air so that both inspiration and expiration are active processes. The mechanical forces are generated by a rapid oscillatory piston pump or by sound waves from a loudspeaker, providing a sinusoidal flow wave.

The system is capable of frequencies from 600 to 3600 cpm (10 to 60 Hz). Tidal volumes are much

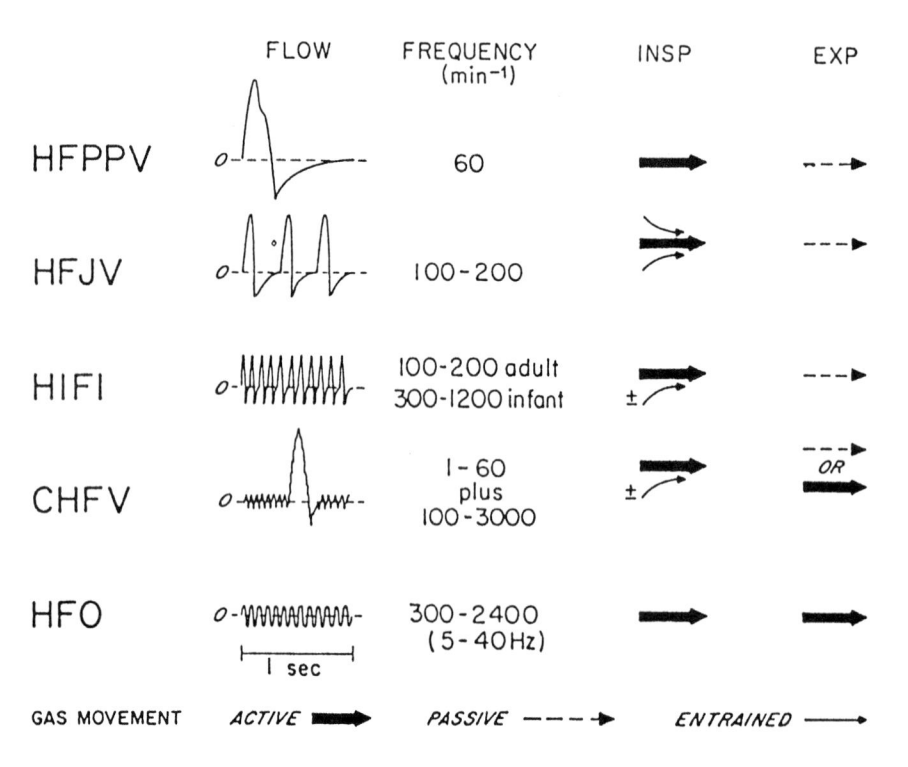

FIG. 23–23. Summary of flow patterns, frequencies and nature of gas movement for several modalities of high-frequency ventilation. From Froese, A.B.: High Frequency Ventilation: Uses and abuses. In ASA Refresher Course, vol 14. Philadelphia, JB Lippincott, 1986.

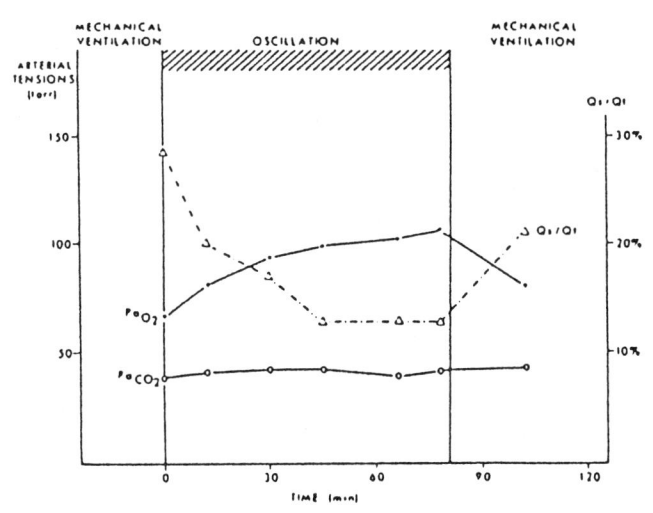

FIG. 23-24. Plot of arterial oxygen and carbon dioxide tensions, and $\dot{Q}s = \dot{Q}t$ vs time in a 74-year-old man with acute chronic respiratory failure secondary to COPD. Baseline values at 0 time were obtained during standard mechanical ventilation. From Butler, W.J., et al: Ventilation by high-frequency oscillation in humans. Anesth. Analg., *59*:577, 1980.

less than dead space volumes and in the range of 1.5 to 3 ml/kg.

Butler has shown that if piston displacement totals 80 ml at 15 Hz, little change in shunt fraction is noted (Fig. 23-24). With piston displacement of 100 to 150 ml at 15 Hz, shunt fraction is greatly reduced from conventional mechanical ventilation of 12% to 8%. Also, in COPD, average shunts of 25% were reduced to 12%. In right-to-left shunts in septic shock, no change in shunt fraction was noted.

Modified HFPPV. The use of a flow interrupter in either the HFPPV or jet system permits frequencies of 60 to 3600 breaths per minute with inspiration active and expiration passive. A rate of 100 to 600 breaths per minute at tidal volumes about one-half to one-fourth dead space is recommended as most effective.[22]

TECHNIQUE OF COMBINING HFPPV AND CONVENTIONAL MODE VENTILATION.[25] A practical mechanical system consists of two Bennett ventilators, one with conventional mode and the other a HFV, with independent fresh gas source for the high-frequency unit. The high-frequency mode may be achieved by using a Bennett MA-2B ventilator by turning both the sensitivity and flow rate buttons to maximal capacity and shutting off the tidal volume button. The outflow of this unit is attached through a Y-connector to the in-flow of the humidifier of the Puritan-Bennett ventilator. The first ventilator provides a rate of 140 to 160 breaths per minute at a tidal volume of 50 to 70 ml each, while the second ventilator provides rates of 2 to 6 breaths per minute at tidal volumes of 10 to 12 ml/kg, according to the patient's ventilatory needs. The oxygen concentration settings for each ventilator is the same. The output of each ventilator is passed through a single delivery tube to the patient's airway (endotracheal tube). An open pore permits free release of overflow, while an exhalatory valve permits ordinary exhalation.

The combined system has been successful in management of flail chest and contused lungs.

COMMENT ON JET VENTILATION.[26] A study of increasing operating jet pressures from 1.3 to 2.3 bars demonstrates that pressure is a main determinant of arterial oxygenation. At the same time, increased operating jet pressures result in lessened carbon dioxide clearance. Besides a small jet catheter through an endotracheal tube, jet ventilation can be accomplished through a tracheostomy tube with a Teflon tube attachment and pulses determined electronically by a solenoid valve.

USES OF HFV.[23]

1. Laryngoscopy and bronchoscopy[1]
2. Management of flail chest (internal pneumatic fixation—concept of Mörch)[27]
3. Respiratory failure
4. In patients with airway disruption—bronchopleural fistulae[22]
5. Alternation with conventional breathing, called *tandem ventilation*, to maintain lung volume and effective gas exchange

PROBLEMS

1. Lower airway pressures, i.e., in trachea, bronchi, and alveoli
2. Upper airway pressures, i.e., an increased end-expiratory pressure or mean airway pressure
3. Effects on circulation
4. Shunt fraction changed in COPD
5. Mechanical systems are complex and cumbersome

Mechanical Ventilator Problems

1. Humidification of gases being delivered remains a major problem
2. Inadvertent PEEP caused by gas trapping or expiratory valve/flow problems
3. Occlusion of expiratory pathway and failure of ventilatory to terminate inspiratory flow
4. "Conventional" ventilator monitoring devices do not work with HFV
5. Ventilator circuits or set-ups are not standardized in most HFVs

ADVANTAGES

1. Low peak and mean airway pressure
2. Minimal cardiovascular interference

3. Good (gas exchange) oxygen delivery and CO_2 washout
4. Patients can be conscious, cooperative, and not uncomfortable, without need for sedatives or narcotics.
5. Avoidance of lung damage in lungs with nonuniform distribution of gas constants—damage to lungs can result in such complications as pneumothorax, pneumomediastinum, and subcutaneous emphysema

REFERENCES

1. Guedel, A.E., and Trewek, D.N.: Ether apneas. Anesth. Analg., 13:263, 1934.
2a. Burstein, C.L., and Rovenstine, E.A.: Apnea during anesthesia. Am. J. Surg., 43:26, 1939.
2b. Harroun, P., Beckert, F.E., and Hathaway, H.R.: Curare and nitrous oxide anesthesia for lengthy operations. Anesthesiology, 7:24, 1946.
3. Cournand, A., et al.: Physiological studies of the effects of intermittent positive pressure breathing on cardiac output in man. Am. J. Physiol., 152:161, 1948.
4. Otis, A.B., Fenn, W.O., and Rahn, H.: The mechanics of breathing in man. J. Appl. Physiol., 2:592, 1950.
5. Rahn, H.: The pressure volume diagram of the thorax and lung. Am. J. Physiol., 146:161, 1946.
6. Mushin, W.W., Rendell-Baker, L., and Thompson, A.W.: Automatic Ventilation of the Lungs, 2nd ed. London, Blackwell Scientific Publications, 1969; 3rd Ed. 1980.
7. Holaday, D.A., and Rattenborg, C.C.: Automatic lung ventilators. Anesthesiology, 23:493, 1962.
7a. Chatburn, R.L.: A new system for understanding mechanical ventilators. Respir. Care, 36:1123, 1991.
8. Barach, A.L., et al.: The physiology of pressure breathing. J. Aviat. Med., 18:73, 1947.
9. Barach, A.L.: Studies on positive pressure respiration. J. Aviat. Med., 17:290, 1946.
10. Barach, A.L.: Physiologic advantages of grunting, groaning and pursed-lip breathing: Adaptive symptoms related to the development of continuous positive pressure breathing. Bull. NY Acad. Med., 49:666, 1973.
11. Barach, A.L., and Swenson, P.: Effect of breathing gases under positive pressure on lumens of small and medium sized bronchi. Arch. Intern. Med., 68:946, 1939.
12. Watrous, W.G., Davis, F.E., and Anderson, B.M.: Manually assisted and controlled respiration: A review. III. Anesthesiology, 12:33, 1949.
13. Motley, H.L.: Intermittent positive pressure breathing. J.A.M.A., 137:37, 1948.
14. Pontoppidan, H.: Terminology. Anesthesiology, 35:439, 1971.
15. Beecher, H.K., Bennett, H.S., and Bassett, D.L.: Circulatory effects of increased pressure in airway. Anesthesiology, 4:612, 1943.
16. Frumin, M.J., Bergman, N.A., and Holaday, D.A.: Alveolar arterial oxygen differences during artificial respiration in man. J. Appl. Physiol., 14:694, 1957.
17. Kirby, R.R., et al.: High level positive end-expiratory pressure (PEEP) in acute respiratory insufficiency. Chest, 67:156, 1975.
18. Nordström, L.: Haemodynamic effects of intermittent positive-pressure ventilation with and without an end-inspiratory pause. Acta Anaesthiol. Scand. Suppl 47, 1972.
19. Gregory, G.A., et al.: Treatment of the idiopathic respiratory distress syndrome with continuous positive airway pressure. N. Engl. J. Med., 284:1133, 1971.
20. Kacmarek, R.M., and Goulet, R.L. (eds): PEEP devices. In Shapiro BA, Cane RD: Positive Airway Pressure Therapy: PPV and PEEP. Anesthesiol. Clin. North Am, vol. 5. Philadelphia, WB Saunders, 1987, pp 757–776.
21. Kacmarek, R.M., et al.: Technical aspects of positive end-expiratory pressure (PEEP). III. Resp. Care, 27:1478, 1982.
22. Maloney, J.V.: Importance of negative pressure phase in mechanical respiration. J.A.M.A., 152:212, 1953.
23. Watson, W.E., Smith, A.C., and Spalding, J.M.K.: Transmural central venous pressure during intermittent positive pressure breathing. Br. J. Anaesth., 34:274, 1962.
24. Prys-Roberts, C. et al.: Circulatory influence of artificial ventilation during nitrous oxide anesthesia in man. Br. J. Anaesth., 39:533, 1967.
25. Norlander, O.P.: Functional analysis of force and power of mechanical ventilators. Acta Anaesthesiol. Scand., 8:57, 1964.
26. Fenn, W.O., and Chadwick, L.E.: Effect of pressure breathing on blood flow through the finger. Am. J. Physiol., 151:220, 1947.
27. Richards, D.W.: Cardiac output by the catheterization technique in various clinical conditions. Fed. Proc., 4:215, 1945.
28. Janeway, H.H.: Simple and complete forms of apparatus for intratracheal anesthesia. Ann. Surg., 59:628, 1914.
29. Fenn, W.O.: Displacement of blood from the lungs by pressure breathing. Am. J. Physiol., 151:258, 1947.
30. Werko, L.: The influence of positive pressure breathing on the circulation in man. Acta Medica Scand., Supp 1947.
30a. Lauson, H.D., Bloomfield, R.A., and Cournand, A.: The influence of the respiration on the circulation in man. Am. J. Med., 86:236, 1953.
31. Kety, S.S., and Schmidt, C.F.: Effects of active and passive hyperventilation on cerebral blood flow, cerebral oxygen consumption, cardiac output and blood pressure of normal young men. J. Clin. Invest., 25:107, 1946.
32. Salem, M.R., et al.: Effect of continuous positive and negative pressure breathing on the urine formation. Fed. Proc., 23:2, 1964.
33. Brecher, G.A.: *Venous Return*. New York, Grune & Stratton, 1956.
34. Hubay, C.A., Brecher, G.A., and Clement, F.L.: Etiological factors affecting pulmonary artery flow with controlled respiration. Surgery, 38:215, 1955.
35. Edwards, W.S.: Effects of Lung Inflation and Epinephrine on Pulmonary Vascular Resistance. Am. J. Physiol., 167:756, 1951.
36. Cournand, A., Motley, H.L., and Werko, L.: Mechanism underlying cardiac output change during intermittent positive pressure breathing. Fed. Proc., 6:92, 1947.
37. Papper, E.M., and Reaves, D.P.: Circulatory depression during controlled respiration. Anesthesiology, 8:407, 1947.
38. Humphreys, G.H., Moore, R.L., and Barkley, H.: Studies of the jugular, carotid and pulmonary pressures of anesthetized dogs during positive inflation of the lungs. J. Thorac. Surg., 8:553, 1939.
39. McIntyre, R.W.: Positive expiratory pressure plateau: Improved gas exchange during mechanical ventilation. Can. Anaesth. Soc. J., 16:477, 1969.
40. Henry J.P., and Pearce, J.W.: The possible role of cardiac atrial stretch receptors in the induction of changes in urine flow. J. Physiol., 131:572, 1956.

41. Gett, P.M., Jones, E.S., and Shephard, G.F.: Pulmonary edema associated with sodium retention during ventilator treatment. Br. J. Anaesth., 43:460, 1971.
42. Henry, J.P.: National Research Council, Division of Medical Sciences Acting for the Committee on Medical Research and the Office of the Scientific Research and Development. Committee on Aviation Medicine Report No. 463 (May 30) 1945.
43. Johnstone, M.: Emphysema and controlled respiration. Anesthesia, 11:165, 1956.
44. Waltz, R.C., et al.: Experimental study of pulmonary histopathology following positive and negative respiration. Surg. Gynecol. Obstet., 99:580, 1954.
45. Adams, W.E.: Differential pressures and reduced lung function in intrathoracic operations. J. Thorac. Surg., 9:254, 1940.
46. Heidrick, A.F., Adams, W.E., and Livingstone, H.M.: Spontaneous pneumothorax following positive pressure intratracheal anesthesia. Arch. Surg., 41:61, 1940.
47. Shapiro, B.A., and Cane, R.D.: Metabolic malfunction of the lung: Non-cardiogenic edema and adult respiratory distress syndrome. Surg. Annu., 13:271, 1981.
48. Katzenstein, A.A., Bloor, C.M., and Leibow, A.A.: Diffuse alveolar damage: The role of oxygen, shock, and related factors. A review. Am. J. Pathol., 85:210, 1976.
49. Fox, R.B., et al.: Pulmonary inflammation due to oxygen toxicity: Involvement of chemotactic factors and polymorphonuclear leukocytes. Am. Rev. Respir. Dis., 123:521, 1981.
50. Petty, T.L., and Ashbaugh, D.G.: The adult respiratory distress syndrome: Clinical features, factors influencing prognosis and principles of management. Chest, 60:233, 1971.
51. Shapiro, B.A., and Cane, R.D.: Acute lung injury and positive and expiratory pressure. In Anesthesiology Clinics of North America, vol. 5. Philadelphia, WB Saunders, 1987.
52. Shapiro, B.A., Cane, R.D., and Harrison, R.A.: Positive end-expiratory pressure in acute lung injury. Chest, 83:558, 1983.
53. Shapiro, B.A., Cane, R.D., and Harrison, R.A.: Positive end-expiratory pressure therapy in adults with special reference to acute lung injury: A review of the literature and suggested clinical correlations. Crit. Care Med., 12:127, 1984.
54. Cane, R.D., and Shapiro, B.A.: Clinical principles of positive pressure ventilation. In Anesthesiology Clinics of North America, vol. 5. Philadelphia, WB Saunders, 1987.
55. Bone, R.C.: The adult respiratory distress syndrome: Treatment in the next decade. Respir. Care, 29:249, 1983.
55a. Hubay, C.A., et al.: Circulatory dynamics of venous return during positive-negative respiration. Anesthesiology, 15:445, 1954.
56. Carr, D.T., Essex, H.E.: Certain effects of positive pressure and respiration on circulatory and respiratory systems. Am. Heart J., 31:53, 1946.
57. Barach, A.L., and Swenson, P.: Effect of breathing gases under positive pressure on lumens of small and medium-sized bronchi. Arch. Intern. Med., 63:946, 1939.
58. Lynch, S., Ellis, K., and Levy, A.: Effects of alternating positive and negative endotracheal pressures on the caliber of the bronchi. Anesthesiology, 20:325, 1959.
59. Gordon, A.S., Frye, C.W., and Langstrom, H.T.: The cardiorespiratory dynamics of controlled respiration in the open and closed chest. J. Thorac. Surg., 32:431, 1956.
60. Etsten, B.: Anesthesia for thoracic surgery. NY State J. Med., 43:1980, 1943.
61. Slocum, H.C., Cooper, B.M., and Allen, C.R.: The control of respiration in anesthesia. Anesthesiology, 11:427, 1950.
62. Burstein, C.L., and Rovenstine, E.A.: Aids in thoracic surgery. NY State J. Med., 46:2142, 1946.
62a. Magill, L.W.: Anesthesia in thoracic surgery with special reference to lobectomy. Proc. Roy. Soc. Med., 29:643, 1936.
63. Holaday, D.A., and Rattenborg, C.C.: Automatic lung ventilators. Anesthesiology, 23:493, 1962.
64. Report of Committee on Pulmonary Nomenclature (Benjamin Burrows, Chairman). Pulmonary terms and symbols. Chest, 67:583, 1975.
65. Montgomery, L.H., and Stephenson, S.: Artificial respiration control. IRE Trans. Med. Electronics, vol. ME-6:29–30, 1959.
66. Frumin, M.J., and Lee, A.: A physiologically oriented artificial respirator which produces $N_2O–O_2$ anesthesia in man. J. Lab. Clin. Med., 49:617, 1957.
67. Mapleson, W.W.: The effect of changes of lung characteristics on the functioning of automatic ventilators. Anesthesia, 17:300, 1962.
68. Fairley, H.B., and Hunter, D.D.: Mechanical ventilators: An assessment of two new machines for use in the operating room. Can. Anesth. Soc. J., 10:364, 1963.
69. Elam, J.O., Kerr, J.H., and Janney, C.D.: Performance of ventilators: Effects of changes in lung thorax compliance. Anesthesiology, 10:56, 1958.
70. Saklad, M.: Ventilators: volume preset vs. pressure preset. Modern Treatment, 6:1, 1969.
71. Elam, J.O., Brown, E.S. and Elder, J.D.: Artificial respiration by mouth-to-mask method. New Engl. J. Med., 250:749, 1954.
72. Brownlee, E.J., and Allbritten, F.F., Jr.: The significance of the lung thorax compliance in ventilation during thoracic surgery. J. Thorac. Surg., 32:454, 1956.
73. Bromage, P.R.: Total respiratory compliance in the anesthetized subjects and modifications produced by noxious stimuli. Clin. Sci., 17:217, 1958.
73a. Bendixen, H.H., et al.: *Respiratory Care*. St. Louis, CV Mosby, 1965.
74. Hodgkin, J.E., Bowser, M.A., and Burton, G.G.: Respiratory weaning. Crit. Care Med., 2:96, 1974.
75. Downs, J.B., et al.: Intermittent mandatory ventilation: A new approach to weaning patients from mechanical ventilators. Chest, 64:331, 1973.
76. Feeley, T.W., and Hedley-White, J.: Weaning from controlled ventilation and supplemental oxygen. New Engl. J. Med., 292:903, 1975.

HIGH-FREQUENCY POSITIVE-PRESSURE VENTILATION

1. Sjöstrand, U.: High frequency positive pressure ventilation (HFPPV): A review. Crit. Care Med., 8:345, 1980.
2. O'Rourke, P.P., and Crone, R.K.: High-frequency ventilation. J.A.M.A., 250:2845, 1983.
3. Meltzer, J.S., and Auer, J.: Continuous respiration without respiratory movements. J. Exp. Med., 11:622, 1909.
4. Enghoff, H., Holmdahl M.H., and Risholm, L.: Diffusion respiration in man. Nature, 168:830, 1951.
5. Holmdahl, M. H.: Pulmonary uptake of oxygen acid-base metabolism, and circulation during prolonged apnoea. Acta Chir. Scand. (Suppl 212), 1:1956.
6. Frumin, M.J., Epstein, R.M., and Cohen, G.: Apneic oxygenation in man. Anesthesiology, 20:789, 1959.
7. Oberg, P.A., and Sjöstrand, U.H.: Studies of blood pressure regulation. I. Common carotid artery clamping in studies of

the carotid sinus baroreceptor control of the systemic blood pressures. Acta Physiol. Scand., 75:276, 1969.
8. Comroe, J.H., et al.: The Lung. Chicago, Year Book Medical Publishers, pp 27–49, 1962.
9. Sjöstrand, U.: Review of the physiological rationale for and development of high frequency positive pressure ventilation—HFPPV. Acta Anaesthesiol. Scand. (Suppl), 64:7, 1977.
10. Chang, H.K.: Mechanisms of gas transport during high frequency oscillation. J. Appl. Physiol., 56:553, 1984.
11. Lehr, J.L., et al.: Photographic measurement of pleural surface motion during long oscillation. J. Appl. Physiol., 59:623, 1985.
12. Fredberg, J.J.: Augmentes diffusion in airways can support pulmonary gas exchange. J. Appl. Physiol., 49:232, 1980.
13. Hazelton, F.R., and Scherer, P.W.: Bronchial bifurcations and respiratory mass transport. Science, 208:69, 1980.
14. Scherer, P.W., et al.: Measurement of axial diffusivities in a model of the bronchial airways. J. Appl. Physiol., 38:719, 1975.
15. Philip, J.R.: Theory of flow and transport processes in pora and porous media in circulatory and respiratory mass transport. London, J & A Churchill Ltd, 1969, pp 25–44.
16. Sjöstrand, U.H., and Eriksson, I.A.: High rates and low volumes in mechanical ventilation—not just a matter of ventilatory frequency. Anesth. Analg. (Cleve), 59:567, 1980.
17. Jonzon, A., et al.: High frequency positive pressure ventilation by endotracheal insufflation. Acta Anaesthesiol. Scand. [Suppl] 43:1–43, 1971.
18. Klain, M., and Smith, R.B.: High frequency percutaneous transtracheal jet ventilation. Crit. Care Med., 5:280, 1977.
19. Carlon, G.C., et al.: Clinical experience with high frequency jet ventilation. Crit. Care Med., 9:1, 1981.
20. Lukenheimer, P.P., et al.: Application of transtracheal pressure: oscillations as a modification of "diffusion respiration." Br. J. Anaesth., 44:627, 1972.
21. Butler, W.J., et al.: Ventilation by high-frequency oscillation in humans. Anesth. Analg., 59:577, 1980.
22. Gillespie D.J. High frequency ventilations: A new concept in mechanical ventilation. Mayo Clin. Proc., 58:187, 1983.
23. Froese, A.B.: High frequency ventilation: Uses and abuses. In ASA Refresher Course, vol 14. Philadelphia. JB Lippincott, 1986.
24. Froese, A.B., and Bryan, A.C.: State of the art: High frequency ventilation. Am. Rev. Resp. Dis., 135:1363, 1987.
25. Barzilay, E., et al.: Combined use of HFPPV with low-rate ventilation in traumatic respiratory insufficiency. Intensive Care Med., 10:197, 1984.
26. Benhamou, D., et al.: Impact of changes in operating pressure during high-frequency jet ventilation. Anesth. Analg., 63:19, 1984.
27. Mörch, E.T.: Controlled ventilation by means of special automatic machines (as used in Sweden and Denmark). Proc. Roy. Soc. Med., 40:603, 1947.

APPENDIX 1. RESPIRATORY THERAPY TERMS

In publications, specific apparatus, as well as time, volume, pressure, and concentration variables, should be indicated when appropriate.*

- *Inspiratory Positive Pressure Breathing (IPPB):* Pressure above atmospheric at the airway opening during inspiration employed to assist ventilation, regardless of apparatus used
- *Positive End-Expiratory Pressure (PEEP):* A residual pressure above atmospheric maintained at the airway opening at the end of expiration. This may be used during spontaneous or mechanical ventilation
- *Constant Positive Pressure Breathing (CPPB)* (Constant Positive Airway Pressure [CPAP]): A pressure above atmospheric maintained at the airway opening throughout the respiratory cycle during spontaneous breathing
- *Negative End-Expiratory Pressure (NEEP):* A pressure below atmospheric maintained at the airway opening at the end of expiration
- *Assisted Ventilation:* Manual or mechanical ventilation in which the patient initiates inspiration and establishes the frequency of breathing
- *Controlled Ventilation:* Manual or mechanical ventilation in which the frequency of breathing is determined by a ventilator according to a preset cycling pattern without initiation by the patient
- *Assist-Control Ventilation:* Manual or mechanical ventilation in which the minimum frequency of breathing is predetermined by the ventilator control, but the patient has the option of initiating inspiration to give a faster rate
- *Intermittent Mandatory Ventilation (IMV):* Periodic controlled ventilation with inspiratory positive pressure, with the patient breathing spontaneously between controlled breaths

* From: ACCP-ATS Joint Committee on Pulmonary Nomenclature: Pulmonary terms and symbols. Chest, 67:5, 1975.

"I procured a large dog, into the veins of which hinder leg we convey'd, by a syringe, a small dose of a warm solution of opium in sac."
Robert Boyle, 1620

HISTORY

1872—Oré of Lyons injected chloral hydrate intravenously
1909—Burkhardt injected chloroform and ether
1909—Bier injected procaine
1909—Krawkow injected hedonal (a urethane derivative)
1913—Noel used paraldehyde
1921—Naragawa injected alcohol
1928—Zerfas and Lundy employed sodium amytal
1929—Kirchner injected Avertin
1930—Pentobarbital sodium was used intravenously
1932—Hexobarbitone was injected intravenously
1934—R.M. Waters' first clinical use of thiopentothal
1934—Lundy (the father of intravenous anesthesia) and Tovell introduced pentothal
1941—Selye reported the anesthetic activity of steroids in experimental animals
1942—Craddock used intravenous alcohol for analgesia
1950—Helrich, Papper, and Rovenstine reported the clinical use of a new thiobarbiturate, thiomylal
1950—Laborit used lytic cocktail for neurolepsis
1954—Stoelting used methohexital
1955—Laubach found hydroxydione, a pregnane derivative, satisfactory for intravenous anesthesia in humans
1962—Janssen used butyrophenone for neurolepsis
1963—Corssen and Domino used fentanyl for neurolepsis

24

BARBITURATE INTRAVENOUS ANESTHETIC AGENTS: THIOPENTAL

DEVELOPMENT OF INTRAVENOUS ANESTHETICS

Many agents have been used intravenously to produce unconsciousness and a safe, reversible anesthetic state. Such is revealed in the history of attempts to produce surgical conditions by this route with limited success.[1] By definition, supplemental agents not intended to produce unconsciousness and those used for relaxation are excluded.

Six groups of compounds have been tested:[2] (1) aliphatic substances, such as alcohol, chloral hydrate, hedonal esters; (2) barbiturates; (3) opiates; (4) steroids; (5) aromatic compounds, such as eugenols, phencyclidines; and (6) neuroleptic drugs, such as phenothiazines and butyrophenones. Only the barbiturates, however, have enjoyed wide clinical utility. Although the phrase *intravenous anesthesia* has become widely used, no single agent has been able to provide all the requisites of the anesthetic state, including analgesia and blockade of the sympathetic nervous system. Agents have been used intravenously to produce unconsciousness, but only produce an apparent anesthetic state allowing brief surgical procedures.[1]

Several intravenous agents are used in the balanced anesthesia technique, each with different effects: hypnotics for unconsciousness; opioids for analgesia; and neurolepts and sympathetic blockers for autonomic nervous system control.

In brief, "intravenous anesthesia" has become synonymous with barbiturate anesthesia and the production of unconsciousness. The subject of intravenous anesthesia will be presented by a detailed representation of thiopental as the paragon of intravenous anesthetics; the other barbiturate agents (Table 24–1) will be discussed and compared with it.

Other agents have a measure of utility when administered by the intravenous route. With the introduction of the lytic cocktail in 1950, combinations of opiates and tranquilizers have been developed to the point of popular clinical utility, ie, neurolept analgesia anesthesia. Since 1965, one phencyclidine (ketamine) has been introduced whose advantages outweigh the side effects. Since 1970 the technique of employing large doses of intravenous morphine has again been found selectively advantageous.

ROLE OF INTRAVENOUS AGENTS. The primary purpose for the use of intravenous agents is the induction of a state of unconsciousness. The intent is to avoid the usual excitatory phenomenon that is encountered with purely inhalation techniques in the absence of adequate preanesthetic medication. It should be appreciated that the potency of these agents is limited largely, with few exceptions, to the development of a state of deep unconsciousness.

TABLE 24–1. INTRAVENOUS BARBITURATES

	Trade Names
THIOBARBITURATES	
Thiopental (thiopentone [U.K.]) (thiopentobarbital; thionembutal) (ethyl-methyl, butyl thiobarbiturate)	Pentothal, Intraval, Trapanal, Hipnopento
Thiamylal (thiosecobarbital; thioseconal) (allylmethyl butyl thiobarbiturate)	Surital
Thialbarbital (thialbarbitone [U.K.]) (5 allyl-5-cyclo-hexenyl, thiobarbiturate)	Kemithal
Thiobutabarbital (ethyl-methylpropyl thiobarbiturate)	Inactin (Germany)
Thioethyamyl* (thioamytal) (isoamyl-ethyl thiobarbiturate)	Venestic
Buthalital† (buthalitone [U.K.]) (allyl-isobutyl thiobarbiturate)	Transital, Baytenal
Methitural (5 methyl-thio-ethyl-5 1 methylbutyl thiobarbiturate)	Nerval, Thiogenal
METHYLATED THIOBARBITURATES	
Methylthiobutabarbital (B 137)—Methylated sulfur analogue of butabarbital methyl thiosoneral (U.K.)	
METHYLATED OXYBARBITURATES	
Methohexital (methohexitone [U.K.]) (methylallyl-methyl pentyl barbiturate)	Brevital, Brietal
Hexobarbital‡ (hexibarbitone [U.K.]) (methyl-cyclohexenyl methylbarbiturate)	Evipal

* Never marketed.
† Withdrawn from market.
‡ Not available in U.S.

Most of the agents, singly or in combination, fail to produce a true state of surgical anesthesia at stage III, planes 1 or 2. With few exceptions, most intravenous agents employed for induction are devoid of analgesic properties. Furthermore, with rare exceptions, they do not provide blockade of stress phenomena. Hence, these agents are, in practice, employed for the production of unconsciousness. They serve to "set the stage" for the establishment of a state in which potent inhalation anesthetic agents that have capacity to produce the full range of surgical anesthesia are then employed, or they are used with adjunctive drugs with opioid and neurolept properties to establish the state of balanced anesthesia.

POTENCY OF INTRAVENOUS AGENTS. Potency and dosage are relative to the end-point chosen. For the intravenous drugs used in anesthesia practice for the induction to a state of general anesthesia, such end-points are:

- The degree of cortical depression (calmness → sedation → drowsiness)[3]
- The minimum amount to produce sleep and unconsciousness (no verbalization) related to time of onset of sleep and failure to respond to verbal commands[4]
- The amount of drug to produce full unconsciousness with depression of some reflexes[5]

Requirements to produce any end-point are related, in part, to body weight, sex, age, metabolic activity, and drug experience. Lean body mass is more significant than total body weight; men usually require a higher dose than women; the young need more than the elderly. Patients accustomed to taking sedatives, including alcohol, analgesics, or narcotics, usually are tolerant to the intravenous agents.

The minimum alveolar concentration (MAC) value for inhalation agents is inappropriate to intravenous agents. Blood levels do not always correlate with the neurologic status, especially when large doses are administered; the phenomenon of acute tolerance ensues.[6]

Concept of UD. In view of these conditions, the concept of UD_{50} and UD_{95} has been proposed by Stella[5] and supported by Clarke.[4] The UD is defined as the dose required to produce full unconsciousness and induce a subject to the state of anesthesia; that is, to the level of stage III, plane 1 in the classic sense. The patient should be asleep and unable to verbalize or respond to auditory stimuli or commands. Certain reflexes, such as eyelid, swallowing, and pharyngeal, should be obtunded but not necessarily absent. Response to a somatic (skin) painful stimulus is still present.

The UD_{50} represents the dose producing the defined level of unconsciousness in 50% of patients not premedicated. An estimated increase by 50% of the dose will approximate the UD for 95% of patients.

For some selected drugs (Table 24–2), the UD_{50} has been determined and a relative potency established.[5]

DEVELOPMENT OF BARBITURATE ANESTHESIA.[1,2] At the dawn of the intravenous barbiturate era, three longer-acting drugs were investigated for clinical use. The first, pernosten, was introduced in 1927 by Bumm. In 1929, amobarbital was introduced as an intravenous anesthetic by Zerfas and Lundy, while in 1931 Lundy experimented with pentobarbital. None of these was satisfactory. Then, the first truly ultra short-acting barbiturate, hexobarbitone (Epival), was discovered by Kropp and Taubb and clinically tested in 1932 by Weese and Scharpff. This drug gave significant impetus to the search for other satisfactory intravenous agents.

Knowledge of short-acting agents was already available because of an important discovery made in 1908 by Einhorn and Diesbach. They determined that barbiturates became less stable and more rapidly destroyed when sulfur was substituted for oxygen on the urea carbon of the barbituric acid molecule.[7] Somewhat later, chemical alteration of secobarbital and pentobarbital by the introduction of sulfur resulted in the clinically useful series of 2-thiobarbiturates. These were first prepared in 1929, thiopental by Taburn and Volweiler and thiamylal by Dox.[6]

In all, 18 thiobarbiturates were synthesized and a classic monograph of this work was published in 1935.[7]

Since then, a voluminous array of clinical reports have appeared. In 1933, both thiopental[7a] and thiamylal[7b] were shown to have anesthetic properties. Thiopental was first used by Ralph M. Waters in 1934. The first report was published by Lundy and Tovell in 1934. Thiopental was then promptly and successfully introduced into clinical practice, due to the efforts of Lundy.[9,9a] Thiamylal was used clinically in 1948 by Seevers.

NOMENCLATURE. In the terminology of the barbiturates, it should be noted that in the United States the ending "-al" is used, whereas in Britain the ending is "-one."

Because effects of the barbiturate class of drugs

TABLE 24–2. RELATIVE POTENCY AND UD_{50} OF SELECTED DRUGS

	Relative Potency*	UD_{50} (Modified)	Dose (mg/kg)
Thiopental	1	2.5	4
Propanidid	1	2.5	4
Ketamine	4	0.6	1
Diazepam	5	0.5	1
Alphaxalone	9	0.2	0.4

* Thiopental is given a value of 1. Other drugs are compared with this value in terms of potency.

656 General Anesthesia

are dose dependent and more specifically related to rate of biotransformation, barbiturates are classified into two large groups: sedative-hypnotic barbiturates and anesthetic barbiturates. On this basis, the groups of drugs under consideration are named the *anesthetic barbiturates* rather than Tatum's classification of ultra-short acting barbiturates.

CHEMICAL CONSIDERATIONS. The barbiturate nucleus (Fig. 24–1) has three common sites for substitution. Changes in the 1 and 2 positions cause significant effects on the quality of action. In position 2 an oxygen atom forms the standard oxybarbiturate; a sulfur atom in this position forms the thiobarbiturate group and results in a rapidly acting drug. In position 1, the introduction of a methyl or ethyl group invariably results in a drug with a more rapid onset of action and more rapid recovery *but a high incidence of excitatory phenomena* such as hypertonus, tremor, and involuntary muscle movements (Table 24–3).

Changes at the 5 carbon position, i.e., 5 and 5′, permits the construction of many congeners, but the effect is largely on the quantitative aspect of action, such as potency. Both positions must be occupied by alkyl or aromatic groups to produce a hypnotic drug.

An increase in the length of one of the side chains in position 5 will progressively increase potency. One side chain must remain short and simple, and together the two side chains should not number more than eight or nine carbons. Thiopental and pentobarbital have the same number of side chain atoms, and there is no appreciable difference in potency.

Removal of one CH$_2$ radical from the long side chain with the production of butabarbital and thiobutabarbital diminishes potency by 25%. Insertion of the amyl side chain producing amobarbital and thioethyamyl diminishes potency by half. The rate of onset, distribution, and recovery, however, are not very different.

Despite the large number of compounds that have been produced, the attempt to obtain a superior agent to thiopental or methohexital has not been successful. As the potency and brevity of action increase, the incidence of side effects increases. Thus, the available intravenous barbiturates may be further classified according to clinical utility (Table 24–4). Five compounds are in use world wide. Of all, thiopental sodium has occupied a preeminent position and has enjoyed both a popularity and the confidence of the medical profession.

STRUCTURE-ACTIVITY RELATIONSHIP.[10] The relationship between structure (Table 24-5) and drug activity has been elucidated, and the story is not complete. Certain generalizations, however, are apparent. In the barbiturates, "hypnophoric" groups consist of the amide and urea groups. They do not confer hypnotic activity but make such possible through linkage with auxiliary structural features

TABLE 24–3. GROUP CHARACTERISTICS

Group	Characteristics
Oxybarbiturates	Delay in onset of action, degree depending on 5 and 5′ side chains; useful as basal hypnotics; prolonged action
Methylated oxybarbiturates	Usually rapidly acting with fairly rapid recovery; high incidence of excitatory phenomena
Thiobarbiturates	Rapidly acting, usually smooth onset of sleep and fairly prompt recovery
Methylated thiobarbiturates	Rapid onset of action and very rapid recovery but with so high an incidence of excitatory phenomena as to preclude use in clinical practice

From Dundee, J.W.: Current views on the clinical pharmacology of the barbiturates. Int. Anesthesiol. Clin., 7:331, 1969.

TABLE 24–4. CLINICAL UTILITY CLASSIFICATION OF BARBITURATES

Classification	Drugs
Equally acceptable drugs	Thiopental
	Thiamylal
	Thialbarbital (UK)
	Thiobutabarbital (Germany)
Drugs whose side effects outweigh their merits	Hexobarbital
	Buthalital (UK)
	Methitural
	All methyl thiobarbiturates
Drugs whose advantages outweigh their side effects	Methohexital

Adapted from Dundee, J.W.: Current views on the clinical pharmacology of the barbiturates. Int. Anesthesiol. Clin., 7:331, 1969.

Group	1	2
(Oxy) barbiturates*	H	O
Methylated barbiturates	CH$_3$	O
Thiobarbiturates	H	S
Methylated thiobarbiturates	CH$_3$	S

FIG. 24–1. The barbiturate nucleus (keto form) and sites of substitution. *None of this group is used for routine intravenous anesthesia. From *The Practitioner*, London, England.

such as branched or unsaturated aliphatic chains or by halogenation.

Hypnotic properties occur if two alkyl groups (not too short) are adjacent to a —CO—NH linkage. Starting with diethyl barbituric acid, hypnotic activity appears and increases with increasing length of chain until a maximum is reached with seven or eight carbon atoms. Exceptions are seen in thialbarbital and methohexital, which have a total of 9 carbons. The overall bulk or molecular weight also increases similarly, but beyond 250 hypnotic activity decreases.

Increasing the length of the alkyl chains also increases the lipophilic character and aids in the distribution of the compound between the aqueous and lipoid phases. To a large extent, the lipophilic property determines the rate at which a compound achieves a critical brain concentration.[10]

ACTION ON SYMPATHETIC GANGLIA. Much evidence exists that barbiturates act postsynaptically to block excitatory transmitter action at both ganglionic and central synapses. At sympathetic ganglia, pentobarbital depresses only the fast nicotinic excitatory postsynaptic potentials (EPSP). It appears that the effect is due to a decrease in sodium conductance. On the other hand, slow excitatory and inhibitory postsynaptic potentials are not blocked. These actions are dependent on a presynaptic release of acetylcholine.[11]

USE OF THIOPENTAL

HISTORICAL BACKGROUND. The use of intravenous thiopental has had three phases of development:

1. When first introduced only air was breathed by the patient and the drug was given for short surgical procedures.[8]
2. In 1938, reports[12,13] appeared on the use of oxygen given continuously by nasal catheter during intravenous anesthesia. The experiences indicated that longer anesthesia could be obtained with a given dose, that muscular relaxation was enhanced and toxic reactions were minimized.
3. Later, Lundy[14] introduced the use of nitrous oxide and oxygen mixtures, usually a 50-50 mixture, administered by inhalation in conjunction with intravenous thiopental. Other combinations were then added such as thiopental plus regional anesthesia,[15] thiopental and spinal analgesia,[16] and intravenous thiopental plus nitrous-oxide–oxygen by inhalation plus intravenous curare.[17]

TECHNIQUE OF ADMINISTRATION. Since 1940, many ingenious mechanical gadgets have been introduced for administering thiopental, but all have been complex and tend to undermine one of the chief advantages of thiopental anesthesia, namely, the simplicity of equipment required for administration—the needle and syringe. There are three modifications that are useful yet simple: (1) the use of a short piece of connecting tubing with syringe and needle for intermittent injection of concentrated solutions of thiopental; (2) the use of a three-way stopcock for longer procedures—through one opening, a physiologic salt solution is administered continuously and through the other thiopental in concentrated solution is injected intermittently; and (3) the ordinary infusion set for the continuous administration of highly dilute solutions.

DISSOCIATION CONSTANT AND DEGREE OF IONIZATION.[18] Thiopental is commercially provided as the sodium salt in a yellow powder form. It behaves as a weak acid. When dissolved in sterile distilled water, a highly alkaline solution is formed (pH 10.5), with most of the drug ionized. As the pH of a solution of a weak acid (barbiturate) is decreased, the amount ionized decreases. The dissociation constant of sodium thiopental is pK_a 7.6, at which only 50% of the substance is ionized and 50% is nonionized. At the pH of plasma (7.4), a larger fraction of sodium thiopental is in the nonionized form and amounts to 60% of the free drug. Also, at the pH of plasma, a larger fraction is unbound to protein and available for dissociation. The nonionized portion of the drug traverses cell membranes.

SOLUBILITY. The sodium salt of thiopental is soluble in distilled water, in saline, and—to a slight extent—in alcohol but not in other organic solvents. Dissolving the drug in 5% dextrose is usually incomplete and results in a sticky solution that is often layered. Mixing of the powder must be vigorous.[5]

PREPARATIONS AND CONCENTRATIONS. The strengths of thiopental solutions currently in use are the 2.5% originally recommended by Lundy,[9] the 5% solution for induction used chiefly in Britain, and the 1% or 0.5 (or 0.4)% solution administered by drip for surgical procedures. With the latter solution, an initial rapid drip rate is used for induction followed by a slow rate for maintenance.[18] Finally, highly dilute solutions, such as the 1:1000 introduced by Lenowitz for sedation and hypnosis particularly, are used as a supplement to spinal and local anesthesia.[19]

MIXTURES WITH RELAXANTS. With the intravenous use of thiopental and curare combinations, it was natural that efforts be made to combine the two in a single solution. Because sodium thiopental produces a highly alkaline solution, e.g., a 2.5% solution has a pH of 10.5 and curare solutions (Intocostrin) have a pH of 5.1, a chemical precipitation of

TABLE 24-5. FORMULAS OF COMMON INTRAVENOUS BARBITURATE AGENTS

Trade Name	Generic Name	Chemical Name and Structural Formula
Pentothal (Abbott)	Thiopental sodium	Na 5-Ethyl-5-(1-Methylbutyl)-2-Thiobarbiturate
Surital (Parke-Davis)	Thiamylal sodium	Na 5-Allyl-5-(1-Methylbutyl)-2-Thiobarbiturate
Brevital (Lilly)	Methohexital sodium	Na 5-(1-Methyl Allyl)-5-(1-Methyl-2-Pentynyl) Barbiturate

Evipal (Evipan-Na) Hexobarbital sodium Na N-Methyl-5-Cyclohexenyl-5-Methyl Barbiturate
(Winthrop-Stearns)

Courtesy of G. Wyant. Comparison of seven anesthetic agents in man. Brit. J. Anaesth. 29:194, 1957.
Note. 1) The official generic name of many barbiturates in Gr. Britain (UK) has the ending **-one**, i.e. thiopental (US) is thiopent*one* in UK. 2) Hexobarbital was used in Europe until 1988 but is now discontinued. It is of historical interest because it was the first successful intravenous barbiturate anesthetic.
Corssen, G., Reves, J.G., and Stanley, T.H.: **Intravenous Anesthesia and Analgesia.** Philadelphia, Lea & Febiger, 1988.

one drug by the other occurs when the two solutions are mixed. A compatible and nonprecipitable combination results when 5 units of curare are present in each milliliter of a 2.5% aqueous thiopental solution. Each milliliter of such a solution contains 25 mg of thiopental and 0.75 mg d-tubocurarine. This solution, prepared by adding 100 units or 15 mg of curare (5 ml Intocostrin) to 0.5 g of thiopental in 15 ml of distilled water, is often called *Baird's solution*.[20,21]

Mixtures of thiopental and gallamine have been used by Evans.[22] A solution of thiopental 500 mg and gallamine 80 mg in 20 ml of water has been used for induction. A mixture of 1 g thiopental plus 240 mg of gallamine may be prepared in 500 ml of 5% dextrose and used for maintenance of a basal state. This dilute solution may be used for induction if a rate of 60 drops per minute is employed. After induction, the rate is slowed to 30 drops per minute or less.

INTERACTION OF BARBITURATES AND RELAXANTS. Barbiturates generally depress muscular function in a complex manner. Initially, there is a mild stimulation of muscle seen with small doses and during induction. This may cause a temporary antagonism to the relaxant drugs. Soon, however, the main effect appears, which is a depression of both the neuromuscular junction and muscular activity. Synergism with all types of relaxants thus occurs. That is, the potency of both competitive curariform agents and depolarizing agents is enhanced. There is no depression of nerve conductivity. Solutions of suxamethonium and thiopentone are not compatible.

SOLUBILITY IN THE PRESENCE OF STEROID-TYPE RELAXANTS.[23] When a solution of pancuronium or one of its analogues is introduced into a solution of 2.5% sodium thiopental, a white flocculent precipitate forms. Often, in rapid-induction techniques, these two drugs are given almost simultaneously. To avoid flocculation, it is necessary to flush the intravenous lines after each drug injection. The nature of the flocculation reaction has been identified as a physiochemical reaction and not one of chemical neutralization. The sodium salt of thiopental is soluble in water and has a pH of 10.6. The solubility in water is maintained as long as there is an alkaline pH greater than 9.9. Pancuronium solutions have a pH of 3.5, and the drug is soluble in water at a wide pH range of 2.0 to 12.0. When pancuronium is added to a thiopental solution, the resultant mixture has a pH of less than 9.25. Because the solubility of sodium thiopental is pH dependent, a decrease in the pH of an aqueous solution decreases its solubility and the drug precipitates out of solution as the white base. As dilution of thiopental is increased and a buffering effect by the blood buffers occurs, thiopental will again leave the flocculent condition and become soluble.

SOLUBILITY WITH SUCCINYLCHOLINE.[23] Due to the marked differences in pH range of aqueous solutions of 2.5% thiopental (10.6) and succinylcholine (3.2-3.5), a white precipitate forms when the solutions are mixed. This precipitate may dissolve if the concentration of thiopental is increased to 5% or more. However, hydrolysis of the succinylcholine is more rapid if the solution is allowed to stand for more than an hour.[23a]

POTENTIATION. The administration of 10% and 15% glucose solutions to patients who had been anesthetized with thiopental potentiates the action and prolongs the duration of narcosis. If patients awaken from thiopental anesthesia and are then given a solution of dextrose, they will become renarcotized. This was reported by Lampson and experimentally demonstrated by Langlais.[24] Two explanations may be considered: (1) that adenosine triphosphate and monophosphate are utilized in the metabolism of these substances but glucose is preferred, allowing thiopental to accumulate; and (2) that the glucose causes a withdrawal of thiopental from the tissues and maintains a high plasma concentration.

Potentiation of the depressant actions of thiopental is also produced by tetraethyl thiuram disulfide (Antabuse) and by alpha tocopherol. These two substances enhance central depression and prolong the recovery time. Antabuse, frequently used in the management of alcoholism, interferes with oxidation of alcohol and therefore acetaldehyde accumulates in the blood stream.[25]

It has been postulated that sodium thiopental, when supplemented by curare, is potentiated as regards depth and duration of anesthesia. Experimental results show that there is little difference in thiopental narcosis alone or supplemented.[26] At the same time it was noted that the only mortality occurred in animals receiving the combined drugs.

Available evidence indicates that chlorpromazine intensifies the action and duration of narcosis produced by the commonly used intravenous barbiturates. With the thiobarbiturates, Dundee[27] has determined the following when phenothiazine derivatives are part of premedication (i.e., chlorpromazine, promethazine): (1) the onset of sleep is hastened; (2) narcosis occurs at a lower plasma level; (3) the period of sleep is prolonged; (4) the effect lasts for 24 hours; and (5) thiamylal narcosis is less affected than that of thiopental.

STABILITY OF SOLUTIONS. Deterioration of solutions of thiopental occurs slowly and steadily.[28] Temperature, light, and concentration are factors in this deterioration. Dilute solutions are less likely to deteriorate, and 0.1% to 0.4% solutions are more stable. It is recommended that 5% solutions be stored at 5° to 6° C but for not more than 7 days. When stored at 18° to 22° C solutions should not be kept for more than 3 days. Undoubtedly, solutions can be kept for longer periods and still be used. Definite changes take place, however, and there is loss of potency of perhaps 10% to 15%. Turbid solutions should also be discarded.

DOSAGE. The dose response of thiopental for induction of general anesthesia in unpremedicated healthy adult patients is set at a range of 3 to 4 mg/kg. This dose range represents an effective dose in most patients and the dose of 4 mg/kg is designated as the UD_{95}, or the dose producing unconsciousness in 95% of subjects. In adult subjects medicated with an opiate, the UD_{95} dose is the lower limit of 3 mg/kg.[29-32] Note that the UD_{50} for thiopental is 2.5 mg/kg (Table 24–2).

In children, the dose range recommended for unpremedicated children is 5 to 6 mg/kg. The UD_{95} is 6 mg/kg. A lower dose of 4 mg/kg is a UD_{95} and appropriate for children receiving an opiate as part of premedication.[33]

Age Effect on Dosage.[34] The dose of thiopental required to induce anesthesia in adults decreases with age.[31,35] An overall reduction in dose of 25% is recommended, particularly in patients over 50 years of age when the decrease is more linear, whereas in the 20 to 40 age group the dose tends to cluster.[31,36]

In nonpremedicated patients, an induction dose for healthy subjects (weighing 60 to 70 kg) 20 to 40 years of age is about 5.4 mg/kg for women and 5.2 mg/kg for men; in healthy subjects 60 to 80 years of age, the dose is about 3 to 4 mg/kg.[31] One explanation for this clinical fact of lower doses is that the older patient is more sensitive to the effects of thiopental and the dose requirement could be attributed to pharmacodynamics; the brain response to a given dose is greater. The evidence at this time, however, clearly demonstrates that pharmacokinetic factors are the determinants (see below).

PHARMACOKINETICS IN ADULTS (TABLE 24–6).[37] After a bolus intravenous injection of thiopental for induction to produce unconsciousness, the serum concentration curve represents a three-compartment model and fits a triexponential equation[38,39] (Figs. 24–2; 24–3). There is an immediate dilution (30 to 60 seconds) in the intravascular compartment (the pi phase), followed by a rapid distribution phase averaging 3 to 6 minutes (alpha), followed by a slower distribution phase averaging 50 to 60 minutes (beta elimination half-time [$t_{\frac{1}{2}}$]). The subsequent elimination phase has a half-life of 12 hours.[39] This elimination coincides with the metabolism and rate of destruction of thiopental of 15%/hr, as classically determined by Mark[6] (Table 24–7).

Ghoneim's[40] studies of patients anesthetized with enflurane–N_2O compared with volunteers not medicated or anesthetized suggest that a simpler model is that of two compartments—a small central compartment and a large peripheral compartment consisting of both rapidly accessible and slowly accessible tissue parts (Fig. 24–4). This represents first-order kinetics, and the early rapid changes in plasma concentration during the first 15 to 20 minutes after administration of the drug. These important early changes—decreasing plasma concentrations—are related to the clinical anesthetic period.

Plasma Concentration (Decay Curve). The early decreases in plasma concentration have been further studied.[38] The fraction of thiopental lost at 1 minute was 0.14 and 0.18 at 15 minutes (Fig. 24–5). Actual concentrations at 0.5 minute were between 90 and 100 μg/ml and at 1 minute were 50 to 60 μg/ml. By 15 minutes, the plasma concentration fell to levels between 6 and 8 μg/ml. The decline in the first few minutes represents the immediate hepatic extraction and early metabolism. The subsequent decline is related to tissue distribution. A continuous ex-

TABLE 24–6. PLASMA LEVELS RELATED TO PHARMACOKINETIC TIME VARIABLES AS DETERMINED BY GHONEIM[40] AND BURCH[39]

	Ghoneim		Burch	
	Time	Plasma Level (μg)	Time	Plasma Level (μg)
Pi phase	0.5 min	30–90*	30 sec	93
"Mixing site" intravascular compartment	1 min	40*	1 min	50
Alpha phase ($t_{\frac{1}{2}}$)	3 min	21	3 min	18*
	7 min	12*	7 min	12
Beta phase ($t_{\frac{1}{2}}$)	48 min	3.8	15 min	7
Gamma phase ($t_{\frac{1}{2}}$)	5 hr	1.34	5 hr	1*
	12 hr	0.5*	12 hr	0.5

* The plasma levels, as determined by Ghoneim and by Burch, are in relative agreement with respect to time after administration. Some of the values are estimated from the pharmacokinetic curves.

Abbreviation: $t_{\frac{1}{2}}$, elimination half-time.

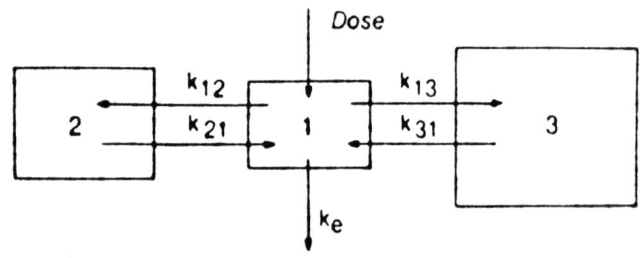

FIG. 24–2. The three-compartment pharmacokinetic model used to characterize thiopental distribution and elimination. The dose is administered into the central compartment (1) and distributed to two peripheral compartments (2, 3). The rate constants of drug transfer between the compartments are k_{12}, k_{21}, k_{13}, and k_{31}. The rate constant for drug elimination from the body is k_e. From Burch, P.G., and Stanski, D.R.: The role of metabolism and protein binding in thiopental anesthesia. Anesthesiology, 58:147, 1983.

traction from hepatic blood and drug metabolism during the elimination phase follows.

Volumes of Distribution (Table 24–7). The volume of the central compartment (V_c) and the volume of distribution at steady state (Vd_{ss}) has been determined as 0.53 L/kg and 2.3 L/kg, respectively.[39] It is noted that Ghoneim places the actual early distribution to highly vascular tissues (brain, heart, lungs, kidneys, liver) at 2.8 minutes, which does not account for dilution (pi) in blood volume.[40] Burch places the time for rapid distribution at 6.8 minutes and includes blood volume and vessel-rich tissues as the V_c.[39]

Clearance and Elimination. Clearance depends on the free fraction of the drug and intrinsic hepatic microsomal enzyme activity. For thiopental, the hepatic extraction ratio of clearance to hepatic blood flow is 0.2 and continues at this low level, providing thiopental to the liver for degradation. This is part of the elimination phase. The return of the drug to the V_c from the deep peripheral compartment becomes the rate-controlling factor in the elimination phase. The adult liver mass is about 2% of body weight, or 1500 g in a 70-kg man, and the blood flow is about 100 ml/min/100 g of tissue.

Plasma Protein Binding. Protein binding of thiopental to plasma protein is substantial. Studies of plasma protein binding show that in healthy subjects 85% of thiopental is bound and 15% is unbound.[41] It is the unbound fraction that penetrates cell membranes and provides the active component. In chromatographic assays, it has been determined that the binding is primarily to the albumin fraction of the plasma protein.[42–45] Differences between children and adults have not been demonstrated. Sorbo[46] has determined that in infants and children, the unbound fraction ranges from 12% to 15% with an average of 13.2% in comparison with the adult free fraction of 12% to 15%, with an average of 13.6% unbound.

Several factors may alter binding. There is a significant increase of unbound drug with age, particularly in the elderly after 50 years of age. Elderly women show a significant increase in the free fraction of thiopental.[47] This is likely related to a lower plasma protein level with aging.[39]

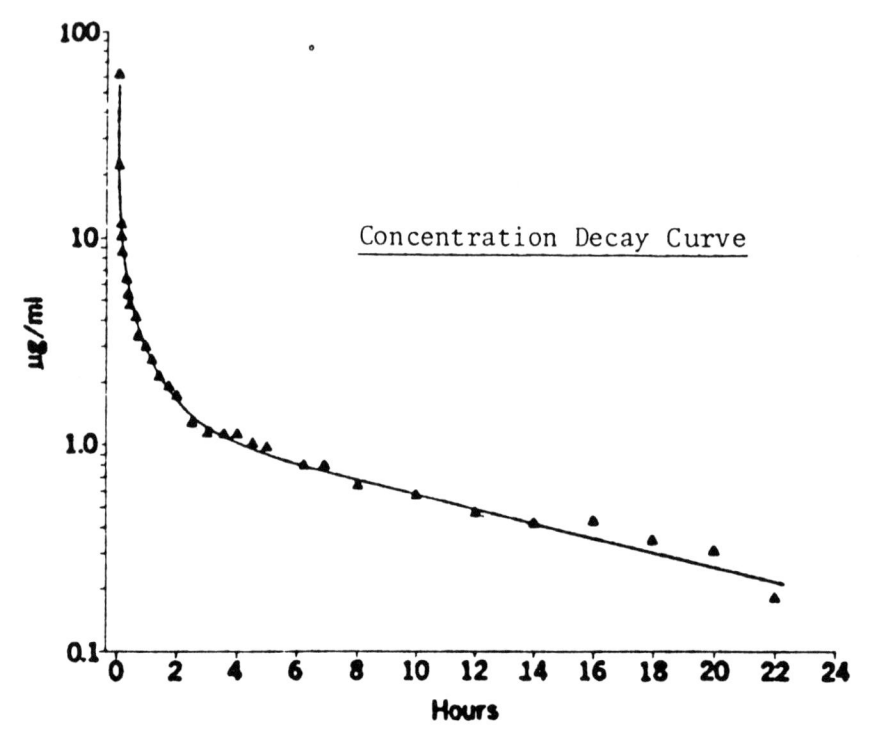

FIG. 24–3. Characteristic triexponential serum concentration decay curve of thiopental. The triangles represent actual total (free and protein bound) thiopental serum levels, while the solid line represents the fitted function characterized by a triexponential equation. From Burch, P.G., and Stanski, D.R.: The role of metabolism and protein binding in thiopental anesthesia. Anesthesiology, 58:148, 1983.

TABLE 24-7. PHARMACOKINETICS OF THIOPENTAL IN SURGICAL PATIENTS

	Rapid Distribution Half-life (min)	Slow Distribution Half-life (min)	Terminal Elimination Half-life (hr)	V_1 (l/kg)	Vd_{ss} (l/kg)	Cl (ml · min^{-1} · kg^{-1})
Mean ± SD	6.8 ± 2.8	59 ± 24	12	0.53 ± 0.18	2.34 ± 0.75	3.4 ± 0.4

Abbreviations: V_1, volume of the central compartment; Vd_{ss}, volume of distribution at steady state; Cl, total body clearance.
From Burch, P.G., and Stanski, D.R.: The role of metabolism and protein binding in thiopental anesthesia. Anesthesiology, 58:146, 1983.

In patients with chronic renal failure, the thiopental free fraction approximates 30% as opposed to 15% in a normal surgical population.[48] Changes in kinetics such as decreased removal from plasma show clearance to rise from 3.2 ml/kl to 4.5 ml/kl/min. This change is secondary to increases in the free fraction in patients with renal failure.[44,45]

In uremic patients and after sulfonamide treatment the amount bound is reduced to 45%, leaving 55% free. Additional studies show that with reduced binding there is an accelerated distribution and increased concentration in the heart and brain.[49] The mechanism of reduced binding in azotemia appears to be an alteration of the albumin molecule by an increase in amino acid alanine of the albumin.[49]

An increase in the free fraction of thiopental has been also observed in patients with alcoholic cirrhosis.[50]

An increase in free fatty acids may displace acidic drugs such as thiopental from their albumin binding.[51]

Binding may also be related to the actual thiopental plasma concentration. Over a concentration range from 93 µg/ml down to 6.9 µg/ml, the percent of plasma protein binding is linear.[48] Morgan[41] has presented evidence that when the thiopental plasma concentration is greater than 100 µg/ml and in the range of 100 to 150 µg/ml, binding is decreased from about 85% to 70%. This indicates that binding is nonlinear under circumstances of high plasma concentrations of thiopental.[52] That is, albumin uptake is complete because binding is concentration dependent. Therefore, at levels of thiopental in excess of 100 µg, the free fraction will be greater and, therefore, the effect of thiopental will be increased and prolonged.

Effects of Age on Pharmacokinetics. Age affects thiopental disposition in adults. A positive correlation exists between age and Vd_{ss}. However, for the initial distribution or "mixing period," V_1 central volume is decreased in the older patient, as dem-

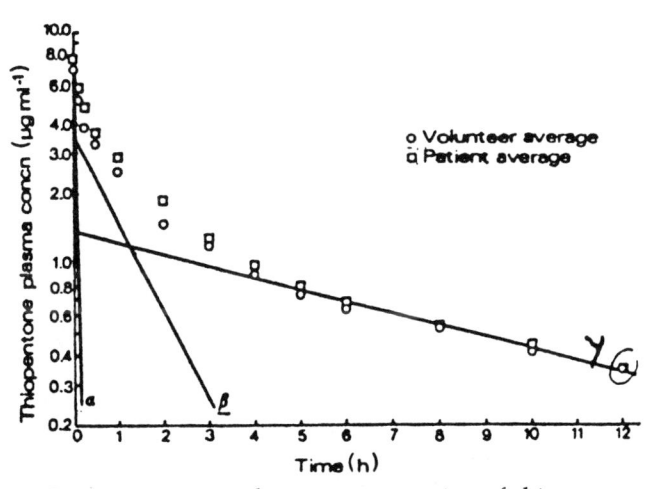

FIG. 24-4. Average plasma concentration of thiopentone in 12 subjects after a dose of 3.5 mg · kg^{-1} iv. The three decay lines were fitted by computer using nonlinear least squares regression analysis. From Ghoneim, M.M., and Van Hamme, M.J.: Pharmacokinetics of thiopentone: Effects of enflurane and nitrous oxide anaesthesia and surgery. Br. J. Anaesth., 50:1239, 1978.

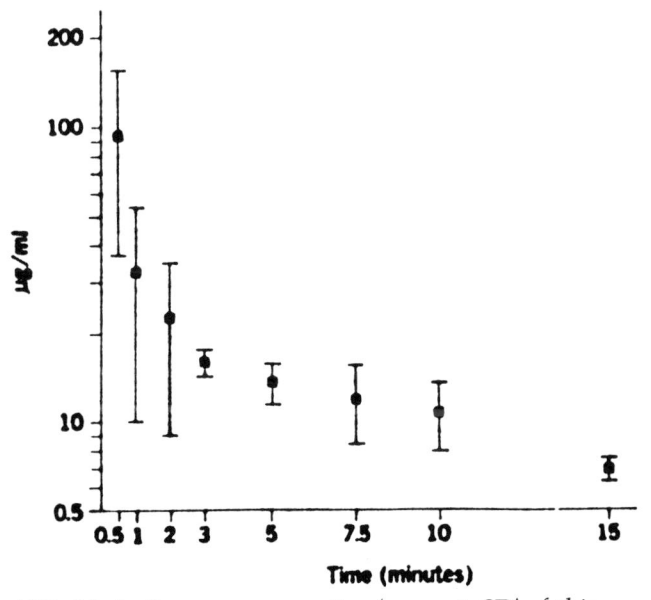

FIG. 24-5. Serum concentration (mean ± SD) of thiopental in arterial blood for the first 15 min after a single bolus iv dose of thiopental for 12 patients. From Burch, P.G., and Stanski, D.R.: The role of metabolism and protein binding in thiopental anesthesia. Anesthesiology, 58:150, 1983.

onstrated by Homer.[36] Christensen[31] found a slight increase in the initial V_1, but stated that it was insignificant. The distribution volumes to rapidly perfused tissues, such as muscle (V_2), were found to be increased with age by most investigators, as was the volume (V_3) distributed to slowly perfused tissues, such as fat.[36]

More frequent blood sampling after drug administration showed a significant reduction in the initial distribution volume. Arterial blood sampling allowed for more accurate distribution data. The initial distribution volume decreased from 15 to 30 L in the 20 to 40-year-old patients to 3 to 7 L in the 60 to 90-year-old patients (Fig. 24–6).

The initial distribution space or central compartment is composed of both the blood volume in the large arterial and venous vessels and the blood in the vessel-rich group of tissues (lungs, heart, brain, liver, and kidney), which rapidly equilibrate with blood. This may be considered as an instantaneous mixing site early after the administration of the drug.

Physiologic factors involved in the reduction of the central volume with age include:[52,53]

- Reduced hepatic blood flow
- Reduce renal blood flow
- Reduced total body water
- Reduced extracellular fluid volume
- Decreased plasma volume
- Reduced size and weight of liver with age, and a progressively smaller portion of body weight

Subsequently, there is a greater relative redistribution to peripheral compartments to the rapidly perfused large compartment (muscle) and to the slowly perfused compartment. No significant change in intercompartmental exchange or clearance has been observed; however, there is an increased volume of distribution of these compartments related to the high water and fat content. At equilibrium, the Vd_{ss} is larger. The increase in body fat with age accounts for a greater uptake of lipid soluble drugs, such as thiopental.

Because the elderly patient has a significant decrease in the initial distribution volume or central compartment, a set dose will provide a higher serum level than in the young subject. A smaller dose will achieve the same end-point of clinical anesthesia and produce electroencephalographic (EEG) suppression. The dose regimen in the older patient is significantly less and decreases with aging.

Influence of Sex on Pharmacokinetics. Elimination half-life increases with age due to an increased Vd_{ss}. Women have a larger volume of distribution than men at all ages. Thus, the elimination half-life is longer in women than in men of the same age.[47]

Novak[52] noted that body fat increases with age and this represents a peripheral storage compartment. For men between 65 and 85 years of age, there is an increase of 18% to 36% (in relation to men aged 18 to 25 years). For women, percentage of body fat is larger than men at all ages and although there is an increase after the age of 45, the percentage is not as great as in men. Ouslander[34] has determined, in contrast to an increase in fat, that by the age of 65 years the lean body mass of women decreases by 5 kg, but in men the decrease approximates 12 kg. Thus, there are differences in size and composition of body compartments according to sex.

With respect to the central compartment, the circulating volume is slightly smaller in women than in men.[32] For the healthy person under 40 years of age, the blood volume of men is approximately 7.5% of body weight and of women 7%. The V_1 as well as the rapidly circulating tissues (heart, brain, liver) is smaller in women than in men. The V_2 distribution volume, largely muscle and splanchnic bed, is larger in men than in women, but unlike V_1, increases with age in both sexes.

The V_3 volume of distribution to poorly circulating tissues, including fat, is larger in women than in men. The V_3 average volume of distribution is almost three times as great in young women as in young men.[31]

From the above pharmacokinetic data, it can be

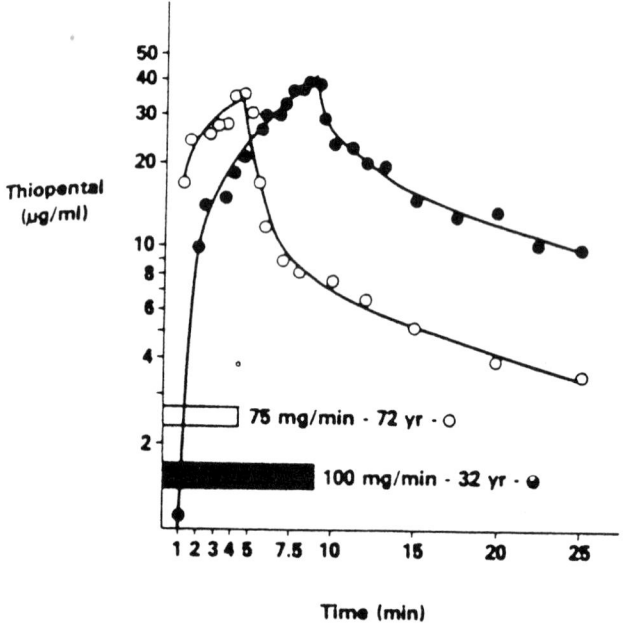

FIG. 24–6. Serum thiopental concentration (*log scale*) versus time in the young (*filled circles and bars*) and the elderly (*unfilled circles and bars*). All of the measured thiopental concentrations for the patients are indicated in this figure. The horizontal bars represent length of the thiopental infusions; solid lines represent fitted data from the pharmacokinetic model. From Homer, T.D., and Stanski, D.R.: The effect of increasing age on thiopental disposition and anesthetic requirement. Anesthesiology, 62:714, 1985.

predicted that the elimination phase is longer for women than for men at all ages.

Influence of Chronic Alcoholism. The requirements for thiopental are usually greater in patients with chronic alcoholism than in otherwise healthy persons. Suggested mechanisms for this include:[54]

1. Cross-tolerance between ethanol and barbiturates[55]
2. An increase in the hepatic rate of breakdown and elimination as a result of enzyme induction by the exposure to ethanol[56]
3. An increase in the volume of distribution of the anesthetic as a result of vasodilatation[57]

In a study of the pharmacokinetics of thiopental in alcoholic patients, the following observations have been determined.[58] Thiopental has a large volume of distribution owing to its lipid solubility; however, there is no difference in the central volume of distribution between alcoholic patients and nonalcoholic persons. Neither the total apparent volume of distribution nor the volume of the central compartment differed. The alpha elimination phase has been set at approximately 15 to 30 minutes and the beta elimination phase is between 680 and 750 minutes. The volume of the central compartment varies from 0.48 L/kg in nonalcoholic persons to 0.66 L/kg in alcoholics, whereas the Vd_{ss} varies between 2.9 and 3.5.

The plasma clearance of thiopental, however, is significantly increased (Fig. 24–7). There is an increase from 3.7 ± 0.9 ml/min/kg in the controls to 5.4 ± 2.2 ml/min/kg in the patients with chronic alcoholism. This change is probably explained by the stimulation of the hepatic monooxygenase system by chronic ethanol consumption.[56] The terminal elimination half-life in the alcoholics is slightly shorter than the values in control subjects—an average of 684 minutes in the alcoholic versus 750 minutes in the control nonalcoholic patients.

Drugs with a high lipid solubility, such as thiopental, will not be significantly influenced by plasma clearance, nor will any changes in plasma clearance significantly affect elimination half-life. The duration of effect and dose requirements are thus likely to be influenced by changes in tissue uptake, so the profile of elimination is mainly influenced by redistribution from deep-tissue depots. The study indicates that there is no pharmacokinetic explanation for the need for a higher initial dose of thiopental in patients with chronic alcoholism.

Because the only change in pharmacokinetics is an increase in plasma clearance, it can be concluded that the requirement for larger doses of thiopental in the presence of chronic alcoholism appears to be a cross-tolerance between alcohol and thiopental and related to more rapid metabolism.[58]

Pharmacokinetics in Children.[46] Infants and children have a large dose requirement for induction of anesthesia.[33] This is explained principally by a twofold increase in clearance rate and a 50% decrease in elimination half-life. The Vd_{ss} is almost identical to that of the adult and apparently is not a factor in the dose requirement. Although the volume of the central compartment is, on the average, larger than that of the adult, it is not statistically significant.

Distribution follows more closely a three-compartment model and is compared to adult values

FIG. 24–7. Mean plasma thiopentone concentrations in control patients (▲) and those with chronic alcoholism (○). The symbols are mean (± SD) of individual concentrations in each group. From Couderc, E., et al: Thiopentone pharmacokinetics in patients with chronic alcoholism. Br. J. Anaesth., 56:1393, 1984.

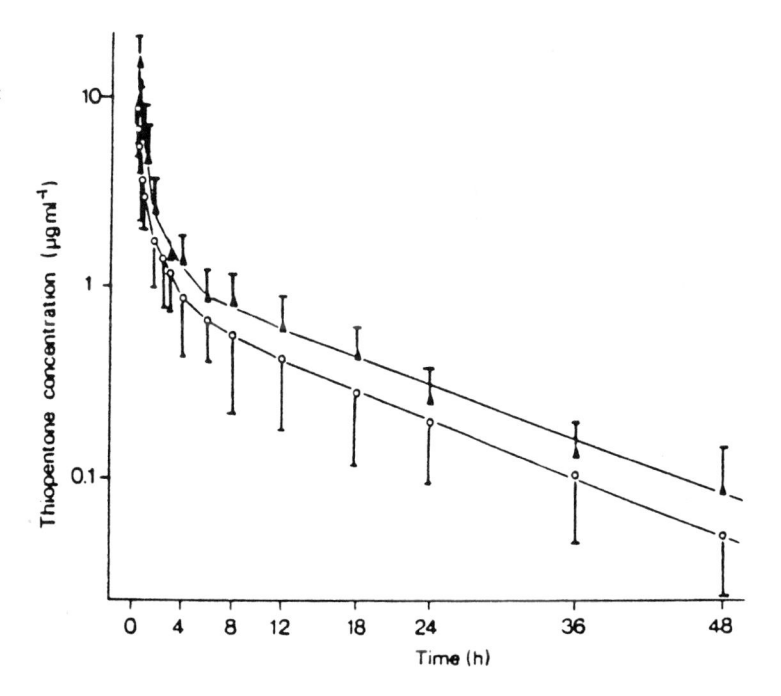

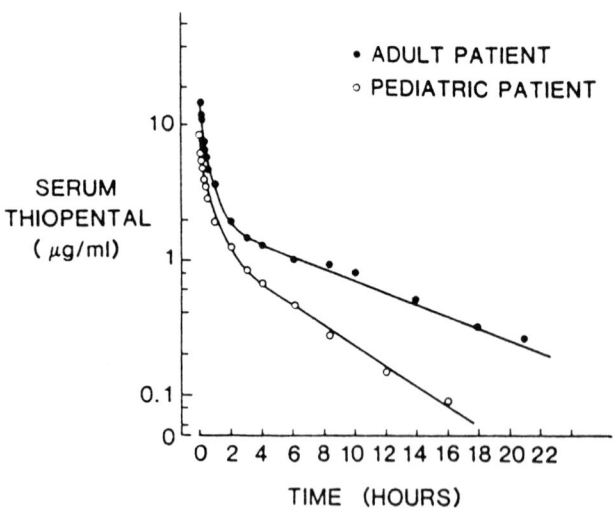

FIG. 24–8. Representative thiopental serum decay curves for a 4-year-old patient given 4 mg · kg^{-1} and a 28-year-old given 6 mg · kg^{-1}, both as an intravenous bolus. The symbols indicate measured serum thiopental levels; the solid line represents a nonlinear regression fit to the data. From Sorbo, S., Hudson, R.J., and Loomis, J.C.: The pharmacokinetics of thiopental in pediatric surgical patients. Anesthesiology, 61:666, 1984.

(Fig. 24–8). The rapid distribution phase (t$_{\frac{1}{2}}$ alpha) was quite variable in Sorbo's studies; the slow tissue distribution phase (t$_{\frac{1}{2}}$ beta) was more rapid than in the adult; and the elimination time (t$_{\frac{1}{2}}$ gamma) was 6 hours, compared with the average adult value of 12 hours. The clearance rate was determined at 6.6 ml/kg/min, which was twice as much as in the adult.

Clearance depends on hepatic blood flow and enzyme activity.[39] Enzyme activity is immature in the neonatal period but rapidly matures.[59] Ordinarily, hepatic blood flow per 100 g of tissue is not too different in infants and adults. The total liver mass of the infant, however, is greater than that of the adult. It varies from a value double that of the adult at birth to a 50% greater mass during infancy and early childhood. The liver mass of the fetus and newborn is about 4% the body weight as compared with 2% in the older child and adult.

TOLERANCE—ACUTE. This phenomenon can be described as the need for greater increments of thiopental to maintain cerebral depression when higher initial doses are administered. Likewise, with higher initial doses, a higher brain concentration is attained and required to maintain the anesthetic state. The blood level at which consciousness is regained is also higher.

PHARMACOLOGIC ACTIONS

CENTRAL NERVOUS SYSTEM. An irregular descending depression occurs, progressing from calmness to complete coma.

As shown by Himwich,[61] oxygen utilization of the various levels of the brain is depressed from above downward. With increasing doses there are increasing degrees of depression of cerebral metabolism. After hypnotic doses, cerebral oxygen consumption is reduced some 21%, from 3.4 ml per 100 g of tissue to 2.7 ml. At the same time, the cerebrovascular resistance is increased and the brain blood flow is reduced from 55 ml/100 g/min to 46 ml. Full anesthetic doses of thiopental lower the oxygen consumption about 36%.

Mitchenfelder[62] has shown that thiopental produces a progressive decrease in cerebral metabolic rate. The oxygen requirement is reduced by 32% when unconsciousness is produced; at the time that pain response is obtunded, the oxygen requirement is reduced by 50% to 55%. Because of this effect, it has been found that thiopental protects against the untoward effects of hypoxia.[63]

The vomiting center shows no direct stimulation. The intracranial pressure is generally decreased.

The anesthetic state may be considered to exist when there is a plasma concentration of 30 μg/ml of thiopental. However, this must be evaluated in terms of the initial dose. Mark[64] has shown that a condition of acute tolerance may exist; if very large doses are administered, awakening may occur when the plasma levels are significantly higher. Thus, a larger dose establishes a higher critical level.

RESPIRATION.[64] Thiopental is a direct depressant to the medullary centers, and both the rate and the amplitude of the respiratory excursion are decreased. In therapeutic doses, respiration is regular and shallow. The chief respiratory drive under thiopental comes from the carotid body and is the drive of reflex anoxia. If just apnea is produced, the rate of destruction or redistribution of thiopental is so rapid that respiration recurs before cyanosis develops. Thiopental also is parasympathomimetic in its action and causes bronchoconstriction.

The respiratory depressant effect is proportional to the dose. With small doses in healthy patients not receiving any opiates, the respiratory depression is minimal. When a total dose of approximately 500 mg is administered as a 0.2% intravenous drip in 25 minutes and an EEG level of 1 or 2 is attained,[65] significant respiratory depressant effects are lacking, and the patient is not anesthetized sufficiently for surgical intervention. The end-expiratory CO$_2$ concentration showed little change from resting values, and the respiratory response to carbon dioxide showed an average increase of 7% over control.[66]

On the other hand, patients receiving an opiate (morphine or meperidine) as part of premedication showed an elevated end expiratory P$_{CO_2}$ value over control and a sharply diminished respiratory response to endogenously accumulated carbon dioxide. The minute volume response to CO$_2$ was reduced about 54%. Thus, in safe clinical anesthesia the major effects on respiration must be attributed to opiates.[67]

Respiratory Response Curve.[68] Careful examination of the response curve to increasing concentrations of inhaled carbon dioxide shows a definite reduction in the slope of the response. Compared to a slope of 1.89 L/min/mm Hg, the administration of thiopental (3.5 mg/kg) flattens the curve to a slope of 1.37 at 1 minute. By 15 minutes, there is recovery to a value of 1.69 L/min/mm Hg. Thus, there is a time course to the ventilatory depression. Of further importance is the effect of chronic obstructive pulmonary disease on response to CO_2 after thiopental administration. In these patients, the response slope goes from 1.53 L/min/mm Hg to a minimum of 0.69 at 30 seconds but shows almost complete recovery of slope to a value of 1.47 by 15 minutes.[68]

CARDIOVASCULAR EFFECTS. The hemodynamic effects of thiopental on the heart and the circulation are summarized in Table 24–8.[69–77]

Myocardial Action. The ultra short-acting barbiturates have a direct weakening effect on myocardium as demonstrated by Johnson.[77] This reduces cardiac output and, in turn, compromises circulation. All properties of heart muscle are directly depressed. There is a reduction of stroke work and stroke power. Sedative doses of 100 to 200 mg may decrease cardiac contractility 10%, whereas light anesthesia may cause a reduction of 20%. Cardiac output is similarly reduced; during deep thiopental anesthesia, this may amount to a 35% reduction.

Circulatory Action. Slight hypotension accompanies thiopental anesthesia. It is pronounced following rapid injection especially of concentrated solution. It is more evident in patients with hypertension.[78] It has also been demonstrated that thiopental and other barbiturates increase cerebrovascular resistance and reduce cerebral blood flow. However, any decrease in circulation is well compensated by the great reduction in cerebral oxygen requirements.[81]

Electrocardiographic Effects. In human subjects there is little effect on the cardiac pacemaker. Stephen[78] has demonstrated that the rate of injection, if rapid, will produce a high incidence of arrhythmias, whereas slow induction produces no electrocardiographic (ECG) changes.

Abnormal ECG changes are not noted during thiopental anesthesia when properly administered.[78] Ectopic beats and arrhythmias of whatever nature that are seen as well as cardiovascular collapse are usually secondary to hypoxemia caused by prolonged respiratory depression.

GASTROINTESTINAL TRACT. Gastrointestinal tone is depressed and amplitude of contractions decreased. There is also diminution in secretory activity throughout the intestinal tract.

EFFECTS ON METABOLISM. Oxygen consumption is lowered by sodium thiopental.[62] Concerning glucose metabolism, Betlach[82] found that the concentration of sugar was somewhat increased but that any hyperglycemic levels were easily controlled. Stern[83]

TABLE 24–8. HEMODYNAMIC EFFECTS OF THIOPENTAL

	Hypnosis (%)	Anesthesia Light (%)	Anesthesia Deep (%)
CARDIAC			
Stroke volume	−5	−20	−35
Cardiac index	−0	−12	−25
Left ventricular work		Decreased	
CIRCULATORY			
Temperature, pulse, respiration	+2	+18	+30
Central venous pressure		Unchanged	
Intrathoracic blood volume	−2	−12	−23
Atrial pressures (right and left)	Unchanged		
Circulation time	Increased	Increased	Increased
Systemic blood pressure	−12	−26	−40
Blood volume[74]		Hemodilution	
Venous O_2 content[79]		−33	
Arterial oxygen content		Decreased	
		Reduced saturation	
Renal and liver[72]		Vasoconstriction	
Capillary circulation[80]		Decreased	
MECHANISM	Redistribution of blood with approximately 60% pooling on venous side accompanied by hemodilution. This decreases venous return and total peripheral resistance increased by direct action. Return of blood depends on feedback mechanism. Pulse rise parallels decrease in cardiac index, stroke, and thoracic blood volume.		

found that the blood sugar concentration under thiopental showed no significant change but that the glucose tolerance was decreased, although this decrease was less under sodium thiopental than during either cyclopropane or spinal anesthesia. These results indicate that sodium thiopental is a superior agent for use in diabetics.

Administration of thiopental to dogs was found to lower liver glycogen.[84] This occurred whether the animals received intravenous glucose prior to anesthesia or during anesthesia, had been on a high carbohydrate diet or had received no supplementary carbohydrates at all. Studies of the relationship of liver function to thiopental anesthesia in rats[85] showed little difference in the duration of anesthesia when a given dose of thiopental was administered first to normal rats and then to the same rats after three fourths of their livers had been removed. If a greater portion (80% to 90%) of the liver of animals is removed, however, there is a significantly prolonged duration of action of thiopental.[86]

Clinically, it has been demonstrated that the liver is of importance in the detoxification of thiopental.[87] Humans given a standard dose of thiopental show a significantly longer duration of action if liver dysfunction exists.[88] Dundee presented evidence that thiopental produces liver dysfunction, especially when doses of 750 mg or more are administered.[89]

RENAL EFFECTS. Renal function shows the stereotypical depression seen with anesthetic agents in general. A decrease in renal plasma flow and glomerular filtration occurs on administration of thiopental even in small sleep doses. A decrease in urine formation is noted; this antidiuretic effect is due to the release of pituitary hormone by thiopental.[90]

EFFECT OF NUTRITION. Nutritional deficiencies are recognized as contributing to increased response to the barbiturates and to a prolongation of action and enhanced toxicity. Weight losses of 10% to 20% result in marked increase in duration of response to thiopental.[91]

Protein and carbohydrate deficiency materially contributes to this enhanced response.[92,93] Conversely, high protein and carbohydrate diets in animals increase the dosage requirements of thiopental for the maintenance of surgical anesthesia. Presumably, this diet improves hepatic function and permits a more rapid transformation of thiopental.

Vitamin levels, especially components of the B complex, are especially important determinants to the manner in which the organism reacts to the barbiturates. Deficiency of riboflavin, pyridoxine, and pantothenic acid results in incoordination, loss of position reflexes, and even anesthesia from doses which in the normal experimental animal do not even have a hypnotic effect. Indeed, the most enhanced response occurred with niacin in one study.[93]

EFFECTS ON MUSCLES. Barbiturates vary in their effect on skeletal muscle contraction. Whether augmentation or depression of contraction occurs depends on the frequency of stimulation.[94] Thus, using single-shock indirect stimulation of the sciatic nerve, an enhancement of the gastrocnemius muscle contraction occurs, whereas with indirect tetanic stimulation, there is a decrease in the amplitude of contraction. The thiobarbiturates produce the greatest depression of contraction to tetanic stimulation and the oxybarbiturates smaller changes. Evidence indicates that the site of action of the barbiturates is the neuromuscular junction. There is no increase in contraction to single stimuli when muscles are stimulated directly by a single shock.

Oxybarbiturates, but not thiobarbiturates, produce depression of myoneural transmission.[95] They also have a direct action on muscle fibers, especially thiobarbiturates, and they prolong contraction time by direct or indirect stimulation.[96] To some extent these two effects offset each other.

AUTONOMIC NERVOUS SYSTEM EFFECT. Induction of anesthesia to the third stage of anesthesia with thiopental is accompanied by decreased sympathetic activity in humans.[97] This blocking of sympathetic activity continues during subsequent administration of inhalation anesthetics. In the technique of administering thiopental in doses of 3 mg/kg to stage III anesthesia and maintenance with a continuous infusion of 0.2 to 0.3 mg/kg/min during administration of 100% oxygen, there is a progressive decrease in norepinephrine plasma concentrations to the extent of 40% by 10 minutes. Levels decrease from about 150 pg/ml to 75 to 90 pg/ml. In techniques employing thiopental for induction, followed by either nitrous oxide–oxygen or halothane for maintenance, there is a trend toward decreased plasma norepinephrine with nitrous oxide, while the plasma norepinephrine remains at control levels during halothane. This contrasts with inhalation induction using halothane–oxygen when the norepinephrine levels increase two- to threefold. No significant effect on epinephrine levels have been noted.[98] Thus, thiopental induction blocks sympathetic activation related to the inhalation of other agents such as nitrous oxide, morphine, or halothane and when narcotic techniques are solely employed.

In experimental studies, Skovsted[99] showed that thiopental inhibits cervical sympathetic preganglionic activity and also blocks baroreceptor activity.

A decrease in sympathetic activity of cutaneous nerves also occurs during induction with thiopental in humans. The decrease is accompanied by vasodilatation of skin vessels.[100]

ENDOCRINE EFFECTS. Antidiuretic hormone is released by thiopental from the pituitary neurohypophysis. Human growth hormone shows little change due to pentothal action. Prolactin release from the anterior pituitary is increased by thiopental. The mechanism for this action involves the hypothalamic-hypophyseal axis. Normally, prolactin secretion is controlled by dopaminergic mechanisms originating in the hypothalamus. An increase in dopamine or dopamine agonists blocks prolactin release by increasing the level of prolactin-inhibiting factor (PIF) in the hypothalamic-hypophyseal axis. Contrariwise, cholinergic action on the dopaminergic system blocks PIF release and allows release of prolactin; pentothal appears to enhance this effect. This pentothal action is reversed by atropine.[101] Bromcriptine, a dopamine agonist, also blocks prolactin release.

Adrenocorticotropic hormone levels and adrenocortical function are diminished. Plasma and urinary 17-OH C5 changes are not observed early but after 30 minutes of thiopental maintained at a constant plasma level of 20 to 40 µg/ml results in a decrease in this element.

Norepinephrine plasma levels are not changed. Sympathoadrenal responses are generally inhibited and stress responses decreased.[102]

MISCELLANEOUS EFFECTS. Barbiturates tend to cause some depression of prothrombin time. It is appreciated in the obstetric situation when infants delivered of mothers given thiopental anesthesia show a greater depression of the prothrombin time. This is usually more pronounced on the second to the fifth day. Vitamin K administration to the mother and the newborn is recommended.[103]

Parasympathomimetic effects are noted in increased bronchiolar tone and in the miotic effect; however, salivary glands are not stimulated. No irritation of mucus membranes is seen.

DISPOSITION OF THIOPENTAL[104,105]

DISTRIBUTION. Quantitative pharmacologic studies with thiopental indicate that there is a rapid initial reduction in plasma level of thiopental but that instead of falling to zero, there is a tapering off of the curve.[106] Thus, the early plasma decline represents a distribution of the thiopental with the establishment of a plasma tissue equilibrium (Fig. 24–9).

A preliminary dilution of a drug occurs when injected intravenously because it mixes with blood in the central pool of the circulation. This comprises the contents of the great vessels, the cardiac chambers, and the pulmonary vasculature. The volume in the human adult is about 1.5 L. An injected drug such as thiopental is mixed almost immediately (30 seconds) and hence, is essentially distributed immediately to tissues to enter the process of plasma tissue equilibration.

Of the circulating thiopental in the plasma, about 75% is bound to nondiffusible constituents, chiefly proteins, presumably by absorption, while 25% is found free and is freely diffusible; presumably, the latter represents the pharmacologically active drug. The drug enters red blood cells, and the concentration represents approximately 40% of the amount in plasma.

Tissue localization of thiopental varies with the tissues involved and the rate of perfusion of the tissue. The distribution and localization of thiopental after a single injection of a given dose appear to occur in three *time phases,* and each phase is associated with a particular tissue reservoir or unit compartment. These compartments represent organs and tissues with similar rates of perfusion per unit mass and similar affinities for thiopental (Fig. 24–10).[104,107,108]

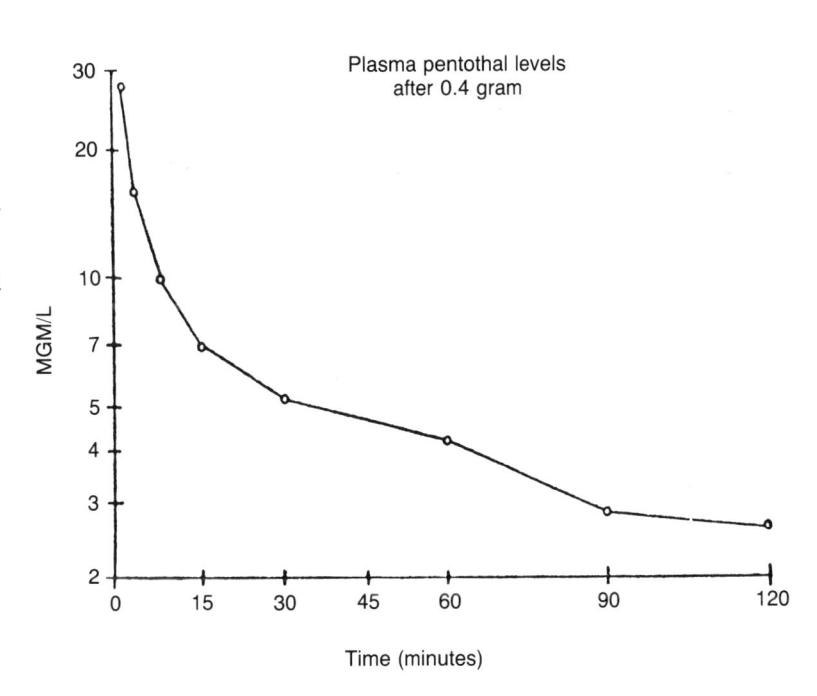

FIG. 24–9. Plasma thiopental decay curve after administration of 0.4 g in 2 minutes. Note the initial rapid fall in plasma level in the first 5 minutes; a somewhat slower fall during the next 20 minutes; and a still slower fall after 30 minutes toward a plateau. At 15 minutes the patient awakened when the plasma level was 7 mg/L. From Brodie, B.B., et al.: The fate of thiopental in man and a method for estimation in biological material. J. Pharmacol. Exp. Ther., 98:85, 1950.

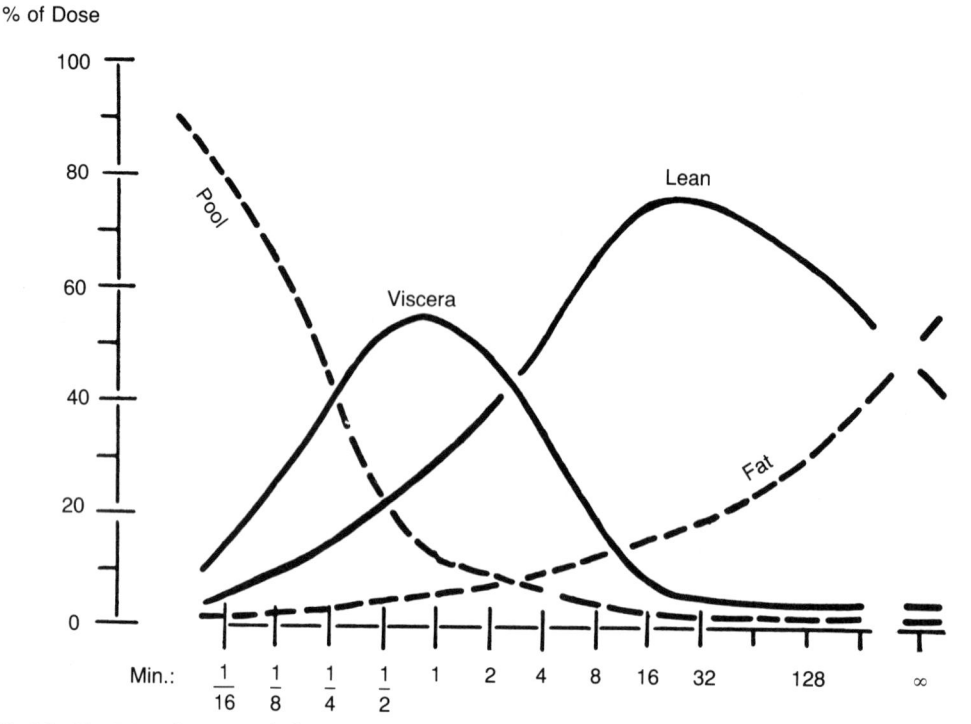

FIG. 24–10. Distribution of thiopental in different bodily tissues and organs at various times after its intravenous injection. The percent of the dose of thiopental contained in different body regions is calculated and plotted against time. Regions specified are four: the blood volume as a central pool; the viscera including the central nervous system, heart, kidney, liver and intestine; the lean extravisceral tissue namely muscle; and the fatty tissues. From Price, H.L., et al.: The uptake of thiopental by body tissue and its relation to the duration of narcosis. Clin. Pharmacol. Ther., 1:16, 1960.

First Phase of Visceral Concentration. The greatest capacity of tissues to equilibrate rapidly with the plasma concentration of drugs resides in those tissues that are rapidly perfused. These tissues include the brain, myocardium, and portal and renal tissues and together form the visceral compartment. Thiopental does not localize in any particular portion of the brain. At 1 minute after injection, the rapidly perfused viscera contain 55% of the dose administered, yet the mass of these tissues is only 6% of body weight. In contrast, the central pool of plasma contains only 12% of the original dose of thiopental, the fat 5%, and the poorly perfused aqueous tissue 28%.

Corroborative evidence of tissue distribution of thiopental is obtained from the study of radioactive thiopental wherein the isotope sulfur 35 is incorporated in the thiopental molecule. The drug is distributed through body tissues within 30 seconds of injection. There is then a rapid initial decline of plasma concentration. Subsequently, there is a slow decline of tissue thiopental.[109]

Aqueous Tissue Compartment (Lean Mass). As time passes, the great initial concentration of drug in the viscera is redistributed to the more slowly perfused aqueous tissue (eg, muscle, connective tissue, bone, lung, skin). These tissues comprise three fourths of body mass but receive only one fourth of the blood flow. As equilibrium is approached, there is a gradient of uptake from the rapidly perfused visceral tissues to the plasma pool to the aqueous compartments. Thus, the rapidly perfused tissues are gradually depleted of drug. At 30 minutes after injection, the rapidly perfused tissues contain only 5% of the injected dose and the fat 18%, but the poorly perfused aqueous tissues contain 75% of the dose. In brief, the brain and other tissues give up thiopental at such a rate that only half the peak content remains at 5 minutes, at the end of 20 minutes only one tenth remains, and at 30 minutes the brain will have given up 96% of its peak concentration.

Fat Compartment.[109,110] In the initial period, fat concentrates thiopental to a small extent. The highest concentrations in the first 30 minutes are only 1.4 times that in the plasma. In fact, the concentration in fat is initially negligible.

Because fat constitutes about one sixth of the body mass, it is evident that the total effect on the process of brain depletion of thiopental is small. In the postanesthetic interval, however, this tissue takes on increasing importance. The fat acquires thiopental principally from the slowly perfused aqueous tissues and part of the first hour the concentration rises rapidly. It finally reaches a maximum in 2.5 to 6 hours (Table 24–9).[110] When equilibrium occurs after more than 8 hours, the fat will contain about 60% of the injected dose, the viscera about 4% and the other aqueous tissues the remainder. Thereafter, the concentration in fat diminishes gradually. The various fat depots in which thiopental is distributed are perirenal fat, omental fat, and lumbodorsal fat.

As long as 2 hours after a single 0.4 g injection of thiopental, a plasma level of about 3 mg/L is detectable. Of interest is the fact that the thiopental concentrations in most organ tissues are higher than in plasma. Also, about 80% of circulating thiopental is bound, presumably by surface absorption to plasma protein.[110]

DESTRUCTION.[104] The destruction of barbiturates is largely determined by their chemical structures. Three chief mechanisms are involved: (1) side chain oxidation; (2) nitrogen dealkylation; and (3) desulfuration of thiobarbiturates.[111]

Drugs with side chains are more easily altered and show less accumulation. Side chains that are branched, unsaturated, or halogenated are more rapidly oxidized or hydrolyzed.[112]

Thiopental is almost completely transformed in the body. The early sharp decline due to tissue distribution does not represent destruction of the drug. A slow, steady, but progressive fall in plasma concentration is observed from 1 to 8 hours and then a still slower decline thereafter. This phase of the curve depends on the rate of drug metabolism. The rate of transformation is slow and has been calculated to be approximately 15% per hour. Thiopental is, thus, not a rapidly destroyed drug and its seemingly short action is due to tissue distribution that is achieved only when small doses are rapidly administered. Successive and large doses, as previously indicated, tend to prolong the somnolent effects, and the drug takes on the characteristics of a long-acting barbiturate.[112]

With increase in anesthetic time, the amount of thiopental required to keep a patient in a state of surgical anesthesia becomes less. As surgery is prolonged, less drug is needed per unit time.[113] These clinical observations support the idea that the rapid destruction of thiopental is only apparent and that a cumulative effect occurs.

Delmonico,[111] investigating sites of detoxification of thiopental in the body, found that the drug is only partially detoxified by the liver and that muscle tissue exerts a detoxicating action as does the blood, presumably by enzymes. A cyclic disappearance and reappearance of thiopental in the blood are related to redistribution in fluid compartments. Richards[112]

TABLE 24–9. DISTRIBUTION OF THIOPENTAL IN BODY TISSUES IN DOGS*

Tissue	Concentration (mg/kg)
Plasma (free and bound drug)	15
Plasma water (free drug)	3.5
Cerebrospinal fluid	3
Liver	28
Brain	24
Muscle	22
Heart	18.5
Kidney	18
Lung	14
Perirenal fat	222
Omental fat	192

* Determination made 2.5 hours after a single injection of 0.65 g thiopental.
Modified from Brodie, B.B., et al: The fate of thiopental in man and a method for estimation in biological material. J. Pharmacol. Exp. Ther., 98:85, 1950.

has shown that on incubation of thiopental with whole blood, there is inhibition and destruction of the drug within 30 minutes.

Two metabolites have been isolated that account for about 30% of the parent drug. They are detectable in the plasma within 1 hour after the start of administration of thiopental and increase progressively in concentration. At first, these metabolites represent about 4% to 5% of the plasma thiopental concentration; in 12 hours some 50% of the plasma drug is the metabolized form. One transformation product is thiopental carboxylic acid. This is probably produced by the oxidation of the alkyl side chain (methyl butyl radical); it has little anesthetic potency. Further metabolism of the parent compound undoubtedly occurs *in vivo* with other products being formed that are not yet defined. In contrast, the oxybarbiturates (pentobarbital) are converted to an alcohol. These barbiturates are metabolized at a much slower rate of 4% per hour.

Some information about the metabolism at the cellular and molecular level is available. It appears that the metabolic breakdown of barbiturates depends on enzymes present in the microsomes of the liver cells. These enzymes need reduced triphosphopyridine nucleolate and oxygen to be active.

ELIMINATION.[104,112] Renal excretion of intact thiopental is negligible. Some of the urine specimens obtained from normal subjects previously given thiopental reveals that only about 0.3% of the administered drug is excreted unchanged. Two transformation products have been isolated from the urine, which accounts for about 30% of the parent drug. Hence, further metabolism undoubtedly occurs *in vivo* with other products being formed that are as yet not definable. After a single injection of thiopental, metabolites are detectable within 1 hour in the plasma. At first these metabolites represent about 4% to 5% of the plasma thiopental concentration and finally represent about 50% of the plasma thiopental concentration in 14 hours.

TOLERANCE. When equivalent large doses are administered at weekly intervals, the plasma concentration at which signs of anesthesia appear and at which recovery occurs are similar and reproducible. Thus, individuals receiving thiopental do not acquire tolerance (in the sense of diminished reactivity to the drug when it is given at later dates).

However, *acute tolerance* occurs in humans. If a high plasma level is maintained by a high dose (10 mg/kg), in contrast to usual doses of 2.0 mg/kg (sleep) or 3 to 5 mg/kg (anesthetic), then signs of recovery appear (conjunctival and corneal reflexes, righting reflexes, eyeball motion, and early orientation) at higher plasma levels of 20 mg/L versus 30 mg/L.[64]

SUMMARY. The tissue localization results in a tissue reservoir from which the blood stream continues to receive a small amount during the so-called postanesthetic interval.

In general, after injection of a single dose, the concentration in organ tissues is higher than in plasma, indicating extensive tissue localization. Initially concentration is highest in viscera than in lean muscle mass, which is dependent on regional perfusion. The tissue that later takes up most thiopental is the body fat. The fat concentration is approximately 10 times that in the brain (Table 24–8).[104,105,112]

Thus, thiopental takes its place with other potent anesthetic agents in showing a definite affinity for lipoid substances.

Destruction of the drug is probably complete. Elimination of products is by the kidneys.

CLINICAL ASPECTS OF THIOPENTAL ANESTHESIA

SIGNS OF BARBITURATE ANESTHESIA.[113] Anesthesia with intravenous thiopental is a modified type of general anesthesia. It should be considered as a state of profound hypnosis. This is related to the lack of selective analgesic action. The stages of anesthesia have been classified on a physiologic basis (Fig. 24–11).

Segmental levels of the brain are affected by thiopental in a sequential manner. Five anatomic areas or segments, called *phyletic areas*, of the brain are identified. These correspond to five levels of function: (1) the oldest area is the medulla in which purely automatic activity such as that concerned with respiration and circulation; (2) the pontine area; (3) the midbrain, in which the centers for specialized sensory and motor nerves are located; (4) the diencephalon, in which there is some organization of sensation and motor activity and a primitive integration of these functions on the instinctive level; and (5) the cerebral cortex, in which all activities are highly integrated, where association, interpretation, and activity is on a conscious level. As the most recently acquired and the most highly developed and sensitive part of the brain, the cortex reacts quickly to stimulants or depressants; it is readily injured by noxious agents.

By studying the oxygen consumption at these levels under thiopental anesthesia, Etsten[113] has shown that there is a descending depression of cerebral oxidation with the medullary centers being the last to be inhibited; when this occurs both respiratory arrest and cardiovascular depression ensue. The sequence of events leading to this stage includes loss of consciousness, a dream state, constriction of the pupils, loss of eyeball activity, loss of pharyngeal reflex, loss of response to cutaneous pain, and later, loss of traction reflexes. All are signs corresponding to Guedel's classification of signs seen under general (ether) anesthesia. That the above sequence can occur under thiopental, however, does not necessarily mean that it is safe or wise to achieve such depth with this drug. Actually, thiopental should be regarded as an impotent drug as far as obtaining planes 3 and 4 of stage III and that these depths are obtained only when doses that may be considered to be in the toxic range are administered.

THE BIOELECTRIC MODEL.[114,115] More detailed and extensive studies of the *initial* effects of low concentration of barbiturates on the central nervous system (CNS) have been performed (Fig. 24–12).

The following sequence in the locus of action in the CNS has been revealed:

1. *Initial Responses*
   a. Initial cortical reaction: denoted by a rapid, large-wave EEG response of cortical cells. Largest in lateral frontal or orbital cortex. The mechanism of this response is *excitation* of subcortical areas, primarily the mesencephalic reticular formation (MRF), which drives the cortex. This drive is propagated upward but does not elicit normal arousal patterns as seen in arousal from ordinary sleep, such as the arousal patterns obtained from the limbic system. However, the high frequency components may contribute to cortical arousal.
   b. Initial thalamic reaction: early and nearly simultaneous excitation of the medial portion of the thalamus with fast *wave* action therein. Similar fast waves appear in the basal ganglia and hypothalamus.
   c. Sensory evoked responses: reticular excitation is also accompanied by an increase of nonspecific sensory evoked responses (SER).

2. *Secondary Response* (spindle formation, slow-wave sequence):

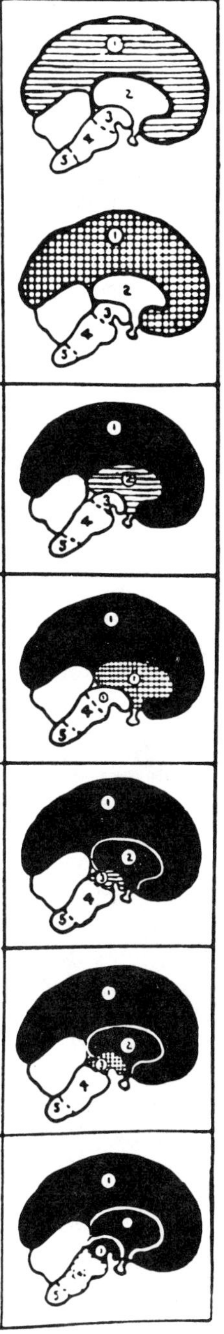

FIG. 24–11. Stages and signs of thiopental anesthesia. The central nervous system characteristics are correlated with regional anesthetic concentration of agent in the brain. From Etsten, B., and Himwich, H.E.: Stages and signs of pentothal anesthesia: Physiologic basis. Anesthesiology, 7:536, 1946.

STAGE	ANESTHESIA	CHARACTERISTICS	SITE of DEPRESSION
I	CLOUDING	EUPHORIA LOSS of DISCRIMINATION TO IMPAIRMENT of ENVIRONMENTAL CONTACT	SLIGHT DEPRESSION of CORTEX TO MODERATE DEPRESSION of CORTEX
II	HYPER-SENSITIVITY	LOSS of CONSCIOUSNESS	PREDOMINANT CONTROL by SUBCORTEX
III Plane I	LIGHT SURGICAL	HYPOACTIVITY to PAINFUL STIMULUS	MODERATE DEPRESSION of SUBCORTEX
Plane II	MODERATE SURGICAL	LOSS of SOMATIC RESPONSE to PAIN	PREDOMINANT CONTROL by MIDBRAIN
Plane III	DEEP SURGICAL	LOSS of VISCERAL RESPONSE to PAIN	MODERATE DEPRESSION of MIDBRAIN
IV	IMPENDING FAILURE	FALL in PULSE PRESSURE	MODERATE DEPRESSION of PONS

a. After initial rapid cortical responses to barbiturates, the EEG develops spindles associated with unconsciousness (later this pattern fades to slow wave activity). A biphasic amplitude is manifest in these spindle waves. A sequence of facilitation followed by depression is displayed by increased followed by decreased amplitude of cortical waves. A slow wave pattern follows spindling. Origin of these spindles and slow waves is the thalamus, which is necessary to drive the cortex and cause spindles to appear. In the absence of the thalamus neither spindles nor slow waves appear.

b. Spindle waves reflect excitability or hypersynchronization of nonspecific thalamic nuclei. Ensuing slow wave phase reflects depression of nonspecific thalamic nuclei.

c. During the phase of hypersynchronization or

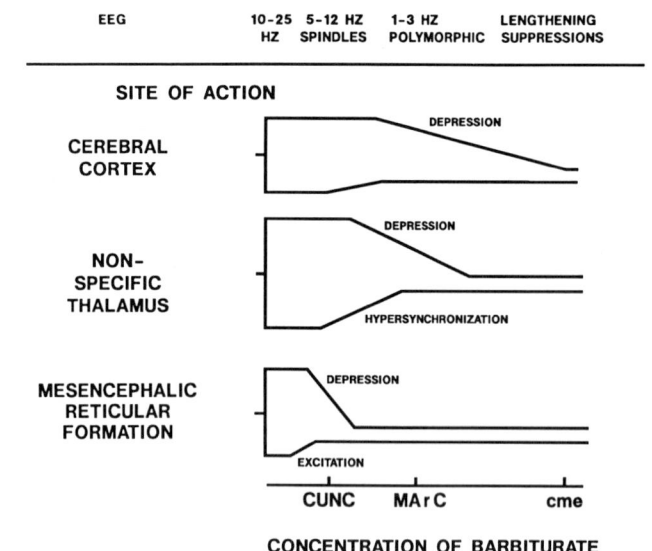

FIG. 24–12. Model of action sequence illustrating bioelectric changes in central nervous system due to barbiturates. *CUNC* = concentration producing unconsciousness; *MArC* = minimal arterial concentration permitting skin incision; *CME* = concentration of maximum efficiency. From Rosner, V., and Clark, L.: In Brain Mechanisms and Unconsciousness. Edited by M.A. Brazier. Oxford, Blackwell Scientific Publications, 1954.

excitation denoted by spindle and slow wave formation, the mesencephalic reticular formation undergoes progressive depression.

d. *Evoked responses*: barbiturates do not reduce specific evoked activity in somatic systems. However, visual responses in humans are easily obtunded.

3. ***Subsequent Responses in EEG*** (suppression): As barbiturate action continues and with larger doses suppression-type activity is manifest in the cortical EEG. This probably represents *both* a loss of incoming impulses from thalamic pathways and direct action of barbiturates on the cortex. This phase is correlated with depression of nonspecific thalamic nuclei. Specific SERs (visual, auditory) continue to be detectable but recovery time lengthens.

A model of action sequence for barbiturates has been developed to illustrate the findings of detailed bioelectric studies of the central nervous system (Fig. 24–12). This differs from the Etsten model (Fig. 24–11), which illustrates a continuous depression in the dose-response curve. Etsten did not study precisely the sequence of the action in the early phases but did provide a broad picture of action. The Rosner model (Fig. 24–12) is an expansion of the initial early phases of barbiturate action. This model may be considered an elucidation of the Etsten sequence.

NATURE OF BARBITURATE ANESTHESIA. Clinically, barbiturates are not suitable as the sole agent for producing anesthesia. Although CNS depression follows the same pattern as with inhalational drugs, the clinical state does not bear a precise relationship with the cerebral depression, especially as related to noxious stimuli. To abolish reflex movements invoked by painful stimuli, it is necessary to produce a state of near apnea by the use of excessively large doses. Thus, the barbiturates provide a basal brain state and are anesthetic adjuncts that must be complemented by agents with more specific analgesia properties. The barbiturates are partial anesthetic agents.

RESPONSE TO PAIN.[116] Barbiturates have little or no direct effects on relieving pain. However, they may modify the pain response or the psychic component of the pain complex.[116] When thiopental is given without opiates in the presence of pain, delirium may result.

Subhypnotic doses of the thiobarbiturates increase the sensitivity to pain. This antianalgesic action applies principally to deep somatic pain, and especially to visceral pain.[117] Small doses may diminish the appreciation of pain from mild superficial skin stimulation, but this is best explained as a result of diminished apprehension and fear and not an analgesic action.

Single injections do produce a state that permits momentary painful manipulations and brief procedures. The surge technique[117a] is employed for dental procedures and for thiobarbiturate anesthesia in cesarean sections lasting less than 9 minutes has been demonstrated.

Clinically, small doses of thiopental antagonize the analgesic action of nitrous oxide or meperidine. Rather than an *antianalgesic* action, the increased sensitivity may be better termed *hyperalgesia*. The mechanism of this phenomenon appears to be the removal of inhibitory systems on painful sensory input. Brazier[115] suggests that an inhibitory system in the diffuse ascending reticular system is blocked, permitting the secondary slow pain impulses to be facilitated.

CLINICAL CRITERIA OF ANESTHESIA[113,118]
(TABLE 24–10)

Stage I. The criteria for this stage are based on responses of the patient at the conscious level.[119] The patients' ability to verbalize is progressively diminished. If asked to count during induction by optimal rates of injection, they begin fairly distinctly, but by the time they reach 15 to 30 words, speech is usually indistinct and muffled. If a person is conversing, suddenly in the midst of the conversation, words become jumbled, mumbled, the patient yawns, and the eyelids close. The patient is usually drowsing but arousable and will respond to a command.

TABLE 24–10. SIGNS OF THIOPENTAL ANESTHESIA*

Stages of Anesthesia	Pupil Size	Pupil Reaction to Light	Pupil Reaction to Pain	Eyeball Activity	Eyelid Tone	Corneal Reflex	Respiration	Muscle Reaction to Pain	Pulse	Blood Pressure
Stage I	4+	4+	4+	Voluntary	4+	4+	N	4+	N	N
Stage II	4+ to 3+	4+	4+	Roving	4+ to 2+	4+ to 0	N	6+	N	N
Stage III										
Plane 1	3+ to 2+	3+ to 1+	3+	Slight	2+ to 0	4+ to 0	Diminished	1+	N	Slight fall
Plane 2	2+ to 1+	0	2+	Deviation then central	2+ to 0	4+ to 0	Depressed	0	I	Varies
Plane 3	1+	0	0	Central	0	0	Depressed to apnea	0	I	Varies
Stage IV	Dilate with anoxia	0	0	Central	0	0	Apnea	0	I	Fall in pulse pressure

* The series of clinical signs are correlated with the four stages of thiopental anesthesia.
Abbreviations: N, normal; I, increased.

Stage II. The dream state or stage of unconsciousness is reached and is passed through quickly. There is usually no excitement. The patient does not verbalize and stops counting. There is no response to a command, such as "open your eyes." The patient has an experience of falling into natural sleep. There is withdrawal reflex from painful stimuli.

Stage III (plane 1; EEG level III). This is the early stage of anesthesia and is achieved quickly. This stage is based on a loss of simple somatic reflexes. Superficial reflexes are diminished and eyeballs are fixed and centered. There is loss of lid tone. Patient may not show withdrawal from minor painful stimuli.

Stage III (plane 2; EEG level IV). Eyelash and eyelid blink reflexes are lost. The corneal reflex may be present, but testing is unnecessary and dangerous. There is relaxation of not only mouth muscles and mastication but also pharyngeal muscles. This relaxation is most profound during the first minutes of anesthesia and tends to be transient.

Swallowing is absent and the gag (base of tongue) and pharyngeal reflex are obtunded sufficiently to permit insertion of an oropharyngeal airway.

A surgical stimulus may be tolerated without withdrawal. Tachycardia and hypertension may be seen, however, because there is no blockade of the sympathetic system.

A further step in depth is usually denoted by a transient state of apnea with recommended doses. When an excessive dose is given, the patient will be rapidly brought to a state of apnea, which is persistent. Administration more rapidly than 50 mg every 5 to 10 seconds results in apnea.

PLASMA CONCENTRATION CORRELATION WITH CLINICAL ANESTHESIA STAGES.[42] Unconsciousness is achieved at plasma levels between 50 and 100 µg/ml. The critical plasma level at which unconsciousness is just maintained is above 40 µg/ml. Patients will respond to commands ("open your eyes") when plasma levels reach between 20 and 30 µg/ml. They are awake usually and verbalize at plasma levels between 5 and 7 µg/ml. This occurs about 15 minutes after a bolus injection of a dose of 4 mg/kg in unmedicated subjects.

These have been duplicated in more recent studies by Hudson[118] and correlated with clinical signs as described. While Kiersey[120] designates the pattern sequence as *levels*, Hudson designates the patterns as *stages*. These levels or stages correspond to the clinical stages.

EEG SIGNS.[118,120] Changes in EEG patterns during thiopental anesthesia were systematically studied by Kiersey[120] in 1951. They classified their findings into four classic patterns and recognized five levels for practical purposes. These have been further confirmed by power spectral analysis by Hudson (Fig. 24–13).[118] The changes in EEG are rapidly achieved and represent equilibrium between blood concentrations and sites of action within the brain. Because other intravenous anesthetics also progressively slow the EEG, the model can be used to characterize their concentration–effect relationship.

Level I (fast). Awake patterns are rapidly replaced by fast waves (10 to 30 cps) of relatively high amplitude (75 to 80 mV).

Level II (complex, rhythmic, and mixed). It is noted that the usual rhythmic pattern produced by the inhalation agents is not readily observed. The transition is evidently too rapid. But slow waves (2 to 4 cps) with an irregular contour and spiky appearance are prominent. The amplitude is high, of the order of 150 mV. Superimposed on these are spiky waves of lower amplitude and of a frequency of 10 cps.

Level III (suppression). A suppression pattern of short duration is soon recognized, i.e., less than 3 seconds. Bursts of activity, described as occurring in two phases, are seen. There is an initial phase of fast frequency 10 cps waves lasting 1 second and a subsequent phase of slower frequency 2 cps waves lasting 2 seconds. The amplitude of these waves is of the order of 60 to 120 mV.

Level IV. This level is denoted by a longer suppression phase lasting 3 to 10 seconds. The waves are similar to those of level III but of lower amplitude.

Level V. Suppression is prolonged to a period of 10 or more seconds. Amplitude is decreased to 25 mV or less. Further suppression is achieved only at the expense of physiologic trespass.

EEG Levels (Stages) Correlated with Dosage. The dose of thiopental required to achieve early burst suppression of the EEG pattern has been studied by Homer.[36] For this depth of thiopental anesthesia (no premedication) in the age group 20 to 40 years, a dose of 10 mg/kg was required. For the age group over 50 years, the average dose was approximately 6 mg/kg. The dose required for burst suppression was found to decrease directly with age (Fig. 24–14). For each 10-year increase in age, the dose required decreased approximately 1 mg/kg. These doses correlated with the clinical signs of unconsciousness and anesthesia and the plasma levels of thiopental, as measured by Becker.[42]

FACTORS INFLUENCING INDUCTION

PREMEDICATION.[29,30,121] The general objectives in preanesthetic medication—to prepare the patient, to achieve a smooth induction and safe anesthetic state—apply to barbiturate anesthesia. In addition, the type of premedication greatly affects the onset of action, the dose of barbiturate, and the incidence of induction complications. Morphine not only reduces the amount of thiopental needed for a given sleep level but significantly reduces the side effects. The usual UD$_{95}$ in unmedicated subjects is 4 to 5 mg/kg with morphine premedication. This is reduced by 20% to 25% to 3 to 4 mg/kg.[110a]

Atropine also limits the incidence of side effects. Other drugs often used, such as scopolamine, meperidine, and promethazine, individually and in combination, increase the incidence of side effects (Table 24–11).

SIDE EFFECTS OF INDUCTION.[122] In the absence of good premedication, three particular types of undesirable effects are associated with induction.

Excitatory Phenomena. This consists principally of tremor, hypertonus, and involuntary muscle movements. Although marked with the methylated thiobarbiturates, these responses are still noted with thiopental and methohexital. The incidence and severity are dose related and are increased by large doses, by antanalgesics such as phenothiazines and scopolamine, and by rapid injection. Opiates and atropine reduce these side effects. A rate of injection of 25 mg/sec (1 ml of a 2.5% solution) appears to be optimal.

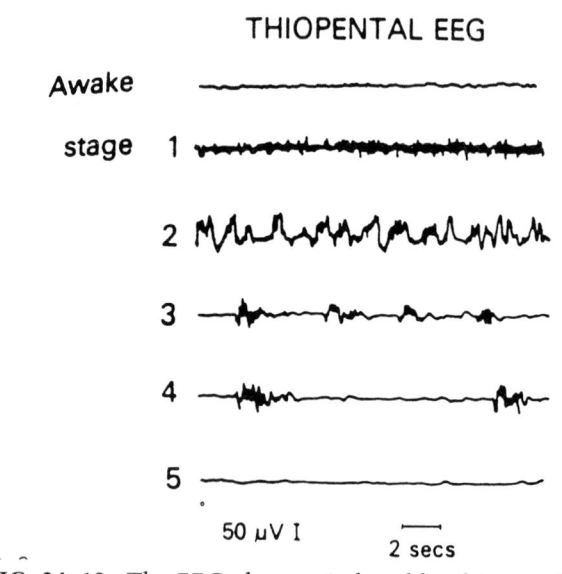

FIG. 24–13. The EEG changes induced by thiopental. Consciousness is lost early in stage 1. Stage 2 represents stage II of anesthesia; stages 3 and 4, surgical anesthesia. From Hudson, R.J., et al.: A model for studying depth of anesthesia and acute tolerance to thiopental. Anesthesiology, 59:302, 1983.

Respiratory Upset. Coughing, sneezing, increased sensitivity of laryngeal reflexes, and hiccoughing occur more frequently with large doses rapidly injected. Doses greater than 3 mg/kg increase the incidence of undesirable respiratory effects. Upsets are especially prone to occur with methohexital and buthalitone. Atropine reduces the occurrence of these undesirable responses.

Apnea is related to large doses or rapidly injected concentrated solutions.

Hypotension. This effect is nonspecific and does not correlate with any particular chemical structure. It is dose dependent. Large doses and rapid rates of injection increase the incidence and severity of hypotension. Normovolemic patients rarely have severe falls in blood pressure. It is more common with less potent congeners where larger doses are required. Thus, it is relatively uncommon with methohexital and thiopental as compared with the other intravenous barbiturates.

SUMMARY OF PREMEDICATION. With proper premedication, the incidence of excitatory responses and respiratory upset is minimized. A combination of atropine and morphine is recommended prior to thiopental administration, whereas a meperidine

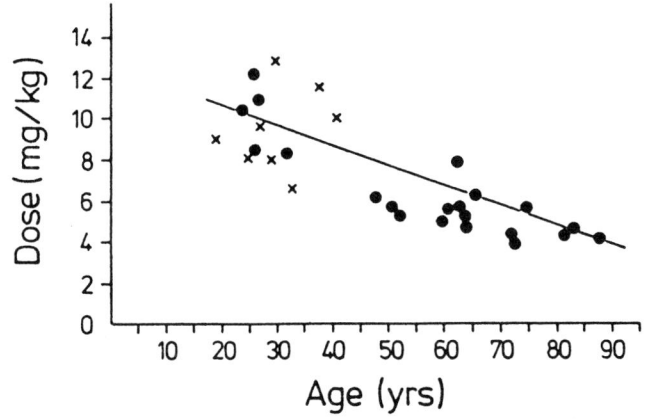

FIG. 24-14. The dose of thiopental needed to reach burst suppression on the EEG decreases with age; ● = surgical patients who underwent arterial blood sampling, whereas X = volunteer subjects who underwent venous blood sampling. The solid line is the regression relationship indicated in the text. From Homer, T.D., and Stanski, D.R.: The effect of increasing age on thiopental disposition and anesthetic requirement. Anesthesiology, 62:714, 1985.

and scopolamine combination is recommended prior to methohexital administration.

SPECIFIC FACTORS OF INDUCTION. Induction of anesthesia may be characterized by its rapidity of onset, attainment of depth, and the presence of undesirable effects. Several specific factors affect these qualities:

1. *Effect of dose:*[29] A short time of onset of action of the intravenous barbiturates is characteristic. Time of onset of sleep action (when patient stops counting) is dose dependent. Varying doses change the average onset time: it is slower with small doses, and 2 mg/kg in 2 to 3 seconds produces sleep in 20 seconds; as the dose increases, doses of 3.5 mg/kg produce a rapid onset of action with an average time of 11 seconds; larger doses do not speed up the induction (Fig. 24-15).

2. *Circulatory state:* A good cardiac output and intact peripheral circulation are necessary for the expected average induction. In cardiac disease, circulatory failure, or shock, onset of action is slow. An intact cerebral circulation is essential.

3. *Forearm blood flow:* An all-important element is the forearm blood flow. An improperly released tourniquet slows the delivery of the drug to the central reservoir; constricted vessels due to pathology (phlebitis), or drug action (vasoconstrictors, fear, cold) delay onset.

4. *Environmental temperature:* Room temperature is of great importance, especially as it affects blood flow to the arm. The effects of two ranges of operating room temperature on thiopental induction were studied by Dundee. A standard sleep dose of thiopental of 3.5 mg/kg was given in 2 to 3 seconds. The following average induction times were determined:

Room Temperature °C (°F)	Thiopental Onset (sec)
22–23 (72)	19.7
29–32 (84)	14.9

The enhanced speed of induction at higher room temperature is related to vasodilatation of the vessels in the arm. An arterial tourniquet released after 1 minute produces a reactive hyperemia, and even in a cool environment the injection of thiopental at this time results in onset of action equal to that at the warmer temperature.

Onset of Action. This is essentially an armbrain circulation time and demonstrates that these drugs are rapid acting. On arrival at the brain, there is immediate penetration of the blood-brain barrier,[29] because of their high lipoid solubility and lack of ionization. The rate of entry is thus dependent on or limited by the cerebral blood flow.

PROCEDURE

ANESTHETIC TECHNIQUE. With intravenous anesthesia, the agent is directly introduced into the blood stream and consequently reaches the CNS quite rapidly. The administration of thiopental is a test of one's ability to judge the capacity of the patient to handle the drug.

As with other techniques, careful consideration must be given to preanesthetic preparation. This includes (1) the evacuation of hollow viscera, the stomach, bladder, and rectum; it is imperative that the stomach be empty (regurgitation and aspiration during thiopental anesthesia occur with ease and hence are pernicious); and (2) proper premedication. It is of great advantage to give to a patient on the evening before operation a barbiturate for sedation, and pentobarbital is highly desirable. This will often bring out any sensitivity to barbiturates on the part of the patient. Preanesthetically, the patient should receive some morphine to depress basal metabolic rate and reduce the thiopental requirement, and it is imperative that atropine be given to every patient in adequate doses before anesthesia is begun.

PREOXYGENATION CONCEPT. The introduction of this concept is related to the basic work carried out by McClure[123] and, subsequently, by Medrado.[124] In the absence of preoxygenation, oxyhemographic studies[123] show that blood oxygen saturation drops to levels of about 60% to 70% on induction with thiopental in healthy patients breathing room air.

TABLE 24–11. PERCENTAGE INCIDENCE OF EXCITATORY PHENOMENA (EP)—TREMOR, SPONTANEOUS INVOLUNTARY MUSCLE MOVEMENT, HYPERTONUS—AND RESPIRATORY UPSET (RU)—COUGH, HICCOUGH, MARKED DEPRESSION—FOUND AFTER EQUIPOTENT DOSES OF THIOPENTAL (4 mg/kg) AND METHOHEXITAL (1.6 mg/kg) GIVEN AFTER VARIOUS PREMEDICANTS

Category	Premedication	Thiopental % EP	Thiopental % RU	Methohexital % EP	Methohexital % RU
N	Atropine 0.6 mg	9	6	33	26
A	Meperidine 100 mg	6	6	7	24
A	Morphine 10 mg	10	5	9	25
AA	Scopolamine 0.4 mg	37	10	52	14
AA	Promethazine 50 mg	23	7	70	37
COMBINATIONS					
A + AA	Meperidine 100 mg/ Scopolamine 0.6 mg	10	3	17	18
A + AA	Meperidine 100 mg/ Promethazine 50 mg	10	6	30	20
AA + AA	Promethazine 50 mg/ Scopolamine 0.4 mg	70	9	100	20

Abbreviations: N, neutral—neither analgesic nor antanalgesic; A, analgesic premedication; AA, antanalgesic premedication; Meperidine, Pethidine, Demerol; Promethazine, Phenergan.
From Dundee, J.W.: Current views on the clinical pharmacology of the barbiturates. Int. Anesthesiol. Clin., 7:331, 1969.

Preoxygenation consists essentially of having the patient breathe 100% oxygen for 2 to 5 minutes with varying ventilatory volumes. In a circle system, a fresh gas flow of 4 liters of oxygen per minute was recommended for 3 or more minutes. This results in elimination of pulmonary nitrogen and maintenance of blood oxygenation. Preoxygenation raises arterial oxygen tension to values above 400 mm Hg. On induction and after 2 minutes of apnea, the arterial oxygen tension is maintained at values around 200 mm Hg. Failure to oxygenate before induction permits falls of arterial oxygen tension below 100 mm Hg (Pa_{O_2} levels of 80), accepted as a critical value during anesthesia.[124]

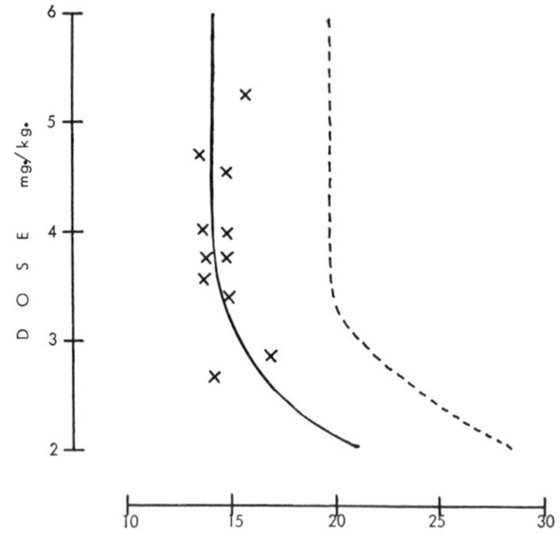

Techniques of Preoxygenation. Oxygenation of blood and nitrogen washout varies with the duration of oxygen administration and the type of breathing. Utilizing a circle system, a fresh gas flow of 4 liters of oxygen per minute for 3 to 4 minutes produced saturation of the blood and resulted in the elimination of 80% of pulmonary nitrogen.[125] A more rapid pulmonary nitrogen washout with effective oxygenation can be obtained if a nonrebreathing system is used and the patient allowed to breath normally for 2 to 3 minutes.[126] However, shorter periods of preoxygenation were suggested by Werner[127] and Gold[128] which would be effective if deep breaths were taken by the patient, although denitrogenation may be incomplete.[125] To this end, an assessment of oxygenation techniques has been carried out by Drummond.[129]

The preliminary administration of oxygen for 2 or 3 minutes, while the patient is breathing at a normal depth and rate, will produce Pa_{O_2} values that will remain satisfactory in most patients for as long as 4 minutes after preoxygenation.[130] It is necessary, of

FIG. 24–15. Time of onset of action of varying doses of thiopental at two environmental temperatures. Solid line = 29–32° C. Dashed line = 22–23° C. X = times recorded during the period of reactive hyperemia that followed release of an arterial tourniquet at 22° C. From Dundee, J.W.: Current views on the clinical pharmacology of the barbiturates. Int. Anesthesiol. Clin., 7:331, 1969.

course, that tracheal intubation be carried out promptly.[131]

In the study by Drummond,[129] the breathing pattern for the inhalation of 100% oxygen involved maximal breaths. It was demonstrated that only 3 or 4 vital capacity breaths in 30 seconds will wash in oxygen more effectively than breaths involving the inspiratory reserve volume only, ie, normal tidal volume breathing.

It is recommended that preoxygenation be accomplished by one of two procedures using a well-fitted and comfortable mask (minimal leaks):

1. By the breathing of 100% oxygen at normal tidal volumes for 3 minutes. This will raise the Pa_{O_2} values to 300 mm Hg or more. This approach is satisfactory in elective surgical procedures.
2. The "four-deep-breaths" technique: There is rapid removal of nitrogen from the lungs and adequate oxygen saturation of the blood resulting in Pa_{O_2} values of 300 mm Hg or more by vital capacity breathing (maximal) with only four respiratory efforts within 30 seconds. This is the recommended technique in emergency circumstances and for rapid-sequence induction.

The four-deep-breaths technique is also useful and recommended in the pregnant patient undergoing emergency delivery or cesarean section, especially when fetal distress is present. Marx[132] has shown that arterial oxygen tension is reduced to a greater extent in the pregnant patient than the nonpregnant patient on rapid induction of anesthesia with intravenous agents. In addition, pregnant patients have decreased functional residual capacity, airway closure also occurs more readily, and in the supine position there are underventilated alveoli. All these changes lead to hypoxemia. Maximal deep breathing for four breaths significantly raises blood saturation and oxygen tension and is recommended in these circumstances.

When these techniques are carried out, there is a persistence of oxygen saturation for 3 or more minutes, even if patients go into apnea.[133] If small leaks about the mask are allowed to exist, oxygenation may not be adequate.[133]

THE TECHNIQUE PROPER. The technique proper may be considered in four phases: (1) preliminary; (2) induction; (3) maintenance; and (4) recovery.

1. *Preliminary.* The administration of oxygen prior to induction is essential. Begin oxygen administration early, continue for 3 to 5 minutes and achieve optimal oxygenation as quickly as possible. Use either spontaneous tidal volume breathing for 3 to 5 minutes or maximal breathing techniques.

    Preliminary to actual induction of a few milliliters of thiopental solution (2.5%) injected as a test dose.[121]

2. *Induction.* Preferably rapid. One should aim at getting the patient asleep. This is accomplished by some anesthetists with a 5% solution of thiopental rapidly injected. This procedure often leads to apnea. More satisfactory is the use of a 2.5% solution injected at a rate of about 10 ml every 15 seconds. An adult male on the average needs at least 0.5 g.

3. *Maintenance.* Once the patient is asleep with constricted pupils and fixed eyeballs, one should wait to observe how well the drug is tolerated. Further doses of 1 to 2 ml are added intermittently according to how the patient reacts. One attempts to administer an amount of thiopental that will balance the constant painful stimulus of surgery.

    It is important to wait at least 5 minutes after the patient is asleep before surgery is begun under ordinary circumstances. This period will allow the various signs of anesthesia to catch up with the concentration of the anesthetic agent that is actually present. It has been found that this short period of watchful waiting will decrease many of the complications, particularly apnea and laryngospasm. This watch period is not followed when the surge technique is used for brief manipulations.

    The administration of oxygen[123] *during* thiopental anesthesia is obviously a necessity. If oxygen other than that in air is not available to the patient, blood oxygen saturation falls to dangerous levels (see earlier discussion). Oxyhemographic studies of thiopental anesthesia reveal the following:

    At least a 40% concentration of oxygen is needed. During prolonged procedures, there is a decreasing tolerance to thiopental preventing adequate blood oxygenation; hence, concentrations of oxygen approaching 100% are indicated for such cases.

    It is important to begin oxygen administration early and to reach maximum oxygenation as soon as possible. It is easier to maintain this level than to bring it about after a period of thiopental anesthesia, when air only is being breathed.

4. *Recovery.* Administration of oxygen should be continued during the postoperative period.

DOSAGE. A general rule regarding barbiturate dosage relates the hypnotic (HD) and anesthetic doses to the lethal dose (LD). This rule is stated as follows: The hypnotic dose (HD_{50}) is approximately equal to one third the anesthetic dose (AD_{50}) and this is approximately equal to one half the lethal dose (LD_{50}).[133,134]

The dose range for the initial hypnotic dose of thiopental is 1 to 2 mg/kg. The initial anesthetic dose range of thiopental is 3 to 4 mg/kg, while the average dose producing a consistent anesthetic sleep level in healthy patients is 3.5 mg/kg.

Current use limits the total dose to a range of 500 to 1000 mg. However, when doses greater than 500 mg are needed, another anesthetic or adjunctive drug should be considered.

Doses over 750 mg in an average surgical experience are considered sufficient to produce liver dysfunction.[89]

It is considered inadvisable to administer thiopental as the principal agent for operations lasting more than 1 hour or that more than 1 g be given to a patient. These limitations have been exceeded by experienced anesthetists. Adams[2] reports one case in which 5.8 g were administered over a period of 8 hours. In a series of maxillofacial injuries undergoing reconstructive surgery, intravenous thiopental with an endotracheal airway was the anesthesia of choice. Doses of 1.5 to 3 g of thiopental were administered in 1 hour without untoward results. Several patients received more than 3 g in 3 hours.[113]

CLINICAL CONSIDERATIONS. Some conditions are considered to be absolute contraindications:[135] (1) the presence of respiratory obstruction; (2) marked cardiovascular instability, shock and myocardial failure; (3) severe asthma and bronchospastic disorders; (4) porphyria. Attention to some of the relative contraindications to thiopental anesthesia is especially important. These are undoubtedly of greater significance than the indications.

Hemorrhage, Shock, and Hypovolemia. Burstein[134] showed experimentally that following hemorrhage the effects of thiopental on the circulatory system are unpredictable, but in general are deleterious. Zweifach[85] showed that the peripheral circulatory dynamics are markedly altered during thiopental anesthesia when associated with shock and hemorrhage. They further found that under such circumstances the response to blood replacement therapy is poor.

Cardiac Insufficiency and Failure. Thiopental has a direct myocardial depressant effect: contractility is impaired, and digitalis effect is reduced.

Airway Problems and Pulmonary Disease. An inadequate airway prior to induction and conditions of hypoxia; any inability to inflate the lungs or provide a free airway.

In status asthmaticus and other bronchospastic disorders, including chronic obstructive emphysema, because of hyperactive laryngeal reflexes and increased bronchomotor tone, the use of thiopental is precluded.

In the presence of acute infections of the neck, inflammation near the carotid sinus depresses the carotid sinus and carotid body reflexes which, when added to the depression of the medullary centers by thiopental, may result in unacceptable respiratory depression.

Effect on Maternal–Fetal Circulation.[132] Thiopental is a myocardial depressant that causes marked decreases in maternal blood pressure when administered rapidly. This compromises uteroplacental perfusion and can result in fetal hypoxemia.

All barbiturates administered to the mother undergo rapid placental transfer. Thiopental easily crosses the placental barrier, and maternal–fetal equilibrium of thiopental is quickly established. Within 1 minute, passage to the fetus begins.

Finster's studies[135] of umbilical vein levels of thiopental at different times (induction delivery times) after administration to the mother show that the highest concentration takes place 2 minutes after a bolus dose to the mother. This concentration parallels the fetal myocardial and liver tissue concentrations and also subjects the fetus to myocardial depression. At the time when delivery has been accomplished, the blood pressure of the baby is lowest; when the infant is born 4 minutes after thiopental administration, over two thirds of the babies are hypotensive. No infants born 4 to 10 minutes after thiopental administration were hypotensive. It is concluded that it takes 4 or more minutes for thiopental to be redistributed and taken up by other fetal tissues, principally the left lobe of the liver,[136] and to decrease fetal myocardial depression. Dreisbach[137] found that fetal respiratory depression is greatest in infants born within 4 minutes and shows continued great depression after 10 minutes. This depression is a direct function of the maternal concentration of the drug and time after administration of thiopental.[138] Doses in excess of 4 mg/kg are associated with greater depression.[139] The "induction–delivery interval" is important, depending on physiologic variables.[132]

Although the cardiocirculatory values are apparently restored by 10 minutes and Apgar scores are over 8 or 9, there remains a prolonged depressant effect, as evidenced by neurobehavioral Scanlon scores.[140] These are depressed in the first few days of life, and the lowest scores are with thiopental when compared to the high scores achieved when delivery has been accomplished with regional anesthesia.[141]

Reflexes. When *potent reflexes* are likely to be initiated or stimulated, thiopental is inadequate. Although curare is administered with thiopental to obtund skeletal muscle responses, the various traction reflexes still produce visceral responses consisting of tachycardia (bradycardia included) and hypertension. If the stimulus is intense, vagal effects may be seen with hypotension. These are mediated via the autonomic nervous system.

When thiopental is used in otolaryngologic procedures, topical anesthesia should be employed, especially in bronchoscopy. The anesthesiologist planning to intubate under thiopental should likewise employ extensive topical anesthesia of the pharynx, the larynx, and the trachea prior to the insertion of an endotracheal airway.

Debility. Barbiturates generally suppress adrenal function.[142] Thiopental depresses adrenal activity, both medullary and cortical. This is clinically evident in a lowered pulse and pressure and constricted pupils. There is also depression of glycogen formation.[143] Epinephrine release is suppressed. In the debilitated patient with a generalized decreased functional activity, thiopental is relatively contraindicated.

Malnutrition. [92] Thiopental is bound to a considerable extent to the albumin fraction of plasma. When hypoproteinemia exists, there will be a larger portion of the injected drug unbound and able to enter the brain.

Anemia. [144] Prolongation of narcosis in patients with hemoglobin below 75% is to be expected. Patients with anemia are prone to greater falls in blood pressure than is expected when thiopental is administered to normochromic patients. Administration of oxygen mixtures above 50% from the beginning of thiopental administration is essential. Otherwise, a fall in oxygen content and in saturation occurs, which is more hazardous in the anemic subject.

Azotemia. [145] Patients having an increased blood urea level demonstrate an increased sensitivity to thiopental. After a standard dose there is a deeper level of anesthesia and an increased sleeping time. Experimental azotemia in animals demonstrated the same results, especially when urethral obstruction exists.

Clinical data indicate that the dose of thiopental needed to maintain an adequate anesthesia is much less in patients with urinary obstruction or with elevated urea levels. In general, the average induction dose should be reduced 25% and the maintenance by 40%.

Metabolic and Electrolyte Disturbances. Any moderate to marked unbalance of electrolytes or fluids is a contraindication. Potassium intoxication is especially hazardous.

In the quiescent phase of porphyria, administration of any barbiturate leads to an acute exacerbation with paralysis, porphyriuria, muscular paralysis, and death.[146]

Endocrine. (a) The action of thiopental is prolonged in patients with Addison's disease. (b) In myxedema overdose is easily achieved. (c) Severe diabetes mellitus is aggravated; glucose tolerance is impaired.[83] (d) Obese subjects retain thiopental for long periods.[148]

Drug Interaction. The dose requirements are usually greater in patients who are chronic alcoholics. Potentiation of action is seen in chronic alcoholic patients being treated with tetraethylthiuran disulfide (Antabuse).[147]

In barbiturate habituation and addiction, unusually large amounts of intravenous barbiturates are needed to produce sleep or a hypnotic effect. Additional doses for maintenance then quickly result in overdose. It is recommended that patients subject to barbiturate drug abuse be given other agents where chronic and acute tolerance may not be manifest.

Miscellaneous. Use should be limited to produce sedation only in patients with myasthenia gravis, hypertensive arteriosclerotic heart disease, raised intracranial pressure, and coronary insufficiency.

ADVANTAGES. There are three advantages of intravenous thiopental anesthesia that have been undisputed:[1,6] (1) simplicity of equipment and administration; (2) nonexplosibility; and (3) ease of administration and rapidity of action.

COMPLICATIONS

Following the disastrous results[150] at Pearl Harbor and again during the North African campaign of World War II, thiopental was held in some disrepute.[149] Thorough investigations revealed its many pharmacologic characteristics, and then proper restrictions were placed on the use of the drug. With the development of caution and respect for the capabilities of the drug and of its contraindications, thiopental has assumed its proper place as one of the more valuable agents in the armamentarium of the trained anesthesiologist.

PRECAUTIONS.[150] Thiopental should not be used by the injudicious or the overconfident because it is a dangerous drug. Once given it cannot be reclaimed or withdrawn from the blood stream by the administrator. There are two safety factors, or two requirements to the use of thiopental: (1) the ability of the administrator to quickly, expertly, and efficiently perform intratracheal intubation and to carry out artificial respiration in accordance with the principles of respiratory physiology; and (2) the presence of a trained physician or anesthesiologist experienced both in cardiovascular and respiratory resuscitation.

VENTILATORY. The well-known complications of apnea and hypoventilation have been observed by all. Apnea usually results from too rapid induction or improper use of concentrated solutions. Treatment consists of establishing an adequate airway and aiding respiration. Laryngospasm due to the drug may be prevented and treated by spraying the pharynx and larynx with cocaine or the administration of 1/75th gr of atropine. If due to reflexes, removal of the stimulus is required. Laryngospasm may also be avoided by allowing at least 5 to 10 minutes to elapse from the time of induction until surgery begins.

RESPIRATORY. Hiccoughing, sneezing, and coughing have been encountered during thiopental anesthesia, and these complications may be combatted by the administration of atropine; spraying the nose, throat, and larynx; changing the anesthetic agent; and, in the case of hiccoughing, increasing the carbon dioxide content through rebreathing, administering curare, and blocking the phrenic nerves.

Premedication with meperidine followed by thiopental represents an adverse drug interaction on occasion. A bizarre, allergic-like phenomenon of the upper airway occurs and edema of the uvula, epiglottis, and glottis has been observed.[152–154]

LOCAL IRRITANT EFFECTS

Pain on Injection.[155] About 10% of patients complain of pain or burning radiating centrally on injection of thiopental or methohexital. This is related to the following factors:

- *Concentration:* A 5% solution doubles the incidence of pain.
- *Rate of injection:* A higher pain response occurs when the 2.5% solution is injected more rapidly than 1 ml/sec.
- *Site of injection:* Pain occurs more frequently following injection into the small veins (back of hand) than into large veins in the antecubital space.[117] The incidence of venous sequelae, however, is greater for injection into the antecubital fossa, i.e., between 3% and 5% for thiopental.[155]

In contrast to a 10% incidence of pain on injection with thiopental, the incidence of pain with diazepam in 40% propylene glycol is 37%, but diazepam is soya bean oil (Diazemils) is 2%. Midazolam has an incidence of 1%, and methohexital has an incidence of 12%.

To avoid pain on injection, the following are recommended:

- The concentration of thiopental should be no more than 2.5%.
- Slow rates of injection (5 ml/10 sec) should be used.
- Use of larger veins is desirable.
- Assure needle placement in lumen of the vein.

Venous Sequelae. Some degree of internal damage occurs in a small percentage of patients. Phlebitis is occasionally seen. It usually appears within 24 hours after injection, but may be delayed. It is seldom severe. Adams[2] sets the incidence of phlebitis at about 1 in 1000 administrations with 5% solution and 1 in 3000 with the 2.5% solution.

Thrombosis is rare and delayed. It may be seen up to 1 week following anesthesia induced with 2.5% thiopental.[155] It is more frequent in the veins of the antecubital fossa.

Instances of pulmonary embolism have been reported but are rare. Usually, they occur 3 to 8 days after injection.[156]

Perivenous Injection. Such injection causes severe local burning pain. Tissue damage may ensue and the extent depends on the amount injected. A large amount may lead to necrosis and tissue slough, including the skin. Early recognition of an extravascular infiltration is important in prevention. If recognized, the injury can be minimized by infiltrating the area with 1% procaine.[157]

EXTRAVASATION. Small quantities of thiopental solution may extravasate when injection of a 2.5% solution is made into superficial veins on the back of the hand, especially near the knuckles. It is more frequent than when injections are made into the antecubital veins. It may not be readily recognized, but it is associated with high-pressure injection. This may cause serious deformities of the metacarpophalangeal joint. The deformity is usually of a flexion type.[155a]

INTRA-ARTERIAL INJECTION.[158,159] This is a serious occasional mishap that is not always recognized. The immediate complaint is of agonizing pain shooting *down* the forearm; withdrawal movements of arm are elicited. Severe arterial spasm with blanching of limb and disappearance of radial pulse ensue. Sequelae include small areas of gangrene, permanent loss of sensation, or loss of fingers or forearm.

The chemical properties of thiopental rather than its alkalinity appear to be the cause of the injury to arterial vessel lining. Intra-arterial thiopental also releases norepinephrine from the arterial vessel walls, which may be responsible for the intense vascular spasm. This may be a singular property because hexobarbital does not cause this release.

Concentration is the single most important determinant of frequency and extent of damage. Incidence of damage increases with increasing concentration as follows: 10% solution—82%; 5% solution—3%; and 2.5% solution—7%. The arterial intima of humans can tolerate safely thiopental concentrations of 25 mg/ml or 2.5% without significant damage, but higher concentrations cause a chemical endarteritis.[158]

Treatment for accidental intra-arterial injection includes:[159] (1) intra-arterial injection of a lidocaine solution, 1 mg/kg, through the same needle; (2) withdrawal of needle; (3) infiltration of tissue about artery with a local anesthetic; (4) anticoagulant therapy (heparinization should be early and adequate); and (5) sympathetic nerve blocks. Somatic peripheral nerve blocks will also afford some interrruption of sympathetic constrictor supply. Note that under general anesthesia, the intensity of vasoconstriction is lessened.

The use of spasmolytic agents and peripheral generalized adrenergic blockade appears to have limited advantages and poor physiologic basis.

ANAPHYLACTOID RESPONSE.[161] The clinical syndrome of human anaphylaxis is mediated by immunoglobulin E (IgE). This is the reagin originally described by Prausnitz and Kustner (Type I hypersensitivity) that has now been isolated and purified. This reagin can be found in all humans and is highly specific.[162,163] Many drugs evoke reactions of the anaphylactic type, including barbiturates. Intravenous thiopental is able to induce fluctuations in total serum IgE levels.[164] Acute hypersensitivity reactions to thiopental have been reported and, although rare, seem to be increasing.[165]

The syndrome includes marked tachycardia, hypotension, and vasodilatation, bronchospasm, erythremia, flushing of skin, urticaria, and cyanosis. Blood studies reveal hypoxemia, hypercarbia, and acidosis (many features of a serotoninergic and bradykinergic reaction.[165,166]

Studies of the anaphylactic reaction involve determination of immunoglobulin by radioimmunoassay. The IgE-membrane complex, or hapten-complex, can combine with an antigen to mobilize histamine-containing granules from the mast cells and basophilic leucocytes.

Immune Complex (Hapten).[162,165] Many drugs with low-molecular-weight that is less than 1000 daltons have been implicated in immunization reactions through the "hapten" mechanism. That is, there is an immune complex that binds firmly to red blood cell membranes, at which the I antigen is attached. At least one report has demonstrated the development of an antibody to thiopental.[167] A drug–antibody complex of this hapten nature can cause hemolysis and a drug-induced hemolytic anemia with concomitant renal failure. The existence of a red blood cell antigen I has been shown in some individuals, to which the thiopental–antibody complex is attached.

Mechanism of Reaction. Histamine is the predominant factor in producing the hypersensitivity reaction. In sensitized subjects, a small dose of 10 µg to 10 mg of thiopental may evoke an immune response. There is an immediate reduction in circulating IgE due to binding with the reaginic substance at the cell surface of the basophil. This is followed by marked stimulation of production and elaboration of antibody to a high IgE level within 1 hour; at the end of 5 hours, there may be a fivefold increase in IgE levels. Other immunoglobulins (IgG, IgA, or IgM) levels are unchanged. Hence, it appears that thiopental may induce an acute hypersensitivity response type I, as well as a pharmacologic type IV response.[161,162]

A proposed clinical test utilizes a radio-allergo sorbent and has been outlined by Etter.[161] An alternative method is to observe the extent of basophilic degranulation before and after a challenging dose of the sensitizing agent.

The potential to release histamine has been tested by means of a preparation of human skin mast cells.[168] Various ascending concentrations of intravenous barbiturates and other drugs are incubated with the preparation and the amount of histamine released is measured and then dose related. Hirshman[168] has demonstrated that thiopental and thiamylal induce a progressive dose-related release in the amount of histamine. In contrast, pentobarbital and methohexital failed to increase histamine above spontaneous levels.

OVERDOSE.[160] In the treatment of inadvertent overdose, the most important procedure is to provide a patent and adequate airway through which oxygen can be administered and artificial ventilation efficiently performed.

ROLE OF ANALEPTICS.[79,169] These drugs have little value in the management of overdose. Schmidt[79] has shown that the injection of analeptics when the respiratory center has been depressed by drugs accompanied by hypoxia, only further depresses the respiratory center causing cellular fatigue. However, one drug may have some value, once adequate oxygenation has been instituted. Doxapram in doses of 2 mg/kg acts as a specific respiratory center stimulant and at this dose level does not stimulate the cortex.

Nutrition and fluid balance in cases of overdose must be supervised with prolonged recovery. Intravenous fluids and alimentation and the administration of liquid feeding mixtures by stomach tube may be instituted. At the same time, excretory requirements must be met.

ABNORMAL MUSCLE MOVEMENTS. Involuntary and aberrant muscle movements are occasionally seen during or soon after the induction of thiopental anesthesia. They are not to be confused with the second stage of anesthesia. These consist of athetoid, twitching, and rolling and jerking movements. A dose–response relationship exists in that a dose twice the sleep dose increases the incidence of occurrence. Inadequate premedication or use of antanalgesics such as tranquilizers (phenothiazines) increases their incidence. Narcotics, especially morphine, prevent their occurrence.

POSTANESTHETIC TREMORS. This postanesthetic phenomenon following thiopental anesthesia occurs frequently. It is seen more often after short anesthesia of 1 to 2 hours. It is manifested by twitching of face muscles and may progress to tremors of arms, head, shoulders, and body muscles. This has been sometimes referred to as the "thiopental shakes." It is not typical shivering.

Sessler[170] has shown that these generalized tremors are a combination of spontaneous clonus and tonic activity. This phenomenon differs from normal shivering. It is also noted that normal thermoregulatory responses to cold are inhibited by the presence of thiopental in the tissues and in the absence of significant residual inhalation agents.[171]

The electromyographic pattern of tremors consists of two parts: irregular tonic contraction of muscle and regular superimposed clonic contractions of the skeletal muscle. In contrast, shivering electromyographic patterns of muscle show 4 to 8 cycles per minute, which wax and wane in amplitude.

The tremors occur more often in the early phase of discontinuing general anesthesia and are related to a cold room environment. There is often a large ventilatory heat and water loss during semiclosed and nonbreathing general anesthesia. An increased oxygen demand of 200% to 300% exists and represents a significant hazard.

Women are more prone to exhibit thiopental shakes during emergence.

Management. Prevention includes humidification of breathing gas mixtures and warming of these mixtures.[172]

It is important to minimize heat loss and to stop shivering, because the oxygen requirements are increased two- to fivefold. Meperidine, in small doses of 10 to 20 mg administered intravenously every 5 minutes until shivering ceases, is the most effective measure. Relief does occur in over 90% of patients.

Other drugs are minimally effective. Morphine provides about a 45% protection and fentanyl 35%.[173] Drugs such as chlorpromazine and dehydrobenzpyridol should not be used.

SPECIAL USES

IN STATUS EPILEPTICUS. Thiopental anesthesia is used with cases of status epilepticus resistant to conventional therapy. A loading dose of 2 to 4 mg/kg of 2.5% thiopental is administered intravenously over a period of 10 minutes; a drip infusion of dilute thiopental (0.2%) solution is then instituted for maintenance. Administration rate should be reduced with time as judged by clinical signs and the need to prevent convulsions. The rate should be adjusted to maintain a blood level of approximately 2 to 4 mg/L and to compensate for the amount metabolized and excreted per hour (15%).

IN CRANIAL TRAUMA.[174] Continuous intravenous thiopental has been used experimentally in the management of acute head trauma. The dosage schedule is similar to that for status epilepticus. Patients have been treated for several days by this method (see Brain Protection).

The effectiveness of this technique is questionable.[175] The time of instituting therapy is an important factor in outcome. Results are not impressive.[176] Following resuscitation from cardiac arrest with persistent coma, a randomized clinical study of thiopental loading has not shown a greater improvement in neurologic function over a standard nonthiopental treatment group.[177]

REFERENCES

1. Keys, T.E.: History of Surgical Anesthesia. Gloucester, MA, Peter Smith, 1945.
2a. Adams, R.C.: Intravenous Anesthesia. New York, Paul B. Hoeber, 1944.
2b. Dundee, J.W., McIlroy, D.A. The history of the barbiturates. Anaesthesia 37:726, 1982.
2c. Dundee, J.W., and Wyant, G.M.: Intravenous Anaesthesia. New York, Churchill Livingstone, 1974.
3. Egbert, L.D., Oech, S.R., and Eckenhoff, J.E.: Comparison of the recovery from methohexital and thiopentone anaesthesia in man. Surg. Gynecol. Obstet., 109:427, 1959.
4. Clarke, R.S., et al.: Clinical studies of induction agents. XXVI: The relative potencies of thiopentone, methohexitone and propanidid. Br. J. Anaesth., 40:593, 1968.
5. Stella, L., Torri, G., and Castiglioni, C.L.: The relative potencies of thiopentone, ketamine, propanidid, alphaxalone and diazepam. Br. J. Anaesth., 51:119, 1979.
6. Mark, L.C.: Archaic classification of barbiturates. Clin. Pharm. Therap., 10:287, 1969.
7a. Tatum, H.L.: The present status of the barbiturate problem. Physiol. Rev., 19:472, 1932.
7b. Grouhzit, O.M., et al.: Pharmacologic study of certain thiobarbiturates. J. Pharmacol. & Exp. Therap. 60:125, 1937.
8. Tabern, D.L., and Volweiler, E.H.: Sulfur containing barbiturate hypnotics. J. Am. Chem. Soc., 51:1961, 1935.
9. Lundy, J.S., and Tovell, R.M.: Some of the newer local and general anesthetic agents. Northwestern Medicine (Seattle), 33:308, 1934.
9a. Lundy, J.S., and Tovell, R.M.: Annual Report for 1934 of Section on Anesthesia, Including Data on Blood Transfusions. Proc. Staff Meet. Mayo Clin., 10:257, 1935.
9b. Tovell, R.M., et al.: A comparative clinical and statistical study of thiopental and thiamylal in human anesthesia. Anesthesiology 16:910, 1955.
10. Burger, A.: Relation of chemical structure of sedative and hypnotic drugs to their activity (symposium). Baltimore, Williams & Wilkins, 1954.
11. Nicoll, R.A.: Pentobarbital: Differential postsynaptic actions on sympathetic ganglion cells. Science, 199:451, 1978.
12. Carraway, B.M., and Carraway, C.V.: Intravenous anesthesia: A clinical study of 1,900 cases. Am. J. Surg., 39:576, 1938.
13. Carraway, B.M.: Pentothal sodium with nasal oxygen: A

report of 3,180 consecutive cases. Anesth. Analg., 18:259, 1939.
14. Lundy, J.S., and Tuohy, E.B.: Newer trends in intravenous anesthesia. Minn. Med., 26:349, 1943.
15. Tuohy, E.B.: Clinical use of intravenous anesthesia alone and in combination with other anesthetics: A method of anesthesia eliminating the hazards of fire and explosion. South. Med. J., 34:42, 1941.
16. Hand, L.V., and Sise, L.F.: Intravenous agents as supplementary anesthesia. Bull. Lahey Clin., 1:18, 1939.
17. Brody, J.: The use of curare in sodium pentothal nitrous oxide anesthesia. Anesthesiology, 6:381, 1945.
18. Brodie, B.B., Kurz, H., and Schanker, L.S.: The importance of dissociation constant and lipid solubility in influencing the passage of drugs into the cerebrospinal fluid. J. Pharmacol. Exp. Ther., 130:22, 1960.
19. Lenowitz, H., Lipson, H.I., and Stevens, E.J.: High dilution pentothal sodium for sedation, narcosis and anesthesia. Anesth. Analg., 23:78, 1941.
20. Baird, J.W.: Pentothal curare mixture. Anesthesiology, 8:75, 1947.
21. Webster, C.F., and Van Bergen, F.H.: Pentothal curare mixture with endotracheal N_2O and O_2 in infants. Bull. Univ. Minnesota Hosp., 20:525, 1949.
22. Evans, F.T., and Gray, P.W.S.: Continuous gallamine and thiopentone mixtures intravenously. Anesthesia, 8:104, 1953.
23. Morton, W.D., and Lerman, J.: The effect of pancuronium on the solubility of aqueous thiopentone. Can. J. Anaesth., 34:87, 1987.
23a. Fraser, P.J.: Hydrolysis of succinylcholine salts. Br. J. Pharmacol., 9:429, 1954.
24. Langlais, K., and Williams, L.: Action of adenosinetriphosphate and adenomonophosphate on thiopental sodium glucose narcosis. J. Pharmacol. Exp. Ther., 103:351, 1951.
25. Musky, J.H., and Giarman, N.J.: Studies on the potentiation of thiopental. J. Pharmacol. Exp. Ther., 114:240, 1955.
26. Paulson, J.A., Lundy, L.S., and Essex, H.E.: Narcosis with pentothal sodium alone compared to narcosis with pentothal sodium combined with curare. Anesthesiology, 10:387, 1949.
27. Dundee, J.W., and Scott, W.E.B.: Effect of phenothorazine on thiobarbiturate narcosis. Anesth. Analg., 37:12, 1958.
28. Robinson, M.H.: Deterioration of solutions of pentothal sodium. Anesthesiology, 8:166, 1947.
29. Dundee, J.W.: Current views on the clinical pharmacology of the barbiturates. Int. Anesthesiol. Clin., 7:331, 1969.
30. Dundee, J.W.: Intravenous Anesthetics. New York, Churchill Livingstone, 1974.
31. Christensen, J.H., Andreasen, F., and Jansen, J.A.: Thiopentone sensitivity in young and elderly women. Br. J. Anaesth., 55:33, 1983.
32. Christensen, J.H., Andreasen, F., and Jansen, J.A.: Influence of age and sex on the pharmacokinetics of thiopentone. Br. J. Anaesth., 53:1189, 1981.
33. Coté, C.J., et al.: The dose response of intravenous thiopental for the induction of general anesthesia in unpremedicated children. Anesthesiology, 55:703, 1981.
34. Ouslander, J.G.: Drug therapy in the elderly. Ann. Intern. Med., 95:711, 1981.
35. Dundee, J.W.: The influence of body weight, sex and age on the dosage of thiopentone. Br. J. Anaesth., 26:164, 1954.
36. Homer, T.D., and Stanski, D.R.: The effect of increasing age on thiopental disposition and anesthetic requirement. Anesthesiology, 62:714, 1985.
37. Stanski, D.R., et al: Pharmacodynamic modelling of thiopental anesthesia. J. Pharmacokinet. Biopharm., 12:223, 1984.
38. Stanski, D.R.: Pharmacokineticic modelling of thiopental (editorial). Anesthesiology, 54:446, 1981.
39. Burch, P.G., and Stanski, D.R.: The role of metabolism and protein binding in thiopental anesthesia. Anesthesiology, 58:146, 1983.
40. Ghoneim, M.M., and Van Hamme, M.J.: Pharmacokinetics of thiopentone: Effects of enflurane and nitrous oxide anaesthesia and surgery. Br. J. Anaesth., 50:1237, 1978.
41. Morgan, D.J., et al.: Pharmacokinetics and plasma binding of thiopental. I. Studies in surgical patients. Anesthesiology, 54:468, 1981.
42. Becker, K.E.: Gas chromatographic assay for free and total plasma levels of thiopental. Anesthesiology, 45:656, 1976.
43. Becker, K.E.: Plasma levels of thiopental necessary for anesthesia. Anesthesiology, 49:192, 1978.
44. Ghonheim, M.N., and Pandya, H.: Plasma protein binding of thiopental in patients with impaired renal or hepatic function. Anesthesiology, 42:545, 1975.
45. Ghonheim, M.N., et al.: Binding of thiopental to plasma proteins: Effects of distribution in brain and heart. Anesthesiology, 45:635, 1976.
46. Sorbo, S., Hudson, R.J., and Loomis, J.C.: The pharmacokinetics of thiopental in pediatric surgical patients. Anesthesiology, 61:666, 1984.
47. Jung, D., et al.: Thiopental disposition as a function of age in female patients undergoing surgery. Anesthesiology, 56:263, 1982.
48. Burch, P.G., and Stanski, D.R.: Decreased protein binding and thiopental kinetics. J. Clin. Pharm. Ther., 32:212, 1981.
49. Boobis, S.W.: Alteration of plasma albumin in relation to decrease in drug binding in uremia. Clin. Pharm. Ther., 22:147, 1977.
50. Pandele, G., et al.: Thiopental pharmacokinetics in patients with cirrhosis. Anesthesiology, 59:123, 1983.
51. Sandor, P., et al: Variations in drug free fraction during alcohol withdrawal. Br. J. Clin. Pharmacol., 15:481, 1983.
52. Novak, L.P.: Aging, total body potassium, fat free mass and cell mass between 18 and 35 years.. J. Gerontol., 27:438, 1972.
53. Bender, A.D.: The effect of increasing age on the distribution of peripheral blood flow in man. J. Am. Geriatr. Soc., 13:192, 1965.
54. Keilty, S.R.: Anesthesia for the alcoholic patient. Anesth. Analg., 48:659, 1969.
55. Loft, S., et al.: Influence of moderate alcohol intake on thiopental anaesthesia. Acta Anaesthesiol. Scand., 26:22, 1982.
56. Rubin, E., and Lieber, C.S.: Hepatic microsomal enzymes in man and rat: Induction and inhibition by ethanol. Science, 162:690, 1968.
57. Sellers, E.M., and Holloway, M.R.: Drug kinetics and alcohol ingestion. Clin. Pharmacokinet., 3:440, 1978.
58. Couderc, E., et al.: Thiopentone pharmacokinetics in patients with chronic alcoholism. Br. J. Anaesth., 56:1393, 1984.
59. Gladtke, E., and Heiman, G.: The rate of development of elimination functions in kidney and liver of young infants, basic and therapeutic aspects of perinatal pharmacology. Edited by P.I. Morselli, S. Garatine, and F. Sereni. New York, Raven Press, 1975, p. 393.

60. Dundee, J.W., Price, H.L., Dripps, R.D.: Acute tolerance to thiopentone in man. Br. J. Anaesth., *28*:344, 1956.
61. Himwich, W.A., et al.: Brain metabolism in man: In anesthesia and in pentothal narcosis. Am. J. Psychiatr., *103*:689, 1947.
62. Mitchenfelder, J.D., and Theye, R.A.: Cerebral protection by thiopental during hypoxia. Anesthesiology, *39*:510, 1973.
63. Smith, A.: Barbiturate protection in cerebral hypoxia. Anesthesiology, *47*:285, 1977.
64a. Mark, L.C., et al.: Quantitative pharmacologic studies with pentothal. N.Y. State J. Med., *49*:1546, 1949.
64b. Richards, C.D.: Actions of general anaesthetics on synaptic transmission in the CNS. Br. J. Anaesth., *55*:201, 1983.
65. Kiersey, E.E., Bickford, R.G., and Faulconer, A.: Electroencephalographic changes during pentothal. Br. J. Anaesth., *23*:141, 1951.
66. Helrich, M., et al.: The influence of opiates on the respiratory response of man to thiopental. Anesthesiology, *17*:459, 1956.
67. Dillon, J.B., and Darsie, M.L.: Oxygen for acute respiratory depression due to administration of thiopental sodium. J.A.M.A., *159*:1115, 1955.
68. Gross, J.B., et al.: Time course of ventilatory depression after thiopental and midazolam in normal subjects and in patients with chronic obstructive pulmonary disease. Anesthesiology, *58*:540, 1983.
69. Etsten, B., and Li, T.H.: Hemodynamic changes during thiopental anesthesia in humans. J. Clin. Invest., *34*:500, 1955.
70. Elder, J.D.: Circulatory changes associated with thiopental anesthesia in man. Anesthesiology, *16*:394, 1955.
71. Collins, V.J.: Evaluation of thiopental anesthesia. Bull. N.Y. Acad. Med., *31*:438, 1955.
72. Papper, E.M., and Bradley, S.E.: Hemodynamic effects of intravenous morphine and pentothal sodium. J. Pharmacol. Exp. Ther., *74*:319, 1942.
73. Price, H.: Hypotensive effects of thiopental. J. Appl. Physiol., *4*:629, 1952.
74. Penrod, K.E., and Hegnauer, A.H.: Effects of pentothal sodium on blood gas transport. Am. J. Physiol., *153*:81, 1948.
75. Hershey, S.G., and Zweifach, B.W.: Peripheral vascular homeostasis in relation to anesthetic agents. Anesthesiology, *11*:145, 1950.
76. Fieldman, E.J., Ridley, R.W., and Wood, E.H.: Hemodynamic studies during thiopental sodium and nitrous oxide anesthesia in humans. Anesthesiology, *16*:473, 1955.
77. Johnson, S.R.: Effect of some anesthetics on circulation in man. Acta Chir. Scand. (Suppl), *158*, 1951.
78. Stephens, C.R., Nowill, W.K., and Martin, R.: Diagnosis and treatment of hypotension during anesthesia. Anesthesiology, *14*:180, 1953.
79. Schmidt, C.: The influence of cerebral blood flow on respiration. Am. J. Physiol., *84*:202, 1928.
80. Zweifach, B.W., et al.: Anesthetic agents as factors in circulatory reactions induced by hemorrhage. Surgery, *19*:48, 1945.
81. McCall, M.L., and Taylor, H.W.: Effects of barbiturate sedation on the brain in toxemia of pregnancy. J.A.M.A., *149*:51, 1952.
82. Clarke, R.S.J.: Anaesthesia and carbohydrate metabolism. Brit. J. Anaesth., *45*:237, 1973.
83. Stern, M., et al.: The effects of anesthesia on glucose tolerance. J. Pharmacol. Exp. Ther., *84*:157, 1945.
84. Booker, W.M.: Observations on the carbohydrate metabolism during prolonged pentothal anesthesia in dogs: The blood sugar and liver glycogen. Anesthesiology, *7*:405, 1946.
85. Schiefley, C.: Pentothal sodium: Its use in the presence of hepatic disease. Anesthesiology, *7*:263, 1946.
86. Shideman, F.E., Kelly, A.R., and Adams, B.J.: The role of the liver in the detoxification of thiopental (pentothal) and two other thiobarbiturates. J. Pharmacol. Exp. Ther., *91*:331, 1947.
87. Shideman, F.E., et al.: The role of the liver in the detoxification of the thiopental (pentothal) by man. Anesthesiology, *10*:421, 1949.
88. Richards, R.K.: Detoxification of pentothal. Anesth. Analg., *20*:64, 1941.
89. Dundee, J.W.: Thiopentone as a factor in the production of liver dysfunction. Br. J. Anaesth., *27*:14, 1955.
90. DeBodo, R.C., and Prescott, K.R.: The antidiuretic action of thiobarbiturates and the mechanism involved. J. Pharmacol. Exp. Ther., *85*:222, 1945.
91. DeBoer, B.: Factors affecting pentothal anesthesia in dogs. Anesthesiology, *8*:375, 1947.
92. Burstein, C.L., and Co, T.: Relationship between hypoproteinemia and toxicity of anesthetic agents. Curr. Res. Anesth. Analg., *27*:287, 1948.
93. Levy, H.A., DiPalma, J.R., and Alper, C.: Effects of nutritional deficiency on response to thiopental. J. Pharmacol. Exp. Ther., *109*:377, 1953.
94. Borgnian, R.L., et al.: Effects of barbiturates on skeletal muscle function. Anesthesiology, *21*:150, 1960.
95. Secher, O.: Pilot investigation into the peripheral action of anaesthetics. Acta Pharmacologica et Toxicologica, *7*:82, 1951.
96. Sirnes, T.B.: Some effects of barbituric acid derivatives on function of mammalian skeletal muscle. Acta Pharmacologica et Toxicologica, *10*:Suppl 1–170, 1954.
97. Joyce, J.T., Roizen, M.F., and Eger, E.I. II: Effect of thiopental induction on sympathetic activity. Anesthesiology, *59*:19, 1983.
98. Joyce, J.T., et al.: Induction of anesthesia with halothane increases plasma norepinephrine concentrations. Anesthesiology, *56*:280, 1982.
99. Skovsted, P., Price, M.L., and Price, H.L.: The effects of short-acting barbiturates on arterial pressure, preganglionic sympathetic activity and barostatic reflexes. Anesthesiology, *33*:10, 1970.
100. Wallin, B.G., and Konig, U.: Changes of skin nerve sympathetic activity during induction of general anesthesia with thiopentone in man. Brain Res., *103*:157, 1976.
101. Kaniaris, P., et al.: Cholinergic action of thiopental on the hypothalamohypophyseal axis. Anesth. Analg., *60*:310, 1981.
102. Price, H.L., et al.: Sympathoadrenal responses to general anesthesia and their relation to hemodynamics. Anesthesiology, *20*:563, 1959.
103. Fitzgerald, J.H., and Webster, A.: Obstetrics: Significance of barbiturates and vitamin K. J.A.M.A., *119*:1082, 1942.
104. Mark, L.C.: The Uptake and Distribution of Anesthetic Agents. New York, McGraw-Hill, 1963.
105. Mark, L.C., et al.: Quantitative pharmacologic studies with pentothal. N. Y. State J. Med., *49*:1546, 1949.
106. Brodie, B.B., et al.: The fate of thiopental in man and a method for estimation in biological material. J. Pharmacol. Exp. Ther., *98*:85, 1950.
107. Price, H.L., Dundee, J.W., and Comer, E.A.: Rates of uptake and release of thiopental by human brain: Relation to kinetics of thiopental anesthesia. Anesthesiology, *18*:171, 1957.

108. Price, H.L., et al.: The uptake of thiopental by body tissue and its relation to the duration of narcosis. Clin. Pharm. Ther., 1:16, 1960.
109. Bollman, J.L., et al.: Tissue distribution with time after a single intravenous administration of pentothal sodium with S^{35}. Anesthesiology, 11:1, 1950.
110. Brodie, B.B., Bernstein, E., and Mark, L.C.: The role of body fat in limiting the duration of action of thiopental. J. Pharm. Exp. Ther., 105:421, 1952.
110a. Dundee, J.W.: Abnormal responses to barbiturates. Br. J. Anaesth., 29:440, 1957.
111. Delmonico, E.J.: Tests for derivatives of barbituric acid. Proc. Staff Meet. Mayo Clin., 14:109, 1939.
112. Richards, R.K.: Inactivation of pentothal. Anesthesiology, 8:90, 1947.
113. Etsten, B., and Himwich, H.E.: Stages and signs of pentothal anesthesia: Physiologic basis. Anesthesiology, 7:536, 1946.
114. Rosner, V., and Clark, L.: In Brain Mechanisms and Unconsciousness. Edited by M.A. Brazier. Oxford, Blackwell Scientific, 1954.
115. Brazier, M.A.: Brain Mechanisms and Unconsciousness. Oxford, Blackwell Scientific, 1954.
116. Clutton-Brock, J.: Pain and the barbiturates. Anaesthesia, 16:80, 1961.
116a. Keats, A.S., Telford, J., and Kurosu, Y.: Studies of analgesic drugs III: Dextromoramide and a comparison of methods of estimating pain relief in man. J. Pharmacol. Exp. Therap., 130:212, 1960.
116b. Beecher, H.K.: Appraisal of drugs intended to alter subjective responses. J.A.M.A., 158:399, 1955.
117. Dundee, J.W.: Alterations in response to somatic pain. Br. J. Anaesth., 32:407, 1960.
117a. Hubbell, A.O., Krogh, H.W.: Management of intravenous anesthesia to control recovery time. J. Oral Surg. Oral Med. Oral Path., 9:403, 1956.
117b. Dundee, J.W., et al.: The induction dose of thiopentone: a method of study. Anaesthesia, 37:1176, 1982.
117c. Hubbell, E., and Krogh, M.: The "surge" technique of thiopental dose for short surgical procedures. J. Oral Surg. Oral Med. Oral Pathol., 9:406, 1956.
118. Hudson, R.J., et al.: A model for studying depth of anesthesia and acute tolerance to thiopental. Anesthesiology, 59:301, 1983.
119. Edwards, R., and Ellis, F.R.: The clinical significance of thiopental binding to haemoglobin and plasma protein. Br. J. Anaesth., 45:811, 1973.
120. Kiersey, E.E., Bickford, R.G., and Faulconer, A.: Electroencephalographic changes during pentothal. Br. J. Anaesth., 23:141, 1951.
121. Dundee, J.W.: Some effects of premedication on the induction characteristics of intravenous anesthetics. Anaesthesia, 20:298, 1965.
122. Schanker, L.S.: Penetration of drugs into central nervous system. In The Uptake and Distribution of Anesthetic Drugs. Edited by E.M. Papper and R. Kitz. New York, McGraw-Hill, 1963.
123. McClure, R.D., Behrmann, V.G., and Hartman, F.W.: The control of anoxemia during surgery anesthesia with the aid of the oxyhemograph. Ann. Surg., 128:685, 1948.
124. Medrado, V., and Stephen, C.R.: Arterial blood gas studies during induction of anesthesia and endotracheal intubation. Surg. Gynecol. Obstet., 123:1275, 1966.
125. Hamilton, W.K., and Eastwood, D.W.: Study of denitrogenation with some inhalation anesthetic systems. Anesthesiology, 16:861, 1955.
126. Berthoud, M., Read, D.H., and Norman, J.: Preoxygenation: How long? Anaesthesia, 38:96, 1983.
127. Werner, H.W., Pratt, T.W., and Tatum, A.L.: A comparative study of several ultrashort acting barbiturates. J. Pharmacol. Exp. Ther., 60:189, 1937.
128. Gold, M.I., Duarte, I., and Muravchick, S.: Arterial oxygenation in conscious patients after 5 minutes and 30 seconds of oxygen breathing. Anesth. Analg., 60:313, 1981.
129. Drummond, G.B., and Park, G.R.: Arterial oxygen saturation before intubation of the trachea: An assessment of oxygenation techniques. Br. J. Anaesth., 56:987, 1984.
130. Heller, M.L., and Watson, T.R.: Polarographic study of arterial oxygenation during apnea in man. N. Engl. J. Med., 264:326, 1961.
130a. Heller, M.L., and Watson, T.R.: The role of preliminary oxygenaton prior to inhalation with high nitrous oxide mixtures: Polarographic Pa$_{O_2}$ study. Anesthesiology, 23:219, 1962.
131. Archer, G.W., and Marx, G.F.: Arterial oxygen tension during apnea in parturient women. Br. J. Anaesth., 46:358, 1974.
132. Marx, G., and Bassell, G.M.: Obstetric Analgesia and Anesthesia. New York, Excerpta Medica, 1980.
133. Norris, M.C., Dewan, D.M.: Preoxygenation for cesarean section: A comparison of two techniques. Anesthesiology, 62:827, 1985.
134. Burstein, C.S., and Hershey, S.G.: Circulatory effects from sodium pentothal administered soon after hemorrhage. Proc. Soc. Exp. Biol. Med., 53:80, 1943.
135. Finster, M., et al.: Plasma thiopental concentration in the newborn following delivery under thiopental-nitrous oxide anesthesia. Am. J. Obstet. Gynecol., 95:621, 1966.
136. Marx, G.F., et al.: Distribution of thiopental in fetal tissues. Anaesthetist, 25:318, 1976.
136a. Finster, M., et al.: Tissue thiopental concentration in the fetus and newborn. Anesthesiology, 36:155, 1972.
137. Dreisbach, R., and Snyder, F.: The effect on the fetus of pentobarbital sodium and pentothal sodium. J. Pharmacol. Exp. Ther., 79:250, 1943.
138. Kosaka, Y., Takahashi, T., and Mark, L.C.: Intravenous barbiturate anesthesia for CS. Anesthesiology, 31:491, 1969.
139. Finster, M., and Mark, L.C.: In Parturition and Perinatology. Edited by G.F. Marx. Philadelphia, F.A. Davis, 1973, p. 63.
140. Scanlon, J.W., et al.: Neurobehavioral responses of newborn infants after maternal epidural anesthesia. Anesthesiology, 40:121, 1974.
141. Hodgkinson, R., et al.: Neonatal neurobehavioral tests following vaginal delivery under ketamine, thiopental and extradural anesthesia. Anesth. Analg., 56:548, 1977.
142. Campbell, P., and Morgan, T.N.: On hyperglycemic action of certain drugs. J. Pharmacol. Exp. Ther., 49:456, 1933.
143. Booker, W.M.: Observations on the carbohydrate metabolism during prolonged pentothal anesthesia in dogs. Anesthesiology, 27:405, 1946.
144. Dundee, J.W.: The use of thiopentone in anemic subjects. J. Irish Med. Assoc., 31:351, 1952.
145. Dundee, J.W., and Richards, R.: Effects of azotemia upon the action of intravenous barbiturate anesthetics. Anesthesiology, 15:333, 1954.
146. Dundee, J.W., and Riding, J.E.: Barbiturates in porphyria. Anaesthesia, 10:55, 1955.
147. Musky, J.H., and Giarman, N.J.: Studies on potentiation of thiopental. J. Pharmacol. Exp. Ther., 114:240, 1955.

148. Jung, D., et al.: Thiopental disposition in lean and obese patients. Anesthesiology, 56:269, 1982.
149. King, E.: The treatment of Army casualties in Hawaii. Army Med. Bull., 61:18, 1942.
150. Ravdin, I.S., and Long, P.H.: The treatment of army casualties in Hawaii. Bull. U.S. Army Med. Dep., 61:1, 1942.
151. Rankin, R.W.: Sodium pentothal anesthesia (Letter) Bull. U.S. Army Med. Dep., March 21, 1944.
152. Burdick, D., and Collins, V.J.: Interaction of meperidine and thiopental. Clin. Anesth. Conf. Bellevue Hospital, September 1947.
153. Scalone, J.B.: Personal communication. 1984.
154. McDermott, F.F., and Papper, E.M.: Respiratory complications associated with demerol. N. Y. State J. Med., 50:1721, 1950.
155. Kawar, P., and Dundee, J.W.: Frequency of pain on injection and venous sequelae following the IV administration of certain anaesthetics and sedatives. Br. J. Anaesth., 54:935, 1982.
155a. Venkateswaran, V.: Flexion deformity of metacarpo-phalangeal joint following extravasation of thiopental. Can. Anesth. Soc. J., 333:827, 1985.
156. Ryan, H.H., and Hickcox, H.H.: Phlebitis and pulmonary embolism following pentothal sodium anaesthesia. N. Y. State J. Med., 47:2102, 1947.
157. Elder, C.K., and Harrison, E.M.: Pentothal sodium slough prevention with procaine. J.A.M.A., 125:116, 1944.
158. Cohen, S.M.: Accidental intra-arterial injection of drugs. Lancet, 2:409, 1948.
159. Stove, H.H., and Donnelly, C.C.: The accidental intra-arterial injection of thiopental. Anesthesiology, 22:995, 1961.
160. Landsberg, J.W.: Treatment of barbiturate overdose (Exhibit) N. Y. State Med. Soc. Meet., May 1948.
161. Etter, M.S., Helrich, M., and MacKenzie, C.F.: Immunoglobulin E fluctuation in thiopental anaphylaxis. Anesthesiology, 42:181, 1980.
162. Ishizaka, K., and Ishizaka, T.: Mechanisms of reaginic hypersensitivity: A review. Clin. Allerg., 1:9, 1971.
163. McFadden, E.R. Jr., and Austin, K.F.: Asthma. *In* Harrison's Principles of Internal Medicine. Edited by G.W. Thorn, R.D. Adams, and E. Braunwald. New York, McGraw-Hill, 1977, pp. 1350–1352.
164. Lilly, J.K., and Hoy, R.H.: Thiopental anaphylaxis and reagin involvement. Anesthesiology, 53:335, 1980.
165. Watkins, J.: Anaphylactoid reaction to IV substances. Br. J. Anaesth., 51:50, 1979.
166. Clarke, R.S.J., Fee, J.H., and Dundee, J.N.: *In* Hypersensitivity Reactions to Drugs. Edited by J.A. Watkins and A.M. Ward. New York, Academic Press, 1978, pp. 41–47.
167. Habibi, B., et al.: Thiopental-related immune hemolytic anemia and renal failure: Specific involvement of red-cell antigen I. N. Engl. J. Med., 312:353, 1985.
168. Hirshman, C.A., et al.: Thiobarbiturate-induced histamine release in human skin mast cells. Anesthesiology, 63:353, 1985.
169. Mousel, L.H., and Essex, H.E.: An experimental study of the effects of respiratory stimulants in animals under pentothal sodium anesthesia. Anesthesiology, 2:272, 1941.
170. Sessler, D.I., et al.: Spontaneous postanesthetic tremor does not resemble thermoregulatory shivering. Anesthesiology, 68:843, 1988.
171. Hammel, H.T.: Anesthetics and body temperature regulation (editorial). Anesthesiology, 68:833, 1988.
172. Pflug, A.E., et al.: Prevention of postanaesthesia shivering. Can. Anaesth. Soc. J., 25:43, 1978.
173. Pauca, A.L., et al.: Effect of pethidine, fentanyl and morphine on postoperative shivering in man. Acta Anaesthesiol. Scand., 28:138, 1984.
174. Miller, S.M., et al.: Cerebral protection by barbiturates and loop diuretics in head trauma: Possible modes of action. Bull. N.Y. Acad. Med., 56:305, 1980.
175. Frost, E.A.: Brain preservation (review). Anesth. Analg., 60:821, 1981.
176. Ping, F.C., and Jenkins, L.C.: Protection of the brain from hypoxia: A Review. Can. Anaesth. Soc. J., 25:468, 1978.
177. Abramson, R. (Brain Resuscitation Clinical Trial I Study Group): Randomized clinical study of thiopental loading in comatose survivors of cardiac arrest. N. Engl. J. Med., 314:397, 1986.

25

INTRAVENOUS ANESTHESIA: THIOPENTAL SUBSTITUTES

Several substitutes of the barbiturate group have been introduced. Some advantages are apparent in each, but significant superiority over thiopental has not been demonstrated except with methohexital (Tables 25–1 and 25–2).

THIAMYLAL

The thiobarbiturate known as *thiamylal* (Surital Sodium) bears the same relationship to secobarbital that thiopental does to pentobarbital. It was synthesized in 1929 at the same time as thiopental and described by Tabern in the classic report of 1935.[1]

CHEMICAL STRUCTURE. Thiamylal is an ultra short-acting thiobarbiturate (Fig. 25–1). In the structure there is (1) an allyl group and (2) a methyl isobutyl group making up the two side chain radicals attached to carbon atom 5. The chemical name is sodium 5-allyl-5'-(1-methylbutyl)-2-thiobarbiturate.

PHARMACOLOGY. Original studies on dogs indicated that thiamylal is about 40% more potent than thiopental. However, careful analysis in humans of doses based on dose per unit weight showed that 6.3 mg/lb for thiopental and 5.9 mg/lb of thiamylal gave essentially the same duration of anesthesia. No statistical significant difference is evident in this data.

Central Nervous System. A descending depression of the central nervous system occurs as the dose administered is increased. Overall effects are similar to thiopental, and the signs of anesthesia are the same. Electroencephalographic (EEG) patterns are indistinguishable from those of thiopental (Fig. 25–2).

Cardiovascular. The development of arrhythmias and the depression of the myocardium are seen and are related (1) to the injection technique and (2) to the agent. Hypertension occurs early in the administration. Decreased saturation of hemoglobin occurs during induction but can be avoided by prior administration of oxygen for 2 to 3 minutes. Rapid

TABLE 25–1. HISTORICAL AND CLINICAL DATA OF THREE CLASSIC INTRAVENOUS BARBITURATES

	Methohexital	Thiamylal	Thiopental
Trade name	Brevital (Eli Lilly)	Surital Sodium (Park-Davis)	Pentothal Sodium (Abbott)
Chemical name	Sodium α-dl-1-methyl-5-allyl-5-(1-methyl-2-pentynyl) oxybarbiturate	5-Allyl-5-(1-Methyl-butyl) 2-Thiobarbiturate	5-Ethyl-5-(1-Methyl-butyl) 2-Thiobarbiturate
Formula	$C_{12}H_{15}N_2O_3Na$	$C_{12}H_{17}N_2O_2SNa$	$C_{11}H_{17}N_2O_2SNa$
Discovery of compound	1954 by Eli Lilly Laboratory	1929 by Dox	1929 by Tabern and Volwiler
Discovery of anesthetic or relaxant properties	1954 by Stoelting	1933 by Gruhzit	1933 by Tatum
First used clinically	1954 by Stoelting	1948 by Seevers	1934 by Lundy
Type of compound	N-methylated oxybarbiturate	5-substituted thiobarbiturate	5-substituted thiobarbiturate
Molecular weight	286.23	276.33	264.23
Buffer employed	6% Sodium carbonate	6% Sodium carbonate	6% Sodium carbonate
Preservative or stabilizing agent used	None	None	None
Thermostability		Precipitates when boiled	Precipitates when boiled
Chemostability	Solution stable for 48 hours	Solution stable for 48–72 hours if tightly stoppered	Solution stable for 48–72 hours if tightly stoppered
Onset of action	15–20 sec	20–30 sec	15–30 sec
Duration of action	5–7 min	8–12 min	10–14 min
Route and or organ of detoxification or elimination	Liver enzymes	Detoxified by the liver and blood	Detoxified by the liver and blood
Usual mode of administration	Intravenous Intramuscular Rectal	Intravenous Rectal	Intravenous Rectal
Specific pharmacologic antagonist	None	Beta-ethyl glutarimide believed to be specific antagonist to the thiobarbiturates	
pH of solution	1% Aqueous—pH 11	2.5%—pH 10.5–11	2.5%—pH 10.5–11

This chart was prepared by University of Tennessee, and modified by V.J. Collins.

induction or use of concentrated solutions predisposes to these complications. Slow induction obviates them, and the avoidance of asphyxia is mandatory since this condition enhances cardiovascular depression.

Comparative Actions. Original clinical claims[2] included a slightly greater potency, more rapid awakening time from a comparable level of anesthesia, and somewhat less a disorientation in recovery, enabling patients to care for themselves more quickly.

A lower incidence and severity of laryngospasm with characteristic tendency for this to be self-limited was observed. An early impression not borne out by subsequent work was that there was less respiratory and circulatory depression.[3]

ADMINISTRATION. The two common intravenous methods of barbiturate drug administration that may be used include the intermittent injection of concentrated solutions and the continuous drip technique with dilute solutions. In the former, the preparation is usually a 2% or 2.5% solution. In Britain, thiamylal is used as a 5% solution similar to their use of thiopental. Sodium carbonate has been added to maintain stability of the concentrated solutions.

The dilute solutions are more commonly used, and a 0.2% to 0.5% concentration is recommended, with the 0.3% or 0.4% being most useful. These dilute solutions are potent enough to induce anesthesia and to provide a light basal state that can be complemented with nitrous oxide-oxygen. When fluid restriction is advisable, e.g., in patients with cardiac disease, the 0.5% solution is recommended.

The most satisfactory solvent is normal or half-normal saline. The drug can be mixed in this diluent and then stored or injected at room temperature. Storage of such solutions can extend for 14 days without change. Precipitation is unlikely if the so-

TABLE 25–2. RELATIONSHIP OF CHEMICAL GROUPING TO CLINICAL ACTION OF BARBITURATES

Group	Substituents Position 1	Substituents Position 2	Group Characteristics When Given IV
Oxybarbiturates	H	O	Delay in onset of action, degree depending on 5 and 5' side chains; useful as basal hypnotics; prolonged action
Methylated barbiturates	CH$_3$	O	Usually rapidly acting with fairly rapid recovery; high incidence of excitatory phenomena
Thiobarbiturates	H	S	Rapidly acting, usually smooth onset of sleep and fairly prompt recovery
Methylated thiobarbiturates	CH$_3$	S	Rapid onset of action and very rapid recovery but with so high an incidence of excitatory phenomena as to preclude use in clinical practice

From Dundee, J., and Wyant, G.: *In* Intravenous Anaesthesia. New York, Churchill Livingstone, 1974.

lutions are made by spinning on the table rather than by vigorous shaking. When distilled water or 5% dextrose is used, cloudy precipitates form on standing.

DOSAGE. The dose ranges are essentially the same as with thiopental. For induction, a range of 50 to 250 mg is usual. For maintenance, 1 g for the first hour and half of the previous dose for each subsequent hour is used.

TECHNIQUES OF USE. These are the same as with thiopental. If the agent is used to induce general anesthesia and then maintenance transferred to other agents, the following are noted: transfer to cyclopropane is more easily accomplished and with smaller doses of thiamylal (3 to 5 ml of 2%); establishment of ether anesthesia requires larger doses 5 to 10 ml of 2% as well as a gradual introduction of the inhalation agent to avoid cough or laryngeal spasm.

The 2.5% solution may be used for crash induction and endotracheal intubation. A dose of 0.5 to 1 g is administered and provides good but transient relaxation of the jaw. The drug must be injected rapidly to produce cerebral flooding with its consequent relaxation. Apnea usually occurs. These aspects are similar to thiopental use.

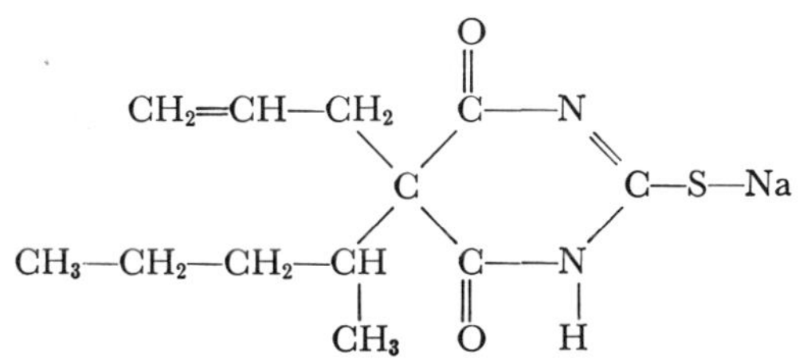

FIG. 25–1. Thiamylal.

COMPLICATIONS. Essentially they are the same as with thiopental; including hypotension, respiratory depression, mild agitation when robust or alcoholic patients are anesthetized, and laryngospasm. Tissue reactions will be noted if extravascular injection occurs.

Contraindications include those to thiopental. Liver disease, asthma, and emphysema with fibrosis are conditions in which complications are likely to ensue.

CONCLUSION. The general conclusion regarding pharmacology is that this drug is similar in most regards to thiopental.[4]

METHITURAL[5,6]

One attempt to provide an ultra short-acting barbiturate with an even shorter duration of action and a more rapidly metabolized molecule than thiopental resulted in methitural (Neraval). This compound is unique among the thiobarbiturates in having a second sulfur atom appearing in the R$_2$ side chain position. The radical is methyl thioethyl.

CHEMISTRY.[7] Methitural is a thiobarbiturate that also has a sulfur atom on its side chain (Fig. 25–3). It is the sodium salt of 5-methyl-thio-ethyl 5 (methylbutyl) thiobarbituric acid. The thio-ethyl radical is present in methionine, which plays an essential role in detoxification processes,[8] and this arrangement is considered to hasten detoxification. It is known that the methyl thio-ethyl group in methionine is responsible for donating methyl in transmethylation processes. It may be that the instability *in vivo* and the special affinity of thio-ethyl group for lipoids account for apparent favorable pharmacologic properties of methitural.[9]

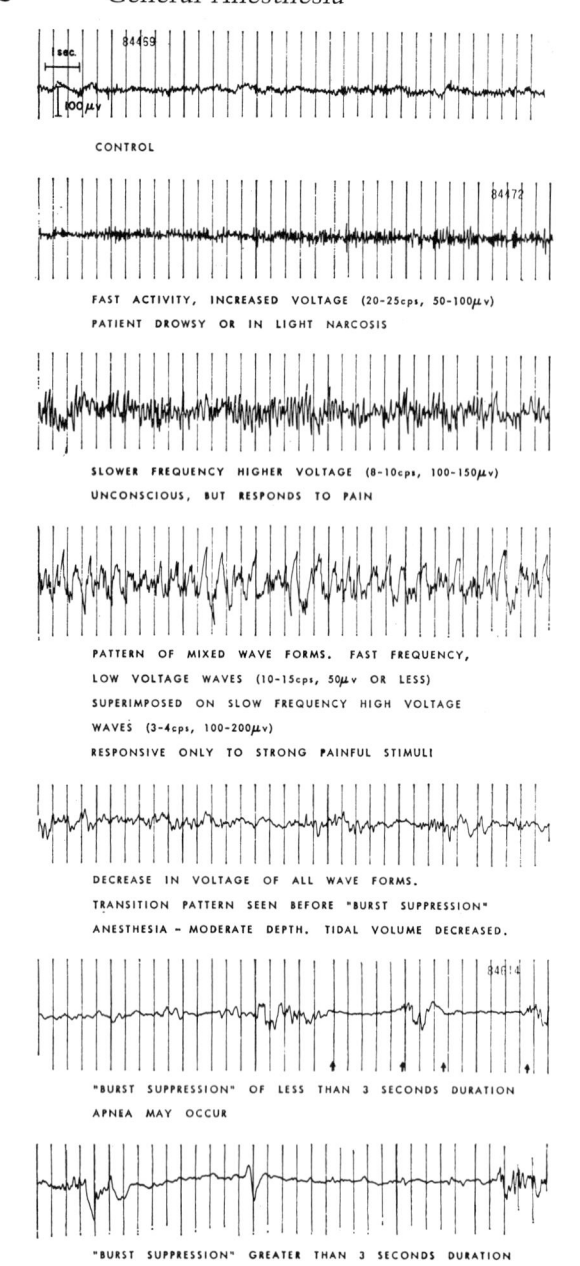

FIG. 25–2. EEG patterns of thiamylal. These patterns are typical of intravenous thiobarbiturate anesthesia.

CONTROL

FAST ACTIVITY, INCREASED VOLTAGE (20-25cps, 50-100μv)
PATIENT DROWSY OR IN LIGHT NARCOSIS

SLOWER FREQUENCY HIGHER VOLTAGE (8-10cps, 100-150μv)
UNCONSCIOUS, BUT RESPONDS TO PAIN

PATTERN OF MIXED WAVE FORMS. FAST FREQUENCY, LOW VOLTAGE WAVES (10-15cps, 50μv OR LESS) SUPERIMPOSED ON SLOW FREQUENCY HIGH VOLTAGE WAVES (3-4cps, 100-200μv)
RESPONSIVE ONLY TO STRONG PAINFUL STIMULI

DECREASE IN VOLTAGE OF ALL WAVE FORMS.
TRANSITION PATTERN SEEN BEFORE "BURST SUPPRESSION"
ANESTHESIA - MODERATE DEPTH. TIDAL VOLUME DECREASED.

"BURST SUPPRESSION" OF LESS THAN 3 SECONDS DURATION
APNEA MAY OCCUR

"BURST SUPPRESSION" GREATER THAN 3 SECONDS DURATION
APNEA IS COMMON

PHARMACOLOGIC ACTION. This agent provides central nervous system depression and is administered intravenously to produce anesthesia. Respiratory depression occurs as does circulatory depression. These effects are no different than with other intravenous thiobarbiturates. They are essentially a function of dose. Parasympathomimetic effects are perhaps more pronounced than with thiopental.

DISPOSITION IN THE BODY.[10] Distribution in the body fluid compartments is the first process of disposition after injection. It is then probably concentrated in most body tissues, especially the brain; finally, it is stored in body fat depots. Subsequently, it is transported to the liver where it undergoes metabolic degradation. This process is more rapid than with thiopental, and excretion of the by-products appears

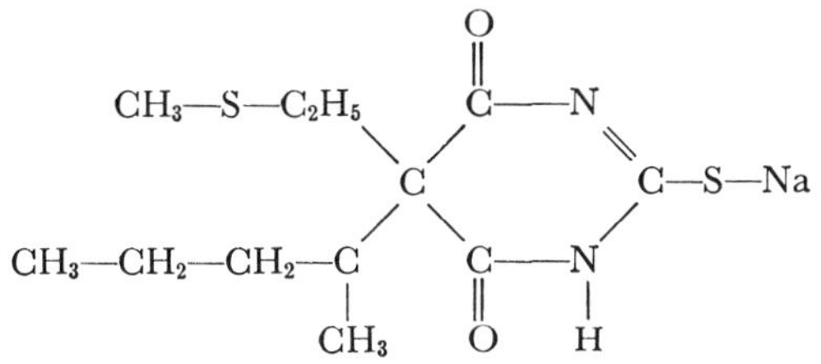

FIG. 25-3. Methitural.

to be more rapid. Hence, cumulative effects are less and awakening is more rapid. There is little of the intact drug excreted in the urine.

ADMINISTRATION AND TECHNIQUE.[11] Preliminary medication is desirable, and all approaches are warranted under specific circumstances. Thus, narcotics, barbiturates, or tranquilizers may be used. Belladonna alkaloids should be administered.

Methitural is administered intravenously, and the techniques are the same as for thiopental. It may be used as the sole anesthetic agent in short procedures but is more commonly employed for induction prior to administration of gaseous anesthetic agents and as a basal supplement for the weaker anesthetic gases. It is also employed like the other intravenous barbiturates to provide hypnosis during regional anesthetic procedures. Anesthetic induction time is longer than with thiopental. Therefore, any instrumentation such as insertion of airways or laryngoscope should not be hurried.

Relaxation is not produced, but the drug is compatible with the curariform agents.

DOSAGE.[7] First, the potency of methitural is one half that of thiopental. Larger doses are required to produce comparable levels of anesthesia. On a weight basis, approximately 50% to 100% more methitural is needed than thiopental.[5] Both the intermittent technique using concentrated solutions and the continuous drip technique using dilute solutions are employed.

For intermittent administration, the most satisfactory concentration is 2.5%. Higher concentrations are quite irritating to veins and tissues. For induction, 4 or 5 ml of this 2.5% solution are injected at intervals of 30 seconds to 1 minute. Usually, a total dose of 200 to 600 mg is sufficient to produce anesthesia in most patients.

The maintenance doses are 2 or 3 ml of the 2.5% solution injected at intervals determined by the signs of diminishing depth of anesthesia.

For continuous administration as a basal and supplemental anesthesia, a 0.5% to 0.8% solution is employed. More dilute solutions will frequently result in the administration of excessive amounts of fluid.

The total dose of methitural should not exceed 2 g in the average patient in good physical status.

COMPLICATIONS.[12] The side effects are those of intravenous barbiturates in general (Table 25-3). The incidence and severity are proportional to the dose and are likely to be seen when excessive doses or overdoses are administered. Included are respiratory depression and apnea, hypoxia, hypotension, laryngospasm, and occasionally excitement. Parasympathomimetic effects such as hiccups, coughing, and laryngospasm are more frequent than with thiopental. Hiccups are particularly disturbing. These effects together with prolonged induction time and more frequent venous irritation constitute disadvantages.

ADVANTAGES. Awakening is slightly faster than from thiopental. Included in the list of advantages are more rapid detoxication; less accumulation; more rapid recovery and quicker return to self-care; and less postanesthetic hangover.

CONTRAINDICATIONS.[13] These are both relative and absolute, depending on patient conditions and are similar to the other barbiturates. The drug should be used cautiously in patients with dyspnea, respiratory obstruction, severe hypotension or hypertension, anemia, and myocardial disease. It is best avoided in patients with emphysema, cardiac decompensation, or extreme obesity. It is contraindicated in patients with severe asthma, shock, or hepatic dysfunction.

CONCLUSION. This intravenous thiobarbiturate has no advantage over thiopental. It is not used in the United States.

HEXOBARBITAL (OXYBARBITURATE)

Hexobarbital (Evipal) was introduced in Germany, and the first clinical report was made by Weese in 1932.[14] It was the first ultra short-acting barbiturate

TABLE 25-3. COMPARISON OF EFFECTS IN HUMANS AFTER A SINGLE 0.5 G DOSE OF FOUR INTRAVENOUS BARBITURATES

	Cough (%)	Hiccoughs (%)	Duration of Sleep (min)	Relative Potency	Onset
Buthalitone	86	50	33	0.37	Fast
Methitural	22	24	30	0.5	Slow
Methohexital	6	12	13	1.5	Very fast
Thiopental	6	12	32	1	Fast

From Wyant, G.M., Dobkin, A.B., and Aascheim, C.M.: Comparison of seven anesthetic agents in man. Br. J. Anaesth., 29:194, 1957.

to be accepted for clinical use and was far superior to any of its predecessors. It differs in formula from the currently used agents in lacking the sulphur atom and being an oxybarbiturate.

COMPLICATIONS. The complications to be found with hexobarbital are those commonly associated with intravenous barbiturates in general, but are significantly more frequent.

1. Respiratory depression, depending on dose
2. Cardiocirculatory depression of varying degrees
3. Muscular twitching in 1% or more of cases
4. Local irritation
5. Hiccoughs and sneezing are common and appear early during the induction period
6. Laryngospasm is more common than with thiopental
7. Excitement on emergence is seen more frequently than with other intravenous barbiturates and is noteworthy in young robust men
8. Depression of the carotid sinus appears to lag behind general anesthesia of the central nervous system.

CONCLUSION. This drug exhibits significant disadvantages. Because both thiopental and methohexital are superior agents, the use of evipal has been discontinued, and it is presented only as a step in the history of intravenous anesthesia.

METHOHEXITAL (A METHYLATED OXYBARBITURATE)

Many attempts have been made, and are continuing, to find an ultra short-acting barbiturate with greater potency and shorter duration of action than thiopental.

In 1954, a new oxybarbiturate was introduced which appeared to have promise as an intravenous agent. It was prepared in the Eli Lilly Laboratories and first clinically investigated by Stoelting.[15] An undesirable effect was the pronounced central nervous stimulation. Further studies revealed that the new agent was composed of two pairs of stereoisomers designated as *alpha* and *beta*. The beta-pair was responsible for the central nervous stimulation and the skeletal muscle activity; on the other hand, the alpha-pair produced excellent anesthesia with few side effects. The sodium salt of the *alpha* isomers is methohexital (Brevital).

CHEMISTRY. This compound is an N-methylated oxybarbiturate (Fig. 25–4). The chemical name of this compound is *alpha* dl-5-(1-methyl allyl) 5-(1-methyl-2-pentynyl) barbituric acid sodium. In contrast to the thiobarbiturates, the oxygen remains attached to 2-carbon. The alpha isomers are the high melting-point isomers.

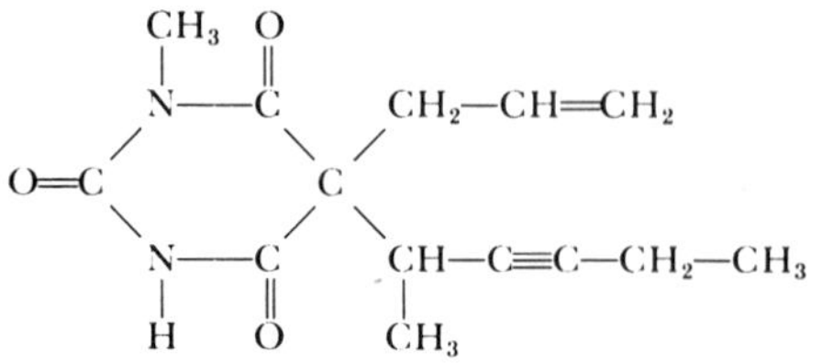

FIG. 25–4. Methohexital.

Methohexital is a white crystalline powder that is readily soluble in water, and such solutions remain stable for at least 6 weeks at room temperature. The pH of the aqueous solution is approximately 11.0% and is highly alkaline.

PREPARATIONS. The common commercial preparation is the powder available in bottles containing 500 mg to which 30 mg of anhydrous sodium carbonate has been added. The agent is employed for intravenous use in either a 1% or 2% solution, and little difference in results can be noted between the use of the two strengths.

The pH of the aqueous solution is highly alkaline (10 to 11) and is hypotonic. After initial dissolving of the powder in distilled water, which may be hazy, the final dilution should preferably be in isotonic saline or 5% dextrose. The final solution should be clear and colorless.

For intramuscular use, a 5% solution in isotonic saline is used. For rectal administration in children, 10% isotonic saline solution is employed.

Ionization Constant.[16] The aqueous solution is almost completely ionized because methohexital, like other barbiturates, is a weak acid. The dissociation constant pKa is 7.9 to 8.3. At this pH, 50% is nonionized and readily crosses cellular membranes such as the blood-brain barrier. At the lower plasma pH of 7.4, methohexital is nonionized, up to 75%, and hence more rapidly crosses cellular membranes.

PHARMACOLOGIC ACTIONS. Central nervous system depression results from the administration of methohexital. Depending on the dose, this effect ranges from sedation through hypnosis to a state of anesthesia. Both respiratory depression and circulatory depression are produced in the typical manner of other barbiturates. The respiratory depression and state of apnea, when produced, are usually not as prolonged.[15a]

The induction of the anesthetic state is more rapid than with thiopental when the end point of sleep achievement for the two are compared.[15b]

The duration of action is shorter by about one half, and the recovery is more rapid than from thiopental. Cumulative effects are much less. In laboratory rats, the lethal dose (LD_{50}) was determined as 31 mg/kg, whereas the anesthetic dose (AD_{50}) was 14 mg/kg.

ENDOCRINE EFFECTS. Most of these changes appear to occur as the anesthetic wears off and the patient recovers.[17]

- A significant increase in epinephrine at end of operation occurs.
- After surgery, the mean cortisol levels increase from about 12 to 20 µg/dl, but by 6 hours postoperatively, the levels decrease to levels of about 10 µg/dl.
- Adrenocorticotrophic hormone levels increase following surgery to 16 pmol/L from 9.0 pmol/L preoperatively. There follows a steady decline to baseline levels, and at 6 hours the average is 12.5 pmol/L and reaches 10 pmol/L by 20 hours.
- Beta-endorphin increases during surgery, and at the end of surgery increases from 6 pmol/L preoperatively to 14 pmol/L. There is a steady decline to baseline levels by 20 hours.

METABOLISM. Liver oxidative enzymes are necessary for the destruction of this compound, with the formation of an alcohol metabolite. Breakdown is more rapid than for thiopental, which accounts for rapid action and recovery. As a first step in biotransformation, hydroxylation occurs at the carbon adjacent to the terminal pentyl side chain.[18] Some N-dealkylation also occurs.

Many of the thiobarbiturates owe their short-acting property principally to tissue distribution. In contrast, the N-methylbarbiturates, such as methohexital, are rapidly metabolized.

ADMINISTRATION AND TECHNIQUES. Preliminary medication with a sedative or hypnotic drug is essential, and a belladonna is a standard component. A combination of meperidine and atropine provides the smoothest induction with the fewest undesirable effects. Patients given inadequate medication frequently develop hiccoughing and mild muscular twitching.

The drug is administered intravenously in the manner of other barbiturates. Both the intermittent techniques with concentrated solutions and the continuous technique with dilute solutions are used, depending on the indications. It may be used as the sole agent for brief procedures or as an induction agent, in which case the concentrated solution is employed.

DOSAGE. All investigations indicate that methohexital is more potent than thiopental; indeed, comparative studies show that it is the most potent intravenous barbiturate, being about three times as potent as thiopental and about four times as potent as thiamylal. Careful measurements show a potency ratio of methohexital to thiopental of 3.3 to 1.[15b,15c]

For intermittent intravenous injection, a 1% solution is sufficient. This is prepared in normal saline (0.5 g in 50 ml). For **induction,** the dose is 1 to 2 mg/kg of body weight, administered at a rate of 1 ml every 5 seconds. This dose provides anesthetic sleep for 5 to 7 minutes. Approximately 50 to 100 mg is needed, with an average dose of 70 mg for a premedicated adult man weighing 70 kg.[19a,19b]

Maintenance by intermittent injection requires the administration of about 10 to 25 mg every 5 minutes. This frequency is largely due to the short duration of action and is somewhat disadvantageous. The continuous drip technique is more convenient.

For sedation anesthesia (basal sleep), continuous drip administration of a 0.1% or 0.2% solution is preferred. This strength is in keeping with the potency of the drug and is effective in attaining any desired state of anesthetization satisfactorily. Induction is accomplished with a rapid rate of drip (a microdrip filter is recommended) until 100 mg has been administered. An effective maintenance dose (ED_{95}) is calculated as 75 µg/kg/min. Maintenance may then be accomplished by administration of 2 to 5 mg/min.

Total dosage recommended is approximately 500 mg for healthy adults with continuous technique.

The intramuscular route is used to produce sedation and basal sleep and is useful in pediatric practice. The dose is 10 mg/kg. For rectal administration to produce sedation, the dose is 25 mg/kg.

PHARMACOKINETICS IN ADULTS.[21–23] The kinetic data for most patients are characterized by a triexponential equation. Mean plasma concentrations versus time provide a representative decay curve, as illustrated in Figure 25–5. Distribution kinetics following a mean dose of 2.4 mg/kg show an initial rapid decline in concentration, with an alpha half-life phase of 5.6 minutes. This includes intravascular mixing, distribution to highly vascular tissues, and localization in such organs as the brain, liver, and heart. This is followed by a slow distribution into tissues with intermediate vascularity, modified by initial drug metabolism, the beta phase with a half-life of almost 60 minutes. The elimination phase represents both redistribution from tissues into the circulation and metabolism, with a half-life of about 4 hours. The kinetic data are summarized in Table 25–4.

The central compartment into which the drug is initially distributed has a value of 0.35 L/kg of body weight. The volume of distribution at steady state has been determined to be 2.2 L/kg after a single bolus dose of methohexital.

Clearance is defined as the volume of plasma from which a drug is completely removed in a unit of time. This affects elimination half-time, which is inversely proportional to clearance. For methohexital, clearance is almost 11 ml/kg/min. This value is similar to previous studies by Breimer,[20] who suggested that the high clearance was due to metabo-

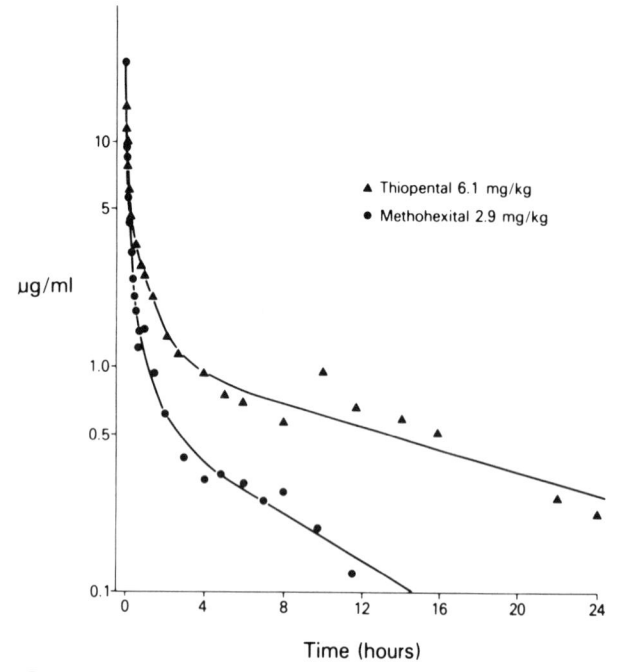

FIG. 25–5. Representative plasma concentration *versus* time curves for methohexital and thiopental. The symbols indicate the measured concentrations; the adjacent lines are the polyexponential functions fit to the data by nonlinear regression. From Hudson, R.J., Stanski, D.R., and Burch, P.G.: Pharmacokinetics of methohexital and thiopental in surgical patients. Anesthesiology, 59:215, 1983.

TABLE 25–4. PHARMACOKINETIC PARAMETERS OF METHOHEXITAL AND THIOPENTAL

	Methohexital*	Thiopental*
Dose (mg · kg^{-1})	2.4 ± 0.4§	6.7 ± 0.7
Distribution half-lives (min)		
Rapid†	5.6 ± 2.7	8.5 ± 6.1
Slow‡	58.3 ± 24.6	62.7 ± 30.4
Elimination half-life (h)	3.9 ± 2.1¶	11.6 ± 6.0
Clearance (ml · kg^{-1} · min^{-1})	10.9 ± 3.0§	3.4 ± 0.5
Vc (L · kg^{-1})	0.35 ± 0.10	0.38 ± 0.09
Vdss (L · kg^{-1})	2.2 ± 0.7	2.5 ± 1.0

* Values are mean ± SD.
† The initial distribution phase for patients with both biexponential and triexponential plasma decay curves.
‡ The slow distribution phase for the three patients given methohexital and the eight patients given thiopental exhibiting triexponential kinetics.
§ $P < 0.001$.
¶ $P < 0.005$.
Abbreviations: Vc, volume of clearance; Vdss, volume of distribution at steady state.
From Hudson, R.J., Stanski, D.R., and Burch, P.G.: Pharmacokinetics of methohexital and thiopental in surgical patients. Anesthesiology, 59:215, 1983.

lism of the drug. It is noted that this clearance is three to four times greater than for thiopental.

Metabolism of methohexital occurs in the liver, and the high clearance is due to a high extraction of the drug from the circulation, indicating rapid metabolism. Because the clearance is dependent directly on blood flow, the extraction ratio for methohexital clearance/hepatic blood flow is about 0.5, indicating that the liver metabolizes one half of the amount of this drug passing through it in a unit of time, as reported by Hudson.[21]

The elimination half-time for methohexital is about 4 hours. This is compared with the elimination phase of thiopental of about 12 hours. Those values indicate the rapid degradation of methohexital and a slower degradation of thiopental.

Termination of the anesthetic effect of barbiturates generally is due to both metabolism and the redistribution of the drug. The cumulative amount of drug removed from the central compartment by metabolism relative to the total amount lost due to both metabolism and redistribution has been calculated by Hudson.[21] At 1 minute, the metabolic loss/total loss ratio for methohexital was about 0.30 and for thiopental about 0.15. At 30 minutes, the ratios were found to be a mean of 0.38 for methohexital and 0.22 for thiopental. Although metabolism plays the major role in the termination of methohexital anesthesia, redistribution of drug from sequestration in peripheral tissues in the brain is a significant factor. The rapid metabolism of methohexital, however, accounts for the more rapid recovery, including psychomotor function.

PHARMACOKINETICS IN CHILDREN

Kinetics of Intravenous Administration.[22] On intravenous administration of a bolus induction dose of 1 to 2 mg/kg methohexital in a 1% solution, studies of kinetics show a three-compartment disposition of the drug (Fig. 25–6). The mean half-life of the initial rapid alpha phase of distribution into the central vascular compartment (a pi phase) and into the vascular-rich tissues was found to be 2.4 minutes.

The mean half-life of the slow beta phase of distribution into tissues with an intermediate vascularity, e.g., muscle, was found to be 23 minutes.

The elimination or terminal half-life was found to be 3.2 hours and designated as the *gamma phase*. This is similar to the time found by Hudson[21] and by Ghoneim[23] of 3.9 hours in adults.

Mean volume of distribution at steady state value was determined to be 2.1 L/kg. This confirms the value reported by others of 2.2 L/kg.[21,23]

Clearance of methohexital in children of about 18 ml/min/kg is considerably higher than the adult clearance of 9 to 11 ml/kg/min.

Kinetics of Intramuscular Administration.[24] Methohexital can be used to provide sedation and basal sleep anesthesia for minor surgical procedures

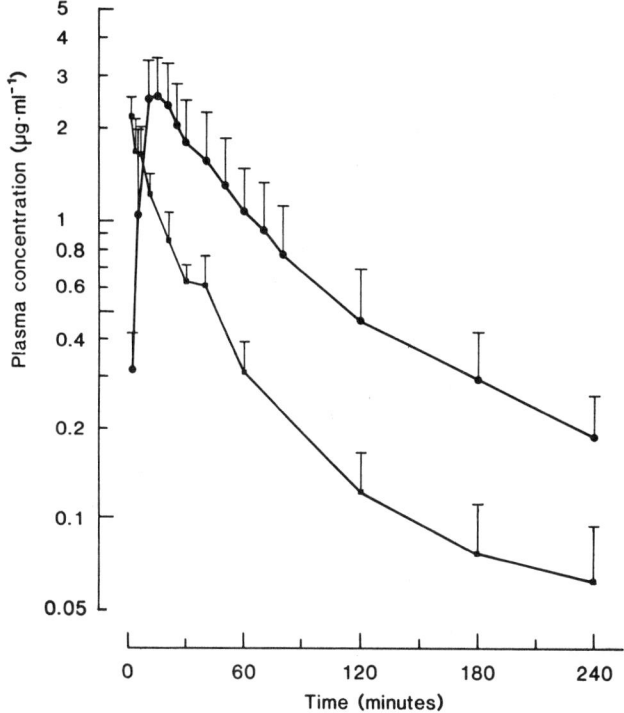

FIG. 25–6. The mean plasma concentration curves of methohexitone after rectal (*upper curve*) or IV (*lower curve*) administration. To permit calculations of means, the plasma concentrations found on IV administration in patients I, V and VI have been corrected for dose by multiplications by 1.5, 0.94, and 0.75, respectively. The bars mark the standard deviation in each point. Because of difficulties in blood sampling before the onset of anesthesia, the first three points in the rectal curve are based on two, five, and six measurements only. From Bjorkman, S., et al: Pharmacokinetics of IV and rectal methohexitone in children. Br. J. Anaesth., 59:1541, 1987.

and permits local anesthetic injection in infants and children where only quiet sleep is needed. A 5% solution (50 mg/ml) is injected into the vastus lateralis muscle. A dose of 10 mg/kg produces the desired effect. Only small volumes are needed with a 5% solution (for a 10-kg infant, 100 mg is the dose, and only 2 ml solution is injected), and the trauma due to relatively large volumes of dilute solutions is eliminated. Sleep and a motionless state are easily achieved. The time from injection to immobilization averages 3 minutes. Time to recovery, denoted by arousal due to stimulation, averaged 50 minutes. An awake and alert state is achieved in about 90 minutes.

Kinetics of Rectal Administration.[22]
This is a well-established technique for children and routine in some practices. A 10% saline solution is used for rectal instillation, and a dose of 25 mg/kg is calculated for induction. The bioavailability of methohexital by this route is 17%, with a sixfold variation among individuals. (For intravenous doses, there is a 2.5-fold difference in bioavailability.) Absorption from the rectum is rapid, with a mean half-time of about 5 minutes (4.6 ± 2.7 minutes).

The kinetic parameters for methohexitone per rectum in children are as follows: $T_{\frac{1}{2}}$ alpha of 4.6 min; $T_{\frac{1}{2}}$ beta of 17 min; and elimination or $T_{\frac{1}{2}}$ gamma of 150 min. At the end of 4 hours, a considerable plasma level is still present, averaging 0.2 μg/ml.

RECOVERY OF FUNCTION. Clinical recovery has been studied by Green.[25a] Immediate recovery of gross functions is relatively rapid—sitting withdrawal reaction, patient's subjective feelings, and opening eyes and response to commands occurs between 6 and 10 minutes with methohexital and 12 and 20 minutes after thiopental.

Measurements by Kortilla[25b] of psychomotor performance including simulated driving, however, show significant impaired performance in the tests of up to 8 hours with either methohexital or thiopental. It is recommended that patients not drive for 24 hours.

COMPLICATIONS. Peculiar to this drug is the frequency of hiccoughing and muscular twitching. When used as the sole agent (no premedication), induction with methohexital is denoted by hiccoughing (41%), coughing (1%), sneezing (5%), and muscle tremors and movements (35%). The incidence is related to the type of preanesthetic medication, the rate of injection, and the induction dose.

Furthermore, inadequate or no premedication seems to predispose to the muscular twitching. These muscular responses and the tremors can usually be controlled by additional amounts of methohexital or by deepening anesthesia with other agents. At no time are they characterized as clonic epileptiform convulsions. They are not to be confused with second-stage signs. A rapid rate of injection predisposes to the above complications. If hypnotic and sleep doses are administered over a period of at least 1 minute, few patients exhibit these untoward effects. A dose-response relationship seems to exist. After atropine premedication, excitatory phenomena occur in twice as many patients given a single initial dose twice the sleep dose.

The usual effects of large doses of barbiturates are to be seen with methohexital, especially on the respiratory system. Because of the great potency of this agent, respiratory depression and apnea are easily produced and are more severe than with thiopental. If these occur when reasonable doses are administered, they are usually transient, lasting up to 3 minutes, and spontaneous respirations are quickly established. In the meantime, intermittent positive pressure breathing is used. Laryngospasm is infrequent.

Adverse cardiovascular effects are minimal. In ordinary doses, little depression of blood pressure is noted.

Pain at the site of injection or along the course of the vein is a complaint in 60% of the patients. The intensity varies but usually evokes bitter complaint from the patient. There seems to be a pronounced amnesia to this side effect, however. High concentrations may cause red blood cell hemolysis, platelet aggregation, and crystal formation. This predisposes to intravascular thrombosis.

INDICATIONS. The indications for methohexital use include the following:

1. For induction, it provides advantages over thiopental of little cumulative effect and minimal hangover.
2. It may be used more safely than other barbiturates for patients in the upright position (neurosurgery; dental surgery) because of minimal *cardiocirculatory depression.*
3. It is preferred over other barbiturates in liver disease because of lack of hepatotoxic responses.
4. It may be given intramuscularly (pediatrics).
5. There is an absence of venous sequelae.
6. It has advantages over other barbiturates as ambulatory surgical anesthesia due to its shorter duration of action.

OTHER ULTRA SHORT-ACTING BARBITURATES

THIALBARBITAL (KEMITHAL). This drug was synthetized in 1938 by Carrington[26] and its pharmacology reviewed in 1946. It is an interesting compound chemically, because one of the radicals attached to the 5 carbon atom of the barbituric acid is a cyclic moiety, a cyclo hexenyl radical (Fig. 25–7). It is a yellow hygroscopic powder that is readily soluble in water.

Pharmacologic actions are similar to thiopental and are about half as potent. Although less respiratory depression is claimed by some, this is not confirmed by blind and other studies. The method of administration is similar to thiopental. The preparation used is a 5% to 10% water solution.

SPIROBARBITURIC ACIDS. In the hope of obtaining an improved drug, a number of spiro derivatives were prepared by Eli Lilly and studied by Swanson.[27] The common barbiturates are disubstitution products in the 5-position of the barbituric acid molecule. These spiro compounds contain a pyrimidine constituent attached to the 5-position carbon of barbituric acid. The nucleus is inactive, but when side chains are attached to the pyrimidine portion, activity develops.

THIOHEXITAL. This is an experimental thiobarbiturate designated as 22,113 Lilly (Fig. 25–8) and has been studied by Mark and Brand.[27a] It is similar to methylhexatone but is a thio derivative without the methyl side chain. It is the most rapidly intravenously metabolized barbiturate. This agent is a racemic mixture of the d- and l-forms. It induces unconsciousness quickly as with other intravenous barbiturates but is denoted by an exceptionally rapid rate of metabolism and rapid reawakening. The rate of metabolism averages 26% per hour (against 15% per hour for thiopental). Thus, it may become a useful agent for ambulatory surgical practice. Some undesirable effects include muscle twitching, tremors and hiccoughs. These are largely obviated by heavier premedication. The agent is administered intermittently or by drip.

These other ultra short-acting barbiturates have hypnotic and some anesthetic action but no analgesic action. They are shorter acting than oxybarbiturates but longer than thiobarbiturates.[28]

A high incidence of bronchospasm has been reported, and at present there are no evident advantages in these drugs and their clinical use has been discontinued (see Table 25–3).

COMPARISON OF INTRAVENOUS BARBITURATES[29,30]

Many new agents of the barbiturate series have been and are being introduced. Claims of advantages over the classic thiopental have been made. It is considered that most of these are only impressions. Two excellent comparative studies have been made, and it is evident that clinical differences between the newer substitutes and thiopental are not marked.

A careful comparison of thiopental and thiamylal in humans revealed the following statistical differences:[4]

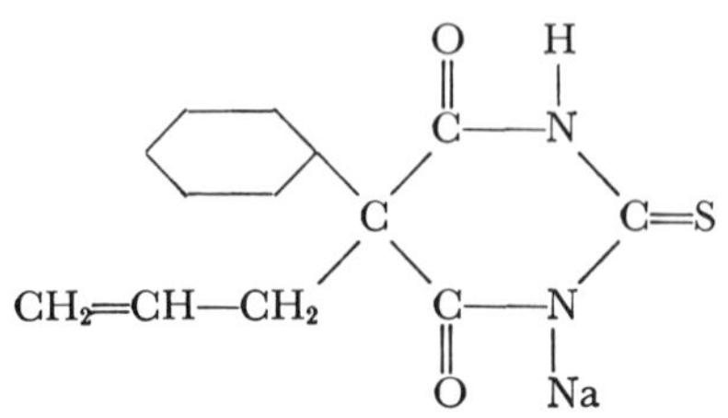

FIG. 25–7. Thialbarbital.

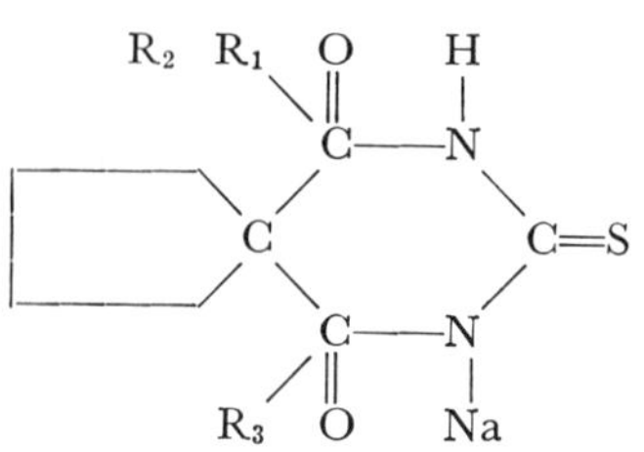

FIG. 25–8. Thiohexital.

TABLE 25-5. COMPARISON OF INTRAVENOUS BARBITURATES

	Cardiac Output (%)	Temperature, Pulse, Respiration (%)	Basal Metabolic Rate (%)
Thiopental (Pentothal)	− 4	−10	−33
Thiamylal (Surital)	+ 6	−12	−29
Hexobarbital (Evipal)	+20	−21	− 6
Methitural (Nerval)	− 6	− 6	−25
Buthalitone (Transital)	−11	+ 3	−23
Methohexital (Brevital)	−15	+17	−25

From Wyant, G.M., Dobkin, A.B., and Aascheim, C.M.: Comparison of seven anesthetic agents in man. Br. J. Anaesth., 29:194, 1957.

1. Greater elevation of blood pressure during maintenance period with thiamylal.
2. A greater amount of thiopental needed for induction to a standard end point, namely, the condition to intubate; however, further analysis based on amount of drug per pound per minute showed little difference.
3. Longer duration of laryngospasm for thiamylal.
4. Higher incidence of dizziness during recovery for thiamylal.

These differences are of little clinical significance.

A careful comparison of seven of the currently popular intravenous agents has been carried out to determine differences (Table 25-5; see also Table 25-3).[30] The following conclusions were reached: Thiopental and thiamylal have almost identical properties and effects. When given in large doses, they are not ultra short-acting barbiturates.

Hexobarbitone, buthalitone, and methitural are markedly shorter-acting agents than the thiopental. The variability in responses, plus the unevenness of the anesthesia, however, represent significant disadvantages. Dolitione, although satisfactory in providing anesthesia, is rather unpredictable and tends to cause phlebitis. It is considered that buthalitone and methitural may have a place in outpatient practice because there is a quicker awakening and absence of disorientation. However, the features of spontaneous muscular movements and hiccoughing are disadvantages that may be tolerated. Hexobarbitone appears to produce the greatest respiratory and cardiovascular changes.

REFERENCES

1. Tabern, D.V., and Volwiler, E.W.: Sulfur-containing barbiturate hypnotics. J. Am. Chem. Soc., 57:1961, 1935.
2. Helrich, M., Papper, E.M., and Rovenstine, E.A.: Surital Sodium: A new anesthetic agent for intravenous use—Preliminary clinical evaluation. Anesthesiology, 11:33, 1950.
3. Stephen, C.R., Martin, R., and Nowill, W.K.: Cardiovascular reactions of Surital, pentothal or Evipal combined with muscle relaxants for rapid anesthesia induction. Anesth. Analg., 32:361, 1953.
4. Tovell, R.M., et al: A comparative clinical and statistical study of thiopental and thiamylal in human anesthesia. Anesthesiology, 16:91, 1955.
5. Boone, J.D., Munoz, R., and Dillon, J.B.: Neraval Sodium: A new ultra short-acting thiobarbiturate—Preliminary clinical investigations. Anesthesiology, 17:284, 1956.
6. Council on Drugs, American Medical Association. Methitural. J.A.M.A., 166:1328, 1958.
7. Miller, E., et al: Thiobarbiturates. J. Am. Chem. Soc., 58:1090, 1930.
8. Richard, R.K., and Taylor, J.D.: Some factors influencing distribution, metabolism and action of barbiturates: A review. Anesthesiology, 17:414, 1956.
9. Zima, O., von Werder, F., and Hotovy, R.: Sodium methylthioethyl-2-pentyl thiobarbiturate (Thiogenal), a new short-acting intravenous anesthetic. Anaesthetist, 3:244, 1954.
10. Blake, M.W., and Perlman, P.L.: Metabolism of the ultra short-acting thiobarbiturate, methitural (Neraval). J. Pharmacol. Exper. Ther., 117:287, 1956.
11. Fitzpatrick, L.J., Clairie, D'A.C., and Mersch, M.A.: Methitural sodium (Neraval Sodium): A new ultra-short-acting intravenous anesthetic. Anesthesiology, 17:684, 1956.
12. Dobkin, A.B., and Wyant, G. M.: The physiological effects of intravenous anesthesia in man. Can. Anaesth. Soc. J., 4:295, 1957.
13. O'Mullane, E.J.: The investigation of a short-acting barbiturate illustrating the fallacies of clinical impression. Br. J. Anaesth., 29:71, 1957.
14. Weese, H., and Scharpff, W.: Evipan, ein neuartiges Einschloffmitte. Deutsche med. Wchnschr., 2:1205, 1932.
15. Stoelting, V.K.: The use of a new intravenous oxygen barbiturate 25398 for intravenous anesthesia: a preliminary report. Anesth. Analg., 36:49, 1957.
15a. Thomas, E.T.: The relative potencies of methohexitone and thiopentone. Anaesthesia, 22:16, 1967.
15b. Clarke, R.S.J., Dundee, J.W., Barron, D.W., et al: Clinical studies of induction agents. XXVI: The relative potencies of thiopentone, methohexitone and propanidid. Br. J. Anaesth., 40:593, 1968.
16. Brodie, B.B., Kurz, H., and Schanker, L.S.: The importance of dissociation constant and lipidsolubility in influencing the passage of drugs into the cerebrospinal fluid. J. Pharmacol. Exp. Ther., 130:22, 1960.
17. Crozier, T.A., et al: Endocrinological changes following etomidate, midazolam, or methohexital. Anesthesiology, 66:628, 1987.
18. Burns, J.J.: Role of Biotransformation. *In* Uptake and Distribution of Anesthetic Agents. New York, McGraw-Hill, 1963.
19a. Taylor, C., and Stoelting, V.K.: Methohexital sodium—a new ultra short-acting barbiturate. Anesthesiology, 21:29, 1960.
19b. Dundee, J.W., Riding, J.E., Barron, D.W., et al: Some factors influencing the induction characteristics of methohexitone anesthesia. Br. J. Anaesth., 33:296, 1961.
20. Bremier, D.D.: Pharmacokinetics of methohexitone following intravenous infusion in humans. Br. J. Anaesth., 48:643, 1976.
21. Hudson, R.J., Stanski, D.R., and Burch, P.G.: Pharmacokinetics of methohexital and thiopental in surgical patients. Anesthesiology, 59:215, 1983.
22. Bjorkman, S., et al: Pharmacokinetics of i.v. and rectal methohexitone in children. Br. J. Anaesth., 59:1541, 1987.
23. Ghoneim, M.M., et al: The pharmacokinetics of metho-

hexital in young and elderly subjects. Acta Anaesthesiol. Scand., 29:480, 1985.
24. Varner, P.D., et al: Methohexital sedation of children undergoing CT scan. Anesth. Analg., 64:643, 1985.
25a. Green, R., Long, H.A., Elliott, C.J.R., et al: A method of studying recovery after anaesthesia: A critical assessment of recovery following methohexitone and thiopentone using a complex performance task. Anaesthesia, 18:189, 1963.
25b. Kortilla, K., et al: Recovery and simulated driving after intravenous anesthesia with thiopental, methohexital, propanidid, or alphadione. Anesthesiology, 43:291, 1975.
26. Carrington, H.C., and Raventos, J.: Kemithal: A new intravenous anesthetic. Br. J. Pharmacol., 1:215, 1946.
27. Swanson, E.E., et al: Pharmacology of spiro-barbituric and spiro-thiobarbituric acids. Curr. Res. Anesth., 29:89, 1950.
27a. Mark, L.C., et al: Studies with thiohexital, an anesthetic barbiturate metabolized with unusual rapidity in man. Anesthesiology, 29:1159, 1968.
28. Volpitto, P.P.: Experiences with ultra short-acting intravenous barbiturates combined with decamethonium bromide for endotracheal intubation. Anesthesiology, 12:648, 1951.
29. Gruber, C.M., et al: Comparison of ultra short-acting barbiturate (22451) with thiobarbiturates during anesthesia. Anesthesiology, 18:50, 1957.
30. Wyant, G.M., Dobkin, A.B., and Aascheim, C.M.: Comparison of seven anesthetic agents in man. Br. J. Anaesth., 29:194, 1957.

26

INTRAVENOUS ANESTHESIA: NARCOTIC AND NEUROLEPTIC–NARCOTIC AGENTS

INTRAVENOUS OPIATES

Opiates may be used intravenously to provide a basal narcotic state or as a supplement to anesthetics with marginal potency, such as nitrous oxide or ethylene. In addition, it is possible to achieve a state of anesthesia sufficient to perform surgical procedures with the opiates alone intravenously.

Of the opiates employed, three have been attended by success. These are (1) morphine, (2) meperidine, and (3) its derivatives including fentanyl, sufentanil, and alfentanil. This chapter concerns the technical application of these drugs intravenously.

ANESTHETIC POTENCY CONCEPT OF OPIOIDS: MIC-BAR. A concept of potency has been proposed by Wynands[1] that is designated *MIC-BAR* (see Inhalation Anesthesia-MAC-BAR Chap. 16)[2] and defined as the minimal (intraarterial) plasma concentration of an opiate that will prevent a hypertensive response to a standard noxious stimulus in 50% of patients.[3,4] This plasma concentration is thus considered to block adrenergic response (BAR) to a stressful surgical stimulus.[5]

The attempt to determine the actual plasma concentration of morphine or fentanyl to achieve the above in patients undergoing aortacoronary artery bypass has failed to establish such a blood level. Even arterial plasma levels of 30 ng/ml after a dose of 50 μg/kg or after doses of 100 μg/kg failed to block adrenergic response in less than 50% of patients. It is considered that narcotics at any dose may not be able to block adrenergic responses.

INTRAVENOUS LOW-DOSE MORPHINE

Morphine has been used intravenously to provide basal narcosis and to supplement impotent inhalation agents. Van Hooersen[6] first described the use of divided doses of morphine as a preanesthetic medication technique to be followed by the administration of nitrous oxide. By this means, a nonasphyxial technique is possible, and mixture of 50% to 75% nitrous oxide with oxygen becomes effective.[7]

ADMINISTRATION. As a supplement, morphine has been most effective and safe when administered by the intermittent method or fractional doses. Clinical experience demonstrates that a basal level can be provided at the beginning and thenceforth little or no additional drugs are required for operations of approximately 3 hours' duration. Brotman[8] found that of the total morphine supplement, over 95% was administered at induction. (In contrast, meperidine requires additional doses for maintenance.) The solution of morphine used as a 0.1% concentration with 1 mg in each ml.

DOSAGE. For basal narcosis in the preanesthetic period, usually two doses are administered. Both may be given slowly intravenously or the first may be given intramuscularly.

1. The first dose varies from 10 to 15 mg administered 1 hour preanesthetically.
2. The second dose is administered intravenously 45 minutes later, and this dose is determined by the status of the patient and the reaction to the first dose.
3. On the patient's arrival in the operating room, an additional intravenous dose may be required.
4. After basal narcosis is established, anesthesia is developed with nitrous oxide and oxygen.

If the interval between doses is at least 20 minutes, there will be no significant overlapping of respiratory depressant effects. It is also noteworthy that when the operation is begun, the respiratory rate invariably resumes a more normal level. The average dose for 3-hour procedures is about 35 mg.

After the establishment of anesthesia, doses of 2 to 5 mg of morphine may be injected intravenously every 45 to 60 minutes. Besides the nitrous oxide–oxygen complement curare or other such agent may be used for relaxation.[9]

DISADVANTAGES. With these doses lack of uniform narcosis, amnesia, and adequate analgesia are the major disadvantage of morphine. Also, there is overlapping of effects, and cumulative effects are observed because the duration of action is relatively long; when given by drip solution, cumulative effects appear. The drug has respiratory and circulatory depressant effects that are pronounced but not as great as with the large-dose technique. Other agents of the meperidine analogues have been investigated.

INTRAVENOUS MEPERIDINE

In 1938, with the development of meperidine as the first completely synthetic narcotic, clinical investigations were initiated to use this agent, instead of morphine, as a basic analgesic for intravenous anesthesia.[10]

PROPERTIES OF MEPERIDINE. Several properties of meperidine make it a desirable agent to be used as a supplement to nitrous oxide. It produces a high degree of analgesia, depresses respiration and circulation less than morphine, and does not have a marked sedative effect. Hence, meperidine allows rapid return to consciousness and mental alertness, has a relatively short duration of the maximal depressant effect (2 hours), and thus offers significant controllability. An adequate anesthetic state can be produced for operations not requiring profound relaxation, and this can be achieved by the administration of nitrous oxide with high concentrations of oxygen (i.e., 25% to 35%).

Return of reflexes is relatively prompt. Postoperatively, pain relief is noted for a long period and the need for additional analgesics in this period is minimized. In addition, the intravenous use of meperidine combined with nitrous oxide–oxygen provides a nonexplosive technique.

ADMINISTRATION. As an intravenous anesthetic supplement, meperidine was first described by Neff in 1947.[10] Clinical experience has established the usefulness of the method; in the United States Brotman[11] and Randal[12] have reported their findings, while in England, Johnson[13] as well as Mushin[14] have noted the advantages. Two methods of administration were advocated: (1) the intermittent or fractional intravenous technique; and (2) continuous drip infusion.

PREPARATION OF SOLUTIONS. For *intermittent injections*, a 1% solution is prepared by diluting 100 mg (2 ml of a 20% ampule) with sterile saline or 5% dextrose up to 10 ml volume in a syringe. This solution contains 10 mg/ml and may be administered through a three-way stopcock or by needle puncture of the sleeve of an intravenous infusion.

For *continuous injection*, a 0.1% solution is prepared by adding 500 mg (or 10 ml of a 20% solution furnished in usual ampules) to 500 ml of 5% dextrose in water. Ausherman[15] recommends the use of a 0.02% to 0.04% solution. This, however, is too dilute and may result in administration of excess fluid.

DOSAGE. In the administration of meperidine to achieve a basal anesthetic state, there are an initial or induction dose and subsequent or maintenance doses.

In general, the dose is determined by patient response and the achievement of the desired effects, namely, adequate surgical working conditions. Also, in general, the continuous drip technique allows better titration of dose against response, which is a refined and more controllable technique, and provides a more uniform level of anesthesia. Experience demonstrates that, for given procedures, the total dose administered will be less by the continuous

TABLE 26–1. DOSAGE OF INTRAVENOUS MEPERIDINE

Method	Induction	Maintenance
Intermittent	50–100 mg (5–10 ml)—average 70 mg	20–40 mg every 20 minutes 100 mg per hr[11]
Continuous	10–50 mg—average 35 mg	0.5 mg per min[10] 30–40 mg per hr[10]

technique as opposed to the fractional (intermittent) method.

TECHNICAL PROCEDURE

1. Premedication consists of:
   a. An intramuscular barbiturate such as sodium amytal 30 minutes to 1 hour preanesthesia.
   b. An intramuscular dose of meperidine according to usual criteria plus appropriate atropine or scopolamine.
2. Establishment of anesthesia
   a. Many clinicians establish anesthesia with an intravenous barbiturate.[7,8,13,14]
   b. Basal analgesia is established by intravenous meperidine, and as the patient becomes drowsy, nitrous oxide–oxygen is administered in a 75–25 mixture.
3. Intravenous meperidine
   a. *Intermittent:* The initial dose is approximately 50 to 100 mg. In healthy patients the larger dose is necessary; in debilitated patients, 50 mg or less may be needed. Nitrous oxide–oxygen mixture is then administered. Maintenance doses are then given every 15 to 20 minutes. An average of about 25 mg should represent a safe single injection.
   b. *Continuous:* The induction dose is administered by allowing the infusion solution to drip at a fast rate until about 25 mg has been introduced in 2 to 3 minutes. The rate is progressively slowed during the next 10 minutes until a maintenance rate of about 0.5 to 1 mg/min is achieved (about 15 drops/min).

INDICATIONS

1. Use in neurosurgery
2. For hip pinning and other orthopedic operations requiring x-ray
3. Cholangiography
4. For operations requiring noninflammable general anesthesia; e.g., cystoscopy
5. For simple operations where intravenous barbiturates are contraindicated
6. In patients with asthma or bronchospastic diseases requiring a mild general anesthesia
7. Intermittent supplementation during cardiac surgery in children[16]
8. Single induction doses for intubation (since laryngospasm and bronchospasm are minimal), and to supplement topical anesthesia for endoscopy[17]
9. In second stage of labor—intermittent intravenous injections 30 to 50 mg in continuous slow infusion of 0.4 mg/min.[18]

INTRAVENOUS ALPHAPRODINE[19]

PROPERTIES. Alphaprodine (Nisentil) is an analogue of meperidine that has a shorter duration of action. The administration of small intravenous doses of alphaprodine reduces the milligrams per minute dose of thiopental and increases the percentage of patients awakening at the end of surgery rather than later.

ANESTHETIC TECHNIQUE. Alphaprodine is administered either by intermittent injection or by continuous drip. The first is more widely used. The dose is calculated as about 1 mg/kg of body weight. After induction of anesthesia with intravenous thiopental, a mixture of nitrous oxide–oxygen is administered by face mask in a semiclosed circuit. Depending on the nature of the surgery, an endotracheal or pharyngeal airway is provided and a relaxant used, if indicated.

The determined dose of alphaprodine is administered. If the depth of anesthesia in 10 minutes is inadequate, additional doses of 5 to 20 mg of alphaprodine are administered 2 to 3 minutes apart until the desired level of anesthesia is obtained. Additional doses are determined by signs of lightening anesthesia (movements of voluntary muscles, breath-holding, irregular breathing, and tachypnea). The interval between supplementary doses of alphaprodine ranges between 10 to 20 minutes.

The mg/min requirement of thiopental is reduced by half when alphaprodine is used as a supplement.

NARCOTIC–BARBITURATE COMBINATION

The use of both a narcotic and a barbiturate such as thiopental (see Chapter 24) to reinforce nitrous oxide–oxygen anesthesia has become a popular technique. It is to be employed where neither the barbiturate nor the narcotic is contraindicated, and this precaution is emphasized. Basically, this combination may be considered a form of anesthesia: hypnosis by barbiturate, analgesia by narcotic, and sleep by anesthesia. Two combinations that have been of value and are more frequently used are thiopental–meperidine–nitrous oxide and thiopental–alphaprodine–nitrous oxide.

TECHNICAL PROCEDURE WITH MEPERIDINE. Premedication is with meperidine in the usual fashion.

1. Induction of anesthesia is accomplished with dilute thiopental solution 0.4% or 0.5% administered by drip. A 2.5% solution may also be used.
2. A basal anesthetic state is maintained by a continuous slow infusion of thiopental or by intermittent injections of small doses.
3. Nitrous oxide–oxygen anesthesia is attained in a 75:25 ratio by semiclosed system or nonrebreathing technique is begun as soon as the patient is asleep from the thiopental.
4. Reinforcement of the nitrous oxide is accomplished by continuous slow infusion of a meperidine drip as previously described. A solution containing 0.5 mg/ml in 5% dextrose is recommended. When the thiopental combination is used simultaneously, the total dose is about 75 mg/hr.[15]

Meperidine administered in this manner enhances the analgesia and definitely reinforces the nitrous oxide. Comparative studies indicate that the amount of thiopental is reduced significantly.

NARCOTIC–ANTAGONIST COMBINATION

Data obtained in animal studies suggest that a narcotic analgesic can be combined with an antagonist in such proportions as will permit the retention of analgesia and the reduction of respiratory depression.[20,21]

In a study of chronic pain, Cullen[22] found that a mixture of 5 mg of levorphan and 0.5 mg of levallorphan provided pain relief with less respiratory depression. Lasagna[23] found that the combination of morphine and nalorphine was less favorable in accomplishing the above goal. Thus, the administration of 10 mg of morphine with 2 mg of nalorphine or 15 mg of morphine and 5 mg of nalorphine did not provide significant attenuation of respiratory depression.

ALPHAPRODINE–LEVALLORPHAN.[24] Respiratory depression is the significant disadvantage of the above technique; however, if the antagonist levallorphan is administered when excessive depression occurs or simultaneously with the initial narcotic dose, there is considerable protection against alphaprodine effects on respiration. The depth of respiration especially is improved. The dose recommended is 0.02 mg/kg of body weight.

The thiopental requirement is two to five times smaller, and there is a reduction in the narcotic requirement when the antagonist is employed.

Significant circulatory changes occur in about 5% of patients chiefly manifested by hypertension. Recovery is fairly rapid, and as expected, patients are free of pain.

LARGE-DOSE INTRAVENOUS MORPHINE TECHNIQUE

The period of 1950 to 1960 was denoted by studies of intravenous meperidine, its analogues, and various combinations. The basic meperidine series of drugs and meperidine combinations itself were unsatisfactory. During the years 1960 to 1970, the development of open cardiac surgery stimulated the need for maintenance of anesthesia during the "pump" period by means other than inhalation anesthetics. Lowenstein[25] introduced the concept that large doses of intravenous morphine could provide a state of anesthesia satisfying the surgical requirements. The technique of large-dose morphine became a popular mode for cardiac surgery anesthesia.[26] A state resembling that of anesthesia was produced without cardiac depression.[27,28]

PREMEDICATION. Patients are premedicated by standard doses of morphine sulfate combined with scopolamine. Such medication is used in patients with heart disease, including valvular disease and coronary artery disease.

DOSAGE. Large doses in the range of 0.5 to 3 mg/kg are employed. The lower dose is used in debilitated patients. The average dose is 1 mg/kg. Doses larger than 3 mg/kg may produce temporary psychotic states.

PHARMACOKINETICS. The pharmacokinetic variables of intravenous morphine are presented in Table 26–2.

ADMINISTRATION. Appropriate monitoring is employed and control base line values determined prior to induction.

Induction. This is accomplished by intravenous administration at a rate of 5 to 10 mg/min. Rates of 10 mg/min or more are associated with hypotension. About half the calculated dose should be administered in the first 3 to 5 minutes and completed in 6 to 30 minutes. Intubation is then accomplished and facilitated with a relaxant. Succinylcholine may be used, combined with pretreatment curare or hexafluorenium, but an antidepolarizing drug is usually

TABLE 26–2. PHARMACOKINETIC VARIABLES
Following Intravenous Morphine

	Stanski	Dahlstrom* (Preoperative) Children
Dilution Phase π (Minutes)	1.25	1.4 ± 0.4
$T_{1/2}$ alpha (minutes)	7.7 (± 1.6)	16 ± 7
$T_{1/2}$ beta (hours)	2.9 hours	3.8 ± 2.3
Total Elimination (hours)	10–44	12–24 hours
Volume Distribution Vd.	3.2 L/kg	6.3 ± 3.L/kg
Clearance Cl_p ml/min/kg	14.7 (± 0.9) (healthy volunteers)	20 ± 7.0
Extraction Ratio	0.7	

*Dahlstroms—Preoperative and postoperative study of effects of anesthesia and surgery. Some significant alteration of clearance; i.e., it is more rapid, but slowed if shock or protracted surgery occurs. Postoperative dynamics show a several-fold variation in morphine analgesic needs.

Data derived from Dahlstrom, B., et al: Morphine kinetics in children. Clin. Pharmacol. Ther., 26:354–365, 1979; Stanski, D.R., et al.: Kinetics of intravenous and intramuscular morphine. Clin. Pharmacol. Ther., 24:52, 1978; and Stanski D.R., et al: Kinetics of high-dose intravenous morphine in cardiac surgery patients. Clin. Pharmacol. Ther., 19:752–756, 1976.

used for maintenance, either *d*-tubocurarine or pancuronium is preferred.

Maintenance. Oxygen up to 100% may be administered without other inhalation anesthetic agents. Nitrous oxide, however, is the principal anesthetic supplement administered by a semiclosed system in a mixture of 60% N_2O–40% oxygen.

Monitoring of both intra-arterial pressure and central venous pressure is mandatory. It is recommended that the central venous catheter actually be placed to measure right ventricular pressure.

For treatment of myocardial insufficiency and hypotension due to the intrinsic cardiac disease, an infusion solution of epinephrine 1 mg in 250 ml isotonic saline should be available and used for most instances of hypotension. The dose is approximately 5 mg/kg.

PHARMACOLOGIC EFFECTS OF LARGE DOSES[25]

1. Profound analgesia occurs not necessarily with loss of consciousness. Good amnesia is induced when adjunctive drugs such as scopolamine and nitrous oxide are added.
2. Liberation of both norepinephrine and epinephrine is increased, which may be salutary in selected debilitated patients with coronary artery disease.
3. No evidence of direct myocardial depression has been adduced. Patients with low cardiac output have improvement in this parameter.
4. Few hemodynamic changes occur, and 1 mg/kg has no significant effect on cardiac output, systemic pulmonary vascular resistance, systemic blood pressure, central venous pressure, or pulse rate in normal healthy subjects.

In severe aortic valvular disease with fixed cardiac output and low cardiac reserve, there is a favorable effect with a decreased systemic vascular resistance and an increased cardiac output. The addition of nitrous oxide modifies the response, however, and a decreased cardiac output occurs along with a decreased systemic vascular resistance.

5. No change in threshold for ectopic ventricular excitation occurs. This is of value in cardiac patients who may need digitalis or cardiac stimulants.

RECOVERY. At the conclusion of surgery, monitoring of all patients must be continued. The following parameters are evaluated.

1. End-tidal CO_2, which should be maintained below 50 mm Hg
2. CO_2 response curve
3. Nerve–muscle response to stimulation
4. Level of consciousness
5. Minute ventilatory value
6. Inspiratory–expiratory force

REVERSAL OF ANESTHETIC DRUGS. Relaxant effects are reversed at the time the anesthesia is discontinued. For curare, the usual effective technique employed is the administration of prostigmine in dose of 4 mg with 1 mg of atropine.

The morphine is reversed by doses of naloxone on the basis of $3–10 \mu g/kg^{-1}$ or a single dose of approximately 0.4 mg.[25a] When given as a single rapid intravenous bolus, diaphoresis, nausea, and vomiting are evoked. Because naloxone duration of action is shorter than that of morphine, two techniques are recommended:[25b]

1. Intermittent: single doses every 1 to 2 hours administered slowly over 1 to 2 minutes
2. Constant infusion: a dilute solution of naloxone of 8 μg/ml is administered. The solution is prepared by adding 4 mg of naloxone (10-ml ampule) to 500 ml of 5% dextrose in water. After an initial or loading dose of 1.5–3.5 $\mu g/kg^{-1}$ in 1 to 2 minutes, the drug is administered at an approximate rate of 3–10 $\mu g/kg^{-1}$/hr. The approximate cumulative requirements for naloxone after 200 mg of morphine are for first hour—0.6 mg; for 6 hours—3 mg; and for 12 hours—6 mg. After 12 hours, little or no naloxone is needed.[25b]

POSTOPERATIVE STATE. Good analgesia and sensory obtundation remain in the postoperative period without circulatory impairment while patient is in the supine position.

ADVANTAGES.

1. No myocardial depression; useful in patients with chronically low cardiac output.
2. Initial dose is sufficient.
3. Ventilation with 100% oxygen is permitted.
4. No potentiation of myocardial irritability occurs.
5. Sympathetic response is intact.
6. Smooth transition to postoperative period is noted.
7. Tolerance of endotracheal tube and easy adaptation to ventilatory control exists for 12 hours.
8. Muscle relaxant effects need not be reversed.
9. Analgesics are rarely needed postoperatively.
10. Morphine is inexpensive.

DISADVANTAGES. Clinical experience revealed significant disadvantages:[25–27]

1. Induction of the morphine "anesthetic state" is slow.
2. Amnesia may not always be complete; scopolamine or a barbiturate may be used to obtund memory in the average patient.[25]
3. Young robust male patients, such as those with coronary artery disease who are to undergo bypass surgery, are not suitable because it is difficult to induce sleep;[29] awareness and memory of the intraoperative events are frequent and disturbing. Doses greater than 3 mg/kg are often needed, and the accompanying physiologic impairment is not acceptable.[25]
4. Inadequate analgesia or suppression of stress responses leads to hypertension.[27]
5. Histamine reactions include cutaneous flushing.
6. Increased airway resistance and bronchoconstriction occur.
7. Cumulative effects include prolonged postoperative respiratory depression.
8. Cardiovascular instability is manifested as frequent bradycardia and hypotension.[27] Hypotension occurs subsequent to head-up posture changes or to rapid rate of injection of the morphine of more than 10 mg/min. In most instances hypotension is related to peripheral vasodilatation and decreased venous return. It is treated by volume fluid infusion.[30]
9. Addition of nitrous oxide increases cardiovascular depression,[28] especially in coronary artery surgery.[29]
10. Intraoperative fluid and blood requirements are increased.[30]
11. Renal disturbances include some reduction of renal blood flow. Any observed diminution of renal function has been temporary. The liberation of antidiuretic hormone appears to be transient and insignificant.
12. Neurologic disturbances include motor movements and temporary but sporadic episodes of memory loss postoperatively. Postoperative psychotic episodes have been noted, but persistent complications have not been observed.

EFFECT OF NARCOTICS OR OPIATES ON STRESS RESPONSES. A stressful stimulus evokes many neuroendocrine responses. These, in turn, produce physiologic reactions. Among the hormones that are released, two of the most important and easily measured are norepinephrine and epinephrine, which produce sympathetic adrenergic reactions.[31] In addition, there is a production of antidiuretic hormone, the arginine vasopressin from the posterior pituitary, and the growth hormone from the posterior pituitary.[31a,31b] Cortisol is released from the adrenal gland,[31b,31c] and there are increases in cyclic adenosine monophosphate and in renin from the kidney.[31d]

Most studies show that none of the neurohormonal responses to a stressful stimulus are completely obtunded by narcotics.[32] (1) Fentanyl doses of 2 to 4 μg/kg as a loading dose does not suppress the increase in plasma vasopressin and the decrease in cortisol that usually occurs consequent to a stressful stimulus.[32a] It has been shown, however, that naloxone does suppress increases in arginine vasopressin.[32b] (2) Large does of fentanyl in the range of 30 to 75 μg/kg of body weight, administered as a loading dose and accompanied by an infusion of 0.3 to 0.75 μg/kg/min, will achieve a plasma fentanyl concentration of 10 to 30 ng/ml or more.[32c] When plasma levels of only 12 to 15 ng/ml are obtained, as by the administration of 30 μg/kg or less, hypertensive episodes are frequent. A dose of 75 μg/kg and a maintenance infusion of 0.75 μg/kg achieve plasma levels of 30 ng/ml or more, and hypertensive episodes are rarely seen during induction of anesthesia. Intubation is usually not accompanied by a hypertensive episode.[5,32c]

Nevertheless, with the large doses of 75 μg/kg and a maintenance dose as previously noted, hypertensive responses are seen on skin incision. Even doses of 100 μg/kg loading and 0.35 μg/kg/min do not decrease the incidence of hypertension during surgery to an incidence below 50%.[1,5]

NEUROLEPTIC–NARCOTIC ANESTHESIA

In 1949, Laborit[34,35] of France challenged the classic concept that general anesthesia can protect an organism from surgical pain by depression of cortical and subcortical centers alone. He introduced a new concept based on selective blocking, not only of the cerebral cortex but of the hypothalamus and of certain cellular, autonomic, and endocrine mechanisms normally activated as a response to stress.[35] Drug combinations consisting of chlorpromazine, promethazine, and meperidine ("lytic cocktail"), capable of causing multifocal inhibition, were used to produce a state of inactivity in such structures as the cerebral cortex, diencephalon, certain hormonal relays, and various ganglionic and terminal synapses. When the use of this method, referred to as *ganglioplegia* or *neuroplegia*, was combined with physical cooling, a state of "artificial hibernation" was produced and surgery could be performed without administering conventional anesthetic agents.

METHOD OF LABORIT.[34] The combination of the drugs in the lytic cocktail may be employed for three purposes: (1) as preoperative medication; (2) intravenously for induction of anesthesia; and (3) for a basal state during maintenance of anesthesia with supplementary nitrous oxide and oxygen. The most widely used mixture is for induction and for fractional doses during maintenance. The composition of the principal mixture is as follows: each 6 ml contains 50 mg chlorpromazine, 50 mg phenergan, and 100 mg meperidine.

Marked circulatory depression often resulted from this induced homeostatic imbalance, which may explain why this technique never reached wide popularity.

DEFINITIONS. *Neurolepsis* is defined as the suppression of cortical and central hypothalamic activity with a minimum of toxic effects.[36,37] The condition of neurolepsis describes a physical state; it differs from anesthesia, which describes a physiologic change.

These terms were coined by Oliver Wendell Holmes in 1846 when he was asked to name the state of narcosis produced by ether. "The state should be called anesthesia. This signifies sensibility to objects of touch. The words antineuritic, aneuritic, neuroleptic, neurolepsia, and neurostasis seem to be anatomical, whereas the change is a physiological one."

Compounds that produced this effect have been made available, first through the introduction of phenothiazines and, second, with the introduction of the butyrophenone derivatives, haloperidole and dehydrobenzperidol.[38,39] These are potent tranquilizers that are also effective alpha-adrenergic blocking agents. When combined with a potent narcotic, a state of neuroleptanalgesia[39] may be produced in which the patient lies at rest and is completely passive.

The term *neuroleptanalgesia* was first proposed by DeCastro[40] to describe a state of indifference and immobilization, termed *mineralization*, that is produced by the combined administration of the neuroleptic (ataractic) drug haloperidol and the narcotic analgesic (narcotic) phenoperidine. Subsequently, the technique underwent several modifications. After 1963, when droperidol (Inapsine) and fentanyl lactate (Sublimaze) were made available, these compounds became the most widely used ataractic and narcotic components of neuroleptanalgesia.

Patients who receive nitrous oxide–oxygen in addition to droperidol and fentanyl not only become analgesic and sedated but also lose consciousness, or, in other words, become anesthetized. The term *neuroleptanesthesia* was proposed to characterize the state of these patients.

CHARACTERISTICS OF NEUROLEPTANALGESIA. The neuroleptanalgesia state is dependent on a neurolept agent (commonly droperidol)* and an opioid analgesic. It is characterized by:

1. Marked tranquility and apparent somnolence (without loss of consciousness); patients are easily aroused
2. Psychic indifference to environmental stimuli
3. Psychomotor placidity or hypokinesis; motor sedation is referred to as *mineralization*
4. Suppressed reflexes
5. Homeostasis—cardiovascular stability
6. Amnesia (may be incomplete)
7. Analgesia
8. Basal anesthesia, on which may be superimposed the effects of inhalation anesthetics to produce full surgical anesthesia.

CHARACTERISTICS OF NEUROLEPTANESTHESIA. This is dependent on the addition of an inhalation anesthetic, usually nitrous oxide, accompanied by an intravenous barbiturate, a benzodiazepine, and a muscle relaxant. By this means, neuroleptanalgesia is converted to neuroleptanesthesia.[41]

---

* Although the phenothiazines are structurally similar, neurolepsis and neuroleptanalgesia imply the use of butyrophenones.

SPECIFIC ANALGESICS. The search for improved means of selectively blocking afferent systems involved in surgical stress led to increased emphasis on analgesia. In 1961, Janssen[42] introduced a series of highly potent piperidine derivatives that were found to render the patient free from pain without affecting certain areas of the central nervous system that are blocked in orthodox anesthesia. These analgesic agents, phenoperidine and fentanyl, are analogues of meperidine and appear to be of particular value for use in anesthesia because of their rapid onset and relatively short duration of action. Fentanyl, in particular, is 100 times as potent as morphine sulphate but has minimal cortical and cardiovascular depressant effects.

COMBINATIONS. The initially proposed combination of haloperidol as the neuroleptic and phenoperidine as the narcotic (DeCastro method[40]) was fraught with serious reactions, including marked circulatory depression, extrapyramidal symptoms, and postoperative psychic changes. The combination of droperidol and fentanyl citrate (Innovar), however, has brought these complications under control.[43]

REFINED CURRENT PREPARATION. The combination of droperidol and fentanyl is the present neuroleptanalgesic of choice. A mixture of these two agents in a preparation with a fixed ratio is available as Innovar. This consists of droperidol, 2.5 mg, and fentanyl, 0.05 mg, in each milliliter of solution.

This represents a ratio of 50:1 of the neurolept to analgesic in a solution buffered with lactic acid and a pH of 3.5. It is supplied in 2 and 5 ml ampules.

Each component may be given separately and accordingly, the total calculated dose of neurolept droperidol is given first, followed by the initial fentanyl and subsequent intermittent maintenance doses of this analgesic as needed.

DROPERIDOL (dehydrobenzeperidol)

CHEMISTRY. Droperidol belongs to the chemical class of butyrophenones. These are substituted piperidines, and this agent is a tetrahydropyridine.

POTENCY.[44,47d] This drug is a major tranquilizer and belongs to the chemical class of butyrophenones (Fig. 26–1). It compares with other tranquilizers and neurolept agents, such as phenothiazine and rauwolfia alkaloids in that it is a more potent and specific drug. It also has significant alpha-adrenergic blocking action. Potentiation of barbiturates, especially thiopental, and narcotic drugs is marked.

PHARMACODYNAMICS.[44] Droperidol has a slow onset of action of 3 to 8 minutes after intravenous injection; peak effect is seen by 15 minutes. A long duration of optimal action of 3 to 6 hours is usual.

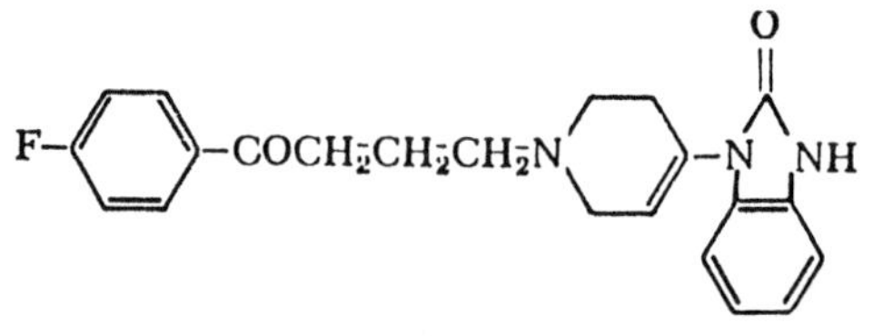

1-{1-[3-(p-fluorobenzoyl)propyl]-1,2,3,6-tetrahydro-4-pyridyl}-2-benzimidazolinone

FIG. 26–1. Structural formula of a butyrophenone derivative with neuroleptic action. Droperidol (Inapsine), or dehydrobenzperidol. From Cutting, W.C.: *In Handbook of Pharmacology.* Csaky, T.Z., and Barnes, B.A., eds., Norwalk, CT, Appleton-Century-Crofts, 1984.

Some mild carryover effect is noted in the postoperative period and may persist for 24 hours. This is minimized with single low doses of 0.15 mg/kg. Doses should be reduced in the elderly, debilitated, and poor-risk patients.

PHARMACOKINETICS.[45] Pharmacokinetic studies of droperidol have been carried out in anesthetized patients receiving single intravenous bolus doses of 150 µg/kg of body weight. A specific radioimmunoassay technique was used to measure plasma concentrations. The kinetics of droperidol can be described according to a three-compartment open model (Table 26–3).[45]

Plasma concentrations of the drug decrease rapidly after injection, and about 90% of an administered dose leaves the plasma within 1 hour. The decline in plasma concentration over a period of time can be expressed as a triexponential equation. The mean half-life for the rapid distribution, $t_{\frac{1}{2}}$ π-phase, and the slow distribution, $t_{\frac{1}{2}}$ α-phase, were determined at 1.4 ± 0.5 minutes and 14.3 ± 6.5 minutes, respectively. The mean elimination half-life, $t_{\frac{1}{2}}$ β-phase, was approximately 100 minutes, while the mean total body clearance was 14.1 ± 4.4 ml · min^{-1} · kg^{-1}. The total apparent volume of distribution was 2.04 ± 0.5 L/kg.

The short terminal half-life of droperidol (Fig. 26–2) is in contrast to the clinical experience of a relatively prolonged duration of optimal pharmacologic action. The total apparent volume of distribution at 2.04 ± 0.5 L/kg was twice the body weight, indicating an extensive uptake of droperidol in tissues and is related to a high liposolubility. Droperidol may be considered to have a high hepatic extraction ratio. The total body clearance is close to the hepatic blood flow. These kinetic values are in keeping with the significant hepatic metabolism.[46]

The plasma concentrations at the π-, α-, and β-phases as first-order constants are noted in Table 26–2. The calculated plasma concentration in the α-phase averages about 143 ng/ml, the plasma concentration in the β-phase averages about 60 ng/ml.

Droperidol is usually used as a neuroleptic in the

TABLE 26–3. DROPERIDOL PHARMACOKINETICS AFTER BOLUS INJECTION

	P (ng/ml)	π (min^{-1})	$t_{1/2}\pi$ (min)	A (ng/ml)	α (min^{-1})	$t_{1/2}\alpha$ (min)	B (ng/ml)	β (min^{-1})	$t_{1/2}\beta$ (min)
Mean ± SD	1033 522	0.58 0.28	1.39 0.52	143 52	0.059 0.027	14.3 6.5	59.1 15.8	0.0069 0.0013	103.8 20.2

P.A.B = ordinal intercepts: π, α, β = first-order rate constants; $t_{1/2}\pi$, $t_{1/2}\alpha$ and $t_{1/2}\beta$ = half-lives for rapid (π) and slow (α) distribution phase and the elimination phase (β). From Fischler, M., et al.: The pharmacokinetics of droperidol in anesthetized patients. Anesthesiology, 64:486, 1986.

neuroleptic–narcotic technique combined with fentanyl. It should be noted that, from this study at least, droperidol has a short elimination half-life of about 104 minutes, whereas fentanyl has a longer half-life, extending from 219 minutes to 522 minutes. Alfentanil, on the other hand, has a half-life elimination time of about 95 minutes. Hence, there is some pharmacokinetic similarity of alfentanil with droperidol. It is suggested by Fischler[45] that perhaps alfentanil and droperidol may represent a better combination.

METABOLIC FATE.[46] Hydrolyzed into p-(fluorobenzoyl)-propionic acid and piperidine, these components are then degraded. Tritium-labeled drug or metabolites are maximally excreted in the urine or feces within 24 hours. About 10% of the intact drug is excreted in the urine.

PHARMACOLOGY

Central Nervous System Effects.[39,43] The effect of a neuroleptic agent must be distinguished from that of classic sedative central nervous system depressants. Marked tranquilization without somnolence is the impressive effect of this drug. There is mental and psychological indifference to environmental stimuli and to sensory input. A behavioral and psychomotor block occurs, which produces a state of catalepsy, and there is an excellent antipsychotic effect. Emotions and affect are reduced. A suppression of spontaneous motor movements occurs, but spinal reflexes are intact.

Extrapyramidal responses—although side effects of most neuroleptics are denoted by abnormal muscular twitching, dyskinesia, or jerks—are rarely produced with droperidol.[41,44]

In rare patients, a state of mental restlessness and agitation may occur. This "inner anxiety" may be marked but later reported as hallucination and a sense of weightlessness. The ability of morphine to provide amnesia is reduced.

Sleep is not produced.[41,44,47] Patients are usually able to respond to verbal commands sluggishly. Some amnesia occurs, but unconsciousness must be produced by an inhalation anesthetic or by an intravenous barbiturate or hypnotic drug.[47] If an inhalation anesthetic is administered before neurolepsis is complete, a stage of delirium is frequently induced. Premature attempts to produce a state of general anesthesia must be avoided.[41]

The alpha rhythm of the electroencephalogram (EEG) is unaltered, but some synchronization is evident. When a narcotic is added, a slow delta rhythm may appear.[48]

Site of Action. Subcortical brain structures are depressed. The limbic, extrapyramidal, nigrostriatal, and hypothalamic systems are blocked, whereas the function of the reticular activating system is maintained. Concentration of the drug occurs in those areas of the brain that are rich in dopaminergic synapses, especially the limbic cortex.[47,49,50] The chemoreceptor trigger zone and the extrapyramidal nuclei are affected.

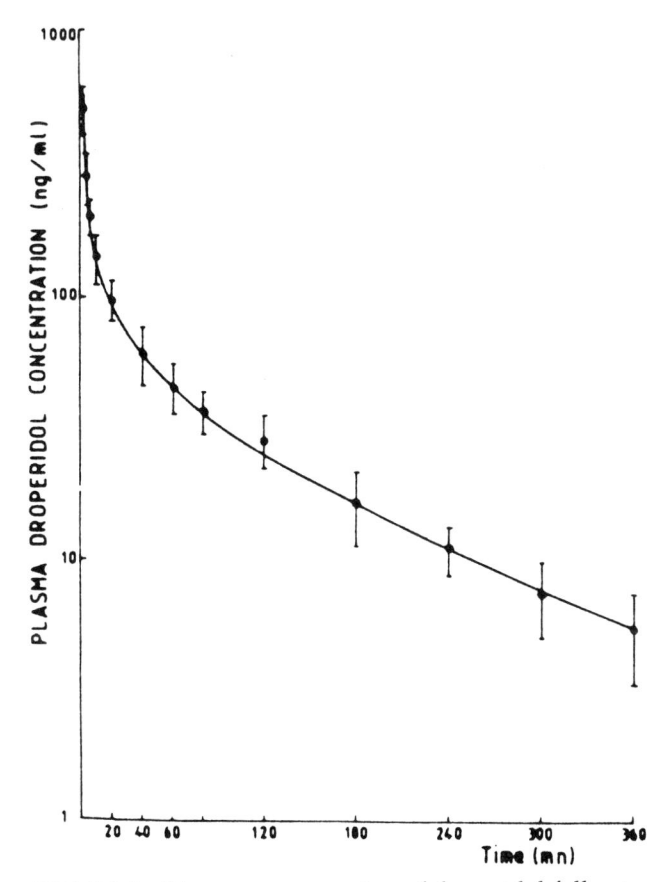

FIG. 26–2. Plasma concentration of droperidol following intravenous injection of 150 μg/kg (mean ± SD) and the fitted curve. From Fischler, M., et al.: The pharmacokinetics of droperidol in anesthetized patients. Anesthesiology, 64:486, 1986.

Mechanism of Action.[51] Mechanism of action is a basic reduction of the permeability of cell membranes in the central nervous system by forming a monolayer. The selected cells are those excited by dopamine, noradrenaline, and 5-hydroxytryptamine. Gamma-aminobutyric acid (GABA) receptors on the postsynaptic membrane are occupied by droperidol, and synaptic transmission is prevented.[39] Reuptake by the presynaptic cells of dopamine and norepinephrine with accumulation of dopamine in the intersynaptic cleft is also inhibited.[51a]

A strong antiemetic effect is apparently due to the depression of the chemoreceptor trigger zone.[52] Ordinary doses of apomorphine do not produce emesis experimentally.[53] Cerebrospinal fluid pressure is reduced in patients either with or without space-occupying lesions.[53]

Cardiovascular Effects. These effects are mainly due to the alpha-adrenergic blocking action.[39,44,50,54] In general, there is stabilization of the cardiovascular functions and homeostatic mechanisms are preserved.[44] Myocardial contractility is not depressed.[44] Cardiac rate increases about 8%, but when accompanied by fentanyl, there is a slowing. After intravenous injection, a 10% fall in systolic pressure occurs, an effect related to peripheral vasodilation, fall in central venous pressure, and decreased venous return.[54] A mild, transient hypotension occurs, and systolic pressure is slightly reduced. An alpha-adrenergic blocking effect is noted and correlates with this fall in pressure.[55] Because some action may continue postoperatively, there are occasional instances of postural hypotension and delay in ambulation. Pulmonary vascular resistance is reduced,[39,50] and pulmonary artery pressure is decreased. Capacitance vessels are dilated.

An additional mechanism for cardiovascular effects is that of a direct action on vascular smooth muscles. The evidence in isolated pulmonary arteries and peripheral veins shows significant depression of the amplitude of spontaneous vessel contraction.[50]

An antiarrhythmic effect is characteristic.[56] Epinephrine-induced arrhythmias are antagonized.[57] This effect is probably related, in part, to a mild beta-receptor blocking action.

Ample evidence exists to show that this drug protects against traumatic and oligemic shock.[58,59] Of importance in this circumstance is the decreased blood viscosity and the increase in blood sugar.[60]

Respiratory Effects. No significant adverse effects on ventilatory parameters or on blood gas composition have been identified following droperidol alone.[61] Following rapid injection or large doses of Innovar, however, some rigidity of the chest wall occurs as a result of enhancement of skeletal muscle tone. The expiratory muscles are principally involved.[62] Functional residual capacity is reduced even when chest wall rigidity is not evident. These effects are due to the fentanyl component.[63,64]

The CO_2 Response Curve. A rightward shift of the CO_2 response curve occurs following Innovar, indicating depression.[65] This is almost identical but less than the response seen with fentanyl alone;[66] hence, this CO_2 response to Innovar is also due to the fentanyl component. It has been suggested by Becker[67] that droperidol attenuates fentanyl induced respiratory depression.

Hypoxic Ventilatory Reflex. In the presence of hypoxia, there is a significant potentiation of the ventilatory responses when droperidol has been previously administered. The chemosensitivity of the carotid body is enhanced, and the mechanism is related to the following: dopamine markedly reduces the hypoxic ventilatory response; because dopamine receptors are readily blocked by droperidol, an increased sensitivity and responsiveness of the carotid body occur.[68]

Endocrine Effects.[69-71] During neuroleptanalgesia, inconsistent results have been found with regard to the effect on plasma levels of catecholamines.[69] Some increases in norepinephrine may occur, but this is most likely caused by the narcotic. Release of epinephrine in small amounts may be evident during surgical stress. A significant increase in rate of urinary excretion of epinephrine occurs, but usually no change in norepinephrine excretion is observed.[72] Adrenocortical function is not impaired.[70,71] An increase in plasma levels of growth hormone occurs. Blood sugar levels increase during droperidol action.[73]

Renal Effects.[74,75] In the neuroleptanalgesia technique, glomerular filtration rate, effective renal plasma flow, insulin and para-aminohippuric acid (PAH) clearance, fractional sodium, fractional osmolal, and fractional water excretion are decreased, while fractional free water reabsorption is increased during anesthesia.

Postanesthetically, renal hemodynamics are promptly restored, whereas fractional sodium and fractional osmolal excretion are unaltered. Urinary excretion is not impaired. It is concluded that neuroleptanalgesia, as far as renal function is concerned, is well suited for the anesthetic management of the poor-risk patient.

The initial hemodynamic renal changes may be attributed to increased sympathetic activity or increased circulatory catecholamines. Adequate doses of droperidol, however, should block this mechanism, and a more likely explanation is the release of renin and increased plasma aldosterone.

Metabolic Effects. The butyrophenones and particularly droperidol reduce total body oxygen consumption by 20% to 30%.[49] Blood viscosity and hematocrit values also decrease.

Hepatic Function.[73] Droperidol has no significant effect on liver function.

Effect on Skeletal Muscles. An increased muscle tone and occasional instance of muscle rigidity may occur following Innovar administration.[76] This is the result of action of the fentanyl component and is discussed in detail under pharmacology of fentanyl.

ADVERSE EFFECTS. Mild to moderate hypotension may be seen. It is usually transient and accompanied by some tachycardia. If persistent, the presence of hypovolemia should be considered.

Extrapyramidal symptoms may appear but are infrequent and usually related to large doses and a resultant dopaminergic block at the striatal level; such symptom complexes are managed by antiparkinson drugs (the dopaminergic-activating drugs).

Dystonia (disordered muscle tone), hyperkinetic locomotion, uncontrolled restlessness, or akathasia symptoms are occasionally seen. These are also related to disturbance at the basal ganglia level but probably result from excessive dopaminergic activity; patients may feel jittery and even apprehensive. These disorders are seen when small doses are employed in otherwise normal patients so that there is excessive dopaminergic activity in the basal ganglia. These symptoms are managed by anticholinergic drugs such as benztropine.[77]

NEUROLEPTIC MALIGNANT SYNDROME

Neuroleptic drugs are used extensively as antipsychotic agents, major tranquilizers, antiemetics, and disassociative anesthesia. One of the unusual complications is a hyperpyrexic condition called the neuroleptic malignant syndrome (NMS).

This syndrome was first described in 1968 by Delay[78] with regard to phenothiazine therapy and was associated with hyperpyrexia and other neurologic abnormalities. Since then, many drugs have been found to be associated with this syndrome, and it is considered that the incidence is estimated to be between 0.5% and 1% of all patients exposed to neuroleptics.

CLINICAL FEATURES. The syndrome effects young men predominantly but may be seen at any age and in both sexes. The syndrome develops typically over a period of 24 to 72 hours and may even be observed several days after discontinuing neuroleptic therapy.

Characteristics of NMS are hyperthermia, hypertonicity of skeletal muscles, variable levels of consciousness, and significant instability of the autonomic nervous system. The common autonomic dysfunctions include pallor, diaphoresis, fluctuating blood pressure, tachycardia, and cardiac dysrhythmias. These signs may occur before other symptoms. The muscular hypertonia is of a "lead-pipe"–type increase in tone. Rigidity and akinesia develop at about the time the temperature elevation is noted.

Laboratory abnormalities are nonspecific. In general, there are a leukocytosis and electrolyte levels, suggesting dehydration; however, this may be a predisposing factor. Liver function abnormalities consist of elevated serum levels of transaminase, lactic dehydrogenase, and alkaline phosphate. The creatine kinase level is often elevated and may exceed 16,000 IU/L.

MECHANISM (DELAY).[78] A drug's potential for inducing NMS appears to parallel its antidopaminergic potency. Discontinuation of antiparkinsonian agents and the use of dopamine-depleting agents can produce NMS. The predisposing factors include exhaustion, dehydration, and, especially, the use of long-acting (depo) neuroleptics.

PRECIPITATING AGENTS. This syndrome has been associated with the following drugs: phenothiazines, butyrophenones, thioxanthenes, and other miscellaneous antipsychotic agents.

Monoamine oxidase inhibitors have also been implicated in the development of hyperthermic reactions. Of significance is the interaction between the monoamine oxidase inhibitors and the reaction seen when synthetic narcotic drugs or additional antidepressants of the tricyclic nature are given together with monoamine oxidase inhibitors.

Of importance to the anesthesiologist is the occurrence of agitation, severe hypotension, delirium, and hyperpyrexia that may occur in patients on monoamine oxidase inhibitors to whom meperidine or dextromethorphan is administered. Deaths have been reported from this combination.

DIFFERENTIAL DIAGNOSIS. Differential diagnosis of NMS includes the heat stroke associated with phenothiazines, which inhibit sweating, central anticholinergic syndrome, and the malignant hyperthermia associated with anesthesia.

TREATMENT.[79] This life-threatening complication of neuroleptic drugs is treated by discontinuance of the neuroleptic and institution of general supportive measures. Specific drug therapy includes dantrolene because of its effectiveness in the treatment of anesthetic malignant hyperthermia. The intravenous dose varies from 2 to 3 mg/kg of body weight per day, followed by oral dosage in the range of 50 to 200 mg/day. Amantadine hydrochloride, a dopamine agonist, has been reported to be successful in the management of NMS.

Bromocriptine, another dopamine agonist, has also been successful in the treatment of NMS. The oral dosage of this drug varies from 2.5 to 10 mg three times per day.

FENTANYL

Fentanyl is an opioid analgesic that is highly potent, with a rapid onset and short duration of activity. Optimal duration of action is about 30 to 60 minutes. This brevity is considered to be the result of rapid redistribution into the fluid compartments of the body.[80,86]

A carryover effect, however, extends for 4 to 6 hours, during which repeat doses or administration of other narcotics becomes cumulative and should be reduced.[81]

CHEMICAL NAME. This drug is related to meperidine series and is named N. (1-phenethyl-4-peperidyl) propionanilide. The structure is illustrated in Figure 26–3.

POTENCY. Compared with morphine, the same degree of analgesia is produced with about 1/100 the dose, i.e., it is 100 times as potent as morphine. In analgesic activity a 100-μg dose of fentanyl is approximately equivalent to 10 mg of morphine sulfate.[82] The mechanism of this action appears to be similar to morphine. The average loading dose in anesthesia practice is 5 μg/kg. Murphy[83,84] has demonstrated a reduction of minimum alveolar concentration (MAC) values of volatile inhalation agents when preceded by a dose of fentanyl.

DOSAGE.[81,82,85] The doses of fentanyl useful as part of premedication or when incorporated in the Innovar preparation are discussed in the section entitled "Technical Procedures."

The doses displayed for the induction or maintenance of an analgesic state and contributing to anesthesia are classed into three categories:

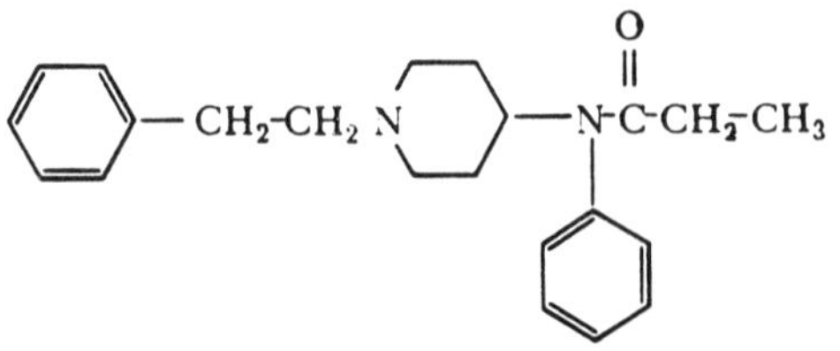

N-(1-phenethyl-4-piperidyl)propionanilide

FIG. 26–3. Structural formula of fentanyl (Sublimaze), a meperidine analogue for analgesia. From Cutting, W.C.: In Handbook of Pharmacology. Csaky, T.Z., and Barnes, B.A. eds. Norwalk, CT, Appleton-Century-Crofts, 1984.

- Low doses ED$_{50}$—2.5 to 10 μg/kg[139]
- Moderate doses—10 to 50 μg/kg[85,113]
- Super doses—50 to 150 μg/kg[85]

PHARMACOKINETICS.[86,87] The plasma decay curve of fentanyl can be described by a three-compartment open system, a central compartment including blood and interstitial locations, and two tissue compartments. Fentanyl is a strong lipophilic drug and rapidly equilibrates with richly vascular tissues, where it becomes highly concentrated. By using radio-labeled drug (^{3}H) and radioimmunoassay techniques, the disposition of fentanyl after a single injection of the drug as shown by plasma levels can be followed.[88]

After a single intravenous dose of 6.4 μg/kg of fentanyl base (10 μg/kg of citrate), the plasma levels fall rapidly and 98.6% of the dose is eliminated from the plasma in 60 minutes. The kinetics of the plasma concentration in humans can be summarized as a three-compartment model (similar to that in the dog) (Fig. 26–4), in which the drug is introduced into the central compartment of the plasma volume and the drug is then distributed to two peripheral compartments. On intravenous injection, fentanyl is immediately diluted and protein bound in the plasma compartment. The half-life of this π-phase has been set at 1.65 minutes and plasma level of 18 ng/ml, and the volume of the central compartment has been calculated as 0.356 L/kg. About 80% of the fentanyl is protein bound at a pH of 7.4, but only about 60% is bound at pH 7.2 (plasma protein 4.7 g/dl); that is, binding is pH dependent. In studies of the radioactive drug (tritiated fentanyl ^{3}H), some metabolites were present at 1.5 minutes after injection and represented 19% of the dose injected (Table 26–4).

Plasma concentrations of fentanyl fall rapidly after injection due to distribution to the peripheral compartments and rapid and extensive uptake by tissues. From a plasma level of about 18 ng/ml at 1.5 minutes, the level declines to about 1.9 ng/ml at 13 to 14 minutes, which represents the α-phase with a half-life ($t_{\frac{1}{2}}$ α) of about 14 minutes. These changes are related to the rapid equilibration with brain and other vascular-rich tissues.

Secondary peaks in plasma concentration have been reported during the elimination phase.[89] Becker has noted this biphasic pattern. A second peak of 20% or more may be seen in plasma fentanyl concentrations about 4 hours postinjection and postoperatively.[90] This second peak is accompanied by a decrease in CO$_2$ response. This depression can be antagonized by small doses of naloxone. It has been shown that 16% of an administered dose will accumulate in the stomach wall by 10 minutes after injection. This may be due to enterosystemic recirculation. Absorption subsequently from the stomach may then cause a secondary rise in plasma fentanyl.

FIG. 26-4. Plasma levels of unchanged ^{3}H-fentanyl, total ^{3}H-radioactivity, and ^{3}H-metabolites in five subjects each given 6.4 µg/kg ^{3}H-fentanyl intravenously. Each data point represents $\bar{x} \pm$ SEM; the standard errors are less than the height of the data points. The nonlinear least-squares line is shown for the β-phase, and the overall curve is represented by the following equation: $Cp(t) = 18 \exp^{-0.43t} + 1.9 \exp^{-0.055t} + 1.4 \exp^{-0.0032t}$. From McClain, D.A., and Hug, C.C., Jr.: Intravenous fentanyl kinetics. Clin. Pharmacol. Ther., 28:106, 1980.

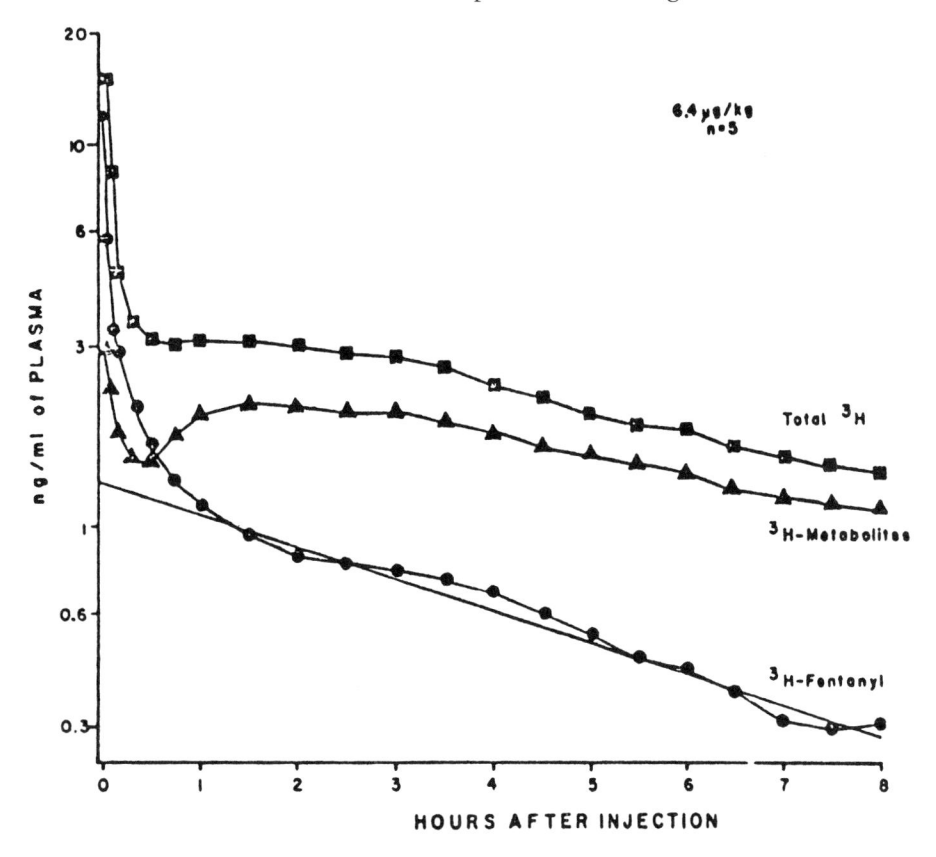

By 60 minutes, 98% of the administered dose is cleared from the plasma, much of which is taken up by the tissues. The terminal elimination phase, however, is prolonged and extends from 20 minutes to 8 hours, with a $t_{\frac{1}{2}}$ β of 219 minutes. This is due to slow reuptake from vascular tissues, including skeletal muscle. The reuptake from these tissues is to the central compartment. Ultimately, this phase is dependent on rapid biotransformation to polar metabolites and excretion by the kidney. The overall apparent volume of distribution has been calculated as 4 L/kg and a clearance rate of 9.56 µg/kg/min.

Large doses of fentanyl on the order of 50 to 100 µg/kg have an extended tissue uptake and elimination phase.[91] In Bovill's study, a bioexponential decay curve was determined after a π-phase of 1.7 minutes. This decay of tissue uptake had a half-life of 69 minutes and a secondary elimination phase of 400 minutes.

AGE EFFECT ON PHARMACOKINETICS.[92] Plasma concentrations of fentanyl are significantly lower in infants and children compared with adults when equipotent doses are administered. The doses for

TABLE 26-4. ^{3}H-FENTANYL PLASMA KINETICS AFTER INTRAVENOUS INJECTION
$Cp(t) = P\exp^{-\pi t} + A\exp^{-\alpha t} + B\exp^{-\beta t}$*

Volunteer	P (ng/ml)	π (min^{-1})	$t_{1/2}$ π (min)	A (ng/ml)	α (min^{-1})	$t_{1/2}\alpha$ (min)	B (ng/ml)	β (min^{-1})	$t_{1/2}\beta$ (min)†
Mean	18.1	0.431	1.65	1.90	0.0549	13.4	1.38	0.00320	219
SEM	±4.1	±0.131	±0.12	±0.50	±0.0065	±1.6	±0.08	±0.00016	+10
3.2 µg/kg									
V$_1$	10.6	0.382	1.82	1.36	0.0433	16.0	0.68	0.00173	399
V$_2$	6.4	0.363	1.69	1.26	0.0646	10.7	0.66	0.00236	293
Mean	8.5	0.373	1.76	1.31	0.0539	13.4	0.67	0.00205	346

* The intercepts and rate constants for the triexponential equation describing fentanyl elimination from plasma were determined by least squares nonlinear regression analysis.

† $r^2 = \dfrac{\Sigma(\text{observed})^2 - \Sigma(\text{deviation})^2}{\Sigma(\text{observed})^2}$

From McClain, D.A., and Hug, C.C., Jr.: Intravenous fentanyl kinetics. Clin Pharmacol. Ther. 28:106, 1980.

infants and children needed to achieve the same clinical analgesia end point are about 50% higher in infants and almost as much in children over the dose for the adult. In a comparative study of plasma concentration in the different age groups, doses of 30 μg/kg were administered to infants and children and 20 μg/kg to adults. Despite the larger doses in infants, the plasma levels in infants were about one half of those of the adult at 2 and 4 minutes after injection—2500 pg/ml versus 5000 pg/ml—and continued significantly lower in the ensuing 60 to 240 minutes. Although the peak plasma levels in children were almost as high as in adults during the first 4 minutes after injection; thereafter, the difference was significantly lower in the children than the adults.

The lower plasma concentrations in infants and children can be related to three factors:[92]

- A larger volume of distribution[93]
- A larger average lipid concentration in infants— 12% in the newborn and 30% of body weight at 10 years;[93] although lipid content decreases with childhood development, it is still higher than in the adult
- A larger free plasma fraction, which equilibrates with other tissues

CLEARANCE. Degradation and elimination of nearly all fentanyl occur in the liver and are dependent on a mixed-function oxidase enzyme system. It is considered that the enzyme system in the neonate and infant period is equal in activity to the adult.[94]

Hepatic blood flow in infants is greater than in children or adults. This can be related to the greater relative liver mass to body mass in the infant of 5% compared with the adult of 2%.[95] The clearance in infants has been determined to be about 18 ml/kg/min compared with about 12 ml in children and 10 ml in adults.[96]

METABOLISM.[97,98] Like most lipophilic drugs, fentanyl is nearly completely metabolized by the liver. Only 6.5% is eliminated unchanged in urine. In a study of patients with cirrhosis of the liver, the average elimination half-life $(t_{\frac{1}{2}}\beta)$ was found to be 304 minutes (control: 263 minutes). The total plasma clearance was 11.3 ml/kg/min (control: 10.8 ml/kg/min), and the volume of distribution was 4.4 L/kg.[97]

It is concluded that the elimination of fentanyl is not primarily dependent on the rate at which it is metabolized in the liver, although there is some delay. Factors that modify clearance in patients with cirrhosis are principally (1) reduced hepatic blood flow; (2) diminished activity of enzymes; and (3) decreased fraction of plasma protein-bound drug.

METABOLITES.[99] Three metabolites have been identified: despropionyl fentanyl, norfentanyl, and despropionyl norfentanyl. High levels of these metabolites appear in the plasma within 20 minutes; that is, during the α-phase while uptake is still progressing. Accounting for 85% of the fentanyl dose, these metabolites are excreted largely in urine; only small amounts of unchanged fentanyl are excreted in the urine, representing about 8% of the total dose. A small portion of the administered dose is also free fentanyl.

PHARMACOLOGY.

Central Nervous System.[81] The site of action is at the thalamic level: hypothalamus, reticular system, and gamma neurons. At the cortical level, some degree of indifference to pain is seen. Pain of both somatic and visceral types is relieved by mesencephalic block. EEG is depressed, and ataxia is seen.

Experimental studies show that fentanyl and alfentanil both suppress brain stem pain transmission.[100] This suppression was determined to be located at the caudate end of the reticular formation, specifically at the nucleus reticularis gigantocellularis.

Additional narcotic features include miosis, euphoria, and respiratory depression. A weak emetic action is noted. As a result of the central action, the probability of habituation and abuse exists.

Other central nervous system depressants are potentiated by this drug, including barbiturates and tranquilizers, whereas there is an additive effect with other analgesics. As expected, fentanyl loading is capable, like other narcotics, of reducing the MAC value of inhalation agents and the UD_{95} dose of intravenous induction agents, such as thiopental.[101] Experimentally, Murphy[84] has shown that the MAC value of enflurane is decreased in proportion to the plasma concentration of fentanyl. In dogs, at high doses, a ceiling effect is evident when the MAC value of enflurane is reduced by 65%. Fentanyl is not recommended in the presence of monoamine oxidase inhibitors. Large doses of 25 μg/kg or more can produce unconsciousnes.[85]

Pharmacodynamics.[102] Onset of pharmacologic effects is noted within 30 to 60 seconds toward the end of a 90-second injection period. By 2 minutes after injection, patients are relaxed and analgesia supervenes. The peak analgesia effect is achieved at a plasma level of 2 ng/ml or above in 3 to 6 minutes. Ventilation is depressed, which is delayed, but peaks between 5 and 15 minutes. As plasma levels fall below 1.9 to 1.5 ng/ml, recovery occurs and adequate spontaneous ventilation returns.[103] Duration of optimal analgesia is about 30 minutes following a dose of 1 to 2 μg/kg. At 60 minutes, only mild sedation and only limited analgesia is present, at which time the plasma level is less than 1.5 ng/ml.

After intramuscular injection, the onset of effects is slower, occurring in 7 to 8 minutes. The duration of effect is longer and approximates 1 to 2 hours.

Respiratory depression may continue for a longer period.

EEG Changes.[104] Fentanyl and its congeners, alfentanil and sufentanil, produce similar EEG changes in humans (Fig. 26–5). With increasing serum concentrations, there is a progressive slowing in the frequency of the EEG pattern. This narcotic effect on the brain has been quantitated using off-line EEG power spectrum analysis. In unpremedicated patients, a continuous infusion of fentanyl at the rate of 150 µg/min was administered until a specific level of EEG depression pattern (delta waves) occurred. This pattern is approximately the third stage of the Kiersey Stage III of central nervous system depression. It is not identical, however, because there is no burst suppression and only the appearance of delta waves. The average dose of fentanyl to achieve the EEG end point was 7 to 8 µg/kg.

The induced peak EEG changes were found to lag distinctly behind peak serum narcotic concentrations with fentanyl.* The steady-state serum concentration of fentanyl that caused this depression was about 25 µg/ml; the time of appearance of third-stage EEG delta was half-time at 6 to 7 minutes. A regular sequence of clinical effects are noted: developing analgesia (at serum concentrations of 2 to 3 ng/ml) is followed by respiratory depression in 3 to 5 minutes and then loss of consciousness 30 to 60 seconds later.[105]

Compared with alfentanil, this lag effect may be due to a larger brain blood partition coefficient for fentanyl. A further comparison with alfentanil indicated that the EEG end point as related to steady-state serum concentration showed the potency ratio to be approximately 75:1. This is in contrast to the dose potency reported in clinical practice that fentanyl is approximately 10 times that of alfentanil. This difference may be explained by alfentanil's smaller initial distribution volume (Fig. 26–6) and less time lag between serum concentration changes and changes in effect.[106]

Cardiovascular Effects. The cardiovascular effects are minimal.[61] Bradycardia that occurs is usually a mild sinus type but is more pronounced when given to patients anesthetized by inhalation agents.[107] A central mechanism is considered the cause of fentanyl-induced bradycardia, because it does not occur after vagotomy.[108] The bradycardia is enhanced following succinylcholine, and asystole has been re-

---

* An hysteresis loop between spectral power EEG changes and serum narcotic concentration is similar to that seen with nondepolarizing muscle relaxants. The two loops are (1) EEG changes versus increasing drug concentrations and (2) EEG changes versus decreasing concentration.

FIG. 26–5. EEG stages for fentanyl and alfentanil. Awake—mixed alpha (8–13 Hz) and beta (>13 Hz) activity. Stage 1—slowing with alpha spindles. Stage 2—more slowing, theta activity present (4–7 Hz). Stage 3—maximal slowing, delta waves present (<4 Hz) with high amplitude. From Scott, J.C., Ponganis, K.V., and Stanski, D.R.: EEG quantitation of narcotic effect: A comparative pharmacodynamic of fentanyl and alfentanil. Anesthesiology, 62:234, 1985.

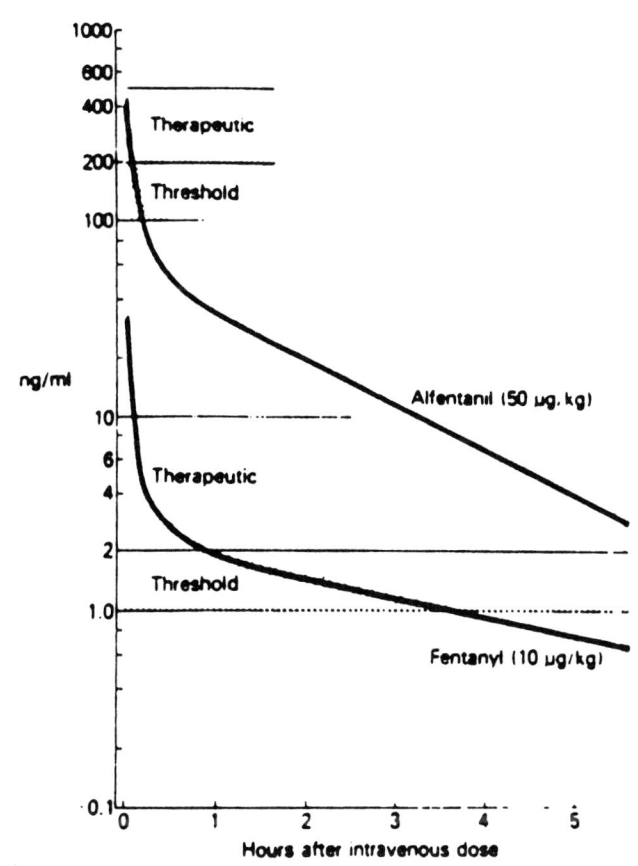

FIG. 26–6. A comparison of the plasma decay curves of a single iv bolus dose of fentanyl and alfentanil. The solid line is the predicted plasma concentration in a single patient with representative pharmacokinetics. While the equivalent alfentanil dose is five times that of fentanyl, during the first 2 h after injection the alfentanil plasma concentrations are 14 to 25 times higher. This is due in part to the smaller volume of distribution of alfentanil. From Stanski, D.R., and Hug, C.C.: Alfentanil: A kinetically predictable narcotic analgesic (editorial). Anesthesiology, 57:435, 1982.

ported.[109] This action is of importance chiefly in patients with conduction defects or recent infarction. Prevention or treatment of this untoward response is best obtained with glycopyrrolate, because atropine frequently produces ventricular beats.[110] High doses of 25 to 100 µg/kg are associated with some cardiovascular changes. Generally, central venous pressure and systemic vascular resistance show no significant changes, but systolic blood pressure and left ventricular stroke work, as well as the index, are decreased significantly after 50 µg/kg.[111] In patients with ischemic coronary artery disease, administration of doses above 30 µg/kg were associated with decreasing left ventricular function, with lowered cardiac index and left ventricular stroke work indexes.[112]

Bazaral[113] has shown that 15 µg/kg is equally effective for induction, compared with 60 µg/kg, without the serious hemodynamics of the larger dose. Chung[114] also has found the low dose to be preferred.

No significant depression of the vascular system is apparent. Slight decreases in systolic pressure may be seen, consistent with sedation and analgesia. In patients with severe hepatic or renal disease, the same caution should be exercised as with other narcotics.

Summary. Bradycardia has been noted, as discussed earlier.[109] With doses greater than 25 µg/kg, significant myocardial depression occurs. Cardiac work index and left ventricular stroke work index are decreased.[111] This depression increases progressively, as the dose extends to 50 µg/kg or more. At this dose level, it is noted that there is a marked decline in plasma norepinephrine and dopamine.[113]

Respiratory Effects.[62,66] In equianalgesic doses, the respiratory depression activity of fentanyl, 2 µg/kg, is similar to meperidine. In large intravenous doses (fentanyl, 2 µg/kg, and meperidine, 2 mg/kg), there is marked depression of the three principal respiratory parameters: rate is reduced by 50% with both drugs; minute volume is reduced to 30 to 40 by both drugs; however, the reduction of tidal volume is greater with fentanyl. Suppression of the cough reflex occurs. There is significant depression in the CO_2 response curve for as long as 2 hours, with a shift to the right.[65]

Ventilation. A dose-dependent and time-dependent ventilatory depression occurs with single bolus doses of 25 µg/kg.[66] This may be evident in the postoperative period, even when the drug has been administered 3 hours previously. Becker[90] has noted this biphasic respiratory depression, which can be related to the secondary plasma concentration peaks. By the CO_2 response test, Cartwright[115] has demonstrated that the depression of ventilation may persist for more than 5 hours after a single bolus dose. In normocapnic patients, a 50% depression of the slope of the ventilation–CO_2 response curve occurs at plasma levels of 2 to 3 ng/ml. At a steady-state plasma concentration of 2.9 ng/ml, there is a significant shift of the response curve to the right and a 45% depression of the response compared to the awake values. In patients who are hyperventilated during anesthesia to hypocapnic levels of Pa_{CO_2} less than 30, there is a greater depression in the postanesthetic period, and the depression is evident at lower plasma levels of fentanyl.

Additionally, hypocapnia–hyperventilation during anesthesia slows the whole-body clearance of fentanyl.[116] This decreased clearance may be related to decreased hepatic blood flow associated with hypocapnia, especially in the elderly. Second, after a period of hypocapnia with depletion of body stores of CO_2, there will be a period of continuing hypocarbia and obligatory hypoventilation until body stores are replenished.[117]

Ventilatory Complications.[118-120] Apnea may develop with larger doses of fentanyl in a significant number of patients (3% to 5%). Other ventilatory difficulties (14%) with or without concomitant apnea include (1) increased tone of the respiratory muscles (stiff chest); (2) laryngeal spasm; and (3) bronchiolar spasm. Neuromuscular blocking drugs (curare) may diminish but do not eliminate the tonic muscular state. However, narcotic antagonists, naloxone (5 µg/kg) or levallorphan (2 µg/kg), rapidly counteract this effect and reestablish spontaneous respiration at the expense of reversing the analgesia. Agonist–antagonist opioids (nalbuphine) are only partially effective and leave significant analgesia. Naloxone may be administered subcutaneously after the initial intravenous injection to obtund the second delayed peak in plasma fentanyl concentration.[120]

Truncal rigidity is seen after large doses.[121] There is decreased pulmonary compliance (Corssen[41] reported 80%) with the classic technique, but separate administration of dehydrobenzperidol (droperidol) and fentanyl reduces the incidence. Usually some stiffness will follow an average dose of 20 µg/kg. The incidence of rigidity varies from 8% to 80%.[118] It can be relieved by small doses of succinylcholine or, preferably, a nondepolarizing relaxant.

Autonomic Nervous System Effects. Vagomimetic properties are noted. Intestinal tone and gastrointestinal motility are increased.

Cholinergic effects are shown, such as nausea, vomiting, hyperhydrosis, and miosis. The sphincter of Oddi is stimulated. These effects are ameliorated by prior administration of the neuroleptic and by atropine.

Metabolic and Hormonal Effects.[122-124] The stress response to surgery and failure to establish an anesthetic state (stage III) even with moderate doses results in catabolic changes. Included are an elevation of blood glucose, an increase in plasma cortisol, growth hormone, and plasma norepinephrine, and dopamine. The increases are small during induction and intubation after doses of 25 μg/kg and are greatly attenuated by doses of 50 μg/kg.[122] On surgical stimulation, such as during sternotomy, bypass procedures, or upper abdominal surgery, however, the increases are greater by two- to three-fold.[123]

Histamine Release. Fentanyl, in doses of 7.5 μg/kg, administered intravenously, causes no elevations of plasma histamine. At 1 minute after injection, plasma histamine remains at a baseline of 0.12 ng/ml and continues so for the duration of action.[125]

Neuromuscular Action. No depressant effect has been determined at the neuromuscular junction of fentanyl (or of droperidol), and neither d-tubocurarine nor succinylcholine action is augmented.

Muscle Rigidity. Occasional rigidity of jaw, neck, chest, and abdominal muscles occurs and is evidenced as a forced and prolonged expiratory effort.[121] This adverse effect follows rapid injection; it is dose-dependent and is more frequent after apneic doses. It appears to be enhanced if not initiated by nitrous oxide, especially when this agent is administered prematurely and aggressively by manual ventilation.[126] It occurs at the time the patient loses consciousness. Rigidity may also become prominent in the postanesthetic period and postanesthesia recovery personnel should be aware of this possibility.[127]

The mechanism is not completely known. In studies of muscle activity as related to nerve stimulation,[128] the initial response is an action potential designated as the *M response* due to the impulse traveling orthodromically; this is followed by a second action potential, due to the same stimulus, producing an impulse that travels centrally and then relayed from the spinal cord back to the muscle. This is called the *H response* (see Hoffman reflex).

Fentanyl and meperidine (morphine in large doses) all cause an increase in the H response and an increase in electromyographic (EMG) activity.[129] Nitrous oxide and droperidol both depress the H response, but simultaneously there is a marked increase in the EMG. Epidural morphine appears not to affect the H reflex.[130]

The studies of Gergis[76] indicate some alteration of the polysynaptic pathways of the spinal cord, independently of the monosynaptic stretch reflex, especially with nitrous oxide, which allows a polysynaptic reflex increase in muscle tone and depression of the H reflex. The origin of expiratory apnea or truncal rigidity may indeed be at higher areas of the central nervous system. The rigidity is effectively treated by narcotic antagonists or d-tubocurarine.

The H Reflex.[128] The H reflex was first described by Hoffman in 1918 and is analogous to the monosynaptic muscle stretch reflex. The afferent impulses arise from stimuli originating in the muscle spindles; they pass centrally to the dorsal roots and then reach the anterior horn nuclei. These cells are activated and the efferent path is over the motoneuron. The testing of this reflex is considered to assess mononeuronal function as well as the integrity of the afferent arc.

Mechanism of Muscle Rigidity.[131] Narcotic-induced muscle rigidity has been observed following various narcotics but has been a prominent observation after the administration of fentanyl and fentanyl derivatives.[132] Rigidity has also been observed following intravenous morphine but has not been a prominent or frequent effect.[129] The rigidity from morphine has been largely of the abdominal musculature.

Consequences. The effect on physiology of muscle rigidity has been studied. The principal hemodynamic change is an immediate marked elevation of central venous pressure. This elevation varies directly with muscle tension, as determined by EMG monitoring. With the onset of rigidity, a rapid metabolic acidosis develops. The arterial oxygen tension decreases, and there is a decrease in the functional residual capacity.[63] Pulmonary compliance is also decreased by a minimum of 16%.[126]

With the rigidity, there is interference with the positive-pressure ventilation. There is a second consequence of importance to anesthesiologists, namely the development of rigidity of neck muscles with flexion of the head toward the chest and difficulty or inability to extend the mandible and maintain an adequate airway.

Clinical studies[131] of EMG records reveal that all muscle groups show increased muscle activity. First, muscle rigidity occurs in the upper body, including the sternocleidomastoid, deltoid, and biceps muscle. This is then followed by the rigidity appearing in the intercostals, the rectus abdominus, and lower extremity muscles.

The physiologic changes, especially the hemodynamic ones, are quite different in time and in sequence to voluntarily increased muscle tone by a maximal voluntary contraction Valsalva maneuver.

Fentanyl and Congeners. The immediate elevation in mean pulmonary artery and central venous pressure is a dominant feature of the rigidity syndrome. With alfentanil, cardiac index, heart rate, and systemic pressure changes are absent or are not impressive. This is in contrast to the changes following a Valsalva maneuver. It is apparent that the increased intramuscular pressure compresses the venous and peripheral arteries at muscle tensions significantly less than those that occur with a Valsalva maneuver.

Mechanism. In view of some of these findings and also the fact that in patients with a pneumatic tourniquet inflated to exclude the narcotic agents from a given extremity, yet that rigidity has still been observed, that a suprasegmental mechanism is involved in the development of rigidity. Further, the rigidity is augmented by a tactile and auditory stimulation, indicating a locus above the spinal cord; therefore, a nonperipheral mechanism is operative.

In fact, it appears that there may be a neurochemical explanation with a common pathway for narcotic rigidity and for drug reactions and a similarity to the motor abnormalities seen in Parkinson's disease. This points toward a basal ganglia locus of action. It is suggested that the rigidity is induced by the action of the narcotics on the μ-receptors located on interneurons in the caudate nucleus.

Seizure Phenomena.[133] Grand mal seizures, types of tonic or myoclonic activity, and cataleptic rigidity have been reported in humans in response to fentanyl.[134,135] In most instances, the seizure-like activity is poorly defined. In general, myoclonic movement disorders can be separated into the epileptic and nonepileptic types, as succinctly reviewed by Durrani.[136] The description in most of the reports seems inconclusive, the EEG activity needs to be available for better definition. In the fentanyl and isoflurane reports, no EEG seizure activity has been reported. It must then be concluded that the type of seizure being reported is a nonepileptic type and is either a mild to a markedly progressive type of myoclonic peripheral muscular activity with intermittent rigidity and loss of rigidity of the skeletal muscle. Full documentation is not available, but the possibility of opiate-induced seizures in subcortical structures such as the hippocampus and amygdala exists. Experimentally high doses of morphine as well as alfentanil have induced abnormal muscle activity and seizures. Seizures have followed subarachnoid morphine and appear to be related to nonopiate mechanisms and are not naloxone reversible.[131] Murkin[137] reports an absence of seizures during induction when high doses of fentanyl are used.

The question of whether the seizure phenomenon related to high doses of fentanyl is a peripheral manifestation of muscle rigidity or a true epileptiform type of seizure, being a central effect, has been further elucidated by other reports.[138] In some instances, the adverse response was delayed but consisted of clonic seizure activity after an initial tonic phase. This, in the experience of neurologists, was diagnosed without doubt as a grand mal seizure. Further, it was terminated by standard antiepileptiform therapy.

Seizures or Myoclonus.[136] Because of the number of reports of perioperative seizure-like phenomena, it is necessary to define terms. This has been clearly outlined by Durrani.[136]

Myoclonus is a movement disorder, and both positive and negative myoclonus can occur from a lesion at any part of the neuraxis. Depending on the EEG findings, myoclonus can be divided into epileptic and nonepileptic types. Epileptic myoclonus, or myoclonic seizures, accompany a distinct group of progressive neurologic disorders that include many chronic viral degenerative and metabolic diseases. Myoclonus is also associated with so-called idiopathic epilepsy and epilepsia partialis continua.

Nonepileptic myoclonus has a variety of presentations, including dystonic myoclonus, periodic tremors of sleep, segmental myoclonus, and multifocal myoclonus. There are specific characteristics in rhythm and frequency, and these may originate either from the brain stem or spinal cord. Spinal segmental myoclonus is produced by unchecked spinal neuronal discharge as a result of lack of inhibition of supraspinal control.

Some agents, such as diethyl ether, enflurane, ketamine, and etomidate, have been shown to produce seizure activity on the EEG and have the potential to initiate a perioperative seizure. On the other hand, fentanyl and isoflurane have been implicated with respect to perioperative seizures, but neither of these agents produce EEG seizure activity.

CLINICAL APPLICATIONS

PREANESTHETIC MEDICATION. The following approaches to preanesthetic medication for neuroleptic analgesia have been practiced:

1. *The sedative approach*—In this approach, one of the following drugs may be injected 1 hour before induction: diazepam, diphenylhydramine (Benadryl, 50 to 150 mg) or promethazine. An anticholinergic, such as scopolamine, is also administered. Foldes[139] considers that drugs with an antihistaminic property are desired to antagonize certain effects of fentanyl. Additionally, the presence of an antihistaminic drug may be useful in combatting some of the undesirable effects of subsequently administered succinylcholine or nondepolarizing muscle relaxants (d-tubocurarine), and may also reduce the occasional parkinsonian effects of the neuroleptic.
2. *The sedative–narcotic approach*—In addition to the sedation as noted above, a narcotic is also employed. Low doses of fentanyl or its congeners (alfentanil or sufentanil) are administered shortly (5 to 15 minutes) before induction. This prevents the psychomotor activity of restlessness, confusion, incoordination, and muscular movements frequently seen.
3. *The neuroleptanalgesic approach*—Premedication can be accomplished with Innovar itself. Small total doses of 0.5 to 2 mg, depending on physical status, age, and weight, are administered for sedative tranquilization. In healthy patients under 50 years of age, an average dose is 0.02 ml/kg; larger doses of 0.02 to 0.95 ml/kg are for a basal state. This premedication dose is about one fifth the induction dose.

Use of only the neuroleptic component as part of premedication is an option. For this purpose, droperidol injectable (Inapsine) is used containing 2.5 mg/ml. In adults, 1 to 4 ml (2.5 to 10 mg) are injected intramuscularly, according to age and physical status. A standard dose of 0.1 mg/kg is recommended. In children, one half this dose is appropriate for this purpose.

TECHNICAL PROCEDURES

Two techniques of neuroleptanalgesia-type anesthesia are currently practiced. The classic technique is that of using the combination of the premixed drugs, whereas the rational recommended technique employs each component separately.

Classic Technique[41,140]

INDUCTION DOSAGE. For anesthesia in children and adults, the dosage of the fixed mixture is set at 1 ml/10 kg (0.1 mg/kg) of body weight (1 ml/20 to 25 lb), each ml containing 2.5 mg droperidol and 0.05 mg fentanyl. In poor-risk, debilitated or elderly patients, this dose should be reduced by one third to one half.[141a]

Dosage on a weight basis of the drug (not ml) is more accurate and appropriate and is represented as follows:

$$\left.\begin{array}{ll}\text{Droperidol} & 0.25 \text{ mg/kg} \\ \text{Fentanyl} & 0.005 \text{ mg/kg}\end{array}\right\} 0.01 \text{ ml/kg}$$

INDUCTION PROCEDURE. Administration of the mixture is by intravenous route in fractional amounts. One half the calculated dose is given as the loading dose at a rate of 1 ml/5 sec. Vital signs are observed and recorded. If after 1 to 2 minutes no significant circulatory or respiratory alterations are noted (faster injections may cause decreased thoracic compliance [stiff chest]), the remainder of the calculated dose is administered at a rate of 0.5 to 1 ml/sec.

Oxygen inhalation by mask prior to and during induction is recommended. With onset of sleep, a general inhalation anesthetic is then administered, usually nitrous oxide–oxygen, 50/50 mixture, in a semiclosed system by mask or via an endotracheal tube.

Intravenous drip of a dilute Innovar solution (10 ml/250 ml of 5% dextrose in water) may be administered rapidly (about 10 ml/min) until sleep is induced, when the drip is slowed or stopped. This provides a slower, cautious injection.

MAINTENANCE. The duration of action of the neuroleptic component is long, about 3 to 6 hours, whereas the analgesic component is 30 to 60 minutes. Therefore, the analgesic state must be maintained by additional doses of fentanyl. Injection is made when signs of lightening anesthesia are noted in response to surgical stress (increased heart rate, elevation of systolic or diastolic pressure, or irregular breathing).

Supplemental doses of fentanyl are about one fourth to one half the original induction dose, or 0.025 to 0.05 mg (0.5 to 1 ml) for an average adult and are also administered intravenously.

Recommended Improved Technique of Foldes

REQUIREMENTS. The recommended technique of neuroleptanalgesia consists of the use of the two principal agents separately according to dose and response activity and *not* together or simultaneously.[139] The requirements of the method are as follows:

1. Appropriate premedication
2. Separate administration of the drugs
3. Neurolepsis with droperidol (slow onset 7 minutes; long duration 3 hours)
4. Analgesia with fentanyl (short duration of 30 minutes)
5. Maintenance by fentanyl alone
6. Anesthesia and unconsciousness with nitrous oxide–oxygen
7. Endotracheal intubation with topical anesthesia and a muscle relaxant
8. Assisted or controlled ventilation

INDUCTION. An infusion should be started in all patients with a 5% dextrose or crystalloidal solution, if not contraindicated. Approximately 300 to 500 ml of solution should be administered before induction. Monitoring procedures are instituted.

Initial Drug and Dose. The initial drug administered is the neuroleptic. Droperidol is injected slowly intravenously in a dose of 0.15 mg/kg. Onset of action is seen in 3 to 5 minutes and full effect in 7 to 10 minutes.

Second Drugs and Dose. Six to eight minutes after the neuroleptic injection, the analgesic is administered intravenously and slowly. A total dose is calculated on the basis of 0.005 mg/kg of fentanyl (5 µg/kg).

A portion of the total dose is administered as a loading dose; the mean loading dose to abolish reaction to a skin incision in about 50% of subjects is approximately 2.5 µg/kg and is administered as follows: (1) the initial fraction of the loading dose of fentanyl is an average of 0.05 mg (50 µg, or 1 ml of the fentanyl preparation) for adults, depending on age, weight, physical status, and presence of other drugs; and (2) increments of 0.01 mg (10 µg) are then administered approximately 2 minutes apart until the patient is well sedated and asleep. At this time, the respiratory rate usually falls to 12 to 16 breaths per minute and there is no response to painful stimulation.

MAINTENANCE BY ANALGESIC DRUG. Whenever the patient shows signs of reacting to surgical stimulation, additional doses of fentanyl are administered. This may be anticipated every 10 to 15 minutes. Supplemental doses are about 0.025 to 0.05 mg (0.5 to 1 ml) every 10 to 15 minutes, or an average of 0.33 µg/kg/min.[139]

Endotracheal intubation, if required, is carried out with the aid of intravenous muscle relaxants in conventional doses. Muscle relaxation, if required, may be provided by use of depolarizing or nondepolarizing muscle relaxants at usual intravenous dosages.

EMERGENCE. Anesthesia is terminated by discontinuing the administration of nitrous oxide and allowing the patient to breathe room air, which results in rapid awakening.

RECOVERY. Recovery is smooth and devoid of nausea or vomiting. Analgesia continues into the postoperative period, and the requirement for narcotics is reduced. Most patients need none for 12 to 14 hours. Routine assessment of vital signs in the recovery period is essential.

Residual action of large doses of the fentanyl may be reversed by use of specific antagonists, levallorphan (5 to 10 mg) or naloxone (0.4 to 0.8 mg). Large doses for induction and maintenance have been employed in cardiac surgery. A dose of 10 to 100 µg/kg has been employed for loading, and the maintenance dose is increased to 0.1 µg/kg.

Induction by Fentanyl (No Neuroleptic)

As a sole agent for the induction of anesthesia, with loss of consciousness and production of amnesia, fentanyl is not a dependable or effective agent. Even the high-dose technique or pretreatment with diazepam does not ensure success.[141] The usual tests of induction of unconsciousness (stage II), namely loss of verbalization and loss of response to verbal commands, have been carefully evaluated following doses of 30 µg/kg, and only about 75% of patients during infusion of fentanyl became anesthetized.[142]

Over 25% of patients require thiopental. These observations are consistent with the central nervous system pharmacodynamics, which do not reveal a significant cortical action.

A comparison of effects of doses of 15 µg/kg against 60 µg/kg for induction shows no substantial advantage of the large dose. In Bazaral's study,[131] the larger dose was associated with initial significant increases in heart rate.

Continuous Infusion Technique

This technique is designed to provide a continuous replacement of fentanyl that is lost or detoxified and to maintain a steady plasma level. Levels of 2 ng/ml or more correlate with analgesia and sedation.[105]

A solution is prepared by diluting 2.5 mg fentanyl in a 500-ml balanced salt solution. This is a 1:2000 dilution and provides 0.5 mg in 100 ml, or 5 µg/ml. More dilute solutions have been proposed, but fluid overload is more likely. The procedure is as follows:

1. An initial or loading dose of fentanyl is calculated according to the classic method of 2.5 to 5 µg/kg of body weight. A concentrated solution containing 50 µg/ml is used. This is administered as bolus fractions over a period of 3 to 4 minutes.
OR The infusion drip may be administered at a rapid rate to introduce 100 µg/min for 3 to 5 minutes (i.e., 10 ml/min), or up to the calculated loading dose.
2. If a high-dose technique is planned, according to either an intermediate dose of 20 to 50 µg/kg or superdoses of 50 to 150 µg/kg,[141] the calculated dose is administered in fractions over a period of 5 to 10 minutes for loading, or until the desired effect is achieved.
3. Maintenance is by continuous drip after loading; a dose one tenth the loading dose is estimated for each 10 min period. Approximately 0.025 to 0.10 µg/kg/min is the approximate range for maintenance, with an average of 0.035 µg/kg/min, which has been determined to provide a continuous state of analgesia.[139]

The rate of flow is determined by calculating the minute dose based on the pharmacokinetics of fentanyl and aimed at maintaining a proper plasma level. A reasonable guide is 2.5 µg/min (0.5 ml/min) for a man weighing 70 kg.

The infusion should be administered as a biologic titration, i.e., the dose is proportional to and determined by the response. When the high-dose technique is used, higher minute doses are required.

The maintenance dose approximates the rate of decline of plasma levels as determined by the clearance value.

Low-Dose Fentanyl–Thiopental Sequence Induction

A low dose of fentanyl administered prior to induction with thiopental provides significant advantages. First, the dose of thiopental required to achieve the proper induction end point is lowered by almost 50%. The end points for induction and the loss of consciousness have been thoroughly standardized and have been defined as the loss of (1) verbalization by the patient, (2) response to a voice command, and (3) eyelid reflex. Second, the usual hemodynamic responses to laryngoscopy and intubation were significantly attenuated but not completely suppressed. Approximately 44% of those pretreated with high doses (20 µg/kg) of fentanyl alone required a volatile agent, such as enflurane, to control the hemodynamic responses. Thus, it is further evident that narcotics at best or even in large doses do not provide a complete anesthetic state.

ADVANTAGES OF NEUROLEPTANALGESIA.

1. The technique is simple, safe, nonexplosive, and economic.
2. Prolonged major surgical procedures can be carried out with a minimum of toxicity exerted by the neuroleptanalgesia agents.
3. Profound analgesia is produced without cardiovascular impairment and cortical depression.
4. Pain relief extends into the postoperative period. Conventional narcotics are rarely needed to control pain during the early postoperative phase. If narcotics are required, their dosage can be cut down to one third or one fourth the usual dose.
5. The adrenergic blocking action of dehydrobenzperidol ensures unusual vascular stability. Its relaxing effect on the peripheral vascular bed provides optimal tissue perfusion, which is of particular significance in the presence of sudden hemorrhage or shock.
6. The antiarrhythmic action of dehydrobenzperidol proves particularly valuable in heart surgery by reducing the incidence of arrhythmias induced by mechanical stimuli such as manipulating the heart, cardiotomy, and so forth. Some electrocardiographic studies indicate that undesirable cardic reflexes and arrhythmias are not completely abolished.

    The antiarrhythmic action has been studied in patients during cyclopropane anesthesia. Ventricular irregularities were produced by intravenous infusion of epinephrine at a slow constant rate. The rate at which an arrhythmia was initiated was defined as the *arrhythmic threshold*. Dehydrobenzperidol (droperidol) in doses of 0.2 mg/kg doubles the arrhythmic threshold.[56]
7. The patient can be awakened during surgery and questioned, which facilitates performing certain neurosurgical procedures, such as excision of epileptogenic foci, hitherto carried out under local anesthesia.
8. Nausea and vomiting during induction maintenance or in the postanesthetic recovery period is rarely seen.
9. There is total amnesia for the induction and the early recovery phase.
10. Fentanyl-induced respiratory depression can readily be counteracted by opiate antagonists.

DISADVANTAGES OF NEUROLEPTANALGESIA.

1. Profound respiratory depression may ensue after completion of the intravenous injection. Hypoventilation or apnea may last from 5 to 12 minutes, after which adequate respiratory exchange is gradually restored.
2. Pulmonary compliance may be lowered during the phase of respiratory depression, making assistance or controlling of respiration difficult. Small amounts of intravenously administered succinylcholine can prevent such development.
3. In the poor-risk patient with marginal compensatory reserves, hypotension may occur during induction. Fluid administration is the preferred method to correct the hypotension. Vasopressors with predominant peripheral action may restore vascular tone.
4. Neuroleptanalgesia does not provide muscle relaxation. Muscle relaxants may, therefore, be required and may have to be administered in higher dosages and at shorter intervals than seen with conventional anesthetic techniques.
5. Large-dose fentanyl techniques are associated with significant vagal-mediated bradycardia.[109]

COMPLICATIONS.

1. Fentanyl-induced respiratory depression may lead to severe hypoxia or asphyxia, if the patient is left unattended or is under the care of a clinician not familiar with the principles of maintaining unobstructed air passages and administering artificial respiration. Reversal agents are useful for management.
2. Inability to inflate the lungs adequately during the respiratory depression phase may result in severe respiratory impairment. Early use of small amounts of intravenous nondepolarizing relaxants will prevent this complication.
3. Narcotic analgesics such as morphine sulphate and meperidine hydrochloride, administered postoperatively for pain relief, can cause severe respiratory depression when given at conventional doses. Opiates antagonists will promptly restore respiratory function under these circumstances.
4. In poor-risk patients or patients of advanced age, hypotension may occur during induction. Such blood pressure reactions promptly respond to small dosages of intravenously administered vasopressors. Hypotensive reactions occur rarely in this type of patient, if the calculated intravenous doses of dehydrobenzperidol and fentanyl are reduced to two thirds or one half.
5. Extrapyramidal-type muscular movements may develop during induction or maintenance of neuroleptanalgesia, which readily respond to intravenously administered atropine sulfate or other antiparkinsonian agents. These movements are not typically parkinsonian and appear to be related to excess cholinergic activity at basal ganglia rather than dopamine deficiency. Hence, atropine is the treatment choice. Among the responses seen are dystonia, akathisia, and oculogyric crisis. Contraction of the muscles of the face, neck, and pharynx and trimus of the jaw may be seen and may persist into the post-

operative period up to 24 hours. Although these effects are rare with droperidol, the use of most neuroleptic agents is contraindicated in Parkinson's disease or other basal ganglia disorders.

6. Infrequent adverse reactions include chills and shivering, blurred vision, muscular hyperactivity, and diaphoresis. Postoperative drowsiness is not expected. Emergence delirium and urticara have been reported.
7. Drug interaction: When fentanyl is used without a neuroleptic, but diazepam and presumably midzolam are administered, significant hemodynamic effects occur. The hypotension is noted especially when the high-dose (750 μg/kg) technique is employed.[141,143]
8. A secondary peaking of fentanyl in plasma can occur 4 to 6 hours after the injection of the drug. This is associated with a biphasic respiratory depression and, when occurring in the postoperative period, represents a considerable hazard. This peaking may be due to increased perfusion of the peripheral compartment, especially skeletal muscle with movement and recovery followed by an increased plasma uptake.
9. Fentanyl high-dose techniques of 25 μg/kg or more, without a concomitant neuroleptic, are associated with some self-limited, abnormal movements. This activity consists of wrist flexion and arm-shoulder twitches; ocular movements are also observed. Rao[133] has described actual seizure-like movements. This phenomenon has also been observed in animals; however, Murkin[137] has studied the EEG changes in patients during induction of a fentanyl state, and although truncal rigidity occurred, no seizure-like waves were noted. In all instances, only diffuse slow-wave EEG activity was noted.
10. Hypersensitivity reactions of type I or type IV anaphylactoid can occur with fentanyl. Such fentanyl allergy has been confirmed by skin testing.[144] Fentanyl, however, is not associated with increases in blood histamine.[145]

NALBUPHINE

This agonist–antagonist opioid has been proposed as the analgesic component of neurolepticopioid anesthesia (balanced), because fentanyl and its congeners have many disadvantages, such as:

- Hypotension, especially in the postanesthetic period and after high doses[146]
- Bradycardia[85]
- Chest wall rigidity[147]
- Postoperative respiratory depression
- Awareness intraoperatively[148]
- Pain and stress reaction[149]

Zsigmond[150] have noted two properties of nalbuphine that make it a suitable agent, especially in cardiac surgery: the drug lacks cardiac depression action[149] and possesses a limit to its respiratory depression, designated as the *ceiling effect*.[151]

The anesthetic procedure is as follows:

- Preoxygenation
- Pretreatment with diazepam 0.4 mg/kg IV
- An intravenous infusion of nalbuphine (loading dose 3 mg/kg over 20 minutes)
- Relaxant with dose of 0.1 mg/kg pancuronium or vecuronium
- *Intubation*, followed by inhalation of N_2O–O_2 50:50
- Maintenance dose of nalbuphine 0.25 mg/kg administered in incremental doses, as indicated by signs of noxious stimulation* and given to maintain a pain- and stress-free state
- Additional doses of muscle relaxant, as needed

Hemodynamic changes at three intraoperative stressful periods of tracheal intubation, skin incision, and sternotomy were not statistically significant. Plasma catecholamines and cortisol levels remained normal. No evidence of histamine release was observed. Postoperative hypnosis, sleep (7 hours), and analgesia were evident. All patients were mechanically ventilated. Nalbuphine is considered an effective and safe alternative to other analgesics and opioids in anesthesia for cardiac surgery and perhaps is preferred to fentanyl.

ALFENTANIL

This ultrashort-acting narcotic analgesic is related to fentanyl and to the meperidine class of narcotics.[152,153] It is about one fifth as potent as fentanyl and with a shorter duration of activity approximating one third to one fourth that of fentanyl. The safety ratio is

$$\frac{LD_{50}}{ED_{50}} = 1000.$$

The chemical structure and comparison with fentanyl is shown in Figure 26–7.

The drug action of a bolus injection lasts for only 3 to 4 minutes and unconsciousness is short. Hence, it is necessary to administer frequent increments or use a continuous infusion. The drug is capable of producing both hypnosis and analgesia and does not affect the cardiovascular system. Large doses can produce respiratory depression, which may continue for more than 20 minutes.

PHARMACOKINETICS.[154,155] The pharmacokinetics of alfentanil have been studied (see Table 26–5 for comparison with fentanyl) and demonstrate that after doses of 25 μg/kg and up to 125 μg/kg as a single

---

* Criteria include (1) increased pupil diameter (> 2 mm); (2) increased right pulmonary pressure (> 20%); and (3) clinical signs: lacrimation, sweating, decreased finger pulse recording, eye movement.

Alfentanil

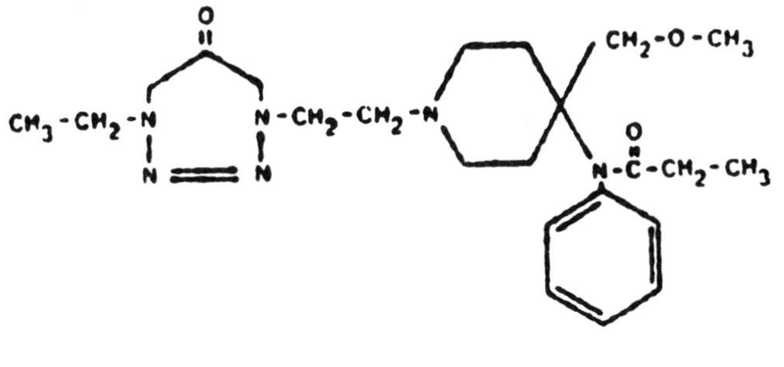

Fentanyl

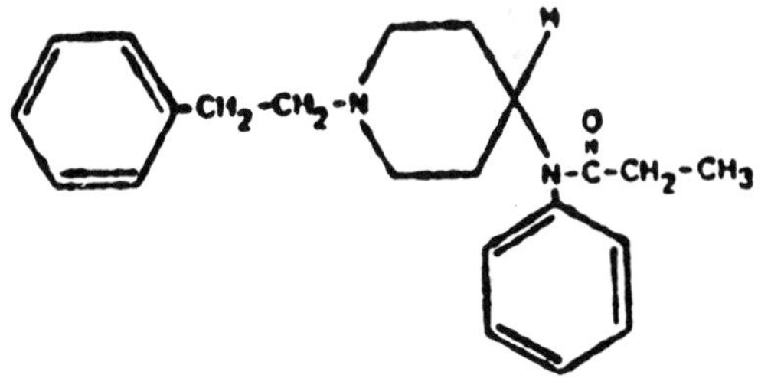

FIG. 26–7. Comparison of the chemical structure of alfentanil and fentanyl. From Bovill, J.G., et al.: The pharmacokinetics of alfentanil (R39209): A new opioid analgesic. Anesthesiology, 57:439, 1982.

intravenous bolus injection, the plasma concentrations decline triexponentially. Indeed, there is a great similarity in the times for either the small or large dose.

The average half-lives were determined as follows:[154] the initial rapid distribution phase, the dilutional phase or $t_{\frac{1}{2}}$ π-phase, approximates 1 to 1.5 minutes. The distribution phase to the body tissues ($t_{\frac{1}{2}}$ α) approximates 12 minutes (11.6 ± 1.6 minutes). The elimination half-life, or $t_{\frac{1}{2}}$ β, approximates 100 minutes (94 ± 6 minutes). The elimination half-life is, therefore, considerably shorter than that of fentanyl (219 minutes) and other opiates. The mean total body clearance is set at 6.5 ml/kg/min, with a volume of distribution at steady state of 0.86 (± 0.19) L/kg. The volume of distribution is about four times smaller than that for fentanyl, while the clearance is one half that of fentanyl.

Fentanyl has a long terminal half-life of 219 to 500 minutes and is eliminated from the body almost entirely by hepatic metabolism. Its short duration of action is related to rapid decline in brain concentrations and redistribution to muscle and fat from which the drug is slowly released to the plasma compartment. Alfentanil has a high degree of plasma protein binding. This is approximately 92%, so that the free fraction is 8%. There is also a lower lipid solubility with a heptane-water partition coefficient of 2.5 as compared to fentanyl with a partition coefficient of 9.0.

POPULATION KINETICS (VARIABLES).[156–158] A careful analysis of several variables from different studies of alfentanil kinetics results in the concept of population kinetics, which tends to affect the pharmacokinetics of a large population of patients undergoing general anesthesia with alfentanil. Such a study reveals the following:

1. *Body weight:* This influences the volume of the central compartment but does not affect clearance. On the basis of weight, the volume of clearance of 0.127 L/kg is larger than when weight is discounted.
2. *Age on clearance:* No influence of age on pharmacokinetics for patients under 40 years of age is evident. But a linearly decreasing function of age for patients more than 40 years of age has been determined. The magnitude of the decrease in clearance is about 30% at a mean age of 77 years. Clearance of drugs from other body compartments also is influenced by age. Thus, there is a slower redistribution from the deep compartments in older patients.
3. *Sex:* Sex has a slight but significant effect on the volume of the central compartment, being about 15% larger in women than in men.

CONCLUSION.[159] Considering the variables, the alfentanil plasma concentration time course of a given dose can be predicted only to the extent of 68%.

TABLE 26–5. PHARMACOKINETIC AND PHYSICOCHEMICAL PROPERTIES OF FENTANYL AND ALFENTANIL

Property	Fentanyl	Alfentanil
Pi phase $t_{1/2}$ π (min)	1.70 ± 0.12	1.2 ± 0.26
Distribution $t_{1/2}$ α (min)	13.4 ± 1.6	11.6 ± 1.6
Elimination $t_{1/2}$ β (h)	3.7 ± 0.4	1.6 ± 0.3
Clearance (ml · kg^{-1} · min^{-1})	11.6 ± 2.6	6.4 ± 1.4
Vd$_{ss}$ (L/kg)	4.2 ± 0.6	0.86 ± 0.62
Free fraction plasma (%)	16	8
pKa	8.4	6.5
Nonionized % at pH 7.4	9.0	89.0
Partition coefficient (octanol/water)	860	130

Modified references 154, 155 and 155a.

The loading dose should be adjusted to body weight, whereas the maintenance dose should be adjusted to age but not to weight. Intersubject variability for clearance is 48% and 33% for the volume of distribution, leaving a residual of 25%. With the analysis of patient factors and variability, the extent of confidence on a chosen dose is approximately 68%.

It is possible to use pharmacokinetic concepts and variables to design drug-administration schemes based on drug disposition and plasma concentrations. Computer-driven infusion pumps use such models.[156,157] Feedback from clinical observations and responses remains necessary to satisfy all individual requirements. Thus, for the present, drug administration in doses must be dependent on clinical end points.

PHARMACOKINETICS IN CHILDREN.[160] A rapid initial disappearance of alfentanil from plasma occurs in children after a bolus dose. A distribution phase of about 5 minutes compares with 10 minutes in adults. The volume of the central compartment has been found to be significantly smaller in children, being about 70 ml/kg versus 190 ml/kg in adults. The total apparent volume of distribution at steady state is also significantly smaller, being about 160 ml/kg compared with 460 ml/kg in adults.

These parameters lead to a shorter elimination half-life in children of about 40 minutes versus 100 minutes in adults.

The total plasma clearance in children and adults is similar (4.7 ± 0.6 versus 4.2 ± 1.7 ml/min/kg).

Infants and Children. No correlation between volume of distribution at steady state and age or weight in children ages 3 months to 14 years has been determined. A weak correlation between clearance and age, however, does exist; that is, the clearance decreases with age, a negative relationship.

Elimination half-life, $t_{\frac{1}{2}}$-β, and the volume of distribution at steady state are not different in infants less than 1 year of age compared with older children.[161]

Clinical Implications. Recovery time after alfentanil administration is more rapid in children than in adults. The small volume of distribution at steady state means that the risk of accumulation is less. Infusion rates to maintain a steady plasma concentration do not differ between children and adults because plasma clearance is smaller. The narcotic effects at the end of an infusion are also terminated more rapidly in children.

EFFECT OF RENAL FAILURE. In chronic renal failure, drug protein binding is decreased. This is especially so for acidic compounds, such as thiopental, but more variable for basic drugs.[162] Alfentanil is a weak based and is ordinarily bound to the extent of 92% to plasma proteins, particularly to alpha$_1$ glycoprotein. Patients with renal failure usually have a reduced protein binding and a high alfentanil plasma free fraction. Corrected kinetic parameters, however, indicate that the unbound volume of distribution and the free drug clearance of this drug are unchanged in patients with renal failure. Thus, the kinetics based on free drug concentrations, i.e., the unbound volume of distribution and the unbound clearance, do not differ significantly in renal failure in patients compared with those with normal renal function. Although there was an associated decrease in alfentanil plasma protein binding, it did not appear to change the clearance kinetics but did increase the volume of distribution at steady state. Hence, there was no increase in the elimination of alfentanil.

MECHANISM OF ACTION. The central nervous system action is similar to that of fentanyl. The low lipid solubility of alfentanil would appear to limit its penetration into cells, especially through the blood-brain barrier. The brain concentration of alfentanil is about one seventh of that in the plasma (fentanyl's brain concentration is 3 to 5 times that of plasma). Although the lipid solubility is low, it is still sufficiently high for the nonionized form in plasma to cross membrane barriers and permit a rapid onset of action and a short duration of action.[163]

The short elimination half-life of alfentanil is explained on the basis of the smaller volume of distribution and the high total clearance. Because of the relatively small volume of distribution, however, the clearance is significantly shorter for the terminal elimination half-life. It is also noted that there is no second peak, so the plasma concentration occurs late in the kinetic pattern of fentanyl.

ANALGESIC PLASMA CONCENTRATIONS.[155] The therapeutic narcotic plasma concentration producing adequate analgesia and providing an anesthetic state with supplemental inhalation anesthetics can be depicted from the plasma decay curves of single intravenous doses of alfentanil (Fig. 26–8). This can also be compared, at the same time, with the decay curve and therapeutic plasma concentration of fentanyl (see Fig. 26–6).

Preliminary investigations[154] indicate that a plasma alfentanil concentration of approximately 300 ng/ml is required to maintain adequate surgical anesthesia using a 40% N_2O–60% O_2 inhalational technique. As plasma levels fall below 300 ng/ml, after approximately 5 minutes following a dose of 50 μg/kg (15 minutes after a dose of 125 μg/kg), analgesia wanes. Inadequate analgesia is evident at 200 ng/ml or below, which may be considered a minimum threshold plasma level.

No secondary peaks of plasma concentration of alfentanil have been determined, in contrast to fentanyl. There is also prompt recovery of the CO_2 response. These observations can be related to a much shorter duration of action of alfentanil.[120]

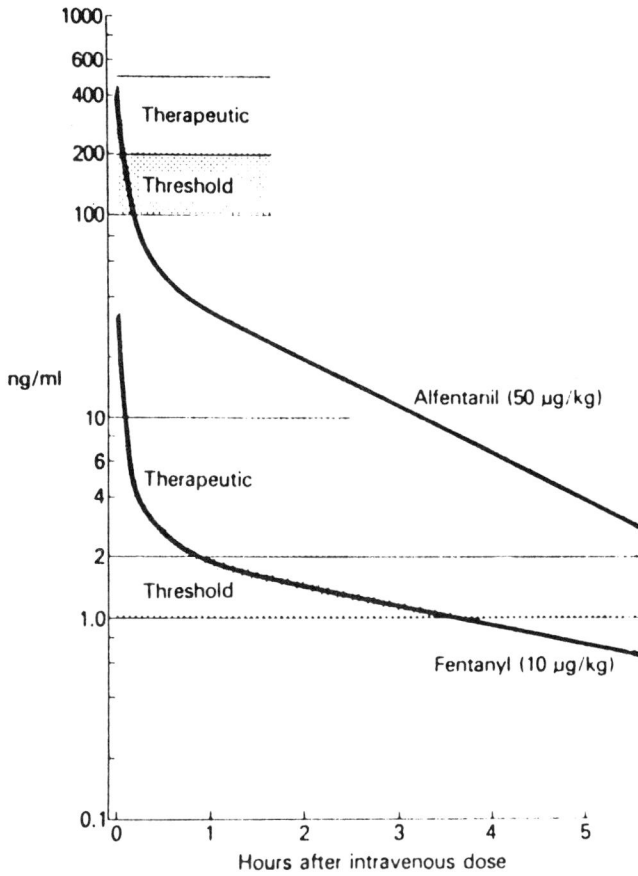

FIG. 26-8. A comparison of the plasma decay curves of a single iv bolus dose of fentanyl and alfentanil. The solid line is the predicted plasma concentration in a single patient with representative pharmacokinetics. While the equivalent alfentanil dose is five times that of fentanyl, during the first 2 h after injection the alfentanil plasma concentrations are 14 to 25 times higher. This is due in part to the smaller volume of distribution of alfentanil. From Stanski, D.R., and Hug, C.C.: Alfentanil—A kinetically predictable narcotic analgesic (editorial). Anesthesiology, 57:435, 1982.

POTENCY. The various congeners of the phenoperidine derivatives can be compared in their potency. The usual bolus dose of alfentanil for induction to unconsciousness is 50 μg/kg, but this will not maintain a state of unconsciousness or analgesia after 5 to 10 minutes. Thus, the potency of alfentanil is about one fifth that of fentanyl. Compared with sufentanil, it is about one fiftieth as potent.

DOSAGE AND ADMINISTRATION.[154,164-166] Two techniques may be used to provide anesthesia. The first is the single or intermittent bolus technique for brief surgical procedures. The dose to achieve anesthesia for a 5 to 10-minute procedure approximates 50 μg/kg of body weight. This dose is effective in the production of unconsciousness but is not quite as rapid as that induced by thiopental and is definitely faster than the onset of action by fentanyl. Supplemental doses may be administered between 5 and 10 minutes to maintain an adequate state of analgesia. The intermittent technique obviously produces a significant fluctuation in the level of the anesthetic narcotic state. It has been proposed by Bovill[154] to use a continuous infusion of alfentanil to provide a more constant plasma concentration in the range of 300 ng/ml and a steady analgesic state. This technique would proceed as follows:

1. An induction dose consisting of 50 μg/kg as a single bolus injection—The onset of unconsciousness and the narcotic anesthetic state is attained at approximately 3 minutes in 66% of patients and lasts approximately 5 minutes.[167] Onset is somewhat more rapid than with fentanyl but is shorter in action. In 35% of subjects, however, double the prescribed dose is necessary to produce unconsciousness. Additional bolus doses of 5 to 15 μg/kg are usually needed to suppress the effects of surgical stimulation in the absence of inhalation anesthetics.[167a,b]
2. Maintenance of analgesia after 4 to 5 minutes by a continuous infusion administration at an average rate of 20 μg/kg/min—It can be estimated that the maintenance dose would approximate one half to one fourth of the loading dose.
3. Preparation—A solution that enables maintenance of the anesthetic state contains 100 mg in 500 ml of Ringer's lactate solution. The rate can be adjusted according to patient response and may be rapid or slow. The administration of 5 ml/min provides a 1-mg dose, which would approximately maintain an adequate plasma level for analgesia.

PHARMACODYNAMICS

Central Nervous System. Unconsciousness is not readily identified. The time to unconsciousness (stage II) is longer and more variable compared with thiopental. Respiratory depression and apnea often precede unconsciousness,[167] but the onset of induction is more rapid than with fentanyl.

Electroencephalographic Changes.[163] EEG changes to doses of alfentanil have been quantitated with steady-state serum concentrations, and these have been compared with the fentanyl EEG changes at a steady-state serum concentration. The steady-state serum concentration causing one half of the maximum EEG slowing was found to be 6.9 ± 1.5 ng/ml for fentanyl; this compares with 520 ± 163 ng/ml for alfentanil, which is then calculated as a fentanyl:alfentanil potency ratio of 75:1. This differs from the clinical dose potency of fentanyl, which has been reported as being seven times as potent as alfentanil. This difference is explained by alfentanil's smaller initial distribution volume and less time lag between serum concentration changes and changes in effect.

Cardiovascular Effects. Studies by Kay[152,153] and Natua[164-166] indicate that alfentanil provides excellent cardiovascular stability, which appears to be better than thiopental, etomidate, midazolam and other intravenous induction agents.

Respiratory Effects. Spontaneous breathing is depressed at plasma levels above 200 ng/ml; apnea may even occur prior to onset of unconsciousness. After the usual induction and maintenance doses, however, spontaneous ventilation will resume within 10 to 20 minutes after discontinuing drug administration at the time when the plasma level declines below 200 ng/ml. This contrasts with fentanyl concentrations, which, when used to supplement inhalation anesthetics at plasma levels of 2 to 10 ng/ml, usually do not permit recovery of spontaneous ventilation until the plasma level approximates 1 ng/ml.[87]

DRUG INTERACTION. Other agents used in anesthesia practice influence alfentanil. There is a prolongation of action by diazepam, as well as by other benzodiazepines and other narcotics.

ADVERSE EFFECTS. It is noted that during induction with alfentanil, as with fentanyl itself, rigidity of the chest may occur. This may be noted in 55% of patients. This rigidity is lessened, but not necessarily obliterated, by the prior administration of diazepam. Pain at the injection site is recognized in about 5% of patients. In the absence of surgical stimulation or blood loss, alfentanil induction doses can cause hypotension and bradycardia. Respiratory depression may occur as with other opioids. It is reversed by opioid antagonists.

ADVANTAGES. This congener of the meperidine series appears to have significant advantages over fentanyl, including rapid production of unconsciousness, minimum cardiovascular depression, minimal respiratory alterations (recovery of CO_2 response occurs early), no alterations of other systemic functions, and short duration of action.

COMMENTARY.[188] Most of the evidence indicates that opiates alone are incapable of preventing neuroendocrine and hemodynamic responses to the somatic and visceral stimulation stress of surgery, no matter what the dose; nor will they appreciably attenuate these responses. Secondly, the parenteral opiates, when used alone, may at best relieve pain but do not prevent the noxious sensory input to the central nervous system. The awakening and awareness phenomena are probably related to this input. Thirdly, the opiates fail to completely obtund the hemodynamic responses to endotracheal intubation or to catheterization, although attenuation is evident. Fourth, amnesia and unconsciousness are incomplete.

In the study by Philbin using large doses of either fentanyl or sufentanil intermittently or by continuous infusion to maintain a high plasma concentration of the opioid did not significantly reduce the *incidence* of responses.[188] It was concluded that "opioids by the nature of their action should not be expected to produce or maintain complete surgical anesthesia" (as defined by the Woodbridge Components).

An editorial view by Hug[189] notes that measurement of actual drug concentrations in blood or other tissues is not necessary because the concentrations do not always correlate with the nervous system effects, reflect the blocking of neuroendocrine responses, or define the therapeutic range of anesthetic goals. In "balanced anesthesia" the continuous titration of dose to the effects desired is necessary and only the ability to test responsiveness is important.[189]

SUFENTANIL

Sufentanil is a synthetic narcotic compound structurally related to fentanyl, and thus belongs to a series of phenylpiperidine derivatives.[168] To some extent, these analogues have been developed to obtain a drug that would indeed produce a "stress-free" state of anesthesia. As yet, no narcotic has been identified that is capable of satisfying the Woodbridge principles of the anesthetic state.

CHEMISTRY. Sufentanil differs from fentanyl structurally in that a thienyl-ethyl group is attached to the nitrogen of the piperdinyl portion of the fentanyl structure (Fig. 26–9).

The drug is available as a citrate salt, and a preservative-free aqueous solution has been prepared at a pH range of 3.5 to 7.5. The concentration is such as to provide 50 μg/ml of the base drug.

DOSE AND POTENCY.[169,170] In anesthesia practice, this opioid analogue, like other narcotics, is administered intravenously. The low-to-moderate-dose technique in noncardiac surgery varies from 1 to 5 μg/kg of body weight as a loading dose, with an

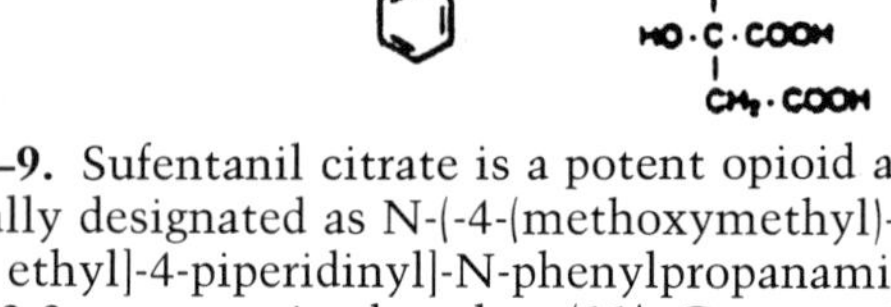

FIG. 26–9. Sufentanil citrate is a potent opioid analgesic chemically designated as N-(-4-(methoxymethyl)-1-[2-(2-thienyl) ethyl]-4-piperidinyl]-N-phenylpropanamide 2-hydroxy-1.2.3-propanetricarboxylate (11). Courtesy Janssen Pharmaceutica Inc., Piscataway, N.J., 1984.

$Ct = 30.3e^{-0.661} + 6.1e^{-0.0491} + 1.0e^{-0.00431}$

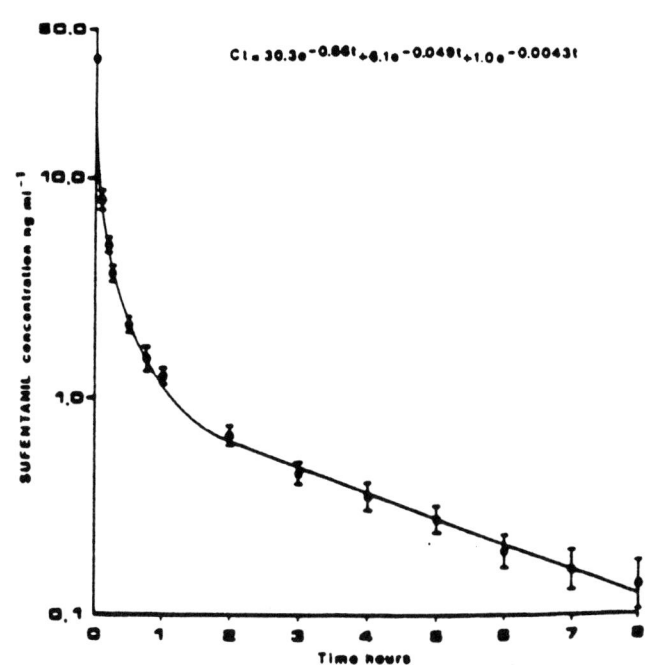

FIG. 26–10. Mean (±SEM) plasma concentrations after bolus intravenous injection of sufentanil 5 μg/kg. The tri-exponential equation describes the line of best fit through the points *(solid line)*. From Bovill, J.G., et al.: Kinetics of alfentanil and sufentanil: A comparison. Anesthesiology, 61:502, 1984.

average of 2.8 μg/kg. Compared with the modified fentanyl technique, this represents a potency ratio of approximately five times that of fentanyl.[171] In the intravenous narcotic or the neuroleptic narcotic techniques, the dose of fentanyl is proposed at 15 μg/kg of body weight.

A high-dose sufentanil technique, employing 15 to 30 μg/kg, has been used for cardiac surgery patients.[172] Although some claims of greater cardiovascular stability have been made for the sufentanil-oxygen technique,[171] most studies show that the cardiovascular stability is only equivalent to that acclaimed for fentanyl. Indeed, Rosow[173] in 1983 found no hemodynamic advantages of this drug over fentanyl. The evidence suggests that narcotic–oxygen anesthesia does not produce dose-related supression of (adverse) cardiovascular reflexes.

Intranasal Sufentanil.[174] The nasal administration of a standard solution of sufentanil by a syringe without a needle has been found effective as a preliminary narcotic preanesthetic medication in children. The dose range is 1.5 to 4.5 μg/kg and the instillation is gradual, over 15 to 20 seconds. Henderson has found this technique is preferred by children to intramuscular or rectal administration of the drug.[174]

PHARMACOKINETICS. A three-compartment model describes the kinetics of sufentanil. (Fig. 26–10) Clinical studies generally support a more rapid onset of analgesic effect and a shorter duration of action compared with fentanyl. A smaller volume of distribution but a similar clearance rate to fentanyl results in a more rapid elimination (Table 26–6).[175–177] Another comparative table (Table 26–7) has been assembled by Murphy.[168]

PHARMACODYNAMICS[168]

1. *Cardiovascular:* Small decreases in systemic blood pressure may be seen following the administration of sufentanil, and this is more pronounced with the higher dose ranges. Modest reductions in central venous pressure are also to be noted; however, there appears to be less hypertension during surgery. Induction of a narcotic-hypnotic state with sufentanil is accompanied by decreases in the mean arterial pressure. Such reduction may continue into the postoperative period, and vasopressor agents may be needed for restoration of normal tension.
2. *Cerebral:* A reduction in cerebral blood flow and a decrease in oxygen utilization occurs at the cerebral level. This is similar to fentanyl.
3. *Seizure Activity:*[170] Abnormal muscular movements of a tonic, chronic type have been reported following sufentanil and considered to represent true seizures. As with the fentanyl reports, however, it is uncertain and poorly documented by means of EEG recordings that these are typical epileptic-type phenomena.

    A review of the types of movements, basically represented as myoclonic seizures, should be classified and defined either as epileptic or non-epileptic myoclonus. This has been further elaborated on in the commentary on fentanyl seizures.[136]
4. *Respiration:* Decreased pulmonary ventilation follows the administration of even small doses. This is related to a decreased respiratory drive. In addition, there is an increased airway resis-

TABLE 26–6. COMPARISON OF FENTANYL AND SUFENTANIL

	$T_{1/2}$ (min) π	$T_{1/2}$ (min) α	$T_{1/2}$ (min) β	V_c (L/kg)	V_o (L/kg)	Cl (ml/min)
Fentanyl	1.7	13	219	0.36	4.0	910
Sufentanil	0.7	14	140	0.10	2.5	793

TABLE 26–7. COMPARATIVE PHARMACOKINETICS IN HUMANS

	Sufentanil	Fentanyl
Distribution half-life ($t_{1/2}\pi$ min)	1.4 ±0.3	1.7 ±0.1
Redistribution half-life ($t_{1/2}\alpha$ min)	17.1 ±2.6	13.4 ±2.0
Elimination half-life ($t_{1/2}\beta$ min)	164.0 ±22.0	219.0 ±10.0
Volume of distribution (v_d L/kg)	2.9 ±0.2	4.0 ±0.2
Plasma clearance (ml/kg/min)	12.7 ±0.8	13.0 ±0.9

From Bovill, J.G., et al.: The pharmacokinetics of sufentanil in surgical patients. Anesthesiology, 61:502, 1984.

tance. With high doses, apnea is often produced. Rigidity of the truncal muscles also occurs as it does with fentanyl, and it is related to both dose and to the speed of injection. It is as frequent as with fentanyl.

5. *Sympathetic Nervous System:*[173,178] Some suppression of the sympathetic outflow occurs with some suppression of catecholamine release and of other hormonal responses to the anesthetic stress, i.e., to endoscopy and intubation; however, suppression is incomplete to surgical stresses. Most studies address the use of the intravenous narcotics to cardiac surgery, especially coronary bypass operations. Bovill[178] and de Lange[179,180] have shown some suppression of the presurgical stress responses. An increase in plasma catecholamine, however, occurs during surgical incision and manipulations.

6. *Hormone:*[181] During coronary bypass procedures, the release of antidiuretic hormone does occur and is sometimes significant.[178–180] The drug thus appears to be no more effective in modifying hormonal responses than is fentanyl.[181a]

7. *Histamine Release:* At low doses, histamine release has not been demonstrated but may be seen with large doses.[182] Histamine levels may increase with surgical incision and with sternotomy.[183]

Sufentanil, in doses of 1.5 µg/kg administered intravenously, results in a slight elevation of plasma histamine at 1.2 minutes after injection. The level rises from a baseline of 0.12 ng/ml to 0.23 ng/ml; at 6 minutes, the level decreases to 0.18 ng/ml.[184]

8. *Choice of Relaxant:* The combination of fentanyl and pancuronium appears to be the satisfactory combination inasmuch as the bradycardia often produced by fentanyl tends to be antagonized by the pancuronium's effect in increasing heart rate. Studies of sufentanil with pancuronium indicate that tachycardia is much greater when sufentanil is the narcotic employed. As a result, it has been recommended by Khoury[185] that metocurine be employed for relaxation during sufentanil–oxygen anesthesia.

COMPARISON AND ADVANTAGES. Comparing sufentanil (20 µg/kg) with morphine (4.4 mg/kg) and fentanyl (100 µg/kg) narcotic techniques with oxygen only for cardiac surgery revealed that sufentanil allowed more rapid induction (failure to respond to command), earlier emergence, and earlier extubation than the other narcotics.[186]

In patients without cardiac disease who are undergoing various general surgical procedures, a sufentanil–N$_2$O–O$_2$ technique showed little intraoperative advantages over fentanyl with regard to suppression of hemodynamic hormonal response to the surgical stress. More rapid recovery from ventilatory depression, however, occurred with sufentanil, and there was greater analgesia in the immediate postoperative period.[187]

REFERENCES

1. Wynands, J.E., et al: Narcotic requirements for intravenous anesthesia. Anesth. Analg, 63:101, 1984.
2. Roizen, M.F., Horrigan, R.W., and Frazer, B.M.: Anesthetic doses (inhalation) blocking adrenergic (stress) and cardiovascular responses to incision—MAC BAR. Anesthesiology, 54:390, 1981.
3. Hardy, J.F., et al: Influence of narcotics on hypertension after coronary artery bypass graft surgery. Can. Anaesth. Soc. J., 30:370, 1983.
4. Lehtinen, A.M., Fyhrquist, F., and Kivalo, I.: The effect of fentanyl on arginine vasopressin and cortisol secretion during anesthesia. Anesth. Analg., 63:25, 1984.
5. Wynands, J.E., et al: Blood pressure response and plasma fentanyl concentrations of high- and very high-dose fentanyl anesthesia for coronary artery surgery. Anesth. Analg., 62:661, 1983.
6. Van Hooersen, B.: Blood urea in scopolamine and atropine and their relation to preoperative medications and pain relief. Texas State J. Med., 34:304, 1938.
7. Cullen, S.C., McQuiston, W.O., and Peterson, V.W.: Nitrous oxide anesthesia for thoraco-plasty. Anesthesiology, 2:310, 1941.
8. Brotman, M., and Cullen, S.C.: Supplementation with demerol during nitrous oxide anesthesia. Anesthesiology, 10:696, 1949.
9. Harroun, P., Beckert, F.E., and Hathaway, H.R.: Curare and nitrous oxide anesthesia for lengthy operations. Anesthesiology, 7:25, 1946.

10. Neff, W., Mayer, E.C., and Perales, M.: Nitrous oxide and oxygen anesthesia with curare relaxation. California Med., 66:67, 1947.
11. Brotman, M., and Cullen, S.C.: Intravenous supplementation during nitrous oxide anesthesia: Comparison of demerol, morphine and a new analgesic. Anesthesiology, 11:527, 1950.
12. Randal, H.S., Belton, K., and Leigh, D.M.: Continuous infusion of demerol during anesthesia. Can. Med. Assoc. J., 67:311, 1952.
13. Johnson, P.D.: Pethidine as an adjunct to nitrous oxide–oxygen anesthesia. Br. Med. J., 2:705, 1951.
14. Mushin, W.W., and Rendell-Baker, L.: Pethidine as a supplement to nitrous oxide anesthesia. Br. Med. J., 2:472, 1949.
15. Ausherman, H.W., Nowilli, W.K., and Stephen, C.R.: Controlled analgesia with continuous drip meperidine. J.A.M.A., 160:175, 1956.
16. Harris, A.J.: The management of anesthesia for congenital heart operations in children. Anesthesiology, 11:328, 1950.
17a. Ruben, H., and Andreassen, A.K.: Intravenous pethidine for laryngoscopy. Br. J. Anaesth., 23:33, 1951.
17b. Ruben, H., and Gammeltoft, A.: Intravenous pethidine for oesophagoscopy and gastroscopy. Anaesthesia, 8:194, 1953.
18. Garcia, C.R., Waltman, R., and Lubin, S.: Continuous intravenous infusion of demerol in labor. Am. J. Obstet. Gynecol., 66:312, 1953.
19. Siker, E.S., et al: Nisentil: A new supplement for nitrous oxide–oxygen thiopentone anaesthesia. Br. J. Anaesth., 26:405, 1954.
20. Yim, G.W., et al: Simultaneous respiratory minute volume and tooth pulp threshold changes following levorphan, morphine and leveorphan–levallorphan mixtures in rabbits. J. Pharmacol. Exp. Ther., 155:96, 1955.
21. Orahovats, P.D., Winter, C.A., and Lehman, E.G.: Pharmacological studies of mixtures of narcotics and N-allylnormorphine. J. Pharmacol. Exp. Ther., 112:246, 1954.
22. Cullen, S.C., and Santos, A.: Analgesics for post-operative pain without respiratory depression. Anesthesiology, 16:674, 1955.
23. Lasagna, L., and Beecher, H.K.: The analgesic effectiveness of nalorphine and nalorphine–morphine combinations in man. J. Pharmacol. Exp. Ther., 112:356, 1954.
24. Foldes, F.F., et al: Levallorphan and alphaprodine in anesthesia. J.A.M.A., 160:168, 1956.
25. Lowenstein, E., et al: Cardiovascular response to large doses of intravenous morphine in man. N. Engl. J. Med., 281:1389, 1969.
25a. Longnecker, D.E., Grazis, P.A., and Eggers, G.N.N.: Naloxone for antagonism of morphine-induced respiratory depression. Anesth. Analg., 52:447, 1973.
25b. Johnston, R.E., Jobes, D.R., Kennell, E.M. et al: Reversal of morphine anesthesia with naloxone. Anesthesiology, 41:361, 1974.
26. Lowenstein, E.: Morphine anesthesia: A perspective (editorial). Anesthesiology, 35:563, 1971.
27a. Hasbrouk, J.D.: Morphine anesthesia for open-heart surgery. Ann. Thorac. Surg., 10:364, 1970.
27b. Stoelting, R.K., and Gibbs, P.S.: Hemodynamic effects of morphine and morphine–nitrous oxide in valvular heart disease and coronary-artery disease. Anesthesiology, 38:45, 1973.
28. McDermott, R.W., and Stanley, T.H.: The cardiovascular effects of low concentrations of nitrous oxide during morphine anesthesia. Anesthesiology, 41:89, 1974.
29. Arens, J.F., et al: Morphine anesthesia for aorto-coronary bypass procedures. Anesth. Analg., 51:901, 1972.
30. Stanley T.H., et al: The effects of high-dose morphine in fluid and blood requirements in open-heart procedures. Anesthesiology, 38:536, 1973.
31. Kopin, I.J., Lake, C.R., and Ziegler, M.: Plasma levels of norepinephrine. Ann. Intern. Med., 88:671, 1978.
31a. Philbin, D.M., and Coggins, C.H.: Plasma antidiuretic hormone levels in cardiac surgical patients during morphine and halothane anesthesia. Anesthesiology, 49:95, 1978.
31b. Reier, C.E., and Kilman, J.W.: Cortisol and growth hormone response to surgical stress during morphine anesthesia. Anesth. Analg. (Cleve.), 52:1003, 1973.
31c. Guillemin, R., et al: β-Endorphin and adrencorticotropin are secreted concomitantly by the pituitary gland. Science, 197:1367, 1977.
31d. Madsen, S.N., et al: Inhibition of plasma cyclic AMP, glucose and cortisol response to surgery by epidural analgesia. Br. J. Surg., 64:669, 1977.
32. Philbin, D.M., et al: Renin, catecholamine, and vasopressin response to the "stress" of anesthesia and surgery. Anesthesiology, 51(3S):S121, 1979.
32a. Lehtinen, A.M.: Opiate action on adenohypophyseal hormone secretion during anesthesia and gynecologic surgery in different phases of the menstrual cycle. Acta Anaesthesiol Scand, 25:73, 1981.
33. Lehtinen, A.M., Fyhrquist, F., and Kivalo, I.: The effect of fentanyl on arginine and cortisol secretion during anesthesia. Anesth. Analg., 63:25, 1984.
34. Laborit H., and Huguenard, P.: Practiquede l'hibernotherapie. Masson Et Cie, Libraries de L'Académie de Médicine, Paris 1954.
35. Laborit, H.: Stress and Cellular Function. Philadelphia, J.B. Lippincott, 1959.
36. Beckett, A.H., and Casey, A.F.: Synthetic analgesics: Stereochemical considerations. J. Pharm. Pharmacol., 6:986, 1954.
37. Beckett, A.H.: Analgesics and their antagonists: Some steric and chemical considerations. I. The dissociation constants of some tertiary amines and synthetic analgesics, the conformations of the methadone-type compounds. J. Pharm. Pharmacol., 8:848, 1956.
38. Janssen, P.A.J.: Vergleichende pharmakologische daten ueber sechs neue basische-4-fluorobutyrophenone-derivative. Arzneim Forsch, 11:819, 1961.
39. Janssen, P.A.J., et al: The pharmacology of dehydrobenzperidol: A new potent and short-acting neuroleptic agent chemically related to haloperidol. Arzneim Forsch, 13:205, 1963.
40. DeCastro, J., and Mundeleer, P.: Die neuroleptanalgesie. Auswahl der praeparate, bedeutung der analgesie und de neurolepsia. Der Anaesthetist 11:10, 1962.
41. Corssen, G., Domino, E.F., and Sweet, R.B.: Neuroleptanalgesia and anesthesia pharmacological and clinical considerations. Anesth. Analg., 43:748, 1964.
42. Janssen, P.A.J., Niemeggers, C.J.E., and Dony, J.G.H.: The inhibitory effect of pentanyl and other morphine-like analgesics on the warm water induced tail withdrawal reflex in rats. Arzneim Forsch, 13:502, 1963.
43. Janssen, P.A.J.: On the pharmacology of analgesics and neuroleptics used for surgical anesthesia. Symposium on Neuroleptanalgesia, First European Congress of Anesthesiology, Vienna, 1962.
44. Yelonsky, J., Katz, R., and Dietrich, E.V.: A study of some of the pharmacologic effects of droperidol. Toxicol. Appl. Pharmacol., 6:37, 1964.
45. Fischler, M., et al: The pharmacokinetics of droperidol in anesthetized patients. Anesthesiology, 64:486, 1986.
46. Cressman, W.A., Plostnieks, J., and Johnson, P.C.: Absorp-

tion, metabolism and excretion of droperidol by human subjects following intramuscular and intravenous administration. Anesthesiology 38:363, 1973.
47. Edmonds-Seal, J., and Prys-Roberts, C.: Pharmacology of drugs used in neuroleptanalgesia. Br. J. Anaesth., 42:207, 1970.
48. Eerola, R., Pontinen, P.J., and Mietlman, P.: Electrocardiographic changes during neuroleptanalgesia. Acta Anaesthesiol. Scand., 7:187, 1963.
49. MacDonald, H.R.: Clinical and circulatory effects of neuroleptanalgesia. Br. Heart J., 28:654, 1966.
50. Muldoon, S.M., et al: Alphaadrenergic blocking properties of droperidol on isolated blood vessels of the dog. Br. J. Anaesth., 49:211, 1977.
51. Hokfelt, T., et al: Dopamine nerve terminals in the rat limbic cortex: Aspects of the dopamine hypothesis of schizophrenia. Science, 184:177, 1974.
51a. Roos, B.E.: Effects of certain tranquilizers on the level of homo-vanillic acid in the corpus stratum. J. Pharm. Pharmacol., 17:280, 1965.
52. Patton, C.M., Moon, M.R., and Dannemiller, F.J. The prophylactic antiemetic effect of droperidol. Anesth. Analg. (Cleve), 53:361, 1974.
53. Fitch, W., et al: The influence of neuroleptanalgesia on cerebrospinal fluid pressure. Br. J. Anaesth., 41:800, 1969.
54. Dixon, S.: Neuroleptanalgesia: Effects of Innovar on myocardial contractility, peripheral vascular resistance and capacitance. Anesth. Analg., 49:331, 1970.
55. Zauder, H.L., et al: Hemodynamics during neuroleptanalgesia. Anesthesiology, 26:266, 1965.
56. Long, G., Dripps, R.D., and Price, H.L.: Measurement of antiarrhythmic potency of drugs in man. Anesthesiology, 28:318, 1967.
57. Bertolo, L., Novakovic, L., and Penna, M.: Antiarrhythmic effect of droperidol. Anesthesiology, 37:529, 1972.
58. Dietzel, W., and Massion, W.H.: The prophylactic effect of Innovar in experimental hemorrhagic shock. Anesth. Analg., 48:968, 1969.
59. Corssen, R., Reves, J.G., and Carter, J.R.: Neurolept dissociative anesthesia and hemorrhage. Int. Anesthesiol. Clin., 12:45, 1974.
60. Aronson, H.B., Mogora, F., and London, M.: The influence of droperidol on blood viscosity in man. Br. J. Anaesth., 42:1089, 1970.
61. Prys-Roberts, C., and Kelman, G.R.: The influence of drugs used in neuroleptanalgesia on cardiovascular and ventilatory function. Br. J. Anaesth., 39:134, 1967.
62. Kallos, T., and Smith, T.C.: The respiratory effects of Innovar given for premedication. Br. J. Anaesth, 41:303, 1969.
63. Kallos, T., Wyche, M.Z., and Garman, J.K.: The effects of Innovar on functional residual capacity and total chest compliance in man. Anesthesiology, 39:558, 1973.
64. Corssen, G., and Kornfeld, T.J.: Comparison of respiratory depressant effect of phentanyl, phentanyl–droperidol and morphine. Anesthesiology, 27:213, 1966.
65. Dunbar, B.S., et al: The respiratory response to carbon dioxide during Innovar–nitrous oxide anesthesia in man. Br. J. Anaesth., 39:861, 1967.
66. Harper, M.H., et al: The magnitude and duration of respiratory depression produced by fentanyl and fentanyl plus droperidol. J. Pharmacol. Exp. Ther., 199:464, 1976.
67. Becker, J.D., et al: Biphasic respiratory depression of fentanyl–droperidol or fentanyl alone used to supplement nitrous oxide anesthesia. Anesthesiology, 44:291, 1976.
68. Ward, D.S.: Stimulation of hypoxic ventilatory drive by droperidol. Anesth. Analg., 63:106, 1984.
69. Oyama, T.: Neuroleptanesthesia. Int. Anesthesiol. Clin., Boston, Little, Brown, 1973.
70. Oyama, T., and Takiguchi, M.: Effect of neuroleptanaesthesia on adrenocortical function in man. Br. J. Anaesth., 42:425, 1970.
71. Oyama, T., and Takiguchi, M.: Effect of neuroleptanaesthesia on plasma levels of growth hormone and insulin in man. Br. J. Anaesth., 42:1105, 1970.
72. Giesecke, A.H., et al: Urinary epinephrine and norepinephrine during Innovar–nitrous oxide anesthesia in man. Anesthesiology, 28:701, 1967.
73. Tornetta, F.J., and Boger, W.P.: Liver function studies in droperidol–fentanyl anesthesia. Anesth. Analg., 43:544, 1964.
74. Gorman, H.M., and Graythorne, N.W.B.: The effects of a new neuroleptanalgesia on renal function in man. Acta Anaesthesiol. Scand. 24(Supp):111, 1966.
75. Jarnberg, P.O., Santesson, J., and Eklund, J.: Renal function during neuroleptanaesthesia. Acta Anaesthesiol. Scand., 22:167, 1978.
76. Gergis, S.D.: Effects of Innovar and Innovar plus nitrous oxide on muscle tone and "H" reflex. Anesth. Analg., 50:743, 1971.
77. Klawans, H.L., et al: Recent advances in the biochemical pharmacology of extrapyramidal movement disorders. Adv. Exp. Med. Biol., 90:21, 1977.
78. Delay, J., and Deniker, P.: Drug-induced extrapyramidal syndromes. In: Vinken P.J., Bruyn G.W., eds. Handbook of Clinical Neurology, Vol. 6. Diseases of the Ganglia. Edited by P.J. Vinken and G.W. Bruyn. Amsterdam, North-Holland Publishing, 1968, 248.
79. Guze, B.H., and Baxter, L.R., Jr.: Neurolept malignant syndrome. N. Engl. J. Med., 313:163, 1985.
80. Hess, R., Herz, A., and Friedel, K.: Pharmacokinetics of fentanyl in rabbits, in view of the importance for limiting the effects. J. Pharmacol. Exp. Ther., 179:474, 1971.
81. Corssen, G., Domino, E.F., and Sweet, R.B.: Neuroleptanalgesia and anesthesia: Pharmacological and clinical considerations. Anesth. Analg., 43:748, 1964.
82. Gardock, J.F., and Yelonsky, J.: A study of pharmacologic action of fentanyl. Toxicol. Appl. Pharmacol., 6:63, 1964.
83. Murphy, M.R., Olson, W.A., and Hug, C.C.: Pharmacokinetics of ^{3}H-fentanyl in the dog anesthetized with enflurane. Anesthesiology, 50:13, 1979.
84. Murphy, M.R., and Hug, C.C.: The anesthetic potency of fentanyl in terms of its reduction of enflurane MAC. Anesthesiology, 57:485, 1982.
85. Stanley, T.H., and Webster, L.R.: Anesthetic requirements and cardiovascular effects of fentanyl–oxygen and fentanyl–diazepam–oxygen anesthesia in man. Anesth. Analg. (Cleve), 57:411, 1978.
86. Hess, R., Stibler, G., and Herz, A.: Pharmacokinetics of fentanyl in man. J. Clin. Pharmacol. Ther., 4:137, 1972.
87. McClain, D.A., and Hug, C.C.: Intravenous fentanyl kinetics. Clin. Pharmacol. Ther., 28:106, 1980.
88. Schleimer, R., et al: Pharmacokinetics of fentanyl as determined by radioimmunoassay. Clin. Pharmacol. Ther., 23:188, 1970.
89. Stoeckel, H., Hengstamm, J.H., and Schuttler, J.: Pharmacokinetics of fentanyl as an explanation for recurrence of respiratory depression. Br. J. Anaesth., 51:741, 1979.
90. Becker, L.D., et al: Biphasic respiratory depression of tentanyl–droperidol or fentanyl alone used to supple-

ment nitrous oxide anesthesia. Anesthesiology, 44:291, 1976.
91. Bovill, J.G., and Sebel, P.S.: Pharmacokinetics of high dose fentanyl. Br. J. Anaesth., 52:795, 1980.
92. Singleton, M.A., Rosen, J.L., and Fisher, D.M.: Plasma concentrations of fentanyl in infants, children and adults. Can. J. Anaesth., 34:152, 1987.
93. Friis-Hansen, B.: Body composition during growth. In-vivo measurements and biochemical data correlated to differential anatomical growth. Pediatrics, 47:264, 1971.
94. Short, C.R., Maines, M.D., and Westfall, B.A.: Postnatal development of drug-metabolizing enzyme activity in liver and extrahepatic tissues of swine. Biol. Neonat., 21:54, 1978.
94a. Tornetta, F.J. and Bolger, W.P.: Liver function studies in droperidol-fentanyl anesthesia. Anesth. Analg., 48:544, 1964.
95. Nayak, N.C., and Ramalingaswami, V.: Normal structure. In The Liver and Biliary Systems in Infants and Children. Chandra, R.K., ed. Edinburgh, Churchill-Livingstone, 1979:1.
96. Johnson, K.L., et al: Fentanyl pharmacokinetics in the pediatric population (abstract). Anesthesiology, 61:A441, 1984.
97. Haberer, J.P., et al: Fentanyl pharmacokinetics in anaesthetized patients with cirrhosis. Br. J. Anaesth., 54:1267, 1982.
98. Gorman, H.M., and Graythorne, N.W.B.: The effects of a new neuroleptanalgesia on renal function in man. Acta Anaesthesiol. Scand. 24 (Supp):111, 1966.
99. Goromaru, T., et al: Identification and quantitative determination of fentanyl metabolites in patients by gas chromatography-mass spectrometry. Anesthesiology, 61:73, 1984.
100. Yuge, O., et al: Fentanyl and alfentanil suppress brain stem pain transmission. Anesth. Analg., 64:597, 1985.
101. Dundee, J.W., et al: Clinical studies of induction agents. XXVI: The relative potencies of thiopentone, methohexitone and propanidid. Br. J. Anaesth., 40:593, 1968.
102. Corssen, G., Domino, E.F., and Sweet, R.B.: Neuroleptanalgesia and anesthesia: Pharmacological and clinical considerations. Anesth. Analg., 43:748, 1964.
103. Cartwright, P., et al: Ventilatory depression related to plasma fentanyl concentrations during and after anesthesia in humans. Anesth. Analg., 62:966, 1983.
104. Scott, J.C., Ponganis, K.V., and Stanski, D.R.: EEG quantitation of narcotic effect: A comparative pharmacodynamic of fentanyl and alfentanil. Anesthesiology, 62:234, 1985.
105. Hug, C.C.: Lipid solubility pharmacokinetics and the EEG: Are you better off today than you were 4 years ago (editorial)? Anesthesiology, 62:221, 1985.
106. Scott, J.C., Ponganis, K.V., and Stanski, D.R.: EEG quantitation of narcotic effect: A comparative pharmacodynamic of fentanyl and alfentanil. Anesthesiology, 62:234, 1985.
107. Graves, C.L., Downs, N.H., and Brownie, A.B.: Cardiovascular effects of minimal analgesic quantities of Innovar, fentanyl and droperidol in man. Anesth. Analg., 54:15, 1975.
108. Reitan, J.A., et al: Central vagal control of fentanyl induced bradycardia during halothane anesthesia. Anesth., Analg., 57:31, 1978.
109. Sorensen, M., et al: Bradycardia and cardiac asystole following a single injection of suxamethonium. Acta Anaesthesiol. Scand., 28:232, 1984.
110. Greenan, J.: Cardiac dysrhythmias and heart rate changes at induction of anesthesia. A comparison of two intravenous anticholinergics. Acta Anaesthesiol. Scand., 28:182, 1984.
111. Quinton, L., et al: High dose fentanyl anesthesia with oxygen for aortocoronary bypass surgery. Can. Anaesth. Soc. J., 28:314, 1981.
112. Hicks, H.C., Mowbray, A., and Yhap, E.O.: Cardiovascular effects of and catecholamine responses to high dose fentanyl–O_2 for induction of anesthesia in patients with ischemic coronary artery disease. Anesth. Analg., 60:563, 1981.
113. Bazaral, M.G., et al: Comparison of the effects of 15 and 60 μg/kg fentanyl used for induction of anesthesia in patients with coronary artery disease. Anesth. Analg., 64:312, 1985.
114. Chung, F., and Evans, D.: Low-dose fentanyl: Haemodynamic response during induction and intubation in geria-
115. Cartwright, P., et al: Ventilatory depression related to plasma fentanyl concentrations during and after anesthesia in humans. Anesth. Analg., 62:966, 1983.
116. Sullivan, S.F., and Patterson, R.W.: Arterial CO_2 tension adjustment rates following hyperventilation. J. Appl. Physiol., 21:247, 1966.
117. Sullivan, S.F., and Patterson, R.W.: Post-hyperventilation hypoxia: Theoretical consideration in man. Anesthesiology, 29:981, 1968.
118. Comstock, M.K., et al: Rigidity and hypercarbia on fentanyl oxygen induction. Anesthesiology, 51:S28, 1979.
119. Comstock, M.K., et al: Rigidity and hypercarbia associated with high-dose fentanyl induction of anesthesia. Anesth. Analg., 60:36, 1981.
120. Valgardsson, A., Werner, O., and Svensson, G.: Antagonism of fentanyl and alfentanil by intravenous plus subcutaneous naloxone. Anaesthesia, 40:772, 1985.
121. Sokoll, M.D., Hoyt, J.L., and Gergis, S.D.: Studies in muscular rigidity, nitrous oxide, and narcotic analgesic agents. Anesth. Analg. (Cleve), 51:16, 1972.
122. Hall, G.M., et al: Substrate mobilization during surgery. Anaesthesia, 33:924, 1978.
123. Stanley, T.H., et al: Plasma catecholamine and cortisol responses to fentanyl–oxygen anesthesia for coronary-artery operations. Anesthesiology, 53:250, 1980.
124. Gieseke, A.H., et al: Urinary epinephrine and norepinephrine during Innovar–nitrous oxide anesthesia in man. Anesthesiology, 28:701, 1967.
125. Flacke, J.W., et al: Histamine release by four narcotics: A doubleblind study in humans. Anesth. Analg., 66:723, 1987.
126. Scamman, F.L.: Fentanyl–O_2–N_2O rigidity and pulmonary compliance. Anesth. Analg., 62:332, 1983.
127. Christian, C.M., Waller, J.L., and Moldenhauer, C.C.: Postoperative rigidity following fentanyl anesthesia. Anesthesiology, 58:275, 1983.
128. Mayer, R.F., and Mawdsley, C.: Studies in man and cat on the significance of the "H" wave. J. Neurol. Neurosurg. Psychiatr., 28:201, 1965.
129. Freund, F.G., et al: Abdominal rigidity induced by morphine and nitrous oxide. Anesthesiology, 38:358, 1973.
130. Grossi, P., and Arner, S.: Effect of epidural morphine on the Hoffman reflex in man. Acta Anaesthesiol. Scand., 28:152, 1984.
131. Benthuysen, J.L., et al: Physiology of alfentanil-induced rigidity. Anesthesiology, 64:440, 1986.
132. Hill, A.P., et al: Prevention of rigidity during fentanyl–

133. Rao, T.L.K., Mummaneni, N., and El-Etr, A.A.: Convulsions: An unusual response to intravenous fentanyl administration. Anesth. Analg., 61:1010, 1982.
134. Sebel, A.M., and Bovill, J.G.: Fentanyl and convulsions. Anesth. Analg., 62:858, 1983.
135. Safat, A.M., and Daniel, D.: Grand mal seizures after fentanyl administration. Anesthesiology, 59:78, 1983.
136. Durrani, Z.: Perioperative myoclonia or seizures (editorial). Anesth. Analg., 66:583, 1987.
137. Murkin, J.M., et al: Absence of seizures during induction of anesthesia with high dose fentanyl. Anesth. Analg., 63:489, 1984.
138. Goroszeniuk, T., Albin, M., and Jones, R.M.: Generalized grand mal seizure after recovery from uncomplicated fentanyl–etomidate anesthesia. Anesth. Analg., 65:979, 1986.
139. Foldes, F.F., et al: A rational approach to neuroleptanesthesia. Anesth. Analg., 45:642, 1975.
140. Corssen, G., Reves, J.G., and Stanley, T.H.: Intravenous Anesthesia and Analgesia. Philadelphia, Lea & Febiger, 1988.
141. Stanley, T.H., and Webster, L.R.: Anesthetic requirements and cardiovascular effects of fentanyl–oxygen and fentanyl–diazepam–oxygen anesthesia in man. Anesth. Analg., 57:411, 1978.
141a. Chung, F., and Evans, D.: Low-dose fentanyl: Haemodynamic response during induction and intubation in geriatric patients. Can. Anaesth. Soc. J., 32:622, 1985.
142. Bailey, P.L., et al: Anesthetic induction with fentanyl. Anesth. Analg., 64:48, 1985.
143. Tomichack, R.C., et al: Diazepam–fentanyl interaction. Anesth. Analg., 62:881, 1983.
144. Bennett, M.J., et al: Anaphylactic reaction during anaesthesia associated with positive intradermal skin test to fentanyl. Can. Anaesth. Soc. J., 33:75, 1986.
145. Rosow, C.E., et al: Histamine release during morphine and fentanyl anesthesia. Anesthesiology, 56:93, 1982.
146. Sebel, P.S., et al: Cardiovascular effects of high dose fentanyl anesthesia. Acta Anaesthesiol. Scand., 26:308, 1982.
147. Corssen, G., et al: Neuroleptanalgesia and anesthesia for open heart surgery. J. Thorac. Cardiovasc. Surg., 49:901, 1965.
148. Mummaneni, N., Rao, T.L.K., and Montoya, A.: Awareness and recall with high-dose fentanyl-oxygen anesthesia. Anesth. Analg., 59:948, 1980.
149. Lee, G., et al: Hemodynamic effects of morphine and nalbuphine in acute myocardial infarction. Clin. Pharmacol. Ther., 27:478, 1981.
150. Zsigmond, E.K., et al: Nalbuphine as an analgesic component in balanced anesthesia for cardiac surgery. Anesth. Analg., 66:1155, 1987.
151. Romagnoli, A., and Keats, A.S.: Ceiling effect for respiratory depression by nalbuphine. Clin. Pharmacol. Ther., 27:478, 1980.
151a. Moldenhauer, C.C., et al: Nalbuphine antagonism of ventilatory depression following high dose fentanyl anesthesia. Anesthesiology, 62:647, 1985.
152. Kay, B., and Stephenson, D.K.: Alfentanil (R39209): Initial clinical experience with a new narcotic analgesic. Anaesthesia, 35:1197, 1980.
153. Kay, B.: Post-operative pain relief: Use of an on-demand analgesia computer (ODAC) and a comparison of the rate of use of fentanyl and alfentanil. Anaesthesia, 36:949, 1981.
154. Bovill, J.G., et al: The pharmacokinetics of alfentanil (R39209): A new opioid analgesic. Anesthesiology, 57:439, 1982.
155. Stanski, D.R., and Hug, C.C., Jr.: Alfentanil: A kinetically predictable narcotic analgesic. Anesthesiology, 57:435, 1982.
155a. Meuldermans, W.E.G., Hurkmans, R.M.A., and Heykants, J.J.P.: Plasma protein binding and distribution of fentanyl, sufentanil, alfentanil and lofentanil in blood. Arch. Int. Pharmacodyn. Ther. 257:4, 1982.
156. Schuttler, J., Schwilden, H., and Stoekel, H.: Pharmacokinetics as applied to total intravenous anaesthesia. Anaesthesia 38(Suppl):53, 1983.
157. Linkens, D.A.: Control technique in drug administration: Mathematical Methods in Medicine. I. Statistical and Analytical Techniques. Edited by D. Ingram and R.F. Bloch. New York, John Wiley, 1984, p. 413.
158. Maitre, P.O., et al: Population pharmacokinetics of alfentanil: The average dose-plasma concentration relationship and interindividual variability in patients. Anesthesiology, 66:3, 1987.
159. Grevel, J., and Whiting, B.: The relevance of pharmacokinetics to optimal intravenous anesthesia (editorial). Anesthesiology, 66:1, 1987.
160. Meistelman, C., et al: A comparison of alfentanil pharmacokinetics in children and adults. Anesthesiology, 66:13, 1987.
161. Goresky, G.V., et al: The pharmacokinetics of alfentanil in children. Anesthesiology, 67:654, 1987.
162. Burch, D.G., and Stanski, D.R.: Decreased protein binding and thiopental kinetics. Clin. Pharmacol. Ther., 32:212, 1982.
163. Scott, S.C., Ponganis, R.V., and Stanski, D.R.: EEG quantitation of narcotic effect; The comparative effects of fentanyl and alfentanil. Anesthesthesiology, 62:235, 1985.
164. Nauta, J., et al: Anesthetic induction with alfentanil: Comparison with thiopental, midazolam and etomidate. Anesthesiology, 55:A255, 1981.
165. Nauta, J., et al: Anesthetic induction with alfentanil: Comparison with thiopental, midazolam and etomidate. Can. Anaesth. Soc. J., 30:53, 1983.
166. Nauta, J., et al: Anesthetic induction with alfentanil: A new short acting narcotic analgesic. Anesth. Analg., 61:267, 1982.
167. Palazzo, M.G.A., Taylor, S., and Strunin, L.: Clinical experience with alfentanil for induction of anesthesia: A comparison with thiopental. Can. Anaesth. Soc. J., 31:517, 1984.
167a. Ausems, M.E., Hug, C.C., Jr., and de Lange, S.: Variable rate infusion of alfentanil as a supplement to nitrous oxide anesthesia for general surgery. Anesth. Analg., 62:982, 1983.
167b. Ausems, M.E., et al: Plasma concentrations of alfentanil required to supplement nitrous oxide anesthesia for general surgery. Anesthesiology, 65:362, 1986.
168. Murphy, M.R.: Clinical pharmacology of alfentanil and sufentanil. Anesthesiol. Rev., 11:17, 1984.
169. Murphy, M.R., and Hug, C.C.: Efficacy of fentanyl in reducing isoflurane MAC: Antagonism by naloxone and nalbuphine. Anesthesiology, 58:A338, 1983.
170. Molbegott, L.P., et al: Probable seizures after sufentanil. Anesth. Analg., 66:91, 1987.
171. Flacke, J.W., et al: Intraoperative effectiveness of sufentanil, fentanyl, meperidine, or morphine in balanced anesthesia: A double-blind study. Anesth. Analg., 62:259, 1983.

172. de Lange, S., et al: Comparison of sufentanil–oxygen and fentanyl–oxygen for coronary artery surgery. Anesthesiology, 56:112, 1982.
173. Rosow, C.E., et al: Sufentanil versus fentanyl. I. Suppression of hemodynamic responses. Anesthesiology, 59:A323, 1983.
174. Henderson, J.M.: ASA Annual Meeting, Atlanta, GA, 1987.
175. McClain, D.A., and Hug, C.C., Jr.: Intravenous fentanyl kinetics. Clin. Pharmacol. Ther., 28:106, 1980.
176. Bovill, J.G., et al: Kinetics of alfentanil and sufentanil: A comparison. Anesthesiology, 55:A174, 1981.
177. Bovill, J.G., et al: The pharmacokinetics of sufentanil in surgical patients. Anesthesiology, 61:502, 1984.
178. Bovill, J.G., et al: The influence of sufentanil on endocrine and metabolic responses to cardiac surgery. Anesth. Analg., 62:391, 1983.
179. de Lange, S., et al: Catecholamine and cortisol responses to high dose sufentanil–O$_2$ and alfentanil–O$_2$ anesthesia during coronary artery surgery. Anesth. Analg., 61:177, 1982.
180. de Lange, S., et al: Antidiuretic and growth hormone responses during coronary artery surgery with sufentanil–oxygen and alfentanil–oxygen anesthesia in man. Anesth. Analg., 61:434, 1982.
181. Sebel, P.S., et al: Hormonal effects of sufentanil anesthesia. Anesth. Analg., 61:214, 1982.
181a. Moldenhauer, C.C.: New narcotics, cardiac anesthesia. II: Cardiovascular pharmacology. Edited by J.A. Kaplan. New York, Grune and Stratton, 1983.
182. Flacke, J.W., et al: Plasma histamine levels during sufentanil anesthesia for coronary bypass graft surgery. Anesth. Analg.. 62:260, 1983.
183. Philbin, D.M., et al: Histamine release during induction with high dose sufentanil. Abstracts of the Sixth European Congress of Anesthesiologists, Paper 611, 1982.
184. Flacke, J.W., et al: Histamine release by four narcotics: A double-blind study in humans. Anesth. Analg. 66:723, 1987.
185. Khoury, G.F., et al: Sufentanil/pancuronium versus sufentanil/metocurine anesthesia for coronary artery surgery. Anesthesiology, 57:A47, 1982.
186. Sanford, T.J., et al: A comparison of morphine, fentanyl, and sufentanil anesthesia for cardiac surgery: Induction, emergence, and extubation. Anesth. Analg., 65:259, 1986.
187. Clark, N.J., et al: Comparison of sufentanil–N$_2$O and fentanyl–N$_2$O in patients without cardiac disease undergoing general surgery. Anesthesiology, 66:130, 1987.
188. Philbin, D.M., et al: Fentanyl and sufentanil anesthesia revisited: How much is enough. Anesthesiology, 73:5, 1990.
189. Hug, C.C., Jr.: Does opioid "anesthesia" exist? (editorial). Anesthesiology, 73:1, 1990.

27

INTRAVENOUS ANESTHESIA: NONBARBITURATES— NON-NARCOTICS

DISSOCIATIVE AGENTS

PHENCYCLIDINES

Cyclohexylamines

Several of a series of cyclohexylamine compounds are able to produce a unique state of analgesia and anesthesia.[1] These compounds are nonnarcotic and nonbarbiturate. Drugs of this series appear to produce a state of sensory dissociation in which the subjects are removed from their environment. The locus of this action may be at cortical or thalamocortical connections.

CHEMISTRY. The fundamental chemical structure of the cyclohexylamines is represented in Figure 27–1. Three analogues have been used clinically, but only one, ketamine, has gained anesthetic utility. The chemical structures of these analogues is shown in Figure 27–2.

Sernyl (CI-395). Greifenstein[2] investigated this compound, which produces analgesia and a disconnected or catatonic state, but a singular disadvantage is the production of marked agitation of the emergence type in 25% of the patients, which occasionally persists for several hours. In addition, hallucinatory phenomena occur in nearly all patients to some degree. These features limit its clinical value. At present this drug is being used in veterinary medicine and animal work as an immobilizer.

CI-400. A second compound of the cyclohexylamine series was introduced with the hope that the disadvantages of the first would be overcome. This compound produces the same degree of sensory blockade with minimal emergence agitation but with some hallucinatory effects[3] in 20% of patients.

Ketamine (CI-581). This compound was first synthesized by Stevens in 1963.[4] This derivative was found to be useful clinically. In early human use, it was found to be effective and without serious adverse side effects.[5]

ABUSE POTENTIAL.[6] The phencyclidine drugs have been abused, especially Sernalyn, which was previously available for the veterinary trade. On the street, this compound is known as *PCP*; other common names include "hog," "angel dust," "peace pill," "crystal," "sheets," "killerweed," and "supergrass." It can be ingested, snorted, (nasal snuffing), or placed in cigarettes ("happy sticks").

Intoxicated persons exhibit bizarre behavior and appear "spaced out" with a blank stare. Confusion with nonsequitor thought is frequent and followed by violent actions giving way to stupor. Large doses cause coma and respiratory depression. All the features of drunkenness are seen, including ataxia and nystagmus. Moderate doses elevate blood pressure and pulse, whereas large doses produce hypertension and sinus tachycardia. Skeletal muscle tone is increased, which progresses to myoclonic jerks. The pupils are normal or constricted, and the eye light reflex is diminished.

Sensation is decreased, especially touch, giving a feeling of floating; hearing, taste, position and muscle-tendon-joint (MTJ) sense are all diminished. Gag and laryngeal reflexes, however, remain active. The electroencephalogram (EEG) shows slow waves or beta activity.

Autonomic responses are exaggerated. The sympathetic responses appear to be mediated by dopamine receptors.

Diazepam has been found effective in controlling agitation in a single dose of 10 mg administered intramuscularly.[7] Halperodal in doses of 2.5 mg IM as well as phentolamine are useful in controlling autonomic responses; diazoxide (0.5 to 1 mg/kg) may be used to control hypertension.

PHENCYCLIDINE DISPOSITION. After intravenous administration of 1 mg of PCP, some 65% is bound to plasma protein. A large volume of distribution indicates extra plasmic binding. Most of the drug is recovered in the urine. Over 75% of the administered dose consists of metabolites and some free drug. About 5% is recoverable in feces, indicating a minor role for biliary excretion. The principal metabolite is a hydroxylated form that is conjugated. A small amount is excreted both by perspiration and in saliva. The terminal phase half-life is 21 hours.[8]

KETAMINE

Extensive laboratory and clinical experience with the phencyclidine derivative, ketamine hydrochloride (CI-581), has been obtained.[5,9] It is unique and unusually safe and effective for a variety of simple surgical and diagnostic procedures. The action of the drug is easy to control and requires a minimum of adjunctives or supportive drugs or devices. This drug

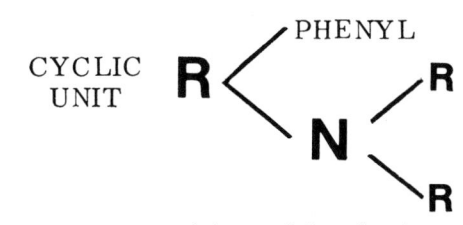

FIG. 27–1. Structure of the Cyclohexylamines.

represents a major step in the development of selectively acting agents.

The anesthetic properties are similar to the earlier compounds, but ketamine is quicker in onset, shorter-acting, and less likely to be followed by psychotic symptoms, particularly in children. In adults, there is less than about a 5% hallucinogenic-type response, which is greatly reduced by premedication.

CHEMISTRY.[1] Chemically, it is d,1-2 (0-chlorphenyl)-2-(methyl amino cyclohexanone hydrochloride) and exists as a white crystalline salt. It is water soluble up to 20% and is clear, colorless, and stable at room temperature.

PREPARATIONS. Ketamine is prepared as a slightly acid (pH 3.5 to 5.5) solution in a concentration of 10, 50, or 100 mg of ketamine as the hydrochloride

FIG. 27–2. Structural formulas for phencyclidine compounds.

salt of the base per ml. A preservative of 1:10,000 benzethonium chloride is included. The 10 mg/ml solution is isotonic with 0.9% of sodium chloride. These formulations are for intramuscular or intravenous injection.

The usual commercial preparation is incompatible with barbiturates, and mixing results in precipitation.

Ketamine is presently available only as a racemic mixture (Fig. 27–3); however, the individual enantiomers have different anesthetic actions. Ketamine's dextro (+) and levo (−) isomers have been investigated by White[10] and are designated as *PK* and *MK*, and the racemic mixture is *RK*. The racemic mixture in saline (Ketalar) has a pH of 3.5 to 5.5.

MECHANISM OF ACTION. Ketamine is a dissociative drug.[9] A peculiar state of unconsciousness is produced in which patients appear not to be asleep or anesthetized but rather "disconnected" from their surroundings. The term *dissociative* is applied to the state of anesthesia. Pharmacologic studies in humans support the observations made in laboratory animals that the anesthetic effect of ketamine is highly selective.

Association pathways in the cortex are apparently blocked first with disruption of environmental contact. The thalamus is also blocked, as are neocortical projection systems. The drug affects these systems intensely and is accompanied by significant obtundation of the medullary reticular activating system. Ketamine also seems capable of stimulating some areas (the limbic system and the hypocampus of the brain) while simultaneously depressing another (cortex). The dissociation is characterized by auditory and somatosensory deprivation while the limbic system is activated, allowing the visual cortex to respond.[9a]

CEREBRAL PATTERNS OF ACTION. Initial studies of EEG patterns by Domino[9] revealed that *ketamine induces* (1) hypersynchronous delta waves in the thalamoneocortical system, and (2) slow theta-arousal waves in the hippocampus and limbic systems.

These changes were interpreted to represent depression of the thalamoneocortical system and concurrent activation of the limbic system; therefore, functional dissociation of two brain areas results.

More explicit information on EEG changes has been obtained in Kayama's EEG studies.[11] After intravenous injection, the usual low-voltage *fast* waves of the sensorimotor and visual cortex first increase in amplitude, become desynchronized, and then hypersynchronize in the form of delta waves. Simultaneously, the ongoing theta waves of the hippocampus are replaced by desynchronization activity to be followed by slow waves. The presence of theta waves signals the presence of full analgesia.[12] Later, seizure activity is manifested in both areas by slow waves, slow waves with spikes, and burst complexes.[12a] During this state of ketamine anesthesia, evoked potentials in the cortex, in response to stimulation of the medial lemniscus, are enhanced and spontaneous single-unit discharges are increased.

Thus, both the thalamoneocortex and the limbic system (hippocampus) activity patterns are *first* strongly desynchronized and then interrupted by *seizure activity*.

The interpretation of Kayama's findings[11] is that ketamine appears to stimulate the thalamoneocortex, and the limbic hippocampus systems concurrently and eventually induces seizure activity. An EEG pattern of seizures interferes with consciousness and produces a state of catalepsy, as in petit mal. A continuum of desynchronization → intermittent hypersynchronization → continuous hypersynchronization → spikes → seizure → silence may be seen in all areas. Kayama[11] considers that Domino[9] did not appreciate the early desynchronization of the neocortex.

SPINAL CORD SUPPRESSION. The analgesic effect of ketamine is rather profound. Besides a central effect, a suppression of neuronal activity in the dorsal horn cells of the spinal cord occurs, which may contribute to the analgesia.

These cells in the dorsal horn are laminated and seem to control selectively the relay of impulses over primary afferents to the spinal lemniscal paths

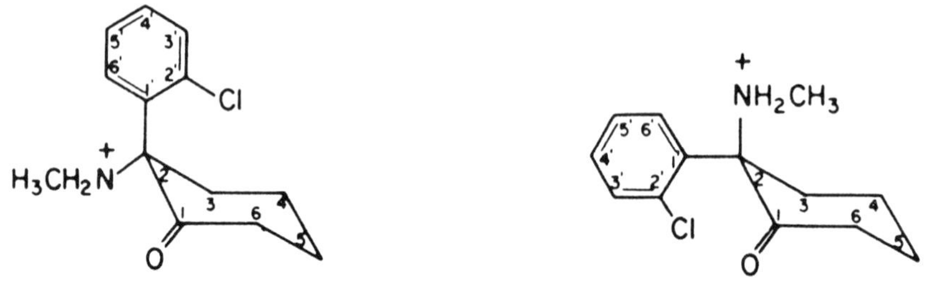

S,(+)-Ketamine hydrochloride   R,(−)-Ketamine hydrochloride

FIG. 27–3. Stereoisomers of ketamine. S(+) ketamine provides most of the physical and pharmacologic properties. The R(−) isomer is associated with more motor activity, psychic emergence reactions, and delirium. From White, P.F., et al.: Pharmacology of ketamine isomers in surgical patients. Anesthesiology, 52:231, 1980.

and then to the cortex. Ketamine selectively suppresses spontaneous and evoked activity of the lamina V cells in the dorsal horn. This area responds to high-threshold cutaneous and visceral afferents. Lamina I cells, which respond to cutaneous and thermal stimulation and receive input from cutaneous A delta fibers, are also suppressed.[13]

SIGNS OF ANESTHESIA.[9,14] As can be expected, the dissociative action of this agent produces a type of surgical anesthesia that is completely different from that produced by traditional anesthetic agents. When entering the *dissociative, cataleptic,* or *unconscious* states, the patient's eyes open widely, and horizontal or vertical nystagmus occurs. Seconds later, the eyeballs become centered and appear to be in a fixed gaze. At this time, the patient is considered to be pharmacologically "isolated." Studies of evoked potentials demonstrate that both visual and somatosensory impulses travel unimpaired from the periphery to the primary sensory cortex, *indicating that sensory isolation occurs within the brain, presumably in the association area.* Under the effect of ketamine, the patient's brain is unable to interpret afferent impulses and make the appropriate response.

Therefore, the patient does not manifest a reaction to light impulses introduced into the eye or pain impulses initiated by procedures such as skin incision or the reduction of a fractured bone.

Signs generally are not classical, because at anesthetic levels, the eyes open even if they close temporarily during induction. As anesthesia is achieved, the blood pressure returns from an elevated to a preinduction level.

PHARMACOLOGIC ACTIONS.[9,15]

1. Profound general analgesia to somatic pain is produced.
2. Respiratory depression is minimal.
3. The cardiovascular system is slightly stimulated.
4. There is no inhibition of reflexes that protect the air passages.
5. A state of dissociation from the environment is produced.

Central Nervous System. The nervous system effects are fascinating and unique. Some areas of the brain, such as the medullary and limbic systems, are stimulated, whereas other areas such as the thalamus, are depressed.

There is a peculiar and progressive loss of consciousness resembling a catatonic state. After the subject appears to go to sleep, the eyelids gradually open. Some upward nystagmus may occur.

Sensation Subjective numbness occurs without blocking touch. Profound somesthetic analgesia is produced; however, visceral sensation and response are obtained.

Mechanism of Analgesia Increased activity of the periaqueductal gray matter occurs, accompanied by theta activity in the EEG.[12] This is correlated with pain relief.[16] This area is one where endogenous peptides and morphine act, in part at the specific opiate receptors located at this point. Increased cerebral metabolic glucose utilization occurs at this site. Even in subanesthetic doses, ketamine appears to be an effective analgesic.[17]

Psychic Effects Changes in body image, mood, and affect do occur. Patients appear subdued. The sensations of weightlessness and "being in space" are often felt.[18]

Amnesia Retrograde amnesia to preoperative events is minimal. The maximum dose that produces some amnesia in 50% of the subjects appears to be about 1 mg/kg as a bolus dose and 1 mg/kg/hr during maintenance.[19] Such amnesia occurs if premedication is heavy. Awareness of procedures during induction or subsequent maintenance when patients are questioned does not occur with ketamine. After recovery from anesthesia, memory of immediate postoperative events is impaired.

Cerebral Hemodynamic Effects Cerebral blood flow increases greatly, by as much as 60% to 80%, but returns to normal within 20 to 30 minutes. The increase is probably the result of increased perfusion pressure that is dependent on increased cerebral vasodilatation and decreased cerebrovascular resistance. There is also an increased cerebral metabolic rate for oxygen. In experimental studies, this amounts to 15% to 20%.[20] Cerebrospinal fluid pressure is also greatly increased to an average of 250 mm H_2O in patients without intracranial disease.[21] In patients with increased intracranial pressure, administration of ketamine can rapidly induce apnea.[22] This increase can be reversed by hyperventilation.

Effect on EEG In humans, ketamine alters the awake alpha activity to a predominant theta (4 to 6 cps) activity. This is often preceded by an unusually brief fast activity of 25 to 35 cps. Appearance of theta activity is accompanied by unconsciousness and analgesia. This is followed by high-voltage complexes superimposed on the theta pattern and signified as a suppression-burst pattern of the spiking type.

In Corrsen's study,[14] seizure discharges were not induced in either normal subjects or in patients with epilepsy and a normal EEG. Rarely, an epileptic with a seizure pattern may have the pattern exaggerated. In patients with seizure disorders, sleep alone may precipitate or aggravate EEG discharges, but the sleep induced by ketamine in these patients decreases the incidence of discharges. Indeed, administrations of ketamine to epileptic subjects may supress or eliminate seizure EEG discharges.[23]

Cardiovascular Effects.[26] Ketamine has both cardiac and peripheral circulatory effects. The cardiovascular stimulatory effects on heart rate, cardiac output, and arterial pressure were first reported by Virtue.[5] These follow a predictable pattern.

In humans, there is an increase in systolic, diastolic, and mean systemic arterial pressures accompanied by an increase in heart rate.[9] These effects occur with small doses of 0.1 mg/kg and in the absence of unconsciousness. Systemic arterial pressures increase further with larger doses up to 0.5 mg/kg. Heart rate also increases progressively up to 33% as doses are increased to this level, but doses larger than 0.5 mg/kg do not produce further changes. Thus, the average intravenous dose used clinically for production of sleep (2 mg/kg) is not associated with tachycardia or pressure change greater than the small dose. The maximum increase is usually seen in 3 to 4 minutes after induction and then subsides.

A variability in response resulting from interaction between the cardiac and vascular actions is seen, depending on the individual's response and the net effect.

Cardiac Effects[10a,24] In normal subjects, ketamine increases heart rate while stroke volume index is maintained. Since Ross[24a] has demonstrated that, in unanesthetized subjects, increasing heart rate causes a decrease in stroke volume with no change in cardiac output, it can be concluded that ketamine has a positive myocardial effect.

Myocardial stimulation may occur from either preloading, using the Frank-Starling mechanism, or by direct increase in myocardial contractility. Both mechanisms have been demonstrated to occur following ketamine.[24] However, decreasing left ventricular end-diastolic pressure (decreasing volume) correlates with a rising cardiac index in most subjects, indicating that the increased contractility effect is the more likely mechanism. Simultaneously, an analysis of the determinants of myocardial oxygen consumption, myocardial wall tension, contractile state, and heart rate demonstrates increased myocardial oxygen demand and muscle work. Rate-pressure product is increased. The coronary flow is increased, but the oxygen extraction fraction does not change.

These effects are dependent on the presence of an intact sympathetic autonomic control. Thus, total epidural block or ganglionic blockade will abolish ketamine-induced pressor effects.[25]

In the absence of sympathetic nervous system activity, most cardiac effects are related to a mild direct myocardial depression, which is usually offset by the reflex pressor action. In high-risk patients in poor physical condition and in those with cardiac disease, depression may predominate and hypotension can develop. Associated with the direct myocardial effect is an antiarrhythmic action. Some experimental animal studies indicate that, in hypovolemic states, ketamine has undesirable cardiovascular and metabolic sequelae.[25a] Compared with low-dose thiopental, however, ketamine is a preferable agent.

Circulation A variable response of systemic vascular resistance occurs. It is a combined result of drug action on peripheral vessels and sympathetic stimulation through action on central nervous system structures and an increased plasma norepinephrine level. There may be either an increase or decrease in systemic vascular resistance but the change is within a range of ± 25% in humans subjects. Generally a maximal peripheral stimulation precedes maximal cardiac response.[26]

Direct Dilation of Vascular Smooth Muscle Direct dilation of vascular smooth muscle occurs.[27] This effect and the sympathetic stimulation, however, represent a dual effect—to some extent, a balancing effect—with the sympathetic action predominating in healthy subjects.[28]

Pulmonary Circulation[29] Pulmonary artery pressure is markedly increased, accompanied by an increase in pulmonary vascular resistance of about 40%. There is a simultaneous increase in right ventricular work. A transient 20% increase in intrapulmonary shunt occurs. These effects can be prevented by prior administration of an alpha-adrenergic blocking agent, such as droperidol.[29a]

Mechanism of Cardiovascular Effect These cardiovascular effects are the result of interaction with the sympathetic nervous system. The pressor response is ascribed to the increase of plasma catecholamines. Direct stimulation of the central sympathetic mechanism has been demonstrated[30] and may also be responsible in part for the release of catecholamines.

The predominant mechanism relates to the increased plasma levels of norepinephrine.[31] Plasma-free norepinephrine may double within the induction period, from 30 to 40 ng/dl to 80 ng/dl.[32] This is because of the ability of ketamine to block norepinephrine reuptake into neuronal sources (Iverson Uptake - 1)[33] and into extraneuronal tissues.[34] (Iverson Uptake - 2).[35] The ketamine block of uptake into neuronal tissues has been ascribed to a cocaine-like effect.[36] But this cocaine mechanism is disrupted. Neuronal block of norepinephrine uptake at vascular smooth muscle is not considered to be the dominant mechanism,[37] but block of disposition and uptake at extraneuronal tissues appears to be the important mechanism increasing circulatory norepinephrine. Miletich[38] has shown experimentally that ketamine blocks uptake by heart muscle. Thus, blockade of both disposition mechanisms allows plasma levels to remain high.[35]

The chronotropic effect and the increased afterload increases cardiac myocardial oxygen demand[24] and produces a dose-related rise in rate-pressure product.[25]

The proposal[39] that depression of baroreceptor activity (desensitization of receptor) causes an increase in sympathetic tone with norepinephrine release has not been supported. Direct stimulation of the baroreceptors during ketamine administration does not further alter the cardiovascular effects.[40]

Respiration.[5,41] During the initial phase of anesthesia, respiration is slightly depressed but a clear airway is well maintained. Tidal volume is usually affected more than rate and is most pronounced in the first minutes after drug injection. The duration of this depression is transient, lasting 1 to 3 minutes.[42] A mild transient reduction in Pa_{O_2} may occur.[43,49]

In the neonatal period and up to 6 months of age respiratory depression is greater and should be anticipated with ordinary doses. Therefore, the usual range of dosage is halved. Overdosage and rapid bolus-type administration may cause profound respiratory depression and apnea.[41]

Effect on Ventilation[43] Ketamine causes a linear dose-related depression of ventilation, determined in volunteers at doses of approximately 3 mg/kg of body weight. The depression is similar to that seen with narcotics, but of a lesser degree. Over a dose range of 0.39 to 3 mg/kg, ketamine causes a log linear dose-related depression of ventilation of a value of 1.6 ± 0.3 L/min for each doubling of the dose. This was determined during isohypercapnic method of Lamberston, an alveolar P_{CO_2} control system that reveals mild degrees of respiratory depression and magnifies any degree of depression.

Effect on CO_2 Response Curve[43] Ketamine alone during isohypercapnia causes a dose-related decrease in ventilation, with a rightward shift of the curve. No detectable change in the slope of the CO_2 response curve after a 3-mg/kg dose of ketamine, however, has been evident.

The respiratory depression can be quantitated either as a 2 mm Hg rightward displacement of the CO_2 response curve or as an isohypercapnic decrease in expired volume of 4 L/min.

Ketamine administered after morphine has an added effect, causing a greater dose-related reduction in expired volume, with a further rightward displacement of the CO_2 response curve.[43]

Ketamine's effect on CO_2-mediated control of respiration, causing a rightward displacement of the CO_2 response curve without a change in the slope, is similar to narcotics in the usual analgesic dose range. This effect differs from all inhalational anesthetics and hypnotics, causing unconsciousness that not only displaces the response curve but decreases the slope. Thus, the maintenance of a normal CO_2 response curve with a rightward shift and without measurable change in slope, yet with a loss of consciousness, is unique.

With a decrease in the level of consciousness with most drugs, there is a decrease in the slope of the CO_2 response curve. This occurs with barbiturates, benzodiazepines, and inhalation anesthetics as well as large-dose opioid anesthesia.

It can be concluded that ketamine is a mild respiratory depressant with effects on the CO_2 response curve that are similar to analgesic doses of morphine.

Effect on Mechanics of Respiratory Muscles Ketamine is unique among anesthetic agents in that skeletal muscle tone is maintained and may even increase.[9] This includes its effects on respiratory muscle mechanics. Diaphragmatic contraction is maintained in spontaneously breathing subjects and may increase with increased demands.[44] The effects are as follows:

- Inspiratory mean flow is maintained as is tidal volume and minute ventilation.[46]
- Occlusion pressure generated by the diaphragm is maintained when the airway is occluded.[45]
- End-expiratory positions of the chest and diaphragm are maintained normally or increased.[45]
- Functional residual capacity does not change during anesthesia and spontaneous breathing in either children[47] or adults.[46] In contrast to volatile agents ketamine has a sparing effect on intercostal muscle activity.
- In computerized tomographic studies of chest measurements and gas exchange values in spontaneously breathing subjects during ketamine anesthesia, no atelectasis was observed and ventillation/perfusion ratios were normal; no abnormal shunts were determined. An increase in rib cage size has been demonstrated[46] and contributes to tidal breathing.

These studies also support the concept that the decrease in chest volume and resultant atelectasis are the result of the loss of skeletal muscle tone of the chest wall and impaired diaphragmatic mechanics.[48]

Pulmonary Effects Rapid administration of ketamine, as a bolus in less than 30 seconds while patients are breathing room air, results in significant reduction in Pa_{O_2}.[49] Preoxygenation limits the fall in arterial oxygen, however, whereas titrated injections to level of unconsciousness timed over a period of 1 minute do not produce arterial hypoxemia.

Bronchial smooth muscle is relaxed by ketamine, and the bronchoconstrictive effects of histamine are antagonized.[50] The degree of spasmolytic effect appears to be dose dependent.[51] Pulmonary compliance is significantly increased, and airway resistance decreased.[52]

Ketamine does not affect the functional residual capacity when compared with the awake state.[47] This is in contrast to the decrease in functional residual capacity with other anesthetic agents. In adults, most induction agents decrease functional residual capacity during spontaneous breathing by an average of 18%; in anesthetized paralyzed mechanically ventilated patients, a reduction of 14% is still present.[47a] Under these circumstances, children have a reduction of 44% in functional residual capacity with agents other than ketamine.[47b] In contrast, the functional residual capacity in children 1 to 8 years of age is not affected by ketamine.

Reflexes. The protective reflexes remain active.[53] Tone of the jaw and tongue muscles is retained. Hence an oropharyngeal airway may not be needed. Cough is present, and gag responses permit self-maintenance of airway. Indeed, attempts to insert an oropharyngeal airway cause gagging and ejection. Swallowing continues so that any mucus, saliva, or regurgitated material is swallowed. Myotactic reflexes are hyperactive.[54]

Laryngeal Competence.[54,54a] Laryngeal competence is retained during ketamine anethesia, although soiling occurs consequent to the instillation of irritants in the pharynx with all agents. Of induction agents studied, the least soiling of the tracheobronchial tree occurs with ketamine (diazepam is almost as protective). The incidence of aspiration, however, is increased with prior sedation or opiate premedication.[54a]

Skeletal Muscle. Muscle tone increases in light anesthesia.[5] Abnormal muscle movements of the extremities are seen during induction and are of a sudden jerking type.[55] Movements during surgery are rarely related to the surgery. Grimacing and pursing of lips, when seen, may indicate lightening of anesthesia.[10a]

In nervous system disorders of the hyperkinetic type (basal ganglia lesions), the drug is not contraindicated.[55a] Ketamine may terminate writhing movements often seen in mental retardation or Down's syndrome (Trisomy 21).[55b]

MISCELLANEOUS ACTIONS.[14] Salivation and tracheal mucus formation are profuse without premedication. Marked lacrimation and profuse sweating occur in many subjects.[42] After intramuscular injection increased salivation is slow to develop and presents few problems during the first 10 to 15 minutes of anesthesia.[14a]

Eye responses follow an interesting course. The immediate induction response is closure of the eyelids, but the lids usually open after the patient is asleep for 0.5 to 1 minute. Closing of the eyes may be a guide to lightening of analgesia. Nystagmus occurs when the eyes are open. Diplopia may occur in the postoperative period.

Uterine Tone. It is evident from studies by Galloon[56] that ketamine has an oxytocic type action. The basal uterine tone during the second trimester of pregnancy is significantly increased by 50% or more after doses of 2 mg/kg of body weight intravenously. At doses of 1.1 mg/kg of body weight, the increase in basal uterine tone averages 20%.[57] It has been estimated that in the third trimester in the patient in labor, the full-term fetus may have some interference with oxygenation because of exaggerated uterine tone and contraction from the ketamine. In studies of Apgar scores following total doses greater than 1 mg/kg of body weight, the scores are unacceptably low. Low doses of 0.3 mg/kg administered to women for normal vaginal delivery did not adversely affect the Apgar scores of the babies.[58] Other studies using ketamine as the primary anesthetic in doses of 0.2 to 0.3 mg/kg for vaginal delivery showed no significant complications in mothers or the newborn.[59] In general, it can be concluded that ketamine must be cautiously used in low doses, otherwise, it is poor choice of agent for obstetric delivery.

If a dose of diazepam (or lorazepam) or a small dose of droperidol-fentanyl is administered, the incidence of awareness is reduced to 2% in mothers and unpleasant dreaming to 3%.[60]

Besides high Apgar scores, Hodgkinson has shown that Scanlon's Neurobehavioral scores are of a high order after ketamine and less depressant than thiopental anesthesia.[60a] Blood gas studies of the newborn infant following ketamine induction anesthesia of the mother for cesarean section show a stable umbilical artery and vein blood P_{O_2} when induction to delivery time (ID time) is 10 minutes or less. P_{CO_2} blood values are lower and the pH values are alkaline. In contrast, a negative correlation has been determined between ID time and umbilical cord blood P_{O_2}. Ketamine is thus a safe agent for obstetric delivery and may be the preferred agent in emergencies when blood loss is significant.[61]

In a study of wakefulness in patients undergoing cesarean section with ketamine–nitrous oxide anesthesia and without prior tranquilizers, neither operative-anesthesia dreams nor recall were evidenced. Compared with thiopental, ketamine was more effective in eliminating awareness.[60]

Metabolic Responses. After induction with 2 mg/kg and establishment of the anesthetic state by a continuous infusion of ketamine 25 μg/kg/min, there are hormonal and metabolic changes evident in blood. There is a significant increase in blood sugar concentration, from 64 mg/dl to 75 mg/dl.[62]

With the onset of surgery, there is a further glycemic response that stabilizes at about 90 mg/dl for 1 to 2 hours of surgery. The cortisol response is similar. After induction of anesthesia, the level rises from control values of about 200 nmol·L^{-1} to 340 nmol. With onset of surgery, the value rises to 500 to 600 nmol for the period of surgery.

Plasma nonesterified fatty acids are decreased by about 13%.[25] Blood lactate and pyruvate concentrations do not change significantly.

It is concluded that ketamine does not exacerbate metabolic responses to surgery.[63]

In animal studies (chicken liver homogenates), ketamine is able to increase alanine synthetase.[64a] It has been used safely, however, in patients with acute intermittent porphyria,[65] as well as in the cutaneous and variegate forms.[65a,65b]

Effect on Catecholamines. Large increases in plasma catecholamine, epinephrine, and norepinephrine levels occur following administration of ketamine. After the intravenous injection of doses of 2 mg/kg, free norepinephrine levels in the plasma rise from a preinjection base level of 0.35 to 0.8 ng/ml by 5 minutes. By 10 minutes, the levels return to control values (Fig. 27–4).[32] Renin activity is not increased. This appears to occur both in human subjects and in animal experiments.[25]

Endocrine Effects. Although thyroxine levels are not altered, ketamine does produce a decrease in T3 plasma levels.[66] The pituitary–adrenal axis is activated, and there is a release of adrenaline and cortisol. Though no change in renin activity has been noted, the response to angiotensin I and angiotensin II is enhanced.

A mild elevation of blood glucose of about 12% follows ketamine administration. This compares with increases after thiopental of 72% and from halothane induction of 55%.[62]

Plasma histamine is not increased by ketamine, and hypersensitivity reactions are rarely seen.[67]

Effect on Neuromuscular Junction. Interference with neuromuscular transmission in a dose-dependent manner has been demonstrated. In low concentration, there is some facilitation of transmission, whereas at high concentration there is blocking.[68,69] Animal experiments indicate that pancuronium block is prolonged following ketamine induction,[68,70] as is vecuronium.[71] The experimental studies indicate some direct postsynaptic effect,[69] although some presynaptic action may occur.[72]

It is suggested that the mechanism is an interference with calcium binding or fluxes in the sarcoplasmic reticulum of the muscle.[73]

Interaction with Relaxants. With the administration of ketamine, there is an initial potentiation of the twitch response to direct muscle stimulation, followed by block of the response.

Clinically, ketamine increases the duration of action of succinylcholine and generally augments nondepolarizing relaxants.[74] In part, this effect is related to an interference with calcium binding[23] and to the inhibition of plasma cholinesterase by ketamine.[75] A slight fall in serum potassium occurs with administration of ketamine. A result of this is a decrease in the incidence and severity of muscle fasciculations induced by succinylcholine.[76] Occasional spasms of muscles in infants have been reported; however, ketamine has been used in myopathic and spastic disorders. It does not appear to trigger malignant hypertension,[77] although it increases creatine phosphokinase levels.[78]

In patients anesthetized with ketamine and nitrous oxide 66% and oxygen 44% with the administration of single doses of either vecuronium or pancuronium at an average ED$_{95}$ (45 μg/kg for vecuronium; 60 μg/kg for pancuronium), the time course of action and reversal kinetics were not different than when other intravenous agents were used. After repeated doses of vecuronium, however, there was prolongation of action.[79] In induction with ketamine and maintenance achieved with inhalation halothane, there is a significant reduction in the dose of pancuronium needed.[74]

CLINICAL CONSIDERATIONS. Ketamine is well established as an intravenous induction agent[80] and is the choice for many unusual medical conditions (Table 27–1).[80]

Ketamine also is of value in the anesthetic management of patients undergoing a variety of surgical

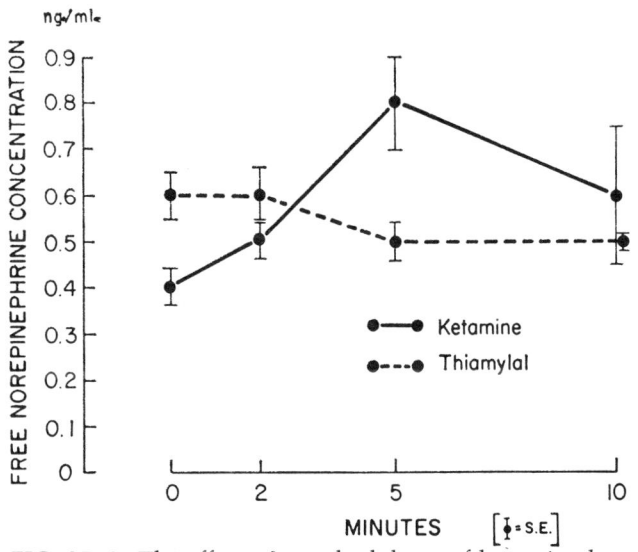

FIG. 27–4. The effect of standard doses of ketamine hydrochloride on free norepinephrine blood levels. Comparison with a barbiturate thiamylal is shown. From Zsigmond, E.K., Kelsch, R.C., and Kothany S.P.: Rise in plasma-free norepinephrine during anesthetic induction with ketamine. Phys. Drug Manual, 6:31, 1974.

TABLE 27–1. SPECIAL INDICATIONS FOR CLINICAL USE OF KETAMINE

- In shock and hypovolemic states[88,89]
- For rapid-sequence induction[114]
- For induction as an alternative to topical awake intubation in presence of full stomach
- For patients with bronchospastic disease: asthma, emphysema[85]
- For management of status asthmaticus[86]
- For patients with acute intermittent porphyria, as well as variegate forms[64,65]
- For prevention and management of priapism[90,91]
- In muscular dystrophy and myopathic disorders (to avoid thiopental use)
- In surgery for malignant hyperpyrexia–susceptible patients—may be a good choice[77]
- As adjunct to regional anesthesia or endoscopic procedures under topical anesthesia
- Anesthetic induction and/or management of mentally retarded patients (Down's syndrome); for cerebral palsy patients and spastic conditions[55b]
- In patients with epidermolysis bullosa (minimal need to lift jaw and manipulate face)[92,93]
- In patients with hereditary angioneurotic edema
- For sedative-analgesia in subanesthetic doses in diagnostic procedures; endoscopy with topical anesthesia[81]
- As an epidural alternative to epidural morphine for postoperative pain[94]
- For uncooperative children or when intravenous access is difficult: give IM[87]
- For patients undergoing repetitive procedures:[87] burn treatment;[87a] plastic and reconstructive surgery[87]

procedures that evoke superficial somatosensory responses (nonvisceral). It is of unique value in managing patients for most diagnostic procedures and for patients undergoing simple repetitive procedures.[81] It is particularly suitable for infants and children. Procedures suitable for ketamine anesthesia include surgery of neck and extremities; those necessitating frequent positional changes or when orthostatic hypotension occurs, and in the treatment of severely burned patients of any age. In eye surgery, upward nystagmus with small doses may interfere with muscle operations.

In patients with acute or chronic bronchial disease, including asthma, the drug protects against bronchospasm and reduces many of the symptoms of acute asthma.

In asthmatic and allergic states, ketamine represents a drug of choice and is indicated as an induction agent.[82] It relieves bronchospasm,[83,84] dilates the bronchial tree,[37] and antagonizes histamine.[50] It is impressively effective in the management of status asthmaticus.[85,86]

In hypovolemic states, an initial variable increase in catecholamines with sympathetic stimulation augments compensatory mechanisms.[25,88,89]

Lack of triggering capacity in malignant hyperthermia-susceptible swine indicates the safety of this agent in patients who are susceptible to malignant hyperthermia.[25,87]

Experience with various types of porphyria shows this drug to be safe in the presence of this disorder.[64,65]

PREMEDICATION.[9] An anticholinergic agent is mandatory.[9,54] This serves to block salivation and mucus formation as well as lacrimation and sweating. Reflex hyperactivity is reduced. Doses should be more generous than when other anesthetics are used (Table 27–2): Atropine 10 µg/kg is effective, or bellafoline 10 µg per kg. Scopolamine is preferred for children in doses of 10 µg/kg. Glycopyrrolate in doses of 8 µg/kg is preferred in adults.

Study of central-acting preanesthetic agents indicates the desirability of an opiate. Morphine sulfate 0.5 mg/10 kg provides a tranquil, acquiescent patient preanesthetically, contributes to the analgesia, and minimizes untoward cardiovascular excitation. Opiates also are more effective in lowering incidence of emergence phenomena.[96]

Tranquilizers as part of preanesthetic medication are advocated.[97] Droperidol and diazepam are useful and superior to barbiturates.[98] An average dose of 5 mg in a 70-kg patient of either drug is administered intramuscularly 1 hour preanesthetically.

ADMINISTRATION AND DOSAGE.[9,14,99,100] Administration is usually by the intravenous route but may be given intramuscularly. Reactions at the site of injection are rare and inconsequential and consist of slight pain and erythema. The drug is best administered slowly; a rate of 10 mg every 15 seconds is an optimal rate and permits evaluation of signs of unconsciousness, especially the eye signs. Six eye signs are to be observed in the following sequence: Blink → Stare → Eyelid closure → Nystagmus → Strabismus → Inactive lid reflex.

Dosage varies with the individual patient according to age, weight, route of administration and other standard factors, including habitus or somatotype. The neonate is more prone to respiratory depression[22] and apnea. Lean body mass is recommended as the preferred basis for calculating dosage.

TABLE 27–2. DOSAGES OF PREANESTHETIC
ANTICHOLINERGICS WHEN USED WITH KETAMINE

Drug Name		Dose
Generic	Chemical	(μg/kg)
Atropine	dl-Hyoscyamine	10–15
Bellafoline	Levo-Hyoscyamine	10
Scopolamine	Levo-Hyoscine	10
Glycopyrrolate	a pyrolidinium derivative	8

Wulfson[99] has proposed that the Weisberg formula be used for determining lean body mass (LBM):

Fat percentage = 90 − 2 × [H − G]
LBM = [100% − Fat %] × Weight

where H is the height in inches and G is girth in inches measured at the umbilical level and at end of expiration. In all persons a fat content is present in body weight. Thin individuals have about 5% to 10% fat, whereas athletic individuals have 10% to 20%, and pyknic individuals 36% or more.

INDUCTION.[99] Intravenous dosage is 2 mg/kg (range of 1.5 to 4 mg/kg) of 1% solution, which produces a rapid onset within 30 seconds. This is a dose empirically arrived at by Corssen[14] but which correlates with lean body mass. The effect lasts 5 to 10 minutes.[101]

The intravenous dose for neonates and infants is recommended at 0.5 to 1 mg/kg.

Intramuscular dosage is 8 to 12 mg/kg of a 5% solution which produces anesthesia after a latent period of 3 to 5 minutes. The effect lasts 10 to 20 minutes.

The endpoint of the sleep or induction dose is the appearance of nystagmus or strabismus, which occurs just before the obliteration of the eyelid reflex.[101] This is followed by abolition of response to verbal commands (Fig. 27–5).

MAINTENANCE.[100] For longer duration of anesthesia, supplementary doses are administered as needed. When intravenous administration is the route, such additions are needed after 10 to 15 minutes.

The maintenance dose averages 1 mg/kg per hour, which may be given in fractions every 15 minutes.[100]

A low-dose continuous infusion technique may also be used.[19,89,101] A mixture of 250 mg in 250 ml of 5% dextrose is employed (0.1% solution) providing 1 mg in each milliliter. The rate of infusion varies between 10 and 50 μg/kg/min. These doses are for body surface operations. Much larger doses are needed for abdominal surgery.[102,103]

PHARMACOKINETICS (Fig. 27–6). Distribution of ketamine in the body is apparently into a three-compartment system and follows a triexponential decay. Initially, there is dilution in the bloodstream; plasma levels then decrease rapidly because of the rapid distribution and uptake by tissues, especially the brain; finally, there is an elimination phase.[104]

In the extracellular–intravascular compartment, one fraction of the drug is protein bound and represents, at physiologic pH of blood, about 12% of the amount injected.[105] The unbound fraction of ketamine is largely ionized; however, there is a continuous, extremely rapid transfer of the nonionized fraction across the blood-brain boundary (no barrier appears to exist). At 2 minutes, the plasma concentration of the unbound fraction represents about 5% to 6% of the total injected dose.

After a dose of 2 mg/kg in humans, plasma levels fall exponentially from 1.49 μg/ml at 4 minutes, to 0.75 μg/ml at 10 minutes, and 0.44 μg/ml at 35 minutes.[105] Peak levels are attained approximately

FIG. 27–5. Cumulative ketamine dose (log scale) vs. response curves for abolition of reaction to verbal commands, eyelash stimulation, and painful stimulation (trapezius squeeze). From Gross, J.B., Caldwell, C.B., and Edwards, M.W.: Induction dose–response curves for midazolam and ketamine in premedication ASA class III and IV patients. Anesth. Analg., 64:795, 1985.

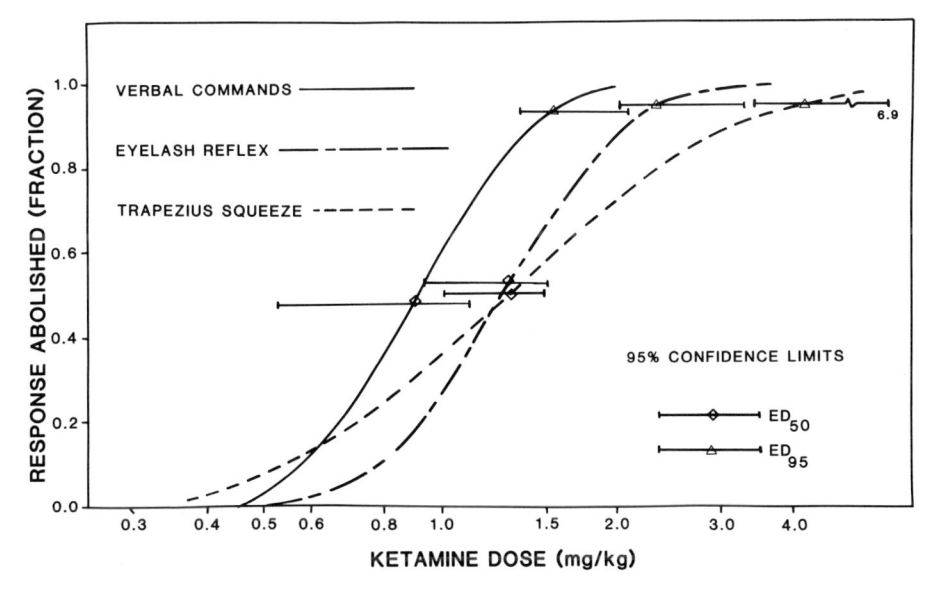

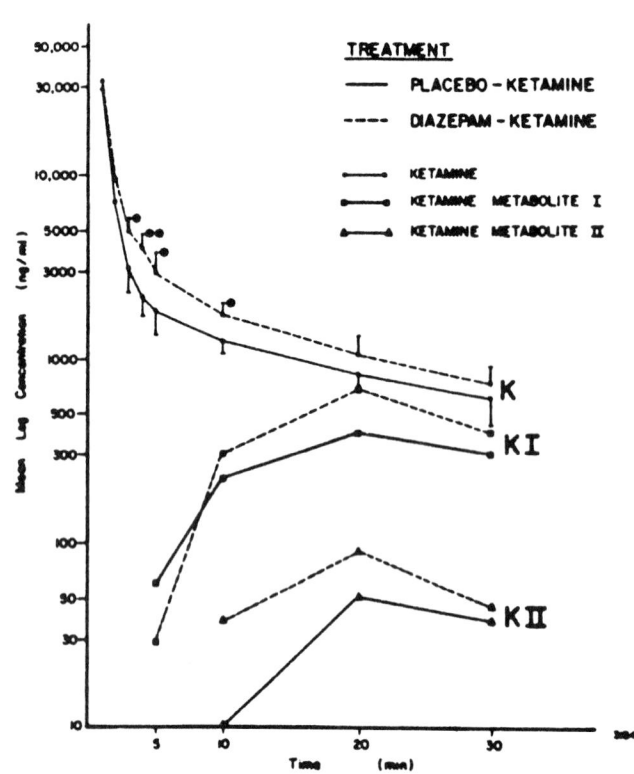

FIG. 27–6. Pharmacokinetics of ketamine and its two major metabolites in the first 30 min following intravenous injection of 2.2 mg/kg dose in healthy volunteers. From Zsigmond, E.K., and Domino, E.T.: Ketamine: Clinical pharmacology, pharmacokinetics, and current use. Anesthesiol. Rev., 7:13, 1980.

2 to 3 minutes after injection. The initial plasma half-life, or pi phase, of plasma dilution is approximately 30 seconds of central dilution. The distribution phase half-life is approximately 8 minutes, and the elimination half-life of an administered dose is 2.2 to 2.9 hours in adults.[106] In humans, consciousness returns at plasma levels of 0.7 to 1 µg/ml.[107] Hence, the duration of anesthetic action, which may be considered the biologic half-life, is less than 10 minutes from a single dose in unmedicated humans. The mean optimal effect for sleep is 7.15 ± 4.56 minutes, whereas the analgesia phase is 2.29 ± (0.64) hours (Table 27–3).

METABOLISM.[107] Metabolic degradation occurs in the liver by two main processes and is nearly complete.[108] It is rapid and accounts for 50% of the administered dose. This biotransformation may play a significant role in the pharmacologic actions of this drug, in contrast to this disposition of thiopental.

Two metabolites have been identified: (1) metabolite I, (norketamine)-[2-amino-2 (0-chlorphenyl) cyclohexanone hydrochloride]—this is the N-dealkylated amine (N-demethylated product)—and (2) metabolite II, (nor-dehydroketamine)-[2-amino-2 (0-chlorphenyl) 3-cyclohexen-1-one hydrochloride].

This is a dehydrated product of the parent ketone after hydroxylation of the cyclohexanone ring.[109] The N-demethylated product, metabolite I, is the major metabolite in humans, and appears in the plasma within 2 to 4 minutes, indicating rapid metabolic degradation. This product also accumulates rapidly in the brain, and its presence there is prolonged and may account for some of the delayed central nervous system actions.[109] The products are mostly conjugated with formation of water-soluble compounds that are excreted in the urine. The unconjugated N-demethylated product (metabolite I) possesses some activity (20–33% of parent compound); the unconjugated demethylated and hydroxylated derivative has 1% the activity of the parent compound.

For metabolite II, significant plasma levels are found after 20 minutes. Maximal concentrations of both metabolites were found at 3 hours to be 4.7 µmol/L for metabolite I and 3.2 µmol/L for metabolite II.[107]

Excretion. About 91% of a given dose is recoverable in the urine as the metabolites. About 3% is excreted in bile and feces. Only a small fraction is recoverable as the unchanged agent.

Acidification of urine as by administration of 0.01% HCl increases the urinary excretion.[106a] The drug can be detected in the urine by gas chromatography.[110]

Brain Uptake.[109] Concerning tissue uptake, studies demonstrate a rapid cortical uptake. By 30 seconds, brain levels reach 7.5% of the total dose administered. Within 1 minute, a peak brain concentration is achieved, and there is equilibration between brain and the serum concentrations. The cerebral cortex retains ketamine preferentially, and redistribution from this site is slow.[109]

Other central nervous system areas, such as the midbrain and brain stem also pick up ketamine; action at basal ganglia produces extrapyramidal effects during the period of loss of consciousness. At any time, the brain/plasma ratio remains at 6.5/1.0. Within 1 hour, peak levels of 0.2 µg/ml occur in cerebrospinal fluid.

Isomers: Pharmacokinetics and Dynamics.[111] As noted earlier, ketamine is a racemic mixture. The isomers have been separated and studied.

The PK (+) isomer provides a more effective anesthesia than either the racemic or MK form. Comparable doses are 1 mg/kg for PK; 2 mg for RM mixture, and 3 mg/kg for MK. The plasma ketamine concentrations and kinetic decay curve show parallel changes with all preparations.

The plasma levels of both isomers show a corresponding course with time with a great increase in the first 30 minutes to a peak level and then a gradual decline. The peak level of metabolites was

TABLE 27-3. KETAMINE KINETICS FOR A THREE-COMPARTMENT OPEN MODEL

	Placebo-ketamine (N = 7)	Diazepam-ketamine (n = 7)
$\pi t_{1/2}$ sec	31.1 ± 16.8 (24.1)	27.2 ± 7.7 (25.0)
$\alpha t_{1/2}$ min	7.79 ± 6.21 (4.68)	6.70 ± 1.72 (6.37)
$\beta t_{1/2}$ hr	2.25 ± .45 (2.17)	2.41 ± .49 (2.32)
$k_{12}*(hr^{-1})$	35.5 ± 20.4	36.4 ± 8.0
$k_{21}*(hr^{-1})$	14.8 ± 9.00	12.0 ± 2.4
$k_{13}*(hr^{-1})$	35.4 ± 27.3	29.6 ± 13.9
$k_{31}*(hr^{-1})$	0.874 ± 0.296	0.707 ± 0.164
$k_{10}*(hr^{-1})$	26.3 ± 23.7	28.2 ± 24.1
$Vd_1^\dagger$ (L/kg)	0.063 ± 0.049	0.043 ± 0.034
$Vd_2^\dagger$ (L/kg)	0.207 ± 0.202	0.132 ± 0.101
$Vd_3^\dagger$ (L/kg)	1.51 ± 0.619	1.34 ± 0.689
$Vd_{ss}^\dagger$ (L/kg)	1.78 ± 0.738	1.517 ± 0.815
Plasma clearance (L/kg/hr)	0.848 ± 0.316	0.719 ± 0.293‡

Data are $\bar{X}$ ± SD. Values in parentheses are harmonic means. All kinetic parameters were calculated from the coefficients and exponents of the least-squares regression analysis of the data in Table 1 of the original article.
* First-order rate parameters.
† Volume of distribution parameters.
‡ P < 0.08 (two-tailed paired comparison Student t test); P < 0.05 (one-tailed test).
From Domino, E.F., et al.: Ketamine kinetics in unmedicated and diazepam premedicated subjects. Clin. Pharmacol. Ther., 36:645, 1984.

highest with the (−) ketamine and RM while significantly lower with (+) ketamine. This course is dose related.

Several pharmacologic differences, however, were noted of the (+) isomer over the RM or the (−) isomer:

- More effective analgesia is provided; there is less postoperative pain—only 1 for PK compared with 10% for RK and 16% for MK
- Dreaming is relatively pleasant with PK, but remains weird after MK or RK; psychic emergence reactions are lowest with PK
- There is little or no delirium or disorientation after PK
- Patient acceptance is best with (+) isomer, and the side effects of illusion, nausea, vomiting, and dizziness are minimal with the dextro form

PHARMACOKINETICS IN CHILDREN.[112] Some differences in the kinetics of ketamine disposition are noted in children in contrast to adults (Table 27-4). After an intravenous injection in children, there is a more rapid onset of action than in adults, with a mean of about 3 minutes. The duration of action is also somewhat shorter. The plasma half-life is approximaely 100 minutes in children and approximately 160 minutes in adults. The clearance of ketamine is slightly more rapid than in adults, whereas the steady state volume is smaller. It is to be noted that the awakening time after an intravenous injection approximates 15 minutes, and the plasma concentration of the ketamine ranges from 1000 to 4000 ng/ml in children. This is in contrast to the awakening plasma concentration of ketamine, which is approximately 600 to 1000 ng/ml in adults.

In the studies by Grant,[112] plasma norketamine

TABLE 27-4. PHARMACOKINETIC VALUES IN CHILDREN AND ADULTS (Mean ± SEM)

Values	Children	Adults
Plasma half-life (min)	100 ± 19	153 ± 27
Clearance (ml · min^{-1} · kg^{-1})	16.8 ± 3.3	12.6 ± 2.2
Steady state volume (L · kg^{-1})	1.9 ± 0.6	2.3 ± 0.4
Mean residence time (min)	108 ± 15	182 ± 25

From Grant, I.S., et al.: Ketamine disposition in children and adults. Br. J. Anaesth. 55:1109, 1983.

concentrations were at all times greater in children. The higher norketamine concentrations in children probably reflect a faster N-demethylation of ketamine and, perhaps, a slowing of the metabolism of norketamine. Norketamine is known to have some anesthetic activity in animals, but such has not been demonstrated in humans.

After intramuscular injection in children, there is a rapid absorption rate, which is much faster and predictable in children than in adults. At 5 minutes after an intramuscular injection, high plasma concentrations of ketamine are determined. Recovery also is faster in children than in adults.

It should be appreciated that the intramuscular injection of ketamine in adults is quite unpredictable. Inasmuch as there is a significant prolonged recovery period as well as a slow onset of action, administration of ketamine by the intramuscular route is unacceptable. In regard to children, a good rule to follow is that the intramuscular dose varies inversely with age.

SPECIAL USES.

Status Asthmaticus Treatment Procedure. In the therapeutic management of patients with status asthmaticus, ketamine has been found to be most effective. It can be used as an adjunct to conventional bronchodilation therapy and may be used to sedate these patients. In addition, when such therapy fails, ketamine has been successful in controlling bronchospasm.[85]

A small loading dose of 50 mg is first administered as a continuous intravenous infusion of an 0.1% solution in Ringer's lactate 1 mg/ml. A dose of approximately 3 mg/kg/hr (40 to 50 µg/kg/min) will suffice to relieve bronchospasm, maintain improved ventilation, and improve blood gases. This infusion can be continued for 6 to 12 hours.[86]

Obstetric Anesthesia (see earlier discussion of uterine tone). As an induction agent, this drug has been widely used for cesarean sections.[113] In a comparison with thiopental, induction before laryngoscopy and intubation did not produce any significant blood pressure change in either the pentothal or the ketamine grouping. When laryngoscopy and intubation were performed, however, mean blood pressures rose between 20% and 30% in both pentothal and ketamine groups. Of equal importance is the fact that with thiopental, the heart rate increased significantly to 20% above preinduction rates, whereas the ketamine heart rate only increased by 15% during laryngoscopy and intubation. Of importance also is that the average maximal rate-pressure product, calculated for thiopental-induced patients, was over 18,000, whereas the rate-pressure product for ketamine was calculated at only 15,000. An examination of the neonatal outcome, including Apgar score and umbilical blood gas analysis, was good and did not differ between the mothers who were induced with pentothal or with ketamine.

Epidural Use for Postoperative Pain. Ketamine may be administered epidurally and has been found to be effective in relieving postoperative pain.[94] This effect is related to the potent analgesic action of this drug; analgesia is achieved at doses of only 4 ml in 5% dextrose administered epidurally and is unrelated to any systemic effect. The drug diffuses readily across the dura and acts directly on the spinal cord, producing segmental analgesia. Kitahata[13] has shown that ketamine produces a lamina-specific inhibition of dorsal horn unit activity and acts in the same manner as opioids on the mu and delta receptors of the spinal cord.[94a]

DISADVANTAGES AND COMPLICATIONS. This anesthetic is not entirely free of undesirable properties.

1. The blood pressure–raising effect may be harmful for patients with a history of cerebral vascular accident, hypertension, or marked cardiac decompensation.[39]
2. During induction, occasional excitatory phenomena are observed in about 6% of patients properly medicated with an opiate-scopolamine combination. Episodes of psychomotor activity may occur in conjunction with premature stimulation, or in patients who are poorly prepared psychologically. They are transitory in most cases and are best controlled by a *short-acting barbiturate.* They are infrequent in infants and children, but adults with emotional problems are prone to this excitation and unpleasant dreams.
3. Short periods of confusion and irrational behavior are occasionally noted in adults and may constitute an unpleasant experience for the patient. Delirium may be observed and consists of purposeless muscular movements. These may border on convulsions, which have been reported.[12] It is not remembered.
4. Respiratory depression is occasionally observed and is unpredictable. Laryngospasm and apnea are rare. Apnea occurs when large doses are injected rapidly or heavy opiate medication is used. Aspiration and depression of laryngeal reflexes have been reported.
5. Miscellaneous adverse effects have been reported and include polyneuropathy, increased intrathecal pressure, and intracranial pressure.[22]
6. A phase of vivid dreaming may occur, with or without psychomotor activity, during emergence from ketamine-induced anethesia.[81]
7. Ketamine does not provide visceral anesthesia. Therefore, the drug is not recommended for use as the sole anesthetic agent in abdominal or thoracic surgery or where visceral pain is expected to occur. To control visceral pain, ketamine must

be supplemented with other general anesthetic agents.
8. Nausea and vomiting are noted in 15% to 20% of patients regardless of premedication but are minimized by antiemetic drugs.
9. Other relative contraindications include allergy, obstructed airway, possible hypertension, prematurity, and neuropsychiatric conditions denoted by fantasy. The administration must always be supervised by an anesthetist.

EMERGENCE. Sequelae of ketamine anesthesia include delirium and unpleasant dreams during emergence in unpremedicated patients. The overall incidence of delirium is about 20%;[96] and of unpleasant dreaming about 33%, of which 10% may be terrifying.[81] This is compared with other anesthetic agents in unpremedicated patients in whom delirium may occur, 5% to 10% usually related to pain.[114] Dreaming may occur in 44% of unpremedicated patients. Twelve percent of the dreams may be unpleasant, but rarely is the dreaming terrifying or persistent as with ketamine.[115]

The incidence of both sequelae is higher (1) when the patient is stimulated, either during induction and before establishment of the anesthetic state or (2) when the patient is stimulated either by attempts at arousal or from pain during recovery.[116] These sequelae are further related to large doses, rapid administration of the drug, and inadequately premedicated patients.

Other phenomena, such as disorientation, depersonalization, derealization, changes in mood and affect, illusions, and hallucinations have also been occasionally reported.[117,118]

Emergence phenomena have also been reported following other general anesthetic procedures.[119] Study of postanesthetic and postoperative behavioral and dreaming phenomena is distorted by the fears that many surgical patients bring with them into the surgical milieu. Such fears as suffocation, disfigurement, cancer and, death have been analyzed by Smaessaert[117] and found to be rather frequent. Furthermore, the various tactile stimulation of presurgical procedures, the administration of medications, as well as the use of intravenous and arterial lines, promote stress changes and abnormal psychological responses.

PREVENTION AND MANAGEMENT. Sklar[120] has demonstrated that psychological techniques including informing the patient of planned procedures and providing reassurance in the preoperative period, are quite effective in abolishing psychic adverse reaction. Proper premedication decreases the occurrence and minimizes the intensity of both emergence sequelae. Several premedication strategies have been advocated.

A morphine-scopolamine combination is one of the most effective approaches in reducing the incidence and terror of unpleasant dreams.[96] On the other hand, a neurolept-narcotic mixture (droperidol-fentanyl) appears to be effective in reducing emergence delirium[98] but may increase the frequency of dreaming.

Diazepam premedication has been reported effective in preventing adverse emergence sequelae,[121] but this has not been a universal finding. The attenuation of undesirable cardiovascular effects of ketamine, however, is usual.

Small doses of ketamine of no more than 1 mg/kg per hour will limit the psychomimetic effects and provide good amnesia and analgesia in 52% of subjects.[19]

Promethazine (35 mg), a tranquilizer, as part of premedication has also been found by most groups to be effective.[95] A combination of promethazine and morphine is more effective in preventing dreaming and in allaying emergence delirium.[95]

A comparative evaluation by Dundee[114] of three benzodiazepines and four other premedication techniques presents well-controlled information. In this study, the benzodiazepines appear to be the most effective generally. Of these agents, lorazepam (4 mg) provided the greatest (followed by flunitrazepam and diazepam) protection against both delirium and unpleasant dreams when given one-half to 1 hour preanesthetically. Also, most patients found the whole anesthetic experience acceptable when the benzodiazepines are used in premedication.

THERAPY AT CONCLUSION OF SURGERY. Diazepam administered in doses of 0.15 mg/kg at the end of an operative procedure under ketamine anesthesia is somewhat effective in taming ketamine emergence.[96] A comparison of diazepam with midazolam and without any other premedication indicates that midazolam 0.07 mg/kg (diazepam 0.12 mg/kg) prior to administration of ketamine showed the midazolam to reduce unpleasant dreams and delirium to one fourth of the incidence with diazepam[122] or to about 5% and may be the preferred approach.

Droperidol will reduce the incidence and severity of psychomimetic effects. A dose of 0.05 mg (50 μg)/kg is effective.[123]

An ideal pharmacologic approach is lacking. Hence, others have used psychological techniques of both reassurance and suggestion. Sklar[120] has been successful in using preanesthetic suggestion. The strategy consists of a compassionate and informative preoperative interview the day before and an explanation that dreaming does occur. Therefore, the patients are asked to think of pleasant experiences and then informed that these would be the content. The anesthetic agent would permit dreaming about their choice of pleasant topics. At the interview, the patients were asked to share their ideas and feelings about the surgery and anesthesia.

White[124] has provided evidence that midazolam, a water-soluble benzodiazepine, as part of a rapid-sequence induction with ketamine (0.15 to 0.75 mg/kg) is more effective in allaying unpleasant psychic effects. Significantly less dreaming or disorientation occurs. Dreams that occurred were not unpleasant.

Comparison of Agents.[125] A comparison of ketamine and thiopental in healthy nonsurgical volunteers has been carefully carried out and involves effects on mental status, mood, and personality. A variety of objective and subjective psychological measures were assessed in the immediate postanesthetic period, 1 day, 2 weeks and 4 months after the administration of anesthesia. Immediately after anesthesia, a significantly greater incidence of abnormalities of mental status, personality, time perception, profile of mood, and other sensory indices were all carefully analyzed. The conclusion from this study was that there is an immediate increase in the number of psychological side effects in normal volunteers following ketamine, and the incidence is significantly greater than with thiopental. The changes found following both drugs, however, were short lived, and no alteration in personality structure was determined. Thus, the ketamine emergence phenomena, as are the thiopental emergence changes, are time limited and do not pose a permanent danger to mental integrity.

Two important concepts emerge from this study: (1) that the patient's mental status before anesthesia is probably an important correlate of mental status during emergence; and (2) that it appears that isolating patients in the recovery room without personal contact results in unpleasant emergence experiences. It is recommended that simple supportive statements, holding of hands, and other measures to assure the patients that they are not isolated but are in fact in a real-life, comfortable reality, be employed.

ABUSE POTENTIAL.[118] Use of ketamine for nonmedical purposes, i.e., recreational, has become widespread. This is related to the production of illusions, dreams, and some hallucinations. Young adults have tended to avoid PCP because of the persistent unpleasant feelings and have found ketamine a satisfactory substitute. Symptoms and general responses, however, are the same as with PCP.

In the drug culture, ketamine is known as "green" (because of the green crystalline appearance of the drug) or "supergrass" as it is often called, when used with marijuana. Common names include "jet," "K," "superacid," "purple," "mauve," and "special coke." The agent should be classified as a controlled substance, Schedule 2, as is PCP.

CONTRAINDICATIONS.[87]

1. Psychiatric disturbances
    a. Questionable in young patients. It is necessary to know precisely the relationship between induced electrical seizure activity and development of brain damage. Repetitive daily subcataleptic doses may induce epileptiform brain-wave patterns.
    b. Stage II anesthesia — delusional-type action is like lysergic acid diethylamide (LSD), which is a street drug of abuse in some countries.
2. Patients on thyroid medication.
3. Major surgery as sole anesthetic.
4. Adjunct in spinal or peridural anesthesia.
5. Neurologic diagnostic procedures (when raised intracranial pressure exists). Ketamine should not be used in neurologic diagnostic procedures or in many neuropsychiatric disturbances:
    a. Many EEG changes similar to those in epilepsy. An epileptiform EEG pattern subject to misinterpretation.
    b. Not in therapeutic neurosurgical procedures if abnormal or bizarre motor activity is present.
6. Clinical circumstances when an increase in arterial pressure is undesirable, as in hypertension; or in patients requiring a pacemaker when an increased afterload would be undesirable. Secondly, in view of the increased MV_{O_2}, it should not be administered to patients with severe myocardial disease, including coronary insufficiency.[26]

ADVANTAGES. This drug has sympathomimetic properties and maintains a satisfactory and supported cardiovascular system. Among the advantages, the following are included:

1. Antihistaminic action
2. Good analgesic effect
3. Antiarrhythmic property
4. Maintenance of circulation in hypotensive states—provides cardiovascular stability
5. Choice in selected medical states (lack of triggering of malignant hyperthermia; (Wadhwa)[77] safe in porphyria[65]
6. Bronchodilation[37] and use in asthma by continuous infusion in status[86]
7. Absence of awareness[60]
8. Usefulness as an induction drug and evidence of great advantage in rapid-sequence induction[124a]
9. Usefulness in cesarean sections compared to thiopental[113]
10. Reduces incidence and severity of succinylcholine fasciculations[126]

THE BENZODIAZEPINES

DIAZEPAM

Diazepam, like most other intravenous nonnarcotic agents, is primarily used as an induction agent for anesthesia.[127,128] It is also used as a soporific during regional and topical anesthesia. It should be considered as a basal hypnotic and should aim to produce a sleep state allowing the administration of other agents or permitting minor manipulations. It is also of value as an anticonvulsant[129] and for preanesthetic medication.[130]

CHEMISTRY. Although drugs of this type were originally synthesized in the 1930s, it was not until the 1950s that a clinically useful benzodiazepine, chlordiazepoxide, was developed by Sternback. Diazepam (Valium) is a benzodiazepine, chemically related to chlordiazepoxide (Librium), and is the prototype of the benzodiazepines (Fig. 27–7). Oxazepam (Serax) is a breakdown product of diazepam resulting from demethylation and hydroxylation.

An electronegative substituent, usually chlorine, in the C-7 position is necessary for anticonvulsant action. Diazepam is a colorless, crystalline compound, insoluble in water, but is highly lipid soluble. It is available commercially in ampules containing 5 mg/ml in an aqueous vehicle containing organic solvents consisting mainly of propylene glycol (40%), ethyl alcohol (10%) as solvents, sodium benzoate and benzoic acid as buffers, and benzyl alcohol (1.5%) as a preservative. This combination produces a slightly viscid solution that requires a large-bore needle for rapid intravenous injection. Diazepam is a weak base with a pKa of 3.3.[132]

Doses of the solvents well in excess of those likely to be injected intravenously are devoid of toxic effects. The pH of the compounded injectable solution is in the 6.4 to 6.9 range. Although transitory cloudiness sometimes occurs when diazepam is diluted with water or saline solution, this does not appear to affect its potency. Dilution of the currently available preparation is not recommended by the manufacturers, because it produces an emulsion of small, particulate matter; furthermore, diazepam should not be mixed with other drugs.

An emulsion of diazepam in soybean oil has been formulated by Mattila[132] (Diazemuls) to minimize phlebitis.

PREANESTHETIC MEDICATION.[130] Diazepam may be used for sedative hypnotic effects in a dose of 10 mg. This dose provides a soporific effect similar to 10 mg of morphine but without any analgesia. For this effect, it may be given orally 1 hour prior to anesthesia or administered intravenously 5 to 10 minutes prior to anesthesia as used in outpatient surgicenters.

When a combination of oral 10 mg diazepam with intramuscular morphine (0.1 to 0.2 mg/kg) is administered 1 hour preanesthetically, an excellent sedative–analgesic effect is achieved.

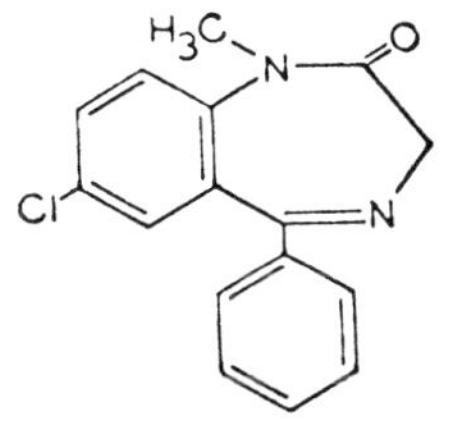

LOCUS OF ACTION.[133–135] The action of diazepam is a dose-dependent reduction in the activity of the central nervous system with decreased anxiety and a calming effect. This is associated with sedation, hypnosis, muscle relaxation, and an anticonvulsant effect.

Specific sites of action in the brain are the limbic system and the amygdala. The latter is a relay area for expression of emotion. The midbrain, hippocampus, and cerebral cortex are also affected.

High-affinity binding sites for benzodiazepines have been demonstrated in these regions, and such receptors are located adjacent to gamma-aminobutyric acid (GABA) receptors. The benzodiazepines appear to act by facilitating the central inhibitory effects of GABA.

Experimentally, small doses of diazepam depress the limbic system of cats without causing cortical depression so that the animals are calm and alert. Aggression, more than activity, is reduced.

DOSAGE AND ADMINISTRATION. Diazepam is an effective oral hypnotic in doses of 20 to 30 mg for adults, producing light sleep; this action is more marked when the drug is given intramuscularly.

Intramuscular administration does not produce a predictable effect because of variable absorption. The oral route appears to be superior (a contrast with short-acting barbiturates). The incidence of pain is about 10% at the intramuscular injection site.[136]

Rectal administration of diazepam is effective in children for premedication. The dose is 0.5 mg/kg. A concentration of 5 mg in 2.5 ml is usually employed and can be available in disposable tubes.[137] An adequate serum concentration is achieved in 5 to 10 minutes after instillation with production of somnolence.

When given intravenously, small doses are employed and a delay of 1 to 2 minutes occurs before maximum depressant action becomes evident; a great individual variation in response to diazepam can be observed. Administration should be slow, about 1 minute for each 1 ml (5 mg).

Choice of veins. The large veins of the forearm should be selected. Small veins such as those on dorsum of hand or wrist must be avoided. Care must be taken to avoid extravasation.

INDUCTION. Induction of anesthesia may result from administration intravenously of a dose of 0.2 mg/kg in patients premedicated with an opiate. A larger dose of 0.45 mg/kg is necessary following premedication with atropine alone; doses up to 0.8 mg/kg may be required to be reasonably certain of in-

FIG. 27–7. Diazepam (Valium)

duction anesthesia, irrespective of the premedication given.

Opiates and barbiturates enhance the hypnotic action of diazepam. The potentiation by diazepam of subsequent doses of barbiturates, i.e., thiopental, is readily observed. Interaction with fentanyl will produce significant depression and apnea.[138]

PHARMACOKINETICS.[139,140] After a single intravenous dose of diazepam, there is a biexponential decline in the plasma levels.* Following a brief pi-phase related to volume of vascular dilution, there is a relatively rapid decline in the plasma level corresponding to the tissue distribution and an alpha-phase of uptake by vascular rich tissues. This elimination half-time alpha-phase varies over 30 to 60 minutes but may extend over a range of 1.1 to 2.8 hours. The drug is widely distributed into body tissues, and the volume of distribution is 1.1 ± 0.3 L/kg, with a range of 0.7 to 1.7 L/kg. It is increased in the aged and in the presence of cirrhosis and hypoalbuminemia.

Subsequently, there is a slow-decline beta-phase corresponding to slow uptake by vascular poor tissues, but largely due to transformation and elimination processes. This is a prolonged phase and has an elimination half-life of 43 ± 13 hours, with a range of 20 to 50 hours. Altough the levels of intact drug rapidly decline, there is a concomitant rise in the plasma demethylated metabolite (Fig. 27–8).

Total clearance rate is slow, at 0.38 ± .06 ml/kg/min, with a range of 0.24 to 0.53 ml/kg/min. The rate increases in hypoalbuminemia and when other drugs that induce metabolic enzymes are present (as in epilepsy). Clearance is decreased in cirrhosis and hepatitis.

The half-life of the parent drug is actually 7 to 10 hours, whereas that of the metabolites is 48 hours or more.[139] Within an hour of administration, the pharmacologically active metabolite desmethyldiazepam appears, and its increasing level mirrors the decline of the parent compound. This metabolite is almost as potent as the parent compound. The subsequent decline of desmethyldiazepam is much slower. Several variables affect diazepam plasma levels.[139-141]

Effect of Binding. Extensive plasma binding occurs. About 98% of the drug is bound; the unbound free fraction range is only from 1% to 3%. In elderly subjects, the unbound fraction is slightly higher. Sex does not affect binding. Binding is decreased in uremia, cirrhosis, neonates, pregnancy, and hypoalbuminemia states.

Effect of Age and Sex.[142] This is evident on clearance studies of the drug. Elderly men have a slower clearance than young men. The elimination half-life increases linearly with age in men. At age 20 years, it is about 20 hours, in subjects of 60 years, it is 75 hours, and at 80 years it is about 100 hours.[142]

In women, age does not significantly effect clearance. The elimination half-life and clearance, however, are similar to that of the elderly man; the elimination half-life is prolonged and is 40 to 80 hours.[139] Smoking influences clearance, and heavy smokers show lower clearance rates.

Effect of Renal Disease.[143] Decreased protein binding results in an increase in the free fraction of drug. The clearance of the unbound fraction is unchanged. But a twofold increase in total clearance occurs (0.94 vs. 0.34 ml/min/kg), accounting for the shortened elimination half-life of 37 hours (versus 92 hours).

Effect of Liver Disease.[142] Duration of action is greatly prolonged. There is decreased protein binding, with an increased volume of distribution and increased free fraction of the agent. Clearance is significantly decreased.

Effect of Race. Kinetic studies also show that the total body clearance rate of diazepam is slower in Asians than whites. Hence, cumulative effects are more likely in Asians.[144]

Circadian Effect. Administration of diazepam orally in the morning is accompanied by high plasma levels for the initial 2 to 3 hours. This is compared with lower levels when the oral dosing is in the evening.[145]

METABOLISM.[141] Diazepam is metabolized exclusively in the liver in humans by microsomal enzymes. Metabolism occurs in three steps: (1) the first biotransformation pathway is by demethylation to N-desmethyldiazepam; this is the major metabolite in plasma and it possesses pharmacologic activity; (2) next, there is slower hydroxylation of desmethyldiazepam to oxazepam, which occurs also in the liver and is also active. The rate of formation of desmethyldiazepam is three times faster than that of the hydroxylation process of desmethyldiazepam to oxazepam; (3) the last step is the conjugation of oxazepam with glucuronide to form the main urinary product; this conjugation is rapid, so that the half-life of oxazepam is 5 to 6 hours. Thus, three metabolites are produced and excreted. Over 70% is recovered in the urine, 20% as unchanged, 10% as N-demethylated, 10% as d-hydroxylated (oxazepam), and 33% as the inactive glucuronide. Diazepam is an hepatic enzyme inducer as it increases the metabolism of other drugs dependent on liver enzymes but also enhances its own destruction.

In patients with liver disease, the rate at both steps of hepatic metabolism, i.e., demethylation and hydroxylation of diazepam, is diminished. These

---

* For subjects with highest lipid solubility, a three-compartment model is more appropriate.[139]

FIG. 27–8. Plasma concentrations of diazepam and its major metabolite, desmethyldiazepam, in representative young and elderly male subjects following intravenous injection of diazepam. Also shown are kinetic functions for diazepam. Note the slower disappearance of diazepam, as well as the slower rate of metabolite formation, in the elderly subject. Both the young and elderly female follow the disappearance curve noted above for the elderly male. (From Greenblatt, D.J., et al: Diazepam disposition determinants. Clin. Pharmacol. Ther., 27:301, 1980.

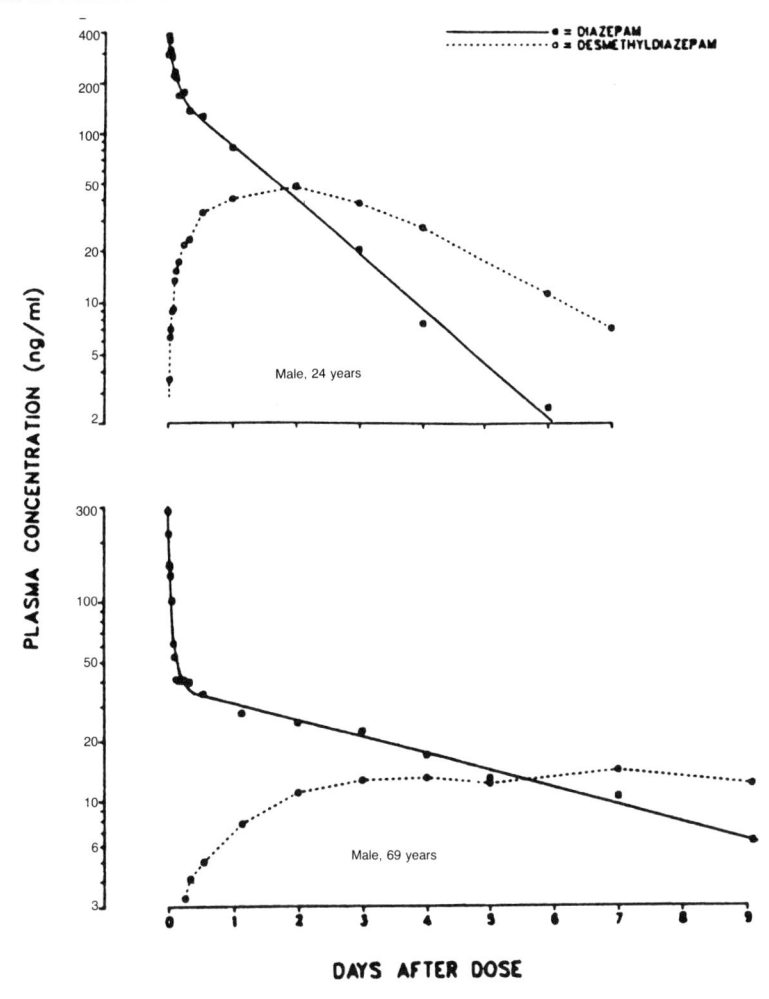

processes are related to the impaired mixed-function oxygenase system. After continuous (chronic) dosage in healthy subjects with diazepam, the transformation to desmethyldiazepam is also slower. This appears to be related to a feedback inhibition of the demethylation process by the metabolite desmethyldiazepam. The last step in metabolism (conjugation of oxazepam), however, is unimpaired in the presence of liver disease. The two active metabolites are separately available as commercial preparations for clinical use.

EXCRETION. Less than 1% of the parent drug is excreted in the urine. The urinary metabolites account for most of the excretion, and the conjugated oxazepam is the major excretory product.[143a]

MECHANISM OF ACTION.[146,147] The central nervous system locus of action has been discussed earlier. The mechanism of action is presumed to be the enhancement of GABA-ergic transmission.

At the spinal cord level, there appears to be increased presynaptic inhibition of afferent neuronal terminals in the posterior gray horns of the primary reflex arc.

BLOOD LEVELS CORRELATED WITH CENTRAL NERVOUS SYSTEM EFFECTS. Sedative effects, impaired mental function, amnesia, blurred vision, and poor muscular coordination are observed at blood levels of diazepam below 400 µg/L. Sleep usually occurs at levels of 1000 µg/L.[143a]

Central Nervous System Pharmacology.[148] Accompanying EEG effects are similar to those produced by chlordiazepoxide and consist of low- to moderate-voltage fast activity that may persist for a week after medication is discontinued. These effects have led to the widespread use of diazepam in psychiatry. It is particularly useful in anxiety–tension states as a preanesthetic medication.

Cerebral Blood Flow and Cerebral Metabolism.[149] Experimental studies show that diazepam causes a moderate decrease (20% to 30%) in cerebral blood flow, but cerebral metabolic rate of oxygen is unchanged or only slightly reduced. When either sedative or sleep doses of diazepam are given and accompanied by nitrous oxide (70%), both cerebral blood flow and cerebral metabolic rate of oxygen are lowered to 60% of control.

Nitrous oxide alone produces only a variable reduction in cerebral metabolic rate of oxygen of an order below 25%.[149a] Thus, a synergistic interaction occurs between diazepam and nitrous oxide.

Amnesia Effect.[127] It would appear that retrograde amnesia—lack of recall of the preinjection period—is not caused regularly by moderate doses of this drug. Memory for subsequent events is markedly reduced when diazepam is given in combination with meperidine or hyoscine but is little affected by 10 mg diazepam alone. About 30% of patients receiving diazepam have retrograde amnesia for the period immediately before injection compared with about 8% of patients induced by thiopental.

ANALGESIC ACTION. Pain studies in humans demonstrate only a slight transient analgesic action following intravenous diazepam.

In contrast to the intravenous barbiturates, this drug does not increase sensitivity to somatic pain. It is not an antianalgesic.

EFFECT ON LARYNGEAL REFLEX.[150] A study of the effect of irritants on the laryngeal reflex, including mechanical as well as chemical, indicates that the sensitivity of the laryngeal reflex is significantly depressed by diazepam.[150] In contrast, lorazepam tends to increase the sensitivity of the laryngeal reflex, whereas midazolam is intermediate and does not significantly depress the reflex to the extent that diazepam does. Hence, diazepam is the choice benzodiazepine for endoscopic procedures.

CARDIOVASCULAR SYSTEM.[127,151] Most investigators find no significant influence on the cardiovascular system.[127] The pulse rate does not change significantly. Blood pressure changes are comparable to those during sleep.[151,159] Normal subjects, given intravenous doses of 40 to 60 mg as preendoscopy medication, experience an increase in heart rate of about 15% within 10 minutes. The systolic pressure falls an average of 12% and diastolic falls 5%. Initially, there is no significant increase in total peripheral resistance, but after 15 minutes it tends to rise about 15% from reflex compensation. Stroke volume falls about 18% within 5 minutes and progressively falls to about 30% in 15 minutes. The left ventricular stroke work falls about 25%. Evidence indicates that there is some negative inotropic effect.

Cardiac output during this period only decreases 15% to 20%. Moderate increases in coronary blood flow are usually seen.[152]

Intravenous diazepam for anesthesia induction shows a minimal hypotensive action. Brown[153] found doses 0.6 to 0.8 mg/kg did not produce a fall in systolic pressure in excess of 20 mm Hg. This effect occurred in fewer than 5% of patients, whereas the incidence was 24% with 4 mg/kg thiopental and 8% after 1.6 mg/kg methohexital in a strictly comparable series of patients.

The cardiovascular effects of tilting in adult men volunteers have been studied before and after intravenous administration of 10 mg diazepam. No changes in blood pressure or pulse rate were produced by the drug.[154]

Clinical reports of a comparison between thiopental and diazepam, when used for cardioversion, show a significantly higher incidence of irregularities with the barbiturate.

Diazepam, when administered with high doses of fentanyl (greater than 50 µg/kg) produces significant hypotension.[155] There ensues a decrease in mean arterial pressure and systemic vascular resistance.[156]

In patients with obstructive lung disease, Rao[151] found no significant cardiovascular changes differing from those with normal pulmonary function. Changes in pulmonary artery pressure and total pulmonary artery resistance are insignificant.[157]

RESPIRATORY EFFECTS.[157-163] Clinical doses of diazepam cause a slight degree of respiratory depression. Following intravenous hypnotic doses of 5 to 15 mg/70 kg, there is significant depression. If given during anesthesia or with an opiate, apnea may ensue. This action may be the result of hypotonia of muscles induced by a central relaxant mechanism. There may also be inhibition of hypoxic respiratory drive.[163] Catchlove,[158] however, did not find significant effects on respiration in patients with obstructive pulmonary disease. Pierce[159] showed that the depression of respiration in patients with chronic obstructive pulmonary disease was comparable with the changes in similar-type patients during sleep.

Diazepam has been noted to increase airway resistance in normal subjects.[160]

Effect on Respiratory CO_2 Response Curve.[161] Most subjects sustain a significant decrease in response to carbon dioxide after hypnotic doses of diazepam. The duration of this effect is about 1 hour, and there is a correlation between the respiratory depression and decreasing levels of consciousness.[161a]

The slope of the curve of the ventilatory response to rebreathing carbon dioxide is depressed by as much as 50% of control. The zero intercept of the curve is also shifted to the left. Bailey[161b] has also noted that there are decreases in resting minute ventilation and an increase in resting CO_2 levels. He recommends that measuring these levels is also a useful procedure.

Reversal of this effect is accomplished by large doses of naloxone. After 15 mg intravenously of diazepam, two doses of 15 mg each (30 minutes apart) of naloxone completely reverses the depression.[161]

PLACENTAL TRANSFER.[162] Diazepam rapidly passes the placental barrier, and within a few minutes equilibrium is reached between maternal and cord blood levels.

CENTRAL MUSCLE-RELAXANT EFFECTS.[163,163a] The benzodiazepines have muscle-relaxant properties and are clinically effective in the treatment of various forms of muscle spasm.

A depressant action occurs on the neurons of the spinal cord. At least part of its beneficial effect is the result of a pharmacologic action on polysynaptic pathways within the spinal cord as well as on supraspinal structures.[163b] In animals, diazepam is about 10 times as effective as meprobamate in suppressing skeletal muscle activity. It is 20 times as effective as chlordiazepoxide in blocking decerebrate rigidity but has only five times the action of the latter drug on the EEG. Its marked antianxiety effect certainly contributes to the muscle-relaxant action observed in dystonic–athetoid children with cerebral palsy.

Action at Neuromuscular Junction.[164] Diazepam in single doses intravenously of 10 mg to adults has little or no discernible effect on the neuromuscular junction. Subsequent gallamine doses, however, show a threefold increase in intensity and duration of block. A twofold increase in block is observed after *d*-turbocurarine. Conversely, succinylcholine block is reduced by 20% to 30%, and a larger dose is required to produce the same degree of blockade. It appears that diazepam may reduce acetylcholine release at the presynaptic membrane.[164] The studies by Feldman[164] indicate some potentiating and additive effects to nondepolarizing muscle relaxants; a mild antagonism to succinylcholine appears to exist.

Abdominal relaxation is not produced by doses of 2.5 to 10 mg, and the dose of tubocurarine required subsequently to produce relaxation is the same as that required in patients who have not had diazepam.[164] Straining on the endotracheal tube occurs during diazepam sleep alone. Curarization is necessary before satisfactory artificial ventilation of the lungs is possible.

EFFECT ON CATECHOLAMINES.[165,166] Significant changes occur in plasma catecholamine levels with the induction of unconsciousness by diazepam. Following intravenous doses between 0.6 and 0.8/kg (as adjunct for endoscopy), the following changes in epinephrine and norepinephrine were determined:[166] epinephrine—a reduction from 140 pg/ml to 75 pg/ml; and norepinephrine—a reduction from 400 pg/ml to 330 pg/ml.

These changes represent a 59% decrease for epinephrine and a significant reduction of 20% to 25% for norepinephrine.

INDICATIONS

As a Tranquilizer. It is an antianxiety agent and has related sedative and soporific actions.

As a Neuroleptic. Diazepam may be employed as part of neuroleptanesthesia, usually combined with meperidine or fentanyl. Diazepam gives some protection from the autonomic effects of reflex stimulation during abnormal surgery.

For a Basal State. Doses of up to 1 mg/kg in an intravenous infusion (80 mg/250 ml) will produce a basal state of sleep. Production of this intensity of hypnotic action depends largely on the rate of infusion; effective doses are given in 5 to 8 minutes (approximately 10 mg/min). Anesthesia is maintained with nitrous oxide and various inhalation supplements along with intravenous opiates.

Surgical Anesthesia. Diazepam is used as an adjunct in balanced-narcotic anesthesia or in inhalation anesthesia. It can be used as a soporific during topical anesthesia or regional anesthesia.

CLINICAL USES

Preanesthetic Medication.[130] Provides an excellent anxiolytic, calming effect with accompanying sedative action.

Induction Agent.[127,153] It is given in doses of 5 to 10 mg at 1- to 2-minute intervals to a total of 0.3 to 0.6 mg/kg. In this instance, the slow onset of action of the drug is obvious, and thickened speech and nystagmus precede the induction of sleep. Anesthesia is continued with standard supplements of inhalation anesthetic drugs.

Dentistry.[167] Ideally, the requirements in dentistry are reduction of nervous tension, blunting of consciousness, minimal suppression of voluntary efforts, neural suppression of reflexes, and pain relief.

The endpoint taken to denote a satisfactory depth of sedation is a drowsy patient who has slurred speech but who is still able to respond to requests.

Although the soporific effects of small doses of diazepam are relatively short lived, the anxiolytic effects seem to last much longer.

In addition, the drug permits opening of the mouth and is useful in treatment of trismus.

Obstetrics.[162] The drug produces no untoward effects on the mothers or infants and markedly reduces apprehension and pain. Furthermore, it blurs the memory for the event. In these doses of 20 to 40 mg intramuscularly, diazepam has no apparent influence on the Apgar score of the neonates or on the length of labor.

Endoscopy.[167a] Diazepam intravenously administered prior to bronchoscopy under local analgesia is an excellent adjunct.[167]

Although diazepam provides muscular relaxation and relief of anxiety, it does not suppress gag and laryngeal reflexes, and when used alone it will not provide suitable conditions for bronchoscopy or esophagoscopy. It will provide good sedation and amnesia, however, and it allows such procedures to be carried out under local topical analgesia.

Tetanus. Action on the spinal internuncial neurones occurs with diazepam.[163b] Hypothermia tends to occur when it is given to neonates.

Although it is effective in controlling the muscle rigidity of tetanus, diazepam is less effective in controlling the muscle spasms in severe cases. It undoubtedly has a place in the treatment of mild or moderate cases, but curarization still appears to be the treatment of choice when the disease is severe.

Convulsive States.[87a] This drug has been found to be effective in abolishing seizure discharges, as an adjunct in treatment of status epilepticus, and in the management of eclampsia.

PRECAUTIONS AND COMPLICATIONS

1. In patients with liver disease, the duration of action is greatly prolonged as a result of altered pharmacokinetics, especially clearance.[141]
2. In patients with renal disease, the pharmacokinetic values are altered because of decreased protein binding and an increase in free fraction; a twofold increase in hepatic clearance occurs, accounting for the shortened elimination half-life.
3. Combination with narcotics in usual doses can cause profound respiratory depression and apnea.[158]
4. The addition of diazepam after large doses of fentanyl or morphine results in significant cardiovascular depression. There is decreased stroke volume, cardiac output, and blood pressure. Cardiac rate may decrease, and bradycardia be observed. Central venous pressure is increased.[155,156]
5. Dizziness persisting for up to 24 hours is an undesirable feature after large doses of diazepam (30 to 50 mg in adults), and occurred in 15% of Brown's patients.[153]
6. Alcohol intake inhibits diazepam metabolism. An increased central nervous system depression occurs. Administration to alcoholics during withdrawal requires high doses to control symptoms and may maintain the dependency on alcohol.[168]
7. Drug interaction—cimetidine impairs hepatic microsomal oxidation of diazepam, reducing its clearance and prolonging elimination half-life. This is of importance in recovery from anesthesia. Side effects and subject performance from long-term use of diazepam, however, have not been demonstrated to be clinically important.[172]
8. Prolonged somnolence and unconsciousness—this may occur unpredictably. Several studies indicate that this sleep state can be reversed by physostigmine.[169] A dose of 40 μg/kg of body weight appears to be optimal.[169a] Occasionally, a muscarinic side effect is noted, but with this dose level it is rare. The mechanism of action is based entirely on inhibition of the central nervous system cholinesterase by physostigmine. Galanthamine has been used as an alternative drug.[170] Aminophylline also is an effective antagonist to diazepam somnolence.[171] A specific antagonist is available, being an imidazodiazepam (flumazenil), which is a competitive inhibitor of the drug at receptors.[173]
9. Judgment and position sense are impaired. On the lateral position, awareness is quite variable in driving and is considerable. It may last for as long as 12 hours.[174]
10. Diazepam–stress reaction—It is paradoxical that the most widely used anxiolytic drug is able to precipitate a "rage reaction." In patients suffering from posttraumatic stress disorder, as seen in Vietnam veterans, the administration of diazepam for supplementary local anesthetic procedures may result in agitation and stress reaction. This may take the form of a full-blown sudden attack of anxiety, fear, or panic, with sleep disturbance, startle response, impaired memory, and disorientation. In one report, the administration of diazepam to Vietnam veterans caused them to relive war experiences; they assumed a belligerent combat-defensive position. This was reversed with aminophylline via a dose of 1 mg/kg intravenously.[175]
11. Pain of injection[176]—The frequency of pain on intravenous injection of diazepam in organic solvent is quite frequent and occurs in 35% to 40% of patients. It is related to rapidity of injection. Pain is frequent, and intensity is greatest with injections in small veins, especially those of the wrist and dorsum of hand.

    Pain is absent with intravenous injections of diazepam in the soybean oil emulsion (Diazemuls) or following midazolam.
12. Thrombophlebitis[177]—Classical signs appear after 2 to 3 days and are maximum at about 7 to 10 days after injection. Pain, swelling, redness, and tenderness are often accompanied by disability. A high frequency is seen with diazepam, when the drug is injected rapidly intravenously into the small veins of the hand.

The frequency varies with the different congeners of diazepam. Midazolam appears to have a low incidence of 1%, flunitrazepam 5%, lorazepam 15%, and diazepam 40%.

It is recommended that injections be made slowly, and into the large antecubital or forearm veins.[176] The fat emulsion of diazepam prepared in soybean oil (Diazemuls) reduces the frequency of thrombophlebitis to approximately 10%, and the pain of injection is absent.

INTOXICATION.[148,178] Benzodiazepines appear to have a low order of toxicity. Alone, they are rarely responsible for serious or fatal intoxication. Of drug intoxication hospital admissions, most are multiple drug overdoses, but 12% to 16% have a benzodiazepine among the drugs. In drug overdose admissions, diazepam implicated alone is less than 1% of patients.[178]

Toxic doses of diazepam usually exceed 250 mg orally. With respect to chlordiazepoxide, acute poisoning is associated with blood concentrations of 20 μg/ml or more, which produce low-grade central nervous system depression with coma or sleep (grade 2 anesthesia), and is related to levels of 60 μg/ml. Ingestion of the benzodiazepines with other central nervous system depressant drugs is a frequent clinical circumstance, and the combination with barbiturates or alcohol is particularly dangerous. Diazepam overdose has been reversed by physostigmine and naloxone.[179,180]

Withdrawal syndrome[178] may be seen after 2 to 3 days of abstinence from several days of relatively high oral dose intake of 15 to 500 mg. After this time, minor manifestations include tremulousness, insomnia, anorexia, anxiety, and even hallucinations. EEG abnormalities are seen, and a rebound increase in rapid-eye-movement sleep occurs. Seizures may occur as late as 7 to 14 days. Auditory hallucinations are common. Disorientation and confusion are present, and patients have autonomic and motor hyperactivity. The onset is delayed when the long-lasting drugs have been used, i.e. diazepam, flurazepam, and others, in contrast to oxazepam and lorazepam. Untreated abstinence syndrome has a substantial morbidity and mortality.

The syndrome is often misdiagnosed as a functional psychosis. Therefore, antipsychotic agents should not be used, because they lower the seizure threshold. Management includes hydration, antianxiety agents, sedation with barbiturates, and careful nutrition.

ADVANTAGES

1. There is an absence of intrinsic cardiovascular toxicity from large doses of diazepam.
2. Detailed liver function tests reveal no abnormalities either in experimental or clinical studies.[127] In the presence of liver disease (alcoholic cirrhosis), however, pharmacokinetic values are altered and duration of action is greatly prolonged.
3. Emetic sequelae are minimal.
4. Anxiolytic action is excellent; amnesic effects are moderate but short lasting usually after intravenous administration.
5. Soporific activity is excellent and is related to the tranquilizing action.

MANAGEMENT OF BENZODIAZEPINE OVERDOSAGE. Supportive measures are the first line of therapy. Drug antagonism, however, is the key to effective management.

Adverse behavioral effects can be reversed by physostigmine.[169,181,182] Aminophylline is also effective.[171,172] Naloxone is effective, especially when narcotic drugs are also present. A specific antagonist, flumazenil, is available for reversing benzodiazepine toxicity.[173]

Flumazenil—The Specific Antagonist. This is an imidazobenzodiazepine, entitled *flumazenil* (RO15–1788), which has been introduced as a competitive antagonist to the benzodiazepines.[173] It has specific activity at the benzodiazepine receptor.[183] The drug itself is devoid of any significant intrinsic action. A preparation is available in a 1-mg dose in 10 ml of sterile solution.

Patients who demonstrate significant central nervous system depression are quite responsive to titrated doses up to 1 mg of the drug.[184] Using a Glasgow Coma Score, with a maximum score of 20 and a minimum score of 4, a variety of patients having taken a benzodiazepine overdose were studied. In all instances, the treated patients responded within 5 minutes and showed an increase in the Glasgow score of approximately 5 units within the 5-minute period.

The most common side effect was a withdrawal reaction on awakening. The milder reaction consisted of anxiety and distress, which may be related to the unfamiliar surroundings of a hospital. These responded to reassurance. A longer-lasting reaction, including hot and cold flashes, included an intense free-floating anxiety.

LORAZEPAM

Lorazepam is a potent benzodiazepine with anxiolytic and amnesic effects. As a result of its subcortical tranquilizing and antianxiety action, there ensues a remarkable state of sedation. The patient is calm and appears to be asleep but can be aroused to answer questions.[185]

ADMINISTRATION AND DOSAGE. Lorazepam can be administered orally, intramuscularly, and intravenously. The dose is calculated on the basis of 0.05 mg/kg (50 μg/kg). The usual doses are 2 to 4 mg and are effective by any of these routes. A dose of 1 mg is equal to 5 mg of diazepam in decreasing anxiety.

This is particularly noted at the 6-hour period after an oral dose.

ABSORPTION AND DISPOSITION.[186] After an oral dose, over 90% is absorbed, but the rate is slower than for diazepam. The peak plasma level is reached in about 1.5 hours.[187]

After intramuscular injection, the absorption is more rapid and the plasma level peaks by 60 minutes. Unlike diazepam, the absorption is extensive and dependable, and there is minimal pain or discomfort by this route.

After intravenous injection, there is a rapid distribution with an alpha half-life of 15 to 20 minutes. About 80% to 90% of the drug is protein bound. The elimination phase extends over 10 to 20 hours and is greatly prolonged in the presence of liver disease.

METABOLISM.[188] Lorazepam is metabolized by conjugation with glucuronide. The product is inactive pharmacologically and is excreted in the urine.

PHARMACOLOGIC EFFECTS. The pharmacologic effects are similar to diazepam but differ pharmacokinetically. The anxiolytic effect is pronounced and renders a patient calm and sedated after intravenous administration within 3 to 4 minutes. The sedative effect, however, is minimal, and it appears that the anxiolytic effect can be dissociated from the sedative effect.[189]

The amnesic action is dose related and is seen with larger doses of at least 4 mg so that patients have little or no recall of perioperative events.[190] The onset of this effect is delayed for 20 minutes, but the effect is prolonged.[191] This lack of recall has been found in 60% to 85% of patients when 4 mg of lorazepam is administered intravenously. Over 80% of patients accepted this drug quite readily. Pentobarbital recall is good and amnesic effects poor. Thus, lorazepam provides a good amnesic effect and is superior to diazepam.[192]

PHARMACOKINETICS. The duration of action of lorazepam is 3 to 4 hours, compared with diazepam's effect of 8 to 12 hours. The distribution half-life is fairly rapid (after intravenous injection, 15 to 20 minutes). The elimination (beta) half-life is approximately 12 to 15 hours for lorazepam compared with that of diazepam of 24 to 38 hours.[193] The peak anxiolytic effect of lorazepam continues for a longer time than that of diazepam.

No correlation has been determined between lorazepam's half-life and the duration of its activity, as manifested by its action at the binding sites of receptors.

CLINICAL USE. Primarily, this drug is useful as part of preanesthetic medication. The doses needed for induction of sleep are larger and the resultant action is too prolonged.

In small doses, lorazepam has been compared with placebo, and it is curious that placebo had an equal degree of antianxiety effect as did the small doses of lorazepam. Patient preference for one or the other was approximately equal.[194] In larger doses, however, most preferred the placebo over the lorazepam, and their liking for the tranquilizer decreased.

Drug abusers usually prefer a quick-acting, short-life high for their "fix" purposes. Placebo was found in this group of patients equal to a dose of 0.5 mg of lorazepam.[194] Either placebo or a small dose of lorazepam, however, was preferred to 1 mg of lorazepam. Aminophylline has been found to be antagonistic to lorazepam as well as to diazepam.[194a]

MIDAZOLAM

Midazolam is a water-soluble benzodiazepine that has similar pharmacologic actions to diazepam but a much shorter duration of action and requires no special solvents. It was synthetized in 1975 by Walser.[195] A significant advantage over diazepam is the lack of tissue and venous irritation, pain, and phlebitis.[176] It is also noted that significant psychomotor impairment only lasts 2 to 8 hours; in contrast, impairment with diazepam continues up to 24 to 48 hours. The major disadvantages of diazepam are avoided.

CHEMISTRY. The maleate salt of midazolam is a colorless crystal. The molecular weight is 362. It is buffered to a pH of 3.5 in the commercial preparation, which keeps the benzodiazepine ring open and maintains its aqueous solubility.[195b] After administration, the physiologic pH of 7.4 (of plasma) induces the closed ring form, which confers high lipophilicity to the drug and is the effective structure. The commercial preparation is compatible with acid salts, such as morphine, atropine, and scopolamine. This drug should not be mixed with or administered with alkaline solutions, such as thiopental, but can be mixed in dextrose or saline and Ringer's lactate solution.

Chemical Formula. This drug is a benzodiazepine with an imidazole ring incorporated (Fig. 27–9). It is named 8-chloro-6-(2-fluorophenyl)-1-methyl-4H-imidazo-[1,5-a] [1,4] benzodiazepine maleate.

PHARMACOLOGY

Central Nervous System.[195] This agent is a typical benzodiazepine. It is a hypnotic-and-anxiolytic drug. Common to the benzodiazepines, it possesses the desirable attributes of benzodiazepines, including sedation, hypnosis, an anticonvulsive action, and skeletal muscle relaxation through blockade of the gamma system. Good antegrade amnesia but no retrograde amnesia is noted. No adverse effects on other functions are noted. The specific amnesic effect is independent of any soporific action.[196] Over

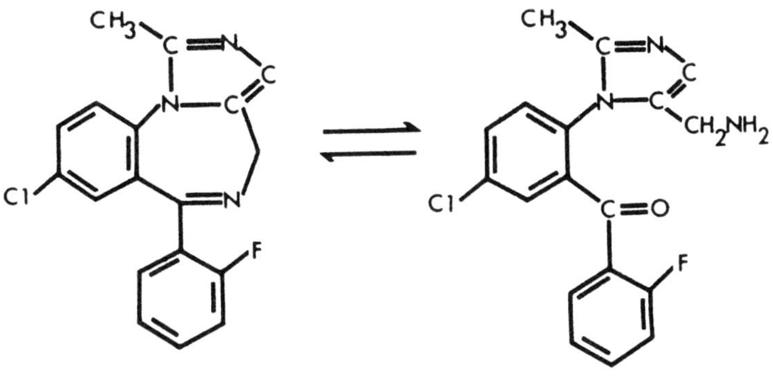

FIG. 27-9. The unique midazolam ring structure. Solubility is pH dependent. At pH less than 4.0 the midazolam is an open ring structure (2) which is the water soluble configuration present in commercial preparations. At a pH above 4.0 the ring closes and becomes lipid soluble: (1) the active lipid soluble ring configuration in blood. (2) the inactive water soluble configuration open ring.
Modified from Stanski, D.R., and Watkins, W.D.: Drug Disposition in Anesthesia. New York, Gruen and Stratton, 1982.

60% of patients have complete amnesia for 10 minutes, and 90% have partial amnesia lasting 30 minutes. This occurs after either intramuscular or intravenous injection and is longer than after diazepam.[197]

At a standard induction dose of 10 to 20 mg, subjects rapidly lose consciousness.[198] Cessation of counting, loss of response to verbal commands, and loss of eyelash and eyelid reflexes occur between 30 and 100 seconds, averaging 1 minute after injection. Invariably, the onset of sleep is accompanied by apnea lasting about 20 seconds. With careful administration for induction, the apnea occurs in about 20% of patients compared with 30% with thiopental. These apneas of induction are more likely in patients premedicated with a narcotic.

Duration of sleep is brief. From the commencement of injection to awakening (opening of eyes on command), the time period is between 4 and 5 minutes. Midazolam lowers MAC values for volatile agents.

Studies of patients with obstructive lung disease show a more profound depression of the response curve than after thiopental.[212] This represents a concern in the postanesthetic period when emergence from general anesthesia is delayed, and patients should be carefully observed. Some observations by Caldwell[199] indicate that this postanesthetic sedation and depression after midazolam can be reversed by physostigmine.

Cardiovascular Effects.[200] Sleep doses for midazolam produce a modest decrease in mean arterial pressure and a decrease in systolic and diastolic arterial pressure.[200] There is a decrease in cardiac output and a decrease in stroke volume index and cardiac index of 15% and 10%, respectively, with no change in the systemic vascular resistance (Table 27-5).[201]

These changes are accompanied by a decrease in whole body oxygen demand (V_{O_2}) and a slight decrease in the arterial-venous oxygen difference

TABLE 27-5. HEMODYNAMIC DATA (mean ± SD) (number of patients = 8)

	Control	5 Minutes	15 Minutes
SAP (mm Hg)	136 ± 31	112 ± 19‡	110 ± 15‡
MAP (mm Hg)	109 ± 20	93 ± 15‡	92 ± 13‡
DAP (mm Hg)	87 ± 16	76 ± 14‡	75 ± 12‡
CI (L · min^{-1} · m^{-2})	3.0 ± 0.5	2.6 ± 0.4*	2.7 ± 0.5*
HR (bts · min^{-1})	81 ± 17	87 ± 16†	87 ± 15.5†
V$_{max}$ (s^{-1})	1.5 ± 0.2	1.6 ± 0.2	1.6 ± 0.3
RAP (mm Hg)	4.5 ± 3.5	3.4 ± 3.4*	3.5 ± 3.5
LVEDP (mm Hg)	7.7 ± 2.7	4.9 ± 2.4*	4.2 ± 2.6†
SI (ml · m^{-2})	37.7 ± 7.3	30.7 ± 5.9‡	31.1 ± 6.3‡
T (ms)	47 ± 3	46 ± 6	46 ± 5
SVR (dyn · cm^{-3} · s)	1530 ± 320	1500 ± 235	1450 ± 270
CSBF (ml · min^{-1})	134 ± 58	104 ± 38†	104 ± 30†
CVR (units)	0.84 ± 0.22	0.92 ± 0.2	0.91 ± 0.19

* $P < 0.05$ *versus* control.
† $P < 0.01$ *versus* control.
‡ $P < 0.001$ *versus* control.

Abbreviations: SAP, systolic arterial pressure; MAP, mean arterial pressure; DAP, diastolic arterial pressure; CI, cardiac index; HR, heart rate; V$_{max}$, maximum velocity of shortening; RAP, right atrial pressure; LVEDP, left ventricular end-diastolic pressure; SI, stroke index; T, relaxation time contant; SVR, systemic vascular resistance; CSBF, coronary sinus blood flow; CVR, coronary vascular resistance.

From Marty, J., et al.: Effects of midazolam on the coronary circulation in patients with coronary artery disease. Anesthesiology, *64:*206, 1986.

$C(A-\bar{V})_{O_2}$. The cardiac index matched the total body oxygen required.

Effects on Myocardial Oxygen Demand.[201] The myocardial oxygen demand (MVO_2) is also markedly decreased and amounts to about 34%. Simultaneously, there was no alteration of myocardial contractility, as evidenced by the maintained maximum velocity of shortening (V_{max}). There is also a decreased left-ventricular end-diastolic pressure (LVEDP), reflecting a decreased preload. This is probably related to increased venous capacitance (Table 27–6).

Coronary Hemodynamics.[201] Coronary vascular resistance (CVR) is not altered. In contrast, a reduction in CVR follows diazapam, which appears to have a coronary artery–dilating effect. This effect may give rise to the coronary steal syndrome and regional ischemia; however, this has not been demonstrated for diazepam.

Coronary perfusion pressure is decreased, as reflected in a fall in diastolic artery pressure (DAP), whereas coronary sinus oxygen tension is increased by about 15% (with a decrease in coronary sinus blood flow of 22%), accompanied by a decreased coronary artery conversion oxygen difference of 10%.

These data indicate a decreased myocardial oxygen demand consequent to the effect of midazolam. Because these studies were conducted on patients with coronary artery disease, it can be concluded that midazolam is a safe induction agent for patients with ischemic heart disease.

Commentary: Cardiovascular Effects Good stability is observed. Systolic and diastolic blood pressure and pulse rates are not significantly altered. There is a decrease in systemic vascular resistance. Hemodynamic changes are more gradual and less pronounced than with equipotent doses of thiopental[200] and are slightly but insignificantly greater than with diazepam.[202] Some direct myocardial depressant effects are noted similar to diazepam. In general, there is less variability in responses than with thiopental or diazepam, and responses are predictable.

Endocrinologic Effects.[203] These are summarized as follows:

- Attenuates stress-related epinephrine increases, which are minimal
- Plasma cortisol decreases from approximately 12.5 to 7.5 µg/dl
- Response to exogenous adrenocorticotropic hormone is unchanged
- Prevents any significant endogenous increase in adrenocorticotropic hormone and beta-endorphins
- Adrenocorticotropic hormone changes are minimal: immediately following surgery, plasma levels change from normal preoperative baseline levels of about 5 pmol/L to 7 pmol/L; at 6 hours, 4 pmol/L; and 5 pmol/L at 20 hours.
- The course of beta-endorphin plasma levels is similar to adrenocorticotropic hormone: preoperative level, 7 pmol/L; at end of surgery, level of 9 pmol/L; at 6 hours, 7 pmol/L; and at 20 hours, 6.5 pmol/L.

Effects on Skeletal Muscle. No influence on the neuromuscular junction has been determined.

Interaction with Muscle Relaxants. Both depolarizing and nondepolarizing muscle relaxants may be safely given. Midazolam does not reinforce or prolong the neuromuscular block.[204]

Exposure of muscle biopsies from malignant-hyperthermia–susceptible patients to midazolam at maximal therapeutic dose concentrations does not result in a detectable muscle contraction on direct stimulation. No interaction or enhancement of the effects of caffeine or halothane are noted.[205]

TABLE 27–6. BLOOD GAS TENSIONS, OXYGEN, AND MYOCARDIAL METABOLISM DATA (mean ± SD) (number of patients = 8)

	Control	5 Minutes	15 Minutes
MVO_2 (ml · min^{-1})	16.8 ± 10.1	11.4 ± 4.4†	11.1 ± 3.6†
$C(a-cs)O_2$ (ml · dl^{-1})	12.1 ± 1.4	10.9 ± 1.5†	10.8 ± 1.3†
Lact(a-cs)/lacta	0.45 ± 0.15	0.52 ± 0.15	0.44 ± 0.2
$PcsO_2$ (mm Hg)	22 ± 3	25 ± 4*	25 ± 4*
pHa	7.41 ± 0.02	7.36 ± 0.02*	7.36 ± 0.02*
Pa_{O_2} (mm Hg)	80 ± 10	70 ± 13*	73 ± 9*
Pa_{CO_2} (mm Hg)	39 ± 4	43 ± 6*	44 ± 5*
$C(a-\bar{v})O_2$ (ml · dl^{-1})	4.5 ± 0.8	4.1 ± 0.4	4.2 ± 0.7
VO_2 (ml · min^{-1} · m^{-2})	133 ± 22	107 ± 8†	108 ± 17*

* $P < 0.05$ versus control.
† $P < 0.01$ versus control.

Abbreviations: MVO_2, myocardial oxygen consumption; VO_2, whole body oxygen consumption.

From Marty, J., et al.: Effects of midazolam on the coronary circulation in patients with coronary artery disease. Anesthesiology, 64:206, 1986.

Respiratory Effect. A modest respiratory depression occurs with midazolam.[207] Apnea may occur on induction, but it is short-lived and is less than that seen after thiopental[195] or after diazepam.[212a] Sedative doses depress hypoxic ventilatory responses.[212a]

Effect on Intraocular and Intracranial Pressure. Midazolam decreases intracranial blood pressure[207] and intraocular pressure.[208] It also decreases cerebral blood flow and cerebral oxygen consumption.

ADMINISTRATION AND DOSAGE

Premedication. Midazolam has been found to be an excellent anxiolytic sedative drug as premedication for regional and other anesthetic procedures. The hypnotic action is especially good, and patients have a high degree of antegrade amnesia—over 90%.[197]

Intramuscular or Intravenous Premedication Injection. As a water-soluble agent, midazolam can be injected intramuscularly and is rapidly absorbed without significant local irritation.[206] The dose for intramuscular or intravenous premedication injection is 0.1 mg/kg of body weight. The sedative and anxiolytic effects are evident within 10 minutes after administration. The maximum effect is usually achieved between 30 and 40 minutes; after intravenous injection, the desired preanesthetic maximum effects are seen within 10 minutes. More than 90% of patients demonstrate good to excellent antegrade amnesia. Recovery from the drug's action is fairly rapid, and patients are in good control within 2 to 3 hours after the administration of the drug. It is recommended that injections be made in the vastus lateralis muscle.

Additional advantages in regional anesthesia are the property of muscle relaxation and the capacity to act as an anticonvulsant.[207]

Induction Dose. This drug is an effective intravenous induction agent. Induction doses should be administered by titration and dose-response to the endpoint noted. In medicated patients, a dose of 0.2 mg/kg (range 0.18 to 0.28 mg) will be adequate for induction to the endpoint of unconsciousness. Fragen[208] determined an average dose to be 0.18 mg/kg as an ED_{50}, but Reves[198] determined the induction dose to be about 0.25 mg/kg (ED_{50}).

A careful study of dose-response for induction of anesthesia reveals that the larger doses are usually required for an effective dose in most patients (ED_{95}) (Fig. 27-10).[198,208] Gross[209] found the values in Table 27-7 in patients premedicated with morphine.

These doses for induction were found to provide hemodynamic stability without tachycardia or hypertensive responses to reflex manipulation. Patients in ASA physical status I and II,[200] as well as physical status III and IV[209,211] were studied. It is also evident that extremely large doses are needed to abolish responses to a painful stimulus and, therefore, this drug is an ineffective analgesic.

A dose of 12.5 to 30 mg appears to be a standard bolus dose for healthy adults weighing between 50 and 80 kg. A 15-mg dose is equivalent to 200 mg of thiopental for induction of sleep to the same endpoint (cessation of counting and loss of eyelid reflex).[195c] Thus, this drug is about 10 to 15 times as potent as thiopental. This is compared with an induction sleep dose of 25 mg for diazepam; hence, midazolam is about twice as potent as diazepam.

The drug is administered over a period of 1 minute. The onset of action is thus rapid because of the

FIG. 27-10. Cumulative midazolam dose (log scale) *vs.* response curves for abolition of reaction to verbal commands, eyelash stimulation, and painful stimulation (trapezius squeeze). Gross, J.B., Caldwell, C.B., and Edwards, M.W.: Induction dose-response curves for midazolam and ketamine in premedicated ASA class III and IV patients: Anesth. Analg., 64:795, 1985.

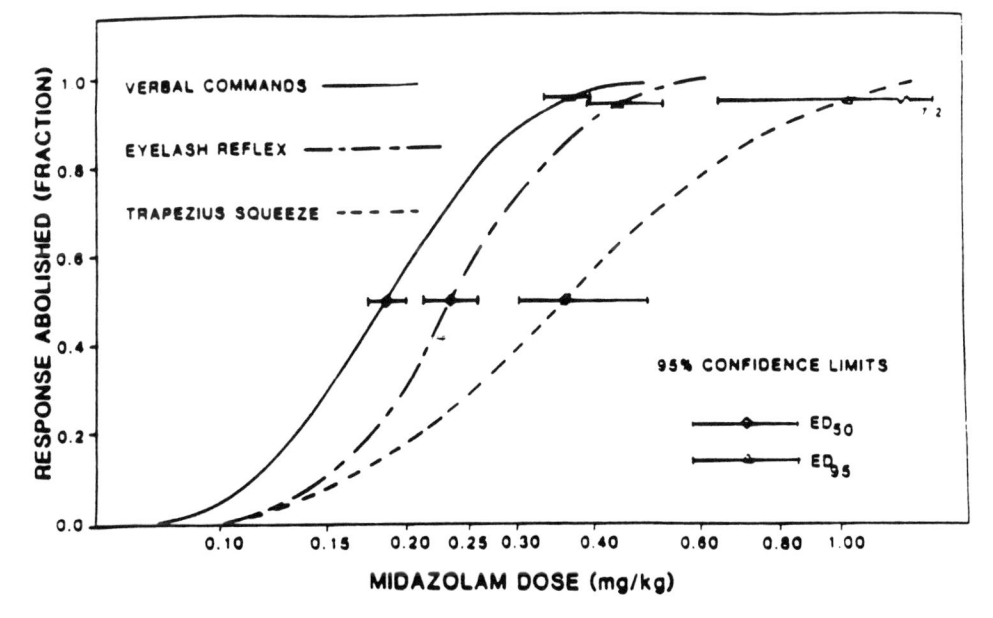

TABLE 27-7. DOSES OF MIDAZOLAM FOR INDUCTION

	ED$_{50}$ Average mg/kg[198,208]	ED$_{95}$ Average mg/kg[209,210]
Loss of verbalization and response to verbal command[208]	0.18	0.3
Loss of eyelash reflex[198]	0.24	0.4
Loss of response to painful stimulation (trapezius squeeze) and pharyngeal stimulation[209]	0.36	1

high lipophilicity at physiologic plasma pH. Induction time and onset of sleep following the bolus injection varies between 60 and 100 seconds.

Compared with a thiopental dose of 3.0 mg/kg (200 mg in a 70-kg man) as a single bolus producing sleep in 30 to 40 seconds in the young and 20 to 30 seconds in the elderly, the induction time of this benzodiazepine is twice as long, requiring about 1 to 1.5 minutes for the onset of sleep. Diazepam's full effect is evidenced at 3 minutes. Emergence may be slightly longer than with thiopental; however, after 3 hours, there is little or no psychomotor impairment.

PHARMACOKINETICS (INTRAVENOUS).[213] Blood levels decrease rapidly (Fig. 27–11). After a single intravenous dose (75 to 100 μg/kg), plasma levels decline in a biexponential manner (Fig. 27–12). A two-compartment model appropriately satisfies the changes in concentration. Table 27–8 presents basic kinetic parameters after immediate plasma dilution.[214,215]

Although most benzodiazepines have a long duration of action because of slow elimination and biologically active metabolites, midazolam is an exception.[216,217] It is rapidly eliminated, as seen by the high clearance rate and relatively shorter beta-phase. Most of the drug is metabolized in the liver by hydroxylation, followed by conjugation with glucuronic acid. Less than 0.5% is excreted unchanged in the urine. Both bound and unbound drug are rapidly degraded by liver enzymes, and the high clearance represents about one third of the total hepatic blood flow. There is extensive first-pass effect after oral administration, which leads to a bioavailability of only 44%.

In Dundee's[195] studies (Table 27–9), blood levels show a progressive decline with time and by 8 hours are not detectable.

Because benzodiazepines and steroids are substrates for the same enzymes, it becomes important in drugs with an overall short duration of action to recognize a circadian influence on elimination. Thus, clearance is slower in the morning when cortisone levels are high; but clearance is more rapid for doses administered in the afternoon or evening.[217]

In the elderly patient, midazolam is a safe and satisfactory intravenous induction agent. The dose should be reduced, and the mean UD$_{95}$ is 0.15 mg/kg in premedicated subjects.[210] In the absence of premedication, a large dose of 0.2 mg/kg may be needed. In any event, titration of incremental doses to central nervous system endpoints is necessary. The onset and duration of action are more predictable than in the younger patient, and apnea is not usually seen. The volume of distribution is greater in the elderly, and there is a longer terminal half-life, but this is much shorter than with diazepam. No observable difference is noted between elderly patients and young women, but there is some difference between the elderly and the young men. Thus, some sex difference exists.[218,219]

Clearance is also sensitive to hepatic blood flow.

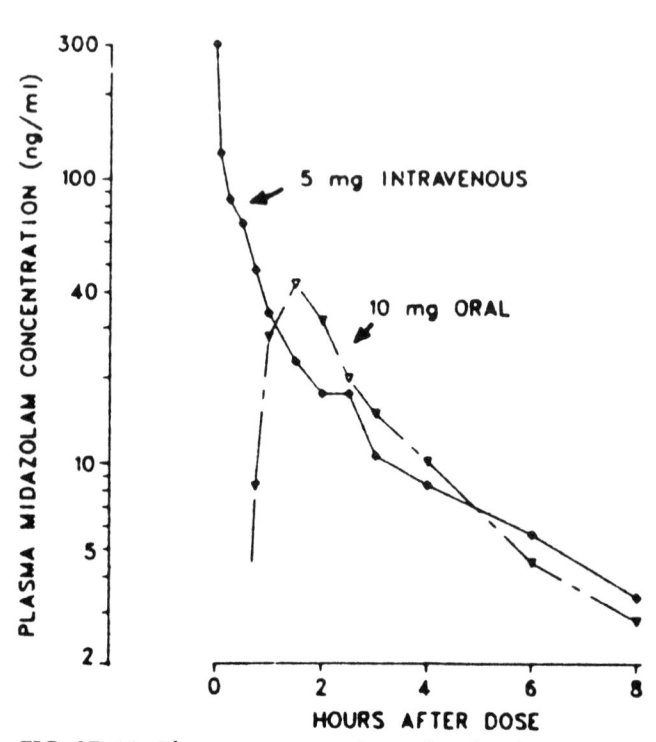

FIG. 27–11. Plasma concentrations of midazolam in a healthy volunteer who received a 5-mg intravenous dose on one occasion and a 10-mg oral dose on another occasion. From Greenblatt, D.J.: Sleep, 5 (Suppl 1): 1982.

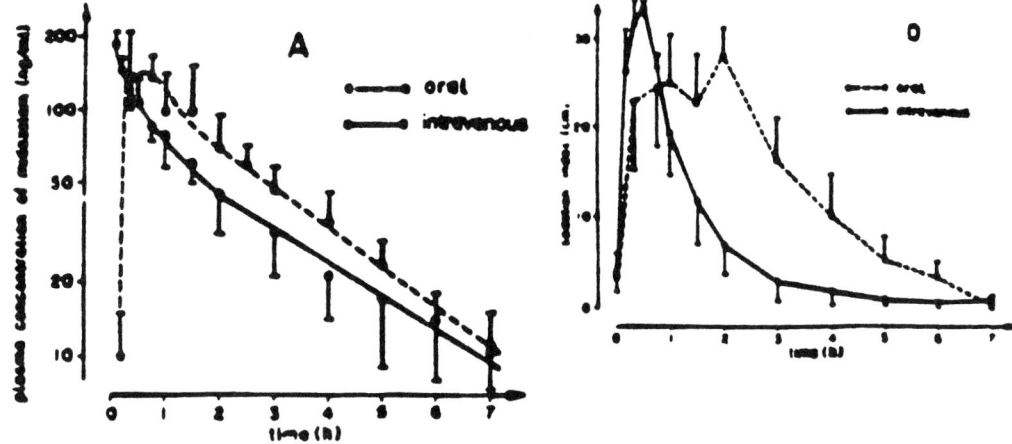

FIG. 27-12. Time courses of plasma levels of midazolam *(A)* and its pharmacologic effects *(B)*. Allonen, H., Ziegler, G., and Klotz, U.: Midazolam kinetics. Clin. Pharmacol. Ther. 30:653, 1981.

Because the hepatic blood flow is greater in the supine position, the clearance is greater in this position. In the evening, the clearance is 500 ml/min, but in the morning it is about 250 ml/min.[217] Clearance is increased in uremia due to increased free fraction and reduced in cirrhosis.

Obesity. In obese subjects, those with greater than 120% of ideal body weight show a significant increase in volume of distribution. This increase is significant even when there is a correction of total body weight, indicating a disproportionate distribution into adipose tissues.[219] Hepatic clearance is not significantly different between obese subjects and those of normal weight.

Critical Illness.[220] In the critically ill patient, such as those with septic shock, multiple trauma, postcardiac arrest, and those with postoperative respiratory failure and/or extensive re-explorations for surgical purposes, the pharmacokinetics of midazolam and its metabolite, α-hydroxymidazolam, are altered. The elimination half-life is significantly increased and generally there is a reduction in plasma clearance. The reduced clearance is largely related to patients in septic shock. This reduced clearance is related to the reduced capacity to form the 1-hydroxymetabolite, which is an active metabolite. As conditions improve and these patients become stable, plasma concentrations of the metabolite increase and overall midazolam clearance returns toward normal. The impaired ability of the critically ill patients in septic shock to metabolize midazolam is probably related to reduced organ perfusion.

Protein Binding.[221,222] Midazolam is highly protein-bound. About 94% is bound mostly to albumin. A direct relationship exists between plasma albumin and onset time. In the elderly, there is a trend toward decreased plasma protein (in the absence of dehydration). Thus, there is usually a higher (free) unbound fraction and onset time may be shortened. The elimination half-life time is increased.

Metabolism.[223] Midazolam is metabolized completely by the liver. Hydroxylation occurs by hepatic microsomal oxidation. The fused imidazole ring is oxidized rapidly, much faster than the methylene group of the diazepam ring of other benzodiazepines. The principal metabolite is α-hydroxymethylmidazolam. Plasma concentrations accumulate over the first 30 minutes after administration and reach the highest concentration in the first 2 hours.[224] It has a beta half-life of 1 hour and has insignificant clinical activity. Other inactive metabolites are 4-hydroxymidazolam and α-4-dihydroxymidazolam.

Excretion. Less than 1% of midazolam is excreted unchanged by the kidney.[224a] The metabolites are conjugated with glucuronic acid and all are excreted as glucuronides. The principal excretory product is the α-hydroxymethylmidazolam glucuronide. Some hepatic elimination occurs but is minimal and flow dependent.

PHARMACODYNAMICS. Rising plasma concentrations correlate with clinical effects. Assessment of effects is carried out progressively as a steady state is achieved; sedation is apparent in 2 to 3 minutes, with a "threshold" plasma concentration of 40 to

TABLE 27-8. PHARMACOKINETICS OF MIDAZOLAM

Variable	Measure
$t_{1/2}$ alpha	12 minutes
$t_{1/2}$ beta	2.4 hours
Plasma binding	94%
Blood/plasma ratio	0.6%
Clearance (ml/min)	
Plasma	283
Free drug	5000
Whole blood	500
Vd_{ss} (L/kg)	0.70

762 General Anesthesia

TABLE 27–9. MIDAZOLAM PLASMA LEVELS (ng/ml)

	5 mg Dose	10 mg Dose
10 minutes	100–250	200–250
30 minutes	75–150	150–175
60 minutes	50–125	100–150
90 minutes	25–100	75–150
3 hours	10–75	20–75
6 hours	0–10	0–15

From Dundee, J.W., Samuel, I.O., and Toner, W.: Midazolam: A water-soluble benzodiazepine. Anaesthesia, 35:454, 1980.

50 ng/ml. At a plasma concentration of 80 ng/ml, hypnotic effects are noted, followed by sleep at 100 ng/ml.[215]

Signs of sedation can be tested by the subject's perception of time and ability to carry out simple intellectual tasks. Amnesia is of a high order with midazolam.

USE. This drug is recommended as a sleep induction agent. It is also recommended as a supplemental agent to nitrous oxide anesthesia for short operative procedures. The onset of unconsciousness and sleep is slightly longer than thiopental. It is an excellent induction agent for outpatient surgery.

Advantages over diazepam include:

- Minimal discomfort or pain at injection site[176]
- Absence of venous thrombosis
- More rapid onset of action
- Predictable dose
- Shorter duration of action
- Shorter time of distribution and of elimination
- More rapid body clearance

Pediatric Preanesthetic Medication. Intramuscular midazolam is an excellent sedative–tranquilizer agent for pediatric preanesthetic medication (Fig. 27–13). It has been found effective at all age levels, especially young children in the 1 to 5-year age group, who are usually more apprehensive and less cooperative.[224] With midazolam premedication, there is an increasing level of sedation as the age of patients increases, and in this regard children can be divided into three age groups: (1) 1–5 years; (2) 6–10 years; and (3) 10–15 years. All patients are more drowsy than with other sedative agents.[208] It is noted, however, that midazolam is a sedative tranquilizer, not a narcotic, and does not provide pain obtundation.

The recommended intramuscular dose has been determined to be between 50 and 100 µg/kg of body weight in children. The average is approximately 80 µg/kg. This average dose has been associated with the following advantages: a smoother inhalation induction of anesthesia, a lower concentration of halothane and other volatile agents, and a shorter length of stay in the recovery room than in control subjects. Compared with morphine, in Rita's study[225] there was a lower incidence of postoperative nausea and vomiting.

Continuous Sedative—Postoperative. Continuous sedation of children in the postoperative period may be a desirable objective.[226] This is important when children are in an intensive care unit after cardiac surgery or when they require artificial ventilation. Recommended dosing is as follows: after an initial bolus dose of 200 µg/kg, midazolam is administered in an infusion at a rate of 2 µg/kg/min. If the patient continues to be restless, the infusion can be increased in steps of $1 \mu g \cdot kg^{-1} \cdot min^{-1}$.

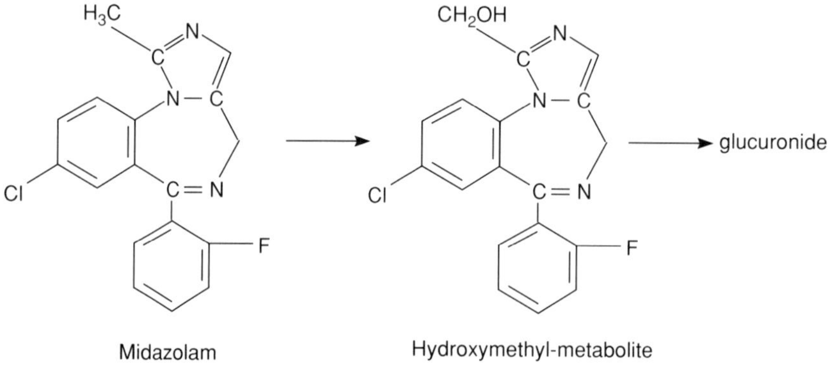

FIG. 27–13. Chemical structure of midazolam and its metabolites. From Gerecke, M. Chemical structure and properties of midazolam. Br. J. Clin. Pharmacol., 16:11S, 1983.

Because midazolam is primarily a sedative–tranquilizer, and in the early postsurgical period analgesia is needed, it too can be provided with an infusion of morphine.[227]

In infants, a satisfactory dosage and rate of morphine infusion is 0.15 μg · kg^{-1} · min^{-1}. In older children over 2 years of age, an infusion dose rate is 0.3 μg · kg^{-1} · min^{-1}.

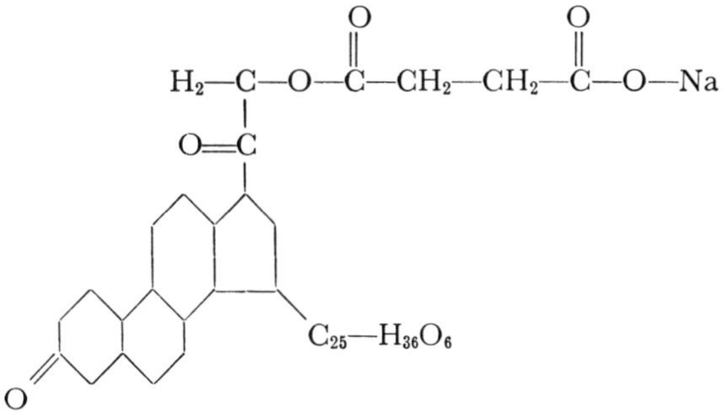

STEROID INTRAVENOUS ANESTHESIA AGENTS

HYDROXYDIONE

In the course of laboratory investigations, endocrinologists have noted the occurrence of drowsiness and even sleep following the administration of steroid compounds. Progesterone possessed this activity to a significant degree. Selye[228–234] reported on this observation in 1941 and noted that the intraperitoneal injection of progesterone in rodents produced sleep. Other steroid compounds were studied, and desoxycorticosterone acetate was also found to have a high degree of activity.[235] In 1950, Hoeffer[236] reported that patients receiving adrenocorticotropic hormone for 3 to 5 days developed EEG changes suggestive of cortical suppression.

Clinical application of these fundamental observations awaited the work of Laubach[237] in 1955. He tested a number of water-soluble steroids and reported that hydroxydione (Viadril) had greatest anesthetic activity with low toxicity and minimal hormonal activity. Gordon[238] first used the agent in humans and, subsequently, Murphy[239] reported clinical observations.

It was noted that resistance would develop to the anesthetic action of the steroids and that it was a pharmacologic adaptation. In addition, the narcotic effect was found to be most pronounced in animals whose nervous system was least developed. On this basis a fish bioassay method of testing anesthetic potency of steroids was developed.

CHEMISTRY. Hydroxydione is the prototype of steroid compounds which possess anesthetic properties. The phenanthrene ring is the basic nucleus and appears in morphine and other important drugs (digitalis). It is synthesized by esterifying 21-hydroxypregnanedione with one of the carboxyl groups of succinic acid. This is then converted to the acid salt by reacting with sodium bicarbonate. The resulting compound is the sodium salt of 21-hydroxy pregnane-3, 20-dione hemisuccinate (empirical formula C_{25}—$H_{36}O_6$) (Fig. 27–14).

Hydroxydione is a white crystalline solid that is nonvolatile (no deliquescence) but soluble in water. The aqueous solution has a pH of 7.8 to 10.2 and is mixed with sodium carbonate and sodium chloride.

FIG. 27–14. Steroid anesthetic—Hydroxydione.

MECHANISM. The exact mechanism of action of the steroid drugs is not known. Explanation of the anesthetic effect and the production of unconsciousness is speculative. Sleep and the anesthetic state are produced and are accomplished through an action on cerebral function. The cerebral metabolic changes are similar to those produced by barbiturates. Cerebral blood flow is reduced,[240] as is the oxygen uptake and the glucose uptake (Kety-Schmidt technique). The decreased metabolism induced by steroids is a physiologic-type inhibition in which there is a steroid "brake" applied to glucose and oxygen uptake. The inhibition of cerebral metabolism is an effect on enzyme systems, and it appears that this is at a different level in the enzyme chain than occurs with barbiturates.

Hydroxydione is distinct from the usual endocrine steroids in that it is inactive for all hormonal actions as tested in animals.[241]

FAT AND EXCRETION. No fat storage of hydroxydione occurs, and there is no tissue reservoir as with the barbiturates that can feed the plasma. Inactivation occurs in the liver by enzymatic reduction. There are conjugated forms of pregnane that are excreted in the urine. Neither liver damage nor nephrectomy affects the duration of activity.[242]

PREMEDICATION. The usual preanesthetic drugs are employed in standard fashion 1 hour prior to induction with hydroxydione. A narcotic is desirable. Meperidine is useful, but morphine seems to offer better results and less tachypnea. Atropine or scopolamine must be given to prevent secretions and obtund reflex vagal excitability.

PREPARATIONS AND DOSAGE.[243] The steroid is freshly prepared either as a concentrated solution of 1% (although Murphy has employed a 2.5% solution)[239] in sterile water, isotonic saline or 5% dextrose *or* as a more dilute 0.1 to 0.4% solution. The 0.4% solution is recommended and is made by dissolving 1 g in 250 ml of 5% dextrose in water. The total recommended dose varies with age, weight, and physical status of the patient and ranges from 500 to 2000 mg. Children may be given 500 mg and young healthy adults 1500 mg. The dose should be reduced for the geriatric patient.

ADMINISTRATION.[243] Administration by continuous intravenous drip is recommended. The initial dose for induction is attained by a relatively rapid rate of infusion and until 250 or 300 mg is given. This should take about 5 minutes (ranges from 2 to 9 minutes). Drowsiness usually appears in 15 minutes, then the rate of infusion is slowed. When a simple rapid injection of the 1% solution is made, 25 ml or 250 mg in 1 minute, the onset of effects is noted in 5 minutes.

Selection of Vein. Venous irritation precludes the use of small veins and veins of the lower extremity. Generally, a forearm or antecubital vein is employed. Extravasation should be avoided, and the small veins on the dorsum of the hand are more frequently the site of irritation.

Supplementation. Hydroxydione is actually a basal anesthetic and requires supplementation with another agent. Nitrous oxide–oxygen in a 70–30 mixture provides the best anesthetic state. Relaxants of both classes can be safely and efficiently used.

Management. Generally, an artificial airway is not required, but the need should always be anticipated. If a narcotic has been used as part of the premedication, the pharyngeal airway can be easily inserted while intubation is accomplished with minimal bucking.

PHARMACOLOGIC PROPERTIES

Central Nervous System.[244] On the intravenous administration of hydroxydione, a progressive depression of the cortex and central nervous system ensues, drowsiness and unconsciousness develop slowly and smoothly without excitement, and progress into the anesthetic state is generally pleasant. Production of this state resembles the onset of ordinary natural sleep.

EEG changes are similar to those produced by the thiobarbiturates and are simply variations of barbiturate changes.[245] All four of the standard EEG patterns can be obtained by increasing the dose. These changes begin to appear within 3 to 4 minutes after the beginning of administration. When EEG level IV is reached, the patient may respond to painful stimuli, such as application of a towel clip. Cortical activity is thus suppressed before surgical anesthesia or analgesia is attained.

Both barbiturates and steroids produce somewhat similar EEG patterns. Both are followed by:[246]

1. Comparable sleep patterns.
2. Progressive disappearance and abolition of standard waking reaction aroused by painful stimulation.
3. Progressive disappearance of the rapid cortical postdischarge evoked by sensory stimulation.
4. Absence of change in the surface positive phase (afferent response) of the primary electrographic complex.
5. Progressive depression of surface negative phase.

Eyeball roving is not usually seen. Eyelid reflex disappears within 6 to 10 minutes from start of injection. The pupillary response to light disappears in deeper levels.[240]

A remarkable feature noted by most clinicians is the early obtundation of the pharyngeal and laryngeal reflexes.[247,248] Insertion of an airway is thus permitted within 10 minutes of induction. Stimulation of the vocal cords evokes a momentary closure but no laryngospasm. Intubation is easily accomplished, and subsequent movement of the endotracheal tube is well tolerated without bucking or bronchospasm and only a few seconds of breath-holding.

RELAXATION. Muscular relaxation is variable. The jaw muscles usually relax, which facilitates opening the mouth and oral instrumentation, including laryngoscopy. Extremity and neck muscles also show adequate relaxation, but the abdominal muscles rarely relax sufficiently to permit abdominal surgery. Relaxant drugs need to be used.

EFFECTS ON RESPIRATION.[249] An overall increase in respiratory rate of approximately 100% is noted in all stages of narcosis. Concomitantly, there is a reduction in tidal volume of about 60%. The resultant minute volume thus shows an increase of 10% to 20%.

Respiratory depression and apnea are not easily produced. Occasionally, when apnea occurs, it is of short duration, i.e., less than 1 minute. Of significance is the ease with which spontaneous respiration can be taken away from the patient and controlled respiration instituted. Resumption of spontaneous respiration often occurs in 30 seconds.

CARDIOVASCULAR EFFECTS.[249] A decrease in stroke cardiac output occurs, amounting to about 25%, whereas cardiac rate increases approximately by one third so that the minute cardiac output and the cardiac index do not change significantly.

By intraarterial measurements, a progressive fall in both systolic and diastolic blood pressures can be demonstrated. The systolic pressure decreases about 25% and the diastolic decreases about 15%. The reduction in pulse pressure is progressive so that in deep narcosis or EEG level 4, it amounts to 35%. The average maximum drop in mean arterial pressure is about 17%.

In clinical practice, hypotension of concern is not seen; the declines in blood pressure are, in part, the typical feature of sleep and, in part, the effect of the agent on the cardiovascular mechanism.

EFFECTS ON RENAL FUNCTION. A mild suppression of renal function and urine output occurs. This is consistent with the stereotyped response that occurs with ether anesthetic agents. Within an hour after discontinuance of the anesthetic, recovery is seen.

Traces of albumin appear in some postoperative urine specimens. Urinary glucuronates are increased and this is probably the result of excretion of conjugated hydroxydione.

RECOVERY. Rapid and smooth recovery is a remarkable feature of hydroxydione administration. Waking time varies from a few minutes to about 20 minutes. It appears to be proportional to the duration of anesthesia and the total dose administered. After only an induction dose, patients will awaken in a few minutes. Maintenance of unconsciousness must be achieved by continuous administration. Eyelid reflex reappears in 5 minutes, response to name in 10 to 15 minutes, and full consciousness in 30 minutes.

COMPLICATIONS AND DISADVANTAGES

1. Inadequate anesthesia.
2. Hypotension—usually mild and self limited. Low pressures are spontaneously rectified. Hence, the hypotension is not significant and is self limited. In circumstances of concern, a dilute solution of a vasopressor may be administered. A dose titrated against a response of phenylephrine or metaraminol are effective.
3. Long onset.

INDICATIONS

1. As a hypnotic—it can be used in minor procedures such as cardiac catheterization and endoscopic and roentgenographic procedures.
2. Ophthalmologic surgery.
3. Minor orthopedic procedures.

ALTHESIN (CT 1341)

Two steroids have been formulated into an injectable preparation known as *CT 1341* (Althesin [Glaxo Inc.]), which has advantages over hydroxydione. This preparation produces rapid induction, stable anesthesia of short duration, and rapid recovery. It has a high therapeutic index and is free from vascular irritation effects. When used as an adjuvant principally for induction, it is compatible with relaxant drugs.[250]

CHEMISTRY. Two pregnanediones are solubilized in cremophor EL (polyoxyethylated castor oil), which is then diluted in water. The 21-acetoxy compound enhances the solubility of the 3-hydroxy compound (Fig. 27–15).

The commercial preparation contains 12 mg total steroid per milliliter, and the preparation is formulated as shown in Table 27–10.

DOSAGE. The activity of a mixture is the result of simple addition of the respective activities of the individual diones. Steroid 1 is the most active, whereas the 21-acetoxy compound is one half as active.

Dosage is conveniently expressed in microliters of solution per kilograms body weight. The induction dose ranges from 40 to 125 μl/kg, with an optimum dose of 60 μl/kg.[250] Doses up to 125 μl/kg have been used by Campbell.[251] Maintenance is achieved with nitrous oxide–oxygen or other inhalational agents. Supplementation of the steroid is accomplished by additional single doses of 100 μl, regardless of body weight.

PHARMACOLOGIC EFFECTS. Mild respiratory stimulation (increased rate) occurs with optimum doses. This is accompanied by a significant fall in Pa_{CO_2} during air breathing.

Mild sinus tachycardia is seen soon after the administration of an induction dose. Total peripheral vascular resistance decreases approximately 20% (unlike pentothal) and hypotension results with a 20% fall in systolic pressure. This is similar to other sleep-induction agents. Cardiac output is unchanged (unlike pentothal).

No effect has been noted at the neuromuscular junction, and there is no interaction with muscle relaxants.

Rate of recovery is faster than with barbiturates, and there is some euphoria on recovery.[251] The mean recovery time is 25 minutes.

Side effects are not serious. Neither nausea nor vomiting has been observed. This preparation does not irritate veins or result in phlebitis. Adverse interactions with succinylcholine, pancuronium, or *d*-tubocurarine have not been observed.

With larger than optimum doses the following may occur:

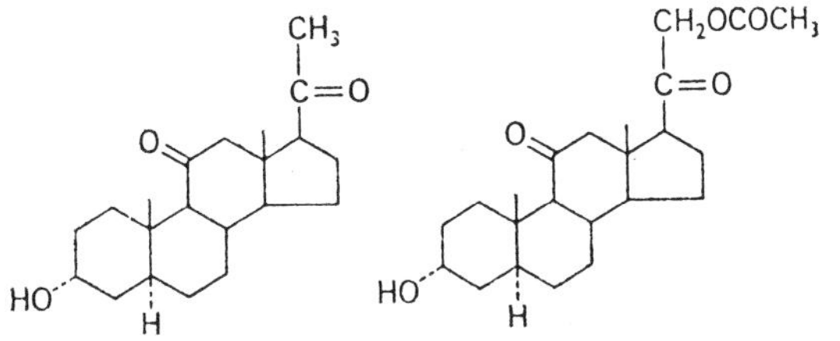

FIG. 27–15. Chemical structure of the two steroids in Althesin.

Steroid I — 3α-hydroxy-5α-pregnane-11,20-dione

Steroid II — 21-acetoxy-3α-hydroxy-5α-pregnane-11,20-dione

TABLE 27-10. FORMULATION OF ALTHESIN

Component	Amount (% weight/volume)
Steroid 1	
3a-hydroxy-5a-pregnane-11,20-dione	0.9
Steroid 2	
21-acetoxy-3a-hydroxy-5a-pregnane-11,20-dione	0.3
Cremophor EL	20.0
Sodium chloride	0.25
Water for injection	to 100

1. Involuntary abnormal muscle movements that are not eliminated by larger doses
2. Severe respiratory depression
3. Intense hypotension

Comment. The steroid drugs represent a unique step in the search for better anesthetic agents. They also represent an unusual mechanism in the production of the anesthetic state. Since their clinical utility has been poor, their use has been discontinued and are of historical interest only. Both have been withdrawn from the market.

NEWER INTRAVENOUS ANESTHETIC AGENTS

INTRAVENOUS ETOMIDATE

Etomidate, an ultrashort-acting hypnotic agent, is used for induction of anesthesia.[252] It has been offered as an alternative to barbiturate induction drugs.[253,254]

CHEMISTRY. Etomidate is an imidazole derivative. Specifically, it is ethylmethylbenzylimidazole-5-carboxylate (Fig. 27-16) that was synthesized in 1972.[252] The salt is a water-soluble compound with a pH of 3.3 and dissolves in cremophor EL propylene glycol and ethanol. The aqueous solution must be freshly prepared. The commercially available agent is in propylene glycol solvent containing 2 mg/ml (0.2% solution). Only the dextroisomer is active as a hypnotic.

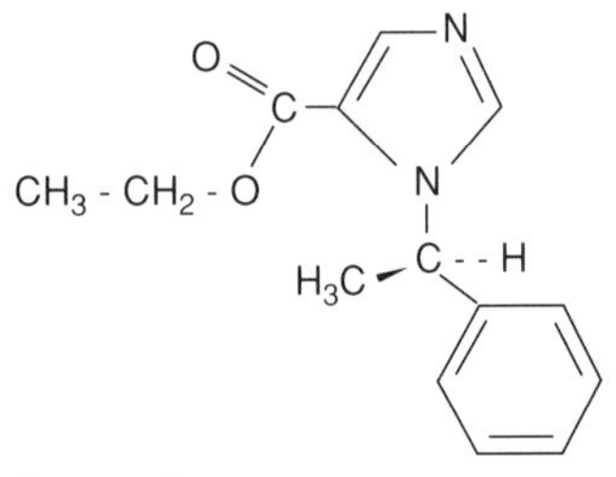

DOSAGE.[254] The usual dose for induction and production of unconsciousness intravenously is approximately 0.3 mg/kg of body weight for a bolus injection.[255] This should be administered over a period of 1 minute. The dose for maintenance of effect is 25 µg/kg/min. The UD_{95} is thus considered to be 0.3 mg/kg. On a w/w basis etomidate is approximately 12 times more potent than thiopental and 5 times more potent than methohexital.

PHARMACOKINETICS. After the administration of an anesthetic dose there is a rapid decline in plasma concentration of unchanged etomidate.[257] This occurs in a biphasic manner and is followed by a slow elimination phase. These changes are consistent with a three-compartment model of distribution.[258] The first phase of distribution in the central compartment has a half-life of about 2.6 minutes, followed by the tissue distribution phase with a half-life of 29 minutes. The third, or beta, phase is prolonged and has a half-life of 4.6 hours.[258] A slow redistribution from the deep tissue compartment accounts for this prolongation.

Protein Binding. At a blood pH of 7.4 etomidate readily binds to human plasma proteins. About 76% is bound to human albumin.[259] Since the unbound fraction exerts a pharmacologic effect any change in albumin concentration will alter potency.

Plasma Clearance. An extensive volume of distribution of 4.5 L/kg accounts for the rapid decline and low plasma levels of etomidate. The plasma clearance rate is of the order of 11.7 ml $\cdot$ kg^{-1} $\cdot$ min^{-1}.[260] Other studies report a greater clearance rate but a marked reduction in the presence of fentanyl.[261]

Metabolism. A rapid destruction of the drug occurs in the liver, by enzymatic hydrolysis at the ester side chain, and terminates the sleep effect of the agent. The hepatic clearance is approximately 15% per hour of the total dose administered.[257] The main metabolite is the carboxylic acid of etomidate, which is pharmacologically inactive.[262] Metabolites accumulate in the plasma over the first 30 minutes after administration and then decrease over the next 3 hours to levels one-half the peak concentration.[260]

Excretion.[257] About 2% of an administered dose is excreted unchanged in the urine. About three-fourths of an administered dose is excreted as the carboxylic acid metabolite in the first 24 hours. About 10% is recovered in the bile, and 13% is found in the feces.[257] There is a definite lack of analgesic action.[263]

In patients with focal epilepsy, enhancement of

FIG. 27-16. Chemical structure of (R)-(+)-etomidate.

both fast activity and epileptogenic discharges has been described. A study of epileptic patients by means of an EEG placed subdurally revealed an increase in epileptiform activity. Such activity is marked in at least one half of the patients.[264]

PHARMACODYNAMICS. The onset of action is rapid, and sleep is produced within a circulation time from the injection site to the brain.[255] The duration of action from a bolus of 0.3 mg/kg of body weight is approximately 3 to 5 minutes.[252] Larger doses may produce longer sleep, and it may be unexpectedly prolonged. Healthy patients quickly awaken. The plasma levels required for hypnosis exceed 0.25 µg/ml in man.[256]

PHARMACOLOGY

Central Nervous System. Sleep is produced by direct cortical action. There appears to be no significant subcortical effect, and dissociative effects or disagreeable dreams are not observed postanesthetically.[252] Patients appear to be fully conscious and alert on recovery.

Cardiopulmonary Effects. These are minimal in healthy patients. Cardic output, systemic blood pressure, and myocardial oxygen consumption remain undisturbed. Some tachycardia is seen after larger doses. Apnea may be produced unexpectedly. Laryngospasm may occur on occasion. In elderly, debilitated, or hypovolemic patients, marked hypotension is likely to occur. This is probably related to the adrenocortical suppression that occurs.

Although some experimental evidence indicates a negative inotropism,[265] the doses needed to produce such an effect are much greater than those used clinically, at least in normal hearts.[265a]

Minimal rate changes occur with ordinary sleep doses. Experiments provide evidence of an increase in central vagal tone; at the least, there is no vagolytic action.[266] Thus, when other drugs with vagomimetic action are also administered, such as succinylcholine, significant bradycardia may ensue.[267]

Effect on Cerebral Metabolism.[268] Continuous infusion of etomidate at a rate of 30 µg/kg/min reduces cerebral metabolic rate about 9%. At an infusion rate of 60 µg/kg/min, a reduction of 30% in cerebral metabolic rate has been observed. The larger dose provides maximal suppression of brain oxygen demands, but at the expense of prolonged postoperative recovery. For neurosurgical purposes, hemodynamic stability is attained with reduced intracerebral blood volume and maintained CO_2 reactivity.

Etomidate has been used both as an induction and maintenance drug, and the effect on cerebral function was observed. Cerebral blood flow is decreased by about 50%. It is of interest that when an infusion of etomidate is preceded by a single bolus loading dose, a greater infusion rate is needed for maximal cerebral metabolic rate suppression. This may represent the phenomenon of acute tolerance, as seen with thiopental.[269]

In intracranial neurosurgery, etomidate may offer several advantages, provided that high dose steroids are given in the immediate postoperative period.[270]

Endocrine Effects. Endocrine effects following infusion of etomidate (induction 0.3 mg/kg; infusion 10 µg/kg/min for 1.5 hours) have been studied (Table 27–11).[271,272] Secretion of cortisol and aldosterone was suppressed for 8 to 22 hours. During the infusion, a study of two precursors showed the following: secretion of 11-deoxycortisol was not inhibited, but after discontinuing etomidate, rose significantly; and 17-alpha-hydroxyprogesterone was suppressed, was elevated for the following 12 hours, but then returned to normal. No effects on levels of plasma estradiol or prolactin were noted. Growth hormone increased during anesthesia, as did adrenocorticotropic hormone (ACTH).[273] At the end of surgery, ACTH levels increased five- to tenfold (from 50 ng/L to 500 ng/L). These studies indicate that etomidate principally influences adrenocortical function. Plasma glucose rose significantly consonant with a stress response but had no clinical sequelae. No evidence of pituitary adverse effects has been demonstrated.

The use for prolonged sedation has been associated with low levels of plasma cortisol and increased mortality.[274] Studies of patients receiving etomidate for induction of anesthesia show marked suppression of adrenocortical function evident for several hours.[275] Usually, the ACTH values are elevated. Despite this, cortisol and aldosterone levels are depressed. Exogenous ACTH produces minimal response. *In vitro* studies reveal a concentration-dependent blockade of the two mitochondrial cytochrome P-450-dependent enzymes and 11-beta-hydroxylase. It is concluded that selected patients who receive etomidate should be treated with corticosteroids. The mortality of patients with multiple trauma requiring mechanical ventilation is increased when etomidate is administered.[276]

Single-bolus doses of 0.3 mg/kg, in contrast to continuous infusions, are able to inhibit 11-beta-hydroxylase[276] and 17-alpha-hydroxylase, which are important in intramitochondrial hydroxylation reactions. This accounts for the accumulation of 11-deoxycorticosterone for as long as 24 hours. The inhibition is partial, because there is only a modest reduction in the plasma concentrations of cortisol or corticosterone, and no discernible increase in ACTH concentrations occurs.[275]

In the opinion of the Committee on Safety of Medicines (Britain, 1983) and the absence of reports of serious adverse effects related to steroidogenesis, the drug has been retained for single-bolus doses in

TABLE 27–11. ENDOCRINOLOGIC EFFECTS OF ETOMIDATE[282]

- A significant increase in epinephrine at end of operative period compared to midazolam
- After surgery, mean cortisol levels decrease from 12.5 to about 6.0 µg/dl; by 6 hours postoperatively, still decreased at about 8 µg/dl
- ACTH endogenous levels increase from 7 to 14 pmol/L and continue to increase to 24 pmol/L at 6 hours postoperatively. Despite these high levels, there is no increase in cortisol levels. At 20 hours postoperatively, the levels of ACTH return to about 14 pmol/L. The high ACTH levels appear to be the result of negative feedback interruption from inhibition of cortisol synthesis by etomidate and resultant low plasma levels; at 20 hours, the ACTH levels are still elevated at 12.5 pmol/L
- Growth hormone is suppressed
- Response to exogenous ACTH unimpaired
- Cortisol secretion is suppressed after etomidate infusion for 8–20 hours
- Spontaneous aldosterone levels are suppressed from about 35 ± 6.7 to 7 pg/ml after surgery, and aldosterone remains suppressed for 20 hours
- β-endorphin increases from a mean of 6 pmol preoperatively to 12 pmol at the end of surgery; a further increase occurs at 6 hours to 20 pmol; at 20 hours, the levels return to baseline.

Modified from Crozier, T.A., et al.: Endocrinological changes following etomidate, midazolam, or methohexital. Anesthesiology, 66:628, 1987.

patients with asthma, drug allergies, and peripheral circulatory failure.[277]

MISCELLANEOUS ACTIONS. Administration to malignant hyperthermia–susceptible pigs does not trigger malignant hyperthermia. It does, however, predispose to a more rapid onset of malignant hyperthermia syndrome triggered by halothane–succinylcholine.[278] The drug should not be considered a safe agent in malignant hypertension–susceptible patients.

A possible use is an alternative to other induction agents to which a patient is sensitive. No significant advantages are otherwise evident over available orthodox induction agents.

It may be a useful drug to enhance epileptogenic activity deliberately in patients with focal epilepsy to identify areas needing cortical resection of epileptogenic tissues.[279]

ADVERSE EFFECTS. Pain on intravenous injection of this drug occurs in approximately 35% (12% to 50%) of patients. Phlebitis, thrombosis, and thrombophlebitis are considered to occur in an unacceptably high incidence.[280,281] Abnormal muscular movements of a myoclonic nature are also seen in about 10% (Fragen 70%)[254] and are disagreeable; these occur in up to 50% of patients. They are partially prevented, however, by opiates or diazepam. Laryngospasm is also seen, as is unexpected apnea.

This drug has been found to inhibit adrenal steroidogenesis.

DISADVANTAGES. Annoying side effects of this agent include the following:

- Pain at the site of injection, attenuated by pretreatment with fentanyl
- Myoclonus, minimized by fentanyl pretreatment
- Nausea and vomiting increased
- Blockade of steroidogenesis
- Laryngospasm and unexpected apnea

PROPOFOL

A series of alkylphenols synthesized by the Pharmaceutical Division of Imperial Chemical Industries was found to have anesthetic properties in animals.[283] The initial solubilization of one of these agents, propofol ICI · 35 868, was in an aqueous cremophor EL castor oil–type mixture and was found to have good anesthetic activity in animals.[284] Using this formulation in 1977, Kay[285] first demonstrated, the anesthetic properties in patients; however, a high incidence of pain on injection, some adverse reactions,[286,287] and the evidence of anaphylactoid reactions related to cremophor EL[288] led to a new formation and the current clinical preparation.[289]

The trade name for propofol in the new formulation is Diprivan. The principal uses are as an induction agent and as a hypnotic drug in balanced anesthesia. It was approved in 1986 for use in England and in the United States in 1988.

CHEMICAL NAME AND STRUCTURE. Propofol is a substituted phenol, designated as 2, 6-diisopropylphenol (Fig. 27–17).[283]

CHEMICAL PROPERTIES. Propofol is a highly lipophilic, highly protein-bound sedative–hypnotic agent of the alkylphenol category. As a substituted phenol, it is insoluble in water and must be reconstituted with an organic solvent to ensure solubility. Fifteen percent cremophor-EL was originally employed for this purpose[284] but after 1982 was no longer used because of its association with anaphylactoid reactions.[286] It is now formulated as a 1%

FIG. 27-17. Chemical structure of propofol (2, 6-diisopropylphenol).

solution in an intralipid emulsion containing 10% soya bean oil, 2.25% glycerol, and 1.2% purified egg phosphatide.[282,289]

DOSAGE.[290] The sleep dose, UD_{50}, is between 1 and 2 mg/kg, whereas the UD_{95} is between 2 to 3 mg/kg in unpremedicated patients; however, the average induction dose, UD_{95}, of 2.5 mg/kg is accompanied by a cardiovascular and respiratory depression.[291] Therefore, for healthy patients under 60 years of age, a dose range of 1.5 to 2 mg/kg is more appropriate and safer. For those over 60 years of age, the dose range should be 1 to 1.5 mg/kg.[290] If unconsciousness does not occur, incremental doses of 20 to 30 mg may be administered to the desired endpoint. Potency is estimated to be less than methohexital, the latter being about 1.5 times more potent than propofol, whereas propofol is about two times more potent than thiopental. As expected, the induction dose is reduced in elderly patients or in those who are premedicated with other central nervous system depressants.

For long procedures, propofol can be used to supplement a nitrous oxide–oxygen inhalation anesthesia.[292,293] The maintenance of a sleep state with propofol requires a two-stage infusion dose schedule after the induction dose.[292] The infusion dose should first be administered at a rate of 150 μg/kg/min (9 mg/kg/h) for 30 minutes; then, administration is slowed to a rate of 100 μg/kg/min for the rest of the operation. To allow a rapid recovery, the infusion should be stopped about 5 minutes before the end of surgery.

PHARMACOKINETICS.[294,295] After a single-bolus dose injection of propofol, the blood concentration declines rapidly because of its extensive distribution and rapid elimination (Figs. 27-18 and 27-19). The distribution half-life (alpha phase) is only 2 to 4 minutes. The elimination half-life (beta phase) is 1 to 3 hours. The drug may accumulate if it is given by repeated bolus injections or if used for anesthesia maintenance as a constant-rate infusion. Propofol is metabolized by the liver.[295] The products of glucuronide conjugation and oxidation are water-soluble glucuronide and sulfate conjugates. Both these products are excreted primarily by the kidneys. Metabolism is rapid, and only about 20% of a bolus dose can be recovered unchanged in 30 minutes. The volume of distribution (Vd_{ss}) is large, approximately 500 L, and clearance of propofol is the highest of any of the currently available intravenous induction agents at 2 L/min, which exceeds the hepatic blood flow and accounts for the rapid elimination half-life (Table 27-12). Plasma protein binding is extensive (98%).

PHARMACODYNAMICS. With an induction dose of 2 to 2.5 mg/kg IV, loss of consciousness occurs in one arm-to-brain circulation time—within 1 minute. The duration of hypnosis ranges from 3 to 10 minutes, and this short time is due to redistribution. Used as a maintenance infusion, a continuous rate

FIG. 27-18. Mean propofol blood concentrations ± SEM as a function of time after cessation of propofol infusions at 3 (·····), 6 (---), or 9 mg · kg^{-1} · hr^{-1} (——). For clarity, SEM of the first 10 min of data are omitted. From Gepts, E., et al.: Disposition of propofol administered as constant rate infusions in humans. Anesth. Analg., 66:1256, 1987.

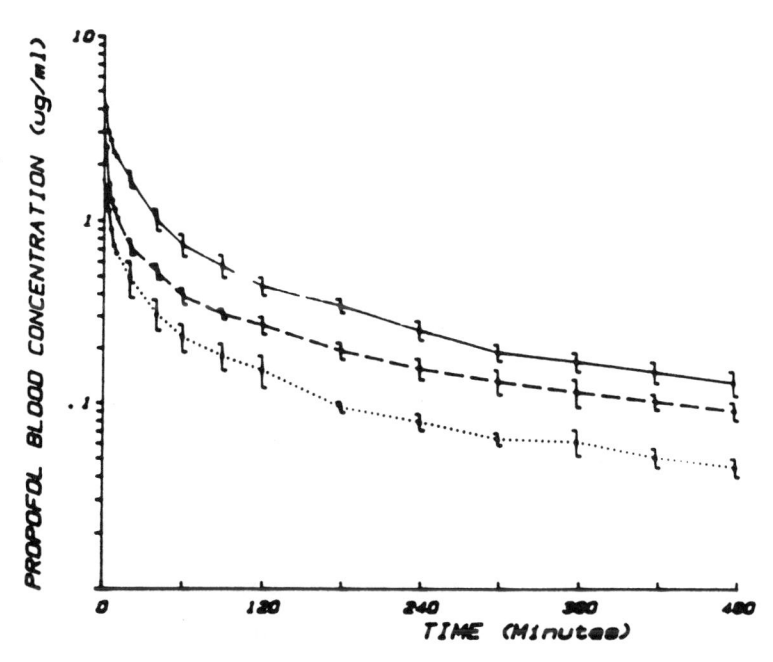

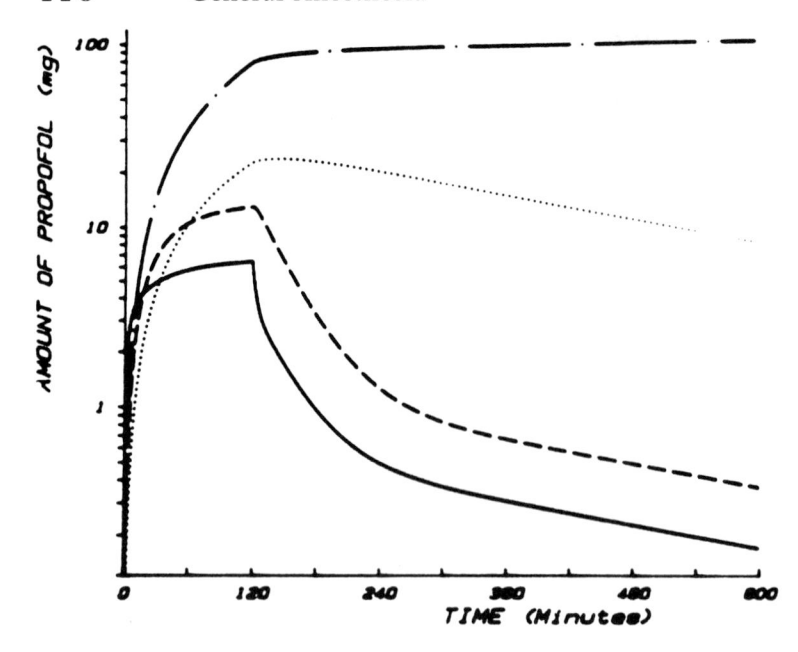

FIG. 27–19. Amount of drug in the central compartment (———), in the second compartment (- - -), in the deep compartment (······) and amount of drug eliminated (-·-·-) during and up to 8 hr after an infusion of propofol for 120 min at a rate of 1 mg/min (computer simulation based on the mean pharmacokinetic parameters of 17 subjects). From Gepts, E., et al.: Disposition of propofol administered as constant rate infusions in humans. Anesth. Analg., 66:1256, 1987.

of 100 to 150 μg/kg/min usually produces a blood concentration of about 3 to 6 μg/ml, which may also be reduced if other general anesthetics are concomitantly administered.[292,295]

The effects of propofol on cerebral hemodynamics are expected to be similar to other intravenous sedative-hypnotics, although such effects have not been clearly delineated with this agent. However, a reduction in intraocular pressure has been demonstrated.[294a]

PHARMACOLOGY

Central Nervous System Effects.[294] Propofol produces a dose-dependent depression of central nervous system function. At low doses, it produces primarily sedation, followed by hypnosis as the dose is increased.

Cardiovascular Effects.[296] Propofol directly depresses the cardiovascular system to at least the same degree as thiopental and probably worse than an equivalent dose of thiopental.[297,297a] There is a 15 to 25% reduction in systolic, diastolic, and mean blood pressures, depending on dose and speed of injection in healthy patients. These blood pressure effects may decrease more than 40% in sick or elderly patients. A dose-related myocardial depression and venodilatation account for these changes.[298]

Heart rate usually remains stable, despite the decrease in arterial pressure,[291] but more frequently slows. The larger doses have a vagotonic effect.[299] This is apparently because this agent does not im-

TABLE 27–12. PROPOFOL PHARMACOKINETIC PARAMETERS DERIVED FROM COMPARTMENTAL (c) AND FROM NONCOMPARTMENTAL (nc) DATA ANALYSIS

Parameters	Propofol rate (mg · kg⁻¹ · hr⁻¹)			
	3 (n = 6)	6 (n = 6)	9 (n = 6)	Mean (n = 18)
$t\frac{1}{2}_\pi$ (c) (min)	3.1 ± 1.1*	3.2 ± 1.1	2.3 ± 1.3	2.8 ± 1.2†
$t\frac{1}{2}_\alpha$ (c) (min)	32.1 ± 15.2	37.5 ± 14.3	24.6 ± 14.2	31.4 ± 14.7
$t\frac{1}{2}_\beta$ (c) (min)	402.7 ± 254.4	385.5 ± 282.2	277.0 ± 138.5	355.0 ± 226.6
MRT (nc) (min)	203.6 ± 155.4	208.5 ± 199.2	117.2 ± 43.4	176.4 ± 145.6
C_{ss} (c) (μg · ml⁻¹)	2.060 ± 0.432†	3.573 ± 0.748†	5.885 ± 0.762†	
(nc) (μg · ml⁻¹)	2.032 ± 0.450†	3.544 ± 0.756†	6.000 ± 0.799†	
V_c (c) (L)	21.350 ± 9.502	16.408 ± 4.350	13.013 ± 3.633	16.924 ± 6.957
V_{ss} (c) (L)	348.333 ± 249.794	331.500 ± 256.932	181.667 ± 73.677	287.167 ± 212.855
(nc) (L)	349.167 ± 203.673	348.333 ± 257.970	175.500 ± 51.177†	
Vd_β (c) (L)	1007.667 ± 451.195	973.333 ± 498.481	598.333 ± 244.213	859.778 ± 432.314
Cl_b (c) (L · min⁻¹)	1.883 ± 0.414	1.864 ± 0.269	1.563 ± 0.181	1.770 ± 0.322
(nc) (L · min⁻¹)	1.927 ± 0.512	1.892 ± 0.298	1.532 ± 0.134	1.781 ± 0.374

* Values are expressed as mean of five values ± SD.
† Statistical difference with the other treatment groups at probability level $P < 0.05$.
Values are expressed as means of 17 values ± SD.
From Gepts, E., et al.: Disposition of propofol administered as constant rate infusions in humans. Anesth. Analg., 66:1256, 1987.

pair baroreflex sensitivity[300] and also probably because central sympatholytic and vagotonic mechanisms are contributory.[299] To offset vagotonic responses to propofol, both atropine and glycopyrrolate are effective when given preinductively.[301]

When used in patients with coronary artery disease, propofol has been shown to increase myocardial lactate production, indicating that the drug may be associated with myocardial ischemia.[302]

Cardiac output and systemic vascular resistance usually decrease by 10% to 20% during both induction of general anesthesia (transiently) as well as during continuous-infusion maintenance anesthesia.[297] A significant decrease in SVR from 1760 to 1260 dyn · S · cm^{-5} or about 30% occurs within 2 minutes of administration and remains below normal for 12 or more minutes. This accounts for the hypotension usually seen.[297b]

Cardiac contractility is impaired. A study of the end-systolic pressure-volume relationship has demonstrated a significant global dose-dependent, negative inotropic property. The stroke volume is reduced. This reduces the systemic arterial pressure.[303]

Respiratory Effects.[296] After intravenous induction doses, transient apnea ensues, which tends to be of longer duration than that of thiopental or methohexital (dose and speed-of-injection dependent). Fong Sung[296] found that 70% of patients receiving propofol for induction of anesthesia had apnea lasting longer than 60 seconds, but only 28.6% of patients receiving induction doses of thiopental had apnea of this duration. If propofol maintenance infusions are employed, the most common finding is an increase in respiratory rate, whereas minute volume of ventilation remains depressed. The CO_2 response curve is depressed by 40% to 60% during propofol infusions. With small doses tidal volume is depressed.[290]

CLINICAL COURSE. Airway reactivity is less than thiopental and may be an alternative induction agent for endoscopic procedures.[304] Induction to unconsciousness is rapid, with progression from the awake state through lack of verbalization, failure to respond to command, and loss of eyelid reflex. The onset process, however, is not significantly different from other customary intravenous induction agents, such as thiopental and methohexital.

RECOVERY. After the administration of induction doses (2 to 2.5 mg/kg IV) of propofol, recovery to awakening is more rapid than after thiopental or thiamylal. The time to orientation and ambulation is about one half as long as compared with thiopental when anesthesia with propofol–N_2O and propofol infusion maintenance are used versus thiopental-isoflurane–N_2O anesthesia.[292,302] Although Gauthier[297] found no difference between the two when used as induction agents for rapidity of spontaneous eye opening, Fong Sung[296] found that the time to awakening after intravenous induction with propofol was only half as long when standard induction doses of thiopental were used. In general, patients are awake within 12 minutes, and motor skills similarly recover in a short time.

SIDE EFFECTS. Propofol, when injected into the smaller veins (as on the dorsum of the hand), is associated with a considerable incidence of burning pain (5% to 6%), more so than that seen after thiopental induction. These effects can be significantly reduced by giving induction doses through larger veins, such as those found in the antecubital fossa. The administration of an opioid, such as a single intravenous dose of fentanyl 100 μg, or alfentanil 500 μg, a few minutes prior to propofol (or 20 mg of lidocaine) minimizes the pain.[305]

There is a low incidence of nausea and vomiting after propofol induction (2% to 5%), which is less than that associated with other intravenous induction agents (10% to 20%). It is considered that propofol has an antiemetic action.[306]

Although hypertension and tachycardia follow laryngoscopy and intubation, propofol attenuates this response to a greater degree than either thiopental or methohexital.[304]

The period of transient apnea accompanying propofol (in doses of less than 2 mg/kg) induction seems to be of longer duration than with thiopental.[296,307] Doses of 2.5 mg/kg produce apnea, with a mean duration of 50 to 60 seconds in 44% of patients.[291]

Myoclonic movements and muscle twitching occur with some frequency and are more common than with thiopental or etomidate. Hiccoughing is seen more than with thiopental but less than with methohexital.[308]

USE IN CHILDREN. Propofol induction in children is accompanied by a significantly greater decrease in blood pressure, particularly in the 1–5 year(s) age group, than that following thiopental or inhalation induction. There was pain on injection (despite the addition of lidocaine) in over half of the children, although it was scored as mild in many patients.[309]

ADVANTAGES AND USES.[308] This is a useful agent for the induction of anesthesia, as well as for the maintenance of anesthesia for short surgical procedures, if complemented with narcotics or nitrous oxide. Its pharmacokinetic data indicate its usefulness as an induction agent in ambulatory surgicenter patients. There is no evidence of histamine release. Its short duration of action and relative lack of nausea and vomiting or other side effects give it some advantage over the currently available induction agents. In fact, the drug appears to have an antiemetic effect.[306] It may find usefulness as an alternative to the benzodiazepines for sedation during regional anesthesia or in the intensive care setting, where it could supplant the use of other sedative–hypnotics.

Propofol, however, is not an amnestic and, in this sense, might not be quite as useful as the benzodiazepines. Propofol has no analgesic properties. Unlike thiopental,[297] it is not an antianalgesic and has no effect on the pain threshold, thus increasing its usefulness during regional anesthesia for sedation.

EUGENOL DERIVATIVES

PROPANIDID

Propanidid is a nonbarbiturate intravenous anesthetic synthesized by Hiltmann and designated as *Bayer 1420*.[310] It is an extremely short-acting agent with minimal undesirable side effects. It was introduced into clinical investigation in 1961.[311] An almost identical drug known as *Propinal G 29,505* has been investigated by Nishimura.[312]

PHYSICAL AND CHEMICAL PROPERTIES. Chemically, the drug is 3-methoxy 4-(N-diethyl-carmidomethoxy) phenylaceticacid-n-propyl ester. Though structurally similar to G 29,505 (see following section), it is not truly a derivative of Eugenol, differing from the Geigy drug by having a propoxy-acyl group in place of the allyl group, as can be seen from the structural formula shown in Figure 27–20.

Bayer 1420 is a yellow oil with a boiling point of 210° C, and it is stable in buffer solutions of pH of 7.0 to 7.4 at body temperature. It has topical and local anesthetic activity and, unlike G 29,505, rarely causes thrombophlebitis. It is insoluble in water but is available in 10-ml vials as a 5% solution in an aqueous solution of 20% cremophor EL.

PHARMACOLOGIC EFFECTS

Toxicity. The LD_{50} in rabbits, cats, and dogs is about 80 mg/kg. No pathologic changes have been noted on gross or microscopic examinations of liver, spleen, kidneys, heart, lungs, thyroid, adrenals, pancreas, brain, bowel, lymph nodes, testes, or ovaries in dogs.[313]

Metabolism. The fate of Bayer 1420 was studied by Putter.[314] It is rapidly inactivated by pseudocholinesterases found in blood and liver. There is an enzymatic splitting at the ester bond so that propanol is split off from the propoxyacetyl group leaving the anesthetically inactive compound known as *HI 1979*. Chemically it is 3-methoxy 4-(N-diethylcarbamidomethoxy)-phenyl-acetic acid.

Central Nervous System.[315] The drug is an extremely rapid-acting agent. It produces unconsciousness and anesthesia. The pupillary, corneal, and laryngeal reflexes usually remain active (or are inactive for a brief period), but the pharyngeal reflex is constantly absent and the mandible relaxed throughout most of the anesthetic period. Thus, laryngoscopy is possible, but intubation may be accompanied by reflex, coughing, bucking, and, rarely, spasm. The average duration of anesthesia provided by 10 mg/kg of Bayer 1420 is about 5 minutes. After 10 to 12 minutes consciousness returns and the patient is well oriented, feels completely normal, and may be expected to leave the operating room without help.

Respiration.[316] Like G 29,505, Bayer 1420 stimulates respiration. Within circulation time after the injection of 10 mg/kg, the tidal volume increases over 300% and the respiratory rate about 50% apparently due to carotid chemoreceptor stimulation. This hyperventilation persists for an average of 40 seconds and is followed by a sudden onset of marked hypoventilation and, frequently, apnea. The period of hypoventilation is similar in duration to the period of hyperventilation. Following the hypoventilation, minute volume respiration returns rather suddenly to control levels. Smaller doses have similar but less pronounced effects on respiration.

Throughout the anesthetic period, oxygen saturation remains at or above normal, so it would appear that the overall effect of Bayer 1420 on respiration is beneficial rather than deleterious.

Cardiovascular System.[315] Simultaneous with the onset of respiratory stimulation, there is a reduction in blood pressure and an increase in pulse rate. The systolic pressure drops an average of 35% and the diastolic 25%, whereas the pulse rises an average of 35%. Infra-red capillary pulse monitoring during this phase of hypotension and tachycardia shows an *increase* in the amplitude of the pulse wave without shift in the position of the dicrotic notch, which would *seem* to indicate an increase in stroke volume rather than a decrease in peripheral resistance.[317]

Liver. No significant hepatotoxic effects have been found with the use of serum transaminase and alkaline phosphatase tests.[318]

Potentiation. Dundee[319] has reported the respiratory depression of succinylcholine to be about twice as long with Bayer 1420 as with thiopental, but there is some evidence presented by Howells,[318] to suggest that this is not a neuromuscular phenomenon.

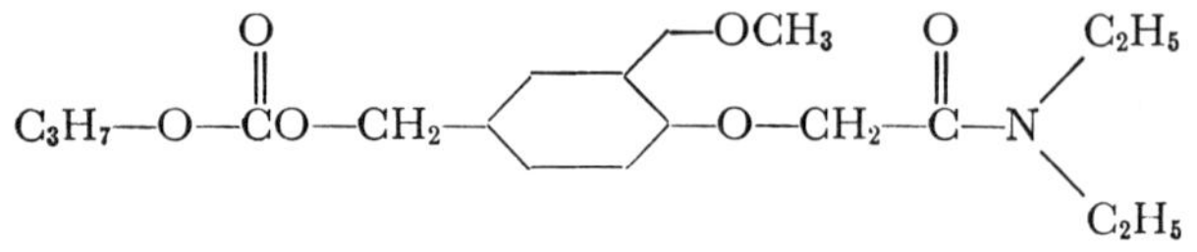

FIG. 27–20. Propanidid (Bayer 1420)

There appears to be no interaction with the nondepolarizing relaxants.

DOSAGE AND ADMINISTRATION.[318,319] The recommended dose is 10 mg/kg as an initial dose, with subsequent doses being 5 mg/kg. Many anesthesiologists in Europe recommend an initial dose of 5 to 7.5 mg/kg. The smaller doses have been used for induction but result in a significant number of inadequately narcotized patients. The 5% solution is somewhat viscous, and it may be desirable after the dose has been calculated to dilute the solutions to 2.5% with normal saline prior to injection.

RECOVERY. The duration of anesthesia with Bayer 1420 is slightly shorter than with G 29,505, but as with the latter drug, when patients open their eyes, full consciousness is apparent. Reflex response to pain returns in 45 seconds, response to command after 1.5 minutes, and the ability to verbalize and perform the Bender Face-Hand test after 3 minutes. After 10 to 12 minutes the patient may be expected to leave the operating room without help.

ANESTHETIC COMPLICATIONS. In premedicated patients, there is a 20% incidence of excitatory phenomena during induction, but this can be abolished with opiate premedication.[319] Involuntary muscle movements of the extremities are frequently seen. About 10% of the patients have hiccoughs, but no hypersecretion, nausea, or vomiting occurs when the drug is used as the sole anesthetic agent.[318] Some postoperative nausea and sickness are seen. The incidence of thrombophlebitis is reported as 0.6%; this represents a significant advantage over G 29,505. Perivascular injection is irritating, and an inflammatory response of the tissues, which is extensive but causes no pain, is completely resolved within 24 to 48 hours. The absence of pain in such red, swollen areas results from the local anesthetic effect of the drug, which may be used to perform painless venipuncture prior to intravenous administration of the anesthetic.

CLINICAL USE. Bayer 1420 has been used as the sole agent in short procedures and as the induction agent in longer cases. It would appear to be superior to G 29,505 in its slightly shorter duration of action, decreased (but significant) respiratory stimulation, and greatly reduced incidence of thrombophlebitis.

SUMMARY.[319] Advantages include brevity of action, rapid clear-headed recovery and use in porphyria. Disadvantages include cardiovascular hypotension, and excitatory effects, high incidence of vomiting and prolongation of succinylcholine. Its use is suggested for minor short procedures (e.g., tooth extraction). It is no longer marketed in Europe and has been abandoned; it was never marketed in North America.

MISCELLANEOUS INTRAVENOUS AGENTS

INTRAVENOUS ETHER (BURKHARDT TECHNIQUE)

In 1908, Burkhardt[321] reported on his experiments with intravenous ether and his clinical use of this method. The preparation used was a 5% volume in volume solution of ether in saline. More concentrated solutions are likely to produce phlebitis and hemoglobinuria. At present, the diluent solution is 5% dextrose. The solution is prepared by dissolving 50 ml of diethyl ether in 1 L of 5% dextrose. Butt[322] has recommended cooling the glucose solution (keeping in refrigerator at 40° F). This facilitates the dissolving of the ether; the ether must be thoroughly dissolved by vigorous shaking.[322]

ADMINISTRATION. The technique of administration consists of establishing an intravenous infusion with a standard Y tube. The prepared anesthetic solution is attached to one arm of the Y and the ether solution is vented to the atmosphere.

Premedication consists of the usual drugs and doses. Induction is accomplished with 300 to 600 ml of the solution (30 to 60 ml/min), taking about 8 to 10 minutes, and the solution is administered from a 1500 ml flask by drip into an arm vein. Induction may also be accomplished to a light sleep state by intravenous thiopental drip, either 2.5% (2 to 5 ml) or by drugs dilute solution (0.1% to 0.4%). Maintenance is achieved by a slower rate of infusion of about 20 ml/min. A 1-hour procedure will require from 1200 to 1500 ml of anesthetic.[323]

EFFECTS. The course is smooth, and little change in pulse occurs. Respiration is increased; postoperative vomiting is rare. Excitement does occur, and Kummell[324] reported frequent thrombosis. Butt[322] has used the method in endoscopic procedures and notes that the anesthetic equipment is conveniently away from the surgical field.

Despite the volumes injected, no cases of pulmonary edema have been reported; however, contraindications as listed by Burkhardt[325] include patients with plethora, anemia, renal disease and arteriosclerosis.

UPTAKE. Eger[326] has used this technique to study the uptake and distribution of ether. Each milliliter of saline-ether solution introduced was converted to milliliters of pure ether vapor at 37° C by multiplying by a factor of 11, based on the fact that a molecular weight of the agent when vaporized occupies 22.4 L.

On this basis, the average uptake of ether is as follows: during the first 5 minutes, about 900 ml of pure vapor per minute (approximately 4 ml liquid ether) enters the peripheral tissues. During the second 5 minutes, this value was halved. During the succeeding 5-minute interval, uptake fell by ever-decreasing amounts so that by the 60th minute only 180 ml/min was required.

GAMMA HYDROXYBUTYRIC ACID

In 1960, Laborit[327] reported on the usefulness of butyric acid to produce protection against stress. This substance is a saturated fatty acid and a natural product of lipid metabolism, administration of which produces sleep and is associated with ketone formation. The basic drug appears to act as a central inhibitory substance. It is related chemically to gamma aminobutyric acid, which is present in the brain in considerable amounts. The latter is an inhibitory material and is capable of preventing convulsions and other central excitatory phenomena but cannot pass the blood-brain barrier. In an attempt to obtain a compound that would penetrate from the blood into the brain and yet not produce ketone bodies, Laborit synthesized gamma hydroxybutyric acid.

CHEMISTRY. This drug is a saturated fatty acid. It is soluble in water and is available as the sodium salt (Fig. 27-21).

PHARMACOLOGY.[327] Sleep is readily produced by this agent, and it is indistinguishable from natural sleep either chemically or by EEG. *Respiration* is slowed with an increased amplitude so that minute volume is near a normal value. Control of respiration is readily achieved especially if there is supplementation with a narcotic or sedative. Periodic Cheyne-Stokes respiration is also occasionally observed. *Cardiovascular* effects observed include bradycardia and a slight elevation of systolic blood pressure.

Relaxation is not sufficient to perform abdominal surgery or to produce a state of good muscular relaxation for late reduction of fractures. Relaxation of the jaw, however, is good and permits easy intubation while the patient is breathing spontaneously.

DOSAGE. This drug is more potent than butyric acid in producing sleep. In many respects its effect resembles the onset of action of rectal tribromethanol. Doses range from 0.65 to 8.0 g. The preparation used is an aqueous solution of 5%. The induction dose is usually 4 to 6 g administered over 20 to 30 minutes, i.e., 1 g every 5 minutes. Supplementary or maintenance doses are difficult to determine.

ADMINISTRATION.[328] Although gamma penetrates the blood-brain boundary, there is a delay of 10 to 15 minutes before effects are noted. Thus, induction is slow and the full onset of action takes from 30 to 45 minutes. Because the induction is so prolonged and time consuming, it does not lend itself to administration by "biologic titration," i.e., by estab-

$$HO-CH_2-CH_2-CH_2-\overset{O}{\underset{\parallel}{C}}-O-Na$$

FIG. 27-21. Gamma hydroxybutyric acid.

lishing a moment-to-moment dose-response relationship. Hence, a predetermined dose is required.

ADVANTAGES. The advantages consist of nonirritation of veins (lack of phlebitis), which distinguishes it from other nonbarbiturates and a mild cardiotonic effect. By potentiating narcotic and hypnotic drugs, it can be considered to have a sparing effect and reduce the amount of other agents. Combination with nitrous oxide is an effective method. Control of respiration is readily achieved while return to spontaneous respiration is rapid. Extrapyramidal gross muscular movements occur when the drug is administered too rapidly. Some use in operations that are expected to be prolonged is merited such as neurosurgery.

DISADVANTAGES. The disadvantages include an unacceptable long induction; lack of easy control in administration and of quick responses so that overdose is possible; and extrapyramidal gross muscular movements, which occur when the drug is administered too rapidly. There appears to be little clinical application. It is of interest with respect to central nervous system mechanisms of drug action.

INTRAVENOUS ETHANOL

Ethanol has several pharmacologic actions that may be useful in the anesthetic management of patients. It has sedative, hypnotic, euphoric, and vasodilator properties. Its use in clinical anesthesia was first reported by Marin of Mexico in 1929.[329]

PHARMACOLOGIC EFFECTS.[330-334] A summary of actions is as follows:

1. Sedation and sleep[330]
2. Cardiovascular stability[335]
3. No demonstrable liver damage but transient liver dysfunction with small doses.[336]
4. Diuresis
5. Hyperglycemia
6. Large doses—produce anuria, intravenous hemolysis
7. Adrenocortical response—rise in blood cortisol with large doses[337]
8. Thrombophlebitis after large doses or concentrated solution

Central Nervous System Effects.[338] The most important effect of alcohol is on the brain. It exerts a form of narcotic depression, which is probably the result of interference with synaptic transmission. Investigations show that the nerve impulses are inhibited and that this effect occurs before any decrease in oxygen consumption. That is, depression of function occurs first and depression of cerebral metabolic rate second.[338,339]

As a central system depressant, alcohol produces signs and symptoms similar to classical general anesthetic agents. The depression is a descending type, and the pattern of depression corresponds to the stages of anesthesia.[334,339]

Stage 1 With small doses of alcohol the higher and complex functions of the cortex, such as judgment, self-control, learning, and discrimination, are diminished. This releases the lower cerebral centers from higher control and inhibition. A form of excitement may be manifest as seen in the induction of anesthesia. At the same time, the patient becomes less aware of his environment. Perception is lessened. Euphoria, loss of inhibition, less efficient hearing, and impaired vision are present. The reaction of a patient is altered, and it is probable that the apparent analgesia produced is the result of a modified appreciation of the pain stimulus so that the pain is considered unimportant.

The blood level of alcohol necessary for these changes is about 0.05% to 0.1%. At a concentration of 0.05% the sensory and association cortical areas are blunted, whereas at a concentration of 0.1% the motor cortical areas are depressed.

Stage 2 With a blood alcohol content between 0.1% and 0.45%, further depression is noted. In addition to the above, motor incoordination now occurs. Voluntary muscles are affected first. Speech is slurred, and muscular incoordination appears. Staggering gait may appear and, subsequently, generalized motor weakness and paralysis. At the same time, the patient becomes progressively stuporous. At the blood level of 0.2%, the entire motor cortical area is depressed and the midbrain is affected. Emotional behavior is changed. At 0.3% the more primitive areas, thalamic and others, are affected. Vomiting may occur at a blood alcohol level of about 0.12%. This emetic effect is central and occurs whether the alcohol is taken orally or intravenously.[340]

Stage 3 Additional doses of alcohol will now produce unconsciousness or coma. It is often said that the person is dead drunk. This occurs at a blood level of 0.5% to 0.6%. Such a level is achieved by the ingestion of one pint of whiskey, or 200 to 250 ml of alcohol, within 1 hour.

Stage 4 Degrees of depression involving paralysis of medullary centers—the respiratory first, followed by the circulatory centers—are not quickly produced. It does occur at levels of alcohol in the blood of 0.6% to 0.7%. This is fatal. It is obvious that the dose capable of producing unconsciousness is near the fatal dose—the dose necessary to induce an anesthetic state approaches the dose producing death. The margin of safety is small and hence alcohol is a poor anesthetic.

Cardiovascular Effects.[335,339,341,342] Although gross hemodynamic measurements of blood pressure are not impressive, there are serious hemodynamic alterations. Low to moderate doses of 0.5 to 1.5 g of ethyl alcohol/kg of body weight cause a rising blood pressure and an increased stroke output. The workload of the heart increases proportionate to the dose, but the functional capacity as measured by the Starling-Sarnoff function curves is markedly reduced.

The oxygen requirement of the myocardium increases proportionately to the work load and correlates linearly with tension-time index.

A redistribution of blood in the peripheral circulatory bed occurs with a significant increase in cutaneous flow. To achieve this effect, a shift away from many viscera occurs.

Cardiac Effects Blood vessels between 85 and 136 mg/100 ml cause an increase in cardiac output at rest because of an increase in heart rate without a change in stroke volume. At rest a small increase in oxygen consumption occurs. During submaximal exercise, there is a comparatively increased oxygen consumption and a decreased mechanical efficiency, but during maximal exercise there are no significant changes.[335,341]

In contrast to normal subjects, the administration of alcohol to patients with a history of chronic intake and evidence of liver impairment causes a significant depression of ventricular function. The arteriovenous oxygen difference is decreased, and the total peripheral resistance is decreased.

Chronic ingestion of excessive amounts of alcohol leads to a syndrome of cardiac myopathy. Triglycerides are used principally as fuel, whereas the use of free fatty acids is decreased.[342,343]

This is mediated partially by norepinephrine release.[337,344] Chronic symptoms include exertional dyspnea and palpitations, reduced exercise tolerance, cardiomegaly, and signs of heart failure. Histochemical studies of the heart reveal deposits of neutral lipids and mitochondrial damage. The sarcoplasmic reticulum is swollen.[342]

The direct effects of alcohol on myocardial structure have been demonstrated.[342,343] Studies reveal a significant myocardiopathy with altered endoplasmic reticulum and mitochondria.

Coronary flow generally is reduced and coronary resistance rises at all dosage levels with moderate doses of alcohol.[335] Russek[341] has demonstrated that the electrocardiographic changes characteristic of ischemia are not prevented in humans by alcohol.[341]

Gastrointestinal Action. Ingestion of alcohol mixtures at concentrations above 20% inhibit gastric secretins locally and cause inflammation of gastric mucosa. Vomiting may be induced. If given intravenously, a blood level of 0.12% also induces a high incidence of vomiting.

METABOLISM OF ALCOHOL.[333,368,344,345] Alcohol is neither selectively excreted nor converted to a storage form in the body. Studies on alcohol labeled with radioactive carbon show that 90% appears as carbon dioxide. Less than 10% of alcohol is eliminated by renal, pulmonary, or cutaneous avenues.[335] After ingestion, blood alcohol rises to a maximum during the absorption phase. As it is distributed to the tissues, the alcohol disappears essentially in a linear fashion from the blood.[345] Alcohol ingested in low concentrations causes a maximal release of the enzyme alcohol dehydrogenase. There is also a release of adrenocorticosteroids[346] and of epinephrine.[347]

Absorption. This is rapid and occurs throughout the gastrointestinal tract. After ingestion it quickly passes down the tract and about 80% is absorbed from the small intestine. There is no limit to rate absorption, which is proportional to its concentration. Concentrations of alcohol of 50% or more have a depressant effect on absorption—a "local narcosis."

Distribution occurs throughout the body and is proportional to the water content of the tissues.[345] Thus, blood, which is 90% water, contains a higher level than the rest of the body tissues, which are about 70% water. Actually, blood contains about 1.25 times as much alcohol per unit mass as do the other body tissues. At equilibrium, organs contain 70% to 80% of the plasma concentration. Plasma levels are determined by many variables; however, the following is a quick approximation: 1 ml (800 mg) of alcohol concentration of about 100 mg/100 ml, or 0.1% in 2 hours (equivalent to 5 ounces of whiskey in a man of 70 kg). It may be stated that each ounce of whiskey (100 proof) will raise the blood level of alcohol approximately 20 mg/100 ml or to 0.02%.

Rate of Metabolism.[345] This is essentially slow. The rate of alcohol metabolism has been estimated to vary between 100 and 200 mg/kg of body weight per hour. (The value 200 mg is equivalent to 0.25 ml of alcohol.) Thus, it is expected that the average man can metabolize about 1 ounce of whiskey per hour. An average man of 70 kg can metabolize 840 ml (about a fifth of whiskey) per day. The actual upper limit appears to be one full quart (or 240 mg/kg per hour).

Factors Influencing Rate.[448,449] Metabolism is essentially linear; however, with higher levels there may be a speed-up of carbohydrate metabolism and the increased pyruvates may participate in coupled oxidation–reduction reactions with alcohol. The rate is insensitive to overall metabolic needs. Hyperthyroidism has no effect. Exposure to cold or muscular exercise does not significantly influence rate. Reducing body temperature slows all body reactions, including alcohol metabolism. The relationship between metabolism and body temperature appears to be the usual one for chemical reactions, namely, a doubling of rate for each 10° rise in temperature.

Proteins effectively increase the rate of metabolism, and alanine and glycine are potent amino acids in this respect.[450]

Substances such as insulin, pyruvate, and fructose have been reported to increase the rate of metabolism, but this is controversial. All three may stimulate a sluggish or minimal initial rate. The phenomenon of tolerance is simply an adaptation of the central nervous system to alcohol, not an alteration in metabolism of alcohol.

PREPARATIONS.[351–353] Solutions of 5% to 10% (w/v) ethanol by weight in isotonic lactated Ringer's solution have been used. The 10% (w/v) solution produces a high incidence of complications, including phlebitis or thrombosis and painful irritation in more than half the subjects, whereas 5% alcohol by volume in a physiologic solution is too dilute and does not readily produce desired anesthetic effects. The ability to get a narcotizing dose of the drug into the circulation is thus limited. In practice, an 8% solution by weight (w/v) is preferred, which is approximately 10% by volume (v/v). This is administered by intravenous drip.

PREANESTHESTIC MEDICATION.[353,354] The control of intravenous ethanol for anesthetic purposes depends on premedication. Without preliminary drugs or with atropine alone, a state of sleep usually cannot be induced with an 8% solution (w/v) with less than 500 ml of solution. Excitement and loss of restraint occur before loss of consciousness. This excitement may be quickly terminated by an intravenous barbiturate.

Preoperative pentobarbital 2.5 to 4 mg/kg (average for an adult—200 mg) will permit quiet induction and use of smaller doses of ethanol. Induction may be accomplished with a dose of thiopental or methohexital followed by ethanol, or the two may be combined. Potentiation of the ethanol occurs with doses of barbiturates, and they prolong recovery. Opiate medication is less satisfactory but does permit smooth induction and use of smaller doses of ethanol, and recovery is not delayed.

Generous doses of atropine, at least 0.6 mg, are needed, especially to combat the salivation induced by the ethanol.

DOSAGE.[353,354] Metabolism and adjunctive drugs determine the dose. Individual variation is great. Without premedication the unpredictability of action and increase in sequelae are great. Following opiate premedication with 100 mg of meperidine or 10 mg of morphine, the range of dosage is 0.5 to 1 g/kg of absolute alcohol (average dosage 0.8 g/kg). This is administration in a period of 10 minutes or less.

ADMINISTRATION. A free-running intravenous infusion must first be assured. *Induction* is then accomplished using the 8% w/v ethanol in isotonic Ringer's lactate solution. In the well-medicated male patient of 70 kg, at least 250 ml of the solution (20 g of ethanol) is administered in 3 to 5 minutes. The rate is about 50 ml/min. Assessment of the patient at this time may indicate additional doses up to a total of 500 ml during the following 5 minutes.

Maintenance is accomplished by administering 2 to 10 ml/min. The amount depends on the rate of metabolism and is determined by observation of the patient's depth of anesthesia. For maintenance dose in the average adult man, the rate of metabolism of ethanol is used as a guide, and in practice is 12 g/h (15 ml) or approximately 0.2 g/min.

USES.[351,352] It is limited, but has advantages in brief and simple procedures. Minor gynecologic procedures and burn debridement or dressings may be performed; however, there is an unacceptable high incidence of undesirable sequelae regardless of the procedure. It is useful in the management of belligerent alcoholics and in those with delirium tremens.

Dilute intravenous alcohol has been used in the postoperative period to provide pain relief, comfort, and the control of excitement.[355,356]

SEQUELAE

Hangover. Hangover is a syndrome following large doses (overindulgence) of ethanol. Hangover occurs in about 33% of patients and is diminished by premedication of chlordiazepoxide (50 mg). The clinical description is that of:

> A physical and emotional state caused by, and following the excessive use of, alcohol. Affects people, particularly of a neurotic nature. The physical reaction (basically psychosomatic) is expressed by symptoms of extreme generalized pain, headache, nausea, and anorexia, jitters, fatigue, extreme thirst, excessive sweating, flushed feelings and marked tremors. All to a large extent due to the toxic effects of alcohol on the body.[345]

Delirium. Emergence reactions are frequent on recovery and occur more frequently when a thiobarbiturate is given as a part of the anesthesia.[351] When promethiazine or pentobarbital are the premedicants, the incidence is low.[358] Control is accomplished by small intravenous doses of diazepam (10 to 20 mg). Benzodiazepams are poor.[359,360]

Amnesia. All depressant premedicant drugs increase the occurrence of amnesia; pentobarbital and opiates are significantly effective. Retrograde amnesia is apparent; and complete memory loss occurs frequently immediately preceding induction. Of patients given methohexital alone, 10% have no memory of this event; when ethanol is given in addition, amnesia is increased to 30%.

Drug Interaction. Potentiation of many central depressants occurs. Barbiturate effects are particularly enhanced. Tranquilizers are synergized.[357,360]

REFERENCES

1. Chen, G., et al.: The pharmacology of 1-(phenylcyclohexyl) piperidine. J. Pharmacol. Exp. Ther., *127*:241, 1959.
2. Greifenstein, F.E., et al.: A study of a 1-aryl cyclohexylamine for anesthesia. Anesth. Analg., *37*:293, 1958.
3. Collins, V.J., Gorospe, C.A., and Rovenstine, E.A.: Intravenous non-barbiturate non-narcotic analgesics. I: Cyclohexylamines. Anesth. Analg., *39*:302, 1960.
4. Stevens, C.L.: Belgium Patents 634, 208, 1963; Parke Davis U.S. Pat. 3,254,124, 1966.
5. Virtue, R.W., et al.: An anesthetic agent; 2-orthochlorophenyl-2-Methylamino-cyclohexanone (CI 581). Anesthesiology, *60*:214, 1967.
6. Showalter, C.W., and Thornton, W.E.: Clinical pharmacology of phencyclidine toxicity. Am. J. Psychiatry, *134*:1234, 1977.
7. Burns, R.S.: Drug abuse and alcoholism. Clin. Toxicol., *9*:477, 1976.
8. Cook, C.E., et al.: Phencyclidine disposition after intravenous and oral doses. J. Clin. Pharm. Ther., *31*:625, 1982.
9. Domino, E.F., Chodoff, P., and Corssen, G.: Pharmacologic effects of CI-581, a new dissociative anesthetic in man. Clin. Pharmacol. Ther., *6*:279, 1965.
9a. Miyasaka, M., Domino, E.F.: Neuronal mechanisms of ketamine induced anesthesia. J. Neuropharmacol., *7*:557, 1968.
10. White, P.F., Ham, J., Way, W. L., and Trevor, A.J.: Pharmacology of ketamine isomers in surgical patients. Anesthesiology, *52*:231, 1980.
10a. White, P.F., Way, W.L., and Trevor, A.J.: Ketamine—Its pharmacology and therapeutic uses. Anesthesiology, *56*:119, 1982.
11. Kayama, Y., and Iwama, K.: The EEG-evoked potentials and single unit activity during ketamine anesthesia in cats. Anesthesiology, *36*:316, 1972.
12. Corssen, G., Domino, E.F., and Bree, R.L.: Electroencephalographic effects of ketamine anesthesia in children. Anesth. Analg., *48*:141, 1969.
12a. Winters, W.G.: Epilepsy or anesthesia with ketamine. Anesthesiology, *36*:309, 1972.
13. Kithata, L.M., Taub, A., and Kosaka, Y.: Lamina-specific suppression of dorsal-horn unit activity by ketamine hydrochloride. Anesthesiology, *38*:4, 1973.
14. Corssen, G., and Domino, E.F.: Dissociative anesthesia: Further pharmacologic studies and first clinical experience with the phencyclidine derivative CI-58L. Anesth. Analg., *45*:29, 1966.
14a. Corssen, G., Reves, J.G., Stanley, T.H.: Intravenous Anesthesia and Analgesia. Philadelphia, Lea & Febiger, 1988.
15. Corssen, G., et al.: Kektamine in the anesthetic management of asthmatic patients. Anesth. Analg., *51*:588, 1972.
15a. Smith, D.J., Westfall, D.P., and Adams, J.D.: Kektamine interacts with opiate receptors as an agonist. Anesthesiology, *53*:85, 1980.
16. Shapiro, H.M., et al.: Local Cerebral Glucose Metabolism During Anesthesia. *In* Blood Flow and Brain Metabolism.

Ed., A.M. Harper, Edinburg, Churchill-Livingstone, 1975, p 942.
16a. Shapiro, H.M., et al.: Local cerebral glucose uptake in awake and halothane-anesthetized primates. Anesthesiology, 48:97, 1978.
17. Sadove, M.S., et al.: Clinical study of droperidol in the prevention of side effects of ketamine anesthesia. Anesth. Analg., 50:562, 1971.
18. Fine, T., and Firestone, S.C.: Sensory disturbances following ketamine anesthesia: Recurrent hallucinations. Anesthesiology, 52:420, 1973.
19. Pandit, S.K., Lothary, S.P., and Kuma, S.M.: Low dose infusion technique with ketamine. Anaesthesia, 35:669, 1980.
20. Dawson, B., Michenfelder D., and Theye, A.: Effects of ketamine on canine cerebral blood flow and metabolism: Modification by prior administration of thiopental. Anesth. Analg., 50:443, 1971.
20a. Takeshita, H., Obuda, Y., and Sari, A.: The effects of ketamine on cerebral circulation and metabolism in man. Anesthesiology, 36:69, 1972.
21. Sari, A., Akuda, Y., and Takashita, H.: The effect of ketamine on cerebrospinal fluid pressure. Anesth. Analg., 51:560, 1972.
21a. Peuler, M., Glass, D.D., and Arens, J.F.: Ketamine and intraocular pressure. Anesthesiology, 43:575, 1975.
22. Lockhart, C.H., and Jenkins, J.J.: Ketamine-induced apnea in patients with increased intracranial pressure. Anesthesiology, 37:92, 1972.
23. Corssen, G., Little, S.G., Tararoli, M.: Ketamine and epilepsy. Anesth. Analg., 53:319, 1974.
23a. Celesia, G.G., Chen, R.C., and Bamforth, B.J.: Effects of ketamine in epilepsy. Neurology, 25:169, 1975.
24. Tweed, W.A., and Mymin, D.: Myocardial force: Velocity relations during ketamine anesthesia at constant heart rate. Anesthesiology, 41:49, 1974.
24a. Ross, J., Linhart, J.W., and Braunwald, E.: Effects of changing heart rate in man by electrical stimulation. Circulation, 32:549, 1965.
25. Traber, D.L., Wilson, R.D., and Priano, L.L: Blockade of the hypertensive response to ketamine. Anesth. Analg., 49:420, 1970.
25a. Weiskopf, R.B., et al.: Cardiovascular and metabolic sequelae of inducing anesthesia with ketamine or thiopental in hypovolemic swine. Anesthesiology, 60:214, 1984.
26. Tweed, W.A., Minuck, M., and Mymin, D.: Circulatory responses to ketamine anesthesia. Anesthesiology, 37:613, 1972.
26a. Pinaud, M., Souron, R., and Nicholas, F.: Ketamine anesthesia for implantation of a permanent pacemaker. Anesth. Analg., 36:531, 1976.
27. Lundey, P.M., Gowdey, C.W., and Calhoun, E.H.: The actions of ketamine on vascular adrenergic neurones. Eur. J. Pharmacol., 23:153, 1973.
28. Liao, J.C., Koethntop, D.E., and Buckley, J.J.: Dual effect of ketamine on the peripheral vasculature. Anesthesiology, 51:S116, 1979.
29. Gooding, J.M., et al.: A physiologic analysis of cardiopulmonary responses to ketamine in non-cardiac patients. Anesth. Analg., 56:813, 1977.
29a. Gassner, S., et al.: The effect of ketamine on pulmonary artery pressure: An experimental and clinical study. Anaesthesia, 29:141, 1974.
30. Wong, D.H.W., and Jenkins, L.C.: An experimental study of the mechanism of action of ketamine on the central nervous system. Can. Anaesth. Soc. J., 21:57, 1974.

31. Bovill, J.G., et al.: Some cardiovascular effects of ketamine in man. Br. J. Pharmacol., 41:411, 1971.
31a. Zsigmond, E.K.: Comment on plasma free norepinephrine during ketamine anesthesia. Anesth. Analg., 51:588, 1972.
32. Zsigmond, E.K., Kelsch, R.C., and Kothany, S.P.: Rise in plasma-free norepinephrine during anesthetic induction with ketamine. Phys. Drug Manual, 6:31, 1974.
33. Iversen, L.L.: Uptake of noradrenaline by the isolated perfused rat heart. Br. J. Pharmacol., 21:523, 1963.
34. Iversen, L.L.: The uptake of catecholamines at high perfusion concentrations in the rat isolated heart: A novel catecholamine uptake process. Br. J. Pharmacol., 25:18, 1965.
35. Salt, P.J., Barnes, P.K., and Besunick, F.J.: Inhibition of neurones and extra neuronal uptake of noradrenaline by ketamine. Br. J. Anaesth., 51:835, 1979.
36. Nedergaard, O.A.: Cocaine-like effect of ketamine on vascular adrenergic neurons. Eur. Pharmacol., 23:153, 1973.
37. Lundey, P.M., Gowdy, C.W., and Colhouhn, E.H.: Tracheal smooth muscle relaxant effect of ketamine. Br. J. Anaesth., 46:333, 1974.
38. Miletich, D.J., et al.: Effect of ketamine on catecholamine metabolism in isolated rat heart. Anesthesiology, 39:271, 1973.
39. Dowdy, E.G., and Kaya, K.: Studies of mechanism of cardiovascular response to CI-581. Anesthesiology, 29:931, 1968.
40. Slogoff, S., and Allen, G.W.: The role of barareceptors in the cardiovascular response to ketamine. Anesth. Analg., 53:704, 1974.
41. Keats, A.S.: The effect of drugs on respiration in man. Annu. Rev. Pharmacol., 25:41, 1985.
42. Stanley, V., et al.: Cardiovascular and respiratory function with CI-581. Anesth. Analg., 47:760, 1968.
42a. Kitamura, S., et al.: Lacrimation under ketamine anesthesia. Jpn. J. Anesth., 20:749, 1971.
43. Bourke, D.L., Malit, L.A., and Smith, T.C.: Respiratory interactions of ketamine and morphine. Anesthesiology, 66:153, 1987.
44. Wilson, A.: Ketamine and muscle relaxants. Br. J. Anaesth., 45:115, 1973.
45. Morel, D.R., Forster, A., and Gemperle, M.: Noninvasive evaluation of breathing pattern and thoraco-abdominal motion following the infusion of ketamine or droperidol in humans. Anesthesiology, 65:392, 1986.
46. Mankikian, B., et al.: Ventilatory pattern and chest wall mechanics during ketamine anesthesia in humans. Anesthesiology, 65:492, 1986.
47. Shulman, D., et al.: The effect of ketamine on the functional residual capacity in young children. Anesthesiology, 62:551, 1985.
47a. Don, H.: The mechanical properties of the respiratory system during anesthesia. Int. Anesthesiol. Clin., 15:113, 1977.
47b. Dobbinson, T.L., Nisbet, H.I.A., Pelton, D.A., Levison, H.: Functional residual capacity and compliance in anaesthetized paralysed children, part II clinical results. Can. Anaesth. Soc. J., 20:322, 1973.
48. Tokics, L., et al.: Computerized tomography of chest and gas exchange measurements during ketamine anesthesia. Acta Anaesthesiol. Scand., 31:684, 1987.
49. Zsigmond, E.K., et al.: Arterial hypoxemia caused by intravenous ketamine. Anesth. Analg., 55:331, 1976.
50. El-Harway, M.B., et al.: Effect of ketamine hydrochloride on the tracheobronchial tree. Mid. East J. Anaesth., 3:445, 1972.

51. Wanna, H.T., and Gergis, S.D.: Procaine, lidocaine, and ketamine inhibit histamine induced contracture of guinea pig tracheal muscle. Anesth. Analg., 57:25, 1978.
52. Huber, F.C., et al.: Ketamine: Its effect on airway resistance. South. Med., J., 65:1176, 1972.
53. Taylor, P.A., and Towey, R.M.: Depression of laryngeal reflexes during ketamine anesthesia. Br. Med. J., 2:668, 1971.
54. Sage, M., and Laird, S.M.: Ketamine and laryngeal reflexes. Br. Med. J., 2:670, 1972.
54a. Carson, I.W., et al.: Laryngeal competence with ketamine and other drugs. Anesthesiology, 38:128, 1973.
55. Radney, P.A., and Badula, R.P.: Generalized extensor spasm in infants following ketamine anesthesia. Anesthesiology, 39:459, 1973.
55a. Schoening, B., Banniza, V., and Koch, H.: Ketamin und diazepam zur anaesthesie bei infantiler cerebral paresc. Anaesthesist, 23:14, 1974.
55b. Bizzari, D.: Experience at N.Y. Hospital Westchester Neuropsychiatric Division. Personal Communication, 1977.
56. Galloon, S.: Ketamine for obstetric delivery. Anesthesiology, 44:522, 1976.
57. Galloon, S.: Ketamine and the pregnant uterus. Can. Anaesth. Soc. J., 20:141, 1973.
58. Janeczka, G.I., El-Etr, A.A., and Younes, A.: Low dose ketamine anesthesia for obstetrical delivery. Anesth. Analg., 53:828, 1974.
59. Akamatsu, T.J., et al.: Experiences with use of ketamine for parturition: I. Primary anesthetic for vaginal delivery. Anesth. Analg., 53:284, 1974.
60. Hill, C.R., et al.: Wakefulness during cesarean section with thiopental, ketamine, or thiopental-ketamine combination (abstract). Anesthesiology, 59:Suppl A419, 1983.
60a. Hodgkinson, K., et al.: Neonatal neurobehavioral tests following vaginal delivery under ketamine, thiopental and extradural anesthesia. Anesth. Analg., 53:824, 1974.
61. Bernstein, K., et al.: Influence of two different anaesthetic agents on the newborn and the correlation between foetal oxygenation and induction-delivery time in elective caesarean section. Acta Anaesthiol. Scand., 29:157, 1985.
62. Kanieris, P., et al.: Serum free fatty acids and blood sugar levels in children under thiopental, halothane and ketamine anesthesia. Can. Anaesth. Soc. J., 22:509, 1975.
63. Lacoumenta, S., et al.: Effects of ketamine anaesthesia on the metabolic response to pelvic surgery. Br. J. Anaesth., 53:493, 1984.
64. Kostrzewska, E., and Gregor, A.: Ketamine in acute intermittent porphyria—dangerous or safe? Anesthesiology, 49:376, 1978.
65. Rizk, S.F.: Ketamine is safe in acute intermittent porphyria. Anesthesiology, 49:376, 1978.
65a. Collins, V.J.: Case reports of 11 patients. Dept. of Anesthesiology, Chicago Cook County Hospital, 1967–1977.
65b. Capouet, B., Dernovoi, B., and Azagra, J.S.: Induction of anaesthesia with ketamine during an acute crisis of hereditary coproporphyria. Can. J. Anaesth., 34:388, 1987.
66. Matuski, A., et al.: Reduced tri-iodothyronine levels during and following-ketamine-N_2O anesthesia in man. Jpn. J. Anaesth., 24:373, 1976.
67. Bovill, J.G., Coppel, D.L., and Dundee, J.W.: Current status of ketamine anesthesia (histamine). Lancet, 1:1285, 1971.
68. Amaki, Y., et al.: Ketamine interaction with neuromuscular blocking agents in the phrenic nerve hemidiaphragm preparation of the rat. Anesth. Analg., 57:238, 1978.
69. Maleque, M.A., Warnick, J.E., and Albuquerque, E.X.: The mechanism and site of action of ketamine on skeletal muscle. J. Pharmacol. Exp. Ther., 219:638, 1981.
70. Bogdan, L.G., Glisson, S.N., and El-Etr, A.A.: The effect of ketamine upon depolarizing and non-depolarizing neuromuscular blockade in rabbit. Nauyn-Scmiedebergs. Arch. Pharmacol., 285:223, 1974.
71. Krieg, N., Crul, J.F., and Booiji, L.H.D.J.: Relative potency of Org NC 45, pancuronium, alcuronium and tubocurarine in anesthetized man. Br. J. Anaesth., 52:783, 1980.
72. Torda, T.A., and Murphy, E.C.: Presynaptic effect of intravenous anesthetic agents at the neuromuscular junction. Br. J. Anaesth., 51:353, 1979.
73. Cronnelly, R., et al.: Ketamine myoneural activity and interaction with neuromuscular blocking agents. Eur. J. Pharmacol., 22:17, 1973.
74. Johnston, R.R., Miller, R.D., and Way, W.L.: The interaction of ketamine with d-tubocurarine, pancuronium and succinylcholine in man. Anesth. Analg., 53:496, 1974.
75. Kothary, S.P., and Zsigmond, E.K.: Prevention of ketamine-induced psychic sequelae by diazepam. Clin. Pharm. Ther., 17:238, 1975.
76. Gal, T.J., and Malit, L.A.: The influence of ketamine induction of potassium changes and fasciculations following suxamethonium. Br. J. Anaesth., 44:1077, 1972.
77. Wadhwa, R.K., and Tantisira, B.: Parotidectomy in a patient with a family history of hyperthermia. Anesthesiology, 40:191, 1974.
78. Meltzer, H.Y., et al.: Effect of ketamine on creatine phosphokinase levels. Lancet, 1:1195, 1975.
79. Engebaek, J., et al.: Dose-response relationships and neuromuscular blocking effects of vecuronium and pancuronium during ketamine anaesthesia. Br. J. Anaesth., 56:953, 1984.
80. Dundee, J.W.: Ketamine: A Preliminary Report on its Use as an Induction Agent. Lancet 1, 1370, 1970.
80a. El-Naggar, M., et al.: Ketamine as an induction agent and adjunct to nitrous oxide-oxygen curare anesthesia sequence. Anesthesiol. Rev., 4:10, 1975.
81. Morgan, M., et al.: Ketamine as the sole anesthetic agent for minor surgical procedures. Anaesthesia, 26:158, 1971.
82. Corssen, G.: Ketamine in the anesthetic management of asthmatic patients. Anesth. Analg., 81:588, 1972.
83. Hirschman, C.A., et al.: Ketamine block of bronchospasm in experimental canine anesthesia. Br. J. Anaesth., 51:713, 1979.
84. Fisher, M.A.: Ketamine hydrochloride in severe bronchospasm. Anaesthesia, 32:771, 1977.
85. Corssen, G., et al.: Ketamine in the anaesthetic management of asthmatic patients. Anesth. Analg., 51:588, 1972.
86. Strube, P.J., and Hallem, P.L.: Ketamine by continuous infusion in status asthmaticus. Anaesthesia, 41:1017, 1986.
87. Corssen, G., Reves, J.G., and Stanley, T.H.: Intravenous Anesthesia and Analgesia. Philadelphia, Lea & Febiger, 1988.
87a. Corssen, G.: Recent developments in anesthetic management of burned patients. J. Trauma, 7:152, 1967.
88. Corssen, G., Reves, J.G., and Carter, J.R.: Neurolept anaesthesia, dissociative anesthesia and hemorrhage. Int. Anesthesiol. Clin., 12:145, 1974.
89. Park, G.R., et al.: Ketamine infusion: Sedative, inotrope and bronchodilator in critically ill patient. Anaesthesia, 42:980, 1987.
90. Gale, A.S.: Ketamine prevention of penile turgescence. J.A.M.A., 219:629, 1972.

90a. Nieder, R.M.: Ketamine treatment of priapism. J.A.M.A., 221:195, 1972.
91. Pietras, J.R., Cromiw, W.J., and Duckett, J.W.: Ketamine as a detumescent during hypospadia repair. J. Urol., 121:654, 1979.
92. Hamann, R.A., and Cohen, P.J.: Anesthetic management of a patient with epidermolysis bullosa dystrophica. Anesthesiology, 34:389, 1971.
93. Lee, C., and Nagel, E.L.: Anesthetic management of a patient with recessive epidermolysis bullosa dystrophica. Anesthesiology, 43:122, 1971.
94. Islas, J.A., Astorga, J., and Laredo, M.: Epidural ketamine for control of postoperative pain. Anesth. Analg., 64:1161, 1985.
94a. Yaksh, T.L.: Spinal opiate analgesia: Characteristics and principles of action. Pain, 11:293, 1981.
95. O'Neill, A.A., et al.: Premedication for ketamine anesthesia: Phase I—the classic drugs. Anesthesiology, 51:475, 1972.
96. Coppel, D.L., Bovill, J.G., and Dundee, J.W.: The taming of ketamine. Anaesthesia, 28:293, 1973.
96a. Coppel, D.L., and Dundee, J.W.: Ketamine anaesthesia for cardiac catheterization. Anaesthesia, 27:25, 1972.
96b. Manners, J.M.: Anaesthesia for diagnostic procedures in cardiac disease. Br. J. Anaesth., 43:276, 1971.
97. Sinclair, M.B.: Ketamine combined with neuroleptanalgesia: A preliminary communication. Anaesthesia, 26:241, 1971.
98. Sadove, M.S., et al.: Clinical study of droperidol in the prevention of side effects of ketamine anesthesia. Anesth. Analg., 50:526, 1971.
99. Wulfsohn, N.L.: Ketamine dosage for induction based on lean body mass. Anesth. Analg., 51:299, 1972.
100. Dundee, J.W.: Ketamine: A preliminary report on its use as an induction agent. Lancet, 1:1370, 1970.
101. Gross, J.B., Caldwell, C.B., and Edwards, M.W.: Induction dose-response curves for midazolam and ketamine in premedication ASA Class III and IV patients. Anesth. Analg., 64:795, 1985.
102. White, P.B.: Use of continuous infusion versus intermittent bolus administration of fentanyl or ketamine during outpatient anesthesia. Anesthesiology, 59:294, 1983.
103. Lilburn, J.K., Dundee, J.W., and Moore, J.: Ketamine infusions: Observations on dosages and cardiovascular effect. Anaesthesia, 33:315, 1978.
104. Zsigmond, E.K., and Domino, E.T.: Ketamine: Clinical pharmacology, pharmacokinetics and current use. Anesthesiol. Rev., 7:13, 1980.
105. Wieber, J., et al.: Pharmacokinetics of ketamine in man. Anaesthetist, 24:260, 1975.
106. Domino, E.F., et al.: Ketamine kinetics in unmedicated and diazepam premedicated subjects. Clin. Pharmacol. Ther., 36:645, 1984.
106a. Domino, E.F.: Effects of urine acidification on plasma and urine epinephrine levels. Clin. Pharmacol. Therap., 22:421, 1977.
107. Idvall, J., et al.: Ketamine infusions: Pharmacokinetics and clinical effects. Br. J. Anaesth., 51:1167, 1979.
108. Little, B., et al.: Study of ketamine as an obstetric anesthetic agent. Am. J. Obstet. Gynecol., 113:247, 1972.
108a. Chang, T., et al.: Metabolic disposition of tritium labeled ketamine (Kelalar: CI 581) in normal human subjects. Clin. Res., 18:597, 1970.
109. Cohen, M.L., et al.: Distribution in the brain and metabolism of ketamine in the rat after intravenous administration. Anesthesiology, 39:370, 1973.
110. Reynolds, D.C.: Detection of phencyclidines. Clin. Toxicol., 9:547, 1976.
110a. Chang, T., and Glazko, J.: A gas chromatographic assay for ketamine. Br. J. Anaesth., 51:835, 1979.
111. White, P.F., et al.: Pharmacology of ketamine isomers in surgical patients. Anesthesiology, 52:231, 1980.
112. Grant, I.S., et al.: Ketamine disposition in children and adults. Br. J. Anaesth., 55:1109, 1983.
113. Schultetus, R.R., Paulus, D.A., and Spohr, G.L.: Haemodynamic effects of ketamine and thiopentone during anaesthetic induction caesarean section. Can. Anaesth. Soc. J., 32:592, 1985.
114. Dundee, J.W., and Lilburn, J.K.: Attenuation of psychic sequelae of ketamine by lorazepam. Anaesthesia, 33:312, 1978.
115. Brice, D.D., Hetherington, R.R., and Utting, J.E.: A simple study of awareness and dreaming during anaesthesia. Br. J. Anaesth., 42:535, 1970.
116. Lilburn, J.K.: et al.: Ketamine sequelae. Anaesthesia, 33:307, 1978.
117. Smaessaert, A., Scher, C.A., and Artusio, J.R., Jr.: Observations in the immediate postanaesthesia period. II: Mode of recovery. Br. J. Anaesth., 32:181, 1960.
118. Fine, T., and Firestone, S.C.: Sensory disturbances following ketamine anaesthesia: Recurrent hallucinations. Anesthesiology, 52:420, 1973.
119. Eckenhoff, J.E., Kneale, D.H., and Dripps, R.D.: The incidence and etiology of postanesthetic excitement. Anesthesiology, 22:667, 1961.
120. Sklar, G.S., Zukin, S., and Rand Reilly, T.A.: Adverse reactions to ketamine anesthesia: Abolition by psychologic technique. Anaesthesia, 36:183, 1981.
121. Kothary, S.P., and Zsigmond, E.K.: Prevention of ketamine-induced psychic sequelae by diazepam. Clin. Pharmacol. Ther., 17:238, 1975.
122. Cartwright, P.D., and Pingel, S.M.: Midazolam and diazepam in ketamine anaesthesia. Anaesthesia, 38:439, 1984.
123. Becsey, L., et al.: Reduction of the psychomimetic and circulatory side-effects of ketamine by droperidol. Anesthesiology, 37:536, 1972.
124. White, P.F.: Comparative evaluation of intravenous agents for rapid sequence induction. Anesthesiology, 57:279, 1982.
124a. Mahisekar, U., Collins, V.J., and Vieira, Z.: Ketamine and vecuronium mixture for rapid sequence induction. In Domino, E.F.: Symposium on Ketamine 25th Anniversary Ed. Ann Arbor Univ. of Michigan Department Pharmacology, N.P. Publisher, 1989.
125. Moretti, R.J., et al.: Comparison of ketamine and thiopental in healthy volunteers: Effects on mental status, mood, and personality. Anesth. Analg., 63:1087, 1984.
126. Gal, T.J., and Malit, L.A.: The influence of ketamine induction on potassium changes and fasciculations following suxamethonium. Br. J. Anaesth., 44:1077, 1972.
127. Dundee, J.W., and Keeilty, S.R.: Diazepam. Int. Anesthesiol. Clin., 7:91, 1969.
127a. Dundee, J.W., et al.: Studies on drugs given before anesthesia XX: diazepam-containing mixtures. Br. J. Anaesth., 42:143, 1970.
128. Fox, G.S., Wynands, J.E., and Bhambhani, M.: A clinical comparison of diazepam and thiopentone as induction agents to general anaesthesia. Can. Anaesth. Soc. J., 15:281, 1968.
129. Chusid, J.G., and Kopeloff, L.M.: Diazepam as anti-convulsant in epileptic and normal monkeys. Fed. Proc., 20:322, 1961.

130. Brandt, A.L., and Oakes, F.D.: Preanaesthesia medication: Double-blind study of a new drug diazepam. Anesth. Analg., 44:125, 1965.
131. Barrett, J., Smyth, W.F., and Davidson, I.E.: An examination of acid-base equilibria of 1,4-benzodiazepines. J. Pharm. Pharmacol., 25:287, 1973.
132. Matilla, M.A.K., et al.: Reduction of venous sequelae of intravenous diazepam with a fat emulsion as a solvent. Br. J. Anaesth., 53:1265, 1981.
133. Costa, E., et al.: New concepts on the mechanism of action of benzodiazepines. Life Sci., 17:167, 1975.
134. Mohler, H., and Okada, T.: Benzodiazepine receptor: Demonstration in the central nervous system. Science, 198:849, 1977.
135. Tallman, J.F., et al.: Receptors for the age of anxiety and pharmacology of the benzodiazepines. Science, 207:274, 1980.
136. Assaf, R.A.E., Dundee, J.W., and Gamble, J.A.S.: The influence of route of administration on clinical action of diazepam. Anaesthesia, 30:152, 1975.
136a. Package insert. Valium injectable (diazepam) Roche. Hoffman-LaRoche, Nutley, N.J., 1983.
137. Mattila, M.A.K., et al.: Diazepam in rectal solutions as premedications in children with special reference to serum concentrations. Br. J. Anaesth., 53:1269, 1981.
137a. Mark, L.C.: The "puff-technique" for IV diazepam. Anesthesiology, 61:631, 1984.
138. Rosht, C.E.: Diazepam fentanyl interaction. Anesth. Analg., 62:821, 1983.
139. Greenblatt, I.J., et al.: Diazepam disposition determinants. Clin. Pharmacol. Ther., 27:301, 1980.
140. Sellers, E.M., et al.: Chlordiazepoxide, oxazepam disposition cirrhosis. Clin. Pharmacol. Ther., 26:240, 1979.
141. Klotz, U., et al.: Disposition of diazepam and its major metabolic desmethyldiazepam in patients with liver disease. Clin. Pharmacol. Ther., 21:430, 1977.
142. Klotz, U., et al.: The effect of age and liver disease on disposition and elimination of diazepam in adult man. J. Clin. Invest., 55:347, 1975.
142a. MacLeod, S.M., et al.: Age- and gender-related differences in diazepam pharmacokinetics. J. Clin. Pharmacol., 19:15, 1979.
143. Ochs, H.R., et al.: Diazepam kinetics in chronic renal failure. Clin. Pharmacol. Ther., 29:270, 1981.
143a. Schwartz, M.A., et al.: Metabolism of diazepam in rat, dog, and man. J. Pharmacol. Exp. Therap., 149:423, 1965.
143b. Reves, J.G.: Benzodiazepines. In Pharmacokinetics in anesthesia. Edited by C. Prys-Roberts and C.C. Hug. Oxford, England, Blackwell, 1984.
144. Ghoneim, M.M., et al.: Diazepam effects and kinetics in caucasians and orientals. Clin. Pharmacol. Ther., 29:757, 1981.
145. Nakano, S., et al.: Circadian stage-dependent changes in diazepam kinetics. Clin. Pharmacol. Ther., 36:271, 1984.
146. Baraldi, M., et al.: GABA receptors in clonal cell lines. Science, 205:821, 1979.
147. Fuxe, K., Agnati, A., and Bolme, D.: The possible involvement of GABA mechanisms in action of benzodiazepines. Psychopharmacol. Bull., 11:55, 1975.
148. Greenblatt, D.J., and Shader, R.: Benzodiazepines. N. Engl. J. Med., 291:1011, 1974.
149. Carlsson, C., et al.: The effects of diazepam on cerebral blood flow and oxygen consumption in rats and its synergestic action with nitrous oxide. Anesthesiology, 45:319, 1976.
149a. Smith, A.L., and Wollman, H.: Cerebral blood flow and metabolism: Effects of anesthetic drugs and techniques. Anesthesiology, 36:378, 1972.
150. Groves, N.D., Rees, J.L., and Rosen, M.: Effects of benzodiazepines on laryngeal reflexes: Comparison of lormetazepam and diazepam. Anaesthesia, 42:808, 1987.
151. Rao, S., et al.: Cardiopulmonary effects of diazepam. Clin. Pharmacol. Ther., 14:182, 1973.
152. Ikram, H., Rubin, A.P., and Jewkes, R.F.: Effect of diazepam on myocardial blood flows of patients with and without coronary artery disease. Br. Heart J., 35:626, 1973.
153. Brown, S.S., and Dundee, J.W.: Clinical studies of induction agents. XXV. Diazepam. Br. J. Anaesth., 40:108, 1968.
154. Katz, N., Fineston, S.C., and Pappas, M.: Circulatory response to tilting after intravenous diazepam in volunteers. Anesth. Analg., 46:243, 1967.
155. Stanley, T.H., Bennett, G.M., and Loeber, E.E.: Cardiovascular effects of diazepam and droperidol during morphine anesthesia. Anesthesiology, 44:255, 1976.
156. Stanley, T.H., and Webster, L.R.: Anesthetic requirements and cardiovascular effects of fentanyl-oxygen and fentanyl-diazepam-oxygen anesthesia in man. Anesth. Analg., 57:411, 1978.
157. Dalen, J.E., et al.: The hemodynamic and respiratory effects of diazepam. Anesthesiology, 30:259, 1969.
158. Catchlove, P.F.H., and Kafer, E.R.: The effects of diazepam on respiration in patients with obstructive pulmonary disease. Anesthesiology, 34:14, 1971.
159. Pierce, A.K., et al.: Respiratory function during sleep in patients with chronic obstructive lung disease. J. Clin. Invest., 45:631, 1966.
160. Cottrell, J.E., Wolfson, B., and Siker, E.S.: Changes in airway resistance following droperidol and diazepam in normal volunteers. Anesth. Analg., 55:18, 1976.
161. Jordan, C., Lehane, J.R., and Jones, J.G.: Respiratory depression following diazepam. Anesthesiology, 23:293, 1980.
161a. Lakshminarayan, S. et al.: Effect of diazepam on ventilatory responses. Clin. Pharmacol. Ther., 20:178, 1976.
161b. Bailey, P.L., et al.: Variability of the respiratory response to diazepam. Anesthesiology, 64:460, 1986.
162. Kerkkola, R., and Kangas, L.: The transfer of diazepam across the placenta during labor. Acta Obstet. Gynecol. Scand., 52:167, 1973.
163. Ngai, S.H., Teng, D.T.C., and Wang, S.C.: Effect of diazepam and other central nervous system depressants on spinal reflexes in cats: A study of site of action. J. Pharmacol. Exp. Ther., 153:344, 1966.
163a. Nathan, P.W.: The action of diazepam in neurological disorders with excessive motor activity. J. Neurol. Sci., 10:33, 1970.
163b. Schlosser, L.: Action of diazepam on the spinal cord. Arch. Int. Pharmacodyn. Ther., 194:93, 1971.
164. Feldman, S.A., and Carwley, B.F.: Interaction of diazepam with muscle relaxants. Br. Med. J., 2:336, 1970.
165. Raza, S.M.A., et al.: Diazepam causes no adverse cardio-circulatory effects in cardiac patients. Clin. Ther., 9:629, 1987.
166. Kumar, S.M., Kothary, S.P., and Zsigmond, E.K.: Plasma free norepinephrine and epinephrine concentrations following diazepam-ketamine induction in patients undergoing cardiac surgery. Acta Anaesthesiol. Scand., 22:593, 1978.
167. Healy, T.E.J., Robinson, J.S., and Vickers, M.D.: Physiological responses to intravenous diazepam as a sedative for conservative dentistry. Br. Med. J., 3:10, 1970.
167a. Waterman, P.H., et al.: The effective use in bronchoscopy. Ann. Otol. Rhinol. Laryngol., 78:499, 1969.

168. Sellers, E.M., et al.: Intravenous diazepam and oral ethanol interaction. Clin. Pharmacol. Ther., 28:638, 1988.
169. Bidwai, A.V., et al.: Reversal of diazepam-induced postanesthetic somnolence with physostigmine. Anesthesiology, 51:256, 1979.
169a. Ruprecht, J., and Dworacek, B.: Central anticholinergic syndrome in anesthesia practice. Acta Anaesthesiol. Belg., 2:45, 1976.
170. Baraka, A.: Personal communication. 1984.
170a. Westra, P., et al.: Pharmacokinetics of galanthamine (a long-lasting anticholinesterase drug) in anesthetized patients. Br. J. Anaesth., 58:1303, 1986.
171. Stirt, J.A.: Aminophylline is a diazepam antagonist. Anesth. Analg., 60:767, 1981.
172. Greenblatt, D.J., et al.: Clinical importance of the interaction of diazepam and cimetidine. N. Engl. J. Med., 310:1639, 1984.
173. Lauven, P.M., et al.: Effects of a benzodiazepine antagonist RO 15-1788. Anesthesiology, 63:61, 1985.
174. O'Hanlon, J.F., et al.: Diazepam impairs lateral position control in highway driving. Science, 217:79, 1982.
175. Cope, D.K., et al.: Diazepam-associated posttraumatic stress reaction. Anesth. Analg., 66:666, 1987.
176. Kawar, P., and Dundee, J.W.: Frequency of pain on injection and venous sequelae following intravenous administration of certain anesthetics and sedatives. Br. J. Anaesth., 54:935, 1982.
177. Hegarty, J., and Dundee, J.W.: Thrombophlebitis incidence after intravenous injection of three benzodiazepines-diazepam lorazepam and flunitrazepam. Br. Med. J., 2:1384, 1977.
178. Greenblatt, D.J., et al.: Acute overdosage with benzodiazepine derivatives. Clin. Pharmacol. Ther., 21:497, 1977.
179. Bell, E.F.: The use of naloxone in the treatment of diazepam poisoning. J. Pediatr., 87:803, 1975.
180. Diliberti, J., O'Brien, M.L., and Turner, T.: The use of physostigmine as an antidote in accidental diazepam intoxication. J. Pediatr., 86:106, 1975.
181. Ruprecht, J.: Physostigmine reversal of diazepam. Anesthesiology, 53:180, 1980.
182. Avant, G.R., et al.: Physostigmine reversal of diazepam-induced hypnosis: A study of human volunteers. Ann. Intern. Med., 91:53, 1979.
183. Mohler, H., and Okada, T.: Benzodiazepine receptor: Demonstration in the central nervous system. Science, 198:849, 1977.
184. O'Sullivan, G.F., and Wade, D.N.: Flumazenil in the management of acute drug overdosage with benzodiazepines and other agents. Clin. Pharmacol. Ther., 42:254, 1987.
185. Ameer, B.O., and Greenblatt, D.J.: Lorazepam: A review of its clinical pharmacological properties and therapeutic uses. Drugs, 21:161, 1981.
186. Dundee, J.W., et al.: Comparison of the actions of diazepam and lorazepam. Br. J. Anaesth., 51:439, 1979.
187. Bradshaw, E.G., et al.: Plasma concentrations and clinical effects of lorazepam after oral administration. Br. J. Anaesth., 52:517, 1981.
188. Elliott, H.W.: Metabolism of lorazepam. Br. J. Anaesth., 48:1017, 1976.
189. Johanson, C.E., and Uhlenhuth, E.H.: Drug preference and mood in humans on diazepam. Psychopharmacology, 71:269, 1980.
190. George, K.A., and Dundee, J.W.: Relative amnesic actions of diazepam, flunitrazepam and lorazepam in man. Br. J. Clin. Pharmacol., 4:45, 1977.
191. Conner, J.T., et al.: Evaluation of lorazepam and pentobarbital as surgical premedicants. J. Pharmacol. Ther., 19:24, 1976.
192. Pandit, S., Heisterkamp, D.V., and Cohen, P.J.: Further studies of the anti-recall effect of lorazepam. Anesthesiology, 45:495, 1976.
193. Greenblatt, D.J., et al.: Pharmacokinetics and bioavailability of intravenous, intramuscular and oral lorazepam in humans. J. Pharm. Sci., 68:57, 1979.
193a. Greenblatt, D.J., et al.: Clinical pharmacokinetics of lorazepam. IV. Long-term oral administration. J. Clin. Pharmacol., 17:495, 1977.
194. Griffiths, R.R., et al.: Drug preference in humans: Double-blind choice comparison of pentobarbital, diazepam and placebo. J. Pharmacol. Exp. Ther., 215:649, 1980.
194a. Wangler, W.A., and Kilpatrick, D.S.: Aminophylline is an antagonist of lorazepam. Anesth. Analg., 64:834, 1985.
195. Dundee, J.W., Samuel, I.O., and Toner, W.: Midazolam: A water-soluble benzodiazepine. Anaesthesia, 35:454, 1980.
195a. Walser, A.: Literature review of RO 21-3981. Basel, Roche Laboratories, Hoffman-LaRoche, 1977–78.
195b. Stanski, D.R., and Watkins, W.D.: Drug Disposition in Anesthesia. New York, Grune & Stratton, 1982.
195c. Sarnquist, F.H., et al.: A bioassay of a water-soluble benzodiazepine against sodium thiopental. Anesthesiology, 42:149, 1980.
196. Dundee, J.W., and Wilson, D.B.: Amnesic action of midazolam. Anaesthesia, 35:459, 1980.
196a. George, K.A., Dundee, J.W.: Relative amnesic actions of diazepam, flunitrazepam, and lorazepam in man. Br. J. Clin. Pharm., 4:45, 1977.
197. Reinhart, K., et al.: Comparison of midazolam, diazepam and placebo i.m. as premedication for regional anaesthesia. Br. J. Anaesth., 57:294, 1985.
198. Reves, J.G., Kissin, I., and Smith, L.R.: The effective dose of midazolam. Anesthesiology, 55:82, 1981.
199. Caldwell, C.M., and Gross, J.B.: Physostigmine reversal of midazolam-induced sedation. Anesthesiology, 57:125, 1982.
200. Leibowitz, P.W., et al.: Comparative cardiovascular effects of midazolam and thiopental in health patients (PS I and II). Anesth. analg., 61:771, 1983.
201. Marty, J., et al.: Effects of midazolam on the coronary circulation in patients with coronary artery disease. Anesthesiology, 64:206, 1986.
202. Samuelson, P.N., et al.: Hemodynamic responses to anesthetic induction with midazolam or diazepam in patients with ischemic heart disease. Anesth. Analg., 60:802, 1981.
203. Crozier, T.A., et al.: Endocrinological changes following etomidate, midazolam, or methohexital. Anesthesiology, 66:628, 1987.
204. Tassonyl, E.: Effects of midazolam on neuromuscular block. Pharmatherapeutica, 3:678, 1984.
205. Fletcher, J.E., Rosenberg, H., and Hilf, M.: Effects of midazolam on directly stimulated muscle biopsies from control and malignant hyperthermia positive patients. Can. Anaesth. Soc., J., 31:377, 1984.
206. Crevoisier, C., et al.: Relation entre l'effet clinique et la pharmacocinetique du midazolam apres l'administration i.v. et i.m. 2e communication: Aspects pharmacocinetiques. Arzneim Forsch, 21:2245, 1981.
207. Nugent, M., Artru, A.A., and Michenfelder, J.D.: Cerebral effects of midazolam. Anesthesiology, 53:5, 1980.
208. Fragen, R.L., Gahl, F., and Caldwell, N.: A water-soluble benzodiazepine, RO 21-3981, for induction of anesthesia. Anesthesiology, 49:41, 1978.
209. Gross, J.B., Caldwell, C.B., and Edwards, M.W.: Induction

dose-response curves for midazolam and ketamine in premedicated ASA class III and IV patients. Anesth. Analg., 64:795, 1985.
210. Kanto, J., et al.: Midazolam as an intravenous induction agent in the elderly: A clinical and pharmacokinetic study. Anesth. Analg., 65:15, 1986.
210a. Dundee, J.W., et al.: The influence of age on the onset of anaesthesia with midazolam. Anaesthesia, 40:441, 1985.
211. Reitan, J.A., and Soliman, I.E.: Comparison of midazolam and diazepam for induction of anesthesia in high risk patients (abstract). Anesthesiology, 59:A378, 1983.
212. Gross, J.B., et al.: Time course of ventilatory depression after thiopental and midazolam in normal subjects and in patients with chronic obstructive pulmonary disease. Anesthesiology, 58:540, 1983.
212a. Forster, A., et al.: Respiratory depression by midazolam and diazepam. Anesthesiology, 53:494, 1980.
212b. Alexander, C.M., and Gross, J.B.: Sedative doses of midazolam depress hypoxic ventilatory responses in humans. Anesth. Analg., 67:377, 1988.
213. Brown, C.R., et al.: Clinical, electroencephalographic, and pharmacokinetic studies of a water-soluble benzodiazepine, midazolam maleate. Anesthesiology, 50:467, 1979.
214. Greenblatt, D.J., et al.: Automated gas chromatograph for studies of midazolam pharmacokinetics. Anesthesiology, 55:176, 1981.
215. Allonen, H., Ziegler, G., and Klotz, U.: Midazolam kinetics. Clin. Pharm. Ther., 30:653, 1981.
216. Hillestad, L., et al.: Diazepam metabolism in normal man. Clin. Pharmacol. Ther., 16:479, 1974.
217. Klotz, U., and Ziegler, G.: Physiologic and temporal variation in hepatic elimination of midazolam. Clin. Pharm. Ther., 32:107, 1982.
218. Avram, M.J., Fragen, R.J., and Caldwell, N.J.: Midazolam kinetics in women of two age groups. Clin. Pharm. Ther., 34:505, 1983.
219. Greenblatt, D.J., et al.: Effect of age, gender and obesity on midazolam kinetics. Anesthesiology, 61:27, 1984.
219a. Collier, P.S. et al.: Influence of age on pharmacokinetics of midazolam. Br. J. Clin. Pharmacol., 13:602, 1981.
220. Shelly, M.P., Mendel, L., and Park, G.R.: Failure of critically ill patients to metabolize midazolam. Anaesthesia, 42:619, 1987.
221. Reves, J.G., Newfeld, P., and Smith, L.R.: Midazolam induction time: Association with serum albumin (abstract). Anesthesiology, 155:A259, 1981.
222. Halliday, N.J., et al.: Influence of plasma proteins on the onset of hypnotic action of intravenous midazolam. Anaesthesia, 40:763, 1985.
223. Woo, G.K., Kolis, S.J., and Schwartz, M.A.: In vitro metabolism of an imidazobenzodiazepine. Pharmacologists, 19:164, 1977.
224. Gerecke, M.: Chemical structure and properties of midazolam compared with other benzodiazepines. Br. J. Clin. Pharmacol., 16:11S, 1983.
224a. Smith, M.T., Eadie, M.J., and Brophy, T.O'R.: The pharmacokinetics of midazolam in man. European J. Clin. Pharmacol., 19:271, 1981.
225. Goulding, R.R., Helliwell, P.J., and Jerr, A.C.: Sedation of children as outpatients for dental operations under general anesthesia. Br. Med. J. 2:855, 1977.
225a. Rita, L., et al.: Intramuscular midazolam for pediatric preanesthetic sedation: A double-blind controlled study with morphine. Anesthesiology, 63:528, 1985.
226. Booker, P.D., et al.: Sedation of children requiring artificial ventilation using an infusion of midazolam. Br. J. Anaesth., 58:1104, 1986.
227. Lloyd-Thomas, A.R., and Booker, P.D.: Infusion of midazolam in pediatric patients after cardiac surgery. Br. J. Anaesth., 58:1109, 1986.
228. Selye, H.: Anesthetic effect of steroid hormones. Proc. Soc. Exper. Biol. Med., 46:116, 1941.
229. Selye, H.: Studies concerning anesthetic action of steroid hormones. J. Pharmacol. Exp. Ther., 73:127, 1941.
230. Selye, H.: Acquired adaptation to anesthetic effect of steroid hormones. J. Immunol., 41:259, 1941.
231. Selye, H.: Correlations between chemical structure and pharmacological actions of steroids. Endocrinology, 30:437, 1942.
232. Selye, H.: Studies concerning correlation between anesthetic potency, hormonal activity and chemical structure among steroid compounds. Anesth. Analg., 21:41, 1942.
233. Selye, H., and Heard, R.D.H.: Fish assay for anesthetic effect of steroids. Anesthesiology, 4:36, 1943.
234. Selye, H., and Stone, H.: Studies concerning the absorption and detoxification of anesthetic steroids. J. Pharmacol. Exp. Ther., 4:386, 1944.
235. Farson, De C.B., Carr, C.J., and Krants, J.C., Jr.: Anesthesia and steroid hormones. Proc. Soc. Exper. Biol. Med., 63:70, 1946.
236. Hoeffer, P.F., and Glaser, G.H.: Effect of pituitary adrenocorticotropic hormones therapy: Electroencephalographic and neuropsychiatric changes in fifteen patients. J.A.M.A., 142:620, 1950.
237. Laubach, G.D., Pan, S.Y., and Rudel, H.W.: Steroid anesthetic agent. Science, 122:78, 1955.
238. Gordon, G.S., et al.: Steroid anesthesia in man: Clinical and cerebral metabolic effects. J. Int. Coll. Surg., 25:9, 1956.
239. Murphy, F.J., Guadagni, N., and DeBon, F.L.: Use of steroid anesthesia in surgery. J.A.M.A., 156:1412, 1955.
240. Gordon, R.A., Lunderville, C.W.P., and Scott, J.W.: Clinical investigation of Viadril. Can. Anaesth. J., 3:335, 1956.
241. Gardock, J.F., P'an, S.Y., and Brown, J.: Hormonal activity of hydroxydione. Endocrinology, 59:129, 1956.
242. Jakoby, W.B., and Tomkins, G.: Enzymatic detoxification mechanism of Viadril. Science, 123:940, 1956.
243. Ansbro, F.P., et al.: Clinical results with Viadril in one thousand cases. J.A.M.A., 164:163, 1957.
244. Howland, W.S., Boyan, C.P., and Wang, K.C.: Use of steroid (Viadril) as anesthetic agent. Anesthesiology, 17:1, 1956.
245. Belleville, J.W., Howland, W.S., and Boyan, C.P.: Comparison of electroencephalographic patterns during steroid and barbiturate narcosis. Br. J. Anaesth., 28:50, 1956.
246. Schneider, J., and Baumgartner, J.: Sleep induced by Viadril and its electroencephalographic patterns. Anesth. Analg., 13:258, 1956.
247. Burstein, C.L.: Utility of Viadril in anesthesia. Anesth. Analg., 35:476, 1956.
248. Mayer, H.D., Cave, H.G., and Burstein, C.L.: Clinical experience with hydroxydione: A new intravenous anesthetic. N.Y. State Med. J., 56:3494, 1956.
249. Montgomery, F.A., et al.: Evaluation of cardiovascular respiratory and general pharmacologic properties of hydroxydione. Anesthesiology, 19:450, 1958.
250. Clarke, R.S.J., et al.: Clinical studies of induction agent XXIX, CT-1341: A new steroid anaesthetic. Br. J. Anaesth., 43:947, 1971.
251. Campbell, D., et al.: A preliminary clinical study of CT-1341—A steroid anaesthetic agent. Br. J. Anaesth., 43:14, 1971.

251a. Tarnow, J., Hess, W., Klein, W.: Etomidate, althesin and thiopental as induction agents for coronary artery surgery. Can. Anaesth. Soc. J., 27:338, 1980.
252. Janssen, P.A.J., et al.: Etomidate, R-(+)-ethyl-1 (alpha-methyl-benzyl) imidazole-5-carboxylate (R 16 659), a potent, short-acting and relatively atoxic intravenous hypnotic agent in rats. Arzneimittelforschung, 21:1234, 1971.
253. Rememan, R.S., and Janssen, D.A.J.: Experimental pharmacology of etomidate. Beerse, Belgium, Janssen Pharmaceutica, 1974.
254. Fragen, R.J., Caldwell, N., and Brunner, E.A.: Clinical use of etomidate for anesthesia induction: A preliminary report. Anesth. Analg., 55:730, 1976.
255. Dundee, J.W., and Wyant, G.M.: Intravenous Anesthesia. 2nd ed. Churchill Livingstone Edinburgh, 1988.
256. Ambre, J.J., et al.: Pharmacokinetics of etomidate, a new intravenous anesthetic. Fed. Proc., 36:997, 1977.
257. Heykants, J.J.P., et al.: Distribution, metabolism and excretion of etomidate, a short-acting hypnotic drug, in the rat. Comparative study of (R)-(+) and (S)-(−) etomidate. Archives Internationales de Pharmacodynamic et de Therapie, 216:113, 1975.
258. Ghoneim, M.M., and Van Hamme, M.J.: Hydrolysis of etomidate. Anesthesiology, 50:227, 1979.
259. Meuldermans, W.E.G., and Heykants, J.J.P.: The plasma protein binding and distribution of etomidate in dog, rat and human blood. Arch. Int. Pharmacodyn. Ther., 221:150, 1976.
260. Van Hamme, M.J., Ghoneim, M.M., and Ambre, J.J.: Pharmacokinetics of etomidate, a new intravenous anesthetic. Anesthesiology, 49:274, 1978.
261. Shuttler, J. et al.: Alterations of the pharmacokinetics of etomidate caused by fentanyl. Anaesthesia, Volume of summaries, Sixth European Congress of Anaesthesiology, London, 1982, Abstract 700, p 368.
262. Hill, R.G., and Taberner, P.V.: Some neuropharmacological properties of the new non-barbiturate hypnotic etomidate (R)+)-ethyl-1-(alpha-methyl-benzyl) imidazole-5-carboxylate). Br. J. Pharmacol., 54:241p, 1975.
263. Gooding, J.M., and Corssen, G.: Etomidate: An ultrashort-acting nonbarbiturate agent for anesthesia induction. Anesth. Analg., 55:286, 1976.
264. Ibrahim, Z.Y., et al.: Effect of etomidate on the electroencephalogram of patients with epilepsy. Anesth. Analg., 65:1004, 1986.
265. Kissin, I., Montomura, A., Ultman, D.F., Reves, S.G.: Inotropic and anesthetic potencies of etomidate and thiopental in dogs. Anesth. Analg., 62:961, 1983.
265a. Komai, H., DeWitt, D.E., and Rusy, B.F.: Negative inotropic effect of etomidate in rabbit papillary muscle. Anesth. Analg., 64:400, 1985.
266. Inoue, K., and Arndt, J.O.: Efferent vagal discharge and heart rate in response to methohexitone, Althesin, ketamine and etomidate in cats. Br. J. Anaesth., 54:1105, 1982.
267. Inoue, K., and Reichelt, W.: Asystole and bradycardia in adult patients after a single dose of suxamethonium. Acta Anaesthesiol. Scand., 30:571, 1986.
268. Cold, G.E., et al.: CBF and CMR_{O_2} during continuous etomidate infusion supplemented with N_2O and fentanyl in patients with supratentorial cerebral tumor: A dose-response study. Acta Anaesthesiol. Scand., 29:490, 1985.
269. Altenburg, B.E., Michenfelder, J.D., and Theye, R.A.: Acute tolerance to thiopental in canine cerebral oxygen consumption. Anesthesiology, 31:443, 1969.
270. Michenfelder, J.: Intelligence reports in anesthesia (commentary). 4:11, 1986.
271. Longnecker, D.E.: Stress free: To be or not to be (editorial). Anesthesiology, 61:643, 1984.
272. Fragen, R.J., et al.: Effects of etomidate on hormonal responses to surgical stress. Anesthesiology, 61:652, 1984.
273. Wagner, R.L., and White, P.F.: Etomidate inhibits adrenocortical function in surgical patients. Anesthesiology, 61:647, 1984.
274. Wagner, R.L., et al.: Inhibition of adrenal steroidogenesis by the anesthetic etomidate. N. Engl. J. Med. 310:1415, 1984.
274a. Wagner, R.L., and White, P.F.: Etomidate inhibits Adrenocortical function in Surgical patients. Anesthesiology, 61:647, 1984.
275. Duthie, D.J.R., Fraser, R., and Nimmo, S.W.: Effect of induction of anaesthesia with etomidate on corticosteroid synthesis in man. Br. J. Anaesth., 57:156, 1985.
276. Owen, H., and Spence, A.A.: Etomidate. Br. J. Anaesth., 56:555, 1984.
277. McDowall, D.G.: Etomidate. Lancet, 2:168, 1985.
278. Suresh, M.S., and Nelson, T.E.: Malignant hyperthermia: Is etomidate safe? Anesth. Analg., 64:420, 1985.
279. Gancher, S., Laxer, K.O., and Krieger, W.: Activation of epileptogenic activity by etomidate. Anesthesiology, 61:616, 1984.
280. Kettler, D., et al: Clinical studies on etomidate. Der Anesthetist 23:116, 1974.
281. Kortilla, K., and Aromaa, U.: Venous complications after intravenous injection of diazepam, flunitrazepam, thiopental and etomidate. Acta Anaesthesiol. Scand., 24:227, 1980.
282. Crozier TA, Beck, D, Schlaeger M, et al: Endocrinological changes following etomidate, midazolam, or methohexital. Anesthesiology, 66:628, 1987.
282a. Moore, R.A., et al.: Perioperative endocrine effects of etomidate. Anaesthesia, 40:124, 1985.
283. James, R., and Glen, J.B.: Synthesis, biological evaluation and preliminary structure-activity considerations of a series of alkylphenols as intravenous anaesthetic agents. J. Med. Chem., 23:1350, 1980.
284. Glen, J.B.: Animal studies of the anaesthetic activity of ICI 35 868. Br. J. Anaesth., 52:731, 1980.
285. Kay, B., and Rolly, G.: ICI 35 868, a new intravenous induction agent. Acta Anaesth. Belg., 28:303, 1977.
286. Briggs, L.P., et al.: Use of diisopropylphenol as main agent for short procedures. Br. J. Anaesth., 53:1197, 1981.
287. Briggs, L.P., and Watkins, J.: An adverse reaction to the administration of disoprofol (Diprivan). Anaesthesia, 37:1099, 1982.
288. Clarke, R.S.J., et al.: Adverse reactions to intravenous anaesthetics: A survey of 100 reports. Br. J. Anaesth., 47:575, 1975.
289. Glen, J.B., and Hunter, S.C.: Pharmacology of an emulsion formation of ICI 35 868. Br. J. Anaesth., 56:617, 1984.
289a. Fragen, R.J.: Diprivan (propofol): A historical perspective. Semin. Anesth., VII (No. 1; Suppl. 1): 1–3, 1988.
290. Dundee, J.W., et al.: Sensitivity to propofol in elderly. Anaesthesia, 41:482, 1986.
291. Cummings, G.C., et al.: Dose requirements for ICI 35, 868 (propofol, Diprivan) in a new formulation for induction of anaesthesia. Anaesthesia, 39:1168, 1984.
292. Youngberg, J.A., et al.: Workshop II overview: The use of Diprivan (propofol) in procedures longer than one hour. Semin. Anesthesia, (Suppl. 1)7:62, 1988.
293. Sear, J.W., et al.: Infusions of propofol to supplement nitrous oxide–oxygen for maintenance of anaesthesia. Anaesthesia, (Suppl.)43:18, 1988.
294. White, P.F.: Propofol: Pharmacokinetics and pharmacodynamics. Semin. Anesthesia, (Suppl. 1)7:4, 1988.

294a. Mirakhur, R.K. and Shepherd, W.F.I.: Intraocular pressure changes with propofol-a comparison with thiopental. Postgrad. Med. J., (Suppl. 3)61:62, 1985.
295. Gepts, E., et al.: Disposition of propofol administered as constant rate infusions in humans. Anesth. Analg., 66:1256, 1987.
296. Fong Sung, Y., Weinstein, M.S., and Biddle, M.R.: Comparison of Diprivan (propofol) and thiopental as intravenous induction agents: Cardiovascular effects, respiratory changes, recovery, and postoperative venous sequelae. Semin. Anesthesia, (Suppl. 1)7:52, 1988.
297. Gauthier, M., Hemmings, G.T., and Bevan, D.R.: A comparison of Diprivan (propofol) and thiopental for induction of anesthesia. Semin. Anesthesia, (Suppl. 1)7:44, 1988.
297a. Youngberg, J.A., and Grogona, A.W.: Comparative evaluation of diprivan, thiopental and thiamylal for induction of anesthesia. Anesthesiology, 63:A365, 1985.
297b. Boer, F., et al.: Effect of propofol on peripheral vascular resistance during cardiopulmonary bypass. Br. J. Anaesth., 65:184, 1990.
298. Coetzee, A., et al.: Effect of various propofol plasma concentrations on regional myocardial contractility and left ventricular afterload. Anesth. Analg., 69:473, 1989.
298a. Morgan, M., and Lunn, J.M.: Experiences with propofol. Anaesthesia, (Suppl.)43, 1988.
299. Baraka, A.: Severe bradycardia following propofol-suxamethonium sequence. Br. J. Anaesth., 61:482, 1988.
300. Cullen, P.M., et al.: Effect of propofol anesthesia on baroreflex activity in humans. Anesth. Analg., 66:1115, 1987.
301. Skues, M.A., et al.: Pre-induction atropine or glycopyrrolate and hemodynamic changes associated with induction and maintenance of anesthesia with propofol and alfentanil. Anesth. Analg., 69:386, 1989.
302. Coates, D.P., et al.: Hemodynamic effects of infusions of the emulsion formulation of propofol during nitrous oxide anesthesia in humans. Anesth. Analg., 66:64, 1987.
303. Mulier, J.P., et al.: Cardiodynamic effects of propofol in comparison with thiopental: Assessment with a transesophageal echocardiographic approach. Anesth. Analg., 72:28, 1991.
304. McKeating, K., Bali, I.M., and Dundee, J.W.: The effects of thiopentone on upper airway integrity. Anaesthesia, 43:638, 1988.
305. Hynynen, M., Korttila, K., and Tammisto, T.: Pain on i.v. injection of propofol (ICI 35 868) in emulsion formulation: Short communication. Acta Anaesthesiol. Scand., 29:651, 1985.
306. McCallum, J.S.C., Milligan, K.R., and Dundee, J.W.: The anti-emetic action of propofol. Anaesthesia, 43:239, 1988.
307. Goodman, N.W., Black, A.M.S., and Carter, J.A.: Some ventilatory effects of propofol as a sole anaesthetic agent. Br. J. Anaesth., 59:1497, 1987.
308. Sebel, P.S., and Lowdon, J.D.: Propofol: A new intravenous anesthetic. Anesthesiology, 71:260, 1989.
309. Morton, N.S., et al.: Propofol for induction of anaesthesia in children: A comparison with thiopentone and halothane inhalational induction. Anaesthesia, 43:350, 1988.
310. Hiltman, R.: Reports on new synthetic intravenous drugs for anesthesia. Farbenfabriken Bayer, Leverkusen, 1961.
311. Raymon, F., Zahony, I., and Collins, V.J.: Bayer 1420: A Preliminary Report. Presented at Iowa Resident Midwest Meeting, May 1963.
312. Nishimura, N.: A preliminary report: A new intravenous non-barbiturate anesthetic. Anesth. Analg., 41:365, 1962.
313. Pallin, I.M., and Lear, E.: Acute toxicity studies with Bayer 1420. Presented at New York State Med. Soc. Meeting, February 11, 1964.
314. Putter, J.: Report on the enzymatic breakdown of Bayer 1420. Farbenfabriken Bayer, Leverkusen Reports, 1962.
315. Dundee, J.W. and Clarke, R.S.J.: Clinical studies of induction agents. I: A comparative study of a new eugenol derivative Br. J. Anaesth., 36:100, 1964.
316. Gordh, T.: Analysis of hyperventilation in propanidid anaesthesia, in Frey, R., Kern, F., and Mayrhofer, O., (eds). Anaesthesiology and Wiederbelebung. Berlin: Springer-Verlag, 1973, pp 131–136.
317. Soga, D., et al.: Die Beeinflussingdes linksventrikularen Myokardkontraktilat und Haemodynamick durch Propanidid beinttand in Anaestheiologie und Wiederbelebung. p. 27–39, ed. Frey, R., Kern, F., and Mayrhofer, O. Berlin: Springer-Verlag, 1973.
318. Howells, T.H., et al.: An introduction to FBA 1420: A new non-barbiturate intravenous anesthetic. Br. J. Anaesth., 36:295, 1964.
319. Dundee, J.W., and Clarke, R.S.J.: Observations of a new propanol derivative FBA 1420: Clinical studies of induction agents. Br. J. Anaesth., 39:236, 1967.
320. Dundee, J.W., and Wyant, G.M.: Intravenous Anaesthesia. 2nd Edition, Edinburgh, Churchill, 1988, pp 318–320.
321. Burkhardt, L.: Uber Chloroform und Athernarkose durch Intravenose Injektion. Arch. Exper. Path. Pharmakol., 61:323, 1909.
322. Butt, H., et al.: Oral and endoscopic survey using intravenous ether anesthetic. Anesthesiology, 44:186, 1965.
323. Sirnes, T.B.: Intravenous ether. Acta Pharm. Tox. Kbh. (Suppl.)10:10, 1954.
324. Kummell, H.: Ueber Intravenouse Aethernarkose. Arch. Clin. Chir., 95:185, 1911.
325. Burkhardt, L.: Ueber Intravenose Narkose. Muenchen. Med. Wschr., 58:778, 1911.
326. Eger, E.I., et al.: The uptake and distribution of intravenous ether. Anesthesiology, 23:647, 1962.
327. Laborit, G., Kind, A., and Regil, C. de L.: 220 Cas d'anesthesia en neurochirurgie avec le 4-hydroxy butyrate de sodium. Presse Med., 69:1216, 1961.
327a. Tsuji, H., Balagot, R.C., and Sadove, M.: Effect of anesthetics on brain gamma aminobutyric and glutamic acid levels. J.A.M.A., 183:659, 1963.
328. Blumenfeld, M., Suntey, R.G., and Harmel, M.: Sodium gamma-hydroxybutyric acid: A new anesthetic adjunct. Anesth. Analg., 41:729, 1962.
329. Marin, M.G.: Application des alkohol ethilico como anesthetico general por via endovenosa Mexico City, F. Mesones, 1929.
330. Behan, R.J.: Ethyl alcohol intravenously as postoperative sedative. Am. J. Surg., 69:227, 1920.
331. Block, M.A.: Alcoholism (editorial) J.A.M.A., 163:550, 1957.
332. Smith, J.J.: The endocrine basis and hormonal therapy of alcoholism. N.Y. State J. Med., 50:1704, 1956.
333. Westerfeld, W.W., and Schulman, M.P.: Metabolism and caloric value of alcohol. J.A.M.A., 170:197, 1959.
334. Harger, R.N.: The pharmacology and toxicology of alcohol. J.A.M.A., 167:2199, 1958.
335. Webb, W.R., and Degerli, I.V.: Ethyl alcohol and the cardiovascular system. J.A.M.A., 191:1055, 1970.
336. Wessler, S., and Avioli, L.V.: Alcoholic hepatitis. J.A.M.A., 203:865, 1968.
337. Jenkins, M., and Sokol, J.K.: Adrenocortical response to ethanol in man. Br. Med. J., 2:804, 1968.
338. Himwich, H.E.: The physiology of alcohol. J.A.M.A., 163:545, 1957.
339. Grollman, A.: Influence of alcohol on circulation. Q.J. Stud. Alcohol, 3:5, 1942.

340. Newman, H.W.: Emetic action of ethyl alcohol. Arch. Intern. Med., 94:417, 1954.
341. Russek, H., Zohman, B., and Dorset, V.: Effects of tobacco and alcohol on cardiovascular system. J.A.M.A., 157:563, 1955.
342. Szanto, P.B., and Meister, H.P.: Alcoholic myocardiopathy. Am. J. Clin. Pathol., 39:294, 1963.
343. Tobin, J.R., et al.: Primary myocardial disease and alcoholism. Circulation, 35:754, 1967.
344. Gordon, J.E.: The Epidemiology of alcoholism. N.Y. State J. Med., 58:1911, 1958.
345. Greenberg, L.A.: Alcohol in the body. Sci. Am., 189:86, 1953.
346. Smith, J.A.: Psychiatric treatment of the alcoholic. N.Y. State J. Med., 58:3157, 1958.
347. Perman, E.A.: Effect of alcohol on secretion of epinephrine. Acta Physiol. Scand., 48:323, 1960.
348. Palthe, P.M., and Van, W.: Ueber Alkoholaergeftung. Deutsch, Z.F., Nerven., 92:791, 1926.
349. Davis, C.W., and Robertson, H.T.: Oxygen in acute alcoholic intoxication. Q.J. Stud. Alcohol, 10:59, 1959.
350. Lewis, A.: The Relation between operative risk and the patient's general condition: Alcohol, other habits of addiction and psychogenic factors. Bull. Soc. Int. Chir., 14:421, 1955.
351. Moore, D.C., and Karp, M.: Intravenous alcohol in the surgical patients. Surg. Gynecol. Obstet., 80:523, 1945.
352. Karp, M., and Sokol, J.K.: Intravenous use of alcohol in the surgical patient. J.A.M.A., 146:21, 1951.
353. Dundee, J.W., and Isaac, M.: Newer intravenous drugs. Int. Anesthesiol. Clin., 7:67, 1969.
354. Isaac, M., et al.: Intravenous ethanol anesthesia. Acta Anaesthesiol. Scand., 15:141, 1971.
355. Rasmussen, N.G.: Dilute alcohol intravenous postoperative. Jackson Clin. Bull., 7:45, 1945.
356. Bronner, B., and Collins, V.J.: Bellevue conferences. May, 1959.
357. Mirsky, J.H., and Giarmiam, N.J.: Studies on potentiation of pentothal. J. Pharm. Exp. Ther., 114:240, 1955.
358. Fazekas, J.: Influence of chlorpromazine and alcohol on cerebral hemodynamics. Am. J. Med. Sci., 230:128, 1955.
359. Hollister, L.E.: Complications of tranquilizing drugs. N. Engl. J. Med., 257:170, 1959.
360. Cooper, V., Slocum, H.C., and Allen, C.: Tetraethylthiuram disulfate and the anesthetic agents. Anesthesiology, 14:29, 1953.

28

INTRAVASCULAR LOCAL ANESTHETICS AND REGIONAL BLOCK

INTRAVENOUS PROCAINE

HISTORY. In 1908 Bier[1] reported on a method of regional anesthesia in the extremities. The technique consisted of injecting procaine into a superficial vein of a limb previously rendered bloodless by bandage or tourniquet. The method was abandoned because there was a sharp increase in mortality accompanying use of local anesthetics presumably because of the concomitant use of epinephrine.[2]

In recent years interest in systemic procaine for various therapeutic purposes has been revived. The conditions for which intravenous procaine has been found effective include the following:

1. Analgesia[3,4]
2. Arrhythmias[5]
3. Arthritis[6,7]
4. Asthma[8–10]
5. Burns—for control of pain[11]
6. Embolus and thrombosis[10]
7. Hiccoughs[12]
8. Obstetric analgesia[13,14]
9. Postoperative pain control[4,15]
10. Pruritis of jaundice[16]
11. Reactions—serum (as an antihistaminic); penicillin; urticaria[17–20]
12. Spasm, muscular, poliomyelitis[21]
13. Trauma[22–24]
14. Vasospasm–peripheral vascular disorder;[25] coronary occlusion

PHARMACOLOGY.[2] Effects of procaine when used for nerve block regional anesthesia are detailed elsewhere. Some of its properties when injected intravenously as a therapeutic agent are outlined in this chapter.

CHEMISTRY AND METABOLISM.[26] Procaine is an ester that is rapidly hydrolyzed in the blood by the enzyme procaine esterase. The enzyme is present in human plasma and in various tissues especially in the liver (in high concentration). It is considered to be identical to plasma cholinesterase.[27]

Two components, an alcohol (diethylaminoethanol) and an acid (para-aminobenzoic acid) are produced.

EXCRETION. Negligible amounts of unaltered procaine are recovered in the urine. Over 80% of the acid is recoverable, but only 30% of the alcohol can be isolated. It is evident, therefore, that the diethylaminoethanol is further metabolized in an undetermined manner.[26a] Also, with continuous intravenous administration of procaine, the concentration of the procaine in plasma does not increase but the alcohol does. This indicates that diethylaminoethanol is the pharmacologically active agent.[26b]

PROPERTIES. Procaine, but more specifically diethylaminoethanol, is a tertiary nitrogenous compound and as such possesses many effects of the tertiary ammonium group, including analgesic, antihistaminic, spasmolytic, and antiarrhythmia (quinidine-like).

Analgesic effects have been well substantiated by the clinical results in the relief of pain from trauma and inflammation. In such conditions as burns, fractures, sprains, and postoperative pain, the results are somewhat spectacular. In arthritis and neuritis, there is less success.

General anesthesia has been produced[3,4] by the intravenous administration of concentrated solutions (1%). When 0.1% solutions were administered, the amount of inhaled anesthetic required is less. It has been demonstrated[30] that there is an elevation of the pain threshold when large amounts of procaine are administered subcutaneously. This effect is presumed to be central; however, methodology in the evaluation of analgesic drugs has been questioned.[26a]

Antihistaminic action has been demonstrated by the efficiency of procaine in the management of allergic states such as serum sickness and reactions to penicillin.

Spasmolytic effects have been used particularly in the diagnosis and treatment of various smooth muscle spasm states and vascular spasm. Following intravenous administration, there is usually a rise in skin temperature accompanied by vasodilatation. Edema and cyanosis tend to be ameliorated. Paresthesias are minimized. All these effects indicate sympathetic blockade. Extensive clinical confirmation is needed.

The antiarrhythmia effect is well established. Procaine acts as a cardiac sedative and as such diminishes cardiac irritability. The specific mechanism of action may be that of a direct protoplasmic depressant, particularly the protoplasm of cardiac muscle. This is similar to the action of quinidine.

PATHOPHYSIOLOGY. In many pathologic conditions, there is an accepted sequence of events that lead to physiologic dysfunction and then anatomic changes. Thus, noxious stimuli applied to an organism not only produce direct mechanical trauma but initiate neural excitation leading to autonomic imbalance. The result is an excessive vascular disturbance with enhanced edema, muscle and blood vessel spasm, and pain. The primary dysfunction is with the capillary unit.[2,6]

The particular dysfunction of the capillary unit of importance is that of increased permeability. The effectiveness of intravenously administered procaine is undoubtedly the result of the ease with which it passes through the walls of injured capillaries. It has been found that intravenous procaine is concentrated from seven to eight times more in traumatized than in normal tissues.[24] On entering the tissue spaces of the injured region, procaine gains access to the irritated nerve endings. These are anesthetized, and relief of spasm occurs. The mode of action of procaine thus appears to be at the receptors of primary neurons in various reflex arcs.[22,24a]

DOSAGE. Dosage is determined on the basis of the initial therapeutic effect and the relevant blood level. The rate of disposition then determines the additional doses needed to maintain the effective level. Significant amounts of procaine will disappear from the blood stream within 20 minutes. From clinical experience it has been determined that 4 mg/kg of body weight gives optimal benefits with minimal toxicity. This dose, when administered during 20 minutes, is called the *procaine unit*.[29] This unit represents a *dose-rate of 0.2 mg (200 µg) per kg of body weight per minute*. A range of 50 to 250 µg/kg/min is recommended. Such doses establish blood levels of about 10 µg/ml.

PREPARATIONS FOR THERAPEUTIC PURPOSES AND ADMINISTRATION. An intravenous drip of a diluted procaine solution, 0.1%, is generally employed.[30] This solution is prepared by adding 5 ml of a 20% procaine solution (1 g) to 1000 ml of isotonic saline or 5% glucose in distilled water. This furnishes a 1:1000 solution, or each milliliter contains 1 mg of procaine.

To facilitate the accurate administration by providing a uniform rate of flow, a Flowrator may be incorporated into an intravenous infusion set.[31]

In general, it is recommended to administer the first 50 ml of a 0.1% solution in 10 minutes to evaluate the patient's response, especially during the first treatment.[32] If signs of toxicity appear, the rate of infusion is slowed or stopped completely, depending on degree of reaction.

ANESTHETIC ADJUNCT.[30,33] For general anesthetic purposes, a more concentrated solution for intravenous drip is employed. This solution is usually 1% procaine and is prepared by dissolving 10 g of procaine in 1000 ml of 5% glucose in distilled water.

The concentrated solution is administered at a rate of 2 to 3 ml/min initially. As further anesthesia is needed, the rate may be increased to 10 to 15 ml/

min. If less anesthesia is desired, maintenance may be obtained with rates of 0.3 to 0.5 ml/min.[30] In this manner from 2 to 5 g of procaine may be given in 1 hour.

No premedication is given, and no preliminary skin test is performed.

Dosage for Anesthesia. Based on the rates of administration the milligram dose of procaine for an anesthetic state is about 2.0 to 3.0 ml/min or 3.5 mg/kg/min in a 70 kg man. Usubiaga studied dosages of intravenous procaine for anesthetic purposes in humans.[34] Based on this work, a dose of 1 to 2 mg/kg/min will produce analgesia and can be used to complement nitrous oxide anesthesia in agreement with Wikinski.[3]

PHARMACOKINETICS.[36] During a continuous infusion of a 1% or 2% procaine solution in 5% dextrose, a steady state is achieved in 20 to 30 minutes at doses of 1 to 2 mg/kg/min. The plasma-level data fit into a two-compartment open pharmacokinetic model with first-order drug elimination. A central and peripheral compartment are recognized, with reciprocal first-order rate drug transfer between the two. Drug elimination is a first-order rate constant from the central compartment.

Plasma levels range from 20 to 65 µg/ml. With termination of infusion, the procaine rapidly disappears and the plasma half-life or $t_{1/2}$ alpha is approximately 2.5 minutes. The elimination half-life $t_{1/2}$ beta is approximately 7.7 minutes (Fig. 28–1).

In these studies, patients were premedicated with thiamylal and diazepam, and no central nervous system (CNS) toxic reactions were noted; however, in medicated human volunteers, Usubiaga[34] found that muscle tremors and convulsions occur with electroencephalographic (EEG) seizure changes at plasma levels of 20 to 80 µg/ml.

RESPONSES AND TOXICITY.[33,34] During the intravenous administration of procaine, certain typical signs and symptoms appear. About 5 minutes after the start of an infusion the patient experiences a general sensation of warmth, often accompanied by a flush of the face and neck. Circumoral pallor also appears (similar to atropine). Next, dryness of the mouth and a metallic taste are noted. Lacrimation and pupillary dilatation follow. Lightheadedness, relaxation, and a sense of well being are felt.[32]

With rapid flow rates or the use of concentrated solutions, certain uncomfortable sensations are manifest. These include, in progressive order, apprehension, dizziness, trembling, drowsiness, and unconsciousness.[33]

In general, the safety of the intravenous administration of procaine for therapy has been attested to by the vast number of administrations without untoward reactions.[30–32] To increase the margin of safety and protect against untoward reactions, it is recommended that vitamin C be administered. This

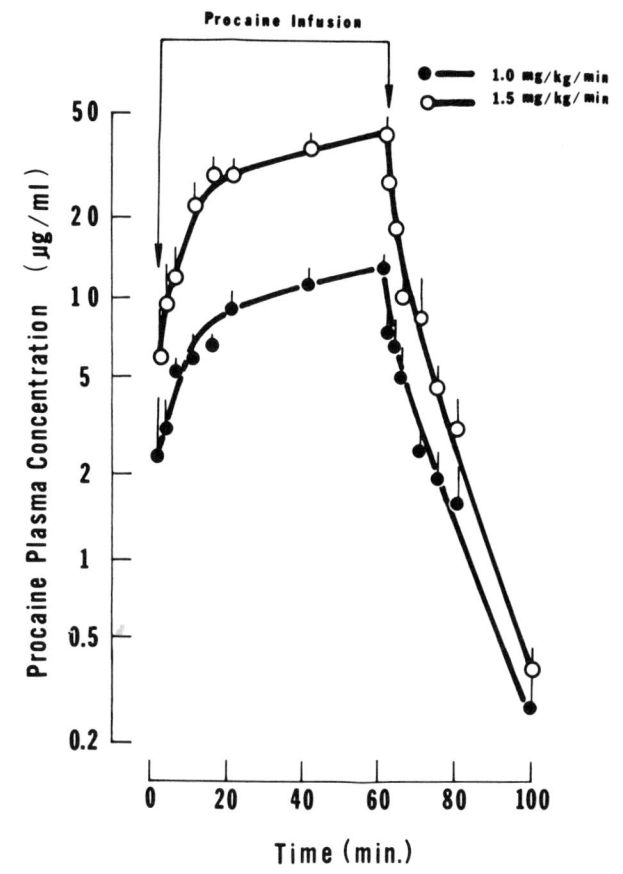

FIG. 28–1. Plasma concentrations of procaine hydrochloride in six patients during and following 60 minutes of infusion at rates of 1 mg/kg/min or 1.5 mg/kg/min (mean ± SEM). From Seifen, A.B., et al.: Pharmacokinetics of intravenous procaine infusion in humans. Anesth. Analg., 58:382, 1979.

can be done by adding 1 g of sodium ascorbate to each 1000 ml of the procaine infusion. Vitamin C has been shown to increase the resistance of patients to the toxic effects of procaine, especially the convulsive action.[37]

Intravenous Procainamide for Arrhythmias

With the demonstration of the effectiveness of bolus doses as well as drip infusion of procaine during World War II[38] a systematic study was undertaken to find a congener with a longer duration of action. Brodie[39] prepared the amide compound of procaine and Mark[40] demonstrated its effectiveness in treating ventricular arrhythmias. The compound also produces its cardiac effect in doses significantly lower than procaine without CNS effects.

Pharmacology.[41] The actions on the heart are similar to those of procaine and are essentially identical to the effects of quinidine. Excitability of the atrial and ventricular muscle is depressed. Conduction is slowed. The effective refractory period is prolonged. Contractility is depressed but much less than with quinidine.

The electrocardiogram (ECG) changes include some variable prolongation of P-R and Q-T intervals, but the widening of QRS complex is consistent. The threshold to ventricular extrasystoles and induced ventricular fibrillation is raised. CNS actions are not prominent.

Pharmacokinetics. [42] Rapid absorption from the gut occurs after oral administration, and maximal plasma concentrations are seen in about 60 minutes. After intramuscular injection, peak plasma concentrations are seen in 30 to 60 minutes, whereas after intravenous administration effective plasma levels are attained in 5 to 15 minutes.[43]

Hydrolysis of the drug is slow and the biological half-life is 3 to 4 hours. Excretion of the drug and its metabolites is by the kidney.

Toxicity. Hypotension occurs after intravenous administration, but this is most likely if the initial pressure is high or the drug is injected rapidly. Troublesome ventricular tachycardia may occur as the atrial rate is reduced; atrioventricular block may occur.

Dosage. [44] The intravenous loading dose is 2.5 to 5 mg/kg administered over a period of 5 minutes. Lima[40] recommends the administration of about 1 g in 1 hour as a loading intravenous infusion dose. Maintenance doses are designed to attain a steady serum concentration of about 6 µg/ml. Doses of 200 mg/hr in a 70-kg man will permit this level to be continued. In patients with renal impairment, the dose should be halved.

Uses. In patients with ventricular arrhythmias who fail to respond to lidocaine, this drug can be safely administered and has been shown to be effective in abolishing serious arrhythmias.[44]

INTRAVENOUS LIDOCAINE ANESTHESIA

As a supplement to general anesthesia, the local anesthetics have been successfully and safely administered intravenously.[45] Lidocaine in combination with nitrous oxide and relaxants has proven particularly adaptable in major surgical procedures.

MECHANISM. Lidocaine produces a central sedative analgesic effect when introduced into the blood stream in appropriate doses.[46] A peripheral tissue effect is also present, which, in part, accounts for the suppression of reflexes[48] and its antiarrhythmic action.[65] This agent is nonallergic. It is detoxified in the liver by oxidation and thus does not depend on plasma cholinesterase.

TECHNIQUE OF USE

Premedication. [45,47] Standard preanesthetic medication is used. An opiate provides a preferred preanesthetic state and contributes to the anesthetic process.

INDUCTION AND DOSAGE. [47] While breathing oxygen, the premedicated patient is given a sleep dose of thiopental. A nitrous oxide-oxygen, 6 L/2 L inhalation mixture, is then administered. After 2 to 5 minutes of a stabilized anesthetic state, a loading dose (initial) of lidocaine in a 2% solution is administered intravenously as a bolus injection.

The loading dose or initial dose is calculated on the basis of 4 mg/kg (original recommendation of Steinhaus[47] is 2 mg/lb). This easily provides a blood level of 10 to 20 µg/ml attained within 5 to 10 minutes. These levels decrease as liver destruction and elimination of the drug proceed.

MAINTENANCE. [49] After the initial dose is distributed in the blood and extracellular fluids, additional doses of lidocaine must be administered to replace the amounts continuously lost by destruction or elimination. These additional doses are designed to maintain the effective blood level.

Maintenance dose rates (replacement doses) are about 100 to 120 µg/kg/min.

The maintenance doses of lidocaine may be administered intravenously, either intermittently as a bolus in a concentrated solution or continuously as a drip of a dilute solution.

The intermittent dose technique (for a 70-kg man) consists of the administration of 2 ml of a 2% solution (40 mg) every 5 minutes during the first hour. During the second hour the dosage is reduced by half to 20 mg every 5 minutes, i.e., 1 ml of the 2% solution; for the third hour, the dosage is again halved to 10 mg every 5 minutes.

A dose rate therefore is provided of 10 µg/kg/min or approximately 8 mg/min in a 70-kg man.

This technique produces fluctuating blood levels and variation in effect.

The continuous drip technique for maintenance is preferred for providing a more even blood level of lidocaine and a smooth effect. It consists of a drip administration of 0.2% solution. This is prepared by dissolving 1 g of lidocaine in 500 ml of dextrose 5% in water flask. Such a solution contains 2 mg/ml. Approximately 4 to 5 ml of this solution should be administered per minute during the first hour and half this amount during the second hour. With standard infusion sets, this is about 40 to 50 drops/minute. Indeed, after the first 30 minutes the rate of infusion can be slowed so that by 1 hour, a rate of 2 ml/min is achieved.

In the aged, toxic patients, and children, the dosage should be reduced by one half. Generally, the administration of lidocaine is accompanied by the administration of thiopental. During maintenance it is common to administer a dose of thiopental equal to the dose of lidocaine.

ADVANTAGES. Several advantages exist for lidocaine as a general anesthetic adjunct. These include (1) analgesia during administration and postoperatively; (2) depression of pharyngeal, laryngeal, and tracheal reflexes; (3) antiarrhythmic action; and (4) suppression of other reflexes, including minimization of nausea and vomiting.

A reduction in the dose requirement of other anesthetic agents occurs when lidocaine is administered as an adjunct.[49] Suppression of pharyngeal and laryngeal reflexes permits the maintenance of airways in light planes of anesthesia.[50] A significant period of postoperative analgesia is produced and may last as long as 8 hours in 60% of the patients. Nausea and vomiting are minimized in the postoperative period. Because of the quick recovery and limited effect on respiration, postoperative pulmonary complications are infrequent.[51]

DISADVANTAGES. The technique requires careful and tedious attention to detail, dosage, and diagnosis of untoward complications. Convulsive manifestations are not unlikely and are the result of overdosage. They occur usually following bolus injections. Twitching of the eyebrows is one of the first signs. An initial fall in blood pressure on skin incision is frequent.

PHARMACOLOGIC EFFECTS. Suppression of reflexes is striking.[48] With respect to cough reflex and using the endotracheal tube as a predictable and effective cough stimulus, cough can be completely suppressed without significant respiratory depression.[52] In comparison with meperidine, it was evident that the opiate usually caused severe respiratory depression before cough suppression. Additional clinical study also demonstrated that intravenous lidocaine definitely contributed to a smoother and shorter induction time with diethylether and with a minimum of irritant effects. It appears that this intravenous local agent provides a type of central nervous system and peripheral depression of reflex paths qualitatively different from the usual central antitussive drug mechanism.

That some respiratory depression occurs is evident when either extremely large doses are employed or when deep anesthesia has been attained by other agents.[51]

A decrease in splanchnic vascular resistance occurs after intravenous administration in humans in doses of 2 to 4 mg per kg of body weight. This decrease in resistance is proportional to the plasma concentration and amounts to about 7%. This results in a decreased portal vein flow. Despite this, there is an active vasodilatation of the hepatic arterial supply and an increase in hepatic blood flow of 17% to 37%.[53]

At larger doses of 4 mg or more of lidocaine per minute in unanesthetized humans, there are significant cardiovascular responses: heart rate, cardiac output (Q̇), and mean arterial blood pressure are increased. Stroke volume increases slightly (4%).[53a] These effects of lidocaine represent a cerebral component of action on vasomotor centers with sympathetic stimulation in the absence of ganglionic blockade or vagolysis.

Direct actions on the electrophysiologic functions of the heart by lidocaine have demonstrated effects important as a basis for the antiarrhythmic action of lidocaine. These include decreased pacemaker activity, shortening of the action potential, and reduced excitability.[53b]

In anesthetized humans, the intravenous administration of lidocaine may be associated with decreases in cardiac output. It has been demonstrated that cardiac output is inversely related to lidocaine blood levels.[53c]

Allergic reactions have not been reported. Other adverse effects are minimal. Rare idiosyncratic reactions, such as tinnitus and dizziness, occur.

EFFECT ON NEUROMUSCULAR JUNCTION.[54] Both procaine and lidocaine are capable of producing neuromuscular blockade.[54] Three possible sites of action of either ester or amide local anesthetics may be considered:

1. In the axon cytoplasm affecting acetylcholine synthesis or at the limiting membrane inhibiting release.
2. At the synaptic cleft affecting acetylcholine or interacting with acetylcholinesterase.[55]
3. Postjunctionally, blocking the action of acetylcholine at the end-plate. Some evidence also exists of a direct muscle membrane action.

From most studies, it appears that the predominant action of the local anesthetics is a postjunctional block attributed to inhibition of acetylcholine action at the end-plate.[50] It can be demonstrated after intra-arterial injection, but it is poorly demonstrated after intravenous injection. It is a nondepolarizing block manifested by twitch depression, poorly sustained tetanus, and post-tetanic facilitation. This block differs from *d*-tubocurarine block, however, because it is not antagonized by the anticholinesterases edrophonium or neostigmine. After intravenous injection of the local agents, blockade is demonstrable only if prior partial block exists with either succinylcholine or *d*-tubocurarine; then, intravenous procaine or lidocaine increases the block.

Depression and abolition of respiration after intravenous procaine or lidocaine and other amide local agents can occur without depression of the neuromuscular junction and is attributable to a depression of the central nervous system.[54]

USES AND ADVANTAGES.

1. Decreases anesthetic requirements; reduces MAC values and potentiates nitrous-oxide–halothane at blood levels of 3 to 6 μg/ml[49]
2. Suppresses cough reflex on intubation[48,50]
3. Suppresses cough during bronchoscopy[52,56]
4. Attenuates circulatory response to intubation[57–59]
5. Prevents increases in intracranial pressure on intubation[60,61]
6. Suppresses increases in intraocular pressure after intubation[62]
7. Controls extubation cough and laryngospasm in children[63] and adults[64]
8. Antiarrhythmia action[65]

Excessive central nervous system sedation and depression postanesthetically as a result of lidocaine or intensive treatment of cardiac dysfunction can be reversed by naloxone.[66]

PHARMACOKINETICS.[67] Lidocaine has a high hepatic extraction ratio and is completely removed after a single pass through the liver. Thus, the hepatic blood flow has an important influence on the rate of removal of lidocaine from the bloodstream. In patients with decreased hepatic blood flow, as in shock or congestive heart failure, a fixed dose may result in high plasma levels.

It has been determined that indocyanine green, an anionic dye, has a high hepatic extraction ratio and provides an index of hepatic blood flow. Because it has a short half-life (45 minutes) and provides a repeatable method, the relation between dye clearance and lidocaine clearance has been found to be linear. In congestive heart failure, the clearing of lidocaine is reduced and plasma levels are quite high.

A steady-state plasma level is achieved quickly if a continuous infusion technique is preceded by a bolus intravenous injection. After discontinuing an infusion, there is a slow decay rate in plasma level; the half-life is about 108 minutes. This slow clearance is related to the drug bound to organs.

SIDE-EFFECTS.[68] Paresthesia, slurred speech, sedation, somnolence, hallucinations, and psychosis have been reported following large doses of lidocaine in the treatment of arrhythmias. Respiratory depression, apnea, and convulsions are also seen. Plasma levels associated with these toxic reactions usually range above 7 μg/ml of blood.[68]

Intravenous Lidocaine for Arrhythmias

MECHANISM. The antiarrhythmic action of lidocaine represents its most important current intravenous use.[69] Blood levels of 2 to 5 μg/ml reduce ventricular irritability, and the diastolic threshold of the myocardial muscle fiber is elevated (at blood levels of 5.2 μg/ml). At these levels there is no depression of conduction in the HisPurkinje system, and there is no vagolytic action.

In general, lidocaine is effective neither in supraventricular arrhythmias nor in the arrhythmias due to digitalis overdose.

INDICATIONS. Clinical indications for intravenous lidocaine are as follows:

1. Suppression of ventricular irritability during cardiac surgery
2. Reduction of cardiac irritability caused by hydrocarbon anesthetics
3. Control of arrhythmias related to cardiac arrest, especially ventricular fibrillation
4. For management of cardiac arrhythmias in patients with coronary artery disease and for coronary occlusion or myocardial infarction
5. Prophylactic use in myocardial infarction

EFFECTIVE DOSES. It is emphasized that the dosages for these patients are one half to one quarter the doses employed for adjunctive anesthetic purposes. Blood levels are directly related to the dose rate, i.e., μg/kg administered per minute (Fig. 28–2). Effective blood levels range between 2 and 5 μg/ml. Lower levels are ineffective.

An effective antiarrhythmic dose is achieved by a loading dose of 1 to 2 mg/kg. This may be repeated once to provide a steady level. Thereafter, a continuous drip technique is employed to maintain a steady state.

When ventricular arrhythmias are refractory (about 20%) to maximum tolerated infusions of lidocaine, the patient may be effectively treated with procainamide. A loading dose of 1,000 mg over one hour is followed by the maintenance dose of 200 mg/hour. This provides a blood level of 6 μg/ml.[70]

One metabolite of lidocaine is active and has an antiarrhythmic effect, namely, monoethyl-glycinexylidide (MEGX). It is about half as potent as the parent lidocaine.[71]

As a potent antiarrhythmic drug, lidocaine has the following effects:

1. Marked suppression of premature ventricular complexes.
2. Decreased atrioventricular conduction, especially in patients with underlying conduction disturbances.
3. Increased ventricular response to atrial flutter or fibrillation.
4. Altered accessory atrioventricular pathways in patients with Wolff-Parkinson-White syndrome.

ADMINISTRATION WITH CONTINUOUS DRIP TECHNIQUE. This is particularly applicable in the management of arrhythmias caused by coronary occlusion and myocardial infarction. Ordinarily, a dilute solution of lidocaine in 5% dextrose and water, ei-

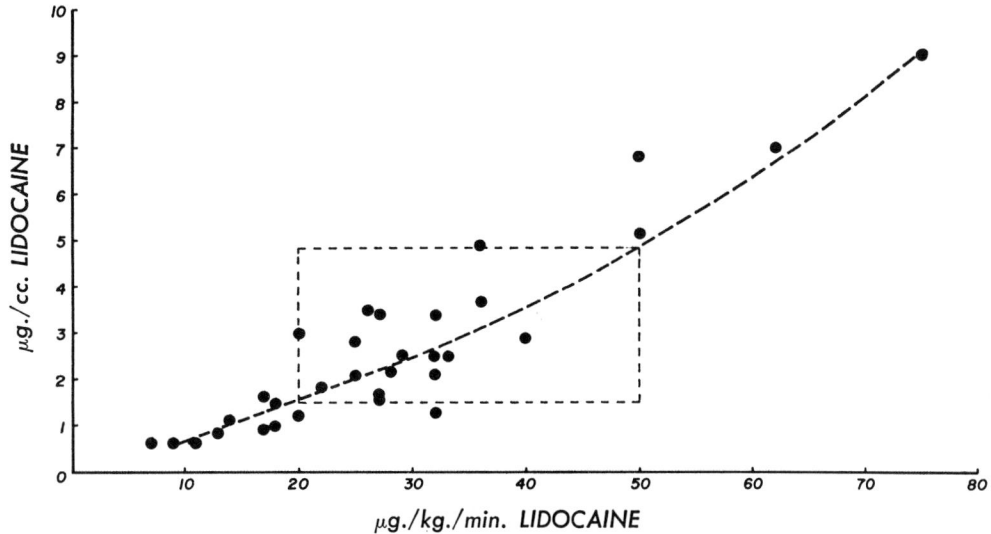

FIG. 28–2. Relation between the rate of infusion and the blood level of lidocaine in 21 patients receiving a constant infusion. All levels were measured after at least two hours of constant infusion. The area enclosed within the rectangle is considered to be the appropriate therapeutic range. From Gianelly, R., et al.: Effect of lidocaine on ventricular arrhythmias in patients with coronary disease. N. Engl. J. Med., 227:1215, 1967.

ther 0.1% or 0.2% (1 or 2 mg/ml) concentration is dripped intravenously. When volume restriction is important, a 1% solution may be employed. Administration is begun slowly and increased gradually to a plateau rate after 60 minutes (Fig. 28–3).

Recommended dose rates are 20 to 55 µg/kg/min. It is recommended that the dose be kept below 55 µg/kg/min (about 4 mg/min in a 70-kg man), which may be considered the maximum minute dose. When rates less than 18 µg/kg/min are administered, there is inadequate or no effect.

Doses greater than the recommended ones and up to 128 µg/kg/min have been administered but produce blood levels greater than 5.3 µg/ml and increase toxic effects.

MULTIPLE BOLUS INJECTION TECHNIQUE.[72] This technique is applicable in emergencies and management of acute arrhythmias resulting from hydrocarbon sensitization of the myocardium during anesthesia (halothane). The single dose range is 1 to 2 mg/kg. It rapidly provides a plasma level of about 2 to 3 µg/ml. A repeat dose may be administered in 5 minutes; subsequent doses should be halved until a maximal dose of 500 mg is administered in 20 minutes. This dose schedule will effectively reduce myocardial irritability and immediately control or progressively reduce the percentage of ectopic beats.

COMPARISON OF ADMINISTRATION TECHNIQUES.[73] The optimal plasma concentration is considered to be between 2 and 4 µg/ml.

1. A conventional technique of administration consists in administering a bolus of 50 to 100 mg in a 2-minute period, followed by a continuous infusion of 2 mg/min. A latency between establishing a stable plasma therapeutic level and effective response is often referred to as a *therapeutic gap*. Subtherapeutic levels are frequent.

2. A second technique is multiple bolus administration. This involves an initial bolus of 100 mg over a 2-minute period, with a maintenance infusion as above, followed by a second bolus dose of 50 mg at 20 minutes and several bolus doses at 5-minute intervals. The inherent danger of overdose is evident.

3. A two-infusion technique: One is a rapid infusion over a period of 15 to 30 minutes at a rate of 8 mg/min, followed by a 2-mg/min maintenance dose. Fluid overload is a chance occurrence.

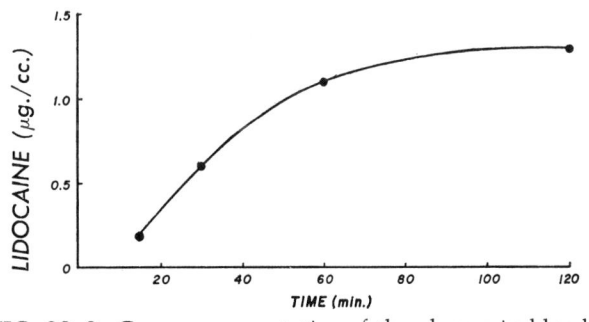

FIG. 28–3. Curve representative of the change in blood lidocaine levels with time, given a constant rate of infusion (27 µg/kg of body weight per minute) starting at zero time. From Gianelly, R., et al.: Effect of lidocaine on ventricular arrhythmias in patients with coronary disease. N. Engl. J. Med., 227:1215, 1967.

4. A three-step technique:[67] (a) a bolus of 100 mg in 2 minutes; (b) an infusion at a rate of 8 mg/min for 25 minutes; (c) the infusion rate is then slowed to 2 mg/min and satisfies pharmacokinetic parameters to achieve a stable 2 to 4 µg/ml plasma level. This appears to provide the best therapeutic plasma level most of the time.

EFFECTS ON CARDIAC FUNCTION. In patients with a myocardial infarction lidocaine infusions of 1 to 3 mg given over 30 to 60 minutes effectively controls arrhythmias and does not interfere with cardiac function. No significant changes in heart rate, mean aortic pressure, systemic vascular resistance, left ventricular, end-diastolic pressure or left ventricular ejection time occurs.[74]

PROPHYLACTIC USE. During the early phases of the diagnosis of myocardial infarction and during prehospital care (i.e., within 6 hours), intramuscular injection of 100 mg of lidocaine is effective for preventing arrhythmias. The incidence of ventricular fibrillation and the mortality rate are significantly reduced (2.5 times).[75]

Immediate institution of continuous drip lidocaine on hospitalization also prevents serious arrhythmias and decreases the mortality.[76]

ADVERSE EFFECTS.[77] Administration of lidocaine to patients with a proven or suspected myocardial infarction as prophylaxis against primary ventricular fibrillation is a widely practiced mode of therapy. Adverse effects to lidocaine are common and range from 7% to 39%. Side effects are high and may be seen in 50% of the reacting patients in the first 12 hours. The major adverse effects include CNS disorders—confusion, slurred speech, tremors, nausea, and vomiting—and sinus bradycardia. Some life-threatening problems are also seen, such as sinus bradycardia of less than 35 bpm, sinus arrest, seizures, coma, and respiratory arrest. Of the adverse responses, more (64%) occurred in patients without infarction than those with infarction (32%). Life-threatening effects occurred in the first 24 hours and predominantly in the first hour of therapy.[77] Lidocaine plasma levels were only weakly associated with adverse effects. Caution in lidocaine use is necessary, and the need for more efficient, minimal-risk, and maximal-effect antiarrhythmic drugs for prophylaxis of ventricular fibrillation is apparent.

INTRAVENOUS REGIONAL ANESTHESIA

Original work by Bier[78–80] in 1908 established the effectiveness of local anesthetics introduced intravenously and localized by appropriate tourniquets to produce extensive regional anesthesia. Bier attempted to alleviate various pain states, and his work is the basis of current techniques. In 1908, Ransohoff[81] applied the method but introduced the agents intra-arterially. Leriche[82] used intravenous local anesthetics in 1935 for the treatment of various vascular disturbances, including arteritis, causalgia and Raynaud's syndrome.[83]

A significant advance was the method of continuous or frequent intermittent injection intravenously of procaine or lidocaine for pain management and surgery.

MECHANISM. An understanding of this method is based on several considerations. Local anesthetics administered intravascularly have a direct action on blood vessel walls and produce vasodilatation. Furthermore, the agent diffuses into tissues and produces anesthetic block of small nerve fibers and large nerve trunks (ulnar, median, and radial). Allen[84] has shown that there is a greater localization of the anesthetic agents in traumatized tissues that is six to eight times greater than in normal tissues. This is presumably the result of ease of diffusion from broken capillaries.

INDICATIONS IN SURGERY.[84–87]

1. Operations below elbow[85–87,88]
2. Operations below knee[89,90]
3. Tendon operations (scar removal; ganglions); hand abscesses; removal of foreign bodies; lacerations; colles fractures; leg; toenails; bunions; amputations (time—100 minutes)
4. Useful in elderly patients and acceptable in children; patients in ASA physical status (PS) I through III are safely managed
5. Patients in PS IV are not usually anesthetized by intravenous regional anesthesia; the method is not recommended in semistuporous or uncooperative patients; infections of the extremity are a contraindication

Resurgence of Use. Althouth Bier and others were successful in applying the technique of intravenous regional anesthesia, most anesthesiologists and surgeons found the technique cumbersome and often inadequate. In 1963, however, Holmes[89] demonstrated great success of the method by careful attention to technical detail and the use of lidocaine as the local anesthetic. Bell[85] likewise demonstrated great success in producing analgesia of the extremities.

TECHNIQUE. Preliminary measurement of blood pressure establishes the systolic pressure and enables the patient to experience the "feel" of an inflated cuff, which provides reassurance (Fig. 28–4).

Localization of an anesthetic agent to an extremity region is achieved in four principal steps:[81,82,84]

1. An intravenous cannula or catheter is inserted into a vein distal to the operative site, usually on the back of the hand or at an ankle vein.

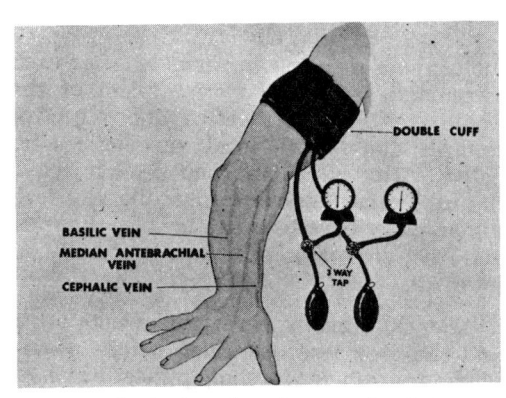

FIG. 28–4. Method of performing routine intravenous regional block with a double cuff. Note surface markings of major superficial veins. From Raj, P.P., et al.: The site of action of intravenous regional anesthesia. Anesth. Analg., 51:776, 1922.

2. Production of an ischemic limb:
   a. By elevation of extremity for 2 to 3 minutes.
   b. By milking or expressing the blood by means of an Esmarch or a Martin bandage wrapped from the distal portion of the limb toward the proximal part.
3. Tourniquet application:
   a. The tourniquet cuff is placed at the proximal end of a limb well above the surgical site.
   b. The cuff is inflated to a level above systolic pressure to prevent re-entry of the blood into the limb.
   c. Note that in the two-cuff technique a secondary tourniquet is placed just distal to the primary cuff, contiguous to the primary cuff.
4. Injection of a dilute solution of a local anesthetic through the "placed" needle or catheter is accomplished.
5. After the onset of anesthesia and before the onset of tourniquet discomfort, the secondary or distal cuff is inflated (the area is now anesthetized) and the primary, or proximal, cuff is deflated (see "two-cuff technique").

IMPORTANT TECHNICAL ASPECTS.[85,89] Several technical details contribute to the effectiveness and success of the intravenous regional anesthetic technique.

Exsanguination. The completeness of exsanguination of the extremity to be anesthetized will provide more complete anesthesia with a more rapid onset. Such exsanguination can be accomplished by a two-step technique: (1) gravity, and (2) Esmarch bandaging. The gravity technique employs the elevation of the extremity for a period of at least 2 minutes. The venous system is relatively well drained but is not completely emptied. It is therefore recommended that the Esmarch bandaging technique then be employed. This simply involves wrapping of the extremity from the distal portion to the proximal portion of the extremity. The Esmarch bandage is a 2- to 3-inch wide rubber bandage that should be applied snugly. This two-step technique will effectively empty out the venous system.[89]

Preinjection Ischemia. Making a limb ischemic, after exsanguination and prior to the injection of the local anesthetic agent, enhances the effectiveness of the regional technique. After exsanguination of the extremity, a tourniquet is applied at the proximal site and inflated well above the systolic pressure. This circumstance continues for 15 to 20 minutes. Harris[91] demonstrated that this ischemic period will minimize the amount of local anesthetic eventually needed. In the study by Bell,[85] complete analgesia resulted from a dose one half of that usually required.

Ischemia of a limb alone is capable of inducing some anesthesia. The pattern of onset is delayed. It is preceded by tingling; the development of numbness and analgesia is slow. Total ischemic anesthesia requires 20 or more minutes.[92]

Site of Injection. The more peripheral the placement of a needle for injection of anesthetic solutions, the more successful the anesthetic procedure. A distal superficial vein is selected for the injection, and it is observed that retrograde dispersion into the tissue occurs. Sorbie[92] has demonstrated that a higher percentage of successful blocks is obtained with needles placed on the dorsum of the hand as compared with the injection made in a forearm or antecubital vein (Table 28–1).

Vascular Engorgement.[93] This condition, when involving an extremity, has been proposed as a feature of the intravenous regional technique. This can be done by *slow inflation* of the tourniquet. Good analgesia with one half the usual volume of anesthetic solution has been reported. In Morrison's studies, 10 to 12 ml of a 2% solution was used instead of 20 to 30 ml of 1% lidocaine. In the amount of local anesthetic drug by weight, there is especially little difference in the total dose employed. Furthermore, most clinicians find that the results have been more variable and success less predictable using this technique.

TABLE 28–1. RELATIONSHIP OF SITE OF ANESTHETIC INJECTION TO SUCCESS OF BIER-TYPE INTRAVENOUS REGIONAL ANESTHESIA

Site of Injection	Percent Failures
Antecubital fossa	22.7
Middle of forearm or leg	18.1
Hand, wrist, or foot	4.1

From Katz, J.: Choice of agents for intravenous regional anesthesia. Reg. Anesth., 4:10, 1979.

TOURNIQUET TIME. Never deflate the tourniquet until at least 20 to 30 minutes have elapsed from the time of injection when lidocaine or procaine has been used. A longer time is advised if bupivacaine is employed. Magora[94] has demonstrated that there is an increase in postdeflation anesthesia.

No tourniquets should remain continuously in place for more than 2 hours. For prolonged surgery, the continuous or intermittent technique can be employed.

SUPPLEMENTAL ANESTHESIA. Some nerves to the arm are poorly anesthetized, namely, the intercostobrachial, the lower lateral, and the posterior cutaneous nerves of the arm. For surgery in these areas of innervation, the nerves must be blocked by local injection to supplement the intravenous regional anesthesia.

TOURNIQUET DISCOMFORT. This may appear in 15 to 20 minutes often as an ache, "tightness," or paresthesia.

If significant, one of the following steps alleviates the condition:

1. The subcutaneous infiltration of a local anesthetic (0.25% lidocaine or mepivacaine) above the tourniquet as a band or armlet around the arm.
2. Application of a second tourniquet cuff just below the first and in the area already anesthetized. The second cuff is applied at the inception of the procedure.

TWO-CUFF TECHNIQUE.[89] In 1963, Holmes introduced the concept of the two-cuff technique to control tourniquet discomfort (Fig. 28–5). The present practice is as follows: Two tourniquet cuffs are applied close together well above the operative site. After producing ischemia of the limb, the upper or proximal cuff is inflated initially and the lower cuff remains deflated; when tourniquet discomfort becomes significant, the lower cuff is rapidly inflated followed by deflation of the upper cuff. Because the lower cuff is in an anesthetized area, little or no discomfort is experienced and an additional hour or more of good anesthesia ensues.

CHOICE OF LOCAL ANESTHETIC AGENTS (TABLE 28–2).[95–97] The most commonly used local anesthetic agent is lidocaine. This was the local anesthetic agent advocated by Holmes[89] in his report when he reintroduced the intravenous regional anesthesia technique, thereby popularizing it. From the experience of most regional anesthetists,[95,96] it is considered that no other agent has been found to be superior. This agent can be used for short procedures and for those procedures lasting over 2 hours by applying the intermittent or continuous technique.[100]

Bupivacaine 0.25% to 0.5% has been used for prolonged surgical procedures.[98,99] An increase in postdeflation sedation and anesthesia occurs.[94] Potentially serious complications have been reported.[101]

Other agents have been used but have undesirable actions; chlorprocaine is associated with a high incidence of thrombophlebitis (5% to 10%),[102] and prilocaine is associated with methemoglobinemia.[103,104] Mepivacaine 0.5% has been used but has no advantages over lidocaine.[105] Tetracaine provides rapid and intense anesthesia.[106]

Prewarming of anesthetic solutions to 30°C or to body temperature is recommended before injection as this results in minimal patient discomfort.[107] There is no diminution of dynamic effect on the onset or the quality of the block. Cold solutions, including those at a room temperature of 22°C, are

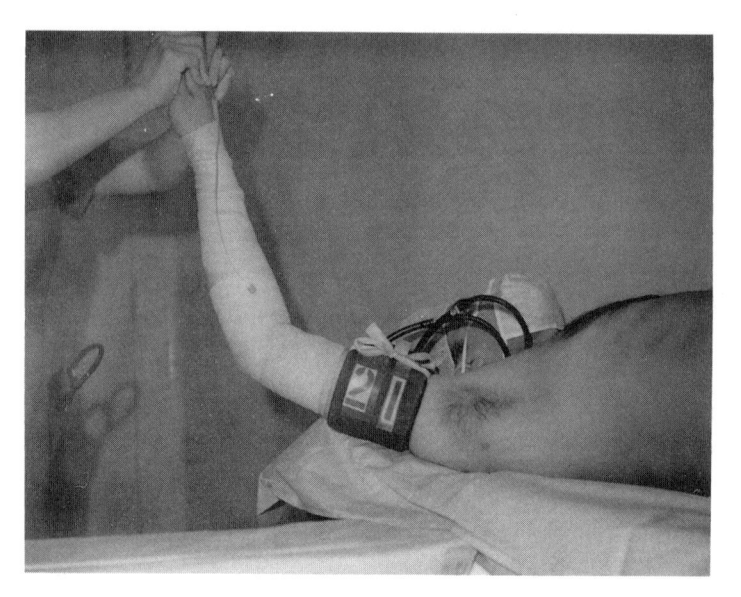

FIG. 28–5. Intravenous regional technique—Continuous two-cuff method. A tourniquet cuff with two inflatable bags labeled *1* and *2* is placed high up on the arm. An elastic ace or Esmarch bandage is wrapped around the arm from the fingers to the tourniquet. Note the tubing of an intravenous catheter that has been inserted in the dorsum of the hand. After "milking" the arm of blood, bag No. 1 is inflated above systolic pressure and the local anesthetic is injected through the catheter to spread through the arm tissues. When the patient experiences discomfort, bag No. 2 is inflated and bag No. 1 is deflated.

TABLE 28-2. CHARACTERISTICS OF THE DIFFERENT LOCAL ANESTHETIC AGENTS USED FOR UPPER EXTREMITY INTRAVENOUS REGIONAL ANESTHESIA

Drug	Usual Concentration (%)	Total Dose (mg/kg)	Time to Surgical Anesthesia (min)	Loss of Volitional Motor Activity (min)	Comment	References
Procaine	0.5	3–4	2	8	The classic drug	74
Chloroprocaine	0.25–2	up to 8	5	15	Thrombophlebitis reported (secondary to preservatives?)	88
Tetracaine	0.2	1–1.5	3–6	8		89
Lidocaine	0.25–0.5	3–4	3–5	15	Most common agent reported	90,91
Mepivacaine	0.5–0.6	2–8	3–4	13	No advantages	92
Bupivacaine	0.2–0.5	1.5–3	2–8	10	Prolonged posttourniquet release; analgesia	87,93
Prilocaine	0.5–1.0	3	4–5	10	Methemoglobinemia	94,95

Modified from Katz, J.: Intravenous regional anesthesia. Semin. Anesthesiol. *11*:50, 1983.

associated with pain injection and often extremely unpleasant sensations.

ALTERNATIVE DRUGS. Ketamine in a 0.5% solution has been used as the agent in the intravenous regional anesthesia technique. A volume of about 40 ml has been effective. The use of this drug is limited by the development of unconsciousness within a few minutes of release of the tourniquet. This state is not antagonized by naloxone.[108]

DOSAGE. A volume–dose relationship is involved in obtaining anesthesia by this method. There must be a volume of solution sufficient to fill the vascular bed, and the concentration must be sufficient to produce anesthesia. The latter is limited by the factor of toxicity.

With regard to regional intravascular anesthesia of the extremities, a large volume of low concentration of the local anesthetic agent is employed. The anesthetic solution is used to replace the blood in the vascular area to be anesthetized. It is thus a volume technique and depends on knowing the vascular volume of the extremities (see below).

To replace the blood volume of an area and also to eliminate the dilution effect of the blood on the anesthetic solution, the selected extremity must be made ischemic.

In general, the total dose of procaine or lidocaine is based on a range of 1.5 to 3 mg/kg of body weight.[109]

For the upper extremity, a dose of 3 mg/kg is used in a 0.5% solution. In most adults a volume of 40 to 50 ml is thus injected.[89] If a preinjection period of ischemia is used, then a smaller volume may be used based on a dose of 1.5 mg/kg or a volume of 20 to 24 ml of an 0.5% solution.[90]

For the lower extremity, the dose is also 3 mg/kg but a solution of 0.25% is used; hence, the volume is doubled.

BLOOD VOLUME IN THE EXTREMITIES. It is essential to know the approximate volume of the extremities for an understanding of the technique of intravenous regional anesthesia. It is also of importance in understanding the loading of central circulation following exsanguination of an extremity and the application of a tourniquet as well as the hypotension that may occur on release of a tourniquet and a reinfusion of an extremity.[110]

From Ebert's investigations,[110] the blood volume in a single upper extremity has been estimated as 3% of the total blood volume. A study by Adams[111] of the blood volume in the lower extremity using Cr-51 tagged red cells reveals a volume of a single lower extremity of about 9% of total blood volume.

For the average man weighing 70 kg, the upper extremity has a blood volume of about 170 ml, and the lower extremity a volume of about 300 ml.[111]

GUIDELINES TO PREVENT LEAKAGE.[112,113] Leakage of anesthetic solutions into the systemic circulation during intravenous regional anesthesia does occur. It has been associated with high plasma levels of the local anesthetic on occasion, which have resulted in significant morbidity and mortality. Seizure phenomena, convulsions, and cardiopulmonary arrest have been reported. The safety of the technique depends on the ability to prevent escape of anesthetic solution into the general circulation by means of an effective tourniquet pressure. An effective tourniquet pressure is one that minimally balances the maximum pressure that is generated in the region of injection of the anesthetic agent into the venous system of the region being anesthetized. An effective tourniquet pressure is not necessarily the gauge pressure. Two considerations thus become important. First are the tourniquet equipment and technique themselves. Second, are the factors related to the maximally developed venous pressure as the anesthetic solution is injected.

The commonly used tourniquet for this procedure consists of two adjacent cuffs, each relatively narrow and 6 cm in width.[114] When either cuff is inflated alone to a gauge pressure of 300 mm Hg, the effective tourniquet pressure may only be 200 mm Hg.[115]

Grice[113] has investigated the various factors affecting venous return. He has used a saline–xenon-133 solution and proper xenon detectors proximal to the tourniquets, enabling identification of solutions leaking past the tourniquet.

Maximum Venous Pressure. The maximum venous pressure that can be developed without leakage has been defined by Grice[113] as the venous pressure above which level there is an associated leakage. Among the factors affecting venous pressure are the following:

1. The venous pressure developed by the force used on injecting the anesthetic solution
2. Venous pressure developed—depends on the site of injection—higher venous pressures are developed when injections are made in the proximal veins
3. The rate of injection—fast rates of injection develop higher pressure

Injections at the elbow result in the passage of the anesthetic solution into the deep venous system in the elbow. It does not traverse readily distally into the distal superficial venous system; there is a limitation by the venous valve system and high syringe pressures are often used. Therefore, at the proximal site, the venous pressure can exceed cuff pressure and produce leakage. Further, the venous system is continuous with the circulation of the forearm bony system, and leakage can occur from the radius to the humerus. It is noted that cuff pressure will not prevent fluid passage through such a pathway.

Venous Pressure Related to Site of Injection. Higher venous pressures are developed when injections are made in the proximal veins. Thus, it is recommended that injections be made in a distal vein at the wrist or in the hand.[115]

Higher pressures develop in the venous system if exsanguination of the arm is incomplete. The filling pressure of the injectate is thus added to the residual venous blood volume and together they provide a greater venous pressure.

Rate of Injection. Higher pressures are developed when the rate of injection is rapid.

Recommendations.

1. The tourniquet pressure should be minimally set at 300 mm Hg.
2. The arm should be exsanguinated by means of an Esmarch bandage.
3. The injection site should be limited to the distal hand or forearm veins.
4. A slow rate of injection is recommended to be approximately 90 seconds.

OBSERVATIONS AND RESPONSES. If exsanguination is excellent, the skin will be pale. If less than perfect, the skin takes on a blotchy appearance ("cutis marmorata") because of blood forced from the deeper vessels into the subcuticular capillaries.

Many patients recognize tightness of the tourniquet; this is usually minor but may subsequently become an ache and uncomfortable.

On the injection of the anesthetic solution, subjects experience some sense of swelling and paresthesia; a feeling of tingling and warmth is common.

Bell[85] recommended a preinjection arterial occlusion. In this, the bandage or tourniquet is inflated and left in place for 20 minutes before the anesthetic solution is injected. This was found to hasten the onset of anesthesia, prolong its duration, and produce more complete anesthesia. Lower doses of the anesthetic agent and smaller volumes of the solution were effective. How this complements the anesthesia is not certain but may be related to the tissue hypoxia or local metabolic changes with elevation of P_{CO_2} and pH changes.

The end point for a completely successful block consists of complete sensory block, motor paralysis of the extremity, and the absence of subjective complaints. Some appropriate preanesthetic medication is an essential part of this as well as the other anesthetic techniques, but it is desirable that the patient be awake and responsive.

KINETICS OF DISTRIBUTION OF THE ANESTHETIC SOLUTION.[109,116] Because the venous system is a one-way flow system on account of valves, an anesthetic solution injected into a peripheral superficial vein travels proximally from the site of injection to the level of the applied inflated tourniquet (Holmes technique). Initially, the solution fills the large superficial veins: radial, ulnar, and median antebrachial. As the full volume of solution is introduced, it concentrates in the region of the elbow, particularly in the anterior part, filling the antecubital veins (basilic, cephalic, and median). This is reasonable, because there are large veins about the elbow with minimal resistance (especially in the collapsed or "milked" state) to the injection of solutions. Small veins in muscles, deep veins, and perforating veins are now filled. As soon as the veins are filled, there is a rapid retrograde filling of venules and capillaries.

Once in the capillaries, there is a diffusion of the drug through the capillary walls into the extravascular space and thence to the tissues. The amount of drug leaving the vascular compartment depends on the original exsanguination of the venous system, the dose of the anesthetic agent, and the volume of the solution.

Human studies with this technique demonstrate that more than 90% of the anesthetic is confined to the region below the tourniquet and remains there until release of the tourniquet (studied with radioactive-tagged lidocaine). Most of the anesthetic drug, i.e., about 70% is rapidly taken up and fixed by the tissues in the region of containment by the tourniquet.[117]

The largest concentration per unit gram of tissue is in the nerve tissue. This is twice the concentration in the skin and four times that of muscle, as determined by radioactive lidocaine uptake.[118]

About 30% of the injected solution remains in the vascular compartment for as long as 30 minutes after the injection and the initial distribution to the local tissues.[116] A gradual decrease occurs thereafter not due to tissue metabolism. If tourniquet release is rapid and occurs within 30 to 50 minutes after injection of the anesthetic solution, a bolus effect may occur from this venous pool, in which appreciable amounts can enter the general circulation and produce toxic reactions.

The amount of drug that enters the general circulation on release of the tourniquet depends on three main factors: the concentration of the anesthetic solution, the volume injected, and the duration of regional vascular containment.

Venous channels distal to the site of injection and toward the fingers are poorly filled. Some diffusion via perforating veins to the interosseous veins also occurs.

Venous Uptake.[116] After the release of a tourniquet, the local anesthetic, which has been confined to the region anesthetized and which now enters the venous circulation, shows a biphasic pattern of venous plasma concentration: (1) an initial immediate peak level within 1 minute due to the uptake of about 30% of the injected drug, and (2) a secondary slower uptake from the remaining portion of injected drug with a gradual decline in plasma concentration during the following 30 minutes. After 30 minutes, about 50% of an injected drug still remains in the anesthetized region and continues to be absorbed at a much slower rate.

KINETICS OF NERVE DISTRIBUTION. The kinetics of nerve distribution of anesthetic solutions in this technique have been studied by Raj.[119] After filling the venous channels around the elbow, which are in proximity to main nerve trunks, smaller vascular channels take the agent to the core of the nerve trunks. Once in the core, the anesthetic diffuses toward the periphery of the nerve. Because fibers to the distal part of the extremity are in the core of the nerve trunk and those to the proximal part of the arm are in the outer nerve layers, it would be expected that the fibers for distal distribution would be blocked first. This is in agreement with the clinical observation that anesthesia develops from the finger tips upward.

Site of Action. Two sites of action for local anesthetics with this technique have been proposed: (1) at the small sensory nerves and the sensory nerve endings (and, presumably, at the neuromuscular junction), and (2) at the nerve trunks. Some conflicting evidence has been adduced.[115] The evidence for an effect at a sensory nerve ending, however, is based on electrophysiologic study of nerve conduction and is so sparse that only the effect on the nerve trunk and its small nerve fibers is admissible.

Bier,[79] in his initial studies, placed two constricting bandages above and below a site of intravenous injection in the arm. A large volume of 80 ml 0.5% procaine was injected between the two tourniquets. He observed rapid onset of anesthesia between the bandages, which he designated as *direct anesthesia*; he noted slower onset of anesthesia in the part of the arm distal to the lower tourniquet. He considered that, because of prompt onset in the area between the bandages, the anesthesia so produced was at the small nerves (and possibly the result of leaking under the lower tourniquet). He designated the block of the distal to the lower tourniquet as *indirect anesthesia* and considered it the result of nerve trunk blockade.

A similar study by Sorbie[92] demonstrated that anesthesia was produced in a nerve trunk distribution. Tourniquets were placed around the upper arm and at the wrist. Injection of 20 ml of 0.5% lidocaine into a forearm vein produced complete anesthesia of the arm and also in the hand beyond the lower tourniquet. Anesthesia developed in a peripheral nerve distribution.

The evidence that the major site of action of intravenous regional anesthesia is at the nerve trunks was accumulated by Raj[119] in three classic experiments:

1. In the first experiment, three tourniquets (the upper tourniquet was double cuffed) were placed on the arm of patients to divide the arm into three compartments on inflation of the tourniquets. A solution of 15 ml of a 0.5% lidocaine–renografin mixture was injected into the medial antecubital vein at the elbow in the upper compartment. The solution was observed to remain in the upper compartment and, after 10 minutes, anesthesia developed in the digits and progressed upward.
2. In a second experiment, with only one tourniquet in the upper arm, a 20-ml solution of 0.5% li-

docaine–renografin mixture was injected into the medial antecubital vein and remained in the upper third of the forearm. Anesthesia again developed from the hand upward.

3. In the third experiment, the arm was again divided into three compartments by tourniquets. After inflation of the tourniquets, 15 ml of the solution of 0.5% lidocaine–renografin mixture (15 ml) was injected into the distal compartment via a cannula placed on the dorsum of the hand, i.e., distal to the wrist tourniquet, preventing the superficial venous drainage. It was observed that the solution travelled to the elbow via deep veins and interosseous veins and promptly reached the superficial veins of the elbow, where it pooled in all the elbow veins. As this pooling occurred, anesthesia of the entire arm distal to the upper tourniquet occurred.

Evidence from these studies supports the view that a major site of action is at nerve trunks, with the onset of anesthesia at the distal portion of the arm.[120] For this to occur, the core fibers of a nerve trunk must initially come in contact with the anesthetic solution. Anatomically, this is accomplished by the anesthetic solution passing retrograde from the elbow vessels into the intrinsic vascular channels inside the nerve trunks. These neurovascular channels have no valves.

The radiopaque contrast medium as a marker for the injected solution has two drawbacks in providing information. It is a hyperosmolar solution and may induce abnormal flow and diffusion in small vasculature. Second, the roentgenography technique may fail to reveal small amounts of the contrast.[115]

Action of Intravenous Regional Anesthetics on Small Nerves.
Convincing evidence of an action on small nerves as one of the sites of action of intravenous regional anesthesia has been adduced by the experiments of Lillie.[121] A radioisotope and a double-blind, placebo-anesthetic controlled study was conducted in healthy volunteers. When a double tourniquet system, one on the upper arm and another at the wrist, was inflated to pressures of 300 mm Hg to isolate the hand from the forearm and a tagged anesthetic solution injected between the cuffs, no radioisotope leakage was found to occur into the general circulation or into the hand. Second, after injection of 40 ml prilocaine 0.5% anesthetic solution into a cubital fossa vein, no anesthesia appeared in the hand, except for a minimal area on the dorsum of the area of sensory distribution of the radial nerve. Finally, while the tourniquets were inflated, cramping pain occurred in the hand. These results indicate that the analgesia obtained with the intravenous regional technique is also caused by blockade of small nerves or, possibly, nerve endings themselves and not in the major trunks at the elbow as was suggested by previous studies of retrograde venous diffusion into the core of the nerve trunks of the ulnar and median nerves.

Multiple Sites of Action Concept.[122]
The conflicting results and conclusions obtained by these different studies have been explained by Rosenberg.[122] He suggested that multiple and complementary mechanisms are probably operative. The intravenous regional technique has assumed that the local anesthetic remains isolated below the proximal tourniquet. However, using radioisotopes, Grice,[113] has clearly demonstrated that injected solutions leak past a properly inflated tourniquet. This may occur even at cuff pressures of 400 mm Hg. Leakage may occur via intertissue diffusion, or there may be a diffusion of the local anesthetic beyond the tourniquet via the intraosseous pathway.

In conclusion, in intravenous regional anesthesia, the site of action most likely occurs at both the smaller nerves and, possibly, the sensory nerve endings, as well as at the main trunks of the ulnar and median nerves.

CLINICAL CONSIDERATIONS. Confining local anesthetics as described to a region of an extremity provides anesthesia lasting 1.5 to 2 hours. Tourniquets are released slowly, and the anesthetic is washed into the general circulation. If a toxic action occurs, symptoms will be seen in 5 to 15 minutes. On release of the tourniquet, recovery is prompt. If the tourniquet has been applied and the anesthetic confined for 1 hour, sensation will return in 2 to 5 minutes.

The method is simple and may be used in various extremity procedures, such as the treatment of fractures, the management of tendon and muscle injuries, and lacerations.

Precautions include the use of low concentrations and careful release of the tourniquet. Provisions must be made to prevent and treat toxic reactions. Oxygen should be administered with a bag-mask system during release of the tourniquet and be readily available for 15 minutes after.

RELEASE OF TOURNIQUET. At the conclusion of surgery, the confining tourniquet is released according to a set plan to avoid high systemic levels of the local anesthetic. Originally, Bier[79] recommended an intermittent release to reduce the likelihood of toxic systemic levels of procaine. A more planned "cyclic," intermittent technique of release is recommended as follows:[123,124]

1. Deflation of tourniquet pressure to zero and immediate reinflation.
2. After 1 minute, a second deflation to zero pressure for 10 seconds and immediate reinflation.
3. After 2 minutes, another deflation to zero for 30 seconds and reinflation.

4. After 3 minutes, another deflation to zero and no reinflation.

During the deflation phases, the operator must observe any complaints, such as buzzing, dizziness, or metallic taste. These symptoms indicate an appreciable blood level and warrant shorter periods of deflation. Variations of intermittent release technique evidently can be used, provided that the objective is understood to be the limitation of plasma levels of the drug.

SYSTEMIC PLASMA LEVELS OF AGENT AFTER TOURNIQUET RELEASE

Effect of Duration of Vascular Occlusion.[116] The duration of vascular occlusion and regional vascular containment of the anesthetic solution significantly affects the concentration of the agent that enters the general circulation on release of the tourniquet. As the time of vascular occlusion increases, there is a steady decrease in the peak systemic arterial plasma concentration (see "Arterial Levels" below).

Venous Levels (Injected Arm). Venous plasma concentrations of the various local anesthetics in the injected arm and in the contralateral arm have been assessed at various periods following tourniquet release. After 20 minutes of vascular occlusion, plasma levels of different anesthetic agents in the venous drainage of the injected arm were observed at 15 to 40 μg/ml two minutes after release of the tourniquet (noncyclic). Lidocaine (0.5% 20 ml) produced the highest concentrations at 40 μg/ml; concentrations of 15 μg/ml were found for etidocaine and prilocaine and 20 μg/ml for bupivacaine. Venous plasma levels from the injected arm progressively decrease but continue to be appreciable for at least 30 minutes. At this time, the lidocaine levels average 10 μg/ml and bupivacaine 1.5 μg/ml.[125]

After 45 minutes of anesthesia, release of tourniquet results in peak venous plasma levels estimated for lidocaine at 7.5 μg/ml, for prilocaine, about 5 μg/ml. For etidocaine and bupivacaine, the venous plasma levels are less than 2 μg/ml (Fig. 28–6).[109,125]

Arterial Levels. The plasma levels in the venous drainage of the injected arm represent the amounts that reach the pulmonary artery and lung. A large proportion of this local anesthetic is taken up by the lung tissue and is also diluted by venous return from other parts of the body.[109] Thus, the arterial level of the anesthetics will be greatly reduced. Peak systemic arterial concentrations are only 30% of the pulmonary arterial plasma levels.[116]

After 10 to 20 minutes of vascular containment using a 1% lidocaine solution (3 mg/kg), the peak arterial plasma concentration of lidocaine was determined at 10.3 μg/ml on the release of the tourniquet. After 45 minutes of occlusion, the plasma arterial concentration of lidocaine is approximately 2.5 μg/ml on the release of tourniquet (Fig. 28–7).[116]

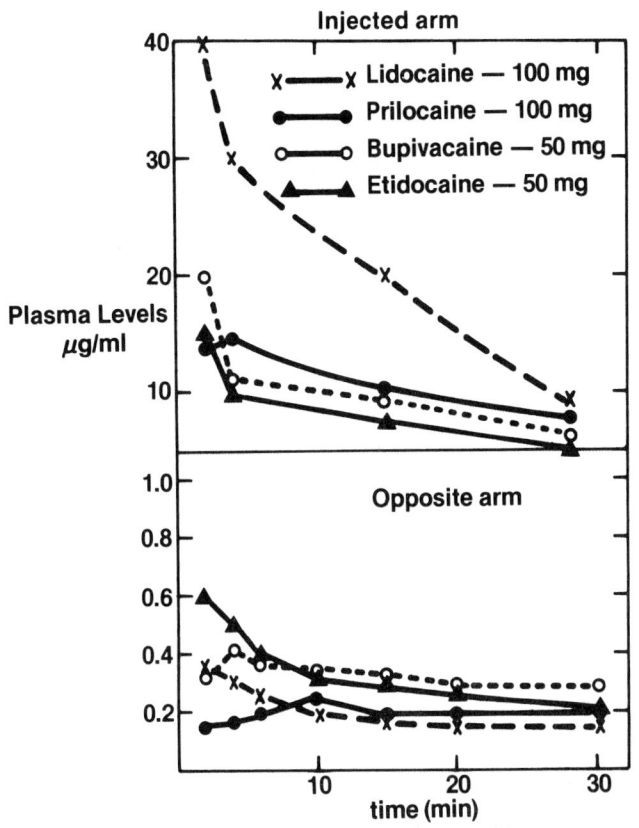

FIG. 28–6. Venous plasma concentrations of lidocaine, prilocaine, bupivacaine, and etidocaine in injected arm and contralateral arm following 20 minutes of tourniquet occlusion. From Covino, B.J.: Pharmacokinetics of intravenous regional anesthesia. Reg. Anesth., 4:5, 1979.

Venous Level (Contralateral Arm). On release of a tourniquet 5 to 10 minutes after the injection of 20 ml of lidocaine 1% anesthetic solution, peak venous concentrations of the local anesthetic are found in the opposite arm of approximately 1 to 2 μg/ml at 1 to 2 minutes after release. This contrasts with the direct intravenous administration of the same dose of the drug as that employed in the regional technique and results in peak levels several times greater in the opposite arm, with peaking at 8 to 10 μg/ml between 4 and 6 minutes.[126]

By 10 to 20 minutes after regional injection, the peak venous blood level in the opposite arm is less than 1 μg/ml on release of the tourniquet.[85] In Evans's studies of several agents,[125] the peak venous concentrations in the contralateral arm after 20 minutes of anesthesia are all under 0.5 μg/ml.

It is evident that not all of the anesthetic is released immediately from the anesthetized region on deflation of the tourniquet but that there is a gradual release from tissues. Thus, tissues tend to retain the anesthetic drug. Exercise of the anesthetized part

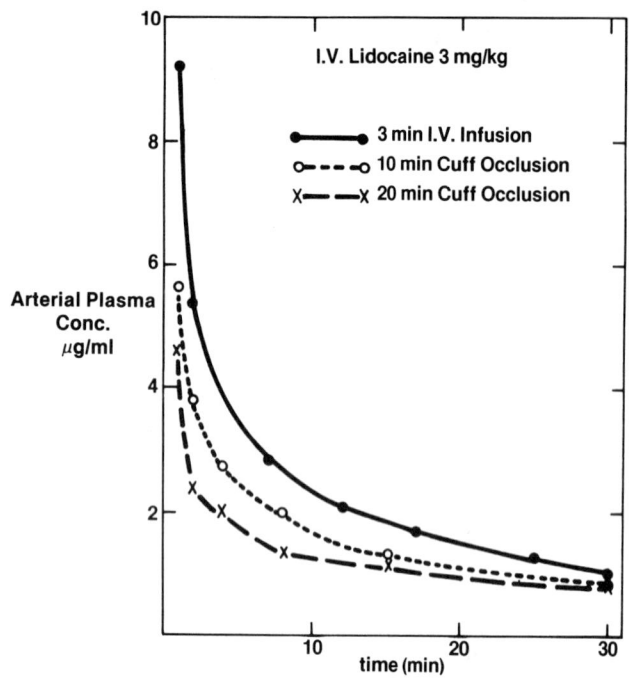

FIG. 28–7. Arterial plasma concentrations of lidocaine in the noninjected arm following direct intravenous administration of 3 mg/kg over 3 minutes and following tourniquet occlusion of 10 and 20 minutes. From Covino, B.J.: Pharmacokinetics of intravenous regional anesthesia. Reg. Anesth., 4:5, 1979.

after tourniquet release, however, will increase the amount removed from the tissues and entering the venous circulation.[127]

Dose Effect. Corresponding levels of lidocaine in the venous blood of the opposite arm in subjects receiving 3 mg/kg reaches a maximum of 1.2 μg/ml when the tourniquet is released 10 to 20 minutes after injection. With a lower dose of 1.5 mg/kg, the plasma concentration never exceeded 1 μg/ml and the average maximum was 0.7 μg/ml.[85]

Concentration Effect. The peak arterial plasma concentration of lidocaine, which occurs following the release of a tourniquet, also depends on the original concentration of the anesthetic solution. As noted above, the systemic arterial plasma concentration from lidocaine 1% after 10 to 20 minutes of occlusion is 10 μg/ml and after 45 minutes of occlusion is 2.5 μg/ml on release of tourniquet. In comparison using 0.5% solution and the same total dosage, much lower arterial plasma concentration occurs at 10 to 20 minutes on release of the tourniquet and is only 5 μg/ml; after 45 minutes, the arterial level is less than 1 μg/ml levels.

It is concluded that larger volumes of dilute solutions, even when the total dosage remains the same, result in lower arterial plasma levels, and toxic reactions are less likely.

STUDY OF CYCLIC DEFLATION–REINFLATION VERSUS NONCYCLIC RELEASE. A second cyclic deflation–reinflation sequence is that of Sukhani's tourniquet deflation to a zero pressure permitted at 10-second intervals (fixed deflation times in a cyclic sequence) (Fig. 28–8). After each 10-second period of deflation, the tourniquet is reinflated. After 1 minute, the cuff is again deflated for 10 seconds. This sequence is repeated a total of three to four times, after which the tourniquet remains deflated. A variation of cyclic deflation–reinflation is to apply a variable deflation time of 0 seconds, 10 seconds, and 30 seconds. An interval of 1 minute is provided between reinflation.[123]

Studies of arterial and venous blood levels of administered lidocaine showed a trend toward lower maximum blood concentrations but a significantly longer time to reach a maximum concentration (Fig. 28–9). A differential between arterial and the ipsilateral venous concentration represents pulmonary uptake of lidocaine. This cyclic deflation technique allows more time for pulmonary extraction to decrease overall lidocaine and results in a gradual rise to a maximum rather than a sudden plasma rise on deflation of the tourniquet. Consequently, toxic reactions are less likely to occur.[124]

RECOVERY. After complete release of the tourniquet, there is rapid return of sensory nerve function within 1 to 5 minutes. Anesthesia is seldom present 10 minutes after release of the tourniquet with most local anesthetic agents. Reactive hyperemia is partially responsible for rapid washout and removal of anesthetic agent.[105]

The return of sensation and activity is equally rapid regardless of the duration of anesthesia and confinement of anesthetic agents by the tourniquet. Curiously, whether the tourniquet is released shortly after injection, i.e., after a period of anesthesia of 15 minutes or less, or after 60 minutes of anesthesia, the return of function still is usually between 1 and 5 minutes.

Bupivacaine is an exception to such rapid returning of sensation. After anesthesia with 0.25% solution, some residual anesthesia continues for 10 to 15 minutes after release of the tourniquet, and this provides significant postoperative advantages.[95]

REACTIONS. Toxic reactions occur when the local anesthetics gain access to the general circulation in critical amounts. These reactions are the same as those that occur after direct intravenous injection.[126]

Most are seen immediately after release of the tourniquet and are related to the plasma level of the drug. The usual proximate causes of the reactions are inadequate occlusion of the confining tourniquet or the release of tourniquets too early or accidentally. Reactions may also occur if excessive doses are employed. In the two-cuff technique, the release of the proximal tourniquet when the distal tourniquet is

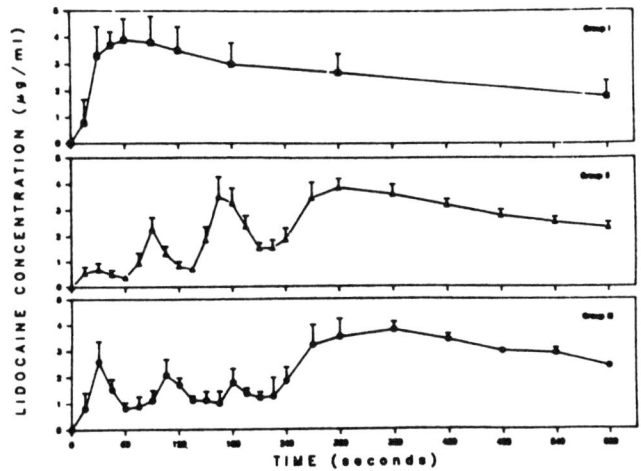

FIG. 28–8. Time course of arterial plasma levels of lidocaine in μg/ml (mean ± SEM) resulting from the three techniques of tourniquet deflation. *Upper,* Noncyclic deflation. *Middle,* Cyclic deflation with variable deflation time (0.10–0.30) and 1-minute intervals. *Lower,* Cyclic deflation with fixed deflation time of 10 seconds and 1-minute intervals. Maximal arterial lidocaine levels did not differ significantly between the three groups. The arterial samples were drawn from the contralateral radial artery. From Sukhani, R., et al.: Lidocaine disposition following intravenous regional anesthesia with different tourniquet deflation techniques. Anesth. Analg., 68:633, 1989.

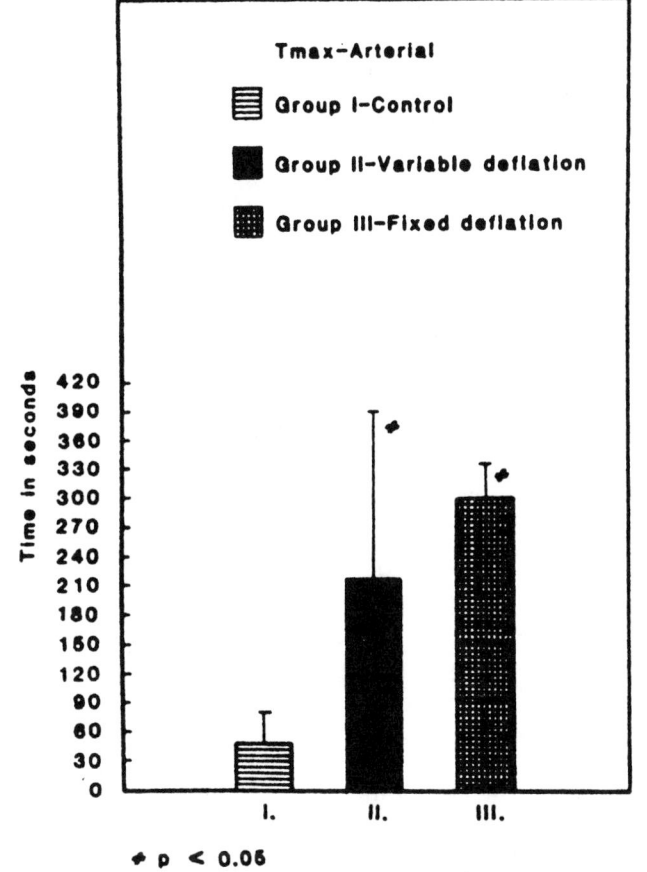

FIG. 28–9. Time (seconds: mean ± SEM) to maximum arterial concentrations of lidocaine in the three groups. Maximum arterial concentration (T_{max}) was significantly longer in both Groups II and III than in Group I; there was no significant difference between Groups II and III. From Sukhani, R., et al: Lidocaine disposition following intravenous regional anesthesia with different tourniquet deflation techniques. Anesth. Analg., 68:633, 1989.

inadequately or not inflated may permit toxic amounts of the local agent to enter the systemic circulation.[85]

Concentrations of radioactive drug remain at the level of injection within the anesthetized limb for 90 minutes or the duration of the vascular occlusion.[117] Only on release of the tourniquet does the drug enter in significant amounts into the systemic circulation. On release, the drug is quickly distributed throughout the body and is found in equal concentrations throughout body tissues within 30 minutes.

When total doses of 3 mg/kg of lidocaine are employed, peak venous systemic plasma concentrations in the opposite arm of up to 1.2 μg/ml are noted only on release of the tourniquet after 10 to 20 minutes. Reactions noted are all mild in about half of the patients at this dose level. With doses of 1.5 mg/kg, venous plasma levels (opposite arm) do not exceed 1 μg/kg on release of tourniquet, and only 6% of patients develop minor complications.[85]

With an average intravenous regional dose of 3 mg/kg of lidocaine, maximum peak venous systemic plasma levels of 1.5 μg/ml on release of the tourniquet after 45 minutes were observed by Mazze.[128] Compared with the plasma levels after axillary and epidural block with the same dose, the intravenous regional technique gave a lesser systemic plasma drug level: 25 μg/ml for axillary block and 3.1 μg/ml after lumbar epidural.

Direct intravenous infusion of lidocaine at a rate of 0.5 mg/min (average total dose of 6.4 mg/kg) gave plasma concentrations of 5.2 μg/ml. This plasma level appears to be the critical one at which CNS symptoms appear.[126,127]

Adverse Effects. In the experience of most clinicians, less than 5% of patients show any significant changes.[128] In recent reports, the overall incidence of adverse effects is about 1.5%.[129]

CNS reactions are mild and consist of temporary dizziness, nystagmus, and drowsiness.[130] Mild seizures and convulsions have been reported, but with intermittent tourniquet release as originally recommended by Bier, these are rarely seen.[129] The incidence rate is calculated as about 1:2000, and is related to technical errors.

Direct intravenous injection (not regional containment) also produces EEG changes consisting of reduction of alpha activity and increase in low-frequency, high-amplitude waves. After intravenous regional anesthesia and the release of the tourniquet, the same type of EEG changes are only occasionally noted. Drowsiness, disorientation, unconsciousness, and some breathing difficulties, lightheadedness, and numbness of the tongue are occasionally seen. These correlate with high blood levels.[130]

CNS toxic reactions can be virtually eliminated by using smaller total doses (1 mg/kg) and by intermittent release of the tourniquet over 2 to 5 min.

ECG Changes. The major changes are mild bradycardia and small decreases in T-wave amplitude; other dysrhythmias have been reported.[129] Pulse and blood pressure changes are insignificant.

Supplemental Medication. Most patients require no additional medication to supplement the preanesthetic medication. About 5% may require some intraoperative heavy sedation. Less than 0.6% may require general anesthesia.[129] This experience is an advantage, for ambulatory surgical procedure patients can be discharged soon after surgery. CNS effects of the local anesthesia are dissipated soon after the surgery and release of the tourniquet.

EFFECT ON NERVE CONDUCTION.[88] During the regional anesthesia produced by localized intravenous injection, the physiology of nerve conduction was investigated by Adams.[88] Time of conduction was greatly increased during induction and after 30 minutes; the median nerve of the arm completely failed to conduct impulses even when the stimulus was greatly increased. After ischemia for 20 minutes and without any anesthetic, measurements showed that the nerve continued to conduct impulses although the conduction time was longer. Thus, hypoxia does not significantly block conduction.

EFFECT ON NEUROMUSCULAR JUNCTION. Local anesthetics produce a definite prejunctional block and a curare-like attachment to cholinergic receptors at the muscle endplate.[88a]

LOWER EXTREMITY BIER-TYPE BLOCK

Intravenous regional anesthesia of the lower extremity is mentioned in the reports of both Holmes[89] and Bell;[85] however, no details of their techniques or results are reported. In 1984, Lehman and Jones[131] used intravenous regional anesthesia for surgical procedures at or distal to the knee. No significant complications occurred, and plasma levels of lidocaine were below the toxic range.

Lehman-Jones (Lower Extremity) Block:

1. Establish IV line in an upper extremity for fluids and drugs.
2. Two standard arterial thigh pneumatic tourniquets are pretested (300 mm Hg for adults; 250 mm Hg for children).
3. Tourniquets are placed adjacent to each other around the thigh as far proximal as possible and over sheet wadding.
4. An intravenous route is established with a 22-gauge plastic needle in the lower extremity at the level of the foot or ankle. The needle is secured with tape.
   a. Dorsum of foot—veins adjacent to dorsalis pedis artery.
   b. Greater saphenous vein just anterior to medial malleolus is the most satisfactory.
5. The lower extremity is elevated for 3 minutes to achieve venous drainage.
6. Exsanguination of the extremity is completed by wrapping the leg from the toes to the level of the tourniquet with an Esmarch bandage. The lower leg should be placed on a pillow.
7. Inflate the upper tourniquet to the preset pressure of 300 mm Hg. Check arterial occlusion by palpating the tibial artery.
8. A lidocaine anesthetic solution of 0.25% or 0.5% concentration is injected into the intravenous line in the lower limb. For the lower concentration, a dose of 3.3 mg/kg of body weight is administered. For a 70-kg man, this amounts to a volume of about 90 ml. This volume should be infused over a period of 3 minutes.
9. Sensory anesthesia develops in 15 to 20 min.
10. At this time, the lower tourniquet is inflated and the upper one deflated.

Comment. A failure rate of about 15% occurs with the thigh tourniquet technique. A thigh tourniquet is attended by significant discomfort. A large volume of solution is required, and because the concentration is low to keep within an 80-ml dose range, the anesthetic block is often incomplete.

Modification for Ankle or Foot Surgery.[132]

1. Establish an intravenous line in an arm for fluids and drugs.
2. Place a standard arterial arm tourniquet around the calf at its widest circumference but at least 3 inches below the head of the fibula to avoid peroneal nerve compression. A double tourniquet on the calf of the lower leg does not evenly fit the curvature of the calf and frequently fails; therefore, it is not used.
3. A standard arterial thigh tourniquet is placed at the midpoint of the thigh as a "back up." This provides an additional means to prevent the anesthetic from entering the systemic circulation in the event of lower tourniquet failure. Both

cuffs are connected to a separate oxygen-powered variable pressure inflation regulator.

4. A 22-gauge plastic needle is inserted into the greater saphenous vein at the ankle just anterior to the medial malleolus for administration of the intravenous anesthetic. The needle is secured and an adapter plug inserted into the needle hub.
5. The lower extremity is elevated for 3 minutes to achieve venous drainage.
6. Exsanguination of the extremity is completed by wrapping the leg from the toes to the level of the tourniquet with an Esmarch bandage. The lower leg should be placed on a pillow.
7. Inflate the calf tourniquet to 300 mm Hg by a pressure-powered regulator.
8. A 0.5% lidocaine anesthetic solution is administered via the ankle plastic needle. The dose of lidocaine is based on the size of the limb and not the patient's weight; it is a volume dose ranging from 40 to 50 ml.
9. A test dose of 10 ml of a 0.5% lidocaine anesthetic solution is injected. The patient is observed for systemic toxicity over a period of 1 minute. In the absence of adverse reactions, the remaining volume is injected.
10. The plastic needle is removed and the extremity surgically prepared. During this time, the adequacy of anesthesia is tested.

Efficiency of Tourniquet.[133] The potential of leaks of anesthetic solution beyond the inflated tourniquet is of concern, because the tourniquet encloses two bones in the distal leg. To study the occurrence of leaks past an intact tourniquet in regional anesthesia of the distal limb of the lower extremity, Davies[133] used a Hoyle double-cuff tourniquet[114] placed around the lower limb above the ankle but just below the bulge of the calf muscle. The cuff gauge pressure required to occlude the dorsalis pedis artery—the occlusion pressure—was determined for both proximal and distal cuffs. The proximal cuff was inflated to the higher of the two cuff pressures plus 100 mm Hg, i.e., to about 450 mm Hg (usually 350 mm Hg is chosen). The technique of block proceeded according to a two-cuff technique: A 1-mm intravenous cannula or needle was inserted on the dorsum of the foot; the foot and ankle were exsanguinated by elevation of leg and wrapping with an Esmarch bandage; then, inflation of the ankle cuff to 100 mm Hg above occlusion pressure and injection of 0.25% bupivacaine, averaging 40 ml (dose of 1.5 mg/kg up to a maximum dose of 100 mg), were performed. Plasma blood samples were taken from an antecubital fossa vein at 1 and 3 minutes after injection, and again when the proximal thigh cuff was inflated and the distal ankle cuff deflated. Bupivacaine was demonstrated in the systemic circulation in all subjects while the tourniquet remained inflated. Drug levels were not in the toxic range. Reasons for leakage included:

- Rapid rate of injection, raising venous pressure
- Fluctuation of systemic arterial pressure
- Passage through interosseous tissues protected by two long bones
- Intraosseous leak

The magnitude of the leak with intravenous regional block of the leg is small, but the incidence is large at 80% to 100% of subjects, compared with leakage in arm intravenous regional block of less than 25%.[134]

Recommendations for tourniquet pressure in intravenous regional anesthesia of the leg are as follows:[135] (1) with tourniquet cuff about the calf, 300 to 400 mm Hg; and (2) with tourniquet about the ankle, 250 mm Hg.

These pressures appear to be occlusion pressures. In accordance with Davies's study,[133] it is recommended that an additional pressure of 100 mm Hg is warranted.

ADVANTAGES OF INTRAVENOUS REGIONAL ANESTHESIA.

- Safe and effective
- Easy to administer
- Reliable
- Low incidence of complication; no mortality following large series in experience to date
- In ambulatory surgery, patients rarely require heavy sedation or general anesthesia; hence, they can safely be discharged from the postanesthesia recovery unit rather promptly
- Any central effects of the local anesthetic agent are rapidly dissipated
- Useful in emergency surgery of the extremities, because patients can remain awake—the danger of aspiration likely with heavy sedation or general anesthesia is minimized

LIMITATIONS AND CONTRAINDICATIONS. Toxic reactions have been reported with doses of 3 mg/kg. The incidence and intensity of these can be reduced by a number of modifications: (1) by using smaller doses and/or volumes of anesthetic solution but within the range of effectiveness; (2) by expressing all the blood from the region to be anesthetized; (3) by maintaining the anesthetic in the localized region for 1 hour; and (4) by preinjection arterial occlusion for 20 minutes.

Contraindications include the usual ones to use of local agents.[126] The technique should not be used in the presence of liver dysfunction or disease. In debilitated and malnourished patients, the toxicity of local agents is greatly increased. A history of drug sensitivity precludes the technique as does any known convulsive disorder. If the peripheral circulation is deficient, it could be further compromised by the tourniquet. Because the local anesthetic esters and amides produce some block of neuromuscular functions, this technique should not be used in myasthenia gravis. Local anesthetic agents also have a quinidine-like action on the heart and, therefore, should not be used in decompensated patients or those on digitalis.

REFERENCES

1. Bier, A.: Uber einen neuen Weg Local anesthesie an den Gliedmassen zu Erzeugen. Arch. klin. Clis., 86:1007, 1908.
2. Graubard, D.J., Robertazzi, R.W., and Peterson, M.C.: Intravenous procaine. N.Y. State J. Med., 47:2187, 1947.
3. Allen, F.M., Crossman, L.W. and Lyons, L.U.: Intravenous procaine analgesia. Anesth. Analg., 25:1, 1946.
4. Kraft, K.A.: Intravenous procaine. Can. Med. Assoc. J., 57:3, 1948.
5. Burstein, C.: Treatment of acute arrhythmias during anesthesia by intravenous procaine. Anesthesiology, 7:113, 1946.
6. Graubard, D.J., and Peterson, M.C.: Intravenous procaine in the management of arthritis. Ct. State Med. J., 8:33, 1949.
7. Graubard, D.J., Kovacs, J., and Ritter, H.H.: The management of destructive arthritis of the hip by means of intravenous procaine. Ann. Intern. Med., 28:1106, 1948.
8. Durieu, H., DeClerco, F., and Duprez, A.: Treatment of asthma with intravenous administration of procaine hydrochloride. Acta Clinica Belgica, 1:150, 1946.
9. Queries and Minor Notes: Procaine and asthma. J.A.M.A., 137:1568, 1948.
10. Ameullie, M.D.: Intravenous procaine. J.A.M.A., 131:699, 1946.
11. Gordon, R.A.: Intravenous novocaine for analgesia in burns. Can. Med. Assoc. J., 49:478, 1943.
12. Gordon, R.A.: Clinical applications for intravenous procaine. Can. Med. Assoc. J., 59:534, 1948.
13. Allen, F.M.: Intravenous obstetrical anesthesia. Am. J. Surg., 70:283, 1945.
14. Johnson, K., and Gilbert, C.R.A.: Intravenous procaine for obstetrical anesthesia. Anesth. Analg., 25:133, 1946.
15. McLachlin, J. A.: The intravenous use of novocaine as a substitute for morphine in postoperative care. Can. Med. Assoc. J., 52:383, 1945.
16. Lundy, J.S.: *Clinical Anesthesia.* Philadelphia, W.B. Saunders, 1942.
17. Dressler, S., and Dwork, R.E.: Reactions to penicillin, J.A.M.A., 133:849, 1947.
18. Cohen, A.E., and Kaufman, J.: Use of procaine in treatment of reactions to penicillin. J. Allergy, 19:68, 1948.
19. State, D., and Wagensteen, O.H.: Procaine intravenously in treatment of delayed serum sickness. J.A.M.A.; 130:990, 1946.
20. Applebaum, E., Abraham, A., and Sinton, W.: A case of serum sickness treated with procaine intravenously. J.A.M.A., 131:1274, 1946.
21. Smith, E., et al.: A new method in the management of acute anterior poliomyelitis. N.Y. State J. Med., 48:2608, 1948.
22. Graubard, D.J., and Ritter, H.H.: Intravenous procaine in the treatment of trauma. Am. J. Surg., 74:765, 1947.
23. Graubard, D.J., Waldman, M.H., and Peterson, M.C.: Intravenous procaine in the management of the injured hand. N.Y. State J. Med., 48:1693, 1948.
24. Graubard, D.J., and Peterson, M.C.: The therapeutic uses of intravenous procaine. Anesthesiology, 10:175, 1949.
24a. Graudard, D.J., Robertazzi, R.W., and Peterson, M.C.: Intravenous procaine. N.Y. State J. Med., 47:2187, 1947.
25. Dodd, R.B., and Pfeffer, C.: Intravenous procaine therapy. Bull. U.S. Army Med. Dept., 8:877, 1948.
26. Brodie, B.B., Lief, P.A., and Poet, R: The fate of procaine in man following intravenous administration. J. Pharmacol. Exper. Therap., 94:359, 1948.
26a. Papper, E.M., et al.: Studies of the pharmacologic properties of procaine and di-ethyl-aminoethanol. N.Y. State J. Med., 48:1711, 1948.
26b. Mark, L.C., et al.: The physiological disposition and cardiac effects of procaine amide. J. Pharmacol. Exp. Ther., 102:5, 1951.
27. Kalow, W.: Hydrolysis of local anesthetics by human serum cholinesterase. J. Pharmacol. Exper. Therap. 104:128, 1952.
28. Bigelow, N., and Harrison, I.: General analgesic effects of procaine. J. Pharmacol. Exp. Ther., 81:368, 1944.
29. Graubard, D.J., Robertazzi, R.W. and Peterson, M.C.: Micro Determination of Blood Levels of Procaine Hydrochloride After Intravenous Injection. Anesthesiology, 8:236, 1947.
30. Graubard, D.J., Robertazzi, R.W., and Peterson, M.C.: One year's experience with intravenous procaine. Anesth. Analg., 27:222, 1948.
31. Graubard, D.J., Robertazzi, R.W., and Peterson, M.C.: Method for Accurately Measuring the Rate of Flow of Intravenous Fluids. Anesthesiology, 8:372, 1947.
32. Keats, A.S., Alessandro G.L., Beecher, H.K.: A Controlled study of pain relief by intravenous procaine. J.A.M.A., 147:1761, 1951.
33. Fraser, R.J., and Kraft, K.A.: Pentothal–procaine analgesia. Anesth. Analg., 27:282, 1948.
34. Usubiaga, J.E., et al.: Local anesthetic induced convulsions in man. Anesth. Analg., 45:611, 1966.
35. Wikinski, J.A., et al.: General anesthesia with intravenous procaine. *In* Aldrete, J.A., and Stanley, T.H., (eds). Trends In Intravenous Anesthesia. Miami, Symposia Specialists, 1980.
36. Seifen, A.B., et al: Pharmacokinetics of intravenous procaine. Anesth. Analg., 58:382, 1979.
37. Richards, R.K.: Effects of vitamin C deficiency and starvation upon the toxicity of procaine. Anesth. Analg., 26:1, 1947.
38. Burstein, C.L.: The utility of intravenous procaine in the anesthetic management of cardiac disturbances. Anesthesiology, 10:133, 1949.
39. Brodie, B.B., et al.: Studies on diethylamino-ethanol: Physiological disposition and action in cardiac arrhythmias. J. Pharmacol. Exp. Ther., 95:18, 1949.
40. Mark, L.C., et al.: Action of procaine-amide on ventricular arrhythmias. J. Pharmacol. Exp. Ther., 98:21, 1950.
41. Koch-Weser, J., Klein, S.W., and Foo-Canto, L.L.: Antiarrhythmic prophylaxis with procainamide in acute myocardial infarction. N. Engl. J. Med., 218:1253, 1969.
42. Koch-Weser, J., and Klein, S.W.: Procainamide dosage schedules, plasma concentrations and clinical effects. J.A.M.A., 215:1454, 1971.
43. Berry, K., Garrett, E.L., and Bellet, S.: The use of pronestyl in treatment of ectopic rhythms: 98 episodes in 78 patients. Am. J. Med., 11:431, 1951.
44. Lima, J.J., et al.: Safety and efficacy of procainamide infusions. Am. J. Cardiol., 43:98, 1979.
45. de Clive-Lowe, S.G., Desmond, J., and North, J.: Intravenous lignocaine anaesthesia. Anaesthesia, 13:138, 1958.
46. Gilbert, C.R.A., and Hanson, I.R.: Intravenous use of xylocaine. Anesth. Analg., 30:301, 1957.

47. Steinhaus, J.E., and Howland, D.E.: Intravenously administered lidocaine as a supplement to nitrous oxide-thiobarbiturate anesthesia. Anesth. Analg., 37:40, 1958.
48. Steinhaus, J.E., and Gaskin, L.: A study of intravenous lidocaine as a suppression of cough reflex. Anesthesiology, 24:285, 1963.
49. Himes, R.S., DiFazio, C.H., and Burney, R.G.: Effects of lidocaine on the anesthetic requirements for nitrous oxide and halothane. Anesthesiology, 47:437, 1977.
50. Poulton, T.J., and James, F.M. III: Cough suppression by lidocaine. Anesthesiology, 50:470, 1979.
51. deKornfeld, T.J., and Steinhaus, J.E.: The effect of intravenously administered lidocaine and succinylcholine on the respiratory activity of dogs. Anesth. Analg., 38:173, 1959.
52. Yukioka, H., et al.: Intravenous lidocaine as a suppressant of coughing during tracheal intubation. Anesth. Analg., 64:1189, 1985.
53. Wiklund, L.: Human hepatic blood flow and its relation to systemic circulation during intravenous infusion of lidocaine. Acta Anaesth. Scand., 21:148, 1977.
53a. McWhirter, W.R., et al.: Cardiovascular effects of controlled lidocaine overdosage in dogs anesthetized with nitrous oxide. Anesthesiology, 39:308, 1973.
53b. Rosen, M.R., Hoffman, B.F., and Wit, A.L.: Electrophysiology and pharmacology of cardiacarrythmias, V. Cardiac antiarrhythmic effects of lidocaine. Am. Heart J., 89:526, 1975.
53c. Stenson, R.E., Constantino, R.T. and Harrison, D.C.: Interrelationships of hepatic blood flow, cardiac output and blood levels of lidocaine in man. Circulation, 43:205, 1971.
54. Katz, R.L., and Gissen, A.J.: Effects of intravenous and intraarterial procaine and lidocaine on neuromuscular transmission in man. Acta Anaesth. Scand., (Suppl.)36:103, 1969.
55. Usubiaga, J.E., and Standaert, F.: The effects of local anesthetics on motor nerve terminals. J. Pharmacol. Exp. Ther., 159:353, 1968.
56. Christensen, V., Ladegaard-Pedersen, H.J., and Skovsted, P.: Intravenous lidocaine as a suppressant of persistent cough caused by bronchoscopy. Acta Anaesth. Scand., (Suppl.) 67:84, 1978.
57. Abou-Madi, M.N., Keszler, H., and Jacoub, J.M.: Cardiovascular reactions to laryngoscopy and tracheal intubation following small and large doses of intravenous lidocaine. Can. Anaesth. Soc. J., 24:12, 1979.
58. Hamill, J.F., et al.: Lidocaine before endotracheal intubation: intravenous or laryngotracheal? Anesthesiology, 55:578, 1981.
59. Tam, S., Chung, F., and Campbell, M.: Intravenous lidocaine: Optimal time of injection before tracheal intubation. Anesth. Analg., 66:1036, 1987.
60. Donegan, M.F., and Bedford, R.F.: Intravenously administered lidocaine prevents intracranial hypertension during endotracheal suctioning. Anesthesiology, 52:516, 1980.
61. Bedford, R.F., et al.: Lidocaine prevents increased ICP after endotracheal intubation. In Intracranial Pressure IV. Schulman K., Mamarou A, Miller J.D. et al., eds. Berlin, Springer, 1980, p 595.
62. Drenger, B., et al.: The effect of intravenous lidocaine on the increase in intraocular pressure induced by tracheal intubation. Anesth. Analg., 64:1121, 1985.
63. Baraka, A.: Intravenous lidocaine controls extubation laryngospasm in children. Anesth. Analg., 57:506, 1978.
64. Wallin, G., et al.: Effects of lidocaine infusion on the sympathetic response to abdominal surgery. Anesth. Analg., 66:1008, 1987.
65. Collinsworth, K.A., Kalman, S.M., and Harrison, D.C.: The clinical pharmacology of lidocaine as an anti-arrhythmic drug. Circulation, 50:1217, 1974.
66. Ackerman, W.E., et al.: Naloxone treatment of intravenous lidocaine-induced central nervous system depression. Anesthesiol. Rev., 14:21, 1987.
67. Greenblatt, D.J., et al.: Pharmacokinetic approach to the clinical use of lidocaine intravenously. J.A.M.A., 236:273, 1976.
68. Zito, R.A., and Reid, P.R.: Lidocaine kinetics predicted by indocyanine green clearance. N. Engl. J. Med., 298:1160, 1978.
69. Gianelly, R., et al.: Effect of lidocaine on ventricular arrhythmias in patients with coronary disease. N. Engl. J. Med., 277:1215, 1967.
70. Lima, J.J., et al.: Safety and efficacy of procainamide infusions. Am. J. Cardiol., 43:98, 1979.
71. Smith, E.R., and Duce, B.R.: The acute anti-arrhythmic and toxic effects in mice and dogs of 2-ethylamino-2',6'-acetoxylidine, a metabolite of lidocaine. J. Pharmacol. Exp. Ther., 179:580, 1971.
72. Wyman, M.G., et al.: Multiple bolus technique for lidocaine administration during the first hours of an acute myocardial infarction. Am. J. Cardiol., 41:313, 1978.
73. Salzer, L.B., et al.: A comparison of methods of lidocaine administration in patients. Clin. Pharmacol. Ther., 29:617, 1981.
74. Rahimtoola, S.H., et al.: Lidocaine infusion in acute myocardial infarction. Arch. Intern. Med., 128:416, 1971.
75. Valentine, P.A., et al.: Lidocaine to prevent death in early phase of acute infarction. N. Engl. J. Med., 291:1327, 1974.
76. Lie, K.I., et al.: Lidocaine in the prevention of primary ventricular fibrillation. N. Engl. J. Med., 291:1324, 1974.
77. Rademaker, A.W., et al.: Character of adverse effects of prophylactic lidocaine in the coronary care unit. Clin. Pharmacol. Ther., 40:71, 1986.
78. Bier, A.: Ueber einen neuen Weg Lokalanaesthesie an den Gliedmaassen zu erzeugen. Verh. dtsch. Ges. Chir., 37:204, 1908.
79. Bier, A.: Uber einen neuen Weg Lokalanesthesia an den Gliedmassen zu Erzeugen. Arch. F. Clin. Chir., 86:1007, 1908.
80. Bier, A.: A new method for local anaesthesia in the extremities. Ann. Surg., 48:780, 1908.
81. Ransohoff, J.L.: Terminal arterial anesthesia. Ann. Surg., 51:453, 1910.
82. Leriche, R.: Intra-arterial therapy of infections and other diseases. Mem. Acad. de Chir., 64:220, 1938.
83. Lundy, J.S.: Clinical Anesthesia. Philadelphia, W.B. Saunders, 1942.
84. Allen, F.M., Crossman, L.W., and Lyons, L.V.: Intravenous procaine analgesia. Anesth. Analg., 25:1, 1946.
85. Bell, H.M., Slater, E.M., and Harris, W.H.: Regional anesthesia with intravenous lidocaine. J.A.M.A., 186:544, 1963.
86. Georgescu, B., et al.: Anesthezia intraosoasa cu novacaina si Flaxedil in chirurgia membrelor. Chirurgia (Buc.), 14:943, 1965.
87. Atiasov, N.E.: Disatiletie metoda vnutrikostnoi anestezii. Ortop, travm. protez. Moskva, 17:96, 1956.
88. Adams, J.P., Dealy, E.J., and Kenmore, P.I.: Intravenous lidocaine for regional anesthesia in selected hand problems. J. Bone Joint Surg. 46:811, 1964.
88a. Usubiaga, J.E. and Standaert, F.: The effects of local anesthetics on motor nerve terminals. J. Pharmacol. Exp. Ther., 159:353, 1968.
89. Holmes, C. McK.: Intravenous regional analgesia: Useful method of producing analgesia of limbs. Lancet, 1:245,

1963.
90. Trias, A.: The use of intravenous regional anaesthesia in orthopedic surgery. Acta Anaesth. Scand., (Suppl.)36:35, 1969.
91. Harris, W.H.: Choice of anaesthetic agents for intravenous regional anaesthesia. Acta Anaesth. Scand., (Suppl.)36:47, 1969.
92. Sorbie, C., and Chacha, P.: Regional anaesthesia by the intravenous route. Br. Med. J. 1:957, 1965.
93. Morrison, J.T.: Intravenous local anaesthesia. Br. J. Surg., 18:641, 1930–31.
94. Magora, F., et al.: Prolonged effects of bupivacaine hydrochloride after cuff release in intravenous regional anaesthesia. Br. J. Anaesth., 52:1131, 1980.
95. Katz, J.: Choice of agents for intravenous regional anesthesia. Reg. Anesth., 4:10, 1979.
96. Brown, E.M.: Intravenous regional anesthesia (Bier block): Review of 20 years' experience. Can. J. Anaesth., 36:307, 1989.
97. Fujita, T., and Miyazaki, M.: A comparative study of various local anesthetic agents in intravenous regional anesthesia. Anesth. Analg., 47:575, 1968.
98. Ware, R.J.: Intravenous regional analgesia using bupivacaine: A double-blind comparison with lignocaine. Anaesthesia, 34:231, 1979.
99. Ware, R.J.: Intravenous regional anesthesia using bupivacaine. Anaesthesia, 34:231, 1981.
100. Katz, J.: Intravenous regional anesthesia. Semin. Anesthesiol., 11:5, 1983.
101. Reynolds, F.: Bupivacaine and intravenous regional anaesthesia. Anaesthesia, 39:105, 1984.
102. Dickler, D.J., Friedman, P.L., and Susman, I.C.: Intravenous regional anesthesia with chlorprocaine. Anesthesiology, 26:244, 1965.
103. Mazze, R.I.: Methemoglobin concentrations following intravenous regional anesthesia. Anesth. Analg., 47:122, 1968.
104. Dunbar, R.W., and Mazze, R.I.: Intravenous regional anesthesia. Anesth. Analg., 46:806, 1967.
105. Atkinson, D.I., Modell, J., and Moya, F.: Intravenous regional anesthesia. Anesth. Analg., 44:313, 1965.
106. Durrani, Z., et al.: Use of tetracaine for intravenous regional anesthesia of upper extremity (abstract). Reg. Anesth., 14:66, 1989.
107. Paul, D.L., Logan, M.R., and Wildsmith, J.A.W.: The effects of injected solution temperature on intravenous regional anaesthesia. Anaesthesia, 43:362, 1988.
108. Amiot, J.F., et al.: Intravenous regional anesthesia with ketamine. Anaesthesia, 40:899, 1985.
109. Covino, B.G.: Pharmacokinetics of intravenous regional anesthesia. Reg. Anesth., 4:5, 1979.
110. Ebert, R.V., and Stead, E.A., Jr.: The effect of application of tourniquets on the hemodynamics of circulation. J. Clin. Invest., 19:561, 1940.
111. Adams, J.P., and Solomon, A.: Use of radioactive chromium to determine blood volume of the extremities. J. Bone Joint Surg., 44:489, 1962.
112. Grice, S.C., et al.: Intravenous regional anesthesia: Evaluation and prevention of leakage under the tourniquet (abstract). Anesthesiology, 63:A221, 1985.
113. Grice, S.C., et al.: Intravenous regional anesthesia: Evaluation and prevention of leakage under the tourniquet. Anesthesia, 65:316, 1986.
114. Hoyle, J.E. A two-compartment cuff intravenous regional anesthesia. Anaesthesia, 19:244, 1964.
115. Grice, S.C., Morell, R.C., and Balestrieri, F.J.: Confusion regarding experimental studies of intravenous regional anesthesia. Anesthesiology, 64:526, 1986.
116. Tucker, G.T., and Boas, R.A.: Pharmacokinetic aspects of intravenous regional anesthesia. Anesthesiology, 34:538, 1971.
117. Knapp, R.B., and Veinberg, M.: Distribution of radioactive local anesthetics following intravenous regional anesthesia. Acta Anaesth. Scand., XXXVI (Suppl.)26:121, 1969.
118. Cotev, S., and Robin, G.C.: Experimental studies on intravenous response analgesia using radioactive lidocaine. Acta Anaesth. Scand. XXXVI (Suppl.)26:127, 1969.
119. Raj, P.P., et al.: The site of action of intravenous regional anesthesia. Anesth. Analg., 51:776, 1972.
120. Raj PP: Site of action of intravenous regional anesthesia. Reg Anesth 4(#1): 8–10, 1979.
121. Lillie, P.E., Glynn, C.J., and Fenwick, D.G.: Site of action of intravenous regional anesthesia. Anesthesiology, 61:507, 1984.
122. Rosenberg, P.H., and Heavner, J.E.: Multiple and complementary mechanisms produce analgesia during intravenous regional anesthesia. Anesthesiology, 62:840, 1985.
123. Sukhani, R., et al.: Arterial blood levels of lidocaine after intravenous regional anesthesia (IVRA): Cyclic versus single deflation of tourniquet (abstract). Reg. Anesth. 11:49, 1986.
124. Sukhani, R., et al: Lidocaine disposition following intravenous regional anesthesia with different tourniquet deflation techniques. Anesth. Analg., 68:633, 1989.
125. Evans, C.J., et al.: Residual nerve block following intravenous regional anaesthesia. Br. J. Anaesth., 46:668, 1974.
126. Foldes, F.F., et al.: Comparison of toxicity of intravenously given local anesthetic agents in man. J.A.M.A., 172:1493, 1960.
127. Hargrove, R.L., et al.: Blood levels of local anesthetics following intravenous regional anesthesia. Acta Anaesth. Scand. (Suppl.)36:115, 1969.
128. Mazze, R.I., and Dunbar, R.W.: Intravenous regional anesthesia—Report of 497 cases with a toxicity study. Acta. Anaesth. Scand., (Suppl.)36:27, 1969.
129. Brown, E.M., McGriff, J.T., and Malinowski, R.W.: Intravenous regional anesthesia (Bier block): Review of 20 years experience. Can. J. Anaesth., 36:307, 1989.
130. Eriksson, E.: The effects of intravenous local anesthetic agents on the central nervous system. Acta Anaesth. Scand., (Suppl.)36:79, 1969.
131. Lehman, W.L., and Jones, W.W.: Intravenous lidocaine for anesthesia in the lower extremity. J. Bone Joint Surg., 66-A:1056, 1984.
132. Nusbaum, L.M., and Hamelberg, W.: Intravenous regional anesthesia for surgery on the foot and ankle. Anesthesiology, 64:91, 1986.
133. Davies, J.A.H., and Walford, A.J.: Intravenous regional anaesthesia for foot surgery. Acta Anaesth. Scand., 30:145, 1986.
134. Davies, J.A.H., Hall, I.D., and Wilkey, A.D.: Bupivacaine leak past inflated tourniquets during intravenous regional analgesia. Anaesthesia, 39:996, 1984.
135. Schwartz, P.S., Newman, A., and Green, A.L.: Intravenous regional anesthesia. J. Am. Pediatr. Med. Assoc., 73:201, 1983.

INDEX

Note: Page numbers in *italics* indicate figures; t indicates tables.

Abdomen
  nerve block. *See* Nerve block, of trunk, abdomen, and perineum.
  during patient repositioning, 201
  reflexes, 1189–1191
    celiac plexus, 1190
    diaphragmatic traction (Brewer-Luckhardt), 1190
    pelvic, 1190
    and pelvic nerve, 1190–1191
    peritoneal and mesenteric, 1190
    renal, 1190
  surgical stress, and spinal anesthesia, 1511
Abducens nerve paralysis, 1565
Abortion, spontaneous, in operating room personnel, 1160
Abscess
  epidural, 1600
  after spinal anesthesia, 1566
Absorption
  alcohol, 776
  carbon dioxide. *See* Carbon dioxide.
  cerebrospinal fluid, 1456–1458
  cocaine, 1248–1249
  epidural anesthesia, 1576–1577
  local anesthetics, 1219, 1243–1245
  lorazepam, 756
  spinal anesthetics, 1474–1475
Abuse potential
  of cyclohexylamines, 735
  of ketamine, 748
Acetone contamination in closed circle system, 427
Acetylcholine, 814–820
  acetylcholinesterase, 819–820, *820, 821*
  chemistry, 814
  choline acetylase, 820, *821*
  end-plate potential and quantal mechanisms, 815–816
    calcium, 815–816, *816*
    magnesium, 816
    potassium, 816
  end-plate receptor, 818
  metabolism, 1221
  in motor nerve endings, 814
  in nerve impulse, 815, 1205
  neuromuscular transmission, 816, 820, 822t
  presynaptic stores, 814
  receptor protein, 817–819, *818*, 818t
  in relaxant reversal. *See* Relaxants, antagonists.
  during sleep, 321
  in synaptic transmission, 816–817, *816, 817*

Acetylcholinesterase, 819–820, *820, 821*
  and anticancer drugs, 259
  pancuronium reversal, 964
  See also Anticholinesterase.
Acetylsalicylic acid, potentiation of action, 1288
Acid-base status
  and muscle relaxants, 877
  and toxicity of local anesthetics, 1299
Acidosis
  from local anesthesia, 1303–1304, *1305*
  and muscle relaxants, 879
Acquired immunodeficiency syndrome (AIDS)
  in anesthesia personnel, 1170–1173
  and spinal anesthesia, 1486
Acrylic bone cement, 256–257
Actinomycin D, pulmonary toxicity, 261
Acupressure, 1638
Acupuncture, 1634–1640
  clinical use, 1639–1640
    anesthesia, 1639–1640
    for pain relief, 1639
    therapeutic, 1639
  complications, 1640
  definition, 1634
  history, 1634–1635
  mechanism of action, 1635–1638
    acupressure, 1638
    analgesia, 1637
    classic meridian theory, 1635
    competitive bombardmenet, 1637
    gate control theory, 1636
    hormonal theory, 1636–1637
    hypnosis and conditioning theory, 1636
    meridans of Ch'i, 1635, *1636*, 1635t
    modes of treatment, 1637–1638
  procedure, 1638
    equipment, 1638
    general guides, 1638
    number and duration of treatments, 1638
    techniques, 1638
Adam's apple. *See* Larynx.
Adapters, endotracheal tube, 494, *495*
Addiction
  cocaine, 1250
  definition, 307
Addison's disease, and thiopental anesthesia, 681
Adenosine, in controlled hypotension, 1085–1086
Adenosine triphosphate (ATP)
  in adenosine-controlled hypotension, 1085–1086

in nerve impulse, 1208
Adhesive arachnoiditis, after spinal anesthesia, 1567
Adrenal gland
  in electroanesthesia, 1122
  in oxygen toxicity, 1147
  and surgical stress, 1508
  thiopental effects, 681
Adrenal nerve, in spinal anesthesia, 1504–1505
Adrenergic blocking drugs, drug interactions, 268
Adrenocorticotropic hormone (ACTH)
  noise effects, 1166–1167
  and surgical stress, 1508
  thiopental effects, 669
Adrenolysis, and controlled hypotension, 1062
Adsorption, heat of, 110, 144–145
Aerosols in breathing systems, 413
Age factors
  alfentanil kinetics, 723
  curare kinetics, 943
  diazepam anesthesia, 750
  and dosage of anesthesia, 289, *289*
  endotracheal anesthesia complications, 578
  in epidural anesthesia, 1577, 1579
  fentanyl kinetics, 713–714
  and gastric contents, 238
  MAC values, 336, 336t
  nitroprusside, 1075, *1075*
  and oculocardiac reflex, 1180
  and operative risk, 38, 44, 46–48, 47t
  oxidative metabolism of inhaled anesthetics, 348
  pain tolerance, 1322
  postspinal headaches, 1557
  and preanesthetic visit, 215
  and pupillary reflex, 366
  and reinfarction risks, 59
  and relaxant action, 847
  in sleep, 320
  and solubility coefficients, 332
  spinal anesthesia, 1476, 1484, 1511–1512, 1552
  succinylcholine, 1010–1011, 1011t
  thiopental dosage and kinetics, 661, 663–664, 676
  and toxicity of local anesthetics, 1299
  and vecuronium kinetics, 975
  See also Elderly.
Air
  conditioning, of operating room, 1165
  convection, in hypothermia, 1109
  density, 107

I-1

Air (Continued)
  embolus, during patient positioning, 196, 200
Airway
  abnormalities, associated syndromes, 560–564
  closure, 169
  complications in infants, 590–591
  in head and neck trauma, 550
  neuromuscular blockade, 851
  obstruction
    in inhalation anesthesia. See Inhalation anesthesia.
  preoperative tests, 226
  positive pressure effects, 624–629
    atrial pressure, 625
    clinical evaluation, 87–88
    hemodynamics, 624–625
    immediate effects on circulation, 624, 625, 626
    IPPV effects, 626–627, 627
    mechanical injury to lungs, 627–628
    metabolic lung injury, 628
    normal ventilation, 624, 625
    oxygen consumption, 625
    precautions, 628
    pressure patterns, 628–629, 629
    pulmonary blood flow, 625–626
    pulmonary ventilation, 626
    renal function, 626
  protection, Sellick maneuver, 529, 548–550
  thiopental effects, 680
  tumors, and extubation, 555
  See also Endotracheal anesthesia.
Alarm systems, anesthesia machines, 141
Alcohol
  endotracheal tube cleaning, 479
  group, of local anesthetics, 1239
  neurolytic agent, 1268
  for pain relief, 4
  paravertebral block, 1436
  subarachnoid neurolysis, 1535–1536
  See also Ethanol.
Alcohol-barbiturate abstinence syndrome, 309
Alcoholism
  acute intoxication, and surgery, 212–213
  enzyme induction, 256
  and MAC values, 339
  and preanesthetic visit, 211–213
  and thiopental, 665, 681
Alcuronium, 951–952, 952, 952t
Aldomet, drug interactions, 267
Alfentanil, 722–726
  advantages, 726
  adverse effects, 726
  analgesia, 724
  chemistry, 723
  dosage and administration, 725
  drug interactions, 726
  EEG changes, 715
  lipid solubility, 1626
  and MAC values, 338
  mechanism of action, 724
  pharmacodynamics, 725–726
  pharmacokinetics, 722–723
    in children, 724
  population kinetics, 723
  potency, 725
  and renal failure, 724
Algorithm, automated oscillometry, 74
Alkalosis, and muscle relaxants, 878–879

Alkylating agents, drug interactions, 260–261
Allen test, direct arterial monitoring, 73
Allergies
  acupuncture, 1639
  to local anesthetics, 1310–1312
    clinical types, 1310–1311
      anaphylactoid reactions, 1310
      cross sensitization, 1310
      delayed reactions, 1310
      delayed tissue sensitization, 1310–1311
      immediate reactions, 1310
    cytotoxic responses, 1312
    differential diagnosis, 1310
    etiology, 1310
    injection pain, 1311–1312
    lidocaine reactions, 1311
    prevention, 1311
    testing methods, 1311
      intracutaneous, 1311
      skin testing, 1311
      transfer of sensitivity, 1311
    treatment, 1311
  relaxant contraindications, 892
  and succinylcholine, 1009
Alopecia
  compression, 194
  from face mask, 431
Alphamethylparatyrosine, drug interactions, 276
Alphaprodine, 703
  and levallorphan, 704
Althesin, 765–766, 765, 766t
  and evoked potentials, 94
Altitude
  and spinal anesthesia, 1560
  See also Climate and altitude effects.
Alveolar ventilation
  capillary flow, 327–328, 327
  and capillary membrane equilibrium, 329–333
    active transport system, 330–331
    blood solubility of anesthetics, 331–332, 331t
    epithelial interface, 330
    passive transport system, 330
    physical transport system, 330
    time requirement, 331
  curve analysis, 325–327, 327
  and pulmonary microcirculation, 164, 164, 327
  second gas effect, 328–329, 329t
  tissue uptake effects, 328, 328, 329
Ambulatory surgery, 1641–1650
  facilities, 1641–1646
    analgesics, 1646
    health-care team, 1642–1643
    monitoring, 1645
    patient selection, 1642–1643
    preanesthetic medication, 291–292, 1645–1646, 292t
    preoperative anesthesia, 1643–1644
  general anesthesia, 1646–1649
    complications, 1649
    muscle relaxants, 1647
    postoperative follow-up, 1649
    recovery and discharge, 1648–1649, 1648t
    regional anesthesia, 1647–1648
  morbidity and mortality, 50, 50t
American Board of Anesthesiology, 20
American Heart Association
  blood pressure standards, 74–75
  sounds of Korotkoff, 72

American Medical Association, anesthesiology as specialty, 20, 21
American National Standards Institute, 469
American Society of Anesthesiologists, 19, 21
  standardization of endotracheal tubes, 469
  waste anesthetic gases, 1164
American Society of Mechanical Engineers, 1136
American Society of Regional Anesthetists, 19
Amide derivatives
  of local anesthetics, 1239, 1256–1266
    bupivacaine, 1259–1262
    dibucaine, 1256–1257
    etidocaine, 1262–1263
    lidocaine, 1257–1258
    mepivacaine, 1258–1259
    propitocaine, 1263–1264
    ropivacaine, 1264–1266
  metabolism, 1221
Aminoglycosides, and organophosphates, 1044
Aminophylline, and nitroprusside action, 1077
Aminopyridine, 1047
  and neuromuscular junction, 885
Amitriptyline (Elavil), drug interactions, 270
Ammonium agents, 1267–1268
  subarachnoid neurolysis, 1536
Amnesia
  definition of, 288
  diazepam effects, 752
  from ethanol, 777
  physostigmine anesthesia, 1033
Amobarbital, 655
Amphetamines
  drug interactions, 275–276
  and MAC values, 337
Amygdala, excitation by local anesthetics, 1303
Amyotrophic lateral sclerosis, and muscle relaxants, 899
Analgesia
  acupuncture, 1637
  in ambulatory surgery, 1646
  definition of, 288
  diazepam effects, 752
  epidural. See Epidural analgesia.
  hyperstimulation, 1344–1345
  music and sound, 1132–1133
  See also Pain.
Analyzers, gas, climate and altitude effects, 445–446
Anaphylaxis
  with local anesthetics, 1270
  and muscle relaxants, 908
  to thiopental, 683
Anatomy
  autonomic reflexes, 1179
  in bone marrow infusions, 298
  bronchial, 599–600
  complications in endotracheal anesthesia. See Endotracheal anesthesia.
  cricothyroid/cricotracheal membrane, 542
  developmental syndromes, and endotracheal anesthesia, 518–519, 522, 560–564
  in epidural anesthesia, 1572–1575, 1572–1574, 1573t

of larynx. *See* Larynx.
nerves. *See* Nerve block.
oculocardiac reflex, 1179–1180
regional anesthesia, 1202–1204
    landmarks, 1202
    nerve fiber structure and histochemistry, 1202–1203, *1203*
    Schwann cells and myelin, 1203, *1204*
    sacrum, 1612–1614, *1612–1614*
    vertebral column, 1445–1446, 1450, *1446*
    vertebral ligaments, 1447–1448
Anemia
    cholinesterase, 839
    and MAC values, 337
    and thiopental anesthesia, 681
Anemometers, 414
Aneroid gauge, 129–130, *132*
Anesthesia
    choice of, 234–236
        general versus regional, 235
        in neonates, 235–236
        principles, 234–235
    during controlled ventilation, 630
    definition of, 288
    and EEG patterns, 93
    general. *See* General anesthesia.
    hazards, 1149–1178
        disinfection procedures, 1174–1175
        environmental, 1149–1173
            chemical, 1158–1165, 1160–1162t
            electricity, 1153–1158, *1153–1156*, 1155t
            fires and explosions, 1149–1151
            noise, 1165–1168, 1166–1167t
            occupational viruses, 1168–1173
            static electricity, 1151–1153
        personnel
            attitudes, 1174
            immunologic profiles, 1173–1174
    in hyperthermia, 1112
    intravenous. *See* Intravenous anesthesia.
    local. *See* Local anesthesia and regional block.
    machines and components, 118–162
        accessories, 138–141
            alarm systems, 141
            anesthetic gas analyzers, 140
            carbon dioxide analyzers, 139–140
            oxygen analyzers, 139
        breathing assembly, 150–157
            breathing bags, 152–153, *153*
            breathing tubing, 150–151
            carbon dioxide absorption, 153–156, *154, 155*
            connection of patient to breathing circuit, 156–157
            gas inflow and pop-off, 156, *156*
            nonrebreathing valves, 151–152, *152*
            respiratory valves, 151, *151*
        checklist, 159
        compressed gas cylinders, 122–128
            color code, 127, *127*
            construction of, 122–123
            conversion factors, 126
            filling limits, 123, 124t
            identification standards, 126–127
            labeling and marking, 123–124, *125*
            pin index system, 127, *128*
            reading, 126
            recommended safe practices, 124–126
            size of, 123, 124t
            standards, 123
            storage of, 127–128
            yokes, 122, *123*
        continuous-flow machines, 121–122, *121, 122,* 122t
        demand (intermittent-flow) machines, 137–138, *129, 130*
        flow controllers, 132–133
            needle valves, 132–133, *136*
        flowmeters, 133–137, *137*
            common manifold, 136–137
            other types, 136
            Thorpe tube, 135–136, *137, 138*
        hazards of, 157–159
            bacterial interactions, 158
            compressed air pipelines, 158
            concentration errors, 157
            contamination of anesthetic mixtures, 157–158
            input carrier gas, 159
            nosocomial infections, 158–159
            recommendations, 158
        historical development, 119–121
        in hyperbaric oxygenation, 1138
        maintenance and service, 138
        manometers, 129–130, *132*
            fail-safe systems (low-pressure cut-off), 130, *133–134*
        pressure regulators, 128–129, *129, 1130*
        valves, 131–132
            check valves, 131, *134*
            cylinder valves, 131
            flush switch, 131–132, *135*
            interlock and switching valves, 131
        vaporization and vaporizers, 141–150
            characteristics of, 141–143, 142t
            chemical heat for crystalization, 145, *145*
            classification, 143–144, 143t
            draw-over methods, 143–144, *144*
            evaporative surface methods, 143, *143*
            direct heating, 144
            heat of adsorption principle, 144–145
            heat transfer, 145
            indirect heat sources, 144
            practical aspects, 141
            process of, 141
            vaporizers, 145–150
                breathe-through or in-circuit, 146–147, *147*
                direct addition of liquid anesthetic, 146
                hazards of, 150
                out-of-circuit, 147
                saturation vaporizers, 147–149, *148,* 148t
                thermally confused vaporizers, 150
                variable bypass vaporizers, 149–150, *149*
        vision considerations, 118–119, *120*
        work station, 118, *119*
    and moving of patient, 171
    potentiation of action, 1282–1290
    topographic landmarks, 1471
    ventilatory support indications, 629–630
    See also specific types of anesthesia.
Anesthesiometer, 12
Anesthetic agents
    absorption, 457, 458t
    density of, 107
    physiochemical properties, 117t
    solubility in blood, 105–106
    See also specific anesthetics.
Anesthetic index
    bupivacaine, 1260
    butacaine, 1256
    definition, 1233
    dibucaine, 1256
    hexylcaine, 1251
    lidocaine, 1257
    mepivacaine, 1259
    propitocaine, 1264
    tetracaine, 1255
Angel dust, 735
Angina treatment, drug interactions, 268
Angiography, coronary, 228
Angiotensin converting enzyme inhibitors, 275
Ankle
    nerve block, 1408–1411, *1410, 1411*
    surgery, regional anesthesia, 804–805
Ankylosis of temporomandibular joint, 524
Anode endotracheal tube, 474–475, *475*
Anoxia, EEG patterns, 93
Antabuse (tetraethyl thiuram disulfide), 272
    and thiopental potentiation, 660, 681
Antacid agents, and anesthetic agents, 237
Antagonists of relaxants. *See* Relaxants, antagonists.
Anterior interosseous nerve syndrome, 203
Antibiotics
    drug interactions, 261–262, 266
    and neuromuscular junction, 884–885, 885t
    and organophosphates, 1043–1044, 1044t
    and pancuronium interaction, 970
    and platelet function, 258
Anticancer agents, cholinesterase inhibition, 840
Anticholinergic drugs
    and MAC values, 339
    in pediatric patients, 302–303
Anticholinesterase, 1028–1032
    acetylcholine binding, 1029, *1030*
    agonist action, 1032
    curare reversal, 948
    mechanism of action, 1029
    muscarinic effects, 1030–1032
    physiologic consequences, 1032
    plasma cholinesterase, 1029–1030
    poisoning, 1048–1050
        azathioprine, 1050
        laboratory diagnosis, 1049
        phosphate-enzyme binding, 1049–1050
        signs and symptoms, 1049
        treatment, 1049
    structure, 1028–1029, *1029*
Anticoagulants
    drug interactions, 262–265
        coumarin derivatives, 262–263
        heparin, 262
        protamine sulfate, 263–265
    protein binding, 254
    and spinal anesthesia, 1487
Anticonvulsant drugs, and neuromuscular blockade, 883–884, 883t

Antidepressant drug interactions
    MAO inhibitors, 269
    tricyclics, 269–272, 270, 271t
Antidiuretic hormone, thiopental effects, 668
Antiestrogenic drugs, and atracurium, 987
Antihistamine
    action of local anesthetics, 1237–1238
    drug interactions, 265–266
Antihypertensive agents
    drug interactions, 266–268
        adrenergic blocking drugs, 268
        guanethidine, 267
        hydralazine and minoxidil, 267–268
        methyldopa, 267
        rauwolfia derivatives, 266–267
    and MAC values, 339
Antiinflammatory agents, renal effects, 258
Antimicrobial action of local anesthetics, 1238
Antioxidants
    enzyme inhibition, 348
    as preservatives, 1312–1313
Antipyrine, enzyme induction, 256
Antithrombotic action of local anesthetics, 1238
Antiviral agents and neuromuscular junction, 884–885
Anxiety
    gastric effects, 238
    and gastrointestinal function, 286
    preanesthetic medication, 285
    preoperative, 208–209
        in cancer patients, 209
        incidence, 209
        reduction of, 210–211
        variables, 209
Aorta transfusion and anesthesia, 299
Apert's syndrome, and endotracheal anesthesia, 518
Apgar scores, ketamine effects, 740, 746
Apnea
    in artificial breathing systems, 619–620
    and barbiturate anesthesia, 676, 681
    in endobronchial anesthesia, 613
    in extubation, 552
    fentanyl effects, 716
    muscle relaxant effects, 905
    postanesthetic Doxapram Test, 860
    and preoxygenation, 424–425
Appendicitis, acupuncture, 1639
Apprehension, in spinal anesthesia, 1546
Aqueous humor, in glaucoma, 277
Arm
    injuries during repositioning, 202–203
    nerve block. See Brachial plexus.
    supports, 175–176, 175, 176
Arnold-Chiari deformity, and endotracheal anesthesia, 519
Arrhythmias, cardiac
    alcoholism effects, 212
    in hyperthermia, 1112–1113
    in hypothermia, 1103
    lidocaine effects, 792–794, 1258
    procainamide effects, 789–790
    with succinylcholine, 1005
Arterial blood pressure. See Blood pressure monitoring.
Arteriosclerosis, and epidural anesthesia, 1581
Arteriotomy, and controlled hypotension, 1061
Arthus-type phenomenon, 1310

Artificial breathing systems. See Breathing systems.
Arytenoid cartilage, 586
Asepsis, for regional anesthesia, 1201–1202
Aspiration
    and full stomach, 438–439
    morbidity and mortality, 50, 51t
    pharyngeal contents, 490
    pneumonitis, 200
Aspirin
    and bleeding time, 1200
    drug interactions, 257–259
Assyrians, methods of anesthesia, 4
Asthma
    acupuncture, 1639
    curare actions, 949
    drug interactions, 275
    ketamine anesthesia, 746
    pancuronium uses, 970
    preoperative evaluation, 232
Athetosis, laryngeal muscles, 467
Atlantoaxial subluxation, 580, 590
Atlanto-occipital distance in endotracheal anesthesia, 519, 521, 525
Atracurium, 834, 981–989
    adverse reactions, 987–988, 988t
    and anticonvulsant drugs, 883
    biodegradation, 985–986
    chemistry, 981–982, 983
    disease states, 984–985
    dosage, 982–984
    drug interactions, 266
    elimination, 986
    for intubation, 984
    isomers, 982
    neuromuscular blockade, 850
    in obesity, 893
    in pediatrics, 988–989, 1045, 988t
    pharmacokinetics, 983, 984t
    pharmacology, 986–989
    plasma binding, 983
    priming action, 868–869
    in rapid sequence induction, 439–440
    reversal, 986
    train-of-four monitoring, 855–856
Atropine
    cholinesterase inhibition, 840
    and MAC values, 339
    and neostigmine, 1034–1035
    parasympathetic blockade, 287
    premedication, and thiopental anesthesia, 676
    sensitivity, and anesthetic risk, 41
Audioanalgesia, 1132–1133
Auditory nerve, after spinal anesthesia, 1565
Auscultatory monitoring, 72–73, 73
Automation
    oscillometers, 74
    record-keeping, 30–32
Autonomic nervous system
    atracurium effects, 986
    curare actions, 945–946, 946t
    in electroanesthesia, 1122
    fentanyl effects, 716
    gallamine effects, 953–954
    in obesity, 217
    pancuronium effects, 967, 967t
    preanesthetic medication, 285
    in spinal anesthesia, 1506–1507
    succinylcholine effects, 1004
    thiopental effects, 668
    See also Ganglionic blockade.
Avogadro's law, 106

Awake patterns
    and general anesthesia, 317
    and MAC values, 340, 340t
Awareness
    during general anesthesia, 316–317, 366–368
    causes, 367
    incidence, 367
    and muscle relaxants, 367
    periods of, 367
    positive suggestions, 368
    postoperative, 367
    prevention of, 368
    recall, 367–368
    tests of, 368
    in hypnosis, 1125
    states of, 287–288, 288t
        amnesia, 288
        analgesia, 288
        anesthesia, 288
        hypnosis, 288
        narcosis, 288
        sedation, 288
    and succinylcholine, 1016–1017
Axillary nerve block, 1369–1374
    advantages and disadvantages, 1370, 1371t
    anatomy, 1370, 1371
    in children, 1374
    indications, 1370–1371
    landmarks, 1370
    techniques, 1371–1373
        classic approach, 1371–1373, 1372
        modified approach, 1373, 1373, 1374
        perivascular, 1375–1376
Axon. See Neuromuscular junction.
Ayre T-tube system, 405–408
    analysis of system, 406–407, 407
    applications, 405–407, 407t
    Baraka double-T-system, 408
    Bisonnette modification, 407–408
    function, 405
Azotemia, and thiopental anesthesia, 681

Backache
    after spinal anesthesia, 1564
    in epidural anesthesia, 1599
    postoperative, 201–202
Bacteria
    anaerobic, hyperbaric oxygenation, 1142
    in anesthesia machines and components, 158
    contamination in breathing systems, 413
    infection
        of endotracheal tubes, 478–479
        prolonged intubation, 587–588, 588t
Bags, breathing, 152–153
Bain circuit, 404, 417–418
Bainbridge reflex, 1193
Baird's solution, 660
Ballistocardiography, 12
Baraka double-T-system, 408
Baralyme, as carbon dioxide absorbent, 453–454
Barbiturates
    abstinence syndrome, 309
    in ambulatory surgery, 1646
    drug interactions, 272–273
    enzyme induction, 256
    intravenous anesthesia, 653–688
        chemistry, 656–657, 656t
        in cranial trauma, 684
        development of, 654–657, 654t
        history, 653

induction, 676–684
  anaphylactoid response, 683
  complications, 681–682
  dosage, 679–680
  extravasation, 682
  intra-arterial injection, 682–683
  muscle movements, 683
  overdose, 683
  postanesthetic tremors, 684
  premedication, 676, 678t
  preoxygenation, 677–679
  procedure, 677–681
  side effects, 676–677
  specific factors, 677, 678
nomenclature, 655–666
pharmacologic actions, 666–669
potency and UD, 655t
in status epilepticus, 684
structure-activity relationships, 656–657, 658t
thiopental. *See* Thiopental.
and narcotic combination, 703–704
poisoning, hyperbaric oxygenation, 1142
premedication for spinal anesthesia, 1458
protein binding, 254, 255
and REM sleep, 322
sensitivity, and anesthetic risk, 41
and toxicity of local anesthetics, 1306
Barbotage, 1465, 1466, 1473
Baric gravity
  of anesthetic solutions, 1466–1468, 1467t
  and spread of injections, 1468
Barometric pressure. *See* Climate and altitude effects.
Baroreceptors
  carotid sinus reflex, 1182, *1182*
  in general anesthesia, 1087–1088
Basal ganglia disorders
  cerebral palsy, 898
  choreoathetosis, 898
  multiple sclerosis, 899
  Parkinsonism, 898
Bayer 1420. *See* Propanidid.
Bedside tests of function, 225–226
  breath-holding test, 225
  respiratory force test, 226
    cough test, 226
  Valsalva test, 226, *227*
Beer's Law, 89
Behavioral disorders, and pain response, 209
Benadryl, drug interactions, 265
Benzocaine
  pharmacology, 1256
  topical anesthesia, 1271–1274
  toxicity, 1296
Benzodiazepines
  in ambulatory surgery, 1645
  and awareness during anesthesia, 368
  drug interactions, 265, 274
  in endotracheal anesthesia, 573
  and neuromuscular transmission, 888
  and REM sleep, 322
  and sleep respiratory patterns, 54
  and toxicity of local anesthetics, 1306, 1309
  See also specific agents.
Bernoulli's Theorem, 116–117, *116*
Beta-adrenergic blockers
  and controlled hypotension, 1069–1070
  during endotracheal anesthesia, 576–577

and oculocardiac reflex, 1180
Bier-type block of lower extremity, 804–806
Binding of drugs, 344
  of etomidate, 766
  of midazolam, 761
  of relaxants, 834, 834t
  plasma proteins, 254
Biochemical differences, and anesthetic risk, 41–42
Biofeedback, pain control, 1344
Biotransformation
  in CSF, 1475
  of curare, 941
  elimination of inhaled anesthetics, 347, 349, 351
  lidocaine, 1257
Bisonnette T-tube system, 407–408
Bisulfite
  and chloroprocaine toxicity, 1254
  in epinephrine solutions, 1284
Bite blocks, in endotracheal anesthesia, 495, *497*
Bladder dysfunction, after epidural anesthesia, 1600
Blanket refrigeration, 1108–1109
Bleeding
  aspirin effect, 1200
  and controlled hypotension, 1057, 1057t
Bleomycin, pulmonary toxicity, 261
Blink reflex, 365–366, 1182
Block, nerve. *See* Nerve block.
Blood
  gases
    analysis, 88–89
    in hyperbaric oxygenation, 1138
    preoperative analysis, 229
    during sleep, 322
  during patient repositioning, 194
  solubility of anesthetics, 105–106, 331–332, 331t
  volume
    and controlled hypotension, 1057–1058
    in extremities, 797
    in obesity, 218
    preoperative screening, 224, 224t
  and transport of anesthetics, 341
Blood-brain barrier
  anticancer drugs, 259–260
  drug uptake, 345–346
  partition coefficient, 105
Blood flow
  cerebral
    diazepam effects, 751–752
    and drug uptake, 345–346
    nitroprusside effects, 1078–1079
    smoking effects, 213
  coronary, in hypothermia, 1102
  hepatic, and toxicity of local anesthetics, 1299
  intestinal, after epidural anesthesia, 1601
  lower limb, in spinal anesthesia, 1505
  and neuromuscular blockade, 850
  positive airway pressure effects, 625
  posture effects. *See* Posture of patient.
  and relaxant action, 863–864
  spinal cord, 1454, 1483–1484, *1454*
  uterine, cocaine effects, 1250
Blood pressure
  and controlled hypotension, 1058, 1059t
  in endotracheal anesthesia, 571
  in hyperbaric oxygenation, 1138

monitoring
  arterial, 71–74
    direct measurement, 78–79
      artery selection and Allen test, 78
      catheters, 78
      complications, 79
      instruments and equipment, 78
      technique, 78–79
    historical aspects, 71
    indirect measurement, 72–77
      auscultatory method, 72–73, *73*
      oscillometry, 73–74, *74*
      palpatory method, 74
      photoplasthysmography, 74
      sphygomanometry, 75–77, *76–78*
    sounds of Korotkoff, 72, *72*
  cardiac output, 85–86
  pulmonary artery, 81–84, *82, 84, 83–85t*
  venous, 79–81, *80*
  posture effects. *See* Posture of patient.
  in spinal anesthesia, 1503–1505
Bloomquist pediatric breathing system, 418
Body build
  complications during endotracheal anesthesia, 578
  and dosage of anesthesia, 289–290
  and hypothermia, 1109
  and relaxant action, 848
Body mass index, 216
  complications in spinal anesthesia, 1552
  and spread of injections, 1470, *1470*
Boiling point, 109
Bone marrow, drug administration, 298–299
  anatomy, 298
  complications, 299
  indications, 298
  materials injected, 299
  needle placement, 298–299
Bonniot's phenomenon, 1585
Bougie guide for transoral intubation, 543–544
Bourdon tube gauge, 129, *132*
Boyle bottle, 150
Boyle's Law, 102, *102*
Braces, 201
Brachial plexus
  injuries during repositioning, 198–199, *198*
  nerve block, 1366–1375
    anatomy, 1366–1367, *1367*
    axillary route, 1369–1374
      advantages and disadvantages, 1370, 1371t
      anatomy, 1370, *1371*
      in children, 1374
      indications, 1370–1371
      landmarks, 1370
      techniques, 1371–1373, *1372–1374*
    perivascular techniques, 1374–1381
      anatomy, 1374–1375
      axillary, 1375–1376
      interscalene, 1379–1381
      subclavian, 1376–1379, *1377, 1378*
    supraclavicular route, 1367–1369
      complications, 1368–1369
      landmarks, 1367, *1369*
      technique, 1367, *1370*
    suprascapular, 1381–1382, *1382*

Bradycardia
  in controlled hypotension, 1070
  fentanyl effects, 715–716
  oculocardiac reflex, 1180
  with succinylcholine, 1005
Bradykinin, pain transmission, 1336
Brain
  drug uptake, 344–346
    exit from CNS, 346
    penetration into CNS, 346
    perfusion, 344–345
    regional cerebral blood flow, 345–346
  in hypnosis, 1127
  ketamine effects, 736
  metabolism, hypothermia effects, 1101
  pain mechanisms, 1331–1333, *1321*
  postural effects, 169–170
  thiopental effects, 672
Brain stem
  and awake period, 321
  evoked potentials, 94
Breasts, during patient repositioning, 200
Breath-holding test, 225, 231, 1441
Breathing assembly. See Anesthesia machines and components.
Breathing bags, 152–153
Breathing patterns during anesthesia. See Respiration.
Breathing systems
  artificial, 618–652
    definitions, 618–620, 652
      apnea, 619–620
      assisted ventilation, 619
      controlled ventilation, 618–619
      depth of anesthesia, 630
      high-frequency positive pressure ventilation, 646–650, *648, 649*
      history, 618
      indications, 620, 629–630
      manual methods, 630–631
        inflation rate, 630
        pressure pattern, 631
        pressure valves, 630
        time sequence of cycle, 630–631
      mechanical ventilation, 631–641
        classification of ventilators, 635–638, *636–638*
        definitions, 631
        discontinuation, 641–646, *644*, 643t, 645t
        representative ventilators, 638–641, *639–641*, 639t, 640t
        ventilator characteristics, 631–635, *633, 634*
      positive airway pressure, 624–629
        atrial pressure, 625
        blood pressure, 625
        hemodynamics, 624–625
        immediate effects on circulation, 624
        IPPV effects, 626–627, *627*
        mechanical injury to lungs, 627–628
        metabolic lung injury, 628
        normal respiration, 624, *625*
        oxygen consumption, 625
        precautions, 628
        pressure patterns, 628–629, *629*
        pulmonary blood flow, 625–626
        renal function, 626
      principles of mechanical pulmonary ventilation, 620–623, *621*
        CPPV, 620–621
        EPI, 623

IPNPV, 623
IPPV, 621
NEEP, 622–623
PEEP, 620–622
pressure sequences, 620
work of ventilation, 623
respiratory therapy terms, 652
variables of ventilation, 623–624
  flow rate and pattern, 624
  pressure, 623
  rate and time sequence, 623–624
  volume, 623
carbon dioxide absorption, 454–455
See also Inhalation anesthesia.
Brewer-Luckhardt reflex, 1190
Broncho-Cath double-lumen tube, 605–606, *607*
Bronchospasm, 569–570
  from cold air, 1187
  curare actions, 949
  definition, 569
  incidence, 570
  mechanism, 570
  muscle relaxant effects, 905
  pancuronium uses, 970
  reflex, 1188–1189
Bucking during extubation, 552–555
  and bronchospasm, 570
Buffers, 1236–1237
  as preservatives, 1313
Bunsen solubility coefficient, 105
Bupivacaine
  cholinesterase inhibition, 840
  and dextrose, in hyperbaric spinal anesthesia, 1523–1524
  drug interactions, 266
  and epinephrine, in obstetrics, 1603–1604
  in isobaric spinal anesthesia, 1524–1526
  metabolism, 1221
  pharmacokinetics, 1485, 1512
  pharmacology, 1259–1262
  potassium effects, 1288, 1480
  pulmonary disposition, 1266
  spread of solution, 1471
  after subarachnoid administration, 1476
  toxicity, 1292, 1296
  See also Local anesthesia; Regional anesthesia.
Buprenorphine, lipid solubility, 1626
Burn patients
  cholinesterases, 839
  curare
    dosage, 949
    protein binding, 941
  hyperkalemia, 874, 915–916
  ketamine anesthesia, 742
  pancuronium effects, 968, 970
  relaxant actions, 865, 895–896, *895*
  succinylcholine, 1015–1016
Busulfan, pulmonary toxicity, 259
Butacaine sulfate pharmacology, 1255–1256
Butesin, 1256
Butorphanol, drug interactions, 266
Butyl-aminobenzoate, 1537

Caffeine, withdrawal headache, 1556, 1562
Calcium
  and end-plate potentials, 815, *816*
  in hypothermia, 1104, 1106
  and relaxant agents, 875–876, 916

Calcium channel blockers
  in controlled hypotension, 1087
  drug interactions, 268
  and neuromuscular junction, 883–884
  and oculocardiac reflex, 1180
  and platelet function, 258
Calorie
  definition, 108
  heat of vaporization, 141
Cancer
  chest radiography, 225
  in operating room personnel, 1159
  preoperative anxiety, 209
  therapy, drug interactions, 259–262
    alkylating agents, 260–261
    antibiotics, 261–262
    antimetabolites, 261
    general effects, 259–260
    vinca alkaloids, 262
Canisters, in carbon dioxide absorption, 454–456
Capillaries
  alveolar. See Alveolar ventilation.
  pulmonary flow, 327–328
Capillary leak syndrome, 257
Capnography, 87
Capsaicin, as local anesthetic, 1274
Captopril, drug interactions, 275
Carbamates, drug interactions, 273
Carbamazepine, and neuromuscular blockade, 883
Carbohydrates
  metabolism, and spinal anesthesia, 1510–1511
  and thiopental anesthesia, 668
Carbon dioxide
  absorption, 153–156, 452–459, *154, 155*
    absorbents, 453–455
      Baralyme, 453–455
      soda lime, 453
    absorber systems, 454–456
      absorber size, 455, 455t
      breathing circuits, 454–455
    absorptive capacity, 454
    canister preparation, 455–456, *456*
    concepts of, 11–12, 14, 18
    indicators, 454
    performance, 456–459
      adsorption of anesthetics, 457
      chemical degradation, 457–459, 458t
      temperature change, 457, *457*
    process of, 453
  analyzers, 139–140
  in brain perfusion, 170–171
  climate and altitude effects, 444
    analyzers, 445–446, 446t
  and curare, 945, 948
  and intraocular pressure, 279
  monitoring, 86–87
  and muscle relaxants, 879–880
  and oculocardiac reflex, 1180
  and pancuronium, 968
  response curve, droperidol effects, 710
  during sleep, 322
  washout methods, 408
  See also Inhalation anesthesia, breathing systems.
Carbon monoxide
  contamination in closed circle system, 427
  poisoning, hyperbaric oxygenation, 1139–1142, 1139–1141t
Carbonated local anesthetics, 1286–1287, 1479

Carbonic acid gas, 10
Carboxyhemoglobin, smoking effects, 213–214
Cardiac arrest
  age factors, 53
  electrical factors, 1155–1156
  in emergency patients, 53
  hypothermia, 1097
  from methylmethacrylate, 257
  psychogenic, 54–55
  in spinal anesthesia, 53–54, 1547
Cardiac output, 85–86
  in spinal anesthesia, 1506
Cardiac rate, in controlled hypotension, 1069–1070
Cardiac Risk Index, 55–57
  correlation with ASA grade, 56
  in noncardiac patients, 56–57, 57t
  predictive value, 56, 227
Cardiac surgery, hyperbaric oxygenation, 1142
Cardiopulmonary resuscitation (CPR), after spinal anesthesia, 54
Cardiovascular drugs, drug interactions, 274
Cardiovascular system
  alcoholism effects, 212
  alfentanil effects, 726
  atracurium effects, 986
  and caudal analgesia, 1615
  cocaine effects, 1250
  curare actions, 949
  dacuronium effects, 971
  diazepam effects, 752
  droperidol effects, 710
  in electroanesthesia, 1122
  in endotracheal anesthesia, 571–573
  ethanol effects, 775
  fentanyl effects, 715–716
  gallamine effects, 954
  hydroxydione effects, 764–765
  in hypothermia, 1101–1104
    arrhythmias, 1103–1104
    bathmotropic action, 1103
    catecholamines, 1102
    coronary blood flow, 1102
    dromotropic action, 1103
    ECG changes, 1103
    venous pressure, 1102
  ketamine effects, 738–739
  metocurine effects, 950
  midazolam effects, 757–758, 757t
  mivacurium effects, 992
  monitoring of, 69–86
    cardiac output, 85–86
    direct arterial monitoring, 78–79, 79t
    electrical cardiac activity, 70–71, 70
    mechanical cardiac activity, 71–86
      arterial blood pressure, 71–74, 72–74
      pulmonary artery pressure, 81–84, 82, 81t
      sphygmomanometry, 74–77, 76–78
      venous pressure, 79–81, 80, 81t
    noise effects, 1167–1168
  in obesity, 216
  pancuronium effects, 964–966
  and patient posture, 163–168
    anesthetic effects, 167–168
    blood flow, 164, 164
    dorsal decubitus position, 164–165, 165t
    gravity effects, 164
    hydrostatic indifferent point (HIP), 164
    hypovolemia, 166
    lateral decubitus position, 166–167
    morphine effects, 167
    prone position, 167–168
    pulmonary vascular pressure and alveolar pressure, 164
    supine-head down tilt, 165–166
    supine-head up tilt, 166
  posture effects. See Posture of patient.
  preanesthetic evaluation, 226–229, 227t
  propanidid effects, 772
  propofol effects, 770–771
  in rapid sequence induction, 440
  relaxant contraindications, 892, 916–917
  smoking effects, 214
  and spinal anesthesia, 1486
  succinylcholine effects, 1004–1005
  thiopental effects, 667, 667t
    substitutes, 689–690
  and toxicity of local anesthetics, 1308–1310
    cardiac effects, 1308–1309
    diazepam effects, 1309
    electrophysiology, 1308, 1308t
    mechanical properties, 1308–1309
    clinical types (syncope), 1309
    treatment, 1309–1310
    mechanism, 1308
    peripheral vascular effects, 1309
  vecuronium effects, 976–977
CARIN (Computerized Anesthesia Recording and Information Network), 31
Carina reflex, 1187
  endobronchial tube, 597, 602–604, 604, 605
Carmustine, pulmonary toxicity, 259
Carotid body, thiopental effects, 666
Carotid sinus
  nerve block, 1359–1361
    anatomy, 1359–1360
    complications, 1360
    indications, 1361
    technique, 1360
  reflex, 1182–1183
Cartilage of larynx. See Larynx.
Case study conferences, intraoperative deaths, 36–37
Catecholamines
  alcoholism effects, 212
  in controlled hypotension, 1089–1090, 1089t
  diazepam effects, 753
  in endotracheal anesthesia, 571
  in hypothermia, 1102
  ketamine effects, 741
  lidocaine effects, 576
  and MAC values, 336
  and muscle relaxants, 917
  noise effects, 1166–1167
  pancuronium effects, 966–967
  and surgical stress, 1508
Catheters
  direct arterial monitoring, 78
  endobronchial. See Endobronchial anesthesia.
  endotracheal tubes, 470–471
  for epidural anesthesia, 1586, 1592–1593, 1596–1597
  indwelling arterial, 78–79
  for insufflation, 411–412
  pulmonary artery pressure monitoring, 81–84
  for retrograde intubation, 542–543
  for spinal anesthesia, 1491
  suction
    during endotracheal intubation, 497, 499–500, 498t, 500–501t
    during extubation, 555, 556t
    pediatric, 509
  venous pressure monitoring, 80–81
Cauda equina syndrome, 1567
Caudal analgesia, 11, 1611–1621
  anatomy of sacrum, 1612–1614, 1612–1614
  complications, 1620–1621, 1620t
  contraindications, 1620t
  disadvantages, 1620
  history, 1611–1612
  indications, 1620
  needle position, 1619–1620
  in pediatrics, 1618–1619, 1619
  physiology, 1614–1615
  technical procedure, 1615–1621
    anesthetic solutions, 1615–1617
    dosage, 1617, 1616
    landmarks, 1615
    techniques, 1617–1618
      continuous, 1617–1618, 1618
      conventional, 1617, 1617
      simplified, 1617, 1618
Celiac plexus reflex, 1190
Central nervous system (CNS)
  in alcoholism, 212
  alfentanil effects, 724–726
  curare actions, 944
  depressants, and sleep, 322
  diazepam effects, 751–752
  diseases, and spinal anesthesia, 1486
  droperidol effects, 709–710
  drug uptake, 345–346
  electrical stimulation, and MAC values, 340
  electroanesthesia, 1120–1122
  ethanol effects, 774–775
  etomidate effects, 767
  fentanyl effects, 714–716
  gallamine effects, 953
  hydroxydione effects, 764
  in hypothermia, 1099
  irritation, in spinal anesthesia, 1546
  ketamine effects, 737–738
  lidocaine effects, 794
  local anesthetics, 803–804
    depression, 1307
    stimulation, 1303–1307
      biochemistry, 1304
      clinical severity, 1305
      comparative toxicity, 1304
      factors, 1303–1304, 1305t
      incidence, 1303
      mechanism, 1303
      prophylaxis and prevention, 1306
      relative toxicity, 1305
      signs and symptoms, 1304–1305, 1305t
      site of action, 1303
      treatment, 1306–1307
  midazolam effects, 756–757
  monitoring of, 90–95
    electroencephalography, 90–94, 92, 93, 91t
    temperature, 94–95
  muscle relaxant effects, 904

I-8 Index

Central nervous system (CNS) (*Continued*)
  oxygen toxicity, 1144–1145
  posture effects. See Posture of patient.
  preanesthetic medication, 284
  propanidid effects, 772
  propofol effects, 770
  regional anesthetic effects, 803–804
  succinylcholine effects, 1004, 1008
  thiopental effects, 666
    bioelectric model, 672–674, *674*
    substitutes, 689, *692*
Cephalosporin drugs, drug interactions, 266
Cerebral cortex, excitation by local anesthetics, 1303
Cerebral palsy
  and muscle relaxants, 898
  potassium release, 915
Cerebrospinal fluid (CSF)
  biotransformation of local anesthetics, 1475
  physiology, 1455–1458
    absorption, 1456–1458
    active secretion, 1456
    circulation, 1458
    composition, 1457, 1457t
    control of production, 1455–1456
    density-specific gravity, 1457, *1458*
    formation, 1455, *1455*, *1456*
    induction drugs, 1457
    volume, 1455
  relaxant effects, 835
  and spinal opioids, 1624–1625
Cerebrovascular disorders
  and muscle relaxants, 896–898
  potassium release, 915
Certificate of death, 37, 37t
Cervical
  injury, during patient positioning, 197–198
  spine, nerve block. See Nerve block, cervical spine.
Cervico (uterine)-laryngeal reflex, 1191
Cesarean section, spinal anesthesia, 1485
Chambers, for hyperbaric oxygenation, 1136–1139
Charles' Law, 102–103, *103*
Chassaignac's tubercle, 1379, 1431
Check valves, 131, *134*
Chemical hazards, 1158–1165
  operating room contamination, 1162, 1162t
  safety measures, 1162–1165
    room air ventilation, 1164–1165
    scavenging circuit gases, 1164, *1165*
    spillage reduction, 1163–1164, *1163–1164*, 1163t
  waste anesthetics and personnel, 1158–1162
    biotransformation, 1161–1162
    blood levels, 1161, 1161t
    cancer and tumors, 1159
    in dentists, 1160–1161, 1161t
    embryo toxicity, 1158
    experimental toxicity studies, 1159
    health effects, 1159
    miscarriages, 1158
    trace concentration effects, 1160t
    urinalysis, 1161
Chemical heat of crystallization, 145, *145*
Chemistry

acetylcholine, 814
althesin, 765, *765*, 766t
barbiturates, 656–657, *656*, 656t
bupivacaine, 1259–1260
butacaine, 1255
chloroprocaine, 1253
cocaine, 1248
cyclohexylamines, 734, *735*
dacuronium, 971, *971*
diazepam, 749, *749*
dibucaine, 1256
edrophonium, *1040*
etidocaine, 1262
etomidate, 766, *766*
fazadinium, 989
gallamine, 952, *953*
gamma hydroxybutyric acid, 774, *774*
hexafluorenium, 1017, *1017*
hexylcaine, 1250–1251
hydroxydione, 763, *763*
ketamine, 735
lidocaine, 1257
local anesthetics, 1234–1236, *1236*
  alcohol group, 1239
  amide derivatives, 1239
  ester compounds, 1239
  mixtures, 1240
  non-esters, 1240
mepivacaine, 1258–1259
methonium compounds, 1065, *1065*
midazolam, 756, *757*
mivacurium, 990, *990*
nitroprusside, 1071, *1071*
pancuronium, 960, *960*
pipecuronium, 980, *980*
procaine, 787–788, 1252
propanidid, 772, *772*
propitocaine, 1263–1264
propofol, 768–769, *769*
relaxants, 828–831, *829–831*
  natural agents, 828–829
  structure and activity, 830–831
  synthetic agents, 829
ropivacaine, 1264
succinylcholine, 1004, *1004*
sufentanil, 726, *726*
tetracaine, 1255
trimethaphan, 1067, *1067*
vecuronium, 972, *972*
Chemoreceptors, carotid body, 467
Chest
  injuries, positioning of patient, 190, 200
  radiography, preoperative, 224–225, 225t
  in cancer patient, 225
Chicken pox, and spinal anesthesia, 1567
Childbirth
  uterine afferent nerve block, 1427
  See also Obstetrics.
Children. See Infants and children.
Chin nerve block, 1351
Chloral hydrate
  protein binding, 254
  and REM sleep, 322
Chloroform
  on cloth, 12
  density, 107
  early uses, 7–9, 119–120
  and EEG patterns, 371
  and intraocular pressure, 279
  solubility coefficient, 332
Chlorprocaine, 796

bacteriostatic action, 1313
metabolism, 1221
pharmacology, 1253–1255
toxicity, 1296
See also Regional anesthesia.
Chlorpromazine
  in alcoholic patient, 213
  cholinesterase inhibition, 840
  drug interactions, 273
  and thiopental potentiation, 660
Choice reaction time, 52
Chokes, in hyperbaric oxygenation, 1143
Cholase, 1048
Cholcystitis, acupuncture, 1639
Choline acetylase, 820, *821*
Cholinesterases, 836–841
  atypical enzymes, 837–838
  biosynthesis, 837
  determination, 841, 841t
  elevated levels, 840–841, 840t
  enzyme identification, 838–839
    dibucaine number, 838
    fluoride number, 838
  inhibitors, 339, 840
  metabolism, 1221
  nomenclature, 836, 837t
  pharmacokinetics, 837
  and succinylcholine, 1010, 1016
  trimethaphan effects, 1068–1069
  variations, 839–840
    acquired deficiency, 839–840, 839t
Chorea, laryngeal muscles, 467
Choreoathetosis, and muscle relaxants, 898
Chronotropism, and toxicity of local anesthetics, 1308–1309
Chymopapain, as local anesthetic, 1270
Cimetidine
  comparison with ranitidine and famitodine, 236–237
  drug interactions, 265
  and succinylcholine, 1016
Circadian rhythm
  and diazepam anesthesia, 750
  pain tolerance, 1322
  of sleep, 320, 321
Circle breathing systems
  closed system, 392–396
    advantages, 392
    carbon dioxide content, 394–395
    contamination, 396, 427–427
    definition, 392
    dilution of anesthetic gas, 395–396
    diffusion loses, 395, 395t, 396t
    leaks, 395–396
    history, 392
    incompatibility of absorption and anesthetics, 396
    requirements, 392
    resistance, 392–393, 393t
    temperature of inspired gases, 393–394
    waste metabolites, 396
    water vapor, 393
  components, 389–390, *389*, *390*
  dead space, 391
  flows and concentrations, 390–391
  function of, 391, *391*
  humidity, 418–420, *419*
  mixing devices, 390
Circle filter system, 12
Circulatory system
  curare actions, 944

maternal-fetal, thiopental effects, 680
nitroprusside effects, 1078
positive airway pressure effects, 624, *625*
of spinal cord, 1450-1455
Circulatory volume loading reflex, 1193
Circumcision
  anesthesia needs, 236
  nerve block, 1426
Cisplatin toxicity, 262
Citanest. *See* Propitocaine.
Cladding, fiberoptic, 544
Classification
  alcoholism, 212
  body build, 210
  breathing systems, 387-389, 423, 388t
  EEG waveforms, 92-93
  endobronchial intubation, 600, 601t
  endotracheal tubes, 471
  glaucoma, 277, 277t
  heart disease, 227t
  hypothermia, 1097, 1098t
  laryngospasm, 567-568
  nerve fibers, 1208, 1499, 1207t, 1500t
  obesity, 216
  operating room deaths, 34-35, 35t
  pain, 1337-1338
  physical status, 38, 39t
  relaxants, 821-828, 823t
    antagonists, 1028, 1028t
    antidepolarizing block, 822-825, *824*, 824t
    depolarizing block, 825-828, *825*
  signs of anesthesia, 361, 361t
  vaporizers, 145
  ventilators, 635-638
Clayton yellow, indicator of carbon dioxide absorption, 454
Cleaning, endotracheal tubes, 478-480
  fiberoptic scope, 547-548
Climate and altitude effects, 444-451
  gas analyzers, 445-446
    carbon dioxide, 445-446, 446t
    oxygen, 445, 446t
    vapor, 446, 447t
  gas density and flow, 447-449, *448*
  minimal alveolar partial pressure, 450, 450t
  oxygen enrichment devices, 449
  partial pressures of gases, 444-445, *445*
  vaporizers, 446-447
Clonidine
  analgesia effects, 1269-1270
  during endotracheal anesthesia, 577-578
  and MAC values, 339
  potentiation of spinal anesthetics, 1480
  preanesthetic medication, 292
Clothing
  flammable, 1150
  static electricity, 1152
Coagulation factors
  after epidural anesthesia, 1601-1602
  in obesity, 217
  preoperative tests, 221-222
Cobefrin, potentiation of action, 1285-1286
Cobra venom, 1271
Cocaine, 1247-1250
  absorption, 1248-1249
  addiction, 1250
  alternatives, 1274

anesthetic properties, 1248
and cardiac function, 1250
chemistry, 1248
during extubation, 554
history, 1247-1248
and MAC values, 339
and nasal mucosa, 1249
pharmacokinetics, 1249
potentiation of action, 1285
preparations, 1248
source, 1248
for surgical anesthesia, 10
and sympathetic nervous system, 1249
toxicity, 1296
and uterine blood flow, 1250
Cognition, pain sensation, 1333
Colchicine
  drug interactions, 268
  and neuromuscular junction, 886
Cold injury, and hypothermia, 915
Cold pressor test, 1442
Cole endotracheal tube, 475-476, *476*
Coley's toxin, 1111
Color codes, compressed gas cylinders, 127
Columbia pediatric breathing system, 418
Comatose patients
  extubation, 555-556
  management and positioning, 189-190
  tactile tracheal intubation, 539
Combustion engines, carbon monoxide, 1139-1140
Compliance
  airway pressure, 88
  in ventilators, 639
Computed tomography, epidural space, 1597-1598
Conduction anesthesia
  definition, 1200
  hexylcaine, 1251
Congenital anomalies, in operating room personnel, 1159-1160
Connectors
  for endobronchial intubation, 600, 607
  endotracheal tube, 493-494, *494*
Conscious patients
  in hypothermia, 1101
  intubation, 539-540
  and ventilators, 641
Consultation, medical, preanesthetic evaluation, 234
Continuous-flow anesthesia machines, 121-122, *121, 122*, 122t
Contraceptives, oral, drug interactions, 275
Contractions
  lower esophageal, 366
  muscle types, 810-811
Conversion factors, compressed gas cylinders, 126
Convulsions, in epidural anesthesia, 1599
Corneal abrasions, during patient repositioning, 194, 195
Coronary artery by-pass surgery
  infarction after, 60
  pancuronium uses, 971
  in smokers, 51
Coronary artery disease
  and endotracheal anesthesia, 571
  perioperative mortality, 58
Corpora cavernosa, transfusion and anesthesia, 299

Cortex, and muscular relaxation, 379
Corticosteroids
  adrenal, drug interactions, 275
  and neuromuscular junction, 886
  and pancuronium interaction, 970
Cortisol
  during sleep, 321-322
  and surgical stress, 1508
Cortisone, drug interactions, 275
Cough
  and bronchospasm, 570
  laryngeal muscles, 468
  reflex, 1187
    lidocaine effects, 791
  and shape of trachea, 487
  test, 226
Coumarin derivatives, drug interactions, 262
CPAP (continuous positive airway pressure), 622
CPPV (continuous positive-pressure ventilation), 620-621, 652
Crack, 1250
Cranial nerves
  palsy, trichloroethylene effects, 458
  after spinal anesthesia, 1564-1566
    abducens nerve paralysis, 1565
    auditory nerve, 1565
    visual disturbances, 1564-1565
  See also Nerve block.
Cranium, during patient positioning, 196
Cricothyroid membrane, 542
Critical flicker fusion frequency, 52
Crossmatching of blood, 221-222
Croup, endotracheal anesthesia complications, 589-590
Crouzon's disease, and endotracheal anesthesia, 518
Cryotherapy, 1097
Crystallization, chemical heat of, 145, *145*
Cuffs
  in blood pressure measurement, 72-75
  for endobronchial intubation, 600
  endotracheal. *See* Endotracheal anesthesia.
Curare, 939-949
  chemistry, 828-829, 939-940, *940*
  clinical uses, 947-949
    administration and dosage, 947-948
    anesthetic state, 947
    drug interactions, 948
    indications, 949
    pharmacodynamics, 948
    plasma concentration, 948
    precautions, 949
    premedication, 947
    recovery and reversal, 948-949
  history, 939
  and MAC values, 338-339
  metabolism, 940-943
    age effects, 943
    biotransformation, 941
    elimination, 942-943, *942-943*
    and liver disease, 943
    pharmacokinetics, 940-941, *941*
    plasma protein binding, 941
    and renal dysfunction, 943
  pharmacologic actions, 944-947
    autonomic nervous system, 945-946, 946t
    cardiac actions, 944-945
    central nervous system, 944
    circulatory system, 944

Curare
  pharmacologic actions (Continued)
    gastrointestinal tract, 946
    histamine release, 946–947
    respiratory system, 945
    skeletal muscle, 944
  protein binding, 254, 255
  and thiopental, 657–660
  See also Relaxants.
Curarine, physicochemical mechanisms of action, 877–881
  acidosis, 879
  alkalosis, 878–879
  carbon dioxide effects, 879–880
  epinephrine, 880
  exercise, 880
  temperature, 880–889
Cushing, Harvey
  ether charts, 11, 29–30, 71
  precordial stethoscopy, 77
Cut-down technique, 295
Cyanide, in nitroprusside treatment, 1073–1074, 1079
Cyclic GMP, in nitroprusside action, 1077
Cyclohexylamines, 734–735
  abuse potential, 735
  chemistry, 734, 735
  CI-400, 734
  disposition, 735
  ketamine. See Ketamine.
  Sernyl (CI-395), 734–735
Cyclooxygenase, aspirin effects, 258
Cyclophosphamide, pulmonary toxicity, 259
Cyclopropane
  alveolar concentration, 328
  and body metabolism, 323
  early uses of, 14, 16, 18
  and EEG patterns, 371
  and intraocular pressure, 279
  solubility coefficient, 332
Cylinders
  compressed gas. See Anesthesia machines and components.
  valves, 131
Cysts, laryngeal, 524
Cytarabine, drug interactions, 261
Cytochrome P-450 system, in drug transformations, 348–349
Cytotoxicity
  bupivacaine, 1261
  chloroprocaine, 1253
  definition, 1233
  hexylcaine, 1251
  lidocaine, 1257
  local anesthetics, 1312
  mepivacaine, 1259
  tetracaine, 1255

Dactinomycin (Actinomycin-D), pulmonary toxicity, 261
Dacuronium, 971–972
Dalton's Law, 104, *104*
Dantrolene, 1018
Datatrac recod system, 31
Daunorubicin toxicity, 261
Dead space, 391–392
Deafness, acupuncture, 1639
Deaths, operating room, 34–38
  accidental and incidental causes, 36
  accuracy of records, 37

anesthesia personnel, 37–38
and anesthetic management, 35
case study conferences, 36–37
causes, 34
classification, 34–35, 35t
death certificate definitions, 37, 37t
equipment failure, 35
patient disease, 35–36
study commissions, 37
surgical factors, 35
Debility
  in hyperthermia, 1113
  relaxant contraindications, 895
Decamethonium compound, 829, 1002–1003, *1003*
Decompression sickness, 1143
Decubitus, 163, 184
Definitions
  acupuncture, 1634
  AIDS, 1170
  alcoholism, 212
  artificial breathing systems, 618–620
  awareness states, 287–288, 288t
  balanced anesthesia, 381–382
  body posture, 163, 184
  bronchospasm, 569
  compressed gas, 122
  drug dependence, 307
  drug evaluation, 303–304
  electroencephalography, 90
  endotracheal anesthesia, 461
  epidural anesthesia, 1571–1572
  general anesthesia, 314
  high-frequency ventilation, 646–647
  hypnosis, 1125–1126
  induction, 424
  inhalation anesthesia breathing systems, 392, 400, 405, 408
  laryngospasm, 567
  local anesthetics, 1233
  malpractice, 61
  mechanical ventilation, 631
  neuroleptic anesthesia, 707
  noise, 1165–1166
  opioid analgesia, 1622–1623
  pain, 1318
  placebo, 305
  regional anesthesia, 1199
  relaxants, 831–832
  respiratory therapy terms, 652
  UD concept, 655
  weaning, 641
Deformities, and preanesthetic visit, 218
Dehydration
  cholinesterases, 839
  and relaxant agents, 872–873
Delirium
  from ethanol, 777
  ketamine anesthesia, 747
  positioning of patient, 190
Delivery systems, spinal opiates, 1627, *1628*
Demand analgesia, 1344
  intermittent-flow machines, 137–138
Denervation sensitivity, 900
Denitrogenation, 425–427, *425*
  tissue desaturation, 426
  uptake of inert gases, 426–427
Density
  of anesthetic solutions, 107, 1466–1468
  definition, 106
Dental anesthesia
  demand machines, 137

diazepam uses, 753
early extractions, 6, 9
flammable substances, 1150
health risks in personnel, 1160–1161
hypnosis, 1131
nerve blocks. See Nerve block.
trauma during endotracheal anesthesia, 496–497
Dentures, during anesthesia, 242
Depolarizing drugs. See Relaxants.
Depressants, drug dependence, 308
Depression in epidural anesthesia, 1599
Desensitization. See Relaxants.
Desipramine, drug interactions, 270
Detoxification of local anesthetics, 1220–1221, 1297–1298
Deuteration, 351
Development of spinal cord, 1448, *1448*
Dextran
  and platelet function, 258
  potentiation of action, 1288–1289
  spinal anesthetics, 1479
Dextrose
  potentiation of spinal anesthetics, 1478–1479
  in spinal anesthesia. See Spinal anesthesia, techniques.
Diabetes mellitus
  in obesity, 217
  stiff joint syndrome, 524
  therapy, drug interactions, 274–275
Diameter Index Safety System (DISS), 130, *134*
Diaphragm
  relaxant actions, 848–849
  traction reflex, 1190
Diazepam, 748–755
  advantages, 755
  in alcoholic patient, 213
  in ambulatory surgery, 1645
  analgesia, 752
  blood level correlation with CNS effects, 751–752
  and cardiovascular system, 752
  and catecholamines, 753
  chemistry, 749, *749*
  clinical uses, 753–754
    convulsive state, 754
    dentistry, 753
    endoscopy, 754
    induction agent, 753
    obstetrics, 753
    precautions and complications, 754–755
    premedication, 749, 753
    tetanus, 754
  dosage and administration, 749
  excretion, 751
  indications, 753
  induction, 749–750
  intoxication, 755
  and intraocular pressure, 279
  and laryngeal reflex, 752
  locus of action, 749
  and MAC values, 338
  mechanism of action, 751
  metabolism, 750–751
  muscle relaxant properties, 753
  and neuromuscular transmission, 888
  overdosage, 755
  pharmacokinetics, 750, *751*
    age and sex effects, 750
    binding effect, 750
    circadian effect, 750

liver disease, 750
race effects, 750
renal disease, 750
placental transfer, 753
respiratory effects, 752
and sleep respiratory patterns, 54
and toxicity of local anesthetics, 1306, 1309
Dibucaine
and dextrose, in hyperbaric spinal anesthesia, 1522
in hypobaric spinal anesthesia, 1527
in isobaric spinal anesthesia, 1524
metabolism, 1221
number, 837–838
pharmacology, 1256–1257
Dichloracetylene, incompatibility in closed circle systems, 396
Dicumarol, drug interactions, 262
Diethylaminoethanol, 788
Diffusion
in closed circle systems, 395
of gases, 107
anesthetic agents, 330–331, 343–344
Diltiazem, drug interactions, 268
Dioscorides, 4
Diphenhydramine (Benadryl), drug interactions, 265
Diphenylhydantoin
enzyme induction, 348
protein binding, 254
Dipyridamole, and platelet function, 258
Disinfectants, chemical
for endotracheal tubes, 479
procedures, 1174
Dissociation constant
regional anesthesia, 1210–1213, 1211t
of thiopental, 657
Distraction in pain control, 1344
Disulfiram
drug interactions, 272
enzyme inhibition, 348
Diuretics, drug interactions, 268–269
Diurnal rhythm
and dosage of anesthesia, 290
and MAC values, 336
Dizziness, after spinal anesthesia, 1564
Doppler piezoelectric microphones, 73
Dorsal decubitus position
cardiovascular system, 164–165, 165t
technical aspects, 177–178, 179
Dosage
in alcoholic patient, 213
alfentanil, 725
althesin, 765
atracurium, 982–984
bupivacaine, 1260–1261
caudal analgesia, 1615
controlled hypotension, 1070
curare, 947–948
dacuronium, 971
diazepam, 749
doxacurium, 994
edrophonium, 1041
epidural. See Epidural anesthesia.
ethanol, 776–777
etidocaine, 1262
etomidate, 766
factors determining, 289–290
age, 289, 289
agents, 290
diseases, 290
diurnal rhythm, 290
emotions, 290

endocrine effects, 290
ethnicity, 289–290
pain, 290
sex, 290
temperature, 290
toxemias, 290
fazadinium, 989
fentanyl, 712, 719
gallamine, 953, 955
gamma hydroxybutyric acid, 774
hydroxydione, 763–764
intravenous regional anesthesia, 797
lidocaine, 792
lorazepam, 755–756
MAC measurement, 334
meperidine, 702, 703t
metocurine, 950
mivacurium, 990–991, 991t
morphine, 702, 704
neostigmine, 1034
nitroglycerin, 1083–1084
nitroprusside, 1071–1072, 1072t
pancuronium, 960
pediatric preanesthetic medication, 301
pipecuronium, 980
procaine, 788–790
propanidid, 773
propofol, 769
pyridostigmine, 1038
ropivacaine, 1265
spinal anesthesia in infants and children, 1533–1534
spinal anesthesia, 1627–1628
spinal opiates, 1627–1628
succinylcholine, 1011–1014
bolus intravenous, 1011–1012
continuous intravenous drip, 1012–1013
intermittent intravenous, 1012
intramuscular, 1013–1014
sufentanil, 726–727
thiopental, 661, 677, 679–680
substitutes, 691, 693, 695
and toxicity of local anesthetics, 1295–1296
vecuronium, 973–974, 973t
Dose potency, in intravenous induction, 428, 428, 429
Dose-response factors of relaxants. See Relaxants.
Double-blind technique, 304–305
Down syndrome
atlantoaxial subluxation, 590
ketamine effects, 740
Doxacurium, 994–995, 994
Doxapram Test, 860
Doxepin, drug interactions, 270
Doxorubicin toxicity, 261
Drapes
flammable, 1150
static electricity, 1153
Dreaming
ketamine anesthesia, 747
perioperative, 367
and REM sleep, 320
and succinylcholine, 1016–1017
Droperidol, 708–711
adverse effects, 711
in ambulatory surgery, 1646
chemistry, 708
and fentanyl, 708
metabolism, 709
pharmacokinetics, 708–709, 709t
pharmacology, 709–711

pharmcodynamics, 708
potency, 708
Drowsiness, in epidural anesthesia, 1599
Drug administration, 292–296
bone marrow infusions, 298–299
hypodermic injection, 293
intramuscular injection, 293–294
intravenous route, 294–296
miscellaneous routes, 299
nasal instillation, 297–298
rectal administration, 298
routes of administration, 293
transbuccal mucosal absorption, 297
transdermal instillation, 298
Drug dependence, 307–309
causes, 307–308
definitions, 307
pathogenesis, 307
pharmacologic considerations, 308–309
alcohol-barbiturate abstinence syndrome, 309
depressants, 308
morphine abstinence syndrome, 308
stimulants, 308
Drug interactions, 253–283
alfentanil and benzodiazepines, 726
atracurium, 987
curare and inhalation agents, 948
ethanol, 777
mechanisms of adverse reactions, 253–256, 243t
enzyme activity
induction, 255–256
inhibition, 256
ionization, 254–255, 255
plasma protein binding, 254
receptor sites, 256
specific interactions, 256–280
acrylic bone cement, 256–257
adrenal corticosteroids, 275
angina therapy, 268
angiotensin converting enzyme inhibitors, 275
antibiotics, 266
anticancer drugs, 259–262, 260t
anticoagulant therapy, 262–265, 264t
antidepressants
MAO inhibitors, 269
tricyclics, 269–272, 271t
antidiabetic drugs, 274–275
antihistaminic agents, 265–266
antihypertensive agents, 266–268
aspirin and aspirin-like drugs, 257–259
asthmatic therapy, 275
barbiturates, 272–273
cardiovascular drugs, 274
disulfiram, 272
diuretics, 268–269
epinephrine reaction with volatile anesthetics, 276
glaucoma treatment, 276–280, 277t
gout therapy, 268
levodopa, 276
lithium salts, 272
pancuronium, 969–970
parasympathetic drugs, 276
psychotropic agents in elderly, 273–274
succinylcholine, 1016
sympathomimetic drugs, 275–276
thyroid preparations, 274

Drug interactions
 specific interactions (*Continued*)
  tranquilizers, 273
 and toxicity of local anesthetics, 1298
Duchenne's dystrophy, 900–901
Dural puncture, in caudal analgesia, 1620
Dynorphins, in pain control, 1335
Dysautonomia, familial, 467
Dyspnea
 affective, in spinal anesthesia, 1507, 1546
 preoperative evaluation, 231–232, 231t
Dysrhythmias, from pulmonary artery catheterization, 83
Dystonia, droperidol effects, 711
Dystrophy
 progressive muscular, 900–901
  Duchenne's, 900–901
  fascio-scapulo-humeral, 901

Ears, during patient repositioning, 194–195
Eating, and solubility coefficients, 332, 337
Echocardiography
 cardiac output, 86, 95
 two-dimensional, heart disease evaluation, 228
Echothiophate, 276, 278, 1043
Eclampsia
 hypothermia, 1097–1098
 magnesium treatment, 876–877
Edema
 airway, in children, 509, *509*
 cerebral, during patient positioning, 196
 laryngeal, during endotracheal anesthesia, 581–582, *582*
 pulmonary
  from methylmethacrylate, 257
  and spinal anesthesia, 1488
 supraglottic obstructive, 582, *583*
Edrophonium, 1039–1041
 clinical uses, 1039–1040
 dose and administration, 1041
 mechanism of action, 1029, 1040–1041
 muscarinic effect, 1041
 pediatric reversal, 1045–1046
 pharmacodynamics, 1041
 priming principle, 1042, 1043t
 screening uses, 1041
 structure, *1040*
Elavil, drug interactions, 270
Elbow nerve block, 1393
 median nerve, 1387–1388
 radial nerve, 1391–1392
 ulnar nerve, 1385–1386
Elderly
 cardiac complications, 57
 complications of anesthesia, 47–48, 215
  over 90 years, 48, 49t
 hemogram, 221
 psychotropic drugs, 273–274
 See also Age factors.
Electrical stimulation
 for acupuncture, 1638
 nerve location, 1224–1225
 pain control, 1337, 1344–1345
Electricity, 1153–1158
 cardiac arrest, 1155–1156
 distribution systems, 1153–1154, *1153*

equipment, 1157
leakage currents, 1154–1155, *1154–1155*, 1155t
macroshock, 1155
mechanical hazards, 1158
microshock, 1156–1157
physiologic effects of shock, 1157, 1157t
references, 1157–1158
safety rules, 1157
static, 1151–1153
 attire and footgear, 1153
 equipment, 1152–1153
 generation of, 1152
 grounding, 1152
 precautions, 1152
Electroanesthesia, 1119–1124, 1345
 clinical uses, 1122
 history, 1119–1120
 magnetic fields, 1122–1123
 mechanism, 1120
 physiology, 1121–1122
 principles, 1120–1121
 procedure, 1121
 site of action, 1120
Electrocardiogram (ECG), 70–71, *70*
 in alcoholism, 212
 in hyperbaric oxygenation, 1138
 in hypothermia, 1103
 preoperative evaluation, 226
 regional anesthetic effects, 804
 in thiopental anesthesia, 667
Electrodes
 blood gas analysis, 88–89
 for EEG, 90–91
 for electroanesthesia, 1121
 in neuromuscular blockade, 859
Electroencephalography (EEG), 90–94
 alfentanil effects, 725
 applications, 93
 classification of patterns, 92–93
 definition, 90
 diazepam effects, 751–752
 etomidate effects, 767
 evoked potentials, 94
 fentanyl effects, 715
 historical aspects, 90, 91t
 hydroxydione effects, 764
 in hyperbaric oxygenation, 1138
 in hyperthermia, 1113
 in hypnosis, 1128–1129
 hypothermia effects, 1100, 1100t
 ketamine effects, 736–738
 limitations, 94
 local anesthetics, 803–804
 measurement systems, 90–91
 as monitor, 93–94
 nitroprusside effects, 1079
 noise effects, 1168
 signs of anesthesia, 369–371
  classification, 370–371, *370*, 370t
  general patterns, 369–370, *369*
  technique, 369
 during sleep, 318–319, 322
 thiopental effects, 672–676, *676*
 waves
  during anesthesia, 92, *93*
  construction of, 91–92
   amplitude, 92
   frequency, 91–92, *92*
   waveforms, 92, *92*
  significance, 91
Electrolytes
 in hypothermia, 1105–1106, 1111

pancuronium effects, 968–969
and relaxant agents, 873–877, 916, 874t
and thiopental anesthesia, 681
Electromagnetic flow probe, 85
Electromyography (EMG)
 relaxant action, 825, 826
 twitch monitoring, 860
Ellis-van Creveld dwarfism, 518–519
Embolism
 air, during patient repositioning, 196, 200
 gas, in hyperbaric oxygenation, 1143
Embryo toxicity, in operating room personnel, 1158
Emergency operations
 cardiac arrest, 53
 mortality risk, 49
 and reinfarction risks, 59
EMLA cream, 1275
EMMA analyzer, 140
Emotions, and dosage of anesthesia, 290
Emphysema
 preoperative evaluation, 232
 subcutaneous and surgical, in epidural anesthesia, 1599–1600
 surgical, 588
Enalapril, drug interactions, 275
Encephalitis, potassium release, 915
End plate
 muscular
  drug actions, 820–821
  histology, 812, *813*
  and quantal mechanisms, 815–816
 relaxant actions, 820–821
  dynamic competition, 821
  physicochemistry, 820–821
  receptor affinity, 821
Endobronchial anesthesia, 597–617
 history, 597–599, *598*
 intubation technique, 599–607
  advantages, 599
  anatomic principles, 599–600, *600*
  anesthesia, 601
  classification, 600, 601t
  indications, 599, 599t
  preparation, 600
  procedure, 601–607
   alternative insertion, 604, 606–607, *605*
   awake intubation, 606–607
   blind technique with single-lumen tube, 601–602, *602*
   Broncho-Cath double-lumen tube, 605–606, *607*
   Carlens catheter method, 602–604, *603–604*
   Robertshaw tube, 604–606, *606*
   White double-lumen catheter, 604, *604*
  tube selection and size, 601, 602t
 physiology of one-lung ventilation, 613–616
  anesthetic effects, 614
  oxygenation efficiency, 614
  PEEP effects, 615–616, *616*
  reflex hypoxic pulmonary vasoconstriction, 614
  shunt, 613–614
  tidal volume, 615, *618*
  ventilation in lateral position, 616
 postintubation management, 607–612
  fiberoptic bronchoscope, 612
  tube position, 607–611, *609–612*

ventilation management, 612–613
Endocrine system
  and dosage of anesthesia, 290
  droperidol effects, 710
  etomidate effects, 767–768
  in hyperbaric oxygenation, 1147
  ketamine effects, 741
  midazolam effects, 758
  noise effects, 1166–1167
  in obesity, 217
  and preanesthetic medication, 285
  and surgical stress. *See* Spinal anesthesia, physiology.
  thiopental effects, 668–669, 681, 695
Endorphins in pain control, 1333–1335
Endoscopy, diazepam anesthesia, 754
Endotracheal anesthesia
  adjunctive equipment, 493–500
    catheters, 497, 499–500, 498t
    connectors and adaptors, 493–494, *494, 495*
    fixation tapes, 498–499
    forceps, 497, *498*
    lubricants, 497–498, 499t
    mouth props, 495–496, *497*
    stylets, 495, *496*
    tooth protectors, 496–497
    tracheal placement, 499
  airways, 437–438
  anatomy of larynx, 461–468
    closure, 468
    compartments, 464, *464*
    framework, 462, *463*
    functions, 465–467
    hyoid bone, 462–464
    membranes and ligaments, 464, *463*
    movement, 467
    muscles, 464–465, 467–468, *466*
    topographic location, 461–462, *462*
  complications, 565–596, 566t, 567t
    clinical description, 565–566
    hemodynamic control, 573–578
      beta-adrenoceptor block, 576–577
      clonidine, 577–578
      fentanyl, 576
      lidocaine, 575–576, 576t
      nitroglycerin, 577
      topical anesthesia, 576
    pathophysiologic and reflex, 566–573
      cardiovascular effects, 571–573, *572–575*
      respiratory effects, 566–571, *568*, 567t
    pediatric, 589–591, 590t
      airway perforation, 591
      atlantoaxial subluxation, 590
      croup, 589–590, 591t
      palatal groove formation, 590–591
      prolonged nasotracheal intubation, 591
    traumatic anatomic complications, 578–585
      arytenoid cartilage dislocation, 586
      assessment of damage, 582–585, 583t, 584t
      atlantoaxial subluxation, 580
      bacteremia, intraoperative, 587–588
      clinical factors, 579
      constitutional factors, 578–579, 578t
      cuff inflation, 586
      edema, laryngeal, 581–582, *582*
      epiglottitis, 580
      granulomas of larynx, 583, *584*
      hypopharyngeal perforation, 585
      laceration and ulceration, 579
      laryngeal nerve paralysis, 585–586
      laryngitis, 580–581
      lingual nerve injury, 585
      mandible dislocation, 579–580
      mucosal denudation of trachea, 586
      nasotracheal intubation, 588–589
      perichondritis of laryngeal cartilage, 583–584
      pulmonary infection, 587
      respiratory tract infection, 586–587
      rupture of trachea, 585
      sore throat, 580
      stenosis, subglottic and tracheal, 584–585
      subglottic membrane, 586
      supraglottic obstructive edema, 582, *583*
      surgical emphysema, 588
      teeth and gum injury, 579
      tension pneumothorax, 588
      tracheitis, 584
      ulcers of larynx, 582, 583t
      vocal cord fusion, 586
  definition, 461
  development, 13, 15, 18
  endotracheal tubes, 468–480
    anode or armored tube, 474–475, *475*
    care of tubes, 478–480
    classification, 471
    Cole tube, 475–476, *476*
    construction materials, 468–469
    endotrol tracheal tube, 476, *476*
    laser-shielded, 477–478, *477*
    length, 472–474, 473t
    Lindholm tube, 476, *476*
    Magill standard tube, 471–472, *472*
    markings, 471
    Murphy type tube, 474, *475*
    for nasal intubation, 474, *472*
    performance criteria, 469–470
    preformed RAE tube, 476–477, *477*
    resistance factors, 470
    selection of, 474, 475t
    sizes, 470, 471t
    standardization, 469
    terminology, 468
    tissue reaction, 478
    tube bore size, 472, 473t
  historical development, 460–461
  laryngoscope, 480–484
    blade tip, 482, *483*
    flange, 482
    handle, 482–483
    lighting, 483–484
    spatula, 481–482, *481*
  leak-proof inhalation systems, 484–493
    inflatable endotracheal cuffs, 484–493
      characteristics, 485
      complications, 490–492
      cuff system, 484–485, *485*
      history, 484
      monitoring of pressure, 488–489, *488*
      performance specifications, 492–493
      pressure regulators, 489–490
      rules for inflation, 488
      special cuffs, 492
      tracheal wall pressures, 485–486, *487*
      types, 485
    pharyngeal packing, 484
  pediatric considerations, 500–510
    airway differences and assessment, 502–503, 505t
    airway edema, 509, *509*
    indications, 504
    laryngoscopy, 508–509
    larynx
      anatomy, 500–501, *502*
      topographic position, 501–502, 503t
    securing of tubes, 509
    stridor, 510, 510t
    suctioning, 509
    tubes, 504–508
      airway resistance, 505
      connectors, 157
      cuffs, 505–506
      dead space, 392
      guidelines, 505
      selection of, 506–508, 507t, 508t
  technical considerations, 518–564
    airway evaluation, 518–525
      anatomic factors, 522, 560–564
      calcified stylohyoid ligaments, 524–525
      diabetic stiff joint syndrome, 524
      epiglottic abnormalities, 523–525
      fibrous dysplasia, 525
      indicators of difficult intubation, 519–521, *522*
      Klippel-Feil syndrome, 525
      laryngeal cysts, 524
      laryngoscopic difficulties, 521–522
      Mallampati score, 522–523, *523*
      paradoxic vocal cord motion, 525
      preintubation evaluation, 518–519, *519–520*
      spine abnormalities, 525
      standard assessment procedure, 519, *521*, 522t
      temporomandibular joint dysfunction, 524
    extubation, 551–556, *552*
      bucking phenomenon, 552–555
      complications, 552
      procedure, 555
      in special conditions, 555–556
      suction catheters, 555
    fiberoptic intubation, 544–548, *544–545*
    indications and advantages, 550–551, 551t
    intubation techniques, 526–551
      bougie guide for transoral intubaiton, 543–544
      cervical fractures, 541
      complications, 542
      in conscious state, 539–540
      cricothyroid/cricotracheal membranes, 542
      direct-vision orotracheal intubation, 526–529
        anesthesia, 526–527
        head position, 527–529, *527–529*
        relaxants, 527
      equipment, 526

I-14 *Index*

Endotracheal anesthesia
   intubation techniques (*Continued*)
      esophageal, 534–536
      laryngoscopy, 529–536
         intubation. See Laryngoscopy.
         operator position, 529–530
         patient position, 530
         procedure, 530
      nasotracheal, 536–538, *536–538*
      in neonate, 540–541
      preintubation preparation, 526
      retrograde intubation, 542–543
      standard methods, 526
      subglottic puncture, 542
      tactile tracheal, 538–539
   protection of airway, Sellick maneuver, 548–550, 549t
Endotrol tracheal tube, 476, *476*
Enflurane
   biotransformation, 349
   and cerebral metabolism of oxygen, 365
   density, 107
   drug interactions, 268, 272
   and evoked potentials, 94
   incompatibility in closed circle systems, 396
   induction in children, 429, 430
   and intraocular pressure, 279
   MAC levels for anesthesia, 363
   metabolism in obese patients, 352
   nephrotoxicity, 350
   in obese patients, 339–340
   platelet aggregation, 263
   postural effects, 167
Enkephalins, in pain control, 1333–1335
Environmental hazards. See Anesthesia, hazards.
Enzymes
   and drug interactions, 255–256
   in drug transformations, 348–349
Ephedrine, and spinal anesthetics, 1481
EPI (end-inspiratory hold plateau), 623
Epidemiology of AIDS, 1170–1171
Epidural anesthesia, 1571–1610
   anatomy, 1572–1575, *1572–1573*
      epidural space, 1573–1574, *1574*
      in children, 1575
      peridural space, 1573, 1573t
   blood patch, 1563
   clinical aspects, 1594
      advantages, 1594
      carbonated local anesthetics, 1286–1287
      indications and contraindications, 1594
      needle position, 1594
   complications, 1594–1602
      abscess, 1600
      backache, 1599
      bladder dysfunction, 1600
      blood coagulation, 1601–1602
      catheters, 1596–1597, 1596t
      computed tomography, 1597–1598
      convulsions and muscular twitching, 1599
      drowsiness and depression, 1599
      dural puncture, 1560, 1594
      emphysema, 1599–1600
      epidural cannulation, 1596
      failures, 1599
      gastric emptying, 1601
      hematoma, 1600
      hypertension, 1598
      hypotension, 1598
      intestinal blood flow, 1601
      intracranial pressure, 1600
      lithotripsy, 1602
      neurologic sequelae, 1599
      pain, 1602
      paralytic ileus, 1601
      potassium, 1601
      rapid injection, 1599
      reactions to local anesthetics, 1599
      respiration, 1602
      shivering, 1600–1601
      subarachnoid block, 1594–1595
      subdural injection, 1595, *1595*
   definition, 1200, 1571–1572
   detection of epidural space, 1582–1585
      confirmation of position, 1585
      fluid choice, 1584
      negative pressure techniques, 1583
      resistance techniques, 1583–1584
      syringe preparation, 1584–1585
   dosage, 1579–1582
      clinical conditions, 1581
      extradural pressure, 1582
      interspace selection, 1579
      position of patient, 1581–1582
      specific gravity of anesthetic, 1582
      speed of injection, 1580–1581
      spread of solutions, 1579–1580
      volume of anesthetic solution, 1579
   etidocaine, 1263
   history, 10–11, 1571
   neurolytic procedure, 1536–1537
   obstetric, 1602–1605
      application, 1602–1603
      epinephrine additive, 1603–1604
      lidocaine, 1604
      mepivacaine, 1604
      morphine, 1604–1605
      narcotics, 1604
      pain in labor, 1602
      postural changes, 1605
   physiology, 1575–1579
      absorption, 1577
      fate of epidural agents, 1576
      pharmacokinetics, 1576
      site of action, 1575, *1576*
      volume capacity, 1578–1579, 1578t
   technical procedure, 1585–1594
      anesthetic solutions, 1588, 1590t
      approach, 1586
      aspiration test, 1588
      catheters, 1592–1593
      cervical injection, 1585
      in children, 1593–1594
      continuous technique, 1592
      injection, 1588–1589
      needle insertion, 1586–1588
         modified pressure, 1586–1587, *1587*
         negative pressure (balloon technique), 1587–1588, *1589*
      needles and catheters, 1586
      paramedian approach, 1591–1592
      position, 1585, *1585*
      preparation, 1586
      site of injection, 1585–1586, 1585t
      test dose, 1589–1591
   vs. spinal anesthesia, 1513
   See also Opioids.
Epidural space. See Epidural anesthesia.
Epiglottis
   anatomy, 462–464
   during endotracheal anesthesia, 580
   intubation difficulties, 523–524
Epilepsy, thiopental anesthesia, 684
Epinephrine
   drug interactions, 276
   and local anesthetics, in obstetrics, 1603–1604
   and muscle relaxants, 880
   potentiation of action, 1282–1285
      absorption, 1285
      contraindications, 1285
      peridural block, 1282–1283
      reactions to, 1284–1285
      uses, 1283–1285
   and spinal anesthesia, 1481, 1512–1513
   toxicity, 1292
Epistaxis, in intubation, 589
Equations
   anesthetic delivered to breathing circuit, 147, 148
   anesthetic inflow, 327
   barometric pressure effects on flowmeter, 448
   caloric heat of vaporization, 141
   carbon dioxide reactions, 453
   cardiac output, 85
   clearance of anesthetic, 328
   diffusion velocity, 330
   dissociation constant, 255
   Henderson-Hasselbalch, 255
   lean body mass, 743
   low-flow liquid injection technique, 398
   oxygen saturation, 88
   resistance to air flow through absorbent, 453
   venous return, 79
   See also Physics of anesthesiology.
Equipment
   direct arterial monitoring, 78
   electrical, 1152–1153, 1157
   for endotracheal anesthesia, 526
   failure, and intraoperative deaths, 35, 43, 44t
   fiberoptic, 545–546
   noise, 1166
   for regional anesthesia, 1201, 1221–1224
Esmarch bandage, 795, 798
Esmolol
   in controlled hypotension, 1086–1087
   during endotracheal anesthesia, 577
Esophagus
   endotracheal tube misplacement, 534–536, 534t
   lower, contractility, 366, 382
   pancuronium effects, 969
   reflexes, 1189
Ester compounds
   metabolism, 1220–1221
   of local anesthetics, 1239
Estrogen
   cholinesterase inhibition, 840
   drug interactions, 275
Ethacrynic acid, protein binding, 254
Ethanol
   contamination in closed circle system, 427
   intravenous anesthesia, 774–777
      administration, 777
      dosage, 776–777

metabolism, 776
pharmacologic effects, 774–776
premedication, 776
preparations, 776
sequelae, 777
uses, 777
Ether
and body metabolism, 323
charts, 11, 29–30
density, 107
diethyl, MAC levels for anesthesia, 363
discovery and controversy, 6–7
early administration devices, 5, 119
and EEG patterns, 371
and intraocular pressure, 279
intravenous (Burkhardt technique), 773–774
solubility coefficient, 332
Ethics of placebo use, 305–306
Ethosuximide, and neuromuscular blockade, 883
Ethyl chloride, solubility coefficient, 332
Ethyl violet, indicator of carbon dioxide absorption, 454
Ethylene
development, 18
solubility coefficient, 332
Etidocaine
metabolism, 1221
pain at injection site, 1311
pharmacology, 1262–1263
See also Regional anesthesia.
Etomidate
in ambulatory surgery, 1646–1647
and evoked potentials, 94
intravenous, 766–768, 766
Eucupin, 1240, 1267
Eugenol derivatives, 772–773
Evaporation
definition, 109
in hypothermia, 1109
Exercise
and muscle relaxants, 880
ventriculography, 228–229
Explosions. See Fires.
Exsanguination, in intravenous regional anesthesia, 795
Extensor-assistant supinator nerve, 199, 203
Extracellular fluid, relaxant distribution, 833
Extracorporeal cooling, 1109–1110
Extravasation, thiopental injection, 682
Extremities
injuries, during patient repositioning, 193, 202–204
intravenous regional anesthesia. See Intravenous anesthesia.
Extubation, 551–556
bucking phenomenon, 552–555
complications, 552, 552t
intraocular pressure, 554
local agents, 554–555
procedure, 555, 547
return to consciousness, 552t
special conditions, 555–556
suction catheters, 555, 556t
timing of, 553
See also Weaning from ventilatory therapy.
Eyelids
nerve block, 1350
reflex, 365–366, 1182

Eyes
eye-roll sign, in hypnosis, 1127
hydroxydione effects, 764
injury during anesthesia, 431–433
drug effects, 431
examination, 431
incidence, 431
lubricants, 432, 432t
protection, 431–432
treatment, 432
types of injury, 431
ketamine effects, 737, 740
muscle systems, succinylcholine effects, 1006–1007
during patient repositioning, 194, 195, 195
relaxant action, 865–866, 867
See also Oculocardiac reflex.

Fabrics
flammable, 1150
static electricity, 1152
Face
blocks, 1350–1351, 1351
mask
application, 430–431
in closed circle systems, 392, 395
dead space, 391–392
facial nerve paralysis, 432–433
in hyperbaric oxygenation, 1138
ocular injury, 431–432
open drop inhalation, 409
and oxygen saturation, 429
neonatal, 503
during patient positioning, 195–196
Facial nerve
muscle stimulation, 859–860
paralysis, during mask anesthesia, 432–433
Familial periodic paralysis, 875, 901
Famitodine, comparison with cimetidine, 236–237
Fasciculation, 811
depolarizing agent complications, 909
succinylcholine effects, 1005, 1009
Fascio-scapulo-humeral dystrophy, 901
Fasting
in children, 241–242
preoperative, 238–240
Fat
embolism, from methylmethacrylate, 257
hydroxydione storage, 763
metabolism, and spinal anesthesia, 1511
storage, in obesity, 216
thiopental concentration, 670–672
Fatigue
of anesthetist, 37, 40, 52–53
muscular, 811
in operating room personnel, 1159
Fatty acids, and thiopental binding, 663
Fazadinium, 989–990, 989
Fear of anesthesia, 207–208, 208t
Femoral nerve block. See Lumbar plexus.
Fentanyl, 712–722
in alcoholic patient, 213
chemistry, 712, 712
clearance, 714
clinical applications, 718–719
complications, 721–722
dosage, 712
during endotracheal anesthesia, 576
epidural, in obstetrics, 1604

and evoked potentials, 94
and intraocular pressure, 279
lipid solubility, 1626
and MAC values, 338
metabolism, 714
pharmacokinetics, 712–713, 713, 713t
age effects, 713–714
pharmacology, 714–718
autonomic nervous system, 716
cardiovascular effects, 715–716
central nervous system, 714–715, 715
and congeners, 717–718
histamine release, 717
metabolic and hormonal effects, 716–717
muscle rigidity, 717
neuromuscular action, 717
respiratory effects, 716
seizures, 718
postural effects, 168
potency, 712
technical procedures, 719–721
classic technique, 719
emergence, 720
Foldes technique, 719–720
induction, 720–721
recovery, 720
Ferguson reflex, 1192
Fertility, in operating room personnel, 1159
Fiberoptic techniques
endobronchial intubation, 608–612
intubation. See Intubation.
Fibers, nerve, spinal anesthesia effects, 1499, 1500t
Fibrillation, muscular, 811
Fibrous dyplasia (polyostotic), 525
Field block definition, 1200
Filters, bacterial, in breathing systems, 413
Fingers
during patient repositioning, 204
spreader - approximator, 199, 203, 200
Fires
in hyperbaric oxygenation, 1137
in operating room, 1149–1151
conditions, 1150–1151
apparatus and agents, 1151
combustible mixtures, 1150
flammable substances, 1150
ignition source, 1150–1151
nonflammable agents, 1151
oxygen supply, 1150
quenching agents and mixtures, 1151
spark-proof equipment, 1151
terminology, 1150
Flexor-pronator-thumb-finger-approximator, 199–200,203
Flow controllers, 132–133, 136
Flowmeters, 133–137, 137
climate and altitude effects, 447–449, 448
common manifold, 136–137
other types, 136
Thorpe tube, 135–136, 137, 138
Fluids
physical properties, 114–117
preanesthetic, 240
and relaxant agents, 872–873
Flumazenil, 755
Fluorides, in drug biotransformation, 349–351

Fluoromar, and EEG patterns, 371
Fluoroxene, solubility coefficient, 332
Flush switch valve, 131–132, *135*
Foot
   nerve block, 1411–1412
   regional anesthesia, 804–805
Forceps, endotracheal, 497, *498*
Forehead nerve block, 1350
Fractures, cervical, and intubation, 541
Frank-Starling curve, 79
Free radicals, in drug metabolism, 351
Fruit extracts, in inhalation anesthesia, 430
Frumin valve, 152
Fungal infections, in anesthesia machines, 158

Gag reflex, 540
   nerve block, 1359
Galanthamine, 1048
Galen, use of anesthesia, 3, 4
Gallamine, 952–956
   chemistry, 952, *953*
   clinical uses, 955–956
   dosage, 953
   and end-plate sensitivity, 817, 824–825
   excretion, 952
   history, 952
   and MAC values, 338–339
   mechanisms of action, 952
   pharmacokinetics, 952–953, *954*
   pharmacology, 953–955
      autonomic nervous system, 953–954
      cardiovascular system, 954, *955*
      central nervous system, 953
      histamine release, 954–955
      respiratory system, 954
   pretreatment for succinylcholine, 1004
   protein binding, 834
   and thiopental, 660
Gamma hydroxybutyric acid, 774
Gamma system, and muscle innervation, 380–381, *381*
Ganglion
   dorsal root, spinal anesthesia effects, 1499
   Gasserian nerve block, 1351–1353
   stellate. *See* Nerve block, paravertebral.
   sympathetic, barbiturate action, 657
Ganglionic blockade
   controlled hypotension, 1064–1070
      methonium compounds, 1065–1066
      pentolinium, 1066–1067
      trimethaphan, 1067–1070
   curare actions, 945–946
Ganglioplegia, 707
Gangrene point, 1440
Gas
   cylinders. *See* Anesthesia machines and components.
   development of anesthesia, 13
   mixtures in endotracheal anesthesia, 487
   partial pressure, climate and altitude effects, 444–445, *445*
   physics of, in high-frequency ventilation, 647
   pulmonary
      distribution, 327
      See also Alveolar ventilation.
   respiratory
      and MAC values, 337

      monitoring of, 86–87
   sterilization of endotracheal tubes, 480
   See also Blood gas; Physics of anesthesiology.
Gas chromatography
   anesthetic and respiratory gas monitoring, 86, 158
   climate and altitude effects, 446
Gasp reflex, 1188
Gastric emptying
   after epidural anesthesia, 1601
   measurement techniques, 238–239
   physiology of, 237–238, *237*
   in pregnancy, 239
   in spinal anesthesia, 1507
Gastritis, acupuncture, 1639
Gastrointestinal tract
   anxiety effects, 286
   and caudal analgesia, 1615
   curare actions, 946
   ethanol effects, 775–776
   preanesthetic evaluation, 236–242
      age factors, 238
      anxiety role, 238
      empty stomach, 236–237
         antacid agents, 237
         cimetidine comparison with ranitidine and famitidine, 236–237
         metoclopramide, 237
      fasting effects, 238–240
      gastric emptying, 237–239, *237*, 238t
      infants and children
         blood glucose, 240–241
         fasting, 241–242
      in pregnancy, 239
   smoking effects, 213
   in spinal anesthesia, 1507
   succinylcholine effects, 1008–1009
   thiopental effects, 667
Gate theory of pain, 1330, 1333, *1330*
   acupuncture, 1636
Gauges on manometers, 129–130
Gay-Lussac's Law, 103, *103*
Gels, electrode, flammability, 1150
General anesthesia
   in ambulatory surgery, 1646–1649
   balanced anesthesia, 381–382
      monitoring of relaxation, 382
      Woodbridge components, 382
   clinical signs, 360–374
      EEG signs, 369–371, 369, 370t, 372t
      history of stages and signs, 360–361
      stage I: induction period, 361
      stage II: unconsciousness, 361–363
      stage III: anesthesia, 363–364
         planes, 364
      stage IV: vital arrest, 364–368
         anesthetic effects, 365
         awareness, 366–368, 369t
         confounding factors, 365
         depth of anesthesia, 364–365
         lower esophageal contractility, 366
         recovery, 366
         reflexes, 365–366
   combinations of techniques and agents, 382–384
      general and regional, 383–384
      general and relaxants, 384
      intravenous-inhalation, 382–383
      large-dose intravenous opiate techniques, 383
      opiate-barbiturate-gas combination, 383

   and controlled hypotension, 1087–1088
   fundamentals, 314–359
      absorption of inhalation agents, 324, 324t
      alveolar-capillary membrane equilibrium, 329–333
         active transport system, 330–331
         alveolar-capillary interface, 330
         blood solubility of anesthetics, 331–332, 331t
         factors modifying solubility, 332–333, 333t
         passive transport system, 330
         physical transport system, 330
         time for, 331
      alveolar concentration of anesthetic, 325–329
         alveolar ventilation effects, 326–327
         curves, 325–326, *326*
         pulmonary capillary flow, 327–328, *327*
         pulmonary gases, 327
         second gas effect, 328–329, 329t
         tissue uptake effects, 328, *328*, *329*
      anesthetic potency, 333–341
         minimum alveolar concentration, 333–338
            adjunctive drug effects, 338–341, 338t
            awake-sleep ratio, 340, *340*
            awake values, 340
            CNS electrical stimulation, 340
            definition, 333–334, *334*
            factors modifying MAC, 335–338, 336t
            MAC-BAR, 335, *335*, 334t
            MAC measure of anesthetic dose, 334
            obesity effect, 339–340
            toxicity, 334–335
      anesthetic state, 322–323
      brain uptake of drugs, 344–346
         drug exit from CNS, 346
         drug penetration into CNS, 346, *346*
         perfusion, 344–345
         regional cerebral blood flow, 345–346
         tissue uptake, 345
      components of, 314–315
         mental block, 315
         motor block, 315
         reflex block, 315
         sensory block, 315
      definition, 314
      elimination of inhaled anesthetics, 347–354
         metabolites, 349–352, 350–351t
         other routes of loss, 353–354, *353*
         oxidative metabolism, 348–349
         pulmonary exhalation, 347–348
         pulmonary recovery of unchanged anesthetic, 352–353
      neural basis, 315, *316*
      partial pressure of inspired agent, 324–325, *325–326*
      sleep, 317–323
         as active phenomenon, 320
         biochemistry, 321–322, *321*, *322*
         classic concept, 318
         and CNS depressants, 322

cyclic aspect of NREM-REM, 320, *320*
  metabolism, 322
  neuroanatomic mechanisms, 320–321
  neurotransmitters, 321
  pacemaker, 320
  physiologic changes, 322
  quantitative aspects, 321
  types, 318–320, 319t
  spinal cord control of sensory input, 315–316, 317t
  tissue concentration of agent, 341–344
    concentration gradient, 342
    drug diffusion, 343–344
    equilibrium between tissue and venous blood, 343, *344*
    membrane boundaries, 343
    regional blood flow, 342, *343*, 342t
    tissue-blood partition coefficient, 342–343, 343t,
    tissue uptake of drugs, 341–342
    transfer systems into cells, 343
    transportation of agents, 341
      blood supply to tissues, 341
      circulatory capacity, 341
  waking state, 316–317, *318*
  and hypothermia, 1107
  physostigmine reversal of, 1033–1034
  respiration, 375–379
    anesthesia effects, 376
    breathing patterns, 376–377, *377*
      apneustic pattern, 377
      expiratory pattern, 377, *378*
    muscle fiber types, 375–376
    muscles, 375, 376t
    muscular relaxation and reflexes, 379–381, 379t
      cortex, 379
      gamma system, 380–381, *381*
      H reflex, 381
      intersegmental neurons, 380
      red nucleus, 380
      spinal center, 380
      tectal nuclei, 379
      vestibular nucleus, 380
    sigh, 378–379
    tracheal tug, 377–378
Genetic studies, cholinesterases, 837–838
Genitalia
  male, during patient repositioning, 194
  monitoring of, 95
  perineal reflexogenic areas, 1191
Georgia valve, 156
Germine diacetate, 1048
Glasgow Coma Scale, mortality risk, 49
Glaucoma, 276–280
  anesthetic effects, 279
  aqueous humor formation, 277
  classification, 277, 277t
  complications of therapy, 278–279
  drug interactions, 278
  pain medication, 432
  physostigmine anesthesia, 1032
  relaxant drugs, 279–280
  therapy, 278
  treatment, drug interactions, 276–280, 277t
Glomerular filtration rate, 95
Glossopharyngeal nerve block, 1358–1359, *1360*
Glucagon, and surgical stress, 1509

Glucocorticoids, noise effects, 1166–1167
Glucose
  and local anesthetics, 1237
  in nerve conduction, 1218
  and potassium potentiation, 1288
  preoperative, in infants and children, 240–241
  and surgical stress, 1509
  and thiopental potentiation, 660
Glucuronic acid conjugation of inhaled anesthetics, 348
Glutaraldehyde, endotracheal tube cleaning, 479
Glutethimide, and REM sleep, 322
Glycopyrrolate
  in children, 1046
  cholinesterase inhibition, 1032
  and neostigmine, 1035
Gout therapy, drug interactions, 268
Graham's Law, 107, *108*
Granules, in carbon dioxide absorption, 453
Granulomas of larynx, 583
Gravitation constant, 108
Gravity
  administration of anesthesia, 411
  and vascular pressures, 164
Greeks, use of anesthesia, 3, 4
Grip strength test, 851
Growth hormone
  during sleep, 322
  thiopental effects, 668
Guanethidine, drug interactions, 267
Guidelines for preanesthetic medication, 290–292, 291t
  clonidine, 292
  evening before surgery, 291
  morning of surgery, 291
  narcotic morphine sulfate, 291
  outpatient anesthesia and surgery, 291–292, 292t
  sedatives and tranquilizers, 291
Guillain-Barré syndrome, and muscle relaxants, 900
Gums, complications during endotracheal anesthesia, 579

H reflex
  fentanyl effects, 717
  and muscle relaxation, 381
Habituation, 307
Hair, and flammable substances, 1150
Hallucination
  perioperative, 366
  preoperative anxiety, 209
Haloperidol, and phenoperidine, 708
Halothane
  in alcoholic patient, 213
  biotransformation, 349
  and body metabolism, 323
  caloric heat of vaporization, 141
  and cerebral metabolism of oxygen, 365
  coefficient of solubility, 105
  density, 107
  drug interactions, 268, 272
  and EEG patterns, 371
  epinephrine interaction, 276
  and evoked potentials, 94
  incompatibility in closed circle systems, 396
  induction in children, 429, 430
  and intraocular pressure, 279

  MAC levels for anesthesia, 363
  metabolism in obese patients, 352
  nephrotoxicity, 350
  platelet aggregation, 263
  and platelet function, 258
  postural effects, 167
  solubility coefficient, 332
Hand nerve block, 1393
Hangover, from ethanol, 777
Head
  elevation positions, 181–183, *182–184*
  holders, 176–177
  injuries
    and hyperkalemia, 915
    positioning of patient, 190, 194–200
  position
    in endotracheal anesthesia, 487
    in inhalation anesthesia, 433–436, *434, 435*
    for laryngoscopy, 527–529, *527–529*
    in nasotracheal intubation, 536
  postural effects, 170
  trauma, thiopental anesthesia, 684
Head-lift test, 851
Head-raising, curare recovery, 949
Headaches
  acupuncture, 1639
  in caudal analgesia, 1621
  after spinal anesthesia, 1555–1564
    age factors, 1557, 1557t
    agent type, 1557
    altitude role, 1560
    bedrest, 1560
    caffeine-sodium benzoate effect, 1562
    continuous anesthesia, 1560
    description, 1556
    differential diagnosis, 1555–1556
    dural puncture, 1560
    epidural blood patch, 1562–1564
    healing of dural holes, 1559–1560
    incidence, 1556
    mechanism, 1560–1561
    and menstruation, 1557
    needles, 1557–1559, 1557t
    onset and duration, 1556
    prevention, 1561
    psychic factor, 1557
    sex differences, 1556–1557
    treatment, 1561–1564
Healing, in regional hypothermia, 1117
Hearing
  during anesthesia, 367
  noise effects, 1168
  after spinal anesthesia, 1565
Heart
  alcoholism effects, 212
  curare actions, 944–945
  lidocaine actions, 1258
  smoking effects, 213
  transfusion and anesthesia, 299
Heart rate
  nitroprusside effects, 1077
  in spinal anesthesia, 1506
Heat
  of adsorption, 144–145
  loss, in anesthetic systems, 412–413
  See also Temperature.
  See also Anesthesia machines and components; Physics of anesthesiology.
Helium
  narcosis, in hyperbaric oxygenation, 1146
  as quenching agent, 1151

Hematology, in hypothermia, 1105–1106
Hematoma
　epidural, 1600
　from regional anesthesia, 263
Hemodynamics
　during endotracheal anesthesia, 573–578
　　beta-adrenoceptors, 576–577
　　clonidine, 577–578
　　fentanyl, 576
　　lidocaine
　　　intravenous, 575–576, 576t
　　　topical, 576
　　　translaryngeal, 576
　　nitroglycerin, topical, 577
　　topical anesthesia, 576
　ketamine effects, 737
　of midazolam, 758
　of pipecuronium, 981, 982t
　positive airway pressure effects, 624–626
　postural changes, 167–168
　in tourniquet deflation, 1550
Hemoglobin, and carbon monoxide, 1139–1141
Hemogram, preoperative, 219–221
　blood indices, 221
　in elderly, 221
　hematocrit, 220–221
　racial differences, 220
Hemorrhage
　from arterial cannulation, 79
　thiopental effects, 680
Hemostasis, and controlled hypotension, 1057, 1057t
Henbane (Hyoscyamus), 4
Henderson-Hasselbalch equation, 255, 1314
Henry's Law, 88, 104, 331, 457
Heparin, drug interactions, 262–265
Hepatitis virus
　and AIDS, 11713
　in anesthesia personnel, 1169–1170
Herb use by Greeks, 3
Hernia block, 1420–1421, *1421*
Herpes simplex virus, in anesthesia personnel, 1168–1169
Heta-starch, and platelet function, 258
Hexafluorenium, 840, 1017–1018
　chemistry, 1017, *1017*
　clinical uses, 1018
　mechanism of action, 1017
　pharmacology, 1017–1018
　and succinylcholine, 1014–1015
Hexamethonium, controlled hypotension, 1062, 1066
Hexobarbital (oxybarbiturate), 693–694
Hexobarbitone, 655
Hexylcaine hydrochloride (cyclaine), 1250–1252, 1251t
　toxicity, 1296
HFV (high-frequency positive-pressure ventilation)
　advantages, 649–650
　classification of ventilators, 647–648, *648*
　　HFJV, 648
　　HFO, 648–649
　　HFPPV, 648
　and conventional ventilation, 649
　definition, 646–647
　history, 647
　jet ventilation, 649
　objectives, 647

physics of gas exchange, 647
uses and problems, 649
Hibernation, 1096, 1110
Hiccoughing, thiopental substitutes, 697–698
Hilar reflex, 1189
Hip surgery, methylmethacrylate complications, 256–257
Hippocampus
　excitation by local anesthetics, 1303
　sleep control, 321
Hippocrates, use of anesthesia, 3
Hirschsprung's disease, 1488
Histamine
　and atracurium, 987
　and curare actions, 946–947
　fentanyl effects, 717
　gallamine effects, 954–955
　and muscle relaxants, 906–908, 907t
　and pancuronium, 969
　and succinylcholine, 1009
　and thiopental anesthesia, 683
　and vecuronium, 977
History of anesthesiology, 3–28
　acupuncture, 1634
　in antiquity, 3–4
　　alcohol, 4
　　cerebral concussion, 4
　　henbane, 4
　　herbs, 3
　　mandrake, 4
　　nerve root compression, 4
　　opium, 4
　　poppy, 3–4
　　strangulation, 4
　apparatus development, 12–13
　　closed inhalers (1876–1906), 12
　　cloth (1846–1850), 12
　　cone inhalers (1850–1876), 12
　　endotracheal anesthesia (1871–1945), 13
　　gas anesthesia (1894–1945), 13
　　open methods (1895–1945), 12
　　semi-open methods (1905–1941), 12
　　vapor methods (1867–1941), 12–13
　artificial breathing methods, 618
　caudal anesthesia, 1611–1612
　clinical signs, 360–361
　early development (1846–1920), 8–11
　　Bert, Paul, and narcosis, 10
　　Bier, August, and spinal anesthesia, 11
　　Cathelin, M., and caudal analgesia, 11
　　Corning, Leonard, and epidural anesthesia, 10–11
　　Halsted, William Stewart, and local anesthesia, 10, *10*
　　nitrous oxide, 9
　　in obstetrics, 9
　　Queen Victoria, 8–9
　　Snow, John, 8–9, *9*
　electroanesthesia, 1119–1120
　electroencephalography, 90
　endobronchial anesthesia, 597–599
　endotracheal anesthesia, 460–461
　epidural anesthesia, 1571, 1622
　ether controversy, 6–7
　　Bigelow, Henry J., 7
　　Holmes, Oliver Wendell, 7
　　Jackson, Charles T., 6–7
　　Long, Crawford W., 6, 7
　　Mitchell, Weir, 6
　　Morton, William T.G., 6–7, *7*

　　Venable, James, 6
　　Wells, Horace, 6
　hypnosis, 1125
　hypotension, controlled, 1056–1057
　hypothermia, 1116
　intravenous barbiturates, 653, 657
　machines and components, 119–121
　military use, 8
　modern anesthesia (1920–1940), 13–20
　　agents and techniques, 18
　　anesthesia as specialty, 20
　　books, 18
　　Bourne, Wesley, 15
　　Buchanan, Thomas Drysdale, 13
　　Griffiths, Harold R., 17–18, *18*
　　Guedel, Arthur E., 14, *14*
　　Gwathmey, James T., 13
　　Lundy, John, 17, *17*
　　Magill, Ivan, 15–16, *15*
　　military aspects, 20
　　organizations, 18–19
　　Rovenstine, Emery A., 16–17, *16*
　　Waters, Ralph, 14–15, *15*
　oxygenation, hyperbaric, 1134–1135
　precursors, 5–6
　　Beddoes, Sir Thomas, 5
　　Davy, Humphrey, 5
　　Faraday, Michael, 5
　　Hickman, Henry Hill, 5
　　mesmerism, 5–6
　present era, 20–26
　　Adriani, John, 25, *25*
　　Apgar, Virginia, 23–25, *24*
　　Beecher, Henry K., 22–23, *23*
　　department of anesthesiology, 21
　　Dripps, Robert D., 25–26, *26*
　　relaxants, 809–810
　　recognition, 21
　　spinal anesthesia, 1445
　　training, 21–22
　techniques and apparatus, 11–12
　　circle system, 12
　　Connell, Karl, 12
　　Foregger, Richard von, 12
　　Heidbrink, Jay A., 11
　　Jackson, Dennis E., 11–12
　　McKesson, E.I., 11
　　monitoring by records, 11
　　pharyngeal airway, 12
　　syringe and needle, 292–293
Hoffman degradation of atracurium, 985–986
Holocaine, 1240
Horner's syndrome, 197
Human error, in critical incidents, 43, 43t
Human immunodeficiency virus (HIV), in anesthesia personnel, 1170–1174
Humidification units, 205
Humidifiers, 413
Humidity, 111
　in breathing systems, 393, 412–413
　of operating room, 1165
　principles and physics, 416–420, *417*, *419*, 416t
Hyaluronidase, 1289
Hydralazine
　in controlled hypotension, 1084–1085
　drug interactions, 267–269
Hydrogen
　contamination in closed circle system, 427
　as quenching agent, 1151

Hydrostatic indifferent point (HIP), 164, 166
Hydroxydione, 763–765
  administration, 764
  chemistry, 763
  complications and disadvantages, 765
  fat and excretion, 763
  indications, 765
  and intraocular pressure, 279
  mechanism of action, 763
  pharmacologic properties, 764–765
  premedication, 763
  preparations and dosage, 763–764
Hyoid bone, 462–464
Hyperalgesia, barbiturate effects, 674
Hyperbaric injections. *See* Oxygenation; Spinal anesthesia, techniques.
Hypercapnia, laryngeal muscles, 468
Hypercarbia, and EEG patterns, 371
Hyperkalemia, and relaxant agents, 873–874, 913–916
Hyperoxia diffusion, during induction, 431
Hyperpyrexia, 711–712
  hypothermia, 1098
  malignant, pancuronium effects, 969, 971
Hypersensitivity reactions
  to local anesthetics, 1310
  and vecuronium, 977–978
Hypertelorism, and endotracheal anesthesia, 518
Hypertension
  and anesthetic risk, 41
  in epidural anesthesia, 1598
  malignant, preoperative screening, 223–224
  and spinal anesthesia, 1485, 1545
  therapy, drug interactions, 266–268
Hyperthermia
  controlled, 1111–1113
  malignant, cholinesterases, 839
Hyperventilation, and pancuronium, 968
Hypnosis, 1125–1133
  and acupuncture, 1636
  applications, 1131–1132
  awakening, 1131
  definition, 288, 1125–1126
  EEG changes, 1128–1129
  history, 1125
  Hypnotic Induction Profile, 1127
  pain control, 1344
  patient selection, 1126
  pediatric preanesthetic medication, 300
  physiology, 1127
  preparation, 1129
  respiratory effects, 1127–1128
  safeguards, 1129–1130
  signs and symptoms, 1129, 1129t
  and sleep, 1128
  stages of, 1129, 1130t
  suggestibility, 1126–1127
  technique, 1130–1131
Hypobaric injections. *See* Spinal anesthesia, techniques.
Hypodermic injection, 293
Hypoglycemics, oral
  drug interactions, 275
  protein binding, 254
Hypokalemia, and relaxant agents, 874–875
Hypopharynx
  obstruction, in inhalation anesthesia, 434, *435*
  perforation, 585
Hypoproteinemia, preoperative screening, 224
Hypotension
  in caudal analgesia, 1621
  controlled, 1056–1095
    autonomic ganglia, 1064–1065
    bleeding during surgery, 1057, 1057t
    complications, 1088–1090, 1088t
      catecholamines, 1089–1090, 1089t
      precautions, 1089
    contraindications, 1060–1061
    ganglionic blocking agents, 1065–1070
      adverse reactions, 1069–1070
      methonium compounds, 1065–1066, *1065*
      pentolinium (ansolysen), 1066–1067
      trimethaphan, 1067–1070, *1067*
    and general anesthesia, 1087–1088
    history, 1056–1057
    indications, 1060, 1061t
    peripheral-acting agents, 1070–1088
      adenosine, 1085–1086
      calcium entry blockers, 1087
      esmolol, 1086–1087
      hydralazine, 1084–1085
      labetalol, 1086
      nitroglycerin, 1082–1084
      nitroprusside. *See* Nitroprusside.
    principles, 1057–1060
    techniques, 1061–1065, 1062t
      block anesthesia, 1063
      monitoring, 1062–1063
      peripheral resistance, 1062
  droperidol effects, 711
  in epidural anesthesia, 1598
  and MAC values, 337, 339
  motion-induced, 193
  oculocardiac reflex, 1180
  pelvic reflexes, 1190
  postural, 193
  in spinal anesthesia, 1505, 1540–1545, 1552
    clinical factors, 1540–1541
    definition, 1540
    mechanism, 1541
    in obstetrics, 1545
    pressor agent, 1544–1545
    prevention, 1541
    symptoms, 1540
    treatment, 1541–1542
    vasoconstrictors, 1544
    vasopressor therapy, 1542–1544
  in thiopental anesthesia, 667, 676
  See also Posture of patient.
Hypothalamus
  and controlled hypotension, 1062
  and sleep, 320–321
  and surgical stress, 1508
Hypothermia
  and cerebral metabolism of oxygen, 365
  controlled, 1096–1115
    clinical applications, 1097–1098
      cardiac and vascular surgery, 1097
      cardiac arrest, 1097
      eclampsia, 1097–1098
      hypopyrexia, 1098
      neurosurgery, 1097
      preferential hypothermia, 1098
    disadvantages and complications, 1110–1111
    extracorporeal technique, 1109–1110
    history, 1096
    indications, 1097
    methods, 1106–1108, 1107t
    pharmacologic, 1110
    physiology, 1098–1106
      blood factors, 1105–1106
      cardiovascular effects, 1101–1104
      cerebral metabolism, 1101
      consciousness levels, 1101
      EEG changes, 1100–1101, 1100t
      liver effects, 1105
      metabolism, 1098–1099
      nervous system effects, 1099–1101, 1100t
      renal effects, 1104–1105
      respiratory effects, 1101
      thermal gradients, 1098
    surface-cooling techniques, 1108–1109
      complications, 1109
      evaporation and air currents, 1109
      immersion, 1108
      pack technique, 1108
      refrigeration blanket, 1108–1109
    terminology, 1096–1097, 1097t
  and EEG patterns, 371
  in hyperbaric oxygenation, 1135
  and MAC values, 337–338
  and muscle relaxants, 880–883
  and neuromuscular blockade, 858
  during patient repositioning, 204–205
  regional, 1116–1118
    clinical uses, 1116–1117
    history, 1116
    physiology, 1116
    techniques, 1117
Hypoventilation syndrome, in obesity, 218
Hypovolemia
  pancuronium uses, 970
  postural effects, 166
  thiopental effects, 680
Hypoxemia
  from methylmethacrylate, 257
  obstructive mechanical, 570–571, *570–572*
  and oculocardiac reflex, 1180
  pediatric, opiate effects, 303
Hypoxia
  diffusion, during induction, 431
  and EEG patterns, 371
  laryngeal muscles, 468
  from local anesthesia, 1303
  reflex pulmonary vasoconstriction, 614
  ventilatory reflex, droperidol effects, 710
Hysterectomy, and spread of injections, 1470–1471

Ibuprofen, renal effects, 258
Ice bags, for hypothermia, 1108
Ideal gas law, 103
Ileus, paralytic
  after epidural anesthesia, 1601
  and spinal anesthesia, 1488
Illusions, preoperative anxiety, 209
Imipramine, drug interactions, 270
Immersion for hypothermia, 1108
Immune complex, thiopental, 683
Immunology of anesthetists, 1173–1174

Immunosuppression, and spinal
    anesthesia, 1486
Impedance cardiography, 85
Implosions, in hyperbaric oxygenation,
    1137
Indicator dilution technique, cardiac
    output, 85
Indicators, of carbon dioxide absorption,
    454, 457
Induction, 428–431
  definition, 424
  diffusion hyperoxia and hypoxia, 431
  by inhalation, 428
    in children, 429–430, 430t
  intravenous, 428, 428t, 429t
  mask application, 430–431
  monitoring of sleep, 428–429
  rapid sequence, 439–440
Infants and children
  alfentanil kinetics, 724
  Apgar score, 24
  aspiration risk, 50
  atracurium, 988–989, 988t
  axillary nerve block, 1374
  cardiac arrest, 53
  caudal analgesia, 1618–1619
  closed circuit breathing systems, 398–
    399, 418–420, 399t
  complications of anesthesia, 47, 48t
  doxacurium, 994, 995t
  endotracheal anesthesia, 500–510
    airway in newborn, 502–503, 505t
    anatomy of larynx, 500–501, 502
    complications, 589–591, 590–591t
    topographic position of larynx, 501–
      502, 503
    tube dimensions, 472–474, 473t
  epidural anesthesia, 1593–1594
  epidural space, 1575
  gasp reflex, 1188
  hernia nerve block, 1421
  inhalation induction, 429–430, 430t
  intercostal nerve block, 1414–1415
  ketamine anesthesia, 742, 745–746,
    745t
  midazolam anesthesia, 762–763
  mivacurium, 991–992
  neonatal
    anesthesia needs, 235–236
    awake laryngoscopy, 540–541
  neuromuscular blockade reversal,
    1045–1047
  preanesthetic medication, 299–303
    advantages, 302
    anticholinergics, 302–303
    medication programs, 299–301
      basal hypnosis, 300
      dosage, 301
      hypnotics, 300
      narcotics, 300–301
      tranquilizers, 301
    midazolam, 301–302
    no medications, 302
    opiate effects on respiratory
      depression and hypoxemia, 303
    regimens, 303t
  preoperative anesthesia, 240–242, 383
  propofol effects, 771
  relaxants
    dose-response, 862–863, 865, 863t
    pretreatment, 913
  sciatic nerve block, 1406–1407
  solubility coefficients, 332

  spinal anesthesia, 1486, 1512, 1532–
    1535
    advantages, 1534
    aseptic preparation, 1532
    drug choice, 1534
    intraoperative care, 1534
    lumbar dura, 1532
    monitoring, 1534
    needle and syringe, 1532
    position, 1532
    premature infants, 1534–1535
    premedication, 1532
    solutions and drug dosage, 1533–
      1534, 1534t
    spinal tap in infant, 1532
  structural deformities, 218
  succinylcholine, 1010–1013, 1011t
  thiopental, 665–666
    substitutes, 696–697
  upper airway
    anatomy, 433
    infections, 232–233
  vecuronium, 973
Infections
  airway, and extubation, 555–556
  anaerobic, hyperbaric oxygenation,
    1142
  from arterial cannulation, 79
  in caudal analgesia, 1621
  complications during endotracheal
    anesthesia, 579
  and hyperkalemia, 915, 915t
  nosocomial, 158–159
  prolonged intubation, 587–588, 588t
  regional hypothermia, 1116–1117
  and spinal anesthesia, 1486, 1566
  during venipuncture, 296
Infiltration anesthesia, 1200
Inflation, during manual artificial
    ventilation, 630
Infrared analysis
  anesthetic and respiratory gas
    monitoring, 86
  carbon dioxide analyzers, 139–140
Infusion techniques, 296
Inguinal paravascular anesthesia, 1398–
    1402
Inhalation anesthesia
  absorption, 324, 324t
  and atracurium, 983–984
  breathing systems, 387–422
    Ayre T-tube system, 405–408
      analysis of system, 406–407, 407
      application, 405–406
      Baraka double-T-system, 408
      Bisonnette modification, 407–408
      clinical application, 407, 407t
      function, 405, 406
    bacterial contamination, 413
    circle systems, 389–391
      components, 389–390, 389, 390
      flows and concentrations, 390–391
      function of, 391, 391
      mixing devices, 390
    classification, 387–389, 423, 388t
    closed circle systems, 392–396
      advantages, 392
      carbon dioxide content, 394–395
      contaminants, 396
      definition, 392
      dilution of anesthetic gases, 395–
        396, 395t, 396t
      history, 392
      incompatibility problems, 396

      requirements, 392
      resistance, 392–393, 394, 393t
      temperature of inspired gases,
        393–394
      waste metabolites, 396
      water vapor, 393
    closed system, to-and-fro, 391, 396–
      397, 397
    dead space, 391–392
    gravity administration, 411
    insufflation, 411–412
    humidity and heat exchange, 412–
      413
    principles and physics, 416–420,
      417, 419, 416t
  iatrogenic problems, 415–416
  low-flow liquid injection technique,
    397–400
    calculation of unit dose, 398
    for children, 398–399, 399t
    dosing intervals, 398
    physiology, 397–398
    precautions, 399–400
  nonrebreathing valvular systems,
    401–402, 402
  open drop inhalation, 408–411
    advantages and disadvantages,
      410–411
    physiology, 410, 410, 411
    procedure and technique, 409–410,
      409
  open systems (carbon dioxide
    washout), 408, 408t
  scavenging of excess gas, 414–415,
    415
  semiclosed single-limb systems:
    Mapleson configurations, 402–
      405, 403
    coaxial Bain circuit, 404
    Jackson-Rees system, 404, 404
    Lack circuit, 404–405
  semiopen systems, 405
  ventilation monitors, 413–414
    anemometers, 414
    volume displacement meters, 414
  and carbon dioxide absorbents, 457
  and intravenous techniques, 382–383
  and MAC values, 337
  and nitroprusside, 1075, 1076
  and pancuronium interaction, 969
  procedures, 423–443
    cardiovascular effects, 440
    choice of breathing system, 423–424
    classification, 423, 388t
    denitrogenation, 425–427, 425
    facial nerve paralysis, 432–433
    induction, 424, 428–431
      in children, 429–430
      diffusion hyperoxia, 431
      diffusion hypoxia, 431
      inhalation method, 428
      intravenous method, 428, 428t
      mask application, 430–431
      sleep monitoring, 428–429
    ocular injury, 431–433
      drug effects, 431
      examination, 431
      incidence, 431
      protection of eye, 431–432, 432t
      treatment, 432
      types, 431
    patient with full stomach, 438–439
    preoxygenation, 424–425
      and alveolar gases, 427–428

rapid sequence induction, 439–440
  relaxants, 440
  single syringe injection, 440
  upper airway obstruction, 433–438
    artificial airways, 436–438, *438*
    head position, 433–434, *434, 435*
    maintenance of airway, 434–436, *436, 437*
    mechanisms, 433, *433*
  records, 34
  and relaxant potency, 861
  and succinylcholine, 1016
Injection site, of local anesthetics, 1226, 1240–1243
Injury Severity Score, 49
Innervation, pelvic viscera, 1191–1192
Inotropism, and toxicity of local anesthetics, 1308–1309
Insecticides, 1048
  and cholinesterases, 839
Insomnia, and CNS depressants, 322
Inspiratory force, 851
Insufflation, 411–412
Insulin
  drug interactions, 274
  and surgical stress, 1509
Intellectual function, after controlled hypotension, 1089
Intensive care unit, 171
Intercostal nerve block, 1413–1419
  anatomy, 1413
  complications, 1415
    subarachnoid injection, 1415
  continuous extrapleural block, 1415–1417, *1416*
  continuous interpleural block, 1417–1418, *1418*
  technique, 1413–1415
    in children, 1414–1415
    posterior block at angle of ribs, 1413–1414, *1414–1415*
Interlock valves, 131
International Association for the Study of Pain, 1318
Intestine
  and muscle relaxants, 909
  neostigmine complications, 1037
Intocostrin. *See* Curare.
Intolerance to local anesthetics, 1310
Intracranial pressure
  atracurium effects, 986–987
  after epidural anesthesia, 1600
  and vecuronium, 978
  See also Pressure.
Intraocular pressure
  atracurium effects, 986–987
  midazolam effects, 759
  and muscle relaxants, 918–919
  and vecuronium, 978
  See also Pressure.
Intravenous drug administration, 294–296
  barbiturates. *See* Barbiturates; Thiopental.
  infection control, 296
  infusion practices, 296
  and inhalation techniques, 382–383
  narcotic and neuroleptic-narcotic agents, 701–733
    alfentanil, 722–726
    fentanyl, 712–722
    nalbuphine, 722
    narcotic-antagonist combination, 704

narcotic-barbiturate combination, 703–704
neuroleptic malignant syndrome, 711–712
neuroleptic-narcotic anesthesia, 707–712
opiates, 701–703
  alphaprodine, 703
  meperidine, 702–703
  morphine, 701–702, 704–707
  potency, 701
sufentanil, 726–728
nonbarbiturates-non-narcotics, 734–786
  benzodiazepines, 748–763
    diazepam, 748–755
    lorazepam, 755–756
    midazolam, 756–763
  dissociative agents, 734–748
    ketamine, 735–748
    phencyclidines, 734–735
  eugenol derivatives, 772–773
  miscellaneous agents, 773–777
    ethanol, 774–777
    ether, 773–774
    gamma hydroxybutyric acid, 774
  newer agents, 766–772
    etomidate, 766–768
    propofol, 768–772
  steroid anesthesia agents, 763–766
    althesin (CT 1341), 765–766
    hydroxydione, 763–765
  thiopental substitutes, 689–700, 690t, 691t
    comparison of, 698–699, 699t
    hexobarbital (oxybarbiturate), 693–694
    methitural, 691–693, *693*
    methohexital, 694–698, *694–697*, 696t
    spirobarbituric acids, 698
    thialbarbital (kemithal), 698, *698*
    thiamylal, 689–691, *691, 692*
    thiohexital, 698, *698*
venipuncture technique, 295–296, *296*
Introducer, for spinal anesthesia, 1463–1464, *1463*, 1463t
Intubation
  airway protection, Sellick maneuver, 548–550
    laryngeal trauma, 549–550
    laser surgery, 549, 549t
    Salem technique, 549
    shared airway, 549
    transtracheal ventilation, 550
  atracurium, 984
  awake neonate and laryngoscopy, 540–541
  bougie guide, 543–544
  and cervical fractures, 541
  in conscious state, 539–540
    gag reflex, 540
    indications, 539–540
    innervation, 539–540
    topical anesthesia, 540
  cricothyroid/cricotracheal membrane anatomy, 542
  direct-vision orotracheal, 526–529
    anesthesia, 526–527, 527t
    head position, 527–529, *527–529*
    relaxants, 527
  endobronchial. *See* Endobronchial anesthesia.
  endotracheal

cough reflex, 1187
indications and advantages, 550–551, 551t
equipment, 526
fiberoptics, 544–548
  care of instrument, 547–548
  complications, 548, 548t
  equipment, 545
  indications, 545
  manipulation of instrument, 545–546, *546–547*
  nasal approach, 547, *547*
  oral approach, 547
  patient preparation, 545
  principles, 544, *544*
  procedure, 546–547
  structure of scope, 544, *545*
laryngoscopy. *See* Laryngoscopy.
nasotracheal
  bacteremia, 587
  epistaxis, 589
  mucosal laceration, 588–589
  nostril stricture, 589
  pediatric, 591
  prohibiting syndromes, 564
  retropharyngeal dissection, 589
  sinusitis, 589
nasotracheal, 536–538
  blind method, 536–538
    advantages and disadvantages, 537–538
    anesthesia, 536
    correction maneuvers, 537
    head position, 536–537
    incorrect placement, 537, *538*
    preparation, 536
    procedure, 536–537, *536–537*
  direct-vision, 536
preintubation preparation, 526
prolonged, and pulmonary infection, 587
retrograde technique, 542–543
standard methods, 526
subglottic puncture, 542
tactile tracheal method, 538–539
technical difficulties, 542
transtracheal technique, 540
Iodophors, endotracheal tube cleaning, 479
Ionization
  drug metabolism, 254–255, 344, *255*
  of thiopental, 657
IPNPV (intermittent positive-negative pressure ventilation), 623, 626–627
IPPV (intermittent positive-pressure ventilation)
  principles of, 620–621
  weaning from, 643–645, 644t
Ischemia
  cerebral, EEG patterns, 93
  in intravenous regional anesthesia, 795
Isobaric injections. *See* Spinal anesthesia, techniques.
Isocarboxide, drug interactions, 269
Isoflurane
  and cerebral metabolism of oxygen, 365
  in controlled hypotension, 1088
  density, 107
  drug interactions, 268, 272
  and evoked potentials, 94
  incompatibility in closed circle systems, 396

Isoflurane (*Continued*)
  induction in children, 429, 430
  metabolism in obese patients, 352
  in obese patients, 339–340
  platelet aggregation, 263

Jackknife positions
  lateral, 186, *186*
  prone, 188–189, *188*
Jet ventilation, 648–649
Journals, early publications, 18

Katharometer, climate and altitude effects, 446, 449
Kelvin temperature scale, 102
Kemithal, 698, *698*
Ketamine, 735–748
  abuse potential, 748
  administration and dosage, 742–743
  advantages, 748
  cerebral actions, 365, 736
  chemistry, 735
  clinical factors, 741–742, 742t
  contraindications, 748
  disadvantages and complications, 746–747
  drug interactions, 266
  emergence, 747
  induction, 743, *743*
  and intraocular pressure, 279
  laryngeal reflex, 1186
  for local anesthesia, 797
  mechanism of action, 736
  metabolism, 744–745
  and neuromuscular transmission, 888
  pharmacokinetics, 743–744, *744*
    in children, 745–746
  pharmacologic effects, 737–741
    cardiovascular, 738–739
    catecholamines, 741
    central nervous system, 737–738
    endocrine, 741
    eye responses, 740
    metabolic responses, 740–741
    neuromuscular junction, 741
    reflexes, 740
    and relaxants, 741
    respiration, 739–740
    salivation, 740
    skeletal muscle, 740
    uterine tone, 740
  premedication, 742, 743t
    in infants, 1532
  preparations, 735–736, *736*
  prevention and management, 747
  in rapid sequence induction, 439–440
  signs of anesthesia, 737
  special uses, 746
    epidural, for postoperative pain, 746
    obstetric anesthesia, 746
    status asthmaticus, 746
  spinal cord suppression, 736–737
    pain pathways, 1330
  therapy at conclusion of surgery, 747–748
Kidney
  alcoholism effects, 212
  alfentanil effects, 724
  aspirin effects, 258
  disease, in operating room personnel, 1160
  droperidol effects, 710
  elimination of inhaled anesthetics, 347–351
  hydroxydione effects, 764–765
  in hypothermia, 1104–1105
  nitroprusside effects, 1078
  in obesity, 216
  and opioid analgesia, 1631
  positive airway pressure effects, 626
  reflexes, 1190
  surgery, lateral flexed position, 186–187
  thiopental effects, 668
  See also Renal.
Kinetics of matter. *See* Pharmacokinetics; Physics of anesthesiology.
Klippel-Feil syndrome, and endotracheal anesthesia, 518, 525
Knee, popliteal nerve block, 1408–1410
Kneeling prone position, 189
Korotkoff sounds, 71, 72, *72*
Kratschmer reflex, 1185–1186
Krypton narcosis, in hyperbaric oxygenation, 1146
Kyphosis, 1450

Labeling of compressed gas cylinders, 123–124, *124*
Labetalol
  in controlled hypotension, 1086
  drug interactions, 268
Labor reflexes, 1192
Laboratory studies and preanesthetic visit, 218–225, 219–220t
  bleeding time and platelet count, 222–223
  blood transfusions, 222
  blood volume, 224, 224t
  chest roentgenogram, 224–225, 225t
  coagulation tests, 221
  crossmatch and screen protocol, 221–222
  fresh frozen plasma, 221
  hemogram, 219–221
    blood indices, 221
    hematocrit, 220–221
  hypoproteinemia, 224
  malignant hypertension susceptibility, 223–224
Lacerations, during endotracheal anesthesia, 579
Lack circuit, 404–405
Lacri-Lube, 432
Laminae, spinal cord pain pathways, 1328–1330
Landmarks for regional anesthesia, 1224
Laplace's Law, 108
Laryngeal nerve
  block, 1361–1362, *1361*, *1362*
  paralysis, 585–586
Laryngeal reflex of Kratschmer, 568
Laryngitis, during endotracheal anesthesia, 580–581
Laryngoscopy
  in awake neonate, 540–541
  in children, 508–509
  components, 481–484, 516–517, *481*
    blade tip, 482, *483*
    flange, 482
    handle, 482–483
    lighting, 483–484
    spatula, 481–482
  head position, 527–529, *527–529*
  history, 480
  intubation, 530–532, *533*
    difficulties, 521–522
  mechanical complications, 533–534
  See also Intubation.
  operator position, 529–530
  patient position, 530
  procedure, 530, *531*
    blade insertion, 530
    epiglottis
      elevation, 530, *532*
      visualization, 530
  See also Endobronchial anesthesia.
Laryngospasm, 567–569, 1186
  causes, 568–569
  classification, 567–568
  definition, 567
  diagnosis, 569
  etomidate anesthesia, 768
  incidence, 567
  management, 569
    complete obstruction, 569
    incomplete, 569
  mechanism, 568
  prevention, 569
  thiopental effects, 681–682
Larynx
  anatomy, 461–468, 542
    compartments, 464, *464*
    framework, 462, *463*
    hyoid bone, 462–464
    in infants and children, 500–501, *502*
    membranes and ligaments, 464, *463*
    muscles
      extrinsic upper airway, 467
      intrinsic, 464–465, *465–467*
      skeletal, 467–468
    topographic location, 461–462, *462*
  closure, 468, *469*
  cysts, 524
  diazepam effects, 752
  edema, 581–582, *582*
  functions, 465–467
  granulomas, 583
  innervation, 539–540
  ketamine effects, 740
  movement, 467
  perichondritis, 583–584
  reflexes, 1185–1186
  trauma evaluation, 549–550
  ulcerations, 582, 583t
Lasers
  anesthetic problems, 549t
  definition, 549
  and endotracheal tubes, 477–478, *477*
  thermal effects, 549
Latency
  definition, 1227
  and toxicity of local anesthetics, 1298
Lateral medullary infarction syndrome, 197
Lateral positions, technical aspects, 183–187
  classic decubitus position, 184–185, *184*, *185*
  flexed positions, 185–187, *186*
  head elevation, 183
  semilateral positions, 185
  Sims' position, 185, *185*
  spinal anesthesia, 185
  terminology, 183–184
  See also Posture of patient.
Laughing gas. *See* Nitrous oxide.
Laundry, HIV prevention, 1174
Lead configuration, for electrocardiography, 70–71, *70*

Leakage
  from anesthesia system, 1163, *1163*
  electrical currents, 1154–1155, *1154–1155*, 1155t
  in intravenous regional anesthesia, 797–798
  in ventilators, 639–640, *641*
Legs, during patient repositioning, 204
Lehman-Jones block, 804
Lemmon technique for spinal anesthesia, 1527
Leukemia, and oxygen requirements, 223
Levallorphan, and alphaprodine, 704
Levodopa
  drug interactions, 276
  and MAC values, 337
Lidocaine
  allergic reactions, 1311
  bacteriostatic action, 1313
  bucking suppression, 553–554
  carbonated, 1286–1287
    in brachial plexus block, 1379
  and dextrose, 1479
    in hyperbaric spinal anesthesia, 1522
  drug interactions, 266
  during endotracheal anesthesia, 575–576, 576t
  and epinephrine, in obstetrics, 1603–1604
  intravenous anesthesia, 790–794
    advantages and disadvantages, 791, 792
    for arrhythmias, 792–794
    induction and dosage, 790
    maintenance, 790–791
    mechanism, 790
    neuromuscular junction, 791
    pharmacokinetics, 792
    pharmacologic effects, 791
    technique, 790
  and MAC values, 338
  metabolism, 1221
  pharmacology, 1257–1258
  potassium effects, 1288, 1479
  pulmonary disposition, 1266
  spinal anesthesia in infants and children, 1534
  in subarachnoid space, 1472–1473
  toxicity, 1292, 1296
  See also Regional anesthesia.
Ligaments
  of larynx. *See* Larynx.
  stylohyoid, intubation difficulties, 524–525
  vertebral
    denticulate, 1449–1450
    interspinous, 1447
    ligamentum flavum, 1447–1448
    supraspinous, 1447
Light, fiberoptic. *See* Intubation.
Lindholm endotracheal tube, 476, *476*
Lingual nerve block, 1358
  injury in intubation, 585
Lipid solubility, 330, 346
  of opioids, 1626
Lips
  neonatal, 503
  nerve block, 1351
Liquids. *See* Physics of anesthesiology.
Lithium
  carbon dioxide absorption, 154
  drug interactions, 272
  and neuromuscular junction, 885
Lithotomy position

discogenic pain, 202
and respiratory function, 169
technical aspects, 179–180, *179, 180*
Lithotripsy, epidural anesthesia, 1602
Litigation, malpractice, 62
Liver
  alcoholism effects, 212
  droperidol effects, 710
  in hypothermia, 1105
  ketamine degradation, 744
  in obesity, 217
  propanidid effects, 772
  thiopental detoxification, 668, 671
Liver disease
  and atracurium, 984–985
  cholinesterases, 839
  curare protein binding, 941, 943
  and diazepam anesthesia, 750–751, 754
  in operating room personnel, 1160
  pancuronium effects, 963
  relaxant contraindications, 894–895, *894*
  and spinal anesthesia, 1485
  and toxicity of local anesthetics, 1299–1300
  and vecuronium kinetics, 975
Local anesthesia
  agents, 1232–1281
    amide derivatives
      bupivacaine, 1259–1262
      dibucaine, 1256–1257
      etidocaine, 1262–1263
      lidocaine, 1257–1258
      mepivacaine, 1258–1259
      propitocaine, 1263–1264
      ropivacaine, 1264–1266
    ammonium agents, 1267–1268
    benzocaine and butesin, 1256
    butacaine sulfate, 1255–1256
    characteristics, 1232
    chemistry, 1238–1240, 1239t
      alcohol group, 1239
      amide derivatives, 1239
      ester compounds, 1239
      mixtures, 1240
      non-esters, 1240
    chloroprocaine, 1253–1255
    chymopapain, 1270–1271
    clonidine, 1269–1270
    cobra venom, 1271
    cocaine, 1247–1250
    comparative pharmacology, 1240–1246, 1241t
      clinical uses, 1246, 1247t
      pharmacodynamics, 1240–1242, *1242, 1243*, 1243t
      pharmacokinetics, 1243–1246, 1246t, 1247t
    definitions, 1233
    eucupin, 1267
    hexylcaine hydrochloride, 1250–1252
    neurolytic agents, 1268–1269
    procaine, 1252–1253
    promethazine, 1270
    pulmonary disposition, 1266–1267, 1267t
    rating of drugs, 1233–1238
      antihistamine activity, 1237–1238
      antimicrobial effect, 1238
      antithrombotic action, 1238
      buffers, 1236–1237
      chemical nature, 1235–1236

glucose and potassium, 1237
molecular configuration, 1234, *1234–1235*
potency, 1234–1235, *1235*
safety factors, 1233
structure activity relations, 1267
tetracaine hydrochloride, 1255
topical anesthetics, 1271–1275
  benzocaine, 1271–1274
  capsaicin, 1274
  EMLA cream, 1275
and neuromuscular blockade, 882–883
potentiation of action
  carbonation, 1286–1287
  pH effects, 1286
reactions to, 1302–1316
  allergic reactions, 1310–1312
    cytotoxic responses, 1312
    differential diagnosis, 1310
    etiology, 1310
    injection pain, 1311–1312
    lidocaine, 1311
    prevention, 1311
    testing methods, 1311
    treatment, 1311
  cardiovascular toxicity, 1308–1310
    cardiac toxicity, 1308–1309
    clinical types, 1309
    mechanism, 1308
    peripheral vascular effects, 1309
    treatment, 1309–1310
  classification, 1302, 1303t
  clinical causes, 1302–1303, 1304t
  CNS depression, 1307
    mechanism, 1307
    psychomotor impairment, 1307
    respiratory control, 1307
    signs and symptoms, 1307
    treatment, 1307
  CNS stimulation, 1303–1307
    biochemisty, 1304
    clinical severity, 1305
    comparative toxicity, 1304
    factors, 1303–1304, *1305*, 1304t
    incidence, 1303
    mechanism, 1303
    prevention, 1306
    prophylaxis, 1306
    relative toxicity, 1305, 1304t
    signs and symptoms, 1304–1305, 1305t
    site of action, 1303
    treatment, 1306–1307
  mechanism of systemic toxicity, 1302
  preservatives, 1312–1314
    antioxidants, 1312–1313
    bacteriostatics, 1313
    buffering, 1313
    sulfites, 1313–1314
and regional block, 787–808
  lidocaine, 790–794
  procaine, 787–790
  regional anesthesia, 794–806
    anesthetic agents, 796–797, 797t
    blood volume in extremities, 797
    clinical uses, 800
    cyclic deflation-reinflation vs. noncyclic release, 802, *803*
    dosage, 797
    ECG changes, 804
    indications, 794
    kinetics of distribution, 798–799

Local anesthesia
    regional anesthesia (Continued)
        leakage prevention, 797–798
        lower extremity Bier-type block, 804–806
        mechanism, 794
        and nerve conduction, 804
        nerve distribution, 799–800
        neuromuscular junction, 804
        plasma levels after tourniquet release, 801–802, 801, 802
        recovery, 802
        technique, 794–795
            exsanguination, 795
            preinjection ischemia, 795
            site of injection, 795, 795t
            vascular engorgement, 795
        tourniquets, 796, 800–801
        toxicity, 802–804
        two-cuff technique, 796, 796
    toxicology, 1291–1301
        adverse response, 1299
        clinical factors, 1296–1299
            detoxification, 1297–1298
            drug interactions, 1298
            latency period, 1298
            nutrition, 1298
            physical status, 1296
            topical anesthesia, 1298–1299
            type of procedure, 1296–1297, 1297
        critical blood levels, 1292–1293, 1292t
        disposition and blood levels
            acid-base status, 1299
            age, 1299
            hepatic blood flow, 1299
            liver disease, 1299–1300
            pregnancy, 1300
            renal disease, 1300
        principles, 1291–1292
        protein binding, 1293–1294, 1294t
        technical factors, 1295–1296
Lofentanyl, lipid solubility, 1626
Lollipop preparations, 297
London Society of Anesthetists, 18
Long Island Society of Anesthetists, 18
Long thoracic nerve of Bell, 198–199
Lorazepam, 755–756
Lordosis, 1450
Lormetazepam, laryngeal reflex, 1186
Lotus as anesthetic, 3
Low-flow liquid anesthesia, 397–400
    calculation of unit dose, 398, 398t
    in children, 398–399, 399t
    dosing intervals, 398
    physiology, 397–398
    precautions, 399–400
Lowe-Aldrete technique, 397–400
Lower extremities nerve block. See Nerve block, lower extremities.
Lubricants
    for endobronchial intubation, 600
    during endotracheal intubation, 497–498, 499t
    for eyes, 432
Lubrifair solution, 432
Lumbar plexus nerve block, 1395–1398
    anatomy, 1395, 1396
    femoral nerve, 1396–1397
    inguinal paravascular technique, 1398–1402
        anatomy, 1399–1400, 1401
        indications, 1401–1402

technique, 1400–1401
lateral femoral cutaneous nerve, 1395–1396, 1398
obturator nerve, 1397–1398
See also Nerve block, paravertebral.
Lumbar puncture in infants and children, 1532
Lungs
    disease, endobronchial anesthesia, 599
    disposition of local anesthetics, 1266–1267, 1267t
    positive airway pressure effects, 625–628
    postural effects, 168–169

MAC-BAR, 335, 334–335t, 335
Machines for anesthesia. See Anesthesia machines and components.
Macroglossia, 562–563
Magill circuit system, 402
Magill endotracheal tube, 471–472, 472
Magnesium
    and end-plate potentials, 816
    and relaxant agents, 876–877
Magnetic fields, and neural structure, 1122–1123
    CNS semiconduction system, 1123
    galvano-magnetic effect, 1123
Maintenance of anesthesia machines, 138
Mallampati score, 522–523
Malnutrition
    and anesthetic risk, 41
    cholinesterases, 839
Malpractice, 61
Mandible
    abnormalities, intubation difficulties, 560–562
        See also Intubation.
    complications during endotracheal anesthesia, 579–580
    in endotracheal anesthesia, 521
    neonatal, 503
    nerve block, 1357–1358
Mandrake (Mandragora officinarum), 4
Manometers, 129–130
    fail-safe systems (low-pressure cut-off), 130, 133
        diameter index safety system, 130, 134
    for oscillometry, 73
Mapleson configurations, 402–405, 403
    coaxial Bain circuit, 404
    Jackson-Rees system, 404, 404
    Lack circuit, 404–405
Marcus Gunn syndrome, 1180–1181
Markings, endotracheal tubes, 471
Mask
    in breathing circuit, 156–157
    See also Face mask.
Mass action law, in regional anesthesia, 1210–1211
Mass balance, pulmonary clearance, 352–353
Mass spectrometry
    anesthetic and respiratory gas monitoring, 86
    oxygen and carbon dioxide measurement, 140–141
Masses, intra-abdominal, during patient repositioning, 201
Mastectomy, brachial plexus nerve block, 1369
Mastocytosis, 265–266

Mattresses, circulating water, 205
Maxilla
    neonatal, 503
    nerve block, 1355–1357
McGill Pain Questionnaire, 209
Mechanical ventilation. See Breathing systems, artificial.
Median nerve
    block, 1386–1389
        anatomy, 1386–1387, 1390
        at elbow, 1387–1388
        at wrist, 1388, 1391
    palsy, 199–200, 203
    solution distribution, 1375
Medicolegal aspects, 61–62
    breach of duty, 61
    duties of physician, 61
Meditation for pain control, 1344
Megacolon, spinal anesthesia, 1488
Melphalan, pulmonary toxicity, 259
Membranes
    capillary. See Alveolar ventilation.
    channel structure, 1213–1214
    subglottic, 586
Memory, after controlled hypotension, 1089
Meninges, of spinal cord, 1448–1449
Meningismus, after spinal anesthesia, 1566–1567
Meningitis, after spinal anesthesia, 1566
Menstrual cycle
    and pain tolerance, 1322
    postspinal headaches, 1557
Mental block, in general anesthesia, 315
Mental function
    noise effects, 1168
    and spinal anesthesia, 1511
Meperidine, 702–703
    administration, 702
    cholinesterase inhibition, 840
    dosage, 702, 703t
    indications, 703
    lipid solubility, 1626
    and MAC values, 338
    and neuromuscular transmission, 887
    preparation, 702
    properties, 702
    for spinal anesthesia, 1530–1532
    technique, 703
Mepivacaine, 796
    in brachial plexus block, 1380–1381
    epidural, in obstetrics, 1604
    pharmacology, 1258–1259
    toxicity, 1292, 1296
    See also Regional anesthesia.
Meprobamate, drug interactions, 273
Meridians of acupuncture, 1635, 1635t
Mesmerism, 5–6
Metabolism, thiopental effects, 667–668, 681
Metaraminol, drug interactions, 273
Meters, of volume displacement, 414
Methadone, lipid solubility, 1626
Methane contamination in closed circle system, 427
Methitural, 691–693
    administration and technique, 693
    advantages, 693
    chemistry, 691, 693
    complications, 693, 693t
    contraindications, 693
    disposition, 692–693
    dosage, 693
    pharmacology, 692

Methohexital, 694–698
  administration and technique, 695
  chemistry, 694, *694*
  complications, 697–698
  dosage, 695
  endocrine effects, 695
  indications, 698
  and MAC values, 338
  metabolism, 695
  pharmacokinetics
    in adults, 695–696, 696t
    in children, 696–697, *697*
  pharmacology, 694
  preparations, 694
    ionization constant, 694
  recovery of function, 697
Methonium compounds, controlled hypotension, 1065–1066, *1065*
Methotrexate, blood-brain barrier, 259–261
Methoxamine, drug interactions, 273
Methoxyflurane
  biotransformation, 349
  and intraocular pressure, 279
  MAC levels for anesthesia, 363
  metabolism in obese patients, 352
  solubility coefficient, 332
Methyldopa (Aldomet)
  drug interactions, 267
  and MAC values, 339
Methylmethacrylate, drug interactions, 256–257
Metoclopramide
  gastrokinetics, 237
  and succinylcholine, 1016
Metocurine, 949–950
  adverse reactions, 950
  chemistry, 949, *950*
  dosage, 950
  in obesity, 893
  pharmacokinetics, 950
  pharmacology, 950
  preparations, 949–950
  priming action, 867
Metoprolol, during endotracheal anesthesia, 576
MIC-BAR concept, 701
Micrognathia, 560–562
Microphones, piezoelectric, blood pressure measurement, 73
Midazolam, 756–763
  administration and dosage, 759–760, *759*, 760t
  in ambulatory surgery, 1645, 1647
  chemistry, 756, *757*
  clinical uses, 762–763
  drug interactions, 265
  and MAC values, 338
  nasal instillation, 297
  and neuromuscular transmission, 888
  pediatric preanesthetic medication, 301–302
  pharmacokinetics, 760–761, *760*
  pharmacology, 756–759
    cardiovascular effects, 757–758, 757t, 758t
    central nervous system, 756–757
    endocrine effects, 758
    and muscle relaxants, 758
    respiratory system, 759
    skeletal muscle, 758
  pharmcodynamics, 761–762
  premedication in infants, 1532
  in rapid sequence induction, 439–440

and sleep respiratory patterns, 54
Migraine, after spinal anesthesia, 1556
Military use of anesthesia, 8, 20
Mimosa Z, 454
Mind-expanding agents, pain control, 1344
Minimum alveolar concentration (MAC), 333–338
  and adjunctive drugs, 338–341
    anticholinergic agents, 339
    antihypertensive drugs, 339
    cholinesterase inhibitors, 339
    clonidine, 339
    fentanyl, 338
    hypotension, deliberate, 339
    lidocaine, 338
    opioids, 338
    relaxant drugs, 338–339
  and alcoholism, 339
  and alveolar partial pressure, 450
  awake-sleep ratio, 340
  awake values, 340, 340t
  and awareness during anesthesia, 367
  and CNS electrical stimulation, 340
  definition, 333–334
  dosage of anesthetic, 334
  MAC-BAR, 335
  median anesthetic dose, 340–341, 341t
  modification factors, 335–338, 336t
    age, 336
    body temperature, 336
    CNS catecholamines, 336–337
    diurnal variation, 336
    electrolytes, 337
    hypotension and anemia, 337
    hypothermia, 337–338
    mixtures of inhalation agents, 337
    respiratory gases, 337
    sex, 336
    and solubility, 337
    thyroid function, 338
  and obesity, 339–340
  and toxicity, 334–335
Minimum anesthetic concentration, local anesthesia, 1215
Minoxidil, drug interactions, 267–268
Miscarriages, in operating room personnel, 1158
Mithramycin toxicity, 261–262
Mitomycin toxicity, 261–262
Mitotane toxicity, 262
Mivacurium, 990–994
  administration and dosage, 990–991, 991t
  chemistry, 990, *990*
  in children, 991–992, 1045
  pharmacodynamics, 992–994
  pharmacokinetics, 992
  pharmacology, 992
Moduless II Anesthesia System, 31
Moisture, in carbon dioxide absorption, 453
Molecular weight of local anesthetics, 1218
Monitoring of anesthetized patient, 67–99
  ambulatory surgery, 1645
  of anesthesia, 51–52
  cardiovascular system, 69–86
    cardiac output, 85–86
    direct arterial monitoring, 78–79, *80*, 79t
    electrical cardiac activity, 70–71, *70*
    mechanical cardiac activity, 71–86

    arterial blood pressure, 71–74
    sphygmomanometry, 74–77, 76–78
    pulmonary artery pressure, 81–84, *82*, 81–83t
    respiratory system, 86–90
    venous pressure monitoring, 79–81, *80*
  central nervous system, 90–95
    electroencephalography, 90–94, *92*, *93*, 91t
    temperature, 94–95
  future systems, 95–96
  genitourinary system, 95
  hyperbaric oxygenation, 1137–1138
  in hyperthermia, 1112
  in hypothermia, 1107–1108
  principles and standards, 69
  single-twitch, 853–854
  of sleep induction, 428–429
  spinal anesthesia in infants and children, 1534
  train-of-four, 826, 827, 854–857
  ventilation, in breathing systems, 413–414
Monoamine oxidase inhibitors
  drug interactions, 269
  and REM sleep, 322
Monoethyl-glycinexylidide, 792
Mood alteration, pain control, 1344
Morbidity and mortality, 42–55
  morbidity complications, 42–44, *43*
    causes of incidents, 43, 43t
    critical incident factor, 42–43, 43t
    timing of incidents, 44, *46*
  mortality rate, 44–46, 46t
    and ASA grade, 45–46, 46–47t
    composite prediction of outcome, 46
    seven-day perioperative mortality, 44–45
    See also Deaths, operating room.
  practice standards, 55, 55t
  preventability, 55
  risk factors, 46–55
    age, 46–48, 47t
      geriatric, 47–48
      infants and children, 47, 48t
      over 90 years, 48, 49t
    ambulatory anesthesia, 50, 50t
    anesthetist fatigue, 52–53
    aspiration, 50–51, 51t
    associated diseases, 49
    cardiac arrest, 53–55
      benzodiazepine effect on sleep respiratory patterns, 54
      psychogenic, 54–55
      in spinal anesthesia, 53–54
    complexity of surgery, 49
    duration of procedure, 48–49, *49*
    emergency operations, 49, *41*
    mode of anesthesia, 51–52
    natural death factor, 49
    relief anesthetist, 53
    sex, 48
    smoking, 51
    traumas, 49–50, 50t
Morphine
  abstinence syndrome, 308
  and cardiovascular positional changes, 167, *168*
  cholinesterase inhibition, 840
  early uses of, 22
  epidural, in obstetrics, 1604–1605
  large-dose intravenous, 704–707

Morphine
  large-dose intravenous (Continued)
    administration, 704–705
    advantages, 706
    disadvantages, 706
    dosage, 704
    pharmacologic effects, 705
    pharmcokinetics, 704, 705t
    postoperative state, 706
    premedication, 704
    recovery, 705
    reversal of, 705–706
  low-dose intravenous technique, 701–702
  and MAC values, 338
  in pain control, 1333–1334
  parasympathetic blockade, 287
  preanesthetic medication, 291
  premedication
    for spinal anesthesia, 1459
    and thiopental anesthesia, 676
  sensitivity, and anesthetic risk, 41
  spinal anesthesia, 1489
  and spinal cord pain pathways, 1329–1330
Motion sickness, and patient transport, 193
Motoneuron disease
  curare actions, 949
  and muscle relaxants, 896–898, 899–900
  in spinal anesthesia, 1507
Mouth
  abnormalities, intubation difficulties, 562–563
  neonatal, 503
  props, endotracheal, 495–496, 497
Mucus, muscle relaxant effects, 905
Multiple sclerosis
  acupuncture, 1639
  after spinal anesthesia, 1567
  and muscle relaxants, 899
Murphy endotracheal tube, 474, 475
Muscle relaxants
  and awareness during anesthesia, 367
  See also Relaxants.
Muscles
  alcoholism effects, 212
  assessment of function
    grip strength test, 851
    head-lift test, 851, 852t
    inspiratory force, 851
    nerve stimulation-response test, 852–854
    respiratory minute volume test, 851
    train-of-four monitoring, 854–857
  fentanyl effects, 717
  injection technique, 293–294
    complications, 294
    deltoid muscle, 293
    gluteal area, 293, 294
    principles, 293
    vastus lateralis muscle site, 293
  of larynx. See Larynx.
  motor block, in general anesthesia, 315
  pulmonary and respiratory, 231–232
  of respiration, 375, 376t
    fiber types, 375–376
  skeletal
    contraction types, 810–811, 812
    curare actions, 944
    depolarizing agent complications, 909

droperidol effects, 711
fibers, 810
ketamine effects, 740
lidocaine actions, 1258
midazolam effects, 758
motor unit, 810, 811
neuromuscular junction, 812
spindle, 810
succinylcholine actions, 1005, 1009
tone, in spinal anesthesia, 1505
ultrastructure, 814, 814
smooth, succinylcholine effects, 1007–1008
and thiopental anesthesia, 668
thiopental effects, 683
Musculocutaneous nerve block, 1393
  solution distribution, 1375
Music
  and awareness during anesthesia, 368
  and sound (audioanalgesia), 1132–1133
Myalgia, depolarizing agent complications, 910–912, 911t
Myasthenia gravis, 901–902
  edrophonium, 1041
  pyridostigmine anesthesia, 1039
Myasthenic syndrome (carcinomatous neuropathy), 902–903
Myelin anatomy, 1203, 1204
Myelitis, after spinal anesthesia, 1567
Myocardial infarction
  perioperative, 57–58, 60–61
    without previous infarction, 58t
  silent, 58
  See also Reinfarction, perioperative.
Myocarditis, hypothermia, 1097
Myocardium
  in hypothermia, 1111
  pancuronium effects, 966
  thiopental effects, 667, 680
Myoclonus, fentanyl effects, 718
Myofascial syndromes, pain control, 1345
Myoglobin, and muscle relaxants, 917–918
Myopathic muscular diseases, 900–903
Myotonia muscular dystrophy, 901
Myxedema, and thiopental anesthesia, 681

Nalbuphine, 722
  and MAC values, 338
Narcosis
  definition of, 288
  and nitrous oxide, 10
Narcotics
  and awareness during anesthesia, 368
  epidural
    in obstetrics, 1604
  and MAC values, 338
  and oculocardiac reflex, 1180
  pediatric preanesthetic medication, 300–301
  in spinal anesthesia, 54
  See also Intravenous anesthesia.
Narkotest, 140
Nasocardiac reflex, 1184–1185
Nasopharyngeal airway, 437
Nasotracheal intubation. See Intubation.
National Bureau of Standards, compressed gas cylinders, 126–127
National Fire Protection Association, 1137, 1157–1158
Natural death factor, 49

Nausea, in spinal anesthesia, 1546
Neck
  in endotracheal anesthesia, 519
  injuries, during patient repositioning, 193–194, 196–198
  positions, and cerebral perfusion, 170
Necrosis of skin, from arterial cannulation, 79
Needles
  for acupuncture, 1638
  and AIDS, 1171–1172
  in bone marrow infusions, 298–299
  for caudal analgesia, 1619–1620
  in drug administration, 292–293
  for epidural anesthesia, 1586–1588, 1587
  filter, in spinal anesthesia, 1537
  and postspinal headaches, 1557–1558, 1561, 1558, 1559, 1557t
  for regional anesthesia, 1223–1224, 1224
  for spinal anesthesia, 1489–1492, 1546, 1490, 1491
    catheters, 1491
    disposable, 1491
    Greene, 1490
    Huber point, 1491
    Hustead, 1491
    Pitkin, 1490
    quality, 1491–1492
    Quincke-Babcock, 1490
    standard, 1490
    Touhy, 1491
    Whitacre, 1490–1491
  valves, 132–133, 136
  in venipuncture, 295–296
NEEP (negative end-expiratory pressure), 622–623, 652
Neoplasia, opioid analgesia, 1630–1631
Neostigmine, 1034–1037
  in bowel, 1037
  chemistry, 1034
  complications, 1037
  depolarizing action, 1036–1037
  dosage, 1034
  glycopyrrolate role, 1035
  mechanism of action, 1029
  metabolism, 1036
  reversal in pediatrics, 1045
  pharmcokinetics, 1035–1036, 1036
  pharmacologic effects, 1035
  priming principle, 1042, 1043t
  in profound block, 1037
  timing, 1034–1035
Nerve block
  cervical spine, 1363–1384
    brachial plexus, 1366–1375
      anatomy, 1366–1367, 1367, 1368, 1368t
      axillary route, 1369–1374, 1371–1374, 1361t
      interscalene technique, 1379–1381
      perivascular techniques, 1374–1381
        axillary, 1375–1376
        subclavian, 1376–1379
      supraclavicular route, 1367–1369, 1369, 1370
      suprascapular, 1381–1382, 1382
    cervical plexus, 1363–1366
      anatomy, 1363–1364, 1364, 1365
      indications, 1364
      landmarks, 1364
      techniques, 1364–1366

Index **I-27**

phrenic nerve block, 1366
clinic, and records, 32–33
clinical order, 1216
cranial nerves, 1350–1362
  carotid sinus block, 1359–1361
  face blocks, 1350–1351, *1351*
    chin, 1351
    eyelids, 1350
    forehead, 1350
    lips, 1351
    nose, 1350–1351
  Gasserian ganglion block, 1351–1353, *1353*
  laryngeal nerve block, 1361–1362, *1361–1362*
  scalp block, 1350, *1351*
  trigeminal block, 1353–1359
    glossopharyngeal, 1358–1359, *1359*
    mandibular division, 1357–1358, *1356*
    maxillary division, 1355–1357, *1356*
    ophthalmic division, 1353–1354, *1354*
  vagus nerve block, 1361, *1359–1360*
definition, 1200
differential, 1215
etidocaine, 1263
failures, 1227
lower extremities, 1395–1412
  lumbar plexus, 1395–1398
    anatomy, 1395, *1396, 1397*
    femoral nerve, 1396–1397, *1399*
    inguinal paravascular technique, 1398–1402, *1401*
    lateral femoral cutaneous nerve, 1395–1396, *1398*
    obturator nerve, 1397–1398, *1400*
  sacral plexus, 1402–1412
    anatomy, 1402–1403, *1401*
    foot innervation, 1411
    popliteal nerve, 1408–1410, *1408–1409*
    sciatic nerve, 1403–1408, *1402–1405*
    tibial nerve, 1410–1411, *1410*
paravertebral, 1429–1437
  alcohol block, 1436
  anatomy, 1429, *1430*
  continuous sympathetic block technique, 1434–1436
  history, 1429
  indications, 1436, 1436t
  somatic block
    in lumbar area, 1430, *1432*
    in thoracic area, 1429–1430, *1430, 1431*
  sympathetic block of stellate ganglion, 1430–1433
    anatomy, 1430, *1432*
    anterior approach, 1431–1433, *1434*
    anterolateral approach, 1431
    complications, 1433
    indications, 1433
  thoracolumbar block, 1433–1434, *1435*
ropivacaine, 1266
transitional, 1216
of trunk, abdomen, and perineum, 1413–1428
  abdominal field block, 1419–1420, *1420*

hernia block, 1420–1421, *1421*
intercostal block, 1413–1419
  anatomy, 1413
  in children, 1414–1415
  complications, 1415
  continuous extrapleural block, 1415–1417
  continuous interpleural block, 1417–1418
  pharmacodynamics, 1419
  pharmacokinetics, 1418–1419
  technique, 1413–1415
perineal anesthesia, 1423–1424, *1423*
presacral block, 1425
pudendal block, 1425–1426, *1426*
splanchnic block, 1421–1423, *1422, 1423*
transsacral block, 1424–1425, *1425*
uterine sympathetic afferent block, 1427
types, 1214
upper extremities, 1385–1394, *1386*
  elbow block, 1393
  hand blocks, 1393
  median nerve, 1386–1389, *1390–1391*
  radial nerve, 1390–1393, *1392–1393*
  ulnar nerve, 1385–1386, *1387–1389*
  wrist block, 1393
Nerves
anesthetic distribution, 799–800
conduction
  and contact of local anesthetic, 1218
  glucose role, 1218
  osmotic effects, 1217–1218
fibers
  anatomy, 1202–1204, *1203*
  classification and function, 1208, 1207t
  comparative sensitivity, 1216–1217
  impulse characteristics, 1205–1208, *1206, 1207*
injuries
  from arterial cannulation, 79
  during repositioning. See Positioning of patient.
  intubation injuries, 585–586
  of oropharynx and larynx, 539–540
  and pain distribution, 1323–1324
  stimulation-response test, 852–854
    block differentiation, 853, *854*
    selection of nerve, 852
    single-twitch monitoring, 853–854
    stimulus frequency, 853, 853t
    twitch vs. tetanus, 854
Neurolepsis, 707
Neuroleptanalgesia, 707
  advantages, 721
  disadvantages, 721
  See also Fentanyl.
Neuroleptanesthesia, 707
Neuroleptic and narcotic anesthesia, 707–712
  characteristics, 707
  combinations, 708
  definitions, 707
  Laborit method, 707
  preparation, 708
  specific analgesics, 708
Neuroleptic malignant syndrome, 711–712
Neurologic complications
  in epidural anesthesia, 1599

after spinal anesthesia, 1566–1568
Neurolysis techniques, 1535–1537
  agents, 1268–1269
    ethyl alcohol, 1268
    phenol solution, 1268–1269
  alcohol neurolysis, 1535–1536, *1536*
  ammonium salts, 1636
  butyl-aminobenzoate, 1537
  epidural procedure, 1536–1537
  phenol neurolysis, 1535
  positioning, 1535
Neuromuscular junction
  acetylcholine transmission, 816, 820
  alcoholism effects, 212
  anatomy, 811–812, *813*
  blockade
    antibiotic effects, 884–885
    and anticonvulsant drugs, 883–884, 883t
    hypothermia effects, 881–882
    and local anesthesia, 882–883
    neostigmine complications, 1037
    and oculocardiac reflex, 1180
    in pediatrics, 1045–1047
    potentiation mechanism, 871
    procaine, 1252
    reversal of. See Relaxants, antagonists.
    train-of-four monitoring, 854–857
  diazepam effects, 753
  disuse sensitivity, 897
  histology, 812, *813*
  ketamine effect, 741
  lidocaine effects, 791
  monitoring
    single twitches technique, 857–860
    block differentiation, 858–859
    electrode placement, 859
    hypothermia effect, 858
    procedure, 858
  pancuronium effects, 964
  refractory period, 825
  regional anesthetic effects, 804
  relaxant uptake, 833
  See also Relaxants.
Neurons, intersegmental, 380
Neuropathies
  in hyperthermia, 1113
  peripheral, after spinal anesthesia, 1567
Neuroplegia, 707
Neurosis of paralysis, 906
Neurosurgery, hypothermia, 1097
Neurotransmitters
  in pain transmission, 1335–1336
  and sleep, 321
  See also Acetylcholine.
New York Heart Association, classification of heart disease, 227t
Nicardipine, in controlled hypotension, 1087
Nicotine, and drug metabolism, 214
Nifedipine, and neuromuscular junction, 883–884
Nisentil, 703
Nitrogen
  monitoring, 86
  narcosis, in hyperbaric oxygenation, 1146
  See also Denitrogenation; Deoxygenation.

Nitroglycerin
  in controlled hypotension, 1082–1084
    administration and uses, 1084
    advantages and disadvantages, 1084
    dosage, 1083–1084
    mechanism of action, 1082–1083
    metabolism, 1083
    pharmacologic effects, 1083
    pharmcokinetics, 1083
  during endotracheal anesthesia, 577
  and platelet function, 258
Nitroprusside
  in controlled hypotension, 1070–1082
    administration and dosage, 1071–1073, 1072t
    age sensitivity, 1075, *1075*
    aminophylline potentiation, 1077
    biotransformation, 1073
    cerebral circulation, 1078–1079
    chemistry, 1071
    complications, 1081–1082
    cyanide levels, 1080–1081, 1080t
    disadvantages, 1082
    history, 1070–1071
    indications and advantages, 1082
    mechanism of action, 1076
    and other agents, 1075–1076
    overdose, 1081
    pharmacokinetics, 1073–1075
    photodegradation, 1071
    physiologic effects, 1077–1078, 1077t
    preparations, 1071
    technique, 1074–1075
    toxicity, 1079–1080, *1080*
  and MAC values, 339
Nitrous oxide
  absorption rate, 426–427
  alveolar concentration, 328
  and cerebral metabolism of oxygen, 365
  climate and altitude effects, 444–445, *445*
  critical conditions, 111–112, *112–113*
  density, 107
  early administration devices, 5–12, 119–120
  and EEG patterns, 371
  and evoked potentials, 94
  monitoring, 86
  platelet aggregation, 263
  solubility coefficient, 332
  and spinal cord pain pathways, 1330
Nodes of Ranvier anatomy, 1203
Noise hazard, 1165–1168
  auditory effects, 1168
  cardiovascular effects, 1167–1168
  definitions, 1165–1166, 1166t
  endocrine effects, 1166–1167
  recommendations, 1168
  sleep and mental function, 1168
  sources, 1166, 1167t
Nomenclature
  barbiturates, 655–656
  cholinesterases, 836, 836t
  common names
    cyclohexylamines, 735
    ketamine, 748
Nonbarbiturate anesthesia. *See* Intravenous anesthesia.
Nonrelaxant anesthetic drugs
  depth of anesthesia, 888–889
  intravenous induction, 888
  premedication, 886–888
  See also Relaxants.
Nonsteroidal antiinflammatory drugs, and platelet function, 258
Noradrenaline
  during sleep, 321
  thiopental effects, 669
Norton spiral metal tube, 477
Nortriptyline, drug interactions, 270
Nose
  drug instillation, 297–298
  membranes, cocaine effects, 1249
  nerve block, 1350–1351
  during patient positioning, 195
Nothria, 315
Nupercaine, dextrose potentiation, 1478
Nutrition
  and thiopental anesthesia, 668, 681
  and toxicity of local anesthetics, 1298

Obesity
  and blood pressure monitoring, 76–77
  kneeling prone position, 189
  and MAC values, 339–340
  metabolism of volatile anesthetics, 352
  and midazolam anesthesia, 761
  and preanesthetic visit, 215–218
  and relaxant kinetics, 892–893
  solubility coefficients, 332
  and spread of injections, 1470, *1470*
  and thiopental anesthesia, 681
  and transport of anesthetics, 341
  and vecuronium kinetics, 975–976
Obstetric anesthesia
  Apgar score, 24
  demand machines, 137
  diazepam uses, 753
  early uses of anesthesia, 9, 13
  epidural anesthesia, 1602–1605
    epinephrine additive, 1603–1604
    lidocaine, 1604
    mepivacaine, 1604
    morphine, 1604–1605
    narcotics, 1604
    pain mechanism in labor, 1602
    postural changes, 1605, *1605*
    technique, 1602–1603
  hypnosis, 1131–1132
  ketamine anesthesia, 740, 746
  lithotomy position, 179
  maternal mortality rates, 50–51
  postspinal headaches, 1556–1557
  reflexes, 1192
  relaxant choice, 891
  and spinal anesthesia, 1485
  uterine afferent nerve block, 1427
Obturator nerve block, 1397–1398, *1400*
Oculocardiac reflex, 1179–1182
  anatomy, 1179–1180
  atypical (Marcus Gunn syndrome), 1180–1181
  clinical aspects, 1180
    nondepolarizing neuromuscular blockers, 1180
    prevention, 1180
  oculo-emetic, 1181, 1181t
  oculorespiratory, 1181–1182
Oil solutions, 1289
Onium compounds, 1048
Open inhalation systems, 408
  classification, 408t
  drop methods, 408–411
    physiology, 410, *410, 411*
    procedure, 409
    technique, 409–410
Operating room environmental hazards. *See* Anesthesia, hazards.
Operative risk, 38–42
  anesthesia factors, 40, 45
  cardiac complications, 55–60
    and ASA grade, 56
    Cardiac Risk Index, 55–57, 56–57t
      predictive value, 56
    coronary disease, 58
    in elderly, 57
    infarction after bypass surgery, 60
    noncardiac surgery, 56–57, 57t
    perioperative myocardial infarction, 57–58, 58t
    reinfarction, perioperative, 58–60, 59t
  physical status
    classification, 38, 45–46, 39t
    and mortality, 40, 41–43t
  race factors, 41–42
  relaxants, 40–41
  surgical factors, 38–40, 45, 40t
Opiates
  in combination anesthesia, 383
  nasal instillation, 297–298
  and neuromuscular transmission, 886–888
  pediatric respiratory depression and hypoxemia, 303
  vs. regional anesthesia, and surgical stress, 1511
  and stress responses, 706–707
  See also Intravenous anesthesia.
Opioids
  and MAC values, 338
  pain modulation and control, 1333–1337
    ascending transmission system, 1336
    descending supraspinal control, 1336–1337
    electrolytes, 1335
    endogenous opioids, 1334–1335
    natural modulation, 1333
    other neurotransmitters, 1335–1336
      serotonin, 1336
      somatostatin, 1336
      substance P, 1335–1336
    receptors, 1333–1334, 1335t
    terminology, 1333
    therapeutic correlates, 1337
  preanesthetic medication, 285, 286
  and spinal cord circulation, 1484
  subarachnoid and epidural analgesia, 1622–1633
    administration routes, 1627
    adverse reactions, 1631, 1631t
    definition, 1622–1623
    dosage, 1627–1628
    history, 1622
    indications, 1629–1631
    mode of action, 1623–1624, 1623t
    narcotic selection, 1626–1627
    opioid selection, 1627
    pharmacodynamics, 1625–1626
    pharmacokinetics, 1624–1625, 1625t
    technical aspects, 1628
    techniques, 1629
    terminology, 1622
    volume of solution, 1628–1629
Opium as anesthetic, 4
Orbital nerve block, 1354–1357
Organizations, early societies, 18–19
Organophosphates, 1043–1045

Index I-29

antagonists, 1044–1045, 1045t
  clinical uses, 1043
  drug interactions, 276, 278
  mechanism of action, 1029
  resistance factors, 1043–1044, 1044t
  reversibility, 1043
Oropharynx
  airway, 437, *438*
  innervation, 539–540
Orotracheal intubation. *See* Intubation.
Orthopedic injuries, positioning of patient, 190
Oscillometry, 73–74, 1439–1440, *74*
  automated, 74
Oscillotonometry, 1440, *1441*
Ostwald solubility coefficient, 105, 331, 342
Otitis media, 233
Ovaries, reflexes, 1190
Overdose, thiopental, 683
Oxalic acid, 349
Oxidation, elimination of inhaled anesthetics, 347–349
Oximetry, 89–90
Oxybarbiturate, 693–694
Oxygen
  analyzers, 139
    climate and altitude effects, 445, 446t
  consumption
    cardiac output, 85
    in hypothermia, 1099
    in low-flow liquid injection technique, 397
    muscle relaxant effects, 904–905
    positive airway pressure effects, 625
    during sleep, 322
    in spinal anesthesia, 1506
    thiopental effects, 667–668
  flammability, 1150
  flushing errors, 157
  high air flow enrichment devices, 449
  in leukemia, 223
  monitoring techniques, 86–87
  supplemental, weaning from, 646
  transcutaneous monitoring, 89–90, 90t
  See also Preoxygenation; Respiratory system.
Oxygenation
  apneic, 613
  hyperbaric, 1134–1148
    chambers, 1136–1139
      anesthesia machines, 1138–1139
      controls, 1137
      design, 1136–1137
      patient monitoring, 1137–1138
      safety conditions, 1137
    complications, 1143–1147, 1143t
      decompression sickness, 1143
      gaseous embolism, 1143
      oxygen toxicity, 1143–1147, *1144*
    history, 1134–1135
    indications, 1139–1143, 1139t
      anaerobic infections, 1142
      barbiturate poisoning, 1142
      carbon monoxide poisoning, 1139–1142, 1139–1141t
      cardiac surgery, 1142
      radiation therapy, 1142
      vascular diseases, 1142–1143
    physiology, 1135–1136, *1136*
  in ventilated lung, 614
Oxyhemoglobin dissociation curve, 88–89

Oxytocin, and succinylcholine, 1016
Pacemaker, for sleep, 320
Packing, pharyngeal, 484
Pain
  acupuncture, 1639
  barbiturate effects, 674
  cervical plexus, 197–198
  discogenic, 202
  and dosage of anesthesia, 290
  and epidural anesthesia, 1602
  evaluation, spinal anesthesia, 1488
  at injection site
    diazepam anesthesia, 754
    local anesthetics, 1311–1312
    thiopental substitutes, 698
  intractable, and MAC values, 340
  mechanism and control, 1317–1349
    ascending pain transmission, 1336
    block peripheral path, 1345, 1346t
    clinical analysis, 1317
    clinical aspects, 1337–1341
      classification, 1337–1338
      injury effects, 1338
      neuronal hyperactivity, 1338
      persistant pain and spasm, 1338
      referred pain, 1338–1340, *1340*
      trigger points, 1340–1341, *1341*
      vascular responses, 1341, *1343*
    definition, 1318
    demand analgesia, 1344
    descending supraspinal control, 1336–1337
    description of, 1317
    hyperstimulation analgesia, 1344–1345
    opioid effects, 1333–1337
      endogenous opioids, 1334–1335, 1335t
      natural modulation, 1333
      neurotransmitters, 1335–1336
        serotonin, 1336
        somatostatin, 1336
        substance P, 1335–1336
      receptors, 1333–1334, 1335t
      terminology, 1333
    pathways, 1324–1333
      central neurophysiologic mechanisms, 1321–1323
        cognition, 1333
        motivation-affective component, 1321–1323
        sensory discrimination, 1321, *1332*
      modulation mechanism, 1330, *1330*
      motor mechanisms, 1333
      multiple gate theory, 1333, *1334*
      somatosensory system, 1324–1330
        drug action on laminae, 1329–1330
        large fibers, 1326, *1327*
        small-diameter fibers, 1326–1328
        somatosensory fibers, 1324–1326
        spinal microanatomy and physiology, 1328–1329, 1329t
    peripheral neurophysiology, 1321
    physiology, 1320
    psychology, 1320–1321, 1344
    quantitation, 1324, 1326t
    raising of threshold, 1341–1344
    receptor mechanism, 1321

    sensory discrimination, 1323, 1324t
    stimulus removal, 1345
    surgical control, 1345–1346
    terminology, 1318, 1319t
    theories, 1318–1320
      patterns, 1319–1320
      primitive, 1318
      specificity, 1318–1319
    therapy, 1341, 1337
    threshold, 1321–1322
      constitutional factors, 1322
      neurologic factors, 1322
      psychological factors, 1322
    tolerance, 1321–1322
    topographical distribution, 1323–1324, *1325*
    transcutaneous electrical nerve stimulation (TENS), 1345
  in neonates, 235
  opioid analgesia, 1630
  and placebo use, 306–307
  postoperative
    depolarizing agent complications, 909–910
    ketamine anesthesia, 746
  prediction, and behavioral disorders, 209
  thiopental injection, 682
  tourniquet, in spinal anesthesia, 1547–1551
Palate
  groove formation in neonates, 590–591
  neonatal, 503
Palatoglossal arch, gag reflex, 540
Palpation of pulse, 74
Pancreatic hormones, and surgical stress, 1509
Pancuronium, 959–971
  administration and dosage, 960, *961*
  and autonomic nervous system, 967
  carbon dioxide effects, 968
  cardiovascular effects, 964–966
  and catecholamines, 966–967, *966*
  chemistry, 960, *960*
  cholinesterase inhibition, 840
  clinical uses, 970–971
  contraindications, 971
  drug interactions, 266, 268, 272, 969–970
  and electrolytes, 968–969
  in hepatic disease, 963
  and histamine release, 969
  history, 959–960
  in hyperventilation, 968
  and intracranial pressure, 969
  and intraocular pressure, 279, 969, 971
  and lower esophageal sphincter, 969
  and MAC values, 339
  in malignant hyperpyrexia, 969, 971
  muscle-sparing action, 967
  neuromuscular junction action, 964
  pediatric reversal, 1045
  pharmacodynamics, 960–961
  pharmacokinetics, 961–964, *962–964*, 962t
  potency, 960
  priming action, 867, 868, 961, *961*
  in rapid sequence induction, 439–440
  recovery and reversal, 963–964
  in renal disease, 963
  site of action, 823
  and thiopental solubility, 660
  See also Relaxants.
Parabens, 1313

Index

Paradoxical reflex, 1188
Paraldehyde, and neuromuscular transmission, 887–888
Paralysis
  bladder and rectal, after spinal anesthesia, 1567
  extubation, 555–556
  facial nerve, during mask anesthesia, 432–433
  familial periodic, 875, 901
  in hyperbaric oxygenation, 1143
  laryngeal nerve, 585–586
  medullary, 364–368
  neurosis of, 906
  and relaxant action, 848–851
    airway muscles, 851
    anatomic differences, 848–849
    blood flow, 850
    depolarizing drugs, 850
    muscle groups, 849–850
    muscle structure, 850–851
    priming principle, 866–869, 867t
    temperature, 851
  skeletal muscle, succinylcholine effects, 1005–1006
  and ventilators, 641
Paraplegia
  acupuncture, 1639
  pain control, 1338, 1345
Parasympathetic agents
  blockade, 287
  drug interactions, 276
Paravertebral nerve block. *See* Nerve block, paravertebral.
Paresthesia
  needling, 1224
  symptoms, 1225
Parkinson's disease
  laryngeal muscles, 467
  and muscle relaxants, 898, 915
Partition coefficient, 105, 353
  of anesthetic gases, 332, 331t
  tissue-blood, 342–343, 342t
Patient
  position. *See* Positioning of patient; Posture.
  selection
    acupuncture, 1639
    ambulatory surgery, 1642–1643
    in hypnosis, 1126
    spinal anesthesia, 1484–1486
Pattern theories of pain, 1319–1320
Pauling paramagnetic analyzer, 87
PCP, 735
Pediatrics. *See* Infants and children.
PEEP (positive end-expiratory pressure)
  in one-lung ventilation, 615–616
  principles of, 620–622, 652
  during thoracic surgery, 613
  weaning from, 645
Penicillin, drug interactions, 266
Penis nerve block, 1426
Pentazocine, and MAC values, 338
Pentobarbital, 655
Pentolinium (ansolysen)
  controlled hypotension, 1066–1067
  and MAC values, 339
Pericardium, reflexes, 1189
Perichondritis, of laryngeal cartilage, 583–584
Perineal anesthesia, 1423–1424, *1423*, *1424*
Periosteal reflex, 1192–1193
Peripheral nervous system
  in hypothermia, 1099–1100
  reflexes, 1192–1193
Peritoneal cavity
  in hypothermia, 1109
  reflexes, 1190
Pernosten, 655
Peroneal nerve block, 1408, *1409*
Persians, use of anesthesia, 4
Personality
  and drug responses, 209, 305
  and physical constitution, 209–210
Personnel, anesthesia, 37–38
  ambulatory surgery, 1642–1643
  biotransformation, 1161–1162
  chemical hazards, 1158–1165
  occupational virus hazards, 1168–1173
    hepatitis, 1169–1170
    herpes simplex virus, 1168–1169
    HIV infection and AIDS, 1170–1173
  during patient repositioning, 194
  static electricity, 1152
Pesticides, enzyme induction, 256, 276
pH
  and buffers, 1236–1237
  and local anesthetic uptake, 1211
  and muscle relaxants, 877
  and pain at injection site, 1312
Phantom limb pain, 1345
Pharmacodynamics
  alfentanil, 725–726
  anticoagulants, 262–263
  atracurium, 983
  bupivacaine, 1261
  curare, 948
  dacuronium, 971
  doxacurium, 994
  droperidol, 708
  edrophonium, 1041
  etidocaine, 1263
  etomidate, 767
  inhalation agents, 429–430, 430t
  local anesthetics, 1218–1219, 1240–1242, 1218t
    administration site, 1240, 1242
    dosage effects, 1240–1242, 1239t
    duration of action, 1242, 1243t
    onset of action, 1240
  meperidine for spinal anesthesia, 1530–1532
  midazolam, 761–762
  mivacurium, 992–994
  opioid analgesia, 1625–1626
  pancuronium, 960–961
  propofol, 769–770
  pyridostigmine, 1038
  ropivacaine, 1265
  succinylcholine, 1010–1011, 1011t
  sufentanil, 727–728
  vecuronium, 976
Pharmacokinetics
  alfentanil, 722–723
    in children, 724
  aminopyridine, 1047
  antidepressants, 270–271
  atracurium, 983
  bupivacaine, 1261, 1485
  cocaine, 1249, 1249t
  curare, 940–941, *941*
  curariform agents, 832–835, *833*
  diazepam, 750, *751*
  droperidol, 708–709, 709t
  edrophonium, 1041
  etidocaine, 1262–1263
  etomidate, 766
  fazadinium, 990
  fentanyl, 712–713
  gallamine, 952–953, 953t
  hydralazine, 1085
  inhaled agents, effect of duration of anesthesia, 353–354
  intercostal nerve block, 1418–1419
  ketamine, 743–745, *744*
  lidocaine, 792
  local anesthetics, 1208–1209, 1219–1221, 1243–1246
    absorption, 1219, 1243–1245
    in brachial block, 1378–1379, 1378–1379t
    destruction, 1220–1221
    disposition, 1219
    distribution, 1245
    elimination, 1221
    excretion, 1246
    gastric fluid levels, 1220
    metabolism, 1245–1246
    plasma protein binding, 1219–1220
    redistribution, 1220, 1220t
  lorazepam, 756
  metoclopramide, 237
  metocurine, 950
  midazolam, 760–761, *760*, 761t
  mivacurium, 992
  neostigmine, 1035–1036
  nitroglycerin, 1083
  nitroprusside, 1073–1075
  opioid analgesia, 1624–1625, 1625t
  pancuronium, 961–964, 962t
  physostigmine, 1033, *1033*
  pipecuronium, 980–981, 981t
  procaine, 790
  propofol, 769, *769*, *770*
  pseudocholinesterases, 837
  pyridostigmine, 1038
  ropivacaine, 1265
  spinal anesthetics, 1476
  succinylcholine, 835–836, *836*, 836t
  sufentanil, 727, 727t, 728t
  thiopental, 661–666, *662–666*, 661t
  substitutes, 695–697
  vecuronium, 974–976, 974–975t
Pharyngeal
  airway, 12
  reflex, 1185
Pharyngitis, during endotracheal anesthesia, 580
Phencyclidines, 734–735
Phenelzine, drug interactions, 269
Phenobarbital
  enzyme induction, 256, 348
  and neuromuscular blockade, 883
Phenol
  endotracheal tube cleaning, 479
  neurolytic agent, 1268–1269
  subarachnoid neurolysis, 1535
Phenthiazine
  drug interactions, 273
  in hypothermia, 1110
Phenylephrine, and spinal anesthetics, 1481
Phenytoin
  enzyme induction, 256
  and neuromuscular blockade, 883
Pheochromocytoma, magnesium treatment, 877
pHisoHex, endotracheal tube cleaning, 479
Phosphaline, 1043
Photodegradation, of nitroprusside, 1071

Photoplethysmography, 74
Phrenic nerve block, 1366
Physical status classification, 38, 39t
   and mortality, 40, 42, 45–46, *41*, 41–42t, 46t
Physics of anesthesiology, 100–117
   critical conditions, 111–114, *112, 113*
   fluids, 114–117, *114*
     flow
       Bernoulli's Theorem, 116–117, *116*, 117t
       nature of, 114–115, *115*
       resistance to, 115–116
      Poiseuille's Law, 114
   gases
     Avogadro's Law, 106
     behavior of, 102–104
       Boyle's Law, 102, *102*
       Charles' Law, 102–103, *103*
       Dalton's Law, 104, *104*
       Gay-Lussac's Law, 103, *103*
       Henry's Law, 104
       ideal gas law, 103
     blood solubility of anesthetics, 105–106, 106t
     density, 106–107
     diffusion, 107, *108*
     Laplace's Law, 108
     solubility in liquids, 104–105, 1–5t
       coefficients of solubility, 105
     specific gravity, 107, 107t
     standard conditions, 106
     surface tension, 107–108
     weight, 106
   heat, 108
   humidity, 111
   molecular theory, 100, *101*
   vapor and gas, 112–114
   vaporization, 108–110, *109*
     latent heat of vaporization, 109–110
     process of, 110–111
     specific heat, 109, 111t
     vapor pressure, 109, *110*
Physostigmine, 1032–1034, *1033*
   mechanism of action, 1029
Pierre-Robin syndrome, and endotracheal anesthesia, 518
Pilocarpine, for glaucoma, 278
Pin index system, compressed gas cylinders, 127
Pineal gland, and sleep, 320–321
Pipecuronium, 979–981, *980*, 981t
Pipelines, compressed air, 158
Piperocaine toxicity, 1295
Pituitary gland
   in acupuncture, 1636–1637
   hormones, and surgical stress, 1509, 1510
   in oxygen toxicity, 1147
Placebo, 305–307
   definition, 305
   ethics, 305–306
   function, 305
   indications, 306
   in pain control, 306–307, 1344
   types, 305
Placenta
   diazepam transfer, 753
   and muscle relaxants, 908–909
   succinylcholine transmission, 1009
   thiopental transfer, 680
Plate, in endotracheal anesthesia, 521
Platelets
   aggregation

     anesthetic effects, 263
     aspirin effects, 258
     preoperative evaluation, 222–223
Plethysmography, 1444
Pleural reflexes, 1189
Pneumocephalus, during patient positioning, 196
Pneumotachography, 88
Pneumothorax, tension, 588
Poiseuille's Law, 114, 295, 470
Poliomyelitis
   and muscle relaxants, 899
   and spinal anesthesia, 1567
Polycythemia, preoperative evaluation, 222–223
Polymixin B, and organophosphates, 1043–1044, 1044t
Pontocaine
   development, 18
   protein potentiation, 1479
Pontogeniculo-occipital activity, 320
Popliteal nerve block, 1408–1410, *1408–1409*
Poppy as anesthetic, 3–4
Positioning of patient
   complications, 192–206
     of abdomen, 201
       intra-abdominal masses, 201
       stabilization braces, 201
       Trendelenburg position, 201
       visceral stomas, 201
     of extremities, 202–204
       arms, 202–203
       fingers, 204
       legs, 204
     of head and neck, 194–200
       brachial plexus injuries, 198–199, *198*
       compression alopecia, 194
       ears, 194–195
       eyes, 195, *195*
       face, 195–196
       intracranial injuries, 196
       neck injuries, 196–198
       nose, 195
       peripheral nerve injuries, 199–200, *200*
     during repositioning, 193–194
       extremity injuries, 193
       miscellaneous injuries, 194
       neck injuries, 193–194
       personnel injuries, 194
       postural hypotension, 193
     of spine, 201–202
       discogenic pain, 202
       lithotomy disengagement, 202
       postoperative backache, 201–202
       unstable spine, 202
     thermal instability, 204–205
     of thorax, 200–201
       aspiration pneumonitis, 200
       breasts, 200
       chest trauma, 200
       venous air embolus, 200–201
     transport, 192–193
       hypotension, 193
       motion sickness, 193
       vital sign monitors, 192–193
     in epidural anesthesia, 1581–1582
     infants and children, 1532
     and preanesthetic visit, 214–215
     and spread of injections, 1469
     technical aspects, 174–191
       chest injuries, 190

       comatose patient, 189–190
       delirium, 190
       head elevation, 181–183
         classic semi-recumbent dorsal decubitus position, 181–182, *182*
         full sitting position, 181
         in lateral decubitus or prone position, 183
         Shapiro's modification for air embolism, 183, *184*
         sidesaddle sitting position, 182–183, *183*
         supine position, 183
       head injuries, 190
       lateral positions, 183–187
         classic decubitus position, 184–185, *184, 185*
         flexed positions, 185–187, *186, 187*
         semilateral positions, 185
         Sims' position, 185, *185*
         spinal anesthesia, 185, 1459–1460, *1460, 1461*
         terminology, 183–184
       lithotomy position, 179–180, *179, 180*
       moving
         and repositioning of patient, 171, 177
         of unconscious patient, 189
       operating table and accessories, 174–177
         arm supports, 175–176, *175, 176*
         head holders, 176–177
         tables, 174–175
         trunk frames, 176, *177, 178*
       orthopedic injuries, 190
       prone positions, 187–190
         jackknife position, 188–189, *188*
         kneeling position, 189
         precautions, 187
         standard position, 187–188, *188*
       supine position, 177–178
       Trendelenburg position, 180, *181*
   See also Posture of patient.
Positive-end expiratory pressure (PEEP), 83
Postanesthetic recovery score, 242–243, *243*
Posture of patient, 163–173
   cardiovascular system, 163–168
     dorsal decubitus position (horizontal), 164–165, 165t
     gravity forces, 164
     hemodynamics on sitting, 167–168
     hypovolemic patients, 166
     lateral decubitus position, 166–167
     lung perfusion, 167
     morphine effects, 167
     prone position, 167–168
     pulmonary vascular pressure and alveolar pressure, 164, *164*
     supine-head down tilt, 165–166
     supine-head up tilt, 166, 165t
   central nervous system, 169–171
     autoregulation, 170
     carbon dioxide role, 170–171
     cerebral perfusion, 170
     head elevation, 170
     head lowering, 170
     neck position, 170
   and controlled hypotension, 1058

Posture of patient (Continued)
  definition, 163
  and epidural pressure, in obstetrics, 1605
  moving anesthetized patient, 171
    during general anesthesia, 171
    during regional anesthesia, 171
    repositioning during surgery, 171
    transportation to intensive care unit, 171
  respiratory system, 168–169
    airway closure, 169
    lateral position, 169
      in lung disease, 169
    lithotomy position, 169
    lung air subdivisions, 168–169
    postoperative posture, 169
    supine position, 168–169
Potassium
  and atracurium, 984–985
  channel structure, 1214
  and end-plate potentials, 816
  after epidural anesthesia, 1601
  in hypothermia, 1105–1106
  and local anesthetics, 1237, 1304
  in nerve impulse, 1205–1208
  pancuronium effects, 968–969
  potentiation of action, 1287–1288
    spinal anesthetics, 1479–1480
  and relaxant agents, 873–875, 913–916
Potency
  bupivacaine, 1260
  chloroprocaine, 1253
  definition, 1233
  etidocaine, 1262
  hexylcaine, 1251
  lidocaine, 1257
  local anesthetics, 1234–1235, 1237
  mepivacaine, 1259
  ropivacaine, 1264–1265
  topical anesthesia, 1272
Potentials
  evoked, 94
  membrane, 828
  motor end-plate (MEPP), 815, 822–824
Potentiation of spinal anesthetics, 1478–1484
  additives, 1478–1480
    carbonated local anesthetics, 1479
    clonidine, 1480
    dextran-40, 1479
    dextrose, 1478–1479
    potassium, 1479–1480
    procaine crystals, 1479
    proteins, 1479
  vasoconstrictors, 1480–1483
    high-dose, 1482–1483
    history, 1480
    neural effect, 1482
    neurologic effects, 1480
    systemic effects, 1481–1482
    techniques, 1481
Pralidoxime, 1049
Prazosin, drug interactions, 268
Preanesthetic
  evaluation and preparation, 207–252
    anesthesia choice, 234–236
      general vs. regional, 235
      in neonates, 235–236
      principles, 234–235
    bedside tests of function, 225–226
      breath-holding test, 225
      cough test, 226
      respiratory force test, 226
      Valsalva test, 226
    cardiovascular evaluation, 226–229
      cardiac disease, 226–227, 227t
      diagnostic studies, 228–229
      specific factors, 227–229
        cardiac performance, 227
        cardiac pump performance, 227–228
    gastrointestinal tract, 236–242
      age factors, 238
      anxiety, 238
      children, 241–242
      empty stomach, 236
      fasting, 238–240
      gastric emptying, 237–238, 237
      gastric volume, 238, 239
      in pregnancy, 239
    general considerations, 215–225
      age, 215
      deformities, 218
      obesity, 215–218
      unusual syndromes, 218
      weight loss, 215
    laboratory studies, 218–225, 219–220t
      bleeding time and platelet count, 222–223
      blood transfusion, 222
      blood volume, 224
      cancer patients, 225
      chest roentgenogram, 224–225
      crossmatch and screen protocol, 221–222
      fresh frozen plasma, 221
      hemogram, 219–221
      hypoproteinemia, 224
      malignant hypertension susceptibility, 223–224
      partial thromboplastin time, 221
    medical consultation, 234
    postanesthetic recovery score, 242–243
    preanesthetic visit, 211–215
      alcoholism, 211–213
      smoking, 213–215
      surgical position, 214–215
    psychological considerations, 207–211
      anxiety, 208–211
      cancer patients, 209
      children, 209
      fear, 207–208, 208t
      pain and behavioral disorders, 209
      personality
        and constitution, 209–210
        and drug responses, 209
      preoperative visit, 208
      sympathetic nervous system, 210
    respiratory evaluation tests, 229–234, 242
      diagnostic pulmonary function tests, 230–231
      dyspnea, 231–232
      forced vital capacity, 229–230
      indications, 229, 229t
      pulmonary diseases, 232–234
        emphysema, 232
        upper respiratory infections, 232–234
      thoracic surgery, 231
      vital capacity, 229–230
    smoking, 213–215
    unconsciousness, 243
    urinary tract, 242
    viability score, 243, 243
  medication principles, 284–313
    alternative routes of administration, 297–299
      bone marrow infusions, 298–299
      nasal instillation, 297–298
      rectal administration, 298
      transbuccal mucosal absorption, 297
      transdermal instillation, 298
    approaches, 286–289
      awareness state, 287
      balanced medication, 286–287
      classic approach, 286
      definitions, 287–288, 288t
      opioid premedications, 286
      parasympathetic blockade, 287
      primary cortical sedation, 286
      subcortical suppression, 286
    dosage factors, 289–290
      age, 289, 289
      agents, 290
      diseases, 290
      diurnal rhythm, 290
      emotions, 290
      endocrine effects, 290
      ethnicity, 289–290
      pain, 290
      sex, 290
      temperature, 290
      toxemias, 290
    drug dependence, 307–309
      definitions, 307
      pathogenesis, 307–308, 307t
      pharmacology, 308–309
    drug evaluation, 303–305
      definitions, 303–304
      double-blind technique, 304–305
      personality and drug reactions, 305
      principles, 304
    guide for medication (adults), 290–292, 291t
      clonidine, 292
      evening before surgery, 291
      morning of surgery, 291
      narcotic morphine sulfate, 291
      outpatient anesthesia and surgery, 291–292
      sedatives and tranquilizers, 291
    objectives, 284–286
      anxiety factors, 285, 285t
      autonomic nervous system, 285
      central nervous system activity, 284
      endocrine system, 285
      gastrointestinal function, 286
      hormonal assessment, 285–286
      opioid reduction of metabolism, 285
      sensory input, 284–285
    parenteral drug administration, 292–296
      hypodermic injection, 293
      intramuscular injection technique, 293–294, 294
      intravenous route, 294–296, 296
      routes of administration, 293
    pediatric, 299–303
      advantages, 302
      anticholinergics, 302–303
      medication programs, 299–301, 301t

midazolam medication, 301–302
no medication, 302
opiate effects, 303
premedication regimens, 303t
placebo, 305–3037
Precipitation, 1236–1237
Pregnancy
chloroprocaine toxicity, 1254
cholinesterases, 839
curare protein binding, 941
gastric emptying, 239
postural changes, 167
pyridostigmine anesthesia, 1039
and spread of injections, 1470–1471
and succinylcholine, 1015
toxemia
magnesium treatment, 876–877
trimethaphan effects, 1068
and toxicity of local anesthetics, 1300
and vecuronium, 978
Premedication
ambulatory surgery, 1645–1646, 1645t
complications in spinal anesthesia, 1552
curare, 947
diazepam, 749, 753
electroanesthesia, 1121
ethanol, 776
ether, intravenous, 773
fentanyl, 718–719
gallamine, 955
hydroxydione, 763
ketamine, 742, 743t
midazolam, 759
muscle relaxants. See Relaxants.
nonrelaxant anesthetic drugs, 886–888
opiates, 886–887
paraldehyde, 887–888
tranquilizers, 887
tribromethanol, 888
regional anesthesia, 1201
spinal anesthesia, 1458–1459
in infants and children, 1532
Preoxygenation, 424–425
and alveolar gases, 427–428
thiopental anesthesia, 677–679
Presacral block, 1425
Preservatives in local anesthetic solutions, 1312–1314, 1312t
antioxidants, 1312–1313
bacteriostatics, 1313
buffering, 1313
sulfites, 1313–1314
Pressure
anterior fontanelle, in neonate, 540–541
critical, 111
intracranial
hydralazine effects, 1085
and muscle relaxants, 919
pancuronium effects, 969
during patient positioning, 196
succinylcholine effects, 1008
and vecuronium, 978
intragastric, 919–920
intraocular
curare actions, 946
during extubation, 554
and muscle relaxants, 918–919
pancuronium effects, 969
succinylcholine effects, 1007
and vecuronium, 978
See also Glaucoma.

during manual artificial ventilation, 630–631
partial, of anesthetic agent, 324, 331, 325–326
regulators, 128–129, 129–131
tracheal wall, 485–487
See also Breathing systems, artificial.
Prilocaine, 796
See also Regional anesthesia.
Procaine
bacteriostatic action, 1313
dissociation constant, 1212
during extubation, 555
in hyperbaric spinal anesthesia, 1521–1522
intravenous anesthesia, 787–790
anesthetic adjunct, 788–789
for arrhythmias, 789–790
chemistry and metabolism, 787–788
dosage, 788
excretion, 788
history, 787
pathophysiology, 788
pharmacokinetics, 789, 789
pharmacology, 787, 1252–1253
preparations, 788
properties, 788
responses and toxicity, 789
metabolism, 1221
potassium potentiation, 1288, 1479
protein potentiation, 1479
in subarachnoid space, 1471–1472
toxicity, 1295
See also Regional anesthesia.
Prolactin, thiopental effects, 669
Promethazine
drug interactions, 265
as local anesthetic, 1270
Prone position
and circulation, 167–168
technical aspects, 187–190
complication and contraindication, 189
jackknife position, 188–189, 188
kneeling position, 189
precautions, 187
standard position, 187–188, 188
Propanidid, 772–773, 772
and neuromuscular transmission, 888
Propitocaine pharmacology, 1263–1264
Propofol, 768–772
advantages, 771–772
in ambulatory surgery, 1647
chemistry, 768–769, 769
in children, 771
clinical uses, 771
dosage, 769
and neuromuscular transmission, 888
pharmacokinetics, 769, 769–770, 770t
pharmacology, 770–771
recovery, 771
side effects, 771
Propranolol
during endotracheal anesthesia, 576
and MAC values, 339
and platelet function, 258
Propylene glycol, potentiation of action, 1289
Prostaglandins, aspirin effects, 258
Protamine sulfate, drug interactions, 263–265
Protein
binding, 254
curare, 941

bupivacaine, 1261
of local anesthetics, 1219–1220, 1293–1294, 1294t
pancuronium, 962
thiopental, 662–663, 668
potentiation of spinal anesthetics, 1288, 1479
Prothrombin time, thiopental effects, 669
Protriptyline, drug interactions, 270
Pseudocholinesterases, 836–841
Pseudomonas aeruginosa, in anesthesia machines, 158
PSV (pressure support ventilation), 622
Psychogalvanic reflex, 1442–1443, 1442
Psychologic factors
of anesthesia, 207–211
anxiety
incidence, 209
reduction measures, 210–211
types, 208
cancer patients, 209
children, 209
fear, 207–208, 208t
pain and behavioral disorders, 209
personality
and drug responses, 209
and physical constitution, 209–210
preoperative visit, 208
sympathetic nervous system, 210
of mask induction, 430
operative risk, 38, 41, 54–55
postspinal headaches, 1557
regional anesthesia, 1200
and spinal anesthesia, 1487
Psychomotor skills
of anesthetist, 52
physostigmine anesthesia, 1033
and toxicity of local anesthetics, 1307
Psychosis, and cholinesterases, 839
Pudendal nerve blocks, 1425–1426
Pulmonary artery pressure monitoring. See Blood pressure monitoring.
Pulmonary function
in endotracheal anesthesia, 571
oxygen toxicity, 1146
preoperative evaluation, 229–232
preoxygenation effect on alveolar gases, 427–428
in smokers, 51
and spinal anesthesia, 1511
See also Carbon dioxide absorption; Ventilation.
Pulse oximetry, 88–90
Punch card systems, 30
Pyridostigmine, 1037–1039, 1038
Pyriform sinus, 585

Quadriplegia vascular injury, during patient positioning, 197
Quanta packets of acetylcholine, 814–815
Quaternaries
endotracheal tube cleaning, 479
ammonium compounds, 260–261, 829–831
Queen Victoria, 8–9
Quenching agents, 1151
Quinidine, drug interactions, 274
Quinine, drug interactions, 274
Quinozolone, and REM sleep, 322

Racial differences
and anesthetic risk, 41–42
cholinesterases, 837
diazepam anesthesia, 750

Radial nerve
 block, 1390–1393
  anatomy, 1390–1391, *1392*
  at elbow, 1391–1392
  at wrist, 1392–1393, *1393*
 palsy, 199, 2–3
 solution distribution, 1376
Radiation therapy, hyperbaric oxygenation, 1142
Radiology in nerve blocks, 1227–1228
RAE endotracheal tubes, 476–477, *477*
Ramon laser scattering, 86
Ranitidine
 comparison with cimetidine, 236–237
 drug interactions, 265
Rapid-eye-movement (REM)
 CNS depressant effects, 322
 neurotransmitters, 321
 and NREM, 319–320
 in paradoxic sleep, 319–320
 physiologic changes, 322
Recall during anesthesia, 366–368
Receptors
 acetylcholine, 817–818
 occupancy in relaxant anesthesia, 871–872
 opiate, 1623
  in spinal cord, 1489
 opioid, 1334
 pain, 1321
Records, anesthetic, 29–34
 character of, 30
 history of, 29–30
 nerve block clinic, 32–33
 purposes of keeping, 29
 resuscitation and inhalation therapy, 34
 transfusion records, 33–34
 types, 30–32, *31*, *32*
  automated systems, 30–32
   CARIN (Computerized Anesthesia Recording and Information Network), 31
   Datatrac system, 31
   Moduless II Anesthesia System, 31
   voice recognition, 31–32
  punch card systems, 30
Recovery score, postanesthetic, 242–243, 243t
Rectal anesthesia, 18
Recto-cardiac reflex, 1191
Recto-laryngeal reflex, 1190–1191
Rectum, drug administration, 298
Red neck syndrome, 266
Red nucleus, 380
Rees breathing system, 404, 418, *404*
Reflex vasodilatation test, 1442
Reflexes
 abdominal, and laryngospasm, 569
 during anesthesia, 365–366
 autonomic, during anesthesia and surgery, 1179–1195
  abdominal, 1189–1191
  bronchospasm, 1188–1189
  carinal, 1187
  carotid sinus mechanisms, 1182–1183
  cough, 1187
  eyelid, 1182
  head's paradoxical, 1188
  innervation of pelvic viscera, 1191–1192
  intrathoracic, 1189
  juxtapulmonary receptor, 1188

  laryngeal, 1185–1186
  obstetrical, 1192
  oculocardiac, 1179–1182
   atypical, 1180–1181
   oculo-emetic, 1181
   oculorespiratory, 1181–1182
  peripheral nerve, 1192–1193
  respiratory tract, 1184–1185, *1184*
  tracheal, 1186–1187
  venous return, 1188
 block, in general anesthesia, 315
 curare actions, 945–946
 hydroxydione effects, 764
 ketamine effects, 740
 lidocaine effects, 791
 thiopental effects, 680–681
 See also Relaxation, muscular; specific reflexes.
Refrigeration, 1096
Regional anesthesia
 in ambulatory surgery, 1647–1648
 caudal. *See* Caudal analgesia.
 drug interactions, 263
 endocrine response, 1509
 principles, 1199–1231
  anatomy, 1202–1204
   landmarks, 1202
   mixed nerve, 1204, *1204*
   myelinated nerve fibers, 1203
   nerve fiber structure and histochemistry, 1202–1203, *1203*
   Schwann cells and myelin, 1203
  definition, 1199
  history, 1199
  humanitarian, 1200–1201
   pre-block evaluation, 1200–1201
   premedication, 1201
   psychological management, 1200
  pharmacology, 1208–1221
   active form, 1213
   block types, 1214
   clinical order of nerve block, 1216, 1216t
   comparative sensitivity, 1216–1217
   diffusion of local anesthetics, 1209, *1209–1211*
   distribution in nerve fiber, 1212
   fixation, 1213
   membrane changes, 1213–1214
   minimum anesthetic concentration, 1215
   penetration process, 1212
   pharmacodynamics, 1218–1221, 1218t
   pharmacokinetics, 1208–1209
   physiochemistry, 1209–1212, 1211t
   unconventional agents, 1214
  physiology, 1204–1208
   action of local anesthetics, 1204
   fiber classification and function, 1208, 1207t
   nerve action potential, 1208
   nerve conduction, 1205
   nerve impulses, 1205–1208
  roentgenographic control, 1227–1229
   indications, 1228
   radiopaque drugs, 1228
   techniques, 1228
  surgical, 1201–1202
   asepsis, 1201–1202
   facilities, 1201

   skin preparation, 1202
   technical considerations, 1221–1227
    failure of block, 1227
    instruments, 1221–1224, *1223*
    nerve site identification, 1224–1226
    procedures, 1226–1227
   types, 1199–1200
  reactions to, 1302–1316
   allergic reactions, 1310–1312
   clinical types, 1310–1311
  See also Local anesthesia and regional block.
Regurgitation
 and full stomach, 438–439
 and pancuronium, 971
Reinfarction, perioperative
 age effect, 59
 characteristics of, 58
 duration of surgery, 59
 emergency surgery, 60
 interval from previous infarction, 59, *61*
 intraoperative medical problem, 59–60
 risk factors, 58–59, 60t
 See also Myocardial infarction.
Relaxants, muscle
 in ambulatory surgery, 1647
 antagonists, 1023–1055
  aminopyridine, 1047
  anticholinesterases, 1028–1032, *1029–1032*
  chemistry, 1024–1025, *1024–1025*
  classification, 1028, 1028t
  deep block, 1027
  to depolarizing agents, 1048–1050
   anticholinesterase poisoning, 1048–1050
   azathioprine, 1050
   cholase, 1048
   onium compounds, 1048
   stilbazoline, 1048
   trimethaphan, 1048
  edrophonium, 1039–1041, *1040*, 1040t
  galanthamine, 1048
  germine diacetate, 1048
  neostigmine, 1034–1037, *1034*
  organophosphates, 1043–1045, 1044t
   irreversible, 1048
  in pediatrics, 1045–1047, *1046*
  physostigmine, 1032–1034, *1033*
  prereversal
   single twitch, 1025–1026
   train-of-four factor, 1026
  priming principle, 1041–1042
  pyridostigmine, 1037–1039, *1038*
  reciprocal, 1027
  recovery rate, 1025
  resistance to, 1027–1028
  reversal objectives, 1023–1024, 1026–1027
  RO1-5733, 1048
  tetraethylammonium, 1047
  timing, 1025
 and apnea, 620
 clinical uses, 847–937
  assessment of relaxation, 851–860
   bedside tests, 851, 851t
   clinical tests, 851, 852t
   electromyography, 860
   monitoring NMJ block, 857–860, *859*

Index **I-35**

nerve stimulation-response test, 852–854, *854*, 853t
pharmacologic test, 860
receptor pool for twitch vs. tetanus response, 854
tetanic stimulation, 857
train-of-four stimulation monitoring, 854–857, *855*
biochemical factors, 872–886
acid-base changes, 877
antibiotics, 844–885, 885t
anticonvulsant drugs, 883–884, 883t
colchicine, 886
corticosteroids, 886
curarine actions, 877–881
electrolytes, 873–877
fluid balance, 872–873, 874t
hypothermia effects, 881–882, *881*, *882*
lithium, 885
local anesthetics, 882–883
complications, 904–909
anaphylaxis, 908
apnea, 905
bronchospasm, 905
CNS effects, 904
of depolarizing agents, 909–912
histamine physiology, 906–908
mucus, 905
neurosis of paralysis, 906
oxygen consumption, 904–905
placental transfer, 908–909
visual disturbances, 905–906
dose-response factors, 860–872
combined relaxants, 869–872, 87t
mechanism of cumulation, 864
pediatric doses, 865
potency, 860–864, 860–864t
prediction of dose, 865–866, *867*
priming for rapid paralysis, 866–869, 868t
indications and contraindications, 890–891, 890–891t
neuromuscular disorders, 896–904
basal ganglia disorders, 898–899
carcinoid tumors, 903
combined relaxants, 904
lower motoneuron disorders, 899–900
myopathic muscular diseases, 900–903
thyroid disease, 903–904
upper motoneuron diseases, 896–898
nonrelaxant anesthetic drugs, 886–890
depth of anesthesia, 888
intravenous induction drugs, 888
premedications, 886–888
volatile anesthesia, 889–890, 889t
physiological factors, 847–851, 848t
age, 847
body build, 848
order of muscular block, 848
paralysis patterns, 848–851, *849*, *850*
sex, 847–848
pretreatment, 912–920
cardiac arrest, 917
cardiac arrhythmias, 916–917
catecholamines, 917
intracranial pressure, 919
intragastric pressure, 919–920

intramuscular succinylcholine, 920
intraocular pressure, 918–919
myoglobinemia, 917–918
pediatric, 913
potassium release, 913–916
timing, 913
sensitivity alterations, 891–896, 891t
allergies, 892
burns, 895–896, *895*
cardio-circulatory diseases, 892
choice of relaxant, 892
debility, 895
hepatic disease, 894–895
obesity, 892–893
renal disease, 893–894
respiratory diseases, 892
trauma, 895
fundamentals, 809–846
chemistry, 828–831, 829t
classification, 821–828, 823t
antidepolarizing block, 822–825, *824*, 825t
depolarizing block, 825–828, *825*
definitions, 831–832, *832*
end-plate reactions, 820–821
history, 809–810
pharmacokinetics
curariform agents, 832–835, *833*, *834*, 834t
succinylcholine, 835–836
physiology, 810–820
acetylcholine, 814–820, *815–823*, 822t
skeletal muscle system, 810–814, *811–814*
pseudocholinesterases, 836–841
for intubation, 526–527
and ketamine interaction, 741
and MAC values, 338–339
midazolam interaction, 758
and morbidity and morality, 40–41
pharmacology and use, 938–1022
alcuronium, 951–952, *952*, 952t
bis-type nondepolarizing, 981–995
atracurium, 981–989
biodegradation, 985–986
chemistry, 981–982, *983*
disease states, 984–985
dosage, 982–984
in pediatrics, 988–989, 988t
pharmacokinetics, 983, 984t
pharmacology, 986–988
doxacurium, 994–995, *994*, 995t
fazadinium, 989–990, *989*
mivacurium, 990–994, *990*, 991t
curare, 939–949
chemistry, 939–940, *940*
clinical use, 947–949
history, 939
mechanism of action, 940
metabolism, 940–943, *941–943*, 944t
pharmacologic actions, 944–947, *945–946*
site of action, 940
depolarizing muscle relaxants, 1002–1018
dantrolene, 1018
decamethonium compound, 1002–1003
hexafluorenium, 1017–1018, *1017*

succinylcholine. *See* Succinylcholine.
gallamine, 952–956, *953–955*, 953t
metocurine, 949–950, *950*
steroid-type nondepolarizing, 959–981
dacuronium, 971–972, *971*
pancuronium. *See* Pancuronium.
pipecuronium, 979–981, *980*
vecuronium, 972–979, *972*, 973–977t
vecuronium analogue ORG 9426, 979
toxiferine, 950–951, *951*
and thiopental, 657–660
Relaxation, muscular
and anesthetic depth, 379t
pain control, 1344
reflexes, 379–381
cortex, 379
gamma system, 380–381, *381*
H reflex, 381
intersegmental neurons, 380
red nucleus, 380
spinal center, 380
tectal nuclei, 379
vestibular nucleus, 380
Renal disease
acupuncture, 1639
and atracurium, 984–985
curare protein binding, 941, 943
and diazepam anesthesia, 750, 754
pancuronium effects, 963, *964*
relaxant contraindications, 893–894
spinal anesthesia, 1485–1486
thiopental binding, 663
and toxicity of local anesthetics, 1300
and vecuronium kinetics, 975
See also Kidney.
Renin-angiotensin, nitroprusside effects, 1078
Repositioning of patient. *See* Positioning of patient.
Reserpine
drug interactions, 266–267
and MAC values, 339
Resistance
in carbon dioxide absorption, 453, 457
closed circle systems, 392–393, *394*, 393t
electrical, of skin, 1441–1442
in endotracheal tubes, 470
pediatric, 505, 509
Respiration
anesthesia effects, 376
sighing, 378–379
tracheal tug, 377–378
breathing patterns during anesthesia, 376–377, *377*
apneustic pattern, 377, *378*
expiratory pattern, 377, *378*
and caudal analgesia, 1615
and controlled hypotension, 1059–1060
in epidural anesthesia, 1602
muscles, 375, 376t
fiber types, 375–376
and opioid analgesia, 1631
pediatric, opiate effects, 303
relaxant contraindications, 892
in spinal anesthesia, 1505, 1546
thiopental effects, 666–667, 676, 682
and toxicity of local anesthetics, 1307

Respiratory bags, 152–153
Respiratory distress syndrome
  extubation, 555–556
  positive airway pressure effects, 628
Respiratory minute volume test, 851
Respiratory system
  alfentanil effects, 726
  complications in endotracheal
      anesthesia, 566–573
    bronchospasm, 569–573
    infections, 586–587
    laryngospasm, 567–569
  curare actions, 945
  dacuronium effects, 971
  diazepam effects, 752
  droperidol effects, 710
  in electroanesthesia, 1122
  elimination of inhaled anesthetics,
      347–348
  fentanyl effects, 716
  gallamine effects, 954
  hydroxydione effects, 764
  in hypnosis, 1127–1128
  in hypothermia, 1101
  ketamine effects, 739–740
  and MAC values, 337
  monitoring of, 86–90
    anesthetic and respiratory gas, 86–
        87, 87
    blood gas analysis, 88–89
    oximetry and transcutaneous
        oxygen, 89–90, 90t
    stethoscope, 86
    ventilation and airway pressure, 87–
        88
  muscles, relaxant actions, 848–849
  nitroprusside effects, 1078
  in obesity, 217–218
  and oculocardiac reflex, 1181–1182
  in oxygen toxicity, 1146
  posture effects. See Posture of patient.
  preanesthetic evaluation, 229–234, 242
    dyspnea, 231–232
    indications, 229, 229t
    pulmonary diseases, 232–234
    pulmonary function tests, 230–231
    thoracic surgery, 231
    vital capacity and forced vital
        capacity, 229–230
  propanidid effects, 772
  propofol effects, 771
  reflexes, 1184–1185
    nasocardiac, 1184–1185
    pharyngeal, 1185
    sternutatory (sneeze), 1185
  succinylcholine actions, 1005
  smoking effects, 213, 214
  See also Pulmonary function.
Respirometers, 88
Resuscitation
  records, 34
  and ventilators, 640
Reticular activating system (RAS), 317,
    322–323, 318
Revell circulator, 390
Reversal of relaxants. See Relaxants,
    antagonists.
Rexed laminae, 315, 317
Rigidity syndrome, fentanyl effects, 717–
    718
Risk factors
  complications in spinal anesthesia,
      1552, 1552t
  for reinfarction, 58–59, 60t

RO1-5733, 1048
Robertshaw endobronchial tube, 604–
    607, 606
Ropivacaine pharmacology, 1264–1266
Rovenstine endobronchial anesthesia,
    597, 598
Rubber, in endotracheal tubes, 478
Ruben valve, 152

Sacral plexus nerve block, 1402–1412
  popliteal nerve, 1408–1410
  tibial nerves, 1410–1411
  See also Sciatic nerve.
Sacrum
  anatomy, 1612–1614, 1612–1614
  nerve block, 1424–1425
  See also Caudal analgesia.
Saddle block, 1469
Salem technique, 529, 548
Salicylates, protein binding, 254
Scalene muscles nerve block, 1379–1381
  complications, 1381
  contralateral block, 1381
  indications and contraindications,
      1381
  mepivacaine levels, 1380–1381
  recommendations, 1381
  technique, 1379–1380
Scalp block, 1350, 1351
Schwann cell anatomy, 1203, 1204
Sciatic nerve
  anatomy, 1402–1403, 1401
  nerve block
    anterior approach, 1406–1407, 1407
    classic technique, 1403–1404, 1404
    lateral approach, 1407–1408
    modified technique, 1404–1405,
        1405–1406
    Rovenstine block, 1404, 1405
Scoliosis, 1450
Scopolamine
  and awareness during anesthesia, 368
  and MAC values, 339
  parasympathetic blockade, 287
  premedication for spinal anesthesia,
      1459
Screen mask, 12
Screening tests, preoperative, 219–222
Scultetus position, 180, 201
Sea level, oxygen pressure, 1135
Sebarese's test, 225
Second gas effect, 328–329, 329t
Sedation
  definition of, 288
  pain control, 1344
  preanesthetic medication, 291
Segmental spinal anesthesia, 1529–1530,
    1530
Seizures
  diazepam anesthesia, 754
  fentanyl effects, 718
Sellick maneuver, 438–439, 529, 548–
    550
Semiclosed circle rebreathing method,
    400–401
  definition, 400
  leaks, 401
  nitrous oxide techniques, 400–401
  principles, 400
Semiclosed single-limb systems, 402–
    405
  See also Mapleson configurations.
Semiopen anesthesia systems, 405
Semon's law, 467

Sensitivity test of succinylcholine,
    1009–1010
Sensory block, in general anesthesia, 315
Serotonin
  pain transmission, 1336
  spinal anesthesia, 1489
Service contracts, anesthesia machines,
    138
Servoflurane, 396
Sex differences
  alfentanil kinetics, 723
  cholinesterase, 847
  diazepam anesthesia, 750
  and dosage of anesthesia, 290
  during endotracheal anesthesia, 578
  MAC values, 336
  operative risk, 38, 44–45, 48
  oxidative metabolism of inhaled
      anesthetics, 348
  pain tolerance, 1322
  postspinal headaches, 1556–1557
  and relaxant action, 847–848
  in spinal anesthesia, 1552
  thiopental distribution, 664
Shivering, after epidural anesthesia,
    1600–1601
Shock
  electrical, 1155–1157
  hypothermia, 1097
  pancuronium uses, 970
  thiopental effects, 680
  and Trendelenburg position, 180
Shoulder pain syndromes, 1340–1341
Shy-Drager syndrome, laryngeal muscles,
    467
Sickle cell disease, 41
Sighing during anesthesia, 378–379
Signs of anesthesia
  classification, 361, 361t
  history, 360–361
  See also General anesthesia.
Silicone rubber absorption, 86
Sims' position, 185, 185
Sinusitis, in intubation, 589
Sitting positions, 181–183, 183–184
Skin
  diseases, and acupuncture, 1639
  electrical resistance, 1441–1442
  injury, in hypothermia, 1111
  patch, transdermal drug
      administration, 298
  penetration by topical anesthesia, 1272
  preparation, for regional anesthesia,
      1201–1202
  temperature, 1438–1439
    in spinal anesthesia, 1516
  testing, allergies to local anesthetics,
      1311
Skin fold test, 216, 216t
Skull, neonatal, 503
Sleep, 317–323
  as active phenomenon, 320
  biochemistry, 321–322, 321, 322
  classic concept, 318
  and CNS depressants, 322
  cyclic aspect of NREM-REM, 320, 320
  and hypnosis, 1128
  induction, monitoring of, 428–429
  laryngeal muscles, 468
  loss, by anesthetist, 52–53
  metabolism, 322
  neuroanatomic mechanisms, 320–321
  neurotransmitters, 321
  noise effects, 1168

pacemaker, 320
physiologic changes, 322
quantitative aspects, 321
respiratory patterns, benzodiazepine effects, 54
types, 318–320, 319t
paradoxic, 319–320
slow-wave, 318–319
See also Awareness.
Smoke, carbon monoxide in, 1139
Smoking
enzyme induction, 256
morbidity and mortality risks, 51
and preanesthetic visit, 213–215
Sneeze reflex, 1185
Soda lime, as carbon dioxide absorbent. *See* Carbon dioxide absorption.
Sodium
channel structure, 1213–1214
in hypothermia, 1105
and MAC values, 337
in nerve impulse, 1205–1208
and relaxant agents, 873
Sodium pentothal
development, 18
and EEG patterns, 371
Solids. *See* Physics of anesthesiology.
Solubility
blood, of anesthetics, 105–106, 331–332, 331t
butacaine, 1255
chloroprocaine, 1253
cocaine, 1248
coefficients, 88, 105, 324
hexylcaine, 1251
lipid, 330, 346
local anesthetics, 1218
and MAC values, 337
procaine, 1252
tetracaine, 1255
thiopental, 657, 660
See also Physics of anesthesiology.
Somatic nerve traction reflex, 1192
Somatosensory system
evoked potentials (SSEP)
ear function during patient positioning, 194–195
during patient positioning, 171
pain pathways, 1324–1330
afferent fibers, 1324–1326
large fibers, 1326
small-diameter fibers, 1326–1328, 1327
spinal microanatomy and physiology, 1328–1329, 1328
Somatostatin, pain transmission, 1336
Sore throat, after endotracheal intubation, 490–491, 497–498, 580, 580t
Specific gravity
anesthetic solutions, 1466–1468
definition, 107
epidural anesthetics, 1582
Specific heat, 109
Sphygmomanometry, 74–77
errors, 76–77
standards, 74–75
technique, 75–76, 76, 77
Spinal anesthesia
cardiac arrest, 53–54
complications, 1540–1554
affective dyspnea, 1546
apprehension, 1546
cardiac arrest, 1547

CNS irritation, 1546
hypertension, 1545
hypotension, 1540–1545
nausea and vomiting, 1546
needle breakage, 1546
puncture difficulty, 1546
respiration, 1546
in subarachnoid block, 1551–1553
tourniquet pain, 1547–1551
and controlled hypotension, 1061
definition, 1200
discovery of, 11
hexylcaine, 1251
lateral position for, 185
physiology, 1498–1520
direct effects, 1498–1503
blockade of different nerve modalities, 1502–1503
dorsal root ganglia, 1499
fiber classification, 1499, 1500t
levels of block, 1499–1501, 1500t
nerve fiber susceptibility, 1499
primary site of action, 1498–1499
spinal cord tracts, 1501–1502
endocrine effects of surgical stress, 1507–1513, 1508t
age effects, 1511–1512
blood loss, 1510
carbohydrate metabolism, 1510–1511
catecholamines, 1508
cortisol, 1508
epinephrine, 1512–1513
fat metabolism, 1511
glucose, 1509
mechanisms, 1507–1508
mental function, 1511
neuroendocrine response, 1509–1510
opiate techniques, 1511
pancreatic hormones, 1509
pituitary hormones, 1509
pulmonary function, 1511
testosterone, 1509
thromboembolism, 1510
thyroid hormones, 1509
upper abdominal surgery, 1511
and epidural anesthesia, 1513
indirect effects, 1503–1507
autonomic nervous system, 1506–1507
blood flow, 1505–1506
blood pressure, 1503–1505
bronchial effect, 1507
cardiac effects, 1506
gastric emptying, 1507
gastrointestinal tract, 1507
hypotension, 1505
motor nerve paralysis, 1507
oxygen utilization, 1506
peripheral circulation, 1505
ventilation, 1507
nerve modalities, 1513–1516
motor block, 1514, 1514t
sensory level of anesthesia, 1513–1514, 1514
skin temperature, 1516
sympathetic block, 1514–1515
sympathogalvanic reflex, 1515–1516
subarachnoid space, 1498
postoperative complications, 1555–1570

cranial nerve disturbance, 1564–1566
abducens nerve paralysis, 1565
auditory nerve, 1565
other nerves, 1566
visual difficulty, 1564–1565
infections, 1566
neurotoxic effects, 1566–1568
adhesive arachnoiditis, 1567
bladder and rectal paralysis, 1567
cauda equina syndrome, 1567
meningismus, 1566–1567
myelitis, 1567
peripheral neuropathies, 1567
spinal cord disease, 1567
postlumbar puncture sequelae, 1555–1564
backache, 1564
dizziness, 1564
headaches, 1555–1562
principles, 1445–1497
anatomy of vertebral column, 1445–1446, 1446
anesthesia levels, 1471
cerebrospinal fluid, 1455–1458, 1455, 1456
circulation of spinal cord, 1450–1455, 1451
contraindications, 1486–1487
definition, 1445
denticulate ligaments, 1449
developmental anatomy of spinal cord, 1448, 1448
diagnosis test, 1488
disadvantages and complications, 1487–1488
elasticity of spinal cord and ligaments, 1449–1450
failures, 1488–1489
fate of injected agents, 1471–1478, 1472
absorption routes, 1474–1475
biotransformation in CSF, 1475
diffusion, 1473
dilution, 1473
distribution, 1473
duration of analgesia, 1476–1477
elimination rate, 1475
pharmacokinetics, 1476
plasma levels after subarachnoid administration, 1475–1476
spread of agents, 1477–1478, 1477
tissue fixation, 1474
tissue uptake, 1473–1474
vascular absorption, 1474
history, 1445
in hyperthyroidism, 1488
indications and patient selection, 1484–1486
ligament anatomy, 1447–1448, 1447
for megacolon, 1488
meninges of spinal cord, 1448–1449
needles and catheters, 1489–1492, 1490, 1491
non-local anesthesia, 1489
pain evaluation, 1488
in paralytic ileus, 1488
potentiation, 1478–1484
additives, 1478–1480
opioid effects, 1484
spinal cord and dural blood flow, 1483–1484, 1484t

Spinal anesthesia
  potentiation (Continued)
    vasoconstrictor agents, 1480–1483
  procedures, 1458–1471
    introducer, 1463–1464
    paramedian approach, 1464
    patient positions, 1459–1460
    premedication, 1458–1459
    puncture technique, 1460–1463, *1461–1463*, 1461t
    spread of solutions, 1464–1470
    Taylor technique, 1464, *1465*
  in pulmonary edema, 1488
  topographic line of Tuffier, 1446–1447
  techniques, 1521–1539
    advantages, 1534
    alcohol neurolysis, 1535–1536
    ammonium salts, 1536
    continuous injection methods, 1527–1532
      continuous drip method, 1529
      intermittent or fractional technique, 1527
      Lemmon technique, 1527, *1528*
      meperidine, 1530
      pharmacodynamics, 1530–1532
      segmental technique, 1529–1530, *1530*
      Touhy technique, 1527–1529
    epidural neurolytic procedure, 1536–1537
    filter needles, 1537
    in infants and children, 1532–1535
      premature infants, 1534–1535
    intraoperative care, 1534
    monitoring, 1534
    neurolysis protocol, 1535
    phenol neurolysis, 1535
    positioning, 1535
    single-injection hyperbaric, 1521–1524
      bupivacaine-dextrose, 1523
      bupivacaine-hyperbaric, 1523–1524
      dibucaine-dextrose, 1522
      lidocaine-dextrose, 1522–1523
      procaine, 1521–1522
      tetracaine-dextrose, 1522
    single-injection hypobaric, 1526–1527
      dibucaine, 1527
      indications, 1526
      tetracaine, 1526
    single-injection isobaric, 1524–1526
      bupicavaine, 1524–1526
      dibucaine, 1524
      tetracaine, 1524
    substitute for alcohol-phenol, 1537
Spinal cord
  abnormalities, and intubation, 525
  cervical injury, during patient positioning, 194, 197–198
  fractures, and intubation, 541
  circulation, 1450–1455
    arterial supply, 1450–1452, *1451*
    blood flow, 1454, *1454*
    regulation, 1454–1455
    veins, 1452, *1452*
  developmental anatomy, 1448, *1448*
  diazepam effects, 753
  ketamine effects, 736–737
  local anesthetic penetration, 1501–1502

meninges, 1448–1449
and muscle relaxants, 899–900
pain pathways, 1328–1329, *1328*
during patient repositioning, 201–202
sensory input, during general anesthesia, 315–316
Spinal fluid, succinylcholine effects, 1008
Spirobarbituric acids, 698
Spirometry
  preoperative, 229
  smoking effects, 214
Splanchnic block, 1421–1423
  anatomy, 1421–1422
  intra-abdominal approach, 1422–1423
  paravertebral technique, 1422, *1423*
Spread of solutions
  amount and volume of drug, 1464–1466
  barbotage, 1466
  baricity, 1468
  in epidural anesthesia, 1579–1580
  injection site, 1466
  needle direction, 1466
  and obesity, 1470
  osmolality factor, 1468
  postinjection position, 1469
  predictability, 1471
  and pregnancy, 1470–1471
  rate of injection, 1466
  sitting position, 1469
  specific gravity, density, and baric gravity, 1466–1468
  temperature, 1469
  venous pressure, 1469–1470
Stages of anesthesia. See General anesthesia.
Standards
  compressed gas cylinders, 123, 126–127
  for monitoring anesthetized patient, 69
Staphylococcus infections, in anesthesia machines, 158–159
Stenosis, subglottic and tracheal, 584–585
Sterilization
  of endotracheal tubes, 478–479
  HIV prevention, 1174
Sternutatory reflex (sneeze), 1185
Steroids, enzyme induction, 256
Stethoscope, 75, 86, 76, 77
  precordial monitoring, 77
Stilbazoline, 1048
Stimulants, drug dependence, 308
Stomach
  age effects, 238
  balloon, in hypothermia, 1109
  fasting effects, 238–240
  full
    and inhalation anesthesia, 438–439
    and pancuronium, 971
  residual volume, 240
  volume, 238, *239*
  See also Gastric emptying; Gastrointestinal tract.
Stomas, visceral, during patient repositioning, 201
Stomatitis, 564
Storage of compressed gas cylinders, 127–128
Stovaine, protein potentiation, 1479
Strangulation anesthesia, 4
Stress
  fentanyl effects, 716–717

hypothermia, 1097, 1110
nitroprusside effects, 1078
opiate effects, 706–707
psychological, and cardiac arrest, 54
surgical, endocrine effects. See Spinal anesthesia, physiology.
tests, heart disease, 227–228
Stridor
  airway obstruction, 525
  endotracheal anesthesia complications, 589–590
  in laryngeal edema, 581
  laryngeal muscles, 468
  pediatric, 510, 510t
Stroke, and muscle relaxants, 896–898
Structure activity relations (SAR), 1267
Study commissions, intraoperative deaths, 37
Stylets
  for endobronchial intubation, 600, 606
  endotracheal, 495, *496*
Subarachnoid anesthesia
  CSF spread, 1478
  diffusion of local anesthetics, 1475
  See also Opioids; Spinal anesthesia.
Subclavian space, perivascular nerve block, 1376–1379, *1377, 1378*
Subneural apparatus of Couteaux, 812
Substance P, in pain control, 1335–1336
Succinylcholine, 1003–1017
  adverse effects, 1017
  in ambulatory surgery, 1647
  chemistry, 829, 1004, *830, 1004*
  clinical uses, 1010–1017
    administration, 1010
    and anticholinesterases, 1016
    burn sensitivity, 1015–1016
    dosage and techniques, 1011–1014
      bolus intravenous dose, 1011–1012
      continuous intravenous drip, 1012–1013
      intermittent intravenous, 1012
      intramuscular, 1013–1014
    dreaming and awareness, 1016–1017
    drug interactions, 1016
    and hexafluorenium, 1014–1015
    and inhalation agents, 1016
    pharmacodynamics-kinetics, 1010–1011
    precautions, 1015
  complications, 1005–1010
    allergic reactions, 1009
    cerebral physiology, 1008
    cholinesterase activity, 1010
    gastrointestinal effects, 1008–1009
    histamine release, 1009
    intracranial pressure, 1008
    intraocular pressure, 1007
    masseter muscle rigidity, 1006
    masticatory muscle stiffness, 1006
    muscle fasciculation and pain, 1009
    ocular muscles, 1006–1007
    placental transmission, 1009
    sensitivity test, 1009–1010
    skeletal muscle paralysis, 1005–1006
    smooth muscle action, 1007–1008
    spinal fluid pressure, 1008
  history, 1003–1004
  intramuscular, 920
  and intraocular pressure, 431
  mechanism of action, 1004
  metabolism, 1004, 1221
  neuromuscular blockade, 850

and pancuronium interaction, 970
pharmacokinetics, 835–836
pharmacology, 1004–1005
and pipecuronium, 980
and pupillary reflex, 366
in rapid sequence induction, 439–440
and thiopental solubility, 660
Sufentanil, 726–728
   advantages, 728
   chemistry, 726
   dose and potency, 726–727
   EEG changes, 715
   intranasal, 727
   lipid solubility, 1626
   pharmacodynamics, 727–728
   pharmacokinetics, 727, 727t, 728t
Suggestibility in hypnosis, 1126–1127
Sulfenetanil, and MAC values, 338
Sulfites as preservatives, 1312–1314
Sulfonamide
   and procaine antagonism, 1252
   and thiopental binding, 663
Supine hypotensive syndrome, 165
Supine position
   head
      down tilt, 165–166
      up tilt, 166
   See also Dorsal decubitus position.
Suprascapular nerve block, 1381–1382
   during repositioning, 198
Surface tension, 107–108
   measurement of, 108
Surgical factors
   cardiac
      hyperbaric oxygenation, 1142
      hypnosis, 1132
      and vascular, hypothermia, 1097
   complexity, and mortality risk, 45, 49
   endocrine effects of stress. See Spinal
      anesthesia.
   pain control, 1345–1346
   and reinfarction risks, 59
   relaxant choice, 891
Susceptibility definition, 307
Swallowing, laryngeal muscles, 468
Sweating tests, 1443–1444, 1443
   cobaltous chloride test, 1444
   starch test, 1444
Switching valves, 131
Sympathetic nervous system
   bupivacaine effects, 1262
   cocaine effects, 1249
   and stress response, 210
   tests of function, 1438–1444, 1439t
      anesthetic effects, 1444, 1443
      breath-holding test, 1441
      electrical skin resistance, 1441–1442
      local temperature
         cold pressor test, 1442
         reflex vsodilatation test, 1442
      oscillometry, 1439–1440
      oscillotonometry, 1440, 1441
      plethysmography, 1444
      psychogalvanic reflex, 1442–1443,
         1442
      skin temperature, 1438–1439, 1440
      sweating tests, 1443–1444
Sympatho-galvanic reflex, in spinal
   anesthesia, 1515–1516
Sympathomimetic drugs, drug
   interactions, 275–276
Syncope, from local anesthetics, 1309
Syringes
   in drug administration, 292–293

for epidural anesthesia, 1584–1585
hypodermic, development of, 10

T tube system. See Ayre T-tube system.
Tables, surgical
   arm supports, 175–176, 175, 176
   head holders, 176–177
   specialized, 175
   standard, 174–175
   trunk frames, 176, 177
   See also Positioning of patient.
Tachycardia
   in controlled hypotension, 1069
   in hyperthermia, 1112
Tamponade, cardiac, positive airway
   pressure effects, 627
Tape, for endotracheal intubation, 498–499
Tears Naturale, 432
Tectal nuclei, 379
Teeth
   during endotracheal anesthesia, 496–497, 519, 579
   neonatal, 503, 505
Temperature
   and blood gas analysis, 88–89
   in carbon dioxide absorption, 457
   in closed circle systems, 393–394
   critical, 111
   and dosage of anesthesia, 290
   and EEG patterns, 93
   ignition, 1150–1151
   local, response of extremity, 1442
   and MAC values, 336
   monitoring of, 94–95, 204–205
   and muscle relaxants, 880–883
      hypothermia effects, 881–882
      mechanisms of action, 881
   and neuromuscular blockade, 851
   of skin, 1438–1439, 1516
   and spread of injections, 1469
   and thiopental induction, 677
   See also Hyperthermia; Hypothermia;
      Physics of anesthesiology.
Temporomandibular joint, intubation
   difficulties, 463–464, 524
Testosterone, and surgical stress, 1509
Tetanus
   diazepam anesthesia, 754
   muscle contraction, 810–811, 826
   and receptor occupancy, 872
Tetracaine (pontocaine), 796
   bacteriostatic action, 1313
   dextrose potentiation, 1478
   in hyperbaric spinal anesthesia, 1522
   during extubation, 554–555
   in hypobaric spinal anesthesia, 1526–1527
   in isobaric spinal anesthesia, 1524
   pharmacology, 1255
   spinal anesthesia in infants and
      children, 1534
   spread of solution, 1471
   toxicity, 1295
   See also Regional anesthesia.
Tetraethyl ammonium derivatives, 1047,
   1268
   controlled hypotension, 1065
Tetrahydrocannabinol
   for glaucoma, 278
   and MAC values, 339
   pain control, 1344
Tetraplegia, midcervical, 197
Theodoric of Lucca, 4

Thermal conductivity, gas analyzers,
   139–140
Thermal gradients, 1098
Thermodilution, cardiac output, 85
Thermography, liquid crystal, 95
Thialbarbital (kemithal), 698, 698
Thiamylal, 689–691
   chemical structure, 689, 691
   pharmacology, 689–690
      administration, 690–691
      cardiovascular system, 689–690
      central nervous system, 689, 692
      complications, 691
      dosage, 691
      techniques of use, 691
Thiobarbiturates
   development, 655
   and EEG patterns, 371
Thiocyanate, in nitroprusside therapy,
   1074, 1079–1081
Thiohexital, 698, 698
Thiopental, 657–666
   administration, 657
   in alcoholic patient, 213
   and body metabolism, 323
   clinical aspects, 672–676
      bioelectric model, 672–674, 674
      criteria of anesthesia, 674–675, 675t
      EEG signs, 675–676, 676, 677
      pain response, 674
      plasma concentration correlation,
         675
      signs of anesthesia, 672, 673
   complications, 681–684
      anaphylactoid reaction, 683
      extravasation, 682
      intra-arterial injections, 682–683
      local irritants, 682
      muscle movements, 683
      overdose, 683
      postanesthetic tremors, 684
      precautions, 681
      respiratory, 682
      ventilatory, 681–682
   in cranial trauma, 684
   destruction, 671
   dissociation constant and ionization
      degree, 657
   distribution, 669–671, 669
      aqueous tissue compartment, 670
      fat compartment, 670–671, 671t
      visceral concentration, 670
   dosage, 661, 655t
      age effect, 661
   elimination, 671–672
   historical background, 657
   induction, 676–684
      circulatory state, 677
      clinical aspects, 680–681
         advantages, 681
         airway problems, 680
         anemia, 681
         azotemia, 681
         cardiac failure, 680
         debility, 681
         drug interaction, 681
         endocrine, 681
         hemorrhage, shock, and
            hypovolemia, 680
         malnutrition, 681
         maternal-fetal circulation, 680
         metabolism and electrolytes, 681
         reflexes, 680–681
      dosage, 677, 679–680

Thiopental
  induction (*Continued*)
    environmental temperature, 677
    forearm blood flow, 677
    premedication, 676, 678t
    procedure, 677–681
      preoxygenation, 677–679
      technique, 677
    side effects, 676
  and intraocular pressure, 279
  and ketamine comparison, 748
  laryngeal reflex, 1186
  and laryngospasm, 568
  and MAC values, 338
  and neuromuscular transmission, 888
  pharmacokinetics, 661–666, 661–663t
    age effects, 663–664, 664
    and alcoholism, 665, 665
    in children, 665–666, 666
    clearance and elimination, 662
    plasma concentration (decay curve), 661–662, 663
    protein binding, 255, 662–663
    sex effects, 664
    tolerance, 666
    volumes of distribution, 662, 663t
  pharmacologic actions, 666–669
    autonomic nervous system, 668
    cardiovascular system, 667, 667t
    central nervous system, 666
    endocrine effects, 668–669
    gastrointestinal tract, 667
    and metabolism, 667–668
    in muscles, 668
    and nutrition, 668
    prothrombin time, 669
    renal effects, 668
    respiration, 666–667
  potentiation, 660
  preparations and concentrations, 657
  and pupillary reflex, 366
  in rapid sequence induction, 439–440
  and relaxant mixtures, 657–660
  solubility, 657
  solution stability, 660–661
  in status epilepticus, 684
  and succinylcholine, 660
  tolerance, 672
Thiophanium, controlled hypotension, 1062
Thompson's disease, 901
Thoracic nerve block. *See* Nerve block, paravertebral.
Thoracic outlet syndrome, 199
Thoracic surgery
  lateral jackknife position, 186
  ventilation management, 612–613
Thoracolumbar sympathetic block, 1433–1434, 1435
Thorax
  during patient repositioning, 200–201
  reflexes, 1189
Thorpe tube flowmeter, 135–136, 137, 138
Threshold, pain, 1321–1322, 1341–1344
Thromboembolism, and regional anesthesia, 1510
Thrombophlebitis
  diazepam anesthesia, 754
  etomidate anesthesia, 768
Thyroid disease
  and muscle relaxants, 903–904
  and spinal anesthesia, 1488
Thyroid gland

hormones
  drug interactions, 274
  and MAC values, 338
  and surgical stress, 1509
  in oxygen toxicity, 1147
Tibial nerve
  block, 1408–1411
  muscle stimulation, 860
Tic douloureux, neuronal hyperactivity, 1338
Tidal volume
  monitoring, 87–88
  in one-lung ventilation, 615, 615
  in positive airway pressure, 628
To-and-fro breathing system, 396–397, 397
  dead space, 391
α-Tocopherol, and thiopental potentiation, 660
Tolerance
  to pain, 1321–1322
  physical, and oxygen toxicity, 1145
  thiopental, 666, 672
Tongue
  in endotracheal anesthesia, 519–521
  neonatal, 503
  nerve block, 1359
Topical anesthesia
  benzocaine, 1271–1274
  capsaicin, 1274
  classification, 1271
  cocaine alternatives, 1274
  definition, 1200
  EMLA cream, 1275
  during endotracheal anesthesia, 576
  hexylcaine, 1251
  innervation, 549–540
  techniques, 540
  toxicity, 1298–1299
Topography, line of Tuffier, 1446–1447
Topping, in vaporization, 111
Touhy technique for spinal anesthesia, 1527–1529
Tourniquets
  for intravenous regional anesthesia, 795–796, 800–801
  pain, in spinal anesthesia, 1547–1551
Toxemias, and dosage of anesthesia, 290
Toxicity
  bupivacaine, 1261
  butacaine, 1256
  caudal analgesia, 1621
  chloroprocaine, 1253–1255
  cocaine, 1248, 1250
  definition, 1233
  diazepam, 755
  dibucaine, 1256
  epinephrine, 1284–1285
  etidocaine, 1262
  hexylcaine, 1251
  lidocaine, 1257
  local anesthetics, 802–804
  and MAC, 334–335
  mepivacaine, 1259
  nitroprusside, 1079–1080
  oxygen, in hyperbaric oxygenation, 1143–1147
  procaine, 789, 790
  propanidid, 772
  propitocaine, 1264
  regional anesthetics, 802–804
  tetracaine, 1255
  tetraethyl ammonium derivatives, 1268

See also Regional anesthesia.
Toxiferine, 828, 950–951, *951*
Trachea
  mucosal denudation, 586, *587*
  reflex, 1186–1187
  rupture in intubation, 585
  tug during anesthesia, 377–378
  See also Endotracheal anesthesia.
Tracheitis, in endotracheal intubation, 584
Tracheobronchial angles, 473–474
Tracheomalacia, 585
Tracheostomy tube removal, 646
Traction reflexes, 1189–1191
Train-of-four monitoring, 854–857
  advantages, 856
  clinical observations, 854–855, *855*
  controlled relaxation, 856
  evaluation, 856
  maintenance of relaxation, 856
  newer relaxants, 855–856
  organophosphates, 1043
  in pediatrics, 1045
  procedure, 854, *855*
  quantitation of block, 855
  and receptor occupancy, 871
  during recovery, 856
  in relaxant antagonism, 1025–1026
  tetanic stimulation, 857
  twitch height, 856–857
  in upper motoneuron disorders, 897
Training programs, 14, 21–22
Tranquilizers
  drug interactions, 273
  and neuromuscular transmission, 887
  pain control, 1344
  pediatric preanesthetic medication, 301
  preanesthetic medication, 291
  and REM sleep, 322
Transbuccal mucosal absorption, 297
Transcutaneous electrical nerve stimulation (TENS), 1337, 1345
Transesophageal echocardiography, cardiac output, 86, 95
Transfusion
  blood, 222
  records, 33–34
Transport
  of anesthetics
    blood supply to tissues, 341
    circulatory capacity, 341
  of patient
    comatose patient, 190
    hypotension, motion-induced, 193
    to intensive care unit, 171
    monitoring loss, 192–193
    motion sickness, 193
    and repositioning, 177
    unconscious patient, 189
Transsacral block, 1424–1425, *1425*
Tranylcypromine (Parnate), drug interactions, 269
Trauma
  cranial, thiopental anesthesia, 684
  dental. *See* Dental anesthesia, trauma.
  laryngeal, 549–550
  mortality risk, 49–50, 50t
  ocular, from face mask, 431–432
  during patient repositioning. *See* Positioning of patient.
  relaxant contraindications, 895
Trauma Score, 49

Treacher-Collins syndrome, and
    endotracheal anesthesia, 518
Tremors, after thiopental anesthesia, 684
Trendelenburg position
  abdominal complications, 201
  cardiovascular effects, 165
  and cerebral perfusion, 170
  compression alopecia, 194
  technical aspects, 180, *181*
Triazolam, drug interactions, 274
Tribromoethanol
  development, 18
  and neuromuscular transmission, 888
Trichloroacetaldehyde, 349
Trichloroethylene
  incompatibility in closed circle
    systems, 396
  and intraocular pressure, 279
  solubility coefficient, 332
Tricyclic antidepressants, drug
    interactions, 269–272
Trifluoroacetic acid, 349
Trifluoroethanol, 349
Trigeminal nerve block, 1353–1359
  mandibular division, 1357–1358
    anatomy, 1357
    techniques, 1357–1358, *1359*
  maxillary division, 1355–1357
    anatomy, 1355
    complications, 1356–1357
    indications, 1357
    infra-orbital branch, 1357, *1357*
    sphenopalatine ganglionic block,
      1357
    techniques, 1355–1356, *1356*
  ophthalmic division, 1353–1354
    anatomy, 1354, *1354*
    landmarks, 1354, *1355*
    supra-orbital branch, 1354
Trigger points, 1340–1341, *1341*
Trimethadione, and neuromuscular
    blockade, 883
Trimethaphan, 1048
  cholinesterase inhibition, 840
  controlled hypotension, 1067–1070
    adjunctive measures, 1068
    advantages, 1069
    chemistry, 1067, *1067*
    continuous technique, 1067
    disadvantages, 1069
    elimination, 1068
    indications, 1068
    intermittent technique, 1067–1068
    mechanism of action, 1067
    physiology, 1068
  and MAC values, 339
  and nitroprusside, 1075–1076
Trisomy 21, atlantoaxial subluxation,
    590
Trunk
  frames, 176, *177*
  nerve block. *See* Nerve block, of
    trunk, abdomen, and perineum.
Tryptophan hydroxylase, during sleep,
    321
Tubal ligation, and spread of injections,
    1470–1471
Tube bag systems, 417–418
Tubes
  in breathing circuits, 150–151
  endobronchial. *See* Endobronchial
    anesthesia.
  endotracheal. *See* Endotracheal
    anesthesia.

Tubocurarine
  and intraocular pressure, 279
  and MAC values, 338–339
  priming action, 868
  See also Curare; Relaxants.
Tumors, carcinoid, and muscle relaxants,
    903
Turbulence, 114–115
Twitch monitoring. *See* Relaxants.

Ulcers
  acupuncture, 1639
  during endotracheal anesthesia, 579,
    582
Ulnar nerve
  block, 1385–1386, *1387*
    at elbow, 1385–1386, *1388*
    at wrist, 1386, *1389*
  paralysis, 199, 202, 203, *200*
  solution distribution, 1375
Ultrasonography, Doppler, cardiac
    output, 85–86
Ultrastructure, neuromuscular junction,
    812, *813*
Ultraviolet analysis
  anesthetic and respiratory gas
    monitoring, 86
  spectrometers, 140
Umbilical cord transfusion and
    anesthesia, 299
Unconsciousness
  in general anesthesia, 361–363
  with ketamine, 736
  thiopental levels, 675
  UD concept, 655
  viability score, 243, 244t
Upper extremities nerve block. *See*
    Nerve block, upper extremities.
Upper respiratory infections,
    preoperative evaluation, 232–
    234
Urinalysis
  output, 95
  preoperative screening, 224
Urologic procedures
  lithotomy position, 179
  preanesthetic evaluation, 242–243
Uterus
  afferent nerve block, 1427
  blood flow, cocaine effects, 1250
  ketamine effects, 740, 746

Vaccines, hepatitis, 1169–1170
Vago-vagal reflex, 1186
Vagus nerve block, 1361, *1359, 1360*
Valium, in ambulatory surgery, 1645
Valsalva test, 225, *226*
Valves
  nonrebreathing, 151–152, 401–402,
    152, 402
  respiratory, 151, *151*
  See also Anesthesia machines and
    components.
van der Waals forces, 108, *109*
Vapor analyzers, climate and altitude
    effects, 446, 447t
Vaporization physics, 108–110
  latent heat of vaporization, 109–110
  process of, 110–111
  specific heat, 109, 111t
  van der Waals forces, 108, *109*
  vapor pressure, 109, *110*
Vaporizers
  climate and altitude effects, 446–447

contaminants, 396
development, 12–13
in hyperbaric oxygenation, 1138
See also Anesthesia machines and
    components.
Vascular system
  in hyperbaric oxygenation, 1142–1143,
    1147
  pain responses, 1341
Vasoconstrictors
  and local anesthetics, 1245
  potentiation of action, 1282–1290
    carbonated local anesthetics, 1286–
      1287
    cobefrin, 1285–1286
    cocaine, 1285
    dextran, 1288–1289
    epinephrine, 1282–1285
    hyaluronidase, 1289
    oil solutions, 1289
    pH of local anesthetics, 1286
    potassium, 1287–1288
  and spinal anesthetics, 1480–1483
  and topical anesthesia, 1273
Vasopressor premedication for spinal
    anesthesia, 1459
Vecuronium, 972–979
  administration and dosage, 973–974
  in ambulatory surgery, 1647
  analogue ORG 9426, 979
  chemistry, 972, *972*
  clinical uses, 973
  drug interactions, 266, 268
  experimental studies, 972–973
  metabolism, 972
  in obesity, 893
  pediatric reversal, 1045
  pharmacodynamics, 976
  pharmacokinetics, 974–976, 974–975t
  pharmacologic actions, 976–979, 977t
  priming action, 867, 868
  in rapid sequence induction, 439–440
  train-of-four monitoring, 855–856
  See also Relaxants.
Venipuncture technique, 295–296
  cut-down, 295
  developing veins, 295
  fluid flow, 295–296
  needle introduction, 295, *296*
  selection of vein, 295
Ventilation
  alveolar. *See* Alveolar ventilation.
  clinical evaluation, 87–88
  fentanyl effects, 716
  laboratory evaluation, 88–89
  monitors, in breathing systems, 413–
    414
  one-lung, physiology of, 613–616
    in lateral position, 616
    oxygenation efficiency, 614
    PEEP effects, 615–616
    reflex hypoxic pulmonary
      vasoconstriction, 614
    shunt, 613–614
    tidal volume, 615, *615*
  pulmonary, in spinal anesthesia, 1507
  room air in operating room, 1164–
    1165
  thiopental effects, 681–682
  during thoracic surgery, 612–613
  transtracheal, 550
  variables of, 623–624
    flow rate and pattern, 624
    pressure, 623

Ventilation
  variables of (Continued)
    rate and time sequence, 623–624
    volume, 623
    work of, 623
  See also Breathing systems, artificial.
Ventilators
  anesthesia requirements, 640
  classification, 635–638
    advantages, 637–638
    constant force generators, 636, 637, 638
    disadvantages, 638
    flow generators (volume preset), 635–636, 636
    humidification, 636–637
    monitoring, 637
  compliance changes, 639, 640t
  construction aspects, 635
  cycling method, 635
  flow control, 635
  high-frequency positive-pressure. See HFV.
  inspiration phase, 634, 633
  leaks, 639–640, 641
  pressure patterns, 634–635, 634
  principles of operation, 631–633
  and pulmonary dysfunction, 640–641, 642t
  resuscitation requirements, 640
  selection of, 638–639, 641, 639t
Ventriculography, exercise, 228–229
Venturi tube, 116–117, 116
Verapamil
  drug interactions, 268
  and neuromuscular junction, 883–884
Vertebral column
  anatomy, 1445–1446, 1446
  veins, 1452–1454, 1453
Vertebrobasilar artery injury, during patient positioning, 197
Vestibular nucleus, 380
Veterinary drugs, 734–735
Viability score, 243, 244t
Vigilance by anesthetist, 52–53

Vinblastine toxicity, 262
Vinca alkaloid toxicity, 262
Vinethene
  density, 107
  development, 18
Virus, occupational hazards, 1168–1173
  hepatitis, 1169–1170
  herpes simplex virus, 1168–1169
  HIV infections and AIDS, 1170–1173
Viscera, pelvic reflexes, 1191–1192
Viscosity definition, 114
Vision
  muscle relaxant effects, 905–906
  after spinal anesthesia, 1564–1565
  work station for anesthetist, 118–119
Vital capacity, preoperative analysis, 229–230
Vital signs, monitoring during patient transport, 192–193
Vitamins, and thiopental anesthesia, 668
Vocal cords
  anatomy, 464, 467
  complications during endotracheal anesthesia, 579
  fusion in intubation, 586
  paradoxic motion, 525
Voice box. See Larynx.
Voice recognition record system, 31–32
Volatile anesthetics
  chemical degradation, 457–458
  and laryngospasm, 568
  and neuromuscular junction, 889–890, 889t
  and vecuronium, 974
Vomiting
  and oculocardiac reflex, 1181
  in spinal anesthesia, 1546

Wakefulness, 287–288, 288t
Warfarin, drug interactions, 262
Washout of anesthetic agent, 325–327
Water
  density, 106
  in hypothermia, 1111
  loss, in anesthetic systems, 412–413

vapor
  open drop inhalation systems, 410
  See also Humidity.
Waves, in electroencephalography, 91–92, 92
Weaning from ventilator therapy, 641–646
  definition, 641
  preparations, 643
  priniciples, 641–643, 643t
  respiratory criteria, 643, 643t
  technique, 643–646, 644
    extubation, 646
    IPPV, 643–645, 645t
    oxygen-enriched atmospheres, 646
    PEEP, 645
Wedensky block, 1216
Weight
  of gas or vapor, 106
  of obese patients, 218
  preanesthetic evaluation, 215
Wheal, intradermal, 1222–1223, 1223
Woodbridge components, in balanced anesthesia, 382
Wooden bowl anesthesia, 4
Work station for anesthetist, 118, 119
World Health Organization (WHO), alcoholism definition, 212
Wound
  healing, lidocaine actions, 1258
  infection, hyperbaric oxygenation, 1142
Wrist nerve block, 1393
  median nerve, 1388
  radial nerve, 1392–1393, 1393
  ulnar nerve, 1386

Xenon narcosis, in hyperbaric oxygenation, 1146
Xylocaine. See Lidocaine.

Yankhauer-Gwathmey mask, 409
Yokes, of compressed gas cylinders, 122, 123

Zero, absolute, 102